CARCINOGENICALLY ACTIVE CHEMICALS

CARCINOGENICALLY ACTIVE CHEMICALS

A Reference Guide

Richard J. Lewis, Sr.

VNR VAN NOSTRAND REINHOLD
_____ New York

Copyright © 1991 by Van Nostrand Reinhold

Library of Congress Catalog Card Number 90-12035
ISBN 0–442–31875–8

Printed in the United States of America

Van Nostrand Reinhold
115 Fifth Avenue
New York, New York 10003

Van Nostrand Reinhold International Company Limited
11 New Fetter Lane
London EC4P 4EE, England

Van Nostrand Reinhold
480 La Trobe Street
Melbourne, Victoria 3000, Australia

Nelson Canada
1120 Birchmount Road
Scarborough, Ontario M1K 5G4, Canada

16 15 14 13 12 11 10 9 8 7 6 5 4 3 2 1

Library of Congress Cataloging-in-Publication Data

Lewis, Richard J., Sr.
   Carcinogenically active chemicals: A reference guide / Richard J. Lewis, Sr.
      p.   cm.
   ISBN 0–442–31875–8
   1. Carcinogens—Handbooks, manuals, etc.   I. Title.
RC268.6.L48   1990
616.99′4071—dc20   90-12035
                                                 CIP

For Mary M. Lewis
who would have loved to see this

CONTENTS

PREFACE

The determination of which substances cause cancer in humans remains a major concern in medical, occupational, and environmental areas. This book provides data to help this determination. It contains data for all substances which are known to produce a carcinogenic effect in humans or animals or are suspected of doing so. Each substance provides references to the experimental literature and publications of scientific review bodies which make carcinogenic determinations.

Three introductory articles discuss the definition of a carcinogen, quantitative risk assessment, and implant carcinogenic effects. They provide a context and framework for the data which follows.

Most of the substances in this book are probably not capable of causing cancer in humans. Fewer than 500 substances are confirmed as human or animal carcinogens by expert review. Another 300 are suspect but lack adequate data for a positive determination. Over 2800 entries list some data, often of poor quality. Expert panels reviewed them because of suspicion based on chemical structure. These are included for completeness and as a signal of past scientific interest.

Classification of Substances

The substance entries are grouped into three classes based on experimental evidence and the opinion of expert review groups. The OSHA, IARC, ACGIH, and DFG MAK decision schedules are not related or synchronized. Thus an entry may have had a recent review by only one group. The most stringent classification of any regulation or expert group is taken as governing.

Class I—Confirmed Carcinogens

These substances are capable of causing cancer in exposed humans. An entry was assigned to this class if it had one or more of the following data items present.

a. An OSHA regulated carcinogen.
b. AN ACGIH assignment as a human or animal carcinogen.
c. A DFG MAK assignment as a confirmed human or animal carcinogen.
d. An IARC assignment of human or animal sufficient evidence of carcinogenicity or higher.
e. NTP Fourth Annual Report on Carcinogens.

Class II—Suspected Carcinogens

These substances may be capable of causing cancer in exposed humans. The evidence is suggestive, but not sufficient to convince expert review committees. Some entries have not yet had expert review, but contain experimental reports of carcinogenic activity. In particular, an entry is included if it has positive reports of carcinogenic endpoint in two species. As more studies are published, many Class II carcinogens will have their carcinogenicity confirmed. On the other hand, some will be judged noncarcinogenic in the future. An entry was assigned to this class if it had one or more of the following data items present.

a. An ACGIH assignment of suspected carcinogen.
b. An DFG MAK assignment of suspected carcinogen.
c. An IARC assignment of human or animal limited evidence.
d. Two animal studies reported positive carcinogenic endpoint in different species.

Class III—Questionable Carcinogens

These entries have minimal published evidence of possible carcinogenic activity. The reported endpoint is often neoplastic growth with no spread or invasion characteristic of carcinogenic pathology. An even weaker endpoint is that of equivocal tumorigenic agent (ETA). Reports are assigned this designation when the study was defective. The report may have lacked control animals, may have used very small sample size, often lack complete pathology reporting, or suffer many other study design defects. Many of these were designed for other than carcinogenic evaluation, and the reported carcinogenic effect is a byproduct of the study, not the goal. The data are presented because some of these substances may be carcinogens. There is insufficient data to affirm or deny the possibility. An entry was assigned to this class if it had one or more of the following data items present.

a. An IARC assignment of inadequate or no evidence.
b. A single human report of carcinogenicity.
c. A single experimental carcinogenic report, or duplicate reports in the same species.
d. One or more experimental neoplastic or equivocal tumorigenic agent report.

Every effort was made to include the most current and complete information. The author welcomes comments or corrections to the data presented.

RICHARD J. LEWIS, SR.

INTRODUCTION

This list of carcinogenically active substances includes drugs, food additives, preservatives, ores, pesticides, dyes, detergents, lubricants, soaps, plastics, extracts from plant and animal sources, plants which are toxic by contact or consumption, and industrial intermediates and waste products from production processes. Some of the information refers to materials of undefined composition. The chemicals included are assumed to exhibit the reported toxic effect in their pure state unless otherwise noted. However, even for a supposedly "pure" chemical, there is usually some degree of uncertainty about its exact composition and the impurities which may be present. This possibility must be considered in attempting to interpret the data presented since a contaminant could cause the toxic effects observed. Some radioactive materials are included but the effect reported is the chemically produced effect rather than the radiation effect.

For each entry the following data are provided when available: the entry number, entry name; CAS number; DOT number; molecular formula; molecular weight; a description of the material and physical properties; and synonyms. After this are listed carcinogenic and mutagenic data with references. Following, where available, are IARC reviews, NTP Carcinogenesis Testing Program results, EPA Extremely Hazardous Substances List, the EPA Genetic Toxicology Program, the Community Right To Know List. The presence of the material on the update of the EPA TSCA Inventory of chemicals in use in the United States is noted. The next grouping consists of the U.S. Occupational Safety and Health Administration's (OSHA) Permissible Exposure Levels, the American Conference of Governmental Industrial Hygienists' (ACGIH) Threshold Limit Values (TLV's), German Research Society's (MAK) values, National Institute for Occupational Safety and Health (NIOSH) Recommended Exposure Levels, and U.S. Department of Transportation (DOT) classifications. Each entry concludes with a Safety Profile, which discusses the carcinogenic, toxic, and other hazards of the entry.

1. *Entry Number* identifies each entry by a unique number consisting of three letters and three numbers, for example, AAA123. The first letter of the entry number indicates the alphabetical position of the entry. Numbers beginning with "A" are assigned to entries indexed with the A's. Entries in the four cross-indexes are referenced to its appropriate entry by the entry number preceded by a Roman numeral indicating the class section containing the entry.

2. *Entry Name* The name of each material is selected, where possible, to be the most commonly used designation.

3. *Chemical Abstracts Service Registry Number (CAS)* is a numeric designation assigned by the American Chemical Society's Chemical Abstracts Service and uniquely identifies a specific chemical compound. This entry allows one to conclusively identify a material regardless of the name or naming system used.

4. *DOT:* indicates a four digit hazard code assigned by the U.S. Department of Transportation. This code is recognized internationally and is in agreement with the United Nations coding

system. The code is used on transport documents, labels, and placards. It is also used to determine the regulations for shipping the material.

5. *Molecular Formula* (*mf:*) or atomic formula (*af:*) designates the elemental composition of the material and is structured according to the Hill System (see *Journal of the American Chemical Society*, 22(8): 478-494, 1900) in which carbon and hydrogen (if present) are listed first, followed by the other elemental symbols in alphabetical order. The formula for compounds that do not contain carbon is ordered strictly alphabetically by element symbol. Compounds such as salts or those containing waters of hydration have molecular formulas incorporating the CAS dot-disconnect convention. In this convention, the components are listed individually and separated by a period. The individual components of the formula are given in order of decreasing carbon atom count, and the component ratios given. A lower case "x" indicates that the ratio is unknown. A lower case "n" indicates a repeating, polymer-like structure. The formula is obtained from one of the cited references or a chemical reference text, or derived from the name of the material.

6. *Molecular Weight* (*mw:*) or atomic weight (*aw:*) is calculated from the molecular formula using standard elemental molecular weights (carbon = 12.01).

7. *Properties* (*PROP:*) are selected to be useful in evaluating the hazard of a material and designing its proper storage and use procedures. A definition of the material is included where necessary. The physical description of the material may include the form, color and odor to aid in positive identification. When available, the boiling point, melting point, density, vapor pressure, vapor density, and refractive index are given. The flash point, autoignition temperature, and lower and upper explosive limits are included to aid in fire protection and control. An indication is given of the solubility or miscibility of the material in water and common solvents. Unless otherwise indicated temperature is given in Celsius, pressure is in millimeters of mercury.

8. *Synonyms* for the entry name are listed alphabetically. Synonyms include other chemical names, common or generic names, foreign names (with the language in parentheses), or codes. Some synonyms consist in whole or in part of registered trademarks. These trademarks are not identified as such. The reader is cautioned that some synonyms, particularly common names, may be ambiguous and refer to more than one material.

9. *Carcinogenic Dose Data* lines include, in sequence, the study result (CAR, NEO, ETA), the route of exposure; the species of animal studied; the toxicity measure; the amount of material per body weight or concentration per unit of air volume and, where applicable, the duration of exposure; a descriptive notation of the type of effect reported; and the reference from which the information was extracted. Only positive test results are cited.

All toxic dose data appearing in the book are derived from reports of the toxic effects produced by individual materials. For human data, a toxic effect is defined as any benign or malignant tumor. There is no qualifying limitation on the duration of exposure or for the quantity or concentration of the material, nor is there a qualifying limitation on the circumstances that resulted from the exposure. Regardless of the absurdity of the circumstances that were involved in a toxic exposure, it is assumed that the same circumstances could recur. For animal data, toxic effects are limited to the production of tumors, benign (neoplastigenesis) or malignant (carcinogenesis). There is no limitation on either the duration of exposure or on the quantity or concentration of the dose of the material reported to have caused these effects.

The report of the lowest total dose administered over the shortest time to produce the toxic effect was given preference, although some editorial liberty was taken so that additional references might be cited.

Each element of the carcinogenic dose line is discussed below:

a. Carcinogenic Study Result. Tumorigenic citations are classified according to the reported results of the study to aid the reader in selecting appropriate references for in-depth review and evaluation. The classification, ETA (equivocal tumorigenic agent), denotes those studies reporting uncertain, but seemingly positive, results. The criteria for the three classifications are listed below. These criteria are used to abstract the data in individual reports on a consistent basis and do not represent a comprehensive evaluation of a material's tumorigenic potential to humans.

The following nine technical criteria are used to abstract the toxicological literature and classify studies that report positive tumorigenic responses. No attempts are made either to evaluate the various test procedures or to correlate results from different experiments.

(1) A citation is coded "CAR" (carcinogenic) when review of an article reveals that all the following criteria are satisfied:

(a) A statistically significant increase in the incidence of tumors in the test animals. The statistical test is that used by the author. If no statistic is reported, a Fisher's Exact Test is applied with significance at the 0.05 level, unless the author makes a strong case for significance at some other level.

(b) A control group of animals is used and the treated and control animals are maintained under identical conditions.

(c) The sole experimental variable between the groups is the administration or non-administration of the test material (see (9) below).

(d) The tumors consist of autonomous populations of cells of abnormal cytology capable of invading and destroying normal tissues, or the tumors metastasize as confirmed by histopathology.

(2) A citation is coded "NEO" (neoplastic) when review of an article reveals that all the following criteria are satisfied:

(a) A statistically significant increase in the incidence of tumors in the test animals. The statistical test is that used by the author. If no statistic is reported, a Fisher's Exact Test is applied with significance at the 0.05 level, unless the author makes a strong case for significance at some other level.

(b) A control group of animals is used, and the treated and control animals are maintained under identical conditions.

(c) The sole experimental variable between the groups is the administration or non-administration of the test material (see (9) below).

(d) The tumors consist of cells that closely resemble the tissue of origin, that are not grossly abnormal cytologically, that may compress surrounding tissues, but that neither invade tissues nor metastasize; or

(e) The tumors produced cannot be classified as either benign or malignant.

(3) A citation is coded "ETA" (equivocal tumorigenic agent) when some evidence of tumorigenic activity is presented, but one or more of the criteria listed in (1) or (2) above is lacking. Thus, a report with positive pathological findings, but with no mention of control animals, is coded "ETA."

(4) Since an author may make statements or draw conclusions based on a larger context than that of the particular data reported, papers in which the author's conclusions differ substantially from the evidence presented in the paper are subject to review.

(5) All doses except those for transplacental carcinogenesis are reported in one of the following formats.

(a) For all routes of administration other than inhalation: cumulative dose in mg (or appropriate unit)/kg/duration of administration.

Whenever the dose reported in the reference is not in the units discussed herein, conversion to this format is made. The total cumulative dose is derived from the lowest dose level that produces tumors in the test group.

(b) For inhalation experiments: concentration in ppm (or mg/m^3)/total duration of exposure. The concentration refers to the lowest concentration that produces tumors.

(6) Transplacental carcinogenic doses are reported in one of the following formats.

(a) For all routes of administration other than inhalation: cumulative dose in mg/kg/(time of administration during pregnancy).

The cumulative dose is derived from the lowest single dose that produces tumors in the offspring. The test chemical is administered to the mother.

(b) For inhalation experiments: concentration in ppm (or mg/m^3)/(time of exposure during pregnancy).

The concentration refers to the lowest concentration that produces tumors in the offspring. The mother is exposed to the test chemical.

(7) For the purposes of this listing, all test chemicals are reported as pure, unless otherwise stated by the author. This does not rule out the possibility that unknown impurities may have been present.

(8) A mixture of compounds whose test results satisfy the criteria in (1), (2), or (3) above is included if the composition of the mixture can be clearly defined.

(9) For tests involving promoters or initiators, a study is included if the following conditions are satisfied (in addition to the criteria in (1), (2), or (3) above):

(a) The test chemical is applied first, followed by an application of a standard promoter. A positive control group in which the test animals are subjected to the same standard promoter under identical conditions is maintained throughout the duration of the experiment. The data are only used if positive and negative control groups are mentioned in the reference.

(b) A known carcinogen is first applied as an initiator, followed by application of the text chemical as a promoter. A positive control group in which the test animals are subjected to the same initiator under identical conditions is maintained throughout the duration of the experiment. The data are only used if positive and negative control groups are mentioned in the reference.

b. Route of Exposure or Administration. Although many exposures to materials in the industrial community occur via the respiratory tract or skin, most studies in the published literature report exposures of experimental animals in which the test materials were introduced primarily through the mouth by pills, in food, in drinking water, or by intubation directly into the stomach. The abbreviations and definitions of the various routes of exposure reported are given in Table 1.

c. Species Exposed. Since the effects of exposure of humans are of primary concern, we have indicated, when available, whether the results were observed in man, woman, child, or infant. If no such distinction was made in the reference, the abbreviation "hmn" (human) is used. However, the results of studies on rats or mice are the most often reported and hence provide the most useful data for comparative purposes. The species and abbreviations used in reporting toxic dose data are listed alphabetically in Table 2.

d. Description of Exposure. In order to better describe the administered dose reported in the literature, six abbreviations are used. These terms indicate whether the dose caused death (LD) or other toxic effects (TD) and whether it was administered as a lethal concentration (LC) or toxic concentration (TC) in the inhaled air. The term "Lo" is used where the number of subjects studied was not a significant number from the population or the calculated percentage of subjects showing an effect was listed as 100. The definition of terms is as follows:

*TDLo—Toxic Dose Low—*the lowest dose of a material introduced by any route, other than inhalation, over any given period of time and reported to produce carcinogenic or neoplastigenic effects in animals or humans.

Table 1. Routes of Administration to, or Exposure of, Animal Species to Toxic Substances

Abbreviation	Route	Definition
Eyes	eye	Administration directly onto the surface of the eye. Used exclusively for primary irritation data. See Ocular
Intraaural	ial	Administration into the ear
Intraarterial	iat	Administration into the artery
Intracerebral	ice	Administration into the cerebrum
Intracervical	icv	Administration into the cervix
Intradermal	idr	Administration within the dermis by hypodermic needle
Intraduodenal	idu	Administration into the duodenum
Inhalation	ihl	Inhalation in chamber, by cannulation, or through mask
Implant	imp	Placed surgically within the body location described in reference
Intramuscular	ims	Administration into the muscle by hypodermic needle
Intraplacental	ipc	Administration into the placenta
Intrapleural	ipl	Administration into the pleural cavity by hypodermic needle
Intraperitoneal	ipr	Administration into the peritoneal cavity
Intrarenal	irn	Administration into the kidney
Intraspinal	isp	Administration into the spinal canal
Intratracheal	itr	Administration into the trachea
Intratesticular	itt	Administration into the testes
Intrauterine	iut	Administration into the uterus
Intravaginal	ivg	Administration into the vagina
Intravenous	ivn	Administration directly into the vein by hypodermic needle
Multiple	mul	Administration into a single animal by more than one route
Ocular	ocu	Administration directly onto the surface of the eye or into the conjunctival sac. Used exclusively for systemic toxicity data
Oral	orl	Per os, intragastric, feeding, or introduction with drinking water
Parenteral	par	Administration into the body through the skin. Reference cited is not specific about the route used. Could be ipr, scu, ivn, ipl, ims, irn, or ice
Rectal	rec	Administration into the rectum or colon in the form of enema or suppository
Subcutaneous	scu	Administration under the skin
Skin	skn	Application directly either intact or abraded. Used for both systemic toxicity and primary irritant effects
Unreported	unr	Dose, but not route, is specified in the reference

TCLo—Toxic Concentration Low—the lowest concentration of a material in air to which humans or animals have been exposed for any given period of time that has produced a carcinogenic or neoplastigenic effect in animals or humans.

LCLo—Lethal Concentration Low—the lowest concentration of a material in air, other than LC50, which has been reported to have caused death in humans or animals.

e. Units of Dose Measurement. As in almost all experimental toxicology, the doses given are expressed in terms of the quantity administered per unit body weight, or quantity per skin surface area, or quantity per unit volume of the respired air. In addition, the duration of time over which the dose was administered is also listed, as needed. Dose amounts are expressed as milligrams (one thousandth of a gram) per kilogram (mg/kg). In some cases, because of dose size and its practical presentation in the file, grams per kilogram (g/kg), micrograms (one millionth of a gram) per kilogram (μg/kg), or nanograms (one billionth of a gram) per kilogram (ng/kg) are used. Volume measurements of dose were converted to weight units by appropriate calculations. Densities were obtained from standard reference texts. Where densities were not readily available,

Table 2. Species (With Assumptions for Toxic Dose Calculation From Non-Specific Data*)

Abbrev.	Species	Age	Weight	Consumption (Approx.) Food g/day	Water mL/day	1 ppm in Food Equals, in mg/kg/day	Approximate Gestation Period days
Bird—type not specified	brd		1 kg				
Bird—wild bird species	bwd		40 gm				
Cat, adult	cat		2 kg	100	100	0.05	64 (59–68)
Child	chd	1–13 Y	20 kg				
Chicken, adult	ckn	8 W	800 gm	140	200	0.175	
Cattle	ctl		500 kg	10,000		0.02	284 (279–290)
Duck, adult (domestic)	dck	8 W	2.5 kg	250	500	0.1	
Dog, adult	dog	52 W	10 kg	250	500	0.025	62 (56–68)
Domestic animals (Goat, Sheep)	dom		60 kg	2,400		0.04	G: 152 (148–156) S: 146 (144–147)
Frog, adult	frg		33 gm				
Guinea Pig, adult	gpg		500 gm	30	85	0.06	68
Gerbil	grb		100 gm	5	5	0.05	25 (24–26)
Hamster	ham	14 W	125 gm	15	10	0.12	16 (16–17)
Human	hmn	Adult	70 kg				
Horse, Donkey	hor		500 kg	10,000		0.02	H: 339 (333–345) D: 365
Infant	inf	0–1 Y	5 kg				
Mammal (species unspecified in reference)	mam		200 gm				

xvi

		Age	Weight				
Man	man	Adult	70 kg	250		0.05	165
Monkey	mky	2.5 Y	5 kg	3	500	0.12	21
Mouse	mus	8 W	25 gm		5		
Non-mammalian species	nml						
Pigeon	pgn		500 gm				
Pig	pig	8 W	60 kg	2,400		0.041	114 (112–115)
Quail (laboratory)	qal		100 gm				
Rat, adult female	rat	14 W	200 gm	10	20	0.05	22
Rat, adult male	rat	14 W	250 gm	15	25	0.06	
Rat, adult	rat	14 W	200 gm	15	25		
Rat, weanling	rat	3 W	50 gm	15	25	0.3	
Rabbit, adult	rbt	12 W	2 kg	60	330	0.03	
Squirrel	sql		500 gm				31
Toad	tod		100 gm				44
Turkey	trk	18 W	5 kg				
Woman	wmn	Adult	50 kg				270

* Values given in Table 2 are within reasonable limits usually found in the published literature and are selected to facilitate calculations for data from publications in which toxic dose information has not been presented for an individual animal of the study. See, for example, *Association of Food and Drug Officials, Quarterly Bulletin*, volume 18, page 66, 1954; Guyton, *American Journal of Physiology*, volume 150, page 75, 1947; *The Merck Veterinary Manual*, 5th Edition, Merck & Co., Inc., Rahway, N.J., 1979; and the UFAW *Handbook on the Care and Management of Laboratory Animals*, 4th Edition, Churchill Livingston, London, 1972. Data for lifetime exposure are calculated from the assumptions for adult animals for the entire period of exposure. For definitive dose data, the reader must review the referenced publication.

all liquids were assumed to have a density of one gram per milliliter. Twenty drops of liquid are assumed to be equal in volume to one milliliter.

All body weights have been converted to kilograms (kg) for uniformity. For those references in which the dose was reported to have been administered to an animal of unspecified weight or a given number of animals in a group (e.g., feeding studies) without weight data, the weights of the respective animal species were assumed to be those listed in Table 2 and the dose is listed on a per-kilogram body weight basis. Assumptions for daily food and water intake are found in Table 2 to allow approximating doses for humans and species of experimental animals where the dose was originally reported as a concentration in food or water. The values presented are selections which are reasonable for the species and convenient for dose calculations.

Concentrations of a gaseous material in air are generally listed as parts of vapor or gas per million parts of air by volume (ppm). However, parts per hundred (pph or percent), parts per billion (ppb), or parts per trillion (ppt) may be used for convenience of presentation. If the material is a solid or a liquid, the concentrations are listed preferably as milligrams per cubic meter (mg/m^3) but may, as applicable, be listed as micrograms per cubic meter ($\mu g/m^3$), nanograms per cubic meter (ng/m^3), or picograms (one trillionth of a gram) per cubic meter (pg/m^3) of air. For those cases in which other measurements of contaminants are used, such as the number of fibers or particles, the measurement is spelled out.

Where the duration of exposure is available, time is presented as minutes (M), hours (H), days (D), weeks (W), or years (Y). Additionally, continuous (C) indicates that the exposure was continuous over the time administered, such as ad libitum feeding studies or 24-hour, 7-day per week inhalation exposures. Intermittent (I) indicates that the dose was administered during discrete periods, such as daily, twice weekly, etc. In all cases, the total duration of exposure appears first after the kilogram body weight and slash, followed by descriptive data; e.g., 10 mg/kg/3W-I indicates ten milligrams per kilogram body weight administered over a period of three weeks, intermittently in a number of separate, discrete doses. This description is intended to provide the reader with enough information for an approximation of the experimental conditions, which can be further clarified by studying the reference cited.

f. Frequency of Exposure. Frequency of exposure to the test material varies depending on the nature of the experiment. Frequency of exposure is given in the case of an inhalation experiment, for human exposures (where applicable), or where CAR, NEO, or ETA is specified as the toxic effect.

g. Duration of Exposure. For assessment of tumorigenic effect, the testing period should be the life span of the animal, or until statistically valid calculations can be obtained regarding tumor incidence. In the toxic dose line, the total dose causing the tumorigenic effect is given. The duration of exposure is included to give an indication of the testing period during which the animal was exposed to this total dose. For multigenerational studies, the time during gestation when the material was administered to the mother is also provided.

h. Notations Descriptive of the Toxicology. The toxic dose line thus far has indicated the route of entry, the species involved, the description of the dose, and the amount of the dose. The next entry found on this line when a toxic exposure (TD or TC) has been listed is the toxic effect. Following a colon will be one of the notations found in Table 3. These notations indicate the organ system affected. No attempt was made to be definitive in reporting these effects because such definition requires much detailed qualification and is beyond the scope of this book. The selection of the dose was based first on the lowest dose producing an effect and second on the latest study published.

10. *Mutation Data* lines include, in sequence, the mutation test system utilized, the species of the tested organism (and where applicable, the route of administration or cell type), the exposure concentration or dose, and the reference from which the information was extracted.

Table 3. Notations Descriptive of the Toxicology

Abbreviation	Definition (not limited to effects listed)
ALR	Allergic systemic reaction such as might be experienced by individuals sensitized to penicillin.
BCM	Blood clotting mechanism effects—any effect which increases or decreases clotting time.
BLD	Blood effects—effect on all blood elements, electrolytes, pH, protein, oxygen carrying or releasing capacity.
BPR	Blood pressure effects—any effect which increases or decreases any aspect of blood pressure.
CAR	Carcinogenic effects—see paragraph 9g in text.
CNS	Central nervous system effects—includes effects such as headaches, tremor, drowsiness, convulsions, hypnosis, anesthesia.
COR	Corrosive effects—burns, desquamation.
CUM	Cumulative effects—where material is retained by the body in greater quantities than is excreted, or the effect is increased in severity by repeated body insult.
CVS	Cardiovascular effects—such as an increase or decrease in the heart activity through effect on ventricle or auricle; fibrillation; constriction or dilation of the arterial or venous system.
DDP	Drug dependence effects—any indication of addiction or dependence.
ETA	Equivocal tumorigenic agent—see text.
EYE	Eye effects—irritation, diploplia, cataracts, eye ground, blindness by affecting the eye or the optic nerve.
GIT	Gastrointestinal tract effects—diarrhea, constipation, ulceration.
GLN	Glandular effects—any effect on the endocrine glandular system.
IRR	Irritant effects—any irritant effect on the skin, eye, or mucous membrane.
MLD	Mild irritation effects—used exclusively for primary irritation data.
MMI	Mucous membrane effects—irritation, hyperplasia, changes in ciliary activity.
MOD	Moderate irritation effects—used exclusively for primary irritation data.
MSK	Musculo-skeletal effects—such as osteoporosis, muscular degeneration.
NEO	Neoplastic effects—see text.
PNS	Peripheral nervous system effects.
PSY	Psychotropic effects—exerting an effect upon the mind.
PUL	Pulmonary system effects—effects on respiration and respiratory pathology.
RBC	Red blood cell effects—includes the several anemias.
REP	Reproductive effects—see text.
SEV	Severe irritation effects—used exclusively for primary irritation data.
SKN	Skin effects—such as erythema, rash, sensitization of skin, petechial hemorrhage.
SYS	Systemic effects—effects on the metabolic and excretory function of the liver or kidneys.
TER	Teratogenic effects—nontransmissible changes produced in the offspring.
UNS	Unspecified effects—the toxic effects were unspecific in the reference.
WBC	White blood cell effects—effects on any of the cellular units other than erythrocytes, including any change in number or form.

A mutation is defined as any heritable change in genetic material. Unlike irritation, reproductive, tumorigenic, and toxic dose data which report the results of whole animal studies, mutation data also include studies on lower organisms such as bacteria, molds, yeasts, and insects, and in vitro mammalian cell cultures. Studies of plant mutagenesis are not included. No attempt is made to evaluate the significance of the data or to rate the relative potency of the compound as a mutagenic risk to man.

Each element of the mutation line is discussed below.

a. Mutation Test System. A number of test systems are used to detect genetic alterations caused by chemicals. Additional ones may be added as they are reported in the literature. Each test system is identified by the 3-letter code shown in parentheses. For additional information about mutation tests, the reader may wish to consult the *Handbook of Mutagenicity Test Procedures*, edited by B. J. Kilbey, M. Legator, W. Nichols, and C. Ramel (Amsterdam: Elsevier Scientific Publishing Company/North-Holland Biomedical Press, 1977).

(1) Mutation in Microorganisms (mmo) System utilizes the detection of heritable genetic alterations in microorganisms which have been exposed directly to the chemical.

(2) Microsomal Mutagenicity Assay (mma) System utilizes an in vitro technique which allows enzymatic activation of promutagens in the presence of an indicator organism in which induced mutation frequencies are determined.

(3) Micronucleus Test (mnt) System utilizes the fact that chromosomes or chromosome fragments may not be incorporated into one or the other of the daughter nuclei during cell division.

(4) Specific Locus Test (slt) System utilizes a method for detecting and measuring rates of mutation at any or all several recessive loci.

(5) DNA Damage (dnd) System detects the damage to DNA strands including strand breaks, crosslinks, and other abnormalities.

(6) DNA Repair (dnr) System utilizes methods of monitoring DNA repair as a function of induced genetic damage.

(7) Unscheduled DNA Synthesis (dns) System detects the synthesis of DNA during usually nonsynthetic phases.

(8) DNA Inhibition (dni) System detects damage that inhibits the synthesis of DNA.

(9) Gene Conversion and Mitotic Recombination (mrc) System utilizes unequal recovery of genetic markers in the region of the exchange during genetic recombination.

(10) Cytogenetic Analysis (cyt) System utilizes cultured cells or cell lines to assay for chromosomal aberrations following the administration of the chemical.

(11) Sister Chromatid Exchange (sce) System detects the interchange of DNA in cytological preparations of metaphase chromosomes between replication products at apparently homologous loci.

(12) Sex Chromosome Loss and Nondisjunction (sln) System measures the nonseparation of homologous chromosomes at meiosis and mitosis.

(13) Dominant Lethal Test (dlt) A dominant lethal is a genetic change in a gamete that kills the zygote produced by that gamete. In mammals, the dominant lethal test measures the reduction of litter size by examining the uterus and noting the number of surviving and dead implants.

(14) Mutation in Mammalian Somatic Cells (msc) System utilizes the induction and isolation of mutants in cultured mammalian cells by identification of the gene change.

(15) Host-Mediated Assay (hma) System uses two separate species, generally mammalian and bacterial, to detect heritable genetic alteration caused by metabolic conversion of chemical substances administered to host mammalian species in the bacterial indicator species.

(16) Sperm Morphology (spm) System measures the departure from normal in the appearance of sperm.

(17) Heritable Translocation Test (trn) Test measures the transmissibility of induced translocations to subsequent generations. In mammals, the test uses sterility and reduced fertility in the progeny of the treated parent. In addition, cytological analysis of the F1 progeny or subsequent progeny of the treated parent is carried out to prove the existence of the induced translocation. In *Drosophila*, heritable translocations are detected genetically using easily distinguishable phenotypic markers, and these translocations can be verified with cytogenetic techniques.

(18) Oncogenic Transformation (otr) System utilizes morphological criteria to detect cytological differences between normal and transformed tumorigenic cells.

(19) Phage Inhibition Capacity (pic) System utilizes a lysogenic virus to detect a change in the genetic characteristics by the transformation of the virus from noninfectious to infectious.

(20) Body Fluid Assay (bfa) System uses two separate species, usually mammalian and bacterial. Test substance is first administered to host, from whom body fluid (e.g., urine, blood) is subse-

quently taken. This body fluid is then tested in vitro, and mutations are measured in the bacterial species.

b. Species. Those test species that are peculiar to mutation data are designated by the 3-letter codes shown below.

	Code	Species
Bacteria	bcs	*Bacillus subtilis*
	esc	*Escherichia coli*
	hmi	*Haemophilus influenzae*
	klp	*Klebsiella pneumoniae*
	sat	*Salmonella typhimurium*
	srm	*Serratia marcescens*
Molds	asn	*Aspergillus nidulans*
	nsc	*Neurospora crassa*
Yeasts	smc	*Saccharomyces cerevisiae*
	ssp	*Schizosaccharomyces pombe*
Protozoa	clr	*Chlamydomonas reinhardi*
	eug	*Euglena gracilis*
	omi	other microorganisms
Insects	dmg	Drosophila melanogaster
	dpo	Drosophila pseudo-obscura
	grh	grasshopper
	slw	silkworm
	oin	other insects
Fish	sal	salmon
	ofs	other fish

If the test organism is a cell type from a mammalian species, the parent mammalian species is reported, followed by a colon and the cell type designation. For example, human leukocytes are coded "hmn:leu." The various cell types currently cited in this edition are as follows:

Designation	Cell Type
ast	Ascites tumor
bmr	bone marrow
emb	embryo
fbr	fibroblast
hla	HeLa cell
kdy	kidney
leu	leukocyte
lng	lung
lvr	liver
lym	lymphocyte
mmr	mammary gland
ovr	ovary
spr	sperm
tes	testis
oth	other cell types not listed above

In the case of host-mediated and body fluid assays, both the host organism and the indicator organism are given as follows: host organism/indicator organism, e.g., "ham/sat" for a test in which hamsters were exposed to the test chemical and *S. typhimurium* was used as the indicator organism.

For in vivo mutagenic studies, the route of administration is specified following the species designation, e.g., "mus-orl" for oral administration to mice. See Table 1 for a complete list of routes cited. The route of administration is not specified for in vitro data.

c. Units of Exposure. The lowest dose producing a positive effect is cited. The author's calculations are used to determine the lowest dose at which a positive effect was observed. If the author fails to state the lowest effective dose, two times the control dose will be used. Ideally, the dose should be reported in universally accepted toxicological units such as milligrams of test chemical per kilogram of test animal body weight. While this is possible in cases where the actual intake of the chemical by an organism of known weight is reported, it is not possible in many systems using insect and bacterial species. In cases where a dose is reported or where the amount can be converted to a dose unit, it is normally listed as milligrams per kilogram (mg/kg). However, micrograms (μg), nanograms (ng), or picograms (pg) per kilogram may also be used for convenience of presentation. Concentrations of gaseous materials in air are listed as parts per hundred (pph), per million (ppm), per billion (ppb), or per trillion (ppt).

Test systems using microbial organisms traditionally report exposure data as an amount of chemical per liter (L) or amount per plate, well, disc, or tube. The amount may be on a weight (g, mg, μg, ng, or pg) or molar (millimole (mmol), micromole (μmol), nanomole (nmol), or picomole (pmol)) basis. These units describe the exposure concentration rather than the dose actually taken up by the test species. Insufficient data currently exist to permit the development of dose amounts from this information. In such cases, therefore, the material concentration units used by the author are reported.

Since the exposure values reported in host-mediated and body fluid assays are doses delivered to the host organism, no attempt is made to estimate the exposure concentration to the indicator organism. The exposure values cited for host-mediated assay data are in units of milligrams (or other appropriate unit of weight) of material administered per kilogram of host body weight or in parts of vapor or gas per million (ppm) parts of air (or other appropriate concentrations) by volume.

11. *Cited Reference* is the final entry of the irritation, mutation, reproductive, tumorigenic, and toxic dose data lines. This is the source from which the information was extracted. All references cited are publicly available. No governmental classified documents have been used for source information. All references have been given a unique six-letter CODEN character code (derived from the American Society for Testing and Materials *CODEN for Periodical Titles* and the CAS *Source Index*), which identifies periodicals, serial publications, and individual published works. For those references for which no CODEN was found, the corresponding six-letter code includes asterisks (*) in the last one or two positions following the first four or five letters of an acronym for the publication title. Following the CODEN designation (for most entries) is the number of the volume, followed by a comma; the page number of the first page of the article, followed by a comma; and a two-digit number, indicating the year of publication in this century. When the cited reference is a report, the report number is listed. Where contributors have provided information on their unpublished studies, the CODEN consists of the first three letters of the last name, the initials of the first and middle names, and a number sign (#). The date of the letter supplying the information is listed. All CODEN acronyms are listed in alphabetical order and defined in the CODEN Section.

12. *Reviews and Status* lines supply additional information to enable the reader to make knowledgeable evaluations of potential chemical hazards. Two types of reviews are listed: (a) International Agency for Research on Cancer (IARC) monograph reviews, which are published by

the United Nations World Health Organization (WHO), and the National Toxicology Program (NTP).

a. Cancer Reviews. In the U.N. International Agency for Research on Cancer (IARC) monographs, information on suspected environmental carcinogens is examined, and summaries of available data with appropriate references are presented. Included in these reviews are synonyms, physical and chemical properties, uses and occurrence, and biological data relevant to the evaluation of carcinogenic risk to humans. The over 43 monographs in the series contain an evaluation of approximately 900 materials. Single copies of the individual monographs (specify volume number) can be ordered from WHO Publications Centre USA, 49 Sheridan Avenue, Albany, New York 12210, telephone (518) 436-9686.

The format of the IARC data line is as follows. The entry 'IARC Cancer Review': indicates that the carcinogenicity data pertaining to a compound has been reviewed by the IARC committee. The committee's conclusion are summarized in three words. The first word indicates whether the data pertains to humans or to animals. The next two words indicate the degree of carcinogenic risk as defined by IARC.

For experimental animals the evidence of carcinogenicity is assessed by IARC and judged to fall into one of four groups defined as follows:

(1) Sufficient Evidence of carcinogenicity is provided when there is an increased incidence of malignant tumors: (a) in multiple species or strains; or (b) in multiple experiments (preferably with different routes of administration or using different dose levels); or (c) to an unusual degree with regard to the incidence, site, or type of tumor, or age at onset. Additional evidence may be provided by data on dose-response effects.

(2) Limited Evidence of carcinogenicity is available when the data suggest a carcinogenic effect but are limited because: (a) the studies involve a single species, strain, or experiment; (b) the experiments are restricted by inadequate dosage levels, inadequate duration of exposure to the agent, inadequate period of follow-up, poor survival, too few animals, or inadequate reporting; or (c) the neoplasms produced often occur spontaneously and, in the past, have been difficult to classify as malignant by histological criteria alone (e.g., lung adenomas and adenocarcinomas, and liver tumors in certain strains of mice).

(3) Inadequate Evidence is available when, because of major qualitative or quantitative limitations, the studies cannot be interpreted as showing either the presence or absence of a carcinogenic effect.

(4) No Evidence applies when several adequate studies are available which show that within the limitations of the tests used, the chemical is not carcinogenic.

It should be noted that the categories Sufficient Evidence and Limited Evidence refer only to the strength of the experimental evidence that these chemicals are carcinogenic and not to the extent of their carcinogenic activity nor to the mechanism involved. The classification of any chemical may change as new information becomes available.

The evidence for carcinogenicity from studies in humans is assessed by the IARC committees and judged to fall into one of four groups defined as follows:

(1) Sufficient Evidence of carcinogenicity indicates that there is a causal relationship between the exposure and human cancer.

(2) Limited Evidence of carcinogenicity indicates that a causal relationship is credible, but that alternative explanations, such as chance, bias, or confounding, could not adequately be excluded.

(3) Inadequate Evidence, which applies to both positive and negative evidence, indicates that one of two conditions prevailed: (a) there are few pertinent data; or (b) the available studies, while showing evidence of association, do not exclude chance, bias, or confounding.

(4) No Evidence applies when several adequate studies are available which do not show evidence of carcinogenicity.

This cancer review reflects only the conclusion of the IARC committee based on the data available for the committee's evaluation. Hence, for some substances there may be a disagreement between the IARC determination and the information on the tumorigenic data lines (see paragraph 10). Also, some substances previously reviewed by IARC may be reexamined as additional data become available. These substances will contain multiple IARC review lines, each of which is referenced to the applicable IARC monograph volume.

An IARC entry indicates that some carcinogenicity data pertaining to a compound has been reviewed by the IARC committee. It indicates whether the data pertain to humans or to animals and whether the results of the determination are positive, suspected, indefinite, negative, or no data.

This cancer review reflects only the conclusion of the IARC Committee based on the data available at the time of the Committee's evaluation. Hence, for some materials there may be disagreement between the IARC determination and the tumorigenicity information in the toxicity data lines.

b. NTP Status. This entry indicates that the material has been tested by the National Toxicology Program (NTP) under its Carcinogenesis Testing Program. These entries are also identified as National Cancer Institute (NCI), which reported the studies before the NCI Carcinogenesis Testing Program was absorbed by NTP. To obtain additional information about NTP, the Carcinogenesis Testing Program, or the status of a particular material under test, contact the Toxicology Information and Scientific Evaluation Group, NTP/TRTP/NIEHS, Mail Drop 18-01, P.O. Box 12233, Research Triangle Park, NC 27709.

c. EPA Extremely Hazardous Substances List. This list was developed by the U.S. Environmental Protection Agency (EPA) as required by the Superfund Amendments and Reauthorization Act of 1986 (SARA). Title III Section 304 requires notification by facilities of a release of certain extremely hazardous substances. These 402 substances were listed by EPA in the *Federal Register* November 17, 1986.

d. Community Right To Know List. This list was developed by the EPA as required by the Superfund Amendments and Reauthorization Act of 1986 (SARA). Title III, Sections 311-312 require manufacturing facilities to prepare Material Safety Data Sheets and notify local authorities of the presence of listed chemicals. Both specific chemicals and classes of chemicals are covered by these Sections.

e. EPA Genetic Toxicology Program (GENE-TOX). This status line indicates that the material has had genetic effects reported in the literature during the period 1969-1979. The test protocol in the literature is evaluated by an EPA expert panel on mutations and the positive or negative genetic effect of the substance is reported. To obtain additional information about this program, contact GENE-TOX program, USEPA, 401 M Street, SW, TS796, Washington, DC 20460, Telephone (202) 382-3513.

f. EPA TSCA Status Line. This line indicates that the material appears on the chemical inventory prepared by the Environmental Protection Agency in accordance with provisions of the Toxic Substances Control Act (TSCA). Materials reported in the inventory include those that are produced commercially in or imported into this country. The reader should note, however, that materials already regulated by EPA under FIFRA and by the Food and Drug Administration under the Food, Drug, and Cosmetic Act, as amended, are not included in the TSCA inventory. Similarly, alcohol, tobacco, and explosive materials are not regulated under TSCA. TSCA regulations should be consulted for an exact definition of reporting requirements. For additional information about TSCA, contact EPA, Office of Toxic Substances, Washington, D.C. 20402. Specific questions about the inventory can be directed to the EPA Office of Industry Assistance, telephone (800) 424-9065.

13. *Standards and Recommendations*. This section contains regulations by agencies of the United States Government or recommendations by expert groups. "OSHA" refers to standards promulgated under Section 6 of the Occupational Safety and Health Act of 1970. "DOT" refers to materials regulated for shipment by the Department of Transportation. Because of frequent changes to and litigation of Federal regulations, it is recommended that the reader contact the applicable agency for information about the current standards for a particular material. Omission of a material or regulatory notation from this edition does not imply any relief from regulatory responsibility.

   a. OSHA Air Contaminant Standards. The values given are for the revised standards which were published in January 13, 1989 and take effect on September 1, 1989 through December 31, 1992. These are noted with the entry "OSHA PEL:" followed by "TWA" or "CL" meaning either time-weighted average or ceiling value, respectively, to which workers can be exposed for a normal 8-hour day, 40-hour work week without ill effects. For some materials, TWA, CL, and Pk (peak) values are given in the standard. In those cases, all three are listed. Finally, some entries may be followed by the designation "(skin)." This designation indicates that the compound may be absorbed by the skin and, even though the air concentration may be below the standard, significant additional exposure through the skin may be possible.

   b. ACGIH Threshold Limit Values. The American Conference of Governmental Industrial Hygienists (ACGIH) Threshold Limit Values are noted with the entry "ACGIH TLV:" followed by "TWA" or "CL" meaning either time-weighted average or ceiling value, respectively, to which workers can be exposed for a normal 8-hour day, 40-hour work week without ill effects. The notation "CL" indicates a ceiling limit which must not be exceeded. The notation "skin" indicates that the material penetrates intact skin, and skin contact should be avoided even though the TLV concentration is not exceeded. STEL indicates a short-term exposure limit, usually a 15-minute time-weighted average, which should not be exceeded. Biological Exposure Indices (*BEI:*) are, according to the ACGIH, set to provide a warning level ". . .of biological response to the chemical, or warning levels of that chemical or its metabolic product(s) in tissues, fluids, or exhaled air of exposed workers. . ."

   The latest annual TLV list is contained in the publication *Threshold Limit Values and Biological Exposure Indices*. This publication should be consulted for future trends in recommendations. The ACGIH TLV's are adopted in whole or in part by many countries and local administrative agencies throughout the world. As a result, these recommendations have a major effect on the control of workplace contaminant concentrations. The ACGIH may be contacted for additional information at 6500 Glenway Ave., Cincinnati, Ohio 45211, USA.

   c. DFG MAK. These lines contain the German Research Society's Maximum Allowable Concentration values. Those materials which are classified as to workplace hazard potential by the German Research Society are noted on this line. The MAK values are also revised annually and discussions of materials under consideration for MAK assignment are included in the annual publication together with the current values. *BAT:* indicates Biological Tolerance Value for a Working Material which is defined as, ". . .the maximum permissible quantity of a chemical compound, its metabolites, or any deviation from the norm of biological parameters induced by these substances in exposed humans." *TRK:* values are Technical Guiding Concentrations for workplace control of carcinogens. For additional information, write to Deutsche Forschungsgemeinschaft (German Research Society), Kennedyallee 40, D-5300 Bonn 2, Federal Republic of Germany. The publication *Maximum Concentrations at the Workplace and Biological Tolerance Values for Working Materials* can be obtained from Verlag Chemie GmbH, Buchauslieferung, P.O. Box 1260/1280, D-6940 Weinheim, Federal Republic of Germany, or Verlag Chemie, Deerfield Beach, Florida.

d. NIOSH REL. This line indicates that a NIOSH criteria document recommending a certain occupational exposure has been published for this compound or for a class of compounds to which this material belongs. These documents contain extensive data, analysis, and references. The more recent publications can be obtained from the National Institute for Occupational Safety and Health, U.S. Department of Health and Human Services, 4676 Columbia Pkwy., Cincinnati, Ohio 45226.

e. DOT Classification. This is the hazard classification according to the U.S. Department of Transportation (DOT) or the International Maritime Organization (IMO.) This classification gives an indication of the hazards expected in transportation, and serves as a guide to the development of proper labels, placards, and shipping instructions. The basic hazard classes include compressed gases, flammables, oxidizers, corrosives, explosives, radioactive materials, and poisons. Although a material may be designated by only one hazard class, additional hazards may be indicated by adding labels or by using other means as directed by DOT. Many materials are regulated under general headings such as "pesticides" or "combustible liquids" as defined in the regulations. These are not noted here as their specific concentration or properties must be known for proper classification. Special regulations may govern shipment by air. This information should serve *only as a guide*, since the regulation of transported materials is carefully controlled in most countries by federal and local agencies. Because of frequent changes to regulations, it is recommended that the reader contact the applicable agency for information about the current standards for a particular material. United States transportation regulations are found in 40 CFR, Parts 100 to 189. Contact the U.S. Department of Transportation, Materials Transportation Bureau, Washington, D.C. 20590.

14. *Safety Profiles* are text summaries of the toxicity of the entry. Carcinogenicity potential is denoted by the words confirmed, suspected, or questionable. Human effects are identified either by human or more specifically by man, woman, child, or infant. The word experimental indicates that the reported effects resulted from a controlled exposure of laboratory animals to the substance. In additional to carcinogenic effects, acute and chronic toxic, reproductive, and irritant effects are also noted. Fire and explosion hazards are briefly summarized in terms of conditions of flammable or reactive hazard.

ACKNOWLEDGMENTS

I wish to thank my wife, Grace, for her constant help and advice in every aspect of writing this work. I extend thanks to Dr. Mark Licker, Executive Editor, Chemistry and Industrial Safety for encouragement. My best to Alberta Gordon and Louise Kurtz for their expert professional advice and assistance in converting the manuscript to this volume.

Special thanks to Ms. Susan H. Munger of The Oldham Publishing Service for her assistance and suggestions.

Section 1

Chapter 1

IDENTIFYING CARCINOGENS

David H. Groth, M.D.
Pathologist and Consultant
Occupational and Environmental Health
Cincinnati, Ohio

INTRODUCTION

It is now generally accepted by the public and most scientists that environmental chemicals can cause and have been shown to cause cancer in humans. It is a common opinion held by most scientists in the field of carcinogenesis that environmental chemicals contribute significantly to the development of cancer in humans and do so to a much greater extent than any other category of agents. It has been estimated that 85% of all cancer is caused by environmental chemicals.

The fact that many different environmental chemicals can cause cancer in humans has been demonstrated in many epidemiological studies. Most of these studies were performed on relatively small groups of workers who were unwittingly exposed to much higher concentrations of carcinogens than was the general public. The chemicals covered in these studies include several aromatic amines (used in making dyes), asbestos, vinyl chloride (used in making polyvinyl chloride, PVC), benzene and arsenic. Other support for the cause and effect relationship between chemical exposure and cancer in humans is derived from epidemiological studies of patients treated with certain pharmaceutical drugs; and the epidemiologic studies on the relationship between cigarette smoking and lung cancer.

At the present time, there are 39 chemicals or mixtures of chemicals and 11 industrial or manufacturing processes for which there is ample evidence of carcinogenicity in humans, based upon epidemiologic studies (IARC, 1987). The data in these studies were compiled by the International Agency for Research on Cancer (IARC) [which is funded by the U.S. National Cancer Institute (NCI)] over a period of 15 years.

Although the ability of environmental chemicals to cause cancer in humans had been known for some time (Pott, 1775: scrotal cancer in chimney sweeps; Harting & Hesse, 1879: lung cancer in miners; Rehn, 1895: bladder cancer in aniline dye workers; Homburger, 1943; lung cancer in asbestos workers), there was very little public interest in controlling the exposure of workers or in identifying and controlling environmental carcinogens in general until the late 1950s. This public interest emerged in the form of a law (Public Law 85–929) commonly known as the Delaney Amendment. Oddly enough, this law concerned food additives and *not* workplace exposures (even though the evidence linking chemical exposures to human cancer was derived from the workplace). This law prohibits the use of any carcinogenic chemical as a food additive. It specifically states, ''That no additive shall be deemed safe if it is found to induce cancer when ingested by man or *animal* . . .''

In the late 1960s and 1970s, public interest in identifying and controlling exposures to environmental chemicals increased, principally because many chemicals were known carcinogens, many others were suspected as probable or possible carcinogens, and by far the majority of environmental chemicals had never even been tested. Several governmental agencies were created by law to do research on the health effects of chemicals and/or to regulate exposures to them. These agencies include the Occupational Safety and Health Administration (OSHA), the National Institute for Occupational Safety and Health (NIOSH), the Environmental Protection Agency (EPA), the Consumer Product Safety Commission (CPSC), the National Institute of Environmental Health Sciences (NIEHS), and the Mine Safety and Health Administration (MSHA). Since EPA was founded, several congressional acts have been passed for which EPA has the administrative responsibilities, namely, the Clean Air Act (CAA), Clean Water Act (CWA), Safe Drinking Water Act (SDWA), Toxic Substance Control Act (TSCA), the Federal Insecticide Fungicide and Rodenticide Act (FIFRA), Resource Conservation and Recovery Act (RCRA), and the Comprehensive Environmental Response, Compensation and Liability Act (CERCLA). The National Toxicology Program (NTP) (administered by NIEHS) has the responsibility for testing chemicals in long-term animal bioassays and for producing the *Annual Report on Carcinogens*.

Many of the chemicals these agencies test and/or regulate are carcinogens or suspected carcinogens. However, there are approximately 60,000 synthetic chemicals used in the United States (Weinstein, 1981). Very few of these chemicals have been tested for their carcinogenic activity in animals and even fewer have been the subjects of epidemiologic study. The task of identifying carcinogens in this sea of chemicals appears rather overwhelming. Nevertheless, there is immense public interest in identifying and regulating carcinogens for the purpose of decreasing the incidence of cancer in the general population and in some occupational groups which are exposed to higher concentrations of these chemicals.

Of the five regulatory agencies responsible for regulating exposures to carcinogens (FDA, OSHA, CPSC, EPA and MSHA), only OSHA has published a complete, formal, carcinogen policy on the identification, classification and regulation of carcinogens (OSHA, 1980). Some of the other agencies have published guidelines on various aspects of these issues, but no detailed policy. The OSHA carcinogen policy was the result of a national forum of scientists and other representatives from government agencies, universities, and industry. It involved years of preparation and months of hearings and testimony, resulting in a 295-page document published in the *Federal Register* on January 22, 1980. It is generally accepted as a milestone in the development of public policy as it relates to the identification and regulation of carcinogens.

However, some people (particularly those with vested economic interests in products labeled as carcinogens) are strongly opposed to many of the criteria used in identifying carcinogens, and to the methods used for regulating exposures to them. It is not uncommon for some people to say, for example, "There is no evidence that this chemical causes cancer in humans," or "I've been using this chemical for 20 years and I don't have cancer," or "Just because it causes cancer in animals doesn't mean it causes cancer in humans," or "You would have to drink 10 gallons of the stuff each day to get cancer." Many of these responses express real concerns based on misinformation, others are ploys used by industry to convince the public there is nothing to worry about so they can protect their economic interests.

This chapter is being written to provide the information needed to understand the process of carcinogen identification and to some extent show how this affects the process of regulation.

WHAT IS A CARCINOGEN?

Simply stated, a *carcinogen* is a substance or agent that causes cancer. This may include a combination of chemical substances or agents. Cancer is a malignant tumor (neoplasm) consisting of a population of abnormal cells which grow and multiply unchecked, invade surrounding tissue and/or metastasize to other sites in the body and, if left untreated, result in the death of the individual.

Various definitions of carcinogens have been published by many advisory committees and agencies. The FDA Advisory Committee on Protocols for Safety Evaluation defined a carcinogen as "a substance that when administered by an appropriate route, causes an increased incidence of malignant tumors in experimental animals as compared with a control series of untreated animals" (FDA, 1971). The National Cancer Advisory Board (NCAB) report of the Subcommittee on Environmental Carcinogenesis stated:

"An agent—which may compromise a combination of chemicals—is carcinogenic in man if it increases the incidence of malignant neoplasms (or a combination of benign and malignant neoplasms) in humans to levels that are significantly higher than those in a comparable group not exposed (or exposed at a lower dose) to the same agent." (NCAB, 1977)

The IARC in the preamble to their monographs on the evaluation of the carcinogenic risk of chemicals to humans states:

"The term 'carcinogen' is used in these monographs to denote an agent that is capable of increasing the incidence of malignant neoplasms; the induction of benign neoplasms may in some circumstances contribute to the judgment that an agent is carcinogenic. . . ."
    "Definitive evidence of carcinogenicity in humans is provided by epidemiological studies. Evidence related to human carcinogenicity may also be provided by experimental studies of carcinogenicity in animals and by other biological data, particularly those relating to humans . . ." (IARC, 1987)

In the *Fourth Annual Report on Carcinogens* prepared by the NTP, it is stated that:

"For the purpose of this report 'known carcinogens' are defined as those substances for which the evidence from human studies indicates that there is a causal relationship between exposure to the substance and human cancer. 'Substances which may reasonably be anticipated to be carcinogens' are defined as those for which there is limited evidence of carcinogenicity in humans or sufficient evidence of carcinogenicity in experimental animals." (NTP, 1985)

In the OSHA carcinogen policy, it is stated:

"A 'potential occupational carcinogen' means any substance, or combination or mixture of substances, which causes an increased incidence of benign and/or malignant neoplasms, or a substantial decrease in the latency period between exposure and onset of neoplasms in humans or in one or more experimental mammalian species as the result of any oral, respiratory, or dermal exposure, or any other exposure which results in the induction of tumors at a site other than the site of administration. This definition also includes any substance which is metabolized into one or more potential occupational carcinogens by mammals."

Accompanying this definition are 295 pages of discussions, recommendations, and conclusions which include almost all the issues related to carcinogen identification (OSHA, 1980).
    In each of the guidelines and the OSHA carcinogen policy statement, several pages of criteria (concerning the types of evidence that are needed to conclude that a substance has been shown to cause cancer in humans or is a potential human carcinogen) are listed and discussed.

HOW IS A CARCINOGEN IDENTIFIED?

The most convincing scientific evidence for proving a substance is carcinogenic in humans is derived from data on human studies. Sufficient evidence has accumulated from such studies to prove a cause and effect relationship between exposure to 50 different chemicals, mixtures of chemicals or industrial processes, and cancer in humans (IARC, 1987). For 28 of these 50, the evidence was derived from studies of people who were exposed to carcinogenic agents in their workplaces. These chemicals (or compounds) include asbestos (four different types), arsenic and arsenic compounds, benzene, benzidine, chromium compounds, nickel and nickel compounds, bis (chloromethyl) ether, vinyl chloride, 4-aminobiphenyl, 2-naphthylamine and talc containing asbestiform fibers. Carcinogens are also identified in well-controlled, laboratory animal experiments. As a matter of record, the carcinogenic effects of several chemicals were first discovered in animals, before they were discovered in humans. The significance of these two approaches (human and animal studies) will be discussed.

HUMAN STUDIES

There are three types of approaches that have been used to identify carcinogens in human populations: the case-cluster, case-control, and cohort studies.

Case Cluster Studies

This method was used to identify almost all of the human carcinogens prior to the development of more formal and methodical epidemiologic approaches. The carcinogenic effects in humans of chimney soot (Pott, 1775); dyes (aromatic amines) (Rehn, 1895); asbestos (Homburger, 1943; Wagner et al. 1960); and vinyl chloride (Creech and Johnson, 1974) were first identified in that way. The conditions under which this particular method was successful in identifying carcinogens were rather unique. The observations were made by one astute physician who was aware of the occupational exposures and/or occupations of his patients, he had an idea of the incidence of the type of cancer under study in other groups of people not so exposed, and the patients experienced a very high relative risk for the type of cancer observed. For example, after Rehn (1895) made the observation that the bladder cancer incidence was much higher in dye-workers (aromatic amines), Case et al. (1954) reported that the relative risk for bladder cancer was up to *61 times* greater in workers exposed to aromatic amines (benzidine, 2-naphthylamine) compared to the general population. After Wagner et al. (1960) first concluded that asbestos caused mesotheliomas (cancer of the lining of the chest and abdomen) in humans (based on a cluster of cases from an asbestos mining district) it was found in several cohort studies that the relative risk for developing mesothelioma in some populations of asbestos workers was more than *1,000 times* that in the general population (Selikoff et al. 1979).

It is quite likely that this case-cluster approach will detect carcinogens in the environment *only* when the relative risks are quite high (at least 5 times greater than the risks experienced in the background or control population). In addition the exposed workers would need to remain in the same community from the time of first exposure until the diagnosis of the disease— typically a period of 15 to 40 years. In many instances the observations appeared somewhat fortuitous and were made only by alert and knowledgeable physicians with an interest in occupational disease.

Case-Control Studies

In case-control studies a group of patients with a specific cancer of interest is studied and their exposure histories are elicited. This group is compared with another group without the cancer and their exposure histories are elicited. If the suspect exposure occurs in significantly higher frequency in the cancer group than in the control group, then inferences can be made regarding the causative agent. This method is not the one most freqently used in epidemiological studies probably because of the difficulties involved in obtaining accurate exposure histories in a random population.

Cohort Studies

These are the most familiar types of analytical epidemiological studies. They involve the comparison of groups of people exposed to the agent or agents of interest to groups of people who are not exposed or are exposed to considerably lower concentrations of the agents of interest. The cancer rates for specific organs in the two groups are compared. These may be retrospective studies (the groups of people have already been exposed for many years and the observations are obtained from historical records) or they may be prospective (the population under study is still alive and the exposure and mortality data are obtained periodically over many years). The control populations used in these types of studies may be the general population of the United States, the state or county in which the exposed group resides or another group of people with similar demographic characteristics, but not exposed (or at much lower levels) to the agents of interest. In all cases the control group must be matched according to age, sex and race.

EVALUATION OF EPIDEMIOLOGICAL STUDIES

The interpretation of the results of epidemiological studies very much depends upon the questions being asked. It must be emphasized that negative (non-positive) epidemiologic studies cannot be used to prove the non-carcinogenicity of a chemical, they can serve only to establish some limits on the nature of the risk (OSTP, 1986; IPC, 1984; IRLG, 1979; NCAB, 1977). Perhaps the single most important reason for this is that the populations studied are not large enough to detect the degree of risk or risks that are of concern. For example, in a study designed to detect an excess incidence of cancer of 1% (1/100) over a background incidence of 5% (5/100) and having a statistical power of 95%, the study population would have to consist of at least 11,182 individuals with the exposure of interest and 11,182 individuals in the control group (Busch and Leidel, 1979). To determine an excess incidence of cancer of 0.1% (1/1,000) over a background incidence of 5% the study population would have to consist of at least 519,000 individuals. Since most occupational exposure cohort mortality studies consist of between 500 and 2,000 people, and the background incidence of lung cancer and breast cancer (in women) is greater than 5%, an excess incidence of 2% of these cancer types would not be detected. Since there are 2-million deaths per year in the U.S., that means that an etiological agent responsible for an excess of 40,000 deaths per year could go undetected using the existing epidemiological methods.

In addition to the number of people in the cohort, there are several other factors that must be considered in evaluating the significance of epidemiological studies. These include the criteria used for selecting the cohort; the characterization of the exposures [e.g., chemical composition of the agent(s), routes of exposure (respiratory, oral, skin) and suitability of measurement methods]; the total dose to which each person is exposed (duration of exposure and concentration of the agent in the air, food and/or water); the length of the latency period (interval between first exposure and the diagnosis of cancer); percentage follow-up (percentage of people that are actually traced from the original defined cohort to the final observation period); suitability of the control group; accuracy of death certificates (cause of death); and the suitability of the classification system used in codifying the cause of death.

Selecting a Cohort

Historically the selection of a cohort was based upon the identification of a group of people who were exposed to a carcinogen that was previously identified by qualitative (descriptive) human studies (i.e., case-clusters, either published or unpublished). Former workers in a factory where the carcinogen was manufactured, mined, or used in the manufacture of other products were then identified, their causes of death determined from death certificates, and comparisons made with a population not so exposed. More recently groups of workers (tradesmen) who worked in a variety of work-sites but with exposure to the same carcinogen (e.g., insulators working with asbestos) have been identified through union records and have been studied. In both methods the selection of the cohorts was based on a high index of suspicion in which the risk ratios in the original study group were likely to be greater than 5 (i.e., a 5-fold greater relative risk for developing cancer in a specific tissue). Using case-cluster studies as the method for selecting a cohort allows for the identification of very few of the suspect or potential carcinogens. More recently, epidemiological studies have been initiated to study factory workers exposed to carcinogens identified on the basis of animal studies (e.g., beryllium, formaldehyde, acrylonitrile). The relative risks experienced by workers exposed to these chemicals were considerably lower than in those cohorts selected for study based on the case-cluster approach (risk ratios around 2 instead of greater than 5).

Another problem in identifying cohorts for study is finding a population that is exposed to one chemical of interest and which is large enough for meaningful statistical analysis. Quite frequently, only a factory or industrial process in which workers are exposed to many different chemicals can be identified. Sorting out which chemical or chemicals are the etiological agents can be an insurmountable task. It is for this reason that IARC lists 11 industries or industrial processes as carcinogenic instead of listing the individual chemicals used in the processes. However, if one or more of the chemicals in those mixed exposures had been tested in animals and were found to be positive, then the human data could be used to verify their carcinogenicity.

Latency Period

Cancer does not usually develop within months after first exposure. Most often in occupational exposures, workers are first exposed in their 20s and are diagnosed with cancer between the ages of 40 and 70. This interval is called the latency period. Typically, in asbestos-exposed workers the latency period for lung cancer is 20 years or more; for mesothelioma, it is 30 years or more. Failure to observe a population of workers for more than 20 years after first exposure can result in erroneous conclusions regarding the carcinogenicity of a chemical. However, there are age groups that are more sensitive to carcinogens, people older than 50 and younger than 15, and in some of those groups the latency periods are shorter. In addition, the higher the dose the more likely the latency period will be shorter.

Dose Estimate

In order to perform quantitative risk assessments the estimation of total dose is critical. Total dose depends on the duration of exposure and the concentration of the chemical in the air, food and/or water and more specifically on the amount that is inhaled, swallowed and/or absorbed through the skin. The exposure measurements available from historical records are very, very sparse. As a consequence, very few quantitative risk-assessments can be based on human exposure data. More often the duration of exposure is used as the sole indicator of dose; and in the case of airborne particulate carcinogens, the degree of dustiness has been used to indicate relative concentrations ("high," "medium," and "low").

However, some people need not be exposed for very long periods of time to receive a sufficient dose to produce cancer. For example, some workers have been exposed for less than six months to asbestos and have died from mesotheliomas more than 35 years later (Morgan and Holmes, 1982; Newhouse and Thompson, 1965). In other instances, people have been exposed to diethylstilbestrol for a few weeks *in utero* and have developed cancer more than 18 years after birth (IARC, 1987, pp. 272–278).

Control Group

In order to determine the carcinogenic effect of an agent, a suitable control group must be selected. Ideally, this control group should be exposed to the same conditions (except for the chemical of interest) as the exposed group, and be matched by age, sex and race. A problem in some studies is the lack of specific exposure data to other carcinogens in either or both the control groups and exposed groups. One of the competing carcinogens to which many people are exposed is cigarette smoke. To obtain a risk ratio that most accurately reflects the carcinogenic potency of the agent under study, data on the smoking histories and exposures to other carcinogens would have to be elicited. However, for most studies it can be safely assumed that the control group is exposed to the same concentration of environmental carcinogens as the exposed group except for the chemical under study.

Manufacturers of industrial carcinogens frequently attribute the carcinogenic effects of their products to cigarette smoke and not to the product itself. However, if the degree or extent of smoking is the same in both the control and exposed groups, then any variation in risk for lung cancer cannot be attributed to cigarette smoking. If the degree of smoking is greater in the exposed group, then part of the increased risk can be attributed to cigarette smoking, but this increased risk is unlikely to exceed 43% (risk ratio of 1.43) of that in the controls. If, on the other hand, the exposed group smokes less than the control group, a carcinogenic effect of the agent of interest will be easily masked and missed (Axelson, 1989). For example, the risk ratios (number of observed cases divided by the number of expected cases) for lung cancer in many of the asbestos-exposed worker populations have exceeded 2, and in some instances have exceeded 10 (Doll, 1955; Dement et al. 1983). It is not possible for those elevated risks to be explained on the basis of different smoking rates between the exposed and control groups. On the other hand, a lower than expected risk ratio for lung cancer was found in one worker population exposed to asbestos (Berry and Newhouse, 1983). It is highly likely that this worker population smoked less than the controls, since smoking in that workplace had been banned since 1931 (Skidmore and Dufficy, 1983). This was not controlled in the epidemiological study.

There are several reasons for developing alternative approaches for identifying carcinogens. These include the many limitations in epidemiological studies and the large number of chemicals in our environment. The most compelling reason, however, is that willful exposure of human populations to untested chemicals and "waiting to see what happens" is irresponsible as well as immoral and unethical.

ANIMAL STUDIES

Tests in experimental animals have been used for many decades for determining toxicities and carcinogenicities of thousands of chemicals which are now in use or considered for use in our society as food additives, pesticides, drugs, and a variety of other commercial products. The addition of a substance that has been found to cause cancer in animals to the human food supply has been prohibited by law since 1958 (Delaney clause in the 1958 Food Additives Amendment to the Food, Drug and Cosmetic Act). All Federal policies accept the use of animal data in predicting human effects and FDA and EPA have *required* industry to conduct carcinogenicity testing of food and color additives, animal drugs, human drugs, pesticides and toxic substances in animals (OTA, 1987). The International Agency for Research on Cancer (IARC) states that "in the absence of adequate data on humans, it is biologically plausible and prudent to regard agents for which there is sufficient evidence of carcinogenicity in experimental animals as if they presented a carcinogenic risk to humans" (IARC, 1987, p. 22).

What evidence do we have that animals can serve as substitutes for humans in reflecting or predicting the carcinogenic potential of a substance? *First,* for several agents (e.g., 4-aminobiphenyl, bis (chloromethyl) ether, diethylstilbestrol, melphalan, 8-methoxypsoralen plus UVR, mustard gas, and vinyl chloride) evidence of carcinogenicity in experimental animals preceded evidence obtained from epidemiological studies in humans. *Second,* of the 44 agents for which there is sufficient or limited evidence of carcinogenicity to humans, *all* 37 that have been adequately tested produce cancer in at least one animal species (IARC, 1987, p. 22). *Third,* the physiological, biochemical and anatomic (gross and microscopic appearance of internal tissues) similarities between different species of mammals are much greater than their differences. Because of these similarities, animals are used in almost every phase of medical research, including genetics and the study of mechanisms of carcinogenesis. These studies have produced the knowledge which has allowed great advances in medicine in the past several decades.

Rodents (rats, mice, and hamsters) are the experimental animals of choice because their biochemical and physiological similarities to humans are close enough to allow them to serve as adequate (not always perfect) substitutes for humans and they are easier and more economical to use than larger species of animals (e.g., monkeys).

Conduct of Animal Experiments

Several government agencies [NCI, NTP, EPA (under TSCA and FIFRA), FDA] and the Pharmaceutical Manufacturers Association (PMA) have developed guidelines for the conduct of animal experiments designed to test the carcinogenic potentials of chemicals (OTA, 1987). They are all in general agreement on several of the critical design parameters. They recommend: 2 species of animals, including mice and rats; both males and females; at least 50 animals/sex/group; 2 or 3 different dose groups plus one control group; one "high dose" group which is described as either slightly below the toxic dose (PMA) or a dose which is predicted not to alter normal longevity of the animals from effects other than carcinogenicity (NTP); dosing the animals 5 or 7 days/week for 2 years; and autopsying animals 1 week to 6 months after the last day of dosing.

Although there is general agreement among the federal agencies and the Pharmaceutical Manufacturers Association on the conduct of animal experiments, some people still take issue with these guidelines and take exception to the use of the maximum tolerated dose ("highest dose"), the use of mice, and the combining of benign tumors with malignant tumors in determining cancer incidence. Other controversial issues include the concept of no threshold for carcinogens and the lack of differentiation between promoters and initiators. These issues will be discussed in the following paragraphs.

Maximum Tolerated Dose (MTD) or Highest Dose (HD)

Because so few animals of any one sex and species are used in bioassay experiments (50 animals per group) and because there is usually a background tumor incidence in various tissues in control animals ranging from 1 to 30%, the system will not detect added increased incidences of tumors of less than about 15% (95% confidence level). Consequently, doses must be given which will cause cancer in 15% or more of the animals, and doses which cause cancer at lower levels must be extrapolated from these higher levels. To increase the number of animals in an experiment in order to test chemicals at doses that would produce cancer in only 0.1% of the population is too expensive and impractical. Frequently, the only dose which will produce a statistically significant increase in cancer incidence in bioassay experiments is the maximum tolerated dose or highest dose (HD). Without the use of such a dose, many carcinogens might not be detected. The definition of the highest dose is the greatest dose which can be delivered to test animals without shortening their life spans from toxic effects other than cancer. In all NTP bioassay studies, this dose is determined from separate sub-chronic (3-month) experiments before the 2-year experiments are begun.

One oft-cited objection to using the highest dose is that the animal's metabolic system is saturated at such doses and either the normal biologic mechanisms cannot inactivate the carcinogen or other products are formed which would not occur at lower doses. In some cases this may be true, but we have no way of knowing what this metabolic threshold is for any one individual. We know that many carcinogens, even when groups of animals are given the highest dose, do not induce cancer in all animals. Apparently, their individual thresholds are different. These differences are much greater in humans who are considerably more heterogeneous with regard to genetic variations, diets, environmental conditions, and exposures to other chemicals. If the degree of binding of carcinogens to DNA in human cells in tissue culture can be used as an indicator of range of variation in susceptibility to carcinogens, there is a greater than 100-fold difference between individuals (Daniel et al. 1984).

For all of the NTP bioassay studies, one other dose scheme, one-half the highest dose, is used as well. The use of a third dosed group, at some lower level, has been recommended, principally to increase the accuracy of the dose-response curve. The cancer incidence data at these doses are then used to plot a curve to determine the risks at lower dose levels, including doses to which humans are exposed. These data are then used to predict risks in various human populations. If the predicted risks exceed a certain predetermined acceptable level of risk, then the chemical may be regulated or banned.

The use of the highest dose in animals has generated considerable debate among scientists and some resistance among the public. It is not uncommon to hear or to read statements like: "You would need to drink 10 gallons of the stuff each day to get cancer." Sometimes in the extrapolation of the doses from the high dose animal studies to humans, the quantities needed to produce the same *incidence* of cancer in humans appear to be ludicrous. However, that is not the reason the substance is being investigated or regulated. It is the incidence of cancer expected at the concentrations to which we are presently being exposed that is of concern. For example, if the ingestion of 10 gallons/day of a substance causes cancer in 50% of subjects, then 1 gallon may cause cancer in 5%, 1 quart in 1.25%, and 1 pint in 0.625%. If the substance is predicted to cause cancer in more than 1 out of 100,000 people at the doses to which the population is exposed, then FDA and EPA, at the present time, either will or should take action.

Benign vs. Malignant Tumors

In all animal experiments, some of the control and exposed animals develop benign tumors as well as malignant tumors (cancer). Most of the agency policies have taken the position that it is appropriate to count both benign and malignant tumors in determining the cancer incidence in animals for purposes of evaluating the carcinogenicity of a substance (OTA, 1987, p. 48). There are several reasons for this.

Malignant tumors (cancers) by definition invade surrounding tissue and/or metastasize to other sites in the body and, if left untreated, will result in death of the individual. *Benign* tumors, on the other hand, grow by expansion and do not invade or metastasize and usually do not result in death of the individual. However, cancer is a multistage process in which the formation of benign tumors frequently precedes the development of cancer. For example, it has been well documented that hepatocellular carcinomas (liver cancer) in rodents arise through a variety of morphological stages. They begin with small cellular foci or clusters of cells (eosinophilic, basophilic or clear cell foci) which progress to larger, more malignant appearing groups of cells (neoplastic nodules) and then to carcinomas (cancers). Also, it is quite likely that benign breast tumors in animals eventually progress to breast cancer. Solleveld et al. (1984) found that the ratio of malignant to benign breast tumors increased when the animals were allowed to live beyond 137 weeks (almost all chronic rodent bioassays are currently terminated after 104 weeks of dosing). Because the NTP animal bioassay experiments are terminated at 104 weeks, the chances of detecting malignant tumors or the transformation of some benign tumors to malignant tumors are reduced. Many benign tumors in humans exhibit similar types of transformation from benign to malignant stages. For example, it is now recognized that colon polyps (benign tumors) eventually progress to colon cancer in humans.

In some instances, benign tumors will compress vital tissues, become hemorrhagic and/or secrete hormones, causing serious illness or death. The animal model does not always reliably predict which organ or tissue will be affected in humans. It is possible that an agent might induce a resectable benign tumor in a non-critical organ or tissue in rodents, but a benign tumor in a critical tissue in humans. For these reasons, it is important to count the benign tumors in the total count of cancers in evaluating the carcinogenic potential of a substance.

Use of Mice in Animal Experiments

The use of mice as test animals in carcinogen bioassays has been criticized because of the relatively high background tumor incidence and high degree of variability in the tumor incidences in control animals between laboratories and between experiments.

The high background incidence of tumors may present a problem because the test might not be sensitive enough to detect small added increased incidences of tumors in the exposed animals. However, using animals that normally rarely develop cancer might result in a test system that is not sensitive to carcinogens.

The high degree of variation in the control tumor incidence is a more significant problem, particularly when the reasons for these variations are unknown. The tumor incidence may vary depending upon the mean survival time of the group, quantity of food eaten, temperature, humidity, lighting, degree of handling, and perhaps the source of the animals. If the exposed and control groups in the same experiment are all derived from the same source and treated in an identical manner under well-controlled conditions, the only reason for differences between exposed and control tumor incidences should be the test chemical exposure. Because of the high degrees of variation in control tumor incidences between laboratories and between experiments in the same laboratory, the only suitable control group in any experiment is the one that is used in the experiment with the exposed group.

Calculations of and intergroup comparisons of mean survival times for each group may be extremely helpful in explaining these differences in tumor incidences. A difference in mean survival of as little as four weeks might very well explain some of this variation. The absence of this kind of information in carcinogen studies makes the interpretation of the data in some experiments very difficult.

Positive vs. Negative (Non-Positive) Results in Animals

All agencies give greater weight to well-conducted positive studies than to negative (non-positive) studies. Usually when a study is repeated in the same way and under the same conditions, the results are the same, i.e., the experiment is reproducible. The most common reasons for non-positive findings in one study and positive results in another with the same agent are: differences in numbers of animals, mean survival times, doses of the agents, and strains of animals. If animals are given a dose which exceeds the MTD, they may die earlier than the controls from toxic effects unrelated to cancer. On the other hand, if the dose is not high enough and/or the group size is not large enough, the carcinogenic effect will not be detected either.

Most policies state that the positive test must be reproducible or be shown to be positive in two different experiments (either two different species, or two sexes, or two different laboratories, or at two different times) in order to label a substance as a carcinogen. However, there are exceptions to this policy if there is other supporting evidence (e.g., positive in vitro tests, structural similarity of the chemical to other known carcinogens, and/or an unusually high incidence of cancer observed). In those instances, one well-conducted positive animal experiment is adequate for proving the carcinogenicity of a substance.

Initiators and Promoters

An initiator is an agent that modifies DNA during the initial step in the induction of cancer. A promoter is an agent that will cause an increased incidence of cancer in animals when applied after the cells have been treated with an initiator. Differentiating between these two classes of carcinogens is frequently difficult because of the number of variables that affect the response, including dose. That is, an initiator may also be a promoter, and a promoter might also act as an initiator under some circumstances. For example, asbestos fibers cause mesotheliomas (cancer of the lining of the chest and abdomen) and lung cancer in experimental animals and humans without the addition of or combination with any other substance. In addition, asbestos dramatically promotes the carcinogenic effect of cigarette smoke in humans and benzo-a-pyrene (a constituent of cigarette smoke) in animals. The designation of an agent as acting solely through an initiation or promotion type mechanism is not currently possible. The Office of Science and Technology Policy commented on this issue by stating:

"At present, given the lack of information on mechanisms of carcinogenesis in humans and the myriad interactions of tissue and the biological effects of promoters demonstrated in experimental systems, it is premature to designate agents as acting through only a promotion-type mechanism . . ." (OSTP, 1986)

Animal Studies: Other Considerations

Almost all the difficulties present in human studies are eliminated in animal studies. For example, the control and exposed groups are identical except for the exposure to the chemical being tested; the dose is precisely known and accurate dose-response calculations can be made; the animals are not lost to follow-up; all animals are autopsied; and accurate, standardized tumor diagnoses are made. One significant problem, however, is the fact that these animals are not exposed to the mixtures of chemicals and other environmental agents to which the average person is exposed. Consequently, any synergistic or additive effects with many of our environmental chemicals will be missed. Another problem is the fact that tested animals do not get the same diseases as humans, e.g., gastric ulcers, colitis, kidney stones—conditions that could very well enhance the carcinogenic potency of a chemical. As a result, the carcinogenic potential and/or potency of a chemical which is based upon animal studies most likely will underestimate the carcinogenic potential and/or potency of that same chemical in humans.

Thresholds or Safe Levels

Is there a "safe level" for carcinogens? Probably no single issue has been so emotionally debated in the field of environmental carcinogenesis as the one on thresholds for carcinogens. The answer at the present time is "no" or "possibly, but no one knows what that level is for any carcinogen." Most of the arguments have been developed (pro and con) on the basis of theoretical concepts. Establishing experimental proof of the threshold concept for one substance requires the utilization of exceptionally large numbers of animals, perhaps as many as 100,000. There is only one published experiment, utilizing thousands of animals, which was designed in an attempt to answer that question (Littlefield et al. 1980). In that experiment, no threshold was demonstrated for the carcinogen, 2-acetylaminofluorene. At the present time, there is insufficient evidence to prove the existence of a threshold for any carcinogen.

Those who favor the threshold theory suggest that defense mechanisms operate to inhibit or inactivate the carcinogenic agents, and it is only when that defense mechanism breaks down that cancer can be initiated and promoted. They also argue that, if a substance operates solely by a promotion-type mechanism, it can be more readily inhibited by these defense mechanisms. The key to their argument appears to be the assumption that as long as everybody has a healthy defense system there will be a threshold. However, there is no way of knowing the adequacy of each person's defense mechanism. In addition, there probably are fluctuations in these defense mechanisms, so at any particular time in life, one might become "defenseless" and the carcinogen would become active at much lower concentrations than predicted.

All federal agencies and the majority of scientists in the field of environmental carcinogenesis agree that there is no evidence to support a threshold concept and assume that none exists.

The Office of Science and Technology Policy (1986) commented on the issue of thresholds by stating:

"Even if the concept of individual thresholds could be supported, the well-recognized genetic variability in the human population would effectively prevent the estimation of a general population threshold value. Moreover, given the high level of background cancer present in the human environment, it seems unlikely that one could rule out the possibility that a new chemical exposure, however limited, might augment an already ongoing mechanistic process and thereby produce a collective or additive exposure that exceeds the unknown threshold level."

In the absence of being able to demonstrate a threshold for a carcinogen, one alternative is to construct dose-response curves for each carcinogen, estimate the risks at "low levels" of exposure, and then evaluate the risks that are probable in our society. A better alternative is to find substitutes for carcinogens and ban their use.

CONCLUSION

We live in an industrialized society that depends upon thousands of chemicals for its growth and success. It is important that we be able to identify those chemicals which are carcinogenic so that exposures to them can be reduced or eliminated. History has taught us that "waiting to see what happens" to relatively small groups of workers who are exposed to untested chemicals can be disastrous to those who are directly exposed as well as to their families. In addition, this approach to testing chemicals is immoral and irresponsible. It may also be economically disastrous to the industries which are responsible for paying for the costs of the diseases incurred.

At the present time, testing in experimental animals provides a very reasonable and valid method for identifying carcinogens. However, it is likely that these animal tests actually underestimate the human cancer risks for many chemicals. It is important, therefore, that research systems be developed to allow more accurate dose-response extrapolations from animal test systems to humans. One other approach is to ban the manufacture and use of all carcinogens.

REFERENCES

Axelson, O. (1989). Confounding from smoking in occupational epidemiology. *Brit. J. Industr. Med.* 46:505–507.

Berry, G. and Newhouse, M. L. (1983). Mortality of workers manufacturing friction materials using asbestos. *Brit. J. Industr. Med.* 40:1–7.

Busch, K. A. and Leidel, N. A. (1979). Statistical design and data analysis requirements. In: *Patty's Industrial Hygiene and Toxicology.* Vol. III. *Theory and Rationale of Industrial Hygiene Practice.* L. J. Cralley and L. V. Cralley, eds. John Wiley & Sons, N.Y. pp. 43–97.

Case, R. A. M., Hosker, M. E. et al. (1954). Tumors of the urinary bladder in workmen engaged in the manufacture and use of certain dyestuff intermediates in the British chemical industry. I. The role of aniline, benzidine, alpha-naphthylamine, and beta-naphthylamine. *Brit. J. Industr. Med.* 11:75–104.

Creech, J. L. and Johnson, M. N. (1974). Angiosarcoma of liver in the manufacture of polyvinyl chloride. *J. Occup. Med.* 16:150–151.

Daniel, F. B., Stoner, G. D. and Schut, H. A. J. Interindividual variation in the DNA binding of chemical genotoxins following metabolism by human bladder and bronchus explants. In *Individual Susceptibility to Genotoxic Agents in the Human Population,* F. J. deSerres and R. W. Pero, eds. Plenum Publishers, 1984, pp. 177–199.

Dement, J., Harris, R. L. et al. (1983). Exposures and mortality among chrysotile asbestos workers. Part II: mortality. *Am. J. Ind. Med.* 4:421–433.

Doll, R. Mortality from lung cancer in asbestos workers (1955). *Brit. J. Industr. Med.* 12:81–86.

FDA (Food and Drug Administration) Advisory Committee on Protocols for Safety Evaluation (1971). Panel on carcinogenesis report on cancer testing in the safety evaluation of food additives and pesticides. *Toxicol. Appl. Pharm.* 20:419–438.

Harting, F. H. and Hesse (1879). Der lungenkrebs die bergkrankheit in den Schneebergen gruben. *Vrtljhrssch, Gerichtl. Med.* 30:296–309; 31:102–132; 313–337.

Homburger, F. (1943). The co-incidence of primary carcinoma of the lungs and pulmonary asbestosis. *Am. J. Path.* 19:797–807.

IARC (International Agency for Research on Cancer) (1987). Overall evaluations of carcinogenicity: An updating of IARC monographs vols. 1–42. Supplement 7. Lyon, France.

IPC (Interdisciplinary Panel on Carcinogenicity) (1984). Criteria for evidence of chemical carcinogenicity. *Science* 225:682–687.

IRLG (Interagency Regulatory Liaison Group) (1979). Scientific bases for identification of potential carcinogens and estimation of risks. *J. Nat. Cancer Inst.* 63(1):241–268.

Littlefield, N. A., Farmer, J. H., et al. (1980). Effects of dose and time in a long-term, low-dose carcinogenicity study. *J. Environ. Pathol. Toxicol.* 3:17–34.

Morgan, A. and Holmes, A. (1982). Concentrations and characteristics of amphibole fibres in the lungs of workers exposed to crocidolite in the British gas-mask factories, and elsewhere, during the Second World War. *Brit. J. Industr. Med.* 39:62–69.

NCAB (National Cancer Advisory Board) (1977). General criteria for assessing the evidence for carcinogenicity of chemical substances: Report of the subcommittee on environmental carcinogenesis. *J. Nat. Cancer Inst.* 58:461–465.

Newhouse, M. L. and Thompson, H. (1965). Mesothelioma of pleura and peritoneum following exposure to asbestos in the London area. *Brit. J. Industr. Med.* 22:261–269.

OSHA (Occupational Safety and Health Administration) (1980). Identification, classification and regulation of potential occupational carcinogens. *Federal Register* 45:5001–5296.

OSTP (Office of Science and Technology Policy, Executive Office, White House) (1986). Chemical carcinogens: A review of the science and its associated principles. *Env. Hlth. Perspec.* 67:201–282.

OTA (Office of Technology Assessment, Congress of the United States) (1987). *Identifying and Regulating Carcinogens—Background Paper.* Superintendent of Documents. U.S. Gov't. Printing Office, Washington, D.C. GPO Stock No. 052–003–01080–1.

Pott, P. (1775). Cancer scroti. In *Chirurgical Observations.* Hawes, Clarke & Collins. London, England. pp. 63–68.

Rehn, L. (1895). Blasengeschwulste bei Anilinarbeitern. *Arch. Klin. Chir.* 50:588–600.

Selikoff, J. J., Hammond, E. C. and Seidman, H. (1979). Mortality of insulation workers in the United States and Canada 1943–1976. *Ann. N.Y. Acad. Sci.* 330:91–116.

Skidmore, J. W. and Dufficy, B. L. (1983). Environmental history of a factory producing friction material. *Brit. J. Industr. Med.* 40:8–12.

Solleveld, H. A., Haseman, J. K. and McConnell, E. E. (1984). Natural history of body weight gain survival and neoplasia in the F344 rat. *J.N.C.I.* 72(1):929–940.

Wagner, J. C., Sleggs, C. A. and Marchand, P. (1960). Diffuse pleural mesothelioma and asbestos exposure in the North-West Cape Province. *Brit. J. Industr. Med.* 17:260–271.

Weinstein, I. B. (1981). The scientific basic for carcinogen detection and primary cancer prevention. *Cancer 47:*1133–1141, 1981.

Wilbourn, J. et al. (1986). Response of experimental animals to human carcinogens: An analysis based upon the IARC monographs program. *Carcinogenesis* 7:1853–1863.

Chapter 2

QUANTITATIVE RISK ASSESSMENT AND CHEMICAL CARCINOGENS IN OCCUPATIONAL ENVIRONMENTS

Melvin E. Andersen, Ph.D.
Risk Assessment Department
Chemical Industry Institute of Toxicology
Research Triangle Park, North Carolina

INTRODUCTION

Quantitative Risk Assessment (QRA), in broad terms, is the marshalling of diverse information to produce an estimate of the quantitative magnitude of the risk posed by a particular activity. Such risks are expressed in various ways: expected fatalities per 100 million passenger miles flown in a new aircraft or expected adverse responses to vaccinations per million treated individuals. This chapter focuses more narrowly on QRA for evaluating the health risks to workers posed by exposure to chemicals known to cause cancer in experimental animals or to chemicals implicated as human carcinogens by observations in occupational populations. In these cases risk assessment is the process by which animal or human toxicity data or human epidemiological observations are factored together to calculate the level of potential risk associated with exposure to a particular chemical. This chapter outlines the methods used in making QRA with occupational carcinogens based primarily on animal testing results and discusses recent advances in incorporating new biological information into these risk assessments.

CHEMICAL CARCINOGENS IN THE OCCUPATIONAL ENVIRONMENT

The ability of occcupational carcinogens to cause cancer was reported over 200 years ago. In 1775 Sir Percival Pott noted the high incidence of scrotum cancer in chimney sweeps in England. Over the years other chemicals have been found to cause cancer after occupational exposures. Among these chemical carcinogens are aromatic amines, asbestos, arsenic, various radioactive materials, benzene, and vinyl chloride. As implemented by the U.S. Environmental Protection Agency (U.S. EPA), QRA has had a very significant impact on control of environmental carcinogens, but as yet has found more limited use in setting occupational exposure limits. However, in the past few years, the Occupational Safety and Health Administration (OSHA) has used risk assessment methods for proposing standards for benzene, asbestos, and formaldehyde. Table 2-1 reproduced from *Managing Carcinogens in the Work Environment* by J. B. Singh (1) contains a list of occupational carcinogens regulated by OSHA.

Table 2-1. OSHA—Regulated Carcinogens

2-Acetylaminofluorene	Ethylene oxide
Acrylonitrile	3-3-Dichlorobenzidine
4-Aminodiphenyl	4-Dimethylaminoazobenzene
Arsenic	Ethyleneimine
Asbestos	4-4'-methylene(bis)2-chloroaniline
Benzene	Methyl chloromethyl ether
Benzidine	Beta-napthylamine
Bis(chloromethyl)ether	Alpha-napthylamine
Beta-propriolactone	4-Nitrobiphenyl
Coal tar pitch volatiles	N-Nitrosodimethylamine
Coke oven emissions	Vinyl chloride
1,2-Dibromo-3-chloropropane	

CANCER TESTING STRATEGIES

There are two aspects important in developing strategies for controlling carcinogenic hazards in the work environment. One is qualitative, that is, what chemicals are potentially capable of causing cancer in exposed workers. The other is quantitative, that is, at what exposure concentration does the risk of cancer become sufficiently great to warrant control of the amount of carcinogen in the work environment? In general, it is much easier to answer the former question, does a chemical have any potential for carcinogenicity, than to give confident guidance on the latter question, what is the proper exposure limit? Frequently, both these qualitative and quantitative questions are examined by conducting toxicity studies with lifetime exposures of animals to test chemicals, and observing these animals for the development of cancer. The overall process of deriving exposure limits for people based on these animal results is a very difficult, but increasingly necessary part of the practice of occupational toxicology.

The difficulty in deriving these human exposure limits from animal results arises from the fact that the animal toxicity tests are conducted under very different exposure conditions than those to which people are exposed. In fact, the animal test system frequently appears to bear almost no relevance at all to human exposure conditions. Test animals are exposed to very high daily doses, sometimes by inappropriate routes of administration, for their entire lifetime. Often a particular animal species is used because it has a higher than normal susceptibility to formation of tumors in particular organs. All of these factors increase the responsiveness of the animal, making it easier to identify those chemicals that have *any potential whatever* to cause tumors in the test animals. At the same time, these same factors make it more difficult to extrapolate the results to predict the human relevance of the toxicity results, that is they obscure the ability to quantify relevant risk to people. In the past quantitative risk assessment approaches have largely ignored these differences between the animal exposure and the expected human exposure conditions and also proceeded to conduct the risk estimation process disregarding the mechanism by which the particular chemical causes cancer.

MECHANISMS BY WHICH CHEMICALS MAY CAUSE CANCER

There are several broad classes of chemical carcinogens, i.e., cancer causing chemicals. So-called genotoxic carcinogens initiate carcinogenic changes by interacting directly with DNA, the genetic material of the cell, to cause mutations during cell division. The second broad group are the non-genotoxic carcinogens. These chemicals do not alter DNA directly, but they have some effects on the growth characteristics of cells. Such chemicals augment the carcinogenic process but do not initiate it. These non-genotoxic carcinogens often cause some change in the cellular environment that enhances tumor formation. Two particular types of non-genotoxic carcinogens are cytotoxicants, like chloroform and carbon tetrachloride, and hormonal analogs such as thyroid suppressants, diethylstillbesterol, and 2,3,7,8-tetrachlorodibenzo-p-dioxin. For regulatory purposes, these different chemicals have all been treated as if they were directly genotoxic, despite recognition of their differing mechanisms of tumor production.

RISK ASSESSMENT IN THE ABSENCE OF ANCILLARY BIOLOGICAL INFORMATION

Just how have risk assessments been carried out for these chemical carcinogens in the past? First, a dose response curve was obtained from the experimental cancer studies relating tumor frequency to the dose given to the animal. In these studies, dose is usually expressed as amount of chemical instilled into the stomach per day or the exposure concentration maintained in the breathing air for some period of time each day. Based on the tissue where the tumor prevalence is highest, a linear correlation through the origin (zero-dose) is used to predict, by appropriate statistical methods, the expected incidence at very low doses. This approach frequently represents an extrapolation over five orders of magnitude in dose. To convert from one dose route to another, certain assumptions are made about breathing rate or amount of water consumed each day, but these corrections are simple relationships to interrelate dose equivalents by the various dose routes. To convert to an allowable dose for humans, a dose correction is used which assumes equivalent toxicity based either on dose expressed as mg/kg/day, a correction favored by the U.S. Food and Drug Administration (FDA), or expressed as mg/unit surface area/day, a correction favored by the U.S. Environmental Protection Agency (EPA). The surface area correction favored by the U.S. EPA implies that humans are always more sensitive to chemicals than are the smaller test animals used in the bioassay studies. In reality, however, these body weight or surface-area correction factors are not well-justified on the basis of any understanding of the tissue dose of chemical substance received by the different animals or of the mechanism of carcinogenic action of the chemical. Today they are justified primarily because they have been used before (i.e., because of tradition). This particular approach to QRA ignores both the mechanism of tumor formation and biological factors which determine tissue dose in different species, at different doses, for different routes of administration. By design this process is almost certain to produce inexact estimates of human risk, but at least the estimates are believed to be conservative (2). Standards set on this basis may well be lower than necessary, but they should clearly be protective of worker health.

Obviously, the implementation of overly conservative approaches to predicting risk has serious drawbacks. Limits set by such approaches greatly restrict commercial operations, decrease our ability to compete in world markets, and lead to large expenditures to change work practices, without concomitant increases in health protection. However, the issue is not that QRA of chemical carcinogens is wrong in principle. It has been damned by its misapplication. Today QRA remains the best approach we have for setting standards for many occupational carcinogens. Genotoxic carcinogens and those chemicals which are metabolized in the body to genotoxic metabolites must be controlled by some decision-making process which includes QRA. The current approach is eminently sensible for these chemicals. But, even with genotoxic carcinogens, QRA will only be effective when the risk estimation processes have a strong basis in biological reality and scientific knowledge instead of upon reliance on conservative assumptions, as is the case now. Indeed, the discipline of quantitative risk assessment for chemical carcinogens—it is now a discipline in its own right—is now rapidly maturing due to incorporation of more realistic biological models for chemical delivery to target tissues and more realistic descriptions of the cellular dynamics of the carcinogenic process itself. These two new initiatives will now be discussed in turn.

PHARMACOKINETICS AND TISSUE DOSE

A complaint frequently heard about the cancer testing program is that the high doses used in animals lead to different distributional behaviors for the chemicals than would be seen at more occupationally realistic exposures. This is clearly true, but it does not mean that the risk assessment is unworkable under these conditions, or that the testing for carcinogenicity at high daily doses is necessarily inappropriate. Instead, it means that our understanding of target tissue does have to be expanded to include the alterations in kinetic behavior that accompany higher administered doses. A quantitative approach to developing a more comprehensive description of target tissue dose at various exposure concentrations has been used in recent years both by chemical engineers studying the distribution of cancer chemotherapy drugs (3) and by toxicologists studying the distribution of volatile solvents (4). This newer approach involves construction of so-called physiologically-based models of pharmacokinetic behavior of toxic chemicals.

Physiologically-based pharmacokinetic models (PB-PK) are based on the structure of the test animal, the known solubilities of chemicals in various tissues, and the known pathways and rates of various metabolic reactions in the test species (Figure 2-1). PB-PK models are extremely versatile and can be used to extrapolate from high doses to more realistic exposure doses, from one route of exposure to another (because the models allow realistic input equations to be incorporated without difficulty), and from one exposure scenario to another (2). Their preeminent strength lies in their ability to support interspecies extrapolation (5). This is possible because the mammalian architecture embedded in a PB-PK model is the same for the human as it is for the test animals. To predict chemical disposition in workers, one simply changes the physiological parameters to those for humans, determines the tissue solubilities in restricted studies with human tissues, and

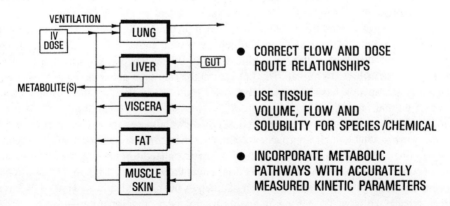

Figure 2-1. A schematic representation of a physiologically-based pharmacokinetic model used with gases and vapors.

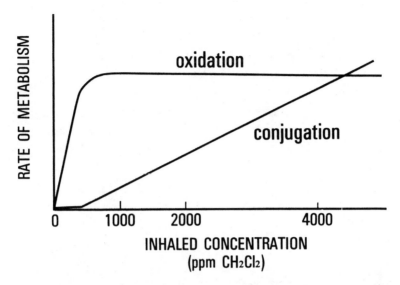

Figure 2-2. Representation of the rate of metabolism of inhaled methylene chloride (CH_2Cl_2) at varying inhaled concentrations. Methylene chloride is metabolized by oxidation and by conjugation with glutathione. These two reaction pathways have different characteristics. At low inhaled concentrations oxidation is the more influential manner of metabolism, but at higher concentrations glutathione conjugation becomes more significant. See Gargas et al. (8) for a more complete description of these results.

incorporates what is known of the metabolism of the test chemical in human tissues. A physiologically-based pharmacokinetic model of this kind has recently been used to improve the quantitative risk assessment process for methylene chloride (6).

Methylene chloride, an important industrial intermediate and commercial solvent, caused lung and liver tumors in mice exposed to 2000 or 4000 ppm for 6 hours per day 5 days per week. Initial risk assessment activities were conducted assuming a direct linear relationship between exposure concentration and tissue dose (7), much as outlined previously. This earlier assessment ignored a great deal of information about the pathways of metabolism of methylene chloride and the contribution of differing pathways as exposure concentration varied. An alternative methylene chloride risk assessment was developed which incorporated biological information about the disposition of methylene chloride in mice and the differences in disposition that would be expected in exposed human subjects (6).

Based on observations in many different studies, methylene chloride is known to be metabolized by two pathways. One, oxidation, is saturated at exposure concentrations above several hundred parts per million in the air. The other, conjugation with glutathione, a natural constituent of the cells in the liver and other organs, is less favored than oxidation, but it contributes increasingly to metabolism as exposure concentration increases (8). Interactions between the two pathways in the living animal lead to nonlinear increases in production of glutathione metabolites with increasing exposure concentration (Figure 2-2).

Once the kinetic characteristics of the two pathways were known, the PB-PK model could easily be used to compute the contribution to metabolism that each pathway makes at the cancer bioassay exposure conditions in mice. The amount metabolized by each pathway could then be compared with the observed tumor prevalence from the bioassay experiments. Tumor incidence was about linearly related to exposure concentration (Table 2-2). As concentration increased from 2000 to 4000 ppm, there was no further increase in the contribution from oxidation. The glutathione pathway contribution did increase between 2000 and 4000 ppm, indicating an associa-

Table 2-2. Methylene Chloride—Dose Response

PPM	TUMOR PREVA-LENCE (%)		MICROSOMAL PATHWAY DOSE	GLUTATHIONE PATHWAY DOSE
	LIVER	LUNG	LIVER(LUNG)	LIVER(LUNG)
0	6%	6%		—
2000	33	63	3575(1531)	851(123)
4000	83	85	3701(1583)	1811(256)

tion between this pathway of metaboilsm and the formation of tumors after methylene chloride exposure. Other experimental work on the ability of methylene chloride and its metabolites to cause bacterial mutations also pointed to glutathione pathway metabolites as part of the carcinogenic process.

For human risk assessment, the model was scaled to represent human parameters and representative human exposure conditions. Then the PB-PK human model was used to calculate expected liver tissue dose of the glutathione metabolite in a "standard person," and the mouse model calculated tissue dose in mice for various exposure concentrations. A standard person is one who weighs 70 kg, has 20% body fat, and has an amount of metabolism determined by average kinetic constants found in studies with human tissues. In Figure 2-3, the curve with the two data points is the liver glutathione pathway dose for mice exposed to various concentrations. The curve is on a log-log scale, and one can appreciate the region over which it is necessary to extrapolate to arrive at relevant occupational or environmental exposures. In addition, the reaction in the mice is nonlinear (that is, it is curved instead of being a straight line) because of dose-dependent interactions between the two pathways of methylene chloride metabolism. Because of the nonlinear behavior, linear extrapolation to low concentrations (the extended straight line) overpredicts tissue dose in the mouse at low exposure concentrations. A similar curve constructed from the human PB-PK model falls below that of the mouse. Thus, humans are expected to have a lower glutathione metabolite tissue exposure for an equivalent atmospheric exposure concentration than will mice. In contrast, the uppermost curve is the human tissue dose derived using the EPA conservative surface area correction factor. The conventional "conservative approach" (top line) and the physiological pharmacokinetic approach (bottom line) which incorporates biological knowledge of tissue disposition differed by 150- to 200-fold (6).

These PB-PK models arc also very effective tools for aiding in the collection of data to be used to validate and refine conclusions drawn from their use to analyze toxicity data. In the case of the methylene chloride studies, it became clear that the measurement of reaction rates for methylene chloride by the glutathione pathway in humans would be critical for developing a fully validated, biologically-realistic model for use in risk assessment. These studies have now been completed using human tissues obtained from accident victims and the data obtained has been used to refine the original risk assessment with methylene chloride (9).

The elaboration of the PB-PK-based methylene chloride risk assessment was narrowly focused on the manner in which data on tissue dose could be incorporated into the risk assessment

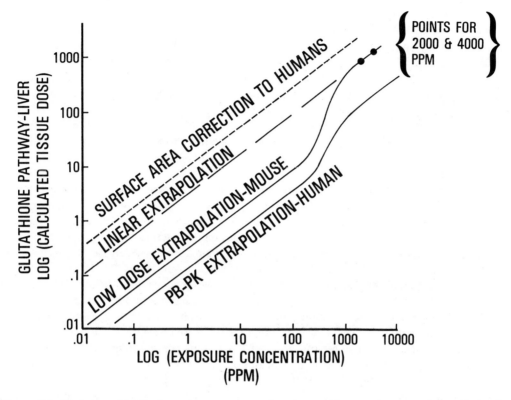

Figure 2-3. Methylene chloride-tissue dose assessment: low dose and interspecies extrapolation. Estimating liver tissue dose for methylene chloride glutathione conjugates with a physiologically-based pharmacokinetic model. See Andersen et al. (6) for a more complete explanation of these curves.

process. The assessment itself was still conducted assuming a linear relationship between expected tissue dose and tumor outcome. This approach, that of linear dependence on appropriate tissue dose with no threshold, seems appropriate for genotoxic carcinogens, but it may not be appropriate for carcinogens acting by other mechanisms.

PHARMACODYNAMIC MODELING OF CHEMICAL CARCINOGENESIS

It is necessary next to examine recently developed biologically-realistic cancer models that promise to allow incorporation of mechanistic data on cancer causation directly into the risk assessment process. Cancer is a complex set of disease processes involving unregulated growth of cells within an individual. A great deal of basic biological research is conducted each year in search of the cause of cancer and of successful treatment strategies. Despite the diversity of the disease process, a compelling, though highly simplified model for cancer has been developed in the past decade by Moolgavkar, Venzon, Knudson, and various colleagues (10, 11). Their model is now referred to as the M-V-K model. It is a form of a two-stage model initially described by Armitage and Doll (12) in the 1950s. The revised two-stage structure is beautiful in its simplicity and surprisingly robust in its ability to explain incidence curves of various human cancers and reconcile various dose response behaviors of environmental carcinogens (14). In its basic elements (Figure 2-4) the M-V-K cancer model explains cancer as the end result of two mutagenic events (μ_1 and μ_2), corresponding to mutations at a single, critical gene locus which in the human is duplicated within the genetic material of the cell. The first event (μ_1) produces an intermediate cell type (N1) that may have different growth characteristics than the normal cell but is not aggressively malignant. A second irreversible event (μ_2) is necessary to complete the cell transformation process, alter the second locus of the critical gene, and obtain the cancer cell (N2) which grows into a tumor. The contribution of Knudson, Moolgavkar and colleagues was the simplicity of the two cell structure for cancer with recognition that variable growth characteristics of the normal and intermediate cells can give rise to many diverse behaviors within the basic description. The M-V-K description includes cell growth parameters explicitly; α_1 and α_2 are birth rates for normal and intermediate cells, and β_1 and β_2 are death rates for these cell types. For the mutation steps, μ_1 and μ_2 are the transition rates. With respect to this model, genotoxicants alter mutation rates, cytotoxicants alter death and birth rates of the normal and intermediate cells, and certain promoters convey growth advantages on the intermediate cell population.

In the occupational environment there are examples of chemicals with widely varying mechanisms of carcinogenesis. Some of them, when examined using even very simple model structures, are likely to have effective thresholds, and others will reveal concentrations below which cancer should not be any problem at all. The cytotoxicants, like chloroform which is metabolized to phosgene (Figure 4), increase the killing of cells. Cell death, if not too extensive, initiates a repair process generating new cells. The mutation rate increases because it is a function of both the mutation frequency, the number of errors per DNA locus per cell division, and the number of divisions per unit time, the birth rate. Mutation rate increases with cytotoxicants because of the net increase in birth rate per time. If concentrations are kept below those that cause overt cytotoxicity, there should be no appreciable cell death, no cell repair to increase birth rate, and no net increase in tumorigenic risk. Thus, there should be an effective threshold for these chemicals and they probably can be regulated on the basis of their cytotoxic thresholds.

Genotoxic agents are more dangerous. In the parlance of the two-stage cancer description, these materials increase the transition rates (μ_1 and μ_2). They presumably do this by forming DNA adducts which increase mutation probability during each cell replication event. This is the

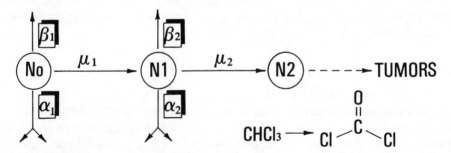

Figure 2-4. Schematic of the two-stage, Moolgavkar-Venzon-Knudson (M-V-K) model for cancer. N0, N1 and N2 are, respectively, normal cells, intermediate cells, with a single mutation at a critical gene locus, and the cancer cell with mutations in both loci of the critical gene. Birth rates of normal and intermediate cells are α_1 and α_2; death rates are β_1 and β_2. Mutation frequencies between cell types are μ_1 and μ_2. Chemicals can enhance cancer causation by affecting any of the various parameters in the model. With a cytotoxicant like chloroform ($CHCl_3$), the phosgene produced by metabolism kills cells. This alters death rates and causes increased birth to restore tissues to normal function.

proposed mechanism of cancer causation for chemicals like vinyl chloride, vinyl bromide, ethylene dibromide, and butadiene. For each of these chemicals metabolites are the presumed mutagenic intermediate. Other occupational chemicals, such as ethylene oxide, are probably directly geno-toxic. The consensus of opinion in the cancer research community is that these chemicals are unlikely to demonstrate a threshold, although they still may show nonlinear effects in terms of dose delivered to target tissues and cells.

Non-genotoxic carcinogens are more difficult to categorize because they are likely to have a wider variety of mechanisms of tumorigenicity. One possible mechanism is the ability of particular chemicals to confer growth advantages on intermediate cells. A growth advantage is simply an increase in the birth/death ($\alpha_2 - \beta_2$) difference. Dioxin appears to act in this manner. It binds to specific cell receptors, the receptor/dioxin complex then enters the nucleus, interacts with DNA, and leads to synthesis of new proteins within the cell. This total sequence of events alters the cell characteristics, conferring a growth advantage on intermediate cells. Important research questions arise regarding the relationship between dioxin dose and the cell response. Is it likely to be linear with dose or is there some dioxin dose that can be tolerated without any cell response (an effective threshold)? With our present state of knowledge, we simply do not know if these kinds of promotional carcinogens have a threshold. A proposal for an occupational exposure limit for dioxin has recently been made (13); however, it relies on safety factors for limit setting instead of the quantitative risk assessment techniques discussed here.

One important consideration with promoters is that they will have an impact only after other factors serve to produce intermediate cells whose growth is favored by the presence of the promoter. Rats and mice used to test for the hepatic carcinogenic potential of dioxin and other chemicals have high natural background tumor rates in the liver, and are expected to be very sensitive to promotion. Humans have a much lower background rate and should be less susceptible. These species differences in background tumor prevalence need to be considered when formulating strategies for quantitative risk analysis of promotional carcinogens found in the occupational environment. To date, they have not been taken into account. Unfortunately, none of these biologically realistic cancer models have been included, to date, for QRA of any occupational carcinogen, although a suggested approach for their incorporation has been outlined by Thorslund et al. (14).

The goal of all these efforts in developing biologically structured models for both the tissue distribution (pharmacokinetics) and the cellular action of carcinogens (pharmacodynamics) is to produce risk assessments that are as accurate as possible, and that are not unnecessarily conservative at each decision point. As these new biologically-based risk assessment technologies mature and risk assessment becomes more grounded in biological reality, the pressures to utilize QRA for standard setting in occupational environments will increase accordingly. More accurate evalua-tion of the risk of carcinogens in the work environment will inexorably lead to a pressing need for policy decisions regarding the "level of risk" from carcinogens that will be tolerated in the workplace. The industrial hygiene profession will have to be prepared to make decisions about using these QRA procedures with chemical carcinogens, and should begin now to consider the impact of thinking about proportionate increase in risk in contrast to thinking about the existence of biological thresholds for all kinds of carcinogens. What does it mean to regulate exposure on the basis of some perceived increase in carcinogenic risk, instead of on the basis of thresholds? And, how do we determine the level of risk which we will tolerate?

TOLERABLE RISKS

All of our everyday activities carry some element of risk: driving to the airport for a business trip, the plane trip itself, and crossing any street at any time. Each of these actions carries a not inconsiderable burden of risk. In our workday activities, there are also numerous risks. Even in what are regarded as safe occupations, such as insurance and real estate, the total lifetime risk for work-related death from all causes is estimateed to be about 1 per 1000 (15). When we talk about risk from chemical carcinogens, we are examining an increase in risk in a particular environment that is not intrinsically risk free. This is true whether we talk about chemical hazards in occupational, home, or recreational environments. There is as yet no general consensus in rule making procedures on the increase in level of risk that will be tolerated. Different federal regulatory agencies have used differing risk levels in their rule making efforts, and the same agency has frequently utilized different risk levels when regulating different chemicals. These regulatory decisions are complex and need to have some flexibility because of the numerous factors involved in the perception of risk. Two elements in this decision-making process deserve brief comment: the uncertainty in the risk assessment process itself and the size of the population at risk.

The use of a risk level of one case per thousand individuals (i.e., 1/1000) has been proposed for the work environment (16). This level seems reasonable when a conventional risk assessment procedure is used that is designed to provide a conservative estimate of risk (i.e., overestimate risk at particular exposure conditions). This type of conservative risk assessment has large uncertainty, but the direction of bias is clearly recognized. It is intended to be conservative. Would this level, 1/1000, still be considered appropriate if the scientific community were to produce more accurate estimates of risk that were quantitatively more correct? Would society fatalistically accept an "accurately" determined random chance of contracting cancer at a level of one in a thousand? In addition, what happens when there are two carcinogens in the workplace, or ten? Do we accept the additive risks or will consideration be given to control mixtures of carcinogens? The industrial hygiene profession and groups like the ACGIH-TLV Committee may well have to address these difficult issues in the near future if they are to maintain their credibility in proposing occupational exposure guidelines for potential human carcinogens. The OSHA-suggested benzene PEL is a case in point. Benzene is a human carcinogen. The risk assessment has been based on both animal bioassay results and on human epidemiology. The risk from the animal study is 1.2/1000 for 1 ppm and 40-year working exposure. Based on human epidemiology studies, the calculated risk would be even higher, about 1/100 (16). The professions of industrial hygiene and occupational health need to examine the biological basis of this QRA for benzene, decide if it is indeed accurate, and then decide on the wisdom of tolerating incremental risks as large as 1/100.

A second issue is the size of the population at risk. Often the acceptable level of risk is determined partially by considering the size of the exposed population. With a smaller population of exposed persons, it takes a larger increase in risk before a statistically significant increase in disease can be observed. Thus, a larger risk is often deemed tolerable in a smaller population. The issue is whether limits should be set to control individual risk or population risk. On the surface, including population size appears to be intended only to protect against any appearance of increased morbidity instead of protecting against the actual risks to exposed individuals. It does make good sense that the population size should be a factor in deciding which chemicals to regulate and study. By focusing on larger exposed populations, scarce resources could be applied to problem areas where large improvements in worker health are most likely to occur. Larger populations thus might deserve more attention. Yet, on the philosophical question, we still have no agreement on whether individual or group risks are the more important in risk assessment decision processes. There are good arguments on both sides of the question regarding the role of population size in tolerable risk calculations. The issue deserves more careful attention than it has received to date.

CONCLUSIONS

The use of quantitative risk assessment is not on the horizon of the occupational environment. It is here now, and is an issue to be reckoned with by everyone in the industrial hygiene profession. With many genotoxic occupational carcinogens, it is simply inappropriate to assume an absolute threshold for carcinogenic effects. Control of these carcinogens will have to be based on quantitative risk assessment and on a more complete understanding of the relationship among test animal bioassays, human epidemiology, expected human toxicity, pharmacokinetics, and cancer pharmacodynamics. If industrial hygienists and occupational toxicologists are not ready to make these QRA decisions, or if they are not willing to develop strategies to make them, then these decisions will surely be made by regulatory agencies with little input from those within these professions.

The quantitative risk assessment process has already been implemented in recent OSHA rulemaking with chemicals such as formaldehyde, asbestos, and benzene. Industrial health professionals have to be ready to tackle these issues of the control of occupational carcinogens responsibly, and today that responsibility includes the task of conducting and understanding quantitative risk assessments with occupational carcinogens. The biologically-based approaches discussed in this chapter will play an increasingly important role in improving the scientific basis of these quantitative risk assessments.

SUGGESTED READING

Hallenback, W. H., Cunningham, K. M. "Quantitative Risk Assessment for Environmental and Occupational Health." Lewis Publishers, Inc., Chelsea, MI (1987).

Paustenbach, D. J. (Ed.). "Risk Assessment of Environmental and Human Health Hazards." John Wiley & Sons, Inc. (1989).

REFERENCES

1. Singh, J. B. "Managing Carcinogens in the Work Environment." *Appl. Ind. Hyg.* 3:58 (1988).
2. Clewell, H. J., III, and Andersen, M. E. "Risk Assessment Extrapolations and Physiological Modeling." *Toxicol. Ind. Health* 1:111 (1985).
3. Gerlowski, L. E., and Jain, R. K. "Physiologically-Based Pharmacokinetic Modeling: Principles and Applications." *J. Pharm. Sci.* 72:1103 (1983).
4. Ramsey, J. C. and Andersen, M. E. "A Physiologically-Based Description of the Inhalation Pharmacokinetics of Styrene in Rats and Humans." *Toxicol. Appl. Pharmacol.* 73:159 (1984).
5. Dedrick, R. L. "Animal Scale-Up." *J. Pharmacokin. Biopharm.* 1:435 (1971).
6. Andersen, M. E., Clewell, H. J., III, Gargas, M. L., et al. "Physiologically-Based Pharmacokinetics and the Risk Assessment Process for Methylene Chloride." *Toxicol. Appl. Pharmacol.* 87:185 (1987).
7. Singh, D. V., Spitzer, H. L., and White, P. D. "Appendum to the Health Assessment Document for Dichloromethane (Methylene Chloride). Updated Carcinogenicity Assessment of Dichloromethane." EPA/600/8–82/004F.
8. Gargas, M. L., Clewell, H. J., III, and Andersen, M. E. "Metabolism of Inhaled Dichloromethanes *in vivo:* Differentiation of Kinetic Constants for Two Independent Pathways." *Toxicol. Appl. Pharmacol.* 87:211 (1986).
9. Reitz, R. H., Mendrala, A. L., Park, C. N., et al. "Incorporation of *in vitro* Enzyme Data into the PB-PK Model for Methylene Chloride (CH_2Cl_2): Implications for Risk Assessment." *Toxicol. Ltrs.* 43:97 (1988).
10. Moolgavkar, S. H. and Venzon, D. J. "Two-Event Models for Carcinogenesis: Incidence Curves for Childhood and Adult Tumors." *Mathematical Biosciences* 47:55 (1979).
11. Moolgavkar, S. H. "Carcinogenesis Modeling: From Molecular Biology to Epidemiology." *Ann. Rev. Public Health.* 7:151 (1986).

12. Armitage, P. and Doll, R. "The Age of Distribution of Cancer and Multistage Theory of Carcinogenesis." *Br. J. Cancer.* 8:1 (1954).

13. Leung, H. W., Murray, F. J., and Paustenbach, D. J. "A Proposed Occupational Exposure Limit for 2,3,7,8-Tetrachlorodibenzo-p-dioxin." *Am. Ind. Hyg. Assoc. J.* 49:000 (1988).

14. Thorslund, T. W., Brown, C. C., and Charnley, G. "Biologically Motivated Cancer Risk Models." *Risk Analysis* 7:109 (1987).

15. Rodricks, J. V., Brett, S. M., and Wrenn, G. C. "Significant Risk Decisions in Federal Regulatory Agencies." *Regulatory Toxicol. Pharmacol.* 7:307 (1987).

16. *Occupational Safety and Health Reporter* pp. 664–678 (September 16, 1987).

Chapter 3

EVALUATION OF IMPLANTED MATERIALS FOR CARCINOGENIC POTENTIAL[1]

Norbert P. Page, DVM, MS
and
Zorach R. Glaser, Ph.D., MPH
Page Associates, Gaithersburg, Maryland and
National Center for Medical Devices and Radiological Health,
U.S. Food and Drug Administration, Rockville, Maryland

INTRODUCTION

Most of the concern regarding carcinogenically hazardous materials has concentrated upon discrete chemicals, radiation, or biological agents which enter the body by ingestion (food, drinking water or medications), inhalation (gases, vapors or particulates), and by skin absorption. Therefore most standard carcinogenicity bioassays have been conducted by oral administration (food, drinking water, or gastric intubation), by inhalation exposure (whole body chambers or nose-only exposures), or by dermal application (skin painting). Since pharmaceuticals and drugs of abuse are often administered to humans by injection, carcinogenicity testing in animals may also include parenteral injections. Solid materials may enter the body because of war injuries or accidents; in addition, solid materials may be intentionally implanted for medical, dental, or cosmetic purposes.

Chemicals that enter the body by gastrointestinal, inhalation, and dermal exposure follow the laws of pharmacokinetics (absorption, distribution, metabolism, and elimination), and chemical interactions with the target tissue or cells can induce a carcinogenic response at virtually any site in the body. In contrast, implanted materials, in some cases, may produce a carcinogenic response unrelated to the chemical, but rather a "physical" effect of the implanted materials. The carcinogenic action of an implanted material may arise from the degradation products or substances that elute from the implant, the solid-state carcinogenic response (a physical effect) of the implant, or a combination of processes. (Goering and Galloway, 1989).

A large volume of literature exists about materials that have been introduced into the body by implantation techniques. In the literature the meaning of the term "implantation" is not consistent among scientists. Some use implantation strictly for surgical implants and others use the term to include any method (surgical and injection) by which materials are deposited in body tissues. For purposes of this review, we have adopted the broader interpretation and include

---

[1] The opinions or assertions contained herein are those of the authors, and not to be construed as official, or as reflecting the views of the Food and Drug Administration. Mention of commercial or trademarked products should not be interpreted as endorsement.

as implantation all methods that have been used to introduce materials into the body excepting inhalation, dermal exposure, ingestion, or intravenous injection. By this definition, the placing (surgically or by injection) of a solid particulate material, such as a polymer or metal, or liquid, into a muscle, dermal or subcutaneous tissue, or elsewhere in the body may result in exposure at the site of injection or systemic exposure, depending upon the physical and chemical properties of the material, and the vascularization and other characteristics of the tissue. For example, some materials may elute from the implant, become phagocytized or otherwise gain entrance into the circulatory and/or lymphatic systems, and be transported to remote sites. In other cases, the material may remain intact at the site of implantation for an indefinite period.

A recent search of the *Registry of Toxic Effects of Chemical Substances* (RTECS, 1989) revealed that 240 chemicals have been tested by surgical implantations. Many more have been tested by injection implantations, particularly subcutaneous, intramuscular, intraperitoneal or intracavity injections.

In some cases, the reason for using surgical or injection implantations has been the ease of administration of the test material in a precise and sufficiently large dose, and the relative sensitivity of the carcinogenicity assay system. In other cases, implantation actually simulates human exposure to materials, such as medical and dental devices, that may be intentionally implanted into the body.

From 1950 to 1970, the implantation of materials by subcutaneous, intramuscular, and intraperitoneal injection was widely used for testing food additives, dyes, and coloring agents for potential carcinogenicity. At about the same time, scientists were also testing polymers and metals by using similar injection techniques, and more sophisticated surgical implantations. Interest in implantation research has continued with the further development of medical and dental devices.

This chapter briefly reviews the types of materials implanted, the methodology employed in implantation studies, and the nature of the tissue reactions associated with the carcinogenic response at the site of implantation.

TYPES OF IMPLANTED MATERIALS

Solid materials may enter the body inadvertently as the result of accidents (automobile, occupational, and hunting) and wartime or crime-related injuries (bullets and shrapnel). Particulates and fibrous materials (asbestos and mineral dusts) may be inhaled, and enter the body via the respiratory tract. However, more people have internally-placed solid materials because of the intentional implantation of medical, dental, and cosmetic devices. Lord (1984) reported that in 1978 alone, one-half to one million cardiovascular devices, one-quarter million partial and total hip joints, more than one-half million intraocular lenses, and well over one-quarter of a million dental implants, finger joints, and mammary prostheses each were implanted. Scheer (1989) reported that 276,000 artificial hips and knees were implanted in 1988, double the number implanted in 1983. It is obvious that the number of implants in humans is steadily increasing, and the number of people with such implants is now in the millions.

Some interesting examples of implant materials are the use of Teflon™ particles to induce tissue buildup or provide constrictions (for cases of urinary incontinence), and polymeric beads and particles for novel drug delivery systems. Some other uses for implants are artificial joints, joint liners and articulating surfaces, breast augmentation, and vascular repairs. Table 3-1 presents a partial list of materials employed in medical and dental devices, and demonstrates the great diversity of materials that may be implanted in the body. A different classification for plastic devices has been compiled by Autian and Lawrence (1972), and is presented in Table 3-2.

Implanted materials may be liquids, dusts, fibers, foams, or dense solid substances. Chemical composition may vary widely, and may include simple chemicals or monomers, synthetic polymers, ceramics, metals, and naturally-occurring complex materials.

TABLE 3-1. Examples of Materials and Devices Which May Be Implanted

Metallic Materials	Bullets and Shell Fragments; Orthopedic Appliances (including pins, nails, screws, and plates); Sutures; Dental Implants and Restorations; Mesh; Foil; Electrodes; Pumps; Pacemakers
Polymeric or Plastic Materials	Gels; Foams; Lubricants; Adhesives; Sponges; Orthopedic Appliances (including pins, plates, clips); Tubing; Patches; Sutures; Coatings, Insulation on Electrodes, Vascular Grafts; Pumps; Filters
Ceramics and Carbon	Dental Restorations; Filters; Cements; Beads; Graphite
Naturally Occurring Biomaterials	Bone; Starch; Dextrin; Cellulose; Collagen; Cartilage; Tendon
Isolates from Tissue and Tissue Products	Elastin; Fibrin; Gut (sutures); Valves; Tissue Grafts; Enzymes; Antibodies; Skin
Minerals and related Inorganic Materials	Carbon, Boron and Other Fibers and Whiskers; Mineral Wool; Glass Fibers; Silica Particles; Fused Silica; Glass Beads; Chalk; Talc
Fibers, Textiles and Composite Materials	Monofilament Suture; Vascular Grafts; Tissue Expanders
Miscellaneous	Dyes; Colors; Pigments; Beads; Contrast Media; Markers; Residue From Processing, Disinfecting, and/or Sterilizing; Lint; Drug Delivery Products; Carriers; Film; Dosimeters; Plasticizers; Accelerators; Retardants; Mold Release Agents; Machining Oils

TABLE 3-2. Plastic Devices Used Medically

Device	Examples
Permanent Implants	Heart Valves, Various Vascular Grafts; Orthopaedic Implants, Implants for Cosmetic Reconstruction; Artificial Organs, etc.
Implants in Contact with Mucosal Tissue	Artificial Eyes, Contact Lenses; Dentures; Intrauterine Devices; Certain Types of Catheters
Corrective, Protective, and Supportive Devices	Splints; Braces; Films; Clothing
Collection and Administration Devices	Blood Transfusion Sets; Various Types of Catheters; Dialysis Units; Hypodermic Devices; Other Injection Devices, etc.
Storage Devices	Bags or Other Containers for Blood; Blood Products; Drug Products; Nutritional Products; Diagnostic Agents, etc.

Source: Autian and Lawrence (1972).

IMPLANTATION TESTING TECHNIQUES

Many testing procedures have been developed to implant materials into body tissues. In some cases, the implant can be made using a large diameter needle, while for other circumstances a surgical procedure is required. Some implantation procedures have been developed as general tests for carcinogenic potential, whereas others attempt to mimic the human exposure situation in which solid materials are implanted in the body. Various forms of materials have been implanted, including materials in liquid vehicles, powders, fibers, whiskers, disks, rods, sheets, and irregular shapes. The materials have been introduced into virtually every location in the body. Historically most testing has involved implantation into the subcutaneous or intramuscular tissues, implantation into body cavities (peritoneal and pleural cavities), implants in the respiratory system, and urinary bladder implants.

As simple general carcinogenicity test systems, the implantation of materials offers a way to introduce large volumes of material into critical target tissues, and may provide for the slow, continuous release of the test substance, simulating a long-term bioassay with minimal effort and cost. Such implantation methods compensate, somewhat, for differences in the pharmacokinetics of absorption between animals and humans. This is particularly true for inhalation testing of particulates in rodents.

Subcutaneous or Intramuscular Routes

Subcutaneous and intramuscular routes were widely used from the 1950s to the 1970s for routine carcinogenicity testing, and were the methods recommended by the International Union Against Cancer (UICC, 1969). Such recommendations were based mainly on the ease of administration of test materials (especially for relatively insoluble substances), the requirement for only small amounts of the test material, and the relative sensitivity of the assay. In addition, subcutaneous and intramuscular administration provided an opportunity to detect systemic carcinogenicity, while avoiding the complications of oral administration, such as poor absorption, and/or decomposition of the substance in the intestinal tract. Also the acute toxicity from the subcutaneous route was generally lower (due to slower absorption) than that which occurred after intraperitoneal or intravenous administration. This allowed for the testing of acutely toxic chemicals and those that could not be effectively tested by oral administration.

Subcutaneous administration appears to be one of the most sensitive routes for tumor induction of some chemicals. In some cases, only a single implant of a rather diverse array of materials, including some aromatic hydrocarbons, some plastics, and a few metal compounds, was necessary to induce cancer. Various solvents or vehicles have been used, including food oils (such as arachnis, corn, and peanut oil) and saline and distilled water. For some chemicals, the test material has been compressed into small pellets for subcutaneous implantation. Diluents such as cholesterol and paraffin have been used to allow slow, continuous release of the chemical from the pellet.

When the subcutaneous and intramuscular assays were introduced into the laboratory array of tests for carcinogenicity, the idea prevailed that carcinogenicity occurred when a chemical interacted with the genetic material of tissue cells, and that the site at which this occurred was of no significance. Cancer induced by a chemical or material at any location was thought to represent the material's inate ability to induce chemical carcinogenicity under any exposure situation. At the time, little was known about a physical mechanism for cancer induction.

The use of the subcutaneous test for carcinogenicity has been highly controversial. Indeed, Page (1977) and the International Agency for Research on Cancer (IARC, 1980), cautioned against the subcutaneous injection assay as a general carcinogenic test method for testing chemicals to which humans are exposed via diet, inhalation, and skin contact. They considered data developed by injection and implantation methods as unreliable for the risk assessment of chemicals entering the body from those means of exposure. They concluded that injection-site tumors alone did not provide sufficient evidence for designating a substance as a systemic carcinogen.

Grasso et al. (1971) conducted a series of studies on factors that were involved in the induction of sarcomas by subcutaneous injections of food additives, including certain dyes and artificial sweeteners. The results of those studies demonstrated that local tissue changes and sarcomas were related to surface activity of the solution injected, and could be modified by the introduction of high concentrations of calcium ions. They concluded that induction of local sarcomas by repeated injections into the same subcutaneous site did not represent a valid index of the carcinogenicity of a chemical.

Support for this general rejection of the subcutaneous route for testing materials intended for ingestion by humans comes from a review of the subcutaneous test results. Local sarcomas have been induced, by subcutaneous or intramuscular injection, by substances normally found in the body, and in a normal diet, such as sucrose and sodium chloride. In addition, many chemicals known to promote the induction of local tumors at the site of subcutaneous or intramuscular injections or implantations have not been demonstrated to have carcinogenic potential by other routes. It is generally assumed that the site-specific sarcoma response is caused by a physical rather than a chemical mechanism, and thus is of little relevance to human exposure at lower dose levels, or from other routes of exposure.

The subcutaneous or intramuscular routes are rarely used now for routine carcinogenicity testing of environmental chemicals, as there is general agreement that the test compound should be administered by a route similar to, or as close as possible to the one by which human exposure occurs. However, for solid materials that will be implanted in humans (e.g., certain medical devices), the subcutaneous and intramuscular routes do indeed simulate a realistic human exposure situation, and for these materials such testing methods are still widely used.

The first report that an implanted solid material could induce tumors at the site of implantation appeared in the studies of Turner (1941) involving Bakelite disks implanted in the subcutaneous tissues of rats. Oppenheimer et al. (1948, 1955) and Heuper (1964), using the same basic technique, induced sarcomas with a variety of polymers and plastics, including cellophane, Dacron™, Teflon™, and many other commonly used polymeric materials. Most of the materials were insoluble; however, some were macromolecules which were water soluble. Apparently an important factor is the storage of the material at the site, and the local tissue response to the foreign material. As the result of the extensive work of Oppenheimer and Turner, the induction of implantation site tumors is often referred to as the "Oppenheimer" or "Oppenheimer-Turner" effect. The nature of this tissue response is described later in this chapter.

Intrapleural/Intraperitoneal Implantations

Many fibrous materials have been assayed for carcinogenicity by surgically implanting the substance on the pleural surfaces of rats. Observation for the development of tumors during the normal lifespan of the animals was then made. Based on the studies of Stanton et al. (1981), several general conclusions can be made which document the importance of fiber dimension and durability, rather than the physicochemical properties of the fibrous material.

The tumors induced in the animal model are pleural sarcomas that resemble the mesenchymal mesotheliomas found in humans following exposure to asbestos. A direct relationship to the dimensions of the material is evident, with an increased probability of cancer induction for long, thin fibers (i.e., 1.5 μm diameter or less, and with a length of 4 μm or greater). Short fibers and large-diameter fibers were inactivated by phagocytosis. Only negligible phagocytosis of the long, thin fibers occurred. These long, thin fibers can also penetrate cells without killing them, although it is unclear if there is a chemical or physical effect. The suggested mechanism is that the progenitor of the cancer cell is not directly affected by the fiber, but that a generalized alteration in the local or systemic environment occurs as a reaction to the fiber, and that this alteration serves to promote existing tumor progenitors.

For intrapleural administration of most materials, a single dose of 10 to 40 mg of material dissolved in 0.5 to 2 ml of saline has been injected through the chest wall into the pleural cavity, and the animal is observed for life. Rats have been routinely used, although mice and hamsters are occasionally the test species for this assay procedure.

Intraperitoneal implantation has also been employed for the testing of solid materials that are intended to be implanted in humans. For example, Autian et al. (1975) studied 17 chemically different polyurethanes for carcinogenic potential in rats. The materials were implanted either in a powder form or as small disks (0.3 cm or less in dimension). It was found that the materials induced a high rate of tumor formation at the site of implantation. Fiber suspensions (2 to 25 mg in 1 to 2 ml of saline) were injected once, and the animals observed for life. In general, the intraperitoneal implantation route has not been as efficient for the production of foreign body tumors as has been the subcutaneous implantation assay, however nearly all of the polyurethanes studied by Autian et al. (1975) induced sarcomas.

Respiratory Tract Implantations

Inhalation is the preferable route for animal bioassay of materials, such as chemical vapors and particulate materials as dusts, and such mineral fibers as asbestos, fibrous glass, silica, and ceramic fibers which are inhaled by humans. Due to technical difficulties in conducting inhalation tests in laboratory rodents, considerable research upon respirable materials has been conducted by artificial exposure methods that deposit greater concentrations of the particulate materials into target tissues than can be achieved by the usual rodent inhalation bioassay. Some of the methods overcome the problems of particle inhalation, deposition, and retention in rodents. Rodents are obligatory nose-breathers, whereas humans inhale through the mouth as well as the nose, and thus in humans, inhaled materials can bypass the nasal filtration process. Since the trachea/bronchi of rodents have a smaller lumen than do those of humans, the particle size distribution reaching the deep lung of the rodent is quite different from the particle size distribution reaching the deep lung of humans. Thus, inhalation tests with rodents fail to mimic the quantitative and qualitative aspects of a human exposure.

In order to detect a minimal carcinogenic response (albeit a response of societal concern, e.g., one induced cancer in 20 animals exposed), animal studies use larger doses of materials than is typical for human exposures, since the animal tests are conducted with small numbers of animals. The use of these higher doses may increase the sensitivity of the carcinogenicity bioassay, however, this may also introduce atypical biological perturbations, such as altered pharmacokinetics or metabolism, that might change the nature of the response. Thus, to achieve the increased sensitivity for detecting a true effect, a reduction in specificity may result. These factors must be considered by the risk assessors.

Other reasons for employing exposure methods, other than standard inhalation chambers, are based on practical or economic considerations. Particle aggregation and other problems arise when high concentrations of particles are generated for inhalation exposure. The high cost of inhalation studies, and the restrictions on the availability of laboratory facilities limit the number of inhalation tests which can be performed.

In order to overcome these testing limitations, methods have been developed which can deposit high volumes of the substance at the target sites of the respiratory tract. In particular, *intratracheal instillation, intrabronchial administration,* and *intrapleural implantations* have been employed. These routes directly expose the various tissues of the respiratory tract and pleural cavity, important "target tissues" for mineral fiber carcinogenicity. By use of these artificial routes of exposure, the fibers are brought into contact with the same target tissues which are important in human exposures.

Other techniques to expose the respiratory tract have been used. For example, threads or pellets impregnated with test substances have been implanted directly into the respiratory tissues (Andervont, 1937, and Kuschner et al. 1957). These techniques have not been widely used, and the three main respiratory tract implantation methods have consisted of intratracheal, intrabronchial, and intrapleural implantation assays.

Intratracheal Instillation

Saffiotti et al. (1968) introduced the intratracheal intubation technique which has been employed by a number of investigators to study respiratory carcinogenicity. The technique involves the administration of the test material once weekly (or at most twice weekly) to Syrian golden hamsters via a catheter passed into the trachea. The test material was deposited on fine metallic carrier dust particles, e.g., ferric oxide, to assure deposition and retention of the material in the respiratory tract. The test material then elutes out of the carrier dust, and can diffuse through the entire lung and bronchi. Intratracheal instillation is considered by IARC (1980) to more closely simulate human inhalation of particulate material than can be accomplished by rodent inhalation studies because of the difference in inhalation kinetics of rodents and humans.

The usual method for intratracheal instillation has been to instill 0.5 to 1 mg of the test material in a particulate/saline carrier material, weekly or biweekly for a period of several weeks (usually 5 to 20 weeks), with lifetime observation (Pott et al. 1987). Rats or hamsters are often used.

Intrabronchial Pellet Implant Technique

Another techique used to study lung cancer etiology was developed by Laskin et al. (1970). This method involves the implantation, using tracheotomy, of pellets containing a test material mixed in cholesterol (1:1 ratio), retained in a stainless steel wire mesh cage, and fastened to the trachea with a spring wire hook. Most studies have been conducted with rats, although hamsters have also been used. Usually 3 to 5 mg of the test substance was impregnated into the cholesterol pellet. This technique provides for a continuous slow release of the test chemical, consistent with the very slow absorption of cholesterol. Among the materials tested have been such potentially carcinogenic materials as 3-methylcholanthrene, chromium compounds, and various radioactive emitters.

Urinary Bladder Implantations

In order to provide for a high concentration of a potential bladder carcinogen, several assays have been developed to inject or implant substances directly in the bladder. The first true bladder implantation method was introduced by Jull in 1951. The technique consists of surgically implanting paraffin or cholesterol pellets containing the test material into the lumen of the bladder of mice. Examination of the animals at various times for hyperplasia and tumor formation, 40, 70, and 110 weeks after implantation, is then conducted. While the technique has identified a number of substances as bladder carcinogens, it is complicated by the instability of some chemicals in the pellet, and the uncertainty of the transfer of the chemical to the bladder epithelium. In addition, the role of urine and foreign bodies complicates the analysis of the bladder implantation data (Clayson et al. 1968). Attempts to use the rat for bladder implantation studies have generally been unsatisfactory, because lesions developed which made interpretation of the results difficult.

Other Implantation Techniques

Numerous other implantation methods are employed, which correspond to the intended use of the material, and the site or tissue that is likely to be in contact with the material or device. The *intraosseous route* has been suggested by Sunderman (1989) as a desirable route for the assay of metal allows that are employed in orthopedic prostheses. *Intravaginal* (and/or *intrauterine*) *implantation* has been used to test certain materials used in IUDs. An example of a novel implantation method is the *cage implant* system developed by Marchant (1989). In this procedure the test material is enclosed in a wire-mesh cylindrical cage and implanted in the subcutaneous tissues of rats. Cellular and molecular interactions can be studied to better define the tissue responses related to implanted materials. Other methods are being evaluated in relation to the site at which the implanted material will be used in humans or animals, e.g., intranasal, intraocular, hepatic, bone, and vascular implants.

Standardization of Implantation Assays

One of the confusing aspects of carcinogenicity testing of implantable materials is the lack of standard methods for the assay procedures. While this promotes the development of new and novel methods, it does not allow for the development of a data base that can be used for comparative toxicity and carcinogenicity evaluations. Government guidelines exist for the testing of environmental agents by ingestion, inhalation, or dermal exposure (U.S. EPA, 1985; Page, 1981), but do not yet exist for other routes of exposure, including implantations. The American Society for Testing and Materials (ASTM, 1987) is developing recommended procedures for the biocompatibility and toxicity testing of implanted materials, however, no ASTM chronic carcinogenicity test method exists now. The longest duration ASTM toxicity method is a 3-month intramuscular test procedure for biocompatibility.

CARCINOGENIC POTENTIAL OF IMPLANTED MATERIALS

The potential of implanted materials or foreign bodies to induce carcinogenicity has been the subject of much investigation. Theoretically, implanted materials can induce a carcinogenic response by the following mechanisms: (a) interaction of chemicals (which may leach from the implant or are degradation products from the implant) with cells and cellular macromolecules near the implant or elsewhere in the body either initiating or promoting a carcinogenic response; (b) physical contact of the material with surrounding cells which might initiate carcinogenicity (transformation of cells to neoplasia) or promote existing preneoplastic cells; and (c) a combination of both chemical and physical mechanisms.

It is now known that many materials which were once thought to be inert will undergo a wide variety of reactions when introduced into the body. Polymers and plastics can become swollen, resulting in dimensional changes and the alteration of chemical and/or physical properties (Moore, et al. 1977). In addition, extraction and loss of plasticizer and/or low molecular weight materials can occur, resulting in changes in thermal, electrical, and mechanical properties, alteration in surface characteristics, depolymerization, and crosslinkage changes (Glaser, 1968, and Glaser and Eirich, 1970). These events may lead to accelerated wear, breakdown, and degradation. Some of the breakdown and wear products have been shown to be quite toxic.

In some of the early polymeric materials which were used in packaging, medical, and dental devices, monomers or additives were found to have diffused from the materials, and represented a source of potential systemic chemical exposure. Metals can be oxidized, reduced, or solvated, and may undergo changes in their chemical and physical properties. Proof that such leaching occurs has been established, because metal ions or monomers have been detected in body fluids.

For example, Sunderman (1989) has reported the finding of serum metallic ions following the implantation of some metallic prostheses into the body. In the situation where chemicals leach from the implant or result from degradation, the carcinogenic responses and the mechanisms for cancer induction are similar to those operative when chemicals enter the body from environmental exposures. The reader is referred to the papers by Groth and Anderson which appear in this book.

On the other hand, implanted materials may also induce a local carcinogenic response unique to implanted materials or inhaled fibrous substances. The mechanism for this type of carcinogenic response is considered a physical phenomenon, with the tumors developing at the implantation sites. As noted earlier, this phenomenon has generally been referred to as a *foreign body tumor* response, with the process designated as *"solid-state carcinogenicity,"* *"physical carcinogenesis,"* or the *"Oppenheimer"* or *"Oppenheimer/Turner effect."* While much of our knowledge of the etiology and pathogenesis of foreign body tumors is derived from experimental animal studies, some evidence is available from clinical studies in humans.

Experimental Studies

The earliest laboratory investigations of the carcinogenicity of foreign bodies were conducted by Turner (1941), and Oppenheimer et al. (1948). Since then, numerous studies have been conducted, as reviewed by Bischoff and Bryson (1964), Brand (1976, 1982), Pedley et al. (1982), and Lawrence (1986). The route of implantation in most studies was subcutaneous, although other routes, e.g., intraperitoneal, intramuscular, and intrauterine implantation, have been employed. In a majority of the studies, sarcomas developed at the site of implantation, and only rarely at some distance from the site. Nearly all of the tumors were sarcomas. It is now realized that the etiology and pathogenesis of foreign body carcinogenesis is more complex than originally thought, and depends primarily on the physical properties of the material rather than its chemical composition.

The response to a material implanted within the body is a typical host response to an invading organism or substance, with the tissue striving to expel or dissolve the foreign material. When that fails, a chronic proliferative process, which attempts to encapsulate and isolate the foreign body follows. As a consequence of these processes, tumors may also be induced and developed at the site of the implant and the surrounding capsule.

The pathogenesis of the neoplastic development at the implant site is not entirely clear, and is the subject of differing viewpoints regarding the cellular and biochemical mechanism(s) that ultimately lead to carcinogenicity. According to Brand (1976), the cells that undergo tumor formation were already pre-neoplastic prior to the introduction of the foreign body and the foreign body merely creates the conditions required for stepwise pre-neoplastic maturation. Kordan (1967) and Ecanow et al. (1977), however, have proposed a direct interaction of the foreign body with cellular macromolecules that can lead to neoplasia. They have speculated that foreign bodies, especially polymers, can undergo molecular binding with the cells, creating physiochemical changes that alter adjacent cellular metabolism and subsequent initiation of neoplasia. It is possible that both of these mechanisms may be involved in some cases of foreign body neoplasia. Lawrence (1986) has speculated that a chemical which can leach from the implant or result from biodegradation may induce a neoplastic change in the adjacent cells and the capsular environment may then promote the initiated cells to become expressed as a true neoplasia. It is also a matter of uncertainty which cells are the progenitor cells that give rise to the foreign body tumor. Early studies seemed to implicate macrophages that invaded the area during the early inflammatory response. This has now been discounted. Some research has suggested that the fibroblast is the progenitor cell, however, it is generally accepted now, based on the studies of Johnson et al. (1973) that the pericyte of the microvasculature (a pleuripotential cell) is the more likely progenitor cell.

Regardless of the actual mechanism(s) or progenitor cells involved, laboratory research has provided considerable insight into the factors that are important in determining the potential for a neoplastic response. Implant size, smoothness and continuity of the surface, and the duration of the implant in the body are of great importance. There are also species differences in response to foreign bodies and induction of foreign body tumors. The chemical composition of the foreign material appears to play only a minor role in the tissue response and induction of a foreign body tumor.

It is clear that the implant must be of a *critical size* to induce the tissue response and neoplasia. Implants of less than 0.5×0.5 cm in rodents have only minor tumorigenic potential; the greater the size above this dimension, the greater the tumor-inducing activity. Bischoff and Bryson (1964) have concluded, however, that the important factor is the number of cells in contact with the unbroken smooth surface of the implant. They conclude that there is a minimum number of cells (threshold), related to the size of the implant, that is required for the cellular activity leading to the neoplastic response.

It is generally accepted, based on studies conducted in 1950–1970, that a smooth, continuous surface promotes the appropriate environment for neoplastic development. Changing the surface by perforations, roughening, woven pattern, or converting the implant to a powder, reduces or eliminates the neoplastic potential.

Materials must remain in place for a minimum duration if neoplasia is to occur. This has been determined to be about 6 months in the rat. A series of studies performed by Oppenheimer et al. (1958) showed that embedded films become enclosed by a connective tissue sheath or pocket, from which, if the film is removed earlier than 6 months after embedding, no tumors are induced. After 6 months, removal of the film does not affect the tumor production if the capsule remains. If the encapsulated pocket is removed, no tumors will occur, regardless of the time of removal, if the tumor has not already developed. The authors considered this evidence that the tumor cells were initially attached to the film, and only at a later stage were they present in the surrounding capsule tissue.

Species differences in the induction of neoplasia with implant materials is quite apparent. Rats and mice are particularly susceptible, but hamsters and dogs are less sensitive. Chickens and guinea pigs are resistant (Brand 1976). The relative sensitivity of humans to rats and mice is not clear. It does not appear that variations in flexibility, irritation from the slight movement of the implants, site of the implant, and the age and sex of the animals will greatly alter the response to the implanted materials.

Most research on implants has involved studies of fibrous materials, plastics, polymers, ceramics, and metals. Asbestos is probably the most studied of the physical carcinogens. Studies have shown that a variety of fibers and dusts (including silica dust, glass fibers, and several forms of asbestos) induced foreign body tumors when implanted in animals, were cytotoxic and transformed cells in culture. The precise mechanism(s) by which fibers exert their carcinogenic effect is not known, although fibrosis precedes the carcinogenic response in all cases. However, since asbestos causes chromosomal changes in cultured cells (Barrett et al. 1983, and Jaurand et al. 1986) the interaction of asbestos with cellular macromolecules cannot be discounted. There is general agreement that the most important determinants of the carcinogenic potential of fibers are fiber length, fiber width, durability and persistence, i.e., the ability of a fiber to remain fixed in a given location in the target tissue for an extended period, and dose to the target organ (IARC 1988). The potency varied considerably, with long, thin fibers, being much more effective than other shapes, whether the material was asbestos or glass fibers (Hesterberg and Barrett, 1984). An increased probability of cancer induction is evident for fibers of 4 μm or greater in length and 1.5 μm or less in diameter. It appears that the carcinogenicity of the longer fibers is related to their resistance to phagocytosis. The most durable and insoluble synthetic man-made fibers are likely to be more hazardous than relatively soluble fibers. Surface properties and chemical leaching, i.e., solubilization of impurities and components, may also contribute to oncogenic potential although this has not been clearly established.

Metallic implants have also induced fibrosarcomas or granulomas when implanted as foils or as particles or powders. The carcinogenicity of metallic powders appears to be associated with specific metals, especially beryllium, cobalt, chromium, and nickel (Sunderman, 1989; Pedley et al. 1982; Furst and Radding, 1984). Other metals, when implanted as foils, can induce the typical foreign body reaction and implantation-site sarcomas. Thus, tumor induction by metals or metal alloys is attributed to both physical and chemical mechanisms. Foils made of gold, silver, steel, Vitallium™, tantalum, iron, and tin induced foreign body tumors, but powders did not. It was concluded that those materials did not induce chemical carcinogenicity, but implants of these materials of sufficient size, rigidity, and a smooth, uninterrupted surface, would induce the typical foreign body response leading to sarcoma induction (Bischoff and Bryson, 1964). Intradermal injections of some metal-containing substances, e.g., zirconium, aluminum, and iron, have induced granulomas.

Most of the research on solid-state carcinogenicity has involved various types of polymers, plastics, and ceramics. As pointed out in the reviews of IARC (1979) and Pedley et al. (1982), some polymers and plastics can release monomers or additives which might induce a chemical carcinogenic response either at the implant site or in other parts of the body. However, nearly all of these materials can induce foreign body tumors if they meet the solid-state criteria for critical size and surface characteristics as previously described.

In summary, the development of implantation site sarcomas has been shown to be related to several factors, especially size of the implant, surface smoothness and continuity, the length of time the implant remains in the tissue, and the species that has been implanted. Generally, large or thick implants produce more sarcomas than do small or thin ones. A continuous surface is more conducive to sarcoma development than is a discontinuous one, or one with perforations. Surfaces with large holes are also less apt to induce sarcomas than surfaces with small holes. Sarcoma induction is also related to the shape of the implant. Disks are particularly effective, as are fibers, films, and sheets. The same material as a powder, a thread, or in a porous form is less likely to induce a sarcoma response. An exception to this is that Ni and Co, in the form of powders, can induce sarcomas at the implant site (Sunderman, 1989).

Solid materials with an uninterrupted surface, with the appropriate size requirements, can produce a fibrous capsule when implanted subcutaneously into rodents. The sarcomas have a long average latent period approaching that of the lifespan of the majority of the animals tested.

Clinical Findings

The experimental evidence for foreign body tumors in laboratory animal experiments is quite substantial. While clinicians have reported cases of tumors associated with the presence of foreign bodies, the number is well below the incidence expected on the basis of the high rate of foreign body tumor induction found in experiments with rodents.

One of the first papers that described cancer in humans at the site of foreign bodies was that of Siddons and MacArthur (1952). They reported two cases of carcinoma of the bronchus which developed at the site of retained metallic objects. They reviewed five other published case reports of similar findings. Five of the seven cases were associated with bullets or shrapnel which had lodged in the body; the other cases involved metal objects that had been accidentally inhaled (a crucifix, and the head of a scarf pin). While the tumor type of the sarcomas varied, they all developed around the object. The latency period was quite long for most of the cases, with an average latency period of 24 years.

Occasional reports of tumors associated with foreign bodies, chronic inflammation, and scars have been reported since 1888. Ott (1970) reported on 24 case studies in which sarcomas had developed in the vicinity of metallic foreign bodies. These studies were described in the literature during the period from 1888 to 1964. Most of the metallic bodies were bullets or shrapnel received during wartime, and which usually were lodged in soft tissues. Again, the latency period generally was long, averaging 25 years (with a range of 2 to 46 years). Sunderman (1989) reviewed the literature for 1956 to 1987 and tabulated a list of 13 patients who developed cancer at the site of metallic orthopedic implants. The latency period was considerably shorter (11 years, with a range of 2 to 30 years) than the two other tabulations described previously. Most of the cases were sarcomas or histiocytomas, and most involved prostheses composed of iron/chromium/nickel (FeCrNi), or cobalt/chromium/molybdenum (CoCrMo) alloys. It is possible that the shorter induction time found by Sunderman can be accounted for by the different location of the implants, in bone rather than soft tissues. Sunderman (1989) also compiled a list of 25 clinical cases, reported by veterinarians, of sarcomas that had developed around implanted orthopedic pins, screws and other metallic implants in dogs.

Tumor induction has been shown to occur with asbestos particles, schistosomiasis, scars, and with chronic inflammation; all such tumor inductions are believed to be the result of similar (or identical) processes. These phenomena have a number of characteristics in common, particularly the induction of a marked fibrotic or foreign body type reaction with a long latency period before the cancer becomes manifest (Brand, 1982).

The probability of cancer in patients who have received implants is unclear at this time. Some scientists, Brand and Brand (1980) and Sunderman (1989), while recognizing that there have been some reports of foreign body tumors in humans, contend that the implantation of polymeric and metallic devices pose an extremely low carcinogenic risk to the implanted patient. These conclusions are based on the small number of clinical reports of implantation-site tumors (as compared to the large number of medical devices that have been implanted) and on the comparatively lower reactivity of human tissues when contrasted with the reaction of the tissues of rodents. While the number of cases of cancer at the site of implanted prosthetic joints are rare, nevertheless it is of concern to the medical community, and the subject of several legal cases (Scheer 1989).

In view of the long latency period for sarcoma development in humans (perhaps as long as 40 years), and the fact that there are several reports in the literature of foreign body tumors in humans, a more cautious position has been proposed by others. Lawrence (1986) suggests that the prudent course is to continue to evaluate new biomaterials by long-term implantation assay with rats. Efforts should continue to find alternative plastics or other materials that do not contain plasticizers or other leachable substances (Autian, 1984), to be used in implanted devices, and to avoid implantations having surface properties that are conducive to foreign-body reactions.

In summary, there can be little doubt that the induction of foreign body tumors is a well-recognized phenomenon in rodents. However, there is considerable uncertainty regarding the relative sensitivity of humans as compared to rodents, and the general applicability of the experimental test results to predict human carcinogenicity.

REFERENCES

Andersen, M. (1990). Quantitative risk assessment and chemical carcinogens in occupational environments. In: *Carcinogenically Active Chemicals: A Reference Guide*, ed. R. Lewis. Van Nostrand Reinhold (Chapter 2, pp. 17–28, this book).

Andervont, H. (1937). Pulmonary tumours in mice: IV. Lung tumours induced by subcutaneous injection of 1,2,4,6-dibenzanthracene in different media and by its direct contact with lung tissue. *Public Health Rep.* 52:1484.

ASTM (1987). Standard Practice for Selecting Generic Biological Test Methods for Materials and Devices. ASTM Committee F-4 on Medical and Surgical Materials and Devices. ASTM vol. 13.01. ASTM, Philadelphia, PA. November 1987.

Autian, J., Singh, R., Turner, J., Hung, W., Nunez, L., and Lawrence W. (1975). Carcinogenesis from polyurethanes. *Cancer Res.* 35:1591–1596.

Autian, J. (1984). Primary toxicological testing as a means of safeguarding the patient. Chapter 11. In: *Contemporary Biomaterials* (J. Boretos and M. Eden, eds.). Noyes Publications, Park Ridge, New Jersey. pp. 180–192.

Autian, J. and Lawrence, W. (1972). Visit to a laboratory. The Materials Science Toxicology Laboratories. U. of Tennessee. *Med. Res. Eng.,* September–October 23–27.

Barrett, J. C., Thomassen, D. G., and Hesterberg, T. H. (1983). Role of chromosomal mutations in cell transformation. *Ann. NY Acad. Sci.,* 407, pp. 291–300.

Bischoff, F. and Bryson, G. (1964). Carcinogenesis through solid state surfaces. *Progr. Exp. Tumor Res.* 5:85–133.

Brand, G. K. (1976). Diversity and complexity of carcinogenic processes: Conceptual inferences from foreign-body tumorigenesis. *J. Natl Cancer Inst.* 57:973–976.

Brand, G. K. (1976). Foreign Body Induced Sarcomas. Chapter 17. In: *Cancer; A Comprehensive Treatise* (F. Beck, ed.). Plenum Press, New York. pp. 485–511.

Brand, G. K. (1982). Cancer associated with asbestosis, schistosomiasis, foreign bodies, and scars. Chapter 19. In: *Cancer: A Comprehensive Treatise.* (F. F. Becker, Ed.). Plenum Publishing Company, New York. pp. 661–692.

Brand, G. K. and Brand, I. (1980). Risk assessment of carcinogenesis at implantation sites. *Plast. Reconstr. Surg.* 66:591–595.

Clayson, D., Pringle, J., Bonser, G., and Wood, M. (1968). The technique of bladder implantation: Further results and assessment. *Brit. J. Cancer* 22:825–832.

Ecanow, B., Gold, B. and Sadove, M. (1977). The role of inert foreign bodies in the pathogenesis of cancer. *Brit. J. Cancer* 36:397.

Furst, A. and Radding, S. (1984). New developments in the study of metal carcinogenesis. *Proc. West. Pharmacol. Soc.* 14:68–71.

Glaser, Z. R. and Eirich, F. R. (1970). Thermal behavior of elastomers at high rates of tensile straining. *J. Polymer Science* (Part C) 31:275–290.

Glaser, Z. R. (1968). Ph.D. Dissertation, Polytechnic Institute of Brooklyn (Polytechnic University of New York). (Advisor: Frederick R. Eirich). Relating macromolecular structure to macroscopic behavior by means of calorimetric and mechanical studies. (Abstract in *Dissertation Abstracts International,* B, 30(6):2643B, 1969).

Goering, P. and Galloway, W. (1989). Toxicology of medical device materials. *Fundament. and Appl. Toxicol.* 13:193–195.

Grasso, P., Gangolli, S., Golberg, L, and Hooson, J. (1971). Physicochemical and other factors determining local sarcoma production by food additives. *Fd. Cosmet. Toxicol.* 9:463–478.

Groth, D. (1990). Federal regulations and the definition of a carcinogen. In: *Carcinogenically Active Chemicals: A Reference Guide,* ed. R. Lewis. Van Nostrand Reinhold (Chapter 1, pp. 3–16, this book).

Heuper, W. (1964). Cancer induction by polyurethane and polysilicone plastics. *J. Natl. Cancer Inst.* 33:1005–1027.

Hesterberg, T. W. and Barrett, J. C. (1984). Dependence of asbestos- and mineral dust-induced transformation of mammalian cells in culture on fiber dimension. *Cancer Res.* 44:2170–2180.

IARC (1979). *Evaluation of Carcinogenic Risks to Humans: Some Monomers, Plastics and Synthetic Elastomers, and Acrolein.* IARC Monographs, Volume 19. International Agency for Research on Cancer, Lyon, France.

IARC (1980). *Long-term and Short-term Screening Assays for Carcinogens: A Critical Appraisal.* IARC Monographs, Supplement 2. International Agency for Research on Cancer, Lyon, France.

IARC (1988). *Evaluation of Carcinogenic Risks to Humans: Man-made Mineral Fibres and Radon.* IARC Monographs, Volume 43. International Agency for Research on Cancer, Lyon, France.

Jaurand, M. C., Kheuang, L., Magne, L., and Bignon, J. (1986). Chromosomal changes induced by chrysotile fibers or benzo-3,4-pyrene in rat pleural mesothelial cells. *Mutation Res.* 169:141–148.

Johnson, K., Ghobrial, H., Buoen, L., Brand, K., and Brand, I. (1973). Nonfibroblastic origin of foreign body sarcomas implicated by histological and electron microscopic studies. *Cancer Res.* 33:3139–3154.

Jull, J. (1951). The induction of tumors of the bladder epithelium in mice by the direct application of a carcinogen. *Brit. J. Cancer* 5:328–330.

Kordan, H. (1967). Localized interfacial forces resulting from implanted plastics as possible physical factors involved in tumor formation. *J. Theoret. Biol.* 17:1–11.

Kuschner, M., Laskin, S., Cristofano, E. and Nelso, N. (1957). Experimental carcinoma of the lung. In: *Proceedings of the 3rd National Cancer Conference,* Philadelphia, Lippincott, pp. 485–495.

Laskin, S., Kuschner, M. and Drew, R. (1970). Studies in pulmonary carcinogenesis. In: *Inhalation Carcinogenesis* (M. Hanna, P. Nettesheim, J. Gilbert, eds.). AEC Sumposium Series 18 (CONF-691001). U.S. Atomic Energy Commission, Washington, D.C. pp. 321–352.

Lawrence, W. H. (1986). Tumor induction. Chapter 17. In: *Handbook of Biomaterials Evaluation. Scientific, Technical, and Clinical Testing of Implant Materials* (ed. A. F. vonRecum). Macmillan Publishing Company, New York. pp. 188–197.

Lord, G. (1984). Safety and risk: Limits of predictability for biomaterials. Chapter 14. In: *Contemporary Biomaterials* (J. Boretos and M. Eden, eds.). Noyes Publications, Park Ridge, New Jersey. pp. 211–218.

Marchant, R. (1989). The cage implant system for determining in vivo biocompatibility of medical device materials. *Fundament. and Appl. Tox.* 13:217–227.

Moore, D., Glaser, Z., Tabacco, M. and Linebaugh, G. (1977). Evaluation of polymeric materials for maxillofacial prosthetics. *J. Prosthetic Dentistry* 38(3):319–326.

Oppenheimer, B., Oppenheimer, E. and Stout, A. (1948). Sarcomas induced in rats by implanting cellophane. *Proc. Soc. Exper. Biol. and Med.* 67:33–34.

Oppenheimer, B., Oppenheimer, E., Stout, A., Willhite, M., and Danishefsky, I. (1958). The latent period in carcinogenesis by plastics in rats and its relation to the presarcomatous stage. *Cancer* 11:204–213.

Oppenheimer, B., Oppenheimer, E., Danishefsky, I., Stout, A., and Eirich, F. (1955). Further studies of polymers as carcinogenic agents in animals. *Cancer Res.* 15:333–340.

Ott, G. (1970). Fremdkorpersarkome. *Exp. Med. Pathol. Klin.* 32:1–118.

Page, N. (1977). Concepts of a bioassay program in environmental carcinogenesis. In: *Environmental Cancer* (H. Kraybill and M. Mehlman, eds.). Vol. 3, Modern Toxicology. Wiley & Sons. pp. 87–141.

Page, N. (1981). *Guidelines for Health Effects Testing.* (N. Page, Chairman, Long-Term Effects Expert Group). In: OECD Testing Guidelines. Organization for Economic Cooperation and Development, Paris, France. ISBN 92–64–1221–4. 175 pp.

Pedley, R., Meachim, G., and Williams, D. (1982). Tumor induction by implant materials. Chapter 10. In: *Fundamental Aspects of Biocompatibility* (D. Williams, ed.). Vol. 2. CRC Press, Boca Raton, Florida. pp. 175–202.

Pott, F., Ziem, U., Reiffer, F., Huth, F., Ernst, H. and Mohr, U. (1987). Carcinogenicity study on fibres, metal compounds, and some other dusts in rats. *Exp. Pathol.* 32:129–152.

RTECS (1989). *Registry of the Toxic Effects of Chemical Substances.* National Institute for Occupational Safety and Health, Atlanta, Georgia.

Saffiotti, U., Cefis, F. and Kilb, L. (1968). A method for the experimental induction of bronchogenic carcinoma. *Cancer Res.* 28:104–124.

Scheer, L. (1989). Asbestos again? Science and Technology, *Forbes Magazine,* June 12, 1989. pp. 162–163.

Siddons, A. and MacArthur, A. (1952). Carcinomata developing at the site of foreign bodies in the lung. *Brit. J. Surgery* 39:542–545.

Stanton, M., Layard, M., Tegeris, A., Miller, E., May, M., Morgan, E., and Smith, A. (1981). Relation of particle dimension to carcinogenicity in amphibole asbestoses and other fibrous minerals. *J. Natl. Cancer Inst.* 67:965–975.

Sunderman, W. (1989). Carcinogenicity of metal alloys in orthopedic prosthesis: Clinical and experimental studies. *Fundam. and Applied Toxicol.* 13:205–216.

Turner, F. (1941). Sarcomas at sites of subcutaneously implanted Bakelite disks in rats. *J. Natl. Cancer Inst.* 2:81–83.

UICC (1969). *Carcinogenicity Testing. A Report of the Panel on Carcinogenicity of the Cancer Research Commission of the UICC.* (I. Berenblum, ed.). UICC Technical Report Series 2. International Union Against Cancer, Geneva, Switzerland.

U.S. EPA (1985). *Final Rule, TSCA Health Effects Testing Guidelines.* 50FR39397. September 27, 1985. U.S. Environmental Protection Agency, Washington, D.C.

Section 2

CLASSIFICATION OF SUBSTANCES

The substance entries are grouped into three classes based on experimental evidence and the opinion of expert review groups. The OSHA, IARC, ACGIH, and DFG MAK decision schedules are not related or synchronized. Thus an entry may have had a recent review by only one group. The most stringent classification of any regulation or expert group is taken as governing.

CLASS I—CONFIRMED CARCINOGENS

These substances are capable of causing cancer in exposed humans. An entry was assigned to this class if it had one or more of the following items present.

- · An OSHA regulated carcinogen.
- · AN ACGIH assignment as a human or animal carcinogen.
- · A DFG MAK assignment as a confirmed human or animal carcinogen.
- · An IARC assignment of human or animal sufficient evidence of carcinogenicity or higher.
- · NTP Fourth Annual Report on Carcinogens.

CLASS II—SUSPECTED CARCINOGENS

These substances may be capable of causing cancer in exposed humans. The evidence is suggestive, but not sufficient to convince expert review committees. Some entries have not yet had expert review, but contain experimental reports of carcinogenic activity. In particular, if an entry has positive reports of carcinogenic endpoint in two species it is included. As more studies are conducted, many Class II carcinogens will have their carcinogenicity confirmed. On the other hand, some will probably be considered non-carcinogenic in the future. An entry was assigned to this class if it had one or more of the following items present.

- · An ACGIH assignment of suspected carcinogen.
- · An DFG MAK assignment of suspected carcinogen.
- · An IARC assignment of human or animal limited evidence.
- · Two animal studies reported positive carcinogenic endpoint in different species.

CLASS III—QUESTIONABLE CARCINOGENS

These entries have minimal published evidence of possible carcinogenic activity. The reported endpoint is often neoplastic growth with no spread or invasion characteristic of carcinogenic pathology. An even weaker endpoint is that of equivocal tumorigenic agent (ETA). Reports are assigned this designation when the study was defective. The report may have lacked control animals, may have very small sample size, often lack complete pathology reporting, or suffer many other study design defects. Many of these were designed for other than carcinogenic evaluation, and the reported carcinogenic effect is a by-product of the study, not the goal. The data are presented because some of these substances may be carcinogens. There is insufficient data to affirm or deny the possibility. An entry was assigned if it had one or more of the following items present.

- An IARC assignment of inadequate or no evidence.
- A single human report of carcinogenicity.
- A single experimental carcinogenic report, or duplicate reports in the same species.
- One or more experimental neoplastic or equivocal tumorigenic agent report.

Key to Abbreviations

abs – absolute
ACGIH – American Conference of Governmental Industrial Hygienists
alc – alcohol
alk – alkaline
amorph – amorphous
anhy – anhydrous
approx – approximately
aq – aqueous
atm – atmosphere
autoign – autoignition
aw – atomic weight
af – atomic formula
BATF – U.S. Bureau of Alcohol, Tobacco, and Firearms
bp – boiling point
b range – boiling range
CAS – Chemical Abstracts Service
cc – cubic centimeter
CC – closed cup
CL – ceiling concentration
COC – Cleveland open cup
conc – concentrated
compd(s) – compound(s)
conc – concentration, concentrated
contg – containing
cryst, crys – crystal(s), crystalline
d – density
D – day(s)
decomp, dec – decomposition
deliq – deliquescent
dil – dilute
DOT – U.S. Department of Transportation
EPA – U.S. Environmental Protection Agency
eth – ether
(F) – Fahrenheit
FCC – Food Chemical Codex
FDA – U.S. Food and Drug Administration
flash p – flash point
flam – flammable
fp – freezing point
g, gm – gram
glac – glacial
gran – granular, granules

GRAS – generally regarded as safe
hygr – hygroscopic
H, hr – hour(s)
HR: – hazard rating
htd – heated
htg – heating
IARC – International Agency for Research on Cancer
incomp – incompatible
insol – insoluble
IU – International Unit
kg – kilogram (one thousand grams)
L,l – liter
lel – lower explosive level
liq – liquid
M – minute(s)
m^3 – cubic meter
mg – milligram
misc – miscible
μ, u – micron
mL, ml – milliliter
mg – milligrams
mm – millimeter
mod – moderately
mp – melting point
mppcf – million particles per cubic foot
mw – molecular weight
mf – molecular formula
mumem – mucous membrane
mw – molecular weight
NIOSH – National Institute for Occupational Safety and Health
ng – nanogram
nonflam – nonflammable
NTP – National Toxicology Program
OC – open cup
org – organic
OSHA – Occupational Safety and Health Administration
PEL – permissible exposure level
petr – petroleum
pg – picogram (one trillionth of a gram)
Pk – peak concentration
pmole – picomole
powd – powder

ppb – parts per billion (v/v)
pph – parts per hundred (v/v) (percent)
ppm – parts per million (v/v)
ppt – parts per trillion (v/v)
prep – preparation
PROP – properties
refr – refractive
rhomb – rhombic
S,sec – second(s)
sl, slt, sltly – slightly
sol – soluble
soln – solution
solv(s) – solvent(s)
spont – spontaneous(ly)
subl – sublimes
TCC – Tag closed cup
tech – technical
temp – temperature
THR – toxic and hazard review
TLV – Threshold Limit Value
TOC – Tag open cup
TWA – time weighted average

U, unk – unknown, unreported
μ, u – micron
uel – upper explosive limits
μg, ug – microgram
ULC, ulc – Underwriters Laboratory Classification
USDA – U.S. Department of Agriculture
vac – vacuum
vap – vapor
vap d – vapor density
vap press – vapor pressure
vol – volume
visc – viscosity
vsol – very soluble
W – week(s)
Y – year(s)
% – percent(age)
> – greater than
< – less than
<= – equal to or less than
=> – equal to or greater than
° – degrees of temperature in Celsius (Centigrade)
(F), °F – temperature in Fahrenheit

Class I/Confirmed Carcinogens

ABC250 CAS: 828-00-2
ACETOMETHOXANE

mf: $C_8H_{14}O_4$ mw: 174.22

PROP: Yellow to amber, clear liquid. Sol in water and org solvents. D: 1.068-1.075 @ 25/25; bp: 66-68° @ 3 mm; fp: $< -25°$.

SYNS: ACETIC ACID-2,6-DIMETHYL-m-DIOXAN-4-YL ESTER ◇ ACETOMETHOXAN ◇ 6-ACETOXY-2,4-DIMETHYL-m-DIOXANE ◇ DDOA ◇ DIMETHOXANE ◇ 2,6-DIMETHYL-m-DIOXAN-4-OL ACETATE ◇ 2,6-DIMETHYL-m-DIOXAN-4-YL ACETATE ◇ DIOXIN (BACTERICIDE) (OBS.) ◇ G1V GARD DXN ◇ NCI-C56213

TOXICITY DATA with REFERENCE
CAR: orl-rat TDLo: 948 g/kg/88W-I JNCIAM 53,791,74
MUT: mma-sat 5500 μg/plate ENMUDM 8(Suppl 7),1,86
MUT: sln-dmg-par 1 pph ENMUDM 7,677,85

CONSENSUS REPORTS: IARC Cancer Review: GROUP 3 IMEMDT 7,56,87; Animal Limited Evidence IMEMDT 15,177,77. NTP Fourth Annual Report On Carcinogens, 1984.

SAFETY PROFILE: Confirmed carcinogen with experimental carcinogenic data. Moderately toxic by ingestion. When heated to decomposition it emits acrid smoke and fumes.

ABG750 CAS: 62-44-2
p-ACETOPHENETIDIDE

mf: $C_{10}H_{13}NO_2$ mw: 179.24

SYNS: 1-ACETAMIDO-4-ETHOXYBENZENE ◇ ACET-p-PHENALIDE ◇ ACET-p-PHENETIDIN ◇ ACETO-4-PHENETIDINE ◇ ACETO-p-PHENALIDE ◇ ACETO-p-PHENETIDIDE ◇ p-ACETOPHENETIDE ◇ ACETOPHENETIDIN ◇ p-ACETPHENETIDIN ◇ ACETOPHENETIDINE ◇ ACETOPHENETIN ◇ ACETPHENETIDIN ◇ ACETYLPHENETIDIN ◇ N-ACETYL-p-PHENETIDINE ◇ ACHROCIDIN ◇ ANAPAC ◇ APC ◇ ASA COMPOUND ◇ BROMO SELTZER ◇ BUFF-A-COMP ◇ CITRA-FORT ◇ CODEMPIRAL ◇ COMMOTIONAL ◇ CONTRADOL ◇ CORICIDIN ◇ CORIFORTE ◇ CORYBAN-D ◇ DAPRISAL ◇ DARVON COMPOUND ◇ DASIKON ◇ EMPIRIN COMPOUND ◇ 4-ETHOXYACETANILIDE ◇ p-ETHOXYACETANILIDE ◇ N-(4-ETHOXYPHENYL)ACETAMIDE ◇ N-p-ETHOXYPHENYLACETAMIDE ◇ FENACETINA ◇ FIORINAL ◇ MELABON ◇ PARACETOPHENETIDIN ◇ PERCOBARB ◇ PERCODAN ◇ p-PHENACETIN ◇ RCRA WASTE NUMBER U187 ◇ SINUTAB ◇ TETRACYDIN ◇ XARIL ◇ ZACTIRIN COMPOUND

TOXICITY DATA with REFERENCE
CAR: orl-hmn TDLo: 57 mg/kg/47Y-I JOURAA 113,653,75
CAR: orl-hmn TDLo: 7300 mg/kg/Y-C SJUNAS 2,145,68
CAR: orl-man TDLo: 57 g/kg/47Y I JOURAA 113,653,75
CAR: orl-man TD: 126 g/kg/25Y-I AIMEAS 93,249,80
CAR: orl-mus TDLo: 1008 g/kg/96W-C IJCNAW 29,439,82
CAR: orl-rat TDLo: 572 g/kg/60W-C GANNA2 70,29,79
CAR: orl-wmn TD: 140 g/kg/13Y-I BJURAN 51,188,79
CAR: orl-wmn TDLo: 80 g/kg/63Y-I JOURAA 113,653,75
NEO: orl-mus TD: 484 g/kg/96W-C IJCNAW 29,439,82
ETA: orl-rat TD: 206 g/kg/2Y-C AMBPBZ 84,375,76
ETA: orl-rat TD: 9450 mg/kg/45W-C ADIRDF 6,139,84
MUT: bfa-rat/sat 800 mg/kg CNREA8 42,3201,82
MUT: cyt-ham: fbr 800 mg/L/48H MUREAV 48,337,77
MUT: cyt-ham: lng 800 mg/L/27H MUREAV 66,277,79
MUT: dnd-mus-ipr 400 mg/kg ATSUDG (5),355,82
MUT: dnd-rat-ipr 165 mg/kg JTEHD6 16,355,85
MUT: dnd-rat-orl 82500 μg/kg JTEHD6 16,355,85
MUT: dni-mus-ipr 20 g/kg ARGEAR 51,605,81
MUT: dni-mus: oth 50 mg/L ONCODU 19,183,80
MUT: dnr-esc 2 mg/well JTEHD6 16,355,85
MUT: hma-rat/sat 200 μg/kg ONCODU 19,183,80

MUT: mma-ham:lng 1 mmol/L   JTEHD6 16,355,85
MUT: mma-sat:333 μg/plate   IARCCD 27,283,80
MUT: orl-hmn TD:28 g/kg/28Y-I:CAR
   ENVRAL 20,192,79
MUT: orl-man TD:27 g/kg/10Y-I:CAR
   AAJRDX 134,1259,80
MUT: sce-mus-ipr 165 mg/kg   JTEHD6 16,355,85

CONSENSUS REPORTS: IARC Cancer Review: GROUP 2A IMEMDT 7,310,87; Animal Inadequate Evidence IMEMDT 13,141,77; Human Limited Evidence IMEMDT 13,141,77; Animal Limited Evidence IMEMDT 24,135,80; Human Limited Evidence IMEMDT 24,135,80. NTP Fourth Annual Report On Carcinogens, 1984. Reported in EPA TSCA Inventory.

SAFETY PROFILE: Confirmed carcinogen producing tumors of the kidney and bladder. Experimental teratogenic data. A human poison by an unspecified route. Poison by intravenous and possibly other routes. Moderately toxic by several routes. Human systemic effects by ingestion: cyanosis, liver damage, and methemoglobinemia-carboxhemoglobinemia. Mutation data reported. Experimental reproductive effects. Chronic effects consist of weight loss, insomnia, shortness of breath, weakness and often aplastic anemia. When heated to decomposition it emits toxic fumes of NO_x.

ADS250   CAS: 79-06-1
ACRYLAMIDE
DOT: 2074
mf: C_3H_5NO mw: 71.09

PROP: White, crystalline solid. Very sol in water, alc, and ether. Mp: 84.5 ± 0.3°, bp: 125° @ 25 mm, d: 1.122 @ 30°, vap press: 1.6 mm @ 84.5°, vap d: 2.45.

SYNS: ACRYLIC AMIDE ◇ AKRYLAMID (CZECH) ◇ ETHYLENECARBOXAMIDE ◇ PROPENAMIDE ◇ 2-PROPENAMIDE ◇ RCRA WASTE NUMBER U007

TOXICITY DATA with REFERENCE
CAR: orl-mus TDLo:300 mg/kg/2W-I
   CALEDQ 24,209,84
CAR: orl-rat TDLo:1456 mg/kg/2Y-C
   TXAPA9 85,154,86
NEO: ipr-mus TD:72 mg/kg/8W-I   CNREA8
   44,107,84
NEO: ipr-mus TDLo:24 mg/kg/8W-I   CNREA8
   44,107,84
MUT: cyt-mus-orl 500 ppm/2W-I   MUREAV
   57,313,78

MUT: dlt-mus-ipr 125 mg/kg   MUREAV 173,35,86
MUT: sce-rat-orl 600 mg/kg/10D-C   ENMUDM
   7(Suppl 3),79,85
MUT: spm-mus-ipr 100 mg/kg   MUREAV 57,313,78

CONSENSUS REPORTS: IARC Cancer Review: GROUP 2B IMEMDT 7,56,87; Animal Sufficient Evidence IMEMDT 39,41,86. EPA Extremely Hazardous Substances List. Community Right-To-Know List. Reported in EPA TSCA Inventory.

OSHA PEL: (Transitional: TWA 0.3 mg/m^3 (skin)) TWA 0.03 mg/m^3 (skin)   ACGIH TLV: Suspected Human Carcinogen, TWA 0.03 mg/m^3 (skin)   DFG MAK: Animal Carcinogen, Suspected Human Carcinogen.   NIOSH REL: TWA 0.3 mg/m^3 DOT Classification: IMO: Poison B; Label: St. Andrews Cross.

SAFETY PROFILE: Confirmed carcinogen with experimental carcinogenic and neoplastigenic data. Poison by ingestion, skin contact, intravenous, intraperitoneal and possibly other routes. Experimental reproductive effects. Mutation data reported. A skin and eye irritant. Intoxication from it has caused a peripheral neuropathy, erythema and peeling of the palms. In industry, intoxication is mainly via dermal route, next via inhalation and last via ingestion. Time of onset varied from 1-24 months to 8 years. Symptoms were, via dermal route, a numbness, tingling and touch tenderness. In a couple of weeks, coldness of extremities; later, excessive sweating, bluish-red and peeling of palms, marked fatigue and limb-weakness. It is dangerous because it can be absorbed through the unbroken skin. From animal experiments it seems to be a central nervous system toxin. Adult rats fed an average of 30 mg/kg for 14 days were all partially paralyzed and had reduced their food consumption by 50 percent. Polymerizes violently at its melting point. When heated to decomposition it emits acrid fumes and NO_x.

ADX500   CAS: 107-13-1
ACRYLONITRILE
DOT: 1093
mf: C_3H_3N mw: 53.07

PROP: Colorless, mobile liquid; mild odor. Sol in water. Mp: −82°, bp: 77.3°, fp: −83°, flash p: 30°F (TCC), lel: 3.1%, uel: 17%, d: 0.806 @ 20°/4°, autoign temp: 898°F, vap press: 100 mm @ 22.8°, vap d: 1.83, flash p: (of 5% aq sol): <50°F.

SYNS: ACRYLNITRIL (GERMAN, DUTCH) ◇ ACRYLONI-
TRILE MONOMER ◇ AKRYLONITRYL (POLISH) ◇ CARBA-
CRYL ◇ CIANURO DI VINILE (ITALIAN) ◇ CYANOETH-
YLENE ◇ CYANURE de VINYLE (FRENCH) ◇ ENT 54
◇ FUMIGRAIN ◇ NITRILE ACRILICO (ITALIAN) ◇ NITRILE
ACRYLIQUE (FRENCH) ◇ PROPENENITRILE ◇ 2-PRO-
PENENITRILE ◇ RCRA WASTE NUMBER U009 ◇ TL 314
◇ VENTOX ◇ VINYL CYANIDE

TOXICITY DATA with REFERENCE
CAR: orl-rat TDLo: 18200 mg/kg/52W C
   FCTOD7 24,129,86
NEO: orl-rat TDLo: 3640 mg/kg/52W-C
   DOWCC* MAR77
ETA: ihl-rat TC : 20 ppm/4H/52W-I   ANYAA9
381,216,82
ETA: ihl-rat TC : 40 ppm/4H/52W-I   ANYAA9
381,216,82
ETA: ihl-rat TCLo: 5 ppm/52W-I   MELAAD
68,401,77
MUT: bfa-mus/sat 30 mg/kg   TXCYAC 16,67,80
MUT: bfa-rat/sat 30 mg/kg   TXCYAC 16,67,80
MUT: dns-rat: lvr 1 mmol/L   PMRSDJ 5,371,85
MUT: mma-sat 2 µL/plate   MUREAV 48,271,77
MUT: mmo-sat 25 µL/plate   NIOSH* 5AUG77
MUT: slt-dmg-orl 1520 µmol/L   PMRSDJ 5,325,85

CONSENSUS REPORTS: IARC Cancer Review: Human Limited Evidence IMEMDT
19,73,79; Animal Limited Evidence IMEMDT
19,73,79. NTP Fourth Annual Report On Carcinogens, 1984. Community Right-To-Know
List. EPA Extremely Hazardous Substances
List. Reported in EPA TSCA Inventory.

OSHA PEL: TWA 2 ppm; CL 10 ppm/15M;
Cancer Hazard.   ACGIH TLV: Suspected Hu-
man Carcinogen, TWA 2 ppm (skin).   DFG
TRK: 3 ppm (7 mg/m^3), Animal Carcinogen,
Suspected Human Carcinogen.   NIOSH REL:
TWA 1 ppm; CL 10 ppm/15M   DOT Classifi-
cation: Flammable Liquid and Poison.

SAFETY PROFILE: Confirmed human carcinogen with experimental carcinogenic, neoplastigenic, tumorigenic, and teratogenic data. Poison
by inhalation, ingestion, skin contact, and other
routes. Human systemic irritant, somnolence,
general anesthesia, cyanosis and diarrhea by
inhalation and skin contact. Human mutation
data reported. Experimental reproductive effects. Dangerous fire hazard when exposed to
heat, flame, or oxidizers. Moderate explosion
hazard when exposed to flame. Can react vigorously with oxidizing materials. To fight fire use

CO_2, dry chemical or alcohol foam. Unstable
and easily oxidized. When heated to decomposition it emits toxic fumes of NO_x and CN^-.

AEB750   CAS: 102488-99-3
ACTINOMYCIN L

SYN: ACTINOMYCIN 2104L

TOXICITY DATA with REFERENCE
NEO: scu-mus TDLo: 4725 µg/kg/35W-I
   BKNJA5 2,105,59

CONSENSUS REPORTS: IARC Cancer Review: Animal Sufficient Evidence IMEMDT
10,29,76

SAFETY PROFILE: Confirmed carcinogen with
experimental neoplastigenic data.

AEC000   CAS: 12623-78-8
ACTINOMYCIN S

SYN: ACTINOMYCIN 1048A

TOXICITY DATA with REFERENCE
NEO: scu-mus TD: 330 µg/kg/22W-I   MJOUAL
8,753,58
NEO: scu-mus TD: 280 µg/kg/18W-I   APJAAG
17,495,67
NEO: scu-mus TDLo: 240 µg/kg/16W-I
   BKNJA5 2,105,59

CONSENSUS REPORTS: IARC Cancer Review: Animal Sufficient Evidence IMEMDT
10,29,76

SAFETY PROFILE: Confirmed carcinogen with
experimental neoplastigenic data.

AES750   CAS: 23214-92-8
ADRIAMYCIN
mf: $C_{27}H_{29}NO_{11}$•ClH   mw: 543.57

PROP: Isolated from cultures of *Streptomyces
peucetius var. Caesius*.

SYNS: ADM ◇ ADRIAMYCIN-HCl ◇ ADRIAMYCIN SEMI-
QUINONE ◇ ADRIBLASTINA ◇ DOXORUBICIN ◇ DX
◇ F.I 106 ◇ 14-HYDROXYDAUNOMYCIN ◇ 14'-HYDROXY-
DAUNOMYCIN ◇ 14-HYDROXYDAUNORUBICINE
◇ KW-125 ◇ NCI-C01514 ◇ NSC-123127

TOXICITY DATA with REFERENCE
CAR: ivn-rat TD: 5 mg/kg   PAACA3 27,238,86
CAR: ivn-rat TD: 8 mg/kg   CNREA8 38,1444,78
CAR: ivn-rat TD: 10 mg/kg   JJIND8 66,81,81
CAR: ivn-rat TD: 10 mg/kg   LAPPA5 38,71,78
CAR: ivn-rat TDLo: 5 mg/kg   CNREA8 43,5248,83

NEO: ivn-rat TD:2 mg/kg   CRNGDP 8,1149,87
NEO: ivn-rat TD:8 mg/kg   EXPEAM 27,1209,71
ETA: ivn-rat TD:5 mg/kg   CNREA8 36,2065,76
ETA: ivn-rat TD:5 mg/kg   PAACA3 21,309,80
MUT: bfa-rat/sat 200 mg/kg   URLRA5 7,119,79
MUT: cyt-ham:ovr 400 µg/L   MUREAV 52,199,78
MUT: cyt-hmn:fbr 10 µg/L/1H   CCPHDZ 3,143,79
MUT: cyt-hmn:lym 20 µg/L   SBJODP 4,1,78
MUT: dnd-hmn:lym 50 µg/L   CJBIAE 58,720,80
MUT: dni-hmn:hla 1 µmol/L   CNREA8 38,4445,78
MUT: mnt-hmn:lym 20 µg/L   SBJODP 4,1,78
MUT: sce-hmn:lym 5 ng/L/48H   ARTODN46,61,80

CONSENSUS REPORTS: IARC Cancer Review: Animal Inadequate Evidence IMEMDT 10,43,76. NTP Fourth Annual Report On Carcinogens, 1984.

SAFETY PROFILE: Confirmed carcinogen with experimental carcinogenic, neoplastigenic, tumorigenic, and teratogenic data. Poison by intraperitoneal, subcutaneous, parenteral and intravenous routes. Experimental reproductive effects. Human mutation data reported. Human systemic effects by intravenous route: cardiac myopathy including infarction, nausea or vomiting, and effects on the hair. When heated to decomposition it emits very toxic fumes of NO_x and HCl.

AET750   CAS: 1402-68-2
AFLATOXIN

TOXICITY DATA with REFERENCE
ETA: mul-mky TDLo:71 mg/kg/6Y-I   FCTXAV 10,519,72
ETA: orl-rat TD:62 mg/kg/37W-C   IJCNAW 4,422,69
ETA: orl-rat TD:66 mg/kg/52W-C   NATUAS 209,90,66
ETA: orl-rat TD:87 mg/kg/52W-C   NATUAS 209,90,66
ETA: orl-rat TDLo:7788 µg/kg/13W-C   NATUAS 202,1016,64
MUT: dlt-mus-ipr 68 mg/kg   NATUAS 219,385,68

CONSENSUS REPORTS: IARC Cancer Review: GROUP 1 IMEMDT 7,83,87; Human Limited Evidence IMEMDT 10,51,76. NTP Fourth Annual Report On Carcinogens, 1984.

SAFETY PROFILE: Confirmed carcinogen with experimental tumorigenic data. Human poison by ingestion. Moderately toxic by other routes. Experimental teratogenic and reproductive effects. Mutation data reported.

AEU250   CAS: 1162-65-8
AFLATOXIN B1
mf: $C_{17}H_{12}O_6$ mw: 312.29

PROP: A metabolite of *Aspergillus flavus link ex fries* (12VXA5 8,24,68). A crystalline material. Mp: 268°.

SYNS: AFBI ◇ AFLATOXIN B

TOXICITY DATA with REFERENCE
CAR: orl-rat TD:8 mg/kg/20W-I   CNREA8 29,2206,69
CAR: orl-rat TD:15 mg/kg/6W-C   FCTXAV 6,135,68
CAR: orl-rat TD:19 mg/kg/15W-I   NEOLA4 28,35,81
CAR: orl-rat TD:1500 µg/kg/7W-I   CNREA8 35,2469,75
CAR: orl-rat TD:2205 µg/kg/21W-C   CNREA8 29,1045,69
CAR: orl-rat TD:8400 µg/kg/20W-C   EXPEAM 34,1069,78
CAR: orl-rat TD:18 mg/kg/43W-C   JNCIAM 55,107,75
CAR: orl-rat TD:1243 µg/kg/71W-C   FCTXAV 12,681,74
CAR: orl-rat TD:2000 µg/kg/4W-I   CNREA8 31,1936,71
NEO: scu-rat TD:1600 µg/kg/20W-I
ETA: mul-mky TDLo:20 mg/kg/4Y-I   JNCIAM 57,67,76
ETA: orl-mky TDLo:168 mg/kg/6Y-C   JNCIAM 57,67,76
MUT: cyt-hmn:lym 19200 nmol/L   TOLED5 7,245,81
MUT: cyt-mus-ipr 5 mg/kg   TOLED5 7,245,81
MUT: dnd-hmn:oth 1 µmol/L   TCMUD8 1,3,80
MUT: dnd-rat:oth 1 µmol/L   TCMUD8 1,3,80
MUT: dni-hmn:hla 50 nmol/L/1H-C   JEPTDQ 2(1),65,78
MUT: sce-hmn:lym 19200 nmol/L   TOLED5 7,245,81   CNREA8 31,1936,71

CONSENSUS REPORTS: IARC Cancer Review: Animal Sufficient Evidence IMEMDT 10,51,76; IMEMDT 1,145,72. NTP Fourth Annual Report On Carcinogens, 1984. EPA Genetic Toxicology Program.

SAFETY PROFILE: Confirmed carcinogen with experimental tumorigenic, neoplastigenic, carcinogenic, and teratogenic data. Acute poison by ingestion, intraperitoneal and possibly other routes. Experimental reproductive effects. Mutation data reported. When heated to decomposition it emits acrid smoke.

AEU750   CAS: 7220-81-7
AFLATOXIN B2
mf: $C_{17}H_{14}O_6$ mw: 314.31

SYN: DIHYDROAFLATOXIN B1

TOXICITY DATA with REFERENCE
ETA: ipr-rat TDLo:600 mg/kg/8W-I   CNREA8
31,1936,71
MUT: dnd-mam:lym 50 μmol/L   CRNGDP
3,423,82
MUT: dnd-rat-par 40 μg/kg/2D-C   BBRCA9
83,1354,78
MUT: dns-rat:lvr 10 μmol/L/1H   CNREA8
37,1845,77
MUT: mma-ham:lng 83 μmol/L   MUREAV
46,27,77
MUT: mma-sat 370 ng/plate   MUREAV 130,79,84
MUT: sce-ham:lng 3100 μg/L   CRNGDP 1,759,80

CONSENSUS REPORTS: IARC Cancer Review: Animal Sufficient Evidence IMEMDT 10,51,76; Animal Limited Evidence IMEMDT 1,145,72. NTP Fourth Annual Report On Carcinogens, 1984.

SAFETY PROFILE: Confirmed carcinogen with experimental tumorigenic data. Poison by ingestion. Mutation data reported. When heated to decomposition it emits acrid smoke and fumes.

AEV000   CAS: 1165-39-5
AFLATOXIN G1
mf: $C_{17}H_{12}O_7$ mw: 328.29

PROP: A metabolite of *Aspergillus flavus link ex fries*.

TOXICITY DATA with REFERENCE
CAR: orl-rat TDLo:5600 μg/kg/2W-I   CNREA8
31,1936,71
CAR: orl-rat TD:24 mg/kg/20W-I   CNREA8
29,2206,69
NEO: scu-rat TDLo:12 mg/kg/30W-I   BJCAAI
19,392,65
NEO: orl-rat TD:8 mg/kg/20W-I   CNREA8
29,2206,69
MUT: cyt-mky:kdy 2 mg/L/2H-C   JNCIAM
48,1647,72
MUT: dni-mky:kdy 2 mg/L/2H-C   JNCIAM
48,1647,72
MUT: dnr-esc 800 μg/L   MUREAV 119,135,83
MUT: mma-sat 31 ng/plate   MUREAV 130,79,84
MUT: mmo-omi 47400 μg/L   JMIMDQ 3,181,85

MUT: sce-ham:lng 2500 μg/L   CRNGDP 1,759,80
MUT: sce-ham:ovr 1 μmol/L   CRNGDP 1,759,80
MUT: spm-oin-par 1600 ng/plate   MYCPAH
88,23,84

CONSENSUS REPORTS: IARC Cancer Review: Animal Sufficient Evidence IMEMDT 10,51,76. NTP Fourth Annual Report On Carcinogens, 1984.

SAFETY PROFILE: Confirmed carcinogen with experimental carcinogenic and neoplastigenic data. Poison by ingestion and intraperitoneal routes. A suspected human carcinogenic. Mutation data reported. When heated to decomposition it emits acrid smoke and irritating fumes.

AEV250
AFLATOXIN G1 mixed with AFLATOXIN B1

PROP: Metabolites of *Aspergillus flavus link ex fries* Aflatoxin G1, 56.4%; Alfatoxin B1, 37.7%.

TOXICITY DATA with REFERENCE
CAR: itr-rat TDLo:72 mg/kg/30W-I   BJCAAI
20,134,66
NEO: scu-mus TDLo:18 mg/kg/23W-I   BJCAAI
19,392,65
NEO: scu-rat TDLo:1760 μg/kg/44W-I   BJCAAI
19,392,65
ETA: orl-rat TDLo:66 mg/kg/66W-C   BJCAAI
20,134,66

CONSENSUS REPORTS: NTP Fourth Annual Report On Carcinogens, 1984.

SAFETY PROFILE: Confirmed carcinogen with experimental carcinogenic, neoplastigenic, and tumorigenic data.

AEV500   CAS: 7241-98-7
AFLATOXIN G2
mf: $C_{17}H_{14}O_7$ mw: 330.31

TOXICITY DATA with REFERENCE
MUT: dns-rat:lvr 10 μmol/L/1H   CNREA8
37,1845,77
MUT: sce-ham:lng 3300 μg/L   CRNGDP 1,759,80

CONSENSUS REPORTS: IARC Cancer Review: Animal Inadequate Evidence IMEMDT 1,145,72. NTP Fourth Annual Report On Carcinogens, 1984. EPA Genetic Toxicology Program.

SAFETY PROFILE: Confirmed carcinogen. Acute poison by ingestion. Mutation data reported. When heated to decomposition it emits acrid smoke and irritating fumes.

AEW000 CAS: 6795-23-9
AFLATOXIN M1
mf: $C_{17}H_{12}O_7$ mw: 328.29

SYN: 4-HYDROXYAFLATOXIN B1

TOXICITY DATA with REFERENCE
ETA: orl-rat TDLo: 8 mg/kg/8W-I FCTXAV 12,381,74
MUT: cyt-rat-orl 1 mg/kg JNCIAM 47,585,71
MUT: dnd-rat-orl 3600 ng/kg CBINA8 32,249,80
MUT: dns-rat: lvr 600 ng/plate TOXID9 1,42,81
MUT: mma-sat 200 ng/plate JEPTDQ 2,1099,79

CONSENSUS REPORTS: IARC Cancer Review: Animal Sufficient Evidence IMEMDT 10,51,76. EPA Genetic Toxicology Program.

SAFETY PROFILE: Confirmed carcinogen with experimental tumorigenic data. Poison by ingestion. Mutation data reported. When heated to decomposition it emits acrid smoke and irritating fumes.

AIB000 CAS: 117-79-3
2-AMINOANTHRAQUINONE
mf: $C_{14}H_9NO_2$ mw: 223.24

PROP: Red needles from alc. Mp: 302°, bp: subl. Insol in water and ether, sol in alc and benzene.

SYNS: 2-AMINO-9,10-ANTHRACENEDIONE ◇ 2-AMINO-9,10-ANTRAQUINONE ◇ β-AMINOANTHRAQUINONE ◇ β-ANTHRAQUINONYLAMINE ◇ NCI-C01876

TOXICITY DATA with REFERENCE
CAR: orl-mus TD: 5600 g/kg/80W-C IARC** 27,191,82
CAR: orl-mus TDLo: 655 g/kg/78W-C NCITR* NCI-CG-TR-144,78
CAR: orl-rat TD: 1890 g/kg/78W-C IARC** 27,191,82
CAR: orl-rat TD: 3780 g/kg/78W-C IARC** 27,191,82
CAR: orl-rat TDLo: 115 g/kg/78W-C NCITR* NCI-CG-TR-144,78
NEO: orl-rat TD: 32 g/kg/77W-C TOLED5 4,71,79
NEO: orl-rat TD: 225 g/kg/78W-C NCITR* NCI-CG-TR-144,78
ETA: orl-mus TD: 2730 g/kg/78W-C IARC** 27,191,82
ETA: orl-mus TD: 330 g/kg/78W-C NCITR* NCI-CG-TR-144,78

MUT: mma-esc 1 mg/plate ENMUDM 7(Suppl 5),1,85
MUT: mma-sat 1 μg/plate ENMUDM 7(Suppl 5),1,85
MUT: mmo-sat 1 mg/plate ENMUDM 7(Suppl 5),1,85

CONSENSUS REPORTS: IARC Cancer Review: GROUP 3 IMEMDT 7,56,87; Animal Limited Evidence IMEMDT 27,191,82. NTP Fourth Annual Report On Carcinogens, 1984. NCI Carcinogenesis Bioassay (feed); Clear Evidence: mouse, rat NCITR* NCI-CG-TR-144,78. Community Right-To-Know List. Reported in EPA TSCA Inventory.

SAFETY PROFILE: Confirmed carcinogen with experimental carcinogenic, neoplastigenic, and tumorigenic data. Moderately toxic via intraperitoneal route. Mutation data reported. When heated to decomposition it emits toxic NO_x.

AIC250 CAS: 97-56-3
2-AMINO-5-AZOTOLUENE
mf: $C_{14}H_{15}N_3$ mw: 225.32

SYNS: AAT ◇ o-AAT ◇ o-AMIDOAZOTOLUOL (GERMAN) ◇ AMINOAZOTOLUENE (INDICATOR) ◇ o-AMINOAZOTOLUENE (MAK) ◇ 4'-AMINO-2,3'-AZOTOLUENE ◇ o-AMINOAZOTOLUENO (SPANISH) ◇ 4'-AMINO-2:3'-AZOTOLUENE ◇ o-AMINOAZOTOLUOL ◇ 4-AMINO-2',3-DIMETHYLAZOBENZENE ◇ 4'-AMINO-2,3'-DIMETHYLAZOBENZENE ◇ o-AT ◇ BRASILAZINA OIL YELLOW R ◇ BUTTER YELLOW ◇ C.I. 11160 ◇ C.I. 11160B ◇ C.I. SOLVENT YELLOW 3 ◇ 2',3-DIMETHYL-4-AMINOAZOBENZENE ◇ FAST GARNET GBC BASE ◇ FAST OIL YELLOW ◇ FAST YELLOW AT ◇ FAST YELLOW B ◇ HIDACO OIL YELLOW ◇ 2-METHYL-4-((2-METHYLPHENYL)AZO)-BENZENAMINE ◇ OAAT ◇ OIL YELLOW 21 ◇ OIL YELLOW 2681 ◇ OIL YELLOW AT ◇ OIL YELLOW ◇ OIL YELLOW A ◇ OIL YELLOW C ◇ OIL YELLOW I ◇ OIL YELLOW 2R ◇ OIL YELLOW T ◇ ORGANOL YELLOW 25 ◇ SOMALIA YELLOW R ◇ SUDAN YELLOW RRA ◇ o-TOLUENEAZO-o-TOLUIDINE ◇ o-TOLUOL-AZO-o-TOLUIDIN (GERMAN) ◇ 5-(o-TOLYLAZO)-2-AMINOTOLUENE ◇ 4-(o-TOLYLAZO)-o-TOLUIDINE ◇ TULABASE FAST GARNET GB ◇ TULABASE FAST GARNET GBC ◇ WAXAKOL YELLOW NL

TOXICITY DATA with REFERENCE
NEO: ipr-mus TDLo: 800 mg/kg GANNA2 58,323,67
NEO: orl-mus TDLo: 480 mg/kg (16-21D post) BEXBAN 85,201,78
NEO: orl-mus TDLo: 480 mg/kg/I BEXBAN 85,201,78
NEO: orl-rat TDLo: 15 g/kg/57W-C BJCAAI 3,387,49
MUT: bfa-rat/sat 500 mg/kg MUREAV 156,131,85

MUT: cyt-ham:lng 15 mg/L/27H   MUREAV 66,277,79
MUT: dnr-esc 25 mg/L   JNCIAM 62,873,79
MUT: dns-ham:lvr 200 nmol/L   MUREAV 136,255,84
MUT: dns-rat-orl 200 mg/kg   ENMUDM 7,101,85
MUT: mma-sat 20 μg/plate   PNASA6 72,5135,75
MUT: mma-sat 25 ng/plate   CNREA8 45,6155,85
MUT: mrc-esc 1 μg/well   MUREAV 46,53,77
CAR: scu-mus TDLo:4000 mg/kg (15-21D post)   BEXBAN 78,1402,74
NEO: scu-mus TDLo:2800 mg/kg/28W-I   JNCIAM 20,431,58
CAR: imp-mus TDLo:80 mg/kg   BJCAAI22,825,68
ETA: mul-mus TDLo:400 mg/kg/I   CNREA8 1,397,41
ETA: orl-dog TDLo:4500 mg/kg/2Y-C   JNCIAM 13,1497,53
ETA: orl-mus TD:5280 mg/kg/88D-C   JNCIAM 16,107,55
ETA: scu-mus TD:4000 mg/kg/39W-I   AJPAA4 51,307,67
ETA: orl-mus TD:80 mg/kg   JNCIAM 7,431,47
ETA: scu-mus TD:80 mg/kg   JNCIAM 7,431,47
ETA: orl-rat TD:31250 mg/kg/35W-C   NIBKAW 24,523,34
ETA: orl-mus TD:3640 mg/kg/25W-C   ASBUAN 56(12),53,39
NEO: orl-mus TD:13440 mg/kg/32W-C   FRPPAO 34,202,79
ETA: imp-mus TD:3200 mg/kg/35W-C   BEBMAE 86,1374,78

CONSENSUS REPORTS: IARC Cancer Review: Animal Sufficient Evidence IMEMDT 8,61,75. Community Right-To-Know List. Reported in EPA TSCA Inventory. EPA Genetic Toxicology Program.

DFG MAK: Animal Carcinogen; Suspected Human Carcinogen.

SAFETY PROFILE: Confirmed carcinogen with experimental carcinogenic, neoplastigenic, and tumorigenic data. Moderately toxic by ingestion and subcutaneous routes. Human mutation data reported. Experimental reproductive effects. When heated to decomposition it emits toxic fumes of NO_x.

AJS100   CAS: 92-67-1
4-AMINODIPHENYL
mf: $C_{12}H_{11}N$ mw: 169.24

PROP: Colorless crystals. Mp. 53°, bp: 302°, d: 1.160 @ 20°/20°, autoign temp: 842°F.

SYNS: p-AMINOBIPHENYL ◇ 4-AMINOBIPHENYL ◇ 4-AMINODIFENIL (SPANISH) ◇ p-AMINODIPHENYL ◇ BIPHENYLAMINE ◇ 4-BIPHENYLAMINE ◇ (1,1′-BIPHE-NYL)-4-AMINE ◇ p-BIPHENYLAMINE ◇ PARAAMINODI-PHENYL ◇ p-PHENYLANILINE ◇ XENYLAMIN (CZECH) ◇ XENYLAMINE

TOXICITY DATA with REFERENCE
CAR: orl-mus TD:5460 μg/kg   EJCAAH 21,865,85
CAR: scu-mus TDLo:216 mg/kg/3D-I   JNCIAM 41,403,68
ETA: orl-dog TD:14 g/kg/3Y-I   IMSUAI 27,25,58
ETA: orl-dog TD:5580 mg/kg/4Y-I   NEOLA4 15,3,68
ETA: orl-dog TD:8200 mg/kg/2Y-I   IMSUAI 27,25,58
ETA: orl-dog TD:8200 mg/kg/90W-I   JAMAAP 172,1611,60
ETA: orl-dog TD:8400 mg/kg/2Y-I   IMSUAI 27,25,58
ETA: orl-dog TD:9600 mg/kg/3Y-I   IMSUAI 27,25,58
ETA: orl-mus TDLo:1520 mg/kg/39W-I   BJCAAI 19,297,65
ETA: orl-rat TDLo:4524 mg/kg/48W-C   ARZNAD 12,270,62
ETA: scu-rat TD:5000 mg/kg/W-I   BMBUAQ 14,141,58
ETA: scu-rat TDLo:4560 mg/kg/44W-I   NATUAS 175,1131,55
MUT: dnd-esc 30 μmol/L   MUREAV 89,95,81
MUT: dnd-rat:lvr 30 μmol/L   SinJF# 26OCT82
MUT: dns-mus-orl 200 mg/kg   MUREAV125,291,84
MUT: mma-sat 2 μg/plate   ENMUDM 5(Suppl 1),3,83
MUT: msc-hmn:fbr 60 mg/L   MUREAV 121,71,83
MUT: orl-mus TD:5460 μg/kg   EJCODS 21,865,85

CONSENSUS REPORTS: IARC Cancer Review: Human Limited Evidence IMEMDT 1,74,72; Animal Sufficient Evidence IMEMDT 1,74,72; Human Sufficient Evidence IMEMDT 28,151,82. NTP Fourth Annual Report On Carcinogens, 1984. Reported in EPA TSCA Inventory. EPA Genetic Toxicology Program. Community Right-To-Know List.

OSHA PEL: Carcinogen   ACGIH TLV: Confirmed Human Carcinogen.   DFG MAK: Human Carcinogen.

SAFETY PROFILE: Confirmed human carcinogen with experimental carcinogenic and tumorigenic data. Poison by ingestion and intraperitoneal routes. Human mutation data reported. An irritant. Effects resemble those of benzidine.

Slight to moderate fire hazard when exposed to heat, flames (sparks), or powerful oxidizers. To fight fire, use water spray, mist, dry chemical. When heated to decomposition it emits toxic fumes of NO_x.

AKP750   CAS: 82-28-0
1-AMINO-2-METHYLANTHRAQUINONE
mf: $C_{15}H_{11}NO_2$ mw: 237.27

SYNS: ACETATE FAST ORANGE R ◇ ACETOQUINONE LIGHT ORANGE JL ◇ 1-AMINO-2-METHYL-9,10-ANTHRACENEDIONE ◇ ARTISIL ORANGE 3RP ◇ CELLITON ORANGE R ◇ C.I. 60700 ◇ C.I. DISPERSE ORANGE 11 ◇ CILLA ORANGE R ◇ DISPERSE ORANGE ◇ DURANOL ORANGE G ◇ 2-METHYL-1-ANTHRAQUINONYLAMINE ◇ MICROSETILE ORANGE RA ◇ NCI-C01901 ◇ NYLOQUINONE ORANGE JR ◇ PERLITON ORANGE 3R ◇ SERISOL ORANGE YL ◇ SUPRACET ORANGE R

TOXICITY DATA with REFERENCE
CAR: orl-mus TDLo:37 g/kg/73W-C   NCITR*
NCI-CG-TR-111,78
CAR: orl-rat TD:1113 g/kg/39W-C   IARC**
27,199,82
CAR: orl-rat TD:60 g/kg/78W-C
NCITR* NCI-CG-TR-111,78
CAR: orl-rat TDLo:30 g/kg/78W-C   NCITR*
NCI-CG-TR-111,78
NEO: orl-rat TD:39 g/kg/77W-C   TOLED5 4,71,79
ETA: orl-mus TD:307 g/kg/73W-C   IARC**
27,199,82
ETA: orl-rat TD:557 g/kg/79W-C   IARC**
27,199,82

CONSENSUS REPORTS: IARC Cancer Review: IMEMDT 7,56,87, Animal Limited Evidence IMEMDT 27,199,82. NTP Fourth Annual Report On Carcinogens, 1984. NCI Carcinogenesis Bioassay (feed); Clear Evidence: mouse, rat NCITR* NCI-CG-TR-111,78. Community Right-To-Know List. Reported in EPA TSCA Inventory.

SAFETY PROFILE: Confirmed carcinogen with experimental carcinogenic, neoplastigenic, and tumorigenic data. When heated to decomposition it emits toxic fumes of NO_x.

AMT500   CAS: 139-13-9
AMINOTRIACETIC ACID
mf: $C_6H_9NO_6$ mw: 191.16

SYNS: N,N-BIS(CARBOXYMETHYL)GLYCINE ◇ NCI-C02766 ◇ NITRILOTRIACETIC ACID ◇ TRIGLYCINE ◇ TRIGLYCOLLAMIC ACID ◇ VERSENE NTA ACID

TOXICITY DATA with REFERENCE
CAR: orl-rat TDLo:430 g/kg/75W-C   NCITR*
NCI-CG-TR-6,77
NEO: orl-mus TDLo:832 g/kg/66W-C   NCITR*
NCI-CG-TR-6,77

CONSENSUS REPORTS: NTP Fourth Annual Report On Carcinogens, 1984. NCI Carcinogenesis Bioassay (feed); Clear Evidence: mouse, rat NCITR* NCI-CG-TR-6,77. Reported in EPA TSCA Inventory. Community Right-To-Know List.

SAFETY PROFILE: Confirmed carcinogen with experimental carcinogenic and neoplastigenic data. Poison by intraperitoneal route. Moderately toxic by ingestion. When heated to decomposition it emits toxic fumes of NO_x.

AMY050   CAS: 61-82-5
AMITROLE
mf: $C_2H_4N_4$ mw: 84.10

SYNS: AMEROL ◇ AMINOTRIAZOLE ◇ 2-AMINOTRIAZOLE ◇ 3-AMINOTRIAZOLE ◇ 3-AMINO-s-TRIAZOLE ◇ 3-AMINO-1,2,4-TRIAZOLE ◇ 2-AMINO-1,3,4-TRIAZOLE ◇ 3-AMINO-1H-1,2,4-TRIAZOLE ◇ AMINOTRIAZOLE (PLANT REGULATOR) ◇ 3-AMINO-1,2,4-TRIAZOLE ◇ AMINO TRIAZOLE WEEDKILLER 90 ◇ AMINOTRIAZOLSPRITZPULVER ◇ AMITOL ◇ AMITRIL ◇ AMITRIL T.L. ◇ AMITROL ◇ AMITROL 90 ◇ AMITROL-T ◇ AMIZOL ◇ AT ◇ ATA ◇ AT LIQUID ◇ AZAPLANT ◇ AZOLAN ◇ AZOLE ◇ CAMPAPRIM A 1544 ◇ CYTROL ◇ DIUROL ◇ DOMATOL ◇ ELMASIL ◇ EMISOL ◇ ENT 25,445 ◇ FENAMINE ◇ FENAVAR ◇ HERBICIDE TOTAL ◇ HERBIZOLE ◇ KLEER-LOT ◇ ORGA-414 ◇ RADOXONE TL ◇ RAMIZOL ◇ RCRA WASTE NUMBER U011 ◇ SIMAZOL ◇ SOLUTION CONCENTREE T271 ◇ TRIAZOLAMINE ◇ 1H-1,2,4-TRIAZOL-3-AMINE ◇ USAF XR-22 ◇ VOROX ◇ WEEDAR ADS ◇ WEEDAZIN ◇ WEEDAZOL ◇ WEEDEX GRANULAT ◇ WEEDOCLOR ◇ X-ALL LIQUID

TOXICITY DATA with REFERENCE
CAR: orl-mus TDLo:113 g/kg/3W-I   JNCIAM
42,1101,69
CAR: orl-rat TD:105 g/kg/60W-C   NMJOAA
23,83,78
CAR: orl-rat TD:122 g/kg/70W-C   JNCIAM
57,861,76
CAR: orl-rat TDLo:4595 mg/kg/2.5Y-C
TXAPA9 69,161,83
NEO: orl-rat TD:3670 mg/kg/2Y-C   SCIEAS
132,296,60
ETA: orl-mus TD:366 g/kg/26W-C   TOLED5
29,145,85
MUT: hma-mus/sat 12 mg/kg   JNCIAM 62,911,79

MUT: mma-sat 50 μg/plate   PMRSDJ 1,351,81
MUT: mrc-asn 600 μg/L   MUREAV 147,288,85
MUT: msc-ham:emb 1 mg/L   MUREAV 140,205,84
MUT: sln-asn 600 μg/L   MUREAV 147,288,85

CONSENSUS REPORTS: IARC Cancer Review: Human Inadequate Evidence IMEMDT 41,293,86; IMEMDT 7,31,74; Animal Sufficient Evidence IMEMDT 7,31,74; IMEMDT 41,293,86. NTP Fourth Annual Report On Carcinogens, 1984. Reported in EPA TSCA Inventory. EPA Genetic Toxicology Program.

OSHA PEL: TWA 0.2 mg/m³   ACGIH TLV: TWA 0.2 mg/m³   DFG MAK: 0.2 mg/m³

SAFETY PROFILE: Confirmed carcinogen with experimental carcinogenic, tumorigenic, neoplastigenic, and teratogenic data. Poison by intraperitoneal route. Moderately toxic by ingestion. Other experimental reproductive effects. Mutation data reported. When heated to decomposition it emits toxic fumes of NO_x. An herbicide and plant growth regulator.

AND250
AMMONIUM CADMIUM CHLORIDE
mf: $4NH_4Cl \cdot CdCl_2$ mw: 397.3

PROP: Colorless, rhombic crystals. D: 2.01; sol in water.

CONSENSUS REPORTS: Cadmium and its compounds are on the Community Right-To-Know List.

OSHA PEL: TWA 0.1 mg(Cd)/m³; CL 0.6 mg(Cd)/m³ (fume)   ACGIH TLV: TWA 0.05 mg(Cd)/m³ (Proposed: TWA 0.01 mg(Cd)/m³ (dust), Human Carcinogen); BEI: 10 μg/g creatinine in urine; 10 μg/L in blood.   DFG BAT: Blood: 1.5 μg/dL; Urine: 15 μg/dL; Suspected Carcinogen.   NIOSH REL: (Cadmium) Reduce to lowest feasible level

SAFETY PROFILE: Confirmed human carcinogen. A poison. When heated to decomposition it emits toxic fumes of NH_3, NO_x and Cl^-.

ANO500   CAS: 135-20-6
AMMONIUM-N-
NITROSOPHENYLHYDROXYLAMINE
mf: $C_6H_6N_2O_2 \cdot H_4N$ mw: 156.19

SYNS: CUPFERRON ◇ N-HYDROXY-N-NITROSO-BENZE-NAMINE, AMMONIUM SALT ◇ KUPFERRON (CZECH) ◇ NCI-C03258 ◇ N-NITROSOFENYLHYDROXYLAMIN AMONNY (CZECH) ◇ N-NITROSOPHENYLHYDROXYLAMIN

AMMONIUM SALZ (GERMAN) ◇ N-NITROSOPHENYLHY-DROXYLAMINE AMMONIUM SALT

TOXICITY DATA with REFERENCE
CAR: orl-mus TDLo:437 g/kg/78W-C   NCITR*
NCI-CG-TR-100,78
CAR: orl-rat TDLo:123 g/kg/78W-C   NCITR*
NCI-CG-TR-100,78
ETA: orl-rat TD:9040 mg/kg/65W-C   ZEKBAI
69,103,67
MUT: cyt-grh-orl 1 ppm   JCGEDO 1,75,66

CONSENSUS REPORTS: NTP Fourth Annual Report On Carcinogens, 1984. NCI Carcinogenesis Bioassay (feed); Clear Evidence: mouse, rat NCITR* NCI-CG-TR-100,78. Reported in EPA TSCA Inventory. Community Right-To-Know List.

SAFETY PROFILE: Confirmed carcinogen with experimental carcinogenic and tumorigenic data. Poison by intravenous route. Powerful eye irritant. Solutions with thorium salts are unstable explosives above 15°C. Solutions with titanium or zirconium salts are unstable explosives above 40°C. When heated to decomposition it emits very toxic NH_3 and NO_x.

AOX250   CAS: 134-29-2
o-ANISIDINE HYDROCHLORIDE
mf: $C_7H_9NO \cdot ClH$ mw: 159.63

SYNS: C.I. 37115 ◇ 2-METHOXYANILINE HYDROCHLO-RIDE ◇ NCI-C03747

TOXICITY DATA with REFERENCE
CAR: orl-mus TD:3605 g/kg/1Y-C   IMEMDT
27,63,82
CAR: orl-mus TDLo:721 g/kg/2Y-C   NCITR*
NCI-CG-TR-89,78
CAR: orl-rat TD:2905 g/kg/83W-C   IMEMDT
27,63,82
CAR: orl-rat TD:5810 g/kg/83W-C   IMEMDT
27,63,82
CAR: orl-rat TD:360 g/kg/78W-C
NCITR* NCI-CG-TR-89,78
CAR: orl-rat TDLo:180 g/kg/2Y-C   NCITR*
NCI-CG-TR-89,78
NEO: orl-mus TD:1803 g/kg/1Y-C   IMEMDT
27,63,82
ETA: orl-mus TD:216 g/kg/78W-C   NCITR*
NCI-CG-TR-89,78
MUT: mmo-sat 333 μg/plate   IARCCD 27,283,80

CONSENSUS REPORTS: IARC Cancer Review: Animal Sufficient Evidence IMEMDT 27,63,82. NTP Fourth Annual Report On Carcinogens, 1984. NCI Carcinogenesis Bioassay (feed); Clear Evidence: mouse, rat NCITR* NCI-CG-TR-89,78. Community Right-To-Know List.

SAFETY PROFILE: Confirmed carcinogen with experimental carcinogenic, neoplastigenic, and tumorigenic data. Mutation data reported. When heated to decomposition it emits very toxic fumes of NO_x and HCl.

AQF000 CAS: 1309-64-4
ANTIMONY OXIDE
mf: O_3Sb_2 mw: 291.50

PROP: White cubes. D: 5.2, mp: 650°, bp: 1550° subl. Very sltly sol in water; sol in KOH and HCl.

SYNS: ANTIMONIOUS OXIDE ◇ ANTIMONY PEROXIDE ◇ ANTIMONY SESQUIOXIDE ◇ ANTIMONY TRIOXIDE (MAK) ◇ ANTIMONY WHITE ◇ C.I. PIGMENT WHITE 11 ◇ DECHLORANE-A-O ◇ DIANTIMONY TRIOXIDE ◇ FLOWERS OF ANTIMONY ◇ NCI-C55152

TOXICITY DATA with REFERENCE
CAR: ihl-rat TCLo: 4200 μg/m³/52W-I AIHAM* 20,1,80
NEO: ihl-rat TD: 1600 μg/m³/52W-I AIHAM* 20,1,80
ETA: ihl-rat TC: 4 mg/m³/1Y-I PESTC* 8,16,80
MUT: mrc-bcs 50 mmol/L MUREAV 77,109,80

CONSENSUS REPORTS: Reported in EPA TSCA Inventory. Antimony and its compounds are on the Community Right-To-Know List.

OSHA PEL: TWA 0.5 mg(Sb)/m3 ACGIH TLV: TWA 0.5 mg(Sb)/m³; Suspected Carcinogen DFG MAK: Animal Carcinogen, Suspected Human Carcinogen. NIOSH REL: TWA 0.5 mg(Sb)/m³

SAFETY PROFILE: Confirmed carcinogen with experimental carcinogenic and neoplastigenic data. Poison by intravenous and subcutaneous routes. Moderately toxic by other routes. Experimental reproductive effects. Mutation data reported. When heated to decomposition it emits toxic Sb fumes. Incompatible with chlorinated rubber and heat of 216°; BrF_3.

AQP000 CAS: 1937-37-7
APOMINE BLACK GX
mf: $C_{34}H_{25}N_9O_7S_2 \cdot 2Na$ mw: 781.78

SYNS: AHCO DIRECT BLACK GX ◇ AIREDALE BLACK ED ◇ AIZEN DIRECT DEEP BLACK GH ◇ AMANIL BLACK GL ◇ APOMINE BLACK GX ◇ ATLANTIC BLACK BD ◇ ATUL DIRECT BLACK E ◇ AZINE DEEP BLACK EW ◇ AZOCARD BLACK EW ◇ AZOMINE BLACK EWO ◇ BELAMINE BLACK GX ◇ BENCIDAL BLACK E ◇ BENZAMIL BLACK E ◇ BENZO DEEP BLACK E ◇ BENZOFORM BLACK BCN-CF ◇ BLACK 2EMBL ◇ BRASILAMINA BLACK GN ◇ CALCOMINE BLACK ◇ CARBIDE BLACK E ◇ CERN PRIMA 38 ◇ CHLORAMINE BLACK C ◇ CHLORAZOL BLACK E (BIOLOGICAL STAIN) ◇ CHLORAZOL BLACK EA ◇ CHLORAZOL BLACK EN ◇ CHROME LEATHER BLACK EM ◇ C.I. 30235 ◇ C.I. DIRECT BLACK 38 ◇ COIR DEEP BLACK C ◇ COLUMBIA BLACK EP ◇ DIACOTTON DEEP BLACK ◇ DIAMINE DEEP BLACK EC ◇ DIAPHTAMINE BLACK V ◇ DIAZINE BLACK E ◇ DIAZOL BLACK 2V ◇ DIPHENYL DEEP BLACK G ◇ DIRECT BLACK A ◇ DIRECT BLACK META ◇ ENIANIL BLACK CN ◇ ERIE BLACK B ◇ FENAMIN BLACK E ◇ FIBRE BLACK VF ◇ FIXANOL BLACK E ◇ FORMALINE BLACK C ◇ FORMIC BLACK C ◇ HISPAMIN BLACK EF ◇ INTERCHEM DIRECT BLACK Z ◇ KAYAKU DIRECT DEEP BLACK EX ◇ LURAZOL BLACK BA ◇ META BLACK ◇ MITSUI DIRECT BLACK EX ◇ NCI-C54557 ◇ NIPPON DEEP BLACK ◇ PAPER BLACK BA ◇ PARAMINE BLACK B ◇ PEERAMINE BLACK E ◇ PHENO BLACK EP ◇ PONTAMINE BLACK E ◇ SANDOPEL BLACK EX ◇ SERISTAN BLACK B ◇ TELON FAST BLACK E ◇ TETRAZO DEEP BLACK G ◇ TERTRODIRECT BLACK E ◇ TETRODIRECT BLACK EFD ◇ UNION BLACK EM ◇ VONDACEL BLACK N

TOXICITY DATA with REFERENCE
CAR: orl-rat TDLo: 6825 mg/kg/13W-C NCITR* NCI-TR-108,78
ETA: imp-mus TDLo: 80 mg/kg TJIDAH 88,467,73
ETA: orl-mus TDLo: 34 mg/kg/60W-C TJIDAH 88,467,73
MUT: bfa-rat: sat 300 mg/kg IAEHDW 49,177,81
MUT: dns-rat-orl 500 mg/kg/12H-C MUREAV 187,227,87
MUT: mma-sat 10 μg/plate TOLED5 4,519,79
MUT: mmo-sat 10 μg/plate TOLED5 4,519,79
MUT: mnt-rat-orl 500 mg/kg/36H-C MUREAV 187,227,87

CONSENSUS REPORTS: IARC Cancer Review: Animal Sufficient Evidence IMEMDT 29,295,82, Human Limited Evidence IMEMDT 29,295,82. NTP Fourth Annual Report On Carcinogens, 1984. Reported in EPA TSCA Inventory. NTP Carcinogenesis Bioassay (feed): Clear Evidence: rat NCICTR* NCI-TR-108,78; No Evidence: mouse NCICTR NCI-TR-108,78. On Community-Right-To-Know List.

SAFETY PROFILE: Confirmed carcinogen with carcinogenic and tumorigenic data. Mutation data reported. When heated to decomposition it emits very toxic fumes of NO_x, Na_2O, and SO_2.

AQY250   CAS: 313-67-7
ARISTOLOCHINE
mf: $C_{17}H_{11}NO_7$ mw: 341.29

PROP: From alcoholic extract of *Aristolochia indico* (CNCRA6 42,35,64).

SYNS: ARISTOLOCHIC ACID ◇ BIRTHWORT ◇ 8-ME-THOXY-6-NITROPHENANTHOL-(3,4-d)-1,3-DIOXOLE-5-CARBOXYLIC ACID ◇ NSC-50413

SAFETY PROFILE: Confirmed carcinogen. From International Register of Potentially Toxic Chemicals: April 1982. Poison by intravenous route. When heated to decomposition it emits toxic fumes of NO_x. Vol 5 No. 1.

ARA750   CAS: 7440-38-2
ARSENIC
DOT: 1558
af: As   aw: 74.92

PROP: Silvery to black, brittle, crystalline and amorphous metalloid. Mp: 814° @ 36 atm, bp: sublimes @ 612°, d: black crystals 5.724 @ 14°; black amorphous 4.7, vap press: 1 mm @ 372° (sublimes). Insol in water; sol in HNO_3.

SYNS: ◇ ARSEN (GERMAN, POLISH) ◇ ARSENICALS ◇ ARSENIC-75 ◇ ARSENIC BLACK ◇ COLLOIDAL ARSENIC ◇ GREY ARSENIC ◇ METALLIC ARSENIC

TOXICITY DATA with REFERENCE
CAR: orl-man TDLo: 76 mg/kg/12Y-I RMCHAW 99,664,71
ETA: imp-rbt TDLo: 75 mg/kg ZEKBAI 52,425,42
MUT: cyt-mus-ipr 4 mg/kg/48H-I EXPEAM 37,129,81

CONSENSUS REPORTS: IARC Cancer Review: Human Sufficient Evidence IMEMDT 23,39,80; Human Inadequate Evidence IMEMDT 2,48,73. NTP Fourth Annual Report On Carcinogens, 1984. Reported in EPA TSCA Inventory. Arsenic and its compounds are on the Community Right-To-Know List.

OSHA PEL: TWA 0.01 mg(As)/m³; Cancer Hazard ACGIH TLV: TWA 0.2 mg(As)/m³ DFG TRK: 0.2 mg/m³ calculated as arsenic in that portion of dust that can possibly be inhaled. NIOSH REL: CL 2 μg(As)/m³ DOT Classification: Poison B; Label: Poison.

SAFETY PROFILE: Confirmed human carcinogen producing liver tumors. Poison by subcutaneous, intramuscular, and intraperitoneal routes. Human systemic skin and gastrointestinal effects by ingestion. Experimental teratogenic and reproductive data. Mutation data reported. Flammable in the form of dust when exposed to heat or flame or by chemical reaction with powerful oxidizers such as bromates; chlorates; iodates; peroxides; lithium; NCl_3; KNO_3; $KMnO_4$; Rb_2C_2; $AgNO_4$; $NOCl$; IF_5; CrO_3; ClF_3; ClO; BrF_3; BrF_5; BrN_3; RbC_3BCH; CsC_3BCH. Slightly explosive in the form of dust when exposed to flame. When heated or on contact with acid or acid fumes, it emits highly toxic fumes; can react vigorously on contact with oxidizing materials. Incompatible with bromine azide; dirubidium acetylide; halogens; palladium; zinc; platinum; NCl_3; $AgNO_3$; CrO_3; Na_2O_2; hexafluoro isopropylideneamino lithium.

ARB000   CAS: 10102-53-1
m-ARSENIC ACID
mf: $AsHO_3$ mw: 123.93

SYN: METAARSENIC ACID

CONSENSUS REPORTS: Reported in EPA TSCA Inventory. Arsenic and its compounds are on the Community Right-To-Know List.

OSHA PEL: TWA 0.01 mg(As)/m³ ACGIH TLV: TWA 0.2 mg(As)/m³ DFG MAK: Human Carcinogen. NIOSH REL: CL 2 μg(As)/m³/15M

SAFETY PROFILE: Confirmed human carcinogen. When heated to decomposition it emits toxic fumes of arsenic.

ARB250   CAS: 7778-39-4
o-ARSENIC ACID
DOT: 1553/1554
mf: AsH_3O_4 mw: 141.95

SYNS: ACIDE ARSENIQUE LIQUIDE (FRENCH) ◇ ARSENATE ◇ ARSENIC ACID, LIQUID (DOT) ◇ ARSENIC ACID, SOLID (DOT) ◇ DESICCANT L-10 ◇ HI-YIELD DESSI-CANT H-10 ◇ ORTHOARSENIC ACID ◇ RCRA WASTE NUMBER P010 ◇ ZOTOX ◇ ZOTOX CRAB GRASS KILLER

TOXICITY DATA with REFERENCE
MUT: cyt-hmn: fbr 100 ppb MUREAV 88,73,81
MUT: cyt-hmn: leu 7200 nmol/L MUREAV 88,73,81

CONSENSUS REPORTS: Reported in EPA TSCA Inventory. Arsenic and its compounds are on the Community Right-To-Know List.

OSHA PEL: TWA 0.01 mg(As)/m^3 ACGIH TLV: TWA 0.2 mg(As)/m^3 DFG MAK: Human Carcinogen. NIOSH REL: CL 2 µg(As)/m^3/15M DOT Classification: Poison B; Label: Poison.

SAFETY PROFILE: Confirmed human carcinogen. Poison by ingestion. An experimental teratogen. Other experimental reproductive effects. Human mutation data reported. When heated to decomposition it emits toxic fumes of arsenic.

ARB750   CAS: 7778-44-1
ARSENIC ACID, CALCIUM SALT (2:3)
DOT: 1573
mf: As$_2$O$_8$•3Ca   mw: 398.08

PROP: Colorless, amorphous powder. D: 3.620. Solubility in water = 0.013/100 @ 25°.

SYNS: ARSENIATE de CALCIUM (FRENCH) ◇ CALCIUM-ARSENAT ◇ CALCIUM ARSENATE (MAK) ◇ CALCIUM ORTHOARSENATE ◇ KALZIUMARSENIAT (GERMAN) ◇ TRICALCIUMARSENAT (GERMAN) ◇ TRICALCIUM ARSENATE

TOXICITY DATA with REFERENCE
NEO: itr-ham TD:214 mg/kg/15W-I   IJCNAW 40,220,87
NEO: itr-ham TDLo:120 mg/kg/15W-C
CALEDQ 27,99,85
ETA: itr-rat TDLo:1600 µg/kg   IJCNAW 24,786,79

CONSENSUS REPORTS: IARC Cancer Review: Human Sufficient Evidence IMEMDT 23,39,80; Animal No Evidence IMEMDT 2,48,73; Animal Inadequate Evidence IMEMDT 23,39,80. Reported in EPA TSCA Inventory. Arsenic and its compounds are on the Community Right-To-Know List. EPA Extremely Hazardous Substances List.

OSHA PEL: TWA 0.01 mg(As)/m^3; Cancer Hazard ACGIH TLV: TWA 0.2 mg(As)/m^3 DFG MAK: Human Carcinogen. NIOSH REL: CL 2 µg(As)/m^3/15M DOT Classification: Poison B; Label: Poison.

SAFETY PROFILE: Confirmed human carcinogen. Poison by ingestion. Moderately toxic by skin contact. When heated to decomposition it emits toxic fumes of arsenic.

ARC000   CAS: 7778-43-0
ARSENIC ACID, DISODIUM SALT
mf: Na$_2$HAsO$_4$•7H$_2$O   mw: 312.01

PROP: Colorless powder, effloresces. D: 1.88, mp: −7H$_2$O @ 130°, bp: decomp @ 150°. Solubility in water = 61/100 @ 15°, sol in glycerol.

SYNS: DISODIUM ARSENATE ◇ DISODIUM ARSENIC ACID ◇ DISODIUM HYDROGEN ARSENATE ◇ DISODIUM HYDROGEN ORTHOARSENATE ◇ DISODIUM MONOHYDROGEN ARSENATE ◇ SODIUM ACID ARSENATE ◇ SODIUM ARSENATE ◇ SODIUM ARSENATE DIBASIC, ANHYDROUS

TOXICITY DATA with REFERENCE
MUT: cyt-hmn:leu 7200 µmol/L   MUREAV 88,73,81
MUT: mrc-bcs 100 mmol/L   MUREAV 77,109,80

CONSENSUS REPORTS: Reported in EPA TSCA Inventory. Arsenic and its compounds are on the Community Right-To-Know List.

OSHA PEL: TWA 0.5 mg(As)/m^3: Cancer Hazard ACGIH TLV: TWA 0.2 mg(As)/m^3 NIOSH REL: CL 2 µg(As)/m^3/15M DFG MAK: Human Carcinogen.

SAFETY PROFILE: Confirmed human carcinogen. Poison by intraperitoneal route. Human mutation data reported. When heated to decomposition it emits toxic fumes of arsenic.

ARC250   CAS: 10048-95-0
ARSENIC ACID, DISODIUM SALT, HEPTAHYDRATE
mf: AsHO$_4$•2Na•7H$_2$O   mw: 312.05

SYNS: DISODIUM ARSENATE, HEPTAHYDRATE ◇ SODIUM ACID ARSENATE, HEPTAHYDRATE ◇ SODIUM ARSENATE, DIBASIC, HEPTAHYDRATE ◇ SODIUM ARSENATE HEPTAHYDRATE

CONSENSUS REPORTS: Arsenic and its compounds are on the Community Right-To-Know List.

OSHA PEL: TWA 0.01 mg(As)/m^3 ACGIH TLV: TWA 0.2 mg(As)/m^3 NIOSH REL: CL 2 µg(As)/m^3/15M DFG MAK: Human Carcinogen.

SAFETY PROFILE: Confirmed human carcinogen. Poison by subcutaneous route. An experimental teratogen. When heated to decomposition it emits toxic fumes of arsenic.

ARC500   CAS: 7774-41-6
o-ARSENIC ACID, HEMIHYDRATE
mf: $AsH_3O_4 \cdot 1/2H_2O$ mw: 150.96

PROP: White, translucent crystals. Mp: 35.5°, bp: $-H_2O$ @ 160°, d: 2.0-2.5.

SYNS: ARSENIC ACID, SOLID (DOT) ◊ ORTHOARSENIC ACID HEMIHYDRATE

CONSENSUS REPORTS: Arsenic and its compounds are on the Community Right-To-Know List.

OSHA PEL: TWA 0.01 mg(As)/m^3 ACGIH TLV: TWA 0.2 mg(As)/m^3 NIOSH REL: CL 2 μg(As)/m^3/15M   DFG MAK: Human Carcinogen.   DOT Classification: Poison B; Label: Poison.

SAFETY PROFILE: Confirmed human carcinogen. Poison by intravenous route. When heated to decomposition it emits toxic fumes of arsenic.

ARC750   CAS: 7645-25-2
ARSENIC ACID, LEAD SALT
mf: $AsH_3O_4 \cdot 7Pb$ mw: 1592.28

SYNS: ARSENIATE de PLOMB (FRENCH) ◊ LEAD ARSENATE

CONSENSUS REPORTS: Arsenic compounds and Lead compounds are on the Community Right-To-Know List.

OSHA PEL: TWA 0.01 mg(As)/m^3; Cancer Hazard   ACGIH TLV: TWA 0.15 mg(Pb)/m^3 NIOSH REL: TWA 0.10 mg(Pb)/m^3; CL 2 μg(As)/m^3/15M   DFG MAK: Human Carcinogen.

SAFETY PROFILE: Confirmed human carcinogen. Poison by ingestion. When heated to decomposition it emits very toxic fumes of lead and arsenic.

ARD000   CAS: 10103-50-1
ARSENIC ACID, MAGNESIUM SALT
DOT: 1622
mf: $AsH_3O_4 \cdot 7Mg$ mw: 312.12

PROP: Monoclinic, white crystals. D: 2.60-2.61.

SYNS: ARSENIATE de MAGNESIUM (FRENCH) ◊ MAGNESIUM ARSENATE ◊ MAGNESIUM ARSENATE PHOSPHOR

CONSENSUS REPORTS: Reported in EPA TSCA Inventory. Arsenic and its compounds are on the Community Right-To-Know List.

OSHA PEL: TWA 0.01 mg(As)/m^3 ACGIH TLV: TWA 0.2 mg(As)/m^3 DFG MAK: Human Carcinogen.   NIOSH REL: CL 2 μg(As)/m^3/15M   DOT Classification: Poison B; Label: Poison.

SAFETY PROFILE: Confirmed human carcinogen. Poison by ingestion. When heated to decomposition it emits toxic fumes of arsenic.

ARD250   CAS: 7784-41-0
ARSENIC ACID, MONOPOTASSIUM SALT
DOT: 1677
mf: $AsH_2O_4 \cdot K$ mw: 180.04

SYNS: MONOPOTASSIUM ARSENATE ◊ MONOPOTASSIUM DIHYDROGEN ARSENATE ◊ MACQUER'S SALT ◊ POTASSIUM ACID ARSENATE ◊ POTASSIUM ARSENATE ◊ POTASSIUM DIHYDROGEN ARSENATE ◊ POTASSIUM HYDROGEN ARSENATE

TOXICITY DATA with REFERENCE
MUT: cyt-hmn:leu 1 μmol/L   CNREA8 25,980,65

CONSENSUS REPORTS: IARC Cancer Review: Human Sufficient Evidence IMEMDT 23,39,80. Reported in EPA TSCA Inventory. Arsenic and its compounds are on the Community Right-To-Know List.

OSHA PEL: TWA 0.01 mg(As)/m^3, Cancer Hazard   ACGIH TLV: TWA 0.2 mg(As)/m^3 NIOSH REL: CL 2 μg(As)/m^3/15M   DOT Classification: Poison B; Label: Poison.

SAFETY PROFILE: Confirmed human carcinogen. Mutation data reported. When heated to decomposition it emits toxic fumes of arsenic.

ARD500   CAS: 15120-17-9
ARSENIC ACID, MONOSODIUM SALT
mf: $AsO_3 \cdot Na$ mw: 145.91

SYNS: ARSENIC ACID, SODIUM SALT (9CI) ◊ SODIUM ARSENATE ◊ SODIUM METAARSENATE ◊ SODIUM MONOHYDROGEN ARSENATE

TOXICITY DATA with REFERENCE
MUT: sln-dmg-orl 2 μmol/L   CNJGA8 11,677,69
MUT: slt-dmg-orl 100 μmol   CNJGA8 17,55,75

CONSENSUS REPORTS: Arsenic and its compounds are on the Community Right-To-Know List.

OSHA PEL: TWA 0.5 mg(As)/m^3: Cancer Hazard   ACGIH TLV: TWA 0.2 mg(As)/m^3 NIOSH REL: CL 2 μg(As)/m^3/15M   DFG MAK: Human Carcinogen.

SAFETY PROFILE: Confirmed human carcinogen. A poison. Mutation data reported. When heated to decomposition it emits toxic fumes of arsenic.

ARD600   CAS: 10103-60-3
ARSENIC ACID, MONOSODIUM SALT
mf: AsH$_2$O$_4$•Na   mw: 163.93

SYNS: MONOSODIUM ARSENATE ◇ SODIUM ARSENATE ◇ SODIUM DIHYDROGEN ARSENATE ◇ SODIUM DIHYDROGEN ORTHOARSENATE

OSHA PEL: TWA 0.5 mg(As)/m^3: Cancer Hazard ACGIH TLV: TWA 0.2 mg(As)/m^3 NIOSH REL: CL 2 μg(As)/m^3/15M DFG MAK: Human Carcinogen.

CONSENSUS REPORTS: Arsenic and its compounds are on the Community Right-To-Know List.

SAFETY PROFILE: Confirmed human carcinogen. Poison by intravenous route. When heated to decomposition it emits toxic fumes of arsenic.

ARD750   CAS: 7631-89-2
ARSENIC ACID, SODIUM SALT
DOT: 1685
mf: AsH$_3$O$_4$•7Na   mw: 202.94

SYNS: SODIUM ARSENATE (DOT) ◇ SODIUM ORTHOARSENATE

TOXICITY DATA with REFERENCE
ETA: ivn-mus TDLo: 10 mg(As)/kg/20W-I
   VDGPAN 55,289,71
ETA: scu-mus TDLo: 10 mg(As)/kg/20D-C
   VDGPAN 55,289,71
ETA: scu-mus TDLo: 10 mg(As)/kg/(1-20D
   VDGPAN 55,289,71
MUT: cyt-hmn: lym 2 μmol/L   ADREDL 267,91,80

CONSENSUS REPORTS: IARC Cancer Review: Human Sufficient Evidence IMEMDT 23,39,80; Animal Inadequate Evidence IMEMDT 2,48,73; IMEMDT 23,39,80. Reported in EPA TSCA Inventory. Arsenic and its compounds are on the Community Right-To-Know List.

OSHA PEL: TWA 0.01 mg(As)/m^3; Cancer Hazard ACGIH TLV: TWA 0.2 mg(As)/m^3 NIOSH REL: CL 2 μg(As)/m^3/15M DOT Classification: Poison B; Label: Poison.

SAFETY PROFILE: Confirmed human carcinogen with experimental tumorigenic data. Poison by ingestion, intravenous, and intraperitoneal routes. Experimental teratogenic and reproductive data. Mutation data reported. When heated to decomposition it emits toxic fumes of As and Na$_2$O.

ARE000   CAS: 64070-83-3
ARSENIC(V) ACID, TRISODIUM SALT, HEPTAHYDRATE (1:3:7)
mf: AsO$_4$•3Na•7H$_2$O   mw: 334.03

SYN: TRISODIUM ARSENATE, HEPTAHYDRATE

CONSENSUS REPORTS: Arsenic and its compounds are on the Community Right-To-Know List.

OSHA PEL: TWA 0.01 mg(As)/m^3; Cancer Hazard ACGIH TLV: TWA 0.2 mg(As)g/m^3 NIOSH REL: CL 2 μg(As)/m^3/15M DFG MAK: Human Carcinogen.

SAFETY PROFILE: Confirmed human carcinogen with experimental carcinogenic data. Poison by intraperitoneal route. When heated to decomposition it emits toxic fumes of arsenic.

ARE750
ARSENICAL FLUE DUST (DOT)

CONSENSUS REPORTS: Arsenic and its compounds are on the Community Right-To-Know List.

OSHA PEL: TWA 0.01 mg(As)/m^3 ACGIH TLV: TWA 0.2 mg(As)/m^3 NIOSH REL: CL 2 μg(As)/m^3/15M DFG MAK: Human Carcinogen. DOT Classification: Poison B; Label: Poison.

SAFETY PROFILE: Confirmed human carcinogen. Poison by inhalation and ingestion.

ARF750
ARSENIC COMPOUNDS

SYN: ARSENICALS

CONSENSUS REPORTS: Arsenic and its compounds are on the Community Right-To-Know List.

OSHA PEL: Inorganic: TWA 0.01 mg(As)/m^3; Cancer Hazard; Organic: TWA 0.5 mg(As)/m^3 ACGIH TLV: TWA 0.2 mg(As)/m^3 NIOSH REL: CL 2 μg(As)/m^3/15M

SAFETY PROFILE: Inorganic compounds are confirmed human carcinogens producing tumors of the mouth, esophagus, larynx, bladder, and para nasal sinus. A recognized carcinogen of the skin, lungs, and liver. Used as insecticides, herbicides, silvicides, defoliants, desiccants and rodenticides. Poisoning from arsenic compounds may be acute or chronic. Acute poisoning usually results from swallowing arsenic compounds; chronic poisoning from either swallowing or inhaling. Acute allergic reactions to arsenic compounds used in medical therapy have been fairly common, the type and severity of reaction depending upon the compound. Inorganic arsenicals are more toxic than organics. Trivalent is more toxic than pentavalent. Acute arsenic poisoning (from ingestion) results in marked irritation of the stomach and intestines with nausea, vomiting, and diarrhea. In severe cases, the vomitus and stools are bloody and the patient goes into collapse and shock with weak, rapid pulse, cold sweats, coma, and death. Chronic arsenic poisoning, whether through ingestion or inhalation, may manifest itself in many different ways. There may be disturbances of the digestive system such as loss of appetite, cramps, nausea, constipation, or diarrhea. Liver damage may occur, resulting in jaundice. Disturbances of the blood, kidneys, and nervous system are not infrequent. Arsenic can cause a variety of skin abnormalities including itching, pigmentation, and even cancerous changes. A characteristic of arsenic poisoning is the great variety of symptoms that can be produced. Dangerous; when heated to decomposition, or when metallic arsenic contacts acids or acid fumes, or when water solutions of arsenicals are in contact with active metals such as Fe; Al; Zn; they emits highly toxic fumes of arsenic.

ARH500   CAS: 1303-28-2
ARSENIC PENTOXIDE
DOT: 1559
mf: As_2O_5 mw: 229.84

PROP: White, amorphous, deliquescent solid. Mp: decomp @ 800°, d: 4.32. Sol in alc. Solubility in water = 65.8/100 @ 20°.

SYNS: ANHYDRIDE ARSENIQUE (FRENCH) ◇ ARSENIC ACID ◇ ARSENIC ACID ANHYDRIDE ◇ ARSENIC ANHYDRIDE ◇ ARSENIC OXIDE ◇ ARSENIC(V) OXIDE ◇ DIARSENIC PENTOXIDE

TOXICITY DATA with REFERENCE
MUT: cyt-hmn:leu 1200 nmol/L   MUREAV 88,73,81
MUT: mrc-bcs 50 mmol/L   MUREAV 77,109,80

CONSENSUS REPORTS: IARC Cancer Review: Human Sufficient Evidence IMEMDT 23,39,80. Reported in EPA TSCA Inventory. Arsenic and its compounds are on the Community Right-To-Know List. EPA Extremely Hazardous Substances List.

OSHA PEL: TWA 0.01 mg(As)/m^3 ACGIH TLV: TWA 0.2 mg(As)/m^3 DFG MAK: Human Carcinogen.   NIOSH REL: CL 2 μg(As)/m^3/15M   DOT Classification: Poison B; Label: Poison.

SAFETY PROFILE: Confirmed human carcinogen. Poison by ingestion and intravenous routes. Mutation data reported. Reacts vigorously with Rb_2C_2. When heated to decomposition it emits toxic fumes of arsenic.

ARI000   CAS: 1303-33-9
ARSENIC SULFIDE
DOT: 1557
mf: As_2S_3 mw: 246.04

PROP: Yellow or red crystals. Bp: 707°, d: 3.43; mp: 312°. Insol in water, sol in alkalies.

SYNS: ARSENIC SESQUISULFIDE ◇ ARSENIC SULFIDE YELLOW ◇ ARSENIC SULPHIDE ◇ ARSENIC TRISULFIDE ◇ ARSENIC YELLOW ◇ ARSENIOUS SULPHIDE ◇ ARSENOUS SULFIDE ◇ C.I. 77086 ◇ DIARSENIC TRISULFIDE ◇ KING'S YELLOW ◇ ORPIMENT

TOXICITY DATA with REFERENCE
ETA: itr-mus TDLo:73885 μg/kg/15W-C   CALEDQ 27,99,85
ETA: scu-rat TDLo:125 mg/kg   BJCAAI 20,190,66

CONSENSUS REPORTS: IARC Cancer Review: Human Sufficient Evidence IMEMDT 23,39,80. Reported in EPA TSCA Inventory. Arsenic and its compounds are on the Community Right-To-Know List.

OSHA PEL: TWA 0.01 mg(As)/m^3; Cancer Hazard   ACGIH TLV: TWA 0.2 mg(As)/m^3 NIOSH REL: CL 2 μg(As)/m^3/15M   DOT Classification: Poison B; Label: Poison.

SAFETY PROFILE: Confirmed human carcinogen with experimental tumorigenic data. A poison. Reacts violently with H_2O_2; (KNO_3 + S).

When heated to decomposition or contact with acid or acid fumes it emits highly toxic fumes of SO_2, H_2S, and As. Reacts with water or steam to emit toxic and flammable vapors.

ARI250   CAS: 7784-35-2
ARSENIC TRIFLUORIDE
mf: AsF_3 mw: 131.92

PROP: Colorless liquid. D: 3.01, mp: −5.95, bp: 51°, vap press: 100 mm @ 13.2°, 400 mm @ 41.5°. Insol in water, sol in alc, benzene, and mercury.

SYNS: ARSENIC FLUORIDE ◇ ARSENOUS FLUORIDE ◇ TRIFLUOROARSINE

CONSENSUS REPORTS: Reported in EPA TSCA Inventory. Arsenic and its compounds are on the Community Right-To-Know List.

OSHA PEL: TWA 0.01 mg(As)/m^3; Cancer Hazard ACGIH TLV: TWA 0.2 mg(As)/m^3 NIOSH REL: CL 2 μg(As)/m^3/15M

SAFETY PROFILE: Confirmed human carcinogen. A poison by inhalation. Strong reaction with P_2O_3. When heated to decomposition it emits very toxic fumes of As and F^-.

ARI750   CAS: 1327-53-3
ARSENIC TRIOXIDE
DOT: 1561
mf: As_4O_6 mw: 395.68

PROP: Colorless, rhombic crystals (dimer, claudetite). D: 4.15, mp: 278°, bp: 460°. Solubility in water = 1.82/100 @ 20°; sol in alc. Cubes: Colorless. D: 3.865, mp: 309°. Solubility in water = 1.2/100 @ 20°.

SYNS: ACIDE ARSENIEUX (FRENCH) ◇ ANHYDRIDE AR-SENIEUX (FRENCH) ◇ ARSENIC BLANC (FRENCH) ◇ ARSENIC OXIDE ◇ ARSENIC(III) OXIDE ◇ ARSENIC SES-QUIOXIDE ◇ ARSENIGEN SAURE (GERMAN) ◇ ARSENIOUS ACID (MAK) ◇ ARSENIOUS OXIDE ◇ ARSENIOUS TRIOXIDE ◇ ARSENOUS ACID ◇ ARSENOUS ACID ANHYDRIDE ◇ ARSENOUS ANHYDRIDE ◇ ARSENOUS OXIDE ◇ ARSENOUS OXIDE ANHYDRIDE ◇ CRUDE ARSENIC ◇ DIARSENIC TRIOXIDE ◇ WHITE ARSENIC

TOXICITY DATA with REFERENCE
NEO: itr-ham TD: 30 mg/kg/15W-I   SAIGBL 24,523,82
NEO: itr-ham TD: 55450 μg/kg/15W-I   CALEDQ 21,141,83
NEO: itr-ham TDLo: 45 mg/kg/15W-I   ARTODN 7,403,84

ETA: itr-ham TD: 40 mg/kg/15W-I   CALEDQ 21,141,83
ETA: itr-ham TD: 39608 μg/kg/24W-I   JOUOD4 5(Suppl),109,83
ETA: itr-ham TD: 55456 μg/kg/24W-I   JOUOD4 5(Suppl),109,83
ETA: itr-rat TD: 75 mg/kg/15W-I   FKIZA471,19,80
ETA: itr-rat TD: 167 mg/kg/15W-I   SAIGBL 20,230,78
ETA: itr-rat TDLo: 16 mg/kg/15W-I   EVHPAZ 19,191,77
MUT: mrc-bcs 50 mmol/L   MUREAV 77,109,80

CONSENSUS REPORTS: IARC Cancer Review: Human Limited Evidence IMEMDT 2,48,73; Human Sufficient Evidence IMEMDT 23,39,80; Animal Inadequate Evidence IMEMDT 2,48,73; IMEMDT 23,39,80. NTP Fourth Annual Report On Carcinogens, 1984. Reported in EPA TSCA Inventory. Arsenic and its compounds are on the Community Right-To-Know List. EPA Extremely Hazardous Substances List.

OSHA PEL: TWA 0.01 mg(As)/m^3: Cancer Hazard ACGIH TLV: Production: Suspected Human Carcinogen DFG MAK: Human Carcinogen. NIOSH REL: CL 2 μg(As)/m^3/15M DOT Classification: Poison B; Label: Poison.

SAFETY PROFILE: Confirmed human carcinogen with experimental neoplastigenic and tumorigenic data. Poison by ingestion, subcutaneous, intradermal, intravenous, and possibly other routes. Human gastrointestinal effects by ingestion. Mutation data reported. Reacts vigorously with Rb_2C_2; ClF_3; F_2; Hg; OF_2; $NaClO_3$.

ARJ000
ARSENIC TRIOXIDE mixed with
SELENIUM DIOXIDE (1:1)

TOXICITY DATA with REFERENCE
ETA: orl-mus TDLo: 16 mg/kg/35W-C   BICHBX 9(3),245,78

CONSENSUS REPORTS: Arsenic and its compounds, as well as selenium and its compounds, are on the Community Right-To-Know List.

OSHA PEL: TWA 0.01 mg(As)/m3; Cancer Hazard ACGIH TLV: TWA 0.2 mg(As)/m3; 0.2 mg(Se)/m3; Suspected Carcinogen

SAFETY PROFILE: Confirmed human carcinogen with experimental tumorigenic data. When heated to decomposition it emits very toxic fumes of As and Se.

ARJ500   CAS: 14060-38-9
ARSENIOUS ACID SODIUM SALT
mf: $AsH_3O_3 \cdot 7Na$ mw: 286.88

PROP: Colorless or grayish-white powder. D: 1.87.

SYNS: ARSONIC ACID, SODIUM SALT (9CI) ◇ ARSENIOUS ACID, SODIUM SALT POLYMERS ◇ NATRIUMARSENIT (GERMAN) ◇ SODIUM ORTHOARSENITE

CONSENSUS REPORTS: Arsenic and its compounds are on the Community Right-To-Know List.

OSHA PEL: TWA 0.01 mg(As)/m^3; Cancer Hazard   ACGIH TLV: TWA 0.2 mg(As)/m^3 NIOSH REL: CL 2 μg(As)/m^3/15M

SAFETY PROFILE: Confirmed human carcinogen. Poison by intraperitoneal and subcutaneous routes. Moderately toxic by ingestion. When heated to decomposition it emits toxic fumes of arsenic.

ARK250   CAS: 7784-42-1
ARSINE
DOT: 2188
mf: AsH_3 mw: 77.95

PROP: Colorless gas, mild garlic odor. D: 2.695 g/L; bp: −62.5°; vap d: 2.66; mp: −116°. Solubility in water = 28 mg/100 @ 20°. Sol in benzene and chloroform.

SYNS: ARSENIC HYDRIDE ◇ ARSENIC TRIHYDRIDE ◇ ARSENIURETTED HYDROGEN ◇ ARSENOUS HYDRIDE ◇ ARSENOWODOR (POLISH) ◇ ARSENWASSERSTOFF (GERMAN) ◇ HYDROGEN ARSENIDE

CONSENSUS REPORTS: IARC Cancer Review: Human Sufficient Evidence IMEMDT 23,39,80. Reported in EPA TSCA Inventory. Arsenic and its compounds are on the Community Right-To-Know List. EPA Extremely Hazardous Substances List.

OSHA PEL: TWA 0.05 ppm   ACGIH TLV: TWA 0.05 ppm   DFG MAK: 0.05 ppm (0.2 mg/m^3)   NIOSH REL: CL 2 μg(As)/m^3/15M   DOT Classification: Poison A; Label: Poison Gas and Flammable Gas.

SAFETY PROFILE: Confirmed human carcinogen. Poison by inhalation. Human red blood

cell, gastrointestinal system, central nervous system, and other systemic effects by inhalation. Flammable when exposed to flame. Moderately explosive when exposed to Cl_2; HNO_3; (K + NH_3); open flame; or powerful shock. Dangerous, more toxic than its oxidation product. When heated to decomposition it emits highly toxic fumes of arsenic.

ARM250   CAS: 1332-21-4
ASBESTOS
DOT: 2212/2590

SYNS: AMIANTHUS ◇ AMOSITE (OBS.) ◇ AMPHIBOLE ◇ ASBEST (GERMAN) ◇ ASBESTOS FIBER ◇ FIBROUS GRUNERITE ◇ NCI CO8991 ◇ SERPENTINE

TOXICITY DATA with REFERENCE
NEO: ipl-rat TD:100 mg/kg   BJCAAI 45,352,82
ETA: ihl-ham TCLo:23 mg/m3/7H/47W-I   ENVRAL 10,368,75
ETA: imp-rat TDLo:750 mg/kg   ZEKBAI 62,561,58
ETA: ipl-ham TDLo:80 mg/kg   43GRAK -,335,79
ETA: ipl-rat TD:300 mg/kg/12W-I   VOONAW 20(4),47,74
ETA: ipl-rat TDLo:100 mg/kg   BJCAAI 41,918,80
ETA: ipr-ham TDLo:200 mg/kg   IAPUDO 30,337,80
ETA: ipr-mus TDLo:80 mg/kg   PAACA3 24,61,83
ETA: ipr-rat TD:100 mg/kg   ENVRAL 29,238,82
ETA: ipr-rat TD:200 mg/kg   STRHAV 39,386,79
ETA: ipr-rat TDLo:50 mg/kg   STRHAV 39,386,79
ETA: ipr-rbt TDLo:25 mg/kg   IAPUDO 30,337,80

CONSENSUS REPORTS: IARC Cancer Review: Human Sufficient Evidence IMEMDT 2,17,73; IMEMDT 14,11,77; Animal Sufficient Evidence IMEMDT 2,17,73; IMEMDT 14, 11,77. NTP Fourth Annual Report On Carcinogens, 1984. Reported in EPA TSCA Inventory. On Community Right-To-Know List. EPA Genetic Toxicology Program.

OSHA PEL: TWA 2 million fb/m^3; CL 10 million fb/m^3; Cancer Hazard   ACGIH TLV: Human Carcinogen, TWA 2 fb/cc   DFG TRK: (Fine dust particles which are able to reach the alveolar area of the lung) crocidolite: 0.05 × 10^6 fibers/m^3 (0.025 mg/m^3) (definition of fiber: length greater than 5 μm; diameter less than 3 μm; length/diameter greater than 3:1, equivalent to 1 fiber/cc); chrysotile, amosite, anthophyllite, tremolite, actinolite: 1 × 10^6 fibers/m^3 (0.05 mg/m^3) applicable when there is more than 2.5% asbestos in the dust; 2.0 mg/m^3 applicable when there is less than or equal to 2.5

wt % asbestos in fine dust.   NIOSH REL: TWA 100,000 fb/m^3 over 5 μm in length   DOT Classification: ORM-C.

SAFETY PROFILE: Confirmed human carcinogen producing lung tumors. Experimental neoplastigenic and tumorigenic data. Human pulmonary system effects by inhalation. Usually at least 4 to 7 years of exposure are required before serious lung damage (fibrosis) results. A common air contaminant.

ARM260   CAS: 77536-66-4
ASBESTOS, ACTINOLITE

SYNS: ACTINOLITE ASBESTOS ◊ ASBESTOS (ACGIH)

CONSENSUS REPORTS: IARC Cancer Review: Animal Sufficient Evidence IMEMDT 14,11,77.

OSHA PEL: TWA 2 million fb/m^3; CL 10 million fb/m^3; Cancer Hazard   ACGIH TLV: Human Carcinogen, TWA 2 fb/cc   DFG TRK: (Fine dust particles which are able to reach the alveolar area of the lung) 1 × 10^6 fibers/m^3 (0.05 mg/m^3) applicable when there is more than 2.5% asbestos in the dust.   NIOSH REL: TWA 100,000 fb/m^3 over 5 μm in length

SAFETY PROFILE: Confirmed human carcinogen.

ARM262   CAS: 12172-73-5
ASBESTOS, AMOSITE

SYNS: AMOSITE ASBESTOS ◊ ASBESTOS (ACGIH)
◊ MYSORITE ◊ NCI C60253A

TOXICITY DATA with REFERENCE
CAR: ihl-man TCLo:400 mppcf/1Y-C:PUL
   AEHLAU 28,61,74
CAR: ihl-rat TCLo:11 mg/m^3/2Y-I   BJCAAI
   29,252,74
CAR: ipl-rat TD:100 mg/kg   BJCAAI 23,567,69
CAR: ipl-rat TDLo:80 mg/kg   TOLED5 13,143,82
CAR: ipr-mus TDLo:80 mg/kg   ENVRAL35,277,84
CAR: scu-mus TDLo:2400 mg/kg/13W-I
   FCTXAV 6,566,68
NEO: ihl-rat TC :12 mg/m^3/13W-I   RRCRBU
   39,37,72
NEO: imp-rat TDLo:200 mg/kg   JJIND8 67,965,81
NEO: ipl-rat TD:200 mg/kg   BJCAAI 28,173,73
NEO: ipl-rat TD:200 mg/kg   JNCIAM 48,797,72
NEO: ipl-rat TD:100 mg/kg   JJIND8 79,797,87
ETA: ihl-rat TC :10 mg/m^3/52W-C   IAPUDO
   30,285,80

ETA: itr-rat TDLo:12 mg/kg/12W-I   TOLED5
   13,143,82
ETA: mul-ham TDLo:290 g/kg/35W-C
   ANYAA9 132,456,65
MUT: cyt-ham:ovr 10 mg/L   CSHCAL 4,941,77
MUT: msc-ham:lng 10 mg/L   MUREAV 68,265,79
MUT: sce-ham:ovr 10 mg/L   JEPTDQ 4(2-3),373,80

CONSENSUS REPORTS: IARC Cancer Review: GROUP 1 IMEMDT 7,106,87; Animal Sufficient Evidence IMEMDT 2,17,73; IMEMDT 14,11,77; Human Sufficient Evidence IMEMDT 2,17,73; IMEMDT 14,11,77. NTP Fourth Annual Report On Carcinogens, 1984. NTP Carcinogenesis Studies (feed); No Evidence: hamster NTPTR* NTP-TR-249,83. EPA Genetic Toxicology Program.

OSHA PEL: TWA 2 million fb/m^3; CL 10 million fb/m^3; Cancer Hazard   ACGIH TLV: Human Carcinogen, TWA 0.5 fb/cc   DFG TRK: (Fine dust particles which are able to reach the alveolar area of the lung) 1 × 10^6 fibers/m^3 (0.05 mg/m^3) applicable when there is more than 2.5% asbestos in the dust.   NIOSH REL: TWA 100,000 fb/m^3 over 5 μm in length

SAFETY PROFILE: Confirmed human carcinogen with experimental carcinogenic, neoplastigenic, and tumorigenic data. Mutation data reported.

ARM264   CAS: 77536-67-5
ASBESTOS, ANTHOPHYLITE

SYNS: ANTHOPHYLITE ◊ ASBESTOS (ACGIH)
◊ AZBOLEN ASBESTOS ◊ FERROANTHOPHYLLITE

TOXICITY DATA with REFERENCE
CAR: ihl-rat TCLo:11 mg/m^3/1Y-I   BJCAAI
   29,252,74
NEO: ipl-ham TDLo:83 mg/kg   31BYAP -,92,74
NEO: ipl-rat TDLo:200 mg/kg   BJCAAI 28,173,73
ETA: ipl-rat TD:2400 mg/kg/34W-I   IAPUDO
   30,343,80
MUT: cyt-ham:ovr 10 mg/L   CSHCAL 4,941,77

CONSENSUS REPORTS: IARC Cancer Review: Animal Sufficient Evidence IMEMDT 2,17,73; IMEMDT 14,11,77; Human Sufficient Evidence IMEMDT 14,11,77. NTP Fourth Annual Report On Carcinogens, 1984. EPA Genetic Toxicology Program.

OSHA PEL: TWA 2 million fb/m^3; CL 10 million fb/m^3; Cancer Hazard   ACGIH TLV: Human Carcinogen, TWA 2 fb/cc   DFG TRK:

(Fine dust particles which are able to reach the alveolar area of the lung) 1×10^6 fibers/m³ (0.05 mg/m³) applicable when there is more than 2.5% asbestos in the dust   NIOSH REL: TWA 100,000 fb/m³ over 5 μm in length

SAFETY PROFILE: Confirmed human carcinogen with experimental carcinogenic, neoplastigenic, and tumorigenic data. Mutation data reported.

ARM266   CAS: 17068-78-9
ASBESTOS, ANTHOPHYLLITE

SYNS: AZBLLEN ASBESTOS ◇ 16 F

ETA: ipr-rat TDLo: 250 mg/kg   ZHYGAM 32,89,86
ETA: ipl-rat TDLo: 300 mg/kg/12W-I
ZHYGAM 32,89,86

SAFETY PROFILE: Confirmed carcinogen with experimental tumorigenic data.

ARM268   CAS: 12001-29-5
ASBESTOS, CHRYSOTILE
DOT: 2590

SYNS: 7-45 ASBESTOS ◇ ASBESTOS (ACGIH) ◇ ASBESTOS, WHITE (DOT) ◇ AVIBEST C ◇ CALIDRIA RG 100 ◇ CALIDRIA RG 144 ◇ CALIDRIA RG 600 ◇ CASSIAR AK ◇ CHRYSOTILE ASBESTOS ◇ CHRYSOTILE (DOT) ◇ HOOKER NO. 1 CHRYSOTILE ASBESTOS ◇ METAXITE ◇ NCI C61223A ◇ PLASTIBEST 20 ◇ SERPENTINE ◇ SERPENTINE CHRYSOTILE ◇ SYLODEX ◇ WHITE ASBESTOS

TOXICITY DATA with REFERENCE
CAR: ihl-man TCLo: 400 mppcf/1Y-C: PUL
AEHLAU 28,61,74
CAR: ihl-rat TC : 11 mg/m³/8H/26W-I   IAPUDO 30,363,80
CAR: ihl-rat TCLo: 11 mg/m³/26W-I   BJCAAI 29,252,74
CAR: ipl-rat TDLo: 100 mg/kg   BJCAAI 23,567,69
CAR: ipr-mus TDLo: 80 mg/kg   ENVRAL 35,277,84
CAR: ipr-rat TDLo: 9 mg/kg   ZHPMAT 162,467,76
CAR: itr-mus TDLo: 200 mg/kg   PAACA3 15,6,74
CAR: orl-rat TDLo: 7100 mg/kg/39W-C
ARGEAR 46,437,76
NEO: ihl-rat TC : 12 mg/m³/13W-I   RRCRBU 39,37,72
NEO: ipl-rat TD: 90 mg/kg   JSOMBS 29,20,79
NEO: ipl-rat TD: 120 mg/kg/2W-I   CALEDQ 17,313,83
NEO: ipl-rat TD: 200 mg/kg   JNCIAM 48,797,72
NEO: ipr-rat TD: 28 mg/kg   NATWAY 59,318,72
NEO: scu-mus TDLo: 2400 mg/kg/13W-I
FCTXAV 6,566,68

ETA: ihl-rat TC : 10 mg/m³/52W-C   IAPUDO 30,285,80
ETA: imp-rat TDLo: 200 mg/kg   IARCCD 8,289,73
ETA: ipr-mus TD: 400 mg/kg   ENVRAL 27,433,82
ETA: ipr-rat TD: 90 mg/kg   ENVRAL 4,496,71
ETA: itr-ham TD: 48 mg/kg/6W-I   IAPUDO 30,305,80
ETA: itr-rat TDLo: 13 mg/kg   ENVRAL 21,63,80
ETA: mul-ham TDLo: 240 g/kg/35W-
ANYAA9 132,456,65
MUT: cyt-ham: emb 100 μg/L   ENVRAL 10,165,75
MUT: oms-ham: ovr 10 mg/L   MUREAV 116,369,83
MUT: oms-hmn: fbr 10 mg/L   MUREAV 116,369,83
MUT: otr-ham: emb 250 ng/cm²   PAACA3 24,96,83
MUT: sce-ham: ovr 100 μg/L   ENVRAL 24,325,81

CONSENSUS REPORTS: IARC Cancer Review: Human Sufficient Evidence IMEMDT 2,17,73; Animal Sufficient Evidence IMEMDT 2,17,73. NTP Fourth Annual Report On Carcinogens, 1984. NTP Carcinogenesis Studies (feed); Some Evidence: rat NTPTR* NTP-TR-295,85. EPA Genetic Toxicology Program.

OSHA PEL: TWA 2 million fb/m³; CL 10 million fb/m³:; Cancer Hazard   ACGIH TLV: Human Carcinogen, TWA 2 fb/cc   DFG TRK: (Fine dust particles which are able to reach the alveolar area of the lung) 1×10^6 fibers/m³ (0.05 mg/m³) applicable when there is more than 2.5% asbestos in the dust.   NIOSH REL: TWA 100,000 fb/m³ over 5 μm in length

SAFETY PROFILE: Confirmed human carcinogen producing tumors of the lung. Human mutation data reported. Poison by intraperitoneal route. Human systemic effects by inhalation: lung fibrosis, dyspnea and cough.

ARM275   CAS: 12001-28-4
ASBESTOS, CROCIDOLITE
DOT: 2212

SYNS: AMORPHOUS CROCIDOLITE ASBESTOS ◇ ASBESTOS (ACGIH) ◇ BLUE ASBESTOS (DOT) ◇ CROCIDOLITE ASBESTOS ◇ CROCIDOLITE (DOT) ◇ FIBROUS CROCIDOLITE ASBESTOS ◇ KROKYDOLITH (GERMAN) ◇ NCI C09007

TOXICITY DATA with REFERENCE
CAR: ihl-rat TCLo: 11 mg/m³/1Y-I   BJCAAI 29,252,74
CAR: ipl-rat TDLo: 100 mg/kg   BJCAAI 23,567,69
CAR: ipr-rat TDLo: 100 mg/kg   PBPHAW 14,47,78
CAR: scu-mus TDLo: 2400 mg/kg/12W-I
FCTXAV 6,566,68

CAR: scu-rat TDLo: 112 mg/kg   ANYAA9 271,431,76

NEO: ihl-rat TC : 12 mg/m^3/13W-I   RRCRBU 39,37,72

NEO: imp-rat TDLo: 200 mg/kg   JJIND8 67,965,81

NEO: ipl-ham TDLo: 83 mg/kg   31BYAP -,92,74

NEO: ipl-rat TD: 10 mg/kg   JNCIAM 48,797,72

ETA: imp-rat TD: 200 mg/kg   IARCCD 8,289,73

ETA: ipl-mus TDLo: 200 mg/kg   31BYAP -,92,74

ETA: ipl-rat TD: 100 mg/kg   IAPUDO 30,311,80

ETA: ipl-rbt TDLo: 8 mg/kg   ENVRAL 4,496,71

ETA: ipr-rat TD: 90 mg/kg   ENVRAL 4,496,71

ETA: ipr-rat TD: 100 mg/kg   ENVRAL 29,238,82

ETA: ipr-rat TD: 125 mg/kg   ENVRAL 29,238,82

ETA: ipr-rat TD: 250 mg/kg   ENVRAL 29,123,82

ETA: itr-dog TDLo: 52 mg/kg/2Y-I   CANCAR 47,1994,81

ETA: scu-mus TD: 1200 mg/kg/10W-I   IJCNAW 2,628,67

ETA: scu-rat TD: 112 mg/kg   PBPHAW 14,47,78

MUT: cyt-ham: emb 2 mg/L   CRNGDP 6,473,85

MUT: dns-ham: oth 1280 ng/cm^2 CNREA8 42,3669,82

MUT: oms-ham: ovr 10 mg/L   MUREAV 116,369,83

MUT: sce-ham: ovr 10 mg/plate   JEPTDQ 4(2-3),373,80

CONSENSUS REPORTS: IARC Cancer Review: Animal Sufficient Evidence IMEMDT 14,11,77, IMEMDT 2,17,73; Human Sufficient Evidence IMEMDT 14,11,77. NTP Fourth Annual Report On Carcinogens, 1984. EPA Genetic Toxicology Program.

OSHA PEL: TWA 2 million fb/m^3; CL 10 million fb/m^3; Cancer Hazard   ACGIH TLV: Human Carcinogen, TWA 0.2 fb/cc   DFG TRK: (Fine dust particles which are able to reach the alveolar area of the lung) crocidolite: 0.05 × 10^6 fibers/m^3 (0.025 mg/m^3) (definition of fiber: length greater than 5 μm; diameter less than 3 μm; length/diameter greater than 3:1, equivalent to 1 fiber/cc). NIOSH REL: TWA 100,000 fb/m^3 over 5 μm in length   DOT Classification: ORM-C; LABEL: none

SAFETY PROFILE: Confirmed human carcinogen with experimental carcinogenic, neoplastigenic, and tumorigenic data by inhalation. Human mutation data reported.

ARM280   CAS: 77536-68-6
ASBESTOS, TREMOLITE

SYNS: ASBESTOS (ACGIH) ◇ FIBROUS TREMOLITE ◇ NCI-C08991 ◇ TREMOLITE ASBESTOS

TOXICITY DATA with REFERENCE

NEO: imp-rat TDLo: 200 mg/kg   JJIND8 67,965,81

NEO: ipl-rat TDLo: 100 mg/kg   BJCAAI 45,352,82

CONSENSUS REPORTS: IARC Cancer Review: Human Sufficient Evidence IMEMDT 14,11,77; Animal Sufficient Evidence IMEMDT 14,11,77. NTP Fourth Annual Report On Carcinogens, 1984.

OSHA PEL: TWA 2 million fb/m^3; CL 10 million fb/m^3; Cancer Hazard   ACGIH TLV: Human Carcinogen, TWA 2 fb/cc   DFG TRK: (Fine dust particles which are able to reach the alveolar area of the lung) 1 × 10^6 fibers/m^3 (0.05 mg/m^3) applicable when there is more than 2.5% asbestos in the dust.

NIOSH REL: TWA 100,000 fb/m^3 over 5 μm in length

SAFETY PROFILE: Confirmed human carcinogen with experimental tumorigenic and neoplastigenic data.

ART250   CAS: 12192-57-3
1-AUROTHIO-d-GLUCOPYRANOSE
mf: C$_6$H$_{11}$O$_5$S•Au   mw: 392.20

SYNS: AUREOTAN ◇ AUROMYOSE ◇ AUROTAN ◇ AUROTHIOGLUCOSE ◇ AURUMINE ◇ AUTHRON ◇ BRENOL ◇ (d-GLUCOPYRANOSYLTHIO)GOLD ◇ (1-d-GLUCOSYLTHIO)GOLD ◇ GLYSANOL B ◇ GOLD THIOGLUCOSE ◇ GTG ◇ ORONOL ◇ ROMOSOL ◇ SOLGANAL ◇ SOLGANAL B ◇ (1-THIO-d-GLUCOPYRA-NOSATO)GOLD ◇ 1-THIO-GLUCOPYRANOSE, MONOGOLD(1+) SALT ◇ THIOGLUCOSE d'OR (FRENCH)

TOXICITY DATA with REFERENCE

CAR: par-mus TD: 750 mg/kg   RFECAC 11,828,66

CAR: par-mus TDLo: 400 mg/kg   PAACA3 3,37,59

NEO: par-mus TD: 750 mg/kg   RFECAC 13,40,68

CONSENSUS REPORTS: IARC Cancer Review: GROUP 1 IMEMDT 7,56,87; Animal Limited Evidence IMEMDT 13,39,77

SAFETY PROFILE: Confirmed carcinogen with experimental carcinogenic, neoplastigenic, and teratogenic data. A deadly human poison by an unspecified route. An experimental poison by intramuscular route. Moderately toxic by subcutaneous and intravenous routes. Other experimental reproductive effects. When heated to decomposition it emits very toxic fumes of SO$_x$. Used to treat rheumatoid arthritis.

ASB250
AZATHIOPRINE

CAS: 446-86-6

mf: $C_9H_7N_7O_2S$ mw: 277.29

SYNS: AZANIN ◇ AZATIOPRIN ◇ AZOTHIOPRINE ◇ BW 57-322 ◇ CCUCOL ◇ IMURAN ◇ IMUREK ◇ IMUREL ◇ METHYLNITROIMIDAZOLYLMERCAPTO-PURINE ◇ 6-(1′-METHYL-4′-NITRO-5′-IMIDAZOLYL)-MER-CAPTOPURINE ◇ 6-(METHYL-p-NITRO-5-IMIDAZOLYL)-THIOPURINE ◇ 6-((1-METHYL-4-NITROIMIDAZOL-5-YL)THIO)PURINE ◇ 6-(1-METHYL-p-NITRO-5-IMIDAZO-LYL)-THIOPURINE ◇ 6-(1-METHYL-4-NITROIMIDAZOL 5 YLTHIO)PURINE ◇ 6-((1-METHYL-4-NITRO-1H-IMIDAZOL-5-YL)THIO)-1H-PURINE ◇ NCI-C03474 ◇ NSC-39084 ◇ RORASUL

TOXICITY DATA with REFERENCE

CAR: ims-mus TDLo:3500 mg/kg/26W-I
  BLOOAW 31,396,68
CAR: orl-man TD:728 mg/kg/43W-C:BLD
  AJMSA9 273,335,77
CAR: orl-man TD:1565 mg/kg/4Y-C:BLD
  AJMEAZ 57,885,74
CAR: orl-man TD:3266 mg/kg/3Y-C:BLD
  AJMEAZ 57,885,74
CAR: orl-rat TD:11 g/kg/W-C   PAACA3 24,91,83
CAR: orl-wmn TD:2 g/kg/3Y-C:BLD
  PGMJAO 53,173,77
CAR: orl-wmn TD:3 g/kg/3.5Y-C:KID
  JAMAAP 237,152,77
CAR: orl-wmn TD:5460 mg/kg/6Y-I:BLD
  AMSVAZ 207,315,80
CAR: orl-wmn TDLo:273 mg/kg/13W-C:
  BLD   BMJOAE 4,235,72
CAR: scu-mus TD:2600 mg/kg/65W-I
  ARZNAD 29,483,79
CAR: scu-mus TDLo:1200 mg/kg/30W-I
  ARZNAD 29,662,79
ETA: ipr-mus TDLo:585 mg/kg/26W-I
  CANCAR 40(Suppl 4),1935,77
ETA: ipr-rat TDLo:360 mg/kg/7W-I   CANCAR
  40(Suppl 4),1935,77
ETA: orl-rat TDLo:1932 mg/kg/46W-C
  ESKHA5 (102),66,84
MUT: cyt-hmn-unr 1074 mg/kg/4Y   MUREAV
  94,501,82
MUT: cyt-hmn:leu 6 mg/L   ZGASAX 9,47,71
MUT: dlt-mus-orl 50 mg/kg/2D   MUREAV 28,87,75
MUT: sce-hmn:lym 100 mg/L   MUREAV 53,215,78
MUT: spm-mus-orl 50 mg/kg/2D   MUREAV
  28,87,75

CONSENSUS REPORTS: IARC Cancer Review: Human Sufficient Evidence IMEMDT 26,47,81; Animal Limited Evidence IMEMDT 26,47,81. NTP Fourth Annual Report On Carcinogens, 1984. NCI Carcinogenesis Studies (ipr); No Evidence: rat CANCAR 40,1935,77; Clear Evidence: mouse CANCAR 40,1935,77. EPA Genetic Toxicology Program.

SAFETY PROFILE: Confirmed human carcinogen producing bladder tumors and leukemia. Poison by subcutaneous, intradermal and intraperitoneal routes. Moderately toxic by ingestion. Other human systemic effects by ingestion and unspecified routes: anemia, bone marrow abnormalities, hair effects, and metabolic effects. An experimental teratogen. Other experimental reproductive effects. Human mutation data reported. When heated to decomposition it emits very toxic fumes of NO_x and SO_x. An immunosuppressant.

BAK250
BARIUM CHROMATE(VI)

CAS: 10294-40-3

mf: $Ba•CrH_2O_4$ mw: 255.36

PROP: Heavy, yellow, crystalline powder. D: 4.498 @ 15°.

SYNS: BARIUM CHROMATE (1:1) ◇ BARIUM CHROMATE OXIDE ◇ BARYTA YELLOW ◇ CHROMIC ACID, BARIUM SALT (1:1) ◇ C.I. 77103 ◇ C.I. PIGMENT YELLOW 31 ◇ LEMON CHROME ◇ LEMON YELLOW ◇ PERMANENT YELLOW ◇ STEINBUHL YELLOW ◇ ULTRAMARINE YELLOW

TOXICITY DATA with REFERENCE
MUT: sce-ham:ovr 100 µg/L   MUREAV 156,219,85

CONSENSUS REPORTS: IARC Cancer Review: Animal Inadequate Evidence IMEMDT 2,100,73; Human Sufficient Evidence IMEMDT 23,205,80. Reported in EPA TSCA Inventory. Barium and its compounds are on the Community Right-To-Know List.

OSHA PEL: TWA 0.1 mg $(C_3O_3)m^3$; 0.5 mg(Ba)/m^3 ACGIH TLV: TWA 0.5 mg(Ba)/m^3; 0.05 mg(Cr)/m^3; Confirmed Human Carcinogen   NIOSH REL: TWA 0.001 mg(Cr (VI))/m^3

SAFETY PROFILE: Confirmed human carcinogen. A poison. Mutation data reported. Used in pyrotechnics and as an explosive initiator.

BAW250
BENZ(e)ACEPHENANTHRYLENE
CAS: 205-99-2

mf: $C_{20}H_{12}$ mw: 252.32

PROP: Mp: 168°.

SYNS: 3,4-BENZ(e)ACEPHENANTHRYLENE ◇ 2,3-BENZ-FLUORANTHENE ◇ 3,4-BENZFLUORANTHENE ◇ BENZO(b)FLUORANTHENE ◇ BENZO(e)FLUORANTHENE ◇ 2,3-BENZOFLUORANTHENE ◇ 3,4-BENZOFLUORANTHENE ◇ 2,3-BENZOFLUORANTHRENE ◇ B(b)F

TOXICITY DATA with REFERENCE
NEO: ipr-mus TDLo: 5046 μg/kg/15D-I CALEDQ 34,15,87
ETA: imp-rat TD: 5 mg/kg 50NNAZ 7,571,83
ETA: scu-mus TDLo: 72 mg/kg/9W-I AICCA6 19,490,63
ETA: skn-mus TD: 72 mg/kg/60W-I CANCAR 12,1194,59
ETA: skn-mus TD: 4037 μg/kg/20D-I CRNGDP 6,1023,85
MUT: mma-sat 31 nmol/plate CRNGDP 6,1023,85
MUT: otr-ham: lng 100 μg/L TXCYAC 17,149,80
MUT: sce-ham-ipr 900 mg/kg/24H MUREAV 66,65,79

CONSENSUS REPORTS: IARC Cancer Review: GROUP 2B IMEMDT 7,56,87, Animal Sufficient Evidence IMEMDT 32,147,83; IMEMDT 3,69,73. NTP Fourth Annual Report On Carcinogens, 1984. EPA Genetic Toxicology Program.

SAFETY PROFILE: Confirmed carcinogen with experimental carcinogenic and tumorigenic data. Mutation data reported. When heated to decomposition it emits acrid smoke and irritating fumes.

BBC250
BENZ(a)ANTHRACENE
CAS: 56-55-3

mf: $C_{18}H_{12}$ mw: 228.30

PROP: Colorless leaflets or plates. Bp: 400°, mp: 160°.

SYNS: BA ◇ BENZANTHRACENE ◇ 1,2-BENZANTHRACENE ◇ 1,2-BENZ(a)ANTHRACENE ◇ 1,2-BENZANTHRAZEN (GERMAN) ◇ BENZANTHRENE ◇ 1,2-BENZANTHRENE ◇ BENZOANTHRACENE ◇ 1,2-BENZOANTHRACENE ◇ BENZO(a)ANTHRACENE ◇ BENZO(a)PHENANTHRENE ◇ BENZO(b)PHENANTHRENE ◇ 2,3-BENZOPHENANTHRENE ◇ 2,3-BENZPHENANTHRENE ◇ NAPHTHANTHRACENE ◇ RCRA WASTE NUMBER U018 ◇ TETRAPHENE

TOXICITY DATA with REFERENCE
CAR: imp-mus TDLo: 80 mg/kg BJCAAI 22,825,68

NEO: skn-mus TD: 240 mg/kg/1W-I BJCAAI 9,177,55
NEO: skn-mus TDLo: 18 mg/kg CNREA8 38,1699,78
ETA: scu-mus TDLo: 2 mg/kg CNREA8 15,632,55
ETA: skn-mus TD: 18 mg/kg CNREA8 38,1705,78
ETA: skn-mus TD: 360 mg/kg/56W-I CNREA8 11,892,51
MUT: dnd-mus-skn 192 μmol/kg CRNGDP 5,231,84
MUT: dnd-sal: tes 5 μg/1H-C BIJOAK 110,159,68
MUT: dni-hmn: oth 10 μmol/L CNREA8 42,3676,82
MUT: dns-hmn: hla 100 μmol/L CNREA8 38,2621,78
MUT: dns-rat: lvr 100 μmol/L ENMUDM 3,11,81
MUT: mma-mus: lym 100 mg/L ENMUDM 8(Suppl 6),13,86
MUT: mma-sat 4 μg/plate CRNGDP 5,747,84
MUT: msc-hmn: lym 9 μmol/L DTESD7 10,277,82

CONSENSUS REPORTS: IARC Cancer Review: GROUP 2A IMEMDT 7,56,87, Animal Sufficient Evidence IMEMDT 32,135,83; IMEMDT 3,45,73. NTP Fourth Annual Report On Carcinogens, 1984. EPA Genetic Toxicology Program. Reported in EPA TSCA Inventory.

SAFETY PROFILE: Confirmed carcinogen with experimental carcinogenic, neoplastigenic, tumorigenic data by skin contact and other routes. Poison by intravenous route. Human mutation data reported. It is found in oils, waxes, smoke, food, drugs. When heated to decomposition it emits acrid smoke and irritating fumes.

BBL250
BENZENE
CAS: 71-43-2

DOT: 1114

mf: C_6H_6 mw: 78.12

PROP: Clear, colorless liquid. Mp: 5.51°, bp: 80.093°-80.094°, flash p: 12°F (CC), d: 0.8794 @ 20°, autoign temp: 1044°F, lel: 1.4%, uel: 8.0%, vap press: 100 mm @ 26.1°, vap d: 2.77, ulc: 95-100.

SYNS: (6)ANNULENE ◇ BENZEEN (DUTCH) ◇ BENZEN (POLISH) ◇ BENZIN (OBS.) ◇ BENZINE (OBS.) ◇ BENZOL (DOT) ◇ BENZOLE ◇ BENZOLENE ◇ BENZOLO (ITALIAN) ◇ BICARBURET of HYDROGEN ◇ CARBON OIL ◇ COAL NAPHTHA ◇ CYCLOHEXATRIENE ◇ FENZEN (CZECH) ◇ MINERAL NAPHTHA ◇ MOTOR BENZOL ◇ NCI-C55276 ◇ NITRATION BENZENE ◇ PHENE ◇ PHENYL HYDRIDE ◇ PYROBENZOL ◇ PYROBENZOLE ◇ RCRA WASTE NUMBER U019

TOXICITY DATA with REFERENCE
CAR: ihl-hmn TC:8 ppb/4W-I:BLD   NEJMAG
316,1044,87
CAR: ihl-hmn TC:10 mg/m^3/11Y-I:BLD
BJIMAG 44,124,87
CAR: ihl-hmn TC:150 ppm/15M/8Y-I:BLD
BLOOAW 52,285,78
CAR: ihl-hmn TCLo:10 ppm/8H/10Y-I:BLD
TRBMAV 37,153,78
CAR: ihl-man TC:600 mg/m^3/4Y-I:BLD
NEJMAG 271,872,64
CAR: ihl-man TCLo:200 mg/m^3/78W-I:BLD
EJCAAH 7,83,71
CAR: ihl-mus TC:300ppm/6H/16W-I   IMMUAM
(3),156,84
CAR: orl-mus TDLo:18250 mg/kg/2Y-C
NTPTR* NTP-TR-289,86
CAR: orl-rat TD:10 g/kg/52W-I   MELAAD
70,352,79
CAR: orl-rat TD:52 g/kg/1Y-I   AJIMD8 4,589,83
CAR: orl-rat TDLo:52 g/kg/52W-I   MELAAD
70,352,79
NEO: ipr-mus TDLo:1200 mg/kg/8W-I
TXAPA9 82,19,86
NEO: orl-mus TD:2400 mg/kg/8W-I   TXAPA9
82,19,86
NEO: skn-mus TDLo:1200 g/kg/49W-I   BJCAAI
16,275,62
ETA: ihl-mus TC:1200ppm/6H/10W-I   PAACA3
25,75,84
ETA: ihl-mus TCLo:300 ppm/6H/16W-I
TXAPA9 75,358,84
ETA: ihl-rat TCLo:1200 ppm/6H/10W-I
PAACA3 25,75,84
ETA: par-mus TDLo:670 mg/kg/19W-I
KLWOAZ 12,109,33
ETA: scu-mus TDLo:600 mg/kg/17W-I
KRANAW 9,403,32
MUT: cyt-ham:lng 550 mg/L   PMRSDJ 5,427,85
MUT: mma-mus:emb 2500 mg/L   PMRSDJ
5,639,85
MUT: oms-hmn:lym 5 μmol/L   CNREA8
45,2471,85
MUT: sln-ham:lvr 62500 μg/L   PMRSDJ 5,397,85
MUT: slt-dmg-orl 11250 μmol/L   PMRSDJ5,325,85

CONSENSUS REPORTS: IARC Cancer Review: GROUP 1 IMEMDT 7,120,87; Human Sufficient Evidence IMEMDT 29,93,82; Human Limited Evidence IMEMDT 7,203,74; Animal Inadequate Evidence IMEMDT 7,203,74; IARC Cancer Review: Animal Limited Evidence IMEMDT 29,93,82. NTP Fourth Annual Report On Carcinogens, 1984. NTP Carcinogenesis Studies (gavage); Clear Evidence: mouse, rat NTPTR* NTP-TR-289,86. EPA Genetic Toxicology Program. Reported in EPA TSCA Inventory. On Community Right-To-Know List.

OSHA PEL: (Transitional: TWA 10 ppm; CL 25 ppm; Pk 50 ppm/10M) TWA 1 ppm; STEL 5 ppm; Pk 5 ppm/15M/8H; Cancer Hazard   ACGIH TLV: TWA 10 ppm; Suspected Human Carcinogen; BEI: 50 mg(total phenol)/L in urine at end of shift recommended as a mean value.   DFG TRK: 5 ppm (16 mg/m^3) Human Carcinogen.   NIOSH REL: TWA 0.32 mg/m^3; CL 3.2 mg/m^3/15M   DOT Classification: Flammable Liquid; Label: Flammable Liquid.

SAFETY PROFILE: Confirmed human carcinogen producing myeloid leukemia, Hodgkin's disease, and lymphomas by inhalation. Experimental carcinogenic, neoplastigenic, tumorigenic, and teratogenic data. A human poison by inhalation. An experimental poison by skin contact, intraperitoneal, intravenous and possibly other routes. Moderately toxic by ingestion and subcutaneous routes. A severe eye and moderate skin irritant. Human systemic effects by inhalation and ingestion: euphoria, somnolence, changes in REM sleep, changes in motor activity, nausea or vomiting, reduced number of blood platelets, other unspecified blood effects, dermatitis, and fever. Other experimental animal reproductive effects. Human mutation data reported. A narcotic. A dangerous fire hazard when exposed to heat or flame. Use with adequate ventilation. To fight fire, use foam, CO$_2$, dry chemical.

BBP750   CAS: 608-73-1
BENZENE HEXACHLORIDE
mf: C$_6$H$_6$Cl$_6$ mw: 290.82

PROP: Technical grade contains 68.7% α-BHC, 6.5% β-BHC and 13.5% γ-BHC (JPFCD2 14,305,79). White, crystalline powder. Mp: 113°, vap press: 0.0317 mm @ 20°.

SYNS: BHC (USDA) ◇ COMPOUND-666 ◇ DBH ◇ ENT 8,601 ◇ GAMMEXANE ◇ HCCH ◇ HEXA ◇ HEXACHLOR ◇ HEXACHLORAN ◇ HEXACHLOROCYCLOHEXANE ◇ 1,2,3,4,5,6-HEXACHLOROCYCLOHEXANE ◇ HEXYLAN

TOXICITY DATA with REFERENCE
CAR: orl-mus TD:12960 mg/kg/26W-C
CMSHAF 1,279,72

CAR: orl-mus TD:21600 mg/kg/52W-C
TUMOAB 69,383,83
CAR: orl-mus TD:12600 mg/kg/30W-C
JCROD7 99,143,81
CAR: orl-mus TDLo:6720 mg/kg/80W-C
JPFCD2 14(3),305,79
NEO: orl-mus TD:5400 mg/kg/13W-C
TUMOAB 69,383,83
ETA: orl-mus TD:9 g/kg/21W-C   AEHLAU
37,156,82
ETA: orl-mus TD:7200 mg/kg/17W-C CMBID4
27,231,81
ETA: orl-mus TD:7200 mg/kg/17W-C   IJEBA6
19,1159,81
ETA: orl-mus TD:10800 mg/kg/26W-C
AEHLAU 37,156,82
ETA: orl-mus TD:10800 mg/kg/26W-C
CMBID4 27,231,81
ETA: orl-mus TD:800 mg/kg/80W-I   JPFCD2
14(3),305,79
ETA: skn-mus TDLo:1600 mg/kg/80W-I
JPFCD2 14(3),305,79
MUT: mmo-omi 100 mg/L   MILEDM 5,103,77
MUT: otr-rat-orl 875 mg/kg/7W-I   CRNGDP
5,479,84

CONSENSUS REPORTS: IARC Cancer Review: Animal Sufficient Evidence IMEMDT 5,47,74

SAFETY PROFILE: Confirmed carcinogen with experimental carcinogenic, neoplastigenic, and tumorigenic data by ingestion and skin contact. Poison by ingestion and subcutaneous routes. Moderately toxic by skin contact. Human systemic effects by inhalation: headache, nausea or vomiting, and fever. Implicated in aplastic anemia. Experimental reproductive effects. Mutation data reported. Lindane is more toxic than DDT or dieldrin. When heated to decomposition it emits highly toxic fumes of phosgene, HCl and Cl⁻. When heated to decomposition it emits highly toxic fumes of phosgene, HCl and Cl⁻.

BBQ000   CAS: 319-84-6
BENZENE HEXACHLORIDE-α-isomer
mf: $C_6H_6Cl_6$ mw: 290.82

SYNS: α-BENZENEHEXACHLORIDE ◊ α-BHC ◊ ENT 9,232 ◊ α-HCH ◊ α-HEXACHLORANE ◊ HEXACHLORCYCLOHEXAN (GERMAN) ◊ α-HEXACHLOROCYCLOHEXANE ◊ α-1,2,3,4,5,6-HEXACHLOROCYCLOHEXANE (MAK) ◊ 1-α,2-α,3-β,4-α,5-β,6-β-HEXACHLOROCYCLOHEXANE ◊ α-LINDANE

TOXICITY DATA with REFERENCE
CAR: orl-mus TD:12960 mg/kg/26W-C
CMSHAF 1,279,72
CAR: orl-mus TD:10 g/kg/24W-C   NAIZAM
25,635,74
CAR: orl-mus TDLo:5 g/kg/24W-C   JNCIAM
51,1637,73
NEO: orl-rat TDLo:20 g/kg/48W-C   JNCIAM
54,801,75
ETA: orl-mus TD:5040 mg/kg/24W-C   SAIGBL
17,54,75
ETA: orl-mus TD:8820 mg/kg/21W-C   JJIND8
71,1307,83
ETA: orl-rat TD:11040 mg/kg/86W-C   CNREA8
41,4140,81
ETA: orl-rat TD:13020 mg/kg/92W-I   CNREA8
41,4140,81
MUT: cyt-rat-orl 756 mg/kg/3W   JNCIAM
54,1245,75
MUT: dns-rat:lvr 1 μmol/L   CNREA8 42,3010,82

CONSENSUS REPORTS: IARC Cancer Review: Animal Sufficient Evidence IMEMDT 20,195,79; IMEMDT 5,47,74. NTP Fourth Annual Report On Carcinogens, 1984. EPA Genetic Toxicology Program. Reported in EPA TSCA Inventory.

DFG MAK: 0.5 mg/m³

SAFETY PROFILE: Confirmed carcinogen with experimental carcinogenic, tumorigenic and neoplastigenic data. Poison by ingestion. Mutation data reported. When heated to decomposition it emits toxic fumes of Cl⁻.

BBQ500   CAS: 58-89-9
BENZENE HEXACHLORIDE-γ isomer
DOT: 2761
mf: $C_6H_6Cl_6$ mw: 290.82

SYNS: AALINDAN ◊ AFICIDE ◊ AGRISOL G-20 ◊ AGROCIDE ◊ AGRONEXIT ◊ AMEISENATOD ◊ AMEISENMITTEL MERCK ◊ APARSIN ◊ APHTIRIA ◊ APLIDAL ◊ ARBITEX ◊ BBH ◊ BEN-HEX ◊ BENTOX 10 ◊ γ-BENZENE HEXACHLORIDE ◊ BEXOL ◊ BHC ◊ γ-BHC ◊ CELANEX ◊ CHLORESENE ◊ CODECHINE ◊ DBH ◊ DETMOL-EXTRAKT ◊ DETOX 25 ◊ DEVORAN ◊ DOL GRANULE ◊ DRILL TOX-SPEZIAL AGLUKON ◊ ENT 7,796 ◊ ENTOMOXAN ◊ EXAGAMA ◊ FORLIN ◊ GALLOGAMA ◊ GAMACID ◊ GAMAPHEX ◊ GAMENE ◊ GAMISO ◊ GAMMA-COL ◊ GAMMAHEXA ◊ GAMMAHEXANE ◊ GAMMALIN ◊ GAMMOPAZ ◊ HCCH ◊ HCH ◊ γ-HCH ◊ HECLOTOX ◊ HEXACHLORAN ◊ γ-HEXACHLORAN ◊ γ-HEXACHLORANE ◊ γ-HEXACHLOROBENZENE ◊ 1-α,2-α,3-β,4-α,5-α,6-β-HEXACHLOROCYCLOHEXANE

◇ γ-HEXACHLOROCYCLOHEXANE (MAK) ◇ 1,2,3,4,5,6-
HEXACHLOROCYCLOHEXANE, γ-ISOMER ◇ HEXATOX
◇ HEXICIDE ◇ HGI ◇ INEXIT ◇ ISOTOX ◇ JACUTIN
◇ KOKOTINE ◇ KWELL ◇ LENDINE ◇ LENTOX
◇ LIDENAL ◇ LINDAGRAIN ◇ LINDANE (ACGIH, DOT,
USDA) ◇ LINTOX ◇ MILBOL 49 ◇ MSZYCOL ◇ NCI-C00204
◇ NEO-SCABICIDOL ◇ NEXIT ◇ NOVIGAM ◇ OVADZIAK
◇ PEDRACZAK ◇ QUELLADA ◇ RCRA WASTE NUMBER
U129 ◇ SANG gamma ◇ STREUNEX ◇ TAP 85 ◇ VITON

TOXICITY DATA with REFERENCE
CAR: orl-mus TDLo:14 g/kg/2Y-C   CRNGDP
8,1889,87
NEO: orl-mus TD:25 g/kg/73W-C   FCTXAV
11,433,73
MUT: cyt-ham:fbr 63 mg/L/48H   MUREAV
48,337,77
MUT: dlt-mus-orl 6720 mg/kg   MUREAV101,315,82
MUT: dnd-rat:lvr 30 μmol/L   SinJF# 26OCT82
MUT: dns-ofs:lvr 45 μmol/L   HKXUDL 4,268,84
MUT: dns-rat:lvr 100 pmol/L   CRNGDP 5,1547,84
MUT: mnt-mus-ipr 100 mg/kg   GISAAA49(5),82,84
MUT: msc-ham:lng 200 mg/L   GISAAA49(5),82,84

CONSENSUS REPORTS: IARC Cancer Review: Animal Sufficient Evidence IMEMDT
5,47,74; IMEMDT 20,195,79. NTP Fourth Annual Report On Carcinogens, 1984. NCI Carcinogenesis Bioassay (feed); No Evidence:
mouse, rat NCITR* NCI-CG-TR-14,77. EPA
Extremely Hazardous Substances List. EPA Genetic Toxicology Program. Community Right-
To-Know List. Reported in EPA TSCA Inventory.

OSHA PEL: TWA 0.5 mg/m³ (skin) ACGIH
TLV: TWA 0.5 mg/m³ (skin)   DFG MAK: 0.5
mg/m³ DOT Classification: ORM-A; Label:
None.

SAFETY PROFILE: Confirmed carcinogen with
experimental carcinogenic neoplastigenic and
teratogenic data. A human systemic poison by
ingestion. Also a poison by ingestion, skin contact, intraperitoneal, intravenous, and intramuscular routes. Human systemic effects by ingestion: convulsions, dyspnea, and cyanosis. Other
experimental animal reproductive effects. Mutation data reported. When heated to decomposition it emits toxic fumes of Cl⁻, HCl, and phosgene.

BBQ750
BENZENEHEXACHLORIDE (mixed
isomers)
mf: C₆H₆Cl₆   mw: 290.82

PROP: Technical BHC contains about 64% α,
10% β, 13% γ, 9% Δ and 1% ε isomers of
1,2,3,4,5,6-hexachlorocyclohexane   (IARC**
5,47,74).

SYNS: BENZAHEX ◇ BENZEX ◇ DOL ◇ DOLMIX
◇ FBHC ◇ FHCH ◇ 1,2,3,4,5,6-HEXACHLOROCYCLOHEX-
ANE (MIXTURE of ISOMERS) ◇ HEXYCLAN ◇ KOTOL
◇ SOPROCIDE ◇ TECHNICAL BHC ◇ TECHNICAL HCH

TOXICITY DATA with REFERENCE
NEO: orl-mus TDLo:13 g/kg/24W-C   GANNA2
62,431,71
ETA: orl-mus TD:11 g/kg/26W-C   TXCYAC
19,31,81

CONSENSUS REPORTS: IARC Cancer Review: Animal Sufficient Evidence IMEMDT
5,47,74; IMEMDT 20,195,79. NTP Fourth Annual Report On Carcinogens, 1984.

SAFETY PROFILE: Confirmed carcinogen with
experimental tumorigenic and neoplastigenic
data. Poison by inhalation and ingestion. Human
systemic effects by an unspecified route: convulsions. When heated to decomposition it emits
highly toxic fumes of Cl⁻, HCl, and phosgene.

BBR000   CAS: 319-85-7
trans-α-BENZENEHEXACHLORIDE
mf: C₆H₆Cl₆   mw: 290.82

SYNS: β-BENZENEHEXACHLORIDE ◇ β-BHC ◇ ENT
9,233 ◇ β-HCH ◇ β-HEXACHLOROBENZENE ◇ 1-α,2-β,3-
α,4-β,5-α,6-β-HEXACHLOROCYCLOHEXANE ◇ β-HEXA-
CHLOROCYCLOHEXANE ◇ β-1,2,3,4,5,6-HEXACHLOROCY-
CLOHEXANE (MAK) ◇ β-ISOMER ◇ β-LINDANE

TOXICITY DATA with REFERENCE
NEO: orl-mus TDLo:18 g/kg/2Y-C   FCTXAV
11,433,73

CONSENSUS REPORTS: IARC Cancer Review: Animal Sufficient Evidence IMEMDT
5,47,74; Animal Limited Evidence IMEMDT
20,195,79. NTP Fourth Annual Report On Carcinogens, 1984. Reported in EPA TSCA Inventory.   DFG MAK: 0.5 mg/m³

SAFETY PROFILE: Confirmed carcinogen with
experimental neoplastigenic data. Mildly toxic
by ingestion. When heated to decomposition
it emits very toxic fumes of Cl⁻, HCl, and
phosgene.

BBX000   CAS: 92-87-5
BENZIDINE
DOT: 1885
mf: C₁₂H₁₂N₂   mw: 184.26

PROP: Grayish-yellow, crystalline powder; white or sltly reddish crystals, powder, or leaf. Mp: 127.5-128.7° @ 740 mm, bp: 401.7°, d: 1.250 @ 20°/4°.

SYNS: BENZIDIN (CZECH) ◇ BENZIDINA (ITALIAN) ◇ BENZYDYNA (POLISH) ◇ p,p-BIANILINE ◇ 4,4′-BIANILINE ◇ (1,1′-BIPHENYL)-4,4′-DIAMINE (9CI) ◇ 4,4′-BIPHENYLDIAMINE ◇ 4,4′-BIPHENYLENEDIAMINE ◇ C.I. 37225 ◇ C.I. AZOIC DIAZO COMPONENT 112 ◇ p,p′-DIAMINOBIPHENYL ◇ 4,4′-DIAMINOBIPHENYL ◇ 4,4′-DIAMINO-1,1′-BIPHENYL ◇ p-DIAMINODIPHENYL ◇ 4,4′-DIAMINODIPHENYL ◇ p,p′-DIANILINE ◇ 4,4′-DIPHENYLENEDIAMINE ◇ FAST CORINTH BASE B ◇ NCI-C03361 ◇ RCRA WASTE NUMBER U021

TOXICITY DATA with REFERENCE
CAR: ihl-man TCLo:17600 µg/m^3/14Y-C: KID AEHLAU 27,1,73
CAR: orl-rat TDLo:108 mg/kg/27D-I CNREA8 28,924,68
CAR: scu-rat TDLo:2025 mg/kg/27W-I CANCAR 3,789,50
ETA: ihl-rat TCLo:10 mg/m^3/56W-I BEXBAN 69,68,70
ETA: itr-rat TDLo:315 mg/kg/34W BEXBAN 69,68,70
ETA: orl-ham TDLo:75 mg/kg/3Y-C 85DAAC 5,129,66
ETA: scu-mus TD:1620 g/kg/45W-I AICCA6 7,46,50
ETA: scu-mus TDLo:8400 mg/kg/35W-I VOONAW 17(5),61,71
ETA: scu-rat TD:800 mg/kg/60W-I VOONAW 20(8),69,74
ETA: scu-rat TD:850 mg/kg/32W-I VOONAW 20(2),53,74
MUT: dnd-hmn:fbr 3 mmol/L ENMUDM 7,267,85
MUT: dnd-rat-ipr 63 mg/kg CRNGDP 6,1285,85
MUT: dns-ham:lvr 20 nmol/L MUREAV 136,255,84
MUT: msc-mus:lym 500 µg/L MUREAV 125,291,84
MUT: oms-dog:oth 100 µmol/L CNREA8 44,1893,84

CONSENSUS REPORTS: IARC Cancer Review: Human Limited Evidence IMEMDT 1,80,72; Human Sufficient Evidence IMEMDT 29,149,82; Animal Sufficient Evidence IMEMDT 1,80,72; IMEMDT 29,149,82. NTP Fourth Annual Report On Carcinogens, 1984. EPA Genetic Toxicology Program. Community Right-To-Know List. Reported in EPA TSCA Inventory.

OSHA: Cancer Suspect Agent ACGIH TLV: Confirmed Human Carcinogen DFG MAK: Human Carcinogen. DOT Classification: Poison B; Label: Poison.

SAFETY PROFILE: Confirmed human carcinogen producing bladder tumors. Experimental carcinogenic and tumorigenic data. Poison by ingestion and intraperitoneal routes. Human mutation data reported. Can cause damage to blood, including hemolysis and bone marrow depression. On ingestion causes nausea and vomiting which may be followed by liver and kidney damage. Any exposure is considered extremely hazardous. When heated to decomposition it emits highly toxic fumes of NO$_x$.

BBY000 CAS: 531-86-2
BENZIDINE SULFATE
mf: C$_{12}$H$_{12}$N$_2$•H$_2$O$_4$S mw: 282.34
SYN: (1,1′-BIPHENYL)-4,4′-DIAMINE SULFATE (1:1)

TOXICITY DATA with REFERENCE
CAR: scu-rat TD:3900 mg/kg/52W-I GTPZAB 19(6),28,75
CAR: scu-rat TDLo:2475 mg/kg/33W-I CANCAR 3,789,50

OSHA: Carcinogen

SAFETY PROFILE: Confirmed human carcinogen with experimental carcinogenic data. When heated to decomposition it emits toxic fumes of SO$_x$ and NO$_x$.

BCJ750 CAS: 207-08-9
BENZO(k)FLUORANTHENE
mf: C$_{20}$H$_{12}$ mw: 252.32
SYNS: 8,9-BENZOFLUORANTHENE ◇ 11,12-BENZOFLUORANTHENE ◇ 11,12-BENZO(k)FLUORANTHENE ◇ 2,3,1′,8′-BINAPHTHYLENE ◇ DIBENZO(b,jk)FLUORENE

TOXICITY DATA with REFERENCE
ETA: imp-rat TDLo:5 mg/kg 50NNAZ 7,571,83
ETA: scu-mus TDLo:72 mg/kg/9W-I AICCA6 19,490,63
ETA: skn-mus TDLo:2820 mg/kg/47W-I CANCAR 12,1194,59
MUT: mma-sat 10 µg/plate CNREA8 40,4528,80

CONSENSUS REPORTS: IARC Cancer Review: Animal Sufficient Evidence IMEMDT 32,163,83

SAFETY PROFILE: Confirmed carcinogen with experimental tumorigenic data. Mutation data reported. When heated to decomposition it emits acrid smoke and irritating fumes.

BCQ500   CAS: 189-55-9
BENZO(rst)PENTAPHENE
mf: $C_{24}H_{14}$ mw: 302.38

PROP: Green-yellow needles. Mp: 280-282°.

SYNS: DB(a,i)P ◇ DIBENZO(a,i)PYRENE ◇ DIBEN-ZO(b,h)PYRENE ◇ 1,2,7,8-DIBENZOPYRENE ◇ 3,4:9,10-DI-BENZOPYRENE ◇ DIBENZ(a,i)PYRENE ◇ 1,2:7,8-DI-BENZPYRENE ◇ 3,4:9,10-DIBENZPYRENE ◇ RCRA WASTE NUMBER U064

TOXICITY DATA with REFERENCE
NEO: scu-ham TDLo: 2 mg/kg   NATUAS 203,308,64
ETA: itr-ham TDLo: 33 g/kg/8W-I   ZKKOBW 82,175,74
ETA: scu-ham TD: 16 mg/kg   PEXTAR 11,384,69
ETA: scu-mus TD: 4 mg/kg   NATUAS 192,286,61
ETA: scu-mus TD: 72 mg/kg/9W-I   COREAF 246,1477,58
ETA: scu-mus TD: 80 mg/kg   IJMRAQ 53,638,65
ETA: scu-mus TD: 4 mg/kg   PAACA3 13,37,72
ETA: scu-mus TDLo: 1000 μg/kg   PEXTAR 11,384,69
ETA: skn-mus TD: 141 mg/kg/47W-I   IJMRAQ 53,638,65
ETA: skn-mus TDLo: 47 mg/kg/39W-I   CANCAR 12,1079,59
MUT: dnd-esc 10 μmol/L   MUREAV 89,95,81
MUT: mma-sat 20 μg/plate   PNASA6 72,5135,75
MUT: mrc-esc 600 μg/well   MUREAV 46,53,77
MUT: msc-ham: lng 30 μg/L   CNREA8 42,1646,82
MUT: otr-ham: kdy 80 μg/L   BJCAAI 37,873,78

CONSENSUS REPORTS: IARC Cancer Review: GROUP 2B IMEMDT 7,56,87; Animal Sufficient Evidence IMEMDT 3,215,73; IMEMDT 32,337,83. NTP Fourth Annual Report On Carcinogens, 1984. EPA Genetic Toxicology Program.

SAFETY PROFILE: Confirmed carcinogen with experimental neoplastigenic and tumorigenic data. Mutation data reported. When heated to decomposition it emits acrid smoke and irritating fumes.

BFL250   CAS: 98-07-7
BENZYL TRICHLORIDE
DOT: 2226
mf: $C_7H_5Cl_3$ mw: 195.47

PROP: Clear, colorless to yellowish liquid; penetrating odor. Mp: −5°, bp: 221°, d: 1.38 @ 15.5°/15.5°, vap d: 6.77.

SYNS: BENZENYL CHLORIDE ◇ BENZENYL TRICHLO-RIDE ◇ BENZOIC TRICHLORIDE ◇ BENZOTRICHLORIDE (DOT, MAK) ◇ BENZYLIDYNE CHLORIDE ◇ CHLORURE de BENZENYLE (FRENCH) ◇ PHENYL CHLOROFORM ◇ PHENYLTRICHLOROMETHANE ◇ RCRA WASTE NUM-BER U023 ◇ TOLUENE TRICHLORIDE ◇ TRICHLOOR-METHYLBENZEEN (DUTCH) ◇ TRICHLORMETHYLBENZOL (GERMAN) ◇ TRICHLOROMETHYLBENZENE ◇ 1-(TRI-CHLOROMETHYL)BENZENE ◇ TRICHLOROPHENYLMETH-ANE ◇ α,α,α-TRICHLOROTOLUENE ◇ φ,φ,φ-TRICHLORO-TOLUENE ◇ TRICLOROMETILBENZENE (ITALIAN) ◇ TRICLOROTOLUENE (ITALIAN)

TOXICITY DATA with REFERENCE
CAR: ipr-mus TDLo: 287 mg/kg/8W-I   CALEDQ 33,167,86
CAR: skn-mus TD: 16320 mg/kg/31W-I   GANNA2 72,655,81
CAR: skn-mus TD: 17600 mg/kg/42W-I   GANNA2 72,655,81
CAR: skn-mus TD: 34000 mg/kg/31W-I   GANNA2 72,655,81
CAR: skn-mus TD: 35200 mg/kg/42W-I   GANNA2 72,655,81
CAR: skn-mus TDLo: 9200 mg/kg/50W-I   GANNA2 72,655,81
ETA: ipr-mus TD: 288 mg/kg/8W-I   PAACA3 27,94,86
ETA: ipr-mus TD: 1440 mg/kg/8W-I   CALEDQ 33,167,86
MUT: mma-esc 500 nmol/plate/20M   MUREAV 54,143,78
MUT: mma-sat 500 nmol/plate/20M   MUREAV 54,143,78
MUT: mma-sat 500 μmol/plate/20M   MUREAV 3,11,81
MUT: mrc-bcs 2600 nmol/disc   MUREAV 54,143,78

CONSENSUS REPORTS: IARC Cancer Review: Human Limited Evidence IMEMDT 29,73,82; Animal Sufficient Evidence IMEMDT 29,73,82. NTP Fourth Annual Report On Carcinogens, 1984. EPA Genetic Toxicology Program. EPA Extremely Hazardous Substances List. Reported in EPA TSCA Inventory.

DFG MAK: Suspected Carcinogen. DOT Classification: IMO: Corrosive Material; Label: Corrosive.

SAFETY PROFILE: Confirmed carcinogen with experimental carcinogenic data by skin contact. Poison by inhalation. Moderately toxic by ingestion and subcutaneous routes. Corrosive to the skin, eyes, and mucous membranes. Large doses can cause central nervous system depression.

Mutation data reported. When heated to decomposition it emits toxic fumes of Cl^-.

BFO250 CAS: 12161-82-9
BERTRANDITE
mf: $H_{10}O_9Si_2 \cdot H_2O \cdot Be_4$ mw: 264.34

SYN: BERYLLIUM SILICATE HYDRATE

CONSENSUS REPORTS: IARC Cancer Review: Animal Sufficient Evidence IMEMDT 1,17,72; Animal Inadequate Evidence IMEMDT 23,143,80. Reported in EPA TSCA Inventory. Beryllium and its compounds are on the Community Right-To-Know List.

OSHA PEL: (Transitional: TWA 0.002 mg(Be)/ m^3; CL 0.005; Pk 0.025/30M/8H) TWA 0.002 mg(Be)/m^3; STEL 0.005 mg(Be)/m^3/30M; CL 0.025 mg(Be)/m^3 ACGIH TLV: TWA 0.002 mg(Be)/m^3, Suspected Human Carcinogen. NIOSH REL: CL not to exceed 0.0005 mg(Be)/m^3

SAFETY PROFILE: Confirmed carcinogen. When heated to decomposition it emits very toxic fumes of BeO.

BFO500 CAS: 1302-52-9
BERYL
mf: $Al_2O_{18}Si_6 \cdot 3Be$ mw: 537.53

PROP: Green, blue, yellow or white crystals. D: 2.63-2.91.

SYNS: BERYL ORE ◇ BERYLLIUM ALUMINOSILICATE ◇ BERYLLIUM ALUMINUM SILICATE

TOXICITY DATA with REFERENCE
NEO: ihl-rat TCLo: 15 mg/m^3/74W-I TXAPA9 15,10,69
MUT: ihl-rat TC: 15 mg/m^3/6H/73W-I

CONSENSUS REPORTS: IARC Cancer Review: GROUP 2A IMEMDT 7,127,87; Animal Sufficient Evidence IMEMDT 23,143,80; IMEMDT 1,17,72. NTP Fourth Annual Report On Carcinogens, 1984. Reported in EPA TSCA Inventory. Beryllium and its compounds are on the Community Right-To-Know List.

OSHA PEL: (Transitional: TWA 0.002 mg(Be)/ m^3; CL 0.005; Pk 0.025/30M/8H) TWA 0.002 mg(Be)/m^3; STEL 0.005 mg(Be)/m^3/30M; CL 0.025 mg(Be)/m^3 ACGIH TLV: TWA 0.002 mg(Be)/m^3, Suspected Human Carcinogen. NIOSH REL: CL not to exceed 0.0005 mg(Be)/m^3

SAFETY PROFILE: Confirmed carcinogen with experimental carcinogenic, neoplastigenic, and tumorigenic data. When heated to decomposition it emits toxic fumes of BeO.

BFO750 CAS: 7440-41-7
BERYLLIUM
DOT: 1567
af: Be aw: 9.01

PROP: A grayish-white, hard, light metal. Mp: 1278°, bp: 2970°, d: 1.85.

SYNS: BERYLLIUM-9 ◇ BERYLLIUM, metal powder (DOT) ◇ GLUCINUM ◇ RCRA WASTE NUMBER P015

TOXICITY DATA with REFERENCE
NEO: itr-rat TDLo: 13 mg/kg ENVRAL 21,63,80
ETA: ivn-rbt TDLo: 20 mg/kg LANCAO 1,463,50
MUT: dnd-esc 30 μmol/L MUREAV 89,95,81
MUT: dnd-hmn: hla 30 μmol/L MUREAV 89,95,81
MUT: dnd-mus: ast 30 μmol/L MUREAV 89,95,81
MUT: dni-nml-ivn 30 μmol/kg PHMCAA 12,298,70

CONSENSUS REPORTS: IARC Cancer Review: GROUP 2A IMEMDT 7,127,87; Human Limited Evidence IMEMDT 23,143,80; Animal Sufficient Evidence IMEMDT 23,143,80; IMEMDT 1,17,72. NTP Fourth Annual Report On Carcinogens, 1984. Beryllium and its compounds are on the Community Right-To-Know List. Reported in EPA TSCA Inventory.

OSHA PEL: (Transitional: TWA 0.002 mg(Be)/ m^3; CL 0.005; Pk 0.025/30M/8H) TWA 0.002 mg(Be)/m^3; STEL 0.005 mg(Be)/m^3/30M; CL 0.025 mg(Be)/m^3 ACGIH TLV: TWA 0.002 mg/m^3, Suspected Human Carcinogen. DFG TRK: Animal Carcinogen, Suspected Human Carcinogen. Grinding of beryllium metal and alloys: 0.005 mg/m^3 calculated as Be in that portion of dust that can possibly be inhaled; other Be compounds: 0.002 mg/m^3 calculated as Be in that portion of dust that can possibly be inhaled NIOSH REL: CL not to exceed 0.0005 mg(Be)/m^3 DOT Classification: Poison B, Flammable Solid Powder and Poison (metal).

SAFETY PROFILE: Confirmed carcinogen with experimental carcinogenic, neoplastigenic, and tumorigenic data. A deadly poison by intravenous route. Human systemic effects by inhalation: lung fibrosis, dyspnea, and weight loss. Human mutation data reported. A moderate fire hazard in the form of dust or powder, or when exposed to flame or by spontaneous chemical reaction. When heated to decomposition in air it emits very toxic fumes of BeO.

BFP000   CAS: 543-81-7
BERYLLIUM ACETATE
mf: $C_4H_6O_4 \cdot Be$ mw: 127.11

PROP: Plates. Mp: decomp @ 300°.

SYN: BERYLLIUM ACETATE, NORMAL

CONSENSUS REPORTS: IARC Cancer Review: Animal Inadequate Evidence IMEMDT 23,143,80. Beryllium and its compounds are on the Community Right-To-Know List.

OSHA PEL: (Transitional: TWA 0.002 mg(Be)/m^3; CL 0.005; Pk 0.025/30M/8H) TWA 0.002 mg(Be)/m^3; STEL 0.005 mg(Be)/m^3/30M; CL 0.025 mg(Be)/m^3 ACGIH TLV: TWA 0.002 mg(Be)/m^3, Suspected Human Carcinogen. DFG MAK: Animal Carcinogen, Suspected Human Carcinogen.   NIOSH REL: CL not to exceed 0.0005 mg(Be)/m^3

SAFETY PROFILE: Confirmed carcinogen. Poison by intraperitoneal route. When heated to decomposition it emits toxic fumes of BeO.

BFP250   CAS: 12770-50-2
BERYLLIUM ALUMINUM ALLOY

PROP: Alloy is 62% beryllium and 38% aluminum (ENVRAL 21,63,80).

SYNS: ALUMINUM ALLOY, Al,Be ◇ ALUMINUM BERYLLIUM ALLOY

TOXICITY DATA with REFERENCE
ETA: itr-rat TDLo: 13 mg/kg   ENVRAL 21,63,80

CONSENSUS REPORTS: IARC Cancer Review: GROUP 2A IMEMDT 7,127,87; Animal Sufficient Evidence IMEMDT 23,143,80. NTP Fourth Annual Report On Carcinogens, 1984. Beryllium and its compounds are on the Community Right-To-Know List.

OSHA PEL: (Transitional: TWA 0.002 mg(Be)/m^3; CL 0.005; Pk 0.025/30M/8H) TWA 0.002 mg(Be)/m^3; STEL 0.005 mg(Be)/m^3/30M; CL 0.025 mg(Be)/m^3 ACGIH TLV: TWA 0.002 mg(Be)/m^3, Suspected Human Carcinogen. DFG MAK: Animal Carcinogen, Suspected Human Carcinogen.   NIOSH REL: CL not to exceed 0.0005 mg(Be)/m^3

SAFETY PROFILE: Confirmed carcinogen with experimental carcinogenic and tumorigenic data. When heated to decomposition it emits very toxic BeO.

BFP500   CAS: 66104-24-3
BERYLLIUM CARBONATE
mf: $C_2H_2Be_3O_8$ mw: 181.07

SYNS: BERYLLIUM CARBONATE, BASIC ◇ BERYLLIUMOXIDE CARBONATE ◇ BIS(CARBONATO(2-)) DIHYDROXYTRIBERYLLIUM

CONSENSUS REPORTS: IARC Cancer Review: GROUP 2A IMEMDT 7,127,87; Animal Sufficient Evidence IMEMDT 23,143,80. Reported in EPA TSCA Inventory. Beryllium and its compounds are on the Community Right-To-Know List.

OSHA PEL: (Transitional: TWA 0.002 mg(Be)/m^3; CL 0.005; Pk 0.025/30M/8H) TWA 0.002 mg(Be)/m^3; STEL 0.005 mg(Be)/m^3/30M; CL 0.025 mg(Be)/m^3 ACGIH TLV: TWA 0.002 mg(Be)/m^3, Suspected Human Carcinogen. DFG MAK: Animal Carcinogen, Suspected Human Carcinogen.   NIOSH REL: CL not to exceed 0.0005 mg(Be)/m^3

SAFETY PROFILE: Confirmed carcinogen. When heated to decomposition it emits toxic BeO dust.

BFP750   CAS: 13106-47-3
BERYLLIUM CARBONATE (1:1)
mf: $CO_3 \cdot Be$ mw: 69.02

SYN: CARBONIC ACID BERYLLIUM SALT (1:1)

CONSENSUS REPORTS: Reported in EPA TSCA Inventory. Beryllium and its compounds are on the Community Right-To-Know List.

OSHA PEL: (Transitional: TWA 0.002 mg(Be)/m^3; CL 0.005; Pk 0.025/30M/8H) TWA 0.002 mg(Be)/m^3; STEL 0.005 mg(Be)/m^3/30M; CL 0.025 mg(Be)/m^3 ACGIH TLV: TWA 0.002 mg(Be)/m^3, Suspected Human Carcinogen. DFG MAK: 50 ppm (90 mg/m^3)   NIOSH REL: CL not to exceed 0.0005 mg(Be)/m^3

SAFETY PROFILE: Confirmed carcinogen. Poison by intraperitoneal route. When heated to decomposition it emits highly toxic fumes of BeO.

BFQ000   CAS: 7787-47-5
BERYLLIUM CHLORIDE
DOT: 1566
mf: $BeCl_2$ mw: 79.91

PROP: Colorless, deliquescent needles. Mp: 440°, bp: 520°, d: 1.899 @ 25°, vap press: 1 mm @ 291° (sublimes).

SYN: BERYLLIUM DICHLORIDE

TOXICITY DATA with REFERENCE
ETA: ihl-rat TCLo: 20 μg/m^3/1H/17W-I
GTPZAB 19(7),34,75
MUT: mmo-esc 10 μmol/L   MUREAV 126,9,84
MUT: msc-ham: lng 2 mmol/L   MUREAV 68,259,79

CONSENSUS REPORTS: IARC Cancer Review: GROUP 2A IMEMDT 7,127,87; Animal Sufficient Evidence IMEMDT 23,143,80. NTP Fourth Annual Report On Carcinogens, 1984. EPA Genetic Toxicology Program. Reported in EPA TSCA Inventory. Beryllium and its compounds are on the Community Right-To-Know List.

OSHA PEL: (Transitional: TWA 0.002 mg(Be)/m^3; CL 0.005; Pk 0.025/30M/8H) TWA 0.002 mg(Be)/m^3; STEL 0.005 mg(Be)/m^3/30M; CL 0.025 mg(Be)/m^3 ACGIH TLV: TWA 0.002 mg(Be)/m^3, Suspected Human Carcinogen. DFG MAK: Animal Carcinogen, Suspected Human Carcinogen.   NIOSH REL: CL not to exceed 0.0005 mg(Be)/m^3 DOT Classification: Poison B; Label: Poison.

SAFETY PROFILE: Confirmed carcinogen with experimental tumorigenic data. Poison by ingestion and intraperitoneal routes. Experimental reproductive effects. Mutation data reported. When heated to decomposition it emits very toxic fumes of BeO and Cl$^-$.

BFQ250   CAS: 13466-27-8
BERYLLIUM CHLORIDE TETRAHYDRATE
mf: BeCl$_2$•4H$_2$O   mw: 151.99

CONSENSUS REPORTS: Beryllium and its compounds are on the Community Right-To-Know List.

OSHA PEL: (Transitional: TWA 0.002 mg(Be)/m^3; CL 0.005; Pk 0.025/30M/8H) TWA 0.002 mg(Be)/m^3; STEL 0.005 mg(Be)/m^3/30M; CL 0.025 mg(Be)/m^3 ACGIH TLV: TWA 0.002 mg(Be)/m^3, Suspected Human Carcinogen. DFG MAK: Animal Carcinogen, Suspected Human Carcinogen.   NIOSH REL: CL not to exceed 0.0005 mg(Be)/m^3

SAFETY PROFILE: Confirmed carcinogen. Poison by intraperitoneal route. When heated to decomposition it emits very toxic Cl$^-$ and BeO.

BFQ500
BERYLLIUM COMPOUNDS
CONSENSUS REPORTS: Beryllium and its compounds are on the Community Right-To-Know List.

OSHA PEL: (Transitional: TWA 0.002 mg(Be)/m^3; CL 0.005; Pk 0.025/30M/8H) TWA 0.002 mg(Be)/m^3; STEL 0.005 mg(Be)/m^3/30M; CL 0.025 mg(Be)/m^3 ACGIH TLV: TWA 0.002 mg/m^3, Suspected Human Carcinogen.   DFG TRK: Animal Carcinogen, Suspected Human Carcinogen. Grinding of beryllium metal and alloys: 0.005 mg/m^3 calculated as Be in that portion of dust that can possibly be inhaled; other Be compounds: 0.002 mg/m^3 calculated as Be in that portion of dust that can possibly be inhaled   NIOSH REL: CL not to exceed 0.0005 mg(Be)/m^3

SAFETY PROFILE: Confirmed carcinogens. Beryllium compounds can enter the body through inhalation of dusts and fumes, and may act locally on the skin. Even alloys of low beryllium content have been shown to be dangerous. In industry, inhalation of the dust can cause severe lung damage with symptoms appearing within months. Effects have been reported in persons living near processing plants and in families of beryllium workers. The fluoride, ammonium fluoride, sulfate, oxide, and hydroxide occur during extraction from beryllium ore. Exposure to the oxide may occur in processing of beryllium alloys and beryllium ceramics.

BFQ750   CAS: 12010-12-7
BERYLLIUM COMPOUND with NIOBIUM (12:1)
mf: Be$_{12}$Nb   mw: 201.03

TOXICITY DATA with REFERENCE
ETA: itr-rat TDLo: 2500 μg/kg   ENVRAL 21,63,80

CONSENSUS REPORTS: Beryllium and its compounds are on the Community Right-To-Know List.

OSHA PEL: (Transitional: TWA 0.002 mg(Be)/m^3; CL 0.005; Pk 0.025/30M/8H) TWA 0.002 mg(Be)/m^3; STEL 0.005 mg(Be)/m^3/30M; CL 0.025 mg(Be)/m^3 ACGIH TLV: TWA 0.002 mg(Be)/m^3, Suspected Human Carcinogen. NIOSH REL: (Beryllium) CL not to exceed 0.005 mg(Be)/m^3

SAFETY PROFILE: Confirmed carcinogen with experimental tumorigenic data. When heated to decomposition in air it emits very toxic fumes of BeO.

BFR000   CAS: 12232-67-6
BERYLLIUM COMPOUND with TITANIUM (12:1)
mf: $Be_{12}Ti$ mw: 156.02

SYN: TITANIUM compounded with BERYLLIUM (1:12)

TOXICITY DATA with REFERENCE
ETA: itr-rat TDLo: 2500 μg/kg   ENVRAL 21,63,80

CONSENSUS REPORTS: Beryllium and its compounds are on the Community Right-To-Know List.

OSHA PEL: (Transitional: TWA 0.002 mg(Be)/m³; CL 0.005; Pk 0.025/30M/8H) TWA 0.002 mg(Be)/m³; STEL 0.005 mg(Be)/m³/30M; CL 0.025 mg(Be)/m³   ACGIH TLV: TWA 0.002 mg(Be)/m³, Suspected Human Carcinogen. NIOSH REL: (Beryllium) CL not to exceed 0.0005 mg(Be)/m³

SAFETY PROFILE: Confirmed carcinogen with experimental tumorigenic data. When heated to decomposition it emits very toxic fumes of BeO.

BFR250   CAS: 12400-16-7
BERYLLIUM COMPOUND with VANADIUM (12:1)
mf: $Be_{12}V$ mw: 159.06

SYN: TITANIUM compd. with BERYLLIUM (1:12)

TOXICITY DATA with REFERENCE
NEO: itr-rat TDLo: 2500 μg/kg   ENVRAL 21,63,80

CONSENSUS REPORTS: Beryllium and its compounds are on the Community Right-To-Know List.

OSHA PEL: (Transitional: TWA 0.002 mg(Be)/m³; CL 0.005; Pk 0.025/30M/8H) TWA 0.002 mg(Be)/m³; STEL 0.005 mg(Be)/m³/30M; CL 0.025 mg(Be)/m³   ACGIH TLV: TWA 0.002 mg(Be)/m³, Suspected Human Carcinogen. NIOSH REL: (Beryllium) CL not to exceed 0.0005 mg(Be)/m³; (REL to Vanadium) 1.0 mg(V)/m³

SAFETY PROFILE: Confirmed carcinogen with experimental tumorigenic data. When heated

to decomposition it emits very toxic fumes of BeO and VO_x.

BFR500   CAS: 7787-49-7
BERYLLIUM FLUORIDE
DOT: 1566
mf: BeF_2 mw: 47.01

PROP: Amorphous, colorless mass. Mp: 800°, d: 1.986 @ 25°.

SYN: BERYLLIUM DIFLUORIDE

TOXICITY DATA with REFERENCE
ETA: ihl-rat TCLo: 20 μg/m³/1H/17W-I
    GTPZAB 19(7),34,75
ETA: ihl-rat TCLo: 49 μg/m³/26W   PEXTAR
    2,203,61

CONSENSUS REPORTS: IARC Cancer Review: GROUP 2A IMEMDT 7,127,87; Animal Sufficient Evidence IMEMDT 23,143,80. NTP Fourth Annual Report On Carcinogens, 1984. Beryllium and its compounds are on the Community Right-To-Know List. Reported in EPA TSCA Inventory.

OSHA PEL: (Transitional: TWA 0.002 mg(Be)/m³; CL 0.005; Pk 0.025/30M/8H) TWA 0.002 mg(Be)/m³; STEL 0.005 mg(Be)/m³/30M; CL 0.025 mg(Be)/m³   ACGIH TLV: TWA 0.002 mg(Be)/m³, Suspected Human Carcinogen; 2.5 mg(F)/m³   NIOSH REL: CL not to exceed 0.0005 mg(Be)/m³   DOT Classification: Poison B; Label: Poison.

SAFETY PROFILE: Confirmed carcinogen with experimental carcinogenic and tumorigenic data by inhalation. Poison by ingestion, subcutaneous, intravenous and intraperitoneal routes. When heated to decomposition, it emits very toxic fumes of BeO and F⁻.

BFR750   CAS: 7787-52-2
BERYLLIUM HYDRIDE
mf: BeH_2 mw: 11.03

PROP: White solid.

CONSENSUS REPORTS: Beryllium and its compounds are on the Community Right-To-Know List.

SAFETY PROFILE: Confirmed carcinogen. A dangerous fire hazard. When heated to 220°C it liberates explosive hydrogen gas. When heated to decomposition it emits toxic fumes of BeO.

BFS000 CAS: 13598-15-7
BERYLLIUM HYDROGEN PHOSPHATE (1:1)
mf: $BeHO_4P$ mw: 104.99

SYNS: BERYLLIUM PHOSPHATE ◇ PHOSPHORIC ACID, BERYLLIUM SALT (1:1) ◇ PHOSPHOROUS ACID, BERYLLIUM SALT

TOXICITY DATA with REFERENCE
ETA: ihl-mky TC:97 mg/m^3/8D-I IMSUAI 3,1,64
ETA: ihl-mky TDLo:900 μg/kg/17W PEXTAR 2,203,61
ETA: ihl-rat TCLo:3571 μg/m^3/17W PEXTAR 2,203,61

CONSENSUS REPORTS: IARC Cancer Review: GROUP 2A IMEMDT 7,127,87; Animal Sufficient Evidence IMEMDT 23,143,80; IMEMDT 1,17,72. NTP Fourth Annual Report On Carcinogens, 1984. Beryllium and its compounds are on the Community Right-To-Know List.

OSHA PEL: (Transitional: TWA 0.002 mg(Be)/m^3; CL 0.005; Pk 0.025/30M/8H) TWA 0.002 mg(Be)/m^3; STEL 0.005 mg(Be)/m^3/30M; CL 0.025 mg(Be)/m^3 ACGIH TLV: TWA 0.002 mg(Be)/m^3, Suspected Human Carcinogen. NIOSH REL: CL not to exceed 0.0005 mg/m^3

SAFETY PROFILE: Confirmed carcinogen with experimental carcinogenic and tumorigenic data. Poison by intravenous route. When heated to decomposition it emits very toxic fumes of BeO and PO$_x$.

BFS250 CAS: 13327-32-7
BERYLLIUM HYDROXIDE
mf: $H_2O_2 \cdot Be$ mw: 43.03

PROP: Amorphous powder or crystals. Mp: decomp @ 138°, d(cr): 1.909.

SYNS: BERYLLIUM DIHYDROXIDE ◇ BERYLLIUM HYDRATE

TOXICITY DATA with REFERENCE
ETA: itr-rat TD:1785 μg/kg/43W-I ENVRAL 21,63,80
ETA: itr-rat TDLo:1125 μg/kg TXAPA9 17,299,70

CONSENSUS REPORTS: IARC Cancer Review: GROUP 2A IMEMDT 7,127,87; Animal Sufficient Evidence IMEMDT 23,143,80. NTP

Fourth Annual Report On Carcinogens, 1984. Beryllium and its compounds are on the Community Right-To-Know List. Reported in EPA TSCA Inventory.

OSHA PEL: (Transitional: TWA 0.002 mg(Be)/m^3; CL 0.005; Pk 0.025/30M/8H) TWA 0.002 mg(Be)/m^3; STEL 0.005 mg(Be)/m^3/30M; CL 0.025 mg(Be)/m^3 ACGIH TLV: TWA 0.002 mg(Be)/m^3, Suspected Human Carcinogen. NIOSH REL: CL not to exceed 0.0005 mg(Be)/m^3

SAFETY PROFILE: Confirmed carcinogen with experimental carcinogenic and tumorigenic data. Poison by intravenous route. When heated to decomposition it emits very toxic fumes of BeO.

BFS750
BERYLLIUM MANGANESE ZINC SILICATE
mf: $BeMnO_4SiZn$ mw: 221.41

SYNS: MANGANESE ZINC BERYLLIUM SILICATE ◇ ZINC MANGANESE BERYLLIUM SILICATE

TOXICITY DATA with REFERENCE
ETA: ihl-rat TCLo:20 mg/m^3/4W PEXTAR 2,203,61
ETA: ivn-rbt TDLo:500 mg/kg/40W-I PEXTAR 2,203,61

CONSENSUS REPORTS: Beryllium, manganese, zinc, and their compounds are on the Community Right-To-Know List.

OSHA PEL: (Transitional: TWA 0.002 mg(Be)/m^3; CL 0.005; Pk 0.025/30M/8H) TWA 0.002 mg(Be)/m^3; STEL 0.005 mg(Be)/m^3/30M; CL 0.025 mg(Be)/m^3 ACGIH TLV: TWA 0.002 mg(Be)/m^3, Suspected Human Carcinogen; TWA 5 mg(Mn)/m^3 NIOSH REL: (Beryllium) CL Not to exceed 0.0005 mg(Be)/m^3

SAFETY PROFILE: Confirmed carcinogen with experimental tumorigenic data. When heated to decomposition it emits very toxic fumes of BeO and ZnO.

BFT000 CAS: 13597-99-4
BERYLLIUM NITRATE
mf: BeN_2O_6 mw: 133.03
DOT: 2464

PROP: White-yellowish crystals, deliquescent. Mp: 60°, bp: decomp @ 100-200°.

SYNS: BERYLLIUM DINITRATE ◇ NITRIC ACID, BERYLLIUM SALT

CONSENSUS REPORTS: Beryllium and its compounds are on the Community Right-To-Know List.

OSHA PEL: (Transitional: TWA 0.002 mg(Be)/m^3; CL 0.005; Pk 0.025/30M/8H) TWA 0.002 mg(Be)/m^3; STEL 0.005 mg(Be)/m^3/30M; CL 0.025 mg(Be)/m^3 ACGIH TLV: TWA 0.002 mg(Be)m^3, Suspected Human Carcinogen. NIOSH REL: CL not to exceed 0.0005 mg(Be)/m^3 DOT Classification: Label: Oxidizer and Poison.

SAFETY PROFILE: Confirmed carcinogen. Poison by intraperitoneal and subcutaneous routes. Experimental reproductive effects. When heated to decomposition it emits very toxic fumes of BeO and NO_x.

BFT250   CAS: 1304-56-9
BERYLLIUM OXIDE
mf: BeO   mw: 25.01

PROP: White, amorphous powder. Mp: 2530° ± 30°, bp: 3900° (approx), d: 3.025.

SYNS: BERYLLIA ◇ BERYLLIUM MONOXIDE ◇ THERMALOX

TOXICITY DATA with REFERENCE
ETA: ihl-rat TCLo: 28 mg/m^3/17W-C   IMSUAI 40,23,71
ETA: ihl-rbt TCLo: 17 mg/m^3/5H/D/48W-I AMPLAO 51,473,51
ETA: imp-rbt TDLo: 10 mg/kg   ARPAAQ 88,89,69
ETA: itr-rat TD: 79 mg/kg/15W-I   SAIGBL 20,230,78
ETA: itr-rat TD: 169 mg/kg/2W-I   AMIHAB 19,190,59
ETA: itr-rat TDLo: 75 mg/kg/15W-I   FKIZA4 71,19,80
ETA: ivn-rbt TD: 500 mg/kg/48W-I   PEXTAR 2,203,61
ETA: ivn-rbt TD: 625 mg/kg/25W-I   AMSHAR 25,99,77
ETA: ivn-rbt TDLo: 500 mg/kg/6W-I   FEPRA7 5,221,46

CONSENSUS REPORTS: IARC Cancer Review: GROUP 2A IMEMDT 7,127,87; Animal Sufficient Evidence IMEMDT 1,17,72; IMEMDT 23,143,80. NTP Fourth Annual Report On Carcinogens, 1984. Beryllium and its compounds are on the Community Right-To-Know List. Reported in EPA TSCA Inventory.

OSHA PEL: (Transitional: TWA 0.002 mg(Be)/m^3; CL 0.005; Pk 0.025/30M/8H) TWA 0.002 mg(Be)/m^3; STEL 0.005 mg(Be)/m^3/30M; CL 0.025 mg(Be)/m^3 ACGIH TLV: TWA 0.002 mg(Be)/m^3, Suspected Human Carcinogen. NIOSH REL: (Beryllium) CL not to exceed 0.0005 mg(Be)/m^3

SAFETY PROFILE: Confirmed carcinogen with experimental tumorigenic data. Experimental reproductive data. When heated to decomposition it emits very toxic fumes of BeO.

BFT500   CAS: 19049-40-2
BERYLLIUM OXYACETATE
mf: $C_{12}H_{18}Be_4O_{13}$ mw: 406.34

SYNS: BERYLLIUM ACETATE, BASIC ◇ BERYLLIUM OXIDE ACETATE ◇ HEXAKIS(μ-ACETATO-O:O'))-μ$^{(4)}$-OXO-TETRABERYLLIUM ◇ HEXAKIS(μ-ACETATO)-μ$^{(4)}$-OXO-TETRABERYLLIUM

CONSENSUS REPORTS: Beryllium and its compounds are on the Community Right-To-Know List.

OSHA PEL: (Transitional: TWA 0.002 mg(Be)/m^3; CL 0.005; Pk 0.025/30M/8H) TWA 0.002 mg(Be)/m^3; STEL 0.005 mg(Be)/m^3/30M; CL 0.025 mg(Be)/m^3 ACGIH TLV: TWA 0.002 mg(Be)/m^3, Suspected Human Carcinogen. NIOSH REL: CL not to exceed 0.0005 mg(Be)/m^3

SAFETY PROFILE: Confirmed carcinogen. When heated to decomposition it emits toxic fumes BeO.

BFT750   CAS: 63990-88-5
BERYLLIUM OXYFLUORIDE
mf: BeF_2O_2 mw: 79.01

CONSENSUS REPORTS: Beryllium and its compounds are on the Community Right-To-Know List.

OSHA PEL: (Transitional: TWA 0.002 mg(Be)/m^3; CL 0.005; Pk 0.025/30M/8H) TWA 0.002 mg(Be)/m^3; STEL 0.005 mg(Be)/m^3/30M; CL 0.025 mg(Be)/m^3 ACGIH TLV: TWA 0.002 mg(Be)/m^3, Suspected Human Carcinogen; 2.5 mg(F)/m^3 NIOSH REL: CL not to exceed 0.0005 mg(Be)/m^3

SAFETY PROFILE: Confirmed carcinogen. Poison by ingestion, subcutaneous, intravenous, and intraperitoneal routes. When heated to decomposition it emits very toxic fumes of BeO and F⁻.

BFU000   CAS: 13597-95-0
BERYLLIUM PERCHLORATE
mf: $Be(ClO_4)_2$ mw: 207.91

PROP: Very hygroscopic crystals, sol in water: 148.6 g/100 mL.

OSHA PEL: (Transitional: TWA 0.002 mg(Be)/m³; CL 0.005; Pk 0.025/30M/8H) TWA 0.002 mg(Be)/m³; STEL 0.005 mg(Be)/m³/30M; CL 0.025 mg(Be)/m³ ACGIH TLV: TWA 0.002 mg(Be)/m³, Suspected Human Carcinogen. NIOSH REL: CL not to exceed 0.0005 mg(Be)/m³

SAFETY PROFILE: Confirmed carcinogen. A powerful oxidant used in propellant and igniter systems. When heated to decomposition it emits toxic fumes of Cl⁻ and BeO.

BFU250   CAS: 13510-49-1
BERYLLIUM SULFATE (1:1)
mf: $O_4S•Be$ mw: 105.07

PROP: Crystals. Mp: 550-600° (decomp), d: 2.443.

SYN: SULFURIC ACID, BERYLLIUM SALT (1:1)

TOXICITY DATA with REFERENCE
ETA: ihl-rat TC:643 μg/m³/39W-I   AMIHAB 19,190,59
ETA: ihl-rat TCLo:432 μg/m³/26W   PEXTAR 2,203,61
ETA: itr-rat TDLo:17 mg/kg/2W-I   AMIHAB 19,190,59
MUT: dnd-ham:emb 560 μmol/L   CNREA8 39,193,79
MUT: mrc-bcs 10 mmol/L   MUREAV 77,109,80
MUT: otr-ham:emb 560 μmol/L   CNREA8 39,193,79
MUT: otr-mus:fbr 200 μg/L   JJIND8 67,1303,81
MUT: otr-rat:emb 60 μg/L   JJIND8 67,1303,81

CONSENSUS REPORTS: IARC Cancer Review: GROUP 2A IMEMDT 7,127,87; Animal Sufficient Evidence IMEMDT 23,143,80. NTP Fourth Annual Report On Carcinogens, 1984. Beryllium and its compounds are on the Community Right-To-Know List. Reported in EPA TSCA Inventory.

OSHA PEL: (Transitional: TWA 0.002 mg(Be)/m³; CL 0.005; Pk 0.025/30M/8H) TWA 0.002 mg(Be)/m³; STEL 0.005 mg(Be)/m³/30M; CL 0.025 mg(Be)/m³ ACGIH TLV: TWA 0.002 mg(Be)/m³, Suspected Human Carcinogen. NIOSH REL: CL not to exceed 0.0005 mg(Be)/m³

SAFETY PROFILE: Confirmed carcinogen with experimental tumorigenic data. Acute poison by inhalation, ingestion, intraperitoneal, subcutaneous, intravenous, and intratracheal routes. Mutation data reported. When heated to decomposition it emits very toxic fumes of SO_x and BeO.

BFU500   CAS: 7787-56-6
BERYLLIUM SULFATE TETRAHYDRATE (1:1:4)
mf: $O_4S•Be•4H_2O$ mw: 177.15

SYNS: BERYLLIUM SULPHATE TETRAHYDRATE ◇ SULFURIC ACID, BERYLLIUM SALT (1:1), TETRAHYDRATE

TOXICITY DATA with REFERENCE
CAR: ihl-rat TCLo:668 μg/m³/40W-C   CNREA8 27,439,67
MUT: cyt-ham:emb 5 mg/L   ENMUDM 3,597,81
MUT: cyt-hmn:lym 5 mg/L   ENMUDM 3,597,81
MUT: mma-sat 3300 ng/plate   ENMUDM 6(Suppl 2),1,84
MUT: sce-ham:emb 1 mg/L   ENMUDM 3,597,81
MUT: sce-hmn:lym 1 mg/L   ENMUDM 3,597,81

CONSENSUS REPORTS: IARC Cancer Review: GROUP 2A IMEMDT 7,127,87; Animal Sufficient Evidence IMEMDT 23,143,80; IMEMDT 1,17,72. NTP Fourth Annual Report On Carcinogens, 1984. Beryllium and its compounds are on the Community Right-To-Know List.

OSHA PEL: (Transitional: TWA 0.002 mg(Be)/m³; CL 0.005; Pk 0.025/30M/8H) TWA 0.002 mg(Be)/m³; STEL 0.005 mg(Be)/m³/30M; CL 0.025 mg(Be)/m³ ACGIH TLV: TWA 0.002 mg(Be)/m³, Suspected Human Carcinogen. NIOSH REL: CL not to exceed 0.0005 mg(Be)/m³

SAFETY PROFILE: Confirmed carcinogen with experimental carcinogenic data by inhalation. Deadly poison by subcutaneous and intravenous routes. Human mutation data reported. When heated to decomposition it emits very toxic fumes of BeO and SO_x.

BFU750
BERYLLIUM TETRAHYDROBORATE
mf: B_2BeH_8 mw: 38.70

CONSENSUS REPORTS: Beryllium and its compounds are on the Community Right-To-Know List.

OSHA PEL: (Transitional: TWA 0.002 mg(Be)/m^3; CL 0.005; Pk 0.025/30M/8H) TWA 0.002 mg(Be)/m^3; STEL 0.005 mg(Be)/m^3/30M; CL 0.025 mg(Be)/m^3 ACGIH TLV: TWA 0.002 mg(Be)/m^3, Suspected Human Carcinogen. NIOSH REL: CL not to exceed 0.0005 mg(Be)/m^3

SAFETY PROFILE: Confirmed carcinogen. Ignites and then explodes in air or on contact with water. Upon decomposition it emits toxic fumes of BeO and BO$_x$.

BFV000
BERYLLIUM TETRAHYDROBORATETRIMETHYL-AMINE
mf: C$_3$H$_{17}$B$_2$BeN   mw: 97.78

CONSENSUS REPORTS: Beryllium and its compounds are on the Community Right-To-Know List.

OSHA PEL: (Transitional: TWA 0.002 mg(Be)/m^3; CL 0.005; Pk 0.025/30M/8H) TWA 0.002 mg(Be)/m^3; STEL 0.005 mg(Be)/m^3/30M; CL 0.025 mg(Be)/m^3 ACGIH TLV: TWA 0.002 mg(Be)/m^3, Suspected Human Carcinogen. NIOSH REL: CL not to exceed 0.0005 mg(Be)/m^3

SAFETY PROFILE: Confirmed carcinogen. It will ignite in contact with air or water. When heated to decomposition it emits toxic fumes of BeO, BO$_x$ and NO$_x$.

BFV250   CAS: 39413-47-3
BERYLLIUM ZINC SILICATE
mf: O$_2$Si•Zn•Be   mw: 134.47

SYN: ZINC BERYLLIUM SILICATE

TOXICITY DATA with REFERENCE
ETA: imp-rbt TDLo: 10 mg/kg   ARPAAQ 88,89,69
ETA: ims-rbt TDLo: 20 mg/kg   BJCAAI 20,778,66
ETA: ivn-rbt TD: 500 mg/kg/6W-I   FEPRA7 5,221,46
ETA: ivn-rbt TD: 500 mg/kg/10W-I   JBJSA3 36B,543,54
ETA: ivn-rbt TDLo: 500 mg/kg/10W-I   JBJSA3 38A,543,54

CONSENSUS REPORTS: IARC Cancer Review: GROUP 2A IMEMDT 7,127,87; Animal

Sufficient Evidence IMEMDT 23,143,80; IMEMDT 1,17,72. NTP Fourth Annual Report On Carcinogens, 1984. Beryllium and its compounds, as well as zinc and its compounds, are on the Community Right-To-Know List.

OSHA PEL: (Transitional: TWA 0.002 mg(Be)/m^3; CL 0.005; Pk 0.025/30M/8H) TWA 0.002 mg(Be)/m^3; STEL 0.005 mg(Be)/m^3/30M; CL 0.025 mg(Be)/m^3 ACGIH TLV: TWA 0.002 mg(Be)/m^3, Suspected Human Carcinogen. NIOSH REL: CL not to exceed 0.0005 mg(Be)/m^3

SAFETY PROFILE: Confirmed carcinogen with experimental tumorigenic data. When heated to decomposition it emits toxic fumes of BeO and ZnO.

BFW135
BETEL TOBACCO EXTRACT

SYN: JAFFNA TOBACCO

TOXICITY DATA with REFERENCE
MUT: mnt-mus: ipr 24 mg/kg   CRNGDP 5,501,84
MUT: msc-ham: lng 5 mg/L   CRNGDP 5,501,84
MUT: otr-ham: emb 50 mg/L   TOLED5 8,17,81
MUT: sce-hmn: lym 10 mg/L   TOLED5 8,17,81

CONSENSUS REPORTS: IARC Cancer Review: Human Sufficient Evidence IMEMDT 37,141,85; Animal Limited Evidence IMEMDT 37,141,85

SAFETY PROFILE: Confirmed human carcinogen. Human mutation data reported.

BGA750   CAS: 1464-53-5
1,1'-BI(ETHYLENE OXIDE)
mf: C$_4$H$_6$O$_2$ mw: 86.10

PROP: Colorless liquid. Bp: 142°, mp: 19°, d: 1.113 @ 18°/4°.

SYNS: BIOXIRANE ◇ 2,2'-BIOXIRANE ◇ BUTADIENDIOXYD (GERMAN) ◇ BUTADIENE DIEPOXIDE ◇ 1,3-BUTADIENE DIEPOXIDE ◇ BUTADIENE DIOXIDE ◇ BUTANE DIEPOXIDE ◇ DEB ◇ DIEPOXYBUTANE ◇ 2,4-DIEPOXYBUTANE ◇ 1,2:3,4-DIEPOXYBUTANE ◇ DIOXYBUTADIENE ◇ ENT 26,592 ◇ ERYTHRITOL ANHYDRIDE ◇ RCRA WASTE NUMBER U085

TOXICITY DATA with REFERENCE
ETA: ipr-rat TDLo: 380 mg/kg/13W-I   BJPCAL 6,235,51
ETA: skn-mus TDLo: 95 g/kg/78W-I   AIHAAP 24,305,63

ETA: unk-mus TDLo: 3400 mg/kg   RARSAM
3,193,63

MUT: cyt-hmn: bmr 100 μg/L   CGCYDF 9,51,83
MUT: mmo-asn 20 μmol/L   MUREAV 132,161,84
MUT: sce-ham: lng 1 mg/L   CNREA8 44,3270,84
MUT: sce-mus-ivn 193 μmol/kg   MUREAV
108,251,83

CONSENSUS REPORTS: NTP Fourth Annual
Report On Carcinogens, 1984. EPA Extremely
Hazardous Substances List. EPA Genetic Toxi-
cology Program. Community Right-To-Know
List. Reported in EPA TSCA Inventory.

SAFETY PROFILE: Confirmed carcinogen with
experimental tumorigenic data. Poison by ingestion, inhalation, skin contact and intraperitoneal
routes. Human mutation data reported. A severe
skin and eye irritant. When heated to decomposition it emits acrid smoke and irritating fumes.

BIE250   CAS: 51-75-2
BIS(β-CHLOROETHYL)METHYLAMINE
mf: $C_5H_{11}Cl_2N$ mw: 156.07

PROP: Dark liquid. Mp: 1° @ 10 mm, d: 1.09
@ 25°, vap press: 0.17 mm @ 25°, vap d:
5.9.

SYNS: BIS(2-CHLOROETHYL)METHYLAMINE ◇ N,N-
BIS(2-CHLOROETHYL)METHYLAMINE ◇ CARYOLYSIN
◇ CHLORMETHINE ◇ CLORAMIN ◇ DICHLOR AMINE
◇ DICHLOREN (GERMAN) ◇ β,β'-DICHLORODIETHYL-N-
METHYLAMINE ◇ DI(2-CHLOROETHYL)METHYLAMINE
◇ 2,2'-DICHLORO-N-METHYLDIETHYLAMINE ◇ EMBI-
CHIN ◇ ENT 25,294 ◇ HN2 ◇ MBA ◇ MECHLORETHAMINE
◇ N-METHYL-BIS-CHLORAETHYLAMIN (GERMAN)
◇ METHYLBIS(β-CHLOROETHYL)AMINE ◇ N-METHYL-
BIS(β-CHLOROETHYL)AMINE ◇ N-METHYL-BIS(2-CHLO-
ROETHYL)AMINE (MAK) ◇ N-METHYL-2,2'-DICHLORODI-
ETHYLAMINE ◇ METHYLDI(2-CHLOROETHYL)AMINE
◇ N-METHYL-LOST ◇ MUSTARGEN ◇ MUSTINE
◇ MUTAGEN ◇ NITROGEN MUSTARD ◇ N-LOST (GERMAN)
◇ NSC 762 ◇ TL 146

TOXICITY DATA with REFERENCE
CAR: ivn-rat TDLo: 5720 μg/kg/1Y-I   ARZNAD
20,1461,70
CAR: skn-man TDLo: 153 mg/kg/3Y-C
ADVEA4 58,421,78
CAR: skn-wmn TD: 256 mg/kg/8.5Y-I   ADVED7
111,127,84
CAR: skn-wmn TDLo: 5840 mg/kg/8Y-I
ADVEA4 58,421,78
NEO: ivn-mus TDLo: 10 mg/kg/42D-I   CNREA8
25,20,65

ETA: ipr-mus TDLo: 69 mg/kg/39W-I   SCIEAS
147,1443,65
ETA: skn-mus TD: 276 mg/kg/23W-I   EXPEAM
36,1211,80
ETA: skn-mus TDLo: 60 mg/kg/14W-I   BJCAAI
9,177,55
MUT: dnr-bcs 10 μg/plate   TAKHAA 44,96,85
MUT: dns-hmn: fbr 160 μg/L   TXCYAC 21,151,81
MUT: sce-hmn: lym 6250 ng/L   CRNGDP5,1637,84

CONSENSUS REPORTS: EPA Genetic Toxicology Program. Reported in EPA TSCA Inventory. EPA Extremely Hazardous Substances
List. Community Right-To-Know List.

DFG MAK: Human Carcinogen.

SAFETY PROFILE: Confirmed human carcinogen producing skin tumors by skin contact. Experimental carcinogenic, tumorigenic, neoplastigenic, and teratogenic data. A deadly poison
by inhalation, ingestion, skin contact and most
other routes. Experimental reproductive effects.
A powerful skin and eye irritant. Human mutation data reported. It has been used as a blistering
agent in chemical warfare. When heated to decomposition it emits very toxic fumes of Cl^-
and NO_x.

BIE500   CAS: 55-86-7
BIS(2-CHLOROETHYL)METHYLAMINE
HYDROCHLORIDE
mf: $C_5H_{11}Cl_2N \cdot ClH$ mw: 192.53

SYNS: ANTIMIT ◇ AZOTOYPERITE ◇ C 6866 ◇ CAROLY-
SINE ◇ CARYOLYSINE ◇ CARYOLYSINE HYDROCHLO-
RIDE ◇ CHLORAMIN ◇ CHLORAMINE ◇ CHLORAMIN HY-
DROCHLORIDE ◇ CHLORETHAMINE ◇ CHLORETHAZINE
◇ CHLORMETHINE HYDROCHLORIDE ◇ CHLORMETHI-
NUM ◇ 2-CHLORO-N-(2-CHLOROETHYL)-N-METHYLETHA-
NAMINE HYDROCHLORIDE ◇ DEMA ◇ DICHLOREN
◇ DICHLOREN HYDROCHLORIDE ◇ β,β'-DICHLORODI-
ETHYL-N-METHYLAMINE HYDROCHLORIDE ◇ DI(2-CHLO-
ROETHYL)METHYLAMINE HYDROCHLORIDE ◇ 1,5-DI-
CHLORO-3-METHYL-3-AZAPENTANE HYDROCHLORIDE
◇ 2,2'-DICHLORO-N-METHYLDIETHYLAMINE HYDRO-
CHLORIDE ◇ DIMITAN ◇ EMBECHINE ◇ EMBICHIN
◇ EMBICHIN HYDROCHLORIDE ◇ EMBIKHINE ◇ ERASOL
◇ ERASOL HYDROCHLORIDE ◇ ERASOL-IDO ◇ HN2.HCl
◇ HN2 HYDROCHLORIDE ◇ KLORAMIN ◇ N-LOST
◇ MBA HYDROCHLORIDE ◇ MEBICHLORAMINE
◇ MECHLORETHAMINE HYDROCHLORIDE ◇ MERCH-
LORETHANAMINE ◇ METHYLBIS(β-CHLORO-
ETHYL)AMINE HYDROCHLORIDE ◇ N-METHYL-BIS-
β-CHLORETHYLAMINE HYDROCHLORIDE ◇ METHYL-
BIS(2-CHLOROETHYL)AMINE HYDROCHLORIDE

◇ N-METHYLBIS(2-CHLOROETHYL)AMINE HYDROCHLORIDE ◇ N-METHYL-2,2'-DICHLORODIETHYLAMINE HYDROCHLORIDE ◇ N-METHYL-DI-2-CHLOROETHYLAMINE HYDROCHLORIDE ◇ METHYLDI(β-CHLOROETHYL)AMINE HYDROCHLORIDE ◇ METHYLDI(2-CHLOROETHYL)AMINE HYDROCHLORIDE ◇ MITOXINE ◇ N-MUSTARD (GERMAN) ◇ MUSTARGEN ◇ MUSTARGEN HYDROCHLORIDE ◇ MUSTINE HYDROCHLOR ◇ MUSTINE HYDROCHLORIDE ◇ NCI-C56382 ◇ NITOL ◇ NITOL "TAKEDA" ◇ NITROGEN MUSTARD HYDROCHLORIDE ◇ NITROGRANULOGEN ◇ NITROGRANULOGEN HYDROCHLORIDE ◇ NSC 762 ◇ NSC-762 HYDROCHLORIDE ◇ PLIVA ◇ STICKSTOFFLOST ◇ ZAGREB

TOXICITY DATA with REFERENCE

CAR: ipr-mus TDLo:6 mg/kg/4W   JNCIAM 36,915,66

CAR: scu-mus TDLo:22 mg/kg/21W-I   BJCAAI 3,118,49

NEO: ivn-mus TDLo:4 mg/kg/6D-I   JNCIAM 11,415,50

NEO: ivn-mus TDLo:4 mg/kg/6D-I   JNCIAM 11,415,50

ETA: scu-mus TD:6 mg/kg/6W-I   JNCIAM 14,131,53

MUT: dlt-dmg-orl 5 mmol/L   MUREAV 95,237,82
MUT: dnd-rat:lvr 30 μmol/L   SinJF# 26OCT82
MUT: dni-hmn:hla 1 μmol/L   MUREAV 92,427,82
MUT: mma-sat 500 μg/plate   BJCAAI 37,873,78
MUT: mmo-asn 2500 μmol/L   SOGEBZ 6,280,70
MUT: msc-mus:lym 20 μg/L   FCTOD7 23,115,85
MUT: otr-ham:kdy 80 μg/L   BJCAAI 37,873,78
MUT: sln-dmg-orl 5 mmol/L   MUREAV 95,237,82

CONSENSUS REPORTS: IARC Cancer Review: GROUP 2A IMEMDT 7,269,87; Animal Sufficient Evidence IMEMDT 9,193,75. NTP Fourth Annual Report On Carcinogens, 1984. EPA Genetic Toxicology Program.

SAFETY PROFILE: Confirmed carcinogen with experimental carcinogenic, neoplastigenic, and tumorigenic data. Deadly poison by ingestion, intravenous, subcutaneous, intraperitoneal, and parenteral routes. Experimental teratogenic data . Human systemic effects by intravenous route: nausea or vomiting, reduction in the number of white blood cells and blood platelates. Other experimental reproductive effects. Human mutation data reported.

BIF250   CAS: 494-03-1
N,N-BIS(2-CHLOROETHYL)-2-NAPHTHYLAMINE
mf: $C_{14}H_{15}Cl_2N$ mw: 268.20

SYNS: 2-BIS(2-CHLOROETHYL)AMINONAPHTHALENE ◇ BIS(2-CHLOROETHYL)-β-NAPHTHYLAMINE ◇ CHLORNAFTINA ◇ CHLORNAPHAZIN ◇ CHLORNAPHTHIN ◇ CHLORONAFTINA ◇ CHLORONAPHTHINE ◇ CLORNAPHAZINE ◇ DICHLOROETHYL-β-NAPHTHYLAMINE ◇ DI(2-CHLOROETHYL)-β-NAPHTHYLAMINE ◇ N,N-DI(2-CHLOROETHYL)-β-NAPHTHYLAMINE ◇ 2-N,N-DI(2-CHLOROETHYL)NAPHTHYLAMINE ◇ ERYSAN ◇ NAPHTHYLAMINE MUSTARD ◇ β-NAPHTHYL-BIS-(β-CHLOROETHYL)AMINE ◇ 2-NAPHTHYLBIS(2-CHLOROETHYL)AMINE ◇ β-NAPHTHYL-DI-(2-CHLOROETHYL)AMINE ◇ NSC-62209 ◇ R48 ◇ RCRA WASTE NUMBER U026

TOXICITY DATA with REFERENCE

CAR: ipr-mus TDLo:330 mg/kg/4W   JNCIAM 36,915,66

CAR: orl-man TDLo:2468 mg/kg/6Y-I   AMSVAZ 176,45,64

CAR: orl-wmn TD:3200 mg/kg/11Y-I   AMSVAZ 185,133,69

CAR: orl-wmn TD:4090 mg/kg/7Y-I   AMSVAZ 176,45,64

CAR: orl-wmn TDLo:3132 mg/kg/10Y-I   AMSVAZ 175,64

CAR: unr-wmn TDLo:3200 mg/kg/11Y-I   AMSVAZ 175,721,64

MUT: dnd-dmg-orl 260 μmol/L   CNREA8 30,195,70
MUT: mma-sat 10 μg/plate   PNASA6 72,5135,75
MUT: mmo-sat 40 μg/plate   CNREA8 37,2209,77

CONSENSUS REPORTS: IARC Cancer Review: GROUP 1 IMEMDT 7,130,87; Animal Sufficient Evidence IMEMDT 4,119,74; Human Sufficient Evidence IMEMDT 4,119,74. NTP Fourth Annual Report On Carcinogens, 1984. EPA Genetic Toxicology Program.

SAFETY PROFILE: Confirmed human carcinogen producing bladder tumors. Human and experimental carcinogenic data. Moderately toxic by intraperitoneal route. When heated to decomposition it emits very toxic fumes of Cl^- and NO_x.

BIF750   CAS: 154-93-8
N,N'-BIS(2-CHLOROETHYL)-N-NITROSOUREA
mf: $C_5H_9Cl_2N_3O_2$ mw: 214.07

SYNS: BCNU ◇ BiCNU ◇ BIS(2-CHLOROETHYL)NITROSOUREA ◇ 1,3-BIS(β-CHLOROETHYL)-1-NITROSOUREA ◇ 1,3-BIS-(2-CHLOROETHYL)-1-NITROSOUREA ◇ BIS-CHLOROETHYLNITROSOUREA ◇ CARMUBRIS ◇ CARMUSTIN ◇ CARMUSTINE ◇ FDA 0345 ◇ NCI-C04773 ◇ NITRUMON ◇ NSC-409962 ◇ SK 27702 ◇ SRI 1720

TOXICITY DATA with REFERENCE

ETA: ipr-mus TDLo: 98 mg/kg/26W-I   CANCAR
40,1935,77

ETA: ipr-rat TDLo: 15 mg/kg/7W-I   CANCAR
40,1935,77

ETA: ivn-rat TD: 26 mg/kg/60W-I   DTESD7
8,273,80

ETA: ivn-rat TD: 45 mg/kg/60W-I   DTESD7
8,273,80

ETA: ivn-rat TD: 51 mg/kg/24W-I   DTESD7
8,273,80

ETA: ivn-rat TDLo: 16 mg/kg/60W-I   DTESD7
8,273,80

ETA: skn-mus TDLo: 276 mg/kg/23W-I
EXPEAM 36,1211,80

MUT: dnd-mam: lym 10 mmol/L   CNREA8
44,1887,84

MUT: dnd-mus-ipr 150 μmol/kg   JCROD7
110,185,85

MUT: mmo-sat 33 μg/plate   TCMUD8 5,319,85

MUT: oms-mus: bmr 40 μmol/L   CNREA8
45,4185,85

MUT: par-ham LD10: 18 mg/kg   JSONAU15,355,80

MUT: sce-hmn: lym 25 μmol/L   CNREA8
45,4798,85

CONSENSUS REPORTS: IARC Cancer Review: GROUP 2A IMEMDT 7,150,87; Human Limited Evidence IMEMDT 26,79,81; Animal Sufficient Evidence IMEMDT 26,79,81. NTP Fourth Annual Report On Carcinogens, 1984. NCI Carcinogenesis Studies (ipr); Some Evidence: rat CANCAR 40,1935,77; Clear Evidence: mouse CANCAR 40,1935,77. EPA Genetic Toxicology Program.

SAFETY PROFILE: Confirmed carcinogen with experimental carcinogenic, tumorigenic and teratogenic data. A human poison by parenteral route. An experimental poison by ingestion, intravenous, intraperitoneal, parenteral and subcutaneous routes. Human systemic effects by parenteral, intravenous and possibly other routes: nausea or vomiting, reduced white blood cell and blood platelet counts, bone marrow damage and potentially fatal respiratory system effects including lung fibrosis, dyspnea, and cyanosis. Other experimental reproductive effects. Human mutation data reported. When heated to decomposition it emits very toxic fumes of Cl^- and NO_x.

BIH250   CAS: 505-60-2
BIS(2-CHLOROETHYL)SULFIDE
mf: $C_4H_8Cl_2S$ mw: 159.08

PROP: Colorless (if pure), to light yellow, oily liquid. Bp: 228°, fp: 14.4°, flash p: 221°F, d: 1.2741 @ 20°/4°, vap d: 5.4, vap press: 0.09 mm @ 30°.

SYNS: BIS(β-CHLOROETHYL)SULFIDE ◇ BIS(2-CHLORO-ETHYL)SULPHIDE ◇ 1-CHLORO-2-(β-CHLOROETHYL-THIO)ETHANE ◇ β,β-DICHLOR-ETHYL-SULPHIDE ◇ 2,2'-DICHLORODIETHYL SULFIDE ◇ DI-2-CHLORO-ETHYL SULFIDE ◇ β,β'-DICHLOROETHYL SULFIDE ◇ 2,2'-DICHLOROETHYL SULPHIDE (MAK) ◇ DISTILLED MUSTARD ◇ KAMPSTOFF "LOST" ◇ MUSTARD GAS ◇ MUSTARD HD ◇ MUSTARD VAPOR ◇ SCHWEFEL-LOST ◇ S-LOST ◇ S MUSTARD ◇ SULFUR MUSTARD ◇ SULFUR MUSTARD GAS ◇ SULPHUR MUSTARD GAS ◇ 1,1'-THIOBIS(2-CHLOROETHANE) ◇ YELLOW CROSS LIQUID ◇ YPERITE

TOXICITY DATA with REFERENCE

CAR: ihl-rat TCLo: 100 μg/m³/1Y-I   NTIS**
AD-A011-260

NEO: ihl-mus TCLo: 1250 mg/m³/15M-C
PSEBAA 82,457,53

NEO: ivn-mus TDLo: 600 mg/kg/6D-I   JNCIAM
11,415,50

ETA: scu-mus TDLo: 6 mg/kg/6W-I   JNCIAM
14,131,53

MUT: cyt-mam: lym 750 nmol/L   CHRTBC
3,162,72

MUT: dnd-ckn: leu 30 mmol/L   TELEAY
(29),2477,75

MUT: dnd-smc 500 μmol/L   CBINA8 44,27,83

MUT: dns-mam: lym 750 nmol/L   CHRTBC
3,162,72

MUT: oms-hmn: hla 75 mg/L   IUSMDJ 9,41,79

CONSENSUS REPORTS: IARC Cancer Review: GROUP 1 IMEMDT 7,259,87; Animal Sufficient Evidence IMEMDT 9,181,75; Human Limited Evidence IMEMDT 9,181,75. NTP Fourth Annual Report On Carcinogens, 1984. EPA Extremely Hazardous Substances List. Community Right-To-Know List. EPA Genetic Toxicology Program. Reported in EPA TSCA Inventory.

DFG MAK: Human Carcinogen.

SAFETY PROFILE: Confirmed human carcinogen with experimental carcinogenic, neoplastigenic, and tumorigenic data. A human poison by inhalation and subcutaneous routes. An experimental poison by inhalation, skin contact, subcutaneous, and intravenous routes. A severe human skin and eye irritant. Human mutation data reported. A military blistering gas. Strongly effects the skin, eyes, lungs, and gastric system. Pulmonary lesions are often fatal. It penetrates the skin deeply and injures blood vessels. Minute amounts can cause inflammation. Secondary infections are common. Combustible when exposed to heat or flame; can be ignited by a large explosive charge. It will react with water or steam to produce toxic and corrosive fumes. To fight fire, use water, foam, CO_2, dry chemical. Dangerous; when heated to decomposition or on contact with acid or acid fumes it emits highly toxic fumes of SO_x and Cl^-.

BIK000   CAS: 542-88-1
BIS(CHLOROMETHYL) ETHER
DOT: 2249
mf: $C_2H_4Cl_2O$ mw: 114.96

PROP: Volatile liquid. Bp: 105°, d: 1.315 @ 20°, vap d: 4.0. flash p: <19°.

SYNS: BCME ◇ BIS-CME ◇ CHLORO(CHLOROMETH-OXY)METHANE ◇ DICHLORDIMETHYLAETHER (GERMAN) ◇ sym-DICHLORODIMETHYL ETHER (DOT) ◇ sym-DICHLO-ROMETHYL ETHER ◇ DIMETHYL-1,1'-DICHLOROETHER ◇ OXYBIS(CHLOROMETHANE) ◇ RCRA WASTE NUMBER P016

TOXICITY DATA with REFERENCE
CAR: ihl-rat TC: 75 ppb/6H/2Y-I   JJIND868,597,82
CAR: ihl-rat TCLo: 100 ppb/6H/4W-I   AEHLAU 30,73,75
CAR: scu-rat TDLo: 375 mg/kg/43W-I   JNCIAM 43,481,69
CAR: skn-mus TD: 11 g/kg/44W-I   JNCIAM 43,481,69
NEO: ihl-mus TCLo: 100 ppb/6H/26W-I   TXAPA9 58,269,81
NEO: ihl-rat TC: 100 ppb/6H/26W-I   TXAPA9 58,269,81
NEO: ipr-mus TDLo: 50 mg/kg/61W-I   CNREA8 35,2553,75
NEO: scu-mus TD: 640 mg/kg/53W-I   CNREA8 35,2553,75
NEO: scu-mus TD: 12500 μg/kg   TXAPA915,92,69
NEO: scu-mus TDLo: 384 mg/kg/42W-I   CNREA8 40,352,80
ETA: ihl-mus TC: 1 ppm/82D-I   AEHLAU22,663,71
ETA: ihl-rat TC: 100 ppb/6H/6W-I   PAACA3 21,106,80
ETA: skn-mus TDLo: 5520 mg/kg/23W-I   AEHLAU 16,472,68
MUT: dni-mus-skn 360 μmol/kg   CNREA8 33,769,73
MUT: dns-hmn: fbr 160 μg/L   TXCYAC 21,151,81

MUT: dns-mus-skn 360 μmol/kgL   CNREA8 33,769,73
MUT: mma-sat 20 μg/plate   BJCAAI 37,873,78
MUT: otr-ham: kdy 80 μg/L   BJCAAI 37,873,78

CONSENSUS REPORTS: IARC Cancer Review: GROUP 1 IMEMDT 7,131,87; Animal Sufficient Evidence IMEMDT 4,231,74; Human Sufficient Evidence IMEMDT 4,231,74. NTP Fourth Annual Report On Carcinogens, 1984. Community Right-To-Know List. EPA Extremely Hazardous Substances List. Reported in EPA TSCA Inventory.

OSHA: Cancer Suspect Agent   ACGIH TLV: TWA 0.001 ppm; Human Carcinogen   DFG MAK: Human Carcinogen.

SAFETY PROFILE: Confirmed human carcinogen with experimental carcinogenic, neoplastigenic, and tumorigenic data. Poison by inhalation, ingestion, and skin contact. Human systemic effects by inhalation: irritation of the conjunctiva, unspecified nasal and respiratory effects. Human mutation data reported. A dangerous fire hazard. When heated to decomposition it emits very toxic fumes of Cl^-.

BIM500   CAS: 72-54-8
1,1-BIS(4-CHLOROPHENYL)-2,2-DICHLOROETHANE
DOT: 2761
mf: $C_{14}H_{10}Cl_4$ mw: 320.04

PROP: Crystalline solid. Mp: 110°, vap d: 11.

SYNS: 1,1-BIS(p-CHLOROPHENYL)-2,2-DICHLORO-ETHANE ◇ 2,2-BIS(p-CHLOROPHENYL)-1,1-DICHLORO-ETHANE ◇ 2,2-BIS(4-CHLOROPHENYL)-1,1-DICHLORO-ETHANE ◇ DDD ◇ p,p'-DDD ◇ 1,1-DICHLOOR-2,2-BIS(4-CHLOOR FENYL)-ETHAAN (DUTCH) ◇ 1,1-DICHLOR-2,2-BIS(4-CHLOR-PHENYL)-AETHAN (GERMAN) ◇ 1,1-DI-CHLORO-2,2-BIS(p-CHLOROPHENYL)ETHANE ◇ 1,1-DI-CHLORO-2,2-BIS(4-CHLOROPHENYL)-ETHANE (FRENCH) ◇ 1,1-DICHLORO-2,2-BIS(p-CHLOROPHENYL)ETHANE (DOT) ◇ 1,1-DICHLORO-2,2-BIS(PARACHLOROPHE-NYL)ETHANE (DOT) ◇ 1,1-DICHLORO-2,2-DI(4-CHLORO-PHENYL)ETHANE ◇ DICHLORODIPHENYL DICHLORO-ETHANE ◇ p,p'-DICHLORODIPHENYLDICHLOROETHANE ◇ 1,1-DICLORO-2,2-BIS(4-CLORO-FENIL)-ETANO (ITALIAN) ◇ DILENE ◇ ENT 4,225 ◇ ME-1700 ◇ NCI-C00475 ◇ RCRA WASTE NUMBER U060 ◇ RHOTHANE ◇ RHO-THANE D-3 ◇ ROTHANE ◇ TDE ◇ p,p'-TDE ◇ TDE (DOT) ◇ TETRACHLORODIPHENYLETHANE

TOXICITY DATA with REFERENCE
NEO: orl-mus TDLo: 39 g/kg/2Y-C   JNCIAM 52,883,74

ETA: orl-rat TDLo:54 g/kg/78W-C NCITR*
NCI-CG-TR-131,78
MUT: cyt-rat:oth 10 μg/L 34LXAP -,555,76
MUT: hma-mus/srm 1500 mg/kg BIZNAT
91,311,72
MUT: otr-mus:emb 28400 nmol/L JNCIAM
54,981,75

CONSENSUS REPORTS: IARC Cancer Review: Animal Sufficient Evidence IMEMDT 5,83,74. NCI Carcinogenesis Bioassay (feed); Clear Evidence: rat NCITR* NCI-CG-TR-131,78; No Evidence: mouse NCITR* NCI-CG-TR-131,78. EPA Genetic Toxicology Program.

DOT Classification: ORM-A; Label: None.

SAFETY PROFILE: Confirmed carcinogen with experimental carcinogenic, neoplastigenic, and tumorigenic data. Poison by ingestion. Moderately toxic by skin contact. Mutation data reported. An insecticide. When heated to decomposition it emits toxic fumes of Cl^-.

BJB500   CAS: 14239-68-0
BIS(DIETHYLDITHIOCARBAMATO) CADMIUM
mf: $C_{10}H_{20}CdN_2S_4$ mw: 408.96

SYNS: CADMIUM DIETHYL DITHIOCARBAMATE ◇ ETHYL CADMATE ◇ ETHYL TUADS

TOXICITY DATA with REFERENCE
ETA: orl-mus TDLo:7100 mg/kg/78W-I
NTIS** PB223-159
ETA: scu-mus TDLo:1000 mg/kg NTIS**PB223-159
MUT: dnd-esc 1 μmol/L ARTODN 46,277,80
MUT: mma-sat 10 μg/plate MUREAV 68,313,79
MUT: mmo-sat 10 μg/plate MUREAV 68,313,79

CONSENSUS REPORTS: Reported in EPA TSCA Inventory. Cadmium and its compounds are on the Community Right-To-Know List.

OSHA PEL: TWA 0.1 mg(Cd)/m³; CL 0.6 mg(Cd)/m³ (fume) ACGIH TLV: TWA 0.05 mg(Cd)/m³ (Proposed: TWA 0.01 mg(Cd)/m³ (dust), Human Carcinogen); BEI: 10 μg/g creatinine in urine; 10 μg/L in blood. DFG BAT: Blood 1.5 μg/dL; Urine 15 μg/dL, Suspected Carcinogen. NIOSH REL: (Cadmium) Reduce to lowest feasible level

SAFETY PROFILE: Confirmed human carcinogen with experimental tumorigenic data. Mutation data reported. When heated to decomposition it emits very toxic fumes of NO_x and SO_x.

BML000
BRACKEN FERN, DRIED

SYNS: 1-CYCLOHEXENE-1-CARBOXYLIC ACID, 3,4,5 ◇ PTERIDIUM AQUILINUM ◇ PTERIS AQUALINA ◇ S. EGRELTRI ATUNUN (TURKISH)

TOXICITY DATA with REFERENCE
CAR: orl-ctl TD:3072 g/kg/3Y-C CNREA8
28,2247,68
CAR: orl-ctl TDLo:600 g/kg/2Y-C VTPHAK
13,110,76
CAR: orl-rat TD:578 g/kg/33W-C BJCAAI
46,423,82
CAR: orl-rat TD:2292 g/kg/55W-C INURAQ
14,213,76
CAR: orl-rat TD:3465 g/kg/33W-C BJCAAI
46,423,82
CAR: orl-rat TD:8800 g/kg/58W-C NUCADQ
3,86,81
CAR: orl-rat TD:6545 g/kg/17W-C GANMAX
17,205,75
CAR: orl-rat TDLo:2209 g/kg/17W-C JNCIAM
45,179,70
NEO: orl-ctl TD:495 g/kg/68W-C CNREA8
27,917,67
NEO: orl-rat TD:4570 g/kg/32W-C AJVRAH
31,191,70
NEO: orl-rat TD:9144 g/kg/73W-C EXPEAM
31,829,75
NEO: orl-rat TD:1350 g/kg/81D-C GANNA2
69,383,78
ETA: orl-mus TDLo:7140 g/kg/17W-C
GANMAX 17,205,75
MUT: bfa-ctl/sat 623 g/kg/2Y-C CNREA8
38,1556,78
MUT: bfa-rat/sat 1000 g/kg JJIND8 65,131,80
MUT: sln-dmg-orl 15 pph MUREAV 92,89,82

CONSENSUS REPORTS: IARC Cancer Review: Human Inadequate Evidence IMEMDT 40,47,86; Animal Sufficient Evidence IMEMDT 40,47,86

SAFETY PROFILE: Confirmed carcinogen with experimental carcinogenic, neoplastigenic, tumorigenic, and teratogenic data. Other experimental reproductive effects. Mutation data reported.

BOP500   CAS: 106-99-0
1,3-BUTADIENE
mf: C_4H_6 mw: 54.10

PROP: Colorless gas; mild aromatic odor. Very reactive. Bp: −4.5°, mp: −113°, fp: −108.9°, flash p: −105°F, lel: 2.0%, uel: 11.5%, d: 0.621 @ 2 0°/4°, autoign temp: 788°F, vap d: 1.87, vap press: 1840 mm @ 21°.

SYNS: BIETHYLENE ◇ BIVINYL ◇ BUTADIEEN (DUTCH) ◇ BUTA-1,3-DIEEN (DUTCH) ◇ BUTADIEN (POLISH) ◇ BUTA-1,3-DIEN (GERMAN) ◇ BUTA-1,3-DIENE ◇ α-γ-BUTADIENE ◇ DIVINYL ◇ ERYTHRENE ◇ NCI-C50602 ◇ PYRROLYLENE ◇ VINYLETHYLENE

TOXICITY DATA with REFERENCE
CAR: ihl-mus TCLo:1250 ppm/6H/60W-I
    SCIEAS 227,548,85
CAR: ihl-rat TC:1000 ppm/6H/2Y-I   AIHAAP
    48,407,87
CAR: ihl-rat TC:8000 ppm/6H/15W-I   EPASR*
    8EHQ-0482-0370
CAR: ihl-rat TCLo:625 ppm/6H/61W   NTPTR*
    NTP-TR-288,84
NEO: ihl-rat TC:8000 ppm/6H/2Y-I   AIHAAP
    48,407,87
MUT: mma-sat 2 pph   TOLED5 6,125,80
MUT: mmo-sat 20 pph/20H-C   TOERD9 3,131,81
MUT: mnt-mus:ihl 100 ppm/6H/2D-C
    ENMUDM 8(Suppl 6),18,86
MUT: msc-mus:lym 20 pph   ENMUDM 8(Suppl
    6),75,86
MUT: sce-mus:ihl 100 ppm/6H/2D-C   ENMUDM
    8(Suppl 6),19,86

CONSENSUS REPORTS: IARC Cancer Review: GROUP 2B IMEMDT 7,136,87; Human Inadequate Evidence IMEMDT 39,155,86; Animal Sufficient Evidence IMEMDT 39,155,86. NTP Carcinogenesis Studies (inhalation); Clear Evidence: mouse NTPTR* NTP-TR-288,84. Reported in EPA TSCA Inventory. Community Right-To-Know List.

OSHA PEL: TWA 1000 ppm   ACGIH TLV: TWA 10 ppm; Suspected Human Carcinogen   DFG MAK: Processing after polymerization and loading: 15 ppm; Others: 5 ppm; Animal Carcinogen, Suspected Human Carcinogen. NIOSH REL: Reduce to lowest feasible level DOT Classification: Flammable Gas; Label: Flammable Gas.

SAFETY PROFILE: Confirmed carcinogen with experimental carcinogenic and neoplastigenic data. Experimental reproductive effects. Mutation data reported. Inhalation of high concentrations can cause unconsciousness and death. Human systemic effects by inhalation: cough, hallucinations, distorted perceptions, changes in the visual field and other unspecified eye effects. The vapors are irritating to eyes and mucous membranes. If spilled on skin or clothing, it can cause burns or frost bite (due to rapid vaporization). Chronic systemic poisoning in humans has not been reported. Dangerous fire hazard when exposed to heat, flame, or powerful oxidizers. Explodes on contact with aluminum tetrahydroborate. To fight fire, stop flow of gas. When heated to decomposition it emits acrid smoke and fumes.

BOT250   CAS: 55-98-1
1,4-BUTANEDIOL DIMETHYL SULFONATE
mf: $C_6H_{14}O_6S_2$ mw: 246.32

PROP: White crystals. Mp: 114-118°.

SYNS: 1,4-BIS(METHANESULFONOXY)BUTANE ◇ (1,4-BIS(METHANESULFONYLOXY)BUTANE) ◇ BISULFAN ◇ BISULPHANE ◇ 1,4-BUTANEDIOL DIMETHANESULPHONATE ◇ BUZULFAN ◇ C.B. 2041 ◇ CITOSULFAN ◇ 1,4-DIMESYLOXYBUTANE ◇ 1,4-DIMETHANESULFONOXYBUTANE ◇ 1,4-DI(METHANESULFONYLOXY)BUTANE ◇ 1,4-DIMETHANESULPHONYLOXYBUTANE ◇ 1,4-DIMETHYLSULFONOXYBUTANE ◇ GT41 ◇ GT 2041 ◇ LEUCOSULFAN ◇ MABLIN ◇ METHANESULFONIC ACID TETRAMETHYLENE ESTER ◇ MIELUCIN ◇ MISULBAN ◇ MITOSTAN ◇ MYELOLEUKON ◇ MYLERAN ◇ NCI-C01592 ◇ NSC-750 ◇ SULPHABUTIN ◇ TETRAMETHYLENE BIS(METHANESULFONATE) ◇ TETRAMETHYLENE DIMETHANE SULFONATE ◇ X 149

TOXICITY DATA with REFERENCE
CAR: orl-man TDLo:5684 μg/kg/21W-C
    BMJOAE 2,1513,77
CAR: orl-wmn TD:1140 mg/kg/9Y-I   AIMDAP
    124,66,69
CAR: orl-wmn TD:16720 μg/kg/2Y-I   JCROD7
    108,362,84
NEO: ivn-mus TDLo:48 mg/kg/42D-I   CNREA8
    25,20,65
ETA: ipr-mus TD:70 mg/kg/6W-I   BLOOAW
    44,49,74
ETA: ipr-mus TD:1200 mg/kg/8W-I   CNREA8
    33,3069,73
MUT: mma-esc 25 μg/plate   TAKHAA 44,96,85
MUT: mma-sat 100 μg/plate   ENMUDM 8(Suppl
    7),1,86
MUT: mmo-sat 333 μg/plate   ENMUDM 8(Suppl
    7),1,86
MUT: sce-ham:ovr 20 mg/L   CNREA8 43,577,83

CONSENSUS REPORTS: IARC Cancer Review: GROUP 1 IMEMDT 7,137,87; Animal

Inadequate Evidence IMEMDT 4,247,74; Human Inadequate Evidence IMEMDT 4,247,74. NTP Fourth Annual Report On Carcinogens, 1984. EPA Genetic Toxicology Program.

SAFETY PROFILE: Confirmed carcinogen producing leukemia, kidney, and uterine tumors. Experimental neoplastigenic and tumorigenic data. Human teratogenic data. Poison by ingestion, subcutaneous, intraperitoneal, intravenous, and possibly other routes. Ingestion by pregnant women can cause cancer of the reproductive system of the fetus including the uterus. Human teratogenic effects by ingestion and possibly other routes include developmental abnormalities of the eye, ear, craniofacial area including the nose and tongue, gastrointestinal system, endocrine system, urogenital system, and other unspecified areas. Other human reproductive effects by ingestion and possibly other routes include: impotence; changes in the uterus, cervix, and vagina; and menstrual cycle disorders. Experimental reproductive effects. Human mutation data reported. When heated to decomposition it emits toxic fumes of SO_x.

BQQ250   CAS: 38252-74-3
N-BUTYL-(3-CARBOXY PROPYL)NITROSAMINE
mf: $C_8H_{16}N_2O_3$ mw: 188.26

SYNS: BCPN ◇ 4-(BUTYLNITROSOAMINO)BUTANOIC ACID ◇ N-NITROSO-N-BUTYL-N-(3-CARBOXYPROPYL)AMINE

TOXICITY DATA with REFERENCE
CAR: orl-rat TDLo: 3760 mg/kg/12W-C
  CRNGDP 4,617,83
ETA: orl-mus TDLo: 7 g/kg/20W-C   GANNA2
  67,175,76
ETA: orl-rat TD: 4375 mg/kg/20W-C   GANNA2
  67,175,76
ETA: orl-rat TD: 4700 mg/kg/14W-C   GANNA2
  63,637,72
MUT: dnd-rat-par 50 mg/kg   CBINA8 29,291,80
MUT: mmo-sat 10 μmol/plate   CNREA8 37,399,77

CONSENSUS REPORTS: IARC Cancer Review: Animal Limited Evidence IMEMDT 17,51,78. NTP Fourth Annual Report On Carcinogens, 1984. EPA Genetic Toxicology Program.

SAFETY PROFILE: Confirmed carcinogen with experimental carcinogenic and tumorigenic

data. Mutation data reported. When heated to decomposition it emits toxic fumes of NO_x.

BRY500   CAS: 924-16-3
n-BUTYL-N-NITROSO-1-BUTAMINE
mf: $C_8H_{18}N_2O$ mw: 158.28

PROP: Pale yellow liquid. Bp: 235°.

SYNS: DBN ◇ DBNA ◇ DI-n-BUTYLNITROSAMIN (GERMAN) ◇ DIBUTYLNITROSOAMINE ◇ DI-n-BUTYLNITROSAMINE ◇ N,N-DI-n-BUTYLNITROSAMINE ◇ N,N-DIBUTYLNITROSOAMINE ◇ NDBA ◇ N-NITROSODIBUTYLAMINE ◇ N-NITROSODI-n-BUTYLAMINE (MAK) ◇ RCRA WASTE NUMBER U172

TOXICITY DATA with REFERENCE
CAR: ivn-mus TDLo: 12 mg/kg/25W-I   IDZAAW
  45,71,70
CAR: orl-rat TD: 648 mg/kg/2Y-I   CALEDQ
  19,207,83
CAR: orl-rat TDLo: 140 mg/kg/4W-C   CNREA8
  46,6160,86
CAR: scu-ham TDLo: 240 mg/kg/8D-I: TER
  ZEKBAI 86,69,76
CAR: scu-mus TDLo: 800 mg/kg/40W-I
  EJCAAH 6,433,70
NEO: ipr-mus TDLo: 240 mg/kg/8W-I   TXAPA9
  82,19,86
NEO: orl-mus TD: 2190 mg/kg/1Y-C   GANNA2
  60,353,69
NEO: orl-mus TDLo: 1200 mg/kg/8W-I
  TXAPA9 82,19,86
NEO: scu-rbt TDLo: 34 g/kg/78W-I   INURAQ
  12,262,75
ETA: ipr-ham TDLo: 200 mg/kg   ZEKBAI
  79,85,73
ETA: orl-gpg TDLo: 24 g/kg/2Y-I   ZEKBAI
  71,183,68
ETA: orl-ham TDLo: 3900 mg/kg/13W-I
  PSEBAA 136,168,71
ETA: orl-rat TD: 64 g/kg/20W-C   GANNA2
  67,825,76
ETA: orl-rat TD: 882 mg/kg/2W-C   JJCREP
  78,227,87
ETA: orl-rat TD: 3640 mg/kg/26W-C   EVHPAZ
  50,169,83
ETA: orl-rat TD: 3900 mg/kg/56W-C   ARZNAD
  19,1077,69
ETA: orl-rat TD: 12600 mg/kg/30W-C   IAPUDO
  41,649,82
ETA: scu-ham TD: 2162 mg/kg/46W-I   JNCIAM
  57,401,76
ETA: scu-mus TD: 3200 mg/kg/30W-I   BECCAN
  46,271,68

ETA: scu-rat TD:7400 mg/kg/37W-I   ARZNAD 19,1077,69

ETA: scu-rat TDLo:8 g/kg/20W-I   XENOBH 3,271,73

MUT: bfa-rat/sat 158 mg/kg   CRNGDP 6,967,85

MUT: dnd-esc 100 nmol/tube   CRNGDP 3,781,82

MUT: dnd-rat:lvr 100 μmol/L   CNREA8 42,2592,82

MUT: dns-hmn:hla 10 μmol/L   CNREA8 38,2621,78

MUT: hma-rat/smc 2912 mg/kg   TCMUD8 3,41,83

MUT: mma-esc 1 μmol/plate   GANNA2 75,8,84

CONSENSUS REPORTS: IARC Cancer Review: GROUP 2B IMEMDT 7,56,87; Animal Sufficient Evidence IMEMDT 28,151,82; IMEMDT 17,51,78; IMEMDT 4,197,74; Human Limited Evidence IMEMDT 17,51,78. NTP Fourth Annual Report On Carcinogens, 1984. Community Right-To-Know List. EPA Genetic Toxicology Program. Reported in EPA TSCA Inventory.

DFG MAK: Animal Carcinogen, Suspected Human Carcinogen.

SAFETY PROFILE: Confirmed carcinogen with experimental carcinogenic, tumorigenic, neoplastigenic, and teratogenic data. Moderately toxic by ingestion, subcutaneous and intraperitoneal routes. Human mutation data reported. When heated to decomposition it emits toxic fumes of NO_x.

CAD000   CAS: 7440-43-9
CADMIUM
af: Cd   aw: 112.40

PROP: Hexagonal crystals, silver-white, malleable metal. Mp: 320.9°, bp: 767 ± 2°, d: 8.642, vap press: 1 mm @ 394°.

SYNS: C.I. 77180 ◇ COLLOIDAL CADMIUM ◇ KADMIUM (GERMAN)

TOXICITY DATA with REFERENCE
CAR: ims-rat TDLo:40 mg/kg/4W-I   JEPTDQ 1(1),51,77

NEO: ims-rat TD:45 mg/kg/4W-I
NCIUS* PH-43-64-886,SEPT,71

ETA: ims-rat TD:63 mg/kg   NATUAS 193,592,62

ETA: ims-rat TD:70 mg/kg   BJCAAI 18,124,64

MUT: cyt-ham:ovr 1 μmol/L   CGCGBR 26,251,80

CONSENSUS REPORTS: IARC Cancer Review: Animal Sufficient Evidence IMEMDT 11,39,76; IMEMDT 2,74,73. NTP Fourth Annual Report On Carcinogens, 1984. Cadmium and its compounds are on the Community Right-

To-Know List. Reported in EPA TSCA Inventory. EPA Genetic Toxicology Program.

OSHA PEL: Fume: TWA 0.1 mg(Cd)/m^3; CL 0.6 mg(Cd)/m^3; Dust: TWA 0.2 mg(Cd)/m^3; CL 0.6 mg(Cd)/m^3 ACGIH TLV: Dust and Salts: TWA 0.05 mg(Cd)/m^3 (Proposed: TWA 0.01 mg(Cd)/m^3 (dust), Human Carcinogen); BEI: 10 μg/g creatinine in urine; 10 μg/L in blood.   DFG BAT: Blood 1.5 μg/dL; Urine 15 μg/dL. MAK: Suspected Carcinogen. NIOSH REL: (Cadmium) Reduce to lowest feasible level

SAFETY PROFILE: Confirmed human carcinogen with experimental carcinogenic, tumorigenic, neoplastigenic, and teratogenic data. A human poison by inhalation and possibly other routes. Poison experimentally by ingestion, inhalation, intraperitoneal, subcutaneous, intramuscular, and intravenous routes. In humans inhalation causes an excess of protein in the urine. Experimental reproductive effects. Mutation data reported. The dust ignites spontaneously in air and is flammable and explosive when exposed to heat, flame, or by chemical reaction. When heated to a high temperature it emits toxic fumes of Cd.

CAD250   CAS: 543-90-8
CADMIUM(II) ACETATE
DOT: 2570
mf: $C_2H_4O_2 \cdot 1/2Cd$ mw: 116.25

PROP: Monoclinic, colorless crystals; odor of acetic acid. Mp: 256°, bp: decomp, d: 2.341.

SYNS: ACETIC ACID, CADMIUM SALT ◇ BIS(ACETOXY)CADMIUM ◇ CADMIUM ACETATE (DOT) ◇ CADMIUM DIACETATE ◇ C.I. 77185

TOXICITY DATA with REFERENCE
MUT: cyt-hmn:lym 10 nmol/L   MUREAV 85,236,81

MUT: dnd-ham:emb 1 μmol/L   CNREA8 39,193,79

MUT: otr-ham:emb 1 μmol/L   CNREA8 39,193,79

CONSENSUS REPORTS: Reported in EPA TSCA Inventory. EPA Genetic Toxicology Program. Cadmium and its compounds are on the Community Right-To-Know List.

OSHA PEL: TWA 0.2 mg(Cd)/m^3; CL 0.6 mg(Cd)/m^3 (dust)   ACGIH TLV: TWA 0.05 mg(Cd)/m^3 (Proposed: TWA 0.01 mg(Cd)/m^3 (dust), Human Carcinogen); BEI: 10 μg/g creatinine in urine; 10 μg/L in blood.   NIOSH REL: (Cadmium) Reduce to lowest feasible level

SAFETY PROFILE: Confirmed human carcinogen. Poison by intraperitoneal route. An experimental teratogen. Other experimental reproductive effects. Human mutation data reported. When heated to decomposition it emits toxic fumes of Cd.

CAD325   CAS: 22750-53-4
CADMIUM AMIDE
mf: CdH_4N_2 mw: 144.46

SYN: CADMIUM DIAMIDE

CONSENSUS REPORTS: Cadmium compounds are on the Community Right-To-Know List.

OSHA PEL: TWA 0.2 mg(Cd)/m^3; CL 0.6 mg(Cd)/m^3 (dust) ACGIH TLV: TWA 0.05 mg(Cd)/m^3 (Proposed: TWA 0.01 mg(Cd)/m^3 (dust), Human Carcinogen); BEI: 10 μg/g creatinine in urine; 10 μg/L in blood. NIOSH REL: (Cadmium) Reduce to lowest feasible level

SAFETY PROFILE: Confirmed human carcinogen. May explode if heated. Reacts violently with water. When heated to decomposition it emits toxic fumes of Cd and NO$_x$.

CAD350   CAS: 14215-29-3
CADMIUM AZIDE
mf: CdN_6 mw: 196.45

SYN: CADMIUM DIAZIDE

CONSENSUS REPORTS: Cadmium compounds are on the Community Right-To-Know List.

OSHA PEL: TWA 0.2 mg(Cd)/m^3; CL 0.6 mg(Cd)/m^3 (dust) ACGIH TLV: TWA 0.05 mg(Cd)/m^3 (Proposed: TWA 0.01 mg(Cd)/m^3 (dust), Human Carcinogen); BEI: 10 μg/g creatinine in urine; 10 μg/L in blood. NIOSH REL: (Cadmium) Reduce to lowest feasible level

SAFETY PROFILE: Confirmed human carcinogen. The dry solid is an unstable heat- and friction-sensitive explosive. When heated to decomposition it emits toxic fumes of NO$_x$ and Cd.

CAD500   CAS: 7495-93-4
CADMIUM BIS(2-ETHYLHEXYL) PHOSPHITE
mf: $C_{32}H_{68}O_6P_2 \cdot Cd$ mw: 723.34

SYN: BIS(2-ETHYLHEXYL) ESTER PHOSPHORUS ACID CADMIUM SALT

CONSENSUS REPORTS: Cadmium and its compounds are on the Community Right-To-Know List.

OSHA PEL: TWA 0.2 mg(Cd)/m^3; CL 0.6 mg(Cd)/m^3 (dust) ACGIH TLV: TWA 0.05 mg(Cd)/m^3 (Proposed: TWA 0.01 mg(Cd)/m^3 (dust), Human Carcinogen); BEI: 10 μg/g creatinine in urine; 10 μg/L in blood. NIOSH REL: (Cadmium) Reduce to lowest feasible level

SAFETY PROFILE: Confirmed human carcinogen. Poison by intraperitoneal route. When heated to decomposition it emits toxic fumes of PO$_x$ and Cd.

CAD750   CAS: 2191-10-8
CADMIUM CAPRYLATE
mf: $C_{16}H_{30}O_4 \cdot Cd$ mw: 398.86

SYN: OCTANOIC ACID, CADMIUM SALT (2:1)

CONSENSUS REPORTS: Reported in EPA TSCA Inventory. Cadmium and its compounds are on the Community Right-To-Know List.

OSHA PEL: TWA 0.2 mg(Cd)/m^3; CL 0.6 mg(Cd)/m^3 (dust) ACGIH TLV: TWA 0.05 mg(Cd)/m^3 (Proposed: TWA 0.01 mg(Cd)/m^3 (dust), Human Carcinogen); BEI: 10 μg/g creatinine in urine; 10 μg/L in blood. NIOSH REL: (Cadmium) Reduce to lowest feasible level

SAFETY PROFILE: Confirmed human carcinogen. Poison by ingestion and intratracheal routes. When heated to decomposition it emits toxic fumes of Cd.

CAE000
CADMIUM CHLORATE
mf: $CdCl_2O_6$ mw: 279.31

PROP: Colorless, deliquescent prisms. Mp: 80°, d: 2.28 @ 18°.

CONSENSUS REPORTS: Cadmium and its compounds are on the Community Right-To-Know List.

OSHA PEL: TWA 0.2 mg(Cd)/m^3; CL 0.6 mg(Cd)/m^3 (dust) ACGIH TLV: TWA 0.05 mg(Cd)/m^3 (Proposed: TWA 0.01 mg(Cd)/m^3 (dust), Human Carcinogen); BEI: 10 μg/g creatinine in urine; 10 μg/L in blood. NIOSH REL: (Cadmium) Reduce to lowest feasible level

SAFETY PROFILE: Confirmed human carcinogen. A powerful oxidizing agent. Flammable by chemical reaction with reducing agents. When heated to decomposition it emits toxic fumes of Cd and Cl$^-$.

CAE250   CAS: 10108-64-2
CADMIUM CHLORIDE
mf: $CdCl_2$ mw: 183.30
DOT: 2570

PROP: Hexagonal, colorless crystals. Mp: 568°, d: 4.047 @ 25°, vap press: 10 mm @ 656°, bp: 960°.

SYNS: CADDY ◇ CADMIUM DICHLORIDE ◇ KADMIUM-CHLORID (GERMAN) ◇ VI-CAD

TOXICITY DATA with REFERENCE
CAR: ihl-rat TC: 41 μg/m^3/23H/78-W-C   JJIND8 70,367,83
CAR: ihl-rat TC: 82 μg/m^3/23H/78W-C   JJIND8 70,367,83
CAR: ihl-rat TCLo: 20 μg/m^3/23H/78W-C   JJIND8 70,367,83
CAR: scu-rat TD: 40770 ng/kg/2D-I   CNREA8 48,4656,88
CAR: scu-rat TD: 7332 μg/kg   PAACA3 24,84,83
CAR: scu-rat TDLo: 3666 μg/kg   PAACA3 24,84,83
NEO: scu-rat TD: 3666 mg/kg   CNREA8 43,4575,83
NEO: scu-rat TD: 5499 μg/kg   PSEBAA 115,653,64
NEO: scu-rat TD: 7332 mg/kg   CNREA8 43,4575,83
ETA: ims-rat TDLo: 4500 μg/kg   ARPAAQ 83,493,67
ETA: par-rat TDLo: 1700 μg/kg   ARPAAQ 83,493,67
ETA: scu-mus TDLo: 5499 μg/kg   JNCIAM 31,745,63
ETA: scu-rat TD: 4500 μg/kg   ARPAAQ 83,493,67
MUT: cyt-ham: ovr 250 μg/L   BECTA6 36,342,86
MUT: cyt-hmn: leu 1 μmol/L   TKIZAM 82,232,74
MUT: cyt-ofs-mul 630 μg/L/4W-C   BECTA6 36,199,86
MUT: dni-hmn: hla 250 μmol/L   MUREAV 92,427,82
MUT: dni-mam: kdy 2 μmol/L   TXCYAC 34,189,85
MUT: oms-ham: ovr 500 μg/L   BECTA6 36,342,86
MUT: ihl-dog LC90: 420 mg/m^3/30M   JIHTAB 29,302,47

CONSENSUS REPORTS: IARC Cancer Review: Animal Sufficient Evidence IMEMDT 11,39,76; IMEMDT 2,74,73. NTP Fourth Annual Report On Carcinogens, 1984. EPA Genetic Toxicology Program. Cadmium and its compounds are on the Community Right-To-Know List. Reported in EPA TSCA Inventory.

OSHA PEL: TWA 0.2 mg(Cd)/m^3; CL 0.6 mg(Cd)/m^3 (dust)   ACGIH TLV: TWA 0.05 mg(Cd)/m^3 (Proposed: TWA 0.01 mg(Cd)/m^3 (dust), Human Carcinogen); BEI: 10 μg/g creatinine in urine; 10 μg/L in blood.   DFG MAK: Animal Carcinogen, Suspected Human Carcinogen.   NIOSH REL: (Cadmium) Reduce to lowest feasible level   DOT Classification: ORM-E; Label: None.

SAFETY PROFILE: Confirmed human carcinogen with experimental carcinogenic, tumorigenic and teratogenic data. Poison by ingestion, inhalation, skin contact, intraperitoneal, subcutaneous, intravenous and possibly other routes. Experimental reproductive effects. Human mutation data reported. When heated to decomposition it emits very toxic fumes of Cd and Cl$^-$.

CAE375   CAS: 72589-96-9
CADMIUM CHLORIDE, DIHYDRATE
mf: $CdCl_2 \cdot 2H_2O$ mw: 219.34

TOXICITY DATA with REFERENCE
ETA: scu-rat TDLo: 6580 μg/kg   ARGEAR 36,119,70

CONSENSUS REPORTS: Cadmium and its compounds are on the Community Right-To-Know List.

OSHA PEL: TWA 0.2 mg(Cd)/m^3; CL 0.6 mg(Cd)/m^3 (dust)   ACGIH TLV: TWA 0.05 mg(Cd)/m^3 (Proposed: TWA 0.01 mg(Cd)/m^3 (dust), Human Carcinogen); BEI: 10 μg/g creatinine in urine; 10 μg/L in blood.   DFG MAK: Animal Carcinogen, Suspected Human Carcinogen.   NIOSH REL: (Cadmium) Reduce to lowest feasible level

SAFETY PROFILE: Confirmed human carcinogen with experimental tumorigenic data. Experimental reproductive effects. When heated to decomposition it emits toxic fumes of Cl$^-$ and Cd.

CAE425   CAS: 7790-78-5
CADMIUM CHLORIDE, HYDRATE (2:5)
mf: $CdCl_2 \cdot 5/2H_2O$ mw: 228.35

TOXICITY DATA with REFERENCE
MUT: dni-hmn: lym 28 μmol/L   IAAAAM 79,83,86

CONSENSUS REPORTS: Cadmium and its compounds are on the Community Right-To-Know List.

OSHA PEL: TWA 0.2 mg(Cd)/m^3; CL 0.6 mg(Cd)/m^3 (dust) ACGIH TLV: TWA 0.05 mg(Cd)/m^3 (Proposed: TWA 0.01 mg(Cd)/m^3 (dust), Human Carcinogen); BEI: 10 μg/g creatinine in urine; 10 μg/L in blood. DFG MAK: Animal Carcinogen, Suspected Human Carcinogen. NIOSH REL: (Cadmium) Reduce to lowest feasible level

SAFETY PROFILE: Confirmed human carcinogen. Poison by intraperitoneal route. Experimental reproductive effects. Human mutation data reported. When heated to decomposition it emits toxic fumes of Cl$^-$ and Cd.

CAE500   CAS: 35658-65-2
CADMIUM CHLORIDE, MONOHYDRATE
mf: CdCl$_2$•H$_2$O   mw: 201.32

TOXICITY DATA with REFERENCE
ETA: orl-rat TDLo:65 mg/kg/2Y-C   CALEDQ
   9,191,80

CONSENSUS REPORTS: Cadmium and its compounds are on the Community Right-To-Know List.

OSHA PEL: TWA 0.2 mg(Cd)/m^3; CL 0.6 mg(Cd)/m^3 (dust) ACGIH TLV: TWA 0.05 mg(Cd)/m^3 (Proposed: TWA 0.01 mg(Cd)/m^3 (dust), Human Carcinogen); BEI: 10 μg/g creatinine in urine; 10 μg/L in blood. DFG MAK: Animal Carcinogen, Suspected Human Carcinogen. NIOSH REL: (Cadmium) Reduce to lowest feasible level

SAFETY PROFILE: Confirmed human carcinogen with experimental tumorigenic data. When heated to decomposition it emits very toxic fumes of Cd and Cl$^-$.

CAE750
CADMIUM COMPOUNDS

TOXICITY DATA with REFERENCE
CAR: ihl-hmn TCLo:1500 μg/m^3/14Y-I:PUL
   ANYAA9 271,273,76

CONSENSUS REPORTS: Cadmium and its compounds are on the Community Right-To-Know List.

OSHA PEL: Fume: TWA 0.1 mg(Cd)/m^3; CL 0.6 mg(Cd)/m^3; Dust: TWA 0.2 mg(Cd)/m^3; CL 0.6 mg(Cd)/m^3 ACGIH TLV: Dust and Salts: TWA 0.05 mg(Cd)/m^3 (Proposed: TWA 0.01 mg(Cd)/m^3 (dust), Human Carcinogen); BEI: 10 μg/g creatinine in urine; 10 μg/L in blood. DFG BAT: Blood 1.5 μg/dL; Urine 15 μg/dL. MAK: Suspected Carcinogen. NIOSH REL: (Cadmium) Reduce to lowest feasible level

SAFETY PROFILE: Confirmed human carcinogen producing lung tumors. Poison by ingestion. The irritating and emetic action is so violent, however, that little of the cadmium has time to be absorbed and fatal poisoning rarely ensues. Experimental carcinogens and teratogens. Cases of human poisoning have been reported from ingestion of food or beverages prepared or stored in cadmium-plated containers. Inhalation of fumes or dusts affects the respiratory tract and the kidneys. Brief exposure to high concentrations may result in pulmonary edema and death. Fatal concentrations may be breathed without sufficient discomfort to warn a workers to leave the exposure. Cadmium oxide fumes can cause metal fume fever resembling that caused by zinc oxide fumes. When heated to decomposition they emit toxic fumes of Cd.

CAF500
CADMIUM DICYANIDE
mf: C$_2$CdN$_2$ mw: 164.44

CONSENSUS REPORTS: Cadmium and its compounds and Cyanide and its compounds are on the Community Right-To-Know List.

OSHA PEL: TWA 0.2 mg(Cd)/m^3; CL 0.6 mg(Cd)/m^3 (dust) ACGIH TLV: TWA 0.05 mg(Cd)/m^3 (Proposed: TWA 0.01 mg(Cd)/m^3 (dust), Human Carcinogen); BEI: 10 μg/g creatinine in urine; 10 μg/L in blood. NIOSH REL: (Cadmium) Reduce to lowest feasible level

SAFETY PROFILE: Confirmed human carcinogen. A poison. When heated to decomposition it emits toxic fumes of Cd and CN$^-$.

CAF750   CAS: 15954-91-3
CADMIUM(II) EDTA COMPLEX

SYN: (ETHYLENEDINITRILO)TETRAACETIC ACID CADMIUM(II) COMPLEX

CONSENSUS REPORTS: Cadmium and its compounds are on the Community Right-To-Know List.

OSHA PEL: TWA 0.2 mg(Cd)/m^3; CL 0.6 mg(Cd)/m^3 (dust) ACGIH TLV: TWA 0.05 mg(Cd)/m^3 (Proposed: TWA 0.01 mg(Cd)/m^3 (dust), Human Carcinogen); BEI: 10 μg/g creatinine in urine; 10 μg/L in blood. NIOSH REL: (Cadmium) Reduce to lowest feasible level

SAFETY PROFILE: Confirmed human carcinogen. Poison by intraperitoneal route. When heated to decomposition it emits toxic fumes of NO_x and Cd.

CAG000   CAS: 14486-19-2
CADMIUM FLUOBORATE
mf: B_2CdF_8 mw: 286.02

SYNS: CADMIUM FLUOROBORATE ◇ TL 1026

CONSENSUS REPORTS: Reported in EPA TSCA Inventory. Cadmium and its compounds are on the Community Right-To-Know List.

OSHA PEL: TWA 0.2 mg(Cd)/m³; CL 0.6 mg(Cd)/m³ (dust); 2.5 mg(F)/m³ ACGIH TLV: TWA 0.05 mg(Cd)/m³ (Proposed: TWA 0.01 mg(Cd)/m³ (dust), Human Carcinogen); BEI: 10 μg/g creatinine in urine; 10 μg/L in blood. NIOSH REL: (Cadmium) Reduce to lowest feasible level

SAFETY PROFILE: Confirmed human carcinogen. Poison by ingestion and inhalation. When heated to decomposition it emits very toxic fumes of Cd and F^-.

CAG250   CAS: 7790-79-6
CADMIUM FLUORIDE
mf: CdF_2 mw: 150.40

PROP: Cubic, white crystals. Mp: 1100°, bp: 1758°, d: 6.64, vap press: 1 mm @ 1112°.

SYN: CADMIUM FLUORURE (FRENCH)

CONSENSUS REPORTS: Reported in EPA TSCA Inventory. Cadmium and its compounds are on the Community Right-To-Know List.

OSHA PEL: TWA 0.2 mg(Cd)/m³; CL 0.6 mg(Cd)/m³ (dust); 2.5 mg(F)/m³ ACGIH TLV: TWA 0.05 mg(Cd)/m³ (Proposed: TWA 0.01 mg(Cd)/m³ (dust), Human Carcinogen); BEI: 10 μg/g creatinine in urine; 10 μg/L in blood. NIOSH REL: (Cadmium) Reduce to lowest feasible level

SAFETY PROFILE: Confirmed human carcinogen. Poison by subcutaneous route. When

heated to decomposition it emits very toxic fumes of Cd and F^-.

CAG500   CAS: 17010-21-8
CADMIUM FLUOSILICATE
mf: CdF_6Si mw: 254.49

PROP: Hexagonal, colorless crystals.

SYN: TL 1070

CONSENSUS REPORTS: Cadmium and its compounds are on the Community Right-To-Know List.

OSHA PEL: TWA 0.2 mg(Cd)/m³; CL 0.6 mg(Cd)/m³ (dust); 2.5 mg(F)/m³ ACGIH TLV: TWA 0.05 mg(Cd)/m³ (Proposed: TWA 0.01 mg(Cd)/m³ (dust), Human Carcinogen); BEI: 10 μg/g creatinine in urine; 10 μg/L in blood. NIOSH REL: (Cadmium) Reduce to lowest feasible level

SAFETY PROFILE: Confirmed human carcinogen. Poison by ingestion and inhalation. When heated to decomposition it emits very toxic fumes of Cd and F^-.

CAG750   CAS: 16039-55-7
CADMIUM LACTATE
mf: $C_6H_{10}O_6 \cdot Cd$ mw: 290.56

PROP: Needles.

SYN: LACTIC ACID, CADMIUM SALT

CONSENSUS REPORTS: Cadmium and its compounds are on the Community Right-To-Know List.

OSHA PEL: TWA 0.2 mg(Cd)/m³; CL 0.6 mg(Cd)/m³ (dust) ACGIH TLV: TWA 0.05 mg(Cd)/m³ (Proposed: TWA 0.01 mg(Cd)/m³ (dust), Human Carcinogen); BEI: 10 μg/g creatinine in urine; 10 μg/L in blood. NIOSH REL: (Cadmium) Reduce to lowest feasible level

SAFETY PROFILE: Confirmed human carcinogen. A poison. When heated to decomposition it emits toxic fumes of Cd.

CAH000   CAS: 10325-94-7
CADMIUM NITRATE
mf: CdN_2O_6 mw: 236.42

PROP: White, prismatic needles; hygroscopic. Mp: 350°.

SYNS: CADMIUM DINITRATE ◇ NITRIC ACID, CADMIUM SALT

TOXICITY DATA with REFERENCE
MUT: mrc-bcs 5 mmol/L   MUREAV 77,109,80

CONSENSUS REPORTS: Reported in EPA TSCA Inventory. EPA Genetic Toxicology Program. Cadmium and its compounds are on the Community Right-To-Know List.

OSHA PEL: TWA 0.2 mg(Cd)/m³; CL 0.6 mg(Cd)/m³ (dust)   ACGIH TLV: TWA 0.05 mg(Cd)/m³ (Proposed: TWA 0.01 mg(Cd)/m³ (dust), Human Carcinogen); BEI: 10 μg/g creatinine in urine; 10 μg/L in blood. NIOSH REL: (Cadmium) Reduce to lowest feasible level

SAFETY PROFILE: Confirmed human carcinogen. Poison by ingestion and possibly other routes. Moderately toxic by inhalation. Mutation data reported. When heated to decomposition it emits very toxic fumes of Cd and NO$_x$.

CAH250   CAS: 10022-68-1
CADMIUM(II) NITRATE TETRAHYDRATE (1:2:4)
mf: N$_2$O$_6$•Cd•4H$_2$O   mw: 308.50

SYNS: DUSICNAN KADEMNATY (CZECH) ◇ NITRIC ACID, CADMIUM SALT, TETRAHYDRATE

TOXICITY DATA with REFERENCE
MUT: mmo-esc 6 μmol/L   ENVRAL 26,279,85

CONSENSUS REPORTS: Cadmium and its compounds are on the Community Right-To-Know List.

OSHA PEL: TWA 0.2 mg(Cd)/m³; CL 0.6 mg(Cd)/m³ (dust)   ACGIH TLV: TWA 0.05 mg(Cd)/m³ (Proposed: TWA 0.01 mg(Cd)/m³ (dust), Human Carcinogen); BEI: 10 μg/g creatinine in urine; 10 μg/L in blood. NIOSH REL: (Cadmium) Reduce to lowest feasible level

SAFETY PROFILE: Confirmed human carcinogen. Poison by ingestion. A severe skin and moderate eye irritant. Mutation data reported. When heated to decomposition it emits very toxic fumes of Cd and NO$_x$.

CAH500   CAS: 1306-19-0
CADMIUM OXIDE
mf: CdO   mw: 128.40

PROP: (1) Amorphous, brown crystals; (2) cubic, brown crystals. Mp (1): <1426°, mp (2): decomp @ 950°, bp: 1559°, d (1): 6.95, d (2): 8.15, vap press: 1 mm @ 1000°.

SYNS: KADMU TLENEK (POLISH) ◇ NCI-C02551

TOXICITY DATA with REFERENCE
NEO: scu-rat TDLo: 90 mg/kg   BJCAAI 20,190,66

CONSENSUS REPORTS: IARC Cancer Review: Human Inadequate Evidence IMEMDT 2,74,73; IMEMDT 11,39,76; Animal Sufficient Evidence IMEMDT 11,39,76; IMEMDT 2, 74,73. Reported in EPA TSCA Inventory. EPA Extremely Hazardous Substances List. Cadmium and its compounds are on the Community Right-To-Know List.

OSHA PEL: TWA 0.2 mg(Cd)/m³; CL 0.6 mg(Cd)/m³ (dust)   ACGIH TLV: TWA 0.05 mg(Cd)/m³ (Proposed: TWA 0.01 mg(Cd)/m³ (dust), Human Carcinogen); BEI: 10 μg/g creatinine in urine; 10 μg/L in blood. DFG MAK: Suspected Carcinogen. NIOSH REL: (Cadmium) Reduce to lowest feasible level

SAFETY PROFILE: Confirmed human carcinogen with experimental neoplastigenic data. Poison by ingestion, inhalation and intraperitoneal routes. Experimental reproductive effects. Human systemic effects by inhalation include: change in the sense of smell, change in heart rate, blood pressure increase, an excess of protein in the urine and other kidney or bladder changes. Mixtures with magnesium explode when heated. When heated to decomposition it emits toxic fumes of Cd.

CAH750
CADMIUM OXIDE FUME
mf: CdO   mw: 128.40

SYN: CADMIUM FUME

CONSENSUS REPORTS: Reported in EPA TSCA Inventory. Cadmium and its compounds are on the Community Right-To-Know List.

OSHA PEL: TWA 0.1 mg(Cd)/m³; CL 0.3 mg(Cd)/m³   ACGIH TLV: TWA 0.05 mg(Cd)/m³ (Proposed: TWA 0.01 mg(Cd)/m³ (dust), Human Carcinogen); BEI: 10 μg/g creatinine in urine; 10 μg/L in blood. NIOSH REL: (Cadmium) Reduce to lowest feasible level

SAFETY PROFILE: Confirmed human carcinogen. Poison by inhalation. Moderately toxic to humans by inhalation. Human pulmonary system effects by inhalation including: coughing, difficult breathing, and cyanosis. A strong irritant via inhalation. When heated to decomposition it emits toxic fumes of Cd.

CAI000   CAS: 13477-17-3
CADMIUM PHOSPHATE
mf: $Cd_3O_8P_2 \cdot 4H_2O$ mw: 599.22

PROP: Amorphous or colorless crystals. Mp: 1500°.

SYN: TL 1182

CONSENSUS REPORTS: Reported in EPA TSCA Inventory. Cadmium and its compounds are on the Community Right-To-Know List.

OSHA PEL: TWA 0.2 mg(Cd)/m^3; CL 0.6 mg(Cd)/m^3 (dust) ACGIH TLV: TWA 0.05 mg(Cd)/m^3 (Proposed: TWA 0.01 mg(Cd)/m^3 (dust), Human Carcinogen); BEI: 10 μg/g creatinine in urine; 10 μg/L in blood. NIOSH REL: (Cadmium) Reduce to lowest feasible level

SAFETY PROFILE: Confirmed human carcinogen. Poison by inhalation. When heated to decomposition it emits toxic fumes of Cd and PO_x.

CAI125   CAS: 12014-28-7
CADMIUM PHOSPHIDE
mf: Cd_3P_2 mw: 399.18

CONSENSUS REPORTS: Cadmium compounds are on the Community Right-To-Know List.

SAFETY PROFILE: Confirmed carcinogen. When heated to decomposition it emits toxic fumes of PO_x and Cd.

CAI250
CADMIUM PROPIONATE
mf: $C_6H_{10}CdO_5$ mw: 258.55

CONSENSUS REPORTS: Cadmium and its compounds are on the Community Right-To-Know List.

SAFETY PROFILE: Confirmed carcinogen. The salt has exploded. When heated to decomposition it emits toxic fumes of Cd.

CAI500
CADMIUM SELENIDE
mf: CdSe   mw: 191.36

PROP: Preparative hazard.

CONSENSUS REPORTS: Cadmium and its compounds as well as Selenium and its com-

pounds are on the Community Right-To-Know List.

SAFETY PROFILE: Confirmed carcinogen. Selenium compounds are considered to be poisons. When heated to decomposition it emits toxic fumes of Cd and Se.

CAI750   CAS: 141-00-4
CADMIUM SUCCINATE
mf: $C_4H_4O_4 \cdot Cd$ mw: 228.48

SYNS: CADMINATE ◇ SUCCINIC ACID, CADMIUM SALT (1:1)

CONSENSUS REPORTS: Reported in EPA TSCA Inventory. Cadmium and its compounds are on the Community Right-To-Know List.

NIOSH REL: (Cadmium) Reduce to lowest possible level.

SAFETY PROFILE: Confirmed carcinogen. Poison by ingestion and intraperitoneal routes. Moderately toxic by ingestion. When heated to decomposition it emits toxic fumes of Cd.

CAJ000   CAS: 10124-36-4
CADMIUM SULFATE (1:1)
mf: $O_4S \cdot Cd$ mw: 208.46

PROP: Rhombic, white crystals. Mp: 1000°, d: 4.691.

SYNS: CADMIUM SULFATE ◇ CADMIUM SULPHATE ◇ SULFURIC ACID, CADMIUM(2+) SALT ◇ SULPHURIC ACID, CADMIUM SALT (1:1)

TOXICITY DATA with REFERENCE
MUT: dnd-rat: lvr 30 μmol/L   MUREAV 113,357,83
MUT: mrc-bcs 5 mmol/L   MUREAV 77,109,80
MUT: msc-mus: lym 150 μg/L   JTEHD6 9,367,82

CONSENSUS REPORTS: IARC Cancer Review: Animal Sufficient Evidence IMEMDT 11,39,76; IMEMDT 2,74,73. Reported in EPA TSCA Inventory. EPA Genetic Toxicology Program. Cadmium and its compounds are on the Community Right-To-Know List.

OSHA PEL: TWA 0.2 mg(Cd)/m^3; CL 0.6 mg(Cd)/m^3 (dust) ACGIH TLV: TWA 0.05 mg(Cd)/m^3 (Proposed: TWA 0.01 mg(Cd)/m^3 (dust), Human Carcinogen); BEI: 10 μg/g creatinine in urine; 10 μg/L in blood. DFG MAK: Suspected Carcinogen. NIOSH REL: (Cadmium) Reduce to lowest feasible level

SAFETY PROFILE: Confirmed human carcinogen with experimental carcinogenic and teratogenic data. Poison by ingestion, subcutaneous and intraperitoneal routes. Experimental reproductive effects. Mutation data reported. When heated to decomposition it emits very toxic fumes of Cd and SO_x.

CAJ250 CAS: 7790-84-3
CADMIUM SULFATE (1:1) HYDRATE (3:8)
mf: $O_4S \cdot Cd \cdot 8/3H_2O$ mw: 256.51

SYNS: CADMIUM SULFATE OCTAHYDRATE ◇ SULFURIC ACID, CADMIUM SALT, HYDRATE

TOXICITY DATA with REFERENCE
NEO: scu-rat TDLo:60 mg/kg/2Y-I AOHYA3 16,111,73
ETA: scu-rat TD:15 mg/kg/2Y-I AOHYA3 16,111,73
MUT: cyt-ham:fbr 10 μmol/L/1H MUREAV 40,125,76
MUT: dnd-esc 3 μmol/L JOBAAY 133,75,78

CONSENSUS REPORTS: IARC Cancer Review: Animal Sufficient Evidence IMEMDT 2,74,73. Cadmium and its compounds are on the Community Right-To-Know List.

OSHA PEL: TWA 0.2 mg(Cd)/m³; CL 0.6 mg(Cd)/m³ (dust) ACGIH TLV: TWA 0.05 mg(Cd)/m³ (Proposed: TWA 0.01 mg(Cd)/m³ (dust), Human Carcinogen); BEI: 10 μg/g creatinine in urine; 10 μg/L in blood. NIOSH REL: (Cadmium) Reduce to lowest feasible level

SAFETY PROFILE: Confirmed human carcinogen with experimental tumorigenic, neoplastigenic, and teratogenic data. Experimental reproductive effects. Mutation data reported. When heated to decomposition it emits very toxic fumes of Cd and SO_x.

CAJ500 CAS: 13477-21-9
CADMIUM SULFATE TETRAHYDRATE
mf: $O_4S \cdot Cd \cdot 4H_2O$ mw: 280.54

SYN: SULFURIC ACID, CADMIUM SALT, TETRAHYDRATE

TOXICITY DATA with REFERENCE
NEO: scu-rat TDLo:20 mg/kg/10W-I BJCAAI 18,667,64

CONSENSUS REPORTS: Cadmium and its compounds are on the Community Right-To-Know List.

OSHA PEL: TWA 0.2 mg(Cd)/m³; CL 0.6 mg(Cd)/m³ (dust) ACGIH TLV: TWA 0.05 mg(Cd)/m³ (Proposed: TWA 0.01 mg(Cd)/m³ (dust), Human Carcinogen); BEI: 10 μg/g creatinine in urine; 10 μg/L in blood. NIOSH REL: (Cadmium) Reduce to lowest feasible level

SAFETY PROFILE: Confirmed human carcinogen with experimental neoplastigenic data. When heated to decomposition it emits very toxic fumes of Cd and SO_x.

CAJ750 CAS: 1306-23-6
CADMIUM SULFIDE
mf: CdS mw: 144.46

PROP: Hexagonal, yellow-orange crystals. Mp: 1750 @ 100 atm, bp: subl in N_2, d: 4.82.

SYNS: AURORA YELLOW ◇ CADMIUM GOLDEN 366 ◇ CADMIUM LEMON YELLOW 527 ◇ CADMIUM ORANGE ◇ CADMIUM PRIMROSE 819 ◇ CADMIUM SULPHIDE ◇ CADMIUM YELLOW ◇ CADMOPUR YELLOW ◇ CAPSEBON ◇ C.I. 77199 ◇ C.I. PIGMENT ORANGE 20 ◇ C.I. PIGMENT YELLOW 37 ◇ FERRO YELLOW ◇ GREENOCKITE ◇ NCI-C02711

TOXICITY DATA with REFERENCE
CAR: scu-rat TDLo:90 mg/kg BJCAAI 20,190,66
ETA: ims-rat TDLo:120 mg/kg BJCAAI 20,190,66
ETA: scu-rat TD:135 mg/kg PBPHAW 14,47,78
ETA: scu-rat TD:250 mg/kg NATUAS 198,1213,63
MUT: cyt-hmn:leu 62 μg/L PJACAW 48,133,72
MUT: dnd-ham:ovr 10 mg/L CRNGDP 3,657,82
MUT: otr-ham:emb 1 mg/L CNREA8 42,2757,82

CONSENSUS REPORTS: IARC Cancer Review: Animal Sufficient Evidence IMEMDT 11,39,76; IMEMDT 2,74,73. NTP Fourth Annual Report On Carcinogens, 1984. EPA Genetic Toxicology Program. Cadmium and its compounds are on the Community Right-To-Know List. Reported in EPA TSCA Inventory.

OSHA PEL: TWA 0.2 mg(Cd)/m³; CL 0.6 mg(Cd)/m³ (dust) ACGIH TLV: TWA 0.05 mg(Cd)/m³ (Proposed: TWA 0.01 mg(Cd)/m³ (dust), Human Carcinogen); BEI: 10 μg/g creatinine in urine; 10 μg/L in blood. DFG MAK: Suspected Carcinogen. NIOSH REL: (Cadmium) Reduce to lowest feasible level

SAFETY PROFILE: Confirmed human carcinogen with experimental carcinogenic and tumorigenic data. Moderately toxic by ingestion and inhalation. Human mutation data reported.

When heated to decomposition it emits very toxic fumes of Cd and SO_x.

CAK000
CADMIUM THERMOVACUUM AEROSOL
mf: Cd   mw: 112.40

SYN: AEROSOL of THERMOVACUUM CADMIUM

CONSENSUS REPORTS: Cadmium and its compounds are on the Community Right-To-Know List.

OSHA PEL: TWA 0.2 mg(Cd)/m³; CL 0.6 mg(Cd)/m³ (dust) ACGIH TLV: TWA 0.05 mg(Cd)/m³ (Proposed: TWA 0.01 mg(Cd)/m³ (dust), Human Carcinogen); BEI: 10 μg/g creatinine in urine; 10 μg/L in blood. NIOSH REL: (Cadmium) Reduce to lowest feasible level

SAFETY PROFILE: Confirmed human carcinogen. Moderately toxic by an unspecified route. When heated to decomposition it emits very toxic fumes of Cd.

CAK250   CAS: 73419-42-8
CADMIUM-THIONEIN
mf: $C_{18}H_{30}N_6O_4S_2$•Cd   mw: 571.06

PROP: Cadmium(II) is bound to the protein thioneine from rat or rabbit liver. (BCPCA6 26,25,77).

CONSENSUS REPORTS: Cadmium and its compounds are on the Community Right-To-Know List.

OSHA PEL: TWA 0.2 mg(Cd)/m³; CL 0.6 mg(Cd)/m³ (dust) ACGIH TLV: TWA 0.05 mg(Cd)/m³ (Proposed: TWA 0.01 mg(Cd)/m³ (dust), Human Carcinogen); BEI: 10 μg/g creatinine in urine; 10 μg/L in blood. NIOSH REL: (Cadmium) Reduce to lowest feasible level

SAFETY PROFILE: Confirmed human carcinogen. Deadly poison by intravenous route. When heated to decomposition it emits very toxic fumes of NO_x, SO_x and Cd.

CAP500   CAS: 13765-19-0
CALCIUM CHROMATE
DOT: 9096
mf: CrO_4•Ca   mw: 156.08

PROP: Monoclinic prisms; yellow color.

SYNS: CALCIUM CHROMATE (VI) ◇ CALCIUM CHROME YELLOW ◇ CALCIUM CHROMIUM OXIDE (CaCrO₄)

◇ CALCIUM MONOCHROMATE ◇ CHROMIC ACID, CALCIUM SALT (1:1) ◇ C.I. 77223 ◇ C.I. PIGMENT YELLOW 33 ◇ GELBIN ◇ RCRA WASTE NUMBER U032 ◇ YELLOW ULTRAMARINE

TOXICITY DATA with REFERENCE
CAR: imp-rat TD: 125 mg/kg   AIHAAP 20,274,59
CAR: imp-rat TD: 10866 μg/kg   BJIMAG 43,243,86
CAR: imp-rat TDLo: 8 mg/kg   CRNGDP 7,831,86
CAR: itr-rat TDLo: 163 mg/kg/130W-I   EXPADD 30,129,86
NEO: ims-rat TD: 216 mg/kg/1Y-I   CNREA8 36,1779,76
NEO: ims-rat TDLo: 76 mg/kg/19W-I   BJCAAI 23,172,69
ETA: imp-rat TD: 50 mg/kg   AEHLAU 5,445,62
MUT: dlt-mus-unr 40 mg/kg   MUREAV 97,180,82
MUT: dnd-ham: ovr 25 μmol/L/1H-C   PAACA3 24,74,83
MUT: mma-esc 100 μg/plate   ENMUDM 6(Suppl 2),1,84
MUT: mmo-sat 50 nmol/plate   CRNGDP 2,283,81
MUT: otr-rat: emb 58 μg/L   JJIND8 67,1303,81
MUT: sce-ham: ovr 100 μg/L   MUREAV 156,219,85

CONSENSUS REPORTS: IARC Cancer Review: Animal Sufficient Evidence IMEMDT 2,100,73; IMEMDT 23,205,80; Human Sufficient Evidence IMEMDT 23,205,80. NTP Fourth Annual Report On Carcinogens, 1984. Reported in EPA TSCA Inventory. EPA Genetic Toxicology Program. Chromium and its compounds are on the Community Right-To-Know List.

OSHA PEL: CL 0.1 mg(CrO_3)/m³ ACGIH TLV: TWA 0.05 mg(Cr)/m³; Confirmed Human Carcinogen; (Proposed: TWA 0.001; Suspected Human Carcinogen) DFG TRK: 0.1 mg/m³ calculated as CrO_3 in that portion of dust that can possibly be inhaled; 0.2 mg/m³ arc-welding by hand; others 0.1 mg/m³. Animal Carcinogen, Suspected Human Carcinogen. NIOSH REL: TWA 0.001 mg(Cr(VI))/m³ DOT Classification: ORM-E; Label: None.

SAFETY PROFILE: Confirmed human carcinogen with experimental carcinogenic, neoplastigenic, and tumorigenic data. Experimental reproductive effects. Mutation data reported. A powerful oxidizer. Mixture with boron burns violently if ignited.

CAP750   CAS: 8012-75-7
CALCIUM CHROMATE(VI) DIHYDRATE
mf: CrO_4•Ca•$2H_2O$ mw: 192.12

SYNS: CALCIUM CHROME YELLOW ◊ CHROMIC ACID, CALCIUM SALT (1:1), DIHYDRATE ◊ C.I. 77223 ◊ C.I. PIGMENT YELLOW 33 ◊ GELBIN YELLOW ULTRAMARINE ◊ PIGMENT YELLOW 33 ◊ STEINBUHL YELLOW

TOXICITY DATA with REFERENCE
CAR: imp-mus TDLo:400 mg/kg   AMIHAB 21,530,60

ETA: scu-mus TDLo:400 mg/kg   AMIHAB 21,530,60

MUT: otr-ham:kdy 250 mg/L   CNREA8 35,1058,75

CONSENSUS REPORTS: IARC Cancer Review: Animal Sufficient Evidence IMEMDT 2,100,72. Chromium and its compounds are on the Community Right-To-Know List.

OSHA PEL: CL 0.1 mg(CrO^3)/m^3 ACGIH TLV: TWA 0.05 mg(Cr)/m^3; Confirmed Human Carcinogen NIOSH REL: (Chromium(VI)) TWA 0.001 mg(Cr(VI))/m^3

SAFETY PROFILE: Confirmed human carcinogen with experimental tumorigenic and carcinogenic data. Poison by ingestion and implant routes. Mutation data reported. A powerful oxidizer.

CBS750   CAS: 63042-08-0
4'-CARBOMETHOXY-2,3'-DIMETHYLAZOBENZENE
mf: $C_{16}H_{16}N_2O_3$ mw: 284.34

SYNS: 4'-CARBOMETHOXY-2,3'-DIMETHYLAZOBENZOL ◊ CARBONIC ACID METHYL-4-(o-TOLYLAZO)-o-TOLYL ESTER ◊ 2,3'-DIMETHYLAZOBENZENE-4'-METHYLCARBONATE

TOXICITY DATA with REFERENCE
ETA: orl-rat TDLo:27 g/kg/43W-C   GANNA2 33,196,39

CONSENSUS REPORTS: NTP Fourth Annual Report On Carcinogens, 1984.

SAFETY PROFILE: Confirmed carcinogen with experimental tumorigenic data. When heated to decomposition it emits toxic fumes of NO_x.

CBY000   CAS: 56-23-5
CARBON TETRACHLORIDE
DOT: 1846
mf: CCl_4 mw: 153.81

PROP: Colorless liquid; heavy, ethereal odor. Mp: $-22.6°$, bp: $76.8°$, fp: $-22.9°$, flash p: none, d: 1.597 @ $20°$, vap press: 100 mm @ $23.0°$.

SYNS: BENZINOFORM ◊ CARBONA ◊ CARBON CHLORIDE ◊ CARBON TET ◊ CZTEROCHLOREK WEGLA (POLISH) ◊ ENT 4,705 ◊ FASCIOLIN ◊ FLUKOIDS ◊ METHANE TETRACHLORIDE ◊ NECATORINA ◊ NECATORINE ◊ PERCHLOROMETHANE ◊ R 10 ◊ RCRA WASTE NUMBER U211 ◊ TETRACHLOORKOOLSTOF (DUTCH) ◊ TETRACHLOORMETAAN ◊ TETRACHLORKOHLENSTOFF, TETRA (GERMAN) ◊ TETRACHLORMETHAN (GERMAN) ◊ TETRACHLOROCARBON ◊ TETRACHLOROMETHANE ◊ TETRACHLORURE de CARBONE (FRENCH) ◊ TETRACLOROMETANO (ITALIAN) ◊ TETRACLORURO di CARBONIO (ITALIAN) ◊ TETRAFINOL ◊ TETRAFORM ◊ TETRASOL ◊ UNIVERM ◊ VERMOESTRICID

TOXICITY DATA with REFERENCE
CAR: scu-rat TD:182 g/kg/70W-I   JJIND8 44,419,70

NEO: orl-mus TD:12 g/kg/88D-I   JJIND8 4,385,44

NEO: orl-mus TD:8580 mg/kg/9W-I   JJIND8 4,385,44

NEO: orl-mus TD:57600 mg/kg/12W-I   JJIND8 2,197,41

NEO: orl-mus TDLo:4400 mg/kg/19W-I   JJIND8 20,431,58

ETA: orl-ham TDLo:9250 mg/kg/30W-I   JJIND8 26,855,61

ETA: par-mus TDLo:305 g/kg/30W-I   BEXBAN 89,845,80

ETA: scu-rat TD:31 g/kg/12W-I   JJIND8 45,1237,70

ETA: scu-rat TD:100 g/kg/25W-I   KRMJAC 12,37,65

ETA: scu-rat TDLo:15600 mg/kg/12W-I   JJIND8 38,891,67

MUT: dnd-esc 300 ppm   MUREAV 89,95,81

MUT: dnr-esc 12500 ng/well   MUREAV 133,161,84

MUT: mmo-asn 5000 ppm   MUREAV 147,288,85

MUT: mmo-sat 20 uL/L   EJMBA2 18,213,83

CONSENSUS REPORTS: IARC Cancer Review: Animal Sufficient Evidence IMEMDT 20,371,79; IMEMDT 1,53,72; Human Inadequate Evidence IMEMDT 1,53,72; Human Limited Evidence IMEMDT 20,371,79. NTP Fourth Annual Report On Carcinogens, 1984. Community Right-To-Know List. EPA Genetic Toxicology Program. Reported in EPA TSCA Inventory.

OSHA PEL: (Transitional: TWA 10 ppm; CL 25 ppm; PK 200 ppm/5 min) TWA 2 ppm ACGIH TLV: TWA 5 ppm; STEL 30 (skin); Suspected Human Carcinogen DFG MAK: 10 ppm (65 mg/m^3); BEI: 1.6 mL/m^3 in alveolar air 1 hour after exposure; Suspected Carcinogen. NIOSH REL: CL 2 ppm/

60M DOT Classification: ORM-A; Label: None; Poison B; Label: Poison.

SAFETY PROFILE: Confirmed carcinogen with experimental carcinogenic, neoplastigenic, tumorigenic, and teratogenic data. A human poison by ingestion and possibly other routes. Poison by subcutaneous and intravenous routes. Mildly toxic by inhalation. Human systemic effects by inhalation and ingestion: nausea or vomiting, pupillary constriction, coma, antipsychotic effects, tremors, somnolence, anorexia, unspecified respiratory system and gastrointestinal system effects. An eye and skin irritant. Damages liver, kidneys, and lungs. Mutation data reported. A narcotic. Individual susceptibility varies widely. Contact dermatitis can result from skin contact. When heated to decomposition it emits toxic fumes of Cl^- and phosgene.

CCL500
CARRAGEENAN, DEGRADED

PROP: Carrageenan derived from *Eucheuma spinosum*, degraded by acid hydrolysis; average molecular weight 20,000-40,000 (CALEDQ 4,171,78).

TOXICITY DATA with REFERENCE
CAR: orl-rat TD: 1080 g/kg/26W-C   CALEDQ
  14,267,81
CAR: orl-rat TD: 1500 g/kg/43W-C   CALEDQ
  4,171,78
CAR: orl-rat TD: 1620 g/kg/39W-C   CALEDQ
  14,267,81
CAR: orl-rat TD: 1700 g/kg/52W-C   CALEDQ
  4,171,78
CAR: orl-rat TD: 4860 g/kg/64W-C   PPTCBY
  9,127,79
CAR: orl-rat TD: 6834 g/kg/73W-C   PPTCBY
  9,127,79
CAR: orl-rat TDLo: 360 g/kg/9W-C   CALEDQ
  14,267,81
NEO: orl-rat TD: 3116 g/kg/77W-C   PPTCBY
  9,127,79
ETA: orl-rat TD: 2250 g/kg/64W-C   PPTCBY
  9,127,79

CONSENSUS REPORTS: IARC Cancer Review: Animal Sufficient Evidence IMEMDT 31,79,83.

SAFETY PROFILE: Confirmed carcinogen with experimental carcinogenic, neoplastigenic, and tumorigenic data. When heated to decomposition it emits toxic fumes of SO_x.

CDO250   CAS: 95-06-7
2-CHLORALLYL
DIETHYLDITHIOCARBAMATE
mf: $C_8H_{14}ClNS_2$ mw: 223.80

PROP: Amber liquid. Bp: 129° @ 1 mm.

SYNS: CDEC ◇ CHLORALLYL DIETHYLDITHIOCARBA-MATE ◇ 2-CHLOROALLYL DIETHYLDITHIOCARBAMATE ◇ 2-CHLOROALLYL-N,N-DIETHYLDITHIOCARBAMATE ◇ 2-CHLORO-2-PROPENE-1-THIOL DIETHYLDITHIOCAR-BAMATE ◇ 2-CHLORO-2-PROPENYL DIETHYLCARBAMO-DITHIOATE ◇ CP 4572 ◇ DIETHYLCARBAMODITHIOIC ACID 2-CHLORO-2-PROPENYL ESTER ◇ DIETHYLDITHIO-CARBAMIC ACID-2-CHLOROALLYL ESTER ◇ NCI-C00453 ◇ SULFALLATE ◇ THIOALLATE ◇ VEGADEX ◇ VEGADEX SUPER

TOXICITY DATA with REFERENCE
CAR: orl-mus TD: 120 g/kg/78W-I
  NCITR* NCI-CG-TR-115,78
CAR: orl-mus TDLo: 59 g/kg/78W-C
  NCITR* NCI-CG-TR-115,78
CAR: orl-rat TD: 11 g/kg/78W-I
  NCITR* NCI-CG-TR-115,78
CAR: orl-rat TDLo: 6825 mg/kg/78W-C
  NCITR* NCI-CG-TR-115,78

MUT: mma-sat 10 uL/plate   PMRSDJ 2,87,81
MUT: mmo-asn 20 uL/plate   JSFAAE 32,826,81
MUT: mmo-omi 1100 μg/plate   PMRSDJ 2,87,81
MUT: mmo-sat 10 uL/plate   PMRSDJ 2,87,81

CONSENSUS REPORTS: IARC Cancer Review: Animal Sufficient Evidence IMEMDT 30,283,83. NTP Fourth Annual Report On Carcinogens, 1984. NCI Carcinogenesis Bioassay (feed); Clear Evidence: mouse, rat NCITR* NCI-CG-TR-115,78. EPA Genetic Toxicology Program.

SAFETY PROFILE: Confirmed carcinogen with experimental carcinogenic data. Moderately toxic by ingestion and skin contact. Mutation data reported. An herbicide. When heated to decomposition it emits very toxic fumes of Cl^-, NO_x, and SO_x.

CDO500   CAS: 305-03-3
CHLORAMBUCIL
mf: $C_{14}H_{19}Cl_2NO_2$ mw: 304.24

SYNS: AMBOCHLORIN ◇ AMBOCLORIN ◇ 4-(BIS(2-CHLOROETHYL)AMINO)BENZENEBUTANOIC ACID ◇ γ-(p-BIS(2-CHLOROETHYL)AMINOPHENYL)BUTYRIC ACID ◇ 4-(p-(BIS(2-CHLOROETHYL)AMINO)PHENYL)BU-TYRIC ACID ◇ 4-(p-BIS(β-CHLOROETHYL)AMINOPHE-NYL)BUTYRIC ACID ◇ CB 1348 ◇ CHLORAMINOPHEN

◇ CHLORAMINOPHENE ◇ CHLOROAMBUCIL ◇ CHLORO-BUTIN ◇ CHLOROBUTINE ◇ N,N-DI-2-CHLOROETHYL-γ-p-AMINOPHENYLBUTYRIC ACID ◇ p-(N,N-DI-2-CHLORO-ETHYL)AMINOPHENYL BUTYRIC ACID ◇ p-N,N-DI-(β-CHLOROETHYL)AMINOPHENYL BUTYRIC ACID ◇ γ-(p-DI(2-CHLOROETHYL)AMINOPHENYL)BUTYRIC ACID ◇ ECLORIL ◇ ELCORIL ◇ LEUKERAN ◇ LEUKERSAN ◇ LEUKORAN ◇ LINFOLIZIN ◇ LINFOLYSIN ◇ NCI-C03485 ◇ NSC-3088 ◇ PHENYLBUTYRIC ACID NITROGEN MUS-TARD ◇ RCRA WASTE NUMBER U035

TOXICITY DATA with REFERENCE
CAR: ipr-mus TDLo:18 mg/kg/4W   JNCIAM 36,915,66

CAR: ipr-rat TD:170 mg/kg/26W-I   RRCRBU 52,1,75

CAR: ipr-rat TDLo:120 mg/kg/26W-I   RRCRBU 52,1,75

CAR: orl-chd TD:108 mg/kg/77W-C:BLD
AFPEAM 36,592,79

CAR: orl-hmn TD:84 mg/kg/3Y-C:BLD
ACCBAT 38,228,83

CAR: orl-hmn TD:180 mg/kg/3Y-I:BLD
AIMDAP 137,355,77

CAR: orl-man TD:59 mg/kg/96W-C:BLD
NPMDAD 10,1717,81

CAR: orl-man TDLo:84 mg/kg/2.5Y-C:BLD
AMSVAZ 199,373,76

CAR: orl-wmn TD:70 mg/kg/94W-C:BLD
ACCBAT 38,228,83

CAR: orl-wmn TD:135 mg/kg/4Y-C:BLD
AIMDAP 137,355,77

CAR: orl-wmn TD:141 mg/kg/5Y-I:BLD
NEJMAG 304,441,81

CAR: orl-wmn TD:200 mg/kg/6Y-C:BLD
ACHAAH 62,283,80

CAR: orl-wmn TD:307 mg/kg/7Y-C:BLD
AIMDAP 134,728,74

CAR: orl-wmn TDLo:101 mg/kg/82W-C:BLD   GYNOA3 6,115,78

CAR: unr-wmn TDLo:161 mg/kg/3Y-I:BLD
SJHAAQ 13,179,74

MUT: dns-hmn:lym 1 μmol/L   JTEHD6 6,1059,80
MUT: mma-sat 100 μg/plate   ENMUDM 8(Suppl 7),1,86
MUT: sce-hmn:lym 150 μg/L   MUREAV 143,225,85
MUT: sln-dmg-orl 2000 ppm   ENMUDM 7,677,85
MUT: trn-dmg-orl 3000 ppm   ENMUDM 7,677,85

CONSENSUS REPORTS: IARC Cancer Review: Human Inadequate Evidence IMEMDT 9,125,75; Human Limited Evidence IMEMDT 26,115,81; Animal Limited Evidence IMEMDT 26,115,81; Animal Sufficient Evidence IMEMDT 9,125,75. NTP Fourth Annual Report On Carcinogens, 1984. EPA Genetic Toxicology Program.

SAFETY PROFILE: Confirmed carcinogen producing leukemia. Experimental carcinogenic, neoplastigenic, and teratogenic data. Poison by ingestion, intravenous, intraperitoneal, and subcutaneous routes. Human respiratory system effects by ingestion: cough, dyspnea, and interstitial fibrosis. Human reproductive effects by ingestion and possibly other routes: changes in spermatogenesis; menstrual cycle changes or disorders; and teratogenic effects of the fetal urogenital system. Human mutation data reported. An anti-neoplastic agent. When heated to decomposition it emits very toxic fumes of Cl^- and NO_x.

CDV100   CAS: 8001-35-2
CHLORINATED CAMPHENE
DOT: 2761
mf: $C_{10}H_{10}Cl_8$ mw: 413.80

PROP: Yellow, waxy solid; pleasant piney odor. Mp: 65-90°. Almost insol in water; very sol in aromatic hydrocarbons.

SYNS: AGRICIDE MAGGOT KILLER (F) ◇ ALLTEX ◇ ALLTOX ◇ ATTAC 6 ◇ ATTAC 6-3 ◇ CAMPHECHLOR ◇ CAMPHOCHLOR ◇ CAMPHOCLOR ◇ CAMPHOFENE HUILEUX ◇ CHEM-PHENE ◇ CHLOROCAMPHENE ◇ CLOR CHEM T-590 ◇ COMPOUND 3956 ◇ CRESTOXO ◇ CRISTOXO 90 ◇ ENT 9,735 ◇ ESTONOX ◇ FASCO-TERPENE ◇ GENIPHENE ◇ GY-PHENE ◇ HERCULES 3956 ◇ HERCULES TOXAPHENE ◇ KAMFOCHLOR ◇ M 5055 ◇ MELIPAX ◇ MOTOX ◇ NCI-C00259 ◇ OCTACHLOROCAMPHENE ◇ PCC ◇ PENPHENE ◇ PHENACIDE ◇ PHENATOX ◇ POLYCHLORCAMPHENE ◇ POLYCHLORINATED CAMPHENES ◇ POLYCHLOROCAMPHENE ◇ RCRA WASTE NUMBER P123 ◇ STROBANE-T-90 ◇ SYNTHETIC 3956 ◇ TOXADUST ◇ TOXAFEEN (DUTCH) ◇ TOXAKIL ◇ TOXAPHEN (GERMAN) ◇ TOXON 63 ◇ TOXYPHEN ◇ TOXAPHENE ◇ VERTAC 90% ◇ VERTAC TOXAPHENE 90

TOXICITY DATA with REFERENCE
CAR: orl-mus TD:13 g/kg/80W-C
NCITR* NCI-CG-TR-37,79

CAR: orl-mus TDLo:6600 mg/kg/80W-C
NCITR* NCI-CG-TR-37,79

ETA: orl-rat TDLo:30 g/kg/80W-C
NCITR* NCI-CG-TR-37,79

MUT: mma-sat 500 μg/plate   SCIEAS 205,591,79
MUT: mmo-sat 100 μg/plate   ENMUDM 8(Suppl 7),1,86
MUT: otr-mus:emb 12400 μg/L   PMRSDJ 5,659,85

MUT: sce-hmn:lym 10 μmol/L   ARTODN
52,221,83

CONSENSUS REPORTS: IARC Cancer Review: Human Limited Evidence IMEMDT 20,327,79; Animal Sufficient Evidence IMEMDT 20,327,79. NTP Fourth Annual Report On Carcinogens, 1984. NCI Carcinogenesis Bioassay (feed); Clear Evidence: mouse, rat NCITR* NCI-CG-TR-37,79.

OSHA PEL: (Transitional: TWA 0.5 mg/m^3 (skin)) TWA 0.5 mg/m^3; STEL 1 mg/m^3 (skin)   ACGIH TLV: TWA 0.5 mg/m^3; STEL 1 mg/m^3 (skin)   DFG MAK: 0.5 mg/m^3 DOT Classification: ORM-A; Label: None.

SAFETY PROFILE: Confirmed carcinogen with experimental carcinogenic, tumorigenic, and teratogenic data. Human poison by ingestion and possibly other routes. Experimental poison by ingestion, intraperitoneal, and possibly other routes. Moderately toxic experimentally by inhalation and skin contact. May be a human carcinogenic. Human systemic effects by ingestion and skin contact: somnolence, convulsions or effect on seizure threshold, coma and allergic skin dermatitis. A skin irritant; absorbed through the skin. Human mutation data reported. Liver injury has been reported. Lethal amounts of toxaphene can enter the body through the mouth, lungs, and skin. Systemic absorption of the insecticide is increased by the presence of digestible oils, and liquid preparations of the insecticide which penetrate the skin more readily than do dusts and wettable powders. When heated to decomposition it emits toxic fumes of Cl$^-$.

CDV625   CAS: 56641-03-3
CHLORINATED POLYETHER POLYURETHAN

PROP: Polymer formed from toluene diisocyanate and 1,4-butanediol and cured with 4,4'-methylenebis(o-chloroaniline)   (CNREA8 36,3973,76).
mf: (C$_{13}$H$_{12}$Cl$_2$N$_2$•C$_9$H$_6$N$_2$O$_2$•(C$_4$H$_8$O)$_n$H$_2$O)$_x$
SYNS: OSTAMER ◇ POLYURETHANE Y-238 ◇ Y-238

TOXICITY DATA with REFERENCE
ETA: imp-rat TD: 293 mg/kg   JNCIAM 33,1005,64
ETA: imp-rat TD: 6750 mg/kg   CNREA8 35,1591,75
ETA: imp-rat TDLo: 20 mg/kg   CNREA8 36,3973,76

CONSENSUS REPORTS: IARC Cancer Review: Animal Sufficient Evidence IMEMDT 19,303,79.

SAFETY PROFILE: Confirmed carcinogen with experimental tumorigenic data. When heated to decomposition it emits toxic fumes of Cl$^-$ and NO$_x$.

CFK125   CAS: 95-83-0
4-CHLORO-1,2-DIAMINOBENZENE
mf: C$_6$H$_7$ClN$_2$ mw: 142.60

SYNS: p-CHLORO-o-PHENYLENEDIAMINE ◇ 4-CHLORO-o-PHENYLENEDIAMINE ◇ 4-CHLORO-1,2-PHENYLENEDIAMINE ◇ 4-Cl-o-PD ◇ 1,2-DIAMINO-4-CHLOROBENZENE ◇ 3,4-DIAMINOCHLOROBENZENE ◇ 3,4-DIAMINO-1-CHLOROBENZENE ◇ NCI-C03292 ◇ URSOL OLIVE 6G

TOXICITY DATA with REFERENCE
CAR: orl-mus TD: 460 g/kg/78W-C   NCITR*
NCI-CG-TR-63,78
CAR: orl-mus TD: 917 g/kg/78W-C   NCITR*
NCI-CG-TR-63,78
CAR: orl-mus TDLo: 324 g/kg/77W-C   CRNGDP
1,495,80
CAR: orl-rat TD: 136 g/kg/78W-C   NCITR*
NCI-CG-TR-63,78
CAR: orl-rat TD: 273 g/kg/78W-C   NCITR*
NCI-CG-TR-63,78
CAR: orl-rat TD: 18750 g/kg/2Y-C   CRNGDP
1,495,80
CAR: orl-rat TDLo: 135 g/kg/77W-C   CRNGDP
1,495,80
NEO: orl-mus TD: 40500 g/kg/96W-C   CRNGDP
1,495,80
MUT: cyt-mus-ipr 100 mg/kg   ENMUDM 8(Suppl 6),53,86
MUT: dnd-hmn:fbr 50 μmol/L   MUREAV
127,107,84
MUT: mma-esc 1 mg/plate   ENMUDM 7(Suppl 5),1,85
MUT: mma-sat 10 μg/plate   ENMUDM 7(Suppl 5),1,85

CONSENSUS REPORTS: IARC Cancer Review: Human Limited Evidence IMEMDT 27,81,82; Animal Sufficient Evidence IMEMDT 27,81,82. NTP Fourth Annual Report On Carcinogens, 1984. NCI Carcinogenesis Bioassay (feed); Clear Evidence: mouse, rat NCITR* NCI-CG-TR-63,78. Reported in EPA TSCA Inventory.

SAFETY PROFILE: Confirmed carcinogen with experimental carcinogenic and neoplastigenic data. Human mutation data reported. When heated to decomposition it emits toxic fumes of Cl$^-$ and NO$_x$.

CGV250   CAS: 13010-47-4
1-(2-CHLOROETHYL)-3-CYCLOHEXYL-1-NITROSOUREA

mf: $C_9H_{16}ClN_3O_2$ mw: 233.73

SYNS: BELUSTINE ◇ CCNU ◇ CECENU ◇ CEENU ◇ CHLOROETHYLCYCLOHEXYLNITROSOUREA ◇ N-(2-CHLOROETHYL)-N'-CYCLOHEXYL-N-NITROSOUREA ◇ ((CHLORO-2-ETHYL)-1-CYCLOHEXYL-3-NITROSOUREA ◇ CINU ◇ (CLORO-2-ETIL)-1-CICLOESIL-3-NITROSOUREA (ITALIAN) ◇ ICIG 1109 ◇ LOMUSTINE ◇ NCI-CO4740 ◇ NSC-79037 ◇ RB 1509 ◇ SRI 2200

TOXICITY DATA with REFERENCE
ETA: ipr-mus TDLo: 98 mg/kg/26W-I   CANCAR 40S,1935,77
ETA: ipr-rat TDLo: 60 mg/kg/7W-I   CANCAR 40(Suppl 4),1935,77
ETA: ivn-rat TD: 127 mg/kg/60W-I   DTESD7 8,273,80
ETA: ivn-rat TD: 178 mg/kg/42W-I   DTESD7 8,273,80
ETA: ivn-rat TDLo: 64 mg/kg/60W-I   DTESD7 8,273,80
ETA: skn-mus TDLo: 276 mg/kg/23W-I   EXPEAM 36,1211,80
MUT: dnd-hmn: emb 100 μmol/L   CNREA8 44,1352,84
MUT: dni-hmn: leu 1 μmol/L   BBACAQ 425,463,76
MUT: dns-hmn: lym 10 mg/L   FRPSAX 36,947,81
MUT: ivn-mus LD10: 40 mg/kg   ANBCB3 23,64,78
MUT: mma-sat 100 nmol/plate   JJIND8 65,149,80
MUT: mmo-esc 500 μmol/L   GANNA2 71,674,80
MUT: msc-ham: lng 10 μmol/L   CNREA8 40,2719,80
MUT: sce-hmn: lym 50 μmol/L   CGCYDF 9,261,83

CONSENSUS REPORTS: IARC Cancer Review: Human Limited Evidence IMEMDT 26,137,81; Animal Sufficient Evidence IMEMDT 26,137,81. NTP Fourth Annual Report On Carcinogens, 1984. NCI Carcinogenesis Studies (ipr); Clear Evidence: mouse CANCAR 40,1935,77; No Evidence: rat CANCAR 40,1935,77. EPA Genetic Toxicology Program.

SAFETY PROFILE: Confirmed carcinogen with experimental carcinogenic, tumorigenic and teratogenic data. Poison by ingestion, intraperitoneal, subcutaneous, intravenous, and possibly other routes. Human systemic effects by ingestion: anorexia, nausea or vomiting, leukopenia (decrease in the white blood cell count), and thrombocytopenia (decrease in the number of blood platelets). Experimental reproductive effects. Human mutation data reported. When heated to decomposition it emits very toxic fumes of Cl^- and NO_x.

CHI900   CAS: 593-70-4
CHLOROFLUOROMETHANE

mf: CH_2ClF mw: 68.48

SYNS: FREON 31 ◇ MONOCHLOROMONOFLUOROMETHANE

TOXICITY DATA with REFERENCE
CAR: orl-rat TDLo: 78 g/kg/1Y-I   TXAPA9 72,15,84
MUT: mma-sat 5 pph   MUREAV 118,277,83
MUT: mmo-sat 5 pph   MUREAV 118,277,83
MUT: msc-ham: ovr 10 pph   EVSRBT 25,91,82
MUT: otr-ham: kdy 100 μmol/L   TXAPA9 72,15,84

CONSENSUS REPORTS: IARC Cancer Review: Animal Limited Evidence IMEMDT 41,229,86.

DFG MAK: Animal Carcinogen, Suspected Human Carcinogen.

SAFETY PROFILE: Confirmed carcinogen with experimental carcinogenic data. Moderately toxic by inhalation. Mutation data reported. When heated to decomposition it emits very toxic fumes of Cl^- and F^-.

CHJ500   CAS: 67-66-3
CHLOROFORM
DOT: 1888
mf: $CHCl_3$ mw: 119.37

PROP: Colorless liquid; heavy, ethereal odor. Mp: −63.5°, bp: 61.26°, fp: −63.5°, flash p: none, d: 1.49845 @ 15°, vap press: 100 mm @ 10.4°, vap d: 4.12.

SYNS: CHLOROFORME (FRENCH) ◇ CLOROFORMIO (ITALIAN) ◇ FORMYL TRICHLORIDE ◇ METHANE TRICHLORIDE ◇ METHENYL TRICHLORIDE ◇ METHYL TRICHLORIDE ◇ NCI-CO2686 ◇ R 20 (REFRIGERANT) ◇ RCRA WASTE NUMBER U044 ◇ TCM ◇ TRICHLOORMETHAAN (DUTCH) ◇ TRICHLORMETHAN (CZECH) ◇ TRICHLOROFORM ◇ TRICHLOROMETHANE ◇ TRICLOROMETANO (ITALIAN)

TOXICITY DATA with REFERENCE
CAR: orl-mus TDLo: 127 g/kg/92W-I   NCITR* NCI-CG-TR-0,76
CAR: orl-rat TD: 7020 mg/kg/78W-I   EVHPAZ 31,171,79
CAR: orl-rat TDLo: 13832 mg/kg/2Y-C   FAATDF 5,760,85

NEO: orl-mus TD:18 g/kg/17W-I   JNCIAM 5,251,45

NEO: orl-rat TD:70 g/kg/78W-I   NCITR* NCI-CG-TR-0,76

NEO: orl-rat TD:98 g/kg/78W-I   NCITR* NCI-CG-TR-0,76

NEO: orl-rat TD:58968 mg/kg/2Y-C   FAATDF 5,760,85

ETA: orl-mus TD:24752 mg/kg/2Y-C   FAATDF 5,760,85

MUT: dnd-mam:lym 1 mmol/L   TOLED5 11,243,82

MUT: dnd-rat-orl 1 μmol/kg   CBINA8 33,301,81

MUT: dns-mus-ipr 50 mg/kg   TOLED5 21,357,84

MUT: oms-grh-ihl 562 mg/L   MUREAV 113,467,83

MUT: sce-hmn:lym 10 mmol/L   ENVRAL 32,72,83

MUT: sce-mus-orl 200 mg/kg/4D-I   ENVRAL 32,72,83

CONSENSUS REPORTS: IARC Cancer Review: Animal Limited Evidence IMEMDT 1,61,72; Human Limited Evidence IMEMDT 20,401,79; Animal Sufficient Evidence IMEMDT 20,401,79. NTP Fourth Annual Report On Carcinogens, 1984. NCI Carcinogenesis Bioassay (gavage); Clear Evidence: mouse, rat NCITR* NCI-CG-TR,1976. EPA Genetic Toxicology Program. EPA Extremely Hazardous Substances List. Community Right-To-Know List. Reported in EPA TSCA Inventory.

OSHA PEL: (Transitional: CL 50 ppm) TWA 2 ppm   ACGIH TLV: TWA 10 ppm; Suspected Human Carcinogen   DFG MAK: Suspected Carcinogen.   NIOSH REL: (Waste Anesthetic Gases and Vapors) CL 2 ppm/1H; (Chloroform) CL 2 ppm/60M   DOT Classification: ORM-A; Label: None; IMO: Poison B; Label: Poison.

SAFETY PROFILE: Confirmed carcinogen with experimental carcinogenic, neoplastigenic, tumorigenic, and teratogenic data. A human poison by ingestion and inhalation. An experimental poison by ingestion and intravenous routes. Moderately toxic experimentally by intraperitoneal and subcutaneous routes. Human systemic effects by inhalation: hallucinations and distorted perceptions, nausea, vomiting, and other unspecified gastrointestinal effects. Human mutation data reported. Nonflammable. When heated to decomposition it emits toxic fumes of Cl⁻.

CIO250   CAS: 107-30-2
CHLOROMETHYL METHYL ETHER
DOT: 1239
mf: C_2H_5ClO mw: 80.52

PROP: Flash p: <73.4°F.

SYNS: CHLORDIMETHYLETHER (CZECH) ◇ CMME ◇ DIMETHYLCHLOROETHER ◇ ETHER METHYLIQUE MONOCHLORE (FRENCH) ◇ METHYLCHLOROMETHYL ETHER ◇ METHYLCHLOROMETHYL ETHER (DOT) ◇ METHYL CHLOROMETHYL ETHER, ANHYDROUS (DOT) ◇ MONOCHLORODIMETHYL ETHER (MAK) ◇ RCRA WASTE NUMBER U046

TOXICITY DATA with REFERENCE

NEO: scu-mus TD:852 mg/kg/71W-I   JNCIAM 48,1431,72

NEO: scu-mus TDLo:312 mg/kg/26W-I   JNCIAM 46,143,71

ETA: ihl-ham TCLo:1 ppm/6H/90D   AEHLAU 30,70,75

ETA: ihl-mus TCLo:2 ppm/82D-I   AEHLAU 22,663,71

ETA: ihl-rat TCLo:1 ppm/6H/72W   AEHLAU 30,70,75

ETA: scu-mus TD:125 mg/kg   TXAPA9 15,92,69

MUT: dni-hmn:lym 5 mL/L   CALEDQ 13,213,81

CONSENSUS REPORTS: IARC Cancer Review: Animal Sufficient Evidence IMEMDT 4,239,74; Human Limited Evidence IMEMDT 4,239,74. NTP Fourth Annual Report On Carcinogens, 1984. EPA Genetic Toxicology Program. Reported in EPA TSCA Inventory. Community Right-To-Know List. EPA Extremely Hazardous Substances List.

OSHA: Carcinogen   ACGIH TLV: Suspected Human Carcinogen.   DFG MAK: Human Carcinogen.   DOT Classification: Flammable Liquid; Label: Flammable Liquid, Poison, anhydrous; IMO: Flammable Liquid; Label: Flammable Liquid.

SAFETY PROFILE: Confirmed human carcinogen with experimental carcinogenic, tumorigenic, and neoplastigenic data. Poison by inhalation. Moderately toxic by ingestion. Human mutation data reported. A very dangerous fire hazard when exposed to heat or flame. To fight fire use alcohol foam, water, CO_2, dry chemical. When heated to decomposition it emits toxic fumes of Cl⁻.

CLK220   CAS: 95-69-2
4-CHLORO-o-TOLUIDINE
mf: C_7H_8ClN mw: 141.61

SYNS: AMARTHOL FAST RED TR BASE ◇ 2-AMINO-5-CHLOROTOLUENE ◇ AZOENE FAST RED TR BASE ◇ AZOGENE FAST RED TR ◇ AZOIC DIAZO COMPONENT

11, BASE ◇ BRENTAMINE FAST RED TR BASE ◇ 5-CHLORO-2-AMINOTOLUENE ◇ 4-CHLORO-2-METHYLANILINE ◇ 4-CHLORO-6-METHYLANILINE ◇ 4-CHLORO-2-METHYL-BENZENEAMINE ◇ 4-CHLORO-2-TOLUIDINE ◇ DAITO RED BASE TR ◇ DEVAL RED K ◇ DEVAL RED TR ◇ DIAZO FAST RED TRA ◇ FAST RED BASE TR ◇ FAST RED 5CT BASE ◇ FAST RED TR ◇ FAST RED TR11 ◇ FAST RED TR BASE ◇ FAST RED TRO BASE ◇ KAKO RED TR BASE ◇ KAMBAMINE RED TR ◇ 2-METHYL-4-CHLOROANILINE ◇ MITSUI RED TR BASE ◇ RED BASE CIBA IX ◇ RED BASE IRGA IX ◇ RED BASE NTR ◇ RED TR BASE ◇ SANYO FAST RED TR BASE ◇ TULABASE FAST RED TR

TOXICITY DATA with REFERENCE
MUT: dnd-ham:lng 3 mmol/L/2H MUREAV 77,317,80
MUT: dnr-esc 2 g/disc JPFCD2 19,95,84
MUT: dnr-sat 250 mg/disc JPFCD2 19,95,84
MUT: mmo-sat 400 µg/plate JPFCD2 19,95,84
MUT: oms-hmn:hla 1 mmol/L BECTA6 11,184,74
MUT: slt-mus-orl 12 g/kg/3D-I MUREAV 135,219,84

CONSENSUS REPORTS: IARC Cancer Review: GROUP 2B IMEMDT 7,56,87; Human Inadequate Evidence IMEMDT 16,277,78; Animal Sufficient Evidence IMEMDT 30,61,83. Reported in EPA TSCA Inventory.

DFG MAK: Human Carcinogen.

SAFETY PROFILE: Confirmed carcinogen. Poison by ingestion and subcutaneous routes. Human mutation data reported. When heated to decomposition it emits toxic fumes of Cl^- and NO_x.

CMI250 CAS: 24613-89-6
CHROMIC CHROMATE
mf: $Cr_3O_{12} \cdot 2Cr$ mw: 452.00

SYNS: CHROMIC ACID, CHROMIUM(3+) SALT (3:2) ◇ CHROMIUM CHROMATE (MAK)

TOXICITY DATA with REFERENCE
NEO: imp-rat TDLo: 112 mg/kg AIHAAP 20,274,59

CONSENSUS REPORTS: IARC Cancer Review: Animal Sufficient Evidence IMEMDT 2,100,73. Reported in EPA TSCA Inventory. Chromium and its compounds are on the Community Right-To-Know List.

OSHA PEL: (Transitional: CL 1 mg/10m³) CL 0.1 mg(CrO_3)/m³ ACGIH TLV: TWA 0.05 mg(Cr)/m³ DFG MAK: Animal Carcinogen, Suspected Human Carcinogen. NIOSH REL: TWA 0.001 mg(Cr(VI))/m³

SAFETY PROFILE: Confirmed carcinogen with experimental carcinogenic and neoplastigenic data. Very powerful oxidizer.

CMI500 CAS: 1308-31-2
CHROMITE (mineral)
mf: Cr_2FeO_4 mw: 223.85

SYNS: CHROME ORE ◇ CHROMITE ◇ CHROMITE ORE ◇ IRON CHROMITE

TOXICITY DATA with REFERENCE
MUT: cyt-ham:ovr 5 mg/L BJCAAI 44,219,81
MUT: cyt-hmn:oth 500 mg/L BJCAAI 44,219,81
MUT: dni-ham:kdy 500 mg/L BJCAAI 44,219,81
MUT: mma-sat 2 mg/plate CRNGDP 3,1331,82
MUT: oms-ham:kdy 500 mg/L BJCAAI 44,219,81
MUT: sce-ham:ovr 10 mg/L CRNGDP 3,1331,82

CONSENSUS REPORTS: IARC Cancer Review: Animal Inadequate Evidence IMEMDT 23,205,80. Chromium and its compounds are on the Community Right-To-Know List.

OSHA PEL: TWA 0.5 mg(Cr)/m³ ACGIH TLV: TWA 0.05 mg/m³ (ore processing); Confirmed Human Carcinogen (ore processing)

SAFETY PROFILE: Confirmed human carcinogen during ore processing. Human mutation data reported.

CMI750 CAS: 7440-47-3
CHROMIUM
af: Cr aw: 52.00

SYN: CHROME

TOXICITY DATA with REFERENCE
ETA: imp-rat TDLo: 1200 µg/kg/6W-I JNCIAM 16,447,55
ETA: imp-rbt TDLo: 75 mg/kg ZEKBAI 52,425,42
ETA: ivn-rat TDLo: 2160 µg/kg/6W-I JNCIAM 16,447,55

CONSENSUS REPORTS: IARC Cancer Review: Animal Inadequate Evidence IMEMDT 23,205,80. NTP Fourth Annual Report On Carcinogens, 1984. Chromium and its compounds are on the Community Right-To-Know List. Reported in EPA TSCA Inventory.

OSHA PEL: TWA 1 mg/m³ ACGIH TLV: TWA 0.5 mg/m³

SAFETY PROFILE: Confirmed carcinogen with experimental tumorigenic data. Human poison by ingestion with gastrointestinal effects. Powder will explode spontaneously in air. Ignites and is potentially explosive in atmospheres of carbon dioxide.

CMK000 CAS: 1333-82-0
CHROMIUM(VI) OXIDE (1:3)
DOT: 1463/1755
mf: CrO_3 mw: 100.00

PROP: Red, rhombic, deliquescent crystals. D: 2.70, mp: 196°, bp: decomp, sol: 61.7 g/100 cc @ 0°, 67.45 g/100 cc @ 100°.

SYNS: ANHYDRIDE CHROMIQUE (FRENCH) ◇ ANIDRIDE CROMICA (ITALIAN) ◇ CHROME (TRIOXYDE de) (FRENCH) ◇ CHROMIC ACID ◇ CHROMIC(VI) ACID ◇ CHROMIC ACID, SOLID (DOT) ◇ CHROMIC ACID, SOLUTION (DOT) ◇ CHROMIC ANHYDRIDE (DOT) ◇ CHROMIC TRIOXIDE (DOT) ◇ CHROMIUM OXIDE ◇ CHROMIUM(VI) OXIDE ◇ CHROMIUM TRIOXIDE ◇ CHROMIUM(6+) TRIOXIDE ◇ CHROMIUM TRIOXIDE, ANHYDROUS (DOT) ◇ CHROMO (TRIOSSIDO di) (ITALIAN) ◇ CHROMSAEUREANHYDRID (GERMAN) ◇ CHROMTRIOXID (GERMAN) ◇ CHROOMTRI-OXYDE (DUTCH) ◇ CHROOMZUURANHYDRIDE (DUTCH) ◇ MONOCHROMIUM OXIDE) ◇ MONOCHROMIUM TRIOX-IDE ◇ PURATRONIC CHROMIUM TRIOXIDE

TOXICITY DATA with REFERENCE
CAR: ihl-ham TCLo: 110 μg/m^3: NOSE,PUL
   AGGHAR 13,528,55
CAR: imp-rat TDLo: 125 mg/kg   AIHAAP 20,274,59
ETA: ihl-mus TCLo: 3480 μg/m^3/2H/1Y-I
   SAIGBL 29,17,87
MUT: cyt-ham: ovr 250 μg/L   TXCYAC 17,219,80
MUT: cyt-hmn: leu 2 mg/L   MUREAV 58,175,78
MUT: dnd-esc 5 mmol/L   CNREA8 40,2455,80
MUT: dnr-sat 50 mmol/L   TOLED5 7,439,81
MUT: mmo-sat 1 mmol/L   TOLED5 8,195,81
MUT: sce-ham: ovr 250 μg/L   TXCYAC 17,219,80

CONSENSUS REPORTS: IARC Cancer Review: Animal Sufficient Evidence IMEMDT 23,205,80. NTP Fourth Annual Report On Carcinogens, 1984. EPA Genetic Toxicology Program. Chromium and its compounds are on the Community Right-To-Know List. Reported in EPA TSCA Inventory.

OSHA PEL: CL 0.1 mg(CrO_3)/m^3 ACGIH TLV: TWA 0.05 mg(Cr)/m^3; Confirmed Human Carcinogen DFG MAK: 0.1 mg/m^3, Suspected Carcinogen.   NIOSH REL: TWA 0.025 mg(Cr(VI))/m^3; CL 0.05/15M   DOT Classification: Oxidizer; Label: Oxidizer, solid; Corrosive Material; Label: Corrosive, solution; Oxidizer; Label: Oxidizer, Corrosive, anhydrous, solid.

SAFETY PROFILE: Confirmed human carcinogen producing nasal and lung tumors. Experimental carcinogenic and tumorigenic data. Poison by ingestion, intraperitoneal, and subcutaneous routes. An experimental carcinogenic and teratogen. Other experimental reproductive effects. Human mutation data reported. Corrosive. Probably a severe eye, skin, and mucous membrane irritant. A powerful oxidizer.

CMK400 CAS: 37224-57-0
CHROMIUM POTASSIUM ZINC OXIDE
SYNS: POTASSIUM ZINC CHROMATE ◇ ZINC POTAS-SIUM CHROMATE

TOXICITY DATA with REFERENCE
CAR: imp-rat TDLo: 10746 μg/kg   BJIMAG 43,243,86

CONSENSUS REPORTS: IARC Cancer Review: Human Sufficient Evidence IMEMDT 23,205,80; Animal Sufficient Evidence IMEMDT 2,100,73. Chromium and its compounds, as well as zinc and its compounds, are on the Community Right-To-Know List.

OSHA PEL: (Transitional: 1 mg(CrO_3)/10m^3) CL 0.1 mg(CrO_3)/m^3 ACGIH TLV: TWA 0.01 mg(Cr)/M^3; Confirmed Human Carcinogen DFG MAK: Human Carcinogen. NIOSH REL: (Chromium (VI)) TWA 0.001 mg(Cr(VI))/m^3

SAFETY PROFILE: Confirmed carcinogen with experimental carcinogenic data. When heated to decomposition it emits toxic fumes of Cr^- and Zn^-.

CMK500 CAS: 15930-94-6
CHROMIUM(6+)ZINC OXIDE HYDRATE (1:2:6:1)
mf: $CrO_4 \cdot H_2O_2 \cdot Zn_2 \cdot H_2O$ mw: 298.78

SYNS: BUTTERCUP YELLOW ◇ CHROMIC ACID, ZINC SALT (1:2) ◇ ZINC CHROMATE HYDROXIDE ◇ ZINC CHRO-MATE (VI) HYDROXIDE ◇ ZINC HYDROXYCHROMATE ◇ ZINC YELLOW

TOXICITY DATA with REFERENCE
MUT: sce-ham: ovr 100 μg/L   MUREAV 156,219,85

CONSENSUS REPORTS: IARC Cancer Review: Human Sufficient Evidence IMEMDT 23,205,80; Animal Sufficient Evidence IMEMDT 2,100,73. Chromium and its compounds, as well as zinc and its compounds, are on the Community Right-To-Know List.

OSHA PEL: (Transitional: 1 mg(CrO$_3$)/10m^3) CL 0.1 mg(CrO$_3$)/m^3 ACGIH TLV: TWA 0.01 mg(Cr)/M^3; Confirmed Human Carcinogen DFG MAK: Human Carcinogen. NIOSH REL: (Chromium (VI)) TWA 0.001 mg(Cr(VI))/m^3

SAFETY PROFILE: Confirmed human carcinogen. Mutation data reported. When heated to decomposition it emits toxic fumes of ZnO.

CML810   CAS: 218-01-9
CHRYSENE
mf: C$_{18}$H$_{12}$ mw: 228.30

PROP: Occurs in coal tar. Is formed during distillation of coal, in very small amount during distillation or pyrolysis of many fats and oils. Orthorhombic bipyramidal plates from benzene. D: 1.274, mp: 254°. Sublimes easily in vacuo, bp: 448°. Sltly sol in alc, ether, carbon bisulfide, and glacial acetic acid; moderately sol in boiling benzene; insol in water. Chrysene is generally only sltly sol in cold organic solvents, but fairly sol in these solvents when hot, including glacial acetic acid.

SYNS: 1,2-BENZOPHENANTHRENE ◇ BENZO(a)PHENAN-THRENE ◇ 1,2-BENZPHENANTHRENE ◇ BENZ(a)PHENAN-THRENE ◇ 1,2,5,6-DIBENZONAPHTHALENE ◇ RCRA WASTE NUMBER U050

TOXICITY DATA with REFERENCE
NEO: skn-mus TD: 23 mg/kg   CNREA8 40,642,80
NEO: skn-mus TDLo: 3600 μg/kg   CNREA8 38,1831,78
ETA: scu-mus TDLo: 200 mg/kg   CNREA8 15,632,55
ETA: skn-mus TD: 40 mg/kg/3W-I   CCSUDL 1,325,76
ETA: skn-mus TD: 99 mg/kg/31W-I   CNREA8 11,301,51
ETA: skn-mus TD: 3600 mg/kg/30W-I   CANCAR 12,1079,59
MUT: dnd-ham:emb 1 mg/L   CRNGDP 3,1051,82
MUT: dnd-mus-skn 192 μmol/kg   CRNGDP 5,231,84
MUT: mma-sat 5 μg/plate   MUREAV 156,61,85
MUT: msc-hmn:lym 6 μmol/L   DTESD7 10,227,82
MUT: msc-hmn:oth 12 μmol/L   MUREAV 130,127,84

CONSENSUS REPORTS: IARC Cancer Review: Animal Limited Evidence IMEMDT 32,247,83; Animal Sufficient Evidence IMEMDT 3,159,73. EPA Genetic Toxicology Program. Reported in EPA TSCA Inventory.

OSHA PEL: 0.2 mg/m^3 ACGIH TLV: Suspected Human Carcinogen DFG MAK: Animal Carcinogen, Suspected Human Carcinogen. NIOSH REL: (Chrysene) To be controlled as a carcinogen.

SAFETY PROFILE: Confirmed carcinogen with experimental carcinogenic, neoplastigenic, and tumorigenic data by skin contact. Human mutation data reported. When heated to decomposition it emits acrid smoke and fumes.

CMO000   CAS: 2602-46-2
C.I. DIRECT BLUE 6, TETRASODIUM SALT
mf: C$_{32}$H$_{20}$N$_6$O$_{14}$S$_4$•4Na   mw: 920.69

PROP: A dye.

SYNS: AIREDALE BLUE 2BD ◇ AIZEN DIRECT BLUE 2BH ◇ AMANIL BLUE 2BX ◇ ATLANTIC BLUE 2B ◇ ATUL DIRECT BLUE 2B ◇ AZOCARD BLUE 2B ◇ AZOMINE BLUE 2B ◇ BELAMINE BLUE 2B ◇ BENCIDAL BLUE 2B ◇ BENZANIL BLUE 2B ◇ BENZO BLUE GS ◇ BLUE 2B ◇ BRASILAMINA BLUE 2B ◇ CALCOMINE BLUE 2B ◇ CHLORAMINE BLUE 2B ◇ CHLORAZOL BLUE B ◇ CHROME LEATHER BLUE 2B ◇ C.I. 22610 ◇ CRESOTINE BLUE 2B ◇ DIACOTTON BLUE BB ◇ DIAMINE BLUE 2B ◇ DIAPHTAMINE BLUE BB ◇ DIAZINE BLUE 2B ◇ DIAZOL BLUE 2B ◇ DIPHENYL BLUE 2B ◇ DIRECT BLUE 6 ◇ ENIANIL BLUE 2BN ◇ FENAMIN BLUE 2B ◇ FIXANOL BLUE 2B ◇ HISPAMIN BLUE 2B ◇ INDIGO BLUE 2B ◇ KAYAKU DIRECT ◇ MITSUI DIRECT BLUE 2BN ◇ NAPHTAMINE BLUE 2B ◇ NB2B ◇ NCI-C54579 ◇ NIAGARA BLUE 2B ◇ NIPPON BLUE BB ◇ PARAMINE BLUE 2B ◇ PHENAMINE BLUE BB ◇ PHENO BLUE 2B ◇ PONTAMINE BLUE BB ◇ SODIUM DIPHENYL-4,4'-BIS-AZO-2''-8''-AMINO-1''-NAPHTHOL-3'',6 '' DISULPHONATE ◇ TERTRODIRECT BLUE 2B ◇ VONDACEL BLUE 2B

TOXICITY DATA with REFERENCE
CAR: orl-rat TDLo: 5250 mg/kg/5W-C   NCITR* NCI-CG-TR-108,78
NEO: orl-rat TD: 2310 mg/kg/4W-C   NCITR* NCI-CG-TR-108,78
ETA: imp-mus TDLo: 80 mg/kg   TJIDAH 88,467,73
ETA: orl-mus TDLo: 34 g/kg/60W-C   TJIDAH 88,467,73
ETA: scu-rat TDLo: 750 mg/kg/27W-I   BJEPA5 38,291,57
MUT: dnd-rat-ipr 61200 μg/kg   TXCYAC 32,315,84
MUT: mma-sat 100 nmol/plate   MUREAV 136,33,94

CONSENSUS REPORTS: IARC Cancer Review: Human Limited Evidence IMEMDT 29,311,82; Animal Sufficient Evidence

IMEMDT 29,311,82. NTP Fourth Annual Report On Carcinogens, 1984. NCI Carcinogenesis Bioassay (feed); Clear Evidence: rat NCITR* NCI-CG-TR-108,78; No Evidence: mouse NCITR* NCI-CG-TR-108,78. Reported in EPA TSCA Inventory. Community Right-To-Know List.

SAFETY PROFILE: Confirmed carcinogen with experimental carcinogenic, neoplastigenic, tumorigenic, and teratogenic data. Other experimental reproductive effects. Mutation data reported. When heated to decomposition it emits very toxic fumes of NO_x, Na_2O and SO_x.

CMY800   CAS: 8007-45-2
COAL TAR
DOT: 1999

SYNS: CARBO-CORT ◇ CRUDE COAL TAR ◇ ESTAR ◇ IMPERVOTAR ◇ LAV ◇ LAVATAR ◇ PIXALBOL ◇ PIX CARBONIS ◇ POLYTAR BATH ◇ SUPERTAH ◇ SYNTAR ◇ TAR ◇ TAR, COAL ◇ TAR, LIQUID (DOT) ◇ ZETAR

TOXICITY DATA with REFERENCE
CAR: skn-mus TDLo: 64 g/kg/36W-I   AMIHBC 4,299,51
ETA: orl-mus TDLo: 12 g/kg/30W-C   AJCAA7 26,552,36
ETA: skn-mus TD: 8400 mg/kg/64W-I   ADMFAU 242,176,72
MUT: mma-esc 50 μg/plate   NTIS** PB84-138973
MUT: mma-sat 10 μg/plate   NTIS** PB84-138973
MUT: mmo-sat 5 μg/plate   NTIS** PB84-138973
MUT: mrc-smc 100 ppm   NTIS** PB84-138973
MUT: oms-hmn-skn 5000 ppm   26UYA8 -,335,71

CONSENSUS REPORTS: IARC Cancer Review: Animal Sufficient Evidence IMEMDT 34,65,84; IMEMDT 35,83,85; IMEMDT 3,22,73; Human Sufficient Evidence IMEMDT 34,65,84; IMEMDT 3,22,73; Human Limited Evidence IMEMDT 35,83,85. NTP Fourth Annual Report On Carcinogens, 1984. Reported in EPA TSCA Inventory.

OSHA PEL: TWA 0.2 mg/m³; Carcinogen DFG MAK: Human Carcinogen. NIOSH REL: TWA 0.1 mg/m³ DOT Classification: Flammable or Combustible Liquid; Label: Flammable Liquid.

SAFETY PROFILE: Confirmed human carcinogen with experimental carcinogenic and tumorigenic data. Mutation data reported. A human and experimental skin irritant. When heated to decomposition it emits acrid smoke and irritating fumes.

CMY825   CAS: 8001-58-9
COAL TAR CREOSOTE
DOT: 1136

SYNS: AWPA #1 ◇ BRICK OIL ◇ COAL TAR OIL ◇ COAL TAR OIL (DOT) ◇ CREOSOTE ◇ CREOSOTE, from COAL TAR ◇ CREOSOTE OIL ◇ CREOSOTE P1 ◇ CREOSOTUM ◇ CRESYLIC CREOSOTE ◇ HEAVY OIL ◇ LIQUID PITCH OIL ◇ NAPHTHALENE OIL ◇ PRESERV-O-SOTE ◇ RCRA WASTE NUMBER U051 ◇ TAR OIL ◇ WASH OIL

TOXICITY DATA with REFERENCE
CAR: skn-mus TDLo: 99 g/kg/33W-I   FAATDF 7,228,86
MUT: bfa-rat/sat 250 mg/kg   IAPUDO 59,279,84
MUT: mma-sat 20 μg/plate   MUREAV 119,21,83

CONSENSUS REPORTS: IARC Cancer Review: Animal Sufficient Evidence, Human Limited Evidence IMEMDT 35,83,85; Animal Sufficient Evicence IMEMDT 3,22,73. NTP Fourth Annual Report On Carcinogens, 1984. Reported in EPA TSCA Inventory.

NIOSH REL: TWA 0.1 mg/m³ DOT Classification: Flammable or Combustible Liquid; Label: Flammable Liquid.

SAFETY PROFILE: Confirmed carcinogen with experimental carcinogenic data. Moderately toxic by ingestion. Experimental reproductive effects. Mutation data reported. When heated to decomposition it emits acrid smoke and fumes.

CMZ100   CAS: 65996-93-2
COAL TAR PITCH VOLATILES

SYNS: PITCH ◇ PITCH, COAL TAR

TOXICITY DATA with REFERENCE
CAR: skn-mus TD: 82 g/kg/52W-I   HYSAAV 33(5),180,68
CAR: skn-mus TDLo: 36 g/kg/18W-I   AJIMD8 2,59,81
NEO: skn-mus TD: 4200 mg/kg/31W-I   TXAPA9 18,41,71

CONSENSUS REPORTS: IARC Cancer Review: Animal Sufficient Evidence, Human Sufficient Evidence IMEMDT 35,83,85; Human Sufficient Evidence IMEMDT 3,22,73. Reported in EPA TSCA Inventory.

OSHA PEL: TWA 0.2 mg/m³; Carcinogen ACGIH TLV: TWA 0.2 mg/m³ (volatile), Confirmed Human Carcinogen NIOSH REL: TWA 0.1 mg/m³ CHE fraction

SAFETY PROFILE: Confirmed carcinogen with experimental carcinogenic and neoplastigenic data by skin contact. When heated to decomposition it emits acrid smoke and fumes.

CNA250   CAS: 7440-48-4
COBALT
af: Co   aw: 58.93

PROP: Gray, hard, magnetic, ductile, somewhat malleable metal. Exists in two allotropic forms. At room temperature, the hexagonal form is more stable than the cubic form; both forms can exist at room temperature. Stable in air or toward water at ordinary temperatures. D 8.92, mp 1493°, bp about 3100°, Brinell hardness: 125, latent heat of fusion 62 cal/g, latent heat of vaporization 1500 cal/g, specific heat (15-100°): 0.1056 cal/g/°C. Readily sol in dil HNO_3; very slowly attacked by HCl or cold H_2SO_4. The hydrated salts of cobalt are red, and the sol salts form red solns which become blue on adding concd HCl.

SYNS: AQUACAT ◇ C.I. 77320 ◇ COBALT-59 ◇ KOBALT (GERMAN, POLISH) ◇ NCI-C60311 ◇ SUPER COBALT

TOXICITY DATA with REFERENCE
NEO: ims-rat TD: 126 mg/kg   BJCAAI 10,668,56
NEO: ims-rat TDLo: 126 mg/kg   NATUAS 173,822,54
ETA: imp-rbt TDLo: 75 mg/kg   ZEKBAI 52,425,42

CONSENSUS REPORTS: Reported in EPA TSCA Inventory. Cobalt and its compounds are on the Community Right-To-Know List.

OSHA PEL: (Transitional: TWA 0.1 mg/m³) TWA 0.05 mg/m³   ACGIH TLV: (metal, dust, and fume) TWA 0.05 mg(Co)/m³   DFG TRK: 0.5 mg/m³ calculated as cobalt in that portion of dust that can possibly be inhaled in the production of cobalt powder and catalysts; hard metal (tungsten carbide) and magnet production (processing of powder, machine pressing, and mechanical processing of unsintered articles); others 0.1 mg/m³ calculated as cobalt in that portion of dust that can possibly be inhaled. Animal Carcinogen, Suspected Human Carcinogen.

SAFETY PROFILE: Confirmed carcinogen with experimental neoplastigenic and tumorigenic data. Poison by intravenous, intratracheal, and

intraperitoneal routes. Moderately toxic by ingestion. Inhalation of the dust may cause pulmonary damage. The powder may cause dermatitis. Ingestion of soluble salts produces nausea and vomiting by local irritation. Powdered cobalt ignites spontaneously in air. Flammable when exposed to heat or flame.

CNA750   CAS: 11114-92-4
COBALT ALLOY, Co, Cr

SYNS: CHROMIUM-COBALT ALLOY ◇ COBALT-CHROMIUM ALLOY ◇ DIN 2.4602 ◇ DIN 2.4964 ◇ HASTELLOY C ◇ HAYNES STELLITE 21 ◇ HEV-4 ◇ VITALLIUM ◇ ZIMALLOY

TOXICITY DATA with REFERENCE
ETA: ims-rat TDLo: 140 mg/kg   LANCAO 1,564,71

CONSENSUS REPORTS: IARC Cancer Review: Animal Limited Evidence IMEMDT 23,205,80. NTP Fourth Annual Report On Carcinogens, 1984. Cobalt and its compounds, as well as chromium and its compounds, are on the Community Right-To-Know List.

OSHA PEL: TWA 1 mg(Cr)/m³; 0.1 mg(Co)/m³ (fume and dust)   ACGIH TLV: TWA 0.5 mg(Cr)/m³

SAFETY PROFILE: Confirmed carcinogen with experimental tumorigenic data.

CNB850
COBALT COMPOUNDS

CONSENSUS REPORTS: Cobalt and its compounds are on the Community Right-To-Know List.

DFG TRK: 0.5 mg/m³ calculated as cobalt in that portion of dust that can possibly be inhaled in the production of cobalt powder and catalysts; hard metal (tungsten carbide) and magnet production (processing of powder, machine pressing, and mechanical processing of unsintered articles); others 0.1 mg/m³ calculated as cobalt in that portion of dust that can possibly be inhaled. Animal Carcinogen, Suspected Human Carcinogen.

SAFETY PROFILE: Confirmed carcinogen with experimental neoplastigenic and tumorigenic data. Cobalt has a low toxicity by ingestion. Ingestion of soluble salts produces nausea and vomiting by local irritation. In animals, administration of cobalt salts produces an increase in the total red cell mass of the blood. In humans, a single case of poisoning with liver and kidney damage has been attributed to cobalt. Locally, cobalt has been shown to produce dermatitis and investigators have been able to demonstrate a hypersensitivity of the skin to cobalt. There have been reports of hematologic, digestive, and pulmonary changes in humans.

CNI750   CAS: 11133-98-5
COPPER-BERYLLIUM ALLOY

SYN: COPPER ALLOY, Cu, Be

CONSENSUS REPORTS: IARC Cancer Review: Animal Inadequate Evidence IMEMDT 23,143,80. Copper and its compounds, as well as beryllium and its compounds, are on the Community Right-To-Know List.

OSHA PEL: (Transitional: TWA 0.002 mg(Be)/m^3; CL 0.005; Pk 0.025/30M/8H) TWA 0.002 mg(Be)/m^3; STEL 0.005 mg(Be)/m^3/30M; CL 0.025 mg(Be)/m^3 ACGIH TLV: TWA 0.002 mg(Be)/m^3, Suspected Human Carcinogen. NIOSH REL: CL not to exceed 0.0005 mg(Be)/m^3

SAFETY PROFILE: Confirmed carcinogen. Cases of berylliosis have been reported from exposure to so called low beryllium alloys. When heated to decomposition it emits very toxic fumes of BeO.

CNJ000   CAS: 55158-44-6
COPPER-COBALT-BERYLLIUM

SYNS: COPPER ALLOY, Cu, Be, Co ◇ BERYLLIUM-COPPER-COBALT ALLOY

CONSENSUS REPORTS: IARC Cancer Review: Animal Inadequate Evidence IMEMDT 23,143,80. Copper, cobalt, and beryllium and their compounds are on the Community Right-To-Know List.

OSHA PEL: (Transitional: TWA 0.002 mg(Be)/m^3; CL 0.005; Pk 0.025/30M/8H) TWA 0.002 mg(Be)/m^3; STEL 0.005 mg(Be)/m^3/30M; CL 0.025 mg(Be)/m^3 ACGIH TLV: TWA 0.002 mg(Be)/m^3, Suspected Human Carcinogen. NIOSH REL: (To Beryllium) CL not to exceed 0.0005 mg(Be)/m^3

SAFETY PROFILE: Confirmed carcinogen. When heated to decomposition it emits very toxic fumes of BeO.

COD750   CAS: 68308-34-9
CRUDE SHALE OILS
DOT: 1288

SYNS: BLUE OIL ◇ GREEN OIL ◇ RAW SHALE OIL ◇ SHALE OIL (DOT) ◇ UNFINISHED LUBRICATING OIL

TOXICITY DATA with REFERENCE
CAR: skn-mus TD: 120 g/kg/30W-I
    NTIS** BNL-51002
CAR: skn-mus TD: 265 g/kg/2Y-I
    NTIS** CONF-801143
CAR: skn-mus TD: 26208 mg/kg/2Y-I
    NTIS** CONF-801143
CAR: skn-mus TD: 31200 mg/kg/2Y-I
    NTIS** CONF-790334-3
CAR: skn-mus TDLo: 20700 mg/kg/69W-I
    EVHPAZ 38,149,81
ETA: skn-mus TD: 168 g/kg/14W-I   BMJOAE
    2,1104,22
ETA: skn-mus TD: 216 g/kg/18W-I   BMJOAE
    2,1104,22
ETA: skn-mus TD: 28800 mg/kg/30W-I
    NTIS** CONF-790334-3
ETA: skn-mus TD: 86400 mg/kg/22W-I
    NTIS** BNL-51002
MUT: cyt-mus-ipr 1500 mg/kg   ENMUDM 4,639,82
MUT: mma-ham: ovr 1 g/L   45KQAH -,173,80
MUT: mmo-sat 1 mg/plate   45KQAH -,173,80
MUT: sce-mus-ipr 1500 mg/kg   ENMUDM 4,408,82
MUT: slt-ham: ovr 1 g/L   NTIS** CONF-800680-3

CONSENSUS REPORTS: IARC Cancer Review: Human Sufficient Evidence IMEMDT 35,161,85; Animal Limited Evidence IMEMDT 35,161,85; Animal Sufficient Evidence IMEMDT 3,22,73.

DOT Classification: Flammable or Combustible Liquid; Label: Flammable Liquid.

SAFETY PROFILE: Confirmed human carcinogen with experimental carcinogenic, neoplastigenic, and tumorigenic data. Mildly toxic by ingestion, skin contact, and intraperitoneal routes. A skin irritant. Mutation data reported. Flammable when exposed to heat and flame. When heated to decomposition it emits acrid smoke and fumes.

COU000   CAS: 14901-08-7
CYCASIN
mf: $C_8H_{16}N_2O_7$ mw: 252.26

SYNS: CYCAS REVOLUTA GLUCOSIDE ◇ CYKAZINE ◇ β-d-GLUCOSYLOXYAZOXYMETHANE ◇ METHYLAZOXYMETHANOL GLUCOSIDE ◇ METHYLAZOXYMETHANOL-β-d-GLUCOSIDE ◇ (METHYL-ONN-AZOXY)METHYL-β-d-GLUCOPYRANOSIDE

TOXICITY DATA with REFERENCE

CAR: orl-ham TDLo: 150 mg/kg   CNREA8 31,283,71

CAR: orl-rat TD: 21 g/kg/3W-C   FEPRA7 23,1386,64

ETA: ipr-rat TDLo: 90 mg/kg   IGKEAO 44,211,74

ETA: orl-mus TDLo: 300 mg/kg   CNREA8 29,1658,69

ETA: orl-rat TDLo: 100 mg/kg   JCROD7 100,231,81

ETA: orl-rat TDLo: 143 mg/kg (8-13D preg) JNCIAM 38,233,67

ETA: orl-rat TDLo: 230 mg/kg (2-5D preg) JNCIAM 38,233,67

ETA: orl-rat TDLo: 480 mg/kg/2D-C   APAVAY 340,151,65

ETA: rec-rat TDLo: 600 mg/kg/11W-I   GANNA2 66,449,75

ETA: scu-mus TDLo: 20 mg/kg/2W-I   RCOCB8 2,627,71

ETA: scu-rat TDLo: 234 mg/kg   JJIND8 74,1275,85

ETA: scu-rat TDLo: 2500 µg/kg   RCOCB82,627,71

MUT: dnd-mus-orl 50 mg/kg   BJCAAI 39,383,79

MUT: dnd-rat-orl 56 mg/kg   MUREAV 54,39,78

MUT: mma-sat 10 µmol/plate   CNREA8 39,3780,79

MUT: mmo-smc 250 µg/L   AEMIDF 45,651,83

MUT: mrc-smc 250 µg/L   AEMIDF 45,651,83

CONSENSUS REPORTS: EPA Genetic Toxicology Program. IARC Cancer Review: Human Inadequate Evidence IMEMDT 10,121,76; Animal Sufficient Evidence IMEMDT 10,121,76; Animal Sufficient Evidence IMEMDT 1,157,72 NTP Fourth Annual Report On Carcinogens, 1984.

SAFETY PROFILE: Confirmed carcinogen with experimental carcinogenic and tumorigenic data. A poison by ingestion. Mutation data reported. When heated to decomposition it emits toxic fumes of NO_x.

CQC675   CAS: 6055-19-2
CYCLOPHOSPHAMIDE HYDRATE
mf: $C_7H_{15}Cl_2N_2O_2P \cdot H_2O$ mw: 279.13

SYNS: 1-BIS(2-CHLOROETHYL)AMINO-1-OXO-2-AZA-5-OXAPHOSPHORIDINE MONOHYDRATE ◇ 2-(BIS(2-CHLOROETHYL)AMINO)-1-OXA-3-AZA-2-PHOSPHOCYCLOHEXANE 2-OXIDE MONOHYDRATE ◇ (BIS(CHLORO-2-ETHYL) AMINO)-2-TETRAHYDRO-3,4,5,6-OXAZAPHOSPHORINE-1,3,2-OXIDE-2-MONOHYDRATE ◇ BIS(2-CHLOROETHYL) PHOSPHORAMIDE CYCLIC PROPANOLAMIDE ESTER MONOHYDRATE ◇ N,N-BIS(β-CHLOROETHYL)-N'-O-PROPYLENEPHOSPHORIC ACID ESTER AMINE MONOHYDRATE ◇ N,N-BIS(2-CHLOROETHYL)TETRAHYDRO-2H-1,3,2-OXA-PHOSPHORIN-2-AMINE-2-OXIDE MONOHYDRATE ◇ N,N-BIS(β-CHLOROETHYL)-N',O-TRIMETHYLENEPHOSPHORIC ACID ESTER DIAMIDE MONOHYDRATE ◇ CB-4564 ◇ CLAFEN ◇ CYCLIC N',O-PROPYLENE ESTER of N,N-BIS(2-CHLOROETHYL)PHOSPHORODIAMIDIC ACID MONOHYDRATE ◇ CYCLOPHOSPHAMIDE MONOHYDRATE ◇ CYCLOPHOSPHAMIDUM ◇ CYCLOPHOSPHAN ◇ CYCLOPHOSPHANE ◇ CYCLOPHOSPHANUM ◇ CYTOPHOSPHAN ◇ CYTOXAN ◇ 2-(DI(2-CHLOROETHYL) AMINO)-1-OXA-3-AZA-2-PHOSPHACYCLOHEXANE-2-OXIDE MONOHYDRATE ◇ N,N-DI(2-CHLOROETHYL)AMINO-N,O-PROPYLENE PHOSPHORIC ACID ESTER DIAMIDE MONOHYDRATE ◇ ENDOXANA ◇ ENDOXAN-ASTA ◇ ENDOXAN MONOHYDRATE ◇ ENDOXAN R ◇ ENDUXAN ◇ GENOXAL ◇ MITOXAN ◇ NSC 26271 ◇ PROCYTOX ◇ SEMDOXAN ◇ SENDOXAN ◇ SENDUXAN

TOXICITY DATA with REFERENCE
MUT: bfa-mus/smc 500 mg/kg   EVSRBT 24,893,81

CONSENSUS REPORTS: IARC Cancer Review: Animal Sufficient Evidence IMEMDT 9,135,75; Human Limited Evidence IMEMDT 9,135,75; Human Sufficient Evidence IMEMDT 26,165,81.

SAFETY PROFILE: Confirmed human carcinogen. Poison by ingestion and intravenous routes. Experimental reproductive effects. Mutation data reported. When heated to decomposition it emits toxic fumes of Cl^-, PO_x, and NO_x.

DAD200   CAS: 50-29-3
DDT
DOT: 2761
mf: $C_{14}H_9Cl_5$ mw: 354.48

PROP: Colorless crystals or white to slightly off-white powder. Odorless or with slight aromatic odor. Mp: 108.5-109°.

SYNS: AGRITAN ◇ ANOFEX ◇ ARKOTINE ◇ AZOTOX ◇ α,α-BIS(p-CHLOROPHENYL)-β,β,β-TRICHLORETHANE ◇ 1,1-BIS-(p-CHLOROPHENYL)-2,2,2-TRICHLOROETHANE ◇ 2,2-BIS(p-CHLOROPHENYL)-1,1,1-TRICHLOROETHANE ◇ BOSAN SUPRA ◇ BOVIDERMOL ◇ CHLOROPHENOTHAN ◇ CHLOROPHENOTHANE ◇ CHLOROPHENOTOXUM ◇ CITOX ◇ CLOFENOTANE ◇ p,p'-DDT ◇ DEDELO ◇ DEOVAL ◇ DETOX ◇ DETOXAN ◇ DIBOVAN ◇ DICHLORODIPHENYLTRICHLOROETHANE ◇ p,p'-DICHLORODIPHENYLTRICHLOROETHANE ◇ 4,4'-DICHLORODIPHENYLTRICHLOROETHANE ◇ DICHLORODIPHENYLTRICHLOROETHANE (DOT) ◇ DICOPHANE ◇ DIDIGAM ◇ DIDIMAC ◇ DIPHENYLTRICHLOROETHANE ◇ DODAT ◇ DYKOL ◇ ENT 1,506

◇ ESTONATE ◇ GENITOX ◇ GESAFID ◇ GESAPON ◇ GESAREX ◇ GESAROL ◇ GUESAPON ◇ GUESAROL ◇ GYRON ◇ HAVERO-EXTRA ◇ HILDIT ◇ IVORAN ◇ IXODEX ◇ KOPSOL ◇ MICRO DDT 75 ◇ MUTOXIN ◇ NCI-C00464 ◇ NEOCID ◇ PARACHLOROCIDUM ◇ PEB1 ◇ PENTACHLORIN ◇ PENTECH ◇ PPZEIDAN ◇ R50 ◇ RCRA WASTE NUMBER U-061 ◇ RUKSEAM ◇ SANTOBANE ◇ TECH DDT ◇ 1,1,1-TRICHLOOR-2,2-BIS(4-CHLOOR FENYL)-ETHAAN (DUTCH) ◇ 1,1,1-TRICHLOR-2,2-BIS(4-CHLOR-PHENYL)-AETHAN (GERMAN) ◇ TRICHLO-ROBIS (4-CHLOROPHENYL) ETHANE ◇ 1,1,1-TRICHLORO-2,2-DI(4-CHLOROPHENYL)-ETHANE ◇ 1,1'-(2,2,2-TRICHLOROETHYLIDENE)BIS(4-CHLOROBENZENE) ◇ 1,1,1-TRICLORO-2,2-BIS(4-CLORO-FENIL)-ETANO (ITAL-IAN) ◇ ZEIDANE ◇ ZERDANE

TOXICITY DATA with REFERENCE
CAR: orl-mus TDLo: 73 mg/kg/26W-C FCTXAV 7,215,69
CAR: orl-rat TDLo: 1225 mg/kg/7W-C
TUMOAB 61,113,75
NEO: orl-mus TD: 5600 mg/kg/80W-I IJCNAW 19,725,77
NEO: orl-mus TD: 7560 mg/kg/90W-C FCTXAV 11,433,73
NEO: orl-mus TDLo: 24 mg/kg (MGN): TER
JNCIAM 51,983,73
NEO: orl-rat TD: 19 g/kg/2Y-C IJCNAW 19,179,77
NEO: orl-rat TD: 438 mg/kg/2Y-C REONBL
26,177,79
NEO: orl-rat TD: 12096 mg/kg/3Y-C TUMOAB 68,11,82
NEO: orl-rat TD: 17976 mg/kg/2Y-C TUMOAB 68,11,82
NEO: orl-rat TD: 24192 mg/kg/3Y-C TUMOAB 68,11,82
NEO: scu-mus TDLo: 370 mg/kg/80W-I
IJCNAW 19,725,77
ETA: orl-ham TDLo: 21280 mg/kg/38W-I:
TER PSEBAA 134,113,70
ETA: orl-mus TD: 3150 mg/kg/15W-C
ZKKOBW 82,25,74
ETA: orl-rat TD: 8100 mg/kg/2Y-C TXAPA9 11,88,67
MUT: cyt-hmn: lym 200 μg/L/72H MUREAV 40,131,76
MUT: dnd-esc 15 μmol/L MUREAV 89,95,81
MUT: dnd-mus: ast 15 μmol/L MUREAV 89,95,81
MUT: dni-dmg: oth 250 ppb EXPEAM 41,745,85
MUT: dni-mus-ipr 20 g/kg ARGEAR 51,605,81
MUT: dns-rat: lvr 100 pmol/L CRNGDP 5,1547,84

CONSENSUS REPORTS: IARC Cancer Review: Animal Sufficient Evidence IMEMDT 5,83,74; Human Inadequate Evidence

IMEMDT 5,83,74. NTP Fourth Annual Report On Carcinogens, 1984. NCI Carcinogenesis Bioassay (feed); No Evidence: mouse, rat NCITR* NCI-CG-TR-131,78. Reported in EPA TSCA Inventory. EPA Genetic Toxicology Program.

OSHA PEL: TWA 1 mg/m³ (skin)   ACGIH TLV: TWA 1 mg/m³   NIOSH REL: (DDT) TWA 0.5 mg/m³; avoid skin contact   DFG MAK: 1 mg/m³   DOT Classification: ORM-A; Label: None.

SAFETY PROFILE: Confirmed carcinogen with experimental carcinogenic, neoplastigenic, tumorigenic, and teratogenic data. Human poison by ingestion and possibly other routes. Experimental poison by ingestion, skin contact, subcutaneous, intravenous, and intraperitoneal routes. Experimental reproductive effects. Human systemic effects by ingestion: anesthetic, convulsions, headache, analgesia, cardiac arrythmias, nausea or vomiting, sweating and unspecified pulmonary changes. Human mutation data reported. An insecticide. When heated to decomposition it emits toxic fumes of Cl⁻.

DAL400   CAS: 23107-12-2
DEHYDRORETRONECINE
mf: $C_8H_{11}NO_2$ mw: 153.20

SYNS: 3,8-DIDEHYDRORETRONECINE ◇ (R)-2,3-DIHY-DRO-1-HYDROXY-1H-PYRROLIZINE-7-METHANOL

TOXICITY DATA with REFERENCE
CAR: scu-mus TDLo: 80 mg/kg/4W-I   JJIND8 61,85,78
CAR: skn-mus TD: 1438 mg/kg/47W-I CALEDQ 17,61,82
CAR: skn-mus TDLo: 120 mg/kg/28W-I JJIND8 61,85,78
NEO: scu-rat TDLo: 350 mg/kg/1Y-I JNCIAM 56,787,76
MUT: dni-rat: lvr 100 μmol/L CBINA8 30,325,80
MUT: mmo-sat 500 μg/plate MUREAV 149,485,85
MUT: oms-rat: lvr 20 μmol/L CBINA8 30,325,80
MUT: otr-ham: kdy 250 μg/L CRNGDP 1,161,80
MUT: sce-hmn: lym 1 μmol/L MUREAV 149,485,85

CONSENSUS REPORTS: IARC Cancer Review: Animal Sufficient Evidence IMEMDT 10,333,76.

SAFETY PROFILE: Confirmed carcinogen with experimental carcinogenic and neoplastigenic data. Poison by intraperitoneal route. Human mutation data reported. When heated to decomposition it emits toxic fumes of NO_x.

DBO000   CAS: 615-05-4
2,4-DIAMINOANISOLE
mf: $C_7H_{10}N_2O$ mw: 138.19

SYNS: C.I. 76050 ◊ C.I. OXIDATION BASE 12 ◊ 2,4-DAA ◊ 2,4-DIAMINEANISOLE ◊ 2,4-DIAMINOANISOL ◊ 2,4-DIAMINOANISOLE BASE ◊ m-DIAMINOANISOLE 1,3-DIAMINO-4-METHOXYBENZENE ◊ 2,4-DIAMINO-1-METHOXYBENZENE ◊ FURRO L ◊ 4-METHOXY-1,3-BENZENEDIAMINE ◊ p-METHOXY-m-PHENYLENEDIAMINE ◊ 4-METHOXY-m-PHENYLENEDIAMINE ◊ 4-MMPD ◊ PELAGOL DA ◊ PELAGOL GREY L ◊ PELAGOL L

TOXICITY DATA with REFERENCE
MUT: dnd-hmn:fbr 50 μmol/L   MUREAV
127,107,84

MUT: dnd-rat:lvr 500 μmol/L   CBINA8 31,35,80
MUT: mma-sat 5 μg/plate   MUREAV 79,289,80
MUT: sce-mus-ipr 12 mg/kg   MUREAV 108,225,83

CONSENSUS REPORTS: IARC Cancer Review: Human Limited Evidence IMEMDT 27,103,82. EPA Genetic Toxicology Program. Reported in EPA TSCA Inventory.

DFG MAK: Animal Carcinogen, Suspected Human Carcinogen. NIOSH REL: (2,4-diaminoanisole) Reduce to lowest feasible level

SAFETY PROFILE: Confirmed carcinogen. Poison by intraperitoneal route. Moderately toxic by ingestion. Human mutation data reported. A skin irritant. When heated to decomposition it emits toxic fumes of NO_x.

DBO400   CAS: 39156-41-7
2,4-DIAMINOANISOLE SULPHATE
mf: $C_7H_{10}N_2O \cdot xH_2O_4S$ mw: 824.75

SYNS: BASF URSOL SLA ◊ C.I. 76051 ◊ C.I. OXIDATION BASE 12A ◊ 2,4-DAA SULFATE ◊ 2,4-DIAMINOANISOLE SULFATE ◊ 2,4-DIAMINO-ANISOL SULPHATE ◊ 2,4-DIAMINO-1-METHOXYBENZENE ◊ 1,3-DIAMINO-4-METHOXYBENZENE SULPHATE ◊ 2,4-DIAMINO-1-METHOXY-BENZENE SULPHATE ◊ 2,4-DIAMINOSOLE SULPHATE ◊ DURAFUR BROWN MN ◊ FOURAMINE BA ◊ FOURRINE SLA ◊ FURRO SLA ◊ 4-METHOXY-1,3-BENZENEDIAMINE SULFATE ◊ 4-METHOXY-1,3-BENZENEDIAMINE SULPHATE ◊ 4-METHOXY-m-PHENYLENEDIAMINE SULFATE ◊ p-METHOXY-m-PHENYLENEDIAMINE SULPHATE ◊ 4-METHOXY-m-PHENYLENEDIAMINE SULPHATE ◊ 4-MMPD SULPHATE ◊ NAKO TSA ◊ NCI-C01989 ◊ OXIDATION BASE 12A ◊ PELAGOL GREY ◊ RENAL SLA ◊ URSOL SLA ◊ ZOBA SLE

TOXICITY DATA with REFERENCE
CAR: orl-mus TDLo: 157 g/kg/78W-C
NCITR* NCI-CG-TR-84,78
CAR: orl-rat TD: 51 g/kg/72W-C
NCITR* NCI-CG-TR-84,78
CAR: orl-rat TD: 689 g/kg/82W-C   IARC**
27,103,82
CAR: orl-rat TD: 1377 g/kg/82W-C   IARC**
27,103,82
CAR: orl-rat TD: 2730 g/kg/78W-C   IARC**
27,103,82
CAR: orl-rat TD: 2870 g/kg/82W-C   IARC**
27,103,82
CAR: orl-rat TDLo: 18 g/kg/10W-C   JJIND8
65,197,80
NEO: orl-mus TD: 1310 g/kg/78W-C   IARC**
27,103,82
ETA: orl-rat TD: 33 g/kg/78W-C
NCITR* NCI-CG-TR-84,78
ETA: orl-rat TD: 350 g/kg/10W-C   IARC**
27,103,82
MUT: mma-sat 1 μg/plate   ENMUDM 7(Suppl 5),1,85
MUT: mrc-smc 500 mg/L   MUREAV 78,243,80
MUT: sln-dmg-orl 15100 μmol/L/3D   MUREAV
48,181,77
MUT: sln-nsc 150 mg/L   MUREAV 167,35,86

CONSENSUS REPORTS: IARC Cancer Review: Animal Sufficient Evidence IMEMDT 27,103,82; Animal Inadequate Evidence IMEMDT 16,51,78. NTP Fourth Annual Report On Carcinogens, 1984. NCI Carcinogenesis Bioassay (feed); Clear Evidence: mouse, rat NCITR* NCI-CG-TR-84,78. Reported in EPA TSCA Inventory. EPA Genetic Toxicology Program. Community Right-To-Know List.

SAFETY PROFILE: Confirmed carcinogen with experimental carcinogenic, neoplastigenic, and tumorigenic data. Poison by intraperitoneal route. Mutation data reported. When heated to decomposition it emits very toxic fumes of NO_x and SO_x.

DCJ200   CAS: 119-90-4
o-DIANISIDINE
mf: $C_{14}H_{16}N_2O_2$ mw: 244.32

PROP: Colorless crystals. Mp: 137-138°, flash p: 403°F, vap d: 8.5.

SYNS: ACETAMINE DIAZO BLACK RD ◊ AMACEL DEVELOPED NAVY SD ◊ AZOENE FAST BLUE BASE ◊ AZOFIX BLUE B SALT ◊ AZOGNE FAST BLUE B ◊ BLUE BN BALSE ◊ BRENTAMINE FAST BLUE B BASE ◊ CELLITAZOL B ◊ C.I. 24110 ◊ C.I. AZOIC DIAZO COMPO

NENT 48 ◇ CIBACETE DIAZO NAVY BLUE 2B ◇ C.I. DIS-
PERSE BLACK 6 ◇ DIACELLITON FAST GREY G
◇ DIACEL NAVY DC ◇ o-DIANISIDIN (CZECH, GERMAN)
◇ o-DIANISIDINA (ITALIAN) ◇ 3,3'-DIANISIDINE
◇ O,O'DIANISIDINE ◇ DIATO BLUE BASE B ◇ 3,3'-DI-
METHOXYBENZIDIN (CZECH) ◇ 3,3'-DIMETHOXYBENZI-
DINE ◇ 3,3'-DIMETOSSIBENZODINA (ITALIAN) ◇ FAST
BLUE B BASE ◇ HILTONIL FAST BLUE B BASE ◇ HILTOSAL
FAST BLUE B SALT ◇ HINDASOL BLUE B SALT
◇ KAKO BLUE B SALT ◇ KAYAKU BLUE B BASE
◇ LAKE BLUE B BASE ◇ MEISEI TERYL DIAZO BLUE HR
◇ MITSUI BLUE B BASE ◇ NAPHTHANIL BLUE B BASE
◇ NEUTROSEL NAVY BN ◇ RCRA WASTE NUMBER U091
◇ SANYO FAST BLUE SALT B ◇ SETACYL DIAZO NAVY
R ◇ SPECTROLENE BLUE B

TOXICITY DATA with REFERENCE
ETA: orl-ham TDLo: 588 g/kg/70W-C   PAACA3
10,78,69
ETA: orl-rat TDLo: 12 g/kg/56W-I   GTPZAB
9,18,65
MUT: dnd-dog: oth 100 μmol/L   CNREA8
44,1893,84
MUT: mma-sat 1 μg/plate   IGAYAY 123,18,82
MUT: mmo-sat 333 μg/plate   ENMUDM 5(Suppl
1),3,83
MUT: oms-dog: oth 100 μmol/L   CNREA8
44,1893,84
MUT: sce-ham: ovr 500 μg/L   ENMUDM 7,1,85

CONSENSUS REPORTS: IARC Cancer Review: Animal Sufficient Evidence IMEMDT
4,41,74. NTP Fourth Annual Report On Carcinogens, 1984. EPA Genetic Toxicology Program. Community Right-To-Know List. Reported in EPA TSCA Inventory.

DFG MAK: Animal Carcinogen, Suspected Human Carcinogen. NIOSH REL: (Benzidine-
based dye) Reduce to lowest feasible level

SAFETY PROFILE: Confirmed carcinogen with
experimental tumorigenic data. Moderately
toxic by ingestion. Mutation data reported.
Combustible when exposed to heat or flame.
When heated to decomposition it emits toxic
fumes of NO_x.

DCP800   CAS: 334-88-3
DIAZOMETHANE
mf: CH_2N_2 mw: 42.05

PROP: Yellow gas at ordinary temp. Mp:
−145°, bp: −23°, d: 1.45.

SYNS: AZIMETHYLENE ◇ DIAZIRINE

TOXICITY DATA with REFERENCE
ETA: ihl-mus TCLo: 272 mg/m^3/26W-I   BJCAAI
16,92,62
ETA: ihl-rat TCLo: 272 mg/m^3/26W-I   BJCAAI
16,92,62
ETA: scu-mus TDLo: 48 g/kg/52W-I   BJCAAI
16,92,62
MUT: mmo-nsc 250 mmol/L   HEREAY 35,521,49

CONSENSUS REPORTS: IARC Cancer Re-
view: GROUP 3 IMEMDT 7,56,87; Animal
Sufficient Evidence IMEMDT 7,223,74. EPA
Genetic Toxicology Program. Community
Right-To-Know List.

OSHA PEL: TWA 0.2 ppm   ACGIH TLV:
TWA 0.2 ppm   DFG MAK: Animal Carcinogen, Suspected Human Carcinogen.

SAFETY PROFILE: Confirmed carcinogen with
experimental tumorigenic data. A poison irritant
by inhalation. A powerful allergen. It can cause
pulmonary edema and frequently causes hypersensitivity leading to asthmatic symptoms. Mutation data reported. Highly explosive when
shocked, exposed to heat or by chemical reaction. When heated to decomposition or on contact with acid or acid fumes it emits highly
toxic fumes of NO_x.

DCS400   CAS: 226-36-8
DIBENZ(a,h)ACRIDINE
mf: $C_{21}H_{13}N$ mw: 279.35

SYNS: 7-AZADIBENZ(a,h)ANTHRACENE ◇ DB(a,h)AC
◇ DIBENZ(a,d)ACRIDINE ◇ 1,2,5,6-DIBENZACRIDINE
◇ 1,2,5,6-DIBENZOACRIDINE ◇ 1,2,5,6-DINAPHTHACRI-
DINE

TOXICITY DATA with REFERENCE
CAR: imp-rat TDLo: 5 mg/kg   CALEDQ 20,97,83
ETA: imp-rat TD: 1500 μg/kg   CALEDQ 20,97,83
ETA: ivn-mus TDLo: 10 mg/kg   JNCIAM 1,225,40
ETA: orl-mus TDLo: 13 g/kg/63W-I   PRLBA4
129,439,40
ETA: scu-mus TD: 1600 mg/kg/24W-I   PRLBA4
129,439,40
ETA: scu-mus TDLo: 430 mg/kg/24W-I
PRLBA4 123,343,37
ETA: skn-mus TD: 790 mg/kg/33W-I   PRLBA4
117,318,35
ETA: skn-mus TDLo: 540 mg/kg/45W-I
ACRSAJ 4,315,56

CONSENSUS REPORTS: IARC Cancer Review: Animal Sufficient Evidence IMEMDT
32,277,83; IMEMDT 3,247,73. NTP Fourth

Annual Report On Carcinogens, 1984. EPA Genetic Toxicology Program.

SAFETY PROFILE: Confirmed carcinogen with experimental carcinogenic and tumorigenic data. When heated to decomposition it emits toxic fumes of NO_x.

DCS600   CAS: 224-42-0
DIBENZ(a,j)ACRIDINE
mf: $C_{21}H_{13}N$ mw: 279.35

SYNS: 7-AZADIBENZ(a,j)ANTHRACENE ◇ DB(a,j)AC ◇ DIBENZ(a,f)ACRIDINE ◇ 1,2,7,8-DIBENZACRIDINE ◇ 3,4,5,6-DIBENZACRIDINE ◇ DIBENZO(a,j)ACRIDINE ◇ 3,4,6,7-DINAPHTHACRIDINE

TOXICITY DATA with REFERENCE
CAR: skn-mus TDLo: 99 mg/kg/99W-I   CALEDQ 37,337,87
ETA: scu-mus TDLo: 40 mg/kg   JNCIAM 1,225,40
ETA: skn-mus TD: 700 mg/kg/29W-I   PRLBA4 117,318,35
ETA: skn-mus TDLo: 590 mg/kg/25W-I   BAFEAG 42,186,55
MUT: dnd-esc 10 μmol/L   PNCCA2 5,39,65
MUT: mma-sat 5 μg/plate   PNASA6 72,5135,75
MUT: pic-esc 50 mg/L   CNREA8 41,532,81

CONSENSUS REPORTS: IARC Cancer Review: Animal Sufficient Evidence IMEMDT 32,283,83; IMEMDT 3,254,73. NTP Fourth Annual Report On Carcinogens, 1984. EPA Genetic Toxicology Program.

SAFETY PROFILE: Confirmed carcinogen with experimental carcinogenic and tumorigenic data. Experimental reproductive effects. Mutation data reported. When heated to decomposition it emits toxic fumes of NO_x.

DCT400   CAS: 53-70-3
DIBENZ(a,h)ANTHRACENE
mf: $C_{22}H_{14}$ mw: 278.36

SYNS: 1,2:5,6-BENZANTHRACENE ◇ DBA ◇ DB(a,h)A ◇ 1,2,5,6-DBA ◇ 1,2,5,6-DIBENZANTHRACEEN (DUTCH) ◇ 1,2:5,6-DIBENZANTHRACENE ◇ 1,2:5,6-DIBENZ(a)AN-THRACENE ◇ DIBENZO(a,h)ANTHRACENE ◇ 1,2:5,6-DI-BENZOANTHRACENE ◇ RCRA WASTE NUMBER U063

TOXICITY DATA with REFERENCE
CAR: imp-mus TD: 100 mg/kg   BMBUAQ 14,147,58
CAR: imp-mus TDLo: 80 mg/kg   BJCAAI 11,212,57
CAR: ims-pgn TDLo: 6 mg/kg   JNCIAM 32,905,64
CAR: orl-mus TD: 4520 mg/kg/36W-C   JNCIAM 1,17,40

CAR: orl-mus TDLo: 4160 mg/kg/26W-I   JPBAA7 49,21,39
CAR: scu-mus TDLo: 6 mg/kg   CRNGDP 4,513,83
CAR: skn-mus TDLo: 1200 mg/kg/50W-I   14JTAF -,275,65
NEO: imp-mus TD: 14 mg/kg   AJPAA4 16,287,40
NEO: imp-mus TD: 200 mg/kg   AJCAA7 36,201,39
NEO: irn-frg TDLo: 12 mg/kg   CNREA8 24,1969,64
NEO: ivn-mus TDLo: 40 mg/kg   PHRPA6 54,1158,39
NEO: scu-mus TD: 78 μg/kg   JNCIAM 3,503,43
NEO: scu-mus TD: 400 mg/kg/10W-I   IJCNAW 2,500,67
NEO: scu-rat TD: 135 mg/kg/9W-I   PSEBAA 68,330,48
NEO: scu-rat TDLo: 2400 μg/kg/50D-I   85DLAB -,-,75
NEO: skn-mus TD: 6 μg/kg   CNREA8 20,1179,60
NEO: skn-mus TD: 400 mg/kg/40W-I   CNREA8 22,78,62
ETA: ivn-gpg TDLo: 30 mg/kg   JNCIAM 13,705,52
ETA: mul-mus TDLo: 40 mg/kg/12D-I   PHRPA6 52,637,37
ETA: scu-gpg TDLo: 250 mg/kg/24D-I   AKBNAE 51,112,38
ETA: scu-mus TD: 6 mg/kg   IJCNAW 32,765,83
MUT: dnd-esc 10 μmol/L   MUREAV 89,95,81
MUT: dnd-hmn: emb 360 nmol/L   CBINA8 22,257,78
MUT: msc-ham: lng 500 μg/L   MUREAV 136,65,84
MUT: msc-mus: lym 4250 μg/L   MUREAV 106,101,82
MUT: otr-rat-orl 200 mg/kg   CNREA8 40,1157,80

CONSENSUS REPORTS: IARC Cancer Review: Animal Sufficient Evidence IMEMDT 32,299,83; IMEMDT 3,178,73. NTP Fourth Annual Report On Carcinogens, 1984. EPA Genetic Toxicology Program. Reported in EPA TSCA Inventory.

SAFETY PROFILE: Confirmed carcinogen with experimental carcinogenic, tumorigenic, and neoplastigenic data. Poison by intravenous route. Human mutation data reported. When heated to decomposition it emits acrid smoke and irritating fumes.

DCY000   CAS: 194-59-2
7H-DIBENZO(c,g)CARBAZOLE
mf: $C_{20}H_{13}N$ mw: 267.34

PROP: Needles. Mp: 158°.

SYNS: 7-AZA-7H-DIBENZO(c,g)FLUORENE ◇ 3,4,5,6-DI-BENZCARBAZOL ◇ 3,4,5,6-DIBENZCARBAZOLE

◇ 3,4,5,6-DIBENZOCARBAZOLE ◇ 3,4,5,6-DINAPHTHA-
CARBAZOLE ◇ 7H-DB(c,g)C

TOXICITY DATA with REFERENCE

CAR: skn-mus TDLo: 99 mg/kg/99W-I   CALEDQ
37,337,87

NEO: itr-ham TDLo: 72 mg/kg/18W-I   JTEHD6
3,935,77

ETA: imp-dog TDLo: 65 mg/kg/52W-I   JPBAA7
68,561,54

ETA: imp-mus TDLo: 40 mg/kg   BJCAAI 6,412,52
ETA: ipr-mus TDLo: 13 mg/kg   BIJOAK 32,1460,38
ETA: ivn-mus TDLo: 10 mg/kg   JNCIAM 1,225,40
ETA: orl-mus TDLo: 280 mg/kg/32W-I   BJCAAI
4,203,50

ETA: orl-mus TDLo: 280 mg/kg/32W-I   BJCAAI
4,203,50

ETA: scu-rat TDLo: 150 mg/kg/17W-I   PRLBA4
122,429,37

ETA: skn-mus TDLo: 90 mg/kg/23W-I   PRLBA4
122,429,37

MUT: dnd-mus-scu 44 μmol/kg   CRNGDP
6,1271,85

CONSENSUS REPORTS: IARC Cancer Review: Animal Sufficient Evidence IMEMDT
32,315,83; IMEMDT 3,260,73. NTP Fourth
Annual Report On Carcinogens, 1984.

SAFETY PROFILE: Confirmed carcinogen with
experimental carcinogenic, neoplastigenic, and
tumorigenic data. Poison by intraperitoneal
route. Mutation data reported. When heated to
decomposition it emits toxic fumes of NO_x.

DDL800   CAS: 96-12-8
1,2-DIBROMO-3-CHLOROPROPANE
DOT: 2872
mf: $C_3H_5Br_2Cl$ mw: 236.35

PROP: Bp: 196°, flash p: 170°F (TOC).

SYNS: BBC 12 ◇ 1-CHLORO-2,3-DIBROMOPROPANE
◇ 3-CHLORO-1,2-DIBROMOPROPANE ◇ DBCP ◇ DIBROM-
CHLORPROPAN (GERMAN) ◇ 1,2-DIBROM-3-CHLOR-PRO-
PAN (GERMAN) ◇ DIBROMOCHLOROPROPANE ◇ 1,2-DI-
BROMO-3-CLORO-PROPANO (ITALIAN) ◇ 1,2-DIBROOM-3-
CHLOORPROPAAN (DUTCH) ◇ FUMAGON ◇ FUMAZONE
◇ NCI-C00500 ◇ NEMABROM ◇ NEMAFUME ◇ NEMAGON
◇ NEMAGONE ◇ NEMAGON SOIL FUMIGANT ◇ NEMANAX
◇ NEMAPAZ ◇ NEMASET ◇ NEMATOCIDE ◇ NEMATOX
◇ NEMAZON ◇ OS 1897 ◇ OXY DBCP ◇ RCRA WASTE
NUMBER 7066 ◇ SD 1897

TOXICITY DATA with REFERENCE

CAR: ihl-mus TC: 3 ppm/6H/2Y-I   JCROD7
98,75,80

CAR: ihl-mus TC: 3 ppm/6H/76W-I   NTPTR*
NTP-TR-206,82

CAR: ihl-mus TC: 600 ppb/6H/76W-I   EVHPAZ
47,365,83

CAR: ihl-mus TC: 600 ppm/6H/2Y-I   NTPTR*
NTP-TR-206,82

CAR: ihl-mus TCLo: 600 ppb/6H/2Y-I   JCROD7
98,75,80

CAR: ihl-rat TC: 3 ppm/6H/2Y-I   BJCAAI
42,772,80

CAR: ihl-rat TC: 3 ppm/6H/84W-I
NTPTR* NTP-TR-206,82

CAR: ihl-rat TC: 600 ppb/6H/2Y-I
NTPTR* NTP-TR-206,82

CAR: ihl-rat TC: 600 ppb/6H/76W-I   EVHPAZ
47,365,83

CAR: ihl-rat TCLo: 600 ppb/6H/2Y-I   BJCAAI
42,772,80

CAR: orl-mus TDLo: 49 g/kg/47W-I
NCITR* NCI-CG-TR-28,78

CAR: orl-rat TD: 9280 mg/kg/64W-I
NCITR* NCI-CG-TR-28,78

CAR: orl-rat TDLo: 5475 mg/kg/73W-I
NCITR* NCI-CG-TR-28,78

CAR: scu-rat TD: 240 mg/kg/12W-I   TOLED5
31(Suppl),202,86

CAR: skn-mus TDLo: 100 g/kg/74W-I   JJIND8
63,1433,79

MUT: dnd-rat-ipr 36 mg/kg   CBTOE2 1,181,85
MUT: dni-hmn: hla 10 mmol/L   MUREAV 92,427,82
MUT: mma-sat 500 ng/plate   ENMUDM 7(Suppl
3),15,85

MUT: sln-dmg-orl 100 ppm/3D   HCKHDV 5(5),7,84
MUT: spm-rat-orl 3560 μg/kg/5D   TXAPA9
48,A46,79

MUT: spm-rbt-orl 375 mg/kg/10W-I   FAATDF
6,628,86

CONSENSUS REPORTS: IARC Cancer Review: Animal Sufficient Evidence IMEMDT
15,139,77; Human Limited Evidence IMEMDT
20,83,79; Animal Sufficient Evidence
IMEMDT 20,83,79. NTP Fourth Annual Report On Carcinogens, 1984. NCI Carcinogenesis
Bioassay Completed; Results Positive: mouse,
rat (NCITR* NCI-CG-TR-28,78). EPA Genetic
Toxicology Program. Community Right-To-
Know List. Reported in EPA TSCA Inventory.

OSHA PEL: TWA 0.001 ppm; Cancer Hazard.   DFG MAK: Animal Carcinogen, Suspected Human Carcinogen.   NIOSH REL: CL
0.01 ppm/30M

SAFETY PROFILE: Confirmed human carcinogen with experimental carcinogenic and terato-

genic data. Poison by ingestion, inhalation, and subcutaneous routes. Moderately toxic by skin contact. An eye and severe skin irritant. A suspected human carcinogenic. Narcotic in high concentrations. Has been implicated in causing human male sterility in factory workers. Human mutation data reported. A soil fumigant. Flammable when exposed to heat or flame. When heated to decomposition it emits toxic fumes of Cl^- and Br^-.

DEN600   CAS: 7572-29-4
DICHLOROACETYLENE
mf: C_2Cl_2 mw: 94.92

SYN: DICHLOROETHYNE

TOXICITY DATA with REFERENCE
CAR: ihl-mus TCLo:2 ppm/24H/77W-I
CRNGDP 5,1411,84
CAR: ihl-rat TCLo:14 ppm/6H/77W-I CRNGDP
5,1411,84
MUT: mma-sat 4000 ppm MUREAV 117,21,83
MUT: mmo-sat 4000 ppm MUREAV 117,21,83

CONSENSUS REPORTS: IARC Cancer Review: Animal Limited Evidence IMEMDT 39,369,86

OSHA PEL: CL 0.1 ppm   ACGIH TLV: CL 0.1 ppm   DFG MAK: Animal Carcinogen, Suspected Human Carcinogen.   DOT Classification: Forbidden.

SAFETY PROFILE: Confirmed carcinogen with experimental carcinogenic data. Poison by inhalation. Central nervous system effects. Can be formed by thermal decomposition ($>70°$) from trichloroethylene. Symptoms include a disabling nausea and intense jaw pain. Strong explosive when shocked or exposed to heat or air. When heated to decomposition or on contact with acid or acid fumes it emits highly toxic fumes of Cl^-.

DEQ600   CAS: 91-94-1
3′,3′-DICHLOROBENZIDINE
mf: $C_{12}H_{10}Cl_2N_2$ mw: 253.14

PROP: Crystals. Mp: 133°; insol in water; sol in alcohol, benzene and glacial acetic acid.

SYNS: C.I. 23060 ◊ CURITHANE C126 ◊ DCB ◊ 4,4′-DIAMINO-3,3′-DICHLOROBIPHENYL ◊ 4,4′-DIAMINO-3,3′-DICHLORODIPHENYL ◊ 3,3′-DICHLORBENZIDIN (CZECH) ◊ 3,3′-DICHLOROBENZIDINA (SPANISH) ◊ DICHLOROBEN-ZIDINE ◊ 3,3′-DICHLOROBENZIDENE ◊ o,o′-DICHLORO-BENZIDINE ◊ DICHLOROBENZIDINE BASE ◊ 3,3′-DI-CHLORO-4,4′-BIPHENYLDIAMINE ◊ 3,3′-DICHLOROBIPHE-NYL-4,4′-DIAMINE ◊ 3,3′-DICHLORO-4,4′-DIAMINOBIPHENYL ◊ 3,3′-DICHLORO-4,4′-DIAMINO(1,1-BIPHENYL) ◊ RCRA WASTE NUMBER U073

TOXICITY DATA with REFERENCE
CAR: orl-rat TD:21 g/kg/50W-C TXAPA9
31,159,75
CAR: orl-rat TDLo:17 g/kg/50W-C TXAPA9
31,159,75
CAR: scu-mus TDLo:320 mg/kg (15-21D preg) BEXBAN 78,1402,75
ETA: orl-dog TDLo:17 g/kg/7Y-I
DUPON* HL.623-74,74
ETA: orl-ham TDLo:176 g/kg/70W-C PAACA3
10,78,69
ETA: orl-mus TDLo:5100 mg/kg/43W-I
VOONAW 5(5),524,59
ETA: orl-rat TD:20 g/kg/52W-I VOONAW
5(5),524,59
ETA: scu-mus TDLo:5200 mg/kg/47W-I
VOONAW 5(5),524,59
ETA: scu-rat TDLo:7 g/kg/43W-I VOONAW
5(5),524,59
MUT: bfa-rat/sat 40 mg/kg SAIGBL 23,426,81
MUT: dnd-mam:lym 25500 nmol/L CBINA8
38,369,82
MUT: dns-hmn:hla 100 nmol/L CNREA8
38,2621,78
MUT: mma-sat 5 μg/plate ENMUDM 6,145,84
MUT: otr-ham:kdy 80 μg/L BJCAAI 37,873,78

CONSENSUS REPORTS: IARC Cancer Review: Human Inadequate Evidence IMEMDT 29,239,82; Animal Sufficient Evidence IMEMDT 29,239,82; IMEMDT 4,49,74. NTP Fourth Annual Report On Carcinogens, 1984. Reported in EPA TSCA Inventory. Community Right-To-Know List. EPA Genetic Toxicology Program.

OSHA PEL: Carcinogen   ACGIH TLV: Suspected Human Carcinogen.   DFG TRK: 0.1 mg/m^3, Animal Carcinogen, Suspected Human Carcinogen.   NIOSH REL: (Benzidine-based Dye) Reduce to lowest feasible level.

SAFETY PROFILE: Confirmed carcinogen with experimental carcinogenic and tumorigenic data. Mildly toxic by ingestion. Human mutation data reported. When heated to decomposition it emits very toxic fumes of Cl^- and NO_x.

DEQ800   CAS: 612-83-9
3,3'-DICHLOROBENZIDINE
DIHYDROCHLORIDE
mf: $C_{12}H_{10}Cl_2N_2 \cdot 2ClH$ mw: 326.06

SYN: 3,3'-DICHLORO-(1,1'-BIPHENYL)-4,4'-DIAMINE
DIHYDROCHLORIDE

TOXICITY DATA with REFERENCE
MUT: mma-sat 1 μg/plate   ENMUDM 5(Suppl 1),3,83
MUT: mmo-sat 10 μg/plate   ENMUDM 5(Suppl
1),3,83

CONSENSUS REPORTS: Reported in EPA
TSCA Inventory.

OSHA PEL: Carcinogen

SAFETY PROFILE: Confirmed carcinogen.
Moderately toxic by ingestion. Mutation data
reported. When heated to decomposition it emits
very toxic fumes of Cl^- and NO_x.

DEV000   CAS: 764-41-0
1,4-DICHLORO-2-BUTENE
mf: $C_4H_6Cl_2$ mw: 125.00

PROP: Colorless liquid. Mp: 1°-3°; bp: 156°;
d: 1.183 @ 25°/4°.

SYNS: DCB ◇ 1,4-DCB ◇ 1,4-DICHLOROBUTENE-2 (MAK)
◇ RCRA WASTE NUMBER U074

TOXICITY DATA with REFERENCE
CAR: ihl-rat TCLo:1 ppm/6H/82W-I
    EPASR* 8EHQ-0985-0567
NEO: ihl-rat TC:100 ppb/6H/82W-I
    EPASR* 8EHQ-0985-0567
MUT: cyt-rat-ihl 1700 μg/m³/30D-I   ZKMAAX
    25,335,85
MUT: mma-sat 1 mmol/L   ARTODN 41,249,79
MUT: mmo-sat 1 mmol/L   ARTODN 41,249,79
MUT: sln-dmg-orl 2 mmol/L/3D-I
    35WYAM -,63,76

CONSENSUS REPORTS: Reported in EPA
TSCA Inventory. EPA Genetic Toxicology Program.

DFG MAK: Animal Carcinogen, Suspected Human Carcinogen.

SAFETY PROFILE: Confirmed carcinogen with
experimental carcinogenic and neoplastigenic
data. Poison by ingestion, inhalation, and intravenous routes. Moderately toxic by skin contact. An experimental teratogen. Mutation data

reported. A severe skin and eye irritant. When
heated to decomposition it emits toxic fumes
of Cl^-.

DFT800   CAS: 1836-75-5
2,4-DICHLORO-4'-NITRODIPHENYL
ETHER
mf: $C_{12}H_7Cl_2NO_3$ mw: 284.10

SYNS: 2,4-DECHLOROPHENYL-p-NITROPHENYL ETHER
◇ 2',4'-DICHLORO-4-NITROBIPHENYL ETHER ◇ 2,4-DI-
CHLORO-1-(4-NITROPHENOXY)BENZENE ◇ 4-(2,4-DICHLO-
ROPHENOXY)NITROBENZENE ◇ 2,4-DICHLOROPHENYL-p-
NITROPHENYL ETHER ◇ 2,4-DICHLOROPHENYL-4-NITRO-
PHENYL ETHER ◇ 2,4,-DICHLORPHENYL-4-
NITROPHENYLAETHER (GERMAN) ◇ FW 925 ◇ MEZOTOX
◇ NCI-C00420 ◇ NICLOFEN ◇ NIP ◇ NITOFEN ◇ NITRAFEN
◇ NITRAPHEN ◇ NITROCHLOR ◇ 4'-NITRO-2,4-DICHLORO-
DIPHENYL ETHER ◇ NITROFEN ◇ NITROFENE (FRENCH)
◇ NITROPHEN ◇ NITROPHENE ◇ PREPARATION 125
◇ TOK ◇ TOK-2 ◇ TOK E ◇ TOK E-25 ◇ TOK E 40
◇ TOKKORN ◇ TOK WP-50 ◇ TRIZILIN

TOXICITY DATA with REFERENCE
CAR: orl-mus TD:47 g/kg/12W-C   JJIND8
    65,937,80
CAR: orl-mus TD:114 g/kg/58W-C
    NCITR* NCI-CG-TR-26,78
CAR: orl-mus TD:200 g/kg/78W-C
    NCITR* NCI-CG-TR-184,79
CAR: orl-mus TD:308 g/kg/78W-C
    NCITR* NCI-CG-TR-26,78
CAR: orl-mus TDLo:24 g/kg/12W-C   JJIND8
    65,937,80
CAR: orl-rat TDLo:42 g/kg/94W-C
    NCITR* NCI-CG-TR-26,78
MUT: mma-sat 10 μg/plate   ENMUDM 7(Suppl
    5),1,85
MUT: mmo-sat 33300 ng/plate   ENMUDM 7(Suppl
    5),1,85
MUT: otr-rat:emb 1500 ng/plate   JJATDK 1,190,81

CONSENSUS REPORTS: IARC Cancer Review: Animal Sufficient Evidence IMEMDT
30,271,83. NCI Carcinogenesis Bioassay
(feed); No Evidence: rat NCITR* NCI-CG-TR-
184,79; Clear Evidence: mouse, rat NCITR*
NCI-CG-TR-26,78; Clear Evidence: mouse
NCITR* NCI-CG-TR-184,79. NTP Fourth
Annual Report On Carcinogens, 1984. EPA Genetic Toxicology Program. Community Right-
To-Know List. Reported in EPA TSCA Inventory.

SAFETY PROFILE: Confirmed carcinogen with
experimental carcinogenic data. Poison by ingestion. Moderately toxic by inhalation and possi-

bly other routes. Mildly toxic by skin contact. An experimental teratogen. Experimental reproductive effects. A skin and severe eye irritant. Mutation data reported. A broad spectrum herbicide. When heated to decomposition it emits very toxic fumes of Cl^- and NO_x.

DGG950   CAS: 542-75-6
1,3-DICHLOROPROPENE
mf: $C_3H_4Cl_2$ mw: 110.97

PROP: Liquid. Bp: 103-110°, flash p: 95°F, d: 1.22, vap d: 3.8.

SYNS: α-CHLOROALLYL CHLORIDE ◇ γ-CHLOROALLYL CHLORIDE ◇ 1,3-DICHLOROPROPENE-1 ◇ α,γ-DICHLORO-PROPYLENE ◇ 1,3-DICHLOROPROPYLENE ◇ NCI-C03985 ◇ RCRA WASTE NUMBER U084 ◇ TELONE ◇ TELONE II SOIL FUMIGANT ◇ VIDDEN D

TOXICITY DATA with REFERENCE
CAR: orl-mus TDLo:31200 mg/kg/2Y-I
    NTPTR* NTP-TR-269,85
CAR: orl-rat TDLo:15600 mg/kg/2Y-I
    NTPTR* NTP-TR-269,85
MUT: mma-sat 1 μmol/plate   ENMUDM 2,59,80
MUT: mmo-sat 33 μg/plate   ENMUDM 5(Suppl 1),3,83
MUT: sce-ham:ovr 900 nmol/L   CNJGA8 22,681,80
MUT: sln-dmg-orl 5750 ppm   ENMUDM 7,325,85

CONSENSUS REPORTS: IARC Cancer Review: Human Inadequate Evidence IMEMDT 41,113,86; Animal Sufficient Evidence IMEMDT 41,113,86. NTP Carcinogenesis Studies (gavage); Clear Evidence: mouse, rat NTPTR* NTP-TR-269,86. Reported in EPA TSCA Inventory. EPA Genetic Toxicology Program. Community Right-To-Know List.

OSHA PEL: TWA 1 ppm (skin)   ACGIH TLV: TWA 1 ppm (skin)   DFG MAK: Animal Carcinogen, Suspected Human Carcinogen.

SAFETY PROFILE: Confirmed carcinogen with experimental carcinogenic data. Poison by ingestion. Moderately toxic by skin contact. Mildly toxic by inhalation. A strong irritant. Mutation data reported. A pesticide. Dangerous fire hazard when exposed to heat, flame or oxidizers. To fight fire, use water, foam, CO_2, dry chemical. When heated to decomposition it emits toxic fumes of Cl^-.

DGH200   CAS: 10061-01-5
cis-1,3-DICHLOROPROPENE
mf: $C_3H_4Cl_2$ mw: 110.97

PROP: Flash point 21°C.

SYNS: (Z)-1,3-DICHLOROPROPENE ◇ cis-1,3-DICHLORO-PROPYLENE

TOXICITY DATA with REFERENCE
NEO: scu-mus TDLo:9240 mg/kg/77W-I
    JJIND8 63,1433,79
MUT: dns-hmn:hla 100 μmol/L   CALEDQ 20,263,83
MUT: mma-sat 20 μg/plate   CNREA8 37,1915,77
MUT: mmo-sat 20 μg/plate   CNREA8 37,1915,77

CONSENSUS REPORTS: EPA Genetic Toxicology Program.

DFG MAK: Animal Carcinogen, Suspected Human Carcinogen.

SAFETY PROFILE: Confirmed carcinogen with experimental neoplastigenic data. Human mutation data reported. A dangerous fire hazard when exposed to heat, flame or oxidizers. When heated to decomposition it emits toxic fumes of Cl^-.

DIV000   CAS: 542-63-2
DIETHYLBERYLLIUM
mf: $C_4H_{10}Be$ mw: 67.13

PROP: Colorless liquid. Mp: 12°; bp: 110° @ 15 mm; vap d: 2.3.

CONSENSUS REPORTS: Beryllium and its compounds are on the Community Right-To-Know List.

OSHA PEL: (Transitional: TWA 0.002 mg(Be)/m³; CL 0.005; Pk 0.025/30M/8H) TWA 0.002 mg(Be)/m³; STEL 0.005 mg(Be)/m³/30M; CL 0.025 mg(Be)/m³   ACGIH TLV: TWA 0.002 mg/m³, Suspected Human Carcinogen.

SAFETY PROFILE: Confirmed human carcinogen. Very poisonous. Dangerous fire hazard when exposed to heat or flame. Spontaneously flammable in air. To fight fire, use special extinguishing agents, dry chemical. Explodes on contact with water. Upon decomposition it emits poisonous fumes of BeO.

DIV800
DIETHYLCADMIUM
mf: $C_4H_{10}Cd$ mw: 170.5

PROP: An oil; decomp by moisture. D: 1.6562, mp: −21°, bp: 64°.

CONSENSUS REPORTS: Cadmium and its compounds are on the Community Right-To-Know List.

OSHA PEL: TWA 0.1 mg(Cd)/m^3; CL 0.6 mg(Cd)/m^3 (fume)   ACGIH TLV: TWA 0.05 mg(Cd)/m^3 (Proposed: TWA 0.01 mg(Cd)/m^3 (dust), Human Carcinogen); BEI: 10 μg/g creatinine in urine; 10 μg/L in blood.   DFG BAT: Blood 1.5 μg/dL; Urine 15 μg/dL, Suspected Carcinogen.   NIOSH REL: (Cadmium) Reduce to lowest feasible level

SAFETY PROFILE: Confirmed human carcinogen. A poison. A dangerous fire and explosion hazard. Explodes when heated rapidly to 130°C. On exposure to air it forms white fumes which turn brown and explode. The vapor explodes when heated to 180°C. When heated to decomposition it emits highly toxic fumes of cadmium.

DKA600   CAS: 56-53-1
DIETHYLSTILBESTEROL
mf: $C_{18}H_{20}O_2$ mw: 268 data.38

PROP: Small crystals. Mp: 171°.

SYNS: ACNESTROL ◇ AGOSTILBEN ◇ ANTIGESTIL ◇ BIO-DES ◇ 3,4-BIS(p-HYDROXYPHENYL)-3-HEXENE ◇ BUFON ◇ CLIMATERINE ◇ COMESTROL ◇ COMESTROL ESTROBENE ◇ CYREN ◇ DAWE'S DESTROL ◇ DEB ◇ DESMA ◇ DES (SYNTHETIC ESTROGEN) ◇ DESTROL ◇ DIASTYL ◇ DIBESTROL ◇ DICORVIN ◇ DI-ESTRYL ◇ trans-4,4'-(1,2-DIETHYL-1,2-ETHENEDIYL)BISPHENOL ◇ 4,4'-(1,2-DIETHYL-1,2-ETHENEDIYL)BIS-PHENOL ◇ α,α'-DIETHYLSTILBENEDIOL ◇ α,α'-DIETHYL-(E)-4,4'-STILBENEDIOL ◇ α,α'-DIETHYL-4,4'-STILBENEDIOL ◇ trans-α,α'-DIETHYL-4,4'-STILBENEDIOL ◇ 2,2'-DIETHYL-4,4'-STILBENEDIOL ◇ trans-DIETHYLSTILBESTEROL ◇ DIETHYLSTILBESTROL ◇ trans-DIETHYLSTILBESTROL ◇ DIETHYLSTILBOESTEROL ◇ trans-DIETHYLSTILBOES-TEROL ◇ DIETILESTILBESTROL (SPANISH) ◇ 4,4'-DIHYDROXYDIETHYLSTILBENE ◇ 4,4'-DIHYDROXY-α,β-DI-ETHYLSTILBENE ◇ 3,4'(4,4'-DIHYDROXYPHENYL)HEX-3-ENE ◇ DISTILBENE ◇ DOMESTROL ◇ DYESTROL ◇ ESTILBEN ◇ ESTRIL ◇ ESTROBENE ◇ ESTROGEN ◇ ESTROMENIN ◇ ESTROSYN ◇ FOLLIDIENE ◇ FONATOL ◇ GRAFESTROL ◇ GYNOPHARM ◇ HIBESTROL ◇ IDROESTRIL ◇ ISCOVESCO ◇ MAKAROL ◇ MENOSTIL-BEEN ◇ MICREST ◇ MICROEST ◇ MILESTROL ◇ NEO-OESTRANOL 1 ◇ NSC-3070 ◇ OEKOLP ◇ OESTROGENINE ◇ OESTROL VETAG ◇ OESTROMENIN ◇ OESTROMENSIL ◇ OESTROMENSYL ◇ OESTROMIENIN ◇ OESTROMON ◇ PABESTROL ◇ PALESTROL ◇ PERCUTATRINE OES-TROGENIQUE ISCOVESCO ◇ PROTECTONA ◇ RCRA WASTE NUMBER U089 ◇ RUMESTROL 1 ◇ RUMESTROL 2 ◇ SEDESTRAN ◇ SERRAL ◇ SEXOCRETIN ◇ SIBOL ◇ SINTESTROL ◇ STIBILIUM ◇ STIL ◇ STILBESTROL ◇ STILBESTRONE ◇ STILBETIN ◇ STILBOEFRAL ◇ STILBOESTROFORM ◇ STILBOESTROL ◇ STILBOFOLLIN ◇ STILBOL ◇ STILKAP ◇ STIL-ROL ◇ SYNESTRIN ◇ SYNTHOESTRIN ◇ SYNTHOFOLIN ◇ SYNTOFOLIN ◇ TAMPOVAGAN STILBOESTROL ◇ TYLOSTERONE ◇ VAGESTROL

TOXICITY DATA with REFERENCE
CAR: imp-ham TD: 160 mg/kg   ZEKBAI 61,1,56
CAR: imp-ham TD: 360 mg/kg/12W-I   CNREA8 43,2678,83
CAR: imp-ham TD: 864 mg/kg/12W-I   CNREA8 43,4638,83
CAR: imp-ham TDLo: 160 mg/kg   BJCAAI 8,451,54
CAR: imp-mky TDLo: 48 mg/kg   LBASAE 23,493,73
CAR: imp-rat TD: 20 mg/kg   CNREA8 43,4781,83
CAR: imp-rat TD: 25 mg/kg   CNREA8 39,773,79
CAR: imp-rat TDLo: 11500 μg/kg   JJIND8 67,455,81
CAR: mul-man TDLo: 25 mg/kg/2Y-C: SKN   UROTAQ 19,180,52
CAR: orl-man TD: 45990 μg/kg/3Y-C: KID   BJURAN 51,6,79
CAR: orl-mus TD: 13 mg/kg/53W-C   JNCIAM 40,225,68
CAR: orl-mus TDLo: 263 μg/kg/50W-C   JNCIAM 33,971,64
CAR: orl-rat TDLo: 103 g/kg/2Y-C   AEHLAU 19,489,69
CAR: orl-wmn TDLo: 7655 μg/kg/4Y-C: TER   BJOGAS 82,417,75
CAR: orl-wmn TDLo: 21 mg/kg (13-15W preg): TER   AJOGAH 137,220,80
CAR: unr-man TDLo: 184 mg/kg/12Y-C: PUL,LIV   JAMAAP 240,1510,78
NEO: orl-ham TD: 69 mg/kg/5Y-C   JOURAA 128,1044,82
NEO: scu-ham TDLo: 816 mg/kg/1Y-I   PSEBAA 66,195,47
NEO: scu-mus TD: 230 mg/kg/39W-I   ZEKBAI 56,482,49
NEO: scu-rat TDLo: 6 μg/kg (15-18D preg)   JTEHD6 5,1059,79
ETA: imp-mus TDLo: 8 mg/kg   JNCIAM 2,65,41
ETA: ivg-mus TDLo: 5280 μg/kg/44W-I   ANYAA9 75,543,59
ETA: par-mus TDLo: 340 mg/kg/34W-I   CNREA8 2,759,42
ETA: scu-dog TDLo: 17 mg/kg/29W-I   AJEBAK 37,549,59
MUT: cyt-ham: lvr 3 mg/L   PMRSDJ 5,397,85
MUT: cyt-hmn: lym 100 μg/L   PMRSDJ 5,457,85

MUT: dnd-hmn:fbr 300 μmol/L ENMUDM 7,267,85

MUT: dnd-hmn:leu 20 μmol/L BCPCA634,3251,85

MUT: mma-esc 50 mg/L MUREAV 130,97,84

MUT: mnt-hmn:lym 5 μmol/L MUREAV 156,199,85

MUT: sce-mus:oth 100 nmol/L JJIND8 75,575,85

CONSENSUS REPORTS: IARC Cancer Review: Human Limited Evidence IMEMDT 6,55,74; IMEMDT 21,173,79; Animal Sufficient Evidence IMEMDT 21,173,79; IMEMDT 6,55,74. NTP Fourth Annual Report On Carcinogens, 1984. EPA Genetic Toxicology Program. Reported in EPA TSCA Inventory.

SAFETY PROFILE: Confirmed carcinogen producing skin, liver, and lung tumors in exposed humans as well as uterine and other reproductive system tumors in the female offspring of exposed women. Experimental carcinogenic, neoplastigenic, tumorigenic, and teratogenic data. A transplacental carcinogen. A human teratogen by many routes. Poison by intraperitoneal and subcutaneous routes. Moderately toxic by ingestion and other routes. It causes glandular system effects by skin contact. Human reproductive effects by ingestion: abnormal spermatogenesis; changes in testes, epididymis and sperm duct; menstrual cycle changes or disorders; changes in female fertility; unspecified maternal effects; developmental abnormalities of the fetal urogenital system; germ cell effects in offspring; and delayed effects in newborn. Implicated in male impotence and enlargement of male breasts. Other experimental reproductive effects. Mutation data reported. When heated to decomposition it emits acrid smoke and fumes.

DKB000　　　　　CAS: 130-80-3
DIETHYLSTILBESTROL DIPROPIONATE
mf: $C_{24}H_{28}O_4$　　mw: 380.52

PROP: Crystals. Mp: 104°.

SYNS: CLINESTROL ◇ CYREN B ◇ DESD ◇ DIBESTIL ◇ trans-4,4'-(1,2-DIETHYL-1,2-ETHENEDIYL)BISPHENOL DIPROPIONATE ◇ α,α'-DIETHYL-4,4'-STILBENEDIOL, DIPROPIONATE ◇ α,α'-DIETHYL-4,4'-STILBENEDIOL trans-DIPROPIONATE ◇ trans-α,α'-DIETHYL-4,4'-STILBENEDIOL DIPROPIONATE ◇ DIETHYLSTILBENE DIPROPIONATE ◇ α,α'-DIETHYL-4,4'-STILBENEDIOL DIPROPIONYL ESTER ◇ DIETHYLSTILBESTEROL DIPROPIONATE ◇ DIETHYLSTILBESTROL PROPIONATE ◇ DIHYDROXYDIETHYLSTILBENE DIPROPIONATE ◇ 4,4'-DIHYDROXY-α,β-DIETHYLSTILBENE DIPROPIONATE ◇ DIPROPIONATO de ESTILBENE

(SPANISH) ◇ p,p'-DIPROPIONOXY-trans-α,β-DIETHYLSTILBENE ◇ DISTILBENE ◇ ESTILBEN ◇ ESTILBIN ◇ ESTROBEN ◇ ESTROBENE ◇ ESTROGENIN ◇ ESTROSTILBEN ◇ EUVESTIN ◇ GYNOLETT ◇ HORFEMINE ◇ NEO-OESTRANOL II ◇ OESTROGYNAEDRON ◇ ORESTOL ◇ PABESTROL ◇ SINCICLAN ◇ STILBESTROL DIETHYL DIPROPIONATE ◇ STILBESTROL DIPROPIONATE ◇ STILBESTROL PROPIONATE ◇ STILBESTRONATE ◇ STILBOESTROL DIPROPIONATE ◇ STILBOFAX ◇ STILRONATE ◇ SYNESTRIN ◇ SYNOESTRON ◇ SYNTESTRIN ◇ SYNTESTRINE ◇ WILLESTROL

TOXICITY DATA with REFERENCE
ETA: imp-ham TDLo:640 mg/kg/38W-I
　　CNREA8 43,5200,83
MUT: cyt-ham:fbr 5 mg/L CRNGDP 3,499,82
MUT: cyt-hmn:lym 1300 nmol/L TGANAK 16(2),24,82
MUT: sce-ham:fbr 5 mg/L CRNGDP 3,499,82
MUT: sln-mus-ipr 50 mg/kg MUREAV 144,27,85

CONSENSUS REPORTS: IARC Cancer Review: Animal Sufficient Evidence IMEMDT 21,173,79. EPA Genetic Toxicology Program.

SAFETY PROFILE: Confirmed carcinogen with experimental tumorigenic data. An experimental teratogen. Other experimental reproductive effects. Human mutagenic data. When heated to decomposition it emits acrid smoke and irritating fumes.

DKB110　　　　　CAS: 64-67-5
DIETHYL SULFATE
DOT: 1594
mf: $C_4H_{10}O_4S$　　mw: 154.20

PROP: Colorless, oily liquid; faint ethereal odor. Mp: −25°, Bp: 209.5° (decomp to ethyl ether), flash p: 220°F (CC), d: 1.172 @ 25°/4°, autoign temp: 817°F, vap press: 1 mm @ 47.0°, vap d: 5.31. Insol in water, decomp by hot water, misc with alcohol and ether.

SYNS: DIAETHYLSULFAT (GERMAN) ◇ DIETHYL ESTER SULFURIC ACID ◇ ETHYL SULFATE

TOXICITY DATA with REFERENCE
CAR: ivn-rat TDLo:85 mg/kg (15D preg)
　　IARCCD 4,45,73
ETA: orl-rat TDLo:3700 mg/kg/81W-I ZEKBAI 74,241,70
ETA: scu-rat TDLo:800 mg/kg/32W-I ZEKBAI 74,241,70
MUT: cyt-mus-ipr 150 mg/kg MUREAV 75,63,80
MUT: mma-sat 5 mg/plate MUREAV 57,141,78
MUT: mmo-sat 5 mg/plate MUREAV 57,141,78
MUT: msc-ham:ovr 1 mmol/L MUREAV 57,217,78

MUT: slt-mus-ipr 100 mg/kg/10W   MUREAV 75,63,80

CONSENSUS REPORTS: IARC Cancer Review: Animal Sufficient Evidence IMEMDT 4,277,74. NTP Fourth Annual Report On Carcinogens, 1984. EPA Genetic Toxicology Program. Community Right-To-Know List. Reported in EPA TSCA Inventory.

DFG TRK: 0.03 ppm; Animal Carcinogen, Human Suspected Carcinogen.

SAFETY PROFILE: Confirmed carcinogen with experimental carcinogenic and tumorigenic data. Poison by inhalation and subcutaneous route. Moderately toxic by ingestion and skin contact. A severe skin irritant. Mutation data reported. To fight fire, use alcohol foam, H_2O foam, CO_2, dry chemicals. When heated to decomposition it emits toxic fumes of SO_x.

DKQ000
DIHYDANTOIN
CAS: 57-41-0

mf: $C_{15}H_{12}N_2O_2$ mw: 252.29

SYNS: ALEVIATIN ◇ ANTISACER ◇ AURANILE ◇ CAUSOIN ◇ CITRULLAMON ◇ COMITAL ◇ CONVUL ◇ DANTEN ◇ DANTINAL ◇ DANTOINAL KLINOS ◇ DANTOINE ◇ DENYL ◇ DIDAN-TDC-250 ◇ DIFENILHIDANTOINA (SPANISH) ◇ DIFENIN ◇ DIFHYDAN ◇ DIHYCON ◇ DI-HYDAN ◇ DILANTIN ◇ DILANTINE ◇ DINTOIN ◇ DIPHANTOIN ◇ DIPHEDAL ◇ DIPHENINE ◇ DIPHENTOIN ◇ DIPHENYLAN ◇ DIPHENYLHYDANTOIN ◇ 5,5-DIPHENYLHYDANTOIN ◇ DIPHENYLHYDANTOINE (FRENCH) ◇ 5,5-DIPHENYLIMIDAZOLIDIN-2,4-DIONE ◇ 5,5-DIPHENYL-2,4-IMIDAZOLIDINEDIONE ◇ DI-PHETINE ◇ DITOINATE ◇ DPH ◇ EKKO CAPSULES ◇ ELEPSINDON ◇ ENKELFEL ◇ EPAMIN ◇ EPANUTIN ◇ EPASMIR '5' ◇ EPDANTOINE SIMPLE ◇ EPELIN ◇ EPIFENYL ◇ EPIHYDAN ◇ EPILAN ◇ EPILANTIN ◇ EPINAT ◇ EPISED ◇ EPTAL ◇ EPTOIN ◇ FENANTOIN ◇ FENIDANTOIN 'S' ◇ FENYLEPSIN ◇ FENYTOINE ◇ GEROT-EPILAN-D ◇ HIDAN ◇ HIDANTILO ◇ HIDANTINA SENOSIAN ◇ HIDANTINA VITORIA ◇ HIDANTOMIN ◇ HYDANTAL ◇ HYDANTOIN ◇ ICTALIS SIMPLE ◇ IDANTOIN ◇ KESSODANTEN ◇ LABOPAL ◇ LEHYDAN ◇ LEPITOIN ◇ LEPSIN ◇ MINETOIN ◇ NCI-C55765 ◇ NEOS-HIDANTOINA ◇ NOVANTOINA ◇ OM-HYDANTOINE ◇ OXYLAN ◇ PHANANTIN ◇ PHENATOINE ◇ RITMENAL ◇ SACERIL ◇ SANEPIL ◇ SILANTIN ◇ SODANTON ◇ SOLANTIN ◇ SYLANTOIC ◇ TACOSAL ◇ THILOPHENYL ◇ TOIN UNICELLES ◇ ZENTRONAL ◇ ZENTROPIL

TOXICITY DATA with REFERENCE
CAR: orl-wmn TD:730 mg/kg/1Y-C:BLD
NKGZAE 43,711,80

CAR: orl-wmn TDLo:730 mg/kg/1Y-C:BLD
NKGZAE 46,1,83
CAR: orl-wmn TDLo:1620 mg/kg (1-39 W post)   JAMAAP 244,1464,80
CAR: orl-wmn TDLo:1620 mg/kg (1-39 W post)   LANCAO 2,481,80
NEO: orl-chd TD:6023 mg/kg/1Y-C: BLD,SKN   AJDEBP 22,28,81
ETA: orl-mus TDLo:5284 mg/kg/17W-C
ZKKOBW 78,290,72
ETA: orl-rat TD:1500 mg/kg/27D-I   CNREA8 28,924,68
ETA: orl-rat TDLo:1500 mg/kg   CNREA8 26,619,66
MUT: cyt-hmn:leu 100 µg/L   AJOGAH 109,961,71
MUT: dnd-esc 50 µmol/L   MUREAV 89,95,81
MUT: dni-hmn:lym 360 µmol/L   TXAPA9 33,38,75
MUT: mnt-mus-ivn 500 µg/kg   MUREAV 141,183,84
MUT: otr-ham:emb 200 mg/L   ENMUDM 8(Suppl 6),4,86
MUT: pic-esc 100 mg/L   VIRLAX 99,257,79

IARC Cancer Review: Human Limited Evidence IMEMDT 13,201,77; Animal Sufficient Evidence IMEMDT 13,201,77. NTP Fourth Annual Report On Carcinogens, 1984. EPA Genetic Toxicology Program.

SAFETY PROFILE: Confirmed carcinogen producing lymphoma, Hodgkin's disease, tumors of the skin and appendages. Experimental carcinogenic, tumorigenic, and teratogen data. A human poison by ingestion. Poison experimentally by ingestion, subcutaneous, intravenous, and intraperitoneal routes. Moderately toxic by an unspecified route. Experimental reproductive effects. Human systemic effects by ingestion: dermatitis, change in motor activity (specific assay), ataxia (loss of muscle coordination), degenerative brain changes, and jaundice. Human teratogenic effects by ingestion and possibly other routes: developmental abnormalities of the central nervous system, cardiovascular (circulatory) system, musculoskeletal system, craniofacial area, skin and skin appendages, eye, ear, other developmental abnormalities. Effects on newborn include abnormal growth statistics (e.g., reduced weight gain), physical abnormalities, other postnatal measures or effects, and delayed effects. Human mutation data reported. A drug for the treatment of grand mal and psychomotor seizures. When heated to decomposition it emits toxic fumes of NO_x.

DNO200 CAS: 15721-33-2
DIISOPROPYLBERYLLIUM
mf: $C_6H_{14}Be$ mw: 95.19

CONSENSUS REPORTS: Beryllium and its compounds are on the Community Right-To-Know List.

OSHA PEL: (Transitional: TWA 0.002 mg(Be)/m^3; CL 0.005; Pk 0.025/30M/8H) TWA 0.002 mg(Be)/m^3; STEL 0.005 mg(Be)/m^3/30M; CL 0.025 mg(Be)/m^3 ACGIH TLV: TWA 0.002 mg/m^3, Suspected Human Carcinogen. DFG TRK: 0.002 mg(Be)/m^3. Animal Carcinogen, Suspected Human Carcinogen.

SAFETY PROFILE: Confirmed human carcinogen. Explosive reaction on contact with water. When heated to decomposition it emits toxic fumes of BeO.

DNU000 CAS: 630-93-3
DILANTIN
mf: $C_{15}H_{11}N_2O_2 \cdot Na$ mw: 274.27

SYNS: ALEPSIN ◇ ANTILEPSIN ◇ ANTISACER ◇ AURANILE ◇ CITRULLAMON ◇ DANTEN ◇ DANTOIN ◇ DENYL ◇ DENYLSODIUM ◇ DERIZENE ◇ DIFENIN ◇ DIFETOIN ◇ DIFHYDAN ◇ DI-HYDAN ◇ DIHYDANTOIN ◇ DILANTIN SODIUM ◇ DI-LEN ◇ DINTOINA ◇ DIPHAN-TOINE SODIUM ◇ DIPHEDAN ◇ DIPHENATE ◇ DIPHENIN ◇ DIPHENINE SODIUM ◇ DIPHENTOIN ◇ DIPHENYLAN SODIUM ◇ DIPHENYLHYDANTOIN SODIUM ◇ 5,5-DIPHE-NYLHYDANTOIN SODIUM ◇ 5,5-DIPHENYL-2,4-IMIDAZO-LIDINE-DIONE, MONOSODIUM SALT ◇ DI-PHETINE ◇ DITOIN ◇ DIVULSAN ◇ DPH ◇ ENKEFAL ◇ EPAMIN ◇ EPANUTIN ◇ EPELIN ◇ EPIFENYL ◇ EPIHYDAN ◇ EPILAN-D ◇ EPILANTIN ◇ EPINAT ◇ EPTOIN ◇ FENANTOIN ◇ FENITOIN ◇ FENYTOINE ◇ HYDANTIN SODIUM ◇ HYDANTOIN SODIUM ◇ IDANTOIL ◇ IDANTOI-NAL ◇ LEPITOIN ◇ LEPITOIN SODIUM ◇ MINETOIN ◇ NOVANTOINA ◇ NOVODIPHENYL ◇ OM-HYDANTOINE SODIUM ◇ PHENYTOIN SODIUM ◇ SACERIL ◇ SDPH ◇ SODANTON ◇ SODIUM DIPHENYLHYDANTOIN ◇ SODIUM DIPHENYL HYDANTOINATE ◇ SODIUM-5,5-DI-PHENYLHYDANTOINATE ◇ SODIUM-5,5-DIPHENYL-2,4-IMIDAZOLIDINEDIONE ◇ SOLANTOIN ◇ SOLANTYL ◇ SOLUBLE PHENYTOIN ◇ SYLANTOIC ◇ TACOSAL ◇ THILOPHENYT ◇ ZENTROPIL

TOXICITY DATA with REFERENCE
MUT: dnd-esc 50 μmol/L MUREAV 89,95,81
MUT: pic-esc 100 mg/L VIRLAX 99,257,79

CONSENSUS REPORTS: IARC Cancer Review: Animal Sufficient Evidence IMEMDT 13,201,77. Reported in EPA TSCA Inventory.

SAFETY PROFILE: Confirmed carcinogen. Experimental teratogen. Poison by ingestion, subcutaneous, intravenous, intraperitoneal, and possibly other routes. Human systemic effects by ingestion: anorexia, respiratory depression, nausea or vomiting, hemorrhage, dermititis, and endocrine effects. Experimental reproductive effects. Mutation data reported. An anticonvulsant and cardiac depressant used for the treatment of grand mal and psychomotor seizures. When heated to decomposition it emits very toxic fumes of NO_x and Na_2O.

DOT300 CAS: 60-11-7
4-DIMETHYLAMINOAZOBENZENE
mf: $C_{14}H_{15}N_3$ mw: 225.32

PROP: Yellow, crystalline tablets; insol in water; sol in strong mineral acids and oils.

SYNS: ATUL FAST YELLOW R ◇ BENZENEAZODI-METHYLANILINE ◇ BRILLIANT FAST YELLOW ◇ BUTTER YELLOW ◇ CERASINE YELLOW GG ◇ C.I. 11020 ◇ C.I. SOLVENT YELLOW 2 ◇ DAB ◇ p-DIMETHYLAMI-NOAZOBENZEN (CZECH) ◇ DIMETHYLAMINOAZOBEN-ZENE ◇ N,N-DIMETHYL-4-AMINOAZOBENZENE ◇ N,N-DIMETHYL-p-AMINOAZOBENZENE ◇ p-DIMETHY-LAMINOAZOBENZENE ◇ 4-(N,N-DIMETHYLAMINO)AZO-BENZENE ◇ DIMETHYLAMINOAZOBENZOL ◇ p-DIMETH-YLAMINO-AZOBENZOL (GERMAN) ◇ 4-DIMETHYLAMI-NOAZOBENZOL ◇ 4-DIMETHYLAMINOPHENYLAZOBEN-ZENE ◇ N,N-DIMETHYL-p-AZOANILINE ◇ N,N-DIMETHYL-p-PHENYLAZOANILINE ◇ N,N-DIMETHYL-4-(PHEN-YLAZO)BENZAMINE ◇ N,N-DIMETHYL-4(PHENYLAZO) BENZENAMINE ◇ DIMETHYL YELLOW ◇ DIMETHYL YELLOW-N,N-DIMETHYLANILINE ◇ DMAB ◇ ENIAL YELLOW 2G ◇ FAST OIL YELLOW B ◇ FAT YELLOW ◇ GRASAL BRILLIANT YELLOW ◇ JAUNE de BEURRE (FRENCH) ◇ METHYL YELLOW ◇ OIL YELLOW ◇ OLEAL YELLOW 2G ◇ ORGANOL YELLOW ADM ◇ ORIENT OIL YELLOW GG ◇ P.D.A.B. ◇ PETROL YELLOW WT ◇ RCRA WASTE NUMBER U093 ◇ RESINOL YELLOW GR ◇ RESOFORM YELLOW GGA ◇ SILOTRAS YELLOW T2G ◇ SOMALIA YELLOW A ◇ STEAR YELLOW JB ◇ SUDAN YELLOW ◇ TOYO OIL YELLOW G ◇ USAF EK-338 ◇ WAXOLINE YELLOW AD ◇ YELLOW G SOLUBLE in GREASE ◇ ZLUT MASELNA (CZECH)

TOXICITY DATA with REFERENCE
CAR: orl-rat TDLo:5426 mg/kg/17W-C
  CBINA8 53,107,85
CAR: scu-mus TDLo:4000 mg/kg (15-21D preg):TER BEXBAN 78,1402,75
NEO: ipr-mus TD:11 mg/kg CNREA8 44,2540,84

NEO: ipr-mus TDLo:3830 μg/kg   CNREA8
44,2540,84

NEO: orl-rat TD:13 g/kg/53W-C   MEXPAG4,1,61

NEO: orl-rat TD:2600 mg/kg/13W-C   CNREA8
17,387,57

NEO: orl-rat TD:3990 mg/kg/19W-C   GANNA2
63,131,72

NEO: orl-rat TD:8316 mg/kg/33W-C   JPBAA7
59,1,47

NEO: orl-rat TD:17200 mg/kg/17W-C   ARPAAQ
81,162,66

NEO: skn-rat TDLo:1440 mg/kg/90W-I
CNREA8 26,2406,66

ETA: mul-mus TDLo:400 mg/kg/I   CNREA8
1,397,41

ETA: orl-dog TDLo:9600 mg/kg/69W-C
JNCIAM 13,1497,53

ETA: orl-ham TDLo:9600 mg/kg/42W-I
ARPAAQ 71,566,61

ETA: orl-rat TD:800 mg/kg/64D-C   ZEKBAI
61,327,56

ETA: orl-rat TD:1800 mg/kg/14W-C   CNREA8
8,141,48

ETA: orl-rat TD:1920 mg/kg/14W-C   CNREA8
5,235,45

ETA: orl-rat TD:2331 mg/kg/7W-I   KTUNAA
32,229,79

MUT: dni-hmn:hla 100 μmol/L   MUREAV
92,427,82

MUT: dnr-esc 80 mg/L   MUREAV 119,135,83

MUT: dns-ham:lvr 1 μmol/L   ENMUDM 5,1,83

MUT: msc-mus:lym 89 μmol/L   MUREAV
110,147,83

MUT: otr-mus:emb 89 μmol/L   MUREAV
152,113,85

CONSENSUS REPORTS: IARC Cancer Review: Animal Sufficient Evidence IMEMDT 8,125,75. NTP Fourth Annual Report On Carcinogens, 1984. EPA Genetic Toxicology Program. Community Right-To-Know List. Reported in EPA TSCA Inventory.

OSHA PEL: Carcinogen

SAFETY PROFILE: Confirmed carcinogen with experimental carcinogenic, neoplastigenic, tumorigenic, and teratogenic data. Poison by ingestion and intraperitoneal routes. Human mutation data reported. When heated to decomposition it emits toxic fumes of NO_x.

DQR200   CAS: 506-63-8
DIMETHYL BERYLLIUM
mf: C_2H_6Be mw: 39.09

PROP: White needles. Bp: sublimes @ 200°.

CONSENSUS REPORTS: Beryllium and its compounds are on the Community Right-To-Know List.

OSHA PEL: (Transitional: TWA 0.002 mg(Be)/m³; CL 0.005; Pk 0.025/30M/8H) TWA 0.002 mg(Be)/m³; STEL 0.005 mg(Be)/m³/30M; CL 0.025 mg(Be)/m³   ACGIH TLV: TWA 0.002 mg/m³, Suspected Human Carcinogen.

SAFETY PROFILE: Confirmed human carcinogen. Λ poison. Flammable when exposed to heat or flame; can react with oxidizing materials. Explosive reaction on contact with water. Ignites on contact with moist air or carbon dioxide. Upon decomposition it emits highly toxic fumes of BeO.

DQR289
DIMETHYLBERYLLIUM-1,2-DIMETHOXYETHANE
mf: $C_2H_6Be \cdot C_4H_{10}O_2$ mw: 129.21

CONSENSUS REPORTS: Beryllium and its compounds are on the Community Right-To-Know List.

SAFETY PROFILE: Confirmed human carcinogen. Ignites spontaneously in air. Upon decomposition it emits highly toxic fumes of BeO.

DQW800   CAS: 506-82-1
DIMETHYLCADMIUM
mf: C_2H_6Cd mw: 142.47

PROP: Oil, decomp by water, foul odor. D: 1.984; mp: −4.5°; bp: 106°.

CONSENSUS REPORTS: Cadmium and its compounds are on Community Right-To-Know List.

OSHA PEL: TWA 0.1 mg(Cd)/m³; CL 0.6 mg(Cd)/m³ (fume)   ACGIH TLV: TWA 0.05 mg(Cd)/m³ (Proposed: TWA 0.01 mg(Cd)/m³ (dust), Human Carcinogen); BEI: 10 μg/g creatinine in urine; 10 μg/L in blood.   DFG BAT: Blood 1.5 μg/dL; Urine 15 μg/dL, Suspected Carcinogen.   NIOSH REL: (Cadmium) Reduce to lowest feasible level

SAFETY PROFILE: Confirmed human carcinogen. Contact with air produces the friction-sensitive explosive dimethyl cadmium peroxide. Explodes when heated above 150°C. Ignition may occur on contact with air if the surface area is large.

DQY950   CAS: 79-44-7
DIMETHYL CARBAMOYL CHLORIDE
DOT: 2262
mf: C_3H_6ClNO mw: 107.55

PROP: Liquid. Mp: $-33°$, bp: 165-167°, d: 1.678 @ 20°/4°, vap d: 3.73.

SYNS: CHLOROFORMIC ACID DIMETHYLAMIDE ◇ DDC ◇ (DIMETHYLAMINO)CARBONYL CHLORIDE ◇ DIMETHYLCARBAMIC ACID CHLORIDE ◇ DIMETHYL-CARBAMIC CHLORIDE ◇ DIMETHYLCARBAMIDOYL CHLORIDE ◇ DIMETHYLCARBAMOYL CHLORIDE ◇ N,N-DIMETHYLCARBAMOYL CHLORIDE (DOT) ◇ DIMETHYLCARBAMYL CHLORIDE ◇ N,N-DIMETHYL-CARBAMYL CHLORIDE ◇ DMCC ◇ RCRA WASTE NUMBER U097 ◇ TL 389

TOXICITY DATA with REFERENCE
CAR: ihl-ham TCLo: 1 ppm/6H/89W-I   JEPTDQ 4(1),107,80
CAR: ihl-rat TCLo: 1 ppm/6H/6W-I   CALEDQ 33,175,86
CAR: scu-mus TDLo: 894 mg/kg/52W-I   JACTDZ 6(4),479,87
CAR: skn-mus TDLo: 17280 mg/kg/72W-I   JACTDZ 6(4),479,87
NEO: ipr-mus TDLo: 2560 mg/kg/64W-I   JNCIAM 53,695,74
NEO: scu-mus TD: 8 g/kg/40W-I   JNCIAM 53,695,74
NEO: scu-mus TD: 5200 mg/kg/26W-I   JNCIAM 48,1539,72
NEO: skn-mus TD: 13 g/kg/55W-I   JNCIAM 53,695,74
NEO: skn-mus TD: 13 g/kg/55W-I   JNCIAM 48,1539,72
ETA: ihl-rat TC: 1 ppm   OHSLAM 6,5,76
ETA: ihl-rat TC: 1 ppm/6H/6W-I   PAACA3 21,106,80
MUT: dns-hmn: fbr 32 μg/L   PMRSDJ 1,528,81
MUT: mma-esc 100 μg/plate   ENMUDM 6(Suppl 2),1,84
MUT: mma-sat 300 ng/plate   ENMUDM 6(Suppl 2),1,84
MUT: mmo-esc 100 μg/plate   ENMUDM 6(Suppl 2),1,84
MUT: mmo-sat 33 μg/plate   ENMUDM 5(Suppl 1),3,83
MUT: sce-ham: lng 100 μmol/L   MUREAV 118,103,83
MUT: sln-dmg-par 10 pph   ENMUDM 7,349,85

CONSENSUS REPORTS: IARC Cancer Review: Animal Sufficient Evidence IMEMDT 12,77,76; Human Inadequate Evidence IMEMDT 12,77,76. NTP Fourth Annual Report On Carcinogens, 1984. EPA Genetic Toxicology Program. Community Right-To-Know List. Reported in EPA TSCA Inventory.

ACGIH TLV: Suspected Human Carcinogen DFG MAK: Animal Carcinogen, Suspected Human Carcinogen. DOT Classification: Corrosive Material; Label: Corrosive.

SAFETY PROFILE: Confirmed carcinogen with experimental carcinogenic, neoplastigenic, and tumorigenic data. Poison by intraperitoneal route. Moderately toxic by inhalation and ingestion. Human mutation data reported. Can cause skin and papillary tumors by skin contact, and squamous cell carcinoma by inhalation. Will react with water or steam to produce toxic and corrosive fumes. A powerful lachrymator. When heated to decomposition it emits very toxic fumes of Cl^- and NO_x.

DSF400   CAS: 57-14-7
1,1-DIMETHYLHYDRAZINE
DOT: 1163
mf: $C_2H_8N_2$ mw: 60.12

PROP: Colorless liquid, ammonia-like odor. Hygroscopic, water-miscible. Bp: 63.3°, fp: $-58°$, flash p: 5°F, d: 0.782 @ 25°/4°, vap press: 157 mm @ 25°, vap d: 1.94, autoign temp: 480°F, lel: 2%, uel: 95%.

SYNS: DIMAZINE ◇ DIMETHYLHYDRAZINE ◇ asym-DI-METHYLHYDRAZINE ◇ N,N-DIMETHYLHYDRAZINE ◇ uns-DIMETHYLHYDRAZINE ◇ unsym-DIMETHYLHYDRA-ZINE ◇ 1,1-DIMETHYLHYDRAZINE (GERMAN) ◇ DI-METHYLHYDRAZINE, unsymmetrical (DOT) ◇ DMH ◇ NIESYMETRYCZNA DWU METYLOHYDRAZYNA (POLISH) ◇ RCRA WASTE NUMBER U098 ◇ UDMH (DOT)

TOXICITY DATA with REFERENCE
CAR: orl-ham TDLo: 228 g/kg/48W-I   CANCAR 40,2427,77
CAR: orl-mus TDLo: 5880 mg/kg/42W-C   JNCIAM 50,181,73
ETA: ipr-mus TDLo: 144 mg/kg/8W-I   JNCIAM 42,337,69
ETA: orl-mus TD: 288 mg/kg/8W-I   JNCIAM 42,337,69
ETA: orl-rat TD: 300 mg/kg/14W-I   NATUAS 246,491,73
ETA: orl-rat TDLo: 150 mg/kg/7W-I   NATUAS 246,491,73

ETA: scu-rat TD:400 mg/kg/20W-I SUFOAX 31,413,80

ETA: scu-rat TDLo:21 mg/kg SUFOAX 31,413,80

MUT: dnd-hmn:fbr 300 μmol/L ENMUDM 7,267,85

MUT: dnd-rat:lvr 30 μmol/L MUREAV 113,357,83

MUT: hma-rat/spt 120 mg/kg/6W-I MUREAV 139,143,84

MUT: msc-ham:lng 5 mmol/L MUREAV 130,121,84

MUT: otr-hmn:fbr 167 μmol/L PNASA6 80,7219,83

MUT: otr-rat-orl 200 μmol/kg CBINA8 43,313,83

CONSENSUS REPORTS: IARC Cancer Review: Animal Sufficient Evidence IMEMDT 4,137,74. NTP Fourth Annual Report On Carcinogens, 1984. EPA Genetic Toxicology Program. Community Right-To-Know List. EPA Extremely Hazardous Substances List. Reported in EPA TSCA Inventory.

OSHA PEL: TWA 0.5 ppm (skin) ACGIH TLV: TWA 0.5 ppm (skin); Suspected Human Carcinogen; (Proposed: TWA 0.01 ppm (skin); Suspected Human Carcinogen) DFG MAK: Animal Carcinogen, Suspected Human Carcinogen. NIOSH REL: (Hydrazines) CL 0.15 mg/m^3/2H DOT Classification: Flammable Liquid; Label: Flammable Liquid and Poison; Flammable Liquid; Label: Flammable Liquid, Corrosive.

SAFETY PROFILE: Confirmed carcinogen with experimental carcinogenic, tumorigenic, and teratogenic data. Poison by ingestion, intraperitoneal, intravenous, and intracerebral routes. Moderately toxic by inhalation and skin contact. Human mutation data reported. A plant growth control agent. Corrosive. A powerful reducing agent. A dangerous fire hazard. It is hypergolic with many oxidants (e.g., dinitrogen tetroxide; hydrogen peroxide; and nitric acid). Dangerous when exposed to heat, flame or oxidizers. To fight fire, use alcohol foam, CO_2, dry chemical. When heated to decomposition it emits highly toxic fumes of NO_x.

DSF600   CAS: 540-73-8
1,2-DIMETHYLHYDRAZINE
DOT: 2382
mf: $C_2H_8N_2$ mw: 60.12

PROP: Clear, colorless, flammable, hygroscopic liquid; fishy ammonia odor. Flash p: <

73.4°F, bp: 81°, mp: −9°, d: 0.8274 @ 20°/4°.

SYNS: N,N′-DIMETHYLHYDRAZINE ◇ sym-DIMETHYLHYDRAZINE ◇ 1,2-DIMETHYLHYDRAZIN (GERMAN) ◇ DIMETHYLHYDRAZINE, SYMMETRICAL (DOT) ◇ DMH ◇ HYDRAZOMETHANE ◇ RCRA WASTE NUMBER U099 ◇ SDMH ◇ SYMETRYCZNA DWUMETYLOHYDRAZYNA (POLISH)

TOXICITY DATA with REFERENCE
CAR: scu-ham TDLo:340 mg/kg/17W-I EXMPA6 27,19,77

CAR: scu-mus TD:300 mg/kg/20W-I JNCIAM 52,999,74

CAR: scu-mus TDLo:200 mg/kg/10W-I JJIND8 63,1081,79

CAR: scu-rat TD:20 mg/kg GANNA2 74,493,83

CAR: scu-rat TD:120 mg/kg/12W-I NASDA6 32,270,81

CAR: scu-rat TD:200 mg/kg/10W-I CRNGDP 3,1097,82

CAR: scu-rat TD:400 mg/kg/10W-I LANCAO 2,1030,80

CAR: scu-rat TD:420 mg/kg/28W-I CRNGDP 4,1175,83

CAR: scu-rat TDLo:90 mg/kg/28W-I BIMDB3 32,41,80

NEO: ipr-mus TDLo:25 mg/kg/24W-I TXAPA9 72,313,84

NEO: orl-mus TDLo:12500 μg/kg/24W-I TXAPA9 72,313,84

NEO: scu-rat TD:42 mg/kg 28W-I BIMDB3 32,41,80

NEO: scu-rat TD:300 mg/kg/11W-I GASTAB 81,475,81

ETA: imp-rbt TDLo: 2 mg/kg CNREA8 35,2292,75

ETA: ipr-rat TDLo:260 mg/kg/13W-I CALEDQ 19,1,83

ETA: orl-rat TDLo:120 mg/kg/4W-I AJCNAC 30,176,77

ETA: par-rat TDLo:160 mg/kg/16W-I PAACA3 21,67,80

ETA: rec-mus TDLo:360 mg/kg/18W-I FEPRA7 34,827,75

ETA: scu-rat TD:80 mg/kg/4W-I CRNGDP 6,637,85

ETA: scu-rat TD:200 mg/kg/20W-I DICRAG 23,137,80

MUT: dnd-ham:lng 2 mmol/L MUREAV 173,157,86

MUT: dns-hmn:lng 100 μL/L NTIS** AD-A041-973

MUT: hma-mus/esc 50 μmol/kg MUREAV 148,1,85

MUT: otr-hmn: fbr 230 μmol/L CALEDQ 29,265,85
MUT: sce-mus-rec 20 mg/kg ENMUDM 8(Suppl 6),41,86

CONSENSUS REPORTS: IARC Cancer Review: Animal Sufficient Evidence IMEMDT 4,145,74. EPA Genetic Toxicology Program.

DFG MAK: Animal Carcinogen, Suspected Human Carcinogen. DOT Classification: Flammable Liquid; Label: Flammable Liquid, Poison.

SAFETY PROFILE: Confirmed carcinogen with experimental carcinogenic, neoplastigenic, tumorigenic, and teratogenic data. Poison by ingestion, intraperitoneal, intravenous, subcutaneous and intramuscular routes. Moderately toxic by inhalation. Experimental reproductive effects. Human mutation data reported. A very dangerous fire hazard when exposed to heat, flame or oxidizers. A high energy propellant for liquid fuelled rockets. When heated to decomposition it emits toxic fumes of NO_x.

DUD100 CAS: 77-78-1
DIMETHYL SULFATE
DOT: 1595
mf: $C_2H_6O_4S$ mw: 126.14

PROP: Colorless, odorless liquid. Mp: −31.8°, bp: 188°, flash p: 182°F (OC), d: 1.3322 @ 20°/4°, vap d: 4.35, autoign temp: 370°F.

SYNS: DIMETHYLESTER KYSELINY SIROVE (CZECH) ◇ DIMETHYL MONOSULFATE ◇ DIMETHYLSULFAAT (DUTCH) ◇ DIMETHYLSULFAT (CZECH) ◇ DIMETILSOLFATO (ITALIAN) ◇ DMS ◇ DMS(METHYL SULFATE) ◇ DWUMETYLOWY SIARCZAN (POLISH) ◇ METHYLE (SULFATE de) (FRENCH) ◇ METHYL SULFATE (DOT) ◇ RCRA WASTE NUMBER U103 ◇ SULFATE de METHYLE (FRENCH) ◇ SULFATE DIMETHYLIQUE (FRENCH) ◇ SULFURIC ACID, DIMETHYL ESTER

TOXICITY DATA with REFERENCE
ETA: ihl-rat TCLo: 17 mg/m³/19W-I ZEKBAI 74,241,70
ETA: scu-rat TDLo: 50 mg/kg ZEKBAI 74,241,70
MUT: cyt-hmn-unr 2 mg/m³ MUREAV 147,301,85
MUT: dnd-ham: lng 800 μmol/L/1H-C CRNGDP 1,795,80
MUT: dnd-hmn: fbr 100 μmol/L CRNGDP 4,559,83
MUT: dnd-hmn: hla 5 μmol/L MUREAV 89,95,81
MUT: dnd-hmn: lym 1 mmol/L JACTDZ 1(3),125,82
MUT: dnd-rat-ivn 80 mg/kg MUREAV 75,63,80
MUT: dnd-rat: lvr 4 mmol/L TCMUD8 1,97,80

MUT: dni-hmn: fbr 75 μmol/L CRNGDP 4,559,83
MUT: dni-hmn: hla 2 mmol/L MUREAV 92,427,82
MUT: dnr-omi 640 μg/plate BIZNAT 95,463,76
MUT: dns-hmn: fbr 50 μmol/L CRNGDP 4,559,83
MUT: dns-hmn: hla 400 μmol/L MUREAV 139,155,84
MUT: dns-rat: lvr 100 μmol/L ENMUDM 3,11,81
MUT: mma-sat 4300 nmol/L/1H PNASA6 75,4465,78
MUT: mmo-sat 10 μmol/plate CBINA8 19,241,77
MUT: sce-hmn: fbr 1 μmol/L MUREAV 75,63,80

CONSENSUS REPORTS: IARC Cancer Review: Animal Sufficient Evidence IMEMDT 4,271,74; Human Inadequate Evidence IMEMDT 4,271,74. NTP Fourth Annual Report On Carcinogens, 1984. EPA Genetic Toxicology Program. Community Right To Know List. EPA Extremely Hazardous Substances List. Reported in EPA TSCA Inventory.

OSHA PEL: (Transitional: TWA 1 ppm (skin)) TWA 0.1 ppm (skin) ACGIH TLV: TWA 0.1 ppm (skin) DFG TRK: Production: 0.02 ppm; Use: 0.04 ppm; Animal Carcinogen, Suspected Human Carcinogen. DOT Classification; Corrosive Material; Label: Corrosive; Poison B; Label: Poison

SAFETY PROFILE: Confirmed carcinogen with experimental carcinogenic, tumorigenic, and teratogenic data. Human poison by inhalation. Experimental poison by ingestion, inhalation, intravenous, and subcutaneous routes. Human mutation data reported. A corrosive irritant to skin, eyes, and mucous membranes. There is no odor or initial irritation to give warning of exposure. On brief, mild exposures, conjunctivitis, catarrhal inflammation of the mucous membranes of the nose, throat, larynx and trachea and possibly some reddening of the skin develop after the latent period. With longer, heavier exposures, the cornea shows clouding, the irritation changes to the nasopharynx are more marked and after 6 to 8 hours pulmonary edema may develop. Death may occur in 3 or 4 days. The liver and kidneys are frequently damaged. Spilling of the liquid on the skin can cause ulceration and local necrosis. In patients surviving severe exposure, there may be serious injury of the liver and kidneys, with suppression of urine, jaundice, albuminuria and hematuria appearing. Death, resulting from the kidney or liver damage, may be delayed for several weeks. Flammable when exposed to heat, flame or oxidizers. To fight fire, use water, foam, CO_2, dry chemical. When heated to decomposition it emits toxic fumes of SO_x.

DVG600   CAS: 25321-14-6
DINITROTOLUENE
DOT: 1600/2038
mf: $C_7H_6N_2O_4$ mw: 182.15

SYNS: DINITROPHENYLMETHANE ◇ DINITROTOL-
UENE, LIQUID (DOT) ◇ DINITROTOLUENE, MOLTEN (DOT)
◇ DINITROTOLUENE, SOLID (DOT) ◇ ar,ar-DINITROTOL-
UENE ◇ METHYLDINITROBENZENE

TOXICITY DATA with REFERENCE
ETA: orl-rat TDLo: 12775 mg/kg/Y-C   PAACA3
24,91,83

MUT: dns-rat-orl 100 mg/kg   CRNGDP 3,241,82

CONSENSUS REPORTS: Reported in EPA TSCA Inventory. EPA Genetic Toxicology Program.

OSHA PEL: TWA 1.5 mg/m^3 (skin) DFG MAK: Animal Carcinogen, Suspected Human Carcinogen. NIOSH REL: (Dinitrotoluene): Reduce to lowest level DOT Classification: ORM-E; Label: None, Liquid and Solid; Poison B; Label: Flammable Liquid and Poison (Liquid); Poison B; Label: Poison (Solid and Molten).

SAFETY PROFILE: Confirmed carcinogen with experimental tumorigenic and teratogenic data. A poison. Experimental reproductive effects. Mutation data reported. Flammable. When heated to decomposition it emits toxic fumes of NO_x.

DVL700   CAS: 117-81-7
DI-sec-OCTYL PHTHALATE
mf: $C_{24}H_{38}O_4$ mw: 390.62

SYNS: BEHP ◇ BIS(2-ETHYLHEXYL)-1,2-BENZENEDI-
CARBOXYLATE ◇ BIS(2-ETHYLHEXYL)PHTHALATE
◇ BISOFLEX 81 ◇ BISOFLEX DOP ◇ COMPOUND 889
◇ DAF 68 ◇ DEHP ◇ DI(2-ETHYLHEXYL)ORTHOPHTHAL-
ATE ◇ DI(2-ETHYLHEXYL)PHTHALATE ◇ DIOCTYL
PHTHALATE ◇ DOP ◇ EHTYLHEXYL PHTHALATE
◇ ERGOPLAST FDO ◇ 2-ETHYLHEXYL PHTHALATE
◇ EVIPLAST 80 ◇ EVIPLAST 81 ◇ FLEXIMEL ◇ FLEXOL
DOP ◇ FLEXOL PLASTICIZER DOP ◇ GOOD-RITE GP 264
◇ HATCOL DOP ◇ HERCOFLEX 260 ◇ KODAFLEX DOP
◇ MOLLAN O ◇ NCI-C52733 ◇ NUOPLAZ DOP ◇ OCTOIL
◇ OCTYL PHTHALATE ◇ PALATINOL AH ◇ PHTHALIC
ACID DIOCTYL ESTER ◇ PITTSBURGH PX-138 ◇ PLATINOL
AH ◇ PLATINOL DOP ◇ RC PLASTICIZER DOP ◇ RCRA

WASTE NUMBER U028 ◇ REOMOL DOP ◇ REOMOL D 79P
◇ SICOL 150 ◇ STAFLEX DOP ◇ TRUFLEX DOP ◇ VESTINOL
AH ◇ VINICIZER 80 ◇ WITCIZER 312

TOXICITY DATA with REFERENCE
CAR: orl-mus TD: 262 g/kg/2Y-C   EVHPAZ
65,271,86
CAR: orl-mus TD: 519 g/kg/2Y-C
NTPTR* NTP-TR-217,82
CAR: orl-mus TDLo: 260 g/kg/2Y-C
NTPTR* NTP-TR-217,82
CAR: orl-rat TD: 524 g/kg/2Y-C   EVHPAZ
65,271,86
CAR: orl-rat TD: 433 g/kg/2Y-C
NTPTR* NTP-TR-217,82
CAR: orl-rat TDLo: 216 g/kg/2Y-C
NTPTR* NTP-TR-217,82
CAR: orl-rat TD: 438 g/kg/2Y-C   CALEDQ38,15,87
ETA: orl-mus TD: 120 g/kg/24W-C   CRNGDP
4,1021,83
MUT: dns-rat: lvr 500 µmol/L   PMRSDJ 5,371,85
MUT: sln-ham: lvr 50 mg/L   PMRSDJ 5,397,85

CONSENSUS REPORTS: IARC Cancer Review: Human Inadequate Evidence IMEMDT 29,269,82; Animal Sufficient Evidence IMEMDT 29,269,82. NTP Fourth Annual Report On Carcinogens, 1984. NTP Carcinogenesis Bioassay (feed); Clear Evidence: mouse, rat NTPTR* NTP-TR-217,82. EPA Genetic Toxicology Program. Reported in EPA TSCA Inventory. Community Right-To-Know List.

OSHA PEL: (Transitional: TWA 5 mg/m^3) TWA 5 mg/m^3; STEL 10 mg/m^3 ACGIH TLV: TWA 5 mg/m^3; STEL 10 mg/m^3 DFG MAK: 10 mg/m^3 NIOSH REL: (DEHP) Reduce to lowest feasible level

SAFETY PROFILE: Confirmed carcinogen with experimental carcinogenic and tumorigenic data. Experimental teratogen data. Poison by intravenous route. Human systemic effects by ingestion: gastrointestinal tract effects. A mild skin and eye irritant. When heated to decomposition it emits acrid smoke.

DVQ000   CAS: 123-91-1
DIOXANE
DOT: 1165
mf: $C_4H_8O_2$ mw: 88.11

PROP: Colorless liquid, pleasant odor. Mp: 12°, bp: 101.1°, lel: 2.0%, uel: 22.2%, flash p: 54°F (CC), d: 1.0353 @ 20°/4°, autoign temp: 356°F, vap press: 40 mm @ 25.2°, vap d: 3.03.

SYNS: DIETHYLENE DIOXIDE ◇ 1,4-DIETHYLENE DIOX-
IDE ◇ DIETHYLENE ETHER ◇ DI(ETHYLENE OXIDE)
◇ DIOKAN ◇ DIOKSAN (POLISH) ◇ DIOSSANO-1,4 (ITAL-
IAN) ◇ DIOXAAN-1,4 (DUTCH) ◇ 1,4-DIOXACYCLOHEX-
ANE ◇ DIOXAN-1,4 (GERMAN) ◇ p-DIOXAN (CZECH)
◇ 1,4-DIOXANE (MAK) ◇ p-DIOXANE ◇ DIOXANNE
(FRENCH) ◇ DIOXYETHYLENE ETHER ◇ GLYCOL ETHYL-
ENE ETHER ◇ NCI-C03689 ◇ RCRA WASTE NUMBER
U108 ◇ TETRAHYDRO-p-DIOXIN ◇ TETRAHYDRO-1,4-
DIOXIN

TOXICITY DATA with REFERENCE
CAR: orl-mus TD:523 g/kg/90W-C
NCITR* NCI-CG-TR-80,78
CAR: orl-mus TDLo:239 g/kg/90W-C
NCITR* NCI-CG-TR-80,78
CAR: orl-rat TD:408 g/kg/2Y-C
NCITR* NCI-CG-TR-80,78
CAR: orl-rat TD:416 g/kg/57W-C BJCAAI
24,164,70
CAR: orl-rat TDLo:185 g/kg/2Y-C
NCITR* NCI-CG-TR-80,78
NEO: ipr-mus TDLo:12 g/kg/8W-I TXAPA9
82,19,86
ETA: ihl-rat TCLo:111 ppm/7H/2Y-C TXAPA9
30,287,74
ETA: orl-rat TD:416 g/kg/57W-C BJCAAI
24,164,70
ETA: orl-rat TD:528 g/kg/63W-I JNCIAM
35,949,65
ETA: skn-mus TDLo:14 g/kg/60W-I EVHPAZ
5,163,73
MUT: dnd-rat:lvr 300 μmol/L SinJF# 26OCT82
MUT: dns-rat-orl 20 mg/kg TXAPA9 60,287,81
MUT: oms-rat-ivn 50 mg/kg ARTODN 49,29,81
MUT: osm-rat-ivn 50 mg/kg ARTODN 49,29,81

CONSENSUS REPORTS: IARC Cancer Review: Animal Sufficient Evidence IMEMDT
11,247,76. NTP Fourth Annual Report On Carcinogens, 1984. NCI Carcinogenesis Bioassay
(oral); Clear Evidence: mouse, rat NCITR*
NCI-CG-TR-80,78. EPA Genetic Toxicology
Program. Glycol ether compounds are on the
Community Right-To-Know List. Reported in
EPA TSCA Inventory.

OSHA PEL: (Transitional: TWA 100 ppm
(skin)) TWA 25 ppm (skin) ACGIH TLV:
TWA 25 ppm (skin) DFG MAK: 50 ppm (180
mg/m^3); Suspected Carcinogen. NIOSH REL:
CL (Dioxane) 1 ppm/30M DOT Classification: Flammable Liquid; Label: Flammable Liquid.

SAFETY PROFILE: Confirmed carcinogen with
experimental carcinogenic, neoplastigenic, tumorigenic, and teratogenic data. Poison by intraperitoneal route. Moderately toxic by ingestion
and inhalation. Mildly toxic by skin contact.
Human systemic effects by inhalation: lachrimation, conjunctiva irritation, convulsions, high
blood pressure, unspecified respiratory and gastrointestinal system effects. Experimental reproductive effects. Mutation data reported. An eye
and skin irritant. The irritant effects probably
provide sufficient warning, in acute exposures,
to enable a worker to leave exposure before
being seriously affected. A very dangerous fire
and explosion hazard when exposed to heat or
flame. To fight fire, use alcohol foam, CO_2,
dry chemical. When heated to decomposition
it emits acrid smoke and irritating fumes.

DXE600 CAS: 144-21-8
DISODIUM METHANEARSENATE
mf: $CH_3AsO_3 \cdot 2Na$ mw: 183.94

PROP: Crystals, water-sol hydrate. Mp: 132-
139°.

SYNS: ANSAR 184 ◇ ANSAR DSMA LIQUID ◇ ARRHENAL
◇ ARSINYL ◇ ARSYNAL ◇ CACODYL NEW ◇ CHIPCO
CRAB KLEEN ◇ CLOUT ◇ CRAB-E-RAD ◇ CRALO-E-RAD
◇ DAL-E-RAD 100 ◇ DIARSEN ◇ DIMET ◇ DINATE
◇ DISODIUM METHANEARSONATE ◇ DISODIUM METH-
YLARSENATE ◇ DISODIUM METHYLARSONATE
◇ DISODIUM MONOMETHYLARSONATE ◇ DISOMAR
◇ DI-TAC ◇ DMA ◇ DREXEL DSMA LIQUID ◇ DSMA LIQUID
◇ JON-TROL ◇ MAA SODIUM SALT ◇ METHAR
◇ METHARSINAT ◇ NAMATE ◇ NEOASYCODILE
◇ SODAR ◇ SODIUM METHANEARSONATE ◇ SODIUM
METHARSONATE ◇ SODIUM METHYLARSONATE
◇ SOMAR ◇ STENOSINE ◇ TONARSEN ◇ VERSAR DSMA
LQ ◇ WEED BROOM ◇ WEED-E-RAD ◇ WEED-HOE

CONSENSUS REPORTS: EPA Genetic Toxicology Program. Arsenic and its compounds
are on the Community Right-To-Know List.

OSHA PEL: TWA 0.5 mg(As)/m^3 ACGIH
TLV: TWA 0.2 mg(As)/m^3

SAFETY PROFILE: Confirmed human carcinogen. Experimental teratogen. Moderately toxic
by ingestion. Experimental reproductive effects.
An herbicide. When heated to decomposition
it emits toxic fumes of As and Na_2O.

EAP000 CAS: 8015-30-3
ENAVID
mf: $C_{21}H_{26}O_2 \cdot C_{20}H_{26}O_2$ mw: 608.93

PROP: Mixture of 98.5% (17-α)-19-norpregn-4-en-20-yn-3-one,17-hydroxy- and 1.5% (17-α)-19-norpregna-1,3,5(10)-trien-20-yn-17-ol,3-methoxy- (IARC** 6,193,74).

SYNS: CONOVID ◇ CONOVID E ◇ ENIDREL ◇ ENOVID ◇ ENOVID-E ◇ ETHINYLESTRADIOL-3-METHYL ETHER and NORETHYNODRED (1:50) ◇ MESTRANOL mixed with NORETHYNODREL ◇ NORETHANDROL ◇ NORETHYNODREL and ETHINYLESTRADIOL-3-METHYL ETHER (50:1) ◇ NORETHYNODREL mixed with MESTRANOL

TOXICITY DATA with REFERENCE

CAR: orl-mus TDLo:207 mg/kg/74W-C
    JNCIAM 43,671,69

NEO: orl-mus TD:1250 mg/kg/89W-I   SCIEAS 154,402,66

NEO: orl-wmn TD:50 mg/kg/5Y-I   LANCAO 2,926,73

NEO: orl-wmn TD:71 mg/kg/7Y-I   LANCAO 2,926,73

NEO: orl-wmn TD:252 mg/kg/10Y-I   LANCAO 1,1251,80

NEO: orl-wmn TDLo:20 mg/kg/2Y-I   LANCAO 2,926,73

NEO: scu-mus TDLo:728 mg/kg/91W-I
    BJCAAI 35,322,77

ETA: orl-mus TD:69 mg/kg/69W-I   PEXTAR 11,440,69

CONSENSUS REPORTS: IARC Cancer Review: Animal Sufficient Evidence IMEMDT 6,191,74. EPA Genetic Toxicology Program.

SAFETY PROFILE: Confirmed carcinogen producing liver tumors in women by ingestion. Experimental carcinogenic, neoplastigenic, and tumorigenic data. Human reproductive effects by ingestion: menstrual cycle changes or disorders; abnormalities of the uterus, cervix, and vagina; and changes in fertility. A human teratogen which causes developmental abnormalities of the urogenital system. Experimental reproductive effects. A steroid. When heated to decomposition it emits acrid smoke and fumes.

EAS500   CAS: 50-18-0
ENDOXAN

mf: $C_7H_{15}Cl_2N_2O_2P$ mw: 261.11

PROP: Crystals. Water-sol, sltly sol in organic solvents. Mp: 41-45°.

SYNS: ASTA ◇ ASTA B518 ◇ B 518 ◇ N,N-BIS-(β-CHLORAETHYL)-N′,O-PROPYLEN-PHOSPHORSAEURE-ESTER-DIAMID (GERMAN) ◇ 2-(BIS(2-CHLOROETHYL)AMINO)-2H-1,3,2-OXAAZAPHOSPHORINE 2-OXIDE ◇ BIS(2-CHLORO ETHYL)PHOSPHORAMIDE-CYCLIC PROPANOLAMIDE ESTER ◇ N,N-BIS(2-CHLOROETHYL)-N′,O-PROPYLENE-PHOSPHORIC ACID ESTER DIAMIDE ◇ N,N-BIS(2-CHLORO-ETHYL)TETRAHYDRO-2H-1,3,2-OXAPHOSPHORIN-2-AMINE-2-OXIDE ◇ N,N-BIS(β-CHLOROETHYL)-N′,O-TRI-METHYLENEPHOSPHORIC ACID ESTER DIAMIDE ◇ N,N-BIS(2-CHLOROETHYL)-N′-(3-HYDROXYPROPYL) PHOSPHORODIAMIDIC ACID intramol. ESTER ◇ CB 4564 ◇ CLAFEN ◇ CLAPHENE ◇ CP ◇ CPA ◇ CTX ◇ CY ◇ CYCLOPHOSPHAMIDE ◇ CYCLOPHOS-PHAMIDUM ◇ CYCLOPHOSPHAN ◇ CYCLOPHOS-PHORAMIDE ◇ CYCLOSTIN ◇ CYTOPHOSPHAN ◇ CYTOXAN ◇ N,N-DI(2-CHLOROETHYL)-N,o-PROPYL-ENE-PHOSPHORIC ACID ESTER DIAMIDE ◇ ENDOXANAL ◇ ENDOXAN-ASTA ◇ ENDOXAN R ◇ GENOXAL ◇ HEXADRIN ◇ MITOXAN ◇ NCI-C04900 ◇ NEOSAR ◇ NSC 26271 ◇ 2-H-1,3,2-OXAZAPHOSPHORINANE ◇ PROCYTOX ◇ RCRA WASTE NUMBER U058 ◇ SEM-DOXAN ◇ SENDUXAN ◇ SK 20501 ◇ ZYKLOPHOSPHAMID (GERMAN)

TOXICITY DATA with REFERENCE

CAR: ivn-rat TDLo:676 mg/kg/1Y-I   ARZNAD 20,1461,70

CAR: orl-hmn TD:920 mg/kg/3Y-C:KID
    AIMEAS 91,221,79

CAR: orl-man TD:1078 mg/kg/3Y-C:KID
    RIHYAC 32,1073,78

CAR: orl-man TD:1190 mg/kg/4Y-I:BLD
    MEDIAV 58,32,79

CAR: orl-man TD:1800 mg/kg/6Y-C:KID
    JOURAA 126,544,81

CAR: orl-man TDLo:2310 mg/kg/4.5Y-C: GIT   BMJOAE 280,524,80

CAR: orl-rat TD:698 mg/kg/89W-I   IJCNAW 23,706,79

CAR: orl-rat TD:1075 mg/kg/86W-I   CANCAR 51,606,83

CAR: orl-rat TD:1270 mg/kg/87W-I   IJCNAW 23,706,79

CAR: orl-rat TDLo:475 mg/kg/100W-I   IJCNAW 23,706,79

CAR: orl-wmn TD:1760 mg/kg/4Y-C:KID
    SJRHAT 12,73,83

CAR: orl-wmn TD:2700 mg/kg/6Y-C:KID
    URGABW 17,105,78

CAR: orl-wmn TDLo:1890 mg/kg/3Y-I:BLD
    JHMJAX 142,211,78

CAR: scu-mus TD:3600 mg/kg/76W-I
    ARHEAW 22,1338,79

CAR: scu-mus TDLo:1352 mg/kg/1Y-I:TER
    ARZNAD 20,1461,70

CAR: unr-man TDLo:857 mg/kg/3Y-C:BLD
    JCPAAK 26,649,73

CAR: unr-wmn TDLo: 1050 mg/kg/69W-C: BLD JCPAAK 26,649,73

NEO: ipr-mus TDLo: 1950 mg/kg/26W-I RRCRBU 52,1,75

MUT: mma-ham: lng 10 mg/L MUREAV 157,189,85

MUT: oms-ckn: emb 3 μg ENMUDM 8,241,86

MUT: par-ham LD10: 110 mg/kg JSONAU 15,355,80

MUT: sce-hmn: fbr 10 μmol/L CNREA8 45,3626,85

MUT: sce-hmn: oth 500 mg/L ENMUDM 7(Suppl 3),26,85

MUT: sce-mky: kdy 100 μmol/l CNREA8 45,3626,85

MUT: sce-rat-orl 240 mg/kg/10D-C ENMUDM 7(Suppl 3),79,85

CONSENSUS REPORTS: IARC Cancer Review: Human Sufficient Evidence IMEMDT 26,165,81; Animal Sufficient Evidence IMEMDT 26,165,81; IMEMDT 9,135,75; Human Limited Evidence IMEMDT 9,135,75. NTP Fourth Annual Report On Carcinogens, 1984. NCI Carcinogenesis Studies (ipr); Clear Evidence: mouse, rat RRCRBU 52,1,75. EPA Genetic Toxicology Program.

SAFETY PROFILE: Confirmed human carcinogen producing leukemia, Hodgkin's disease, gastrointestinal, and bladder tumors. Experimental carcinogenic, neoplastigenic, and teratogenic data. A human poison by ingestion and many other routes. Human systemic effects by ingestion, intravenous, intraperitoneal, subcutaneous, and possibly other routes: kidney changes (hepatic dysfunction), leukopenia (reduced white blood cell count), nausea and alopecia (loss of hair). Human reproductive and teratogenic effects by multiple routes: spermatogenesis, testical changes, epididymis and sperm duct changes, menstrual cycle changes; fetal developmental abnormalities of the craniofacial area, musculoskeletal and cardiovascular systems. Experimental reproductive effects. Human mutation data reported. A powerful skin irritant. Used as an immunosuppressive agent in non-malignant diseases. When heated to decomposition it emits highly toxic fumes of PO_x, NO_x and Cl^-.

EAZ500
EPICHLOROHYDRIN
CAS: 106-89-8
DOT: 2023
mf: C_3H_5ClO mw: 92.53

PROP: Colorless, mobile liquid, irritating chloroform-like odor. Bp: 117.9°, fp: − 57.1°, flash p: 105.1°F (OC) (40°C), mp -25.6°C, d: 1.1761 @ 20°/20°, vap press: 10 mm @ 16.6°, vap d: 3.29.

SYNS: 1-CHLOOR-2,3-EPOXY-PROPAAN (DUTCH) ◇ 1-CHLOR-2,3-EPOXY-PROPAN (GERMAN) ◇ 1-CHLORO-2,3-EPOXYPROPANE ◇ 3-CHLORO-1,2-EPOXYPROPANE ◇ epi-CHLOROHYDRIN ◇ (CHLOROMETHYL)ETHYLENE OXIDE ◇ CHLOROMETHYLOXIRANE ◇ 2-(CHLORO-METHYL)OXIRANE ◇ CHLOROPROPYLENE OXIDE ◇ γ-CHLOROPROPYLENE OXIDE ◇ 3-CHLORO-1,2-PROPYL-ENE OXIDE ◇ 1-CLORO-2,3-EPOSSIPROPANO (ITALIAN) ◇ ECH ◇ EPICHLOORHYDRINE (DUTCH) ◇ EPICHLOR-HYDRIN (GERMAN) ◇ EPICHLORHYDRINE (FRENCH) ◇ α-EPICHLOROHYDRIN ◇ (dl)-α-EPICHLOROHYDRIN ◇ EPICHLOROHYDRYNA (POLISH) ◇ EPICHLOROPHYDRIN ◇ EPICLORIDRINA (ITALIAN) ◇ 1,2-EPOXY-3-CHLOROPRO-PANE ◇ 2,3-EPOXYPROPYL CHLORIDE ◇ GLYCEROL EPI-CHLORHYDRIN ◇ RCRA WASTE NUMBER U041 ◇ SKEKhG

TOXICITY DATA with REFERENCE

CAR: ihl-rat TCLo: 100 ppm/6H/30D-C JJIND8 65,751,80

CAR: orl-rat TDLo: 60 g/kg/81W-I GANNA2 71,922,80

NEO: ipr-mus TDLo: 2400 mg/kg/8W-I TXAPA9 82,19,86

NEO: orl-rat TD: 85050 mg/kg/81W-C NAIZAM 32,270,81

NEO: scu-mus TD: 2760 mg/kg/69W-I JNCIAM 53,695,74

ETA: ihl-rat TC: 100 ppm CHWKA9 123,25,78

ETA: ihl-rat TC: 100 ppm/6H/6W-I PAACA3 21,106,80

ETA: ihl-rat TD: 30 ppm/6H/57W-I JJIND8 65,751,80

ETA: orl-rat TD: 36 g/kg/81W-I GANNA2 71,922,80

ETA: orl-rat TD: 5150 mg/kg/2Y-I TXCYAC 36,325,85

ETA: orl-rat TD: 42525 mg/kg/81W-C NAIZAM 32,270,81

ETA: scu-mus TDLo: 720 mg/kg/18W-I JNCIAM 48,1431,72

ETA: unk-mus TDLo: 19 mg/kg RARSAM 3,193,63

MUT: cyt-mus-ihl 5 mg/m^3 MUREAV 85,287,81

MUT: dni-hmn: hla 2700 μmol/L MUREAV 92,427,82

MUT: dns-hmn: fbr 32 μg/L PMRSDJ 1,528,81

MUT: mmo-klp 200 μmol/L MUREAV 89,269,81

MUT: sce-hmn: lym 10 nmol/L CARYAB 34,261,81

MUT: spm-mus-ihl 5 mg/m^3 MUREAV 85,287,81

CONSENSUS REPORTS: IARC Cancer Review: Animal Sufficient Evidence IMEMDT

11,131,76. NTP Fourth Annual Report On Carcinogens, 1984. EPA Genetic Toxicology Program. Community Right-To-Know List. EPA Extremely Hazardous Substances List. Reported in EPA TSCA Inventory.

OSHA PEL: (Transitional: TWA 5 ppm (skin)) TWA 2 ppm (skin) ACGIH TLV: TWA 2 ppm (skin) DFG TRK: 3 ppm; Animal Carcinogen, Suspected Human Carcinogen. NIOSH REL: Minimize exposure DOT Classification: Flammable Liquid; Label: Flammable Liquid; IMO: Poison B; Label: Poison, Flammable Liquid.

SAFETY PROFILE: Confirmed carcinogen with experimental carcinogenic, neoplastigenic, tumorigenic, and teratogenic data. Poison by ingestion, intravenous, intraperitoneal, parenteral, and subcutaneous routes. Moderately toxic by skin contact and inhalation. Human mutation data reported. Human systemic effects by inhalation: unspecified effects on the respiratory system, sense of smell, and eyes. A skin and eye irritant. A sensitizer. Flammable when exposed to heat or flame. When heated to decomposition it emits toxic fumes of Cl^-.

ECU750   CAS: 12126-59-9
EQUIGYNE

PROP: Conjugated forms of natural mixed estrogens, principally sodium estrone sulfate and sodium equilin sulfate, or synthetic estrogen piperazine estrone sulfate (IMEMDT** 21, 147,79).

SYNS: AMNESTROGEN ◇ CES ◇ CLIMESTRONE ◇ CO-ESTRO ◇ CONEST ◇ CONESTRON ◇ CONJES ◇ CONJUGATED ESTROGENS ◇ CONJUTABS ◇ ESTRATAB ◇ ESTRIFOL ◇ ESTROATE ◇ ESTROCON ◇ ESTROMED ◇ ESTROPAN ◇ EVEX ◇ FEMACOID ◇ FEMEST ◇ FEM H ◇ FEMOGEN ◇ FORMATRIX ◇ GANEAKE ◇ GENISIS ◇ GLYESTRIN ◇ KESTRIN ◇ MENEST ◇ MENOGEN ◇ MENOTAB ◇ MENOTROL ◇ MILPREM ◇ MSMED ◇ NEO-ESTRONE ◇ NOVOCONESTRON ◇ OESTRILIN ◇ OESTRO-FEMINAL ◇ OESTROPAK MORNING ◇ OVEST ◇ PALOPAUSE ◇ PAR ESTRO ◇ PMB ◇ PREMARIN ◇ PRESOMEN ◇ PROMARIT ◇ SK-ESTROGENS ◇ SODESTRIN-H ◇ TAG-39 ◇ THEOGEN ◇ TRANSANNON ◇ TROCOSONE ◇ ZESTE

TOXICITY DATA with REFERENCE
CAR: orl-wmn TDLo:108 mg/kg/4Y-C:
    CVS,LIV   AIMDAP 137,357,77
NEO: orl-wmn TD:27 mg/kg/3Y-C:LIV
    NYSJAM 78,1933,78

CONSENSUS REPORTS: IARC Cancer Review: Animal Inadequate Evidence IMEMDT 21,147,79; Human Limited Evidence IMEMDT 21,147,79. NTP Fourth Annual Report On Carcinogens, 1984.

SAFETY PROFILE: Confirmed human carcinogen producing tumors of the vascular system and liver. Human reproductive effects by ingestion and possibly other routes: changes in female fertility. When heated to decomposition it emits toxic fumes of Na_2O.

EDC650   CAS: 66733-21-9
ERIONITE (CaKNa (Al₂Si₇O₁₈)₂·14H₂O)
mf: $Al_2O_{18}Si_7 \cdot 1/2Ca \cdot 7H_2O \cdot 1/2Na$
    mw: 715.68

TOXICITY DATA with REFERENCE
CAR: ipr-mus TD:20 mg/kg   ENVRAL 35,277,84
CAR: ipr-mus TDLo:400 mg/kg   JACTDZ
    4(1),225,85
ETA: ipl-rat TD:125 mg/kg   ENVRAL 29,238,82
ETA: ipl-rat TDLo:100 mg/kg   ENVRAL 29,238,82
ETA: ipr-mus TD:400 mg/kg   ENVRAL 27,433,82
ETA: ipr-mus TDLo:20 mg/kg   PAACA3 24,61,83

CONSENSUS REPORTS: IARC Cancer Review: Animal Sufficient Evidence, Human Sufficient Evidence IMEMDT 42,225,87.

SAFETY PROFILE: Confirmed carcinogen with experimental carcinogenic and tumorigenic data.

EDO000   CAS: 50-28-2
ESTRADIOL
mf: $C_{18}H_{24}O_2$ mw: 272.42

PROP: Needles out of benzene, acetone. Mp: 173-179°, bp: decomp. Sol in dioxone, alc and ether.

SYNS: ALTRAD ◇ BARDIOL ◇ DIHYDROFOLLICULAR HORMONE ◇ DIHYDROFOLLICULIN ◇ DIHYDROMENFORMON ◇ DIHYDROTHEELIN ◇ 3,17-β-DIHYDROXYESTRA-1,3,5(10)-TRIENE ◇ 3,17-β-DIHYDROXY-1,3,5(10)-ESTRA-TRIENE ◇ DIHYDROXYESTRIN ◇ 3,17-β-DIHYDROXYOES-TRA-1,3,5-TRIENE ◇ 3,17-β-DIHYDROXY-1,3,5(10)-OESTRATRIENE ◇ DIHYDROXYOESTRIN ◇ DIMENFOR-MON ◇ DIMENFORMON PROLONGATUM ◇ DIOGYN ◇ DIOGYNETS ◇ E² ◇ 3,17-EPIDIHYDROXYESTRATRIENE ◇ 3,17-EPIDIHYDROXYOESTRATRIENE ◇ ESTRADIOL-17-β ◇ α-ESTRADIOL ◇ β-ESTRADIOL ◇ 3,17-β-ESTRADIOL ◇ 17-β-ESTRADIOL ◇ cis-ESTRADIOL ◇ d-ESTRADIOL ◇ d-3,17-β-ESTRADIOL ◇ ESTRALDINE ◇ ESTRA-1,3,5(10)-TRIENE-3,17-β-DIOL ◇ 17-β-ESTRA-1,3,5(10)-TRIENE-3,17-

DIOL ◇ 1,3,5-ESTRATRIENE-3,17-β-DIOL ◇ ESTROVITE ◇ FEMESTRAL ◇ FEMOGEN ◇ GYNERGON ◇ GYNESTREL ◇ GYNOESTRYL ◇ LAMDIOL ◇ MACRODIOL ◇ MACROL ◇ MICRODIOL ◇ NORDICOL ◇ NSC-9895 ◇ OESTERGON ◇ OESTRADIOL ◇ α-OESTRADIOL ◇ β-OESTRADIOL ◇ 3,17-β-OESTRADIOL ◇ cis-OESTRADIOL ◇ d-OESTRADIOL ◇ d-3,17-β-OESTRADIOL ◇ OESTRADIOL R ◇ OESTRADIOL-17-β ◇ OESTRA-1,3,5(10)-TRIENE-3,17-β-DIOL ◇ 17-β-OESTRA-1,3,5(10)-TRIENE-3,17-DIOL ◇ OESTROGLANDOL ◇ OESTROGYNAL ◇ 17-β-OH-ESTRADIOL ◇ 17-β-OH-OESTRADIOL ◇ OVAHORMON ◇ OVASTEROL ◇ OVASTEVOL ◇ OVOCICLINA ◇ OVOCYCLIN ◇ OVOCYCLINE ◇ OVOCYLIN ◇ PRIMOFOL ◇ PROFOLIOL ◇ PROGYNON ◇ PROGYNON-DH ◇ SYNDIOL

TOXICITY DATA with REFERENCE

CAR: imp-ham TD: 360 mg/kg/15W-I   MOPMA3 23,278,83

CAR: imp-ham TD: 547 mg/kg/12W-I   CNREA8 43,4638,83

CAR: imp-ham TDLo: 286 mg/kg   CNREA8 12,274,52

CAR: imp-rat TDLo: 100 mg/kg/52W-C   JJCREP 78,134,87

NEO: orl-mus TDLo: 58 mg/kg/82W-C   BJCAAI 35,322,77

ETA: imp-gpg TD: 40 mg/kg   LANCAO 1,1313,39
ETA: imp-gpg TD: 100 mg/kg   LANCAO 1,1313,39
ETA: imp-gpg TD: 2400 μg/kg   BSBSAS 8,142,51
ETA: imp-gpg TDLo: 1200 μg/kg   RCBIAS 3,108,44

ETA: imp-ham TD: 160 mg/kg   CANCAR 10,757,57
ETA: imp-mus TD: 30 mg/kg   REEBB3 16,425,71
ETA: imp-mus TD: 34 mg/kg   EJCAAH 11,39,75
ETA: imp-mus TDLo: 100 μg/kg   BIMDB3 29,45,78

ETA: imp-rat TD: 62500 μg/kg/36W-I   JJIND8 73,123,84

ETA: ipr-rat TDLo: 1400 mg/kg/13W-I   NIGHAE 52,655,83

ETA: orl-mus TD: 44 mg/kg/52W-C   JEPTDQ 1,1,77

ETA: scu-gpg TDLo: 7 mg/kg/12W-I   CRSBAW 130,9,39

MUT: cyt-ham: ovr 50 μmol/L   TOLED5 29,201,85

MUT: dni-hmn: lym 10 μmol/L   PSEBAA 146,401,74

MUT: dns-hmn: mmr 10 nmol/L   CNREA8 45,1644,85

MUT: dns-rat-par 10 μg/k   ACHCBO 18,213,85

MUT: dns-rbt: oth 100 nmol/L   CRNGDP 3,703,82

MUT: mnt-hmn: lym 5 μmol/L   MUREAV 156,199,85

CONSENSUS REPORTS: IARC Cancer Review: Human Limited Evidence IMEMDT 21,279,79; Animal Sufficient Evidence IMEMDT 21,279,79; IMEMDT 6,99,74. NTP Fourth Annual Report On Carcinogens, 1984. EPA Genetic Toxicology Program.

SAFETY PROFILE: Confirmed carcinogen with experimental carcinogenic, neoplastigenic, tumorigenic, and teratogenic data. A promoter. Human reproductive effects by ingestion: fertility effects. Experimental reproductive effects. Human mutation data reported. A steroid hormone much used in medicine. When heated to decomposition it emits acrid smoke and irritating fumes.

EDP000   CAS: 50-50-0
ESTRADIOL-3-BENZOATE
mf: $C_{25}H_{28}O_3$ mw: 376.53

PROP: White or slightly yellow to brownish crystalline powder, odorless. Almost insol in water; sol in alcohol, acetone, and dioxane; sparingly sol in vegetable oils; sltly sol in ether. Mp: 191-196°

SYNS: BENOVOCYLIN ◇ BENZHORMOVARINE ◇ BENZOATE d'OESTRADIOL (FRENCH) ◇ BENZOESTROFOL ◇ BENZOFOLINE ◇ BENZO-GYNOESTRYL ◇ BENZOIC ACID ESTRADIOL ◇ DIFFOLLISTEROL ◇ DIFOLLICULINE ◇ DIHYDROESTRIN BENZOATE ◇ DIHYDROFOLLICULIN BENZOATE ◇ DIMENFORMON BENZOATE ◇ DIMENFORMONE ◇ DIOGYN B ◇ EBZ ◇ ESTON-B ◇ ESTRADIOL BENZOATE ◇ ESTRADIOL-17-β-BENZOATE ◇ ESTRADIOL-17-β-3-BENZOATE ◇ β-ESTRADIOL BENZOATE ◇ β-ESTRADIOL-3-BENZOATE ◇ 17-β-ESTRADIOL BENZOATE ◇ 17-β-ESTRADIOL-3-BENZOATE ◇ ESTRADIOL MONOBENZOATE ◇ 17-β-ESTRADIOL MONOBENZOATE ◇ ESTRA-1,3,5(10)-TRIENE-3,17-DIOL (17-β)-3-BENZOATE ◇ ESTRA-1,3,5(10)-TRIENE-3,17-β-DIOL, 3-BENZOATE ◇ 1,3,5(10)-ESTRATRIENE-3,17-β-DIOL 3-BENZOATE ◇ FEMESTRONE ◇ FOLLICORMON ◇ FOLLIDRIN ◇ GRAAFINA ◇ de GRAAFINA ◇ GYNECORMONE ◇ GYNFORMONE ◇ HIDROESTRON ◇ HORMOGYNON ◇ HYDROXYESTRIN BENZOATE ◇ MEE ◇ ODB ◇ OESTRADIOL BENZOATE ◇ OESTRADIOL-3-BENZOATE ◇ β-OESTRADIOL BENZOATE ◇ β-OESTRADIOL-3-BENZOATE ◇ 17-β-OESTRADIOL-3-BENZOATE ◇ OESTRADIOL MONOBENZOATE ◇ OESTRAFORM (BDH) ◇ 1,3,5(10)-OESTRATRIENE-3,17-β-DIOL 3-BENZOATE ◇ OVAHORMON BENZOATE ◇ OVASTEROL-B ◇ OVEX ◇ OVOCYCLIN BENZOATE ◇ OVOCYCLIN M ◇ OVOCYCLIN-MB ◇ PRIMOGYN B ◇ PRIMOGYN BOLEOSUM ◇ PRIMOGYN I ◇ PROGYNON B ◇ PROGYNON BENZOATE ◇ RECTHORMONE OESTRADIOL ◇ SOLESTRO ◇ UNISTRADIOL

TOXICITY DATA with REFERENCE

CAR: scu-mus TD:38 mg/kg/39W-I   CNREA8
8,337,48

CAR: scu-mus TDLo:24 mg/kg/36W-I   CNREA8
8,337,48

NEO: imp-rat TDLo:25 mg/kg   EJCAAH13,1437,77

ETA: imp-gpg TD:50 mg/kg   CNREA8 1,367,41

ETA: imp-gpg TD:100 mg/kg   CNREA8 1,367,41

ETA: imp-gpg TDLo:3000 μg/kg   RCBIAS
3,108,44

ETA: imp-ham TDLo:80 mg/kg:TER   JPBAA7
56,1,44

ETA: imp-mus TD:80 mg/kg   CNREA8 1,290,41

ETA: imp-mus TDLo:60 mg/kg   CNREA81,290,41

ETA: imp-rat TD:30 mg/kg   NATUAS 175,724,55

ETA: imp-rat TD:100 mg/kg   JPTLAS 141,29,83

ETA: par-mus TDLo:38 mg/kg/57W-I   CNREA8
1,359,41

ETA: scu-gpg TD:4 mg/kg/9W-I:TER
CRSBAW 130,9,39

ETA: scu-gpg TDLo:240 μg/kg/8W-I:TER
LANCAO 1,1313,39

ETA: scu-mus TD:15 mg/kg/22W-I   CNREA8
1,345,41

ETA: scu-mus TD:4790 μg/kg/36W-I   YJBMAU
12,213,39

ETA: scu-mus TDLo:23 mg/kg/36W-I   YJBMAU
17,75,44

MUT: dni-rat-scu 10 μg/kg   JOENAK 65,45,75

CONSENSUS REPORTS: IARC Cancer Review: Animal Sufficient Evidence IMEMDT 21,279,79.

SAFETY PROFILE: Confirmed carcinogen with experimental carcinogenic, tumorigenic, and teratogenic data. Human reproductive effects by intramuscular route: menstrual cycle changes and disorders. Experimental reproductive effects. Mutation data reported. A steroid. When heated to decomposition it emits acrid smoke and irritating fumes.

EDR000   CAS: 113-38-2
ESTRADIOL DIPROPIONATE
mf: $C_{24}H_{32}O_4$ mw: 384.56

SYNS: AGOFOLLIN ◇ DIMENFORMON DIPROPIONATE ◇ DIOVOCYCLIN ◇ DIOVOCYLIN ◇ DIPROPIONATE d'OESTRADIOL (FRENCH) ◇ DIPROSTRON ◇ ENDOFOLLICOLINA D.P. ◇ ESTRADIOL-3,17-DIPROPIONATE ◇ β-ESTRADIOL DIPROPIONATE ◇ β-ESTRADIOL-3,17-DIPROPIONATE ◇ 3,17-β-ESTRADIOL DIPROPIONATE ◇ 17-β-ESTRADIOL DIPROPIONATE ◇ ESTRA-1,3,5(10)-TRIENE-3,17-DIOL (17-β)-DIPROPIONATE ◇ 1,3,5(10)-ESTRATRIENE-3,17-β-DIOL

DIPROPIONATE ◇ ESTROICI ◇ ESTRONEX ◇ FOLLICYCLIN P ◇ NACYCLYL ◇ OESTRADIOL DIPROPIONATE ◇ OESTRADIOL-3,17-DIPROPIONATE ◇ β-OESTRADIOL DIPROPIONATE ◇ 3,17-β-OESTRADIOL DIPROPIONATE ◇ 17-β-OESTRADIOL DIPROPIONATE ◇ OVOCYCLIN DIPROPIONATE ◇ OVOCYCLIN-P ◇ PROGYNON-DP

TOXICITY DATA with REFERENCE

ETA: imp-gpg TDLo:2200 μg/kg   RCBIAS
3,108,44

ETA: par-rat TDLo:40 mg/kg/26W-I   CNREA8
2,632,42

ETA: scu-mus TD:54 mg/kg/27W-I   YJBMAU
12,213,39

ETA: scu-mus TD:3000 mg/kg/25W-I   JPBAA7
51,9,40

ETA: scu-mus TDLo:36 mg/kg/36W-I   YJBMAU
12,213,39

CONSENSUS REPORTS: IARC Cancer Review: Animal Sufficient Evidence IMEMDT 21,279,79. EPA Genetic Toxicology Program.

SAFETY PROFILE: Confirmed carcinogen with experimental carcinogenic, tumorigenic, and teratogenic data. A poison by intravenous and parenteral routes. Experimental reproductive effects. A drug for the treatment of menopause. When heated to decomposition it emits acrid smoke and irritating fumes.

EDS000   CAS: 28014-46-2
ESTRADIOL POLYESTER with PHOSPHORIC ACID
mf: $(C_{18}H_{24}O_2 \cdot H_3O_4P)_x$

SYNS: ESTRADIOL PHOSPHATE POLYMER ◇ ESTRADURIN ◇ (17-β)-ESTRA-1,3,5(10)-TRIENE-3,17-DIOL POLYMER with PHOSPHORIC ACID ◇ OESTRADIOL PHOSPHATE POLYMER ◇ OESTRADIOL POLYESTER with PHOSPHORIC ACID ◇ PEP ◇ POLY(ESTRADIOL PHOSPHATE) ◇ POLYOESTRADIOL PHOSPHATE

TOXICITY DATA with REFERENCE

CAR: ims-wmn TDLo:173 mg/kg/9Y-I:LIV
ACLRBL 7,287,75

CONSENSUS REPORTS: IARC Cancer Review: Animal Sufficient Evidence IMEMDT 21,279,79.

SAFETY PROFILE: Confirmed carcinogen producing liver tumors. An experimental teratogen. A drug used in cancer treatment. When heated to decomposition it emits toxic fumes of PO_x.

EDV000   CAS: 53-16-7
ESTRONE
mf: $C_{18}H_{22}O_2$ mw: 270.40

PROP: White crystals. Mp: 254°. Insol in water, sol in alc, benzene, ether and chloroform.

SYNS: AQUACRINE ◊ CRINOVARYL ◊ CRISTALLOVAR ◊ CRYSTOGEN ◊ DESTRONE ◊ DISYNFORMON ◊ E¹ ◊ ENDOFOLLICULINA ◊ ESTERONE ◊ 1,3,5-ESTRA-TRIEN-3-OL-17-ONE ◊ 1,3,5(10)-ESTRATRIEN-3-OL-17-ONE ◊ Δ-1,3,5-ESTRATRIEN-3-β-OL-17-ONE ◊ ESTRIN ◊ ESTROL ◊ ESTRON ◊ ESTRONA (SPANISH) ◊ ESTRO-NE-A ◊ ESTRUGENONE ◊ ESTRUSOL ◊ FEMESTRONE IN-JECTION ◊ FEMIDYN ◊ FOLIKRIN ◊ FOLIPEX ◊ FOLISAN ◊ FOLLESTRINE ◊ FOLLICULAR HORMONE ◊ FOLLICULIN ◊ FOLLICULINE BENZOATE ◊ FOLLICUNODIS ◊ FOLLI-DRIN ◊ GLANDUBOLIN ◊ HIESTRONE ◊ HORMOFOLLIN ◊ HORMOVARINE ◊ 3-HYDROXYESTRA-1,3,5(10)-TRIEN-17-ONE ◊ 3-HYDROXY-17-KETO-ESTRA-1,3,5-TRIENE ◊ 3-HYDROXY-17-KETO-OESTRA-1,3,5-TRIENE ◊ 3-HY-DROXY-OESTRA-1,3,5(10)-TRIEN-17-ONE ◊ 3-HYDROXY-1,3,5(10)-OESTRATRIEN-17-ONE ◊ KESTRONE ◊ KETO-DESTRIN ◊ KETOHYDROXY-ESTRATRIENE ◊ KETOHY-DROXYESTRIN ◊ KETOHYDROXYOESTRIN ◊ KOLPON ◊ MENAGEN ◊ MENFORMON ◊ Δ-1,3,5-OESTRATRIEN-3-β-OL-17-ONE ◊ 1,3,5-OESTRATRIEN-3-OL-17-ONE ◊ 1,3,5(10)-OESTRATRIEN-3-OL-17-ONE ◊ OESTRIN ◊ OESTROFORM ◊ OESTRONE ◊ OESTROPEROS ◊ OVEX ◊ OVIFOLLIN ◊ PERLATAN ◊ SOLLICULIN ◊ THEELIN ◊ THELESTRIN ◊ THELYKININ ◊ THYNES-TRON ◊ TOKOKIN ◊ UNDEN ◊ WNYESTRON

TOXICITY DATA with REFERENCE
NEO: orl-mus TDLo: 11 mg/kg/68W-C BIMDB3 29,45,78

NEO: scu-mus TDLo: 108 mg/kg/90W-I ZEKBAI 56,482,49

ETA: imp-gpg TD: 2 mg/kg: TER RBBIAL 5,1,45

ETA: imp-gpg TD: 1800 µg/kg RCBIAS 3,108,44

ETA: imp-gpg TDLo: 640 µg/kg: TER BSBSAS 8,142,51

ETA: imp-ham TD: 640 mg/kg/38W-I CNREA8 43,5200,83

ETA: imp-ham TDLo: 320 mg/kg/59W-C NCIMAV 1,1,59

ETA: imp-mus TDLo: 48 mg/kg YJBMAU 17,75,44

ETA: imp-rat TD: 80 mg/kg PCCRA4 6,50,66

ETA: imp-rat TDLo: 16 mg/kg CNREA8 13,147,53

ETA: par-mus TDLo: 1200 µg/kg/W-I COREAF 195,630,32

ETA: scu-gpg TDLo: 40 mg/kg/18W-I: TER CRSBAW 130,9,39

ETA: scu-mus TD: 48 mg/kg/24W-I JNCIAM 1,119,40

MUT: cyt-ham: ovr 50 µmol/L TOLED5 29,201,85

MUT: cyt-rat-ipr 10 mg/kg CUSCAM 50,425,81

MUT: dnd-rat-orl 870 nmol/kg CBINA8 23,13,78

CONSENSUS REPORTS: IARC Cancer Review: Human Limited Evidence IMEMDT 21,343,79; Animal Sufficient Evidence IMEMDT 6,123,74; IMEMDT 21,343,79. NTP Fourth Annual Report On Carcinogens, 1984. Reported in EPA TSCA Inventory.

SAFETY PROFILE: Confirmed carcinogen with experimental carcinogenic, neoplastigenic, tumorigenic, and teratogenic data. A poison by intraperitoneal and subcutaneous routes. Human reproductive effects by implantation: spermatogenesis and impotence. Mutation data reported. A steroid drug for the treatment of menopause and ovariectomy symptoms. When heated to decomposition it emits acrid smoke and irritating fumes.

EEH500 CAS: 57-63-6
ETHINYL ESTRADIOL
mf: $C_{29}H_{24}O_2$ mw: 296.44

SYNS: 3,17-β-DIHYDROXY-17-α-ETHYNYL-1,3,5(10)-ES-TRATRIENE ◊ 3,17-β-DIHYDROXY-17-α-ETHYNYL-1,3,-5(10)-OESTRATRIENE ◊ ESTROGEN ◊ 17-α-ETHINYL-3,17-DIHYDROXY-Δ¹,³,⁵-ESTRATRIENE ◊ 17-α-ETHINYL-3,17-DIHYDROXY-Δ¹,³,⁵-OESTRATRIENE ◊ 17-ETHINYLESTRA-DIOL ◊ 17-ETHINYL-3,17-ESTRADIOL ◊ 17-α-ETHINYLESTRADIOL ◊ 17-α-ETHINYL-17-β-ESTRADIOL ◊ 17-α-ETHINYLESTRA-1,3,5(10)-TRIENE-3,17-β-DIOL ◊ ETHINYLESTRIOL ◊ ETHINYLOESTRADIOL ◊ 17-ETHI-NYL-3,17-OESTRADIOL ◊ ETHINYL-OESTRANOL ◊ 17-α-ETHINYLOESTRA-1,3,5(10)-TRIENE-3,17-β-DIOL ◊ 17-α-ETHINYL-Δ(SUP 1,3,5(10))OESTRATRIENE-3,17-β-DIOL ◊ ETHINYLOESTRIOL ◊ 17-ETHYNYL-3,17-DIHY-DROXY-1,3,5-OESTRATRIENE ◊ ETHYNYLESTRADIOL ◊ 17-α-ETHYNYLESTRADIOL ◊ 17-α-ETHYNYLESTRA-DIOL-17-β ◊ 17-α-ETHYNYL-1,3,5(10)-ESTRATRIENE-3,17-β-DIOL ◊ 17-α-ETHYNYLESTRA-1,3,5(10)-TRIENE-3,17-β-DIOL ◊ ETHYNYLOESTRADIOL ◊ 17-ETHYNYLOESTRA-DIOL ◊ 17-α-ETHYNYLOESTRADIOL ◊ 17-α-ETHYNYL-17-β-OESTRADIOL ◊ 17-α-ETHYNYLOESTRADIOL-17-β ◊ 17-ETHYNYLOESTRA-1,3,5(10)-TRIENE-3,17-β-DIOL ◊ 17-α-ETHYNYL-1,3,5-OESTRATRIENE-3,17-β-DIOL ◊ 17-α-ETHYNYL-1,3,5(10)-OESTRATRIENE-3,17-β-DIOL ◊ 17-α-ETHYNYLOESTRA-1,3,5(10)-TRIENE-3,17-β-DIOL ◊ 19-NOR-17-α-PREGNA-1,3,5(10)-TRIEN-2-YNE-3,17-DIOL ◊ (17-α)-19-NORPREGNA-1,3,5(10)-TRIEN-20-YNE-3,17,-DIOL

TOXICITY DATA with REFERENCE
CAR: imp-rat TDLo: 5 mg/kg JJIND8 67,455,81

CAR: orl-wmn TD: 102 mg/kg/5Y-I LANCAO 1,273,80

CAR: orl-wmn TDLo: 2738 µg/kg/10Y-I MJAUAJ 1,473,81

NEO: imp-ham TDLo:621 mg/kg   CNREA8
12,274,52

ETA: imp-ham TD:800 mg/kg/34W-I   CNREA8
43,5200,83

ETA: imp-rat TD:5 mg/kg   CTRRDO 63,1180,79

ETA: orl-rat TD:245 mg/kg/35W-C   EMSUA8
22,28,64

ETA: orl-rat TDLo:6 μg/kg/2Y-C   JTEHD6
6,885,80

MUT: dni-hmn:lym 50 μmol/L   PSEBAA
146,401,74

MUT: mmo-ssp 50 μg/plate   EGJBAY 20,29,79

CONSENSUS REPORTS: IARC Cancer Review: Human Limited Evidence IMEMDT 21,233,79; Animal Sufficient Evidence IMEMDT 6,77,74; IMEMDT 21,233,79. NTP Fourth Annual Report On Carcinogens, 1984. Reported in EPA TSCA Inventory.

SAFETY PROFILE: Confirmed human carcinogen producing liver tumors. Experimental carcinogenic, tumorigenic, and neoplastigenic data. Moderately toxic by ingestion. Human systemic effects by ingestion: glandular effects. Experimental reproductive effects. Human mutation data reported. When heated to decomposition it emits acrid smoke and irritating fumes.

EFU000   CAS: 64-17-5
ETHYL ALCOHOL
DOT: 1170
mf: C_2H_6O mw: 46.08

PROP: Clear, colorless liquid; fragrant odor and burning taste. Bp: 78.32°, ULC: 70, lel: 3.3%, uel: 19% @ 60°, fp: $< -130°$, flash p: 55.6°F, d: 0.7893 @ 20°/4°, autoign temp: 793°F, vap press: 40 mm @ 19°, vap d: 1.59, refr index: 1.364. Misc in water, alc, chloroform, and ether.

SYNS: ABSOLUTE ETHANOL ◇ AETHANOL (GERMAN) ◇ AETHYLALKOHOL (GERMAN) ◇ ALCOHOL ◇ ALCOHOL, ANHYDROUS ◇ ALCOHOL, DEHYDRATED ◇ ALCOOL ETHYLIQUE (FRENCH) ◇ ALCOOL ETILICO (ITALIAN) ◇ ALGRAIN ◇ ALKOHOL (GERMAN) ◇ ALKOHOLU ETYLOWEGO (POLISH) ◇ ANHYDROL ◇ COLOGNE SPIRIT ◇ COLOGNE SPIRITS (ALCOHOL) (DOT) ◇ ETANOLO (ITALIAN) ◇ ETHANOL (MAK) ◇ ETHANOL 200 PROOF ◇ ETHANOL SOLUTION (DOT) ◇ ETHYLALCOHOL (DUTCH) ◇ ETHYL ALCOHOL ANHYDROUS ◇ ETHYL HYDRATE ◇ ETHYL HYDROXIDE ◇ ETYLOWY ALKOHOL (POLISH) ◇ FERMENTATION ALCOHOL ◇ GRAIN ALCOHOL ◇ JAYSOL ◇ JAYSOL S ◇ METHYLCARBINOL ◇ MOLASSES ALCOHOL ◇ NCI-C03134 ◇ POTATO ALCOHOL ◇ SD ALCO-

HOL 23-HYDROGEN ◇ SPIRITS of WINE ◇ SPIRIT ◇ TECSOL

TOXICITY DATA with REFERENCE
ETA: orl-mus TD:400 g/kg/57W-I   ZIETA2
59,203,28

ETA: orl-mus TDLo:320 mg/kg/50W-I
CALEDQ 13,345,81

ETA: rec-mus TDLo:120 g/kg/18W-I   ZIETA2
59,203,28

MUT: cyt-hmn:fbr 12000 ppm   ACYTAN 16,41,72

MUT: cyt-hmn:leu 1 pph/72H-C   TSITAQ
20,421,78

MUT: cyt-hmn:lym 1160 g/L   AEMBAP 85A,25,77

MUT: cyt-mus-orl 40 g/kg   NATUAS 302,258,83

MUT: dni-hmn:lym 220 mmol/L   PNASA6
79,1171,82

MUT: mmo-asn 20 pph   MUREAV 48,51,77

MUT: mmo-esc 140 g/L   MUREAV 130,97,84

CONSENSUS REPORTS: IARC Cancer Review: Human Sufficient Evidence IMEMDT 44,259,88. Reported in EPA TSCA Inventory. EPA Genetic Toxicology Program.

OSHA PEL: TWA 1000 ppm   ACGIH TLV: TWA 1000 ppm   DFG MAK: 1,000 ppm $(1,900 \text{ mg/m}^3)$ DOT Classification: Flammable Liquid; Label: Flammable Liquid; Flammable or Combustible Liquid; Label: Flammable Liquid.

SAFETY PROFILE: Confirmed human carcinogen for ingestion of beverage alcohol. Experimental tumorigenic and teratogenic data. Moderately toxic to humans by ingestion. Moderately toxic experimentally by intravenous and intraperitoneal routes. Mildly toxic by inhalation and skin contact. Human systemic effects by ingestion and subcutaneous route: sleep disorders, hallucinations, distorted perceptions, convulsions, motor activity changes, ataxia, coma, antipsychotic, headache, pulmonary changes, alteration in gastric secretion, nausea or vomiting, other gastrointestinal changes, menstrual cycle changes and body temperature decrease. Can also cause glandular effects in humans. Human reproductive effects by ingestion, intravenous, and intrauterine routes: changes in female fertility index. Effects on newborn include: changes in apgar score, neonatal measures or effects and drug dependence. Experimental reproductive effects. Human mutation data reported. An eye and skin irritant. Flammable liquid when exposed to heat or flame.

EIY500 CAS: 106-93-4
1,2-ETHYLENE DIBROMIDE
DOT: 1605
mf: $C_2H_4Br_2$ mw: 187.88

PROP: Colorless, heavy liquid; sweet odor. Bp: 131.4°, fp: 9.3°, flash p: none, d: 2.172 @ 25°/25°, 2.1707 @ 25°/4°, vap press: 17.4 mm @ 30°, vap d: 6.48.

SYNS: AETHYLENBROMID (GERMAN) ◊ BROMOFUME ◊ BROMURO di ETILE (ITALIAN) ◊ CELMIDE ◊ DBE ◊ 1,2-DIBROMAETHAN (GERMAN) ◊ 1,2-DIBROMOETANO (ITALIAN) ◊ 1,2-DIBROMOETHANE (MAK) ◊ α,β-DIBRO-MOETHANE ◊ sym-DIBROMOETHANE ◊ DIBROMURE d'ETHYLENE (FRENCH) ◊ 1,2-DIBROOMETHAAN (DUTCH) ◊ DOWFUME 40 ◊ DOWFUME EDB ◊ DOWFUME W-8 ◊ DWUBROMOETAN (POLISH) ◊ EDB ◊ EDB-85 ◊ E-D-BEE ◊ ENT 15,349 ◊ ETHYLENE BROMIDE ◊ FUMO-GAS ◊ GLYCOL BROMIDE ◊ GLYCOL DIBROMIDE ◊ ISCOBROME D ◊ KOPFUME ◊ NCI-C00522 ◊ NEPHIS ◊ PESTMASTER ◊ PESTMASTER EDB-85 ◊ RCRA WASTE NUMBER U067 ◊ SOILBROM-40 ◊ SOILBROM-85 ◊ SOILFUME ◊ UNIFUME

TOXICITY DATA with REFERENCE
CAR: ihl-mus TDLo:40 ppm/6H/90W-I
CALEDQ 12,121,81
CAR: ihl-rat TC:20 ppm/7H/78W-I   TXAPA9 63,155,82
CAR: ihl-rat TC:40 ppm/6H/88W-I   NCITR* NCI-CG-TR-201,82
CAR: ihl-rat TCLo:10 ppm/6H/2Y-I   NCITR* NCI-CG-TR-201,82
CAR: ihl-rat TCLo:10 ppm/6H/2Y-I   NTPTR* NTP-TR-201,82
CAR: orl-mus TD:23 g/kg/53W-I   NCITR* NCI-CG-TR-86,78
CAR: orl-mus TD:28 g/kg/53W-I   NCITR* NCI-CG-TR-86,78
CAR: orl-mus TDLo:16 g/kg/53W-I   NCITR* NCI-CG-TR-86,78
CAR: orl-rat TD:16 g/kg/61W-I   NCITR* NCI-CG-TR-86,78
CAR: orl-rat TD:18 g/kg/44W-I   NCITR* NCI-CG-TR-86,78
CAR: orl-rat TD:24 g/kg/57W-I   NCITR* NCI-CG-TR-86,78
CAR: orl-rat TD:6630 mg/kg/34W-I   NCITR* NCI-CG-TR-86,78
CAR: orl-rat TD:7000 mg/kg/47W-I   NCITR* NCI-CG-TR-86,78
CAR: orl-rat TDLo:540 mg/kg /78W-C
BANRDU 5,279,80
NEO: ipr-mus TDLo:840 mg/kg/8W-I   TXAPA9 82,19,86

NEO: skn-mus TDLo:190 g/kg/62W-I   JJIND8 63,1433,79
MUT: mma-esc 333 μg/plate   ENMUDM 7(Suppl 5),1,85
MUT: mmo-sat 1 μg/plate   ENMUDM 7(Suppl 5),1,85
MUT: msc-hmn:lym 5 mg/L   MUREAV 142,133,85
MUT: sce-hmn:lym 10 nmol/L   MUREAV 97,188,82

CONSENSUS REPORTS: IARC Cancer Review: Animal Sufficient Evidence IMEMDT 15,195,77. NTP Fourth Annual Report On Carcinogens, 1984. NCI Carcinogenesis Bioassay (gavage); Clear Evidence: mouse, rat NCITR* NCI-CG-TR-86,78; NTP Carcinogenesis Bioassay (inhalation); Clear Evidence: mouse, rat NTPTR* NTP-TR-210,82. EPA Genetic Toxicology Program. Community Right-To-Know List. Reported in EPA TSCA Inventory.

OSHA PEL: TWA 20 ppm; CL 30 ppm; Pk 50 ppm/5M/8H   ACGIH TLV: Suspected Human Carcinogen   DFG TRK: 0.1 ppm; Animal Carcinogen, Suspected Human Carcinogen. NIOSH REL: (EDB) 0.045 ppm; CL 1 mg/m³/15M   DOT Classification: ORM-A; Label: None; Poison B; Label: Poison.

SAFETY PROFILE: Confirmed carcinogen with experimental carcinogenic, neoplastigenic, and teratogenic data. Human poison by ingestion. Experimental poison by ingestion, skin contact, intraperitoneal and possibly other routes. Moderately toxic by inhalation and rectal routes. Experimental reproductive effects. Human mutation data reported. A severe skin and eye irritant. An experimental eye irritant. Implicated in worker sterility. When heated to decomposition it emits toxic fumes of Br^-.

EIY600 CAS: 107-06-2
ETHYLENE DICHLORIDE
DOT: 1184
mf: $C_2H_4Cl_2$ mw: 98.96

PROP: Colorless, clear liquid; pleasant odor, sweet taste. Bp: 83.5°, ULC: 60-70, lel: 6.2%, uel: 15.9%, fp: −35.7°, flash p: 56°F, d: 1.257 @ 20°/4°, autoign temp: 775°F, vap press: 100 mm @ 29.4°, vap d: 3.35, refr index: 1.445 @ 20°. Sol in alc, ether, acetone, carbon tetrachloride; sltly sol in water.

SYNS: AETHYLENCHLORID (GERMAN) ◊ BICHLORURE d'ETHYLENE (FRENCH) ◊ BORER SOL ◊ BROCIDE ◊ CHLORURE d'ETHYLENE (FRENCH) ◊ CLORURO di ETHENE (ITALIAN) ◊ 1,2-DCE ◊ DESTRUXOL BORER-SOL

◇ 1,2-DICHLOORETHAAN (DUTCH) ◇ 1,2-DICHLOR-
AETHAN (GERMAN) ◇ DICHLOREMULSION ◇ DI-CHLOR-
MULSION ◇ DICHLORO-1,2-ETHANE (FRENCH) ◇ 1,2-DI-
CHLOROETHANE ◇ α,β-DICHLOROETHANE ◇ sym-DI-
CHLOROETHANE ◇ DICHLOROETHYLENE ◇ 1,2-DICLO-
ROETANO (ITALIAN) ◇ DUTCH LIQUID ◇ DUTCH OIL
◇ EDC ◇ ENT 1,656 ◇ ETHANE DICHLORIDE ◇ ETHYLEEN-
DICHLORIDE (DUTCH) ◇ ETHYLENE CHLORIDE
◇ 1,2-ETHYLENE DICHLORIDE ◇ GLYCOL DICHLORIDE
◇ NCI-C00511 ◇ RCRA WASTE NUMBER U077

TOXICITY DATA with REFERENCE
CAR: orl-mus TD:38 g/kg/78W-I:TER   NCITR*
NCI-CG-TR-55,78
CAR: orl-mus TD:76 g/kg/78W-I:TER   NCITR*
NCI-CG-TR-55,78
CAR: orl-mus TDLo:3536 mg/kg/78W-I
BANRDU 5,35,80
CAR: orl-rat TD:18 g/kg/78W-I   NCITR* NCI-
CG-TR-55,78
CAR: orl-rat TD:38 g/kg/78W-I   NCITR* NCI-
CG-TR-55,78
CAR: orl-rat TDLo:5286 mg/kg/69W-I
BANRDU 5,35,80
NEO: skn-mus TDLo:1120 g/kg/74W-I   JJIND8
63,1433,79
ETA: ihl-mus TCLo:5 ppm/7H/78W-I   BANRDU
5,3,80
ETA: ihl-rat TCLo:5 ppm/7H/78W-I   BANRDU
5,3,80
MUT: mmo-sat 40 μmol/plate   CBINA8 20,1,78
MUT: msc-hmn:lym 100 mg/L   MUREAV
142,133,85
MUT: otr-ham:emb 200 μL/plate   EVSRBT
25,75,82
MUT: slt-mus-ipr 300 mg/kg   MUREAV 117,201,83

CONSENSUS REPORTS: IARC Cancer Review: Human Limited Evidence IMEMDT
20,429,79; Animal Sufficient Evidence
IMEMDT 20,429,79. NTP Fourth Annual Report On Carcinogens, 1984. NCI Carcinogenesis
Bioassay (gavage); Clear Evidence: mouse-rat
NCITR* NCI-CG-TR-55,78. EPA Genetic Toxicology Program. Reported in EPA TSCA Inventory.

OSHA PEL: (Transitional: TWA 50 ppm; CL
100 ppm; PK 200 ppm/5M)) TWA 1 ppm; STEL
2 ppm   ACGIH TLV: TWA 10 ppm   DFG
MAK: 20 ppm (80 mg/m³); Suspected Carcinogen.   NIOSH REL: TWA 1 ppm; CL 2 ppm/
15M   DOT Classification: Flammable Liquid;
Label: Flammable Liquid; IMO: Flammable
Liquid; Label: Flammable Liquid, Poison.

SAFETY PROFILE: Confirmed carcinogen with
experimental carcinogenic, neoplastigenic, tumorigenic, and teratogenic data. An experimental transplacentral carcinogen. A human poison
by ingestion. Poison experimentally by intravenous and subcutaneous routes. Moderately toxic
by inhalation, skin contact, and intraperitoneal
routes. Human systemic effects by ingestion and
inhalation: flaccid paralysis without anesthesia
(usually neuromuscular blockade), somnolence,
cough, jaundice, nausea or vomiting, hypermotility, diarrhea, ulceration or bleeding from the
stomach, fatty liver degeneration, change in cardiac rate, cyanosis and coma. It may also cause
dermatitis, edema of the lungs, toxic effects
on the kidneys, and severe corneal effects. A
strong narcotic. Experimental reproductive effects. A skin and severe eye irritant, and strong
local irritant. Its smell and irritant effects warn
of its presence at relatively safe concentrations.
Human mutation data reported. Flammable liquid. To fight fire, use water, foam, CO₂, dry
chemicals. When heated to decomposition it
emits highly toxic fumes of Cl⁻ and phosgene.

EJM900   CAS: 151-56-4
ETHYLENEIMINE
DOT: 1185
mf: C_2H_5N mw: 43.08

PROP: Oily, water-white liquid. Pungent am-
moniacal odor. Bp: 55-56°, fp: −71.5°, flash
p: 12°F, d: 0.832 @ 20°/4°, autoign temp:
608°F, vap press: 160 mm @ 20°, vap d: 1.48,
lel: 3.6%, uel: 46%.

SYNS: AETHYLENIMIN (GERMAN) ◇ AMINOETHYLENE
◇ AZACYCLOPROPANE ◇ AZIRANE ◇ AZIRIDIN (GERMAN)
◇ AZIRIDINE ◇ DIHYDROAZIRENE ◇ DIHYDRO-1H-AZI-
RINE ◇ DIMETHYLENEIMINE ◇ DIMETHYLENIMINE
◇ EI ◇ ENT 50,324 ◇ ETHYLEENIMINE (DUTCH)
◇ ETHYLENE IMINE, INHIBITED (DOT) ◇ ETHYLENIMINE
◇ ETHYLIMINE ◇ ETILENIMINA (ITALIAN) ◇ RCRA WASTE
NUMBER P054 ◇ TL 337

TOXICITY DATA with REFERENCE
CAR: orl-mus TDLo:235 mg/kg/76W-C
JNCIAM 42,1101,69
CAR: orl-mus TDLo:6500 μg/kg/5D-I
VOONAW 27(5),88,81
NEO: scu-rat TDLo:20 mg/kg/67D-I   BJPCAL
9,306,54
ETA: scu-rat TD:10 mg/kg/8W-I   BJPCAL9,306,54
MUT: cyt-hmn:lng 1 μmol/L   EVSRBT 24,433,81
MUT: dlt-mus-ipr 5 mg/kg   EVSRBT 24,943,81

MUT: dns-mus-par 5 mg/kg   EVSRBT 24,943,81
MUT: mnt-nml-mul 5000 ppm/8D-C   MUREAV 125,275,84
MUT: msc-ham:ovr 2 mg/L   MUREAV 94,449,82
MUT: sln-dmg-mul 1 pph/8H-C   GNKAA5 21,958,85

CONSENSUS REPORTS: IARC Cancer Review: GROUP 3 IMEMDT 7,56,87; Animal Sufficient Evidence IMEMDT 9,37,75. Community Right-To-Know List. EPA Extremely Hazardous Substances List. Reported in EPA TSCA Inventory. EPA Genetic Toxicology Program.

OSHA PEL: TWA 1 mg/m^3 (skin); Carcinogen ACGIH TLV: TWA 0.5 ppm (skin) DFG TRK: 0.5 ppm; Animal Carcinogen, Suspected Human Carcinogen. DOT Classification: Flammable Liquid; Label: Flammable Liquid and Poison.

SAFETY PROFILE: Confirmed carcinogen with experimental carcinogenic, neoplastigenic, tumorigenic, and teratogenic data. Poison by ingestion, skin contact, inhalation, intraperitoneal, and possibly other routes. Human mutation data reported. A skin, mucous membrane, and severe eye irritant. An allergic sensitizer of skin. A very dangerous fire and explosion hazard. To fight fire, use alcohol foam, CO_2, dry chemical. When heated to decomposition it emits acrid smoke and irritating fumes.

EJN500
ETHYLENE OXIDE
CAS: 75-21-8
DOT: 1040
mf: C_2H_4O mw: 44.06

PROP: Colorless gas at room temperature. Mp: −111.3°, bp: 10.7°, ULC: 100, lel: 3.0%, uel: 100%, flash p: −4°F, d: 0.8711 @ 20°/20°, autoign temp: 804°F, vap press: 1095 mm @ 20°, vap d: 1.52. Misc in water and alc; very sol in ether.

SYNS: AETHYLENOXID (GERMAN) ◇ AMPROLENE ◇ ANPROLENE ◇ ANPROLINE ◇ DIHYDROOXIRENE ◇ DIMETHYLENE OXIDE ◇ ENT 26,263 ◇ E.O. ◇ 1,2-EPOXYAETHAN (GERMAN) ◇ EPOXYETHANE ◇ 1,2-EPOXYETHANE ◇ ETHENE OXIDE ◇ ETHYLEENOXIDE (DUTCH) ◇ ETHYLENE (OXYDE d') (FRENCH) ◇ ETILENE (OSSIDO di) (ITALIAN) ◇ ETO ◇ ETYLENU TLENEK (POLISH) ◇ FEMA No. 2433 ◇ MERPOL ◇ NCI-C50088 ◇ OXACYCLOPROPANE ◇ OXANE ◇ OXIDOETHANE ◇ α,β-OXIDOETHANE ◇ OXIRAAN (DUTCH) ◇ OXIRANE ◇ OXYFUME ◇ OXYFUME 12 ◇ RCRA WASTE NUMBER U115 ◇ STERILIZING GAS ETHYLENE OXIDE 100% ◇ T-GAS

TOXICITY DATA with REFERENCE
CAR: ihl-rat TC:33 ppm/6H/2Y-I   FCTOD7 24,145,86
CAR: ihl-rat TC:50 ppm/7H/2Y-I   TXAPA9 76,69,84
CAR: ihl-rat TCLo:33 ppm/6H/2Y-I   TXAPA9 75,105,84
CAR: orl-rat TD:5112 mg/kg/2Y-I   BJCAAI 46,924,82
CAR: orl-rat TDLo:1186 mg/kg/2Y-I   BJCAAI 46,924,82
CAR: scu-mus TD:908 mg/kg/95W-I   ZHPMAT 174,383,81
CAR: scu-mus TD:2576 mg/kg/95W-I   ZHPMAT 174,383,81
CAR: scu-mus TDLo:292 mg/kg/95W-I   ZHPMAT 174,383,81
NEO: scu-mus TD:1090 mg/kg/91W-I   BJCAAI 39,588,79
ETA: ihl-rat TC:33 ppm/6H/2Y-I   NRTXDN 6,117,85
MUT: dlt-mus-ihl 500 ppm/6H/4D-C   ENMUDM 8,1,86
MUT: dnd-mus-ipr 100 mg/kg   ENMUDM 8(Suppl 6),74,86
MUT: dns-hmn:leu 4 mmol/L   CBINA8 47,265,83
MUT: mmo-omi 540 mg/L   47YKAF 8,273,84
MUT: sce-hmn:lym 4 pph   TCMUD8 6,15,86
MUT: sce-hmn:lym 10 mg/L   PHMGBN 25,214,82

CONSENSUS REPORTS: IARC Cancer Review: Animal Inadequate Evidence IMEMDT 11,157,76; Human Inadequate Evidence IMEMDT 36,189,85; Animal Sufficient Evidence IMEMDT 36,189,85. NTP Fourth Annual Report On Carcinogens, 1984. Community Right-To-Know List. EPA Extremely Hazardous Substances List. Reported in EPA TSCA Inventory. EPA Genetic Toxicology Program.

OSHA PEL: TWA 1 ppm; Cancer Hazard ACGIH TLV: TWA 1 ppm; Suspected Human Carcinogen. DFG TRK: 3 ppm; Animal Carcinogen, Suspected Human Carcinogen. NIOSH REL: (Oxirane) TWA 0.1 ppm; CL 5 ppm/10M/D DOT Classification: Flammable Liquid; Label: Flammable Liquid; Flammable Gas; Label: Poison Gas and Flammable Gas.

SAFETY PROFILE: Confirmed human carcinogen with experimental carcinogenic, tumorigenic, neoplastigenic, and teratogenic data. Poison by ingestion, intraperitoneal, subcutaneous, intravenous, and possibly other routes. Moderately toxic by inhalation. Human systemic effects by inhalation: convulsions, nausea, vomiting, olfactory and pulmonary changes. Experimental reproductive effects. Mutation data reported. A skin and eye irritant. An irritant to mucous membranes of respiratory tract. Highly flammable liquid or gas. When heated to decomposition it emits acrid smoke and irritating fumes.

ENV000   CAS: 759-73-9
1-ETHYL-1-NITROSOUREA
mf: $C_3H_7N_3O_2$ mw: 117.13

PROP: Pale yellow crystals. Mp: 103° (decomp) 1% water soln @ 20°.

SYNS: AENH (GERMAN) ◊ AETHYLNITROSO-HARN-STOFF (GERMAN) ◊ ENU ◊ N-ETHYL-N-NITROSOCAR-BAMIDE ◊ ETHYLNITROSOUREA ◊ N-ETHYL-N-NITRO-SO-UREA ◊ NEU ◊ NITROSOETHYLUREA ◊ NSC 45403 ◊ RCRA WASTE NUMBER U176

TOXICITY DATA with REFERENCE
CAR: ipr-mus TD:30 mg/kg   CALEDQ 18,131,83
CAR: ipr-mus TDLo:20 mg/kg (19D preg):
    TER   VOONAW 23(3),41,77
CAR: ipr-rat TDLo:10 mg/kg (15D preg):TER
    SCIEAS 218,682,82
CAR: ipr-rat TDLo:45 mg/kg   ANTRD4 4,5,84
CAR: ivn-rat TDLo:50 mg/kg (15D preg):TER
    ZEKBAI 73,371,70
CAR: orl-rat TDLo:10 mg/kg (19D preg):TER
    CALEDQ 2,93,76
CAR: orl-rat TDLo:374 mg/kg/2W-C   JJIND8
    75,743,85
CAR: par-mus TDLo:58565 µg/kg (18D
    preg):TER   JNCIAM 51,1965,73
CAR: scu-rat TDLo:5 mg/kg   CRNGDP 6,769,85
CAR: skn-mus TDLo:375 mg/kg/40W-I
    JCROD7 102,13,81
NEO: ipr-ham TDLo:274 mg/kg   CNREA8
    43,829,83
NEO: ipr-ham TDLo:800 mg/kg (16D preg):
    TER   ZKKOBW 90,233,77
NEO: ipr-mus TD:240 mg/kg   BIJOAK 174,1031,78
NEO: ipr-mus TDLo:234 mg/kg   CBINA83,117,71
NEO: ipr-rat TD:10 mg/kg (21D preg):TER
    JSONDX 5,396,84
NEO: ipr-rbt TDLo:100 mg/kg (15-24D preg):
    TER   JJIND8 65,607,80
NEO: ivn-rbt TDLo:80 mg/kg (25D preg):TER
    BEXBAN 85,369,78
NEO: orl-mus TDLo:20 mg/kg/24W-I   TXAPA9
    72,313,84

NEO: skn-ham TDLo:107 mg/kg/20W-C
    ZKKOBW 90,233,77
ETA: ipr-dog TDLo:100 mg/kg (53D preg):
    TER   CALEDQ 12,161,81
ETA: ivn-dog TDLo:30 mg/kg (59D preg):
    TER   ZAPPAN 121,54,77
ETA: ivn-ham TDLo:80 mg/kg (15D preg):
    TER   ZAPPAN 121,54,77
ETA: ivn-mky TDLo:610 mg/kg/2Y-I   PAACA3
    18,53,77
ETA: ivn-pig TDLo:120 mg/kg (20-31D preg):
    TER   ARGEAR 34,25,69
ETA: ivn-rat TD:10 mg/kg (16D preg):TER
    ANPTAL 34,21,76
ETA: ivn-rat TD:20 mg/kg (17D preg):TER
    CALEDQ 1,345,76
ETA: ivn-rat TD:20 mg/kg/(12D preg):TER
    NAGZAC 54,130,79
ETA: ivn-rbt TD:70 mg/kg (25D preg):TER
    NEOLA4 25,453,78
ETA: ivn-rbt TD:150 mg/kg (8-10D preg):
    TER   ZKKOBW 89,331,77
ETA: orl-rat TD:180 mg/kg   ANYAA9 381,250,82
ETA: orl-rat TD:520 mg/kg/1Y-I   PPTCBY2,73,72
ETA: par-mus TDLo:100 mg/kg/(18D preg):
    TER   PAACA3 17,122,76
ETA: par-rbt TDLo:160 mg/kg (25D preg):
    TER   ZAPPAN 121,54,77
ETA: skn-rat TDLo:350 mg/kg (16-22D preg):
    TER   ZKKOBW 81,169,74
ETA: unr-rat TDLo:5 mg/kg (13D preg):TER
    XENOBH 3,271,73
MUT: cyt-ham-orl 100 mg/kg   TRENAF 36,396,85
MUT: dnd-hmn:lym 1 mmol/L   JACTDZ
    1(3),125,82
MUT: dni-hmn:hla 100 µmol/L   MUREAV
    92,427,82
MUT: dns-rbt:oth 15 µmol/L   CRNGDP 6,661,85
MUT: sce-ham:emb 3 mmol/L   CRNGDP6,1565,85
MUT: sln-dmg-orl 30 µmol/L   ENMUDM 6,483,84

CONSENSUS REPORTS: IARC Cancer Review: Human Limited Evidence IMEMDT 17,191,78; Animal Sufficient Evidence IMEMDT 17,191,78; IMEMDT 1,135,72. NTP Fourth Annual Report On Carcinogens, 1984. EPA Genetic Toxicology Program. Community Right-To-Know List. Reported in EPA TSCA Inventory.

SAFETY PROFILE: Confirmed carcinogen with experimental carcinogenic, neoplastigenic, tumorigenic, and teratogenic data. Poison by ingestion, subcutaneous, and intravenous routes. Moderately toxic by intraperitoneal route. Human mutation data reported. When heated to decomposition it emits toxic fumes of NO_x.

FDR000 CAS: 53-96-3
N-FLUOREN-2-YL ACETAMIDE
mf: $C_{15}H_{13}NO$ mw: 223.29

SYNS: AAF ◊ 2-AAF ◊ 2-ACETAMIDOFLUORENE ◊ 2-ACETAMINOFLUORENE ◊ ACETOAMINOFLUORENE ◊ 2-ACETYLAMINO-FLUOREN (GERMAN) ◊ N-ACETYL-2-AMINOFLUORENE ◊ 2-ACETYLAMINOFLUORENE (OSHA) ◊ AZETYLAMINOFLUOREN (GERMAN) ◊ FAA ◊ 2-FAA ◊ 2-FLUORENYLACETAMIDE ◊ N-2-FLUORENYLACET-AMIDE ◊ RCRA WASTE NUMBER U005

TOXICITY DATA with REFERENCE
CAR: ipr-rat TDLo: 192 mg/kg/4W-I   CNREA8 32,1554,72

CAR: itr-ham TDLo: 8800 mg/kg/73W-I
JNCIAM 50,503,73

CAR: orl-ham TDLo: 9240 mg/kg/44W-C
GANNA2 59,239,68

CAR: orl-mus TD: 13 g/kg/53W-C   JCPCBR 19,591,79

CAR: orl-mus TD: 13140 mg/kg/1Y-C   TXAPA9 41,535,77

CAR: orl-mus TDLo: 7840 mg/kg/49W-C
EJCAAH 5,41,69

CAR: orl-rat TD: 1220 mg/kg/19W-C   CNREA8 22,1002,62

CAR: orl-rat TD: 1344 mg/kg/16W-C   TXAPA9 19,687,71

CAR: orl-rat TD: 2100 mg/kg/25W-C   CALEDQ 19,55,83

CAR: orl-rat TD: 2100 mg/kg/30W-C   TXAPA9 5,526,63

CAR: orl-rat TD: 2610 mg/kg/23W-C   JNCIAM 10,1201,50

CAR: orl-rat TD: 2940 mg/kg/35W-C   TXAPA9 19,687,71

CAR: orl-rat TDLo: 672 mg/kg/8W-C   TXAPA9 74,63,84

CAR: orl-rbt TD: 14 g/kg/56W-I: TER   CNREA8 27,838,67

CAR: orl-rbt TDLo: 6500 mg/kg/65W-I
PAMIAD 32,177,68

CAR: skn-rat TD: 2590 mg/kg/23W-I   CNREA8 28,234,68

CAR: skn-rat TDLo: 260 mg/kg/71W-I   JNCIAM 10,1201,50

NEO: ipr-mus TDLo: 60 mg/kg/2W-I   TXAPA9 82,19,86

NEO: orl-dog TDLo: 2625 mg/kg/25W-C
CNREA8 10,266,50

ETA: imp-mus TDLo: 96 mg/kg   GMCRDC 17,383,75

ETA: imp-rat TDLo: 22 mg/kg   CNREA8 33,2489,73

ETA: ipr-rbt TDLo: 3600 mg/kg/40W-I   CNREA8 27,838,67

ETA: mul-ham TDLo: 3370 mg/kg/37W-I
INURAQ 14,206,76

ETA: orl-cat TDLo: 11 g/kg/69W-C   CNREA8 11,280,51

ETA: orl-ckn TDLo: 2800 mg/kg/13W-I   BJCAAI 9,163,55

ETA: par-ckn TDLo: 3430 mg/kg/3Y   BJCAAI 8,147,54

ETA: par-rat TDLo: 1700 mg/kg/17W-I
CNREA8 6,617,46

ETA: scu-mus TDLo: 400 mg/kg (15D preg): TER   IJCNAW 20,293,77

MUT: dnd-hmn: fbr 1 mmol/L   ENMUDM 7,267,85

MUT: dnr-esc 5 μmol/L   MUREAV 89,95,81

MUT: mmo-sat 100 μg/plate   CBINA8 22,297,78

MUT: otr-rat: emb 100 μg/L   JJIND8 67,1303,81

MUT: otr-rat: lvr 100 μmol/L   CNREA8 43,5087,83

MUT: sce-hmn: lym 4400 μg/L   CNREA8 40,4775,80

MUT: sce-mus-ipr 20 mg/kg   MUREAV 157,181,85

CONSENSUS REPORTS: NTP Fourth Annual Report On Carcinogens, 1984. Community Right-To-Know List. EPA Genetic Toxicology Program. Reported in EPA TSCA Inventory.

OSHA PEL: Carcinogen

SAFETY PROFILE: Confirmed human carcinogen with experimental carcinogenic, neoplastigenic, tumorigenic, and teratogenic data. Moderately toxic by ingestion and intraperitoneal routes. Experimental reproductive effects. Human mutation data reported. When heated to decomposition it emits toxic fumes of NO_x.

FMV000 CAS: 50-00-0
FORMALDEHYDE
DOT: 1198/2209
mf: CH_2O mw: 30.03

PROP: Clear, water-white, very sltly acid gas or liquid; pungent odor. Pure formaldehyde is not available commercially because of its tendency to polymerize. It is sold as aqueous solutions containing from 37% to 50% formaldehyde by weight and varying amounts of methanol. Some alcoholic solns are used industrially and the physical properties and hazards may be greatly influenced by the solvent. Lel: 7.0%, uel: 73.0%, autoign temp: 806°F, d: 1.0, bp:

−3°F, flash p: (37% methanol-free): 185°F, flash p: (15% methanol-free): 122°F.

SYNS: ALDEHYDE FORMIQUE (FRENCH) ◇ ALDEIDE FORMICA (ITALIAN) ◇ BFV ◇ FA ◇ FANNOFORM ◇ FORMALDEHYD (CZECH, POLISH) ◇ FORMALDEHYDE, solution (DOT) ◇ FORMALIN ◇ FORMALIN 40 ◇ FORMALIN (DOT) ◇ FORMALINA (ITALIAN) ◇ FORMALINE (GERMAN) ◇ FORMALIN-LOESUNGEN (GERMAN) ◇ FORMALITH ◇ FORMIC ALDEHYDE ◇ FORMOL ◇ FYDE ◇ HOCH ◇ IVALON ◇ KARSAN ◇ LYSOFORM ◇ METHANAL ◇ METHYL ALDEHYDE ◇ METHYLENE GLYCOL ◇ METHYLENE OXIDE ◇ MORBOCID ◇ NCI-C02799 ◇ OPLOSSINGEN (DUTCH) ◇ OXOMETHANE ◇ OXY-METHYLENE ◇ PARAFORM ◇ POLYOXYMETHYLENE GLYCOLS ◇ RCRA WASTE NUMBER U122 ◇ SUPERLYSO-FORM

TOXICITY DATA with REFERENCE
CAR: ihl-rat TC:14 ppm/6H/84W-I   JJIND8 68,597,82
CAR: ihl-rat TC:15 ppm/6H/2Y-I   CIIT** DOCKET #10992,82
CAR: ihl-rat TC:15 ppm/6H/78W-I   CNREA8 49,3398,80
CAR: ihl-rat TC:15 ppm/6H/86W-I   TXAPA9 81,401,85
CAR: ihl-rat TCLo:14300 ppb/6H/2Y-I   CNREA8 43,4382,83
ETA: ihl-mus TC:15 ppm/6H/104W-I   EVSRBT 25,353,82
ETA: ihl-mus TCLo:14300 ppb/6H/2Y-I   CNREA8 43,4382,83
ETA: ihl-rat TC:6 ppm/6H/2Y-I   EVSRBT 25,353,82
ETA: ihl-rat TC:5600 ppb/6H/2Y-I   CNREA8 43,4382,83
ETA: ihl-rat TC:14300 ppb/6H/2Y-I   50EXAK -,111,83
ETA: ihl-rat TC:18750 μg/m³/2Y-I   GISAAA 48(4),60,83
ETA: scu-rat TD:350 mg/kg/78W-I   FAONAU 50A,77,72
ETA: scu-rat TDLo:1170 mg/kg/65W-I   GANNA2 45,451,54
MUT: dnd-hmn:fbr 100 μmol/L   ENMUDM 7,267,85
MUT: dnd-rat:oth 500 μmol/L   ENMUDM 8(Suppl 6),11,86
MUT: dni-esc 5 mmol/L   MUREAV 156,153,85
MUT: mma-mus:lym 25 mg/L   FCTOD7 23,115,85
MUT: mma-sat 5 μL/plate   BIMADU 6,129,85
MUT: sce-ham:lng 67 μmol/L   ARTODN 58,10,85
MUT: sln-dmg-par 2000 ppm   ENMUDM 7,677,85

CONSENSUS REPORTS: IARC Cancer Review: Human Inadequate Evidence IMEMDT 29,345,82; Animal Sufficient Evidence IMEMDT 29,345,82. NTP Fourth Annual Report On Carcinogens, 1984. EPA Genetic Toxicology Program. Reported in EPA TSCA Inventory.

OSHA PEL: TWA 1 ppm; STEL 2 ppm (For certain industries: TWA 3 ppm; CL 5 ppm; Pk 10 ppm/30M   ACGIH TLV: TWA 1 ppm; Suspected Human Carcinogen (Proposed: CL 0.3 ppm; Suspected Human Carcinogen)   DFG MAK: 0.5 ppm (0.6 mg/m³); Suspected Carcinogen.   NIOSH REL: (Formaldehyde) Limit to lowest feasible level.   DOT Classification: Combustible Liquid; Label: None; ORM-A; Label: None; Flammable or Combustible Liquid; Label: Flammable Liquid.

SAFETY PROFILE: Confirmed carcinogen with experimental carcinogenic, tumorigenic, and teratogenic data. Human poison by ingestion. Experimental poison by ingestion, skin contact, inhalation, intravenous, intraperitoneal, and subcutaneous routes. Human systemic effects by inhalation: lacrimation, olfactory changes, aggression and pulmonary changes. Experimental reproductive effects. Human mutation data reported. A human skin and eye irritant. Combustible liquid when exposed to heat or flame. To fight fire, stop flow of gas (for pure form); alcohol foam for 37 percent methanol-free form. When heated to decomposition it emits acrid smoke and fumes.

FOM050   CAS: 1332-10-1
FOWLER'S SOLUTION

SYNS: ARSENICAL SOLUTION ◇ POTASSIUM ARSENITE SOLUTION

CONSENSUS REPORTS: IARC Cancer Review: GROUP 1 IMEMDT 7,100,87.

SAFETY PROFILE: Confirmed carcinogen.

HAO875   CAS: 1317-60-8
HEMATITE

PROP: Consists mainly of Fe_2O_3 (IARC** 1,29,71).

SYNS: BLOOD STONE ◇ HAEMATITE ◇ IRON ORE ◇ RED IRON ORE

CONSENSUS REPORTS: NTP Fourth Annual Report on Carcinogens. IARC Cancer Review:

Group 3, Indefinite IMSUPP 4,254,82. Reported in EPA TSCA Inventory.

SAFETY PROFILE: Confirmed carcinogen.

HCB000   CAS: 13007-92-6
HEXACARBONYLCHROMIUM
mf: C_6CrO_6 mw: 220.06

SYN: CHROMIUM CARBONYL (MAK) ◇ CHROMIUM CARBONYL (OC-6-11) (9CI) ◇ CHROMIUM HEXACARBONYL ◇ HEXACARBONYL CHROMIUM

TOXICITY DATA with REFERENCE
ETA: imp-rat TDLo: 75 mg/kg   CNREA8 37,1476,77

CONSENSUS REPORTS: IARC Cancer Review: Animal Inadequate Evidence IMEMDT 23,205,80; Chromium and its compounds are on the Community Right-To-Know List. Reported in EPA TSCA Inventory.

OSHA PEL: CL 0.1 mg(CrO_3)/m^3 ACGIH TLV: TWA 0.05 mg(Cr)/m^3; Confirmed Human Carcinogen; (Proposed: TWA 0.001; Suspected Human Carcinogen)   DFG TRK: 0.1 mg/m^3 calculated as CrO_3 in that portion of dust that can possibly be inhaled; 0.2 mg/m^3 arc-welding by hand; others 0.1 mg/m^3. Animal Carcinogen, Suspected Human Carcinogen.   NIOSH REL: TWA 0.001 mg(Cr(VI))/m^3

SAFETY PROFILE: Confirmed carcinogen with experimental tumorigenic data. Poison by intravenous route. Explodes at 210°C. See also CHROMIUM COMPOUNDS and CARBONYLS.

HCC500   CAS: 118-74-1
HEXACHLOROBENZENE
DOT: 2729
mf: C_6Cl_6 mw: 284.76

PROP: Monoclinic prisms. Mp: 231°, bp: 323-326°, flash p: 468°F, vap press: 1 mm @ 114.4°, vap d: 9.8. D: 2.44. Insol in water, sol in benzene, very sltly sol in hot alcohol, sol in hot ether and chloroform.

SYNS: AMATIN ◇ ANTICARIE ◇ BUNT-CURE ◇ BUNT-NO-MORE ◇ CO-OP HEXA ◇ ESACHLOROBENZENE (ITALIAN) ◇ GRANOX NM ◇ HCB ◇ HEXA C.B. ◇ HEXACHLORBENZOL (GERMAN) ◇ JULIN'S CARBON CHLORIDE ◇ NO BUNT LIQUID ◇ PENTACHLOROPHENYL CHLORIDE ◇ PERCHLOROBENZENE ◇ PHENYL PERCHLORYL ◇ RCRA WASTE NUMBER U127 ◇ SAATBEIZ-FUNGIZID (GERMAN) ◇ SANOCIDE ◇ SMUT-GO ◇ SNIECIOTOX

TOXICITY DATA with REFERENCE
CAR: orl-ham TDLo: 1000 mg/kg/18W-C
   NATUAS 269,510,77
CAR: orl-rat TD: 5475 mg/kg/2Y-C   PAACA3 24,59,83
CAR: orl-rat TD: 6300 mg/kg/90W-C   CRNGDP 6,631,85
CAR: orl-rat TDLo: 2738 mg/kg/2Y-C   PAACA3 24,59,83
NEO: orl-ham TD: 3360 mg/kg/80W-C:CAR
   TXAPA9 41,155,77
NEO: orl-mus TDLo: 6972 mg/kg/83W-C
   IJCNAW 23,47,79
NEO: orl-rat TD: 1050 mg/kg/30W-C   CALEDQ 11,169,80
MUT: dnd-esc 20 μmol/L   MUREAV 89,95,81
MUT: mmo-smc 100 ppm   RSTUDV 6,161,76

CONSENSUS REPORTS: IARC Cancer Review: Animal Sufficient Evidence IMEMDT 20,155,79; Human Limited Evidence IMEMDT 20,155,79. NTP Fourth Annual Report On Carcinogens, 1984. Community Right-To-Know List. Reported in EPA TSCA Inventory. EPA Genetic Toxicology Program.

DFG MAK: BAT: 15 μg/dL in plasma/serum. DOT Classification: IMO: Poison B; Label: St. Andrews Cross.

SAFETY PROFILE: Confirmed carcinogen with experimental carcinogenic, neoplastigenic, and teratogenic data. A human poison by an unspecified route. A suspected human carcinogenic. Experimental reproductive effects. Mildly toxic experimentally by inhalation. Mutation data reported. A fungicide. Combustible when exposed to heat or flame. To fight fire, use CO_2, dry chemical. When heated to decomposition it emits highly toxic fumes of Cl^-.

HEK000   CAS: 680-31-9
HEXAMETHYL PHOSPHORAMIDE
mf: $C_6H_{18}N_3OP$ mw: 179.24

PROP: Clear, colorless, mobile liquid, spicy odor. Bp: 233°, fp: 6°, d: 1.024 @ 25°/25°, vap d: 6.18.

SYNS: ENT 50,882 ◇ HEXAMETAPOL ◇ HEXAMETHYL-PHOSPHORIC ACID TRIAMIDE (MAK) ◇ HEXAMETHYL-PHOSPHORIC TRIAMIDE ◇ N,N,N,N,N,N-HEXAMETHYL-PHOSPHORIC TRIAMIDE ◇ HEXAMETHYLPHOS-PHOROTRIAMIDE ◇ HEXAMETHYLPHOSPHOTRIAMIDE ◇ HEXMETHYLPHOSPHORAMIDE ◇ HMPA ◇ HMPT ◇ HPT ◇ MEMPA ◇ PHOSPHORIC TRIS(DIMETHYL-AMIDE) ◇ PHOSPHORYL HEXAMETHYLTRIAMIDE

◇ TRI(DIMETHYLAMINO)PHOSPHINEOXIDE ◇ TRIS(DI-METHYLAMINO)PHOSPHINE OXIDE ◇ TRIS(DI-METHYLAMINO)PHOSPHORUS OXIDE

TOXICITY DATA with REFERENCE
CAR: ihl-rat TC:100 ppb/6H/26W-I   JJIND8
68,157,82
CAR: ihl-rat TC:100 ppb/26W-C   AJPAA4
106,8,82
CAR: ihl-rat TC:400 ppb/6H/43W-I   JJIND8
68,157,82
CAR: ihl-rat TC:400 ppb/35W-I   SCIEAS
190,422,75
CAR: ihl-rat TC:4000 ppb/39W-C   AJPAA4
106,8,82
CAR: ihl-rat TCLo:50 ppb/52W-C   AJPAA4
106,8,82
ETA: ihl-rat TC:50 ppb/6H/52W-I   ENVRAL
33,106,84
ETA: ihl-rat TD:50 ppb/6H/52W-I   TXAPA9
62,90,82
ETA: ihl-rat TD:100 ppb/6H/26W-I   TXAPA9
62,90,82
MUT: cyt-hmn:lym 500 mg/L   MUREAV 156,19,85
MUT: dns-hmn:hla 125 mg/L   PMRSDJ 5,375,85
MUT: otr-ham:emb 400 mg/L   PMRSDJ 5,665,85
MUT: sce-rat:lvr 2 g/L   PMRSDJ 5,287,85
MUT: slt-dmg-orl 560 μmol/L   PMRSDJ 5,313,85

CONSENSUS REPORTS: IARC Cancer Review: Animal Sufficient Evidence IMEMDT 15,211,77. NTP Fourth Annual Report On Carcinogens, 1984. Community Right-To-Know List. Reported in EPA TSCA Inventory. EPA Genetic Toxicology Program.

ACGIH TLV: Suspected Human Carcinogen. DFG MAK: Animal Carcinogen, Suspected Human Carcinogen.

SAFETY PROFILE: Confirmed carcinogen with experimental carcinogenic and tumorigenic data. Moderately toxic by ingestion, skin contact, intraperitoneal, and intravenous routes. Experimental reproductive effects. Human mutation data reported. When heated to decomposition it emits very toxic fumes of phosphine, PO_x, and NO_x.

HGS000   CAS: 302-01-2
HYDRAZINE
DOT: 2029/2030
mf: H_4N_2 mw: 32.06

PROP: Colorless, oily, fuming liquid or white crystals. Mp: 1.4°, bp: 113.5°, flash p: 100°F

(OC), d: 1.1011 @ 15° (liquid), autoign temp: can vary from 74°F in contact with iron rust, 270°F in contact with black iron, 313°F in contact with stainless steel, 518°F in contact with glass. Vap d: 1.1; lel: 4.7%, uel: 100%.

SYNS: ANHYDROUS HYDRAZINE (DOT) ◇ DIAMIDE ◇ DIAMINE ◇ HYDRAZINE, ANHYDROUS (DOT) ◇ HYDRAZINE, AQUEOUS SOLUTION (DOT) ◇ HYDRAZINE BASE ◇ HYDRAZYNA (POLISH) ◇ RCRA WASTE NUMBER U133

TOXICITY DATA with REFERENCE
CAR: ihl-rat TCLo:5 ppm/6H/1Y-I   FAATDF
5,1050,85
CAR: ipr-mus TDLo:400 mg/kg/5W-I   UICMAI
7,180,67
NEO: orl-mus TDLo:1951 mg/kg/2Y-C
IJCNAW 9,109,72
ETA: ihl-ham TCLo:1 ppm/6H/1Y-I   .FAATDF
5,1050,85
ETA: ihl-ham TCLo:5 ppm/6H/1Y-I   PAACA3
21,74,80
ETA: ihl-mus TCLo:1 ppm/6H/1Y-I   PAACA3
21,74,80
ETA: ihl-rat TC:5 ppm/6H/1Y-I   PAACA321,74,80
ETA: ihl-rat TCLo:1 ppm/6H/1Y-I   PAACA3
21,74,80
MUT: dnd-ham:orl 15 mg/kg   PAACA3 24,59,83
MUT: dnd-rat:lvr 3 mmol/L   MUREAV 113,357,83
MUT: dni-hmn:hla 50 μmol/L   CNREA8 44,59,84
MUT: dni-rat-orl 60 mg/kg   CRNGDP 4,953,83
MUT: mmo-omi 70 μg/L   MUREAV 173,233,86
MUT: msc-mus:lym 1 mmol/L   MUREAV89,321,81
MUT: otr-ham:kdy 80 μg/L   BJCAAI 37,873,78
MUT: sce-ham:lng 1 mmol/L   HUGEDQ 54,155,80

CONSENSUS REPORTS: IARC Cancer Review: Animal Sufficient Evidence IMEMDT 4,127,74. NTP Fourth Annual Report On Carcinogens, 1984. EPA Extremely Hazardous Substances List. Community Right-To-Know List. Genetic Toxicology Program. Reported in EPA TSCA Inventory.

OSHA PEL: (Transitional: TWA 1 ppm (skin)) TWA 0.1 ppm (skin)   ACGIH TLV: TWA 0.1 ppm (skin); Suspected Human Carcinogen; (Proposed: 0.01 ppm (skin); Suspected Human Carcinogen) DFG TRK: 0.1 ppm; Animal Carcinogen, Suspected Human Carcinogen. NIOSH REL: (Hydrazines) CL 0.04 mg/m³/2H DOT Classification: Flammable Liquid; Label: Flammable Liquid and Poison; Corrosive Material; Label: Corrosive, aqueous solution.

SAFETY PROFILE: Confirmed carcinogen with experimental carcinogenic, neoplastigenic, and tumorigenic data. A poison by ingestion, skin contact, intraperitoneal, intravenous and possibly other routes. Moderately toxic by inhalation. An experimental teratogen. Other experimental reproductive effects. Human mutation data reported. A powerful reducing agent which is corrosive to the eyes, skin, and mucous membranes. Flammable liquid. The vapor will burn without air. It is a powerful explosive. It is very sensitive and must not be used without full and complete instructions from the manufacturer for handling, storage and disposal. Dangerous; when heated to decomposition it emits highly toxic fumes of NO_x and NH_3.

HGW500 CAS: 10034-93-2
HYDRAZINE SULFATE (1:1)
mf: $H_4N_2 \cdot H_2O_4S$ mw: 130.14

PROP: Colorless crystals. D: 1.378, mp: 85°. Sol in water, insol in alcohol. Very sol in hot water.

SYNS: HYDRAZINE HYDROGEN SULFATE ◇ HYDRAZINE MONOSULFATE ◇ HYDRAZINE SULPHATE ◇ HYDRAZINIUM SULFATE ◇ HYDRAZONIUM SULFATE ◇ HS ◇ IDRAZINA SOLFATO (ITALIAN) ◇ NSC-150014 ◇ SIRAN HYDRAZINU (CZECH)

TOXICITY DATA with REFERENCE
CAR: orl-mus TD: 18524 mg/kg/84W-I JCROD7 105,258,83
CAR: orl-mus TDLo: 19 g/kg/61W-C JNCIAM 41,331,68
CAR: orl-rat TDLo: 43 g/kg/85W-C JNCIAM 41,331,68
NEO: orl-mus TD: 226 mg/kg TUMOAB 72,125,86
NEO: orl-mus TD: 1280 mg/kg/4W-I BJCAAI 18,543,64
NEO: orl-mus TD: 1664 mg/kg/8W-I JNCIAM 42,337,69
NEO: orl-mus TD: 18480 mg/kg/84W-I JCROD7 105,258,83
NEO: orl-rat TD: 38 g/kg/68W-I JNCIAM41,331,68
ETA: ipr-mus TD: 475 mg/kg/5W-I IJCNAW 4,318,69
ETA: ipr-mus TD: 950 mg/kg/10W-I IJCNAW 4,318,69
ETA: ipr-mus TDLo: 832 mg/kg/8W-I JNCIAM 42,337,69
ETA: orl-mus TD: 11 g/kg/46W-I NATUAS 194,488,62
ETA: orl-mus TD: 14080 mg/kg/64W-I CALEDQ 17,75,82

MUT: cyt-ham: ovr 1167 mg/L PMRSDJ 1,551,81
MUT: dnd-ham-orl 1035 mg/kg/9W-I TXAPA9 70,324,83
MUT: dnr-bcs 20 μL/disc MUREAV 97,1,82
MUT: dns-hmn: fbr 1 mg/L PMRSDJ 1,528,81
MUT: mmo-omi 1500 μg/L MUREAV 173,233,86
MUT: otr-ham: kdy 2500 μg/L PMRSDJ 1,638,81
MUT: sce-ham: lng 100 nmol/L MUREAV 118,103,83

CONSENSUS REPORTS: IARC Cancer Review: Animal Sufficient Evidence IMEMDT 4,127,74. NTP Fourth Annual Report On Carcinogens, 1984. Community Right-To-Know List. Reported in EPA TSCA Inventory. EPA Genetic Toxicology Program.

NIOSH REL: (Hydrazines) CL 0.04 mg/m^3/2H

SAFETY PROFILE: Confirmed carcinogen with experimental carcinogenic, neoplastigenic, and tumorigenic data. A poison by ingestion and intraperitoneal routes. Human systemic effects by ingestion: paresthesia (abnormal sensations), somnolence, nausea or vomiting. Human mutation data reported. An eye irritant. A reducing agent. When heated to decomposition it emits very toxic fumes of SO_x and NO_x.

HHG000 CAS: 122-66-7
HYDRAZOBENZENE
mf: $C_{12}H_{12}N_2$ mw: 184.26

PROP: Light or yellow crystals from ethanol. D: 1.58, mp: 131°, bp: decomp. Very sltly sol in water, insol in acetylene.

SYNS: N,N'-BIANILINE ◇ sym-DIPHENYLHYDRAZINE ◇ 1,2-DIPHENYLHYDRAZINE ◇ HYDRAZOBENZEN (CZECH) ◇ HYDRAZODIBENZENE ◇ NCI-C01854 ◇ RCRA WASTE NUMBER U109

TOXICITY DATA with REFERENCE
CAR: orl-mus TDLo: 26 g/kg/78W-C NCITR* NCI-CG-TR-92,78
CAR: orl-rat TD: 9820 mg/kg/78W-C NCITR* NCI-CG-TR-92,78
CAR: orl-rat TDLo: 2620 mg/kg/78W-C NCITR* NCI-CG-TR-92,78
ETA: orl-rat TD: 36 g/kg/53W-I: TER VOONAW 20(4),53,74
ETA: scu-mus TDLo: 8400 mg/kg/38W-I VOONAW 20(4),53,74
ETA: scu-rat TD: 16 g/kg/1Y-I CANCAR 3,789,50
ETA: scu-rat TDLo: 6 g/kg/27W-I: TER VOONAW 20(4),53,74
ETA: skn-mus TDLo: 5280 mg/kg/26W-I VOONAW 20(4),53,74

MUT: dni-mus-ipr 100 mg/kg   MUREAV 46,305,77
MUT: mma-sat 10 ng/plate   ENMUDM 7(Suppl 5),1,85

CONSENSUS REPORTS: NTP Fourth Annual Report On Carcinogens, 1984. NCI Carcinogenesis Bioassay (feed); Clear Evidence: mouse, rat NCITR* NCI-CG-TR-92,78. Community Right-To-Know List. Reported in EPA TSCA Inventory.

SAFETY PROFILE: Confirmed carcinogen with experimental carcinogenic and tumorigenic data. Poison by ingestion. Mutation data reported. When heated to decomposition it emits toxic fumes of NO_x.

HJQ350   CAS: 3817-11-6
4-HYDROXYBUTYLBUTYLNITRO-SAMINE
mf: $C_8H_{18}N_2O_2$ mw: 174.28

SYNS: BBN ◇ BBNOH ◇ BHBN ◇ BUTANOL (4)-BUTYL-NITROSAMINE ◇ BUTYL-BUTANOL(4)-NITROSAMIN ◇ BUTYL-BUTANOL-NITROSAMINE ◇ N-BUTYL-N-(4-HYDROXYBUTYL)NITROSAMINE ◇ n-BUTYL-(4-HYDROXYBUTYL)NITROSAMINE ◇ 4-(BUTYLNITROSAMINO)-1-BUTANOL ◇ 4-(n-BUTYLNITROSAMINO)-1-BUTANOL ◇ DIBUTYLAMINE, 4-HYDROXY-N-NITROSO- ◇ HBBN ◇ NBHA ◇ N-NITROSO-n-BUTYL-(4-HYDROXYBUTYL)A-MINE ◇ OH-BBN

TOXICITY DATA with REFERENCE
CAR: orl-dog TDLo: 10 g/kg/2Y-C   CNREA8 41,1958,81
CAR: orl-mus TD: 1200 mg/kg/10W-I   CRNGDP 2,251,81
CAR: orl-mus TD: 1820 mg/kg/26W-C   CNREA8 46,2001,86
CAR: orl-mus TD: 2400 mg/kg/8W-I   CRNGDP 3,1473,82
CAR: orl-mus TDLo: 800 mg/kg/10W-I   CRNGDP 2,251,81
CAR: orl-rat TD: 12 g/kg/43W-C   ARPTAF 41(12),23,79
CAR: orl-rat TD: 280 mg/kg/4W-C   CRNGDP 4,895,83
CAR: orl-rat TD: 1348 mg/kg/8W-C   BJCAAI 45,474,82
CAR: orl-rat TD: 1400 mg/kg/8W-C   NASDA6 33,1,82
CAR: orl-rat TD: 1638 mg/kg/20W-C   JJIND8 79,263,87
CAR: orl-rat TD: 2100 mg/kg/6W-C   URLRA5 3,73,75
CAR: orl-rat TD: 2800 mg/kg/8W-C   GTKRDX 9,836,82

CAR: orl-rat TDLo: 560 mg/kg/8W-C   GANNA2 71,138,80
CAR: scu-ham TDLo: 22500 mg/kg/75W-I   CDPRD4 4,79,81
NEO: scu-ham TDLo: 100 mg/kg (14D post)   ZEKBAI 90,119,77
MUT: cyt-ham: lng 900 mg/L/27H   MUREAV 66,277,79
MUT: mma-sat 10 μmol/plate   MUREAV 140,147,84
MUT: sce-rat: lvr 1500 μmol/L   MUREAV 93,409,82

CONSENSUS REPORTS: IARC Cancer Review: Animal Sufficient Evidence IMEMDT 17,51,78

SAFETY PROFILE: Confirmed carcinogen with experimental carcinogenic and neoplastigenic data. Moderately toxic by ingestion. Mutation data reported. When heated to decomposition it emits toxic fumes of NO_x.

HKC500   CAS: 124-65-2
HYDROXYDIMETHYLARSINE OXIDE, SODIUM SALT
DOT: 1688
mf: $C_2H_6AsO_2 \cdot Na$ mw: 159.99

SYNS: ALKARSODYL ◇ ANSAR 160 ◇ ARSECODILE ◇ ARSYCODILE ◇ BOLLS-EYE ◇ CACODYLATE de SODIUM (FRENCH) ◇ CACODYLIC ACID SODIUM SALT ◇ CHEMAID ◇ ((DIMETHYLARSINO)OXY)SODIUM-As-OXIDE ◇ DUTCH-TREAT ◇ PHYTAR 560 ◇ RAD-E CATE 16 ◇ SILVISAR ◇ SODIUM CACODYLATE (DOT) ◇ SODIUM DIMETHYLAR-SINATE ◇ SODIUM DIMETHYLARSONATE ◇ SODIUM SALT of CACODYLIC ACID

CONSENSUS REPORTS: Arsenic and its compounds are on the Community Right-To-Know List. EPA Extremely Hazardous Substances List. Reported in EPA TSCA Inventory.

OSHA PEL: TWA 0.5 mg(As)/m^3 ACGIH TLV: TWA 0.2 mg(As)/m^3 DOT Classification: IMO: Poison B; Label: Poison.

SAFETY PROFILE: Confirmed human carcinogen. Poison by ingestion. Moderately toxic by subcutaneous route. Experimental teratogenic and other reproductive effects. When heated to decomposition it emits toxic fumes of As and Na_2O.

IAQ000   CAS: 96-45-7
2-IMIDAZOLIDINETHIONE
mf: $C_3H_6N_2S$ mw: 102.17

PROP: White crystals. Water solubility: 9 g/100 mL @ 30°. Often occurs as a main degradation product of the metal salts of ethylene bis-dithiocarbamic acid.

SYNS: 4,5-DIHYDROIMIDAZOLE-2(3H)-THIONE ◇ ETHYLENE THIOUREA ◇ N,N'-ETHYLENETHIOUREA ◇ 1,3-ETHYLENE-2-THIOUREA ◇ l'ETHYLENE THIOUREE (FRENCH) ◇ ETU ◇ 2-MERCAPTOIMIDAZOLINE ◇ 2-MER-KAPTOIMIDAZOLIN (CZECH) ◇ NA-22 ◇ NCI-C03372 ◇ PENNAC CRA ◇ RCRA WASTE NUMBER U116 ◇ RODANIN S-62 (CZECH) ◇ SODIUM-22 NEOPRENE AC-CELERATOR ◇ 2-THIOL-DIHYDROGLYOXALINE ◇ USAF EL-62 ◇ VULKACIT NPV/C2 ◇ WARECURE C

TOXICITY DATA with REFERENCE
CAR: orl-mus TDLo:77 g/kg/82W-C   JNCIAM 42,1101,69
CAR: orl-rat TD:44 g/kg/2Y-C:TER   EJTXAZ 9,303,76
CAR: orl-rat TD:146 g/kg/2Y-C   EJTXAZ9,303,76
CAR: orl-rat TD:9125 mg/kg/2Y-C   FCTXAV 13,493,75
CAR: orl-rat TD:11466 mg/kg/78W-C   JJIND8 67,75,81
CAR: orl-rat TDLo:5306 mg/kg/77W-C   JNCIAM 49,583,72
MUT: dnd-bcs 2 mg/disc   PMRSDJ 1,175,81
MUT: mma-esc 200 mg/L   PMRSDJ 1,396,81
MUT: mma-sat 3333 μg/plate   ENMUDM 8(Suppl 7),1,86
MUT: otr-ham:kdy 80 μg/L   BJCAAI 37,873,78

CONSENSUS REPORTS: IARC Cancer Review: Animal Sufficient Evidence IMEMDT 7,45,74. NTP Fourth Annual Report On Carcinogens, 1984. Community Right-To-Know List. EPA Genetic Toxicology Program. Reported in EPA TSCA Inventory.

NIOSH REL: (ETU) Use encapsulated form; minimize exposure.

SAFETY PROFILE: Confirmed carcinogen with experimental carcinogenic data. Poison by ingestion and intraperitoneal routes. Experimental teratogenic and reproductive effects. Mutation data reported. An eye irritant. When heated to decomposition it emits very toxic fumes of NO_x and SO_x.

IBA000　　　CAS: 2465-27-2
4,4'-(IMIDOCARBONYL)BIS(N,N-DIMETHYLAMINE) MONOHYDROCHLORIDE
mf: $C_{17}H_{21}N_3 \cdot ClH \cdot H_2O$　　mw: 321.89

SYNS: ADC AURAMINE O ◇ AIZEN AURAMINE ◇ AURAMINE (MAK) ◇ AURAMINE HYDROCHLORIDE

◇ AURAMINE O (BIOLOGICAL STAIN) ◇ AURAMINE YELLOW ◇ 4,4'-BIS(DIMETHYLAMINO)BENZHYDRYL-IDENIMINE HYDROCHLORIDE ◇ 4,4'-BIS(DIMETHYL-AMINO)BENZOPHENONE-IMINE HYDROCHLORIDE ◇ 1,1-BIS(p-DIMETHYLAMINOPHENYL)METHYL-ENIMINEHYDROCHLORIDE ◇ CALCOZINE YELLOW OX ◇ 4,4'-CARBONIMIDOYLBIS(N,N-DIMETHYL-BENZENAMINE)MONOHYDROCHLORIDE ◇ C.I. 41000 ◇ C.I. BASIC YELLOW 2 ◇ C.I. BASIC YELLOW 2, MONO-HYDROCHLORIDE ◇ MITSUI AURAMINE O

TOXICITY DATA with REFERENCE
NEO: orl-mus TDLo:73 g/kg/52W-C   BJCAAI 16,87,62
NEO: orl-rat TDLo:40 g/kg/87W-C   BJCAAI 16,87,62
ETA: scu-rat TDLo:440 mg/kg/21W-I   BJCAAI 16,87,62
MUT: dnd-esc 30 ppm   MUREAV 89,95,81
MUT: dnd-hmn:fbr 300 μmol/L   JTEHD69,941,82
MUT: dnd-rat:lvr 3 μmol/L   SinJF# 26OCT82
MUT: mma-sat 2 mg/plate   CRNGDP 2,1317,81
MUT: sce-mus-ipr 7500 μg/kg   JTEHD6 9,941,82

CONSENSUS REPORTS: Reported in EPA TSCA Inventory. EPA Genetic Toxicology Program.

DFG MAK: Animal Carcinogen, Suspected Human Carcinogen.

SAFETY PROFILE: Confirmed carcinogen with experimental neoplastigenic and tumorigenic data. Poison by skin contact, ingestion, and intraperitoneal routes. Human mutation data reported. A chelating agent which might disturb trace element metabolism if taken into the body. Used as a biological stain. When heated to decomposition it emits very toxic fumes of NO_x and HCl.

IBB000　　　CAS: 492-80-8
4,4'-(IMIDOCARBONYL)BIS(N,N-DIMETHYLANILINE)
mf: $C_{17}H_{21}N_3$　　mw: 267.41

PROP: Yellow needles. Mp: 136°. Insol in water.

SYNS: APYONINE AURAMINE BASE ◇ AURAMINE (MAK) ◇ AURAMINE BASE ◇ BIS(p-DIMETHYLAMINOPHE-NYL)METHYLENEIMINE ◇ BRILLIANT OIL YELLOW ◇ 4,4'-CARBONIMIDOYLBIS(N,N-DIMETHYLBENZEN-AMINE) ◇ C.I. 41000B ◇ C.I. BASIC YELLOW 2, FREE BASE ◇ C.I. SOLVENT YELLOW 34 ◇ 4,4'-DIMETHY-LAMINOBENZOPHENONIMIDE ◇ GLAURAMINE ◇ RCRA WASTE NUMBER U014 ◇ TETRAMETHYL-

DIAMINODIPHENYLACETIMINE ◇ WAXOLINE
YELLOW O ◇ YELLOW PYOCTANINE

TOXICITY DATA with REFERENCE
NEO: orl-mus TDLo:29 g/kg/52W   BJCAAI
10,653,56
ETA: orl-mus TD:42 g/kg/50W-C   AICCA6
19,483,63
ETA: orl-rat TDLo:37 g/kg/87W-C   AICCA6
19,483,63
ETA: scu-rat TDLo:263 mg/kg/21W-C   AICCA6
19,483,63
MUT: dns-hmn:fbr 20 mg/L   TXCYAC 21,151,81
MUT: mma-sat 250 μg/plate   PMRSDJ 1,333,81
MUT: otr-ham:emb 2 mg/L   NCIMAV 58,243,81
MUT: otr-ham:kdy 13100 μg/L   PMRSDJ 1,626,81
MUT: otr-rat-orl 150 mg/kg   CNREA8 40,1157,80

CONSENSUS REPORTS: IARC Cancer Review: Human Sufficient Evidence IMEMDT 1,69,72; Animal Sufficient Evidence IMEMDT 1,69,72. Community Right-To-Know List. Reported in EPA TSCA Inventory.

DFG MAK: Animal Carcinogen, Suspected Human Carcinogen.

SAFETY PROFILE: Confirmed human carcinogen with experimental carcinogenic, neoplastigenic, and tumorigenic data. Poison by intraperitoneal route. Human mutation data reported. Used as an antiseptic. When heated to decomposition it emits toxic fumes of NO_x.

IBZ000   CAS: 193-39-5
INDENO(1,2,3-cd)PYRENE
mf: $C_{22}H_{12}$ mw: 276.34

SYNS: 2,3-PHENYLENEPYRENE ◇ 2,3-o-PHENYLENEPYRENE ◇ 1,10-(o-PHENYLENE)PYRENE ◇ 1,10-(1,2-PHENYLENE)PYRENE ◇ RCRA WASTE NUMBER U137

TOXICITY DATA with REFERENCE
CAR: imp-rat TD:20750 μg/kg   JJIND8 71,539,83
CAR: imp-rat TDLo:4150 μg/kg   JJIND8 71,539,83
CAR: scu-mus TDLo:72 mg/kg/9W-I   AICCA6
19,490,63
ETA: imp-rat TD:5 mg/kg   50NNAZ 7,571,83
ETA: skn-mus TDLo:40 mg/kg/20D-I   CRNGDP
7,1761,86
MUT: mma-sat 3 μg/plate/48H   FCTXAV 17,141,79
MUT: otr-ham:lng 100 μg/L   TXCYAC 17,149,80

CONSENSUS REPORTS: IARC Cancer Review: Animal Sufficient Evidence IMEMDT 32,373,83; IMEMDT 3,229,73. NTP Fourth Annual Report On Carcinogens, 1984. Reported in EPA TSCA Inventory.

SAFETY PROFILE: Confirmed carcinogen with experimental carcinogenic and tumorigenic data. Mutation data reported. When heated to decomposition it emits acrid smoke and fumes.

IGM000   CAS: 10102-50-8
IRON(II) ARSENATE (3:2)
DOT: 1608
mf: $As_2O_8 \cdot 3Fe$ mw: 445.39

SYNS: ARSENATE of IRON, FERROUS ◇ FERROUS ARSENATE (DOT) ◇ FERROUS ARSENATE, SOLID (DOT) ◇ IRON ARSENATE (DOT)

CONSENSUS REPORTS: Arsenic and its compounds are on the Community Right-To-Know List.

OSHA PEL: TWA 0.01 mg(As)/m³; Cancer Hazard   ACGIH TLV: TWA 0.2 mg(As)/m³; TWA 1 mg/(Fe)/m³   NIOSH REL: (Inorganic Arsenic) CL 0.002 mg(As)/m³/15M   DOT Classification: Poison B; Label: Poison.

SAFETY PROFILE: Confirmed human carcinogen. A deadly poison by various routes. A pesticide. When heated to decomposition it emits toxic fumes of As.

IGN000   CAS: 10102-49-5
IRON(III) ARSENATE (1:1)
DOT: 1606
mf: $AsO_4 \cdot Fe$ mw: 194.77

SYNS: ARSENATE of IRON, FERRIC ◇ FERRIC ARSENATE, SOLID (DOT)

CONSENSUS REPORTS: Arsenic and its compounds are on the Community Right-To-Know List.

OSHA PEL: TWA 0.01 mg(As)/m³; Cancer Hazard   ACGIH TLV: TWA 0.2 mg(As)/m³; TWA 1 mg/(Fe)/m³   NIOSH REL: (Inorganic Arsenic) CL 0.002 mg(As)/m³/15M   DOT Classification: Poison B; Label: Poison.

SAFETY PROFILE: Confirmed human carcinogen. A deadly poison. A pesticide. When heated to decomposition it emits toxic fumes of As.

IGO000   CAS: 63989-69-5
IRON(III)-o-ARSENITE PENTAHYDRATE
DOT: 1607
mf: $As_2Fe_2O_6 \cdot Fe_2O_3 \cdot 5H_2O$ mw: 607.34

PROP: Brown-yellow powder.

SYNS: FERRIC ARSENITE, BASIC ◇ FERRIC ARSENITE, SOLID (DOT)

CONSENSUS REPORTS: Arsenic and its compounds are on the Community Right-To-Know List.

OSHA PEL: TWA 0.01 mg(As)/m³; Cancer Hazard ACGIH TLV: TWA 0.2 mg(As)/m³; TWA 1 mg/(Fe)/m³ NIOSH REL: (Inorganic Arsenic) CL 0.002 mg(As)/m³/15M DOT Classification: Poison B; Label: Poison.

SAFETY PROFILE: Confirmed human carcinogen. A deadly poison. When heated to decomposition it emits toxic fumes of As.

IGS000   CAS: 9004-66-4
IRON-DEXTRAN COMPLEX

PROP: For human use, it is a sterile dark brown colloidal solvent, water-soluble. Approximate molecular weight is 180,000 (IARC** 2, 161,72).

SYNS: A 100 (PHARMACEUTICAL) ◇ CHINOFER ◇ DEXTRAN ION COMPLEX ◇ DEXTROFER 75 ◇ EISENDEXTRAN (GERMAN) ◇ Fe-DEXTRAN ◇ FENATE ◇ FERDEX 100 ◇ FERRIC DEXTRAN ◇ FERRIDEXTRAN ◇ FERRODEXTRAN ◇ FERROFLUKIN 75 ◇ FERROGLUCIN ◇ FERROGLUKIN 75 ◇ IMFERON ◇ IMPOSIL ◇ IRO-JEX ◇ IRON DEXTRAN ◇ IRON DEXTRAN INJECTION ◇ IRON HYDROGENATED DEXTRAN ◇ IRONORM INJECTION ◇ MYOFER 100 ◇ POLYFER ◇ PROLONGAL ◇ RCRA WASTE NUMBER U139 ◇ URSOFERRAN

TOXICITY DATA with REFERENCE
CAR: ims-wmn TD:52 mg(Fe)/kg/6W-I
   BMJOAE 1,1411,60
CAR: scu-rat TD:1500 mg(Fe)/kg/8W-I
   IJCNAW 2,370,67
CAR: scu-rat TD:2400 mg(Fe)/kg/24W-I
   BJCAAI 18,801,64
CAR: scu-rat TDLo:750 mg(Fe)/kg/4W-I
   IJCNAW 2,370,67
NEO: ims-rat TD:3760 mg(Fe)/kg/47W-I
   BMJOAE 1,947,59
NEO: ims-rat TDLo:1150 mg/kg/17W-I
   BJCAAI 15,838,61
NEO: ims-wmn TDLo:20 mg/kg/3Y-I   BMJOAE
   2,277,73
ETA: ims-mus TDLo:2 g(Fe)/kg/9W-I   BJCAAI
   21,448,67
ETA: ims-rbt TDLo:28 g/kg/27W-I   BMJOAE
   1,1593,67
ETA: scu-ham TDLo:40 g/kg/10W-I   JNCIAM
   24,109,60
ETA: scu-mus TD:104 mg/kg/13W-I   JNCIAM
   24,109,60

ETA: scu-mus TD:1120 mg(Fe)/kg/28W-I
   BMJOAE 1,1800,62
ETA: scu-mus TDLo:2300 mg/kg/I   BECCAN
   40,30,62
ETA: scu-rat TD:104 g/kg/26W-I   JNCIAM
   24,109.60

CONSENSUS REPORTS: IARC Cancer Review: Human Inadequate Evidence IMEMDT 2,161,73; Animal Sufficient Evidence IMEMDT 2,161,73. NTP Fourth Annual Report On Carcinogens, 1984.

SAFETY PROFILE: Confirmed carcinogen producing tumors at site of application. Experimental carcinogenic, neoplastigenic, tumorigenic, and teratogenic data. Moderately toxic by ingestion and several other routes. Other experimental reproductive effects.

IHE000
IRON OXIDE, CHROMIUM OXIDE, and NICKEL OXIDE FUME

PROP: Fume composed of iron(+3) oxide: chromium(+3) oxide:nickel(+2)oxide, 6:1:1 (BJIMAG 29,169,72).

SYNS: CHROMIUM OXIDE, NICKEL OXIDE, and IRON OXIDE FUME ◇ NICKEL OXIDE, IRON OXIDE, and CHROMIUM OXIDE FUME

CONSENSUS REPORTS: Nickel and its compounds, as well as chromium and its compounds, are on the Community Right-To-Know List.

OSHA PEL: TWA 1 mg(Ni)/m³; CL 0.1 mg (CrO₃)/m³ ACGIH TLV: TWA 1 mg(Ni)/m³; (Proposed: TWA 0.05 mg(Ni)/m³; Human Carcinogen); 0.05 mg(Cr)/m³ NIOSH REL: (Chromium (VI)) TWA 0.025 mg(Cr(VI))/m³; CL 0.05/15M; (Inorganic Nickel) TWA 0.015 mg(Ni)/m³

SAFETY PROFILE: Confirmed human carcinogen. Human systemic effects by inhalation: cough.

IHG000   CAS: 8047-67-4
IRON OXIDE, SACCHARATED

PROP: Saccharated oxide of iron (JNCIAM 24,109,60).

SYNS: COLLIRON I.V. ◇ FEOJECTIN ◇ FERRIC OXIDE, SACCHARATED ◇ FERRIC SACCHARATE IRON OXIDE (MIX.) ◇ FERRIVENIN ◇ IRON SACCHARATE ◇ IRON SUGAR ◇ IVIRON ◇ NEO-FERRUM ◇ PROFERRIN

◇ SACCHARATED FERRIC OXIDE ◇ SACCHARATED IRON ◇ SUCROFER

TOXICITY DATA with REFERENCE

NEO: ims-rat TDLo: 148 g/kg/74W   BMJOAE 1,947,59

ETA: scu-mus TD: 150 g/kg/I   BECCAN 40,30,62

ETA: scu-mus TDLo: 104 g/kg/13W-I   JNCIAM 24,109,60

CONSENSUS REPORTS: IARC Cancer Review: Animal Sufficient Evidence IMEMDT 2,161,73.

SAFETY PROFILE: Confirmed carcinogen with experimental neoplastigenic and tumorigenic data. A poison by intravenous route.

ISR000   CAS: 62-56-6
ISOTHIOUREA
DOT: 2877

mf: CH_4N_2S mw: 76.13

PROP: White powder or crystals. Mp: 177°, bp: decomp, d: 1.405.

SYNS: PSEUDOTHIOUREA ◇ RCRA WASTE NUMBER U219 ◇ SULOUREA ◇ THIOCARBAMATE ◇ THIOCAR-BAMIDE ◇ β-THIOPSEUDOUREA ◇ THIOUREA (DOT) ◇ 2-THIOUREA ◇ THU ◇ TSIZP 34 ◇ USAF EK-497

TOXICITY DATA with REFERENCE

CAR: mul-rat TDLo: 151 g/kg/52W-I   CNREA8 17,302,57

CAR: orl-rat TDLo: 78 g/kg/56W-C   CNREA8 17,302,57

NEO: orl-rat TD: 18 g/kg/2Y-C   SCIEAS 108,626,48

ETA: mul-rat TD: 179 g/kg/1Y-I   CNREA8 14,494,54

ETA: orl-rat TD: 40 g/kg/2Y-C   SCIEAS 108,626,48

ETA: orl-rat TD: 90 g/kg/1Y-I   BJEPA5 28,46,47

ETA: orl-rat TD: 1950 mg/kg/2Y-C   TXAPA9 11,88,67

MUT: dnd-esc 20 μmol/L   MUREAV 89,95,81

MUT: dni-hmn: lym 20 mmol/L   PNASA6 79,1171,82

MUT: hma-mus/sat 125 mg/kg   JNCIAM 62,911,79

MUT: mmo-sat 150 μg/plate   ABCHA6 44,3017,80

MUT: mmo-smc 52600 μmol/L   MGGEAE 174,39,79

MUT: msc-ham: lng 10 mmol/L   ARTODN 58,5,85

MUT: orl-rat TD: 90 g/kg/1Y-I   BJEPA5 28,46,47

CONSENSUS REPORTS: IARC Cancer Review: Animal Sufficient Evidence IMEMDT 7,95,74. NTP Fourth Annual Report On Carcinogens, 1984. EPA Genetic Toxicology Program. Reported in EPA TSCA Inventory.

DOT Classification: Poison B; Label: St. Andrews Cross.

SAFETY PROFILE: Confirmed carcinogen with experimental carcinogenic, neoplastigenic, and tumorigenic data. A human poison by an unspecified route. An experimental poison by ingestion and intraperitoneal routes. Human mutation data reported. Human systemic effects by ingestion: hemorrhage, granulocytopenia (reduction in number of granulocytes), and changes in cell count (unspecified). May cause depression of bone marrow with anemia, leukopenia, and thrombocytopenia. May also cause allergic skin eruptions. Experimental teratogenic and reproductive effects. When heated to decomposition it emits very toxic fumes of NO_x and SO_x.

KEA000   CAS: 143-50-0
KEPONE
DOT: 2761

mf: $C_{10}Cl_{10}O$ mw: 490.60

PROP: A chlorinated polycyclic ketone, a crystalline material, sltly water-sol, sol in alc, ketones and acetic acid. Mp: decomp @ 350°. Readily hydrates on exposure to room temperature and humidity; normally used as a mono- to trihydrate (NCIPR*).

SYNS: CHLORDECONE ◇ CIBA 8514 ◇ COMPOUND 1189 ◇ 1,2,3,5,6,7,8,9,10,10-DECACHLORO(5.2.1.0$^{(2,6)}$.0$^{(3,9)}$. 0$^{(5,8)}$)DECANO-4-ONE ◇ DECACHLOROKETONE ◇ DECACHLORO-1,3,4-METHENO-2H-CYCLOBUTA (cd)PENTALEN-2-ONE ◇ DECACHLOROOCTAHYDRO-KEPONE-2-ONE ◇ DECACHLOROOCTAHYDRO-1,3,4-METHENO-2H-CYCLOBUTA(cd)PENTALEN-2-ONE ◇ 1,1a,3,3a,4,5,5,5a,5b,6-DECACHLOROOCTAHYDRO-1,3,4-METHENO-2H-CYCLOBUTA(cd)PENTALEN-2-ONE ◇ DECACHLOROPENTACYCLO(5.2.1.0$^{(2,6)}$.0$^{(3,9)}$.0$^{(5,8)}$)DE-CAN-4-ONE ◇ DECACHLOROPENTACYCLO(5.3.0.0$^{(2,6)}$. 0$^{(4,10)}$.0$^{(5,9)}$)DECAN-3-ONE ◇ DECACHLOROTETRA-CYCLODECANONE ◇ DECACHLOROTETRA-HYDRO-4,7-METHANOINDENEONE ◇ ENT 16,391 ◇ GENERAL CHEMICALS 1189 ◇ MEREX ◇ NCI-C00191 ◇ RCRA WASTE NUMBER U142

TOXICITY DATA with REFERENCE

CAR: orl-mus TD: 1340 mg/kg/80W-C   AIHAAP 37,680,76

CAR: orl-mus TD: 1550 mg/kg/80W-C   AIHAAP 37,680,76

CAR: orl-mus TDLo: 1200 mg/kg/80W-I NCITR* NCI-CG-TR-b,76

CAR: orl-rat TD: 670 mg/kg/80W-I   NCITR* NCI-CG-TR-b,76

CAR: orl-rat TDLo:200 mg/kg/2Y-C   NEOLA4
26,231,79

MUT: spm-qal-orl 200 ppm/42D-C   TXAPA9
43,535,78

CONSENSUS REPORTS: IARC Cancer Review: Human Limited Evidence IMEMDT 20,67,79; Animal Sufficient Evidence IMEMDT 20,67,79. NTP Fourth Annual Report On Carcinogens, 1984. EPA Genetic Toxicology Program.

DFG MAK: Suspected Carcinogen. NIOSH REL: (Kepone) CL 0.001 mg/m³/15M DOT Classification: ORM-E; Label: None.

SAFETY PROFILE: Confirmed carcinogen with experimental carcinogenic data. Poison by ingestion, skin contact, and possibly other routes. Experimental teratogenic and reproductive effects. Mutation data reported. Inhalation, absorption or ingestion by humans can lead to central nervous system, liver and kidney damage, including bizarre symptoms caused by damage to the nervous system. Usually, the symptoms are tremors, ataxia, skin changes, hyperexcitability, hyperactivity, muscle spasms, testicular atrophy, low sperm count, estrogenic effects, sterility, breast enlargement, liver lesions and cancer. An insecticide and fungicide. Registration suspended by the USEPA.

KHU000   CAS: 74278-22-1
KROMAD

PROP: Contains 5% cadmium sebacate, 5% potassium chromate, 1% malachite green and 16% thiram (FMCHA2-,D176,80).

CONSENSUS REPORTS: Cadmium and its compounds, as well as chromium and its compounds, are on the Community Right-To-Know List.

OSHA PEL: TWA 0.1 mg(Cd)/m³; CL 0.6 mg(Cd)/m³ (fume)   ACGIH TLV: TWA 0.05 mg(Cd)/m³ (Proposed: TWA 0.01 mg(Cd)/m³ (dust), Human Carcinogen); BEI: 10 μg/g creatinine in urine; 10 μg/L in blood.   DFG BAT: Blood 1.5 μg/dL; Urine 15 μg/dL, Suspected Carcinogen. NIOSH REL: (Cadmium) Reduce to lowest feasible level.

SAFETY PROFILE: Confirmed human carcinogen. Poison by ingestion. Moderately toxic by skin contact. When heated to decomposition it emits toxic fumes of K_2O, Cd, and Cr.

LAH000   CAS: 64059-26-3
LACTIC ACID, BERYLLIUM SALT

SYN: BERYLLIUM LACTATE

CONSENSUS REPORTS: Beryllium and its compounds are on The Community Right-To-Know List.

OSHA PEL: (Transitional: TWA 0.002 mg(Be)/m³; CL 0.005; Pk 0.025/30M/8H) TWA 0.002 mg(Be)/m³; STEL 0.005 mg(Be)/m³/30M; CL 0.025 mg(Be)/m³   ACGIH TLV: TWA 0.002 mg(Be)m³, Suspected Carcinogen NIOSH REL: CL (Beryllium) not to exceed 0.0005 mg(Be)/m³.

SAFETY PROFILE: Confirmed carcinogen. Poison by intravenous route. When heated to decomposition it emits very toxic fumes of Be.

LCG000   CAS: 301-04-2
LEAD ACETATE
DOT: 1616
mf: $C_4H_6O_4 \cdot Pb$ mw: 325.29

PROP: Trihydrate: colorless crystals or white granules or powder. Sltly acetic odor, slowly effloresces. D: 2.55, mp: 75° (when rapidly heated), decomp above 200°. Very sol in glycerol.

SYNS: ACETATE de PLOMB (FRENCH) ◇ ACETIC ACID LEAD (2+) SALT ◇ BLEIACETAT (GERMAN) ◇ DIBASIC LEAD ACETATE ◇ LEAD (2+) ACETATE ◇ LEAD(II) ACETATE ◇ LEAD DIACETATE ◇ LEAD DIBASIC ACETATE ◇ NORMAL LEAD ACETATE ◇ PLUMBOUS ACETATE ◇ RCRA WASTE NUMBER U144 ◇ SALT of SATURN ◇ SUGAR of LEAD

TOXICITY DATA with REFERENCE
NEO: orl-rat TD:7560 mg/kg/72W-C   ENVRAL
24,391,81
NEO: orl-rat TD:9150 mg/kg/44W-C   AJPAA4
50,571,67
NEO: orl-rat TDLo:900 mg/kg/60D-C   ENVRAL
24,391,81
ETA: orl-rat TD:138 g/kg/76W-C   TOPADD
13,50,85
ETA: orl-rat TD:218 g/kg/1Y-C   BECTA6
23,464,79
ETA: orl-rat TD:250 g/kg/47W-C   BJCAAI
16,283,62
ETA: orl-rat TD:2430 mg/kg/23W-C   ENVRAL
24,391,81
ETA: orl-rat TD:4605 mg/kg/44W-C   ENVRAL
24,391,81

MUT: cyt-hmn:lym 1 mmol/L/24H TXCYAC
10,67,78
MUT: cyt-rat-ipr 51800 μg/kg AEHLAU 40,144,85
MUT: cyt-rat-unr 9 mg/kg/26W-C GISAAA
49(3),15,84
MUT: mnt-rat-ipr 51800 μg/kg AEHLAU 40,144,85
MUT: oms-rat-ipr 10400 μg/kg AEHLAU 40,144,85
MUT: otr-rat:emb 200 mg/L JJIND8 67,1303,81
MUT: sln-smc 250 μmol/L MUTAEX 1,21,86

CONSENSUS REPORTS: IARC Cancer Review: GROUP 3 IMEMDT 7,230,87; Animal Sufficient Evidence IMEMDT 23,325,80; IMEMDT 1,40,72; Human Limited Evidence IMEMDT 23,325,80. NTP Fourth Annual Report On Carcinogens, 1984. Lead and its compounds are on the Community Right-To-Know List. Reported in EPA TSCA Inventory. EPA Genetic Toxicology Program.

OSHA PEL: TWA 0.05 mg(Pb)/m^3 ACGIH TLV: TWA 0.15 mg(Pb)/m^3 NIOSH REL: (Inorganic Lead) TWA 0.10 mg(Pb)/m^3 DOT Classification: ORM-E; Label: None; Poison B; Label: St. Andrews Cross.

SAFETY PROFILE: Confirmed carcinogen with experimental carcinogenic, neoplastigenic, tumorigenic, and teratogenic data. Poison by ingestion, intraperitoneal, subcutaneous, and intravenous routes. Experimental reproductive effects. Human mutation data reported. Used as a color additive in hair dyes, an insecticide, an astringent, and sedative. When heated to decomposition it emits toxic fumes of Pb.

LCJ000   CAS: 6080-56-4
LEAD ACETATE(II), TRIHYDRATE
mf: $C_4H_6O_4 \cdot Pb \cdot 3H_2O$ mw: 379.35

SYNS: ACETIC ACID, LEAD(+2) SALT TRIHYDRATE ◇ BIS(ACETATO)TRIHYDROXYTRILEAD ◇ BLEIAZETAT (GERMAN) ◇ LEAD ACETATE TRIHYDRATE ◇ LEAD DIACETATE TRIHYDRATE ◇ PLUMBOUS ACETATE

TOXICITY DATA with REFERENCE
CAR: orl-rat TDLo:8524 mg/kg/78W-C:TER
ZAPPAN 111(1),1,68
MUT: dni-mus-ipr 20 g/kg ARGEAR 51,605,81

CONSENSUS REPORTS: IARC Cancer Review: Animal Sufficient Evidence IMEMDT 1,40,72. EPA Genetic Toxicology Program. Lead and its compounds are on the Community Right-To-Know List.

OSHA PEL: TWA 0.05 mg(Pb)/m^3 NIOSH REL: (Inorganic Lead) TWA 0.10 mg(Pb)/m^3

SAFETY PROFILE: Confirmed carcinogen with experimental carcinogenic and teratogenic data. Poison by intraperitoneal route. Moderately toxic by subcutaneous route. Experimental reproductive effects. Mutation data reported. When heated to decomposition it emits toxic fumes of Pb.

LCK000   CAS: 7784-40-9
LEAD ACID ARSENATE
DOT: 1617
mf: $AsHO_4 \cdot Pb$ mw: 347.12

PROP: White crystals.

SYNS: ACID LEAD ARSENATE ◇ ACID LEAD ORTHOARSENATE ◇ ARSENATE of LEAD ◇ ARSINETTE ◇ DIBASIC LEAD ARSENATE ◇ GYPSINE ◇ LEAD ARSENATE ◇ LEAD ARSENATE, SOLID (DOT) ◇ LEAD ARSENATE (STANDARD) ◇ ORTHO L10 DUST ◇ ORTHO L40 DUST ◇ SCHULTENITE ◇ SECURITY ◇ SOPRABEL ◇ STANDARD LEAD ARSENATE ◇ TALBOT

CONSENSUS REPORTS: IARC Cancer Review: Human Sufficient Evidence IMEMDT 23,39,80; Animal Inadequate Evidence IMEMDT 1,40,72; IMEMDT 1,40,72. Arsenic and its compounds, as well as lead and its compounds, are on the Community Right-To-Know List. Reported in EPA TSCA Inventory.

OSHA PEL: TWA 0.05 mg(Pb)/m^3; 0.01 mg(As)/m^3 ACGIH TLV: TWA 0.15 mg(Pb)/m^3; 0.2 mg(As)/m^3 NIOSH REL: (Inorganic Lead) TWA 0.10 mg(Pb)/m^3; (Inorganic Arsenic) CL 0.002 mg(As)/m^3/15M DOT Classification: Poison B; Label: Poison.

SAFETY PROFILE: Confirmed human carcinogen. A poison by ingestion. Moderately toxic to humans by an unspecified route. Used as an insecticide and herbicide. When heated to decomposition it emits very toxic fumes of As and Pb.

LCL000   CAS: 10031-13-7
LEAD(II) ARSENITE
DOT: 1618
mf: $As_2O_4 \cdot Pb$ mw: 421.03

PROP: White powder. D: 5.85. Insol in water; sol in dil HNO_3.

SYN: LEAD ARSENITE, SOLID (DOT)

CONSENSUS REPORTS: Arsenic and its compounds, as well as lead and its compounds, are on the Community Right-To-Know List.

OSHA PEL: TWA 0.05 mg(Pb)/m^3; 0.01 mg(As)/m^3; Cancer Hazard ACGIH TLV: TWA 0.15 mg(Pb)/m^3; 0.2 mg(As)/m^3 NIOSH REL: (Inorganic Lead) TWA 0.10 mg(Pb)/m^3; (Inorganic Arsenic) CL 0.002 mg(As)/m^3/15M DOT Classification: Poison B; Label: Poison.

SAFETY PROFILE: Confirmed human carcinogen. A poison. When heated to decomposition it emits very toxic fumes of Pb and As.

LCR000 CAS: 7758-97-6
LEAD CHROMATE
mf: CrO$_4$•Pb   mw: 323.19

PROP: Yellow or orange-yellow powder. One of the most insol salts. Insol in acetic acid; sol in solns of fixed alkali hydroxides, dil HNO$_3$. Mp: 844°. Bp: decomp, d: 6.3.

SYNS: CANARY CHROME YELLOW 40-2250 ◇ CHROMATE de PLOMB (FRENCH) ◇ CHROME GREEN ◇ CHROME LEMON ◇ CHROME YELLOW ◇ CHROMIC ACID, LEAD(2+) SALT (1:1) ◇ CHROMIUM YELLOW ◇ C.I. 77600 ◇ C.I. PIGMENT YELLOW 34 ◇ COLOGNE YELLOW ◇ C.P. CHROME YELLOW LIGHT ◇ CROCOITE ◇ DAINICHI CHROME YELLOW G ◇ GIALLO CROMO (ITALIAN) ◇ KING'S YELLOW ◇ LEAD CHROMATE(VI) ◇ LEIPZIG YELLOW ◇ LEMON YELLOW ◇ PARIS YELLOW ◇ PIGMENT GREEN 15 ◇ PLUMBOUS CHROMATE ◇ PURE LEMON CHROME L3GS

TOXICITY DATA with REFERENCE
NEO: ims-rat TDLo: 324 mg/kg/39W-I   CNREA8 36,1779,76
NEO: scu-rat TDLo: 135 mg/kg   TUMOAB 57,213,71
ETA: scu-rat TD: 135 mg/kg   PBPHAW 14,47,78
MUT: cyt-ham: ovr 5 mg/L   BJCAAI 44,219,81
MUT: cyt-hmn: lym 13 μmol/L   MUREAV 77,157,80
MUT: dni-ham: kdy 150 mg/L   BJCAAI 44,219,81
MUT: ipr-gpg LD75: 156 mg/kg   MEIEDD 10,777,83
MUT: mnt-mus-ipr 500 mg/kg   TJEMAO 146,373,85
MUT: oms-ham: kdy 150 mg/L   BJCAAI 44,219,81
MUT: sce-ham: ovr 100 μg/L   MUREAV 156,219,85
MUT: sce-hmn: lym 20 μmol/L   MUREAV 77,157,80

CONSENSUS REPORTS: IARC Cancer Review: Animal Inadequate Evidence IMEMDT 2,100,73; Animal Sufficient Evidence IMEMDT 23,205,80; Human Sufficient Evidence IMEMDT 23,205,80. NTP Fourth Annual Report On Carcinogens, 1984. Lead and its compounds, as well as chromium and its compounds, are on the Community Right-To-Know List. Reported in EPA TSCA Inventory. EPA Genetic Toxicology Program.

OSHA PEL: TWA 0.05 mg(Pb)/m^3; CL 0.1 mg(CrO$_3$)/m^3 ACGIH TLV: 0.05 mg(Cr)/m^3; Human Carcinogen; (Proposed: TWA 0.05 ppm (Pb), 0.012 ppm (Cr); Suspected Human Carcinogen) DFG MAK: Suspected Carcinogen. NIOSH REL: (Chromium(VI)) TWA 0.001 mg(Cr(VI))/m^3; (Inorganic Lead) TWA 0.10 mg(Pb)/m^3.

SAFETY PROFILE: Confirmed carcinogen with experimental neoplastigenic and tumorigenic data. Poison by intraperitoneal route. Mildly toxic by ingestion. Human mutation data reported. When heated to decomposition it emits toxic fumes of Pb.

LCS000 CAS: 18454-12-1
LEAD CHROMATE, BASIC
mf: CrO$_4$Pb•OPb   mw: 546.38

PROP: Red, amorphous or crystalline solid. Mp: 920°.

SYNS: ARANCIO CROMO (ITALIAN) ◇ AUSTRIAN CINNABAR ◇ BASIC LEAD CHROMATE ◇ CHINESE RED ◇ CHROME ORANGE ◇ CHROMIUM LEAD OXIDE ◇ C.I. 77601 ◇ C.I. PIGMENT ORANGE 21 ◇ C.I. PIGMENT RED ◇ C.P. CHROME ORANGE DARK 2030 ◇ C.P. CHROME LIGHT 2010 ◇ C.P. CHROME ORANGE MEDIUM 2020 ◇ DAINICHI CHROME ORANGE R ◇ GENUINE ACETATE CHROME ORANGE ◇ GENUINE ORANGE CHROME ◇ INDIAN RED ◇ INTERNATIONAL ORANGE 2221 ◇ IRGACHROME ORANGE OS ◇ LEAD CHROMATE OXIDE (MAK) ◇ LEAD CHROMATE, RED ◇ LIGHT ORANGE CHROME ◇ NO. 156 ORANGE CHROME ◇ ORANGE CHROME ◇ ORANGE NITRATE CHROME ◇ PALE ORANGE CHROME ◇ PERSIAN RED ◇ PURE ORANGE CHROME M ◇ RED LEAD CHROMATE ◇ VYNAMON ORANGE CR

TOXICITY DATA with REFERENCE
CAR: scu-rat TDLo: 135 mg/kg   ANYAA9 271,431,76
NEO: scu-rat TD: 135 mg/kg   TUMOAB 57,213,71
ETA: scu-rat TD: 135 mg/kg   PBPHAW 14,47,78
MUT: cyt-ham: ovr 5 mg/L   BJCAAI 44,219,81
MUT: cyt-hmn: oth 500 mg/L   BJCAAI 44,219,81
MUT: dni-ham: kdy 150 mg/L   BJCAAI 44,219,81
MUT: oms-ham: kdy 150 mg/L   BJCAAI 44,219,81
MUT: oms-hmn: oth 500 mg/L   BJCAAI 44,219,81
MUT: sce-ham: ovr 1 mg/L   ENMUDM 7,185,85

CONSENSUS REPORTS: IARC Cancer Review: Human Sufficient Evidence IMEMDT 23,205,80; Animal Limited Evidence IMEMDT 23,205,80. NTP Fourth Annual Report On Carcinogens, 1984. Lead and its compounds, as well as chromium and its compounds are on the Community Right-To-Know List. Reported in EPA TSCA Inventory.

OSHA PEL: TWA 0.05 mg(Pb)/m^3; CL 0.1 mg(CrO$_3$)/m^3 ACGIH TLV: TWA 0.05 mg(Cr)/m^3; TWA 0.15 mg(Pb)/m^3 DFG MAK: Suspected Carcinogen. NIOSH REL: (Chromium(VI)) TWA 0.001 mg(Cr(VI))/m^3; (Inorganic Lead) TWA 0.10 mg(Pb)/m^3.

SAFETY PROFILE: Confirmed human carcinogen with experimental carcinogenic, neoplastigenic, and tumorigenic data. Human mutation data reported. When heated to decomposition it emits very toxic fumes of Pb.

LDU000   CAS: 7446-27-7
LEAD(II) PHOSPHATE (3:2)
mf: O$_8$P$_2$•3Pb   mw: 811.51

PROP: Hexagonal, colorless crystals or white powder. Mp: 1014, d: 6.9-7.3. Insol in water, alc; sol in HNO$_3$, fixed alkali hydroxides.

SYNS: BLEIPHOSPHAT (GERMAN) ◇ C.I. 77622 ◇ LEAD ORTHOPHOSPHATE ◇ LEAD PHOSPHATE ◇ LEAD PHOSPHATE (3:2) ◇ LEAD (2+) PHOSPHATE ◇ NORMAL LEAD ORTHOPHOSPHATE ◇ PHOSPHORIC ACID, LEAD (2+) SALT (2:3) ◇ PLUMBOUS PHOSPHATE ◇ TRILEAD PHOSPHATE

TOXICITY DATA with REFERENCE
CAR: par-rat TDLo: 580 mg/kg/34W-I   BJCAAI 19,860,65
ETA: scu-rat TDLo: 540 mg/kg/6W-I   APAVAY 323,694,53

CONSENSUS REPORTS: IARC Cancer Review: Animal Sufficient Evidence IMEMDT 23,325,80; IMEMDT 1,40,72; Human Limited Evidence IMEMDT 23,325,80. NTP Fourth Annual Report On Carcinogens, 1984. Lead and its compounds are on the Community Right-To-Know List. Reported in EPA TSCA Inventory.

OSHA PEL: TWA 0.05 μg(Pb)/m^3 ACGIH TLV: TWA 0.15 mg(Pb)/m^3 NIOSH REL: TWA 0.10 mg(Pb)/m^3

SAFETY PROFILE: Confirmed carcinogen with experimental carcinogenic and tumorigenic data. A suspected human carcinogen. When heated to decomposition it emits very toxic fumes of Pb and PO$_x$.

MDF350   CAS: 7784-37-4
MERCURY(II) ORTHOARSENATE
DOT: 1623
mf: AsHO$_4$•Hg   mw: 340.52

PROP: Yellow powder. Mp: decomp. Insol in water, sol in HCl or HNO$_3$.

SYN: MERCURIC ARSENATE

CONSENSUS REPORTS: Mercury and its compounds, as well as arsenic and its compounds, are on the Community Right-To-Know List.

OSHA PEL: 0.01 mg(As)/m^3; Cancer Hazard; (Transitional: CL 1 mg(Hg)/10m^3) CL 0.1 mg(Hg)/m^3 (skin) ACGIH TLV: TWA 0.1 mg(Hg)/m^3 (skin) NIOSH REL: TWA 0.05 mg(Hg)/m^3; CL 2 μg/m^3/15M DOT Classification: Poison B; Label: Poison.

SAFETY PROFILE: Confirmed human carcinogen. A poison. When heated to decomposition it emits very toxic fumes of Hg and As.

MGO750   CAS: 120-71-8
5-METHYL-o-ANISIDINE
mf: C$_8$H$_{11}$NO   mw: 137.20

SYNS: m-AMINO-p-CRESOL, METHYL ESTER ◇ 3-AMINO-p-CRESOL METHYL ESTER ◇ 1-AMINO-2-METHOXY-5-METHYLBENZENE ◇ 3-AMINO-4-METHOXYTOLUENE ◇ 2-AMINO-4-METHYLANISOLE ◇ AZOIC RED 36 ◇ C.I. AZOIC RED 83 ◇ CRESIDINE ◇ p-CRESIDINE ◇ KRESIDIN ◇ KREZIDINE ◇ 2-METHOXY-5-METHYLANILINE ◇ 2-METHOXY-5-METHYL-BENZENAMINE (9CI) ◇ 4-METHOXY-m-TOLUIDINE ◇ 4-METHYL-2-AMINOANISOLE ◇ NCI-C02982

TOXICITY DATA with REFERENCE
CAR: orl-mus TD: 1607 g/kg/2Y-C   IMEMDT** 27,91,82
CAR: orl-mus TD: 2961 g/kg/92W-C   IMEMDT** 27,91,82
CAR: orl-mus TDLo: 355 g/kg/92W-C   NCITR* NCI-CG-TR-142,79
CAR: orl-rat TD: 364 g/kg/2Y-C   ANTRD41,279,81
CAR: orl-rat TD: 437 g/kg/2Y-C   ANTRD41,279,81
CAR: orl-rat TD: 3640 g/kg/2Y-C   IMEMDT** 27,91,82
CAR: orl-rat TD: 7280 g/kg/2Y-C   IMEMDT** 27,91,82

CAR: orl-rat TDLo: 364 g/kg/2Y-C   NCITR*
NCI-CG-TR-142,79

NEO: orl-rat TD: 182 g/kg/2Y-C   NCITR* NCI-
CG-TR-142,79

MUT: mma-esc 2 mg/plate   ENMUDM 7(Suppl
5),1,85

MUT: mma-sat 3330 ng/plate   ENMUDM 7(Suppl
5),1,85

MUT: mmo-sat 62500 ng/plate   ENMUDM 7(Suppl
5),1,85

MUT: otr-rat: emb 31 μg/plate   JJATDK 1,190,81

CONSENSUS REPORTS: IARC Cancer Review: Human Limited Evidence IMEMDT 27,91,82; Animal Sufficient Evidence IMEMDT 27,91,82. NTP Fourth Annual Report On Carcinogens, 1984. NCI Carcinogenesis Bioassay (feed); Clear Evidence: mouse, rat NCITR* NCI-CG-TR-142,79. Reported in EPA TSCA Inventory. Community Right-To-Know List.

SAFETY PROFILE: Confirmed carcinogen with experimental carcinogenic and neoplastigenic data. Moderately toxic by ingestion. Mutation data reported. When heated to decomposition it emits toxic fumes of NO_x.

MHY550   CAS: 7568-37-8
METHYL CADMIUM AZIDE
mf: CH_3CdN_3 mw: 97.13

CONSENSUS REPORTS: Cadmium and its compounds are on the Community Right-To-Know List.

OSHA PEL: TWA 0.1 mg(Cd)/m³; CL 0.6 mg(Cd)/m³ (fume)   ACGIH TLV: TWA 0.05 mg(Cd)/m³ (Proposed: TWA 0.01 mg(Cd)/m³ (dust), Human Carcinogen); BEI: 10 μg/g creatinine in urine; 10 μg/L in blood.   DFG BAT: Blood 1.5 μg/dL; Urine 15 μg/dL, Suspected Carcinogen.   NIOSH REL: (Cadmium) Reduce to lowest feasible level

SAFETY PROFILE: Confirmed human carcinogen. When heated to decomposition it emits toxic fumes of Cd and NO_x.

MJM200   CAS: 101-14-4
4,4′-METHYLENE BIS(2-CHLOROANILINE)
mf: $C_{13}H_{12}Cl_2N_2$ mw: 267.17

SYNS: BIS AMINE ◇ CURALIN M ◇ CURENE 442 ◇ CYANASET ◇ DI(-4-AMINO-3-CHLOROPHENYL)METHANE ◇ DI-(4-AMINO-3-CLOROFENIL)METANO (ITALIAN) ◇ 4,4′-DIAMINO-3,3′-DICHLORODIPHENYLMETHANE ◇ 3,3′-DICHLOR-4,4′-DIAMINODIPHENYLMETHAN (GERMAN) ◇ 3,3′-DICHLORO-4,4′-DIAMINODIPHENYLMETHANE ◇ 3,3′-DICLORO-4,4′-DIAMINODIFENILMETANO (ITALIAN) ◇ MBOCA ◇ 4,4′-METHYLENE(BIS)-CHLOROANILINE ◇ METHYLENE-4,4′-BIS(o-CHLOROANILINE) ◇ p,p′-METHYLENEBIS(α-CHLOROANILINE) ◇ 4,4′-METHYLENEBIS(o-CHLOROANILINE) ◇ p,p′-METHYLENEBIS(o-CHLOROANILINE) ◇ 4,4′-METHYLENEBIS-2-CHLOROBENZENAMINE ◇ METHYLENE-BIS-ORTHOCHLOROANILINE ◇ 4,4-METILENE-BIS-o-CLOROANILINA (ITALIAN) ◇ MOCA ◇ RCRA WASTE NUMBER U158

TOXICITY DATA with REFERENCE
CAR: orl-rat TD: 11 g/kg/2Y-C   JEPTDQ 2,149,78
CAR: orl-rat TD: 16 g/kg/77W-C   JEPTDQ 2(1),149,78
CAR: orl-rat TD: 21 g/kg/60W-C   TXAPA9 31,159,75
CAR: orl-rat TD: 24 g/kg/57W-C   TXAPA9 31,159,75
CAR: orl-rat TD: 27 g/kg/65W-C   JEPTDQ 2(1),149,78
CAR: orl-rat TD: 27 g/kg/78W-C   TXAPA9 31,159,75
CAR: orl-rat TD: 34 g/kg/80W-C   TXAPA9 31,159,75
CAR: orl-rat TD: 8100 mg/kg/77W-C   JEPTDQ 2(1),149,78
CAR: orl-rat TDLo: 4050 mg/kg/77W-C   JEPTDQ 2(1),149,78
CAR: scu-rat TDLo: 25 g/kg/89W-C   NATWAY 58,578,71
ETA: orl-rat TD: 27 g/kg/79W-C   NATWAY 58,578,71
MUT: dns-ham: lvr 10 μmol/L   TXAPA9 58,231,81
MUT: dns-rbt: lvr 10 μmol/L   CNREA8 43,3120,83
MUT: otr-ham: kdy 80 μg/L   BJCAAI 37,873,78
MUT: otr-mus: fbr 10 μg/L   JJIND8 67,1303,81
MUT: sce-ham: ovr 500 μg/L   ENMUDM 7,1,85

CONSENSUS REPORTS: IARC Cancer Review: Animal Sufficient Evidence IMEMDT 4,65,74. NTP Fourth Annual Report On Carcinogens, 1984. EPA Genetic Toxicology Program. Community Right-To-Know List. Reported in EPA TSCA Inventory.

OSHA PEL: TWA 0.02 ppm (skin)   ACGIH TLV: TWA 0.02 ppm (skin); Suspected Human Carcinogen.   DFG MAK: Animal Carcinogen, Suspected Human Carcinogen.   NIOSH REL: (MOCA) Lowest detectable limit.

SAFETY PROFILE: Confirmed carcinogen with experimental carcinogenic and tumorigenic data. Poison by intraperitoneal route. Moderately toxic by ingestion. Mutation data reported. When heated to decomposition it emits very toxic fumes of Cl^- and NO_x.

MJN000   CAS: 101-61-1
4,4'-METHYLENE BIS(N,N'-DIMETHYLANILINE)
mf: $C_{17}H_{22}N_2$ mw: 254.41

SYNS: p,p'-BIS(DIMETHYLAMINO)DIPHENYLMETHANE ◇ 4,4'-BIS(DIMETHYLAMINO)DIPHENYLMETHANE ◇ BIS(p-DIMETHYLAMINOPHENYL)METHANE ◇ BIS(p-(N,N-DIMETHYLAMINO)PHENYL)METHANE ◇ p,p'-BIS(N,N-DIMETHYLAMINOPHENYL)METHANE ◇ p,p-DI-METHYLAMINODIPHENYLMETHANE ◇ METHANE BASE ◇ 4,4'-METHYLENEBIS(N,N-DIMETHYL)BENZENAMINE ◇ MICHLER'S BASE ◇ MICHLER'S HYDRIDE ◇ MICHLER'S METHANE ◇ NCI-C01990 ◇ TETRA-BASE ◇ TETRAMETHYLDIAMINODIPHENYLMETHANE ◇ 4,4'-TETRAMETHYLDIAMINODIPHENYLMETHANE ◇ p,p-TETRAMETHYLDIAMINODIPHENYLMETHANE

TOXICITY DATA with REFERENCE
CAR: orl-mus TD:683 g/kg/78W-C   IARC** 27,119,82
CAR: orl-mus TD:1365 g/kg/78W-C   IARC** 27,119,82
CAR: orl-rat TD:27 g/kg/2Y-C   TOLED5 6,391,80
CAR: orl-rat TD:310 g/kg/59W-C   IARC** 27,119,82
CAR: orl-rat TD:15488 mg/kg/59W-C   JJIND8 72,1457,84
CAR: orl-rat TDLo:8500 mg/kg/59W-C   NCITR* NCI-CG-TR-186,79
NEO: orl-mus TD:164 g/kg/78W-C   NCITR* NCI-CG-TR-186,79
NEO: orl-mus TDLo:82 g/kg/78W-C   NCITR* NCI-CG-TR-186,79
ETA: orl-rat TD:14 g/kg/2Y-C   TOLED5 6,391,80
ETA: orl-rat TD:155 g/kg/59W-C   IARC** 27,119,82
ETA: orl-rat TD:7744 g/kg/59W-C   JJIND8 72,1457,84
MUT: dnr-esc 20 mg/L   JNCIAM 62,873,79
MUT: dns-rat:lvr 5 mg/L   MUREAV 97,359,82
MUT: hma-mus/sat 125 mg/kg   JNCIAM 62,911,79
MUT: mma-sat 10 μg/plate   IARCCD 27,283,80
MUT: sce-rbt:lym 50 mg/L   MUREAV 89,197,81

CONSENSUS REPORTS: IARC Cancer Review: Animal Limited Evidence IMEMDT 27,119,82. NTP Fourth Annual Report On Carcinogens, 1984. NCI Carcinogenesis Bioassay (feed); Clear Evidence: mouse, rat NCITR*

NCI-CG-TR-186,79. EPA Genetic Toxicology Program. Reported in EPA TSCA Inventory. Community Right-To-Know List.

DFG MAK: Suspected Carcinogen.

SAFETY PROFILE: Confirmed carcinogen with experimental carcinogenic, neoplastigenic, and tumorigenic data. Moderately toxic by ingestion. Mutation data reported. When heated to decomposition it emits toxic fumes of NO_x.

MJO250   CAS: 838-88-0
4,4'-METHYLENEBIS(2-METHYLANILINE)
mf: $C_{15}H_{18}N_2$ mw: 226.35

PROP: Mp: 149°.

SYNS: BIS-4-AMINO-3-METHYLFENYLMETHAN (CZECH) ◇ 3,3'-DIMETHYL-4,4'-DIAMINODIPHENYLMETHANE ◇ MBOT ◇ ME-MDA ◇ 4,4'-METHYLENEBIS(2-METHYL-BENZENAMINE) ◇ 4,4'-METHYLENE DI-o-TOLUIDINE

TOXICITY DATA with REFERENCE
CAR: orl-dog TDLo:4900 mg/kg/4Y-I   JEPTDQ 1,339,78
CAR: orl-rat TD:4820 mg/kg/69W-C   TXAPA9 31,159,75
CAR: orl-rat TD:6500 mg/kg/26W-I   TXAPA9 31,159,75
CAR: orl-rat TDLo:4656 mg/kg/55W-C   TXAPA9 31,159,75
MUT: mma-sat 1 mg/plate   ARTODN 49,185,82

CONSENSUS REPORTS: IARC Cancer Review: Animal Limited Evidence IMEMDT 4,73,74. Reported in EPA TSCA Inventory.

DFG MAK: Animal Carcinogen; Suspected Human Carcinogen.

SAFETY PROFILE: Confirmed carcinogen with experimental carcinogenic data. Moderately toxic by ingestion. An eye irritant. Mutation data reported. When heated to decomposition it emits toxic fumes of NO_x.

MJQ000   CAS: 101-77-9
4,4'-METHYLENEDIANILINE
DOT: 2651
mf: $C_{13}H_{14}N_2$ mw: 198.29

PROP: Tan flakes or lumps; faint amine-like odor. Mp: 90°, flash p: 440°F.

SYNS: 4-(4-AMINOBENZYL)ANILINE ◇ BIS-p-AMINO-FENYLMETHAN (CZECH) ◇ BIS(p-AMINOPHENYL)METH-ANE ◇ BIS(4-AMINOPHENYL)METHANE ◇ CURITHANE

◇ DDM ◇ p,p'-DIAMINODIFENYLMETHAN (CZECH)
◇ 4,4'-DIAMINODIPHENYLMETHAN (GERMAN) ◇ DI-
AMINODIPHENYLMETHANE ◇ p,p'-DIAMINODIPHENYL-
METHANE ◇ 4,4'-DIAMINODIPHENYLMETHANE
◇ DI-(4-AMINOPHENYL)METHANE ◇ DIANALINE-
METHANE ◇ 4,4'-DIPHENYLMETHANEDIAMINE
◇ EPICURE DDM ◇ MDA ◇ METHYLENEBIS(ANILINE)
◇ 4,4'-METHYLENEBISANILINE ◇ METHYLENEDI-
ANILINE ◇ p,p'-METHYLENEDIANILINE ◇ NCI-C54604
◇ TONOX

TOXICITY DATA with REFERENCE
ETA: orl-rat TDLo: 320 mg/kg/I   NATUAS
219,1162,68
ETA: scu-rat TDLo: 1410 mg/kg/I   NATWAY
57,247,70
MUT: dnd-rat-ipr 370 μmol/kg   CRNGDP2,1317,81
MUT: mma-sat 50 μg/plate   MUREAV 67,123,79
MUT: mmo-sat 250 μg/plate   MUREAV 67,123,79
MUT: sce-mus-ipr 9 mg/kg   MUREAV 108,225,83

CONSENSUS REPORTS: IARC Cancer Review: Animal Sufficient Evidence IMEMDT 39,347,86; Animal Inadequate Evidence IMEMDT 4,79,74. NTP Fourth Annual Report On Carcinogens, 1984. Community Right-To-Know List. Reported in EPA TSCA Inventory.

ACGIH TLV: TWA 0.1 ppm (skin); Suspected Human Carcinogen.   DFG MAK: Animal Carcinogen, Suspected Human Carcinogen.   DOT Classification: Poison B; Label: St. Andrews Cross.

SAFETY PROFILE: Confirmed carcinogen with experimental tumorigenic data. Poison by ingestion, subcutaneous, and intraperitoneal routes. Human systemic effects by ingestion: rigidity, jaundice, other liver changes. An eye irritant. Mutation data reported. It is not rapidly absorbed through the skin. Combustible when exposed to heat or flame. When heated to decomposition it emits highly toxic fumes of aniline and NO_x.

MJQ100   CAS: 13552-44-8
4,4'-METHYLENEDIANILINE DIHYDROCHLORIDE
mf: $C_{13}H_{14}N_2 \cdot 2ClH$ mw: 271.21
SYN: NCI-C54604

TOXICITY DATA with REFERENCE
CAR: orl-mus TD: 21630 mg/kg/2Y-C   JJIND8
72,1457,84
CAR: orl-mus TD: 43800 mg/kg/2Y-C   NTPTR*
NTP-TR-248,83
CAR: orl-mus TDLo: 21900 mg/kg/2Y-C
NTPTR* NTP-TR-248,83

CAR: orl-rat TD: 21630 mg/kg/2Y-C   JJIND8
72,1457,84
CAR: orl-rat TD: 21900 mg/kg/2Y-C   NTPTR*
NTP-TR-248,83
CAR: orl-rat TDLo: 10950 mg/kg/2Y-C   NTPTR*
NTP-TR-248,83
NEO: orl-rat TD: 10815 mg/kg/2Y-C   JJIND8
72,1457,84

CONSENSUS REPORTS: IARC Cancer Review: Animal Sufficient Evidence IMEMDT 39,347,86. NTP Fourth Annual Report On Carcinogens, 1984. NTP Carcinogenesis Studies (oral); Clear Evidence: mouse, rat NTPTR* NTP-TR-248,83. Reported in EPA TSCA Inventory.

SAFETY PROFILE: Confirmed carcinogen with experimental carcinogenic and neoplastigenic data. When heated to decomposition it emits toxic fumes of NO_x and HCl.

MKB000   CAS: 10595-95-6
N,N-METHYLETHYLNITROSAMINE
mf: $C_3H_8N_2O$ mw: 88.13

SYNS: ETHYLMETHYLNITROSAMINE ◇ METHYL-
AETHYLNITROSAMIN (GERMAN) ◇ METHYLETHYLNI-
TROSAMINE ◇ N-METHYL-N-NITROSO-ETHAMINE
◇ N-METHYL-N-NITROSOETHYLAMINE ◇ NEMA
◇ N-NITROSOETHYLMETHYLAMINE ◇ N-NITROSO-
METHYLETHYLAMINE (MAK) ◇ NMEA

TOXICITY DATA with REFERENCE
CAR: orl-rat TDLo: 600 mg/kg/15W-I   CNREA8
46,2252,86
ETA: orl-ham TD: 360 mg/kg/20W-I   CNREA8
47,3968,87
ETA: orl-rat TD: 700 mg/kg/30W-I   CNREA8
47,3968,87
ETA: orl-rat TD: 72 mg/kg/30W-I   CNREA8
40,19,80
ETA: orl-rat TD: 90 mg/kg/30W-I   FCTOD7
21,601,83
ETA: orl-rat TD: 360 mg/kg/30W-I   JJIND8
68M681,82
ETA: orl-rat TD: 420 mg/kg/71W-C   ZEKBAI
69,103,67
ETA: orl-rat TD: 600 mg/kg/15W-C   PAACA3
25,126,84
ETA: orl-rat TD: 2250 mg/kg/30W-C   CALEDQ
14,297,81
MUT: hma-mus/sat 22500 μg/kg   MUREAV
110,9,83
MUT: mma-esc 5 mmol/L   MUREAV 89,209,81
MUT: mma-sat 500 μg/plate   CRNGDP 5,1091.84

MUT: pic-esc 100 mg/L   TCMUE9 1,91,84
MUT: slt-dmg-orl 100 μmol/L   ENMUDM 5,455,83

CONSENSUS REPORTS: IARC Cancer Review: Animal Limited Evidence IMEMDT 17,221,78. EPA Genetic Toxicology Program.

DFG MAK: Animal Carcinogen, Suspected Human Carcinogen.

SAFETY PROFILE: Confirmed carcinogen with experimental carcinogenic and tumorigenic data. Poison by ingestion. Mutation data reported. When heated to decomposition it emits toxic fumes of NO_x.

MKB750   CAS: 72-33-3
3-METHYLETHYNYLESTRADIOL
mf: $C_{21}H_{26}O_2$ mw: 310.47

SYNS: COMPOUND 33355 ◇ DELTA-MVE ◇ 17-α-ETHINYL ESTRADIOL 3-METHYL ETHER ◇ ETHINYLESTRADIOL-3-METHYL ETHER ◇ 17-α-ETHINYL OESTRADIOL-3-METHYL ETHER ◇ ETHINYLOESTRADIOL-3-METHYL ETHER ◇ ETHYNYLESTRADIOL-3-METHYL ETHER ◇ 17-ETHYNYLESTRADIOL-3-METHYL ETHER ◇ 17-α-ETHYNYLESTRADIOL-3-METHYL ETHER ◇ (+)-17-α-ETHYNYL-17-β-HYDROXY-3-METHOXY-1,3,5(10)-ESTRATRIENE ◇ (+)-17-α-ETHYNYL-17-β-HYDROXY-3-METHOXY-1,3,-5(10)-OESTRATRIENE ◇ 17-α-ETHYNYL-3-METHOXY-1,-3,5(10)-ESTRATRIEN-17-β-OL ◇ 17-ETHYNYL-3-METHOXY-1,3,5(10)-ESTRATRIEN-17-β-OL ◇ 17-α-ETHYNYL-3-METHOXY-17-β-HYDROXY-Δ-1,3,5(10)-ESTRATRIENE ◇ 17-α-ETHYNYL-3-METHOXY-17-β-HYDROXY-Δ-1,3,5(10)-OESTRATRIENE ◇ 17-ETHYNYL-3-METHOXY-1,3,5(10)-OESTRATIEN-17-β-OL ◇ ETHYNYLOESTRADIOL METHYL ETHER ◇ 17-ETHYNYLOESTRADIOL-3-METHYL ETHER ◇ 17-α-ETHYNYLOESTRADIOL-3-METHYL ETHER ◇ 17-α-ETHYNYLOESTRADIOL METHYL ETHER ◇ MESTRANOL ◇ MESTRENOL ◇ 3-METHOXY-17-α-ETHINYLESTRADIOL ◇ 3-METHOXY-17-α-ETHINYLOESTRADIOL ◇ 3-METHOXYETHYNYLESTRADIOL ◇ 3-METHOXY-17-α-ETHYNOESTRADIOL ◇ 3-METHOXY-17-α-ETHYNYLESTRADIOL ◇ 3-METHOXYETHYNYLOESTRADIOL ◇ 3-METHOXY-17-ETHYNYLOESTRADIOL-17-β ◇ 3-METHOXY-17-α-ETHYNYL-1,3,5(10)-ESTRATRIEN-17-β-OL ◇ 3-METHOXY-17-α-ETHYNYL-1,3,5(10)-OESTRATRIEN-17-β-OL ◇ 3-METHOXY-19-NOR-17-α-PREGNA-1,3,5(10)-TRIEN-10-YN-17-OL ◇ 3-METHOXY-17-α-19-NORPREGNA-K,3,5(10)-TRIEN-20-YN-17-OL ◇ (17-α)-3-METHOXY-19-NORPREGN-1,3,5(10)-TRIEN-20-YN-17-OL ◇ 3-METHYLETHYNYLOESTRADIOL

TOXICITY DATA with REFERENCE
NEO: orl-mus TD: 20 mg/kg/28W-C   REEBB3 16,425,71

NEO: orl-mus TDLo: 19 mg/kg/30W-C   CRSBAW 168,1190,74
ETA: ipr-rat TDLo: 61 mg/kg/84W-C   ONCOAR 20(4),93,87
ETA: orl-rat TDLo: 2400 μg/kg/17W-C   PAACA3 21,76,80
MUT: oms-mus-scu 120 μg/kg   AJOGAH 120,390,74

CONSENSUS REPORTS: IARC Cancer Review: Human Limited Evidence IMEMDT 21,257,79; Animal Sufficient Evidence IMEMDT 6,87,74; IMEMDT 21,257,79. NTP Fourth Annual Report On Carcinogens, 1984.

SAFETY PROFILE: Confirmed carcinogen with experimental neoplastigenic, tumorigenic, and teratogenic data. Human reproductive effects by ingestion: changes in ovaries and fallopian tubes, fertility effects. Experimental reproductive effects. Mutation data reported. An FDA proprietary drug. A steroid used in oral contraceptives. When heated to decomposition it emits acrid smoke and irritating fumes.

MKW200   CAS: 74-88-4
METHYL IODIDE
DOT: 2644
mf: CH_3I mw: 141.94

PROP: Colorless liquid, turns brown on exposure to light. Mp: −66.4°, bp: 42.5°, d: 2.279 @ 20°/4°, vap press: 400 mm @ 25.3°, vap d: 4.89. Sol in water @ 15°, misc in alc and ether.

SYNS: IODOMETHANE ◇ IODOMETANO (ITALIAN) ◇ IODURE de METHYLE (FRENCH) ◇ JOD-METHAN (GERMAN) ◇ JOODMETHAAN (DUTCH) ◇ METHYLJODID (GERMAN) ◇ METHYLJODIDE (DUTCH) ◇ METYLU JODEK (POLISH) ◇ MONOIODURO di METILE (ITALIAN) ◇ RCRA WASTE NUMBER U138

TOXICITY DATA with REFERENCE
NEO: ipr-mus TDLo: 44 mg/kg/8W-I   CNREA8 35,1411,75
ETA: scu-rat TDLo: 50 mg/kg   ZEKBAI 74,241,70
MUT: dnd-esc 1 μmol/L   ARTODN 46,277,80
MUT: mma-mus: lym 50 mg/L/4H   MUREAV 59,61,79
MUT: mmo-esc 20 μmol/L   ARTODN 46,277,80
MUT: msc-mus: lym 3600 μg/L   ENMUDM 7,523,85
MUT: slt-hmn: ovr 1500 μg/L   MUREAV 136,137,84

CONSENSUS REPORTS: IARC Cancer Review: GROUP 3 IMEMDT 7,56,87; Animal Limited Evidence IMEMDT 41,213,86. NTP

Fourth Annual Report On Carcinogens, 1984. Community Right-To-Know List. EPA Genetic Toxicology Program. Reported in EPA TSCA Inventory.

OSHA PEL: (Transitional: TWA 5 ppm (skin)) TWA 2 ppm (skin) ACGIH TLV: TWA 2 ppm (skin); Suspected Human Carcinogen. DFG MAK: Animal Carcinogen, Suspected Human Carcinogen. NIOSH REL: (Methylbromide) Reduce to lowest level. DOT Classification: Poison B; Label: Poison.

SAFETY PROFILE: Confirmed carcinogen with experimental neoplastigenic and tumorigenic data. A poison by ingestion, intraperitoneal and subcutaneous routes. Moderately toxic by inhalation and skin contact. A human skin irritant. Human mutation data reported. When heated to decomposition it emits toxic fumes of I^-.

MMN250 CAS: 443-48-1
2-METHYL-5-NITROIMIDAZOLE-1-ETHANOL
mf: $C_6H_9N_3O_3$ mw: 171.18

SYNS: ACROMONA ◇ ANAGIARDIL ◇ ATRIVYL ◇ BAYER 5360 ◇ BEXON ◇ CLONT ◇ CONT ◇ DANIZOL ◇ DEFLAMON-WIRKSTOFF ◇ EFLORAN ◇ ELYZOL ◇ ENTIZOL ◇ 1-(β-ETHYLOL)-2-METHYL-5-NITRO-3-AZA-PYRROLE ◇ EUMIN ◇ FLAGEMONA ◇ FLAGESOL ◇ FLAGIL ◇ FLAGYL ◇ GIATRICOL ◇ GINEFLAVIR ◇ 1-(β-HYDROXYETHYL)-2-METHYL-5-NITROIMIDAZOLE ◇ 1-(2-HYDROXYETHYL)-2-METHYL-5-NITROIMIDAZOLE ◇ 1-HYDROXYETHYL-2-METHYL-5-NITROIMIDAZOLE ◇ 1-(2-HYDROXY-1-ETHYL)-2-METHYL-5-NITROIMIDA-ZOLE ◇ KLION ◇ MERONIDAL ◇ 2-METHYL-1-(2-HYDROX-YETHYL)-5-NITROIMIDAZOLE ◇ 2-METHYL-3-(2-HYDROX-YETHYL)-4-NITROIMIDAZOLE ◇ METRONIDAZ ◇ METRONIDAZOL ◇ METRONIDAZOLO ◇ MONAGYL ◇ NALOX ◇ NEO-TRIC ◇ NIDA ◇ NOVONIDAZOL ◇ NSC-50364 ◇ ORVAGIL ◇ 1-(β-OXYETHYL)-2-METHYL-5-NITROIMIDAZOLE ◇ RP 8823 ◇ SANATRICHOM ◇ SC 10295 ◇ TRICHAZOL ◇ TRICHOCIDE ◇ TRICHOMOL ◇ TRICHOMONACID "PHARMACHIM" ◇ TRICHOPOL ◇ TRICOM ◇ TRICOWAS B ◇ TRIKOJOL ◇ TRIMEKS ◇ TRIVAZOL ◇ VAGILEN ◇ VAGIMID ◇ VERTISAL

TOXICITY DATA with REFERENCE
CAR: orl-mus TD:1680 mg/kg:REP JCREA8 112,135,86
CAR: orl-mus TD:21800 mg/kg/2Y-I JCREA8 112,135,86
CAR: orl-mus TDLo:181 g/kg/72W-C JNCIAM 48,721,72
CAR: orl-rat TDLo:219 g/kg/35W-C JJIND8 63,863,79

NEO: orl-mus TD:8 g/kg/14W-C TUMOAB 69,379,83
NEO: orl-rat TD:3 g/kg/14W-C TUMOAB 70,307,74
ETA: orl-rat TDLo:27 g/kg/35W-C:TER JNCIAM 51,403,73
MUT: bfa-hmn/sat 10 mg/kg MUREAV 77,357,80
MUT: bfa-rat/sat 800 mg/kg MUREAV 97,171,82
MUT: cyt-hmn:lym 500 mg/L ENMUDM 6,467,84
MUT: dnd-rat:lvr 3 mmol/L SinJF# 26OCT82
MUT: dnr-esc 2 mg/L MUREAV 164,9,86
MUT: hma-mus/esc 4 mg/kg/2H MUREAV 164,9,86
MUT: sce-ham-orl 125 mg/kg BLFSBY 29B,613,83

CONSENSUS REPORTS: IARC Cancer Review: Animal Sufficient Evidence IMEMDT 13,113,77. NTP Fourth Annual Report On Carcinogens, 1984. EPA Genetic Toxicology Program.

SAFETY PROFILE: Confirmed carcinogen with experimental carcinogenic, neoplastigenic, tumorigenic, and teratogenic data. Moderately toxic by ingestion, intraperitoneal and subcutaneous routes. Human systemic effects by ingestion: paresthesia, nerve or sheath structural changes, eye changes, tremors, fever, jaundice and other liver changes. Experimental reproductive effects. Human mutation data reported. When heated to decomposition it emits toxic fumes of NO_x.

MMU250 CAS: 614-00-6
N-METHYL-N-NITROSOANILINE
mf: $C_7H_8N_2O$ mw: 136.17

SYNS: N-METHYL-N-NITROSOBENZENAMINE ◇ METHYLPHENYLNITROSAMINE ◇ MNA ◇ NITROSO-METHYLANILINE ◇ N-NITROSO-N-METHYLANILINE ◇ N-NITROSOMETHYLPHENYLAMINE (MAK) ◇ NMA ◇ PHENYLMETHYLNITROSAMINE

TOXICITY DATA with REFERENCE
CAR: orl-rat TD:500 mg/kg/20W-I CNREA8 46,2252,86
CAR: orl-rat TD:4050 mg/kg/29W-C BJCAAI 18,265,64
CAR: orl-rat TDLo:61 mg/kg/29W-C CALEDQ 1,215,76
CAR: scu-rat TDLo:78 mg/kg/39W-I CALEDQ 1,215,76
NEO: orl-mus TDLo:2744 mg/kg/28W-C JNCIAM 46,1029,71
ETA: orl-rat TD:500 mg/kg/20W-C PAACA3 25,126,84

ETA: orl-rat TD: 1000 mg/kg/50W-I   CRNGDP 4,157,83

ETA: orl-rat TD: 1250 mg/kg/50W-I   CRNGDP - 4,157,83

ETA: orl-rat TD: 3400 mg/kg/35W-C   ARZNAD 19,1077,69

ETA: orl-rat TD: 3400 mg/kg/35W-C   ZEKBAI 69,103,67

MUT: dni-mus-ipr 20 g/kg   ARGEAR 51,605,81

MUT: mma-esc 50 nmol/plate   GANNA2 75,8,84

MUT: mma-sat 735 nmol/plate   CALEDQ 15,289,82

MUT: mrc-smc 2500 mg/L   IAPUDO 57,721,84

CONSENSUS REPORTS: Reported in EPA TSCA Inventory. EPA Genetic Toxicology Program.

DFG MAK: Animal Carcinogen, Suspected Human Carcinogen.

SAFETY PROFILE: Confirmed carcinogen with experimental carcinogenic, neoplastigenic, tumorigenic, and teratogenic data. Poison by ingestion and intraperitoneal routes. Experimental reproductive effects. Mutation data reported. When heated to decomposition it emits toxic fumes of NO_x.

MNA750   CAS: 684-93-5
N-METHYL-N-NITROSOUREA
mf: $C_2H_5N_3O_2$ mw: 103.10

SYNS: METHYLNITROSO-HARNSTOFF (GERMAN) ◇ N-METHYL-N-NITROSO-HARNSTOFF (GERMAN) ◇ METHYLNITROSOUREA ◇ 1-METHYL-1-NITROSOUREA ◇ METHYLNITROSOUREE (FRENCH) ◇ MNU ◇ N-NITROSO-N-METHYLCARBAMIDE ◇ N-NITROSO-N-METHYL-HARNSTOFF (GERMAN) ◇ NITROSOMETHYLUREA ◇ N-NITROSO-N-METHYLUREA ◇ 1-NITROSO-1-METHYLUREA ◇ NMH ◇ NMU ◇ NSC 23909 ◇ RCRA WASTE NUMBER U177 ◇ SKI 24464 ◇ SRI 859

TOXICITY DATA with REFERENCE

CAR: ipr-gpg TDLo: 180 mg/kg/18W-I   NEOLA4 24,57,77

CAR: ipr-mus TD: 12500 μg/kg   GERNDJ 28,114,82

CAR: ipr-mus TDLo: 50 mg/kg   BJCAAI 24,588,70

CAR: ipr-rat TDLo: 20 mg/kg (18D post)   IJCNAW 15,385,75

CAR: ipr-rat TDLo: 100 mg/kg   ENDOAO 107,1218,80

CAR: itr-ham TD: 300 mg/kg/15W-I   PEXTAR 24,345,79

CAR: itr-ham TDLo: 36 mg/kg/26W-I   IJCNAW 6,217,70

CAR: ivn-mus TD: 50 mg/kg   JCREA8 108,214,84

CAR: ivn-mus TDLo: 50 mg/kg   BJCAAI 30,325,74

CAR: ivn-rat TD: 25 mg/kg/8D-I   NATUAS 267,620,77

CAR: ivn-rat TD: 50 mg/kg   JJIND8 71,625,83

CAR: ivn-rat TD: 100 mg/kg/2W-I   EXPADD 19,81,81

CAR: ivn-rat TDLo: 20 mg/kg   CRNGDP 3,1473,82

CAR: mul-rat TDLo: 150 mg/kg/30W-I   ZAPPAN 114,447,71

CAR: orl-gpg TDLo: 440 mg/kg/44W-I   CNREA8 35,2269,75

CAR: orl-ham TDLo: 20 mg/kg/5W-I   AOBIAR 25,623,80

CAR: orl-rat TDLo: 6 mg/kg   CNREA8 45,4827,85

CAR: par-rat TD: 7500 μg/kg   BJCAAI 42,129,80

CAR: par-rat TD: 7500 μg/kg/3W-I   CALEDQ 8,3,79

CAR: par-rat TDLo: 5 mg/kg/2W-I   BJCAAI 45,337,82

CAR: rec-mus TDLo: 360 mg/kg/2W-I   PSEBAA 148,166,75

CAR: rec-rat TD: 60 mg/kg/3W-I   CNREA8 38,4427,78

CAR: rec-rat TDLo: 32 mg/kg/11D-I   BBACAQ 574,423,79

CAR: scu-ham TDLo: 146 mg/kg/41W-I   JNCIAM 51,1295,73

CAR: scu-mus TDLo: 75 mg/kg (14-19D post)   VOONAW 17(8),75,71

CAR: scu-rat TDLo: 1250 μg/kg   CRNGDP 6,769,85

CAR: skn-mus TDLo: 306 mg/kg/7W-I   CNREA8 44,1027,84

CAR: skn-rat TDLo: 576 mg/kg/24W-I   ARGEAR 55,117,85

CAR: unr-ham TDLo: 400 mg/kg/10W-I   PEXTAR 24,330,79

CAR: unr-rat TDLo: 10 mg/kg   40RMA7 -,64,78

CAR: unr-rat TDLo: 20 mg/kg (21D post)   VOONAW 20(12),76,74

CAR: unr-rat TDLo: 20 mg/kg (21D post)   VOONAW 20(12),76,74

NEO: ipr-ham TD: 71 mg/kg   CNREA8 43,829,83

NEO: ipr-ham TDLo: 30 mg/kg   CNREA8 43,829,83

NEO: ivn-grb TDLo: 38 mg/kg/15W-I   JNCIAM 55,637,75

NEO: ivn-mus TDLo: 50 mg/kg (15D post)   SEIJBO 21,261,81

NEO: ivn-rbt TDLo: 40 mg/kg (25D post)   BEXBAN 85,369,78

NEO: orl-mus TDLo: 300 mg/kg/8W-I   TXAPA9 82,19,86

NEO: rec-gpg TDLo: 168 mg/kg/42W-I   JNCIAM 54,785,75

ETA: imp-dog TDLo: 183 mg/kg/21W-C   JJIND8
65,921,80

ETA: ivn-dog TDLo: 240 mg/kg/52W-I
EXPEAM 26,303,70

ETA: ivn-ham TDLo: 60 mg/kg/13W-I   KGGZAL
25,262,68

ETA: ivn-rat TDLo: 10 mg/kg (15D post)
KFIZAO 84,23,75

ETA: ivn-rat TDLo: 20 mg/kg (22D post)
IARCCD 4,127,73

ETA: ivn-rbt TDLo: 150 mg/kg/30W-I   ZSNUAI
198,65,70

ETA: ocu-rat TDLo: 800 μg/kg   EXERA6 42,83,86

ETA: orl-mky TDLo: 20 g/kg/6Y-I   CANCAR
40,1950,77

ETA: orl-pig TDLo: 1170 mg/kg/5Y-I   REXMAS
169,33,76

ETA: par-dog TDLo: 3009 mg/kg/34W-I   JJIND8
65,921,80

ETA: par-rat TDLo: 5 mg/kg (21D post)   IARCCD
4,1,73

ETA: par-rat TDLo: 80 mg/kg/2W-I   SHKKAN
25,819,83

ETA: skn-ham TDLo: 155 mg/kg/13W-I
NATUAS 214,611,67

MUT: cyt-hmn: lym 4 μmol/L   MUREAV 160,95,86

MUT: msc-hmn: fbr 200 μmol/L   PAACA3
25,102,84

MUT: oms-mam: lym 1 mmol/L   CBINA846,179,83

MUT: sce-mus: mmr 1 μmol/L   MUREAV
147,165,85

MUT: sln-dmg-par 1 mmol/L   MUREAV 149,193,85

CONSENSUS REPORTS: IARC Cancer Review: Human Limited Evidence IMEMDT 17,227,78; Animal Sufficient Evidence IMEMDT 17,227,78, IMEMDT 1,125,72. NTP Fourth Annual Report On Carcinogens, 1984. EPA Genetic Toxicology Program. Community Right-To-Know List. Reported in EPA TSCA Inventory.

SAFETY PROFILE: Confirmed carcinogen with experimental carcinogenic, neoplastigenic, tumorigenic, and teratogenic data. Poison by ingestion, implant, intraperitoneal, subcutaneous and intravenous routes. Experimental reproductive effects. Human mutation data reported. Explodes at room temperature. Can detonate with (KOH + CH_2Cl_2). When heated to decomposition it emits toxic fumes of NO_x.

MQS500   CAS: 90-94-8
MICHLER'S KETONE
mf: $C_{17}H_{20}N_2O$ mw: 268.39

PROP: Leaves from ethanol. Mp: 172°, bp: >360° decomp. Insol in water, very sol in benzene, sol in alc, very sltly sol in ether.

SYNS: p,p′-BIS(N,N-DIMETHYLAMINO)BENZOPHENONE ◇ 4,4′-BIS(DIMETHYLAMINO)BENZOPHENONE ◇ BIS(p-(N,N-DIMETHYLAMINO)PHENYL)KETONE ◇ BIS(4-(DIMETHYLAMINO)PHENYL)METHANONE ◇ p,p′-MICHLER'S KETONE ◇ NCI-C02006 ◇ TETRAMETHYLDIAMINO-BENZOPHENONE

TOXICITY DATA with REFERENCE
CAR: orl-mus TD: 164 g/kg/78W-C   NCITR*
NCI-TR-181,79

CAR: orl-mus TDLo: 82 g/kg/78W-C   NCITR*
NCI-TR-181,79

CAR: orl-rat TD: 27 g/kg/78W-C   NCITR* NCI-TR-181,79

CAR: orl-rat TDLo: 15 g/kg/78W-C   NCITR*
NCI-TR-181,79

NEO: orl-rat TD: 8 g/kg/78W-C   NCITR* NCI-TR-181,79

MUT: cyt-ham: fbr 1500 μg/L   MUTAEX 1,17,86

MUT: dns-rat-orl 200 mg/kg   ENMUDM 7(Suppl 3),73,85

MUT: mma-sat 33300 ng/plate   ENMUDM 7(Suppl 5),1,85

CONSENSUS REPORTS: NCI Carcinogenesis Bioassay (feed); Clear Evidence: mouse, rat NCITR* NCI-CG-TR-181,79. NTP Fourth Annual Report On Carcinogens, 1984. Reported in EPA TSCA Inventory. EPA Genetic Toxicology Program.

DFG MAK: Suspected Carcinogen.

SAFETY PROFILE: Confirmed human carcinogen with experimental carcinogenic and neoplastigenic data. Poison by ingestion. Mutation data reported. When heated to decomposition it emits toxic fumes of NO_x.

MQV755   CAS: 64741-49-7
MINERAL OIL, PETROLEUM CONDENSATES, VACUUM TOWER

SYNS: CONDENSATES (PETROLEUM), VACUUM TOWER (9CI) ◇ VACUUM RESIDUUM

CONSENSUS REPORTS: IARC Cancer Review: GROUP 1 IMEMDT 7,252,87; Animal Sufficient Evidence IMEMDT 33,87,84. Reported in EPA TSCA Inventory.

SAFETY PROFILE: Confirmed carcinogen. When heated to decomposition it emits acrid smoke and irritating fumes.

MQV760   CAS: 64742-18-3
MINERAL OIL, PETROLEUM DISTILLATES, ACID-TREATED HEAVY NAPHTHENIC

SYNS: ACID-TREATED HEAVY NAPHTHENIC DISTIL-LATE ◇ DISTILLATES (PETROLEUM), ACID-TREATED HEAVY NAPHTHENIC (9CI)

CONSENSUS REPORTS: IARC Cancer Review: GROUP 1 IMEMDT 7,252,87; Animal Sufficient Evidence IMEMDT 33,87,84. Reported in EPA TSCA Inventory.

SAFETY PROFILE: Confirmed carcinogen. When heated to decomposition it emits acrid smoke and irritating fumes.

MQV765   CAS: 64742-20-7
MINERAL OIL, PETROLEUM DISTILLATES, ACID-TREATED HEAVY PARAFFINIC

SYNS: ACID-TREATED HEAVY PARAFFINIC DISTILLATE ◇ DISTILLATES (PETROLEUM), ACID-TREATED HEAVY-PARAFFINIC (9CI)

CONSENSUS REPORTS: IARC Cancer Review: GROUP 1 IMEMDT 7,252,87; Animal Sufficient Evidence IMEMDT 33,87,84. Reported in EPA TSCA Inventory.

SAFETY PROFILE: Confirmed carcinogen. When heated to decomposition it emits acrid smoke and irritating fumes.

MQV770   CAS: 64742-19-4
MINERAL OIL, PETROLEUM DISTILLATES, ACID-TREATED LIGHT NAPHTHENIC

SYNS: ACID-TREATED LIGHT NAPHTHENIC DISTILLATE ◇ DISTILLATES (PETROLEUM), ACID-TREATED LIGHT NAPHTHENIC (9CI)

CONSENSUS REPORTS: IARC Cancer Review: GROUP 1 IMEMDT 7,252,87; Animal Sufficient Evidence IMEMDT 33,87,84. Reported in EPA TSCA Inventory.

SAFETY PROFILE: Confirmed carcinogen. When heated to decomposition it emits acrid smoke and irritating fumes.

MQV775   CAS: 64742-21-8
MINERAL OIL, PETROLEUM DISTILLATES, ACID-TREATED LIGHT PARAFFINIC

SYNS: ACID-TREATED LIGHT PARAFFINIC DISTILLATE ◇ DISTILLATES (PETROLEUM), ACID-TREATED LIGHT PARAFFINIC (9CI)

CONSENSUS REPORTS: IARC Cancer Review: GROUP 1 IMEMDT 7,252,87; Animal Sufficient Evidence IMEMDT 33,87,84. Reported in EPA TSCA Inventory.

SAFETY PROFILE: Confirmed carcinogen. When heated to decomposition it emits acrid smoke and irritating fumes.

MQV780   CAS: 64741-53-3
MINERAL OIL, PETROLEUM DISTILLATES, HEAVY NAPHTHENIC

SYNS: DISTILLATES (PETROLEUM), HEAVY NAPHTHENIC (9CI) ◇ HEAVY NAPHTHENIC DISTILLATE ◇ HEAVY NAPHTHENIC DISTILLATES (PETROLEUM)

TOXICITY DATA with REFERENCE
NEO: skn-mus TDLo:216 g/kg/36W-I   EPASR* 8EHQ-0887-0691S
MUT: mmo-sat 5 µL/plate   CBTOE2 2,63,86

CONSENSUS REPORTS: IARC Cancer Review: GROUP 1 IMEMDT 7,252,87; Animal Sufficient Evidence IMEMDT 33,87,84. Reported in EPA TSCA Inventory.

SAFETY PROFILE: Confirmed carcinogen with experimental neoplastigenic data. Mutation data reported. When heated to decomposition it emits acrid smoke and irritating fumes.

MQV785   CAS: 64741-51-1
MINERAL OIL, PETROLEUM DISTILLATES, HEAVY PARAFFINIC

SYNS: DISTILLATES (PETROLEUM), HEAVY PARAFFINIC (9CI) ◇ HEAVY PARAFFINIC DISTILLATE

TOXICITY DATA with REFERENCE
MUT: mmo-sat 3 uL/plate   CBTOE2 2,63,86

CONSENSUS REPORTS: IARC Cancer Review: GROUP 1 IMEMDT 7,252,87; Animal Sufficient Evidence IMEMDT 33,87,84. Reported in EPA TSCA Inventory.

SAFETY PROFILE: Confirmed carcinogen. Mutation data reported.

MQV790 CAS: 64742-52-5
MINERAL OIL, PETROLEUM DISTILLATES, HYDROTREATED HEAVY NAPHTHENIC

SYNS: DISTILLATES (PETROLEUM), HYDROTREATED HEAVY NAPHTHENIC (9CI) ◇ HYDROTREATED HEAVY NAPHTHENIC DISTILLATE ◇ HYDROTREATED HEAVY NAPHTHENIC DISTILLATES (PETROLEUM) ◇ PETROLEUM DISTILLATES, HYDROTREATED HEAVY NAPHTHENIC

TOXICITY DATA with REFERENCE
NEO: skn-mus TDLo: 480 g/kg/80W-I EPASR*
   8EHQ-0887-0691S
ETA: skn-mus TD: 402 g/kg/78W-I BJCAAI
   48,429,83
ETA: skn-mus TDLo: 398 g/kg/22W-I BJCAAI
   48,429,83
MUT: mmo-sat 10 μL/plate CBTOE2 2,63,86

CONSENSUS REPORTS: IARC Cancer Review: GROUP 1 IMEMDT 7,252,87; Animal Inadequate Evidence IMEMDT 33,87,84. Reported in EPA TSCA Inventory.

SAFETY PROFILE: Confirmed carcinogen with experimental tumorigenic data. Mutation data reported. When heated to decomposition it emits acrid smoke and irritating fumes.

MQV795 CAS: 64742-54-7
MINERAL OIL, PETROLEUM DISTILLATES, HYDROTREATED HEAVY PARAFFINIC

SYNS: DISTILLATES (PETROLEUM), HYDROTREATED HEAVY PARAFFINIC (9CI) ◇ HYDROTREATED HEAVY PARAFFINIC DISTILLATE

CONSENSUS REPORTS: IARC Cancer Review: GROUP 1 IMEMDT 7,252,87; Animal Inadequate Evidence IMEMDT 33,87,84. Reported in EPA TSCA Inventory.

SAFETY PROFILE: Confirmed carcinogen. When heated to decomposition it emits acrid smoke and irritating fumes.

MQV800 CAS: 64742-53-6
MINERAL OIL, PETROLEUM DISTILLATES, HYDROTREATED LIGHT NAPHTHENIC

SYNS: DISTILLATES (PETROLEUM), HYDROTREATED LIGHT NAPHTHENIC (9CI) ◇ HYDROTREATED LIGHT NAPHTHENIC DISTILLATE ◇ HYDROTREATED LIGHT NAPHTHENIC DISTILLATES (PETROLEUM)

TOXICITY DATA with REFERENCE
NEO: skn-mus TDLo: 480 g/kg/80W-I EPASR*
   8EHQ-0887-0691S

CONSENSUS REPORTS: IARC Cancer Review: GROUP 1 IMEMDT 7,252,87; Animal Sufficient Evidence IMEMDT 33,87,84. Reported in EPA TSCA Inventory.

SAFETY PROFILE: Confirmed carcinogen with experimental neoplastigenic data. When heated to decomposition it emits acrid smoke and irritating fumes.

MQV805 CAS: 64742-55-8
MINERAL OIL, PETROLEUM DISTILLATES, HYDROTREATED LIGHT PARAFFINIC

SYNS: DISTILLATES (PETROLEUM), HYDROTREATED LIGHT PARAFFINIC (9CI) ◇ HYDROTREATED LIGHT PARAFFINIC DISTILLATE

CONSENSUS REPORTS: IARC Cancer Review: GROUP 1 IMEMDT 7,252,87; Animal Sufficient Evidence IMEMDT 33,87,84 Reported in EPA TSCA Inventory.

SAFETY PROFILE: Confirmed carcinogen. When heated to decomposition it emits acrid smoke and irritating fumes.

MQV810 CAS: 64741-52-2
MINERAL OIL, PETROLEUM DISTILLATES, LIGHT NAPHTHENIC

SYNS: DISTILLATES (PETROLEUM), LIGHT NAPHTHENIC (9CI) ◇ LIGHT NAPHTHENIC DISTILLATE ◇ LIGHT NAPHTHENIC DISTILLATES (PETROLEUM)

TOXICITY DATA with REFERENCE
NEO: skn-mus TDLo: 480 g/kg/80W-I EPASR*
   8EHQ-0887-0691S

CONSENSUS REPORTS: IARC Cancer Review: GROUP 1 IMEMDT 7,252,87; Animal Sufficient Evidence IMEMDT 33,87,84. Reported in EPA TSCA Inventory.

SAFETY PROFILE: Confirmed carcinogen with experimental neoplastigenic data. When heated to decomposition it emits acrid smoke and irritating fumes.

MQV815 CAS: 64741-50-0
MINERAL OIL, PETROLEUM DISTILLATES, LIGHT PARAFFINIC

SYNS: DISTILLATES (PETROLEUM), LIGHT PARAFFINIC (9CI) ◇ LIGHT PARAFFINIC DISTILLATE

TOXICITY DATA with REFERENCE
MUT: mmo-sat 5 uL/plate   CBTOE2 2,63,86

CONSENSUS REPORTS: IARC Cancer Review: GROUP 1 IMEMDT 7,252,87; Animal Sufficient Evidence IMEMDT 33,87,84. Reported in EPA TSCA Inventory.

SAFETY PROFILE: Confirmed carcinogen. Mutation data reported. When heated to decomposition it emits acrid smoke and irritating fumes.

MQV835   CAS: 64742-64-9
MINERAL OIL, PETROLEUM DISTILLATES, SOLVENT-DEWAXED LIGHT NAPHTHENIC

SYNS: DISTILLATES (PETROLEUM), SOLVENT-DE-WAXED LIGHT NAPHTHENIC (9CI) ◊ SOLVENT-DEWAXED LIGHT NAPHTHENIC DISTILLATE

CONSENSUS REPORTS: IARC Cancer Review: GROUP 1 IMEMDT 7,252,87; Animal Sufficient Evidence IMEMDT 33,87,84. Reported in EPA TSCA Inventory.

SAFETY PROFILE: Confirmed carcinogen. When heated to decomposition it emits acrid smoke and irritating fumes.

MQV840   CAS: 64742-56-9
MINERAL OIL, PETROLEUM DISTILLATES, SOLVENT-DEWAXED LIGHT PARAFFINIC

SYNS: DISTILLATES (PETROLEUM), SOLVENT-DE-WAXED LIGHT PARAFFINIC (9CI) ◊ SOLVENT-DEWAXED LIGHT PARAFFINIC DISTILLATE

CONSENSUS REPORTS: IARC Cancer Review: GROUP 1 IMEMDT 7,252,87; Animal Sufficient Evidence IMEMDT 33,87,84. Reported in EPA TSCA Inventory.

SAFETY PROFILE: Confirmed carcinogen. When heated to decomposition it emits acrid smoke and irritating fumes.

MQV852   CAS: 64741-97-5
MINERAL OIL, PETROLEUM DISTILLATES, SOLVENT-REFINED LIGHT NAPHTHENIC

SYNS: DISTILLATES (PETROLEUM), SOLVENT-REFINED LIGHT NAPHTHENIC (9CI) ◊ SOLVENT-REFINED LIGHT NAPHTHENIC DISTILLATE

CONSENSUS REPORTS: IARC Cancer Review: GROUP 1 IMEMDT 7,252,87; Animal

Sufficient Evidence IMEMDT 33,87,84. Reported in EPA TSCA Inventory.

SAFETY PROFILE: Confirmed carcinogen. When heated to decomposition it emits acrid smoke and irritating fumes.

MQV855   CAS: 64741-89-5
MINERAL OIL, PETROLEUM DISTILLATES, SOLVENT-REFINED LIGHT PARAFFINIC

SYNS: DISTILLATES (PETROLEUM), SOLVENT REFINED LIGHT PARAFFINIC (9CI) ◊ SOLVENT-REFINED LIGHT PARAFFINIC DISTILLATE

CONSENSUS REPORTS: IARC Cancer Review: GROUP 1 IMEMDT 7,252,87; Animal Sufficient Evidence IMEMDT 33,87,84. Reported in EPA TSCA Inventory.

SAFETY PROFILE: Confirmed carcinogen. When heated to decomposition it emits acrid smoke and irritating fumes.

MQV859   CAS: 64742-04-7
MINERAL OIL, PETROLEUM EXTRACTS, HEAVY PARAFFINIC DISTILLATE SOLVENT

SYNS: EXTRACTS (PETROLEUM), HEAVY PARAFFINIC DISTILLATE SOLVENT (9CI) ◊ HEAVY PARAFFINIC DISTIL-LATE, SOLVENT EXTRACT

CONSENSUS REPORTS: IARC Cancer Review: GROUP 1 IMEMDT 7,252,87; Animal Sufficient Evidence IMEMDT 33,87,84. Reported in EPA TSCA Inventory.

SAFETY PROFILE: Confirmed carcinogen. When heated to decomposition it emits acrid smoke and irritating fumes.

MQV857   CAS: 64742-11-6
MINERAL OIL, PETROLEUM EXTRACTS, HEAVY NAPHTHENIC DISTILLATE SOLVENT

SYNS: EXTRACTS (PETROLEUM), HEAVY NAPHTHENIC DISTILLATE SOLVENT (9CI) ◊ HEAVY NAPHTHENIC DIS-TILLATE SOLVENT EXTRACT

CONSENSUS REPORTS: IARC Cancer Review: GROUP 1 IMEMDT 7,252,87; Animal Sufficient Evidence IMEMDT 33,87,84. Reported in EPA TSCA Inventory.

SAFETY PROFILE: Confirmed carcinogen. Experimental reproductive data. When heated to decomposition it emits acrid smoke and irritating fumes.

MQV860   CAS: 64742-03-6
MINERAL OIL, PETROLEUM EXTRACTS, LIGHT NAPHTHENIC DISTILLATE SOLVENT

SYNS: EXTRACTS (PETROLEUM), LIGHT NAPHTHENIC DISTILLATE SOLVENT (9CI) ◊ LIGHT NAPHTHENIC DISTILLATE, SOLVENT EXTRACT

CONSENSUS REPORTS: IARC Cancer Review: GROUP 1 IMEMDT 7,252,87; Animal Sufficient Evidence 33,87,84. Reported in EPA TSCA Inventory.

SAFETY PROFILE: Confirmed carcinogen. When heated to decomposition it emits acrid smoke and irritating fumes.

MQV862   CAS: 64742-05-8
MINERAL OIL, PETROLEUM EXTRACTS, LIGHT PARAFFINIC DISTILLATE SOLVENT

SYNS: EXTRACTS (PETROLEUM), LIGHT PARAFFINIC DISTILLATE SOLVENT (9CI) ◊ LIGHT PARAFFINIC DISTILLATE, SOLVENT EXTRACT

CONSENSUS REPORTS: IARC Cancer Review: GROUP 1 IMEMDT 7,252,87; Animal Sufficient Evidence IMEMDT 33,87,84. Reported in EPA TSCA Inventory.

SAFETY PROFILE: Confirmed carcinogen. When heated to decomposition it emits acrid smoke and irritating fumes.

MQV863   CAS: 64742-10-5
MINERAL OIL, PETROLEUM EXTRACTS, RESIDUAL OIL SOLVENT

SYNS: EXTRACTS (PETROLEUM), RESIDUAL OIL SOLVENT (9CI) ◊ RESIDUAL OIL SOLVENT EXTRACT

CONSENSUS REPORTS: IARC Cancer Review: GROUP 1 IMEMDT 7,252,87; Animal Sufficient Evidence IMEMDT 33,87,84. Reported in EPA TSCA Inventory.

SAFETY PROFILE: Confirmed carcinogen. When heated to decomposition it emits acrid smoke and irritating fumes.

MQV865   CAS: 64742-68-3
MINERAL OIL, PETROLEUM NAPHTHENIC OILS, CATALYTIC DEWAXED HEAVY

SYNS: CATALYTIC-DEWAXED HEAVY NAPHTHENIC DISTILLATE ◊ NAPHTHENIC OILS (PETROLEUM), CATALYTIC DEWAXED HEAVY(9CI)

CONSENSUS REPORTS: IARC Cancer Review: GROUP 1 IMEMDT 7,252,87; Animal Sufficient Evidence IMEMDT 33,87,84. Reported in EPA TSCA Inventory.

SAFETY PROFILE: Confirmed carcinogen. When heated to decomposition it emits acrid smoke and irritating fumes.

MQV867   CAS: 64742-69-4
MINERAL OIL, PETROLEUM NAPHTHENIC OILS, CATALYTIC DEWAXED LIGHT

SYNS: CATALYTIC-DEWAXED LIGHT NAPHTHENIC DISTILLATE ◊ NAPHTHENIC OILS (PETROLEUM), CATALYTIC DEWAXED LIGHT (9CI)

CONSENSUS REPORTS: IARC Cancer Review: GROUP 1 IMEMDT 7,252,87; Animal Sufficient Evidence IMEMDT 33,87,84. Reported in EPA TSCA Inventory.

SAFETY PROFILE: Confirmed carcinogen. When heated to decomposition it emits acrid smoke and irritating fumes.

MQV868   CAS: 64742-70-7
MINERAL OIL, PETROLEUM PARAFFIN OILS, CATALYTIC DEWAXED HEAVY

SYNS: CATALYTIC-DEWAXED HEAVY PARAFFINIC DISTILLATE ◊ PARAFFIN OILS (PETROLEUM), CATALYTIC DEWAXED HEAVY (9CI)

CONSENSUS REPORTS: IARC Cancer Review: GROUP 1 IMEMDT 7,252,87; Animal Sufficient Evidence IMEMDT 33,87,84. Reported in EPA TSCA Inventory.

SAFETY PROFILE: Confirmed carcinogen. When heated to decomposition it emits acrid smoke and irritating fumes.

MQV870   CAS: 64742-71-8
MINERAL OIL, PETROLEUM PARAFFIN OILS, CATALYTIC DEWAXED LIGHT

SYNS: CATALYTIC-DEWAXED LIGHT PARAFFINIC DISTILLATE ◊ PARAFFIN OILS (PETROLEUM), CATALYTIC DEWAXED LIGHT (9CI)

CONSENSUS REPORTS: IARC Cancer Review: GROUP 1 IMEMDT 7,252,87; Animal Sufficient Evidence IMEMDT 33,87,84. Reported in EPA TSCA Inventory.

SAFETY PROFILE: Confirmed carcinogen. When heated to decomposition it emits acrid smoke and irritating fumes.

MQV872   CAS: 64742-17-2
MINERAL OIL, PETROLEUM RESIDUAL OILS, ACID-TREATED

SYNS: ACID-TREATED RESIDUAL OIL ◇ RESIDUAL OILS (PETROLEUM), ACID-TREATED (9CI)

CONSENSUS REPORTS: IARC Cancer Review: GROUP 1 IMEMDT 7,252,87; Animal Sufficient Evidence IMEMDT 33,87,84.

SAFETY PROFILE: Confirmed carcinogen. When heated to decomposition it emits acrid smoke and irritating fumes.

MQV875   CAS: 8042-47-5
MINERAL OIL, SLAB OIL

SYNS: SLAB OIL (9CI) ◇ WHITE MINERAL OIL

CONSENSUS REPORTS: IARC Cancer Review: GROUP 1 IMEMDT 7,252,87; Animal Inadequate Evidence IMEMDT 33,87,84. Reported in EPA TSCA Inventory.

SAFETY PROFILE: Confirmed carcinogen. When heated to decomposition it emits acrid smoke and irritating fumes.

MQW500   CAS: 2385-85-5
MIREX
mf: $C_{10}Cl_{12}$ mw: 545.50

PROP: Very white, odorless crystals. Decomp @ 485°. Water-insol, sol in dioxane and benzene.

SYNS: BICHLORENDO ◇ CG-1283 ◇ DECHLORANE 4070 ◇ DODECACHLOROOCTAHYDRO-1,3,4-METHENO-2H-CYCLOBUTA(c,d)PENTALENE ◇ 1,1a,2,2,3,3a,4,5,5,5a,5b,6-DODECACHLOROOCTAHYDRO-1,3,4-METHENO-1H-CYCLOBUTA(c,d)PENTALENE ◇ DODECACHLOROPENTACYCLODECANE ◇ DODECACHLOROPENTACYCLO(3,2,2,0^{2,6},0^{3,9},0^{5,10})DECANE ◇ ENT 25,719 ◇ FERRIAMICIDE ◇ HEXACHLOROCYCLOPENTADIENEDIMER ◇ 1,2,3,4,5,5-HEXACHLORO-1,3-CYCLOPENTADIENE DIMER ◇ HRS 1276 ◇ NCI-C06428 ◇ PERCHLORODIHOMOCUBANE ◇ PERCHLOROPENTACYCLODECANE ◇ PERCHLOROPENTACYCLO(5.2.1.0^{2,6}.0^{3,9}.0^{5,8})DECANE

TOXICITY DATA with REFERENCE
CAR: orl-mus TDLo: 2222 mg/kg/58W-C
  JNCIAM 42,1101,69
ETA: orl-rat TDLo: 2340 mg/kg/56W-C
  EXMPA6 38,271,83
MUT: oms-rat-orl 100 mg/kg   TOLED5
  23,127,84

CONSENSUS REPORTS: IARC Cancer Review: Human Limited Evidence IMEMDT 20,283,79; Animal Sufficient Evidence IMEMDT 20,283,79; IMEMDT 5,203,74. NTP Fourth Annual Report On Carcinogens, 1984. EPA Genetic Toxicology Program.

SAFETY PROFILE: Confirmed carcinogen with experimental carcinogenic, tumorigenic, and teratogenic data. Poison by ingestion. Moderately toxic by inhalation and skin contact. Experimental reproductive effects. Mutation data reported. A persistent insecticide which is toxic to non-target species. It can bioaccumulate.

NBE000   CAS: 134-32-7
1-NAPHTHYLAMINE
DOT: 2077
mf: $C_{10}H_9N$ mw: 143.20

PROP: White crystals, reddening on exposure to air; unpleasant odor. Mp: 50°, bp: 300.8°, flash p: 315°F, d: 1.131, vap press: 1 mm @ 104.3°, vap d: 4.93. Sublimes, volatile with steam. Sol in 590 parts water; very sol in alc, ether. Keep well closed and away from light.

SYNS: ALFANAFTILAMINA (ITALIAN) ◇ ALFA-NAFTYLOAMINA (POLISH) ◇ 1-AMINONAFTALEN (CZECH) ◇ 1-AMINONAPHTHALENE ◇ C.I. AZOIC DIAZO COMPONENT 114 ◇ 1-NAFTILAMINA (SPANISH) ◇ α-NAFTYLAMIN (CZECH) ◇ 1-NAFTYLAMINE (DUTCH) ◇ NAPHTHALIDINE ◇ 1-NAPHTHYLAMIN (GERMAN) ◇ α-NAPHTHYLAMINE ◇ RCRA WASTE NUMBER U167

TOXICITY DATA with REFERENCE
ETA: ipr-rat TDLo: 1300 mg/kg/13W-I   CNREA8
  28,535,68
MUT: dnd-dog-orl 60 μmol/kg   EVHPAZ 49,125,83
MUT: dnd-rat:lvr 3 mmol/L   SinJF# 26OCT82
MUT: dns-ham:lvr 10 μmol/L   ENMUDM 6,1,84
MUT: mma-sat 10 μg/plate   ENMUDM 6,497,84
MUT: mmo-sat 50 μg/plate   PMRSDJ 1,261,81
MUT: sce-mus-ipr 38 mg/kg   MUREAV 108,225,83

CONSENSUS REPORTS: IARC Cancer Review: Animal Inadequate Evidence IMEMDT 4,87,74; Human Limited Evidence IMEMDT 4,87,74. EPA Genetic Toxicology Program.

Community Right-To-Know List. Reported in EPA TSCA Inventory.

OSHA PEL: Carcinogen   DOT Classification: Poison B; Label: St. Andrews Cross.

SAFETY PROFILE: Confirmed carcinogen with experimental tumorigenic data. Along with β-naphthylamine and benzidine, it has been incriminated as a cause of urinary bladder cancer. Poison by subcutaneous and intraperitoneal routes. Moderately toxic by ingestion. Mutation data reported. Combustible when exposed to heat or flame. To fight fire, use dry chemical, CO_2, mist, spray. When heated to decomposition it emits toxic fumes of NO_x.

NBE500
β-NAPHTHYLAMINE
CAS: 91-59-8
DOT: 1650
mf: $C_{10}H_9N$ mw: 143.20

PROP: White to faint pink, lustrous leaflets; faint aromatic odor. Mp: 111.5°, d: 1.061 @ 98°/4°, vap press: 1 mm @ 108.0°. Bp: 306° also listed as 294°. Sol in hot water, alc, ether.

SYNS: 2-AMINONAFTALEN (CZECH) ◇ 2-AMINO-NAPHTHALENE ◇ BETA-NAFTYLOAMINA (POLISH) ◇ C.I. 37270 ◇ FAST SCARLET BASE B ◇ NA ◇ β-NAFTYL-AMIN (CZECH) ◇ β-NAFTILAMINA (ITALIAN) ◇ 2-NAFTYL-AMINE (DUTCH) ◇ β-NAFTYLOAMINA (POLISH) ◇ 2-NAPHTHALAMINE ◇ 2-NAPHTHALENAMINE ◇ β-NAPHTHYLAMIN (GERMAN) ◇ 2-NAPHTHYLAMIN (GERMAN) ◇ 6-NAPHTHYLAMINE ◇ 2-NAPHTHYLAMINE ◇ 2-NAPHTHYLAMINE MUSTARD ◇ RCRA WASTE NUMBER U168 ◇ USAF CB-22

TOXICITY DATA with REFERENCE
CAR: orl-dog TD:94500 mg/kg/9Y-I   BJCAAI 44,892,81
CAR: orl-dog TDLo:18 g/kg/2Y-I   JNCIAM 49,193,72
CAR: orl-ham TD:365 g/kg/43W-C   IMSUAI 35,564,66
CAR: orl-ham TDLo:217 mg/kg/45W-C 85DAAC 5,129,66
CAR: orl-rat TDLo:17100 mg/kg/57W-I BJCAAI 46,646,82
CAR: orl-rbt TDLo:40 g/kg/5Y   LANCAO 2,286,51
CAR: par-mus TDLo:18 mg/kg   BECCAN 40,42,62
NEO: ipr-mus TDLo:1500 mg/kg/8W-I   JJIND8 67,1299,81
NEO: orl-mus TDLo:600 mg/kg/8W-I   TXAPA9 82,19,86
NEO: orl-rat TD:16 g/kg/52W-I   CNREA8 37,2943,77

ETA: imp-mus TDLo:100 mg/kg   BJCAAI 10,539,56
ETA: ipr-rat TDLo:1300 mg/kg/13W-I   CNREA8 28,535,68
ETA: mul-dog TD:4379 mg/kg/80W-C   JIHTAB 20,46,38
ETA: mul-dog TD:5169 mg/kg/91W-C   JIHTAB 20,46,38
ETA: orl-dog TD:108 mg/kg/4Y   LANCAO 2,236,51
ETA: orl-mky TDLo:17 g/kg/5Y-I   JNCIAM 42,825,69
ETA: orl-mus TD:31 g/kg/2Y   LANCAO 2,286,51
ETA: orl-rat TD:13 g/kg/1Y-I:TER   JNCIAM 41,985,68
ETA: orl-rbt TD:30 g/kg/5Y   LANCAO 2,286,51
ETA: scu-mus TD:80 mg/kg   ZEKBAI 58,56,51
ETA: scu-mus TDLo:1600 mg/kg/40W-I   VOONAW 15(2),71,69
ETA: scu-rat TDLo:6 g/kg/60W-I   VOONAW 20(8),69,74
ETA: unr-dog TDLo:40 g/kg/81W   VOONAW 15(2),71,69
MUT: dnd-dog-orl 60 μmol/kg   EVHPAZ 49,125,83
MUT: dnd-hmn:fbr 50 μmol/L   MUREAV 127,107,84
MUT: dnd-rat:lvr 300 μmol/L   MUREAV 113,357,83
MUT: dns-ham:lvr 50 μmol/L   MUREAV 136,255,84
MUT: mmo-sat 2500 ng/plate   PMRSDJ 1,261,81
MUT: sce-mus-ipr 100 mg/kg   MUREAV 108,225,83

CONSENSUS REPORTS: IARC Cancer Review: Animal Sufficient Evidence IMEMDT 4,97,74; Human Sufficient Evidence IMEMDT 4,97,74. NTP Fourth Annual Report On Carcinogens, 1984. Community Right-To-Know List. EPA Genetic Toxicology Program. Reported in EPA TSCA Inventory.

OSHA PEL: Carcinogen   ACGIH TLV: Confirmed Human Carcinogen.   DFG MAK: Human Carcinogen.   DOT Classification: Poison B; Label: Poison.

SAFETY PROFILE: Confirmed carcinogen with experimental neoplastigenic, tumorigenic, and teratogenic data. Long and continued exposure to even small amounts may produce tumors and cancers of the bladder. Poison by intraperitoneal route. Moderately toxic by ingestion and possibly other routes. Human mutation data reported. A very toxic chemical in any of its physical forms, such as flake, lump, dust, liquid, or vapor. It can be absorbed into the body through the lungs, the gastrointestinal tract, or the skin.

Combustible when exposed to heat or flame. At elevated temperatures it evolves a vapor which is flammable and explosive. When heated to decomposition it emits toxic fumes of NO_x.

NBJ500   CAS: 7090-25-7
1-NAPHTHYL METHYLNITROSOCARBAMATE
mf: $C_{12}H_{10}N_2O_3$ mw: 230.24

SYNS: DENAPON, NITROSATED (JAPANESE) ◊ METHYL-NITROSOCARBAMIC ACID-1-NAPHTHYL ESTER ◊ 1-NAPHTHYL-N-METHYL-N-NITROSOCARBAMATE ◊ N-NITROSOCARBARYL ◊ NITROSO-NAC

TOXICITY DATA with REFERENCE
CAR: orl-rat TDLo: 600 mg/kg/10W-I   EESADV 2,413,78
CAR: skn-mus TDLo: 921 mg/kg/50W-I   JCREA8 102,13,81
NEO: scu-rat TDLo: 1000 mg/kg   FCTXAV 13,365,75
ETA: orl-rat TD: 600 mg/kg/10W-I   IARCCD 19,495,78
ETA: orl-rat TD: 2500 mg/kg/10W-I   CALEDQ 1,275,76
ETA: orl-rat TD: 6203 mg/kg/24W-I   IARCCD 14,429,76
MUT: cyt-ham:lng 10 μmol/L   IAPUDO 31,797,80
MUT: dnr-hmn:fbr 10 μmol/L   MUREAV 44,1,77
MUT: mmo-asn 1 μg/plate   MUREAV 97,293,82
MUT: mmo-sat 500 ng/plate   IGMPAX 78,301,82
MUT: mnt-nml-mul 5000 ppb/8D-C   MUREAV 125,275,84
MUT: sce-ham:lng 10 μmol/L   IAPUDO 31,797,80

CONSENSUS REPORTS: IARC Cancer Review: Animal Sufficient Evidence IMEMDT 12,37,76. EPA Genetic Toxicology Program.

SAFETY PROFILE: Confirmed carcinogen with experimental carcinogenic, neoplastigenic, and tumorigenic data. Human mutation data reported. When heated to decomposition it emits toxic fumes of NO_x.

NCW500   CAS: 7440-02-0
NICKEL
af: Ni   aw: 58.71

PROP: A silvery-white, hard, malleable and ductile metal. D: 8.90 @ 25°, vap press: 1 mm @ 1810°. Crystallizes as metallic cubes. Mp: 1455°, bp: 2730°. Stable in air at room temp.

SYNS: C.I. 77775 ◊ Ni 270 ◊ NICKEL 270 ◊ NICKEL (DUST) ◊ NICKEL (ITALIAN) ◊ NICKEL PARTICLES

◊ NICKEL SPONGE ◊ Ni 0901-S ◊ Ni 4303T ◊ NP 2 ◊ RANEY ALLOY ◊ RANEY NICKEL

TOXICITY DATA with REFERENCE
CAR: imp-rat TDLo: 250 mg/kg   JNCIAM 16,55,55
CAR: ims-rat TD: 1 g/kg/17W-I   PAACA3 9,28,68
CAR: ims-rat TDLo: 56 mg/kg   IAPUDO 53,127,84
NEO: imp-rbt TDLo: 165 mg/kg/2Y-I: TER   JNCIAM 16,55,55
NEO: ims-mus TD: 800 mg/kg/13W-I   NCIUS* PH 43-64-886,JUL,68
NEO: ims-mus TDLo: 200 mg/kg   NCIUS* PH 43-64-886,SEPT,70
NEO: ims-rat TD: 125 mg/kg/13W-I   NCIUS* PH 43-64-886,JUL,68
NEO: ims-rat TD: 200 mg/kg/21W-I   PWPSA8 14,68,71
ETA: ihl-gpg TCLo: 15 mg/m^3/91W-I   AMPLAO 65,600,58
ETA: imp-rat TD: 23 mg/kg   JNCIAM 16,55,55
ETA: ims-ham TDLo: 200 mg/kg/21W-I   PWPSA8 14,68,71
ETA: ims-rat TD: 58 mg/kg   PAACA3 17,11,76
ETA: ims-rat TD: 90 mg/kg/18W-I   NCIUS* PH 43-64-886,AUG,69
ETA: ims-rat TD: 889 μg/kg   JPTLAS 97,375,69
ETA: ipl-rat TD: 125 mg/kg/21W-I   PWPSA8 16,150,73
ETA: ipl-rat TD: 1250 mg/kg/17W-I   TRBMAV 10,167,52
ETA: ipl-rat TDLo: 100 mg/kg/21W-I   PWPSA8 16,150,73
ETA: par-rat TDLo: 40 mg/kg/52W-I: TER   AEHLAU 5,445,62
ETA: scu-rat TDLo: 3000 mg/kg/6W-I   JNCIAM 16,55,55
MUT: otr-ham:emb 5 μmol/L   TOXID9 1,132,81
MUT: otr-ham:kdy 400 mg/L   IAPUDO 53,193,84

CONSENSUS REPORTS: IARC Cancer Review: Animal Sufficient Evidence IMEMDT 11,75,76; Animal Inadequate Evidence IMEMDT 2,126,73. NTP Fourth Annual Report On Carcinogens, 1984. Community Right-To-Know List. Reported in EPA TSCA Inventory.

OSHA PEL: TWA Soluble: Compounds: 0.1 mg(Ni)/m^3; Insoluble Compounds: 1 mg(Ni)/m^3 ACGIH TLV: TWA 1 mg(Ni)/m^3; (Proposed: TWA 0.05 mg(Ni)/m^3; Human Carcinogen)   DFG TRK: 0.5 mg/m^3; Human Carcinogen.   NIOSH REL: (Inorganic Nickel) TWA 0.015 mg(Ni)/m^3

SAFETY PROFILE: Confirmed carcinogen with experimental carcinogenic, neoplastigenic, tumorigenic, and teratogenic data. Poison by ingestion, intratracheal, intraperitoneal, subcutaneous, and intravenous routes. Experimental reproductive effects. Ingestion of soluble salts causes nausea, vomiting, diarrhea. Mutation data reported. Powders may ignite spontaneously in air.

NCX000   CAS: 373-02-4
NICKEL(II) ACETATE (1:2)
mf: $C_4H_6O_4 \cdot Ni$ mw: 176.81

PROP: Green prisms. Mp: decomp, d: 1.798.

SYNS: ACETIC ACID, NICKEL(2+) SALT ◇ NICKELOUS ACETATE

TOXICITY DATA with REFERENCE
NEO: ims-rat TDLo: 420 mg/kg/47W-I
    NCIUS* PH 43-64-886,JUL,68
NEO: ipr-mus TDLo: 360 mg/kg/8W-I   CNREA8
    36,1744,76
ETA: imp-rat TDLo: 95 mg/kg/78W-C   PAACA3
    5,50,64
ETA: ims-rat TD: 225 mg/kg/46W-I
    NCIUS* PH 43-64-886,AUG,69
MUT: dns-rat-ipr 129 μmol/kg/5D-I   CRNGDP
    6,1819,85
MUT: otr-ham:kdy 225 mg/L   IAPUDO 53,193,84
MUT: pic-esc 160 μmol/L   ENMUDM 6,59,84

CONSENSUS REPORTS: IARC Cancer Review: GROUP 1 IMEMDT 7,264,87. Nickel and its compounds are on the Community Right-To-Know List. Reported in EPA TSCA Inventory.

OSHA PEL: (Transitional: TWA 1 mg/m³) TWA 0.1 mg (Ni)/m³   ACGIH TLV: TWA 0.1 mg(Ni)/m³; (Proposed: TWA 0.05 mg(Ni)/m³; Human Carcinogen)   NIOSH REL: (Inorganic Nickel) TWA 0.015 mg(Ni)/m³

SAFETY PROFILE: Confirmed carcinogen with experimental neoplastigenic and tumorigenic data. Poison by ingestion, intraperitoneal, and subcutaneous routes. Experimental reproductive effects. Mutation data reported. When heated to decomposition it emits irritating fumes.

NCY125   CAS: 12255-10-6
NICKEL ARSENIDE SULFIDE
mf: AsNiS   mw: 165.69

SYN: NICKEL SULFARSENIDE

TOXICITY DATA with REFERENCE
CAR: ims-rat TDLo: 158 mg/kg   IAPUDO53,127,84

NEO: irn-rat TDLo: 79022 μg/kg   CRNGDP
    5,1511,84

OSHA: Cancer Hazard

SAFETY PROFILE: Confirmed human carcinogen with experimental carcinogenic and neoplastigenic data. When heated to decomposition it emits toxic fumes of Ni, As, and SO_x.

NCY500   CAS: 3333-67-3
NICKEL(II) CARBONATE (1:1)
mf: $CNiO_3$ mw: 118.72

PROP: Rhombic, light green crystals. Mp: decomp.

SYNS: BASIC NICKEL CARBONATE ◇ CARBONIC ACID, NICKEL SALT (1:1) ◇ C.I. 77779 ◇ NICKELOUS CARBONATE

TOXICITY DATA with REFERENCE
ETA: imp-rat TDLo: 95 mg/kg/78W-C   PAACA3
    5,50,64
MUT: dnd-rat-ipr 10 mg/kg/3H   CNREA8
    42,3544,82
MUT: oms-rat-ipr 40 mg/kg   CNREA8 44,3892,84
MUT: sce-ham:ovr 400 nmol/L   ENMUDM
    7,381,85

CONSENSUS REPORTS: IARC Cancer Review: Animal Sufficient Evidence IMEMDT 11,75,76. NTP Fourth Annual Report On Carcinogens, 1984. Nickel and its compounds are on the Community Right-To-Know List. Reported in EPA TSCA Inventory.

OSHA PEL: TWA 1 mg(Ni)/m³   ACGIH TLV: TWA 1 mg(Ni)/m³; (Proposed: TWA 0.05 mg(Ni)/m³; Human Carcinogen)   DFG TRK: 0.5 mg/m³; Human Carcinogen.   NIOSH REL: (Inorganic Nickel) TWA 0.015 mg(Ni)/m³

SAFETY PROFILE: Confirmed carcinogen with experimental carcinogenic and tumorigenic data. Poison by subcutaneous route. Mutation data reported.

NCZ000   CAS: 13463-39-3
NICKEL CARBONYL
DOT: 1259
mf: C_4NiO_4 mw: 170.75

PROP: Colorless, volatile liquid or needles. Bp: 43°, mp: −19.3°, lel: 2% @ 20°, d: 1.3185 @ 17°, vap press: 400 mm @ 25.8°, flash p: <−4°. Oxidizes in air. Sol in alc, benzene, chloroform, acetone, carbon tetrachloride.

SYNS: NICKEL CARBONYLE (FRENCH) ◇ NICHEL TETRACARBONILE (ITALIAN) ◇ NICKEL TETRACARBONYL

◇ NICKEL TETRACARBONYLE (FRENCH) ◇ NIKKELTET-
RACARBONYL (DUTCH) ◇ RCRA WASTE NUMBER P073

TOXICITY DATA with REFERENCE
CAR: ivn-rat TDLo:54 mg/kg/20W-I   CNREA8
32,2253,72
ETA: ihl-rat TC:4 ppm/30M/2Y-I   AJPAA4
46,1027,65
ETA: ihl-rat TCLo:250 mg/m^3/30M/1Y   AJCPAI
35,203,61

CONSENSUS REPORTS: IARC Cancer Review: Animal Limited Evidence IMEMDT
2,126,73; IMEMDT 11,75,76. NTP Fourth Annual Report On Carcinogens, 1984. EPA Extremely Hazardous Substances List. Nickel and
its compounds are on the Community Right-
To-Know List. Reported in EPA TSCA Inventory.

OSHA PEL: TWA 0.001 ppm (Ni)   ACGIH
TLV: TWA 0.05 ppm (Ni); (Proposed: TWA
0.05 mg(Ni)/m^3; Human Carcinogen) DFG
TRK: 0.1 ppm; Animal Carcinogen, Suspected
Human Carcinogen. NIOSH REL: (Nickel
Carbonyl) TWA 0.001 ppm   DOT Classification: Poison B; Label: Poison, Flammable Liquid; Flammable Liquid; Label: Flammable Liquid and Poison.

SAFETY PROFILE: Confirmed carcinogen with
experimental carcinogenic, tumorigenic, and
teratogenic data. Chronic exposure may cause
cancer of the lungs, nasal sinuses. A human
poison by inhalation. Poison experimentally by
inhalation, intravenous, subcutaneous, and intraperitoneal routes. Experimental reproductive
effects. Human systemic effects by inhalation:
somnolence, fever and other pulmonary
changes. Vapors may cause coughing, dyspnea
(difficult breathing), irritation, congestion and
edema of lungs, tachycardia (rapid pulse), cyanosis, headache, dizziness, weakness. A very
dangerous fire hazard when exposed to heat,
flame, or oxidizers. To fight fire, use water,
foam, CO$_2$, dry chemical. When heated to decomposition or on contact with acid or acid
fumes it emits highly toxic fumes of carbon
monoxide.

NDA500   CAS: 1271-28-9
**NICKEL, COMPOUND with
pi-CYCLOPENTADIENYL (1:2)**
mf: C$_{10}$H$_{10}$•Ni   mw: 188.91

SYNS: pi-CYCLOPENTADIENYL COMPOUND with NICKEL
◇ DI-pi-CYCLOPENTADIENYLNICKEL ◇ NICKEL BISCY-
CLOPENTADIENE ◇ NICKELOCENE

TOXICITY DATA with REFERENCE
NEO: ims-ham TDLo:200 mg/kg   PWPSA8
14,68,71
NEO: ims-rat TD:600 mg/kg/47W-I
NCIBR* PH43-64-886,JUL68
NEO: ims-rat TD:650 mg/kg/1Y-I   PWPSA8
14,68,71
NEO: ims-rat TD:1260 mg/kg/56W-I
NCIUS* PH 43-64-886,DEC,68
NEO: ims-rat TDLo:600 mg/kg/52W-I
NCIBR* PH43-64-886,DEC65
ETA: ims-rat TD:50 mg/kg
NCIUS* PH-43-64-886,SEPT,65

CONSENSUS REPORTS: IARC Cancer Review: Animal Sufficient Evidence IMEMDT
11,75,76; Animal Inadequate Evidence
IMEMDT 2,126,73. NTP Fourth Annual Report
On Carcinogens, 1984. Nickel and its compounds are on the Community Right-To-Know
List. Reported in EPA TSCA Inventory.

NIOSH REL: TWA 15 μg(Ni)/m^3

SAFETY PROFILE: Confirmed carcinogen with
experimental carcinogenic, neoplastigenic, and
tumorigenic data. Poison by intraperitoneal and
intramuscular routes. Moderately toxic by ingestion. When heated to decomposition it emits
acrid smoke and irritating fumes.

**NDB000
NICKEL COMPOUNDS**

CONSENSUS REPORTS: Nickel and its compounds are on the Community Right-To-Know
List.

OSHA PEL: TWA Soluble: Compounds: 0.1
mg(Ni)/m^3; Insoluble Compounds: 1 mg(Ni)/
m^3 ACGIH TLV: TWA 1 mg/m^3; (Proposed:
TWA 0.05 mg(Ni)/m^3; Human Carcinogen)
DFG MAK: Human Carcinogen. NIOSH
REL: (Inorganic Nickel) TWA 0.015 mg(Ni)/m^3

SAFETY PROFILE: Many are human carcinogens by inhalation. Nickel and many of its compounds are poisons and carcinogens. All airborne nickel contaminating dusts are regarded
as carcinogenic by inhalation. Nickel carbonyl
is probably the most hazardous compound of
nickel in the workplace. It is carcinogenic and
highly irritating to the lungs and can produce

asphyxia by decomposing to form carbon monoxide. Nickel chloride ($NiCl_2$), sulfate ($NiSO_4 \cdot 6H_2O$), nitrate [$Ni(NO_3)_2 \cdot 6H_2O$], carbonate ($NiCO_3$), hydroxide [$Ni(OH)_2$] and acetate [$Ni(COOCH_3)_2$] are the salts of greatest commercial importance.

Nickel refinery workers experience increased mortality rates from cancer of the lungs and nasal cavities attributed to inhalation of airborne nickel compounds. Cancer develops in rodents after administration of Ni_3S_2, NiO, and $Ni(CO)_4$. Nickel chloride, sulfate, carbonate, and carbonyl are experimental teratogens.

NDE000   CAS: 12054-48-7
NICKEL(II) HYDROXIDE
DOT: 9140
mf: H_2NiO_2 mw: 92.73

PROP: Light green crystals or amorphous.

SYNS: NICKEL HYDROXIDE (DOT) ◇ NICKELOUS HYDROXIDE

TOXICITY DATA with REFERENCE
CAR: ims-rat TDLo: 480 µg/kg   CRNGDP 4,275,83
ETA: ims-rat TD: 60 mg/kg   45ICAX -,59,80

CONSENSUS REPORTS: IARC Cancer Review: Animal Sufficient Evidence IMEMDT 11,75,76. Nickel and its compounds are on the Community Right-To-Know List. Reported in EPA TSCA Inventory.

OSHA PEL: (Transitional: TWA 1 mg/m³) TWA 0.1 mg (Ni)/m³ ACGIH TLV: TWA 0.1 mg(Ni)/m³; (Proposed: TWA 0.05 mg(Ni)/m³; Human Carcinogen) NIOSH REL: (Inorganic Nickel) TWA 0.015 mg(Ni)/m³ DOT Classification: ORM-E; Label: None.

SAFETY PROFILE: Confirmed carcinogen with experimental carcinogenic and tumorigenic data. Poison by subcutaneous route.

NDF500   CAS: 1313-99-1
NICKEL MONOXIDE
mf: NiO   mw: 74.71

PROP: Cubic, green-black crystals; yellow when hot. Mp: 1900°, d: 7.45. Insol in water; sol in acids.

SYNS: BUNSENITE ◇ C.I. 77777 ◇ GREEN NICKEL OXIDE ◇ NICKELOUS OXIDE ◇ NICKEL OXIDE (MAK) ◇ NICKEL(II) OXIDE (1:1) ◇ NICKEL PROTOXIDE

TOXICITY DATA with REFERENCE
CAR: ims-rat TDLo: 71264 µg/kg   IAPUDO 53,127,84

ETA: imp-rat TDLo: 95 mg/kg/78W-C   PAACA3 5,50,64
ETA: ims-mus TDLo: 400 mg/kg   CNREA8 22,158,62
ETA: ims-rat TD: 180 mg/kg   CNREA8 22,158,62
ETA: ipl-rat TDLo: 40 mg/kg   55DXAE-,37,85
ETA: itr-rat TDLo: 90 mg/kg   VOONAW 24(4),44,78
MUT: otr-ham:kdy 100 mg/L   IAPUDO 53,193,84
MUT: otr-mus:emb 500 µmol/L   PAACA3 24,100,83

CONSENSUS REPORTS: IARC Cancer Review: Animal Inadequate Evidence IMEMDT 2,126,73; Animal Sufficient Evidence IMEMDT 11,75,76. NTP Fourth Annual Report On Carcinogens, 1984. Nickel and its compounds are on the Community Right-To-Know List. Reported in EPA TSCA Inventory.

OSHA PEL: TWA 1 mg(Ni)/m³ ACGIH TLV: TWA 1 mg(Ni)/m³; (Proposed: TWA 0.05 mg(Ni)/m³; Human Carcinogen) DFG TRK: 0.5 mg/m³; Human Carcinogen. NIOSH REL: (Inorganic Nickel) TWA 0.015 mg(Ni)/m³

SAFETY PROFILE: Confirmed carcinogen with experimental carcinogenic and tumorigenic data. Poison by intratracheal, intravenous, and subcutaneous routes. Mutation data reported.

NDI500
NICKEL REFINERY DUST

PROP: *Analysis:* Cupric oxide (3.4%), nickel sulfate (20.0%), nickel sulfide (57.0%), nickel oxide (6.3%), cobalt oxide (1.0%), ferric oxide (1.8%), silicon dioxide (1.2%), misc. (2.0%), water (7.3%) (CNREA8 22,158,62).

TOXICITY DATA with REFERENCE
CAR: ims-rat TDLo: 90 mg/kg   CNREA8 22,152,62
NEO: ims-mus TDLo: 135 mg/kg   CNREA8 22,152,62

CONSENSUS REPORTS: IARC Cancer Review: Human Sufficient Evidence IMEMDT 2,126,73. Nickel and its compounds are on the Community Right-To-Know List.

OSHA PEL: TWA 1 mg(Ni)/m³ ACGIH TLV: TWA 1 mg(Ni)/m³; (Proposed: TWA 0.05 mg(Ni)/m³; Human Carcinogen) NIOSH REL: (Inorganic Nickel) TWA 0.015 mg (Ni)/m³

SAFETY PROFILE: Confirmed carcinogen with experimental carcinogenic and neoplastigenic data. A human carcinogenic. Moderately toxic by intramuscular route. When heated to decomposition it emits toxic fumes of SO_x.

NDJ399   CAS: 12255-80-0
NICKEL SUBARSENIDE
mf: As_2Ni_5 mw: 443.39

SYN: NICKEL ARSENIDE (As_2-Ni_5)

TOXICITY DATA with REFERENCE
CAR: ims-rat TDLo: 443 mg/kg   IAPUDO53,127,84

OSHA: Cancer Hazard

SAFETY PROFILE: Confirmed human carcinogen with experimental carcinogenic data. Moderately toxic by ingestion. When heated to decomposition it emits toxic fumes of As.

NDJ400   CAS: 12256-33-6
NICKEL SUBARSENIDE
mf: As_8Ni_{11} mw: 1245.17

SYN: NICKEL ARSENIDE (As_8-Ni_{11})

TOXICITY DATA with REFERENCE
CAR: ims-rat TDLo: 108 mg/kg   IAPUDO53,127,84

OSHA: Cancer Hazard

SAFETY PROFILE: Confirmed human carcinogen with experimental carcinogenic data. When heated to decomposition it emits toxic fumes of As.

NDJ475   CAS: 12137-13-2
NICKEL SUBSELENIDE
mf: Ni_3Se_2 mw: 334.05

SYNS: NICKEL SELENIDE ◇ NICKEL SELENIDE (3:2) CRYSTALLINE

TOXICITY DATA with REFERENCE
CAR: ims-rat TDLo: 319 mg/kg   IAPUDO53,127,84
MUT: otr-ham: emb 5 μmol/plate   TOXID9 1,132,81

OSHA PEL: TWA Soluble: Compounds: 0.1 mg(Ni)/m³; Insoluble Compounds: 1 mg(Ni)/m³; TWA 0.2 mg(Se)/m³   ACGIH TLV: TWA 1 mg(Ni)/m³; (Proposed: TWA 0.05 mg(Ni)/m³; Human Carcinogen); TWA 0.2 mg(Se)/m³   DFG TRK: 0.5 mg/m³; Human Carcinogen.   NIOSH REL: (Inorganic Nickel) TWA 0.015 mg(Ni)/m³

SAFETY PROFILE: Confirmed carcinogen with experimental carcinogenic data. Mutation data reported.

NDJ500   CAS: 12035-72-2
NICKEL SUBSULFIDE
mf: Ni_3S_2 mw: 240.25

SYNS: HEAZLEWOODITE ◇ NICKEL SUBSULPHIDE ◇ NICKEL SULFIDE ◇ α-NICKEL SULFIDE (3:2) CRYSTALLINE ◇ NICKEL SULPHIDE ◇ NICKEL TRITADISULPHIDE

TOXICITY DATA with REFERENCE
CAR: ihl-rat TCLo: 970 μg/m³/6H/76W-I
   JNCIAM 54,1165,75
CAR: ims-ham TDLo: 80 mg/kg   AEMBAP91,57,78
CAR: ims-rat TD: 10 mg/kg   CRNGDP 4,461,83
CAR: ims-rat TD: 229 mg/kg   IAPUDO 53,127,84
CAR: ims-rat TD: 4800 μg/kg   CRNGDP 4,461,83
CAR: ims-rat TDLo: 100 mg/kg   CRNGDP 8,1005,87
CAR: ims-rat TDLo: 115 mg/kg   CRNGDP4,275,83
CAR: irn-rat TDLo: 25 mg/kg   LAINAW 35,71,76
CAR: irn-rat TDLo: 45 mg/kg   JEPTDQ 2,1511,79
CAR: ivn-rat TDLo: 10 mg/kg   FEPRA7 39(3,Pt.1),330
CAR: ocu-rat TD: 10 mg/kg   IOVSDA 22,768,82
CAR: ocu-rat TDLo: 2500 μg/kg
   NTIS** DOE/EV/03140-5
CAR: par-rat TDLo: 40 mg/kg   CNREA8 38,268,78
NEO: ims-ham TD: 40 mg/kg   AEMBAP 91,57,78
NEO: ims-ham TD: 20 mg/kg   RCOCB8 14,319,76
NEO: irn-rat TD: 23 mg/kg   JEPTDQ 2,1511,79
NEO: mul-ham TDLo: 272 g/kg/18W-I   AEMBAP 91,57,78
ETA: imp-rat TDLo: 95 mg/kg/78W-C   PAACA3 5,50,64
ETA: imp-rbt TDLo: 27 mg/kg   EJCBDN 19,276,79
ETA: ims-mus TDLo: 200 mg/kg   CNREA8 22,158,62
ETA: itt-rat TD: 40 mg/kg: TER   PAACA3 18,52,77
ETA: itt-rat TDLo: 5 mg/kg   PAACA3 18,52,77
ETA: scu-rat TDLo: 25 mg/kg   JJCREP 79,212,88
ETA: scu-rat TDLo: 125 mg/kg   BJCAAI 20,190,66
MUT: dnd-ham: ovr 10 mg/L   CRNGDP 3,657,82
MUT: dnd-mam: lym 4800 mg/L   BICHAW 21,771,82
MUT: dnd-rat: lvr 3 mmol/L   SinJF# 26OCT82
MUT: dns-ham: emb 10 mg/L   CALEDQ 17,273,83
MUT: otr-ham: emb 5 μmol/plate   TOXID9 1,132,81
MUT: sce-hmn: lym 1 mg/L   CNREA8 41,4136,81

CONSENSUS REPORTS: IARC Cancer Review: Animal Sufficient Evidence IMEMDT 2,126,73, IMEMDT 11,75,76. NTP Fourth Annual Report On Carcinogens, 1984. Nickel and its compounds are on the Community Right-

To-Know List. Reported in EPA TSCA Inventory.

OSHA PEL: TWA 1 mg(Ni)/m^3 ACGIH TLV: TWA 1 mg(Ni)/m^3; (Proposed: TWA 0.05 mg(Ni)/m^3; Human Carcinogen) NIOSH REL: TWA 0.015 mg(Ni)/m^3

SAFETY PROFILE: Confirmed carcinogen with experimental carcinogenic, neoplastigenic, tumorigenic, and teratogenic data. Poison by intraperitoneal route. Experimental reproductive effects. Human mutation data reported. When heated to decomposition it emits toxic fumes of SO$_x$.

NDL100   CAS: 11113-75-0
NICKEL SULFIDE
mf: NiS   mw: 90.77

SYNS: NICKEL MONOSULFIDE ◇ NICKELOUS SULFIDE ◇ NICKEL(II) SULFIDE ◇ α-NICKEL SULFIDE (1:1) CRYSTALLINE

TOXICITY DATA with REFERENCE
CAR: ims-rat TDLo: 86585 μg/kg   IAPUDO 53,127,84
NEO: irn-rat TDLo: 43290 μg/kg   CRNGDP 5,1511,84
MUT: cyt-ham: ovr 5 mg/L   CNREA8 45,2320,85
MUT: cyt-mus: mmr 1 mmol/L/48H   MUREAV 67,221,79
MUT: cyt-rat: oth 1 mg/L   LAINAW 19,663,68
MUT: dnd-ham: ovr 1 mg/L   CALEDQ 15,35,82
MUT: dns-ham: ovr 1 mg/L   CALEDQ 17,273,83
MUT: otr-ham: emb 5 μmol/plate   TOXID9 1,132,81

CONSENSUS REPORTS: Nickel and its compounds are on the Community Right-To-Know List.

OSHA PEL: TWA 1 mg(Ni)/m^3 ACGIH TLV: TWA 1 mg(Ni)/m^3; (Proposed: TWA 0.05 mg(Ni)/m^3; Human Carcinogen) DFG TRK: 0.5 mg/m^3; Human Carcinogen. NIOSH REL: TWA 0.015 mg(Ni)/m^3

SAFETY PROFILE: Confirmed carcinogen with experimental carcinogenic and neoplastigenic data. Mutation data reported. When heated to decomposition it emits toxic fumes of SO$_x$.

NEJ500   CAS: 602-87-9
5-NITROACENAPHTHENE
mf: C$_{12}$H$_9$NO$_2$ mw: 199.22

SYNS: 1,2-DIHYDRO-5-NITRO-ACENAPHTHYLENE ◇ 5-NAN ◇ NCI-C01967 ◇ 5-NITROACENAPHTHYLENE ◇ 5-NITROACENAPTHENE ◇ 5-NITRONAPHTHALENE ETHYLENE

TOXICITY DATA with REFERENCE
CAR: orl-mus TD: 80 g/kg/78W-C: TER   NCITR* NCI-TR-118,78
CAR: orl-mus TDLo: 33 g/kg/78W-C   NCITR* NCI-TR-118,78
CAR: orl-rat TD: 60 g/kg/70W-C   NCITR* NCI-TR-118,78
CAR: orl-rat TD: 61 g/kg/17W-C   SAIGBL 15,495,73
CAR: orl-rat TD: 120 g/kg/17W-C   TJIDAH 89,475,74
CAR: orl-rat TDLo: 40 g/kg/78W-C   NCITR* NCI-TR-118,78
ETA: imp-mus TDLo: 160 mg/kg   NEZAAQ 24,263,69
ETA: ipr-mus TDLo: 3744 mg/kg/78W-I   NEZAAQ 24,263,69
MUT: mma-esc 10 μg/plate   ENMUDM 7(Suppl 5),1,85
MUT: mma-sat 300 ng/plate   ENMUDM 7(Suppl 5),1,85
MUT: mmo-sat 30 ng/plate   ENMUDM 7(Suppl 5),1,85

CONSENSUS REPORTS: IARC Cancer Review: Animal Sufficient Evidence IMEMDT 16,319,78. NCI Carcinogenesis Bioassay (feed); Clear Evidence: mouse, rat NCITR* NCI-CG-TR-118,78. Reported in EPA TSCA Inventory. EPA Genetic Toxicology Program.

DFG MAK: Animal Carcinogen, Suspected Human Carcinogen.

SAFETY PROFILE: Confirmed carcinogen with experimental carcinogenic, neoplastigenic, and teratogenic data. Mutation data reported. When heated to decomposition it emits toxic fumes of NO$_x$.

NFQ000   CAS: 92-93-3
4-NITROBIPHENYL
mf: C$_{12}$H$_9$NO$_2$ mw: 199.22

PROP: Needles from alc. Mp: 113-114°, bp: 340°. Insol in water; sltly sol in cold alc; very sol in ether.

SYNS: 4-NITROBIPHENYL ◇ p-NITRODIPHENYL ◇ p-NITRODIPHENYL ◇ p-PHENYL-NITROBENZENE ◇ 4-PHENYL-NITROBENZENE ◇ PNB

TOXICITY DATA with REFERENCE
NEO: orl-dog TDLo: 7000 mg/kg/2Y-I   JAMAAP 172,1611,60

ETA: orl-dog TD:7000 mg/kg/3Y-I   IMSUAI
27,634,58
MUT: dnd-rat:lvr 300 μmol/L   SinJF# 26OCT82
MUT: dns-rat:lvr 100 μmol/L   ENMUDM 3,11,81
MUT: mma-mus:lym 77600 μl/L   MUREAV
97,49,82
MUT: mmo-bcs 50 mmol/L   EXPEAM 39,530,83
MUT: otr-ham:kdy 80 μg/L   BJCAAI 37,873,78

CONSENSUS REPORTS: IARC Cancer Review: Animal Limited Evidence IMEMDT 4,113,74. Reported in EPA TSCA Inventory.

OSHA: Carcinogen.   ACGIH TLV: Confirmed Human Carcinogen.   DFG MAK: Animal Carcinogen, Suspected Human Carcinogen.

SAFETY PROFILE: Confirmed carcinogen with experimental carcinogenic, neoplastigenic, and tumorigenic data. Poison by intraperitoneal route. Moderately toxic by ingestion. Mutation data reported. When heated to decomposition it emits toxic fumes of NO_x.

NHQ500   CAS: 581-89-5
2-NITRONAPHTHALENE
mf: $C_{10}H_7NO_2$ mw: 173.18

PROP: Colorless in ethanol. Mp: 79°, bp: 165° @ 15 mm. Insol in water, very sol in alc and ether.

SYN: β-NITRONAPHTHALENE

TOXICITY DATA with REFERENCE
ETA: orl-dog TDLo:2400 mg/kg/34/W-I
XPHCI* 17DEC76
ETA: orl-mky TDLo:340 g/kg/5Y-C   GANNA2
61,79,70
MUT: dnr-esc 5 mg/L   JJIND8 62,873,79
MUT: hma-mus/sat 125 mg/kg   JJIND8 62,911,79
MUT: mma-sat 100 μg/plate   PNASA6 72,5135,75
MUT: mmo-sat 1 μg/plate   MUREAV 122,243,83
MUT: mrc-smc 1 pph   JJIND8 62,901,79
MUT: otr-ham:emb 1 mg/L   IJCNAW 19,642,77

CONSENSUS REPORTS: EPA Genetic Toxicology Program.

DFG TRK: 0.035 ppm; Animal Carcinogen, Suspected Human Carcinogen.

SAFETY PROFILE: Confirmed carcinogen with experimental tumorigenic data. Moderately toxic by ingestion and intraperitoneal routes. Mutation data reported. A skin and lung irritant. Combustible when exposed to heat or flame. When heated to decomposition it emits toxic fumes of NO_x.

NIY000   CAS: 79-46-9
2-NITROPROPANE
DOT: 2608
mf: $C_3H_7NO_2$ mw: 89.11

PROP: Colorless liquid. Bp: 120°, fp: −93°, flash p: 82°F (TCC), d: 0.992 @ 20°/20°, autoign temp: 802°F, vap press: 10 mm @ 15.8°, vap d: 3.06, lel: 2.6%. Misc with organic solvents; sol in water, alc, and ether.

SYNS: DIMETHYLNITROMETHANE ◇ ISONITROPROPANE ◇ NIPAR S-20 ◇ NIPAR S-20 SOLVENT ◇ NIPAR S-30 SOLVENT ◇ NITROISOPROPANE ◇ β-NITROPROPANE ◇ 2-NP ◇ RCRA WASTE NUMBER U171

TOXICITY DATA with REFERENCE
CAR: ihl-rat TCLo:207 ppm/7H/26W-I   JEPTDQ
2(5),233,79
CAR: orl-rat TDLo:4277 mg/kg/16W-I
CRNGDP 8,1947,87
ETA: ihl-rat TC:207 ppm/26W-I   XPHCI*25APR77
MUT: dnd-sat 50 mg/L   MUREAV 104,49,82
MUT: mma-sat 1 mg/plate   ENMUDM 5(Suppl 1),3,83
MUT: mmo-sat 1 mg/plate   ENMUDM 5(Suppl 1),3,83

CONSENSUS REPORTS: IARC Cancer Review: Human Inadequate Evidence IMEMDT 29,331,82; Animal Sufficient Evidence IMEMDT 29,331,82. NTP Fourth Annual Report On Carcinogens, 1984. Community Right-To-Know List. EPA Genetic Toxicology Program. Reported in EPA TSCA Inventory.

OSHA PEL: (Transitional: TWA 25 ppm) TWA 10 ppm   ACGIH TLV: TWA 10 ppm; Suspected Human Carcinogen.   DFG TRK: 5 ppm; Animal Carcinogen, Suspected Human Carcinogen.   DOT Classification: Flammable or Combustible Liquid; Label: Flammable Liquid.

SAFETY PROFILE: Confirmed carcinogen with experimental carcinogenic, tumorigenic, and teratogenic data. Poison by intraperitoneal route. Moderately toxic by ingestion and inhalation. Human systemic effects by inhalation: anorexia, hypermotility, diarrhea, nausea or vomiting. Experimental reproductive effects. Mutation data reported. Can cause liver and kidney injury, methemoglobinemia, and cyanosis. Very dangerous fire hazard when exposed to heat, open flame, or oxidizers. To fight fire, use alcohol foam, CO_2, dry chemical, water spray. When heated to decomposition it emits toxic fumes of NO_x.

NJH000
NITROSAMINES

PROP: Compounds which have the chemical group $=N-N=O$ attached to an alkyl or aryl group. They are formed by reaction between an amine and NO_x or nitrites.

SAFETY PROFILE: Confirmed carcinogen of the lung, nasal sinus, brain, esophagus, stomach, liver, bladder, and kidney. They are often produced in food as by-products from processing and preparation. They are found in whisky, herbicides, and cosmetics as well as in tanneries, rubber factories, and iron foundries. They can be formed within the body by reaction of amine-containing foods or drugs with the nitrites resulting from bacterial conversion of nitrates.

NJT500
NITROSO COMPOUNDS

PROP: Compounds of the form $C-N=O$ or $N-N=O$. Organic nitrogen compounds.

SAFETY PROFILE: Usually highly toxic carcinogens, teratogens, and mutagens by almost all routes of exposure. Some of these compounds may have hazardous instabilities under the appropriate conditions. When heated to decomposition they emit very toxic fumes of NO_x.

NJT550
N-NITROSO COMPOUNDS

PROP: A class of organic compounds of the form $R_2-N-N=O$ or $R=N-N=O$.

SAFETY PROFILE: Many members of this class are toxins, carcinogens, teratogens and mutagens. Sources of exposure to N-nitroso compounds are: formation in the environment and absorption from food, water, air, or industrial and consumer products; formation in the body from precursors in food, water or air; from tobacco; and from naturally occurring compounds. Some are used in the production of rubber and they may be formed as by-products in industrial processes. Nitrosamines have been found in food and cosmetics. N-nitroso compounds can be formed from the reaction of nitrates with nitrite under acidic conditions. These conditions can occur in the environment, mouth and stomach. Nitrites are formed in the mouth by the action of bacteria on nitrates. Nitrosatable substances in the environment include secondary and tertiary amines, quaternary ammonium compounds, ureas, carbamates, and guanidines. Many of the resulting N-nitroso compounds are experimental carcinogens and mutagens.

NJW500   CAS: 55-18-5
N-NITROSODIETHYLAMINE
mf: $C_4H_{10}N_2O$ mw: 102.16

PROP: Yellow oil. D: 0.9422 @ 20°/4°, bp: 47° @ 5 mm, bp: 176.9°. Sol in water, alc, and ether.

SYNS: DANA ◇ DEN ◇ DENA ◇ DIAETHYLNITROSAMIN (GERMAN) ◇ DIETHYLNITROSAMINE ◇ N,N-DIETHYLNI-TROSAMINE ◇ DIETHYLNITROSOAMINE ◇ N-ETHYL-N-NI-TROSO-ETHANAMINE ◇ NDEA ◇ N-NITROSODIAETHYLA-MINE (GERMAN) ◇ NITROSODIETHYLAMINE ◇ RCRA WASTE NUMBER U174

TOXICITY DATA with REFERENCE
CAR: ipr-mus TDLo: 90 mg/kg   CALEDQ 1,249,76
CAR: ivn-grb TDLo: 50 mg/kg   ZEKBAI 83,233,75
CAR: ivn-rat TDLo: 80 mg/kg   JNCIAM 49,1729,72
CAR: ivn-rat TDLo: 150 mg/kg (22D post):
   TER   IARCCD 4,45,73
CAR: orl-ham TDLo: 480 mg/kg/20W-I
   IAPUDO 30,305,80
CAR: orl-mus TD: 75 mg/kg/30W-C   VOONAW 11(6),74,65
CAR: orl-mus TD: 330 mg/kg/7W-C   FCTXAV 12,367,74
CAR: orl-mus TDLo: 57 mg/kg/10D-C   IJCNAW 5,119,70
CAR: orl-rat TDLo: 119 mg/kg/3.3Y-C
   CRNGDP 8,1635,87
CAR: orl-rat TDLo: 150 mg/kg (22D post):
   TER   IARCCD 4,92,73
CAR: orl-rbt TDLo: 1250 mg/kg/52W-I   JNCIAM 34,453,65
CAR: scu-grb TDLo: 198 mg/kg/33W-I   ZEKBAI 83,233,75
CAR: scu-ham TD: 700 mg/kg/21W-I   BTPGAZ 151,134,74
CAR: scu-ham TDLo: 336 mg/kg/12W-I
   IAPUDO 30,305,80
CAR: scu-mus TDLo: 104 mg/kg/52W-I
   IAPUDO 31,813,80
NEO: ipr-mus TD: 40 mg/kg/24W-I   TXAPA9 72,313,84
NEO: ipr-mus TD: 50 mg/kg   PAACA3 25,79,84
NEO: ipr-mus TDLo: 120 mg/kg (21D post):
   REP   VOONAW 17(1),45,71
NEO: ipr-rat TDLo: 390 mg/kg/26W-I   RRCRBU 52,1,75
NEO: itr-ham TD: 60 mg/kg/15W-I   SAIGBL 24,523,82

NEO: itr-ham TDLo: 104 mg/kg/52W-I PEXTAR 24,162,79

NEO: orl-cat TDLo: 870 mg/kg/78W-I IJCNAW 22,552,78

NEO: orl-rat TD: 55 mg/kg/2Y-I ARTODN 4,29,80

NEO: scu-ham TD: 60 mg/kg/11W-I CNREA8 28,2197,68

NEO: scu-ham TD: 2500 μg/kg JCREA8 94,1,79

NEO: scu-ham TDLo: 1250 μg/kg (15D post): TER CNREA8 47,5112,87

NEO: scu-mus TDLo: 80 mg/kg (15-20D post): REP ZEKBAI 67,152,65

NEO: skn-mus TDLo: 800 mg/kg/20W-I EJCAAH 16,695,80

ETA: idr-ham TDLo: 588 mg/kg/21W-I ARPAAQ 78,189,64

ETA: ihl-ham TDLo: 216 mg/kg/9W-I ZEKBAI 64,499,62

ETA: ims-brd TDLo: 540 mg/kg/27W-I NATWAY 53,437,66

ETA: ims-ckn TDLo: 400 mg/kg/20W-I IJCNAW 22,552,78

ETA: ipr-ham TDLo: 30 mg/kg (15D post): TER ZAPPAN 121,82,77

ETA: ipr-ham TDLo: 272 mg/kg/17W-I ARPAAQ 78,189,64

ETA: ipr-mky TDLo: 280 mg/kg/60W-I PAACA3 25,74,84

ETA: mul-dog TDLo: 560 mg/kg/26W EXPEAM 23,497,67

ETA: orl-dog TDLo: 210 mg/kg/5W-C ARZNAD 14,73,64

ETA: orl-gpg TDLo: 172 mg/kg/12W-C EXPEAM 25,296,69

ETA: orl-ham TDLo: 150 mg/kg (post): REP PSEBAA 136,1007,71

ETA: orl-mky TDLo: 5140 mg/kg/2Y-I JNCIAM 36,323,66

ETA: orl-pig TD: 1400 mg/kg/45W EXPEAM 23,497,67

ETA: orl-pig TDLo: 750 mg/kg/67W-C ZEKBAI 72,102,69

ETA: rec-rat TDLo: 633 mg/kg/28W-C ZEKBAI 65,529,63

ETA: scu-rat TDLo: 480 mg/kg (10-21D post) NATWAY 54,47,67

ETA: scu-rat TDLo: 480 mg/kg/12D-I: TER NATWAY 54,47,67

ETA: skn-ham TDLo: 5600 mg/kg/26W-I ARPAAQ 78,189,64

MUT: cyt-hmn: hla 500 mg/L MUREAV 57,369,78

MUT: cyt-rat-ipr 1 mg/kg MUREAV 140,181,84

MUT: dni-rat: lvr 100 μmol/L CNREA8 45,337,85

MUT: dns-hmn: lvr 5 mmol/L CRNGDP 4,683,83

MUT: dns-hmn: lym 10 mmol/L BTERDG 5,331,83

MUT: dns-hmn: oth 100 μmol/L JJIND8 69,557,82

MUT: dns-hmn: oth 450 mg/L CRNGDP 6,1079,85

MUT: dns-rat: lvr 10 μmol/L MUREAV 144,197,85

CONSENSUS REPORTS: IARC Cancer Review: Animal Sufficient Evidence IMEMDT 1,107,72, IMEMDT 17,83,78, IMEMDT 28,151,82; Human Limited Evidence IMEMDT 17,83,78. NTP Fourth Annual Report On Carcinogens, 1984. NCI Carcinogenesis Studies (ipr); Clear Evidence: mouse, rat RRCRBU 52,1,75. Reported in EPA TSCA Inventory. Community Right-To-Know List.

DFG MAK: Animal Carcinogen, Suspected Human Carcinogen.

SAFETY PROFILE: Confirmed carcinogen with experimental carcinogenic, neoplastigenic, tumorigenic, and teratogenic data. Poison by ingestion, intravenous, intraperitoneal, subcutaneous, and possibly other routes. Experimental reproductive effects. Human mutation data reported. A transplacental carcinogen. When heated to decomposition it emits toxic fumes of NO_x.

NKA000   CAS: 601-77-4
N-NITROSODIISOPROPYLAMINE
mf: $C_6H_{14}N_2O$ mw: 130.22

SYNS: DIISOPROPYLNITROSAMIN (GERMAN) ◇ N-NITROSODI-i-PROPYLAMINE (MAK)

TOXICITY DATA with REFERENCE

CAR: orl-rat TDLo: 14 g/kg/110W-C ZEKBAI 69,103,67

ETA: orl-rat TD: 1800 mg/kg/50W-I JJIND8 62,407,79

DFG MAK: Animal Carcinogen, Suspected Human Carcinogen.

SAFETY PROFILE: Confirmed carcinogen with experimental carcinogenic and tumorigenic data. Moderately toxic by ingestion. When heated to decomposition it emits toxic fumes of NO_x.

NKA600   CAS: 62-75-9
N-NITROSODIMETHYLAMINE
mf: $C_2H_6N_2O$ mw: 74.10

PROP: Yellow liquid; sol in water, alcohol and ether. Bp: 152°, d: 1.005 @ 20°/4°.

SYNS: DIMETHYLNITROSAMIN (GERMAN) ◇ DIMETHYLNITROSAMINE ◇ N,N-DIMETHYLNITROSAMINE

◇ DIMETHYLNITROSOAMINE ◇ DMN ◇ DMNA ◇ N-METHYL-N-NITROSOMETHANAMINE ◇ NDMA ◇ NITRO-SODIMETHYLAMINE ◇ RCRA WASTE NUMBER P082

TOXICITY DATA with REFERENCE

CAR: ihl-rat TCLo: 200 μg/m³/45W-C
VOONAW 21(6),107,75

CAR: ipr-mus TDLo: 7 mg/kg IJCNAW 28,199,81
CAR: ipr-rat TD: 20 mg/kg JSONAU 8,539,76
CAR: ipr-rat TD: 30 mg/kg CRNGDP 5,1003,84
CAR: ipr-rat TD: 40 mg/kg BJEPA5 51,587,70
CAR: ipr-rat TDLo: 30 mg/kg CNREA8 30,2796,70
CAR: orl-mus TD: 370 mg/kg/56W-C JNCIAM 41,1213,68
CAR: orl-mus TDLo: 80 mg/kg/8W-C IJCNAW 28,199,81
CAR: orl-rat TD: 42 mg/kg/30W-I CNREA8 41,4997,81
CAR: orl-rat TDLo: 23 mg/kg/2Y-I CNREA8 41,4997,81
CAR: scu-ham TD: 74200 μg/kg/53W-I CALEDQ 31,181,86
CAR: scu-ham TDLo: 62 mg/kg/44W-I JNCIAM 51,1295,73
CAR: scu-mus TDLo: 38 mg/kg (17-19D post): TER VOONAW 17(8),75,71
NEO: ihl-mus TCLo: 200 μg/m³/45W-C VOONAW 21(6),107,75
NEO: ipr-ham TDLo: 20 mg/kg CRNGDP 1,91,80
NEO: ipr-mus TD: 7 mg/kg CBINA8 1,395,69/70
NEO: orl-mus TD: 11 mg/kg/16W-C PAACA3 25,98,84
NEO: orl-mus TDLo: 140 μg/kg (4 W pre-3 W post): TER JJIND8 62,1553,79
NEO: orl-rat TD: 114 mg/kg/81W-I GISAAA 48(3),19,83
NEO: orl-rat TD: 336 mg/kg/2W-C TOLED5 18(Suppl 1),115,83
NEO: scu-ham TDLo: 12 mg/kg (14D post) ZEKBAI 90,79,77
NEO: scu-mus TDLo: 70 mg/kg/1W-C BJCAAI 20,871,66
NEO: skn-mus TDLo: 800 mg/kg/20W-I EJCAAH 16,695,80
NEO: unr-rat TDLo: 7 mg/kg (15-21D post): TER IARCCD 4,1,73
ETA: ims-rat TDLo: 18 mg/kg INURAQ 4,39,66
ETA: irn-rat TDLo: 20 mg/kg JJIND8 71,787,83
ETA: ivn-rat TDLo: 18 mg/kg INURAQ 4,39,66
ETA: mul-rat TDLo: 420 mg/kg/2W-C APHGBP 23,87,73
ETA: orl-ham TDLo: 13 mg/kg BJCAAI 46,985,82
ETA: orl-rat TDLo: 30 mg/kg (21D post): TER BEXBAN 78,1308,74

ETA: orl-rbt TDLo: 325 mg/kg/37W-C BJCAAI 23,125,69
ETA: orl-uns TDLo: 49 mg/kg/71W-C IARCCD 14,443,76
ETA: scu-rat TDLo: 24466 μg/kg/20W-I CNREA8 46,498,86
MUT: dnd-mam: lym 430 μmol/L MUREAV 135,87,84
MUT: dns-hmn: hla 100 mmol/L/1H-C BANRDU 13,101,82
MUT: dns-mus: lvr 10 μmol/L TOPADD 12,119,84
MUT: dns-ofs: lvr 100 μmol/L NCIMAV 65,163,84

CONSENSUS REPORTS: IARC Cancer Review: Animal Sufficient Evidence; IMEMDT 17,125,78, IMEMDT 1,95,72; Human Limited Evidence IMEMDT 17,125,78; Human Inadequate Evidence IMEMDT 1,95,72. Reported in EPA TSCA Inventory. EPA Genetic Toxicology Program. Community Right-To-Know List. EPA Extremely Hazardous Substances List.

OSHA PEL: Carcinogen ACGIH TLV: Suspected Human Carcinogen DFG MAK: Animal Carcinogen, Suspected Human Carcinogen.

SAFETY PROFILE: Confirmed carcinogen with experimental carcinogenic, neoplastigenic, tumorigenic, and teratogenic data. A transplacental carcinogen. Human poison by ingestion. Experimental poison by ingestion, inhalation, intraperitoneal, subcutaneous, intravenous, and possibly other routes. Human systemic effects by ingestion: ulceration or bleeding from small intestine, nausea or vomiting, and fever. Experimental reproductive effects. Human mutation data reported. Has caused fatal liver disease in humans. When heated to decomposition it emits toxic fumes of NO_x.

NKB500 CAS: 156-10-5
p-NITROSODIPHENYLAMINE
mf: $C_{12}H_{10}N_2O$ mw: 198.24

PROP: Green plates with bluish luster (from benzene) or steel blue prisms or plates (from ether + H_2O). Mp: 144-145°. Sltly sol in water or petr ether; very sol in alc, ether, benzene, chloroform.

SYNS: NAUGARD TKB ◇ NCI-C02244 ◇ p-NITROSODI-FENYLAMIN (CZECH) ◇ 4-NITROSODIPHE-NYLAMINE ◇ p-NITROSO-N-PHENYLANILINE ◇ 4-NITROSO-N-PHENYLANILINE ◇ 4-NITROSO-N-PHENYL-BENZENAMINE ◇ N-PHENYL-p-NITROSOANILINE ◇ TKB

TOXICITY DATA with REFERENCE

CAR: orl-mus TD:1698 g/kg/57W-C   IARC**
27,227,82

CAR: orl-mus TD:3150 g/kg/50W-C   IARC**
27,227,82

CAR: orl-mus TDLo:204 g/kg/57W-C
NCITR* NCI-CG-TR-190,79

CAR: orl-rat TD:2730 g/kg/78W-C   IARC**
27,227,82

CAR: orl-rat TDLo:1365 g/kg/78W-C   IARC**
27,227,82

NEO: orl-mus TD:378 g/kg/50W-C
NCITR* NCI-CG-TR-190,79

NEO: orl-rat TD:82 g/kg/78W-C
NCITR* NCI-CG-TR-190,79

NEO: orl-rat TD:164 g/kg/78W-C
NCITR* NCI-CG-TR-190,79

MUT: dns-mus:ast 50 μmol/L   MUREAV 89,95,81

MUT: mma-sat 200 μg/plate   ENMUDM
5(Suppl 1),3,83

CONSENSUS REPORTS: IARC Cancer Review: Animal Inadequate Evidence IMEMDT 27,227,82. NTP Fourth Annual Report On Carcinogens, 1984. NCI Carcinogenesis Bioassay (feed); Clear Evidence: mouse, rat NCITR* NCI-CG-TR-190,79. Community Right-To-Know List. Reported in EPA TSCA Inventory.

SAFETY PROFILE: Confirmed carcinogen with experimental carcinogenic and neoplastigenic data. Poison by intravenous route. Moderately toxic by ingestion. Mutation data reported. An eye irritant. When heated to decomposition it emits toxic fumes of NO_x.

NKB700   CAS: 621-64-7
N-NITROSODI-N-PROPYLAMINE
mf: $C_6H_{14}N_2O$ mw: 130.22

SYNS: DI-n-PROPYLNITROSAMINE ◇ DIPROPYLNITRO-SOAMINE ◇ DPN ◇ DPNA ◇ NDPA ◇ N-NITROSODIPRO-PYLAMINE ◇ N-NITROSO-N-DIPROPYLAMINE ◇ N-NITRO-SO-N-PROPYL-1-PROPANAMINE ◇ N-NITROSO-N-PROPYL-PROPANAMINE ◇ RCRA WASTE NUMBER U111

TOXICITY DATA with REFERENCE

CAR: orl-rat TD:1056 mg/kg/30W-I   CALEDQ
19,207,83

CAR: orl-rat TDLo:660 mg/kg/60W-I   CALEDQ
19,207,83

CAR: scu-ham TDLo:1760 mg/kg/27W-I
ZKKOBW 90,141,77

CAR: scu-mus TDLo:1516 mg/kg/44W-I
ZKKOBW 90,253,77

NEO: scu-ham TD:100 mg/kg   ZKKOBW 90,79,77

NEO: scu-ham TDLo:100 mg/kg (14D preg):
TER   ZKKOBW 90,79,77

NEO: scu-rat TDLo:926 mg/kg/38W-I   JNCIAM
54,937,75

ETA: orl-mus TDLo:120 mg/kg/50W-I   IAPUDO
41,643,82

ETA: orl-rat TD:675 mg/kg/30W-C   CALEDQ
14,297,81

ETA: orl-rat TD:1150 mg/kg/30W-C   ARZNAD
19,1077,69

ETA: orl-rat TD:1350 mg/kg/30W-I   EESADV
2,421,78

ETA: orl-rat TD:1880 mg/kg/30W-I   JJIND8
62,407,79

ETA: scu-ham TD:143 mg/kg/38W-I   JNCIAM
51,1019,73

MUT: dnd-rat:lvr 30 μmol/L   CNREA8 42,2592,82

MUT: dns-hmn:hla 100 μmol/L   CNREA8
38,2621,78

MUT: dns-rat:lvr 1 mmol/L   MUREAV 144,197,85

MUT: mma-esc 1 μmol/plate   GANNA2 75,8,84

MUT: mma-sat 1 μmol/plate   GANNA2 75,8,84

MUT: msc-mus:lym 500 mg/L   MUREAV
106,305,82

CONSENSUS REPORTS: IARC Cancer Review: Animal Sufficient Evidence IMEMDT 17,177,78; Human Limited Evidence IMEMDT 17,177,78. NTP Fourth Annual Report On Carcinogens, 1984. EPA Genetic Toxicology Program. Community Right-To-Know List. Reported in EPA TSCA Inventory.

DFG MAK: Animal Carcinogen, Suspected Human Carcinogen.

SAFETY PROFILE: Confirmed carcinogen with experimental carcinogenic, neoplastigenic, tumorigenic, and teratogenic data. Moderately toxic by ingestion and subcutaneous routes. Experimental reproductive effects. Human mutation data reported. When heated to decomposition it emits toxic fumes of NO_x.

NKD000   CAS: 612-64-6
N-NITROSO-N-ETHYL ANILINE
mf: $C_8H_{10}N_2O$ mw: 150.20

PROP: Yellow oil. D: 1.087 @ 20°/4°, bp: 119-120° @ 15 mm. Insol in water.

SYNS: ETHYLNITROSOANILINE ◇ N-ETHYL-N-NITRO-SOBENZENAMINE ◇ NEA ◇ NITROSOETHYLANILINE ◇ N-NITROSOETHYLPHENYLAMINE (MAK)

TOXICITY DATA with REFERENCE
MUT: otr-ham:emb 6300 μg/L   JJIND8 67,1303,81

MUT: otr-mus:fbr 400 μg/L JJIND8
67,1303,81

CONSENSUS REPORTS: EPA Genetic Toxicology Program.

DFG MAK: Animal Carcinogen, Suspected Human Carcinogen.

SAFETY PROFILE: Confirmed carcinogen. Poison by ingestion and intraperitoneal routes data. An experimental teratogen. Experimental reproductive effects. Mutation data reported. Many N-nitroso compounds are carcinogens. When heated to decomposition it emits toxic fumes of NO_x.

NKM000 CAS: 1116-54-7
NITROSOIMINO DIETHANOL
mf: $C_4H_{10}N_2O_3$ mw: 134.16

SYNS: BIS(β-HYDROXYAETHYL)NITROSAMIN (GERMAN) ◇ BIS(β-HYDROXYETHYL)NITROSAMINE ◇ DIAETHANOLNITROSAMIN (GERMAN) ◇ DIETHANOLNITROSOAMINE ◇ 2,2'-DIHYDROXY-N-NITROSODIETHYLAMINE ◇ 2,2'-IMINODI-N-NITROSOETHANOL ◇ NCI-C55583 ◇ NDELA ◇ N-NITROSOAMINODIETHANOL ◇ N-NITROSOBIS(2-HYDROXYETHYL)AMINE ◇ N-NITROSODIAETHANOLAMIN (GERMAN) ◇ N-NITROSODIETHANOLAMINE (MAK) ◇ 2,2'-(NITROSOIMINO)BISETHANOL ◇ RCRA WASTE NUMBER U173

TOXICITY DATA with REFERENCE
CAR: orl-ham TDLo:21600 mg/kg/45W-I
CNREA8 43,2521,83
CAR: orl-rat TD:8 g/kg/50W-I FCTOD7 22,23,84
CAR: orl-rat TD:10 g/kg/50W-C CRNGDP
5,167,84
CAR: orl-rat TD:12 g/kg/75W-I FCTOD7 22,23,84
CAR: orl-rat TD:100 g/kg/1Y-I CNREA8
42,5167,82
CAR: orl-rat TD:3450 mg/kg/2Y-I CNREA8
42,5167,82
CAR: orl-rat TDLo:855 mg/kg/2Y-I CNREA8
42,5167,82
CAR: scu-ham TD:15 g/kg/5W-I CALEDQ4,55,77
CAR: scu-ham TD:7200 mg/kg/27W-I IAPUDO
41,299,82
CAR: scu-ham TD:10500 mg/kg/42W-I
CALEDQ 14,23,81
CAR: scu-ham TD:17920 mg/kg/27W-I
CNREA8 43,2521,83
CAR: scu-ham TDLo:6080 mg/kg/27W-I
CNREA8 43,2521,83
NEO: skn-ham TDLo:21600 mg/kg/36W-I
IAPUDO 41,299,82
ETA: orl-rat TD:1202 mg/kg/2Y-C IAPUDO
41,591,82

MUT: hma-mus/esc 450 μmol/kg CRNGDP
2,909,81
MUT: mma-sat 100 μmol/plate MUREAV
158,141,85
MUT: mmo-sat 100 μmol/plate MUREAV
158,141,85
MUT: mrc-smc 17 g/L IAPUDO 57,721,84
MUT: otr-rat-orl 8400 mg/kg/6W-C CRNGDP
5,725,84
MUT: sln-dmg-skn 2 mmol/L TCMUD8 4,437,84

CONSENSUS REPORTS: IARC Cancer Review: Animal Sufficient Evidence IMEMDT 17,77,78; Human Limited Evidence IMEMDT 17,77,78. NTP Fourth Annual Report On Carcinogens, 1984. Reported in EPA TSCA Inventory.

DFG MAK: Animal Carcinogen, Suspected Human Carcinogen.

SAFETY PROFILE: Confirmed carcinogen with experimental carcinogenic, neoplastigenic, and tumorigenic data. Mildly toxic by ingestion. Mutation data reported. When heated to decomposition it emits toxic fumes of NO_x.

NKZ000 CAS: 59-89-2
4-NITROSOMORPHOLINE
mf: $C_4H_8N_2O_2$ mw: 116.14

SYNS: N-NITROSOMORPHOLIN (GERMAN) ◇ NITROSOMORPHOLINE ◇ N-NITROSOMORPHOLINE (MAK) ◇ NMOR

TOXICITY DATA with REFERENCE
CAR: orl-ham TDLo:365 mg/kg/61W-C
CALEDQ 17,333,83
CAR: orl-rat TD:80 g/kg/50W-I CRNGDP3,911,82
CAR: orl-rat TD:200 g/kg/50W-I CRNGDP
3,911,82
CAR: orl-rat TDLo:320 mg/kg JCROD7 94,233,79
CAR: scu-ham TD:1514 mg/kg/32W-I JNCIAM
51,1295,73
CAR: scu-ham TDLo:861 mg/kg35W-I JNCIAM
51,1295,73
NEO: orl-mus TD:5600 mg/kg/50W-C ZEKBAI
66,303,64
NEO: orl-mus TDLo:3140 mg/kg/28W-C
JNCIAM 46,1029,71
ETA: ivn-rat TD:290 mg/kg/58W-I ZEKBAI
69,103,67
ETA: ivn-rat TDLo:286 mg/kg/57W-I ZEKBAI
66,138,64
ETA: orl-ham TD:1080 mg/kg/26W-I CRNGDP
5,875,84

ETA: orl-ham TD: 1161 mg/kg/35W-I IAPUDO 57,617,84

ETA: orl-rat TD: 180 mg/kg/I ZEKBAI 66,1,64

ETA: orl-rat TD: 420 mg/kg/4W-C GANNA2 65,123,74

ETA: orl-rat TD: 600 mg/kg/34W-C FCTXAV 10,887,72

MUT: dns-hmn: fbr 160 μg/L PMRSDJ 1,528,81

MUT: mma-esc 100 μg/plate PMRSDJ 1,387,81

MUT: mmo-asn 10 μL/plate MUREAV 80,265,81

MUT: mmo-sat 20 μg/plate IAPUDO 31,677,80

MUT: msc-ham: ovr 500 μmol/L TCMUE9 1,129,84

MUT: sce-mus-ipr 37500 μg/kg ENMUDM 6,408,84

MUT: slt-dmg-orl 210 μmol/kg MUREAV 144,177,85

CONSENSUS REPORTS: IARC Cancer Review: Animal Sufficient Evidence IMEMDT 17,263,78; Human Limited Evidence IMEMDT 17,263,78. Community Right-To-Know List. EPA Genetic Toxicology Program.

DFG MAK: Animal Carcinogen, Suspected Human Carcinogen.

SAFETY PROFILE: Confirmed carcinogen with experimental carcinogenic, neoplastigenic, and tumorigenic data. Poison by ingestion, intraperitoneal, subcutaneous, and intravenous routes. Moderately toxic by inhalation. Human mutation data reported. When heated to decomposition it emits toxic fumes of NO_x.

NLD500 CAS: 16543-55-8
N'-NITROSONORNICOTINE
mf: $C_9H_{11}N_3O$ mw: 177.23

SYNS: 1'-NITROSO-1'-DEMETHYLNICOTINE ◇ 1-NITROSO-2-(3-PYRIDYL)PYRROLIDINE ◇ 3-(1-NITROSO-2-PYRROLIDINYL)PYRIDINE ◇ (S)-3-(1-NITROSO-2-PYRROLIDINYL)PYRIDINE ◇ NNN

TOXICITY DATA with REFERENCE

CAR: ipr-ham TD: 2850 mg/kg/25W-I CNREA8 41,2849,81

CAR: ipr-ham TDLo: 1422 mg/kg/25W-I CNREA8 41,2849,81

CAR: scu-rat TD: 3160 mg/kg/20W-I CNREA8 40,298,80

CAR: scu-rat TDLo: 567 mg/kg/22W-I CNREA8 44,2285,84

CAR: unr-ham TDLo: 2836 mg/kg/25W- IAPUDO 41,635,82

NEO: ipr-mus TD: 3300 mg/kg/41W-I NATUAS 202,1126,64

NEO: ipr-mus TDLo: 880 mg/kg/7W-I JNCIAM 60,819,78

NEO: scu-ham TD: 1290 mg/kg/6W-I CNREA8 41,2386,81

NEO: scu-ham TD: 3100 mg/kg/25W-I CALEDQ 2,169,77

NEO: scu-ham TDLo: 1288 mg/kg/6W-I IAPUDO 41,309,82

NEO: unr-ham TD: 1418 mg/kg/25W-I IAPUDO 41,635,82

ETA: ipr-rat TDLo: 880 mg/kg/8W-I CALEDQ 6,365,79

ETA: orl-ham TDLo: 2694 mg/kg/31W-C CALEDQ 20,333,83

ETA: orl-rat TD: 3 g/kg/30W-I JNCIAM 54,1237,75

ETA: orl-rat TDLo: 2552 mg/kg/36W-C CALEDQ 20,333,83

ETA: scu-rat TD: 1640 mg/kg/14W-I IAPUDO 41,499,82

MUT: dnd-rat-ivn 360 μg/kg CNREA8 42,2877,82

MUT: mma-sat 50 μg/plate MUREAV 40,19,76

MUT: mmo-esc 50 μg/plate MUREAV 40,19,76

MUT: mrc-bcs 20 μg/disc/24H MUREAV 40,19,76

CONSENSUS REPORTS: IARC Cancer Review: Animal Sufficient Evidence IMEMDT 17,281,78; Human Limited Evidence IMEMDT 17,281,78. NTP Fourth Annual Report On Carcinogens, 1984. Community Right-To-Know List. EPA Genetic Toxicology Program.

SAFETY PROFILE: Confirmed carcinogen with experimental carcinogenic, neoplastigenic, and tumorigenic data. Mutation data reported. When heated to decomposition it emits toxic fumes of NO_x.

NLJ500 CAS: 100-75-4
N-NITROSOPIPERIDINE
mf: $C_5H_{10}N_2O$ mw: 114.17

PROP: Light yellow oil. D: 1.063 @ 18.5°/4°, bp: 217-218°. Sol in water, very sol in acid solns.

SYNS: HEXAHYDRO-N-NITROSOPYRIDINE ◇ NITROSOPIPERIDIN (GERMAN) ◇ N-NITROSO-PIPERIDIN (GERMAN) ◇ 1-NITROSOPIPERIDINE ◇ N-N-PIP ◇ NPIP ◇ NO-PIP ◇ RCRA WASTE NUMBER U179

TOXICITY DATA with REFERENCE

CAR: ivn-rat TDLo: 400 mg/kg/40W-I NATWAY 50,100,63

CAR: orl-gpg TDLo: 1326 mg/kg/52W-I IAPUDO 41,665,82

CAR: orl-ham TDLo: 206 mg/kg/1Y-C CALEDQ 21,219,83

CAR: orl-mus TDLo: 2160 mg/kg/1Y-C
NATWAY 56,142,69

CAR: orl-rat TD: 840 mg/kg/56W-I   IAPUDO
31,657,80

CAR: orl-rat TD: 1400 mg/kg/30W-C   CRNGDP
2,1045,81

CAR: orl-rat TDLo: 350 mg/kg/2Y-I   IAPUDO
31,657,80

CAR: orl-rat TDLo: 3915 mg/kg/29W-I   BJCAAI
18,265,64

CAR: scu-ham TDLo: 1245 mg/kg/25W-I
CALEDQ 2,169,77

NEO: orl-rat TD: 1400 mg/kg/28W-I   CALEDQ
12,99,81

NEO: scu-ham TD: 100 mg/kg   ZKKOBW 90,71,77

NEO: scu-ham TD: 623 mg/kg/44W-I   JNCIAM
51,1295,73

NEO: scu-ham TD: 1047 mg/kg/37W-I   JNCIAM
51,1295,73

ETA: orl-mky TDLo: 540 g/kg/5Y-I   27CWAL
3(Pt.3),216,72

ETA: orl-rat TD: 504 mg/kg/4W-C   GANNA2
65,123,74

ETA: scu-rat TD: 850 mg/kg/52W-I   ARZNAD
19,1077,69

ETA: scu-rat TD: 900 mg/kg/1Y-I   ZEKBAI
66,138,64

ETA: scu-rat TDLo: 680 mg/kg/34W-I   XENOBH
3,217,73

MUT: dnd-hmn: lng 100 μmol/plate   JNCIAM
59,1401,77

MUT: dnd-rat-ipr 50 mg/kg   CNREA8 33,3209,73

MUT: dnr-esc 25 μL/well   CBINA8 15,219,76

MUT: mma-ham: emb 1 mg/L   MUREAV 129,111,84

MUT: mma-smc 50 mmol/L/24H   MUREAV
57,155,78

MUT: msc-ham: lng 10 μmol/L/18H   CNREA8
40,406,80

CONSENSUS REPORTS: IARC Cancer Review: Human Limited Evidence IMEMDT 17,287,78; Animal Sufficient Evidence IMEMDT 17,287,78; IMEMDT 28,151,82. NTP Fourth Annual Report On Carcinogens, 1984. Community Right-To-Know List. EPA Genetic Toxicology Program. Reported in EPA TSCA Inventory.

DFG MAK: Animal Carcinogen, Suspected Human Carcinogen.

SAFETY PROFILE: Confirmed carcinogen with experimental carcinogenic, neoplastigenic, and tumorigenic data. Poison by ingestion, intravenous, and subcutaneous routes. Experimental reproductive effects. Human mutation data reported. When heated to decomposition it emits toxic fumes of NO_x.

NLM500   CAS: 39603-53-7
1-(NITROSOPROPYLAMINO)-2-PROPANOL

mf: $C_6H_{14}N_2O_2$ mw: 146.22

SYNS: β-HYDROXYPROPYLPROPYLNITROSAMINE ◇ (2-HYDROXYPROPYL)PROPYLNITROSOAMINE ◇ N-NITROSO-2-HYDROXY-N-PROPYL-N-PROPYLAMINE

TOXICITY DATA with REFERENCE
CAR: scu-ham TDLo: 2630 mg/kg/36W-I
ZKKOBW 90(3),141,77

CAR: scu-mus TD: 4800 mg/kg/39W-I
ZKKOBW 91,189,78

CAR: scu-mus TDLo: 3272 mg/kg/53W-I
ZKKOBW 91,189,78

CAR: scu-rat TDLo: 3500 mg/kg/55W-I
JNCIAM 54,937,75

ETA: scu-ham TD: 1150 mg/kg/23W-I   JNCIAM
51,287,73

MUT: mma-sat 500 nmol/plate   ZKKOBW86,293,76

CONSENSUS REPORTS: IARC Cancer Review: Animal Sufficient Evidence IMEMDT 17,177,78.

SAFETY PROFILE: Confirmed carcinogen with experimental carcinogenic and tumorigenic data. Moderately toxic by subcutaneous route. Experimental reproductive effects. Mutation data reported. When heated to decomposition it emits toxic fumes of NO_x.

NLP500   CAS: 930-55-2
N-NITROSOPYRROLIDINE

mf: $C_4H_8N_2O$ mw: 100.14

SYNS: N-NITROSOPYRROLIDIN (GERMAN) ◇ 1-NITROSOPYRROLIDINE ◇ NO-PYR ◇ N-N-PYR ◇ NPYR ◇ RCRA WASTE NUMBER U180 ◇ TETRAHYDRO-N-NITROSOPYRROLE

TOXICITY DATA with REFERENCE
CAR: ipr-ham TDLo: 1602 mg/kg/25W-I
CNREA8 41,2849,81

CAR: orl-ham TD: 704 mg/kg/39W-C   JCROD7
104,75,82

CAR: orl-ham TD: 1049 mg/kg/64W-C   JCROD7
104,75,82

CAR: orl-ham TDLo: 465 mg/kg/52W-C
JCROD7 104,75,82

CAR: orl-rat TD: 792 mg/kg/2Y-I   IJCNAW
26,47,80

CAR: orl-rat TD: 1599 mg/kg/76W-C   ZKKOBW 90,161,77

CAR: orl-rat TD: 2250 mg/kg/50W-I   CALEDQ 12,99,81

CAR: orl-rat TD: 4033 mg/kg/62W-C   IARCCD 14,429,76

CAR: orl-rat TD: 4380 mg/kg/52W-C   YKKZAJ 97,320,77

CAR: orl-rat TDLo: 685 mg/kg/98W-C   ZKKOBW 90,161,77

CAR: unr-ham TDLo: 1602 mg/kg/25W-I   IAPUDO 41,635,82

NEO: ipr-ham TD: 798 mg/kg/25W-I   CNREA8 41,2849,81

NEO: orl-mus TDLo: 3235 mg/kg/92W-C   85DUA4 -,129,70

NEO: scu-mus TDLo: 396 mg/kg/72W-I   85DUA4 -,129,70

ETA: orl-rat TD: 1350 mg/kg/30W-C   PAACA3 25,126,84

MUT: dnd-hmn: lng 100 μmol/plate   JNCIAM 59,1401,77

MUT: dns-rat: lvr 500 μmol/L   ENMUDM 3,11,81

MUT: mma-esc 7500 μmol/L   IAPUDO 41,543,82

MUT: mma-ham: lng 10 mmol/L   CNREA8 37,1044,77

MUT: mma-sat 100 μg/plate   MUREAV 67,21,79

MUT: mrc-esc 400 μg/well   MUREAV 46,53,77

MUT: msc-rat: lvr 100 μmol/L   MUREAV 130,53,84

CONSENSUS REPORTS: IARC Cancer Review: Animal Sufficient Evidence IMEMDT 17,313,78; Human Limited Evidence IMEMDT 17,313,78. NTP Fourth Annual Report On Carcinogens, 1984. EPA Genetic Toxicology Program. Reported in EPA TSCA Inventory.

DFG MAK: Animal Carcinogen, Suspected Human Carcinogen.

SAFETY PROFILE: Confirmed carcinogen with experimental carcinogenic, neoplastigenic, and tumorigenic data. Poison by ingestion and subcutaneous routes. Human mutation data reported. When heated to decomposition it emits toxic fumes of NO_x.

NLR500   CAS: 13256-22-9
N-NITROSOSARCOSINE
mf: $C_3H_6N_2O_3$ mw: 118.11

SYNS: N-METHYL-N-NITROSOGLYCINE ◇ N-NITROSO-METHYLGLYCINE ◇ NITROSO SARKOSIN (GERMAN)

TOXICITY DATA with REFERENCE
ETA: orl-mus TDLo: 118 g/kg/56W-C   FEPRA7 33,596,74

ETA: orl-rat TDLo: 29 g/kg/41W-C   ARZNAD 19,1077,69

CONSENSUS REPORTS: IARC Cancer Review: Animal Sufficient Evidence IMEMDT 17,327,78; Human Limited Evidence IMEMDT 17,327,78. NTP Fourth Annual Report On Carcinogens, 1984.

SAFETY PROFILE: Confirmed carcinogen with experimental tumorigenic data. Mildly toxic by ingestion. When heated to decomposition it emits toxic fumes of NO_x.

NMP500   CAS: 99-55-8
5-NITRO-o-TOLUIDINE
mf: $C_7H_8N_2O_2$ mw: 152.17

SYNS: 2-AMINO-4-NITROTOLUENE ◇ AZOFIX SCARLET G SALT ◇ AZOGENE FAST SCARLET G ◇ C.I. 37105 ◇ C.I. AZOIC DIAZO COMPONENT 12 ◇ DAINICHI FAST SCARLET G BASE ◇ DAITO SCARLET BASE G ◇ DEVOL SCARLET B ◇ DIABASE SCARLET G ◇ DIAZO FAST SCARLET G ◇ FAST RED SG BASE ◇ FAST SCARLET G ◇ HILTONIL FAST SCARLET G BASE ◇ KAYAKU SCARLET G BASE ◇ LAKE SCARLET G BASE ◇ LITHOSOL ORANGE R BASE ◇ 6-METHYL-3-NITROANILINE ◇ 2-METHYL-5-NITRO-BENZENEAMINE ◇ MITSUI SCARLET G BASE ◇ NAPHTHANIL SCARLET G BASE ◇ NAPHTOELAN FAST SCARLET G SALT ◇ NCI-C01843 ◇ 4-NITRO-2-AMINO-TOLUENE (MAK) ◇ PNOT ◇ RCRA WASTE NUMBER U181 ◇ SCARLET BASE CIBA II ◇ SUGAI FAST SCARLET G BASE ◇ SYMULON SCARLET G BASE

TOXICITY DATA with REFERENCE
CAR: orl-mus TDLo: 150 g/kg/78W-C   NCITR* NCI-CG-TR-107,78

MUT: mma-sat 33300 ng/plate   ENMUDM 7(Suppl 5),1,85

MUT: mmo-sat 10 μg/plate   ENMUDM 4,163,82

MUT: otr-rat: emb 41 μg/plate   JJATDK 1,190,81

CONSENSUS REPORTS: NCI Carcinogenesis Bioassay (feed); Clear Evidence: mouse NCITR* NCI-CG-TR-107,78. Reported in EPA TSCA Inventory.

DFG MAK: Animal Carcinogen, Suspected Human Carcinogen.

SAFETY PROFILE: Confirmed carcinogen with experimental carcinogenic data. Moderately toxic by ingestion. Mutation data reported. Decomposes exothermically when heated to 150°C. When heated to decomposition it emits toxic fumes of NO_x.

NNP500 CAS: 68-22-4
19-NORETHISTERONE
mf: $C_{20}H_{26}O_2$ mw: 298.46

SYNS: 17-α-ETHINYLESTRA-4-EN-17-β-OL-3-ONE ◇ 17-α-ETHINYL-17-β-HYDROXY-Δ:4-ESTREN-3-ONE ◇ 17-α-ETHINYL-19-NORTESTOSTERONE ◇ 17-α-ETHYNYL-4-ESTREN-17-OL-3-ONE ◇ 17-α-ETHYNYL-17-HYDROXY-4-ESTREN-3-ONE ◇ 17-α-ETHYNYL-17-β-HYDROXY-19-NORANDROST-4-EN-3-ONE ◇ 17-α-ETHYNYL-19-NORANDROST-4-EN-17-β-OL-3-ONE ◇ 17-α-ETHYNYL-19-NOR-4-ANDROSTEN-17-β-OL-3-ONE ◇ 17-α-ETHYNYL-19-NORTESTOSTERONE ◇ (17-α)-17-HYDROXY-19-NORPREGN-4-EN-20-YN-3-ONE ◇ 17-β-HYDROXY-19-NORPREGN-4-EN-20-YN-3-ONE ◇ 17-HYDROXY-19-NOR-17-α-PREGN-4-EN-20-YN-3-ONE ◇ 19-NOR-ETHINYL-4,5-TESTOSTERONE ◇ 19-NOR-17-α-ETHYNYLANDROSTEN-17-β-OL-3-ONE ◇ 19-NOR-17-α-ETHYNYL-17-β-HYDROXY-4-ANDROSTEN-3-ONE ◇ 19-NOR-17-α-ETHYNYLTESTOSTERONE ◇ NORLUTIN

TOXICITY DATA with REFERENCE
ETA: imp-mus TDLo: 166 mg/kg/77W-C
  NATUAS 212,686,66
ETA: scu-mus TDLo: 163 mg/kg/78W-C
  BJCAAI 21,153,67
MUT: cyt-mam: oth 100 μg/kg AJOGAH 120,390,74
MUT: dni-hmn: lym 50 μmol/L PSEBAA 146,401,74
MUT: oms-dom: oth 100 μg/L AJOGAH 120,390,74
MUT: oms-mam: oth 100 μg/L AJOGAH 120,390,74
MUT: oms-mus: oth 10 μg/L AJOGAH 120,390,74

CONSENSUS REPORTS: IARC Cancer Review: Animal Limited Evidence IMEMDT 21,441,79; Animal Sufficient Evidence IMEMDT 6,179,74. NTP Fourth Annual Report On Carcinogens, 1984. EPA Genetic Toxicology Program.

SAFETY PROFILE: Confirmed carcinogen with experimental carcinogenic, tumorigenic, and teratogenic data. Mildly toxic by ingestion. Human systemic effects by ingestion: dermatitis and androgenic effects. Human reproductive effects by ingestion, implant, and possibly other routes: spermatogenesis; testes, epididymis, sperm duct changes; impotence; male breast development; other male effects; ovaries, fallopian tube changes; menstrual cycle changes or disorders uterus, cervix, vagina effects; postpartum effects; changes in female fertility. Human teratogenic effects by ingestion and possibly other routes: developmental abnormalities of the musculoskeletal system and urogenital system; and behavioral effects in the newborn. Experimental reproductive effects. Human mutation data reported. When heated to decomposition it emits acrid smoke and irritating fumes.

OAT000 CAS: 2223-93-0
OCTADECANOIC ACID, CADMIUM SALT
mf: $C_{36}H_{72}O_4 \cdot Cd$ mw: 681.48

SYNS: CADMIUM STEARATE ◇ KADMIUMSTEARAT (GERMAN) ◇ STEARIC ACID, CADMIUM SALT

CONSENSUS REPORTS: EPA Extremely Hazardous Substances List. Cadmium and its compounds are on the Community Right-To-Know List. Reported in EPA TSCA Inventory.

OSHA PEL: TWA 0.1 mg(Cd)/m³; CL 0.6 mg(Cd)/m³ (fume) ACGIH TLV: TWA 0.05 mg(Cd)/m³ (Proposed: TWA 0.01 mg(Cd)/m³ (dust), Human Carcinogen); BEI: 10 μg/g creatinine in urine; 10 μg/L in blood. DFG BAT: Blood 1.5 μg/dL; Urine 15 μg/dL, Suspected Carcinogen. NIOSH REL: (Cadmium) Reduce to lowest feasible level

SAFETY PROFILE: Confirmed carcinogen. Poison by inhalation. Moderately toxic by ingestion. Human systemic effects by inhalation: hallucinations or distorted perceptions; nausea or vomiting, other gastrointestinal effects; weight loss or decreased weight gain; cardiac effects. When heated to decomposition it emits toxic fumes of Cd.

OPM000 CAS: 101-80-4
4,4'-OXYDIANILINE
mf: $C_{12}H_{12}N_2O$ mw: 200.26

PROP: Colorless crystals. Mp: 187°, bp: >300°.

SYNS: p-AMINOPHENYL ETHER ◇ 4-AMINOPHENYL ETHER ◇ BIS(4-AMINOPHENYL)ETHER ◇ BIS(p-AMINOPHENYL)ETHER ◇ DADPE ◇ 4,4'-DIAMINOBIPHENYLOXIDE ◇ DIAMINODIPHENYL ETHER ◇ 4,4-DIAMINODIPHENYL ETHER ◇ p,p'-DIAMINODIPHENYL ETHER ◇ 4,4'-DIAMINODIPHENYL OXIDE ◇ 4,4'-DIAMINOPHENYL ETHER ◇ NCI-C50146 ◇ OXYBIS(4-AMINOBENZENE) ◇ 4,4'-OXYBISANILINE ◇ p,p'-OXYBIS(ANILINE) ◇ 4,4'-OXYBISBENZENAMINE ◇ OXYDIANILINE ◇ p,p'-OXYDIANILINE ◇ 4,4'-OXYDIPHENYLAMINE ◇ OXYDI-p-PHENYLENEDIAMINE

TOXICITY DATA with REFERENCE
CAR: orl-mus TD: 69216 mg/kg/2Y-C JJIND8 72,1457,84

CAR: orl-mus TDLo: 13 g/kg/2Y-C
NCITR* NCI-CG-TR-205,80

CAR: orl-rat TD: 8652 mg/kg/2Y-C
JJIND8 72,1457,84

CAR: orl-rat TDLo: 8652 mg/kg/2Y-C   NCITR*
NCI-CG-TR-205,80

NEO: orl-mus TD: 12978 mg/kg/2Y-C   JJIND8
72,1457,84

ETA: orl-mus TD: 11 g/kg/30W-I   VOONAW
21(3),69,75

ETA: orl-rat TD: 19 g/kg/77W-I   VOONAW
21(3),69,75

ETA: scu-mus TDLo: 7000 mg/kg/39W-I
VOONAW 21(8),54,77

ETA: scu-rat TDLo: 8550 mg/kg/76W-I
VOONAW 21(3),69,75

MUT: dnd-rat-ipr 3640 μmol/kg   CRNGDP
2,1317,81

MUT: mma-sat 10 μg/plate   MUREAV 143,11,85

MUT: mmo-sat 250 μg/plate   MUREAV 67,123,79

CONSENSUS REPORTS: IARC Cancer Review: Animal Sufficient Evidence IMEMDT 29,203,82; Animal Inadequate Evidence IMEMDT 16,301,78. NCI Carcinogenesis Bioassay (feed); Clear Evidence: mouse, rat NCITR* NCI-CG-TR-205,80. Reported in EPA TSCA Inventory.

DFG MAK: Animal Carcinogen, Suspected Human Carcinogen.

SAFETY PROFILE: Confirmed carcinogen with experimental carcinogenic, neoplastigenic, and tumorigenic data. Poison by intraperitoneal route. Moderately toxic by ingestion. Mutation data reported. Experimental reproductive effects. Mutation data reported. When heated to decomposition it emits toxic fumes of NO_x.

PAN100   CAS: 434-07-1
PAVISOID
mf: $C_{21}H_{32}O_3$ mw: 332.53

PROP: Crystals from ethyl acetate. Mp: 178-180°.

SYNS: ADROIDIN ◇ ADROYD ◇ ANADROL ◇ ANADROYD ◇ ANAPOLON ◇ ANASTERON ◇ ANASTERONAL ◇ ANASTERONE ◇ BECOREL ◇ CI-406 ◇ 4,5-DIHYDRO-2-HYDROXYMETHYLENE-17-α-METHYLTESTOSTERONE ◇ DYNASTEN ◇ HMD ◇ 17-β-HYDROXY-2-HYDROXYMETHYLENE-17-α-METHYL-3-ANDROSTANONE ◇ 17-β-HYDROXY-2-(HYDROXYMETHYLENE)-17-α-METHYL-5-α-ANDROSTAN-3-ONE ◇ 17-β-HYDROXY-2-(HYDROXY-METHYLENE)-17-METHYL-5-α-ANDROSTAN-3-ONE

◇ 17-HYDROXY-2-(HYDROXYMETHYLENE)-17-METHYL-5-α-17-β-ANDROST-3-ONE ◇ 2-HYDROXYMETHYLENE-17-α-METHYL-5-α-ANDROSTAN-17-β-OL-3-ONE ◇ 2-HYDROXYMETHYLENE-17-α-METHYL-DIHYDROTESTOSTERONE ◇ 2-(HYDROXYMETHYLENE)-17-α-METHYLDIHYDROTESTOSTERONE ◇ 2-HYDROXYMETHYLENE-17-α-METHYL-17-β-HYDROXY-3-ANDROSTANONE ◇ METHABOL ◇ 17-α-METHYL-2-HYDROXYMETHYLENE-17-HYDROXY-5-α-ANDROSTAN-3-ONE ◇ NASTENON ◇ NSC-26198 ◇ OXIMETHOLONUM ◇ OXIMETOLONA ◇ OXITOSONA-50 ◇ OXYMETHALONE ◇ OXYMETHENOLONE ◇ OXYMETHOLONE ◇ PARDROYD ◇ PLENASTRIL ◇ PROTANABOL ◇ ROBORAL ◇ SYNASTERON ◇ ZENALOSYN

TOXICITY DATA with REFERENCE
CAR: orl-chd TD: 3735 mg/kg/3Y-C   LANCAO
2,1273,72

CAR: orl-chd TDLo: 270 mg/kg/9W-C   NEJMAG
296,1411,77

CAR: orl-man TDLo: 2336 mg/kg/2Y-C
CANCAR 43,440,79

CAR: unr-chd TDLo: 3050 mg/kg/3Y-C
JOPDAB 87,122,75

CONSENSUS REPORTS: IARC Cancer Review: Human Inadequate Evidence IMEMDT 13,131,77. NTP Fourth Annual Report On Carcinogens, 1984.

SAFETY PROFILE: Confirmed human carcinogen producing liver tumors. Human systemic effects by ingestion: impaired liver function. An experimental teratogen. Experimental reproductive effects. When heated to decomposition it emits acrid smoke and irritating fumes.

PDC250   CAS: 136-40-3
PHENAZOPYRIDINIUM CHLORIDE
mf: $C_{11}H_{11}N_5$•ClH   mw: 249.73

PROP: Red crystals; sltly bitter taste. Sltly sol in cold water, alc; sol in acetic acid; insol in acetone, benzene, chloroform, ether.

SYNS: AZODINE ◇ AZODIUM ◇ AZODYNE ◇ AZO GANTRISIN ◇ AZO GASTANOL ◇ AZO-MANDELAMINE ◇ AZOMINE ◇ AZO-STANDARD ◇ AZO-STAT ◇ AZOTREX ◇ BARIDIUM ◇ BISTERIL ◇ CYSTAMINE "MCCLUNG" ◇ CYSTOPYRIN ◇ CYSTURAL ◇ 2,6-DIAMINO-3-PHENYLAZOPYRIDINE HYDROCHLORIDE ◇ 2,6-DIAMINO-3-(PHENYLAZO)PYRIDINE MONOHYDROCHLORIDE ◇ DI-AZO ◇ DIRIDONE ◇ DOLONIL ◇ EUCISTIN ◇ GIRACID ◇ MALLOFEEN ◇ MALLOPHENE ◇ NC 150 ◇ NCI-C01672 ◇ NEFRECIL ◇ PAP ◇ PDP ◇ PHENAZO ◇ PHENAZODINE ◇ PHENAZOPYRIDINE HYDROCHLORIDE ◇ PHENYLAZO-DIAMINOPYRIDINE HYDROCHLORIDE ◇ β-PHENYLAZO-α,α′-DIAMINOPYRIDINE HYDROCHLORIDE ◇ 3-PHENYL-AZO-2,6-DIAMINOPYRIDINE HYDROCHLORIDE ◇ PHE-NYLAZO-α,α′-DIAMINOPYRIDINE MONOHYDROCHLO-RIDE ◇ PHENYLAZOPYRIDINE HYDROCHLORIDE ◇ 3-(PHENYLAZO)-2,6-PYRIDINEDIAMINE, HYDRO-CHLORIDE ◇ PHENYLAZO TABLETS ◇ PHENYL-IDIUM ◇ PHENYL-IDIUM 200 ◇ PIRID ◇ PIRIDACIL ◇ PYRAZO-DINE ◇ PYRAZOFEN ◇ PYREDAL ◇ PYRIDACIL ◇ PYRIDENAL ◇ PYRIDENE ◇ PYRIDIATE ◇ PYRIDIUM ◇ PYRIDIVITE ◇ PYRIPYRIDIUM ◇ PYRIZIN ◇ SEDURAL ◇ SULADYNE ◇ SULODYNE ◇ THIOSULFIL-A FORTE ◇ URAZIUM ◇ URIDINAL ◇ URIPLEX ◇ UROBIOTIC-250 ◇ URODINE ◇ UROFEEN ◇ UROMIDE ◇ UROPHENYL ◇ UROPYRIDIN ◇ UROPYRINE ◇ UTOSTAN ◇ VESTIN ◇ W 1655

TOXICITY DATA with REFERENCE
CAR: orl-mus TDLo:81 g/kg/80W-C
  NCITR* NCI-CG-TR-99,78
CAR: orl-rat TDLo:225 g/kg/78W-C
  NCITR* NCI-CG-TR-99,78
ETA: orl-mus TD:40 g/kg/78W-C
  NCITR* NCI-CG-TR-99,78
ETA: orl-rat TD:110 g/kg/78W-C
  NCITR* NCI-CG-TR-99,78

CONSENSUS REPORTS: IARC Cancer Review: Animal Sufficient Evidence IMEMDT 24,163,80; Human Limited Evidence IMEMDT 24,163,80; Animal Inadequate Evidence IMEMDT 8,117,75. NTP Fourth Annual Report On Carcinogens, 1984. NCI Carcinogenesis Bioassay (feed); Clear Evidence: mouse, rat NCITR* NCI-CG-TR-99,78.

SAFETY PROFILE: Confirmed carcinogen with experimental carcinogenic and tumorigenic data. A poison by intraperitoneal and intravenous routes. Moderately toxic by ingestion. Human systemic effects by ingestion: somnolence, cyanosis, diarrhea, nausea or vomiting, anuria or decreased urine volume, normocytic anemia, methemoglobinemia-carboxhemoglobinemia, dehydration, changes in blood sodium levels. When heated to decomposition it emits very toxic fumes of NO_x and HCl.

PDT250   CAS: 59-96-1
N-PHENOXYISOPROPYL-N-BENZYL-β-CHLOROETHYLAMINE
mf: $C_{18}H_{22}ClNO$ mw: 303.86

SYNS: A 688 ◇ BENSYLYTE ◇ 2-(N-BENZYL-2-CHLORO-ETHYLAMINO)-1-PHENOXYPROPANE ◇ BENZYL(2-CHLO-ROETHYL)-(1-METHYL-2-PHENOXYETHYL)AMINE

◇ BENZYLT ◇ N-(2-CHLOROETHYL)-N-(1-METHYL-2-PHENOXYETHYL)BENZENEMETHANAMINE ◇ N-(2-CHLO-ROETHYL)-N-(1-METHYL-2-PHENOXYETHYL)BENZYLA-MINE ◇ DIBENYLIN ◇ DIBENYLINE ◇ DIBENZYLINE ◇ NSC 37448 ◇ PHENOXYBENZAMINE

TOXICITY DATA with REFERENCE
NEO: ipr-mus TDLo:100 mg/kg/8W-I   CNREA8
  33,3069,73

CONSENSUS REPORTS: IARC Cancer Review: Animal Sufficient Evidence IMEMDT 24,185,80; Animal Limited Evidence IMEMDT 9,223,75

SAFETY PROFILE: Confirmed carcinogen with experimental carcinogenic and neoplastigenic data. Poison by intravenous and intracerebral routes. Moderately toxic by ingestion. Human reproductive effects by ingestion: spermatogenesis. Experimental reproductive effects. When heated to decomposition it emits very toxic fumes of Cl^- and NO_x.

PED750   CAS: 148-82-3
l-PHENYLALANINE MUSTARD
mf: $C_{13}H_{18}Cl_2N_2O_2$ mw: 305.23

SYNS: ALANINE NITROGEN MUSTARD ◇ ALKERAN ◇ AT-290 ◇ l-3-p-(BIS(2-CHLOROETHYL)AMINO)PHE-NYL)ALANINE ◇ p-N-BIS(2-CHLOROETHYL)AMINO-l-PHENYLALANINE ◇ 3-(p-(p-(BIS(2-CHLOROETHYL)AMINO)PHENYL)-l-ALANINE ◇ 4-(BIS(2-CHLORO-ETHYL)AMINO)-l-PHENYLALANINE ◇ CB 3025 ◇ p-N-DI(CHLOROETHYL)AMINOPHENYLALANINE ◇ p-DI-(2-CHLOROETHYL)AMINO-l-PHENYLALANINE ◇ 3-p-(DI(2-CHLOROETHYL)AMINO)-PHENYL-l-ALANINE ◇ MELPHA-LAN ◇ NCI-CO4853 ◇ NSC-8806 ◇ l-PAM ◇ PHENYLALA-NINE NITROGEN MUSTARD ◇ RCRA WASTE NUMBER U150 ◇ l-SARCOLYSIN ◇ p-l-SARCOLYSIN ◇ SK-15673

TOXICITY DATA with REFERENCE
CAR: ipr-mus TDLo:60 mg/kg/26W-I   RRCRBU
  52,1,75
CAR: orl-man TD:17 mg/kg/4Y-I   AMSVAZ
  211,203,82
CAR: orl-man TD:34 mg/kg/2Y-I   SJHAAQ
  8,375,71
CAR: orl-man TD:66 mg/kg/4Y-I   BLOOAW
  44,333,74
CAR: orl-man TDLo:57 μg/kg/D-C   BLOOAW
  41,17,73
CAR: orl-wmn TD:12 mg/kg/3Y-I   ONCOBS
  40,268,83
CAR: orl-wmn TD:23 mg/kg/2Y-I   AMSVAZ
  211,203,82

CAR: orl-wmn TDLo:80 μg/kg/D-C   BLOOAW
41,17,73
CAR: unr-wmn TDLo:26 mg/kg/2Y-C   JCPAAK
26,649,73
NEO: ipr-mus TD:15 mg/kg/6W-I   CNREA8
37,317,77
NEO: ipr-rat TDLo:70 mg/kg/26W-I   RRCRBU
52,1,75
ETA: skn-mus TDLo:58 mg/kg/9W-I   BJCAAI
10,363,56
MUT: dnr-esc 100 μg/disc   CNREA8 34,1658,74
MUT: mmo-sat 100 μg/plate   ONCODU 18,95,79

CONSENSUS REPORTS: IARC Cancer Review: Animal Sufficient Evidence; Human Limited Evidence IMEMDT 9,167,75. NTP Fourth Annual Report On Carcinogens, 1984. NCI Carcinogenesis Studies (ipr); Clear Evidence: mouse, rat RRCRBU 52,1,75. EPA Genetic Toxicology Program.

SAFETY PROFILE: Confirmed human carcinogen producing leukemia and Hodgkin's disease. Poison by ingestion, intravenous, and intracerebral routes. An experimental carcinogenic. Human systemic effects by ingestion: nausea. Human reproductive effects by ingestion: menstrual changes. Mutation data reported. A skin irritant. Used as a poison gas. When heated to decomposition, it emits toxic fumes of Cl^- and NO_x.

PJL750   CAS: 1336-36-3
POLYCHLORINATED BIPHENYLS
DOT: 2315

PROP: Bp: 340-375°, flash p: 383°F (COC), d: 1.44 @ 30°. A series of technical mixtures consisting of many isomers and compounds that vary from mobile oily liquids to white crystalline solids and hard noncrystalline resins. Technical products vary in composition, in the degree of chlorination and possibly according to batch (IARC** 7,262,74).

SYNS: AROCLOR ◇ CHLOPHEN ◇ CHLOREXTOL ◇ CHLORINATED BIPHENYL ◇ CHLORINATED DIPHENYL ◇ CHLORINATED DIPHENYLENE ◇ CHLORO BIPHENYL ◇ CHLORO-1,1-BIPHENYL ◇ CLOPHEN ◇ DYKANOL ◇ FENCLOR ◇ INERTEEN ◇ KANECHLOR ◇ MONTAR ◇ NOFLAMOL ◇ PCB (DOT, USDA) ◇ PHENOCHLOR ◇ POLYCHLORINATED BIPHENYL ◇ POLYCHLOROBIPHE-NYL ◇ PYRALENE ◇ PYRANOL ◇ SANTOTHERM ◇ SOVOL ◇ THERMINOL FR-1

TOXICITY DATA with REFERENCE
CAR: orl-mus TDLo:1250 mg/kg/25W-I
FCTOD7 21,688,83

CAR: orl-rat TD:1250 mg/kg/25W-I
FCTOD7 21,688,83
ETA: orl-ratTDLo:16800mg/kg/2Y-C   TOERD9
1,159,78

CONSENSUS REPORTS: IARC Cancer Review: GROUP 2A IMEMDT 7,322,87; Human Limited Evidence IMEMDT 18,43,78. NTP Fourth Annual Report On Carcinogens, 1984. EPA Extremely Hazardous Substances List. Reported in EPA TSCA Inventory.

DFG MAK: Suspected Carcinogen. NIOSII REL: TWA (Polychlorinated Biphenyls) 0.001 mg/m³ DOT Classification: ORM-E; Label: None.

SAFETY PROFILE: Confirmed carcinogen with carcinogenic and tumorigenic data. Moderately toxic by ingestion. Some are poisons by other routes. Experimental reproductive effects. Combustible when exposed to heat or flame. When heated to decomposition they emit highly toxic fumes of Cl^-.

PKL750   CAS: 25931-01-5
POLYURETHANE Y-195
mf: $(C_{15}H_{10}N_2O_2 \cdot C_6H_{10}O_4 \cdot C_2H_6O_2)_x$

SYNS: ADIPIC ACID, POLYMER with ETHYLENE GLYCOL and METHYLENEDI-p-PHENYLENE ISOCYANATE ◇ AMCHEM R 14 ◇ HEXANEDIOIC ACID, POLYMER with 1,3-ETHANEDIOL and 1,1'-METHYLENEBIS(4-ISOCYANA-TOBENZENE) ◇ MUL F 66 ◇ R 14 ◇ Y 195

TOXICITY DATA with REFERENCE
ETA: imp-rat TDLo:6750 mg/kg   CNREA8
35,1591,75

CONSENSUS REPORTS: IARC Cancer Review: Animal Sufficient Evidence IMEMDT 19,303,79. Reported in EPA TSCA Inventory.

SAFETY PROFILE: Confirmed carcinogen with experimental tumorigenic data. When heated to decomposition it emits toxic fumes of NO_x.

PKM000
POLYURETHANE Y-217

TOXICITY DATA with REFERENCE
ETA: imp-rat TDLo:6750 mg/kg   CNREA8
35,1591,75

CONSENSUS REPORTS: IARC Cancer Review: Animal Sufficient Evidence IMEMDT 19,303,79.

SAFETY PROFILE: Confirmed carcinogen with experimental tumorigenic data. When heated to decomposition it emits very toxic fumes of NO_x and CN^-.

PKM250 CAS: 26375-23-5
POLYURETHANE Y-218
mf: $(C_{15}H_{10}N_2O_2 \cdot C_6H_{10}O_4 \cdot C_4H_{10}O_2)_x$

SYNS: ADIPIC ACID, POLYMER with 1,4-BUTANEDIOL and METHYLENEDI-p-PHENYLENE ISOCYANATE ◇ HEXANEDIOIC ACID, POLYMER with 1,4-BUTANEDIOL and 1,1'-METHYLENEBIS(4-ISOCYANATOBENZENE) ◇ PANDEX ◇ TEXIN 445D ◇ TPU 10M ◇ Y 218

TOXICITY DATA with REFERENCE
ETA: imp-rat TDLo:6750 mg/kg   CNREA8
35,1591,75

CONSENSUS REPORTS: IARC Cancer Review: Animal Sufficient Evidence IMEMDT 19,303,79.

SAFETY PROFILE: Confirmed carcinogen with experimental tumorigenic data. When heated to decomposition it emits very toxic fumes of CN^- and NO_x.

PKM500 CAS: 32238-28-1
POLYURETHANE Y-221
mf: $(C_{15}H_{10}N_2O_2 \cdot C_{10}H_{14}O_4 \cdot C_6H_{10}O_4 \cdot C_4H_{10}O_2)_x$

SYNS: ADIPIC ACID, POLYMER with 1,4-BUTANEDIOL, METHYLENEDI-p-PHENYLENE ISOCYANATE and 2,2'-(p-PHENYLENEDIOXY)DIETHANOL ◇ Y 221

TOXICITY DATA with REFERENCE
ETA: imp-rat TDLo:6750 mg/kg   CNREA8
35,1591,75

CONSENSUS REPORTS: IARC Cancer Review: Animal Sufficient Evidence IMEMDT 19,303,79. Reported in EPA TSCA Inventory.

SAFETY PROFILE: Confirmed carcinogen with experimental tumorigenic data. When heated to decomposition it emits very toxic fumes of CN^- and NO_x.

PKM750
POLYURETHANE Y-222
TOXICITY DATA with REFERENCE
ETA: imp-rat TDLo:6750 mg/kg   CNREA8
35,1591,75

CONSENSUS REPORTS: IARC Cancer Review: Animal Sufficient Evidence IMEMDT 19,303,79.

SAFETY PROFILE: Confirmed carcinogen with experimental tumorigenic data. When heated to decomposition it emits very toxic fumes of CN^- and NO_x.

PKN000 CAS: 52292-20-3
POLYURETHANE Y-223
SYNS: TECOFLEX HR ◇ Y-223

TOXICITY DATA with REFERENCE
ETA: imp-rat TDLo:6750 mg/kg   CNREA8
35,1591,75

CONSENSUS REPORTS: IARC Cancer Review: Animal Sufficient Evidence IMEMDT 19,303,79. Reported in EPA TSCA Inventory.

SAFETY PROFILE: Confirmed carcinogen with experimental tumorigenic data. When heated to decomposition it emits very toxic fumes of CN^- and NO_x.

PKN250
POLYURETHANE Y-224
TOXICITY DATA with REFERENCE
ETA: imp-rat TDLo:6750 mg/kg   CNREA8
35,1591,75

CONSENSUS REPORTS: IARC Cancer Review: Animal Sufficient Evidence IMEMDT 19,303,79.

SAFETY PROFILE: Confirmed carcinogen with experimental tumorigenic data. When heated to decomposition it emits very toxic fumes of CN^- and NO_x.

PKN500 CAS: 56779-19-2
POLYURETHANE Y-225
SYN: 1,4-BUTANEDIAMINE, 2-METHYL-, POLYMER with α-HYDRO-omega-HYDROXYPOLY(OXY-1,4-BUTANEDIYL) and 1,1'-METHYLENEBIS(4-ISOCYANATOCYCLOHEXANE)

TOXICITY DATA with REFERENCE
ETA: imp-rat TDLo:6750 mg/kg   CNREA8
35,1591,75

CONSENSUS REPORTS: IARC Cancer Review: Animal Sufficient Evidence IMEMDT 19,303,79.

SAFETY PROFILE: Confirmed carcinogen with experimental tumorigenic data. When heated to decomposition it emits very toxic fumes of CN^- and NO_x.

PKN750   CAS: 56386-98-2
POLYURETHANE Y-226

TOXICITY DATA with REFERENCE
ETA: imp-rat TDLo:6750 mg/kg   CNREA8
35,1591,75

CONSENSUS REPORTS: IARC Cancer Review: Animal Sufficient Evidence IMEMDT 19,303,79.

SAFETY PROFILE: Confirmed carcinogen with experimental tumorigenic data. When heated to decomposition it emits very toxic fumes of CN^- and NO_x.

PKO000   CAS: 56631-46-0
POLYURETHANE Y-227

TOXICITY DATA with REFERENCE
ETA: imp-rat TDLo:6750 mg/kg   CNREA8
35,1591,75

CONSENSUS REPORTS: IARC Cancer Review: Animal Sufficient Evidence IMEMDT 19,303,79.

SAFETY PROFILE: Confirmed carcinogen with experimental tumorigenic data. When heated to decomposition it emits very toxic fumes of CN^- and NO_x.

PKO500   CAS: 27083-55-2
POLYURETHANE Y-290
mf: $(C_{15}H_{10}N_2O_2 \cdot C_6H_{10}O_4 \cdot C_4H_{10}O_2 \cdot C_2H_6O_2)_x$

SYNS: E6 ◇ PPE201 ◇ P07 ◇ TEXIN 192A ◇ TPU 2T

TOXICITY DATA with REFERENCE
ETA: imp-rat TDLo:6750 mg/kg   CNREA8
35,1591,75

CONSENSUS REPORTS: IARC Cancer Review: Animal Sufficient Evidence IMEMDT 19,303,79.

SAFETY PROFILE: Confirmed carcinogen with experimental tumorigenic data. When heated to decomposition it emits very toxic fumes of CN^- and NO_x.

PKP000   CAS: 25805-16-7
POLYURETHANE Y-302
mf: $(C_{15}H_{10}N_2O_2 \cdot C_4H_{10}O_2)_x$

SYNS: 1,4-BUTANEDIOL POLYMER with 1,1'-METHYLENEBIS(4-ISOCYANATOBENZENE) ◇ ISOCYANIC ACID, METHYLENEDI-p-PHENYLENE ESTER, POLYMER with 1,4-BUTANEDIOL ◇ SANPRENE LQX 31 ◇ Y 302

TOXICITY DATA with REFERENCE
ETA: imp-rat TDLo:6750 mg/kg   CNREA8
35,1591,75

CONSENSUS REPORTS: IARC Cancer Review: Animal Sufficient Evidence IMEMDT 19,303,79.

SAFETY PROFILE: Confirmed carcinogen with experimental tumorigenic data by implant route. When heated to decomposition it emits very toxic fumes of CN^- and NO_x.

PKP250   CAS: 25036-33-3
POLYURETHANE Y-304

TOXICITY DATA with REFERENCE
ETA: imp-rat TDLo:6000 mg/kg   CNREA8
35,1591,75

CONSENSUS REPORTS: IARC Cancer Review: Animal Sufficient Evidence IMEMDT 19,303,79.

SAFETY PROFILE: Confirmed carcinogen with experimental tumorigenic data. When heated to decomposition it emits very toxic fumes of CN^- and NO_x.

PKV500   CAS: 10124-50-2
POTASSIUM ARSENITE
DOT: 1678
mf: $AsH_3O_3 \cdot xK$ mw: 399.65

PROP: White, hygroscopic powder. Sol in water.

SYNS: ARSENENOUS ACID, POTASSIUM SALT ◇ ARSENITE de POTASSIUM (FRENCH) ◇ ARSONIC ACID, POTASSIUM SALT ◇ KALIUMARSENIT (GERMAN) ◇ NSC 3060 ◇ POTASSIUM METAARSENITE

TOXICITY DATA with REFERENCE
CAR: orl-chd TD:390 mg/kg/3Y-C:SKN
AIMEAS 61,296,64
CAR: orl-man TD:441 mg/kg/3W-C:SKN
ANSUA5 99,348,34
CAR: orl-man TD:7560 mg/kg/26W-C:SKN
ANSUA5 99,348,34
CAR: orl-man TDLo:214 mg/kg/15Y-C:LIV
GASTAB 68,1582,75
ETA: skn-mus TDLo:576 mg/kg/12W-I
BMJOAE 2,1107,22
MUT: cyt-hmn:leu 1 μmol/L/48H   CNREA8
25,980,65

CONSENSUS REPORTS: Human Sufficient Evidence IMEMDT 23,39,80; Animal Inadequate Evidence IMEMDT 23,39,80, IMEMDT 2,48,73. EPA Extremely Hazardous Substances List. Arsenic and its compounds are on the Community Right-To-Know List.

OSHA PEL: TWA 0.01 mg(As)/m³; Cancer Hazard ACGIH TLV: TWA 0.2 mg(As)/m³ NIOSH REL: CL (Inorganic Arsenic) 0.002 mg(As)/m³/15M DOT Classification: Poison B; Label: Poison.

SAFETY PROFILE: Confirmed human carcinogen producing skin and liver tumors. Poison by ingestion, skin contact, subcutaneous, and intravenous routes. Human mutation data reported. Human systemic effects: dermatitis, liver changes. When heated to decomposition it emits toxic fumes of As and K_2O. Used in veterinary medicine and for chronic dermatitis in humans.

PLW500 CAS: 11103-86-9
POTASSIUM ZINC CHROMATE HYDROXIDE
mf: $Cr_2HO_9Zn_2 \cdot K$ mw: 418.85

SYNS: BUTTERCUP YELLOW ◇ CHROMIC ACID, POTASSIUM ZINC SALT (2:2:1) ◇ CITRON YELLOW ◇ POTASSIUM ZINC CHROMATE ◇ ZINC CHROME ◇ ZINC YELLOW

CONSENSUS REPORTS: IARC Cancer Review: Animal Inadequate Evidence IMEMDT 23,205,80. Chromium and its compounds, as well as zinc and its compounds, are on the Community Right-To-Know List. Reported in EPA TSCA Inventory.

OSHA PEL: (Transitional: 1 mg(CrO_3)/10m³) CL 0.1 mg(CrO_3)/m³ ACGIH TLV: TWA 0.01 mg(Cr)/M³; Confirmed Human Carcinogen DFG MAK: Human Carcinogen. NIOSH REL: (Chromium (VI)) TWA 0.001 mg(Cr(VI))/m³

SAFETY PROFILE: Confirmed carcinogen. When heated to decomposition it emits toxic fumes of ZnO and K_2O. Used as a corrosion inhibiting pigment and in steel priming.

PMB000 CAS: 12126-59-9
PREMARIN

SYNS: CEE ◇ CONJUGATED EQUINE ESTROGEN

TOXICITY DATA with REFERENCE
ETA: orl-rat TDLo:51 mg/kg/2Y-C   TXAPA9 11,489,67

CONSENSUS REPORTS: IARC Cancer Review: Human Limited Evidence IMEMDT

21,147,79; Animal Inadequate Evidence IMEMDT 21,147,79. NTP Fourth Annual Report On Carcinogens, 1984.

SAFETY PROFILE: Confirmed carcinogen with experimental tumorigenic data. Human reproductive effects by ingestion: changes in female fertility. Experimental teratogenic effects. A steroid. When heated to decomposition it emits acrid smoke and irritating fumes.

PME250 CAS: 671-16-9
PROCARBAZINE
mf: $C_{12}H_{19}N_3O$ mw: 221.34

SYNS: IBENZMETHYZINE ◇ 2-(p-ISOPROPYL CARBAMOYL BENZYL)-1-METHYLHYDRAZINE ◇ N-ISOPROPYL-α-(2-METHYLHYDRAZINO)-p-TOLUAMIDE ◇ MATULANE ◇ 4-((2-METHYLHYDRAZINO)METHYL)-N-ISOPROPYLBENZAMIDE ◇ 1-METHYL-2-(-ISOPROPYLCARBAMOYL)BENZYL)HYDRAZINE ◇ MIH ◇ NATULAN ◇ NSC-77213 ◇ PCB ◇ RO 4-6467

TOXICITY DATA with REFERENCE
CAR: ivn-rat TDLo:1250 mg/kg/1Y-I   ARZNAD 20,1461,70
NEO: ipr-mus TDLo:1200 mg/kg/4W-I   JNCIAM 59,423,77
ETA: ivn-rat TDLo:125 mg/kg (22D preg)   IARCCD 4,92,73
ETA: orl-mky TDLo:7 g/kg/7Y-I   CANCAR 40,1950,77
MUT: cyt-ham:ovr 25 mmol/L   MUREAV 74,77,80
MUT: cyt-mus-unk 50 mg/kg   MUREAV 74,77,80
MUT: dlt-dmg-unk 20 mmol/L   MUREAV 74,77,80
MUT: dns-rbt-ivn 5 mg/kg   ARTODN 46,139,80
MUT: mma-ham:lng 500 μmol/L   MUREAV 74,77,80
MUT: mmo-asn 10 mg/plate   MUREAV 80,265,81
MUT: mmo-smc 12 g/L   BSIBAC 56,1322,80
MUT: mnt-mus-unk 15 mg/kg   MUREAV 74,77,80
MUT: sce-ham-unk 25 mg/kg   MUREAV 74,77,80
MUT: sce-ham:ovr 50 μmol/L   MUREAV 74,77,80
MUT: sce-mus-unk 50 mg/kg   MUREAV 74,77,80
MUT: sln-dmg-orl 10 mmol/L   ENMUDM 2,515,80
MUT: sln-dmg-unk 500 μmol/L   MUREAV 74,77,80
MUT: slt-mus-ipr 20 mg/kg   SCIEAS 209,299,80
MUT: slt-mus-ivn 20 mg/kg   SCIEAS 209,299,80
MUT: slt-mus-orl 20 mg/kg   SCIEAS 209,299,80
MUT: spm-mus-ipr 120 mg/kg   CNREA8 42,122,82

CONSENSUS REPORTS: NTP Fourth Annual Report On Carcinogens, 1984.

SAFETY PROFILE: Confirmed carcinogen with experimental carcinogenic, neoplastigenic, tumorigenic, and teratogenic data. Poison by intravenous route. Moderately toxic by intraperitoneal route. Has been implicated as a brain carcinogen. Experimental reproductive effects. Mutation data reported. When heated to decomposition it emits toxic fumes of NO_x.

PME500   CAS: 366-70-1
PROCARBAZINE HYDROCHLORIDE
mf: $C_{12}H_{19}N_3O \cdot ClH$ mw: 257.80

PROP: Crystals. Mp: 223-236°.

SYNS: IBENZMETHYZINE HYDROCHLORIDE ◇ IBENZ-
METHYZIN HYDROCHLORIDE ◇ IBZ ◇ 1-(p-ISOPROPYL-
CARBAMOYLBENZYL)-2-METHYLHYDRAZINE HYDRO-
CHLORIDE ◇ 2-(p-(ISOPROPYLCARBAMOYL)BENZYL)-1-
METHYLHYDRAZINE HYDROCHLORIDE ◇ N-ISOPROPYL-
p-(2-METHYLHYDRAZINOMETHYL)BENZAMIDEHYDRO-
CHLORIDE ◇ N-ISOPROPYL-α-(2-METHYLHYDRAZINO)-p-
TOLUAMIDE HYDROCHLORIDE ◇ MATULANE ◇ MBH
◇ N-(1-METHYLETHYL)-4-((2-METHYLHYDRAZINO)
METHYL)BENZAMIDE MONOHYDROCHLORIDE ◇ p-(N'-
METHYLHYDRAZINOMETHYL)-N-ISOPROPYL)BENZ-
AMIDE ◇ p-(N'-METHYLHYDRAZINOMETHYL)-N-ISOPRO-
PYLBENZAMIDE HYDROCHLORIDE ◇ 1-METHYL-2-p-
(ISOPROPYLCARBAMOYL)BENZOHYDRAZINE
HYDROCHLORIDE ◇ 1-METHYL-2-(p-ISOPROPYL-
CARBAMOYLBENZYL)HYDRAZINE HYDROCHLORIDE
◇ MIH HYDROCHLORIDE ◇ NATHULANE ◇ NATUŁAN
◇ NATULANAR ◇ NATULAN HYDROCHLORIDE
◇ NCI-C01810 ◇ NSC-77213 ◇ PCB HYDROCHLORIDE
◇ PROCARBAZIN (GERMAN) ◇ RO 4-6467

TOXICITY DATA with REFERENCE
CAR: ipr-mus TD:4680 mg/kg/52W-I
  NCITR* NCI-CG-TR-19,79
CAR: ipr-mus TDLo:2340 mg/kg/42W-I
  NCITR* NCI-CG-TR-19,79
CAR: ipr-rat TD:2340 mg/kg/26W-I
  NCITR* NCI-CG-TR-19,79
CAR: ipr-rat TD:4680 mg/kg/26W-I   RRCRBU
  52,1,75
CAR: ipr-rat TDLo:1170 mg/kg/26W-I
  NCITR* NCI-CG-TR-19,79
CAR: orl-mus TDLo:2 g/kg/8W-I   JNCIAM
  42,337,69
CAR: scu-rat TDLo:300 mg/kg   CALEDQ21,155,83
NEO: ipr-mus TD:1136 mg/kg/8W-I   JNCIAM
  42,337,69
NEO: ipr-mus TD:1950 mg/kg/26W-I   RRCRBU
  52,1,75
NEO: ipr-mus TD:2560 mg/kg/8W-I   CNCRA6
  39,77,64
NEO: orl-mus TD:2 g/kg/8W-I   CNCRA6 39,77,64

ETA: ipr-mky TDLo:4088 mg/kg/5Y-I
  BCSYDM 3,239,82
ETA: ipr-rat TD:500 mg/kg   JNCIAM
  40,1027,68
ETA: mul-mky TD:20 g/kg/8Y-I   BCSYDM
  3,239,82
ETA: mul-mky TDLo:3270 mg/kg/69W-I
  CNREA8 38,2125,78
ETA: orl-rat TD:1200 mg/kg/14W-C   ONCOBS
  41,106,84
ETA: orl-rat TDLo:500 mg/kg   JNCIAM40,1027,68
MUT: dnd-rat-ipr 25 mg/kg   ENMUDM 7,563,85
MUT: hma-mus/esc 100 mg/kg   MUREAV164,19,86
MUT: mma-esc 78 μg/well   CRNGDP 4,347,83
MUT: slt-ham:ovr 600 mg/L   MUREAV 136,137,84

CONSENSUS REPORTS: IARC Cancer Review: Human Limited Evidence IMEMDT 26,311,81; Animal Sufficient Evidence IMEMDT 26,311,81. NTP Fourth Annual Report On Carcinogens, 1984. NCI Carcinogenesis Bioassay (ipr); Clear Evidence: mouse, rat NCITR* NCI-CG-TR-19,79; (ipr); Clear Evidence: mouse, rat RRCRBU 52,1,75. EPA Genetic Toxicology Program.

SAFETY PROFILE: Confirmed carcinogen with experimental carcinogenic, neoplastigenic, tumorigenic, and teratogenic data. Poison by an unspecified route. Moderately toxic by ingestion, subcutaneous, intravenous, intraperitoneal and possibly other routes. Experimental reproductive effects. Mutation data reported. When heated to decomposition it emits very toxic fumes of NO_x and HCl. Used as a chemotherapeutic agent.

PMH500   CAS: 57-83-0
PROGESTERONE
mf: $C_{31}H_{30}O_2$ mw: 314.51

PROP: A female sex hormone. White, crystalline powder; odorless. D: 1.166 @ 23°, mp: 127-131°. Practically insol in water; sol in alc, acetone, and dioxane; sparingly sol in oils.

SYNS: CORLUTIN ◇ CORLUVITE ◇ CORPORIN
◇ CORPUS LUTEUM HORMONE ◇ CYCLOGEST ◇ Δ⁴-PREG-
NENE-3,20-DIONE ◇ GLANDUCORPIN ◇ HORMOFLAVEINE
◇ HORMOLUTON ◇ LINGUSORBS ◇ LIPO-LUTIN
◇ LUCORTEUM SOL ◇ LUTEAL HORMONE ◇ LUTEOHOR-
MONE ◇ LUTEOSAN ◇ LUTEX ◇ LUTOCYCLIN ◇ LUTRO-
MONE ◇ NALUTRON ◇ NSC-9704 ◇ PERCUTACRINE
◇ PIAPONON ◇ 3,20-PREGNENE-4 ◇ PREGNENEDIONE
◇ PREGNENE-3,20-DIONE ◇ PREGN-4-ENE-3,20-DIONE
◇ 4-PREGNENE-3,20-DIONE ◇ PROGEKAN ◇ PROGES-

TEROL ◇ β-PROGESTERONE ◇ PROGESTERONUM ◇ PROGESTIN ◇ PROGESTONE ◇ PROLIDON ◇ SYNGES-TERONE ◇ SYNOVEX S ◇ SYNTOLUTAN

TOXICITY DATA with REFERENCE

NEO: imp-mus TD:14 g/kg/77W-C NATUAS 212,686,66

NEO: imp-mus TD:1300 mg/kg/78W-I BJCAAI 21,144,67

NEO: imp-mus TD:2592 mg/kg/77W-C NATUAS 212,686,66

NEO: imp-mus TDLo:1296 mg/kg/77W-C NATUAS 212,686,66

NEO: scu-mus TD:9500 mg/kg/19W-I BJCAAI 19,824,65

NEO: scu-mus TDLo:40 mg/kg BJCAAI 19,824,65

ETA: imp-dog TDLo:270 mg/kg/78W 36PYAS -,145,77

ETA: imp-mus TD:19 g/kg/77W-C NATUAS 212,686,66

ETA: imp-mus TD:216 mg/kg/77W-C NATUAS 212,686,66

ETA: imp-mus TD:648 mg/kg/77W-C NATUAS 212,686,66

ETA: ims-dog TDLo:26643 mg/kg/4Y-I FESTAS 31,340,79

ETA: scu-mus TD:200 mg/kg/5W-I IJCAAR 9,244,72

MUT: cyt-hmn:kdy 100 μg/L CNJGA8 10,299,68
MUT: cyt-mus:emb 1 mg/L DANKAS 282,173,85
MUT: dni-hmn:kdy 100 μg/L CNJGA8 10,299,68
MUT: dni-hmn:lym 5 μmol/L PSEBAA 146,401,74
MUT: otr-rat:emb 2600 μg/L JJIND8 67,1303,81

CONSENSUS REPORTS: IARC Cancer Review: Animal Limited Evidence IMEMDT 21,491,79; Animal Sufficient Evidence IMEMDT 6,135,74. NTP Fourth Annual Report On Carcinogens, 1984. EPA Genetic Toxicology Program. Reported in EPA TSCA Inventory.

SAFETY PROFILE: Confirmed carcinogen with experimental carcinogenic, neoplastigenic, tumorigenic, and teratogen data. Poison by intravenous and intraperitoneal routes. Human teratogenic effects by ingestion, parenteral, and possibly other routes: developmental abnormalities of the urogenital system. Human male reproductive effects by intramuscular route: changes in spermatogenesis, the prostate, seminal vesicle, Cowper's gland, and accessory glands; impotence, and breast development. Human female reproductive effects by ingestion, parenteral and intravaginal routes: fertility changes;

menstrual cycle changes and disorders; uterus, cervix, and vagina changes. Experimental reproductive effects. Human mutation data reported. When heated to decomposition it emits acrid smoke and irritating fumes.

PML400 CAS: 1120-71-4
PROPANE SULTONE
mf: $C_3H_6O_3S$ mw: 122.15

SYNS: 3-HYDROXY-1-PROPANESULFONIC ACID γ-SULTONE ◇ 3-HYDROXY-1-PROPANESULPHONIC ACID SULFONE ◇ 3-HYDROXY-1-PROPANESULPHONIC ACID SULTONE ◇ 1,2-OXATHIOLANE-2,2-DIOXIDE ◇ 1-PROPANESULFONIC ACID-3-HYDROXY-γ-SULTONE ◇ 1,3-PROPANE SULTONE (MAK) ◇ RCRA WASTE NUMBER U193

TOXICITY DATA with REFERENCE

CAR: ivn-rat TDLo:20 mg/kg/(15D preg): TER ZEKBAI 75,69,70

CAR: orl-rat TD:12 g/kg/60W-C JJIND8 67,75,81
CAR: orl-rat TD:13 g/kg/32W-C JJIND8 67,75,81
CAR: orl-rat TDLo:7840 mg/kg/60W-I NATUAS 230,460,71

CAR: skn-mus TD:50 mg/kg/W-I TXAPA9 37,93,76

CAR: skn-mus TDLo:1000 mg/kg TXCYAC 6,139,76

NEO: scu-mus TDLo:756 mg/kg/63W-I JNCIAM 46,143,71

ETA: orl-rat TD:1100 mg/kg/37W-I ZEKBAI 75,69,70

ETA: scu-rat TD:166 mg/kg INTSAO 66,161,81
ETA: scu-rat TD:434 mg/kg/15W-I INTSAO 66,161,81
ETA: scu-rat TD:559 mg/kg/17W-I INTSAO 66,161,81
ETA: scu-rat TDLo:10 mg/kg ZEKBAI 75,69,70

MUT: cyt-hmn:lym 1 mmol/L TOLED5 28,139,85
MUT: dnd-esc 10 μmol/L MUREAV 89,95,81
MUT: otr-hmn:oth 7500 μg/L CNREA8 41,5096,81
MUT: otr-mus:emb 50 mg/L TOLED5 9,301,81
MUT: otr-mus:fbr 30 μg/L CRNGDP 3,377,82
MUT: sce-hmn:lym 500 μmol/L TOLED5 28,139,85

CONSENSUS REPORTS: IARC Cancer Review: Animal Sufficient Evidence IMEMDT 4,253,74. NTP Fourth Annual Report On Carcinogens, 1984. Community Right-To-Know List. Reported in EPA TSCA Inventory. EPA Genetic Toxicology Program.

ACGIH TLV: Suspected Human Carcinogen. DFG MAK: Animal Carcinogen, Suspected Human Carcinogen.

SAFETY PROFILE: Confirmed carcinogen with experimental carcinogenic, neoplastigenic, tumorigenic, and teratogenic data. Poison by subcutaneous route. Moderately toxic by skin contact and intraperitoneal routes. Experimental reproductive effects. Human mutation data reported. Implicated as a human brain carcinogen. A skin irritant. When heated to decomposition it emits toxic fumes of SO_x.

PMT100
β-PROPIOLACTONE
CAS: 57-57-8

mf: $C_3H_4O_2$ mw: 72.07

SYNS: BETAPRONE ◇ BPL ◇ HYDRACRYLIC ACID β-LACTONE ◇ 3-HYDROXYPROPIONIC ACID LACTONE ◇ PROPANOLIDE ◇ PROPIOLACTONE ◇ β-PROPIOLACTONE ◇ 1,3-PROPIOLACTONE ◇ 3-PROPIOLACTONE ◇ β-PROPIONOLACTONE ◇ β-PROPRIOLACTONE (OSHA) ◇ β-PROPROLACTONE

TOXICITY DATA with REFERENCE
CAR: ihl-rat TCLo: 5 ppm/6H/30D-I   JJIND8 79,285,87
CAR: orl-mus TDLo: 3080 mg/kg/77W-I   JJIND8 63,1433,79
CAR: orl-rat TDLo: 2868 mg/kg/1Y-I   BJCAAI 46,924,82
CAR: scu-rat TD: 1080 mg/kg/54W-I   JNCIAM 39,1213,67
CAR: scu-rat TDLo: 22 mg/kg/25W-I   BMBUAQ 20,96,64
CAR: skn-mus TD: 11 g/kg/56W-I   TXCYAC 6,139,76
CAR: skn-mus TD: 37772 mg/kg/2Y-I
CAR: skn-mus TDLo: 6200 mg/kg/15W-I   BJCAAI 9,177,55
NEO: scu-mus TD: 408 mg/kg/34W-I   JNCIAM 53,695,74
NEO: scu-mus TD: 648 mg/kg/54W-I   JJIND8 63,1433,79
NEO: scu-mus TD: 1168 mg/kg/40W-I   JNCIAM 37,825,66
NEO: scu-mus TDLo: 69 mg/kg/43W-I   BJCAAI 19,392,65
NEO: scu-rat TD: 50 mg/kg/25W-I   BJCAAI 15,85,61
ETA: itr-rat TDLo: 72 mg/kg/30W-I   BJCAAI 20,134,66
ETA: itr-rat TDLo: 72 mg/kg/30W-I   BJCAAI 20,134,66
ETA: ivn-mus TDLo: 40 mg/kg   BJCAAI 10,357,56
ETA: orl-mus TD: 320 mg/kg/8W-I   CNREA8 43,4747,83

ETA: orl-rat TDLo: 3050 mg/kg/61W-I   JNCIAM 37,825,66
ETA: skn-gpg TDLo: 56 mg/kg/141W-I   BJCAAI 20,200,66
ETA: skn-mus TD: 8100 mg/kg/27W-I   BJCAAI 10,357,56
MUT: dnd-hmn: lym 1 mmol/L   JACTDZ 1(3),125,82
MUT: otr-hmn: fbr 28 μmol/L   PNASA6 80,7219,83
MUT: otr-mus: fbr 500 μg/L   JJIND8 69,503,82
MUT: sce-ham: lng 100 μmol/L   MUREAV 118,103,83
MUT: slt-dmg-orl 200 mmol/L   ENMUDM 6,153,84

CONSENSUS REPORTS: IARC Cancer Review: Animal Sufficient Evidence IMEMDT 4,259,74. NTP Fourth Annual Report On Carcinogens, 1984. EPA Genetic Toxicology Program. Community Right-To-Know List. EPA Extremely Hazardous Substances List. Reported in EPA TSCA Inventory.

OSHA: Carcinogen.   ACGIH TLV: TWA 0.5 ppm; Suspected Human Carcinogen. DFG MAK: Animal Carcinogen, Suspected Human Carcinogen.

SAFETY PROFILE: Confirmed carcinogen with experimental carcinogenic, neoplastigenic, and tumorigenic data. Poison by inhalation. Moderately toxic by intraperitoneal route. An initiator. Human mutation data reported. When heated to decomposition it emits acrid smoke and irritating fumes.

PNL400
PROPYLENE IMINE
CAS: 75-55-8

DOT: 1921
mf: C_3H_7N mw: 57.11

PROP: Liquid. Vap d: 2.0, flash p: 14°F.

SYNS: 2-METHYLAZACYCLOPROPANE ◇ 2-METHYLAZIRIDINE ◇ METHYLETHYLENIMINE ◇ 2-METHYLETHYLENIMINE ◇ 1,2-PROPYLENEIMINE ◇ PROPYLENE IMINE, INHIBITED (DOT) ◇ RCRA WASTE NUMBER P067

TOXICITY DATA with REFERENCE
CAR: orl-rat TD: 3920 mg/kg/27W-C   JJIND8 67,75,81
CAR: orl-rat TD: 4129 mg/kg/58W-C   JJIND8 67,75,81
CAR: orl-rat TDLo: 1120 mg/kg/28W-I   NATUAS 230,460,71
MUT: mma-esc 10 μg/plate   ENMUDM 6(Suppl 2),1,84

MUT: mma-sat 3300 ng/plate ENMUDM
6(Suppl 2),1,84

MUT: mmo-esc 1 μg/plate ENMUDM6(Suppl2),1,84

MUT: mmo-sat 3300 ng/plate ENMUDM
6(Suppl 2),1,84

CONSENSUS REPORTS: IARC Cancer Review: Animal Limited Evidence IMEMDT 9,61,75. NTP Fourth Annual Report On Carcinogens, 1984. EPA Genetic Toxicology Program. Reported in EPA TSCA Inventory. EPA Extremely Hazardous Substances List. Community Right-To-Know List.

OSHA PEL: TWA 2 ppm (skin) ACGIH TLV: TWA 2 ppm (skin), Suspected Human Carcinogen. DFG MAK: Animal Carcinogen, Suspected Human Carcinogen. DOT Classification: Flammable Liquid; Label: Flammable Liquid.

SAFETY PROFILE: Confirmed carcinogen with experimental carcinogenic data. Poison by ingestion and skin contact. Moderately toxic by inhalation. Mutation data reported. Severe eye irritant. Implicated as a brain carcinogen. A very dangerous fire hazard when exposed to heat or flame; can react vigorously with oxidizing materials. When heated to decomposition it emits toxic fumes of NO_x.

PNL600 CAS: 75-56-9
PROPYLENE OXIDE
DOT: 1280
mf: C_3H_6O mw: 58.09

PROP: Colorless liquid; ethereal odor. Bp: 33.9°, lel: 2.8%, uel: 37%, fp: −104.4°, flash p: −35°F (TOC), d: 0.8304 @ 20°/20°, vap press: 400 mm @ 17.8°, vap d: 2.0. Sol in water, alc, and ether.

SYNS: EPOXYPROPANE ◇ 1,2-EPOXYPROPANE ◇ 2,3-EPOXYPROPANE ◇ METHYL ETHYLENE OXIDE ◇ METHYL OXIRANE ◇ NCI-C50099 ◇ OXYDE de PROPYLENE (FRENCH) ◇ PROPENE OXIDE ◇ PROPYLENE EPOXIDE ◇ 1,2-PROPYLENE OXIDE

TOXICITY DATA with REFERENCE
CAR: ihl-mus TCLo:400 ppm/6H/2Y-I
NTPTR* NTP-TR-267,85

CAR: orl-rat TDLo:10798 mg/kg/2Y-I BJCAAI
46,924,82

CAR: scu-mus TD:868 mg/kg/95W-I ZHPMAT
174,383,81

CAR: scu-mus TD:2912 mg/kg/95W-I ZHPMAT
174,383,81

CAR: scu-mus TD:6616 mg/kg/95W-I ZHPMAT
174,383,81

CAR: scu-mus TDLo:272 mg/kg/95W-I
ZHPMAT 174,383,81

NEO: ihl-rat TCLo:100 ppm/7H/2Y-I TXAPA9
76,69,84

NEO: scu-mus TD:3640 mg/kg/91W-I BJCAAI
39,588,79

ETA: ihl-rat TC:400 ppm/6H/2Y-I JJIND8
77,573,86

ETA: orl-rat TD:2714 mg/kg/2Y-I BJCAAI
46,924,82

ETA: scu-rat TDLo:1500 mg/kg/46W-I
ANYAA9 68,750,58

MUT: cyt-rat:lvr 25 mg/L MUREAV 153,57,85

MUT: dnd-esc 1 μmol/L ARTODN 46,277,80

MUT: mmo-omi 25 mmol/L MUREAV 73,1,80

MUT: mmo-sat 350 μg/plate ABCHA6 47,2461,83

MUT: sce-hmn:lym 25000 ppm ENMUDM-
7(Suppl 3),48,85

MUT: sln-dmg-ihl 645 ppm/24H-C MUREAV
117,337,83

CONSENSUS REPORTS: IARC Cancer Review: Human Inadequate Evidence IMEMDT 36,227,85; Animal Sufficient Evidence IMEMDT 36,227,85; Animal Limited Evidence IMEMDT 11,191,76. Carcinogenesis Studies (inhalation); Some Evidence: rat NTPTR* NTP-TR-267,85; Clear Evidence: mouse NTPTR* NTP-TR-267,85. Reported in EPA TSCA Inventory. EPA Genetic Toxicology Program. Community Right-To-Know List. EPA Extremely Hazardous Substances List.

OSHA PEL: (Transitional: TWA 100 ppm) TWA 20 ppm ACGIH TLV: TWA 20 ppm DFG MAK: Animal Carcinogen, Suspected Human Carcinogen. DOT Classification: Flammable Liquid; Label: Flammable Liquid.

SAFETY PROFILE: Confirmed carcinogen with experimental carcinogenic, neoplastigenic, and tumorigenic data. Poison by intraperitoneal route. Moderately toxic by ingestion, inhalation, and skin contact. Experimental reproductive effects. Human mutation data reported. A severe skin and eye irritant. Flammable liquid. A very dangerous fire and explosion hazard when exposed to heat or flame. Keep away from heat and open flame. To fight fire, use alcohol foam, CO_2, dry chemical. When heated to decomposition it emits acrid smoke and fumes.

PNX000 CAS: 51-52-5
6-PROPYL-2-THIOURACIL
mf: $C_7H_{10}N_2OS$ mw: 170.25

PROP: White, bitter, crystalline powder. Mp: 219-221°. Insol in ether, chloroform, benzene; very sol in aq solns of ammonia; very sltly sol in water.

SYNS: 2,3-DIHYDRO-6-PROPYL-2-THIOXO-4(1H)-PY-RIMIDINONE ◊ 2-MERCAPTO-4-HYDROXY-6-N-PROPYLPY-RIMIDINE ◊ 2-MERCAPTO-6-PROPYL-4-PYRIMIDONE ◊ 2-MERCAPTO-6-PROPYLPYRIMID-4-ONE ◊ PROCASIL ◊ PROPACIL ◊ PROPILTHIOURACIL ◊ 6-PROPIL-TIOURA-CILE (ITALIAN) ◊ PROPYCIL ◊ 6-PROPYL-2-THIO-2,-4(1H,3H)PYRIMIDINEDIONE ◊ PROPYL-THIORIST ◊ PROPYLTHIOURACIL ◊ 4-PROPYL-2-THIOURACIL ◊ 6-N-PROPYLTHIOURACIL ◊ 6-N-PROPYL-2-THIOURACIL ◊ PROPYL-THYRACIL ◊ PROPYTHIOURACIL ◊ PROTHI-UCIL ◊ PROTHIURONE ◊ PROTHYCIL ◊ PROTHYRAN ◊ PROTIURAL ◊ PTU (THYREOSTATIC) ◊ 2-THIO-4-OXO-6-PROPYL-1,3-PYRIMIDINE ◊ 2-THIO-6-PROPYL-1,3-PY-RIMIDIN-4-ONE ◊ 6-THIO-4-PROPYLURACIL ◊ THIURAGYL ◊ THYREOSTAT II ◊ T 72

TOXICITY DATA with REFERENCE
CAR: orl-ham TDLo: 653 g/kg/70W-C   CANCAR 21,952,68
NEO: orl-gpg TDLo: 37 g/kg/2Y-C   GROWAH 27,305,63
ETA: orl-mus TDLo: 600 g/kg/73W-C   PSEBAA 112,365,63
MUT: dni-hmn: lym 100 mg/L   JCEMAZ 43,1046,76
MUT: mmo-smc 1 g/L   CHINAG (21),847,80

CONSENSUS REPORTS: IARC Cancer Review: Animal Sufficient Evidence IMEMDT 7,67,74. NTP Fourth Annual Report On Carcinogens, 1984. Reported in EPA TSCA Inventory.

SAFETY PROFILE: Confirmed carcinogen with experimental carcinogenic, neoplastigenic, tumorigenic, and teratogenic data. Poison by an unspecified route. Moderately toxic by ingestion. Human teratogenic effects by ingestion: developmental abnormalities of the endocrine system and changes in newborn viability. Experimental reproductive effects. Human mutation data reported. When heated to decomposition it emits very toxic fumes of SO_x and NO_x.

POD500
PROTACTINIUM
af: Pa   aw: 231.036

PROP: A bright, lustrous metal. Mp: 1600°, d: 15.37, vap press: 5×10^{-5} mm @ 1927°. Natural isotope ^{231}Pa (Actinium series), $T_{0.5}$ = 3×10^4 Y., decays to radioactive ^{227}Ac by alphas of 5.0 MeV. Artificial isotope ^{233}Pa (Neptunium Series), $T_{0.5}$ = 27D, decays to radioactive ^{233}U by betas of 0.15 (37%), 0.26 (58%), 0.57 (5%) MeV; emits gammas of 0.02-0.42 MeV. Natural isotope ^{234}Pa (Uranium Series), $T_{0.5}$ = 6.7H, decays to radioactive 234U by betas of 0.23-1.36 MeV, emits gammas of 0.04-0.8 MeV.

SAFETY PROFILE: Confirmed carcinogen. A highly radiotoxic metallic element. An alpha emitter. It is a general hazard if absorbed systemically. The dust and fumes are hazardous if inhaled. A severe radiation hazard.

SAD000   CAS: 94-59-7
SAFROL
mf: $C_{10}H_{10}O_2$ mw: 162.20

PROP: Colorless liquid or crystals; sassafras odor. Mp: 11°, bp: 234.5°, d: 1.0960 @ 20°, vap press: 1 mm @ 63.8°. Insol in water; very sol in alc; misc with chloroform, ether.

SYNS: 5-ALLYL-1,3-BENZODIOXOLE ◊ ALLYLCATE-CHOL METHYLENE ETHER ◊ ALLYLDIOXYBENZENE METHYLENE ETHER ◊ 1-ALLYL-3,4-METHYLENEDIOXY-BENZENE ◊ 4-ALLYL-1,2-METHYLENEDIOXYBENZENE ◊ m-ALLYLPYROCATECHIN METHYLENE ETHER ◊ 4-ALLYLPYROCATECHOL FORMALDEHYDE ACETAL ◊ ALLYLPYROCATECHOL METHYLENE ETHER ◊ 1,2-METHYLENEDIOXY-4-ALLYLBENZENE ◊ 3,4-METHYL-ENEDIOXY-ALLYBENZENE ◊ 5-(2-PROPENYL)-1,3-BENZO-DIOXOLE ◊ RCA WASTE NUMBER U203 ◊ RHYUNO OIL ◊ SAFROLE ◊ SAFROLE MF ◊ SHIKIMOLE ◊ SHIKOMOL

TOXICITY DATA with REFERENCE
CAR: orl-mus LDLo: 22 g/kg/90W-I   CNREA8 39,4378,79
CAR: orl-mus TD: 121 g/kg/36W-C   JJIND8 67,365,81
CAR: orl-mus TD: 132 g/kg/81W-I   JNCIAM 42,1101,69
CAR: orl-mus TD: 175 g/kg/52W-C   JJIND8 67,365,81
CAR: orl-mus TD: 187 g/kg/56W-C   CNREA8 33,590,73
CAR: orl-mus TD: 212 g/kg/1Y-C   CNREA8 43,1124,83
CAR: orl-mus TD: 252 g/kg/75W-C   JJIND8 67,365,81
CAR: orl-mus TD: 82602 mg/kg/81W-C   DIGEBW 19,42,79
CAR: orl-rat TD: 183 g/kg/2Y-C   FEPRA7 20,287,61

CAR: orl-rat TDLo:200 g/kg/94W-C   CNREA8
37,1883,77

NEO: orl-mus TD:56 g/kg/52W-C   CNREA8
43,5163,83

NEO: orl-mus TD:210 g/kg/52W-C   CNREA8
37,1883,77

NEO: orl-mus TDLo:480 mg/kg (12-18D post)
CNREA8 39,4378,79

MUT: cyt-ham:lng 75 mg/L   PMRSDJ 5,427,85
MUT: dns:hmn:hla 10 µL/L   PMRSDJ 5,347,85
MUT: otr-ham:kdy 80 µg/L   BJCAAI 37,873,78
MUT: otr-mus:emb 100 mg/L   PMRSDJ 5,659,85
MUT: sce-ham:lng 500 µmol/L   PMRSDJ 5,469,85

CONSENSUS REPORTS: IARC Cancer Review: GROUP 3 IMEMDT 7,56,87; Animal Sufficient Evidence IMEMDT 10,231,76, IMEMDT 1,169,72. NTP Fourth Annual Report On Carcinogens, 1984. Community Right-To-Know List. EPA Genetic Toxicology Program. Reported in EPA TSCA Inventory.

SAFETY PROFILE: Confirmed carcinogen with experimental carcinogenic and neoplastigenic data. Poison by intraperitoneal and intravenous routes. Moderately toxic by ingestion and subcutaneous routes. Experimental reproductive effects. Human mutation data reported. A skin irritant. Combustible when exposed to heat or flame. When heated to decomposition it emits acrid smoke and irritating fumes.

SBT000   CAS: 7446-34-6
SELENIUM MONOSULFIDE
mf: SSe   mw: 111.02

PROP: Orange-yellow tablets or powder. Mp: 111.03°, bp: decomp @ 118-119°, d: 3.056 @ 0°.

SYNS: NCI-C50033 ◇ SELENIUM SULFIDE ◇ SELENIUM SULPHIDE ◇ SELENSULFID (GERMAN) ◇ SULFUR SELENIDE

TOXICITY DATA with REFERENCE
CAR: orl-mus TDLo:72 g/kg/2Y-C
NCITR* NCI-CG-TR-194,80
CAR: orl-rat TDLo:11 g/kg/2Y-C
NCITR* NCI-CG-TR-194,80

CONSENSUS REPORTS: NTP Fourth Annual Report On Carcinogens, 1984. NCI Carcinogenesis Bioassay (dermal); Inadequate Studies: mouse NCITR* NCI-CG-TR-197,80; (gavage); Clear Evidence: mouse, rat NCITR* NCI-CG-TR-194,80. Selenium and its compounds are on the Community Right-To-Know List.

OSHA PEL: TWA 0.2 mg(Se)/m^3 ACGIH TLV: TWA 0.2 mg(Se)/m^3

SAFETY PROFILE: Confirmed carcinogen with experimental carcinogenic data. Poison by ingestion. When heated to decomposition it emits very toxic fumes of SO_x and Se.

SCJ000   CAS: 14464-46-1
SILICA, CRYSTALLINE-CRISTOBALITE
mf: O_2Si mw: 60.09

PROP: White, cubic-system crystals formed from quartz at temperatures above 1000°C (NTIS** PB246-697).

SYNS: CALCINED DIATOMITE ◇ CRISTOBALITE

TOXICITY DATA with REFERENCE
CAR: ipl-rat TDLo:90 mg/kg   JNCIAM 57,509,76
ETA: ipl-rat TD:100 mg/kg   BJCAAI 41,908,80

CONSENSUS REPORTS: IARC Cancer Review: Animal Sufficient Evidence IMEMDT 42,209,88; Human Limited Evidence IMEMDT 42,209,88. Reported in EPA TSCA Inventory.

OSHA PEL: (Transitional: TWA Respirable Fraction: (10 mg/m^3/2(%SiO_2+2)); Total Dust: 30 mg/m^3/2(%SiO_2+2)) TWA Respirable Fraction: 0.05 mg/m^3 ACGIH TLV: TWA Respirable Fraction: 0.05 mg/m^3 DFG MAK: 0.15 mg/m^3 NIOSH REL: TWA 50 µg/m^3

SAFETY PROFILE: Confirmed carcinogen with experimental carcinogenic and tumorigenic data. Poison by intratracheal route. Human systemic effects by inhalation: cough, dyspnea, fibrosis. About twice as toxic as silica in causing silicosis.

SCJ500   CAS: 14808-60-7
SILICA, CRYSTALLINE-QUARTZ
mf: O_2Si mw: 60.09

PROP: Mp: 1710°, bp: 2230°, d: 2.6.

SYNS: AGATE ◇ AMETHYST ◇ CHALCEDONY ◇ CHERTS ◇ FLINT ◇ ONYX ◇ PURE QUARTZ ◇ QUARTZ ◇ QUAZO PURO (ITALIAN) ◇ ROSE QUARTZ ◇ SAND ◇ SILICA FLOUR (powdered crystalline silica) ◇ SILICIC ANHYDRIDE

TOXICITY DATA with REFERENCE
CAR: ihl-rat TCLo:50 mg/m^3/6H/71W-I
ENVRAL 40,499,86
CAR: ipl-rat TD:100 mg/kg   BJCAAI 41,908,80
CAR: ipl-rat TDLo:90 mg/kg   JNCIAM 57,509,76
CAR: ipr-rat TDLo:45 mg/kg   ZHPMAT 162,467,76

CAR: itr-rat TDLo: 111 mg/kg   CNREA8 2,243,86
NEO: imp-rat TDLo: 900 mg/kg   AICCA6 10,119,54
NEO: ipl-ham TDLo: 83 mg/kg   31BYAP -,97,74
NEO: ipl-rat TD: 100 mg/kg   JJIND8 79,797,87
NEO: ipr-rat TD: 450 mg/kg/4W-I   NATWAY 59,318,72
ETA: imp-mus TDLo: 4000 mg/kg   BJCAAI 22,825,68
ETA: imp-rat TD: 4554 mg/kg   CORTBR 88,223,72
ETA: ipl-rat TD: 100 mg/kg   AIHAAP 41,836,80
ETA: ipl-rat TD: 200 mg/kg   JNCIAM 48,797,72
ETA: ipr-rat TD: 90 mg/kg/4W-I   JNCIAM 57,509,76
ETA: itr-rat TDLo: 100 mg/kg/19W-I   EVHPAZ 34,47,80
ETA: ivn-rat TDLo: 90 mg/kg   JNCIAM 57,509,76

CONSENSUS REPORTS: IARC Cancer Review: Animal Sufficient Evidence IMEMDT 42,209,88; Human Limited Evidence IMEMDT 42,209,88. Reported in EPA TSCA Inventory.

OSHA PEL: (Transitional: TWA Respirable Fraction: 10 mg/m^3/2(%SiO$_2$+2); Total Dust: 30 mg/m^3/2(%SiO$_2$+2)) TWA Respirable Fraction: 0.1 mg/m^3 ACGIH TLV: TWA Respirable Fraction: 0.1 mg/m^3 DFG MAK: 0.15 mg/m^3 NIOSH REL: TWA 50 μg/m^3; 3000000 fibers/m^3

SAFETY PROFILE: Confirmed carcinogen with experimental carcinogenic, tumorigenic, and neoplastigenic data. Experimental poison by intratracheal and intravenous routes. Human systemic effects by inhalation: cough, dyspnea, liver effects.

SCK000   CAS: 15468-32-3
SILICA, CRYSTALLINE-TRIDYMITE
mf: O$_2$Si   mw: 60.09

PROP: White or colorless platelets or orthorhombic (crystals) formed from quartz @ temperatures >870° (NTIS** PB246-697).

SYNS: TRIDIMITE (FRENCH) ◇ TRIDYMITE

TOXICITY DATA with REFERENCE
ETA: ipl-rat TDLo: 100 mg/kg   BJCAAI 41,908,80
ETA: itr-mus TDLo: 400 mg/kg   PAACA3 15,6,74

CONSENSUS REPORTS: IARC Cancer Review: Animal Sufficient Evidence IMEMDT 42,209,88; Human Limited Evidence IMEMDT 42,209,88.

OSHA PEL: (Transitional: TWA Respirable: 10 mg/m^3/2(%SiO$_2$+2); Total Dust: TWA 30

mg/m^3/2(%SiO$_2$+2))   TWA   0.05   mg/m^3 ACGIH TLV: TWA Respirable Fraction: 0.05 mg/m^3 DFG MAK: 0.15 mg/m^3 NIOSH REL: TWA 50 μg/m^3

SAFETY PROFILE: Confirmed carcinogen with experimental tumorigenic data. Poison by intratracheal route. Human systemic effects by inhalation: cough, dyspnea. About twice as toxic as silica in causing silicosis.

SCK600   CAS: 60676-86-0
SILICA, FUSED
mf: O$_2$Si   mw: 60.09

PROP: Made up of spherical submicroscopic particles under 0.1 micron in size (AMIHBC 9,389,54).

SYNS: AMORPHOUS FUSED SILICA ◇ FUSED QUARTZ ◇ FUSED SILICA (ACGIH) ◇ QUARTZ GLASS ◇ SILICA, AMORPHOUS FUSED ◇ SILICA, VITREOUS ◇ SILICON DIOXIDE ◇ VITREOUS QUARTZ

CONSENSUS REPORTS: IARC Cancer Review: Animal Sufficient Evidence IMEMDT 42,209,88; GROUP 2A IMEMDT 7,341,87; Human Limited Evidence IMEMDT 42,209,88. Reported in EPA TSCA Inventory.

OSHA PEL: (Transitional: TWA Respirable: 10 mg/m^3/2(%SiO$_2$+2); Total Dust: TWA 30 mg/m^3/2(%SiO$_2$+2))   TWA   0.1   mg/m^3 ACGIH TLV: TWA Respirable Fraction: 0.1 mg/m^3

SAFETY PROFILE: Confirmed carcinogen. Poison by intraperitoneal, intravenous and intratracheal routes.

SDW000
SILVER PEROXYCHROMATE
mf: AgCrO$_5$ mw: 239.87

CONSENSUS REPORTS: Silver and its compounds, as well as chromium and its compounds, are on the Community Right-To-Know List.

SAFETY PROFILE: Confirmed carcinogen. An oxidant. When mixed with H$_2$SO$_4$ @ −80° it explodes on slow warming to −30°.

SEC000
SMOKE CONDENSATE, CIGARETTE

SYNS: CIGARETTE SMOKE CONDENSATE ◇ CSC ◇ TOBACCO SMOKE CONDENSATE ◇ TOBACCO TAR

TOXICITY DATA with REFERENCE

CAR: skn-mus TD:408 g/kg/2Y-I BJCAAI 38,250,78

CAR: skn-mus TD:499 g/kg/2Y-I TXCYAC 23,177,82

CAR: skn-mus TD:624 g/kg/2Y-I TXCYAC 23,177,82

CAR: skn-mus TDLo:374 g/kg/2Y-I TXCYAC 23,177,82

NEO: ihl-rat TCLo:360 g/kg/2Y-I JJIND8 64,383,80

NEO: skn-mus TD:656 g/kg/82W-I JNCIAM 47,235,71

NEO: skn-mus TD:656 mg/kg/82W-I JNCIAM 47,235,71

NEO: skn-mus TD:1450 g/kg/26W-I CNREA8 28,2363,68

ETA: scu-rat TDLo:160 mg/kg/64W-I ARZNAD 18,814,68

ETA: skn-mus TD:168 g/kg/56W-I BJCAAI 21,56,67

ETA: skn-mus TD:282 g/kg/47W-I PEXTAR 26,128,83

ETA: skn-mus TD:326 g/kg/68W-I NATUAS 194089,62

ETA: skn-mus TD:336 g/kg/56W-I BJCAAI 21,56,67

MUT: bfa-hmn/sat 44 cigarettes/D PNASA6 74,3555,77

MUT: dni-hmn:fbr 10 mg/L LIFSAK 17,767,75

MUT: mma-sat 300 μg/plate ENMUDM 7,471,85

MUT: mmo-esc 10 g/L MUREAV 130,97,84

MUT: sce-hmn-ihl 10 cigarettes/D HEREAY 88,147,78

MUT: sce-hmn:lym 10 mg/L CRNGDP 4,227,83

CONSENSUS REPORTS: IARC Cancer Review: Human Sufficient Evidence IMEMDT 38,309,86, Animal Sufficient Evidence IMEMDT 38,309,86.

SAFETY PROFILE: Confirmed carcinogen with experimental carcinogenic, neoplastigenic, and tumorigenic data. Experimental reproductive effects. Human mutation data reported.

SED400
SMOKELESS TOBACCO

PROP: A variety of habituating substances containing tobacco as the major ingredient and used without burning. Tobacco is a product of the leaves and stems of two species of Nicotiana, *N. Tabacum* (grown in North America and Western Europe) and *N. Rustica* (grown in the USSR and India). There is considerable evidence that many if not all of the forms of smokeless tobacco are human carcinogens.

The smokeless tobaccos are introduced into the body through the mouth (chewing tobacco, snuff, misshri, gudakhu, shammah, khaini, nass, naswar or in combination with betel quid) or nose (snuff).

The various smokeless tobacco products are:

Chewing Tobacco is placed between the cheek and gum and chewed slowly. There are 3 main types: plug, twist/roll, and loose-leaf.

Fine-Cut Tobacco was formerly classified in the United States as chewing tobacco and is now placed in the category of moist fine-cut snuff.

Gudakhu is a paste of powdered tobacco, molasses and other ingredients used in parts of India to clean teeth.

Khaini is a mixture of tobacco and lime formed into a ball and placed in the mouth.

Kiwam is made from processed tobacco leaves. After the stalks and stems are removed, the leaves are soaked and boiled in water with flavorings and spices, crushed, then strained, leaving a paste which is chewed.

Loose-Leaf Tobacco is prepared from fermented cigar leaves, sweetened with sugars, syrups, liquors, and other flavoring materials. It is packaged as batches of loose pieces or cut strips.

Mainpuri Tobacco is a chewed mixture of tobacco with slaked lime, areca nut, camphor, and cloves. It is used in India.

Mishri is prepared from roasted or half-burnt tobacco which has been baked till black on a hot metal plate and then powdered. It is used primarily to clean teeth but is also used as chewing tobacco. Synonyms are masheri and misheri.

Nass is a mixture of tobacco, lime, wood-ash, and cottonseed oil, chewed in Iran and the central Asian region of the USSR.

Naswar is a mixture of powdered tobacco, slaked lime, and indigo placed on the bottom of the mouth or behind the lower lip. It is used in Afghanistan and Pakistan.

Pattiwala Tobacco is a sun-cured tobacco leaf chewed with or without lime. It is used in India.

Pill is dried and pelleted Kiwam paste.

Plug Tobacco is made from enriched to

bacco leaves or leaf fragments wrapped in fine tobacco and pressed into flat bars or rolls. It is chewed.

Shammah is a mixture of powdered tobacco leaves with calcium or sodium carbonate and other materials, including ash, placed in the cheek or behind the lower lip. It is used in southern Saudi Arabia.

Snuff is taken through the mouth or the nose. Moist snuff is finely cut tobacco plus flavorings with a moisture content of up to 50 percent. It is placed in the cheek. Dry snuff has a moisture content of less than 10 percent and may have flavorings. It may be sniffed through the nose, placed behind the lower lip or in the cheek. Oriental snuff is about 50 percent heated calcium carbonate and calcium phosphate with some powdered cuttle-fish bone. In southern Africa, snuff is made from powdered tobacco leaves, plant ash, and sometimes oils, lemon juice, and herbs. In the United States, ''dipping'', refers to the ingestion use of snuff.

Twist/Roll Tobacco is stripped tobacco leaves rolled or twisted like a length of rope.

Zarda is tobacco leaf broken into small pieces and boiled in water with lime and spices to dryness and then colored with vegetable dyes. It is usually chewed mixed with areca nut and spices.

SYNS: CHEWING TOBACCO ◇ GUDAKHU (INDIA) ◇ KHAINI (INDIA) ◇ KIWAM (INDIA) ◇ MASHERI (INDIA) ◇ MISHERI (INDIA) ◇ MISHRI (INDIA) ◇ NASS (IRAN) ◇ NASWAR (PAKISTAN and AFGHANISTAN) ◇ PILLS (INDIA) ◇ SHAMMAH (SAUDI ARABIA) ◇ SNUFF ◇ ZARDA (INDIA)

SAFETY PROFILE: Tobaccos contain from 0.5-5% alkaloids predominantly as l-nicotine (>85%). Nicotine is strongly addictive and is the chief cause of tobacco dependence. It is a mild stimulant. It readily forms salts with most acids. These salts are poorly absorbed through the mucous membranes whereas the base is easily absorbed. This explains the practice of combining lime or other alkali in conjunction with ingestion tobacco use. Nicotine and some of the other tobacco alkaloids are experimental teratogens and mutagens.

There are several known classes of carcinogens present in the smokeless tobaccos: N-nitrosamines, polynuclear aromatic hydrocarbons (PAH's), heavy metals (arsenic trioxide, lead, cadmium and nickel compounds), and radionuclides (^{226}Ra, ^{210}Pb and ^{210}Po). Of these, nitro-

samines are present in the highest concentration (in the range of mg/kg). The concentrations of the nitrosamines are 100 times higher in tobacco than in other consumer products. Nitrosamine concentrations are higher in chewing tobacco than in cigarette smoke. The major nitrosamines in tobacco are N'-nitrososonornicotine (NNN), 4-(methylnitrosamine)-1-(3-pyridyl)-1-butanone (NNK) and N'-nitrosoanatabine (NAT). They are probably generated during curing, fermentation and aging of the tobacco leaf from the tobacco alkaloids: nicotine, nornicotine, anatabine, anabasine, continine, myosmine, 2,3'-dipyridyl and N'-formyl-nornicotine. They may also form in the mouth.

There is sufficient evidence that the ingestion use of snuff, chewing tobacco, and tobacco mixed with lime is carcinogenic to humans. Evidence suggests that the ingestion use of other smokeless tobacco preparations and the nasal use of snuff is carcinogenic to humans. Oral precancerous lesions are commonly observed in smokeless tobacco users.

SEY500   CAS: 7784-46-5
SODIUM ARSENITE
mf: AsO$_2$•Na   mw: 129.91
DOT: 1686/2027

PROP: White or grayish white powder. Commercially: 95%-98% pure. Very sol in water; sltly sol in alc.

SYNS: ARSENENOUS ACID, SODIUM SALT (9CI) ◇ ARSENIOUS ACID, SODIUM SALT ◇ ARSENITE de SODIUM (FRENCH) ◇ ATLAS ''A'' ◇ CHEM PELS C ◇ CHEM-SEN 56 ◇ KILL-ALL ◇ PENITE ◇ PRODALUMNOL ◇ PRODALUMNOL DOUBLE ◇ SODANIT ◇ SODIUM ARSENITE, liquid (solution) (DOT) ◇ SODIUM ARSENITE, solid (DOT) ◇ SODIUM METAARSENITE

TOXICITY DATA with REFERENCE
MUT: cyt-hmn:fbr 1 nmol/L   AEMBAP 91,117,78
MUT: cyt-hmn:leu 1 nmol/L   AEMBAP 91,117,78
MUT: cyt-hmn:lym 1 mg/L   ENMUDM 3,597,81
MUT: dnr-esc 63 μg/well   ENMUDM 3,429,81
MUT: mmo-smc 100 mmol/L   MUREAV 117,149,83
MUT: oms-hmn:lym 700 nmol/L   SWEHDO 7,277,81
MUT: sce-ham:emb 800 nmol   CRNGDP 6,1421,85
MUT: sce-ham:fbr 1 mg/L   MUREAV 104,141,82
MUT: sce-hmn:leu 100 μg/L   ENMUDM 3,597,81
MUT: sce-hmn:lym 3900 nmol/L   SWEHDO 7,277,81

CONSENSUS REPORTS: IARC Cancer Review: Animal Inadequate Evidence IMEMDT

23,39,80; Human Sufficient Evidence IMEMDT 23,39,80; Animal No Evidence IMEMDT 2,48,73. Arsenic and its compounds are on the Community Right To Know List. Reported in EPA TSCA Inventory. EPA Genetic Toxicology Program. EPA Extremely Hazardous Substances List.

OSHA PEL: TWA 0.01 mg(As)/m^3 ACGIH TLV: TWA 0.2 mg(As)/m^3 NIOSH REL: CL (Inorganic Arsenic) 0.002 mg(As)/m^3/15M DOT Classification: Poison B; Label: Poison

SAFETY PROFILE: Confirmed human carcinogen. Human poison by ingestion. Experimental poison by ingestion, skin contact, intravenous, intramuscular, and intraperitoneal routes. An experimental teratogen. Experimental reproductive effects. Human mutation data reported. Used as a herbicide and pesticide. When heated to decomposition it emits toxic fumes of As and Na$_2$O.

SEZ000 CAS: 7784-46-5
SODIUM ARSENITE (liquid)

CONSENSUS REPORTS: Arsenic and its compounds are on the Community Right To Know List. Reported in EPA TSCA Inventory. NIOSH REL: CL 2 μg/m^3/15M DOT Classification: Poison B; Label: Poison.

SAFETY PROFILE: Confirmed human carcinogen. A deadly poison. When heated to decomposition it emits toxic fumes of As and Na$_2$O.

SFB500 CAS: 63915-76-4
SODIUM BERYLLIUM MALATE
mf: C$_8$H$_6$Be$_4$Na$_2$O$_{12}$•7H$_2$O mw: 502.30

CONSENSUS REPORTS: Beryllium and its compounds are on the Community Right To Know List.

OSHA PEL: (Transitional: TWA 0.002 mg(Be)/m^3; CL 0.005; Pk 0.025/30M/8H) TWA 0.002 mg(Be)/m^3; STEL 0.005 mg(Be)/m^3/30M; CL 0.025 mg(Be)/m^3 ACGIH TLV: TWA 0.002 mg(Be)/m^3, Suspected Carcinogen NIOSH REL: CL (Beryllium) not to exceed 0.0005 mg(Be)/m^3

SAFETY PROFILE: Confirmed carcinogen. Poison by intravenous route. When heated to decomposition it emits toxic fumes of BeO and Na$_2$O.

SFC000 CAS: 63915-77-5
SODIUM BERYLLIUM TARTRATE
mf: C$_8$H$_4$Be$_4$Na$_2$O$_{13}$•10H$_2$O mw: 570.34

CONSENSUS REPORTS: Beryllium and its compounds are on the Community Right To Know List.

OSHA PEL: (Transitional: TWA 0.002 mg(Be)/m^3; CL 0.005; Pk 0.025/30M/8H) TWA 0.002 mg(Be)/m^3; STEL 0.005 mg(Be)/m^3/30M; CL 0.025 mg(Be)/m^3 ACGIH TLV: TWA 0.002 mg(Be)/m^3, Suspected Carcinogen NIOSH REL: CL (Beryllium) not to exceed 0.0005 mg(Be)/m^3

SAFETY PROFILE: Confirmed carcinogen. Poison by subcutaneous and intravenous routes. When heated to decomposition it emits toxic fumes of BeO and Na$_2$O.

SFW500 CAS: 13517-17-4
SODIUM CHROMATE DECAHYDRATE
mf: CrO$_4$2Na•10H$_2$O mw: 342.18

SYN: CHROMIC ACID, DISODIUM SALT, DECAHYDRATE

CONSENSUS REPORTS: Chromium and its compounds are on the Community Right To Know List.

OSHA PEL: CL 0.1 mg(CrO$_3$)/m^3 ACGIH TLV: TWA 0.05 mg(Cr)/m^3 NIOSH REL: TWA 0.025 mg(Cr(VI))/m^3; CL 0.05 mg/m^3/15M

SAFETY PROFILE: Confirmed human carcinogen. When heated to decomposition it emits toxic fumes of Na$_2$O.

SGI000 CAS: 10588-01-9
SODIUM DICHROMATE
DOT: 1479
mf: Cr$_2$O$_7$•2Na mw: 261.98

PROP: Anhydrous. Mp: 356.7°, decomp @ about 400°, d: 2.35 @ 13°. Very sol in water.

SYNS: BICHROMATE de SODIUM (FRENCH) ◊ BICHROMATE of SODA ◊ CHROMIC ACID, DISODIUM SALT ◊ CHROMIUM SODIUM OXIDE ◊ DISODIUM DICHROMATE ◊ NATRIUMBICHROMAAT (DUTCH) ◊ NATRIUMDICHROMAAT (DUTCH) ◊ NATRIUMDICHROMAT (GERMAN) ◊ SODIO (DICROMATO di) (ITALIAN) ◊ SODIUM BICHROMATE ◊ SODIUM CHROMATE ◊ SODIUM DICHROMATE(VI) ◊ SODIUM DICHROMATE de (FRENCH)

TOXICITY DATA with REFERENCE
ETA: ihl-rat TCLo: 252 μg/m^3/78W-I TXCYAC 42,219,86
ETA: ipl-rat TDLo: 160 mg/kg/69W-I AEHLAU 5,445,62

MUT: cyt-hmn: lym 2 μmol/L   CARYAB 33,239,80
MUT: dnd-rat-ipr 20 mg/kg   JBCHA3 256,3623,81
MUT: dnd-rat: lvr 3 mmol/L   SinJF# 26OCT82
MUT: mma-sat 30 μg/plate   PCBRD2 109,453,82
MUT: sce-ham: lng 35 μg/L   CRNGDP 4,605,83
MUT: slt-dmg-orl 2340 μmol/L   MUREAV
   157,157,85

CONSENSUS REPORTS: IARC Cancer Review: GROUP 1 IMEMDT 7,165,87; Animal Inadequate Evidence IMEMDT 2,100,73; IMEMDT 23,205,80; Human Inadequate Evidence IMEMDT 23,205,80. Chromium and its compounds are on the Community Right To Know List. Reported in EPA TSCA Inventory. EPA Genetic Toxicology Program.

OSHA PEL: CL 0.1 mg/(CrO$_3$)/m^3 ACGIH TLV: TWA 0.05 mg(Cr)/m^3 NIOSH REL: TWA 0.025 mg(Cr(VI))/M^3; CL 0.05 mg/M^3/ 15M   DOT Classification: ORM-A; Label: None

SAFETY PROFILE: Confirmed carcinogen with experimental tumorigenic data. Poison by ingestion, skin contact, intravenous, intraperitoneal, and subcutaneous routes. Human systemic effects by ingestion: cough, nausea or vomiting, and sweating. Human mutation data reported. A caustic and irritant. A powerful oxidizer. When heated to decomposition it emits toxic fumes of Na$_2$O.

SID000   CAS: 57-30-7
SODIUM LUMINAL
mf: C$_{12}$H$_{11}$N$_2$O$_3$•Na   mw: 254.24
PROP: White crystals.
SYNS: 5-ETHYL-5-PHENYLBARBITURIC ACID SODIUM ◇ 5-ETHYL-5-PHENYLBARBITURIC ACID SODIUM SALT ◇ 5-ETHYL-5-PHENYL-2,4,6-(1H,3H,5H)PYRIMIDINE-TRIONE MONOSODIUM SALT ◇ GARDENAL SODIUM ◇ LUMINAL SODIUM ◇ PBS ◇ PHENEMALUM ◇ PHENOBAL SODIUM ◇ PHENOBARBITAL ELIXIR ◇ PHENOBARBITAL Na ◇ PHENOBARBITAL SODIUM ◇ PHENOBARBITAL SODIUM SALT ◇ PHENOBARBITONE SODIUM ◇ PHENOBARBITONE SODIUM SALT ◇ PHENYLETHYLBARBITURIC ACID, SODIUM SALT ◇ SODIUM 5-ETHYL-5-PHENYLBARBITURATE ◇ SODIUM PHENOBARBITAL ◇ SODIUM PHENOBARBITONE ◇ SODIUM PHENYLETHYLBARBITURATE ◇ SODIUM PHENYLETHYLMALONYLUREA ◇ SOL PHENOBARBITAL ◇ SOL PHENOBARBITONE ◇ SOLUBLE PHENOBARBITAL ◇ SOLUBLE PHENOBARBITONE

TOXICITY DATA with REFERENCE
NEO: orl-rat TDLo: 25 g/kg/2Y-C   IJCNAW
   19,179,77

ETA: orl-rat TD: 11650 mg/kg/33W-C   JJIND8
   71,815,83
MUT: dni-mus-ipr 20 g/kg   ARGEAR 51,605,81
MUT: dnr-esc 400 μg/well   ENMUDM 3,429,81
MUT: msc-mus: lym 5 mmol/L   MUREAV
   110,147,83

CONSENSUS REPORTS: IARC Cancer Review: Animal Sufficient Evidence IMEMDT 13,157,77. EPA Genetic Toxicology Program.

SAFETY PROFILE: Confirmed carcinogen with experimental carcinogenic, neoplastigenic, tumorigenic, and teratogenic data. Poison by ingestion, intravenous, intraperitoneal, intraduodenal, and subcutaneous routes. Human systemic effects by ingestion: nausea or vomiting and coma. Experimental reproductive effects. Mutation data reported. Used to treat epilepsy, as an hypnotic and sedative. When heated to decomposition it emits toxic fumes of NO$_x$ and Na$_2$O.

SKF000   CAS: 12206-14-3
SODIUM TETRAPEROXYCHROMATE
mf: CrNa$_3$O$_8$ mw: 248.97

CONSENSUS REPORTS: Chromium and its compounds are on the Community Right To Know List.

OSHA PEL: CL 0.1 mg(CrO$_3$)/m^3 ACGIH TLV: TWA 0.05 mg(Cr)/m^3 NIOSH REL: TWA 0.025 mg(Cr(VI))/m^3; CL 0.05 mg/m^3/ 15M

SAFETY PROFILE: Confirmed human carcinogen. Explodes when heated to 115°C. When heated to decomposition it emits toxic fumes of Na$_2$O.

SKS750
SOOT

PROP: Soot is defined as a brown-to-black substance incidentally produced during the incomplete and uncontrolled combustion of any carbonaceous material. It is a mixture of colloidal carbon, organic tars and refractory inorganics whose composition depends on combustion conditions. It is not unusual for the tarry component to account for more than 50 wt% of the soot, particularly, when produced by inefficient combustion of coal or wood. Can be distinguished from carbon black on the basis of differences in physical and chemical properties.

SAFETY PROFILE: Confirmed human carcinogen producing skin, scrotum, or lung tumors.

The tarry component and, to a lesser extent, trace inorganic impurities, are believed responsible for the known health hazards attributed to soot, i.e., chronic contact or long-term inhalation can lead to cancer.

SMD000 CAS: 18883-66-4
STREPTOZOTICIN
mf: $C_8H_{15}N_3O_7$ mw: 265.26

PROP: Plateletes. Mp: 115° (decomp).

SYNS: 2-DEOXY-2-(((METHYLNITROSOAMINO)CARBONYL)AMINO)-d-GLU-COPYRANOSE ◇ 2-DEOXY-2-(3-METHYL-3-NITROSO-UREIDO)-d-GLUCOPYRANOSE ◇ 2-DEOXY-2-(3-METHYL-3-NITROSOUREIDO)-α(and β)-d-GLUCOPYRANOSE ◇ N-d-GLUCOSYL(2)-N′-NITROSOMETHYLHARNSTOFF (GERMAN) ◇ N-d-GLUCOSYL-(2)-N′-NITROSOMETHYL-UREA ◇ NCI-C03167 ◇ NSC 85598 ◇ NSC-85998 ◇ RCRA WASTE NUMBER U206 ◇ STR ◇ STREPTOZOCIN ◇ STRZ ◇ STZ ◇ U-9889 ◇ ZANOSAR

TOXICITY DATA with REFERENCE
CAR: ivn-mus TDLo: 250 mg/kg   CNREA8 45,703,85
NEO: ipr-mus TDLo: 470 mg/kg/26W-I   RRCRBU 52,1,75
NEO: ipr-rat TDLo: 470 mg/kg/26W-I   RRCRBU 52,1,75
NEO: ivn-rat TD: 30 mg/kg   CNREA8 38,2144,78
NEO: ivn-rat TD: 30 mg/kg   NNGZAZ 54,1070,78
NEO: ivn-rat TD: 50 mg/kg   CNCRA6 52,563,68
NEO: ivn-rat TD: 50 mg/kg   PSEBAA 151,356,76
NEO: ivn-rat TDLo: 25 mg/kg   BJCAAI 36,692,7
ETA: ipr-ham TDLo: 100 mg/kg/I   JNCIAM 51,1287,73
ETA: ivn-rat TD: 50 mg/kg   CCROBU 59,891,75
ETA: ivn-rat TD: 65 mg/kg   EXPEAM 38,129,82
ETA: ivn-rat TD: 65 mg/kg   GANNA2 68,397,77
ETA: ivn-rat TD: 65 mg/kg   NNGZAZ 54,1290,78
ETA: ivn-rat TD: 65 mg/kg   TRPLAU 24,152,77
MUT: cyt-hmn: lng 500 mg/L   MUREAV 12,183,71
MUT: dni-hmn: lng 1 g/L/3H-C   MUREAV 12,183,71
MUT: dnr-bcs 2500 ng/plate   TAKHAA 44,96,85
MUT: dns-rat-ipr 250 mg/kg   ENMUDM 7,889,85
MUT: dns-rat: lvr 50 μmol/L   ENMUDM 3,11,81
MUT: mmo-esc 20 ng/plate   TAKHAA 44,96,85
MUT: mmo-sat 20 ng/plate   TAKHAA 44,96,85
MUT: msc-ham: lng 500 μmol/L   CNREA8 40,2719,80
MUT: msc-mus: lym 10 mg/L   MUREAV 125,291,84

CONSENSUS REPORTS: IARC Cancer Review: Human Limited Evidence IMEMDT 17,337,78; Animal Sufficient Evidence IMEMDT 17,337,78. NTP Fourth Annual Report On Carcinogens, 1984. NCI Carcinogenesis Studies (ipr); Clear Evidence: mouse, rat RRCRBU 52,1,75. EPA Genetic Toxicology Program.

SAFETY PROFILE: Confirmed carcinogen with experimental carcinogenic, neoplastigenic, tumorigenic, and teratogenic data. Experimental poison by ingestion, intravenous, parenteral, subcutaneous, and intraperitoneal routes. Moderately toxic to humans by intravenous route. Human systemic effects by ingestion and intravenous routes: nausea or vomiting, impaired liver function and kidney changes. Human mutation data reported. Experimental reproductive effects. When heated to decomposition it emits toxic fumes of NO_x.

SME500 CAS: 91724-16-2
STRONTIUM ARSENITE
DOT: 1691
mf: As_2O_4Sr mw: 301.46

PROP: White powder.

SYNS: ARSENIOUS ACID, STRONTIUM SALT ◇ STRONTIUM ARSENITE, SOLID (DOT)

CONSENSUS REPORTS: Arsenic and its compounds are on the Community Right To Know List.

OSHA PEL: TWA 0.01 mg(As)/m³; Cancer Hazard   NIOSH REL: CL 0.002 mg(As)/m³/ 15M   DOT Classification: Poison B; Label: Poison

SAFETY PROFILE: Confirmed human carcinogen. A deadly poison. When heated to decomposition it emits toxic fumes of As.

SMH000 CAS: 7789-06-2
STRONTIUM CHROMATE (1:1)
DOT: 9149
mf: $CrO_4 \cdot Sr$ mw: 203.62

PROP: Monoclinic, yellow crystals. D: 3.895 @ 15°.

SYNS: CHROMIC ACID, STRONTIUM SALT (1:1) ◇ C.I. PIGMENT YELLOW 32 ◇ DEEP LEMON YELLOW ◇ STRONTIUM CHROMATE (VI) ◇ STRONTIUM CHROMATE 12170 ◇ STRONTIUM YELLOW

TOXICITY DATA with REFERENCE
ETA: imp-rat TDLo: 125 mg/kg   AIHAAP 20,274,59

ETA: itr-rat TDLo:40 mg/kg/34W-I   AEHLAU
  5,445,62

MUT: mmo-sat 800 ng/plate   MUREAV 156,219,85
MUT: sce-ham:ovr 100 μg/L   MUREAV 156,219,85

CONSENSUS REPORTS: IARC Cancer Review: Animal Sufficient Evidence IMEMDT 2,100,73; IMEMDT 23,205,80; Human Sufficient Evidence IMEMDT 23,205,80. NTP Fourth Annual Report On Carcinogens, 1984. Chromium and its compounds are on the Community Right To Know List. Reported in EPA TSCA Inventory.

OSHA PEL: CL 0.1 mg(CrO_3)/m^3 ACGIH TLV: TWA 0.05 mg(Cr)/m^3; Confirmed Human Carcinogen; (Proposed: TWA 0.001 mg(Cr)/m^3; Suspected Human Carcinogen) DFG TRK: 0.1 mg/m^3; Animal Carcinogen, Suspected Human Carcinogen. NIOSH REL: TWA 0.0001 mg(Cr(VI))/m^3 DOT Classification: ORM-E; Label: None

SAFETY PROFILE: Confirmed human carcinogen with experimental carcinogenic and tumorigenic data. Moderately toxic by ingestion. Mutation data reported.

SOP500   CAS: 140-57-8
SULFUROUS ACID, 2-(p-tert-BUTYLPHENOXY)-1-METHYLETHYL-2-CHLOROETHYL ESTER
mf: $C_{15}H_{23}ClO_4S$ mw: 334.89

PROP: Liquid. D: 1.145-1.1620, mp: −31.7°, bp: 175° @ 0.1 mm, vap press: <10 mm @ 25°. Misc with many organic solvents; insol in water.

SYNS: ACARACIDE ◇ ARACIDE ◇ ARAMITE ◇ ARAMI-TEARARAMITE-15W ◇ ARATRON ◇ BUTYLPHENOXYISO-PROPYL CHLOROETHYL SULFITE ◇ 2-(p-BUTYLPHE-NOXY)ISOPROPYL 2-CHLOROETHYL SULFITE ◇ 2-(p-tert-BUTYLPHENOXY)ISOPROPYL 2′-CHLOROETHYL SUL-PHITE ◇ 2-(p-BUTYLPHENOXY)-1-METHYLETHYL 2-CHLO-ROETHYL SULFITE ◇ 2-(p-tert-BUTYLPHENOXY)-1-METH-YLETHYL 2-CHLOROETHYL ESTER of SULPHUROUS ACID ◇ 2-(p-tert-BUTYLPHENOXY)-1-METHYLETHYL-2-CHLORO-ETHYL SULFITE ESTER ◇ 2-(4-tert-BUTYLPHENOXY)ISO-PROPYL-2-CHLOROETHYL SULFITE ◇ 2-(p-tert-BUTYLPHE-NOXY)-1-METHYLETHYL 2′-CHLOROETHYL SULPHITE ◇ 2-(p-tert-BUTYLPHENOXY)-1-METHYLETHYL SULPHITE of 2-CHLOROETHANOL ◇ 1-(p-t-BUTYLPHENOXY)-2-PRO-PANOL-2-CHLOROETHYL SULFITE ◇ CES ◇ 2-CHLORO-ETHANOL-2-(p-t-BUTYLPHENOXY)-1-METHYLETHYL SUL-FITE ◇ 2-CHLOROETHANOL ESTER with 2-(p-t-BUTYL-PHENOXY)-1-METHYLETHYL SULFITE ◇ β-CHLORO-ETHYL-β′-(p-tert-BUTYLPHENOXY)-α′- METHYLETHYL SULFITE ◇ β-CHLOROETHYL-β-(p-tert-BUTYLPHEN-OXY)-α-METHYLETHYL SULPHITE ◇ 2-CHLOROETHYL 1-METHYL-2-(p-tert-BUTYLPHENOXY)ETHYL SUL-PHATE ◇ 2-CHLOROETHYL SULFUROUS ACID-2-(4-(1,1-DI-METHYLETHYL)PHENOXY)-1-METHYLETHYL ESTER ◇ 2-CHLOROETHYL SULPHITE of 1-(p-tert-BUTYLPHE-NOXY)-2-PROPANOL ◇ COMPOUND 88R ◇ ENT 16,519 ◇ NIAGARAMITE ◇ ORTHO-MITE ◇ 88-R

TOXICITY DATA with REFERENCE
CAR: orl-mus TDLo:130 g/kg/80W-C   JNCIAM
  42,1101,69
CAR: orl-rat TDLo:21900 mg/kg/2Y-C
  TXAPA9 2,441,60
NEO: orl-rat TDLo:15 g/kg/2Y-C   CANCAR
  13,1035,60
ETA: orl-dog TDLo:20 g/kg/2Y-C   CANCAR
  13,780,60
ETA: orl-rat TD:8100 mg/kg/2Y-C   TXAPA9
  11,88,67

CONSENSUS REPORTS: IARC Cancer Review: Animal Sufficient Evidence IMEMDT 5,39,74. NTP Fourth Annual Report On Carcinogens, 1984.

SAFETY PROFILE: Confirmed carcinogen with experimental carcinogenic, neoplastigenic, and tumorigenic data. Experimental poison by intraperitoneal route. Moderately toxic to humans by ingestion. Moderately toxic experimentally by ingestion. Experimental reproductive effects. A pesticide and a chlorinated hydrocarbons. When heated to decomposition it emits toxic fumes of Cl^- and SO_x.

TAB775   CAS: 14807-96-6
TALC, containing asbestos fibers
mf: H_2O_2Si•3/4Mg   mw: 96.33

TOXICITY DATA with REFERENCE
ETA: ipr-rat TDLo:200 mg/kg   JJIND8 67,965,81

CONSENSUS REPORTS: IARC Cancer Review: Human Sufficient Evidence IMEMDT 42,185,87; Reported in EPA TSCA Inventory.

ACGIH TLV: Human Carcinogen; TWA > 2 mg/m^3, Respirable Dust

SAFETY PROFILE: Confirmed human carcinogen with experimental tumorigenic data.

TAI000   CAS: 1746-01-6
TCDD
mf: $C_{12}H_4Cl_4O_2$ mw: 321.96

PROP: Colorless needles. Mp: 305°.

SYNS: 2,3,7,8-CZTEROCHLORODWUBENZO-p-DWUOK-SYNY (POLISH) ◇ DIOKSYNY (POLISH) ◇ DIOXINE ◇ DIOXIN (herbicide contaminant) ◇ NCI-C03714 ◇ TCDBD ◇ 2,3,7,8-TCDD ◇ 2,3,7,8-TETRACHLORODIBEN-ZO(b,e)(1,4)DIOXAN ◇ 2,3,6,7-TETRACHLORODIBENZO-p-DIOXIN ◇ 2,3,7,8-TETRACHLORODIBENZO-p-DIOXIN ◇ 2,3,7,8-TETRACHLORODIBENZO-1,4-DIOXIN ◇ TETRA-DIOXIN

TOXICITY DATA with REFERENCE

CAR: orl-mus TDLo: 52 μg/kg/2Y-I
  NTPTR* NTP-TR-209,82

CAR: orl-rat TD: 73 μg/kg/2Y-C   ANYAA9
  320,397,78

CAR: orl-rat TDLo: 52 μg/kg/2Y-I
  NTPTR* NTP-TR-209,82

CAR: skn-mus TDLo: 62 μg/kg/2Y-I
  NCITR* NCI-CG-TR-201,82

NEO: orl-mus TD: 36 μg/kg/52W-I   NATUAS
  278,548,79

ETA: orl-mus TD: 1 μg/kg/2Y-I
  NTPTR* NTP-TR-209,82

ETA: orl-rat TD: 1 μg/kg/2Y-I
  NTPTR* NTP-TR-209,82

ETA: orl-rat TD: 27 μg/kg/65W-C   FEPRA7
  36,396,77

ETA: orl-rat TD: 137 μg/kg/65W-C   FEPRA7
  36,396,77

ETA: orl-rat TD: 328 μg/kg/78W-C   PESTC*
  5,12,77

ETA: skn-mus TD: 80 μg/kg   BECTA6 18,552,77

MUT: dni-hmn: oth 10 nmol/L   TXAPA9 77,434,85

MUT: hma-mus/smc 25 μg/kg   CMSHAF 12,549,83

MUT: mmo-smc 10 mg/L   CMSHAF 12,549,83

MUT: oms-mus: oth 1 nmol/L   JBCHA3
  259,12357,84

CONSENSUS REPORTS: IARC Cancer Review: Human Inadequate Evidence IMEMDT 15,41,77; Animal Inadequate Evidence IMEMDT 15,41,77. NTP Fourth Annual Report On Carcinogens, 1984. NTP Carcinogenesis Bioassay (gavage); Clear Evidence: mouse, rat NTPTR* NTP-TR-209,82; (dermal). EPA Genetic Toxicology Program.

DFG MAK: Animal Carcinogen, Suspected Human Carcinogen.   NIOSH REL: (Dioxin) Reduce to lowest feasible level.

SAFETY PROFILE: Confirmed carcinogen with experimental carcinogenic, neoplastigenic, tumorigenic, and teratogenic data. One of the most toxic synthetic chemicals. A deadly experimen-

tal poison by ingestion, skin contact, intraperitoneal, and possibly other routes. Human systemic effects by skin contact: allergic dermatitis. Experimental reproductive effects. Human mutation data reported. An eye irritant. When heated to decomposition it emits toxic fumes of Cl^-.

TBF500   CAS: 58-22-0
TESTOSTERONE
mf: $C_{19}H_{28}O_2$ mw: 288.47

PROP: Crystals. Mp: 155°. Insol in water; sol in alc and ether.

SYNS: ANDROLIN ◇ ANDRONAQ ◇ ANDROST-4-EN-17β-OL-3-ONE ◇ Δ⁴-ANDROSTEN-17(β)-OL-3-ONE ◇ ANDRUSOL ◇ CRISTERONE T ◇ GENO-CRISTAUZ GREMY ◇ HOMO-STERONE ◇ 17-β-HYDROXY-Δ⁴-ANDROSTEN-3-ONE ◇ 17-β-HYDROXYANDROST-4-EN-3-ONE ◇ 17-β-HY-DROXY-4-ANDROSTEN-3-ONE ◇ 17-HYDROXY-(17-β)-AND-ROST-4-EN-3-ONE ◇ 7-β-HYDROXYANDROST-4-EN-3-ONE ◇ MALESTRONE (AMPS) ◇ MERTESTATE ◇ NEO-TESTIS ◇ ORETON-F ◇ ORQUISTERONE ◇ PERANDREN ◇ PERCUTACRINE ANDROGENIQUE ◇ PRIMOTEST ◇ PROMOTESTON ◇ SUSTANONE ◇ SYNANDROL F ◇ TESLEN ◇ TESTANDRONE ◇ TESTICULOSTERONE ◇ TESTOBASE ◇ TESTOPROPON ◇ TESTOSTEROID ◇ trans-TESTOSTERONE ◇ TESTOSTERONE HYDRATE ◇ TESTOSTOSTERONE ◇ TESTOVIRON SCHERING ◇ TESTOVIRON T ◇ TESTRONE ◇ TESTRYL ◇ VIRORMONE ◇ VIROSTERONE

TOXICITY DATA with REFERENCE

NEO: imp-mus TDLo: 400 mg/kg/50D-C
  CNREA8 48,2788,88

NEO: orl-mus TDLo: 6240 mg/kg/52D-C
  CNREA8 48,2788,88

NEO: scu-mus TDLo: 30 mg/kg/5D-I: TER
  JNCIAM 39,75,67

MUT: cyt-hmn: kdy 100 μg/L   CNJGA8 10,299,68

MUT: dnd-mam: lvr 1 μmol/L   ENZYAS 41,183,71

MUT: dnd-mam: lym 10 μmol/L   ENZYAS
  41,183,71

MUT: dnd-mus: lvr 100 μmol/L   ENZYAS
  41,183,71

MUT: dni-hmn: kdy 100 μg/L   CNJGA8 10,299,68

MUT: dni-hmn: lym 50 μmol/L   PSEBAA
  146,401,74

MUT: dns-rat-par 10 mg/kg   ACHCBO 18,213,85

MUT: spm-nml-par 12 mg/8W-I   JEZOAO
  205,403,78

CONSENSUS REPORTS: IARC Cancer Review: Animal Sufficient Evidence IMEMDT 6,209,74, IMEMDT 21,519,79; Human Limited Evidence IMEMDT 21,519,79. Reported in EPA TSCA Inventory. EPA Genetic Toxicology Program.

SAFETY PROFILE: Confirmed carcinogen with experimental neoplastigenic and teratogenic data. Poison by intraperitoneal route. Human teratogenic effects by unspecified route: developmental abnormalities of the urogenital system. Experimental reproductive effects. Human mutation data reported. Workers engaged in manufacture and packaging have shown effects from this hormone, i.e., enlargement of the breasts in male workers. A promoter. When heated to decomposition it emits acrid smoke and irritating fumes. Used as a drug for the treatment of hypogonadism and metastatic breast cancer.

TBG000   CAS: 57-85-2
TESTOSTERONE PROPIONATE
mf: $C_{22}H_{32}O_3$ mw: 344.54

SYNS: AGOVIRIN ◇ ANDROGEN ◇ ANDROSAN ◇ Δ^4-ANDROSTENE-17-β-PROPIONATE-3-ONE ◇ ANDROTESTON ◇ ANDROTEST P ◇ ANDRUSOL-P ◇ ANERTAN ◇ AQUAVIRON ◇ BIO-TESTICULINA ◇ ENARMON ◇ HOMANDREN (amps) ◇ HORMOTESTON ◇ MASENATE ◇ NASDOL ◇ NEO-HOMBREOL ◇ NSC 9166 ◇ OKASA-MASCUL ◇ ORCHIOL ◇ ORCHISTIN ◇ ORETON ◇ ORETON PROPIONATE ◇ 17-(1-OXOPROPOXY)-(17-β)-ANDROST-4-EN-3-ONE ◇ PANESTIN ◇ PERANDREN ◇ PROPIOKAN ◇ RECTHORMONE TESTOSTERONE ◇ STERANDRYL ◇ SYNANDROL ◇ SYNERONE ◇ TELIPEX ◇ TESTAFORM ◇ TESTEX ◇ TESTODET ◇ TESTODRIN ◇ TESTOGEN ◇ TESTONIQUE ◇ TESTORMOL ◇ TESTOSTERON PROPIONATE ◇ TESTOSTERONE-17-PROPIONATE ◇ TESTOSTERONE-17-β-PROPIONATE ◇ TESTOVIRON ◇ TESTOXYL ◇ TESTREX ◇ TOSTRIN ◇ TP ◇ UNITESTON ◇ VULVAN

TOXICITY DATA with REFERENCE
NEO: scu-rat TDLo: 10 mg/kg   JSONDX 5,396,84
ETA: imp-ham TDLo: 360 mg/kg   CNREA8 25,141,65
ETA: imp-mus TDLo: 5200 mg/kg/65W-I   NATUAS 192,1303,61
ETA: imp-rat TDLo: 432 mg/kg/48W-C   CNREA8 37,1929,77
MUT: cyt-ofs-unr 500 μg   BEXBBO 15,329,80
MUT: dnd-rat: lvr 300 μmol/L   SinJF# 26OCT82
MUT: spm-ofs-unr 500 μg   BEXBBO 15,329,80
MUT: spm-rat-scu 10 mg/kg   AMTUA3 8,68,71

CONSENSUS REPORTS: IARC Cancer Review: Animal Sufficient Evidence IMEMDT 21,519,79. Reported in EPA TSCA Inventory.

SAFETY PROFILE: Confirmed carcinogen with experimental neoplastigenic, tumorigenic, and teratogenic data. Moderately toxic by ingestion and intraperitoneal routes. Human male reproductive effects by intramuscular and parenteral routes: changes in spermatogenesis, testes, epididymis, and sperm duct. Human female reproductive effects by intramuscular and parenteral routes: menstrual cycle changes or disorders and effects on fertility. Experimental reproductive effects. Mutation data reported. When heated to decomposition it emits acrid smoke and irritating fumes.

TFA000   CAS: 62-55-5
THIOACETAMIDE
mf: C_2H_5NS mw: 75.14

PROP: Colorless leaflets; mercaptan odor. Mp: 113°. Very sol in water; sltly sol in alc and ether.

SYNS: ACETOTHIOAMIDE ◇ ETHANETHIOAMIDE ◇ RCRA WASTE NUMBER U218 ◇ TAA ◇ THIACETAMIDE ◇ USAF CB-21 ◇ USAF EK-1719

TOXICITY DATA with REFERENCE
CAR: orl-rat TDLo: 7350 mg/kg/40W-C   JJIND8 79,1047,87
NEO: orl-mus TDLo: 10 g/kg/39W-C   BJCAAI 24,498,70
ETA: orl-mus TD: 7956 mg/kg/32W-C   JNCIAM 56,493,76
ETA: orl-mus TD: 18360 mg/kg/73W-C   IJCAAR 9,154,72
ETA: orl-rat TD: 1008 mg/kg/9W-C   NATUAS 175,257,55
ETA: orl-rat TD: 1600 mg/kg/12W-C   CNREA8 28,1703,68
ETA: orl-rat TD: 4320 mg/kg/34W-C   ECEBDI 45,34,77
ETA: orl-rat TD: 5140 mg/kg/47W-C: TER   JPBAA7 72,415,56
ETA: orl-rat TD: 6000 mg/kg/43W-C   ONCOBS 38,249,81
ETA: orl-rat TD: 7200 mg/kg/51W-C   ONCOBS 38,249,81
ETA: orl-rat TD: 7665 mg/kg/1Y-C   JJIND8 71,553,83
ETA: orl-rat TD: 9900 mg/kg/71W-C   ONCOBS 38,249,81
MUT: cyt-hmn: fbr 1 g/L   BJCAAI 42,112,80
MUT: cyt-rat-ipr 150 mg/kg   JNCIAM 46,49,71
MUT: dnd-rat-ipr 60 mg/kg   CNREA8 36,4647,76
MUT: hma-mus/sat 125 mg/kg   JJIND8 62,911,79

MUT: mmo-smc 19900 μmol/L   MGGEAE 174,39,79

MUT: mrc-smc 3000 ppm   JJIND8 62,901,79

MUT: otr-rat:emb 30 mg/L   JJIND8 67,1303,81

MUT: sln-dmg-orl 100 ppm/24H   MUREAV 58,259,78

MUT: sln-dmg-par 2500 ppm   MUREAV 58,259,78

CONSENSUS REPORTS: IARC Cancer Review: Animal Sufficient Evidence IMEMDT 7,77,74. NTP Fourth Annual Report On Carcinogens, 1984. EPA Genetic Toxicology Program. Community Right-To-Know List. Reported in EPA TSCA Inventory.

SAFETY PROFILE: Confirmed carcinogen with experimental carcinogenic, neoplastigenic, tumorigenic, and teratogenic data. Poison by ingestion and intraperitoneal routes. Moderately toxic by subcutaneous route. Human mutation data reported. Experimental reproductive effects. Exposure has caused liver damage. When heated to decomposition it emits very toxic fumes of NO_x and SO_x.

TFI000   CAS: 139-65-1
4,4'-THIODIANILINE
mf: $C_{12}H_{12}N_2S$ mw: 216.32

PROP: Needles. Mp: 108°.

SYNS: BIS(p-AMINOPHENYL)SULFIDE ◇ BIS(4-AMINO-PHENYL) SULFIDE ◇ BIS(p-AMINOPHENYL)SULPHIDE ◇ BIS(4-AMINOPHENYL) SULPHIDE ◇ p,p'-DIAMINODIPHE-NYL SULFIDE ◇ 4,4'-DIAMINODIPHENYL SULFIDE ◇ p,p'-DIAMINODIPHENYL SULPHIDE ◇ DI(p-AMINOPHE-NYL) SULFIDE ◇ DI(p-AMINOPHENYL)SULPHIDE ◇ NCI-C01707 ◇ THIOANILINE ◇ 4,4'-THIOANILINE ◇ 4,4'-THIOBIS(ANILINE) ◇ 4,4'-THIOBISBENZENAMINE ◇ p,p-THIODIANILINE ◇ THIODI-p-PHENYLENEDIAMINE

TOXICITY DATA with REFERENCE
CAR: orl-mus TD:328 g/kg/70W-C
    NCITR* NCI-CG-TR-47,78

CAR: orl-mus TD:963 g/kg/77W-I   IARC** 27,147,82

CAR: orl-mus TD:1925 g/kg/77W-I   IARC** 27,147,82

CAR: orl-mus TDLo:113 g/kg/54W-C
    NCITR* NCI-CG-TR-47,78

CAR: orl-rat TD:37 g/kg/70W-C
    NCITR* NCI-CG-TR-47,78

CAR: orl-rat TD:74 g/kg/70W-C
    NCITR* NCI-CG-TR-47,78

CAR: orl-rat TD:510 g/kg/68W-I   IARC** 27,147,82

CAR: orl-rat TD:1020 g/kg/68W-I   IARC** 27,147,82

CAR: orl-rat TDLo:3600 mg/kg/27D-I   CNREA8 28,924,68

ETA: orl-rat TD:1500 mg/kg/30D-I   IARC** 27,147,82

ETA: orl-rat TD:2000 mg/kg/30D-I   IARC** 27,147,82

MUT: mma-sat 10 μg/plate   MUREAV 67,123,79

MUT: mmo-sat 10 μg/plate   MUREAV 67,123,79

CONSENSUS REPORTS: IARC Cancer Review: Human Limited Evidence IMEMDT 27,147,82; Animal Sufficient Evidence IMEMDT 27,147,82; Animal Limited Evidence IMEMDT 16,343,78. NCI Carcinogenesis Bioassay (feed); Clear Evidence: mouse, rat NCITR* NCI-CG-TR-47,78. Reported in EPA TSCA Inventory. Community Right-To-Know List.

DFG MAK: Animal Carcinogen, Suspected Human Carcinogen.

SAFETY PROFILE: Confirmed carcinogen with experimental carcinogenic and tumorigenic data. Poison by intravenous route. Moderately toxic by ingestion. May be a human carcinogenic. Experimental reproductive effects. Mutation data reported. When heated to decomposition it emits very toxic fumes of NO_x and SO_x.

TFQ750   CAS: 52-24-4
THIOTRIETHYLENEPHOSPHORAMIDE
mf: $C_6H_{12}N_3PS$ mw: 189.24

SYNS: CBC 806495 ◇ GIROSTAN ◇ NCI-C01649 ◇ NSC-6396 ◇ ONCOTEPA ◇ ONCOTIOTEPA ◇ 1,1',1''-PHOSPHINOTHIOYLIDYNETRISAZIRIDINE ◇ PHOSPHORO-THIOIC ACID TRIETHYLENETRIAMIDE ◇ SK 6882 ◇ TESPAMINE ◇ THIOFOZIL ◇ THIOPHOSPHAMIDE ◇ THIO-TEP ◇ TIOFOSFAMID ◇ TIOFOZIL ◇ TRIAZIRIDI-NYLPHOSPHINE SULFIDE ◇ N,N',N''-TRI-1,2-ETHANE-DIYLPHOSPHOROTHIOIC TRIAMIDE ◇ N,N',N''-TRI-1,2-ETHANEDIYLTHIOPHOSPHORAMIDE ◇ TRI(ETHYLENE-IMINO)THIOPHOSPHORAMIDE ◇ N,N',N''-TRIETHYLENE-PHOSPHOROTHIOIC TRIAMIDE ◇ N,N',N''-TRIETHYLENE-THIOPHOSPHAMIDE ◇ N,N',N''-TRIETHYLENETHIO-PHOSPHORAMIDE ◇ TRIETHYLENETHIOPHOSPHOROTRI-AMIDE ◇ TRIS(1-AZIRIDINYL)PHOSPHINE SULFIDE ◇ TRIS(ETHYLENIMINO)THIOPHOSPHATE ◇ TSPA

TOXICITY DATA with REFERENCE
CAR: ipr-mus TD:360 mg/kg/1Y-I
    NCITR* NCI-CG-TR-58,78

CAR: ipr-rat TD:218 mg/kg/1Y-I
    NCITR* NCI-CG-TR-58,78

CAR: ipr-rat TDLo:218 mg/kg/1Y-I
NCITR* NCI-CG-TR-58,78
CAR: ivn-rat TDLo:52 mg/kg/1Y-I   ARZNAD
20,1461,70
CAR: par-man TDLo:33 mg/kg/3Y-I:BLD
CMAJAX 129,578,83
CAR: unr-wmn TDLo:17 mg/kg/56W-I:BLD
LANCAO 2,775,70
NEO: ipr-mus TD:47 mg/kg/8W-I   CNREA8
33,3069,73
ETA: skn-mus TDLo:10 g/kg/17W-I   GANNA2
57,295,66
MUT: cyt-ham-unr 150 μg/kg   MUREAV 74,166,80
MUT: cyt-ham:lng 330 μmol/L/2H   HEREAY
94,21,81
MUT: cyt-hmn:leu 10 mg/L   MUREAV 14,345,72
MUT: cyt-hmn:lym 52 μmol/L   SOGEBZ
10,1580,74
MUT: cyt-mus-par 2500 μg/kg   IJEBA6 18,866,80
MUT: cyt-rbt-ivn 3 mg/kg   BEXBAN 94,1118,82
MUT: dnr-esc 600 μmol/L   ZKKOBW 92,177,78
MUT: dns-hmn:lym 1 mg/L   TGANAK 17(2),58,83
MUT: mmo-sat 100 μg/plate   TAKHAA 44,96,85
MUT: mnt-mus-ipr 1 mg/kg   GNKAA5 20,365,84
MUT: otr-mus:emb 500 μg/L   CNREA8 37,2202,77
MUT: sce-ham-unr 150 μg/kg   MUREAV 74,166,80
MUT: sce-ham:oth 400 ng/L   GNKAA5 16,2164,80
MUT: sce-hmn:lym 1 mg/L   TGANAK 16(2),34,82

CONSENSUS REPORTS: IARC Cancer Review: Human Limited Evidence IMEMDT 9,85,75; Animal Sufficient Evidence IMEMDT 9,85,75. NTP Fourth Annual Report On Carcinogens, 1984. NCI Carcinogenesis Bioassay (ipr); Clear Evidence: mouse, rat NCITR* NCI-CG-TR-58,78. EPA Genetic Toxicology Program.

SAFETY PROFILE: Confirmed human carcinogen producing leukemia. Poison by ingestion, intraperitoneal, intravenous, and subcutaneous routes. Experimental teratogenic data. Human systemic effects by parenteral and possibly other routes: paresthesia, bone marrow changes and leukemia. Experimental reproductive effects. Human mutation data reported. When heated to decomposition it emits very toxic fumes of PO_x, SO_x, and NO_x.

TFT750   CAS: 1314-20-1
THORIUM OXIDE
mf: O_2Th mw: 264.00

PROP: Heavy, white crystalline powder. D: 9.7, mp: 3390°. Insol in water, alkalies; slowly

sol in acids. Sterile contrast medium made up of 24-26% stabilized colloidal thorium dioxide in 25% aqueous dextrin and 0.15% methyl parasept as preservative (CNREA8 22,152,62).

SYNS: THORIA ◇ THORIUM DIOXIDE ◇ THOROTRAST ◇ THORTRAST ◇ UMBRATHOR

TOXICITY DATA with REFERENCE
CAR: iat-hmn TD:1302 mg/kg:LIV   BJCAAI
41,446,80
CAR: iat-hmn TDLo:490 mg/kg   ANYAA9
145,776,67
CAR: iat-man TD:1190 mg/kg:LIV,BLD
APMIAL 53,147,61
CAR: iat-wmn TD:2 g/kg   ANYAA9 145,776,67
CAR: par-wmn TD:2350 mg/kg:KID   EUURAV
3,69,77
CAR: par-wmn TDLo:1 g/kg:LIV   ANYAA9
145,700,67
CAR: unr-ham TDLo:2 g/kg   GANNA2 57,431,66
NEO: par-hmn TD:700 mg/kg:LIV,BLD
ANYAA9 145,676,67
NEO: par-hmn TD:1260 mg/kg:LIV,BLD
ANYAA9 145,676,67
NEO: unr-hmn TDLo:2880 mg/kg:LIV
AJRRAV 83,163,60
ETA: ims-mus TDLo:400 mg/kg   CNREA8
22,152,62
ETA: ivn-mus TD:10 mg/kg   BJCAAI 9,253,55
ETA: ivn-mus TDLo:10 g/kg   BJCAAI 10,527,56
ETA: ivn-rat TDLo:160 mg/kg   ANYAA9
145,738,67
ETA: ivn-rbt TD:300 mg(Th)/kg/2Y-I   AICCA6
16,425,60
ETA: ivn-rbt TD:3600 mg/kg   PAMIAD 25,27,62
ETA: ivn-rbt TDLo:1500 mg/kg   ANYAA9
145,724,67
ETA: par-gpg TDLo:4 g/kg/15W-I   AJCAA7
35,363,39
ETA: scu-mus TDLo:20 g/kg   JNCIAM 1,349,40

CONSENSUS REPORTS: NTP Fourth Annual Report On Carcinogens, 1984. Community Right-To-Know List. Reported in EPA TSCA Inventory.

SAFETY PROFILE: Confirmed human carcinogen producing angiosarcoma, liver and kidney tumors, lymphoma and other tumors of the blood system, and tumors at the application site.

TFU500   CAS: 299-75-2
I-THREITOL-1,4-
BISMETHANESULFONATE
mf: $C_6H_{14}O_6S_2$ mw: 246.32

SYNS: CB 2562 ◊ 1,4-DIMETHANESULFONATE THREITOL ◊ (2s,3s)-1,4-DIMETHANESULFONATE TREITOL ◊ NSC-39069 ◊ TREOSULFAN ◊ TRESULFAN

TOXICITY DATA with REFERENCE
MUT: sce-hmn-unr 28 mg/kg/D   EJCODS 18,979,82
MUT: sce-hmn:lym 4500 μg/L   EJCODS 18,979,82
MUT: sln-dmg-par 160 mmol/L   GENTAE 46,447,61
MUT: sln-dmg-unr 160 mmol/L   ANYAA9 160,228,69

CONSENSUS REPORTS: IARC Cancer Review: Human Sufficient Evidence IMEMDT 26,341,81. EPA Genetic Toxicology Program.

SAFETY PROFILE: Confirmed carcinogen. Poison by intravenous route. Human mutation data reported. When heated to decomposition it emits toxic fumes of SO$_x$.

TGI100
TOBACCO PLANT

PROP: Large annual or perennial shrubs with leaves that are often broad, hairy, and sticky. The trumpet-shaped flowers are white, yellow, green-yellow or red. The seed capsule holds many small seeds. *N. tabacum* is the principal commercial tobacco in the western countries. *N. rustica*, native to South America, is found sporadically across the United States and is the most widely cultivated tobacco in the Orient. *N. longiflora* is commonly cultivated as a garden ornamental. *N. attenuata* grows in the region bounded by Idaho, Baja California, and Texas. *N. glauca* is native to South America and now grows in the southwestern United States, Hawaii, Mexico, and the West Indies.

SYNS: NICOTIANA ATTENUATA ◊ NICOTIANA GLAUCA ◊ NICOTIANA LONGIFLORA ◊ NICOTIANA RUSTICA ◊ NICOTIANA TABACUM ◊ PAKA (HAWAII) ◊ TABAC (FRENCH) ◊ TABACO (SPANISH)

SAFETY PROFILE: Confirmed human carcinogen by several routes. The whole plant contains poisonous nicotine and other chemically related alkaloids. The primary alkaloid in *N. tabacum* is nicotine. The primary alkaloid in *N. glauca* is anabasine. Ingestion of any part of the plant can cause salivation, nausea, vomiting, distorted perceptions, convulsions vasomotor collapse and respiratory failure. Most serious poisonings result from ingestion of the leaves in salad, use of infusions as enemas, or skin absorption of alkaloids during commercial harvesting.

TGJ750
o-TOLIDINE
CAS: 119-93-7

mf: C$_{14}$H$_{16}$N$_2$ mw: 212.32

PROP: White to reddish crystals. Mp: 129-131°C. Very sltly sol in water; sol in alc, ether, acetic acid.

SYNS: BIANISIDINE ◊ 4,4'-BI-o-TOLUIDINE ◊ C.I. 37230 ◊ C.I. AZOIC DIAZO COMPONENT 113 ◊ (4,4'-DIAMINE-3,3'-DIMETHYL(1,1'-BIPHENYL) ◊ 4,4'-DIAMINO-3,3'-DIMETHYLBIPHENYL ◊ 4,4'-DIAMINO-3,3'-DIMETHYLDIPHENYL ◊ DIAMINODITOLYL ◊ 3,3'-DIMETHYLBENZIDIN ◊ 3,3'-DIMETHYLBENZIDINE ◊ 3,3'-DIMETHYL-4,4'-BIPHENYLDIAMINE ◊ 3,3'-DIMETHYLBIPHENYL-4,4'-DIAMINE ◊ 3,3'-DIMETHYL-(1,1'-BIPHENYL)-4,4'-DIAMINE ◊ 3,3'-DIMETHYL-4,4'-DIPHENYLDIAMINE ◊ 3,3'-DIMETHYLDIPHENYL-4,4'-DIAMINE ◊ 4,4'-DI-o-TOLUIDINE ◊ FAST DARK BLUE BASE R ◊ RCRA WASTE NUMBER U095 ◊ o-TOLIDIN ◊ 2-TOLIDIN (GERMAN) ◊ 2-TOLIDINA (ITALIAN) ◊ TOLIDINE ◊ o-TOLIDINE ◊ 3,3'-TOLIDINE ◊ o,o'-TOLIDINE ◊ 2-TOLIDINE

TOXICITY DATA with REFERENCE
CAR: orl-rat TDLo:4500 mg/kg/27D-I   CNREA8 28,924,68
ETA: imp-rat TDLo:5040 mg/kg/1Y-I   JNCIAM 45,283,70
ETA: scu-rat TD:9 g/kg/51W-I   CANCAR 3,789,50
ETA: scu-rat TD:3240 mg/kg/34W-I   JNCIAM 45,283,70
ETA: scu-rat TD:5040 mg/kg/56W-I   GTPZAB 9(7),18,65
ETA: scu-rat TDLo:1650 mg/kg/33W-I   VOONAW 20(2),53,74
MUT: bfa-rat/sat 10 μg/plate   MUREAV 79,173,80
MUT: dns-ham:lvr 1 μmol/L   MUREAV 136,255,84
MUT: dns-hmn:hla 1 μmol/L   CNREA8 38,2621,78
MUT: dns-rat:lvr 1 μmol/L   MUREAV 136,255,84
MUT: hma-rat/sat 50 μg/plate   MUREAV 79,173,80
MUT: otr-ham:kdy 80 μg/L   BJCAAI 37,873,78
MUT: sce-rbt:lym 50 mg/L   MUREAV 89,197,81

CONSENSUS REPORTS: IARC Cancer Review: Animal Limited Evidence IMEMDT 1,87,72. NTP Fourth Annual Report On Carcinogens, 1984. EPA Genetic Toxicology Program. Community Right-To-Know List. Reported in EPA TSCA Inventory.

ACGIH TLV: Suspected Human Carcinogen DFG MAK: Animal Carcinogen, Suspected Human Carcinogen. NIOSH REL: (o-Toluidine) CL 0.02 mg/m^3/60M; avoid skin contact.

SAFETY PROFILE: Confirmed carcinogen with experimental carcinogenic and tumorigenic data. Poison by intraperitoneal route. Moderately toxic by ingestion. Human mutation data reported. When heated to decomposition it emits toxic fumes of NO_x.

TGL750   CAS: 95-80-7
TOLUENE-2,4-DIAMINE
mf: $C_7H_{10}N_2$ mw: 122.19
DOT: 1709

PROP: Prisms. Mp: 99°, bp: 280°, vap press: 1 mm @ 106.5°.

SYNS: 3-AMINO-p-TOLUIDINE ◇ 5-AMINO-o-TOLUIDINE ◇ AZOGEN DEVELOPER H ◇ BENZOFUR MT ◇ C.I. 76035 ◇ C.I. OXIDATION BASE ◇ DEVELOPER H ◇ 1,3-DIAMINO-4-METHYLBENZENE ◇ 2,4-DIAMINO-1-METHYLBENZENE ◇ 2,4-DIAMINOTOLUEN (CZECH) ◇ DIAMINOTOLUENE ◇ 2,4-DIAMINOTOLUENE ◇ 2,4-DIAMINO-1-TOLUENE ◇ 2,4-DIAMINOTOLUOL ◇ EUCANINE GB ◇ FOURAMINE ◇ FOURRINE M ◇ META TOLUYLENE DIAMINE ◇ 4-METHYL-1,3-BENZENEDIAMINE ◇ 4-METHYL-m-PHENYLENEDIAMINE ◇ MTD ◇ NAKO TMT ◇ NCI-C02302 ◇ PELAGOL GREY J ◇ PONTAMINE DEVELOPER TN ◇ RCRA WASTE NUMBER U221 ◇ RENAL MD ◇ TDA ◇ 2,4-TOLAMINE ◇ m-TOLUENEDIAMINE ◇ 2,4-TOLUENE-DIAMINE ◇ m-TOLUYLENDIAMIN (CZECH) ◇ m-TOLUYLENEDIAMINE ◇ 2,4-TOLUENEDIAMINE (DOT) ◇ m-TOLYENEDIAMINE ◇ m-TOLYLENEDIAMINE ◇ TOLYLENE-2,4-DIAMINE ◇ 2,4-TOLYLENEDIAMINE ◇ 4-m-TOLYLENEDIAMINE ◇ ZOBA GKE ◇ ZOGEN DEVELOPHER H

TOXICITY DATA with REFERENCE
CAR: orl-mus TD: 17 g/kg/2Y-C
  NCITR* NCI-CG-TR-162,79
CAR: orl-mus TD: 8400 mg/kg/2Y-C   GANNA2
70,453,79
CAR: orl-mus TD: 16800 mg/kg/2Y-C   GANNA2
70,453,79
CAR: orl-mus TDLo: 8050 mg/kg/101W-C
  NCITR* NCI-CG-TR-162,79
CAR: orl-rat TD: 5030 mg/kg/84W-C
  NCITR* NCI-CG-TR-162,79
CAR: orl-rat TD: 9000 mg/kg/36W-C   CNREA8
29,1137,69
CAR: orl-rat TDLo: 2100 mg/kg/90W-C   JJIND8
62,1107,79
MUT: dnd-hmn: fbr 100 μmol/L   MUREAV
127,107,84
MUT: dnd-rat-ipr 37 mg/kg   CRNGDP 6,1285,85
MUT: dns-hmn: lvr 1 mmol/L   PAACA3 24,69,83
MUT: mma-sat 50 μg/plate   ENMUDM 7,535,85
MUT: msc-mus: lym 198 mg/L   MUREAV
135,115,84

CONSENSUS REPORTS: IARC Cancer Review: Animal Sufficient Evidence IMEMDT 16,83,78. NTP Fourth Annual Report On Carcinogens, 1984. NCI Carcinogenesis Bioassay (feed); Clear Evidence: mouse, rat NCITR* NCI-CG-TR-162,79. Community Right-To-Know List. Reported in EPA TSCA Inventory. EPA Genetic Toxicology Program.

DFG MAK: Animal Carcinogen, Suspected Human Carcinogen.   DOT Classification: Poison B; Label: St. Andrews Cross.

SAFETY PROFILE: Confirmed carcinogen with experimental carcinogenic data. Poison by ingestion, intraperitoneal, and subcutaneous routes. Experimental reproductive effects. Human mutation data reported. A skin and eye irritant. This material has a marked toxic action upon the liver and can cause fatty degeneration of that organ. When heated to decomposition it emits toxic fumes of NO_x.

TGM740   CAS: 26471-62-5
TOLUENE-1,3-DIISOCYANATE
DOT: 2078
mf: $C_9H_6N_2O_2$ mw: 174.17

SYN: BENZENE-, 1,3-DIISOCYANATOMETHYL- ◇ DESMODUR T100 ◇ DIISOCYANATOMETHYLBENZENE ◇ DIISOCYANATOTOLUENE ◇ HYLENE-T ◇ ISOCYANIC ACID, METHYLPHENYLENE ESTER ◇ METHYL-meta-PHENYLENE DIISOCYANATE ◇ METHYLPHENYLENE ISOCYANATE ◇ MONDUR-TD ◇ MONDUR-TD-80 ◇ NACCONATE-100 ◇ NIAX ISOCYANATE TDI ◇ RCRA WASTE NUMBER U223 ◇ RUBINATE TDI ◇ RUBINATE TDI 80/20 ◇ T 100 ◇ TDI ◇ TDI-80 ◇ TDI 80-20 ◇ TOLUENE DIISOCYANATE ◇ TOLYLENE DIISOCYANATE ◇ TOLYLENE ISOCYANATE

TOXICITY DATA with REFERENCE
CAR: orl-mus TDLo: 63 g/kg/2Y-I
  NTPTR* NTP-TR-251,86
CAR: orl-rat TDLo: 31800 mg/kg/2Y-I
  NTPTR* NTP-TR-251,86
NEO: orl-rat TD: 63600 mg/kg/2Y-I
  NTPTR* NTP-TR-251,86
MUT: cyt-ham: ovr 800 mg/L   SCIEAS 236,933,87
MUT: cyt-hmn: lyms 92 mg/L   TOLED5 36,37,87
MUT: mma-mus: lyms 50 mg/L   SCIEAS 236,933,87
MUT: mma-sat 100 μg/plate   ENMUDM
9(Suppl 9),1,87
MUT: msc-mus: lyms 50 mg/L   SCIEAS 236,933,87
MUT: sce-ham: ovr 50 mg/L   SCIEAS 236,933,87

CONSENSUS REPORTS: IARC Cancer Review: GROUP 2B IMEMDT 7,56,87, Animal

Sufficient Evidence IMEMDT 39,287,86; Human Inadequate Evidence IMEMDT 39,287,86. NTP Fourth Annual Report On Carcinogens, 1984. NTP Carcinogenesis Studies (gavage): Clear Evidence: mouse, rat NTPTR* NTP-TR-251,86. Reported in EPA TSCA Inventory.

NIOSH REL: TDI-air:10H TWA 0.005 ppm;CL 0.02 ppm/10M DOT Classification: Poison B; LABEL: Poison

SAFETY PROFILE: Confirmed carcinogen with experimental carcinogenic and neoplastigenic data. Poison by inhalation. Moderately toxic by ingestion. Severe skin irritant. Human mutation data reported. Capable of producing severe dermatitis and bronchial spasm. A common air contaminant. Combustible when exposed to heat or flame. Explosive in the form of vapor when exposed to heat or flame. To fight fire, use dry chemical, CO_2. Storage in polyethylene containers is hazardous due to absorption of water through the plastic. When heated to decomposition it emits highly toxic fumes of NO_x.

TGM750 CAS: 584-84-9
TOLUENE-2,4-DIISOCYANATE
mf: $C_9H_6N_2O_2$ mw: 174.17

PROP: Clear, faintly yellow liquid; sharp, pungent odor. Mp: 19.5-21.5°, d (liquid): 1.2244 @ 20/4°, bp: 251°, flash p: 270°F (OC), vap d: 6.0, lel: 0.9%, uel: 9.5%. Misc with alc (decomp), ether, acetone, carbon tetrachloride, benzene, chlorobenzene, kerosene, olive oil.

SYNS: CRESORCINOL DIISOCYANATE ◇ DESMODUR T80 ◇ DI-ISOCYANATE DE TOLUYLENE ◇ DI-ISO-CYANATO-LUENE ◇ 2,4-DIISOCYANATO-1-METHYLBENZENE (9CI) ◇ 2,4-DIISOCYANATOTOLUENE ◇ DIISOCYANAT-TOLUOL ◇ ISOCYANIC ACID, METHYLPHENYLENE ESTER ◇ ISOCYANIC ACID, 4-METHYL-m-PHENYLENE ESTER ◇ HYLENE T ◇ HYLENE TCPA ◇ HYLENE TLC ◇ HYLENE TM ◇ HYLENE TM-65 ◇ HYLENE TRF ◇ 4-METHYL-PHE-NYLENE DIISOCYANATE ◇ 4-METHYL-PHENYLENE ISO-CYANATE ◇ MONDUR TD ◇ MONDUR TD-80 ◇ MONDUR TDS ◇ NACCONATE IOO ◇ NCI-C50533 ◇ NIAX TDI ◇ NIAX TDI-P ◇ RCRA WASTE NUMBER U223 ◇ RUBI-NATE TDI 80/20 ◇ TDI ◇ 2,4-TDI ◇ TDI-80 ◇ TDI (OSHA) ◇ TOLUEEN-DIISOCYANAAT ◇ TOLUEN-DISOCIANATO ◇ TOLUENE DIISOCYANATE ◇ TOLUENE-2,4-DIISOCYA-NATE ◇ 2,4-TOLUENEDIISOCYANATE ◇ TOLUILENOD-WUIZOCYJANIAN ◇ TULUYLENDIISOCYANAT ◇ TOLUYL-ENE-2,4-DIISOCYANATE ◇ TOLYENE 2,4-DIISOCYANATE ◇ meta-TOLYLENE DIISOCYANATE ◇ TOLYLENE-2,4-DIISOCYANATE ◇ 2,4-TOLYLENEDIISOCYANATE

TOXICITY DATA with REFERENCE
MUT: mma-sat 100 μg/plate ENMUDM 9(Suppl 9),1,87

CONSENSUS REPORTS: NTP Fourth Annual Report On Carcinogens, 1984. IARC Cancer Review: Human Inadequate Evidence IMEMDT 39,287,86; Animal Sufficient Evidence IMEMDT 39,287,86. Community Right-To-Know List. EPA Extremely Hazardous Substances List. Reported in EPA TSCA Inventory.

OSHA PEL: (Transitional: CL 0.02 ppm) TWA 0.005 ppm; STEL 0.02 ppm ACGIH TLV: TWA 0.005 ppm; STEL 0.02 ppm DFG MAK: 0.01 ppm (0.07 mg/m^3 NIOSH REL: (Diisocyanates) TWA 0.005 ppm; CL 0.02 ppm/10M DOT Classification: Poison B; Label: Poison.

SAFETY PROFILE: Confirmed carcinogen. Poison by ingestion, inhalation, and intravenous routes. Human systemic effects by inhalation: unspecified changes to the eyes and sense of smell, respiratory obstruction, cough, sputum, and other pulmonary and gastrointestinal changes. Mutation data reported. A severe skin and eye irritant. Capable of producing severe dermatitis and bronchial spasm. A common air contaminant. Combustible when exposed to heat or flame. Explosive in the form of vapor when exposed to heat or flame. To fight fire, use dry chemical, CO_2. Reaction with water releases carbon dioxide. Storage in polyethylene containers is hazardous due to absorption of water through the plastic. When heated to decomposition it emits highly toxic fumes of NO_x.

TGQ750 CAS: 95-53-4
o-TOLUIDINE
mf: C_7H_9N mw: 107.17
DOT: 1708

PROP: Colorless liquid. Mp: −16.3°, bp: 200-202°, ULC: 20-25, flash p: 185° (CC), d: 1.004 @ 20/4°, autoign temp: 900°F, vap press: 1 mm @ 44°, vap d: 3.69. Sltly sol in water, dilute acid; sol in alc and ether.

SYNS: 1-AMINO-2-METHYLBENZENE ◇ 2-AMINO-1-METHYLBENZENE ◇ o-AMINOTOLUENE ◇ 2-AMINOTOL-UENE ◇ C.I. 37077 ◇ 1-METHYL-2-AMINOBENZENE ◇ 2-METHYL-1-AMINOBENZENE ◇ o-METHYLANILINE ◇ 2-METHYLANILINE ◇ o-METHYLBENZENAMINE ◇ 2-METHYLBENZENAMINE ◇ o-TOLUIDIN (CZECH) ◇ 2-TOLUIDINE ◇ o-TOLUIDYNA (POLISH) ◇ o-TOLYLAMINE

TOXICITY DATA with REFERENCE

NEO: orl-rat TDLo:109 g/kg/2Y-C   FCTOD7 25,619,87

NEO: scu-mus TDLo:320 mg/kg (15-21D preg):REP   BEXBAN 78,1402,74

ETA: orl-rat TDLo:7250 mg/kg/23W-C   APMIAL 26,447,49

ETA: scu-rbt TDLo:840 mg/kg/14W-I   IARC** 27,155,82

MUT: dns-hmn:hla 50 uL/L   PMRSDJ 5,347,85

MUT: msc-mus:lym 10 mg/L   PMRSDJ 5,587,85

MUT: otr-mus:emb 500 mg/L   PMRSDJ 5,659,85

MUT: sce-ham:lng 2500 μmol/L   PMRSDJ 5,469,85

MUT: slt-dmg-orl 1 mmol/L   PMRSDJ 5,313,85

CONSENSUS REPORTS: IARC Cancer Review: Human Inadequate Evidence IMEMDT 16,349,78; Human Limited Evidence IMEMDT 27,155,82; Animal Inadequate Evidence IMEMDT 16,349,78. NTP Fourth Annual Report On Carcinogens, 1984. EPA Genetic Toxicology Program. Community Right-To-Know List. Reported in EPA TSCA Inventory.

OSHA PEL: TWA 5 ppm (skin)   ACGIH TLV: TWA 2 ppm (skin); Suspected Human Carcinogen.   DFG MAK: Animal Carcinogen, Suspected Human Carcinogen.   DOT Classification: Poison B; Label: Poison.

SAFETY PROFILE: Confirmed carcinogen with experimental neoplastigenic and tumorigenic data. Poison by ingestion and intraperitoneal routes. Moderately toxic by skin contact. Human systemic effects by inhalation: urine volume increase, hematuria and blood methemoglobinemia-carboxhemoglobinemia. Human mutation data reported. A skin and eye irritant. Human mucous membrane effects. Flammable when exposed to heat or flame. To fight fire, use foam, CO_2, dry chemical. When heated to decomposition it emits highly toxic fumes of NO_x.

TGS500   CAS: 636-21-5
o-TOLUIDINE HYDROCHLORIDE
mf: $C_7H_9N \cdot ClH$ mw: 143.63

PROP: Monoclinic prisms. Mp: 218-220°, bp: 242°. Sol in water; sltly sol in alc.

SYNS: 1-AMINO-2-METHYLBENZENE HYDROCHLORIDE ◇ 2-AMINO-1-METHYLBENZENE HYDROCHLORIDE ◇ 2-AMINOTOLUENE HYDROCHLORIDE ◇ o-AMINOTOLUENE HYDROCHLORIDE ◇ 1-METHYL-2-AMINOBENZENE HYDROCHLORIDE ◇ 2-METHYL-1-AMINOBENZENE HYDROCHLORIDE ◇ o-METHYLANILINE HYDROCHLORIDE ◇ 2-METHYLANILINE HYDROCHLORIDE ◇ o-METHYLBENZENAMINE HYDROCHLORIDE ◇ 2-METHYLBENZENAMINE HYDROCHLORIDE ◇ NCI-C02335 ◇ RCRA WASTE NUMBER U222 ◇ 2-TOLUIDINE HYDROCHLORIDE ◇ o-TOLYLAMINE HYDROCHLORIDE

TOXICITY DATA with REFERENCE

CAR: orl-mus TD:262 g/kg/2Y-C   NCITR* NCI-CG-TR-153,79

CAR: orl-mus TD:1210 g/kg/78W-C   JEPTDQ 2(2),325,78

CAR: orl-mus TD:2142 g/kg/2Y-C   IARC** 27,155,82

CAR: orl-mus TD:12936 g/kg/77W-C   IARC** 27,155,82

CAR: orl-mus TDLo:146 g/kg/2Y-C   NCITR* NCI-CG-TR-153,79

CAR: orl-rat TD:125 g/kg/73W-C   CALEDQ 16,103,82

CAR: orl-rat TD:159 g/kg/2Y-C   NCITR* NCI-CG-TR-153,79

CAR: orl-rat TD:233 g/kg/101W-C   NCITR* NCI-CG-TR-153,79

CAR: orl-rat TD:2121 g/kg/2Y-C   IARC** 27,155,82

CAR: orl-rat TD:4242 g/kg/2Y-C   IARC** 27,155,82

CAR: orl-rat TD:12936 g/kg/77W-C   IARC** 27,155,82

CAR: orl-rat TDLo:117 g/kg/101W-C   NCITR* NCI-CG-TR-153,79

MUT: dnd-bcs 20 μL/disc   PMRSDJ 1,175,81

MUT: dnr-esc 500 mg/L   PMRSDJ 1,195,81

MUT: mma-sat 50 μg/plate   PMRSDJ 1,351,81

MUT: sln-smc 50 mg/L   PMRSDJ 1,468,81

CONSENSUS REPORTS: IARC Cancer Review: Animal Sufficient Evidence IMEMDT 27,155,82. NTP Fourth Annual Report On Carcinogens, 1984. NCI Carcinogenesis Bioassay (feed); Clear Evidence: mouse, rat NCITR* NCI-CG-TR-153,79. EPA Genetic Toxicology Program. Community Right-To-Know List. Reported in EPA TSCA Inventory.

SAFETY PROFILE: Confirmed carcinogen with experimental carcinogenic data. Poison by intraperitoneal route. Moderately toxic by ingestion. Mutation data reported. When heated to decomposition it emits very toxic fumes of HCl and NO_x.

THV500   CAS: 73941-35-2
2,4,5-TRIBROMOIMIDAZOLE CADMIUM SALT (2:1)
mf: $C_6Br_6N_4 \cdot Cd$ mw: 719.96

SYN: CADMIUM salt of 2,4-5-TRIBROMOIMIDAZOLE

CONSENSUS REPORTS: Cadmium and its compounds are on the Community Right-To-Know List.

OSHA PEL: TWA 0.2 mg(Cd)/m^3; CL 0.6 mg(Cd)/m^3 (dust) ACGIH TLV: TWA 0.05 mg(Cd)/m^3 (Proposed: TWA 0.01 mg(Cd)/m^3 (dust), Human Carcinogen); BEI: 10 μg/g creatinine in urine; 10 μg/L in blood. NIOSH REL: (Cadmium) Reduce to lowest feasible level.

SAFETY PROFILE: Confirmed human carcinogen. Poison by intravenous route. When heated to decomposition it emits very toxic fumes of Br$^-$, Cd, and NO$_x$.

TIH000 CAS: 12380-95-9
TRICADMIUM DINITRIDE
mf: Cd$_3$N$_2$ mw: 365.21

SYN: CADMIUM NITRIDE

CONSENSUS REPORTS: Cadmium compounds are on the Community Right-To-Know List.

OSHA PEL: TWA 0.2 mg(Cd)/m^3; CL 0.6 mg(Cd)/m^3 (dust) ACGIH TLV: TWA 0.05 mg(Cd)/m^3 (Proposed: TWA 0.01 mg(Cd)/m^3 (dust), Human Carcinogen); BEI: 10 μg/g creatinine in urine; 10 μg/L in blood. NIOSH REL: (Cadium) Reduce to lowest feasible level.

SAFETY PROFILE: Confirmed human carcinogen. Many cadmium compounds are poisons. Explodes violently on shock or heating. Explodes on contact with water, acids, or bases. When heated to decomposition it emits very toxic fumes of NO$_x$ and Cd.

TIL360 CAS: 2431-50-7
2,3,4-TRICHLOROBUTENE-1
mf: C$_4$H$_5$Cl$_3$ mw: 159.44

SYN: 1-BUTENE, 2,3,4-TRICHLORO-

CONSENSUS REPORTS: Reported in EPA TSCA Inventory.

DFG MAK: Animal Carcinogen; Suspected Human Carcinogen.

SAFETY PROFILE: Confirmed carcinogen. Poison by ingestion. When heated to decomposition it emits toxic fumes of Cl$^-$.

TIW000 CAS: 88-06-2
2,4,6-TRICHLOROPHENOL
mf: C$_6$H$_3$Cl$_3$O   mw: 197.44

PROP: Colorless needles or yellow solid; strong phenolic odor. Mp: 68°, bp: 244.5°, fp: 62°, d: 1.490 @ 75/4°, vap press: 1 mm @ 76.5°. Sol in water; very sol in alc, ether.

SYNS: DOWICIDE 2S ◇ NCI-C02904 ◇ OMAL ◇ PHENA-CHLOR ◇ RCRA WASTE NUMBER U231 ◇ 2,4,6-TRICHLOR-FENOL (CZECH)

TOXICITY DATA with REFERENCE
CAR: orl-mus TD:882 g/kg/2Y-C
  NCITR* NCI-CG-TR-155,79
CAR: orl-mus TDLo:441 g/kg/2Y-C
  NCITR* NCI-CG-TR-155,79
CAR: orl-rat TD:374 g/kg/2Y-C
  NCITR* NCI-CG-TR-155,79
CAR: orl-rat TDLo:185 g/kg/2Y-C
  NCITR* NCI-CG-TR-155,79

CONSENSUS REPORTS: IARC Cancer Review: Animal Inadequate Evidence IMEMDT 20,349,79; Human Limited Evidence IMEMDT 41,319,86. NTP Fourth Annual Report On Carcinogens, 1984. NCI Carcinogenesis Bioassay (feed); Clear Evidence: mouse, rat NCITR* NCI-CG-TR-155,79. Chlorophenol compounds are on the Community Right-To-Know List. Reported in EPA TSCA Inventory. EPA Genetic Toxicology Program.

SAFETY PROFILE: Confirmed carcinogen with experimental carcinogenic data. Poison by intraperitoneal route. Moderately toxic by ingestion and skin contact. A skin and severe eye irritant. When heated to decomposition it emits toxic fumes of Cl$^-$. Used as a germicide and preservative.

TLG250 CAS: 137-17-7
2,4,5-TRIMETHYLANILINE
mf: C$_9$H$_{13}$N   mw: 135.23

SYNS: 1-AMINO-2,4,5-TRIMETHYLBENZENE ◇ psi-CUMIDINE ◇ NCI-C02299 ◇ PSEUDOCUMIDINE ◇ 1,2,4-TRI-METHYL-5-AMINOBENZENE ◇ 2,4,5-TRIMETHYLANILIN (CZECH) ◇ 2,4,5-TRIMETHYLBENZENAMINE

TOXICITY DATA with REFERENCE
CAR: orl-mus TD:68 g/kg/2Y-C
  NCITR* NCI-CG-TR-160,79
CAR: orl-mus TD:35350 mg/kg/2Y-C   IARC**
  27,177,82
CAR: orl-mus TD:70700 mg/kg/2Y-C   IARC**
  27,177,82
CAR: orl-mus TDLo:17 g/kg/2Y-C
  NCITR* NCI-CG-TR-160,79

CAR: orl-rat TD: 28 g/kg/2Y-C
NCITR* NCI-CG-TR-160,79
CAR: orl-rat TD: 566 g/kg/2Y-C   IARC**27,177,82
CAR: orl-rat TDLo: 7000 mg/kg/101W-C
NCITR* NCI-CG-TR-160,79
ETA: orl-rat TD: 141 g/kg/2Y-C   IARC**27,177,82
MUT: dnd-ham: lng 10 mmol/L   MUREAV
77,317,80
MUT: mma-sat 10 μg/plate   ENMUDM
8(Suppl 7),1,86

CONSENSUS REPORTS: IARC Cancer Review: Animal Limited Evidence IMEMDT 27,177,82. NCI Carcinogenesis Bioassay (feed); Clear Evidence: mouse, rat NCITR* NCI-CG-TR-160,79.

DFG MAK: Animal Carcinogen, Suspected Human Carcinogen.

SAFETY PROFILE: Confirmed carcinogen with experimental carcinogenic and tumorigenic data. Moderately toxic by ingestion. Mutation data reported. When heated to decomposition it emits toxic fumes of NO_x. Used as a dye, pigment and printing ink.

TLY000   CAS: 64047-30-9
TRIMETHYL-2-OXEPANONE
(mixed isomers)
mf: $C_9H_{16}O_2$ mw: 156.25

SYN: TRIMETHYL-ε-LACTONE (mixed isomers)

CONSENSUS REPORTS: IARC Cancer Review: Animal Sufficient Evidence IMEMDT 19,303,79.

SAFETY PROFILE: Confirmed carcinogen. Mildly toxic by ingestion and skin contact. When heated to decomposition it emits acrid smoke and irritating fumes.

TNC500   CAS: 126-72-7
TRIS
mf: $C_9H_{15}Br_6O_4P$ mw: 697.67

PROP: Crystals. D: 2.24, flash p: > 112°.

SYNS: ANFRAM 3PB ◇ APEX 462-5 ◇ BROMKAL P 67-6HP ◇ 2,3-DIBROMO-1-PROPANOL, PHOSPHATE (3:1) ◇ 2,3-DIBROMO-1-PROPANOL PHOSPHATE ◇ (2,3-DIBROMOPROPYL) PHOSPHATE ◇ FIREMASTER T23P-LV ◇ FLACAVON R ◇ FLAMMEX AP ◇ FYROL HB32 ◇ NCI-C03270 ◇ PHOSPHORIC ACID, TRIS(2,3-DIBROMOPROPYL) ESTER ◇ RCRA WASTE NUMBER U235 ◇ TDBP (CZECH) ◇ TRIS(DIBROMOPROPYL)PHOSPHATE ◇ TRIS(2,3-DIBROMOPROPYL) PHOSPHATE ◇ TRIS(2,3-DI-

BROMOPROPYL) PHOSPHORIC ACID ESTER ◇ TRIS-2,3-DIBROMPROPYL ESTER KYSELINY FOSFORECNE (CZECH) ◇ TRIS (FLAME RETARDANT) ◇ USAF DO-41 ◇ ZETIFEX ZN

TOXICITY DATA with REFERENCE
CAR: orl-mus TD: 43 g/kg/103W-C
NCITR* NCI-CG-TR-76,78
CAR: orl-mus TD: 87 g/kg/103W-C
NCITR* NCI-CG-TR-76,78
CAR: orl-mus TDLo: 39 g/kg/92W-C
NCITR* NCI-CG-TR-76,78
CAR: orl-rat TDLo: 1330 mg/kg/76W-C
NCITR* NCI-CG-TR-76,78
CAR: skn-mus TDLo: 85 g/kg/71W-I   CNREA8
38,3236,78
NEO: orl-rat TD: 26 g/kg/52W-I   LAINAW44,74,81
NEO: orl-rat TD: 1800 mg/kg/103W-C
NCITR* NCI-CG-TR-76,78
NEO: orl-rat TD: 3600 mg/kg/103W-C
NCITR* NCI-CG-TR-76,78
ETA: orl-rat TD: 1820 mg/kg/2Y-C   FCTXAV
18,743,80
ETA: orl-rat TD: 43680 mg/kg/2Y-C   FCTXAV
18,743,80
MUT: dnd-hmn: oth 2 mg/L   MUREAV 56,89,77
MUT: dnr-esc 10 μg/plate   MUREAV 74,107,80
MUT: dns-rat: lvr 50 μmol/L   MUREAV 124,213,83
MUT: mma-esc 100 μg/plate   ENMUDM
7(Suppl 5),1,85
MUT: msc-ham: lng 20 μmol/L   MUREAV
124,213,83

CONSENSUS REPORTS: IARC Cancer Review: Animal Sufficient Evidence IMEMDT 20,575,79; Human Limited Evidence IMEMDT 20,575,79. NTP Fourth Annual Report On Carcinogens, 1984. NCI Carcinogenesis Bioassay (feed); Clear Evidence: mouse, rat NCITR* NCI-CG-TR-76,78. Community Right-To-Know List. Reported in EPA TSCA Inventory. EPA Genetic Toxicology Program.

SAFETY PROFILE: Confirmed carcinogen with experimental carcinogenic, neoplastigenic, tumorigenic, and teratogenic data. Poison by intraperitoneal route. Moderately toxic by ingestion and possibly other routes. Experimental reproductive effects. Human mutation data reported. An eye and severe skin irritant. Can cause testicular atrophy and sterility. Once used as a flame retardant additive to synthetic textiles and plastics, particularly in children's sleepwear. Use discontinued because it can be absorbed by human skin, or chewed or sucked off of sleepwear by infants. May be flammable when exposed to heat or flame. When heated to decomposition it emits very toxic fumes of Br^- and PO_x.

UVA000
URETHANE
CAS: 51-79-6

mf: $C_3H_7NO_2$ mw: 89.11

PROP: Colorless, odorless crystals. Mp: 49°, bp: 184°, d: 0.9862, vap press: 10 mm @ 77.8°, vap d: 3.07. Very sol in water, alc, ether.

SYNS: A 11032 ◊ AETHYLCARBAMAT (GERMAN) ◊ AETHYLURETHAN (GERMAN) ◊ CARBAMIC ACID, ETHYL ESTER ◊ CARBAMIDSAEURE-AETHYLESTER (GERMAN) ◊ ESTANE 5703 ◊ ETHYL CARBAMATE ◊ ETHYL-URETHAN ◊ ETHYL URETHANE ◊ o-ETHYLURETHANE ◊ LEUCETHANE ◊ LEUCOTHANE ◊ NSC 746 ◊ PRACARBAMIN ◊ PRACARBAMINE ◊ RCRA WASTE NUMBER U238 ◊ U-COMPOUND ◊ URETAN ETYLOWY (POLISH) ◊ URETHAN

TOXICITY DATA:
CAR: ipr-mus TD:880 mg/kg/7W-I   CNREA8 40,1194,80
CAR: ipr-mus TDLo:7 mg/kg/39W-I   SCIEAS 147,1443,65
CAR: orl-mus TD:1200 mg/kg/4W-I   BJCAAI 15,322,61
CAR: orl-mus TD:1280 mg/kg/4W-I   BJCAAI 15,322,61
CAR: orl-mus TDLo:12 g/kg/15D-C   TUMOAB 53,81,67
CAR: scu-mus TDLo:1000 mg/kg (15D preg): TER   CNREA8 34,2217,74
CAR: skn-ham TDLo:1000 mg/kg/W-I   CRSBAW 158,440,64
CAR: skn-mus TDLo:90 g/kg/56W-I   CRNGDP 5,911,84
NEO: ihl-mus TCLo:138 ppm/130D-I   AEHLAU 22,663,71
NEO: ipr-mus TD:10 mg/kg   CNREA8 33,3069,73
NEO: ipr-mus TD:400 mg/kg   CNREA8 35,1411,75
NEO: ipr-mus TD:500 mg/kg   CNREA8 44,107,84
NEO: ipr-mus TD:800 mg/kg   CNREA8 36,1744,76
NEO: ipr-mus TD:4990 μg/kg   CNREA843,1124,83
NEO: ipr-mus TDLo:500 mg/kg (19D preg): TER   CNREA8 38,137,78
NEO: ipr-rat TDLo:500 mg/kg   RRCRBU 52,29,75
NEO: ivn-mus TDLo:1000 mg/kg (18D preg): TER   JNCIAM 8,63,47
NEO: orl-ham TDLo:55 g/kg/64W-C   EJCAAH 5,165,69

NEO: scu-mus TD:500 mg/kg   CNREA833,1677,73
NEO: scu-mus TDLo:200 mg/kg:TER   CNREA8 34,2217,74
ETA: orl-mky TDLo:325 g/kg/5Y-I   PAACA3 21,78,80
ETA: orl-rat TDLo:30 g/kg/52W-C   CNREA8 7,107,47
ETA: scu-ham TDLo:1 g/kg   IJCNAW 6,63,70
ETA: scu-rat TDLo:8 g/kg/8W-I   JNCIAM 43,749,69
ETA: unr-mus TDLo:1 g/kg (17D preg):TER   BCSTB5 2,710,74
MUT: cyt-mus-scu 20 mg/kg   JJCREP 76,1141,85
MUT: dnd-hmn:fbr 3 mmol/L   ENMUDM 7,267,85
MUT: dns-hmn:fbr 20 mg/L   TXCYAC 21,151,81
MUT: mnt-rat-ipr-15 g/kg/10W-I   MUREAV 127,169,84
MUT: otr-mus:emb 1100 μmol/L   MUREAV 152,113,85
MUT: sce-ham-ipr 400 mg/kg   MUREAV126,159,84
MUT: sce-hmn:lym 10 μmol/L   MUREAV89,75,81
MUT: sce-rat-ipr 400 mg/kg   MUREAV 126,159,84

CONSENSUS REPORTS: IARC Cancer Review: Animal Sufficient Evidence IMEMDT 7,111,74. NTP Fourth Annual Report On Carcinogens, 1984. Community Right-To-Know List. Reported in EPA TSCA Inventory. EPA Genetic Toxicology Program.

DFG MAK: Animal Carcinogen, Suspected Human Carcinogen.

SAFETY PROFILE: Confirmed carcinogen with experimental carcinogenic, neoplastigenic, and tumorigenic data. A transplacental carcinogen. Moderately toxic by ingestion, intraperitoneal, subcutaneous, intramuscular, parenteral, intravenous, and possibly other routes. Experimental reproductive effects. A powerful teratogen in mice. Human mutation data reported. Causes depression of bone marrow and occasionally focal degeneration in the brain. Can also produce central nervous system depression, nausea and vomiting. Has been found in over 1000 beverages sold in the United States. The most heavily contaminated liquors are bourbons, sherries, and fruit brandies (some had 1,000 to 12,000 ppb urethane). Many whiskeys, table and dessert wines, brandies and liqueurs contain potentially hazardous amounts of urethane. The allowable limit for urethane in alcoholic beverages is 125 ppb. It is formed as a side product during processing. When heated it emits toxic fumes of NO_x. Used as an intermediate in the manufacture of pharmaceuticals, pesticides and fungicides.

VMP000
VINYL BROMIDE
CAS: 593-60-2

DOT: 1085

mf: C_2H_3Br mw: 106.96

PROP: A gas. Mp: $-138°$, bp: $15.6°$, d: 1.51. Insol in water; misc in alc, ether.

SYNS: BROMOETHENE ◇ BROMOETHYLENE ◇ BRO-MURE de VINYLE (FRENCH) ◇ VINILE (BROMURO di) (ITAL-IAN) ◇ VINYLBROMID (GERMAN) ◇ VINYL BROMIDE, in-hibited (DOT) ◇ VINYLE (BROMURE de) (FRENCH)

TOXICITY DATA with REFERENCE
CAR: ihl-rat TC:52 ppm/6H/2Y-I   TXAPA9 64,367,82

CAR: ihl-rat TCLo:10 ppm/6H/2Y-I   TXAPA9,64,367,82

NEO: ihl-rat TCLo:250 ppm/1Y   CHWKA9 121(20),40,77

ETA: ihl-rat TC:10 ppm   CHWKA9 123(24),25,78

MUT: mma-sat 2 pph/16H   ARTODN 41,249,79

MUT: mmo-sat 2 pph/16H   ARTODN 41,249,79

MUT: otr-rat-ihl 2000 ppm/14W-I   ARTODN 47,71,81

CONSENSUS REPORTS: IARC Cancer Review: GROUP 2A IMEMDT 7,56,87; Animal Sufficient Evidence IMEMDT 39,133,86; Animal Inadequate Evidence IMEMDT 19,367,79. Community Right-To-Know List. Reported in EPA TSCA Inventory. EPA Genetic Toxicology Program.

OSHA PEL: TWA 5 ppm   ACGIH TLV: TWA 5 ppm; Suspected Human Carcinogen.   DFG MAK: Human Carcinogen.   NIOSH REL: (Vinyl Bromide) Lowest Detectable Level   DOT Classification: Flammable Gas; Label: Flammable Gas.

SAFETY PROFILE: Confirmed carcinogen with experimental carcinogenic, neoplastigenic, and tumorigenic data. Moderately toxic by ingestion. Mutation data reported. A very dangerous fire hazard when exposed to heat or flame. Can react violently with oxidizing materials. May polymerize in sunlight. To fight fire, use CO_2, dry chemical or water spray. When heated to decomposition it emits toxic fumes of Br^-

VNP000
VINYL CHLORIDE
CAS: 75-01-4

DOT: 1086

mf: C_2H_3Cl mw: 62.50

PROP: Colorless liquid or gas (when inhibited); faintly sweet odor. Mp: $-160°$; bp: $-13.9°$, lel: 4%, uel: 22%; flash p: 17.6°F (COC), fp: $-159.7°$, d (liquid): 0.9195 @ 15/4°, vap press: 2600 mm @ 25°, vap d: 2.15, autoign temp: 882°F. Sltly sol in water; sol in alc; very sol in ether.

SYNS: CHLORETHENE ◇ CHLORETHYLENE ◇ CHLO-ROETHENE ◇ CHLOROETHYLENE ◇ CHLORURE de VINYLE (FRENCH) ◇ CLORURO di VINILE (ITALIAN) ◇ ETHYLENE MONOCHLORIDE ◇ MONOCHLOROETHENE ◇ MONO-CHLOROETHYLENE (DOT) ◇ RCRA WASTE NUMBER U043 ◇ TROVIDUR ◇ VC ◇ VCM ◇ VINILE (CLORURO di) (ITAL-IAN) ◇ VINYLCHLORID (GERMAN) ◇ VINYL CHLORIDE MONOMER ◇ VINYL C MONOMER ◇ VINYLE(CHLORURE de) (FRENCH) ◇ WINYLU CHLOREK (POLISH)

TOXICITY DATA with REFERENCE
CAR: ihl-ham TCLo:50 ppm/4H/30W-I   APDCDT 3,216,76

CAR: ihl-hmn TC:300 mg/m^3/W-C:BLD   GTPZAB 26(1),28,82

CAR: ihl-man TCLo:200 ppm/14Y-I:LIV   VAPHDQ 372,195,76

CAR: ihl-mus TC:50 ppm/4H/30W-I   CSHCAL 4,119,77

CAR: ihl-mus TC:50 ppm/6H/4W-I   JTEHD6 7,909,81

CAR: ihl-mus TC:50 ppm/47W-I   JTEHD6 4,15,78

CAR: ihl-mus TCLo:50 ppm/30W-I   ANYAA9 271,431,76

CAR: ihl-rat TC:5 ppm/4H/52W-I   EVHPAZ 41,3,81

CAR: ihl-rat TC:50 ppm/6H-43W-I   JTEHD6 7,909,81

CAR: ihl-rat TC:50 ppm/7H/26W-C   TXAPA9 68,120,83

CAR: ihl-rat TC:100 ppm/7H/26W-C   TXAPA9 68,120,83

CAR: ihl-rat TC:250 ppm/2Y-I   AANLAW 56,1,74

CAR: ihl-rat TCLo:1 ppm/4H/52W-I   EVHPAZ 41,3,81

CAR: orl-rat TD:34 g/kg/3Y-I   EVHPAZ 21,1,77

CAR: orl-rat TDLo:3463 mg/kg/52W-I   EVHPAZ 41,3,81

ETA: ipr-rat TDLo:21 mg/kg/65W-I   APDCDT 3,216,76

ETA: scu-rat TDLo:21 mg/kg/67W-I   APDCDT 3,216,76

MUT: cyt-hmn:hla 10 mmol/L   TXCYAC 9,21,78

MUT: cyt-man-unr 25 ppm/10Y   MUREAV 51,271,78

MUT: dns-rat:lvr 2100 μmol/L   CRNGDP 5,1629,84

MUT: mma-sat 1 pph   CBTOE2 1,159,85
MUT: msc-ham:ovr 10 pph   EVSRBT 25,91,82
MUT: otr-mus:emb 75 mg/L   CALEDQ 28,85,85

CONSENSUS REPORTS: IARC Cancer Review: Animal Sufficient Evidence IMEMDT 19,377,79; IMEMDT 7,291,74; Human Limited Evidence IMEMDT 7,291,74; Human Sufficient Evidence IMEMDT 19,377,79. NTP Fourth Annual Report On Carcinogens, 1984. Community Right-To-Know List. Reported in EPA TSCA Inventory. EPA Genetic Toxicology Program.

OSHA PEL: TWA 1 ppm; CL 5 ppm/15M; Cancer Suspect Agent   ACGIH TLV: TWA 5 ppm; Human Carcinogen.   DFG TRK: Existing installations: 3 ppm, Human Carcinogen; Others: 2 ppm.   NIOSH REL: (Vinyl Chloride) Lowest Detectable Level   DOT Classification: Flammable Gas; Label: Flammable Gas.

SAFETY PROFILE: Confirmed human carcinogen producing liver and blood tumors. Poison by inhalation. Moderately toxic by ingestion. Experimental teratogenic data. Human reproductive effects by inhalation: changes in spermatogenesis. Human mutation data reported. A severe irritant to skin, eyes, and mucous membranes. Causes skin burns by rapid evaporation and consequent freezing. In high concentration it acts as an anesthetic. A very dangerous fire hazard when exposed to heat, flame or oxidizers. To fight fire, stop flow of gas. When heated to decomposition it emits highly toxic fumes of Cl^-.

VOA000   CAS: 106-87-6
VINYL CYCLOHEXENE DIOXIDE
mf: $C_8H_{12}O_2$ mw: 140.20

PROP: Colorless liquid. D: 1.098 @ 20/20°, bp: 227°, flash p: 230°F.

SYNS: CHISSONOX 206 ◇ EP-206 ◇ 1,2-EPOXY-4-(EPOXY-ETHYL)CYCLOHEXANE ◇ 1-EPOXYETHYL-3,4-EPOXYCY-CLOHEXANE ◇ 3-(EPOXYETHYL)-7-OXABICY-CLO(4.1.0)HEPTANE ◇ 3-(1,2-EPOXYETHYL)-7-OXA-BICYCLO(4.1.0)HEPTANE ◇ 4-(1,2-EPOXYETHYL)-7-OXABICYCLO(4.1.0)HEPTANE ◇ 4-(EPOXYETHYL)-7-OXABICYCLO(4.1.0)HEPTANE ◇ ERLA-2270 ◇ ERLA-2271 ◇ 1-ETHYLENEOXY-3,4-EPOXYCYCLOHEXANE ◇ NCI-C60139 ◇ 3-OXIRANYL-7-OXABICYCLO(4.1.0)HEPTENE ◇ UCET TEXTILE FINISH 11-74 (OBS.) ◇ UNOX EPOXIDE 206 ◇ VINYL CYCLOHEXENE DIEPOXIDE ◇ 4-VINYLCY-CLOHEXENE DIEPOXIDE ◇ 4-VINYL-1-CYCLOHEXENE DI-EPOXIDE ◇ 4-VINYL-1,2-CYCLOHEXENE DIEPOXIDE ◇ 1-VINYL-3-CYCLOHEXENE DIOXIDE ◇ 4-VINLYCYCLO-HEXENE DIOXIDE ◇ 4-VINYL-1-CYCLOHEXENE DIOXIDE (MAK)

TOXICITY DATA with REFERENCE
CAR: skn-mus TDLo:56 g/kg/47W-I   JNCIAM 31,41,63
ETA: ipr-rat TDLo:5000 mg/kg/10W-I   BJPCAL 6,235,51
ETA: skn-mus TD:12 g/kg/9W-I   BJPCAL6,235,51
ETA: skn-mus TD:90 g/kg/74W-I   AIHAAP 24,305,63
ETA: unr-mus TDLo:2800 mg/kg   RARSAM 3,193,63
MUT: mmo-klp 1 mmol/L   MUREAV 89,269,81
MUT: mmo-smc 25 mmol/L   BSIBAC 56,1803,80
MUT: mrc-smc 25 mmol/L   BSIBAC 56,1803,80

CONSENSUS REPORTS: IARC Cancer Review: GROUP 3 IMEMDT 7,56,87; Animal Sufficient Evidence IMEMDT 11,141,76. Reported in EPA TSCA Inventory.

OSHA PEL: TWA 10 ppm (skin)   ACGIH TLV: TWA 10 ppm (skin); Suspected Human Carcinogen.   DFG MAK: Animal Carcinogen, Suspected Human Carcinogen.

SAFETY PROFILE: Confirmed carcinogen with experimental carcinogenic and tumorigenic data. Poison by unspecified route. Moderately toxic by ingestion and skin contact. Mildly toxic by inhalation. Mutation data reported. A severe skin irritant. Combustible when exposed to heat or flame. To fight fire, use water, foam, dry chemical. When heated to decomposition it emits acrid smoke and irritating fumes.

XDJ000   CAS: 298-81-7
XANTHOTOXIN
mf: $C_{12}H_8O_4$ mw: 216.20

SYNS: AMMOIDIN ◇ 6-HYDROXY-7-METHOXY-5-BEN-ZOFURANACRYLIC ACID Δ-LACTONE ◇ MELADININ ◇ MELADININE ◇ MELOXINE ◇ METHOXA-DOME ◇ METHOXSALEN ◇ 8-METHOXY-(FURANO-3'.2':6.7-COU-MARIN) ◇ 9-METHOXY-7H-FURO(3,2-g)BENZOPYRAN-7-ONE ◇ 8-METHOXY-2',3',6,7-FUROCOUMARIN ◇ 8-ME-THOXY-4',5',6,7-FUROCOUMARIN ◇ 8-METHOXYPSORA-LEN ◇ 9-METHOXYPSORALEN ◇ 8-MOP ◇ 8-MP ◇ NCI-C55903 ◇ OXSORALEN ◇ OXYPSORALEN ◇ PRORALONE-MOP

TOXICITY DATA with REFERENCE
MUT: cyt-hmn:lym 100 μmol/L   PLMEAA 42,333,81

MUT: dnd-esc 20 μmol/L   CBINA8 21,103,78
MUT: dnd-mam:lym 20 μmol/L   CBINA8
  21,103,78
MUT: dnd-omi 20 μmol/L   CBINA8 21,103,78
MUT: dnd-sal:spr 20 μmol/L   CBINA8 21,103,78
MUT: dns-rat:lvr 100 μmol/L   ENMUDM 3,11,81
MUT: msc-mus:lym 20 mg/L   CEDEDE 5,147,80
MUT: sce-hmn:lym 100 μmol/L   PLMEAA
  42,333,81

CONSENSUS REPORTS: IARC Cancer Review: GROUP 1 IMEMDT 7,243,87; Human Inadequate Evidence IMEMDT 24,101,80; Animal Inadequate Evidence IMEMDT 24,101,80. Reported in EPA TSCA Inventory. EPA Genetic Toxicology Program.

SAFETY PROFILE: Confirmed carcinogen. Poison by intraperitoneal route. Moderately toxic by ingestion and subcutaneous routes. Human mutation data reported. When heated to decomposition it emits acrid smoke and irritating fumes. A drug used to treat skin diseases.

ZDJ000   CAS: 1303-39-5
ZINC ARSENATE
DOT: 1712
mf: $As_4O_{15} \cdot 5Zn$ mw: 866.53

PROP: White, odorless powder.

SYNS: ARSENIC ACID, ZINC SALT ◇ ZINC ARSENATE, BASIC ◇ ZINC ARSENATE, SOLID (DOT)

CONSENSUS REPORTS: Arsenic and its compounds, as well as zinc and its compounds, are on the Community Right-To-Know List.

OSHA PEL: TWA 0.01 mg(As)/m^3; Cancer Hazard NIOSH REL: CL 0.002 mg(As)/m^3/15M   DOT Classification: Poison B; Label: Poison.

SAFETY PROFILE: Confirmed human carcinogen. A poison. When heated to decomposition it emits toxic fumes of As and ZnO.

ZDS000   CAS: 10326-24-6
ZINC-m-ARSENITE
DOT: 1712
mf: $AsHO_2 \cdot 1/2Zn$ mw: 140.61

PROP: A white powder.

SYNS: ARSENIOUS ACID, ZINC SALT ◇ ZINC ARSENITE, SOLID (DOT) ◇ ZINC METAARSENITE ◇ ZINC METHARSENITE ◇ ZMA

CONSENSUS REPORTS: Arsenic and its compounds, as well as zinc and its compounds, are on the Community Right-To-Know List.

OSHA PEL: TWA 0.01 mg(As)/m^3: Cancer Hazard   ACGIH TLV: TWA 0.2 mg(As)/m^3 NIOSH REL: (Inorganic Arsenic) CL 0.002 mg(As)/m^3/15M   DOT Classification: Poison B; Label: Poison.

SAFETY PROFILE: Confirmed human carcinogen. A poison. When heated to decomposition it emits toxic fumes of As and ZnO.

ZFJ100   CAS: 13530-65-9
ZINC CHROMATE
mf: $CrH_2O_4 \cdot Zn$ mw: 183.39

SYNS: BASIC ZINC CHROMATE ◇ BUTTERCUP YELLOW ◇ CHROMIC ACID, ZINC SALT ◇ CHROMIUM ZINC OXIDE ◇ C.I. 77955 ◇ C.I. PIGMENT YELLOW 36 ◇ CITRON YELLOW ◇ C.P. ZINC YELLOW X-883 ◇ PRIMROSE YELLOW ◇ PURE ZINC CHROME ◇ ZINC CHROMATE(VI) HYDROXIDE ◇ ZINC CHROME YELLOW ◇ ZINC CHROMIUM OXIDE ◇ ZINC HYDROXYCHROMATE ◇ ZINC TETRAOXYCHROMATE 76A ◇ ZINC YELLOW

TOXICITY DATA with REFERENCE
CAR: ihl-man TCLo:5 mg/m^3/8H/7Y-I:PUL
  BJIMAG 32,62,75
CAR: imp-rat TDLo:12928 μg/kg   BJIMAG
  43,243,86
ETA: scu-rat TDLo:135 mg/kg   PBPHAW 14,47,78
MUT: cyt-ham:ovr 5 mg/L   BJCAAI 44,219,81
MUT: mma-sat 1600 ng/plate   MUREAV 156,219,85
MUT: mmo-sat 800 ng/plate   MUREAV 156,219,85
MUT: oms-ham:kdy 50 mg/L   BJCAAI 44,219,81
MUT: oms-hmn:oth 500 mg/L   BJCAAI 44,219,81
MUT: sce-ham:ovr 100 μg/L   MUREAV 156,219,85

CONSENSUS REPORTS: IARC Cancer Review: Human Sufficient Evidence IMEMDT 23,205,80; Animal Sufficient Evidence IMEMDT 23,205,80. NTP Fourth Annual Report On Carcinogens, 1984. EPA Genetic Toxicology Program. Reported in EPA TSCA Inventory. Zinc and chromium and their compounds, are on the Community Right-To-Know List.

OSHA PEL: (Transitional: 1 mg(CrO$_3$)/10m^3) CL 0.1 mg(CrO$_3$)/m^3 ACGIH TLV: TWA 0.01 mg(Cr)/M^3; Confirmed Human Carcinogen   DFG TRK: 0.1 mg/m^3; Human Carcinogen.   NIOSH REL: (Chromium (VI)) TWA 0.001 mg(Cr(VI))/m^3

SAFETY PROFILE: Confirmed human carcinogen producing lung tumors. A poison via in travenous route. Human mutation data reported.

ZFJ120   CAS: 37300-23-5
ZINC CHROMATE with ZINC HYDROXIDE and CHROMIUM OXIDE (9:1)
mf: $CrO_4 \cdot Zn \cdot H_4O_2Zn \cdot CrO_3$ mw: 183.39

SYN: ZINC YELLOW

TOXICITY DATA with REFERENCE
MUT: mmo-sat 90 nmol/plate   CRNGDP
   2,283,81

CONSENSUS REPORTS: Reported in EPA TSCA Inventory.

OSHA PEL: (Transitional: 1 $mg(CrO_3)/10m^3$) CL 0.1 $mg(CrO_3)/m^3$ ACGIH TLV: TWA 0.01 $mg(Cr)/M^3$; Confirmed Human Carcinogen DFG TRK: 0.1 mg/m^3; Human Carcinogen. NIOSH REL: (Chromium (VI)) TWA 0.001 $mg(Cr(VI))/m^3$

SAFETY PROFILE: Confirmed human carcinogen producing lung tumors. Mutation data reported.

ZFJ150
ZINC CHROMATE, POTASSIUM DICHROMATE and ZINC HYDROXIDE (3:1:1)
mf: $CrK_2O_4 \cdot 3CrO_4Zn \cdot H_2O_2Zn$ mw: 837.70

SYN: POTASSIUM DICHROMATE, ZINC CHROMATE and ZINC HYDROXIDE (1:3:1)

TOXICITY DATA with REFERENCE
CAR: imp-rat TDLo: 8 mg/kg   CRNGDP 7,831,86

OSHA PEL: (Transitional: 1 $mg(CrO_3)/10m^3$) CL 0.1 $mg(CrO_3)/m^3$ ACGIH TLV: TWA 0.01 $mg(Cr)/M^3$; Confirmed Human Carcinogen DFG TRK: 0.1 mg/m^3; Human Carcinogen. NIOSH REL: (Chromium (VI)) TWA 0.001 $mg(Cr(VI))/m^3$

SAFETY PROFILE: Confirmed human carcinogen with experimental carcinogenic data.

ZJA000   CAS: 22323-45-1
ZINC MERCURY CHROMATE COMPLEX
mf: $7ZnO \cdot 2HgO \cdot 2CrO_3 \cdot 7H_2O$ mw: 1328.91

SYNS: CHROMIC ACID, MERCURY ZINC COMPLEX
◇ EXPERIMENTAL FUNGICIDE 224 (UNION CARBIDE)
◇ MERCURY ZINC CHROMATE COMPLEX

CONSENSUS REPORTS: Zinc, mercury, chromium and their compounds are on the Community Right-To-Know List.

OSHA PEL: (Transitional: 1 $mg/10m^3$) CL 0.1 $mg(CrO_3)/m^3$ ACGIH TLV: TWA 0.05 $mg(Cr)/m^3$, Confirmed Human Carcinogen. DFG MAK: Animal Carcinogen, Suspected Human Carcinogen. NIOSH REL: TWA 0.025 $mg(Cr(VI))/m^3$; CL 0.05/15M; 0.05 $mg(Hg)/m^3$

SAFETY PROFILE: Confirmed carcinogen. Moderately toxic by ingestion. When heated to decomposition it emits very toxic fumes of Hg and ZnO.

Class II/Suspected Carcinogens

AAG250
ACETALDEHYDE
CAS: 75-07-0

DOT: 1089
mf: C_2H_4O mw: 44.06

PROP: Colorless, fuming liquid; pungent, fruity odor. Mp: −123.5°, bp: 20.8°, lel: 4.0%, uel: 57%, flash p: −36°F (CC), d: 0.804 @ 0°/20°, autoign temp: 347°F, vap d: 1.52. Misc in water, alc, and ether.

SYNS: ACETALDEHYD (GERMAN) ◇ ACETIC ALDEHYDE ◇ ALDEHYDE ACETIQUE (FRENCH) ◇ ALDEIDE ACETICA (ITALIAN) ◇ ETHANAL ◇ ETHYL ALDEHYDE ◇ FEMA No. 2003 ◇ NCI-C56326 ◇ OCTOWY ALDEHYD (POLISH) ◇ RCRA WASTE NUMBER U001

TOXICITY DATA with REFERENCE
CAR: ihl-rat TCLo: 735 ppm/6H/2Y-I   TXCYAC 41,213,86
ETA: ihl-ham TCLo: 2040 ppm/7H/52W-I   EJCAAH 18,13,82
ETA: ihl-rat TCLo: 1410 ppm/6H/65W-I   TXCYAC 31,123,84
MUT: dnd-mam: lym 1 mol/L/30M   MUREAV 58,115,78
MUT: dnr-esc 10 µL/plate   EVHPAZ 21,79,77
MUT: mma-sat 10 µL/plate   EVHPAZ 21,79,77
MUT: sce-ham: cvr 5 ppm/9D   MUREAV 56,211,77
MUT: sce-hmn: ipr 500 µg/kg   MUREAV 88,389,81

CONSENSUS REPORTS: IARC Cancer Review: GROUP 2B IMEMDT 7,77,87; Animal Sufficient Evidence IMEMDT 36,101,85; Human Inadequate Evidence IMEMDT 36,101,85. On Community Right-To-Know List. Reported in EPA TSCA Inventory. EPA Genetic Toxicology Program.

OSHA PEL: (Transitional: TWA 200 ppm) TWA 100 ppm; STEL 150 ppm   ACGIH TLV: TWA 100 ppm; STEL 150 ppm   DFG MAK: 50 ppm (90 mg/m³), Suspected Carcinogen. DOT Classification: Flammable Liquid; LABEL: Flammable Liquid

SAFETY PROFILE: Suspected carcinogen with experimental carcinogenic and tumorigenic data. Poison by intratracheal and intravenous routes. A human systemic irritant by inhalation. A narcotic. Human mutation data reported. An experimental teratogen. Other experimental reproductive effects. A skin and severe eye irritant. A common air contaminant. Highly flammable liquid. When heated to decomposition it emits acrid smoke and fumes.

AAI000
ACETAMIDE
CAS: 60-35-5

mf: C_2H_5NO mw: 59.08

PROP: Colorless crystals; mousey odor. Mp: 81°, bp: 221.2°, d: 1.159 @ 20°/4°, vap press: 1 mm @ 65°. Decomp in hot water.

SYNS: ACETIC ACID AMIDE ◇ ACETIMIDIC ACID ◇ AMID KYSELINY OCTOVE ◇ ETHANAMIDE ◇ METHANECARBOXAMIDE ◇ NCI-C02108

TOXICITY DATA with REFERENCE
CAR: orl-mus TDLo: 517 g/kg/1Y-C   JEPTDQ 3(5-6),149,80
CAR: orl-rat TDLo: 431 g/kg/1Y-C   JEPTDQ 3(5-6),149,80
NEO: orl-rat TD: 546 g/kg/52W-C   TXAPA9 14,163,69
MUT: oms-mus/ast 10 pph   IDZAAW 51,53,76
MUT: otr-ham: emb 1 mg/L   IJCNAW 19,642,77

CONSENSUS REPORTS: IARC Cancer Review: GROUP 2B IMEMDT 7,56,87; Animal Sufficient Evidence IMEMDT 7,389,87. On Community Right-To-Know List. Reported in EPA TSCA Inventory.

DFG MAK: Suspected Carcinogen.

SAFETY PROFILE: Suspected carcinogen with experimental carcinogenic, neoplastigenic, and teratogenic data. Moderately toxic by intraperitoneal and possibly other routes. Other experimental reproductive effects. Mutation data reported. When heated to decomposition it emits toxic fumes of NO_x.

AAL750   CAS: 531-82-8
2-ACETAMIDO-4-(5-NITRO-2-FURYL)THIAZOLE
mf: $C_9H_7N_3O_4S$ mw: 253.25

SYNS: 2-ACETAMINO-4-(5-NITRO-2-FURYL)THIAZOLE ◇ 2-ACETYLAMINO-4-(5-NITRO-2- FURYL)THIAZOLE ◇ N-(4-(5-NITRO-2-FURANYL)-2-THIAZOLYL)ACETAMIDE ◇ N-(4-(5-NITRO-2-FURYL)-2-THIAZOLYL)ACETAMIDE ◇ N-(4-(5-NITRO-2-FURYL)THIAZOL-2-YL)ACETAMIDE

TOXICITY DATA with REFERENCE
CAR: orl-ham TDLo: 26 g/kg/48W-C   JNCIAM 51,941,73
CAR: orl-mus TD: 12 g/kg/14W-C   CNREA8 33,1593,73
CAR: orl-mus TD: 6000 mg/kg/14W-C   CNREA8 38,1398,78
CAR: orl-mus TDLo: 2400 mg/kg/14W-C   CNREA8 30,2320,70
CAR: orl-rat TDLo: 43 g/kg/46W-C   CNREA8 30,936,70
NEO: orl-rat TD: 47 g/kg/46W-C   JNCIAM 54,841,75
NEO: orl-rat TD: 52 g/kg/46W-C   JNCIAM 54,841,75
ETA: orl-dog TDLo: 27 g/kg/2Y-C   JNCIAM 45,535,70
MUT: dnr-sat 500 nmol/well   CNREA8 34,2266,74
MUT: mma-sat 100 ng/plate   MUREAV 40,9,76
MUT: mmo-esc 300 nmol/well   CNREA8 34,2266,74
MUT: mrc-esc 500 nmol/well   CNREA8 34,2266,74

CONSENSUS REPORTS: IARC Cancer Review: GROUP 2B IMEMDT 7,56,87; Animal Sufficient Evidence IMEMDT 1,181,72; IMEMDT 7,185,74

SAFETY PROFILE: Suspected carcinogen with experimental carcinogenic, neoplastigenic, and tumorigenic data. Mutation data reported. When heated to decomposition it emits very toxic fumes of SO_x and NO_x.

AAQ250   CAS: 2832-40-8
ACETAMINE YELLOW CG
mf: $C_{15}H_{15}N_3O_2$ mw: 269.33

SYNS: ACTIOQUINONE LIGHT YELLOW ◇ AMACEL YELLOW G ◇ CALCOSYN YELLOW GC ◇ CELLITON FAST YELLOW G ◇ C.I. 11855 ◇ CIBACET YELLOW GBA ◇ C.I. DISPERSE YELLOW 3 ◇ HISPERSE YELLOW G ◇ N-(4-((2-HYDROXY-5-METHYLPHENYL)AZO)PHENYL)ACETAMIDE

◇ 4'-((6-HYDROXY-m-TOLYL)AZO)ACETANILIDE ◇ INTRASPERSE YELLOW GBA EXTRA ◇ MICROSETILE YELLOW GR ◇ NACELAN FAST YELLOW CG ◇ NCI-C53781 ◇ YELLOW Z

TOXICITY DATA with REFERENCE
CAR: orl-mus TDLo: 433 g/kg/2Y-C   NTPTR* NTP-TR-222,82
CAR: orl-rat TD: 216 g/kg/2Y-C   NTPTR* NTP-TR-222,82
CAR: orl-rat TDLo: 180 g/kg/2Y-C   NTPTR* NTP-TR-222,82
ETA: orl-mus TD: 216 g/kg/2Y-C   NTPTR* NTP-TR-222,82
MUT: cyt-frg-par 2800 μL/7D   CYTBAI 25,175,79

CONSENSUS REPORTS: Community Right-To-Know List. Reported in EPA TSCA Inventory. IARC Cancer Review: Animal Inadequate Evidence IMEMDT 8,97,75; NTP Carcinogenesis Bioassay (feed); Clear Evidence: mouse, rat NTPTR* NTP-TR-222,82

SAFETY PROFILE: Suspected carcinogen with experimental tumorigenic and carcinogenic data. An allergen. Mutation data reported. When heated to decomposition it emits toxic fumes of NO_x.

AAW000   CAS: 56856-83-8
ACETIC ACID METHYLNITROSAMINOMETHYL ESTER
mf: $C_4H_8N_2O_3$ mw: 132.14

SYNS: α-ACETOXY DIMETHYLNITROSAMINE ◇ N-α-ACETOXYMETHYL-N-METHYLNITROSAMINE ◇ ACETOXYMETHYL-METHYL-NITROSAMIN (GERMAN) ◇ ACETOXYMETHYL METHYLNITROSAMINE ◇ 1-ACETOXY-N-NITROSODIMETHYLAMINE ◇ AMMN ◇ ANN (GERMAN) ◇ DMN-OAC ◇ MAMN ◇ METHYL(ACETOXYMETHYL)NITROSAMINE ◇ N-NITROSO-N-(ACETOXY)METHYL-N-METHYLAMINE ◇ N-NITROSO-N-METHYL-N-ACETOXYMETHYLAMINE

TOXICITY DATA with REFERENCE
CAR: ipr-rat TD: 13 mg/kg   CNREA8 39,1462,79
CAR: ipr-rat TD: 13 mg/kg   JJIND8 63,93,79
CAR: ipr-rat TDLo: 13 mg/kg   JJIND8 63,93,79
CAR: orl-ham TDLo: 20 mg/kg/21W-I   JJIND8 73,737,84
CAR: orl-rat TD: 70 mg/kg/20W-I   ZEKBAI 85,47,76
CAR: orl-rat TDLo: 13 mg/kg   JJIND8 63,93,79
CAR: rec-rat TDLo: 112 mg/kg/16W-I   ZKKOBW 92,105,78
CAR: scu-rat TD: 50 mg/kg/10W-I   IAPUDO 41,619,82

CAR: scu-rat TDLo:50 mg/kg/10W-I   JCROD7
104,13,82

NEO: ipr-rat TD:13 mg/kg   PAACA3 16,32,75
NEO: ipr-rat TD:13 mg/kg   VTPHAK 16,574,79
ETA: ihl-rat TCLo:2600 µg/m^3/5H/7W-I
TXCYAC 27,139,83

ETA: ivn-rat TD:90 mg/kg/37W-I   ZEKBAI
91,217,78

ETA: ivn-rat TDLo:13 mg/kg   JJIND8 63,93,79

ETA: orl-rat TD:60 mg/kg/90D-I   ZKKOBW
91,317,78

ETA: rec-rat TD:20 mg/kg/10W-I   JCROD7
104,115,82

ETA: rec-rat TD:20 mg/kg/10W-I   TJEMAO
144,237,84

ETA: rec-rat TDLo:12 mg/kg/46W-I   HEGAD4
30,30,83

MUT: cyt-dmg-par 100 µmol/L   CNREA8
35,3780,75

MUT: cyt-hmn:hla 10 µmol/L   TXCYAC 9,21,78

MUT: dnr-bcs 500 nmol/plate   GANNA2 70,663,79

MUT: mmo-esc 25 µmol/plate   GANNA2 70,663,79

MUT: mmo-sat 5 µmol/plate   GANNA2 70,663,79

MUT: msc-ham:lng 100 µmol/L   GANNA2
72,531,81

MUT: oms-omi 3 mmol/L   CBINA8 14,1,76

MUT: sln-dmg-par 100 µmol/L   CBINA8 14,21,76

MUT: slt-dmg-par 100 µmol/L   CNREA835,3780,75

SAFETY PROFILE: Suspected carcinogen with experimental carcinogenic, neoplastigenic, tumorigenic and teratogenic data. Poison by ingestion, subcutaneous, intravenous, and intraperitoneal routes. Human mutation data reported. When heated to decomposition it emits toxic fumes of NO$_x$.

AAX175   CAS: 9003-22-9
ACETIC ACID, VINYL ESTER, POLYMER with CHLOROETHYLENE
mf: $(C_4H_6O_2 \cdot C_2H_3Cl)n$

SYNS: ACETIC ACID ETHENYL ESTER POLYMER with CHLORETHENE (9CI) ◇ A 15 (POLYMER) ◇ BAKELITE LP 70 ◇ BAKELITE VLFV ◇ BAKELITE VMCC ◇ BAKELITE VYNS ◇ BREON 351 ◇ CHLOROETHYLENEVINYL ACETATE POLYMER ◇ CORVIC 236581 ◇ DENKALAC 61 ◇ DIAMOND SHAMROCK 744 ◇ EXON 450 ◇ EXON 454 ◇ GEON 135 ◇ HOSTAFLEX VP 150 ◇ LEUCOVYL PA 1302 ◇ NORVINYL P 6 ◇ OPALON 400 ◇ PLIOVAC AO ◇ POLYVINYL CHLORIDE-POLYVINYL ACETATE ◇ PVC CORDO ◇ RHODOPAS 6000 ◇ SARPIFAN HP 1 ◇ SCONATEX ◇ SOLVIC 523KC ◇ SUMILIT PCX ◇ TENNUS 0565 ◇ TYGON ◇ VAGD ◇ VINNOL H 10/60 ◇ VINYL ACETATE-VINYL CHLORIDE COPOLYMER ◇ VINYL ACETATE-VINYL CHLORIDE

POLYMER ◇ VINYL CHLORIDE-VINYL ACETATE POLYMER ◇ VINYLITE VYDR 21 ◇ VLVF ◇ VMCC ◇ VYNW

TOXICITY DATA with REFERENCE
ETA: imp-mus TDLo:1200 mg/kg   JNCIAM
58,1443,77

CONSENSUS REPORTS: IARC Cancer Review: Animal Limited Evidence IMEMDT 19,377,79. Reported in EPA TSCA Inventory.

SAFETY PROFILE: Suspected carcinogen with experimental tumorigenic data. When heated to decomposition it emits toxic fumes of HCl.

ABU000   CAS: 51-98-9
17-ACETOXY-19-NOR-17-α-PREGN-4-EN-20-YN-3-ONE
mf: $C_{22}H_{28}O_3$ mw: 340.50

SYNS: 17-β-ACETOXY-19-NOR-17-α-PREGN-4-EN-20-YN-3-ONE ◇ (17-α)-17-(ACETYLOXY)-19-NORPREGN-4-EN-20-YN-3-ONE ◇ 17-ACETYLOXY(17-α)-19-NORPREGN-4-ES-TREN-17-β-OL-ACETATE-3-ONE ◇ 17-ENT ◇ 17-α-ETHINYL-19-NORTESTOSTERONE ACETATE ◇ 17-α-ETHINYL-19-NORTESTOSTERONE-17-β-ACETATE ◇ 17-α-ETHYNYL-17-β-ACETOXY-19-NORANDROST-4-EN-3-ONE ◇ 17-α-ETHYNYL-17-HYDROXYESTR-4-EN-3-ONE ACETATE ◇ 17-α-ETHYNYL-19-NORTESTOSTERONE ACETATE ◇ 17-HY-DROXY-19-NOR-17-α-PREGN-4-EN-20-YN-3-ONE ACETATE ◇ 17-β-HYDROXY-19-NOR-17-α-PREGN-4-EN-20-YN-3-ONE ACETATE ◇ NORETHINDRONE-17-ACETATE ◇ 19-NOR-ETHISTERONE ACETATE ◇ 19-NORETHYNYLTESTOSTER-ONE ACETATE ◇ NORETHYSTERONE ACETATE ◇ NORLUTATE ◇ NORLUTINE ACETATE ◇ ORLUTATE

TOXICITY DATA with REFERENCE
ETA: orl-rat TDLo:303 µg/kg/2Y-C   JTEHD6
6,895,80

MUT: dlt-mus-orl 1120 mg/kg/4W   MUREAV
26,535,74

MUT: spm-mus-orl 11200 mg/kg/4W   MUREAV
26,535,74

CONSENSUS REPORTS: IARC Cancer Review: Animal Limited Evidence IMEMDT 21,441,79; Animal Sufficient Evidence IMEMDT 6,179,74 EPA Genetic Toxicology Program.

SAFETY PROFILE: Suspected carcinogen with experimental tumorigenic and teratogenic data. Human reproductive effects by ingestion and implant routes: menstrual cycle changes, postpartum effects and changes in fertility. A human teratogen by an unspecified route with developmental abnormalities of the urogenital system.

Other experimental animal reproductive effects. Mutation data reported. When heated to decomposition it emits acrid smoke and irritating fumes. Used in the treatment of menstrual disorders and uterine bleeding.

AEW500
AFLATOXIN Ro
CAS: 29611-03-8

mf: $C_{17}H_{14}O_6$ mw: 314.31

SYN: AFLATOXICOL

TOXICITY DATA with REFERENCE
CAR: orl-rat TDLo: 1092 g/kg/1Y-C   JJIND8 66,1159,81

MUT: mma-sat 25 ng/plate   PNASA6 73,2241,76

SAFETY PROFILE: Suspected carcinogen with experimental carcinogenic data. Mutation data reported. When heated to decomposition it emits acrid smoke and irritating fumes.

AFM250
ALIPHATIC and AROMATIC EPOXIDES

SAFETY PROFILE: Suspected carcinogen with experimental tumors of the skin, lung, and blood-forming tissues.

AGB250
ALLYL CHLORIDE
CAS: 107-05-1

DOT: 1100
mf: C_3H_5Cl mw: 76.53

PROP: Colorless liquid. Mp: $-136.4°$, bp: 44.6°, d: 0.938 @ 20°/4°, flash p: $-25°F$, lel: 2.9%, uel: 11.2%, autoign temp: 905°F, vap d: 2.64. Solubility = <0.1 in water.

SYNS: ALLILE (CLORURO DI) (ITALIAN) ◊ ALLYLCHLORID (GERMAN) ◊ ALLYLE (CHLORURE D') (FRENCH) ◊ CHLORALLYLENE ◊ CHLOROALLYLENE ◊ 3-CHLOROPRENE ◊ 3-CHLORO-1-PROPENE ◊ 3-CHLOROPROPENE ◊ 1-CHLORO PROPENE-2 ◊ 1-CHLORO-2-PROPENE ◊ α-CHLOROPROPYLENE ◊ 3-CHLORO-1-PROPYLENE ◊ 3-CHLOROPROPYLENE ◊ 3-CHLORPROPEN (GERMAN) ◊ 2-PROPENYL CHLORIDE ◊ NCI-C04615

TOXICITY DATA with REFERENCE
ETA: ipr-mus TDLo: 5880 mg/kg/8W-I   CNREA8 39,391,79

ETA: orl-mus TD: 78 g/kg/78W-I   NCITR* NCI-CG-TR-73,78

ETA: orl-mus TDLo: 50 g/kg/78W-I   NCITR* NCI-CG-TR-73,78

MUT: mmo-esc 20 μL/plate   MUREAV 153,57,85

MUT: mmo-omi 10 μL/plate   CBINA8 30,9,80

CONSENSUS REPORTS: IARC Cancer Review: Animal Inadequate Evidence IMEMDT 36,39,85; NCI Carcinogenesis Bioassay (gavage); No Evidence: rat NCITR* NCI-CG-TR-73,78; Clear Evidence: mouse NCITR* NCI-CG-TR-73,78. Reported in EPA TSCA Inventory. EPA Genetic Toxicology Program. Community Right-To-Know List.

OSHA PEL: (Transitional: TWA 1 ppm) TWA 1 ppm; STEL 2 ppm   ACGIH TLV: TWA 1 ppm; STEL 2 ppm   DFG MAK: 1 ppm (3 mg/m^3), Suspected Carcinogen.   NIOSH REL: TWA 1 ppm; CL 3 ppm/15M   DOT Classification: Flammable Liquid; Label: Flammable Liquid.

SAFETY PROFILE: Suspected carcinogen with experimental tumorigenic and teratogenic data. Poison by ingestion, intraperitoneal, and intravenous routes. Moderately toxic by inhalation and skin contact. Experimental reproductive effects. Human mutation data reported. A skin, eye, and mucous membrane irritant. Chronic exposure may cause liver and kidney damage. The vapors of allyl chloride are quite irritating to the eyes, nose, and throat. Dangerous fire and explosion hazard when exposed to heat, flame or oxidizers. To fight fire, use CO_2, alcohol foam, dry chemical.

AGJ250
ALLYL ISOTHIOCYANATE
CAS: 57-06-7

DOT: 1545
mf: C_4H_5NS mw: 99.16

PROP: Colorless to pale yellow liquid; irritating odor with mustard taste. Mp: $-80°$, bp: 150.7°, flash p: 115°F, d: 1.013-1.016 @ 25°/25°, vap press: 10 mm @ 38.3°, vap d: 3.41, refr index: 1.527-1.531. Misc with alc, carbon disulfide, and ether.

SYNS: AITC ◊ ALLYL ISORHODANIDE ◊ ALLYL ISOSULFOCYANATE ◊ ALLYL ISOTHIOCYANATE, stabilized (DOT) ◊ ALLYL MUSTARD OIL ◊ ALLYLSENFOEL (GERMAN) ◊ ALLYL SEVENOLUM ◊ ALLYL THIOCARBONIMIDE ◊ ARTIFICIAL MUSTARD OIL ◊ CARBOSPOL ◊ FEMA No. 2034 ◊ ISOTHIOCYANATE d'ALLYLE (FRENCH) ◊ 3-ISOTHIOCYANATO-1-PROPENE ◊ MUSTARD OIL ◊ NCI-C50464 ◊ OIL of MUSTARD, ARTIFICIAL ◊ OLEUM SINAPIS VOLATILE ◊ 2-PROPENYL ISOTHIOCYANATE ◊ REDSKIN ◊ SENF OEL (GERMAN) ◊ SYNTHETIC MUSTARD OIL ◊ VOLATILE OIL of MUSTARD

TOXICITY DATA with REFERENCE

NEO: orl-rat TDLo: 12875 mg/kg/2Y-I   NTPTR*
NTP-TR-234,82

MUT: cyt-ham: fbr 4 mg/L   FCTOD7 22,623,84

MUT: mma-esc 5 mmol/L   FOMIAZ 27,25,82

MUT: mma-sat 1 μmol/plate   CBINA8 38,303,82

MUT: mmo-esc 5 μg/plate   KEKHB8 (9),11,79

MUT: mmo-sat 100 μg/plate   ABCHA6 44,4017,80

MUT: otr-ham: fbr 5 nmol/L   JTSCDR 10,177,85

MUT: sln-dmg-ihl: 100 ppm/8M   PREBA3
62B,284,46,47

CONSENSUS REPORTS: IARC Cancer Review: Animal Limited Evidence IMEMDT 36,55,85; NTP Carcinogenesis Bioassay (gavage); No Evidence: mouse NTPTR* NTP-TR-234,82; Clear Evidence: rat NTPTR* NTP-TR-234,82. Reported in EPA TSCA Inventory.

SAFETY PROFILE: Suspected carcinogen with experimental neoplastigenic, tumorigenic, and teratogenic data. Poison by ingestion, skin contact, intravenous, subcutaneous, and intraperitoneal routes. Other experimental reproductive effects. An allergen. May cause contact dermatitis. Mutation data reported. Combustible liquid. To fight fire, use foam, CO_2, dry chemical.

AHK500   CAS: 50-07-7
AMETYCIN
mf: $C_{15}H_{18}N_4O_5$ mw: 334.37

SYNS: 7-AMINO-9-α-METHOXYMITOSANE ◇ MIT-C ◇ MITO-C ◇ MITOCIN-C ◇ MITOMYCIN ◇ MITOMYCIN-C ◇ MITOMYCINUM ◇ MMC ◇ MUTAMYCIN ◇ MUTAMYCIN (MITOMYCIN for INJECTION) ◇ MYTOMYCIN ◇ NCI-C04706 ◇ NSC 26980 ◇ RCRA WASTE NUMBER U010

TOXICITY DATA with REFERENCE

CAR: ivn-rat TDLo: 2600 μg/kg/8W-I   ARZNAD
20,1461,70

CAR: scu-mus TDLo: 280 μg/kg/18W-I
APHGBP 17,495,67

NEO: ipr-rat TDLo: 3000 μg/kg/26W-I   RRCRBU
52,1,75

MUT: cyt-hmn: fbr 100 μg/L   TRBMAV 27,409,69

MUT: cyt-hmn: hla 10 μmol/L   TXCYAC 51,181,65

MUT: cyt-hmn: leu 100 μg/L/24H   GENTAE
51,181,65

MUT: sce-hmn: leu 100 μg/L   GENTAE 9,21,78

CONSENSUS REPORTS: IARC Cancer Review: GROUP 2B IMEMDT 7,56,87; Animal Sufficient Evidence IMEMDT 10,171,76; NCI Carcinogenesis Studies (ipr); Clear Evidence:

rat RRCRBU 52,1,75; No Evidence: mouse RRCRBU 52,1,75. EPA Extremely Hazardous Substances List. EPA Genetic Toxicology Program. Reported in EPA TSCA Inventory.

SAFETY PROFILE: Suspected carcinogen with experimental carcinogenic, neoplastigenic, and teratogenic data. Poison by ingestion, subcutaneous, intravenous, and intraperitoneal routes. Human systemic effects by intravenous route: dyspnea and lung fibrosis. Experimental reproductive effects. Human mutation data reported. When heated to decomposition it emits toxic fumes of NO_x.

AJD750   CAS: 26148-68-5
AMINO-α-CARBOLINE
mf: $C_{11}H_9N_3$ mw: 183.2

SYNS: 2-AMINO-α-CARBOLINE ◇ 2-AMINO-9H-PYRIDO(2,3-B)INDOLE

TOXICITY DATA with REFERENCE

CAR: orl-mus TD: 41400 mg/kg/98W-C
EVHPAZ 67,129,86

CAR: orl-mus TD: 44712 mg/kg/89W-C
CRNGDP 5,815,84

CAR: orl-mus TD: 50424 mg/kg/82W-C
CRNGDP 5,815,84

CAR: orl-mus TDLo: 37600 mg/kg/98W-C
EVHPAZ 67,129,86

MUT: dnr-bcs 10 uL/plate   ABCHA6 45,2031,81

MUT: mma-sat 1 μg/plate   CALEDQ 10,141,80

MUT: sce-hmn: lym 4000 μg/L   MUREAV 77,65,80

MUT: slt-dmg-orl 400 ng/kg   JJCREP 76,468,85

CONSENSUS REPORTS: Cancer Review: GROUP 2B IMEMDT 7,56,87; Animal Sufficient Evidence IMEMDT 40,245,86

SAFETY PROFILE: Suspected carcinogen with experimental carcinogenic data. Human mutation data reported. When heated to decomposition it emits toxic fumes of NO_x.

AJQ675   CAS: 77500-04-0
2-AMINO-3,8-DIMETHYLIMIDAZO(4,5-f)
QUINOXALINE
mf: $C_{11}H_{11}N_5$ mw: 213.27

SYNS: 2-AMINO-3,8-DIMETHYL-3H-IMIDAZO(4,5-f)QUINOXALINE ◇ 3,8-DIMETHYL-3H-IMIDAZO(4,5-f)QUINOXALIN-2-AMINE

TOXICITY DATA with REFERENCE

CAR: orl-mus TDLo: 42336 mg/kg/84W-C
CRNGDP 8,665,87

CAR: orl-rat TDLo:8580 mg/kg/61W-C
CRNGDP 9,71,88
MUT: mma-sat 5 ng/plate   MUREAV 144,131,85
MUT: msc-ham:ovr 300 mg/L   MUTAEX 2,483,87
MUT: slt-dmg-orl 100 ng/kg   JJCREP 76,468,85

CONSENSUS REPORTS: IARC Cancer Review: GROUP 3 IMEMDT 7,56,87; Animal Inadequate Evidence IMEMDT 40,283,86

SAFETY PROFILE: Suspected carcinogen with experimental carcinogenic data. Mutation data reported. When heated to decomposition it emits toxic fumes of NO_x.

AJR500   CAS: 68808-54-8
3-AMINO-1,4-DIMETHYL-5H-
PYRIDO(4,3-b)INDOLE ACETATE
mf: $C_{13}H_{13}N_3 \cdot C_2H_4O_2$ mw: 271.35

SYN: 1,4-DIMETHYL-5H-PYRIDO(4,3-b)INDOL-3-AMINE ACETATE ◇ 1,4-DIMETHYL-5H-PYRIDO(4,3-b)INDOL-3-AMINE MONOACETATE ◇ TRP-P-1 (ACETATE)

TOXICITY DATA with REFERENCE
CAR: orl-mus TDLo:11 g/kg/89W-C   SCIEAS
213,346,81
CAR: orl-rat TDLo:1539 mg/kg/29W-C
MUT: mma-sat 1 μg/plate   CPBTAL 26,611,78
MUT: slt-dmg-orl 200 ppm   MUREAV 122,315,83

SAFETY PROFILE: Suspected carcinogen with experimental carcinogenic data. Mutation data reported. When heated to decomposition it emits toxic fumes of NO_x.

AJV000   CAS: 132-32-1
3-AMINO-9-ETHYLCARBAZOLE
mf: $C_{14}H_{14}N_2$ mw: 210.30

PROP: In cancer bioassay both free amine and hydrochloride salt used (NCITR* NCI-CG-TR-93,78).

SYN: 3-AMINO-N-ETHYLCARBAZOLE

TOXICITY DATA with REFERENCE
CAR: orl-mus TDLo:87 g/kg/78W-C   NCITR*
NCI-CG-TR-93,78
CAR: orl-rat TDLo:33 g/kg/78W-C   NCITR*
NCI-CG-TR-93,78

CONSENSUS REPORTS: Reported in EPA TSCA Inventory.

DFG MAK: Suspected Carcinogen.

SAFETY PROFILE: Suspected carcinogen with experimental carcinogenic data. Poison by ingestion and intraperitoneal routes. When heated to decomposition it emits toxic fumes of NO_x.

AJV250   CAS: 6109-97-3
3-AMINO-9-
ETHYLCARBAZOLEHYDROCHLORIDE
mf: $C_{14}H_{14}N_2 \cdot ClH$ mw: 246.76

PROP: In cancer bioassay both free amine and hydrochloride salt used (NCITR* NCI-CG-TR-93,78).

SYN: NCI-C03043

TOXICITY DATA with REFERENCE
CAR: orl-mus TDLo:87 g/kg/78W-C   NCITR*
NCI-CG-TR-93,78
CAR: orl-rat TDLo:33 g/kg/78W-C   NCITR*
NCI-CG-TR-93,78
MUT: mma-sat 1 μg/plate   ENMUDM 5(Suppl 1),3,83

CONSENSUS REPORTS: NCI Carcinogenesis Bioassay Completed; Results Positive: mouse, rat (NCITR* NCI-CG-TR-93,78).

SAFETY PROFILE: Suspected carcinogen with experimental carcinogenic data. Poison by ingestion. Mutation data reported. When heated to decomposition it emits very toxic fumes of NO_x and HCl.

AKS250   CAS: 67730-11-4
2-AMINO-6-METHYLDIPYRIDO
(1,2-a:3',2'-d)IMIDAZOLE
mf: $C_{11}H_{10}N_4$ mw: 198.25

SYNS: GLU-P-I ◇ 6-ME-GLU-P-2 ◇ 6-METHYL DIPYRIDO(1,2-a:3',2'-d)IMIDAZOL-2-AMINE

TOXICITY DATA with REFERENCE
CAR: orl-mus TD:17512 mg/kg/57W-C
CRNGDP 5,815,84
CAR: orl-mus TDLo:15200 mg/kg/58W-C
EVHPAZ 67,129,86
CAR: orl-mus TDLo:17212 mg/kg/47W-C
CRNGDP 5,815,84
CAR: orl-rat TDLo:9100 mg/kg/68W-C
EVHPAZ 67,129,86
MUT: dnd-mam:lym 10 μmol/L   BBRCA9
96,611,80
MUT: dnd-mus-ipr 10 mg/kg   JJCREP 76,835,85
MUT: dnd-mus:lvr 50 μmol/L   JJCREP 76,835,85
MUT: mma-sat 250 ng/plate   JJCREP 76,835,85
MUT: msc-ham:lng 250 mg/L   MUREAV 118,91,83
MUT: pic-sat 10 nmol/plate   PPTCBY 9,337,79
MUT: sce-hmn:lym 1000 μg/L   MUREAV 77,65,80

CONSENSUS REPORTS: IARC Cancer Review: GROUP 2B IMEMDT 7,56,87; Animal Sufficient Evidence IMEMDT 40,223,86

SAFETY PROFILE: Suspected carcinogen with experimental carcinogenic data. Human mutation data reported. When heated to decomposition it emits toxic fumes of NO_x.

AKT600   CAS: 76180-96-6
2-AMINO-3-METHYLIMIDAZO (4,5-f)QUINOLINE

mf: $C_{11}H_{10}N_4$ mw: 198.25

TOXICITY DATA with REFERENCE
CAR: orl-mus TD:25 g/kg/96W-C   CRNGDP 5,921,84
CAR: orl-mus TD:29 g/kg/96W-C   CRNGDP 5,921,84
CAR: orl-mus TDLo:20800 mg/kg/97W-C
    EVHPAZ 67,129,86
CAR: orl-rat TDLo:4300 mg/kg/56W-C
    EVHPAZ 67,129,86
ETA: orl-rat TD:1050 mg/kg/2W-C   JJCREP 79,691,88
ETA: orl-rat TD:3600 mg/kg/43W-C   GANNA2 75,467,84
MUT: dnd-mus-ipr 10 mg/kg   JJCREP 76,835,85
MUT: dnd-mus:leu 100 μmol/L   MUREAV 144,57,85
MUT: dnd-mus:lvr 100 μmol/L   JJCREP 76,835,85
MUT: dns-ham:lng 3 μmol/L   ENMUDM 7,245,85
MUT: hma-mus/sat 198 μg/kg   MUREAV 156,93,85
MUT: sln-dmg-orl 1 mmol/L   MUREAV 156,93,85
MUT: slt-dmg-orl 100 ng/kg   JJCREP 76,468,85

CONSENSUS REPORTS: IARC Cancer Review: GROUP 2B IMEMDT 7,56,87; Animal Sufficient Evidence IMEMDT 40,261,86

SAFETY PROFILE: Suspected carcinogen with experimental carcinogenic and tumorigenic data. Mutation data reported. When heated to decomposition it emits toxic fumes of NO_x.

ALD500   CAS: 62450-07-1
3-AMINO-1-METHYL-5H-PYRIDO (4,3-b)INDOLE

mf: $C_{12}H_{11}N_3$ mw: 197.26

SYNS: 3-AMINO-1-METHYL-γ-CARBOLINE ◇ 1-METHYL-3-AMINO-5H-PYRIDO(4,3-b)INDOLE ◇ TRP-P-2 ◇ TRYPTOPHAN P2

TOXICITY DATA with REFERENCE
CAR: imp-mus TDLo:40 mg/kg   CALEDQ 17,101,82
CAR: orl-mus TDLo:9648 mg/kg/57W-C
    EVHPAZ 67,129,86
CAR: scu-mus TD:12500 μg/kg   CRNGDP 8,1721,87

CAR: scu-mus TDLo:12500 μg/kg   PPTCBY 37,193,85
NEO: orl-rat TDLo:4350 mg/kg/2Y-C   CALEDQ 13,23,81
NEO: scu-mus TD:12500 μg/kg   CRNGDP 8,1721,87
MUT: dnd-mus-ipr 10 mg/kg   JJCREP 76,835,85
MUT: dnd-mus:lvr 50 μmol/L   JJCREP 76,835,85
MUT: dnd-sat 1 μg/plate   ENMUDM 6,437,84
MUT: mma-sat 50 ng/plate   CRNGDP 5,505,84
MUT: mmo-sat 50 ng/plate   CRNGDP 5,505,84

CONSENSUS REPORTS: IARC Cancer Review: GROUP 2B IMEMDT 7,56,87; Animal Sufficient Evidence IMEMDT 31,255,83. EPA Genetic Toxicology Program.

SAFETY PROFILE: Suspected carcinogen with experimental carcinogenic and neoplastigenic data. Mutation data reported. When heated to decomposition it emits toxic fumes of NO_x.

ALD750   CAS: 68006-83-7
2-AMINO-3-METHYL-9H-PYRIDO (2,3-b)INDOLE

mf: $C_{12}H_{11}N_3$ mw: 197.2

SYN: 2-AMINO-3-METHYL-α-CARBOLINE

TOXICITY DATA with REFERENCE
CAR: orl-mus TD:37380 mg/kg/64W-C
    CRNGDP 5,815,84
CAR: orl-mus TDLo:35424 mg/kg/70W-C
    CRNGDP 5,815,84
MUT: dnr-bcs 10 μL/plate   ABCHA6 45,2031,81
MUT: mma-sat 10 ng/plate   CALEDQ 10,141,80
MUT: mmo-sat 1 μg/plate   ABCHA6 43,1155,79
MUT: slt-dmg-orl 400 ng/kg   JJCREP 76,468,85

CONSENSUS REPORTS: IARC Cancer Review: GROUP 2B IMEMDT 7,56,87; Animal Sufficient Evidence IMEMDT 40,253,86

SAFETY PROFILE: Suspected carcinogen with experimental carcinogenic data. Mutation data reported. When heated to decomposition it emits toxic fumes of NO_x.

ALL750   CAS: 5307-14-2
4-AMINO-2-NITROANILINE

mf: $C_6H_7N_3O_2$ mw: 153.16

SYNS: C.I. 76070 ◇ C.I. OXIDATION BASE 22 ◇ 1,4-DIAMINO-2-NITROBENZENE ◇ DURAFUR BROWN ◇ DURAFUR BROWN 2R ◇ DYE GS ◇ FOURAMIEN 2R ◇ FOURRINE 36 ◇ FOURRINE BROWN 2R ◇ NCI-C02222 ◇ 2NDB ◇ 2-NITRO-1,4-BENZENEDIAMINE ◇ 2-NITRO-1,4-

DIAMINOBENZENE ◇ NITRO-p-PHENYLENEDIAMINE
◇ o-NITRO-p-PHENYLENEDIAMINE (MAK) ◇ 2-NITRO-1,4-
PHENYLENEDIAMINE ◇ 2-NITRO-p-PHENYLENEDIAMINE
◇ 2-NP ◇ 2-NPPD ◇ 2-N-p-PDA ◇ OXIDATION BASE 22
◇ URSOL BROWN RR ◇ ZOBA BROWN RR

TOXICITY DATA with REFERENCE
NEO: orl-mus TDLo:288 g/kg/78W-C   NCITR*
NCI-CG-TR-169,79
ETA: orl-mus TD:144 g/kg/78W-C   NCITR*
NCI-CG-TR-169,79
MUT: cyt-hmn:lym 50 mg/L/24H   NATUAS
255,506,75
MUT: dns-rat:lvr 100 mg/L   MUREAV 97,359,82
MUT: mmo-sat 5 μg/plate   NATUAS 255,506,75
MUT: otr-ham:emb 500 μg/L   NCIMAV 58,243,81
MUT: sce-ham-orl 125 mg/kg   BLFSBY 29B,613,83

CONSENSUS REPORTS: IARC Cancer Review: Animal Inadequate Evidence IMEMDT
16,73,78. NCI Carcinogenesis Bioassay (feed);
No Evidence: rat NCITR* NCI-CG-TR-169,79;
Clear Evidence: mouse NCITR* NCI-CG-TR-
169,79. Reported in EPA TSCA Inventory. EPA
Genetic Toxicology Program.

DFG MAK: Suspected Carcinogen.

SAFETY PROFILE: Suspected carcinogen with
experimental carcinogenic, neoplastigenic, and
teratogenic data. Poison by intraperitoneal
route. Moderately toxic by ingestion. Other experimental reproductive effects. Mutation data
reported. When heated to decomposition it emits
toxic fumes of NO_x.

AOL000   CAS: 13256-07-0
n-AMYL-N-METHYLNITROSAMINE
mf: $C_6H_{14}N_2O$ mw: 130.22

SYNS: AMN ◇ METHYLAMYLNITROSAMIN (GERMAN)
◇ METHYLAMYLNITROSAMINE ◇ METHYL-N-AMYLNI-
TROSAMINE ◇ N-METHYL-N-NITROSOPENTYLAMINE
◇ METHYL-N-PENTYLNITROSAMINE ◇ N-NITROSO-N-
METHYL-N-AMYLAMINE ◇ NITROSOMETHYL-N-PENTYL-
AMINE

TOXICITY DATA with REFERENCE
CAR: orl-rat TD:168 mg/kg/8W-C   NIPAA4
82,1293,85
CAR: orl-rat TDLo:168 mg/kg/8W-C   NIPAA4
78,1889,81
CAR: par-rat TDLo:75 mg/kg/3W-C   JJIND8
74,1283,85
CAR: scu-rat TD:384 mg/kg/32W-I   CCLCDY
2,263,80

CAR: scu-rat TDLo:240 mg/kg/40W-I   CCLCDY
2,263,80
NEO: ipr-rat TDLo:50 mg/kg   CNREA8 39,3644,79
ETA: ipr-rat TD:150 mg/kg   CNREA8 45,577,85
ETA: orl-rat TD:192 mg/kg/90D-C   GANNA2
71,94,80
ETA: orl-rat TD:330 mg/kg/31W-C   ARZNAD
19,1077,69
ETA: scu-rat TD:310 mg/kg/31W-I   ZEKBAI
69,103,67
MUT: dnr-esc 25 μL/well   CBINA8 15,219,76
MUT: mma-esc 1 μmol/plate   GANNA2 75,8,84
MUT: mma-sat 10 μg/plate   TCMUE9 1,13,84

CONSENSUS REPORTS: EPA Genetic Toxicology Program.

SAFETY PROFILE: Suspected carcinogen with
experimental carcinogenic, neoplastigenic, and
tumorigenic data. Poison by ingestion, subcutaneous, and intraperitoneal routes. Mutation data
reported. When heated to decomposition it emits
toxic NO_x.

AOQ000   CAS: 62-53-3
ANILINE
DOT: 1547
mf: C_6H_7N mw: 93.14

PROP: Colorless, oily liquid; characteristic
odor. Bp: 184.4°, lel: 1.3%, ulc: 20-25, flash
p: 158°F (CC), fp: −6.2°, d: 1.02 @ 20°/4°,
autoign temp: 1139°F, vap press: 1 mm @ 34.8°,
vap d: 3.22.

SYNS: AMINOBENZENE ◇ AMINOPHEN ◇ ANILIN
(CZECH) ◇ ANILINA (ITALIAN, POLISH) ◇ ANILINE OIL
◇ BENZENAMINE ◇ BLUE OIL ◇ C.I. 76000 ◇ HUILE d'ANI-
LINE (FRENCH) ◇ NCI-CO3736 ◇ PHENYLAMINE

TOXICITY DATA with REFERENCE
NEO: orl-rat TD:72800 mg/kg/2Y-C   FCTOD7
25,619,87
NEO: orl-rat TDLo:11 g/kg/29W-C   APMIAL
26,473,49
MUT: bfa-rat/sat 300 mg/kg   MUREAV 79,173,80
MUT: dnr-esc 25 μL/well/16H   CBINA8 15,219,76
MUT: mma-sat 100 μg/plate   PJABDW 53,34,77

CONSENSUS REPORTS: IARC Cancer Review: Animal Inadequate Evidence IMEMDT
4,27,74; Human No Evidence IMEMDT 4,
27,74. EPA Extremely Hazardous Substances
List. Community Right-To-Know List. Reported in EPA TSCA Inventory.

OSHA PEL: (Transitional: TWA 5 ppm (skin))
TWA 2 ppm (skin)   ACGIH TLV: TWA 2

ppm (skin) (Proposed: BEI: 50 mg/L total p-aminophenol in urine at end of shift. DFG MAK: 2 ppm (8 mg/m³), Suspected Carcinogen; BAT: 1 mg/L in urine at end of shift. DOT Classification: Label: Poison B.

SAFETY PROFILE: Suspected carcinogen with experimental neoplastigenic data. A human poison by an unspecified route. Poison experimentally by most routes including inhalation and ingestion. A skin and severe eye irritant, and a mild sensitizer. In the body, aniline causes formation of methemoglobin, resulting in prolonged anoxemia and depression of the central nervous system; less acute exposure causes hemolysis of the red blood cells, followed by stimulation of the bone marrow. The liver may be affected with resulting jaundice. Long-term exposure to aniline dye manufacture has been associated with malignant bladder growths. A common air contaminant. Moderately flammable when exposed to heat or flame. To fight fire, use alcohol foam, CO_2, dry chemical. It can react vigorously with oxidizing materials. When heated to decomposition it emits highly toxic fumes of NO_x.

AOV900   CAS: 90-04-0
o-ANISIDINE
DOT: 2431
mf: C_7H_9NO mw: 123.17

SYNS: o-AMINOANISOLE ◇ 2-AMINOANISOLE ◇ 1-AMINO-2-METHOXYBENZENE ◇ 2-ANISIDINE ◇ o-ANISYLAMINE ◇ 2-METHOXY-1-AMINOBENZENE ◇ o-METHOXYANILINE ◇ 2-METHOXY-BENZENAMINE (9CI) ◇ o-METHOXYPHENYLAMINE

TOXICITY DATA with REFERENCE
MUT: dni-mus-orl 200 mg/kg   MUREAV 46,305,77
MUT: mma-sat 333 μg/plate   IMEMDT 27,63,82

CONSENSUS REPORTS: IARC Cancer Review: GROUP 2B IMEMDT 7,56,87; Human Limited Evidence IMEMDT 27,63,82. EPA Genetic Toxicology Program. Reported in EPA TSCA Inventory. Community Right-To-Know List.

OSHA PEL: TWA 0.5 mg/m³ ACGIH TLV: TWA 0.5 mg/m³ (skin) DFG MAK: 0.1 ppm (0.5 mg/m³) DOT Classification: DOT-IMO: Poison B; Label: St. Andrews Cross.

SAFETY PROFILE: Suspected carcinogen. Moderately toxic by ingestion. Mutation data reported. When heated to decomposition it emits toxic fumes of NO_x.

APG000   CAS: 613-13-8
2-ANTHRACENAMINE
mf: $C_{14}H_{11}N$ mw: 193.26

PROP: Yellow leaflets from alc. Mp: 238°; bp: subl @ 93° @ 9 mm. Insol in water, sltly sol in alc and ether.

SYNS: β-AMINOANTHRACENE ◇ 2-AMINOANTHRACENE ◇ 2-ANTHRACYLAMINE ◇ 2-ANTHRAMINE ◇ 2-ANTHRYLAMINE

TOXICITY DATA with REFERENCE
CAR: imp-mus TDLo: 50 mg/kg   BJCAAI 12,222,58
CAR: orl-rat TD: 100 mg/kg   CNREA8 26,619,66
CAR: orl-rat TDLo: 45 mg/kg/30D-I   CNREA8 28,924,68
CAR: skn-mus TD: 624 mg/kg/2Y-I   NTIS** CONF-801143
CAR: skn-mus TDLo: 62 mg/kg/2Y-I   NTIS** CONF-801143
ETA: imp-mus TD: 96 mg/kg/   BMBUAQ 14,147,58
ETA: skn-ham TDLo: 1200 mg/kg/55W-I   CNREA8 20,100,60
ETA: skn-mus TD: 800 μg/kg/20W-I   BJCAAI 9,631,55
ETA: skn-rat TD: 46800 mg/kg/26W-I   ONCOAR 17,236,64
ETA: skn-rat TDLo: 260 μg/kg/33W-I   BJCAAI 9,631,55
MUT: dnr-esc 100 mg/L   JNCIAM 62,873,79
MUT: hma-mus/sat 125 mg/kg   JNCIAM 62,911,79
MUT: mma-sat 2 μg/plate   PNASA6 72,5135,75
MUT: mmo-sat 6 nmol/plate   BBRCA9 89,259,79

SAFETY PROFILE: Suspected carcinogen with experimental carcinogenic and tumorigenic data. Mutation data reported. When heated to decomposition it emits toxic fumes of NO_x.

API750   CAS: 87-29-6
ANTHRANILIC ACID, CINNAMYL ESTER
mf: $C_{16}H_{15}NO_2$ mw: 253.32

PROP: Reddish yellow powder; balsamic odor. Mp: 60°, flash p: +212°F. Sol in alc, chloroform, ether; insol in water.

SYNS: 2-AMINOBENZOIC ACID-3-PHENYL-2-PROPENYL ESTER ◇ CINNAMYL ALCOHOL ANTHRANILATE ◇ CINNAMYL-2-AMINOBENZOATE ◇ CINNAMYL-o-AMINOBENZOATE ◇ CINNAMYL ANTHRANILATE (FCC) ◇ FEMA No. 2295 ◇ NCI-C03510 ◇ 3-PHENYL-2-PROPENYLANTHRANILATE ◇ 3-PHENYL-2-PROPEN-1-YL ANTHRANILATE

TOXICITY DATA with REFERENCE
CAR: orl-mus TD:2621 g/kg/2Y-C NCITR*
NCI-TR-196,80
CAR: orl-mus TDLo:1310 g/kg/2Y-C NCITR*
NCI-TR-196,80
CAR: orl-rat TD:1092 g/kg/2Y-C NCITR* NCI-
TR-196,80
CAR: orl-rat TDLo:546 g/kg/2Y-C NCITR*
NCI-TR-196,80
NEO: ipr-mus TDLo:12 g/kg/8W-I CNREA8
33,3069,73

CONSENSUS REPORTS: IARC Cancer Review: GROUP 3 IMEMDT 7,56,87; Animal Limited Evidence IMEMDT 31,133,83; Animal Inadequate Evidence IMEMDT 16,287,78; NCI Carcinogenesis Bioassay (feed); Clear Evidence: mouse, rat NCITR* NCI-CG-TR-196,80. Reported in EPA TSCA Inventory.

SAFETY PROFILE: Suspected carcinogen with experimental carcinogenic and neoplastigenic data. Combustible liquid. When heated to decomposition it emits toxic fumes of NO_x.

ARO500
ASPHALT
CAS: 8052-42-4
DOT: 1999

PROP: Black or dark brown mass. Bp: <470°, flash p: 400+°F (CC), d: 0.95−1.1, autoign temp: 905°F.

SYNS: ASPHALTUM ◇ BITUMEN (MAK) ◇ JUDEAN PITCH ◇ MINERAL PITCH ◇ PETROLEUM PITCH ◇ ROAD ASPHALT (DOT) ◇ ROAD TAR (DOT)

TOXICITY DATA with REFERENCE
CAR: skn-mus TDLo:130 g/kg/81W-I HYSAAV
33(4-6),180,68
ETA: skn-mus TD:69 g/kg/43W-I HYSAAV
33(4-6),180,68

CONSENSUS REPORTS: IARC Cancer Review: Human Inadequate Evidence IMEMDT 35,39,85. Reported in EPA TSCA Inventory.

ACGIH TLV: TWA 5 mg/m³ DFG MAK: Suspected Carcinogen. NIOSH REL: CL 5 mg/m³/15M DOT Classification: ORM-C; Label: None.

SAFETY PROFILE: Suspected carcinogen with experimental carcinogenic and tumorigenic data. A moderate irritant. May contain carcinogenic components. Combustible when exposed to heat or flame. To fight fire, use foam, CO_2, or dry chemical.

ASA500
AZASERINE
CAS: 115-02-6

mf: $C_5H_7N_3O_4$ mw: 173.15

PROP: Produced by the strain *Streptomyces fragilis* (85ERAY 2,1249,78)

SYNS: AZASERIN ◇ l-AZASERINE ◇ AZS ◇ CI-337 ◇ CL 337 ◇ CN-15,757 ◇ DIAZOACETATE (ESTER)-l-SERINE ◇ l-DIAZOACETATE (ESTER) SERINE ◇ DIAZO-ACETIC ACID ESTER with SERINE ◇ o-DIAZOACETYL-l-SERINE ◇ NSC-742 ◇ P-165 ◇ RCRA WASTE NUMBER U015 ◇ l-SERINE DIAZOACETATE ◇ l-SERINE DIAZOACETATE (ester)

TOXICITY DATA with REFERENCE
CAR: ipr-rat TDLo:260 mg/kg/26W-I CNREA8
35,2249,75
NEO: ipr-mus TDLo:30 mg/kg/8W-I TXAPA9
82,19,86
NEO: ipr-rat TD:120 mg/kg/24W-I CALEDQ
4,229,78
NEO: ipr-rat TD:150 mg/kg/5W-I JJIND8
62,1269,79
NEO: ipr-rat TD:210 mg/kg/6W-I CANCAR
47,1562,81
NEO: ipr-rat TDLo:120 mg/kg/24W-I GANNA2
69,633,78
NEO: orl-mus TDLo:150 mg/kg/8W-I TXAPA9
82,19,86
NEO: orl-rat TDLo:150 mg/kg/5W-C CANCAR
47,1562,81
ETA: ipr-rat TD:30 mg/kg/6W-I FEPRA7
34,827,75
ETA: ipr-rat TD:50 mg/kg CALEDQ 9,43,80
ETA: ipr-rat TD:60 mg/kg/6W-I PAACA3
21,109,80
ETA: ipr-rat TD:150 mg/kg/15W-I AJPAA4
105,94,81
ETA: ipr-rat TD:440 mg/kg/13W-I CNREA8
40,592,80
MUT: dnd-hmn:fbr 10 mmol/L ENMUDM7,267,85
MUT: dnr-esc 50 μg/plate CNREA8 34,1658,74
MUT: dns-rat-ipr 100 mg/kg ENMUDM 7,889,85
MUT: dns-rat:oth 100 μmol/L ENMUDM6,321,84
MUT: mma-sat 200 ng/plate PNASA6 72,5135,75
MUT: mmo-bcs 500 μmol/L EXPEAM 39,530,83
MUT: mmo-esc 100 μg/disc APMBAY 6,23,58
MUT: mmo-sat 10 μL/plate ANYAA9 76,475,58

CONSENSUS REPORTS: IARC Cancer Review: GROUP 2B IMEMDT 7,56,87; Animal Limited Evidence IMEMDT 10,73,76. EPA Genetic Toxicology Program.

SAFETY PROFILE: Suspected carcinogen with experimental carcinogenic, neoplastigenic, and tumorigenic data. Poison by ingestion, intra-peritoneal, and subcutaneous routes. Experimental teratogenic and reproductive effects. Human mutation data reported. When heated to decomposition it emits toxic fumes of NO_x.

ASP250   CAS: 25843-45-2
AZOXYMETHANE
mf: $C_2H_6N_2O$ mw: 74.10

SYN: AOM

TOXICITY DATA with REFERENCE
CAR: ims-rat TDLo:22 mg/kg/11W-I   JJIND8
73,1297,84
CAR: ivn-rat TDLo:20 mg/kg (22D post)
IARCCD 4,45,73
CAR: rec-gpg TDLo:104 mg/kg/33W-I   JNCIAM
56,653,76
CAR: scu-rat TD:45 mg/kg/3W-I   JJIND8
75,791,85
CAR: scu-rat TD:64 mg/kg/8W-I   JJIND8
73,275,84
CAR: scu-rat TD:80 mg/kg/10W-I   CNREA8
38,4427,78
CAR: scu-rat TD:80 mg/kg/10W-I   JJIND8
66,553,81
CAR: scu-rat TD:192 mg/kg/24W-I   JJIND8
62,1097,79
CAR: scu-rat TD:208 mg/kg/26W-I   JNCIAM
54,439,75
CAR: scu-rat TD:312 mg/kg/39W-I   DICRAG
16,438,73
CAR: scu-rat TDLo:3200 μg/kg   VTPHAK
12,165,75
ETA: ipr-mus TDLo:96 mg/kg/13W-I   JAVMA4
164,729,74
ETA: orl-ham TDLo:60 mg/kg/20W-I   CNREA8
47,3968,87
ETA: orl-rat TDLo:16 mg/kg   23HZAR -,267,70
ETA: orl-rat TDLo:20 mg/kg/(22D   XENOBH
3,271,73
ETA: rec-rat TDLo:200 mg/kg/20W-I   CNREA8
35,287,75
ETA: scu-rat TD:12 mg/kg   FEPRA7 31,1482,72
ETA: scu-rat TD:20 mg/kg   JJIND8 72,745,84
ETA: scu-rat TD:37 mg/kg/10W-I   JAVMA4
164,729,74
MUT: dnd-rat-scu 30 mg/kg   CNREA8 38,1589,78
MUT: mma-sat 13600 μmol/L/20M   CNREA8
38,4585,78
MUT: sln-dmg-unk 1 mmol/L/3D-C   DRISAA
50,138,73

SAFETY PROFILE: Suspected carcinogen with experimental carcinogenic and tumorigenic data. Poison by subcutaneous route. Mutation data reported. When heated to decomposition it emits toxic fumes of NO_x.

BAY300   CAS: 98-87-3
BENZAL CHLORIDE
DOT: 1886
mf: $C_7H_6Cl_2$ mw: 161.03

PROP: Very refractive liquid. Mp: −16°, bp: 214°, d: 1.29.

SYNS: BENZYL DICHLORIDE ◇ BENZYLENE CHLORIDE ◇ BENZYLIDENE CHLORIDE (DOT) ◇ CHLORURE de BEN-ZYLIDENE (FRENCH) ◇ α,α-DICHLOROTOLUENE ◇ RCRA WASTE NUMBER U017

TOXICITY DATA with REFERENCE
CAR: skn-mus TDLo:9200 mg/kg/50W-I
GANNA2 72,655,81
NEO: skn-mus TD:35200 mg/kg/42W-I
GANNA2 72,655,81
MUT: mma-esc 600 nmol/plate/20M   MUREAV
54,143,78
MUT: mma-sat 600 nmol/plate/20M   MUREAV
54,143,78
MUT: mrc-bcs 31 μmol/disc   MUREAV 54,143,78

CONSENSUS REPORTS: IARC Cancer Review: Human Inadequate Evidence IMEMDT 29,65,82; Animal Limited Evidence IMEMDT 29,65,82. Reported in EPA TSCA Inventory. EPA Genetic Toxicology Program. EPA Extremely Hazardous Substances List. Community Right-To-Know List.

DFG MAK: Suspected Carcinogen. DOT Classification: Poison B; Label: Poison.

SAFETY PROFILE: Suspected carcinogen with experimental carcinogenic and neoplastigenic data. Poison by inhalation. Moderately toxic by ingestion. A suspected human carcinogenic. A strong irritant and lachrymator. Causes central nervous system depression. Mutation data reported. When heated to decomposition it emits toxic fumes of Cl^-.

BBL000   CAS: 142-04-1
BENZENAMINE HYDROCHLORIDE
DOT: 1548
mf: $C_6H_7N \cdot ClH$ mw: 129.60

PROP: Crystals. Vap d: 4.46, d: 1.22, mp: 198°, bp: 245°, flash p: 380°F (OC).

SYNS: ANILINE CHLORIDE ◊ ANILINE HYDROCHLO-
RIDE (DOT) ◊ "ANILINE SALT" ◊ ANILINIUM CHLORIDE
◊ CHLORHYDRATE d'ANILINE (FRENCH) ◊ CHLORID ANI-
LINU (CZECH) ◊ NCI-CO3736 ◊ PHENYLAMINE HYDRO-
CHLORIDE ◊ SUL ANILINOVA (CZECH) ◊ USAF EK-442

TOXICITY DATA with REFERENCE
CAR: orl-rat TD:238 g/kg/2Y-C   NCITR* NCI-
CG-TR-130,78
CAR: orl-rat TD:2163 g/kg/2Y-C   IARC**
27,39,82
CAR: orl-rat TD:4326 g/kg/2Y-C   IARC**
27,39,82
CAR: orl-rat TDLo:130 g/kg/2Y-C   NCITR*
NCI-CG-TR-130,78
ETA: orl-rat TD:137 g/kg/60W-C   IARC**
27,39,82
MUT: otr-rat:emb 79500 ng/plate   JJATDK
1,190,81
MUT: sce-ham:fbr 10 μmol/L   JNCIAM 58,1635,77
MUT: sce-hmn:lym 50 μmol/L   BLFSBY
29b,561,84

CONSENSUS REPORTS: IARC Cancer Review: Animal Limited Evidence IMEMDT
27,39,82. NCI Carcinogenesis Bioassay Completed; Results Positive: rat (NCITR* NCI-CG-
TR-130,78); Results Negative: Mouse (NCITR*
NCI-CG-TR-130,78). Reported in EPA TSCA
Inventory. EPA Genetic Toxicology Program.

DOT Classification: DOT-IMO: Poison B; Label: St. Andrews Cross.

SAFETY PROFILE: Suspected carcinogen with
experimental carcinogenic, tumorigenic, and
teratogenic data. Poison by intraperitoneal
route. Moderately toxic by ingestion. Human
mutation data reported. A skin and eye irritant.
Combustible when exposed to heat or flame.
When heated to decomposition or on contact
with acid or acid fumes, it emits highly toxic
fumes of aniline and chlorine compounds. To
fight fire, use water, CO_2, water mist or spray,
dry chemical.

BBX750   CAS: 531-85-1
BENZIDINE HYDROCHLORIDE
mf: $C_{12}H_{12}N_2 \cdot 2ClH$ mw: 257.18

SYNS: (1,1'-BIPHENYL)-4,4'-DIAMINE, DIHYDROCHLO-
RIDE ◊ DIHIDROCLORURO de BENZIDINA (SPANISH)

TOXICITY DATA with REFERENCE
CAR: ipr-rat TDLo:62 mg/kg/4W-I   CRNGDP
2,747,81
CAR: orl-mus TD:5040 mg/kg/60W-C   TXAPA9
64,171,82

CAR: orl-mus TD:8064 mg/kg/80W-C   EJCAAH
16,1205,80
CAR: orl-mus TDLo:3360 mg/kg/80W-C
TXAPA9 64,171,82
ETA: orl-ham TDLo:75 mg/kg/3Y-C   85DAAC
5,129,66
ETA: orl-mus TD:1600 mg/kg/84W-C   CNREA8
35,2814,75
ETA: orl-mus TD:1680 mg/kg/40W-C   TOPADD
9,1,81
ETA: orl-mus TD:13440 mg/kg/1Y-C   FAATDF
4,69,84
MUT: dnd-esc 20 μmol/L   MUREAV 89,95,81
MUT: dnd-hmn:hla 20 μmol/L   MUREAV 89,95,81
MUT: mma-sat 100 nmol/plate   MUREAV 136,33,84
MUT: mmo-sat 100 nmol/plate   MUREAV 136,33,84
MUT: sce-ham-ipr 12500 μg/kg   MUREAV
113,33,83
MUT: sce-ham-orl 12500 μg/kg   MUREAV
113,33,83

CONSENSUS REPORTS: Reported in EPA
TSCA Inventory. EPA Genetic Toxicology Program.

SAFETY PROFILE: Suspected carcinogen with
experimental carcinogenic and tumorigenic
data. Human mutation data reported. When
heated to decomposition it emits very toxic
fumes of HCl and NO_x.

BBY300
BENZIDINE SULPHATE and
HYDRAZINE-BENZENE
mf: $C_6H_8N_2 \cdot C_{12}H_{12}N_2 \cdot H_2O_4S$ mw: 390.50

SYN: HYDRAZINE-BENZENE and BENZIDINE SULFATE

TOXICITY DATA with REFERENCE
CAR: scu-rat TDLo:9100 mg/kg/52W-I
GTPZAB 19(6),28,75

SAFETY PROFILE: Suspected carcinogen with
experimental carcinogenic data. When heated
to decomposition it emits toxic fumes of NO_x
and SO_x.

BCE500   CAS: 81-07-2
1,2-BENZISOTHIAZOL-3(2H)-ONE-1,1-
DIOXIDE
mf: $C_7H_5NO_3S$ mw: 183.19

PROP: White crystals or powder; odorless with
sweet taste. Mp: 228° (decomp), bp: sublimes.
Sol in water, alc, chloroform, and ether.

SYNS: ANHYDRO-o-SULFAMINE BENZOIC ACID
◊ 3-BENZISOTHIAZOLINONE-1,1-DIOXIDE ◊ o-BENZOIC

SULPHIMIDE ◇ o-BENZOSULFIMIDE ◇ BENZOSULPHIMIDE ◇ BENZO-2-SULPHIMIDE ◇ o-BENZOYL SULFIMIDE ◇ o-BENZOYL SULPHIMIDE ◇ 1,2-DIHYDRO-2-KETOBENZI-SOSULFONAZOLE ◇ 1,2-DIHYDRO-2-KETOBENZISOSUL-PHONAZOLE ◇ 2,3-DIHYDRO-3-OXOBENZISOSULFONA-ZOLE ◇ 2,3-DIHYDRO-3-OXOBENZISOSULPHONAZOLE ◇ GARANTOSE ◇ GLUCID ◇ GLUSIDE ◇ HERMESETAS ◇ 3-HYDROXYBENZISOTHIAZOL-S,S-DIOXIDE ◇ INSOLU-BLE SACCHARINE ◇ KANDISET ◇ NATREEN ◇ RCRA WASTE NUMBER U202 ◇ SACARINA ◇ SACCAHARIMIDE ◇ SACCHARINA ◇ SACCHARIN ACID ◇ SACCHARINE ◇ SACCHARINOL ◇ SACCHARINOSE ◇ SACCHAROL ◇ SAXIN ◇ SUCRE EDULCOR ◇ SUCRETTE ◇ o-SULFOBEN-ZIMIDE ◇ o-SULFOBENZOIC ACID IMIDE ◇ 2-SULPHOBEN-ZOIC IMIDE ◇ SYKOSE ◇ SYNCAL ◇ ZAHARINA

TOXICITY DATA with REFERENCE
NEO: imp-mus TDLo: 80 mg/kg   BJCAAI 11,212,57
ETA: orl-mus TDLo: 548 g/kg/1Y-C   IJEBA6 24,197,86
ETA: orl-rat TDLo: 2008 g/kg/2Y-C   JAPMA8 40,583,51
ETA: skn-mus TDLo: 9600 mg/kg/10W-I   BJCAAI 10,363,56
MUT: cyt-smc 200 mg/L   NATUAS 294,263,81
MUT: dnd-mus-ipr 100 mg/kg   ATSUDG (5),355,82
MUT: dnd-rat: lvr 3 mmol/L   SinJF# 26OCT82
MUT: dns-rat: lvr 100 pmol/L   CRNGDP 5,1547,84
MUT: sce-ham: lng 100 mg/L   BJCAAI 45,769,82

CONSENSUS REPORTS: IARC Cancer Review: GROUP 2B IMEMDT 7,334,87; Human Inadequate Evidence IMEMDT 22,111,80; Animal Sufficient Evidence IMEMDT 22,111,80. EPA Genetic Toxicology Program. Reported in EPA TSCA Inventory. Community Right-To-Know List.

SAFETY PROFILE: Suspected carcinogen with experimental neoplastigenic, tumorigenic, and teratogenic data. Mild acute toxicity by ingestion. Experimental reproductive effects. Mutation data reported. When heated to decomposition it emits toxic NO_x and SO_x.

BCJ000   CAS: 5208-87-7
1,3-BENZODIOXOLE-5-(2-PROPEN-1-OL)
mf: $C_{10}H_{10}O_3$ mw: 178.20

SYNS: 1'-HYDROXYSAFROLE ◇ 1,2-METHYLENEDIOXY-4-(1-HYDROXYALLYL)BENZENE ◇ α-VINYLPIPERONYL ALCOHOL

TOXICITY DATA with REFERENCE
CAR: ipr-mus TDLo: 17820 μg/kg   CNREA8 47,2275,87

CAR: orl-mus TD: 230 g/kg/52W-C   CNREA8 37,1883,77
CAR: orl-mus TDLo: 206 g/kg/56W-C   CNREA8 33,590,73
CAR: orl-rat TD: 79 g/kg/34W-C   CNREA8 33,590,73
CAR: orl-rat TDLo: 77 g/kg/73W-C   CNREA8 37,1883,77
CAR: scu-rat TDLo: 1426 mg/kg/10W-I   CNREA8 43,1124,83
NEO: orl-mus TD: 61 g/kg/52W-C   CNREA8 43,5163,83
NEO: orl-mus TD: 117 g/kg/52W-C   CNREA8 43,5163,83
ETA: orl-mus TD: 117 g/kg/1Y-C   PAACA3 24,79,83
ETA: scu-rat TD: 265 mg/kg/10W-I   CNREA8 33,590,73
MUT: dnd-ham-ipr 100 mg/kg   CNREA8 36,1686,76
MUT: dnd-mus-ipr 100 mg/kg   CNREA8 36,1686,76
MUT: dnd-rat-ipr 100 mg/kg   CNREA8 36,1686,76
MUT: dns-hmn: fbr 10 mmol/L   IJCNAW 16,284,75
MUT: mma-sat 1 μmol/plate   MUREAV 60,143,79
MUT: mmo-sat 1 μmol/plate   MUREAV 60,143,79
MUT: oms-mus-ipr 400 μmol/kg   CNREA8 41,2664,81

SAFETY PROFILE: Suspected carcinogen with experimental carcinogenic, neoplastigenic, and tumorigenic data. Human mutation data reported. When heated to decomposition it emits acrid smoke and irritating fumes.

BCJ500   CAS: 205-82-3
BENZO(j)FLUORANTHENE
mf: $C_{20}H_{12}$ mw: 252.32

SYNS: 10,11-BENZFLUORANTHENE ◇ BENZ(j)FLUO-ROANTHRENE ◇ BENZO(1)FLUORANTHENE ◇ 7,8-BENZO-FLUORANTHENE ◇ B(j)F ◇ DIBENZO(a,jk)FLUORENE

TOXICITY DATA with REFERENCE
CAR: imp-rat TDLo: 25 mg/kg   JJIND8 71,539,83
NEO: ipr-mus TDLo: 11102 μg/kg/15D-I   CALEDQ 34,15,87
ETA: imp-rat TD: 5 mg/kg   50NNAZ 7,571,83
ETA: skn-mus TDLo: 312 mg/kg/26W-I   CANCAR 12,1194,59
MUT: dnd-mus-skn 3760 nmol/kg   PAACA3 25,121,84
MUT: mma-sat 10 μg/plate   CNREA8 40,4258,80

CONSENSUS REPORTS: IARC Cancer Review: GROUP 2B IMEMDT 7,56,87; Animal Limited Evidence IMEMDT 3,82,73; Animal Sufficient Evidence IMEMDT 32,155,83

SAFETY PROFILE: Suspected carcinogen with experimental carcinogenic, neoplastigenic, and tumorigenic data. Mutation data reported. When heated to decomposition it emits acrid smoke and irritating fumes.

BCS750
BENZO(a)PYRENE
CAS: 50-32-8

mf: $C_{20}H_{12}$ mw: 252.32

PROP: Yellow crystals. Mp: 179°, bp: 312° @ 10 mm. Insol in water; sol in benzene, toluene, and xylene.

SYNS: BENZO(d,e,f)CHRYSENE ◇ 3,4-BENZOPIRENE (ITALIAN) ◇ 3,4-BENZOPYRENE ◇ 6,7-BENZOPYRENE ◇ 3,4-BENZPYREN (GERMAN) ◇ BENZ(a)PYRENE ◇ 3,4-BENZ(a)PYRENE ◇ 3,4-BENZYPYRENE

TOXICITY DATA with REFERENCE

CAR: imp-mus TDLo: 200 mg/kg   BJCAAI 39,761,79

CAR: imp-rat TD: 500 µg/kg   CALEDQ 20,97,83

CAR: imp-rat TDLo: 150 µg/kg   JJIND8 72,733,84

CAR: ims-rat TD: 3150 µg/kg   PAACA3 21,72,80

CAR: ims-rat TDLo: 2400 µg/kg   NTIS** DOE/ EV/03140-5

CAR: ipr-mus TDLo: 300 mg/kg (16-18D post) JTEHD6 6,569,80

CAR: itr-ham TD: 360 mg/kg/36W-I   CNREA8 32,28,72

CAR: itr-ham TDLo: 64 mg/kg   CALEDQ 3,231,77

CAR: itr-rat TD: 200 mg/kg/15W-I 31BYAP-,199,74

CAR: itr-rat TDLo: 68 mg/kg/15W-I 85AGAF-,480,76

CAR: orl-mus TDLo: 700 mg/kg/75W-I GISAAA 45(12),14,80

CAR: orl-rat TDLo: 15 mg/kg   EXPTAX 18,288,80

CAR: rec-mus TD: 560 mg/kg/14W-I   CALEDQ 20,117,83

CAR: rec-mus TDLo: 200 mg/kg   ONCOBS 37,77,80

CAR: scu-mus TD: 8 mg/kg   CNREA8 12,657,52

CAR: scu-mus TD: 12 mg/kg   GANNA2 62,309,71

CAR: scu-mus TDLo: 9 mg/kg   JJIND8 71,309,83

CAR: scu-mus TDLo: 480 mg/kg (11-15D post) PSEBAA 135,84,70

CAR: skn-mus TD: 12 mg/kg/20D-I   CRNGDP 6,1483,85

CAR: skn-mus TD: 18 mg/kg/73W-I   EVHPAZ 38,149,81

CAR: skn-mus TD: 26 mg/kg/65W-I   AJPAA4 102,381,81

CAR: skn-mus TDLo: 25 ng/kg/110W-I ARGEAR 50,266,80

CAR: skn-mus TDLo: 120 mg/k (multi) BEXBAN 71,677,71

CAR: skn-mus TDLo: 164 mg/kg/36W-I DTESD7 10,321,82

NEO: ipr-mus TDLo: 10 mg/kg ARTODN 4,74,80

NEO: itr-ham TDLo: 120 mg/kg/17W-I CALEDQ 25,271,85

NEO: itr-mus TDLo: 200 mg/kg/10W-I   PWPSA8 22,269,79

NEO: ivn-rbt TDLo: 30 mg/kg (25D post) BEXBAN 85,369,78

NEO: scu-rat TDLo: 455 µg/kg/60D-I   CBINA8 29,159,80

ETA: ice-rat TDLo: 22 mg/kg   CNREA8 29,1927,69

ETA: ihl-ham TCLo: 9500 µg/m³/4H/96W-I JJIND8 66,575,81

ETA: ihl-mus TCLo: 200 ng/m³/6H/13W-I GISAAA 47(7),23,82

ETA: imp-dog TDLo: 651 mg/kg/21W-C JJIND8 65,921,80

ETA: imp-frg TDLo: 45 mg/kg   EXPEAM 20,143,64

ETA: ipr-rat TDLo: 16 mg/kg   BJCAAI 12,65,58

ETA: itr-rbt TDLo: 145 mg/kg/2Y-I   GANNA2 71,197,80

ETA: ivn-mus TDLo: 10 mg/kg   JNCIAM 1,225,40

ETA: ivn-rat TDLo: 39 mg/kg/6D-I   CNREA8 29,506,69

ETA: orl-ham TDLo: 420 mg/kg/21W-I   ZEKBAI 65,56,62

ETA: par-dog TDLo: 819 mg/kg/26W-I   JJIND8 65,921,80

ETA: scu-ham TDLo: 4000 µg/kg   CNREA8 32,360,72

ETA: scu-mky TDLo: 40 mg/kg   PSEBAA 127,594,68

ETA: skn-rbt TDLo: 17 mg/kg/57W-I   HSZPAZ 236,79,35

ETA: unr-mus TDLo: 80 mg/kg/8D-I   BEBMAE 88(11),592,79

MUT: bfa-mus/sat 100 mg/kg   CNREA8 38,4478,78

MUT: cyt-ham-ipr 200 mg/kg   TOLED5 2,277,78

MUT: dnd-hmn: oth 1500 nmol/L   TCMUD8 1,3,80

MUT: dns-rbt-skn 100 µg/L   PAACA3 21,94,80

MUT: hma-mus/lng 25 mg/kg   PSEBAA 158,269,78

MUT: mnt-mus-scu 100 mg/kg   EXPEAM 36,297,80

MUT: msc-ham-ipr 200 mg/kg   TOLED5 2,277,78

MUT: sce-ham: lng 1 µg/L   JCINAO 64,1245,79

MUT: slt-mus-orl 80 mg/kg   ARTODN 38,99,77

CONSENSUS REPORTS: IARC Cancer Review: GROUP 2A IMEMDT 7,56,87; Animal Sufficient Evidence IMEMDT 32,211,83;

IMEMDT 3,91,73. Reported in EPA TSCA Inventory.

OSHA PEL: TWA 0.2 mg/m^3

SAFETY PROFILE: Suspected carcinogen with experimental carcinogenic, neoplastigenic, tumorigenic, and teratogenic data. A poison via subcutaneous, intraperitoneal and intrarenal routes. Other experimental reproductive effects. Human mutation data reported. A common air contaminant of water, food, and smoke. When heated to decomposition it emits acrid smoke and fumes.

BCV250   CAS: 21247-98-3
BENZO(a)PYRENE-6-METHANOL
mf: $C_{21}H_{14}O$ mw: 282.35

SYN: 6-HYDROXYMETHYLBENZO(a)PYRENE

TOXICITY DATA with REFERENCE
CAR: scu-rat TDLo: 100 mg/kg/40D-I   JMCMAR 16,714,73
CAR: skn-mus TDLo: 180 mg/kg/20W-I   CBINA8 22(1),53,78
NEO: scu-mus TDLo: 20 mg/kg   BJCAAI 26,506,72
NEO: scu-rat TD: 508 μg/kg/60D-I   CBINA8 29,159,80
NEO: skn-mus TD: 4510 μg/kg   CCSUDL 3,371,78
ETA: skn-mus TD: 180 mg/kg/20W-I   PAACA3 18,59,77
MUT: bfa-rat/sat 1mg/kg   MUREAV 173,251,86
MUT: dnd-mam: lym 500 mg/L   CBINA8 25,35,79
MUT: dnd-omi 30 μmol/L   CBINA8 31,51,80
MUT: dnd-rat: lym 500 mg/L   CBINA8 25,35,79
MUT: mma-ham: lng 3600 nmol/L   PNASA6 73,607,76
MUT: mma-sat 500 ng/plate   PNASA6 72,5135,75
MUT: sln-dmg-par 5 mmol/L   CNREA8 33,302,73

CONSENSUS REPORTS: EPA Genetic Toxicology Program.

SAFETY PROFILE: Suspected carcinogen with experimental carcinogenic, neoplastigenic, and tumorigenic data. Mutation data reported. When heated to decomposition it emits acrid smoke and fumes.

BDF000   CAS: 149-30-4
2-BENZOTHIAZOLETHIOL
mf: $C_7H_5NS_2$ mw: 167.25

PROP: Light yellow powder. Mp: 170°, d: 1.42 @ 25°.

SYNS: CAPTAX ◇ MBT ◇ MERCAPTOBENZOTHIAZOLE ◇ 2-MERCAPTOBENZOTHIAZOLE ◇ 2-MERKAPTOBENZO-

TIAZOL (POLISH) ◇ NCI-C56519 ◇ PENNAC MBT POWDER ◇ ROKON ◇ ROTAX ◇ SULFADENE ◇ USAF GY-3 ◇ USAF XR-29

TOXICITY DATA with REFERENCE
CAR: orl-rat TDLo: 195 g/kg/2Y-I   NTPTR* NTP-TR-332,88
CAR: scu-mus TDLo: 215 mg/kg   NTIS** PB223-159
ETA: orl-mus TD: 195 g/kg/2Y-I   NTPTR* NTP-TR-332,88
ETA: orl-mus TDLo: 35 g/kg/78W-I   NTIS** PB223-159

CONSENSUS REPORTS: NTP Carcinogenesis Studies (gavage); Some Evidence rat NTPTR* NTP-TR-332,88: (gavage); Equivocal Evidence: mouse NTPTR* NTP-TR-332,88. Reported in EPA TSCA Inventory.

SAFETY PROFILE: Suspected carcinogen with experimental carcinogenic, tumorigenic, and teratogenic data. Poison by intraperitoneal routes. Moderately toxic by ingestion. Other experimental reproductive effects. When heated to decomposition or on contact with acids or acid fumes it emits toxic SO_x and NO_x.

BEE375   CAS: 100-44-7
BENZYL CHLORIDE
mf: C_7H_7Cl mw: 126.59
DOT: 1738

PROP: Colorless liquid, very refractive; irritating, unpleasant odor. Mp: −43°, bp: 179°, lel: 1.1%, flash p: 153°F, d: 1.1026 @ 18/4°, autoign temp: 1085°F, vap d: 4.36.

SYNS: BENZILE (CLORURO di) (ITALIAN) ◇ BENZYL-CHLORID (GERMAN) ◇ BENZYLE (CHLORURE de) (FRENCH) ◇ CHLOROMETHYLBENZENE ◇ CHLOROPHE-NYLMETHANE ◇ α-CHLOROTOLUENE ◇ φ-CHLOROTOL-UENE ◇ α-CHLORTOLUOL (GERMAN) ◇ CHLORURE de BENZYLE (FRENCH) ◇ NCI-C06360 ◇ RCRA WASTE NUMBER P028 ◇ TOLYL CHLORIDE

TOXICITY DATA with REFERENCE
CAR: orl-mus TDLo: 31 g/kg/2Y-I   JJIND8 76,1231,86
ETA: scu-rat TD: 2100 mg/kg/53W-I   ZEKBAI 74,241,70
ETA: scu-rat TDLo: 50 mg/kg   FCTXAV 6,576,68
ETA: skn-mus TDLo: 9200 mg/kg/50W-I   GANNA2 72,655,81
MUT: cyt-rat: oth 120 μmol/L   PMRSDJ 4,247,82
MUT: dnd-hmn: fbr 1 mmol/L   MUREAV 145,209,85
MUT: dnd-hmn: oth 1 mmol/L   MUREAV 145,209,85

MUT: dns-hmn:hla 50 μmol/L CALEDQ20,263,83
MUT: otr-ham:emb 1600 μg/L CRNGDP1,323,80

CONSENSUS REPORTS: Animal Limited Evidence IMEMDT 29,49,82; Animal Sufficient Evidence IMEMDT 11,217,76; Human Inadequate Evidence IMEMDT 29,49,82. EPA Genetic Toxicology Program. Community Right-To-Know List. Reported in EPA TSCA Inventory. EPA Extremely Hazardous Substances List.

OSHA PEL: TWA 1 ppm ACGIH TLV: TWA 1 ppm DFG MAK: 1 ppm (5 mg/m^3); Suspected Carcinogen. NIOSH REL: (Benzyl Chloride) CL 5 mg/m^3/15M DOT Classification: Corrosive Material; Label: Corrosive.

SAFETY PROFILE: Suspected carcinogen with experimental carcinogenic and tumorigenic data. Poison by inhalation. Moderately toxic by ingestion and subcutaneous routes. Experimental reproductive effects. Human mutation data reported. A corrosive irritant to skin, eyes, and mucous membranes. Flammable and moderately explosive when exposed to heat or flame. Can react vigorously with oxidizing materials. When heated to decomposition it emits toxic fumes of Cl$^-$.

BFW000   CAS: 39323-48-3
BETEL NUT

PROP: Mottled brown with fawn color. Extract of 50 g sun-dried betel nut in 100 mL boiling water (IJCNAW 17,469,76).

SYNS: ARECA CATECHU ◇ ARECA CATECHU Linn., fruit extract ◇ ARECA CATECHU Linn., nut extract ◇ BN ◇ PINANG ◇ POOGIPHALAM, nut extract ◇ SUPARI, nut extract

TOXICITY DATA with REFERENCE
CAR: orl-mus TDLo:340 g/kg/17W-I BJCAAI 40,922,79
CAR: scu-mus TDLo:1728 mg/kg/13W-I IJEBA6 18,1159,80
NEO: scu-mus TD:48 g/kg/5W-I IJCNAW 17,469,76
NEO: scu-rat TDLo:2016 mg/kg/42W-I JNCIAM 60,683,78
MUT: mnt-mus-ipr 1600 mg/kg CRNGDP5,501,84
MUT: msc-ham:lng 5 mg/L CRNGDP 5,501,84
MUT: sce-mus-ipr 62500 μg/kg/5D-C CRNGDP 7,37,86

CONSENSUS REPORTS: IARC Cancer Review: Animal Limited Evidence IMEMDT 37,141,85

SAFETY PROFILE: Suspected carcinogen with experimental carcinogenic, neoplastigenic, and teratogenic data. Moderately toxic by intraperitoneal route. Other experimental reproductive effects. When heated to decomposition it emits toxic fumes of NO$_x$.

BFW125
BETEL QUID EXTRACT

TOXICITY DATA with REFERENCE
CAR: scu-mus TDLo:3376 mg/kg/13W-I IJEBA6 18,1159,80
ETA: skn-mus TD:2920 g/kg/2Y-C BJCAAI 14,597,60
ETA: skn-mus TDLo:720 g/kg/26W-C BJCAAI 14,597,60
MUT: dni-hmn:lym 25000 ppm CNREA8 39,4802,79
MUT: dni-mus:fbr 25000 ppm CNREA839,4802,79
MUT: dni-rat:mmr 25000 ppm CNREA839,4802,79

CONSENSUS REPORTS: IARC Cancer Review: Human Inadequate Evidence IMEMDT 37,141,85; Animal Limited Evidence IMEMDT 37,141,85

SAFETY PROFILE: Suspected carcinogen with experimental carcinogenic and tumorigenic data by skin contact. Human mutation data reported.

BFX000   CAS: 613-35-4
4′,4′′′-BIACETANILIDE
mf: C$_{16}$H$_{16}$N$_2$O$_2$ mw: 268.34

PROP: Mp: 329°.

SYNS: N,N′-(1,1′-BIPHENYL)-4,4′-DIYLBIS-ACETAMIDE 4′,4′′′-BIACETANILIDE ◇ N,N′-4,4′-BIPHENYL-YLENEBISACETAMIDE ◇ 4,4′-DIACETYLAMINOBI-PHENYL ◇ N,N′-DIACETYL BENZIDINE ◇ 4,4′-DI-ACETYLBENZIDINE

TOXICITY DATA with REFERENCE
CAR: ipr-rat TDLo:64 mg/kg/4W-I CRNGDP 2,747,81
NEO: ipr-rat TD:900 mg/kg ARPAAQ 81,146,66
NEO: scu-rat TDLo:900 mg/kg ARPAAQ81,146,66
ETA: orl-rat TDLo:6300 mg/kg/35W-C CNREA8 16,525,56
ETA: scu-rat TD:4350 mg/kg/39W-I VOONAW 8(11),11,62
MUT: dnd-rat:lvr 100 mg/L CRNGDP 5,407,84
MUT: mma-sat 5 μg/plate ENMUDM 6,145,84

CONSENSUS REPORTS: IARC Cancer Review: GROUP 2B IMEMDT 7,56,87, Animal

Sufficient Evidence IMEMDT 16,293,78. Reported in EPA TSCA Inventory.

SAFETY PROFILE: Suspected carcinogen with experimental carcinogenic, neoplastigenic, and tumorigenic data. Mutation data reported. When heated to decomposition it emits toxic fumes of NO_x.

BGJ750   CAS: 132-27-4
2-BIPHENYLOL, SODIUM SALT
mf: $C_{12}H_9O \cdot Na$ mw: 192.20

SYNS: BACTROL ◇ D.C.S. ◇ DORVICIDE A ◇ DOWICIDE ◇ 2-HYDROXYDIPHENYL SODIUM ◇ MIL-DU-RID ◇ MYSTOX WFA ◇ NATRIPHENE ◇ OPP-Na ◇ ORPHENOL ◇ o-PHENYLPHENOL SODIUM SALT ◇ 2-PHENYLPHENOL SODIUM SALT ◇ PREVENTOL-ON ◇ SODIUM-2-HYDROXY-DIPHENYL ◇ SODIUM-o-PHENYLPHENATE ◇ SODIUM-2-PHENYLPHENATE ◇ SODIUM-o-PHENYLPHENOLATE ◇ SODIUM-o-PHENYLPHENOXIDE ◇ SOPP ◇ STOMOLD B ◇ TOPANE

TOXICITY DATA with REFERENCE
CAR: orl-rat TD: 126 g/kg/13W-C   FCTXAV 19,303,81
CAR: orl-rat TDLo: 109 g/kg/13W-C   FCTOD7 24,207,86
NEO: orl-rat TD: 223 g/kg/26W-C   FCTOD7 25,359,87
ETA: orl-rat TD: 269 g/kg/32W-C   GANNA2 74,625,83
ETA: orl-rat TD: 486 g/kg/2Y-C   NAIZAM 37,270,86
MUT: mmo-asn 16 μmol/L   PHYTAJ 66,217,76
MUT: sln-asn 52 μmol/L   EVHPAZ 31,81,79

CONSENSUS REPORTS: IARC Cancer Review: Animal Limited Evidence IMEMDT 30,329,83. Reported in EPA TSCA Inventory.

SAFETY PROFILE: Suspected carcinogen with experimental carcinogenic, neoplastigenic, and tumorigenic data. Moderately toxic by ingestion. An experimental teratogen. Other experimental reproductive effects. A human skin irritant. A severe skin irritant to experimental animals. When heated to decomposition it emits toxic fumes of Na_2O.

BGP250   CAS: 304-28-9
2,7-BIS(ACETAMIDO)FLUORENE
mf: $C_{17}H_{16}N_2O_2$ mw: 280.35

SYNS: 2,7-DIACETAMIDOFLUORENE ◇ 2,7-DIACE-TYLAMINOFLUORENE ◇ 2,7-FAA ◇ 2,7-FLUORENYLBIS-ACETAMIDE ◇ N,N'-FLUOREN-2,7-YLBISACETAMIDE

◇ N,N'-FLUOREN-2,7-YLENEBISACETAMIDE ◇ N,N'-2,7-FLUORENYLENEBISACETAMIDE ◇ N,N'-(FLUOREN-2,7-YLENE)BIS(ACETYLAMINE) ◇ N,N'-2,7-FLUORENYLENE-DIACETAMIDE

TOXICITY DATA with REFERENCE
CAR: ipr-rat TDLo: 2044 mg/kg/29W-I   JNCIAM 29,977,62
CAR: orl-mus TD: 7668 mg/kg/30W-C   ONCOBS 41,101,84
CAR: orl-mus TDLo: 2100 mg/kg/13W-C   JNCIAM 40,629,68
CAR: orl-rat TDLo: 4830 mg/kg/46W-C   GANNA2 60,211,69
NEO: orl-mus TD: 6480 mg/kg/26W-C   NAIZAM 33,545,83
ETA: ipr-rat TD: 8 mg/kg   JJIND8 71,211,83
ETA: orl-rat TD: 228 g/kg/26W-C   APHGBP 22,477,72
ETA: orl-rat TD: 1830 mg/kg/32W-C   NCIMAV 5,85,61
ETA: orl-rat TD: 2035 mg/kg/34W-C   NCIMAV 5,1,61
ETA: orl-rat TD: 2060 mg/kg/34W-C   JNCIAM 29,977,62
ETA: orl-rat TD: 2250 mg/kg/21W-C   GANNA2 62,471,71
ETA: orl-rat TD: 2800 mg/kg/32W-C   APHGBP 26,341,76
ETA: orl-uns TDLo: 1200 mg/kg/34W-C   JJIND8 74,909,85
MUT: cyt-rat-orl 315 mg/kg/3W   JNCIAM 54,1245,75
MUT: dns-rat: lvr 500 nmol/L   ENMUDM 3,11,81
MUT: mma-sat 10 μg/plate   PNASA6 72,5135,75
MUT: mmo-sat 100 μg/plate   PNASA6 69,3128,72

CONSENSUS REPORTS: EPA Genetic Toxicology Program.

SAFETY PROFILE: Suspected carcinogen with experimental carcinogenic, neoplastigenic, and tumorigenic data. Mutation data reported. When heated to decomposition it emits toxic fumes of NO_x.

BGT000   CAS: 28434-86-8
BIS(4-AMINO-3-CHLOROPHENYL) ETHER
mf: $C_{12}H_{10}Cl_2N_2O$ mw: 269.14

SYNS: 3,3'-DICHLOR-4,4'-DIAMINO-DIPHENYLAETHER (GERMAN) ◇ 3,3'-DICHLORO-4,4'-DIAMINODIPHENYL ETHER ◇ 4,4'-OXYBIS(2-CHLOROANILINE) ◇ 4,4'-OXYBIS(2-CHLORO-BENZENAMINE)

TOXICITY DATA with REFERENCE
CAR: scu-rat TD:14 g/kg/96W-I NATWAY 64,394,77
CAR: scu-rat TDLo:11 g/kg/27W-I NATWAY 57,676,70

CONSENSUS REPORTS: IARC Cancer Review: GROUP 2B IMEMDT 7,56,87; Animal Sufficient Evidence IMEMDT 16,309,78

SAFETY PROFILE: Suspected carcinogen with experimental carcinogenic data. When heated to decomposition it emits toxic fumes of Cl^- and NO_x.

BHB000 CAS: 64092-23-5
BIS(2-BENZOYLBENZOATO)BIS(3-(1-METHYL-2-PYRROLIDINYL)PYRIDINE) NICKEL TRIHYDRATE
mf: $C_{48}H_{46}N_4NiO_6 \cdot 3H_2O$ mw: 887.75

SYN: NICOTINE, COMPOUND, with NICKEL(II)-o-BEN-ZOYL BENZOATE TRIHYDRATE (2:1)

CONSENSUS REPORTS: Nickel and its compounds are on The Community Right-To-Know List.

OSHA PEL: (Transitional: TWA 1 mg/m^3) TWA 0.1 mg (Ni)/m^3 ACGIH TLV: TWA 0.1 mg (Ni)/m^3; (Proposed: TWA 0.05 mg(Ni)/m^3; Human Carcinogen) NIOSH REL: (Inorganic Nickel) TWA 0.015 mg(Ni)/m^3

SAFETY PROFILE: Suspected carcinogen. Poison by ingestion and intraperitoneal routes. When heated to decomposition it emits toxic fumes of NO_x.

BHT750 CAS: 531-76-0
dl-3-(p-(BIS(2-CHLOROETHYL)AMINO)PHENYL) ALANINE
mf: $C_{13}H_{18}Cl_2N_2O_2$ mw: 305.23

SYNS: 4-(BIS(2-CHLOROETHYL)AMINO)-dl-PHENYLALA-NINE ◇ 3-(p-(BIS(2-CHLOROETHYL)AMINO)PHENYL)ALA-NINE ◇ CB-3307 ◇ p-DI-(2-CHLORAETHYL)-AMINO-dl-PHE-NYL-ALANIN (GERMAN) ◇ p-DI(2-CHLOROETHYL)AMINO-dl-PHENYLALANINE ◇ MERFALAN ◇ MERPHALAN ◇ o-MERPHALAN ◇ NCI-CO4944 ◇ NSC-14210 ◇ PHENYL-ALANIN-LOST (GERMAN) ◇ dl-PHENYLALANINE MUS-TARD ◇ SAKOLYSIN (GERMAN) ◇ SARCOCLORIN ◇ dl-SARCOLYSIN ◇ dl-SARCOLYSINE

TOXICITY DATA with REFERENCE
ETA: ipr-mus TDLo:98 mg/kg/26W-I CANCAR 40S,1935,77

MUT: mmo-omi 10 mmol/L MUREAV 23,5,74
MUT: pic-esc 200 mg/L ARMKA7 51,9,65
MUT: pic-omi 5 mmol/L MUREAV 1,355,64
MUT: sln-dmg-par 4500 µmol/L GENRA81,173,60

CONSENSUS REPORTS: IARC Cancer Review: GROUP 2B IMEMDT 7,56,87; Animal Limited Evidence IMEMDT 9,167,75; NCI Carcinogenesis Studies (ipr); Clear Evidence: mouse CANCAR 40,1935,77; No Evidence: rat CANCAR 40,1935,77

SAFETY PROFILE: Suspected carcinogen with experimental tumorigenic data. A poison by ingestion, intraperitoneal, intravenous, and intracerebral routes. Other experimental reproductive effects. Mutation data reported. An antineoplastic agent. When heated to decomposition it emits very toxic fumes of Cl^- and NO_x.

BIA250 CAS: 66-75-1
5-(BIS(2-CHLOROETHYL)AMINO)URACIL
mf: $C_8H_{11}Cl_2N_3O_2$ mw: 252.12

SYNS: AMINOURACIL MUSTARD ◇ 5-(BIS(2-CHLORO-ETHYL)AMINO)-2,4(1H,3H)PYRIMIDINEDIONE ◇ 5-N,N-BIS(2-CHLOROETHYL)AMINOURACIL ◇ CB-4835 ◇ CHLORETHAMINACIL ◇ DEMETHYLDOPAN ◇ DES-METHYLDOPAN ◇ 5-(DI-(β-CHLOROETHYL)AMINO)URA-CIL ◇ 5-(DI-2-CHLOROETHYL)AMINOURACIL ◇ 2,6-DIHY-DROXY-5-BIS(2-CHLOROETHYL)AMINOPYRAMIDINE ◇ ENT 50,439 ◇ NCI-CO4820 ◇ NORDOPAN ◇ NSC-34462 ◇ RCRA WASTE NUMBER U237 ◇ SK-19849 ◇ U-8344 ◇ URACILLOST ◇ URACILMOSTAZA ◇ URACIL MUSTARD ◇ URAMUSTIN ◇ URAMUSTINE

TOXICITY DATA with REFERENCE
CAR: ipr-mus TD:30 mg/kg/39W-I SCIEAS 147,1443,65
CAR: ipr-mus TDLo:240 µg/kg/4W JNCIAM 36,915,66
NEO: ipr-mus TD:8 mg/kg/3W-I CNREA8 33,3069,73
NEO: ipr-mus TD:9500 µg/kg/26W-I RRCRBU 52,1,75
NEO: ipr-rat TDLo:1000 µg/kg/26W-I RRCRBU 52,1,75
MUT: dnd-dmg-par 2 mmol/L CNREA8 30,195,70
MUT: dnr-esc 25 mg/L JNCIAM 62,873,79
MUT: hma-mus/sat 12 mg/kg JNCIAM 62,911,79
MUT: mma-mus:lym 200 µg/L/4H MUREAV 59,61,79
MUT: mma-sat 100 µg/plate PNASA6 72,5135,75
MUT: mmo-sat 125 µg/plate JNCIAM 62,893,79
MUT: mrc-smc 5 pph JNCIAM 62,901,79

MUT: msc-mus:lym 150 µg/L/2H   MUREAV 59,61,79

CONSENSUS REPORTS: IARC Cancer Review: GROUP 2B IMEMDT 7,370,87; Animal Sufficient Evidence IMEMDT 9,235,75; NCI Carcinogenesis Studies (ipr); Clear Evidence: mouse, rat RRCRBU 52,1,75. EPA Genetic Toxicology Program.

SAFETY PROFILE: Suspected carcinogen with experimental carcinogenic and neoplastigenic data. A deadly poison by ingestion and intraperitoneal routes. Mutation data reported. When heated to decomposition it emits very toxic fumes of Cl^- and NO_x.

BIM750   CAS: 72-55-9
2,2-BIS(p-CHLOROPHENYL)-1,1-DICHLOROETHYLENE
mf: $C_{14}H_8Cl_4$ mw: 318.02

SYNS: DDE ◇ p,p'-DDE ◇ DDT DEHYDROCHLORIDE ◇ 1,1-DICHLORO-2,2-BIS(p-CHLOROPHENYL)ETHYLENE ◇ p,p'-DICHLORODIPHENYL DICHLOROETHYLENE ◇ 1,1'-DICHLOROETHENYLIDENE)BIS(4-CHLOROBENZENE) ◇ NCI-C00555

TOXICITY DATA with REFERENCE
CAR: orl-mus TD:17 g/kg/78W-C   NCITR* NCI-TR-131,78
CAR: orl-mus TDLo:9700 mg/kg/78W-C   NCITR* NCI-TR-131,78
NEO: orl-ham TD:41 g/kg/97W-C   CNREA8 43,776,83
NEO: orl-ham TD:57 g/kg/68W-C   CNREA8 43,776,83
NEO: orl-ham TD:81 g/kg/97W-C   CNREA8 43,776,83
NEO: orl-ham TDLo:36 g/kg/86W-C   CNREA8 43,776,83
NEO: orl-mus TD:28 g/kg/80W-C   JNCIAM 52,883,74
MUT: cyt-rat:oth 10 µg/L   34LXAP -,555,76
MUT: dnd-rat:lvr 300 µmol/L   SinJF# 26OCT82
MUT: msc-mus:lym 40 mg/L/4H   MUREAV 59,61,79
MUT: sln-dmg-orl 1 pph   ENMUDM 7,325,85
MUT: slt-ham:ovr 25 mg/L   MUREAV 136,137,84

CONSENSUS REPORTS: IARC Cancer Review: Animal Limited Evidence IMEMDT 5,83,74. NCI Carcinogenesis Bioassay (feed); Clear Evidence: mouse NCITR* NCI-CG-TR-131,78; No Evidence: rat NCITR* NCI-CG-TR-131,78. EPA Genetic Toxicology Program.

SAFETY PROFILE: Suspected carcinogen with experimental carcinogenic and neoplastigenic data. Poison by ingestion. Experimental reproductive effects. Mutation data reported. An insecticide. When heated to decomposition it emits very toxic fumes of Cl^-.

BIX500   CAS: 15442-77-0
BIS(3,4-DICHLOROBENZOATO)NICKEL
mf: $C_{14}H_6Cl_4NiO_4$ mw: 438.71

CONSENSUS REPORTS: Nickel and its compounds are on The Community Right-To-Know List.

OSHA PEL: (Transitional: TWA 1 mg/m³) TWA 0.1 mg (Ni)/m³   ACGIH TLV: TWA 0.1 mg(Ni)/m³; (Proposed: TWA 0.05 mg(Ni)/m³; Human Carcinogen)   NIOSH REL: (Inorganic Nickel) TWA 0.015 mg(Ni)/m³

SAFETY PROFILE: Suspected carcinogen. Poison by intravenous route. When heated to decomposition it emits toxic fumes of Cl^-.

BKF250   CAS: 2784-94-3
N',N'-BIS(2-HYDROXYETHYL)-N-METHYL-2-NITRO-p-PHENYLENEDIAMINE
mf: $C_{11}H_{17}N_3O_4$ mw: 255.31

SYNS: HC BLUE 1 ◇ NCI-C04159

TOXICITY DATA with REFERENCE
CAR: orl-mus TD:131 g/kg/2Y-C   NTPTR* NTP-TR-271,85
CAR: orl-mus TDLo:98280 mg/kg/39W-C   FCTOD7 25,703,87
CAR: orl-rat TDLo:66 g/kg/2Y-C   NTPTR* NTP-TR-271,85
MUT: dns-rat:lvr 50 mg/L   NTPTR* NTP-TR-271,85
MUT: mma-sat 100 µg/plate   NTPTR* NTP-TR-271,85
MUT: mmo-sat 333 µg/plate   NTPTR* NTP-TR-271,85
MUT: msc-mus:lym 30 mg/L   NTPTR* NTP-TR-271,85

CONSENSUS REPORTS: NTP Carcinogenesis Studies (feed); Some Evidence: rat NTPTR* NTP-TR-271,85;(feed); Clear Evidence: mouse NTPTR* NTP-TR-271,85. Reported in EPA TSCA Inventory.

SAFETY PROFILE: Suspected carcinogen with experimental carcinogenic data. Mutation data reported. When heated to decomposition it emits toxic fumes of NO_x.

BKH500   CAS: 794-93-4
BIS(HYDROXYMETHYL)FURATRIZINE
mf: $C_{11}H_{11}N_5O_5$ mw: 293.27

SYNS: 3-BIS(HYDROXYMETHYL)AMINO-6-(5-NITRO-2-FURYLETHENYL)-1,2,4-TRIAZINE ◇ DHNT ◇ 3-DI(HYDROXYMETHYL)AMINO-6-(5-NITRO-2-FURYLETHNEYL)-1,2,4-TRIAZINE ◇ 3-DI(HYDROXYMETHYL)AMIMO-6-(2-(5-NITRO-2-FURYL)VINYL)-1,2,4-TRIAZINE ◇ DIHYDROXY-METHYL FURATRIZINE ◇ FURATONE ◇ FURATONE-S ◇ N-(6-(5-NITROFURFURYLIDENEMETHYL)-1,2,4-TRIAZIN-3-YL)IMINODIMETHANOL ◇ 6-(5-NITRO-2-FURYLVINYL)-3-(DIHYDROXYDIMETHYLAMINO)-1,2,4-TRIAZENE ◇ N-(6-(2-(5-NITRO-2-FURYL)VINYL)-1,2,4-TRIAZIN-3-YL)IMINODIMETHANOL ◇ ((6-(2-(5-NITRO-2-FURYL)-VINYL)-as-TRIAZIN-3-YL)IMINO)DIMETHANOL ◇ PAN-FURAN-S

TOXICITY DATA with REFERENCE
CAR: orl-mus TDLo:12740 mg/kg/35W-C
    NAIZAM 31,31,80
CAR: orl-rat TD:26 g/kg/35W-C   GANNA2
    68,371,77
CAR: orl-rat TD:27 g/kg/36W-C   JNCIAM
    60,1339,78
CAR: orl-rat TD:27 g/kg/37W-C   IGAYAY
    108,96,79
CAR: orl-rat TDLo:25725 mg/kg/35W-C
    NAIZAM 31,31,80
MUT: dnd-esc 500 μg/L   MIIMDV 21,481,77
MUT: dni-esc 500 μg/L   MIIMDV 21,481,77
MUT: dni-omi 1 mg/L   NKRZAZ 22,1159,74
MUT: dnr-esc 20 μg/L   NKRZAZ 22,1159,74
MUT: mmo-esc 125 μg/L   MUREAV 146,243,85
MUT: oms-omi 1 mg/L   NKRZAZ 22,1159,74
MUT: orl-mus TD:10290 mg/kg/35W-C
    ONKOD2 2,41,79
MUT: orl-mus TD:20580 mg/kg/35W-C
    ONKOD2 2,41,79
MUT: orl-rat TD:63210 mg/kg/43W-C   EXPADD
    26,213,84
MUT: pic-esc 800 μg/L   MUREAV 146,243,85

CONSENSUS REPORTS: IARC Cancer Review: GROUP 2B IMEMDT 7,56,87; Animal Sufficient Evidence IMEMDT 24,77, 80

SAFETY PROFILE: Suspected carcinogen with experimental carcinogenic and tumorigenic data. Moderately toxic by ingestion, intraperitoneal, and subcutaneous route. Mutation data reported. An antibacterial agent. When heated to decomposition it emits toxic fumes of NO_x.

BLS250   CAS: 14264-16-5
BIS(TRIPHENYLPHOSPHINE) DICHLORONICKEL
mf: $C_{24}H_{54}P_2 \cdot Cl_2Ni$ mw: 534.33

SYNS: BIS(TRI-N-BUTYLPHOSPHINE)DICHLORONICKEL ◇ TRIBUTYL-PHOSPHINE compd. with NICKELCHLORIDE (2:1)

CONSENSUS REPORTS: Reported in EPA TSCA Inventory. Nickel and its compounds are on the Community Right-To-Know List.

OSHA PEL: (Transitional: TWA 1 mg/m³) TWA 0.1 mg (Ni)/m³   ACGIH TLV: TWA 0.1 mg(Ni)/m³; (Proposed: TWA 0.05 mg(Ni)/m³; Human Carcinogen)   NIOSH REL: TWA 0.015 mg/(Ni)/m³

SAFETY PROFILE: Suspected carcinogen. Poison by intravenous route. When heated to decomposition it emits very toxic fumes of Cl^- and PO_x.

BLV250   CAS: 13394-86-0
(m,o'-BITOLYL)-4-AMINE
mf: $C_{14}H_{15}N$ mw: 197.30

SYNS: 2',3-DIMETHYL-4-AMINOBIPHENYL ◇ 3,2'-DIMETHYL-4-AMINOBIPHENYL ◇ 3,2'-DIMETHYL-4-AMINO-DIPHENYL ◇ 3,2'-DIMETHYL-4-BIPHENYLAMINE ◇ 3,2'-DMAB

TOXICITY DATA with REFERENCE
CAR: scu-ham TD:1095 mg/kg/37W-I   CALEDQ
    20,349,83
CAR: scu-ham TD:4440 mg/kg/77W-I   JJIND8
    67,481,81
CAR: scu-ham TDLo:2300 mg/kg/37W-I
    JNCIAM 48,1733,72
CAR: scu-rat TD:960 mg/kg/21W-I   ANZJA7
    29,38,59
CAR: scu-rat TD:1000 mg/kg/20W-I   CNREA8
    41,1363,81
CAR: scu-rat TD:1000 mg/kg/20W-I   JJIND8
    71,419,83
CAR: scu-rat TD:1100 mg/kg/31W-I   CNREA8
    27,708,67
CAR: scu-rat TD:1400 mg/kg/14W-I   ANSUA5
    161,309,65
CAR: scu-rat TD:2200 mg/kg/22W-I   ANSUA5
    161,309,65
CAR: scu-rat TD:2300 mg/kg/36W-I   BJCAAI
    9,170,55
CAR: scu-rat TD:10400 mg/kg/2Y-I   CANCAR
    28,29,71

CAR: scu-rat TDLo:680 mg/kg/I   ARPAAQ 86,475,68

ETA: par-rat TDLo:280 mg/kg/14W-I 23HZAR-,280,70

MUT: cyt-mus-orl 50 mg/kg   JJIND8 71,133,83

MUT: dns-rat:lvr 10 μmol/L   CALEDQ 4,69,78

MUT: mma-sat 10 μg/plate   PNASA6 72,5135,75

MUT: otr-ham:emb 100 μg/L   NCIMAV 58,243,81

CONSENSUS REPORTS: EPA Genetic Toxicology Program.

SAFETY PROFILE: Suspected carcinogen with experimental carcinogenic and tumorigenic data. Moderately toxic by intraperitoneal route. Mutation data reported. When heated to decomposition it emits toxic fumes of NO_x.

BLY000   CAS: 11056-06-7
BLEOMYCIN

PROP: A group of related glycopeptide antibiotics isolated from *Streptomyces verticillus* (12VXA5 9, 171,76).

SYNS: BLEO ◇ BLENOXANE ◇ BLEOCIN ◇ BLM

TOXICITY DATA with REFERENCE

MUT: cyt-mus:oth 4 nmol/L   IPPABX 20,1,84

MUT: dnd-hmn:fbr 10 mg/L   ENMUDM 7,267,84

MUT: dns-hmn:hla 110 μmol/L   CRNGDP 7,77,86

MUT: mnt-hmn:lym 1250 μg/L   MUREAV 130,395,84

MUT: sce-ham-ipr 7500 ug/kg   CNREA8 43,577,83

CONSENSUS REPORTS: IARC Cancer Review: GROUP 2B IMEMDT 7,134,87, Human Inadequate Evidence IMEMDT 26,97,81. EPA Genetic Toxicology Program.

SAFETY PROFILE: Suspected carcinogen. A human poison by intravenous route; moderately toxic to humans by intramuscular route. Poison experimentally by intravenous and intraperitoneal routes. Human systemic effects by ingestion and intramuscular routes: dyspnea and fibrosing alveolitis (lung). Experimental reproductive effects. Human mutation data reported. When heated to decomposition it emits toxic fumes of NO_x.

BND500   CAS: 75-27-4
BROMODICHLOROMETHANE
mf: $CHBrCl_2$ mw: 163.83

PROP: Colorless liquid. Bp: 89.2−90.6°, d: 1.971 @ 25°/25°.

SYNS: BDCM ◇ DICHLOROBROMOMETHANE ◇ NCI-C55243

TOXICITY DATA with REFERENCE

CAR: orl-mus TD:38250 mg/kg/2Y-C   NTPTR* NTP-TR-321,87

CAR: orl-mus TDLo:25500 mg/kg/2Y-C NTPTR* NTP-TR-321,87

CAR: orl-rat TD:51 g/kg/2Y-C   NTPTR* NTP-TR-321,87

CAR: orl-rat TDLo:25500 mg/kg/2Y-C   NTPTR* NTP-TR-321,87

MUT: mmo-sat 50 μL/plate   DHEFDK FDA-78-1046,78

MUT: sce-hmn:lym 400 μmol/L   ENVRAL 32,72,83

MUT: sce-mus-orl 200 mg/kg/4D-I   ENVRAL 32,72,83

CONSENSUS REPORTS: NTP Carcinogenesis Studies (gavage): Clear Evidence: rat, mouse NTPTR* NTP-TR-321,87. EPA Genetic Toxicology Program. Community Right-To-Know List. Reported in EPA TSCA Inventory.

SAFETY PROFILE: Suspected carcinogen with experimental carcinogenic data. Moderately toxic by ingestion. Human mutation data reported. When heated to decomposition it emits very toxic fumes of Br^- and Cl^-.

BOP750   CAS: 30031-64-2
l-BUTADIENE DIEPOXIDE
mf: $C_4H_6O_2$ mw: 86.10

SYNS: (S-(R*,R*))-2,2'-BIOXIRANE ◇ (2S,3S)-DIEPOXYBUTANE ◇ l-DIEPOXYBUTANE ◇ l-1,2:3,4-DIEPOXYBUTANE ◇ (2S,3S)-1,2:3,4-DIEPOXYBUTANE ◇ NSC-32606

TOXICITY DATA with REFERENCE

NEO: ipr-mus TDLo:110 mg/kg/4W   JNCIAM 36,915,66

NEO: par-mus TDLo:192 mg/kg/4W-I   NCISA* PH-43-62-483

MUT: dnd-omi 5 mmol/L   BBACAQ 228,400,71

MUT: mmo-ssp 31 mmol/L   ADWMAX -,193,62

CONSENSUS REPORTS: IARC Cancer Review: GROUP 2B IMEMDT 7,56,87; Animal Sufficient Evidence IMEMDT 11,115,76. EPA Genetic Toxicology Program.

SAFETY PROFILE: Suspected carcinogen with experimental neoplastigenic data. Poison by intraperitoneal route. Mutation data reported. When heated to decomposition it emits acrid and irritating fumes.

BOU250   CAS: 1633-83-6
BUTANE SULTONE
mf: $C_4H_8O_3S$ mw: 136.18

SYNS: BUTANESULFONE ◇ Δ-BUTANE SULTONE ◇ 1,4-BUTANESULTONE (MAK) ◇ 1,4-BUTYLENE SULFONE ◇ Δ-VALEROSULTONE

TOXICITY DATA with REFERENCE

ETA: orl-rat TDLo:1300 mg/kg/1Y-I   ZEKBAI 75,69,70

ETA: scu-mus TDLo:1680 mg/kg/42W-I   JNCIAM 53,695,74

ETA: scu-rat TDLo:2280 mg/kg/76W-I   ZEKBAI 75,69,70

MUT: dnr-esc 10 μL/disc   JNCIAM 62,873,79

MUT: hma-mus/sat 138 mg/kg   JNCIAM 62,911,79

MUT: mma-sat 100 μL/plate   JNCIAM 62,873,79

MUT: mmo-sat 100 μg/plate   JNCIAM 62,893,79

MUT: mmo-ssp 331 mmol/L   CBINA8 14,195,76

MUT: mrc-smc 1 pph   JNCIAM 62,901,79

MUT: otr-ham:emb 5 mg/L   IJCNAW 19,642,77

MUT: otr-ham:kdy 80 μg/L   ARTODN 33,225,75

CONSENSUS REPORTS: EPA Genetic Toxicology Program. Reported in EPA TSCA Inventory.

DFG MAK: Suspected Carcinogen.

SAFETY PROFILE: Suspected carcinogen with experimental tumorigenic data. Poison by subcutaneous, intravenous and intraperitoneal routes. Moderately toxic by ingestion. Human mutation data reported. When heated to decomposition it emits toxic fumes of SO_x.

BQI000   CAS: 25013-16-5
BUTYLATED HYDROXYANISOLE
mf: $C_{11}H_{16}O_2$ mw: 180.27

PROP: White waxy solid; faint characteristic odor. Mp: 48-63°. Sol in alc and propylene glycol; insol in water.

SYNS: ANTRANCINE 12 ◇ BHA (FCC) ◇ BUTYLHYDROXYANISOLE ◇ tert-BUTYLHYDROXYANISOLE ◇ tert-BUTYL-4-HYDROXYANISOLE ◇ 2(3)-tert-BUTYL-4-HYDROXYANISOLE ◇ BUTYLOHYDROKSYANIZOL (POLISH) ◇ EMBANOX ◇ FEMA No. 2183 ◇ NIPANTIOX 1-F ◇ PREMERGE PLUS ◇ SUSTANE ◇ SUSTANE 1-F ◇ TENOX BHA ◇ VERTAC

TOXICITY DATA with REFERENCE

CAR: orl-ham TDLo:437 g/kg/1Y-C   JJCREP 77,1083,86

CAR: orl-rat TD:269 g/kg/32W-C   CRNGDP 4,895,83

CAR: orl-rat TD:728 g/kg/2Y-C   TOLED5 31(Suppl),207,86

CAR: orl-rat TD:874 g/kg/1Y-C   JJCREP 77,1083,86

CAR: orl-rat TD:874 g/kg/2Y-C   GANNA2 73,332,82

CAR: orl-rat TD:876 g/kg/2Y-C   JJIND8 70,343,83

CAR: orl-rat TDLo:728 g/kg/2Y-C   GANNA2 73,332,82

NEO: orl-ham TD:202 g/kg/24W-C   GANNA2 74,459,83

NEO: orl-rat TD:202 g/kg/24W-C   JJCREP 77,854,86

NEO: orl-rat TD:4200 mg/kg/10W-C   CNREA8 46,165,86

ETA: orl-mus TDLo:874 g/kg/1Y-C   JJCREP 77,1083,86

ETA: orl-rat TD:182 g/kg/2Y-C   GANNA2 73,332,82

ETA: orl-rat TD:218 g/kg/2Y-C   GANNA2 73,332,82

MUT: mmo-omi 12500 μg/L   FMLED7 14,183,82

MUT: sce-ham:fbr 100 μmol/L   JNCIAM 58,1635,77

CONSENSUS REPORTS: IARC Cancer Review: GROUP 2B IMEMDT 7,56,87; Animal Sufficient Evidence IMEMDT 40,123,86. Reported in EPA TSCA Inventory. EPA Genetic Toxicology Program.

SAFETY PROFILE: Suspected carcinogen with experimental carcinogenic, neoplastigenic, and tumorigenic data. Moderately toxic by ingestion and intraperitoneal routes. Experimental reproductive effects. Mutation data reported. When heated to decomposition it emits acrid and irritating fumes.

BRF500   CAS: 50-33-9
4-BUTYL-1,2-DIPHENYL-3,5-DIOXO PYRAZOLIDINE
mf: $C_{19}H_{20}N_2O_2$ mw: 308.41

SYNS: ALINDOR ◇ ALKABUTAZONA ◇ ALQOVERIN ◇ ANERVAL ◇ ANPUZONE ◇ ANTADOL ◇ ANUSPIRAMIN ◇ ARTIZIN ◇ ARTRIZONE ◇ ARTROPAN ◇ AZDID ◇ AZOBUTYL ◇ AZOLID ◇ BENZONE ◇ BETAZED ◇ BIZOLIN 200 ◇ B.T.Z. ◇ BUSONE ◇ BUTACOMPREN ◇ BUTACOTE ◇ BUTADION ◇ BUTADIONA ◇ BUTAGESIC ◇ BUTALAN ◇ BUTALGINA ◇ BUTALIDON ◇ BUTALUY ◇ BUTAPHEN ◇ BUTAPIRAZOL ◇ BUTAPYRAZOLE ◇ BUTARECBON ◇ BUTARTRIL ◇ BUTARTRINA ◇ BUTAZINA ◇ BUTAZOLIDIN ◇ BUTAZONA ◇ BUTAZONE ◇ BUTE ◇ BUTIDIONA ◇ BUTIWAS-SIMPLE ◇ BUTONE ◇ BUTOZ ◇ 4-BUTYL-1,2-DIPHENYLPYRAZOLIDINE-3,5-DIONE ◇ 4-BUTYL-1,2-DIPHENYL-3,5-PYRAZOLIDINE-

DIONE ◇ BUTYLPYRIN ◇ BUVETZONE ◇ BUZON
◇ CHEMBUTAZONE ◇ FA-192 ◇ DIGIBUTINA ◇ DIOSSI-
DONE ◇ 3,5-DIOXO-1,2-DIPHENYL-4-N-BUTYLPYRAZOLI-
DENE ◇ 3,5-DIOXO-1,2-DIPHENYL-4-N-BUTYL-PYRAZOLI-
DIN ◇ 3,5-DIOXO-1,2-DIPHENYL-4-N-BUTYL-
PYRAZOLIDINE ◇ DIOZOL ◇ DIPHEBUZOL ◇ DIPHENYL-
BUTAZONE ◇ 1,2-DIPHENYL-4-BUTYL-3,5-DIOXOPYRAZO-
LIDINE ◇ 1,2-DIPHENYL-4-BUTYL-3,5-PYRAZOLIDINE-
DIONE ◇ 1,2-DIPHENYL-3,5-DIOXO-4-
BUTYLPYRAZOLIDINE ◇ 1,2-DIPHENYL-2,3-DIOXO-4-N-
BUTYLPYRAZOLINE ◇ ECOBUTAZONE ◇ ELMEDAL
◇ EQUI BUTE ◇ ERIBUTAZONE ◇ ESTEVE ◇ FBZ
◇ FEBUZINA ◇ FENARTIL ◇ FENIBUTASAN ◇ FENIBUTA-
ZONA ◇ FENIBUTOL ◇ FENILBUTAZONA ◇ FENILBUTINE
◇ FENILIDINA ◇ FENOTONE ◇ FENYLBUTAZON
◇ FLEXAZONE ◇ IA-BUT ◇ INTALBUT ◇ INTRABUTAZONE
◇ IPSOFLAME ◇ KADOL ◇ LINGEL ◇ MALGESIC
◇ MEPHABUTAZONE ◇ MERIZONE ◇ NADAZONE
◇ NADOZONE ◇ NCI-C56531 ◇ NEO-ZOLINE ◇ NOVOPHE-
NYL ◇ PBZ ◇ PHEBUZIN ◇ PHEBUZINE ◇ PHEN-BUTA-
VET ◇ PHENBUTAZOL ◇ PHENOPYRINE ◇ PHENYLBUTAZ
◇ PHENYLBUTAZON (GERMAN) ◇ PHENYLBUTAZONE
◇ PHENYLBUTAZONUM ◇ PHENYL-MOBUZON ◇ PIRAR-
REUMOL 'B'' ◇ PRAECIRHEUMIN ◇ PYRABUTOL
◇ PYRAZOLIDIN ◇ RECTOFASA ◇ REUDO ◇ REUDOX
◇ REUMASYL ◇ REUMAZIN ◇ REUMAZOL ◇ REUPOLAR
◇ ROBIZON-V ◇ RUBATONE ◇ R-3-ZON ◇ SCANBUTA-
ZONE ◇ SCHEMERGIN ◇ SHIGRODIN ◇ TAZONE
◇ TETNOR ◇ TEVCODYNE ◇ THERAZONE ◇ TICINIL
◇ TODALGIL ◇ USAF GE-15 ◇ UZONE ◇ VAC-10
◇ WESCOZONE ◇ ZOLAPHEN ◇ ZOLIDINUM ◇ ZORANE

TOXICITY DATA with REFERENCE
CAR: mul-wmn TDLo: 4200 mg/kg/77W-I
  BMJOAE 2,1569,61
CAR: orl-man TD: 140 mg/kg/3W-C: BLD
  BMJOAE 2,1552,60
CAR: orl-man TDLo: 4368 mg/kg/4Y-C: BLD
  BMJOAE 1,744,64
MUT: cyt-ham-orl 25 mg/kg   MUREAV 13,377,71
MUT: cyt-ham:fbr 1 g/L   ESKHA5 96,55,78
MUT: mnt-mus-ipr 50 mg/kg   IJEBA6 18,869,80
MUT: mnt-mus-orl 75 mg/kg   IJEBA6 18,869,80
MUT: oms-hmn:emb 20 mg/L   BEXBAN 74,828,72

CONSENSUS REPORTS: IARC Cancer Review: GROUP 3 IMEMDT 7,316,87; Human Inadequate Evidence IMEMDT 13,183,77. EPA Genetic Toxicology Program. Reported in EPA TSCA Inventory.

SAFETY PROFILE: Suspected human carcinogen producing leukemia. A human poison by parenteral route. An experimental poison by ingestion, intraperitoneal, subcutaneous, intravenous and intramuscular routes. Human systemic effects by ingestion and possibly other routes: fever, blood pressure increase, other unspecified vascular effects, damage to kidney tubules and glomeruli, decreased urine volume, blood in the urine, reduction in the number of white blood cells, and agranulocytosis. An experimental teratogen. Experimental reproductive effects. Human mutation data reported. An eye irritant. An anti-inflammatory agent. When heated to decomposition it emits toxic fumes of NO_x.

BSA250   CAS: 869-01-2
n-BUTYLNITROSOUREA
mf: $C_5H_{11}N_3O_2$ mw: 145.19

SYNS: BNU ◇ BUTYLNITROSOHARNSTOFF (GERMAN)
◇ N-n-BUTYL-N-NITROSOUREA ◇ 1-BUTYL-1-NITRO-
SOUREA ◇ N-NITROSOBUTYLUREA

TOXICITY DATA with REFERENCE
CAR: orl-mus TDLo: 2800 mg/kg/10W-C
  GANNA2 68,281,77
CAR: orl-rat TDLo: 4867 mg/kg/24W-I
  GANNA2 67,33,76
CAR: orl-rat TDLo: 16512 mg/kg/50W-I
  JCROD7 107,32,84
ETA: orl-dog TDLo: 960 mg/kg/81W-I   PARPDS
  164,216,79
ETA: orl-mus TD: 2800 mg/kg/10W-C   PPTCBY
  6,57,76
ETA: orl-mus TDLo: 3360 mg/kg/12W-C
  GANNA2 61,287,70
ETA: orl-rat TD: 200 mg/kg   GANNA2 66,615,75
ETA: orl-rat TD: 300 mg/kg   GMCRDC 12,283,72
ETA: orl-rat TD: 1050 mg/kg/5W-C   BIHAA2
  (40),107,73
ETA: orl-rat TD: 2400 mg/kg/17W-I   GANNA2
  62,557,71
ETA: orl-rat TD: 2505 mg/kg/24W-C   GANNA2
  60,237,69
ETA: orl-rat TD: 2505 mg/kg/24W-C
  25NJAN -,24,70
ETA: scu-rat TD: 450 mg/kg   ANYAA9 381,250,82
ETA: scu-rat TDLo: 300 mg/kg   GMCRDC
  12,283,72
ETA: skn-mus TDLo: 581 mg/kg/50W-I
  JCROD7 102,13,81
MUT: cyt-ham-ipr 240 mg/kg   MUREAV 81,117,81
MUT: dnd-mam:lym 10 mmol/L   CRNGDP
  5,621,84
MUT: mmo-sat 1 μg/plate   MUREAV 68,1,79
MUT: pic-esc 2 mg/L   TCMUE9 1,91,84
MUT: sce-ham:fbr 500 μmol/L   CNREA8
  44,3270,84

CONSENSUS REPORTS: EPA Genetic Toxicology Program.

SAFETY PROFILE: Suspected carcinogen with experimental carcinogenic, tumorigenic, and teratogenic data. An poison by ingestion. Moderately toxic by subcutaneous route. Mutation data reported. When heated to decomposition it emits toxic fumes of NO_x.

BSS500
1-BUTYLUREA and SODIUM NITRITE (2:1)

TOXICITY DATA with REFERENCE
CAR: orl-mus TD:421 g/kg/46W-C   IJCNAW
23,253,79
CAR: orl-mus TDLo:380 g/kg/42W-C   IJCNAW
23,253,79
CAR: orl-rat TD:170 g/kg/37W-C   IJCNAW
23,253,79
CAR: orl-rat TDLo:126 g/kg/33W-C   IJCNAW
23,253,79
ETA: orl-rat TDLo:1350 mg/kg (13-21D preg):REP   GANNA2 68,81,77
NEO: orl-rat TD:27500 mg/kg/50D-C   ZAPPAN
121,61,77

SAFETY PROFILE: Suspected carcinogen with experimental carcinogenic, neoplastigenic, and tumorigenic data. When heated to decomposition it emits toxic fumes of NO_x.

BSX000   CAS: 3068-88-0
β-BUTYROLACTONE
mf: $C_4H_6O_2$ mw: 86.10

SYNS: 3-HYDROXYBUTANOIC ACID-β-LACTONE ◇ HYDROXYBUTYRIC ACID LACTONE ◇ 3-HYDROXYBUTYRIC ACID LACTONE ◇ 4-METHYL-2-OXETANONE

TOXICITY DATA with REFERENCE
CAR: scu-rat TDLo:38 g/kg/78W-I   JNCIAM
39,1213,67
CAR: skn-mus TD:80 g/kg/67W-I   14JTAF
-,275,64
CAR: skn-mus TDLo:59 g/kg/49W-I   JNCIAM
35,707,65
NEO: scu-mus TDLo:12 g/kg/30W-I   JNCIAM
37,825,66
ETA: orl-rat TDLo:31 g/kg/61W-I   JNCIAM
37,825,66
ETA: skn-mus TD:43 g/kg/36W-I   JNCIAM
39,1217,67
MUT: dnd-mam:lym 10 mmol/L   BBACAQ
138,611,67

MUT: oms-mam:lym 286 nmol/L   CBINA8
34,323,81

CONSENSUS REPORTS: IARC Cancer Review: GROUP 2B IMEMDT 7,56,87, Animal Sufficient Evidence IMEMDT 11,225,76. Reported in EPA TSCA Inventory.

SAFETY PROFILE: Suspected carcinogen with experimental carcinogenic, neoplastigenic, and tumorigenic data. Mildly toxic by ingestion. A moderate skin irritant. Mutation data reported. When heated to decomposition it emits acrid and irritating fumes.

CBF250   CAS: 302-22-7
CAP
mf: $C_{23}H_{29}ClO_4$ mw: 404.97

SYNS: 17-ACETOXY-6-CHLORO-6-DEHYDROPROGESTERONE ◇ 17-α-ACETOXY-6-CHLORO-6-DEHYDROPROGESTERONE ◇ 17-α-ACETOXY-6-CHLORO-6,7-DEHYDROPROGESTERONE ◇ 17-α-ACETOXY-6-CHLORO-4,6-PREGNADIENE-3,20-DIONE ◇ 17-α-ACETOXY-6-CHLOROPREGNA-4,6-DIENE-3,20-DIONE ◇ 17-(ACETYLOXY)-6-CHLOROPREGNA-4,6-DIENE-3,20-DIONE ◇ CHLORMADINON ACETATE ◇ CHLORMADINONE ACETATE ◇ CHLORMADINONU (POLISH) ◇ 6-CHLORO-17-α-ACETOXY-4,6-PREGNADIENE-3,20-DIONE ◇ Δ⁶-6-CHLORO-17-α-ACETOXYPROGESTERONE ◇ 6-CHLORO-Δ⁶-17-ACETOXYPROGESTERONE ◇ 6-CHLORO-Δ⁶-(17-α)ACETOXYPROGESTERONE ◇ 6-CHLORO-Δ⁶-DEHYDRO-17-ACETOXYPROGESTERONE ◇ 6-CHLORO-6-DEHYDRO-17-α-ACETOXYPROGESTERONE ◇ 6-CHLORO-6-DEHYDRO-17-α-HYDROXYPROGESTERONE ACETATE ◇ 6-CHLORO-17-α-HYDROXYPREGNA-4,6-DIENE-3,20-DIONE ACETATE ◇ 6-CHLORO-17-α-HYDROXY-Δ⁶-PROGESTERONE ACETATE ◇ CHLOROMADINONE ACETATE ◇ 6-CHLORO-Δ⁴,⁶-PREGNADIENE-17-α-OL-3,20-DIONE-17-ACETATE ◇ 6-CHLORO-PREGNA-4,6-DIEN-17-α-OL-3,20-DIONE ACETATE ◇ CLORDION ◇ CMA ◇ C-QUENS ◇ 6-DEHYDRO-6-CHLORO-17-α-ACETOXYPROGESTERONE ◇ LORMIN ◇ LUTINYL ◇ NSC-92338 ◇ RS 1280 ◇ SKEDULE ◇ ST 155

TOXICITY DATA with REFERENCE
ETA: orl-dog TDLo:182 mg/kg/2Y-C   JAMAAP
219,1601,72
ETA: orl-dog TDLo:639 mg/kg/7Y-C   JTEHD6
3,167,77

CONSENSUS REPORTS: IARC Cancer Review: Animal Limited Evidence IMEMDT 21,365,79; Animal Sufficient Evidence IMEMDT 6,149,74.

SAFETY PROFILE: Suspected carcinogen with experimental carcinogenic, tumorigenic, and teratogenic data. Moderately toxic by intraperitoneal route. Human maternal and reproductive effects by ingestion, intramuscular, and possibly other routes: ovary, uterus, cervix, vagina, and fallopian tube changes; menstrual cycle changes or disorders; changes in fertility; and other unspecified female effects. A human teratogen which causes developmental abnormalities of the endocrine system in the fetus. Experimental reproductive effects. An oral contraceptive. When heated to decomposition it emits toxic fumes of Cl⁻.

CBN375
CARBENDAZIM and SODIUM NITRITE (5:1)

SYNS: METHYL-2-BENZIMIDAZOLE CARBAMATE and SODIUM NITRITE ◇ SODIUM NITRITE and CARBENDAZIM (1:5) ◇ SODIUM NITRITE and METHYL-2-BENZIMIDAZOLE CARBAMATE

TOXICITY DATA with REFERENCE
CAR: orl-mus TD:88 g/kg/12W-I   MGONAD
19,175,75
CAR: orl-mus TDLo:31 g/kg/26W-I   IJCNAW
15,830,75
CAR: orl-mus TDLo:3000 mg/kg (7-14D preg)
IJCNAW 17,742,76

SAFETY PROFILE: Suspected carcinogen with experimental carcinogenic data. When heated to decomposition it emits toxic fumes of Na_2O and NO_x.

CDP250   CAS: 56-75-7
CHLORAMPHENICOL
mf: $C_{11}H_{12}Cl_2N_2O_5$ mw: 323.15

PROP: Crystalline. Mp: 151°. Sltly sol in water.

SYNS: ALFICETYN ◇ AMBOFEN ◇ AMPHENICOL ◇ AMPHICOL ◇ AMSECLOR ◇ ANACETIN ◇ AQUAMYCETIN ◇ AUSTRACIL ◇ AUSTRACOL ◇ BIOCETIN ◇ BIOPHENICOL ◇ CAF ◇ CAM ◇ CAP ◇ CATILAN ◇ CHEMICETIN ◇ CHEMICETINA ◇ CHLOMIN ◇ CHLOMYCOL ◇ CHLORAMEX ◇ CHLORAMFICIN ◇ CHLORAMFILIN ◇ d-CHLORAMPHENICOL ◇ d-threo-CHLORAMPHENICOL ◇ CHLORAMSAAR ◇ CHLORASOL ◇ CHLORA-TABS ◇ CHLORICOL ◇ CHLORNITROMYCIN ◇ CHLOROCAPS ◇ CHLOROCID ◇ CHLOROCIDIN C TETRAN ◇ CHLOROCOL ◇ CHLOROJECT L ◇ CHLOROMAX ◇ CHLOROMYCETIN ◇ CHLORONITRIN ◇ CHLOROPTIC ◇ CHLOROVULES ◇ CIDOCETINE ◇ CIPLAMYCETIN ◇ CLORAMIDINA ◇ CLOROAMFENICOLO (ITALIAN) ◇ CLOROMISAN

◇ CLOROSINTEX ◇ COMYCETIN ◇ CPH ◇ CYLPHENICOL ◇ DESPHEN ◇ DETREOMYCINE ◇ DEXTROMYCETIN ◇ d-(−)-threo-2-DICHLOROACETAMIDO-1-p-NITROPHENYL-1,3-PROPANEDIOL ◇ d-threo-N-DICHLOROACETYL-1-p-NITROPHENYL-2-AMINO-1,3-PROPANEDIOL ◇ d-(−)-threo-2,2-DICHLORO-N-(β-HYDROXY-α-(HYDROXYMETHYL))-p-NITROPHENETHYLACETAMIDE ◇ d-(−)-2,2-DICHLORO-N-(β-HYDROXY-α-(HYDROXYMETHYL)-p-NITROPHENYL-ETHYL)ACETAMIDE ◇ d-threo-N-(1,1'-DIHYDROXY-1-p-NITROPHENYLISOPROPYL)DICHLOROACETAMIDE ◇ DOCTAMICINA ◇ ECONOCHLOR ◇ EMBACETIN ◇ EMETREN ◇ ENICOL ◇ ENTEROMYCETIN ◇ ERBAPLAST ◇ ERTILEN ◇ FARMICETINA ◇ FENICOL ◇ GLOBENICOL ◇ GLOROUS ◇ HALOMYCETIN ◇ HORTFENICOL ◇ I 337A ◇ INTRAMYCETIN ◇ ISMICETINA ◇ ISOPHENICOL ◇ ISOPTO FENICOL ◇ KAMAVER ◇ KEMICETINE ◇ LEUKOMYAN ◇ LEVOMYCETIN ◇ LOROMISIN ◇ MASTIPHEN ◇ MEDIAMYCETINE ◇ MICOCHLORINE ◇ MICROCETINA ◇ MYCHEL ◇ MYCINOL ◇ NCI-C55709 ◇ d-(−)-threo-1-p-NITROPHENYL-2-DICHLORACETAMIDO-1,3-PROPANEDIOL ◇ d-threo-1-(p-NITROPHENYL)-2-(DI-CHLOROACETYLAMINO)-1,3-PROPANEDIOL ◇ NORIMYCIN V ◇ NOVOCHLOROCAP ◇ NOVOMYCETIN ◇ NOVOPHENICOL ◇ NSC 3069 ◇ OFTALENT ◇ OLEOMYCETIN ◇ OPTHOCHLOR ◇ OTOPHEN ◇ PANTOVERNIL ◇ PARAXIN ◇ PETNAMYCETIN ◇ QUEMICETINA ◇ RIVOMYCIN ◇ ROMPHENIL ◇ SEPTICOL ◇ SINTOMICETINA ◇ STANOMYCETIN ◇ SYNTHOMYCINE ◇ TEVCOCIN ◇ TIFOMYCINE ◇ TREOMICETINA ◇ U-6062 ◇ UNIMYCETIN ◇ VETICOL

TOXICITY DATA with REFERENCE
CAR: orl-man TD:434 mg/kg/W-C:BLD
ACHAAH 66,267,81
CAR: orl-wmn TD:1680 mg/kg/6W-I:BLD
NEJMAG 277,1003,67
CAR: orl-wmn TDLo:300 mg/kg/60W-I:BLD
NEJMAG 277,1003,67
MUT: cyt-hmn:lym 500 mg/L   HUMAA7 7,305,69
MUT: dni-hmn:bmr 1500 μmo/L   46GFA5 -,17,81
MUT: oms-bcs 10 mg/L   MGGEAE 189,73,83
MUT: spm-mus-ipr 500 mg/kg   FOBLAN 21,60,75

CONSENSUS REPORTS: IARC Cancer Review: Human Limited Evidence IMEMDT 10,85,76. Reported in EPA TSCA Inventory. EPA Genetic Toxicology Program.

SAFETY PROFILE: Suspected human carcinogen producing leukemia, aplastic anemia, and other bone marrow changes. Experimental tumorigenic and teratogenic data. Poison by intraperitoneal, intravenous, and subcutaneous routes. Moderately toxic by ingestion. Human systemic effects by an unknown route: changes in plasma or blood volume, unspecified liver effects, and hemorrhaging. Other experimental reproductive effects. Human mutation data reported. An antibiotic. When heated to decomposition it emits very toxic fumes of NO_x and Cl^-.

CDR750 CAS: 57-74-9
CHLORDANE
DOT: 2762
mf: $C_{10}H_6Cl_8$ mw: 409.76

PROP: Colorless to amber; odorless, viscous liquid. Bp: 175°, d: 1.57-1.63 @ 15.5°/15.5°.

SYNS: ASPON-CHLORDANE ◇ BELT ◇ CD 68 ◇ CHLOORDAAN (DUTCH) ◇ CHLORDAN ◇ γ-CHLORDAN ◇ CHLORDANE, LIQUID (DOT) ◇ CHLORINDAN ◇ CHLOR KIL ◇ CHLORODANE ◇ CHLORTOX ◇ CLORDAN (ITALIAN) ◇ CORODANE ◇ CORTILAN-NEU ◇ DICHLORO-CHLORDENE ◇ DOWCHLOR ◇ ENT 9,932 ◇ ENT 25,552-X ◇ HCS 3260 ◇ KYPCHLOR ◇ M 140 ◇ M 410 ◇ NCI-C00099 ◇ NIRAN ◇ 1,2,4,5,6,7,8,8-OCTACHLOOR-3a,4,7,7a-TETRAHYDRO-4,7-endo-METHANO-INDAAN (DUTCH) ◇ OCTACHLOR ◇ OCTACHLORODIHYDRODICYCLO-PENTADIENE ◇ 1,2,4,5,6,7,8,8-OCTACHLORO-2,3,3a,-4,7,7a-HEXAHYDRO-4,7-METHANOINDENE ◇ 1,2,4,5,6,-7,8,8-OCTACHLORO-2,3,3a,4,7,7a-HEXAHYDRO-4,7-METHANO-1H-INDENE ◇ 1,2,4,5,6,7,8,8-OCTA-CHLORO-3a,4,7,7a-HEXAHYDRO-4,7-METHYLENE INDANE ◇ OCTACHLORO-4,7-METHANOHYDROINDANE ◇ OCTA-CHLORO-4,7-METHANOTETRAHYDROINDANE ◇ 1,2,-4,5,6,7,8,8-OCTACHLORO-4,7-METHANO-3a,4,7,7a-TETRAHYDROINDANE ◇ 1,2,4,5,6,7,8,8-OCTACHLORO-3a,-4,7,7a-TETRAHYDRO-4,7-METHANOINDAN ◇ 1,2,4,5,6,7,8,8-OCTACHLORO-3a,4,7,7a-TETRA-HYDRO-4,7-METHANOINDANE ◇ 1,2,4,5,6,7,10,10-OCTA-CHLORO-4,7,8,9-TETRAHYDRO-4,7-METHYLENEIN-DANE ◇ 1,2,4,5,6,7,8,8-OCTACHLOR-3a,4,7,7a-TETRA-HYDRO-4,7-endo-METHANO-INDAN (GERMAN) ◇ OCTA-KLOR ◇ OKTATERR ◇ ORTHO-KLOR ◇ 1,2,4,5,6,7,8,8-OTTOCHLORO-3A,4,7,7A-TETRAIDRO-4,7-endo-METANO-INDANO (ITALIAN) ◇ RCRA WASTE NUMBER U036 ◇ SD 5532 ◇ SHELL SD-5532 ◇ SYNKLOR ◇ TAT CHLOR 4 ◇ TOPICHLOR 20 ◇ TOPICLOR ◇ TOPICLOR 20 ◇ TOXICHLOR ◇ VELSICOL 1068

TOXICITY DATA with REFERENCE
CAR: orl-mus TD: 3780 mg/kg/80W-C NCITR* NIC-CG-TR-8,77
CAR: orl-mus TDLo: 2020 mg/kg/80W-C NCITR* NCI-CG-TR-8,77
MUT: dns-hmn: fbr 1 μmol/L MUREAV 42,161,77
MUT: msc-ham: lng 10 μmol/L CBINA8 19,369,77

MUT: sce-hmn: lym 10 μmol/L ARTODN 52,221,83
MUT: sce-ofs-mul 54 pmol/L MUREAV 118,61,83

CONSENSUS REPORTS: IARC Cancer Review: GROUP 3 IMEMDT 7,146,87; Human Inadequate Evidence IMEMDT 20,45,79; Animal Sufficient Evidence IMEMDT 20,45,79. NCI Carcinogenesis Bioassay (feed); Clear Evidence: mouse NCITR* NCI-CG-TR-8,77; No Evidence: rat NCITR* NCI-CG-TR-8,77. EPA Genetic Toxicology Program. Community Right-To-Know List. EPA Extremely Hazardous Substances List.

OSHA PEL: TWA 0.5 mg/m³ (skin) ACGIH TLV: TWA 0.5 mg/m³ (skin) DFG MAK: Suspected Carcinogen. DOT Classification: Combustible Liquid; Label: None; Flammable Liquid; Label: Flammable Liquid.

SAFETY PROFILE: Suspected carcinogen with experimental carcinogenic and teratogenic data. Poison to humans by ingestion and possibly other routes. An experimental poison by ingestion, inhalation, intravenous, and intraperitoneal routes. Moderately toxic by skin contact. Human systemic effects by ingestion or skin contact: tremors, convulsions, excitement, ataxia (loss of muscle coordination), and gastritis. Other experimental reproductive effects. Human mutation data reported. Combustible liquid. It is no longer permitted for use as a termiticide in homes. When heated to decomposition it emits toxic fumes of Cl^-.

CDS000 CAS: 115-28-6
CHLORENDIC ACID
mf: $C_9H_4Cl_6O_4$ mw: 388.83

SYNS: 1,4,5,6,7,7-HEXACHLORO-5-NORBORNENE-2,3-DICARBOXYLIC ACID ◇ KYSELINA 3,6-ENDOMETHYLEN-3,4,5,6,7,7-HEXACHLOR-Δ⁴-TETRAHYDROFTALOVA (CZECH) ◇ KYSELINA HET (CZECH) ◇ NCI-C55072

TOXICITY DATA with REFERENCE
CAR: orl-mus TDLo: 108 g/kg/2Y-C NTPTR* NTP-TR-304,87
CAR: orl-rat TDLo: 45063 mg/kg/2Y-C NTPTR* NTP-TR-304,87
MUT: msc-mus: lyms 1700 mg/L NTPTR* NTP-TR-304,87

CONSENSUS REPORTS: NTP Carcinogenesis Studies (feed): Clear Evidence: mouse, rat NTPTR* NTP-TR-304,87. Reported in EPA TSCA Inventory.

SAFETY PROFILE: Suspected carcinogen with experimental carcinogenic data. A severe eye and mild skin irritant. When heated to decomposition it emits toxic fumes of Cl⁻.

CDV250
CHLORINATED HYDROCARBONS, ALIPHATIC

SYN: ALIPHATIC CHLORINATED HYDROCARBONS ◊ CHLORINATED HC, ALIPHATIC

SAFETY PROFILE: Suspected carcinogen with experimental tumors of the liver, lung, skin, and blood-forming tissues. The substitution of a chlorine (or other halogen) atom for a hydrogen greatly increases the anesthetic action of the aliphatic hydrocarbons and increases the range of their systemic effects. In many cases, the chlorine derivative is quite toxic. In general, the unsaturated chlorine derivatives are more narcotic but less toxic than the saturated derivatives. In the saturated group, the narcotic effect is proportional to the number of chlorine atoms. This relationship is not true for toxicity.

CFA750   CAS: 302-70-5
2-CHLORO-N-(2-CHLOROETHYL)-N-METHYLETHANAMINE-N-OXIDE HYDROCHLORIDE
mf: $C_5H_{11}Cl_2NO \cdot ClH$ mw: 208.53

SYNS: CHLORMETHINE-N-OXIDE HYDROCHLORIDE ◊ 2,2'-DICHLORO-N-METHYLDIETHYLAMINE N-OXIDE HYDROCHLORIDE ◊ HN₂ OXIDE HYDROCHLORIDE ◊ MBAO HYDROCHLORIDE ◊ MECHLORETHAMINE OXIDE HYDROCHLORIDE ◊ METHYL-BIS-(β-CHLORAETHYL)-AMIN-N-OXYD-HYDROCHLORID (GERMAN) ◊ METHYL-BIS(β-CHLOROETHYL)AMINE-N-OXIDE HYDROCHLORIDE ◊ N-METHYLBIS(2-CHLOROETHYL)AMINE-N-OXIDE HYDROCHLORIDE ◊ N-METHYL-2,2'-DICHLORODIETHYL-AMINE-N-OXIDE HYDROCHLORIDE ◊ METHYLDI(2-CHLOROETHYL)AMINE-N-OXIDE HYDROCHLORIDE ◊ MITO-MEN ◊ MUSTRON ◊ NITROGEN MUSTARD OXIDE ◊ NITROGEN MUSTARD-N-OXIDE ◊ NITROGEN MUSTARD-N-OXIDE HYDROCHLORIDE ◊ NITROMIM ◊ NITROMIN HYDROCHLORIDE ◊ N-OXYD-LOST ◊ NSC-10107 ◊ OSSIAMINA ◊ OSSICHLORIN ◊ OXYAMINE ◊ SK-598 ◊ XA 2

TOXICITY DATA with REFERENCE
ETA: mul-rat TDLo: 1300 mg/kg/93W-I
    ZEKBAI 62,112,57

MUT: bfa-rat/sat 250 mg/kg   URLRA5 7,119,79
MUT: cyt-slw-par 1670 μL   ZEVBA5 89,216,58

MUT: mmo-sat 500 μg/plate   URLRA5 7,119,79
MUT: pic-esc 200 mg/L   ARMKA7 51,9,65

CONSENSUS REPORTS: IARC Cancer Review: GROUP 2B IMEMDT 7,56,87; Animal Sufficient Evidence IMEMDT 9,209,75; EPA Genetic Toxicology Program.

SAFETY PROFILE: Suspected carcinogen with experimental tumorigenic data. Poison by ingestion, subcutaneous, intravenous, and intraperitoneal routes. Human systemic effects by an unspecified route: convulsions and unspecified changes in bone marrow. Mutation data reported. An antineoplastic agent. When heated to decomposition it emits toxic fumes of Cl⁻ and NO_x.

CHD250   CAS: 13909-09-6
1-(2-CHLOROETHYL)-3-(4-METHYL-CYCLOHEXYL)-1-NITROSOUREA
mf: $C_{10}H_{18}ClN_3O_2$ mw: 247.76

SYNS: 1-(2-CHLOROETHYL)-3-(trans-4-METHYL-CYCLO-HEXYL)-1-NITROSOUREA ◊ N-(2-CHLOROETHYL)-N'-(trans-4-METHYLCYCLOHEXYL)-N-NITROSOUREA ◊ ME-CCNU ◊ METHYL-CCNU ◊ trans-METHYL-CCNU ◊ METHYL-LO-MUSTINE ◊ NCI-C04955 ◊ NSC-95441 ◊ SEMUSTINE

TOXICITY DATA with REFERENCE
CAR: ipr-mus TDLo: 117 mg/kg/26W-I
    CANCAR 40(Suppl 4),1935,77
CAR: ipr-rat TDLo: 30 mg/kg/7W-I   CANCAR 40(Suppl 4),1935,77
CAR: orl-hmn TDLo: 22 mg/kg/60W-C
    NEJMAG 309,1079,83
CAR: orl-wmn TD: 73 mg/kg/3Y-I   NEJMAG 302,120,80
ETA: ivn-rat TD: 64 mg/kg/60W-I   DTESD7 8,273,80
ETA: ivn-rat TD: 127 mg/kg/60W-I   DTESD7 8,273,80
ETA: ivn-rat TD: 203 mg/kg/48W-I   DTESD7 8,273,80
ETA: ivn-rat TDLo: 32 mg/kg/60W-I   DTESD7 8,273,80
MUT: dnd-esc 50 μmol/L   MUREAV 89,95,81
MUT: dni-mus: oth 10 μmol/L   CNREA8 43,5837,83
MUT: ipr-mus LD10: 37 mg/kg   CNREA8 34,194,74
MUT: mma-sat 100 nmol/plate   JJIND8 65,149,80
MUT: mmo-sat 100 nmol/plate   JJIND8 65,149,80

CONSENSUS REPORTS: NCI Carcinogenesis Studies (ipr); Clear Evidence: rat CANCAR 40,1935,77; No Evidence: mouse CANCAR 40,1935,77.

SAFETY PROFILE: Suspected human carcinogen producing leukemia. Experimental carcinogenic and tumorigenic data. Poison by ingestion, intraperitoneal, intravenous, and other possibly other routes. Mutation data reported. Human systemic effects by ingestion: nausea or vomiting, damage to kidney tubules and glomeruli, and hematuria (blood in the urine). When heated to decomposition it emits very toxic fumes of Cl^- and NO_x.

CIR250   CAS: 94-74-6
(4-CHLORO-2-METHYLPHENOXY)ACETIC ACID
mf: $C_9H_9ClO_3$ mw: 200.63

SYNS: AGRITOX ◇ AGROXONE ◇ ANICON KOMBI ◇ ANICON M ◇ BH MCPA ◇ BORDERMASTER ◇ BROMINAL M & PLUS ◇ B-SELEKTONON M ◇ CHIPTOX ◇ 4-CHLORO-o-CRESOXYACETIC ACID ◇ 4-CHLORO-o-TOLOXYACETIC ACID ◇ ((4-CHLORO-o-TOLYL)OXY)ACETIC ACID ◇ CHWASTOX ◇ CORNOX-M ◇ DED-WEED ◇ DICO-PUR-M ◇ DICOTEX ◇ DOW MCP AMINE WEED KILLER ◇ EMCEPAN ◇ EMPAL ◇ HEDAPUR M 52 ◇ HERBICIDE M ◇ HORMOTUHO ◇ 4K-2M ◇ KILSEM ◇ KREZONE ◇ LEGUMEX DB ◇ LEUNA M ◇ LEYSPRAY ◇ LINORMONE ◇ M 40 ◇ 2M-4C ◇ MCP ◇ MCPA ◇ MEPHANAC ◇ METAXON ◇ METHOXONE ◇ 2-METHYL-4-CHLORO-PHENOXYACETIC ACID ◇ 2-METHYL-4-CHLORPHEN-OXYESSIGSAEURE (GERMAN) ◇ 2M-4KH ◇ NETAZOL ◇ OKULTIN M ◇ PHENOXYLENE SUPER ◇ RAPHONE ◇ RAZOL DOCK KILLER ◇ RHOMENE ◇ RHONOX ◇ SEPPIC MMD ◇ SHAMROX ◇ SOVIET TECHNICAL HERBI-CIDE 2M-4C ◇ TRASAN ◇ U 46 M-FLUID ◇ USTINEX ◇ VACATE ◇ VERDONE ◇ VESAKONTUHO MCPA ◇ WEEDAR MCPA CONCENTRATE ◇ WEEDONE MCPA ES-TER ◇ WEED-RHAP ◇ ZELAN

TOXICITY DATA with REFERENCE
MUT: dns-mus-orl 200 mg/kg   MUREAV 55,197,78
MUT: hma-mus/sat 200 mg/kg   ECBUDQ 27,182,78
MUT: mmo-smc 30 μmol/L/3H   MUREAV 60,291,79
MUT: sce-ham:ovr 10 μmol/L/1H   CRNGDP 5,703,84
MUT: sln-dmg-orl 5 mmol/L   EXPEAM 30,621,74

CONSENSUS REPORTS: IARC Cancer Review: GROUP 2B IMEMDT 7,156,87; Animal Inadequate Evidence IMEMDT 30,255,83; Human Inadequate Evidence IMEMDT 30,255,83; Human Limited Evidence IMEMDT 41,357,86. Reported in EPA TSCA Inventory. EPA Genetic Toxicology Program.

SAFETY PROFILE: Suspected carcinogen. Poison by subcutaneous and intravenous routes. Moderately toxic by ingestion. Human systemic effects by ingestion: blood pressure decrease and coma. An experimental teratogen. Other experimental reproductive effects. Mutation data reported. An herbicide. When heated to decomposition it emits toxic fumes of Cl^-.

CIR500   CAS: 93-65-2
4-CHLORO-2-METHYLPHENOXY-α-PROPIONIC ACID
mf: $C_{10}H_{11}ClO_3$ mw: 214.66

SYNS: ACIDE 2-(4-CHLORO-2-METHYL-PHENOXY)PRO-PIONIQUE (FRENCH) ◇ ACIDO 2-(4-CLORO-2-METIL-FEN-OSSI)-PROPIONICO (ITALIAN) ◇ BH MECOPROP ◇ CHIPCO TURF HERBICIDE MCPP ◇ 2-(4-CHLOOR-2-METHYL-FENOXY)-PROPIONZUUR (DUTCH) ◇ 2-(4-CHLOR-2-METHYL-PHENOXY)-PROPIONSAEURE (GERMAN) ◇ 2-(4-CHLORO-2-METHYLPHENOXY)PROPIONIC ACID ◇ (+)-α-(4-CHLORO-2-METHYLPHENOXY) PROPIONIC ACID ◇ 2-(4-CHLOROPHENOXY-2-METHYL)PROPIONIC ACID ◇ 2-(p-CHLORO-o-TOLYLOXY)PROPIONIC ACID ◇ CMPP ◇ COMPITOX ◇ FBC CMPP ◇ HEDONAL MCPP ◇ ISO-CORNOX ◇ KILPROP ◇ LIRANOX ◇ 2M-4CP ◇ MCPP ◇ 2-MCPP ◇ MCPP 2,4-D ◇ MCPP-D-4 ◇ MCPP-K-4 ◇ MECOMEC ◇ MECOPEOP ◇ MECOPER ◇ MECOPEX ◇ MECOPROP ◇ MECOTURF ◇ MECPROP ◇ MEPRO ◇ METHOXONE ◇ α-(2-METHYL-4-CHLOROPHEN-OXY)PROPIONIC ACID ◇ 2-(2-METHYL-4-CHLOROPHEN-OXY)PROPIONIC ACID ◇ 2-METHYL-4-CHLOROPHENOXY-α-PROPIONIC ACID ◇ 2-(2-METHYL-4-CHLORPHENOXY)-PROPIONSAEURE (GERMAN) ◇ 2M 4KHP ◇ N.B. MECOPROP ◇ PROPAL ◇ PROPONEX-PLUS ◇ RANKOTEX ◇ RUNCATEX ◇ RD 4593 ◇ U 46 ◇ U 46 KV-ESTER ◇ U 46 KV-FLUID ◇ VI-PAR ◇ VI-PEX

TOXICITY DATA with REFERENCE
MUT: dns-mus-orl 100 mg/kg   MUREAV 55,197,78
MUT: mrc-smc 742 ppm   MUREAV 21,83,73

CONSENSUS REPORTS: IARC Cancer Review: GROUP 2B IMEMDT 7,156,87; Human Limited Evidence IMEMDT 41,357,86. EPA Genetic Toxicology Program. Reported in EPA TSCA Inventory.

SAFETY PROFILE: Suspected carcinogen. Moderately toxic by ingestion, skin contact, intraperitoneal, and possibly other routes. An experimental teratogen. Other experimental results. Mutation data reported. An herbicide. When heated to decomposition it emits toxic fumes of Cl^-.

CIU750   CAS: 563-47-3
3-CHLORO-2-METHYLPROPENE
DOT: 2554
mf: C_4H_7Cl mw: 90.56

PROP: Colorless, volatile liquid, disagreeable
odor. Bp: 72.17°, lel: 2.3%, uel: 9.3%, fp:
$< -80°$, d: 0.9257 @ 20°/4°, vap press: 101.7
mm @ 20°, vap d: 3.12, flash p: −10°. Misc
in alc, ether.

SYNS: 3-CHLOR-2-METHYL-PROP-1-EN (GERMAN)
◊ γ-CHLOROISOBUTYLENE ◊ 3-CHLORO-2-METHYL-1-
PROPENE ◊ CHLORURE de METHALLYLE (FRENCH)
◊ 3-CLORO-2-METIL-PROP-1-ENE (ITALIAN) ◊ CLORURO
di METALLILE (ITALIAN) ◊ ISOBUTENYL CHLORIDE
◊ METHALLYL CHLORIDE ◊ α-METHALLYL CHLORIDE
◊ 2-METHYL-ALLYLCHLORID (GERMAN) ◊ β-METHYLAL-
LYL CHLORIDE ◊ 2-METHYLALLYL CHLORIDE
◊ METHYL ALLYL CHLORIDE (DOT) ◊ NCI-C54820

TOXICITY DATA with REFERENCE
CAR: orl-mus TDLo:51500 mg/kg/2Y-I
  NTPTR* NTP-TR-300,86
CAR: orl-rat TDLo:77250 mg/kg/2Y-I   NTPTR*
  NTP-TR-300,86
NEO: orl-rat TD:77250 mg/kg/2Y-I   NTPTR*
  NTP-TR-300,86
ETA: orl-mus TDLo:51500 mg/kg/2Y-I
  PAACA3 26,95,85
ETA: orl-rat TDLo:38625 mg/kg/2Y-I   PAACA3
  26,95,85
MUT: dns-hmn:hla 1 mmol/L   CALEDQ 20,263,83
MUT: mma-sat 6 μmol/plate   BCPCA6 29,2611,80
MUT: mmo-sat 6 μmol/plate   BCPCA6 29,2611,80

CONSENSUS REPORTS: NTP Carcinogenesis Studies (gavage); Clear Evidence: mouse,
rat NTPTR* NTP-TR-300,86. Reported in EPA
TSCA Inventory.

DOT Classification: IMO: Flammable Liquid;
Label: Flammable Liquid.

SAFETY PROFILE: Suspected carcinogen with
experimental carcinogenic, neoplastigenic, and
tumorigenic data. Mildly toxic to humans by
inhalation. An irritant. Human mutation data
reported. Very dangerous fire hazard when exposed to heat, flame, or oxidizers. Moderately
explosive when exposed to heat or flame. Can
react vigorously with oxidizing materials. To
fight fire, use alcohol foam, CO_2, dry chemical.
When heated to decomposition it emits toxic
fumes of Cl^-.

CIV000   CAS: 6959-48-4
**3-(CHLOROMETHYL) PYRIDINE
HYDROCHLORIDE**
mf: $C_6H_6ClN \cdot ClH$ mw: 164.04

SYN: NCI-C03838

TOXICITY DATA with REFERENCE
CAR: orl-mus TDLo:49 g/kg/81W-I   NCITR*
  NCI-CG-TR-95,78
CAR: orl-rat TDLo:37 g/kg/83W-I   NCITR*
  NCI-CG-TR-95,78
MUT: mma-esc 1 mg/plate   ENMUDM 7(Suppl
  5),1,85
MUT: mma-sat 33300 ng/plate   ENMUDM 7(Suppl
  5),1,85
MUT: mmo-sat 333 μg/plate   IARCCD 27,283,80
MUT: otr-rat:emb 640 ng/plate   JJATDK 1,190,81

CONSENSUS REPORTS: NCI Carcinogenesis Bioassay (gavage); Clear Evidence: mouse,
rat NCITR* NCI-CG-TR-95,78. EPA Genetic
Toxicology Program.

SAFETY PROFILE: Suspected carcinogen with
experimental carcinogenic data. Poison by ingestion. Mutation data reported. When heated
to decomposition it emits very toxic fumes of
NO_x and Cl^-.

CJL000
CHLOROPHENOLS

CONSENSUS REPORTS: Chlorophenol compounds are on the Community Right-To-Know
List.

SAFETY PROFILE: Many are suspected experimental carcinogens. Most are strong eye and
skin irritants. They are systemic irritants by inhalation, ingestion, and skin contact. Generally
mutagenic. Pentachlorophenol is a poison by
several routes. A teratogen and mutagen. When
heated to decomposition they emit toxic fumes
of Cl^-.

CJS125   CAS: 5131-60-2
4-CHLORO-m-PHENYLENEDIAMINE
mf: $C_6H_7ClN_2$ mw: 142.60

PROP: Mp: 90°.

SYNS: C.I. 76027 ◊ 4-CHLORO-1,3-BENZENEDIAMINE
◊ 1-CHLORO-2,4-DIAMINOBENZENE ◊ 4-CHLOROPHENE-
1,3-DIAMINE ◊ 4-CHLOROPHENYLENE-1,3-DIAMINE
◊ 4-CHLORO-1,3-PHENYLENEDIAMINE ◊ 4-Cl-M-PD
◊ NCI-C03305

TOXICITY DATA with REFERENCE

CAR: orl-mus TD:764 g/kg/78W-C NCITR* NCI-CG-TR-85,78

CAR: orl-mus TD:3745 g/kg/78W-C IARC** 27,81,82

CAR: orl-mus TD:7140 g/kg/78W-C IARC** 27,81,82

CAR: orl-mus TD:16200 g/kg/96W-C CRNGDP 1,495,80

CAR: orl-mus TDLo:648 g/kg/77W-C CRNGDP 1,495,80

CAR: orl-rat TD:1092 g/kg/78W-C IARC** 27,81,82

CAR: orl-rat TD:2184 g/kg/78W-C IARC** 27,81,82

CAR: orl-rat TD:5460 g/kg/78W-C IARC** 27,81,82

CAR: orl-rat TD:7500 g/kg/2Y-C CRNGDP 1,495,80

CAR: orl-rat TDLo:164 g/kg/78W-C NCITR* NCI-CG-TR-85,78

NEO: orl-rat TD:108 g/kg/77W-C CRNGDP 1,495,80

ETA: orl-mus TD:917 g/kg/78W-C NCITR* NCI-CG-TR-85,78

MUT: mma-sat 10 μg/plate ENMUDM 7(Suppl 5),1,85

MUT: mmo-sat 1 mg/plate ENMUDM 7(Suppl5),1,85

CONSENSUS REPORTS: IARC Cancer Review: Animal Inadequate Evidence IMEMDT 27,81,82. NCI Carcinogenesis Bioassay (feed); Clear Evidence: mouse, rat NCITR* NCI-CG-TR-85,78. Reported in EPA TSCA Inventory.

SAFETY PROFILE: Suspected carcinogen with experimental carcinogenic, neoplastigenic, and tumorigenic data. Mutation data reported. When heated to decomposition it emits toxic fumes of Cl^- and NO_x.

CLK225   CAS: 95-79-4
5-CHLORO-o-TOLUIDINE
mf: C_7H_8ClN mw: 141.61

PROP: Solid. Bp: 241°, mp: 29°.

SYNS: ACCO FAST RED KB BASE ◇ 1-AMINO-3-CHLORO-6-METHYLBENZENE ◇ 2-AMINO-4-CHLOROTOLUENE ◇ ANSIBASE RED KB ◇ AZOENE FAST RED KB BASE ◇ AZOIC DIAZO COMPONENT 32 ◇ 4-CHLORO-2-AMINOTOLUENE ◇ 3-CHLORO-6-METHYLANILINE ◇ 5-CHLORO-2-METHYLANILINE ◇ FAST RED KB AMINE ◇ FAST RED KB BASE ◇ FAST RED KB SALT ◇ FAST RED KB SALT SUPRA ◇ FAST RED KBS SALT ◇ GENAZO RED KB SOLN ◇ HILTONIL FAST RED KB BASE ◇ LAKE RED KB BASE ◇ METROGEN RED FORMER KB SOLN ◇ NAPHTHOSOL

FAST RED KB BASE ◇ NCI-CO2051 ◇ PHARMAZOID RED KB ◇ RED KB BASE ◇ SPECTROLENE RED KB ◇ STABLE RED KB BASE

TOXICITY DATA with REFERENCE

CAR: orl-mus TD:262 g/kg/78W-C NCITR* NCI-CG-TR-187,79

CAR: orl-mus TDLo:131 g/kg/78W-C NCITR* NCI-CG-TR-187,79

ETA: orl-rat TDLo:164 g/kg/78W-C NCITR* NCI-CG-TR-187,79

MUT: dni-mus-orl 200 mg/kg MUREAV 46,305,77

CONSENSUS REPORTS: NTP Carcinogenesis Bioassay (feed): Clear Evidence: mouse NCITR* NCI-TR-187,79; (feed): Inadequate Studies: rat NCITR* NCI-TR-187,79. Reported in EPA TSCA Inventory. EPA Genetic Toxicology Program.

DFG MAK: Suspected Carcinogen.

SAFETY PROFILE: Suspected carcinogen with experimental carcinogenic and tumorigenic data. Moderately toxic by ingestion. When heated to decomposition it emits very toxic fumes of Cl^- and NO_x.

CLK235   CAS: 3165-93-3
4-CHLORO-2-TOLUIDINE
HYDROCHLORIDE
DOT: 1579
mf: $C_7H_8ClN \cdot ClH$ mw: 178.07

SYNS: AMARTHOL FAST RED TR BASE ◇ AMARTHOL FAST RED TR SALT ◇ 2-AMINO-5-CHLOROTOLUENE HYDROCHLORIDE ◇ AZANIL RED SALT TRD ◇ AZOENE FAST RED TR SALT ◇ AZOGENE FAST RED TR ◇ AZOIC DIAZO COMPONENT 11 BASE ◇ BRENTAMINE FAST RED TR SALT ◇ CHLORHYDRATE de 4-CHLOROORTHOTOLUIDINE (FRENCH) ◇ 5-CHLORO-2-AMINOTOLUENE HYDROCHLORIDE ◇ 4-CHLORO-2-METHYLANILINE HYDROCHLORIDE ◇ 4-CHLORO-6-METHYLANILINE HYDROCHLORIDE ◇ 4-CHLORO-2-METHYLBENZENEAMINE HYDROCHLORIDE ◇ 4-CHLORO-o-TOLUIDINE HYDROCHLORIDE ◇ 4-CHLORO-o-TOLUIDINE HYDROCHLORIDE (DOT) ◇ C.I. 37085 ◇ C.I. AZOIC DIAZO COMPONENT 11 ◇ DAITO RED SALT TR ◇ DEVOL RED K ◇ DEVOL RED TA SALT ◇ DEVOL RED TR ◇ DIAZO FAST RED TR ◇ DIAZO FAST RED TRA ◇ FAST RED 5CT SALT ◇ FAST RED SALT TR ◇ FAST RED SALT TRA ◇ FAST RED SALT TRN ◇ FAST RED TR SALT ◇ HINDASOL RED TR SALT ◇ KROMON GREEN B ◇ 2-METHYL-4-CHLORO-ANILINE HYDROCHLORIDE ◇ NATASOL FAST RED TR SALT ◇ NCI-C02368 ◇ NEUTROSEL RED TRVA ◇ OFNA-PERL SALT RRA ◇ RCRA WASTE NUMBER U049

◇ RED BASE CIBA IX ◇ RED BASE IRGA IX ◇ RED SALT CIBA IX ◇ RED SALT IRGA IX ◇ RED TRS SALT ◇ SANYO FAST RED SALT TR

TOXICITY DATA with REFERENCE
CAR: orl-mus TD:97 g/kg/78W-C   JEPTDQ
2(2),325,78
CAR: orl-mus TD:104 g/kg/99W-C   NCITR*
NCI-CG-TR-165,78
CAR: orl-mus TD:108 g/kg/78W-C   JEPTDQ
2(2),325,78
CAR: orl-mus TD:216 g/kg/78W-C   JEPTDQ
2(2),325,78
CAR: orl-mus TDLo:49 g/kg/78W-C   JEPTDQ
2(2),325,78

CONSENSUS REPORTS: IARC Cancer Review: Animal Inadequate Evidence, Human Inadequate Evidence IMEMDT 16,277,78. NCI Carcinogenesis Bioassay (Feed); Clear Evidence: Mouse; No Evidence: Rat (NCITR* NCI-CG-TR-165,79). Reported in EPA TSCA Inventory.

DOT Classification: Poison B; Label: Poison; DOT-IMO: Poison B; Label: St. Andrews Cross.

SAFETY PROFILE: Suspected carcinogen with experimental carcinogenic data. Moderately toxic by intraperitoneal route. When heated to decomposition it emits toxic fumes of NO_x and Cl^-.

CLO750   CAS: 569-57-3
CHLOROTRIANISENE
mf: $C_{23}H_{21}ClO_3$ mw: 380.89

SYNS: ANISENE ◇ CHLORESTROLO ◇ 1,1′,1′′-(1-CHLORO-1-ETHENYL-2-YLIDENE)-TRIS(4-METHOXYBENZENE) ◇ CHLOROTRIANIZEN ◇ CHLOROTRISIN ◇ CHLOROTRIS(p-METHOXYPHENYL)ETHYLENE ◇ CHLORTRIANISEN ◇ CLORESTROLO ◇ CLOROTRISIN ◇ CTA ◇ HORMONISENE ◇ KHLORTRIANIZEN ◇ MERBENTUL ◇ METACE ◇ NSC-10108 ◇ RIANIL ◇ TACE ◇ TACE-FN ◇ TRI-p-ANISYLCHLOROETHYLENE ◇ TRIS(p-METHOXYPHENYL)CHLOROETHYLENE

TOXICITY DATA with REFERENCE
ETA: orl-rat TDLo:37 mg/kg/2Y-C   TXAPA9
11,489,67
ETA: scu-mus TDLo:180 mg/kg/89W-I
AMPLAO 50,750,50

CONSENSUS REPORTS: IARC Cancer Review: Animal Inadequate Evidence IMEMDT 21,139,79; Human Limited Evidence IMEMDT 21,139,79.

SAFETY PROFILE: Suspected human carcinogen with experimental tumorigenic data. Human reproductive effects by ingestion: changes in fertility. Used in cancer treatment. When heated to decomposition it emits very toxic fumes of Cl^-.

CLW250   CAS: 50892-23-4
(4-CHLORO-6-(2,3-XYLIDINO)-2-PYRIMIDINYLTHIO)ACETIC ACID
mf: $C_{14}H_{14}ClN_3O_2S$ mw: 323.82

SYNS: ((4-CHLORO-6-((2,3-DIMETHYLPHENYL)AMINO)-2-PYRIMIDINYL)THIO)ACETIC ACID ◇ WY-14,643

TOXICITY DATA with REFERENCE
CAR: orl-mus TDLo:37 g/kg/62W-C   CNREA8
39,152,79
CAR: orl-rat TD:46 g/kg/65W-C   CRNGDP
2,645,81
CAR: orl-rat TDLo:29 g/kg/69W-C   CNREA8
39,152,79
ETA: orl-rat TD:27 g/kg/64W-C   CALEDQ
32,33,86
MUT: dni-mus:oth 100 μmol/L   CNREA8
40,36,80
MUT: dns-rat:lvr 1 mmol/L   CALEDQ 24,147,84

SAFETY PROFILE: Suspected carcinogen with experimental carcinogenic and tumorigenic data. Mutation data reported. When heated to decomposition it emits very toxic fumes of Cl^-, NO_x, and SO_x.

CLW500   CAS: 65089-17-0
2-((4-CHLORO-6-(2,3-XYLIDINO)-2-PYRIMIDINYL)THIO)-N-(2-HYDROXYETHYL)ACETAMIDE
mf: $C_{16}H_{19}ClN_4O_2S$ mw: 366.90

SYNS: BR-931 ◇ PIRINIXIL

TOXICITY DATA with REFERENCE
CAR: orl-mus TDLo:137 g/kg/81W-C   NATUAS
283,397,80
CAR: orl-rat TDLo:17 g/kg/81W-C   NATUAS
283,397,80
MUT: dni-mus:oth 25 μmol/L   CNREA8 40,36,80
MUT: dns-rat:lvr 100 μmol/L   CALEDQ
24,147,84

SAFETY PROFILE: Suspected carcinogen with experimental carcinogenic data. Mutation data reported. When heated to decomposition it emits very toxic fumes of Cl^-, NO_x and SO_x.

CME250 CAS: 3546-10-9
CHOLESTERYL-p-BIS(2-CHLOROETHYL)AMINO PHENYLACETATE
mf: $C_{39}H_{59}Cl_2NO_2$ mw: 644.89

SYNS: (p-BIS(2-CHLOROETHYL)AMINO)PHENYL)ACE-TATE CHOLESTEROL ◇ (p-(BIS(2-CHLOROETHYL)AMINO) PHENYL)ACETIC ACID CHOLESTEROL ESTER ◇ (4-(BIS(2-CHLOROETHYL)AMINO)PHENYL)ACETIC ACID CHOLES-TERYL ESTER ◇ 5-CHOLESTEN-3-β-OL 3-(p-(BIS(2-CHLORO-ETHYL)AMINO)PHENYL)ACETATE ◇ FENESTERIN ◇ FENESTRIN ◇ NCI-C01558 ◇ NSC 104469 ◇ PHEN-ESTERINE ◇ PHENESTRIN

TOXICITY DATA with REFERENCE
CAR: orl-mus TD:2340 mg/kg/1Y-I NCITR* NCI-CG-TR-60,78
CAR: orl-mus TD:4680 mg/kg/1Y-I NCITR* NCI-CG-TR-60,78
CAR: orl-mus TDLo:1092 mg/kg/1Y-I NCITR* NCI-CG-TR-60,78
CAR: orl-rat TD:1560 mg/kg/1Y-I NCITR* NCI-CG-TR-60,78
CAR: orl-rat TDLo:780 mg/kg/52W-I NCITR* NCI-CG-TR-60,78
NEO: ipr-mus TDLo:2400 mg/kg/8W-I CNREA8 33,3069,73

CONSENSUS REPORTS: NCI Carcinogen-esis Bioassay (gavage); Clear Evidence: mouse, rat NCITR* NCI-CG-TR-60,78.

SAFETY PROFILE: Suspected carcinogen with experimental carcinogenic and neoplastigenic data. When heated to decomposition it emits very toxic fumes of Cl^- and NO_x.

CMJ500
CHROMIUM COMPOUNDS

CONSENSUS REPORTS: Chromium and its compounds are on the Community Right-To-Know List.

SAFETY PROFILE: Chromate salts are sus-pected human carcinogens producing tumors of the lungs, nasal cavity, and paranasal sinus. Chromic acid and its salts have a corrosive action on the skin and mucous membranes. The lesions are confined to the exposed parts, affecting chiefly the skin of the hands and forearms and the mucous membranes of the nasal septum. The characteristic lesion is a deep, penetrating ulcer, which, for the most part, does not tend to suppurate, and which is slow in healing. Small ulcers, about the size of a matchhead, may be found, chiefly around the base of the nails, on the knuckles, dorsum of the hands and forearms. These ulcers tend to be clean and progress slowly. They are frequently painless, even though quite deep. They heal slowly and leave scars. On the mucous membranes of the nasal septum, the ulcers are usually accompanied by purulent discharge and crusting. If exposure continues, perforation of the nasal septum may result but produces no deformity of the nose. Hexavalent compounds are more toxic than the trivalent. Eczematous dermatitis due to trivalent chromium compounds has been reported.

CMJ900 CAS: 1308-38-9
CHROMIUM(III) OXIDE (2:3)
mf: Cr_2O_3 mw: 152.00

SYNS: ANADOMIS GREEN ◇ ANIDRIDE CROMIQUE (FRENCH) ◇ CASALIS GREEN ◇ CHROME GREEN ◇ CHROMIC ACID ◇ CHROME OCHER ◇ CHROME OXIDE ◇ CHROME OXIDE GREEN ◇ CHROMIA ◇ CHROMIC ACID GREEN ◇ CHROMIC OXIDE ◇ CHROMIUM OXIDE ◇ CHROMIUM(III) OXIDE ◇ CHROMIUM(3+) OXIDE ◇ CHROMIUM SESQUIOXIDE ◇ CHROMIUM(3+) TRIOXIDE ◇ C.I. 77288 ◇ C.I. No. 77278 ◇ C.I. PIGMENT GREEN 17 ◇ DICHROMIUM TRIOXIDE ◇ 11661 GREEN ◇ GREEN CHROME OXIDE ◇ GREEN CHROMIC OXIDE ◇ GREEN CIN-NABAR ◇ GREEN ROUGE ◇ GUIGNER'S GREEN ◇ LEAF GREEN ◇ LEVANOX GREEN GA ◇ OIL GREEN ◇ OXIDE of CHROMIUM ◇ ULTRAMARINE GREEN

TOXICITY DATA with REFERENCE
ETA: ipr-rat TDLo:90 mg/kg VOONAW 13(11),57,67
ETA: ipl-rat TDLo:45 mg/kg VOONAW 13(11),57,67
ETA: itr-rat TDLo:90 mg/kg VOONAW 13(11),57,67
MUT: dnd-esc 5 mmol/L CNREA8 40,2455,80
MUT: dnr-sat 50 mmol/L TOLED5 7,439,81
MUT: mmo-sat 1 mmol/L TOLED5 8,195,81
MUT: sce-ham:lng 34 mg/L CRNGDP 4,605,83

CONSENSUS REPORTS: IARC Cancer Re-view: Animal Inadequate Evidence IMEMDT 23,205,80. Reported in EPA TSCA Inventory. Chromium and its compounds are on the Com-munity Right-To-Know List.

OSHA PEL: TWA 0.5 mg(Cr)/m^3 ACGIH TLV: TWA 0.5 mg(Cr)/m^3 DFG MAK: Sus-pected Carcinogen.

SAFETY PROFILE: Suspected carcinogen with experimental tumorigenic data. Mutation data reported. Probably a severe eye, skin, and mucous membrane irritant. A powerful oxidizer.

CMO250   CAS: 72-57-1
C.I. DIRECT BLUE 14, TETRASODIUM SALT
mf: $C_{34}H_{28}N_6O_{14}S_4 \cdot 4Na$ mw: 964.88

SYNS: AMANIL SKY BLUE ◇ AMIDINE BLUE 4B ◇ AZIDINE BLUE 3B ◇ AZURRO DIRETTO 3B ◇ BENCIDAL BLUE 3B ◇ BENZAMINE BLUE ◇ BENZO BLUE ◇ BLEU DIAMINE ◇ BLUE EMB ◇ BRASILAMINA BLUE 3B ◇ CENTRALINE BLUE 3B ◇ CHLORAMINE BLUE ◇ CHLORAZOL BLUE 3B ◇ CHROME LEATHER BLUE 3B ◇ C.I. 23850 ◇ C.I. DIRECT BLUE 14 ◇ CONGOBLAU 3B ◇ CONGO BLUE ◇ CRESOTINE BLUE 3B ◇ DIAMINE BLUE 3B ◇ DIANILBLAU ◇ DIANIL BLUE ◇ DIAZINE BLUE 3B ◇ DIPHENYL BLUE 3B ◇ DIRECT BLUE 14 ◇ HISPAMIN BLUE 3BX ◇ NAPHTAMINE BLUE 2B ◇ NAPHTHYLAMINE BLUE ◇ NCI C61289 ◇ NIAGARA BLUE ◇ ORION BLUE 3B ◇ PARAMINE BLUE 3B ◇ PARKIBLEU ◇ PARKIPAN ◇ PONTAMINE BLUE 3BX ◇ PYRAZOL BLUE 3B ◇ PYROTROPBLAU ◇ RCRA WASTE NUMBER U236 ◇ RENOLBLAU 3B ◇ SODIUM DITOLYLDIAZOBIS-8-AMINO-1-NAPHTHOL-3,6-DISULFONATE ◇ SODIUM DI-TOLYLDIAZOBIS-8-AMINO-1-NAPHTHOL-3,6-DISULPHO-NATE ◇ TB ◇ TRIANOL DIRECT BLUE 3B ◇ TRIPAN BLUE ◇ TRYPANBLAU (GERMAN) ◇ TRYPAN BLUE ◇ TRYPAN BLUE SODIUM SALT

TOXICITY DATA with REFERENCE
CAR: scu-rat TDLo: 630 mg/kg/43W-I   BJEPA5 33,524,52
NEO: scu-rat TD: 7500 mg/kg/86W-I   LAINAW 12,1221,63
ETA: par-rat TD: 620 mg/kg/31W-I   GANNA2 48,573,57
ETA: par-rat TDLo: 250 mg/kg/10W-I   CANCAR 5,792,52
ETA: scu-mus TD: 1275 mg/kg/34W-I   APHGBP 33,1,53
ETA: scu-rat TD: 300 mg/kg/6W-I   AJPAA4 106,326,82
ETA: scu-rat TD: 1300 mg/kg/1Y-I   AJPAA4 106,326,82
ETA: unr-rat TD: 700 mg/kg/4W-I   FZPAAZ 75,74,66
MUT: bfa-rat/sat 500 mg/kg   MUREAV 156,131,85
MUT: dnd-esc 20 μmol/L   MUREAV 89,95,81
MUT: dns-ham:lvr 100 μmol/L   MUREAV 136,255,84
MUT: dns-rat:lvr 10 μmol/L   MUREAV 136,255,84
MUT: mma-sat 250 μg/plate   MUREAV 56,249,78

CONSENSUS REPORTS: IARC Cancer Review: GROUP 2B IMEMDT 7,56,87; Animal Sufficient Evidence IMEMDT 8,267,75. EPA Genetic Toxicology Program. Reported in EPA TSCA Inventory.

SAFETY PROFILE: Suspected carcinogen with experimental carcinogenic, neoplastigenic, tumorigenic, and teratogenic data. Poison by intraperitoneal, intravenous, and subcutaneous routes. Other experimental reproductive effects. Mutation data reported. When heated to decomposition it emits very toxic fumes of NO_x, Na_2O and SO_x.

CMO750   CAS: 16071-86-6
C.I. DIRECT BROWN
mf: $C_{31}H_{20}N_6O_9S \cdot Cu \cdot 2Na$ mw: 762.15

SYNS: AIZEN PRIMULA BROWN BRLH ◇ AMANIL SUPRA BROWN LBL ◇ ATLANTIC RESIN FAST BROWN BRL ◇ BENZAMIL SUPRA BROWN BRLL ◇ CALCODUR BROWN BRL ◇ CHLORAMINE FAST BROWN BRL ◇ CHROME LEATHER BROWN BRLL ◇ C.I. 30145 ◇ DERMA FAST BROWN W-GL ◇ DIPHENYL FAST BROWN BRL ◇ DIRECT BROWN 95 ◇ NCI-C54568 ◇ SATURN BROWN LBR ◇ SOLAR BROWN PL ◇ TETRAMINE FAST BROWN BRS

TOXICITY DATA with REFERENCE
NEO: orl-rat TDLo: 2625 mg/kg/5W-C   NCITR* NCI-CG-TR-108,78
MUT: dns-rat-orl 100 mg/kg   MUREAV 136,147,84
MUT: mma-sat 30 nmol/plate   MUREAV 136,147,84
MUT: mmo-sat 100 nmol/plate   MUREAV 136,147,84

CONSENSUS REPORTS: IARC Cancer Review: Animal Limited Evidence IMEMDT 29,321,82; Human Limited Evidence IMEMDT 29,321,82; NCI Carcinogenesis Bioassay (feed); Clear Evidence: rat NCITR* NCI-CG-TR-108,78; No Evidence: mouse NCITR* NCI-CG-TR-108,78. Reported in EPA TSCA Inventory. Community Right-To-Know List.

SAFETY PROFILE: Suspected carcinogen with experimental carcinogenic and neoplastigenic data. Mutation data reported. When heated to decomposition it emits very toxic fumes of Na_2O, SO_x, and NO_x.

CMP800
CIGARETTE REFINED TAR

SYNS: TAR, FROM TOBACCO ◇ CIGARETTE TAR ◇ COLOMBIAN BLACK TOBACCO CIGARETTE REFINED TAR ◇ TOBACCO REFINED TAR ◇ TOBACCO TAR ◇ U.S. BLENDED LIGHT TOBACCO CIGARETTE REFINED TAR

TOXICITY DATA with REFERENCE
CAR: ivg-mus TDLo: 1320 mg/kg/44W-I
JNCIAM 23,1,59
CAR: skn-mus TD: 235 g/kg/52W-I CANCAR
21,376,68
CAR: skn-mus TD: 390 g/kg/65W-I AJPAA4
102,381,81
CAR: skn-mus TDLo: 118 g/kg/52W-I CANCAR
21,376,68
MUT: cyt-ham: lng 10 mg/L BJCAAI 25,574,71
MUT: mmo-sat 1 mg/L GANNA2 69,85,78
MUT: otr-ham: emb 1 mg/L GANNA2 69,85,78
MUT: otr-ham: lng 10 mg/L BJCAAI 25,574,71

SAFETY PROFILE: Suspected carcinogen with experimental carcinogenic data. Mutation data reported.

CMY625
COAL CONVERSION MATERIALS, SRC-II HEAVY DISTILLATE

SYN: SRC-II HEAVY DISTILLATE

TOXICITY DATA with REFERENCE
CAR: skn-mus TD: 285 g/kg/2Y-I NTIS** CONF-801143
CAR: skn-mus TD: 28704 mg/kg/2Y-I NTIS** CONF-801143
CAR: skn-mus TDLo: 2870 mg/kg/2Y-I NTIS** CONF-801143

SAFETY PROFILE: Suspected carcinogen with experimental carcinogenic data by skin contact.

COB250
CROTONALDEHYDE
CAS: 4170-30-3
DOT: 1143
mf: C_4H_6O mw: 70.09

PROP: Water-white, mobile liquid; pungent suffocating odor. Bp: 104°, fp: −76.0°, lel: 2.1%, uel: 15.5%, flash p: 55°F, d: 0.853 @ 20°/20°, vap d: 2.41, autoign temp: 405°F.

SYNS: 2-BUTENAL ◇ CROTONIC ALDEHYDE ◇ KROTO-NALDEHYD (CZECH) ◇ β-METHYL ACROLEIN ◇ RCRA WASTE NUMBER U053

TOXICITY DATA with REFERENCE
CAR: orl-rat TDLo: 2664 mg/kg/2Y-C CNREA8
46,1285,86
MUT: dnd-mam: lym 21500 mg/L/16H CNREA8
44,990,84
MUT: mmo-sat 250 μmol/L ENMUDM 7(Suppl 3),56,85

MUT: sln-dmg-par 3500 ppm ENMUDM 7,677,85
MUT: trn-dmg-par 3500 ppm ENMUDM 7,677,85

CONSENSUS REPORTS: EPA Extremely Hazardous Substances List. Reported in EPA TSCA Inventory.

OSHA PEL: TWA 2 ppm DFG MAK: Suspected Carcinogen. DOT Classification: Flammable Liquid; Label: Flammable Liquid and Poison.

SAFETY PROFILE: Suspected carcinogen with experimental carcinogenic data. Poison by ingestion and inhalation. Mutation data reported. An eye, skin, and mucous membrane irritant. A lachrymating material which can cause corneal burns and is very dangerous to the eyes. Caution: Keep away from heat and open flame. Keep container closed. Use with adequate ventilation. Extremely irritating to eyes, skin, mucous membranes. When necessary, the lacrimatory effect of the vapors may be counteracted by ammonia fumes. Dangerous fire hazard when exposed to heat or flame; can react with oxidizing materials. To fight fire, use alcohol foam, CO_2, dry chemical. When heated to decomposition it emits acrid smoke and fumes.

CPQ625
CAS: 100-88-9
N-CYCLOHEXYLSULPHAMIC ACID
mf: $C_6H_{13}NO_3S$ mw: 179.26

PROP: Crystals; sweet-sour taste. Mp: 169-170°. Fairly strong acid. Very sparingly soluble in water. Slowly hydrolyzed by hot water.

SYNS: CYCLAMATE ◇ CYCLAMIC ACID ◇ CYCLOHEXA-NESULPHAMIC ACID ◇ CYCLOHEXYLAMIDOSULPHURIC ACID ◇ CYCLOHEXYLAMINESULPHONIC ACID ◇ CYCLO-HEXYLSULFAMIC ACID (9CI) ◇ CYCLOHEXYLSULPHAMIC ACID ◇ HEXAMIC ACID ◇ SUCARYL ◇ SUCARYL ACID

TOXICITY DATA with REFERENCE
CAR: orl-man TD: 131 g/kg/5Y-C: KID
JOURAA 118,258,77
CAR: orl-man TD: 164 g/kg/6Y-C: KID
JOURAA 118,258,77
CAR: orl-man TDLo: 22 g/kg/77W-C: KID
JOURAA 118,258,77

CONSENSUS REPORTS: Reported in EPA TSCA Inventory.

SAFETY PROFILE: Suspected human carcinogen producing bladder tumors. Poison by intravenous route. Mildly toxic by ingestion. When heated to decomposition it emits toxic fumes of SO_x and NO_x.

CQN000   CAS: 4465-94-5
CYTOXAL ALCOHOL
mf: $C_7H_{17}Cl_2N_2O_3P \cdot C_6H_{13}N$ mw: 378.33

SYNS: 2-(BIS(2-CHLOROETHYL)AMINO)TETRAHYDRO-OXAZAPHOSPHORINE CYCLOHEXYLAMINE SALT ◇ N,N-BIS(2-CHLOROETHYL)-N'-(3-HYDROXY-PROPYL)PHOSPHORODIAMIDATE, CYCLOHEXYLAM-MONIUM SALT ◇ N,N-BIS(2-CHLOROETHYL)-N'-3-PHOS-PHORODIAMIDIC ACID HYDROXYLPROPYLCYCLOHEXY-LAMINE SALT ◇ CYTOXYL ALCOHOL CYCLOHEXYLAM-MONIUM SALT ◇ NCI-C04922 ◇ NSC-52695

TOXICITY DATA with REFERENCE
CAR: ipr-rat TDLo:2900 mg/kg/26W-I
    RRCRBU 52,1,75
ETA: ipr-mus TDLo:3900 mg/kg/26W-I
    CANCAR 40S,1935,77
MUT: dni-hmn:lym 500 μmol/L   AGACBH
    4,117,74
MUT: mma-sat 100 μg/plate   NTPTB* JAN82
MUT: mmo-sat 100 μg/plate   NTPTB* JAN82

CONSENSUS REPORTS: NCI Carcinogenesis Studies (ipr); Clear Evidence: mouse, rat RRCRBU 52,1,75.

SAFETY PROFILE: Suspected carcinogen with experimental carcinogenic, tumorigenic, and teratogenic data. Poison by intravenous route. Moderately toxic by ingestion and subcutaneous routes. Experimental reproductive effects. Human mutation data reported. When heated to decomposition it emits very toxic fumes of NO_x, NH_3, PO_x, and Cl^-.

DAA800   CAS: 94-75-7
2,4-D
DOT: 2765
mf: $C_8H_6Cl_2O_3$ mw: 221.04

PROP: White powder. Mp: 141°; bp: 160° @ 0.4 mm; vap d: 7.63.

SYNS: ACIDE-2,4-DICHLORO PHENOXYACETIQUE (FRENCH) ◇ ACIDO (2,4-DICLORO-FENOSSI)-ACETICO (ITALIAN) ◇ AGROTECT ◇ AMIDOX ◇ AMOXONE ◇ AQUA-KLEEN ◇ BH 2,4-D ◇ CHIPCO TURF HERBICIDE "D" ◇ CHLOROXONE ◇ CROP RIDER ◇ CROTILIN ◇ D 50 ◇ DACAMINE ◇ 2,4-D ACID ◇ DEBROUSSAILLANT 600 ◇ DECAMINE ◇ DED-WEED ◇ DED-WEED LV-69 ◇ DESORMONE ◇ (2,4-DICHLOOR-FENOXY)-AZIJNZUUR (DUTCH) ◇ DICHLOROPHENOXYACETIC ACID ◇ 2,4-DI-CHLOROPHENOXYACETIC ACID (DOT) ◇ 2,4-DICHLOR-PHENOXYACETIC ACID ◇ (2,4-DICHLOR-PHENOXY)-ES-SIGSAEURE (GERMAN) ◇ DICOPUR ◇ DICOTOX ◇

◇ DINOXOL ◇ DMA-4 ◇ DORMONE ◇ 2,4-DWUCHLOROFE-NOKSYOCTOSY KWAS (POLISH) ◇ EMULSAMINE BK ◇ EMULSAMINE E-3 ◇ ENT 8,538 ◇ ENVERT 171 ◇ ENVERT DT ◇ ESTERON ◇ ESTERON 99 ◇ ESTERON 76 BE ◇ ESTERON BRUSH KILLER ◇ ESTERON 99 CONCEN-TRATE ◇ ESTERONE FOUR ◇ ESTERON 44 WEED KILLER ◇ FARMCO ◇ FERNESTA ◇ FERNIMINE ◇ FERNOXONE ◇ FOREDEX 75 ◇ FORMOLA 40 ◇ HEDONAL (The herbicide) ◇ HERBIDAL ◇ IPANER ◇ KROTILINE ◇ LAWN-KEEP ◇ MACRONDRAY ◇ MIRACLE ◇ MONOSAN ◇ MOXONE ◇ NETAGRONE 600 ◇ NSC 423 ◇ PENNAMINE ◇ PHENOX ◇ PIELIK ◇ PLANOTOX ◇ PLANTGARD ◇ RCRA WASTE NUMBER U240 ◇ RHODIA ◇ SALVO ◇ SPRITZ-HORMIN/2,4-D ◇ SUPER D WEEDONE ◇ SUPERORMONE CONCEN-TRE ◇ TRANSAMINE ◇ TRIBUTON ◇ TRINOXOL ◇ U 46 ◇ U-5043 ◇ U 46DP ◇ VERGEMASTER ◇ VERTON D ◇ VIDON 638 ◇ VISKO-RHAP DRIFT HERBICIDES ◇ WEED-AG-BAR ◇ WEEDAR-64 ◇ WEED-B-GON ◇ WEEDEZ WONDER BAR ◇ WEEDONE LV4 ◇ WEED TOX ◇ WEEDTROL

TOXICITY DATA with REFERENCE
MUT: cyt-rat-ipr 2500 μg/kg   RABIDH 32,265,83
MUT: dni-ham:ovr 1 mmol/L   TOLED5 29,137,85
MUT: sce-ham:orl 900 mg/kg/9D-I   CRNGDP
    5,703,84
MUT: sce-ham:ovr 10 μmol/L/1H   CRNGDP
    5,703,84
MUT: sce-hmn:lym 10 mg/L   JOHEA8
    73,224,82

CONSENSUS REPORTS: IARC Cancer Review: Human Limited Evidence IMEMDT 41,357,86; Animal Inadequate Evidence IMEMDT 15,111,77; Human Inadequate Evidence IMEMDT 15,111,77. EPA Genetic Toxicology Program. Reported in EPA TSCA Inventory. Community Right-To-Know List.

OSHA PEL: TWA 10 mg/m^3 ACGIH TLV: TWA 10 mg/m^3 DFG MAK: 10 mg/m^3 DOT Classification: ORM-A; Label: None.

SAFETY PROFILE: Suspected human carcinogen. Experimental teratogenic data. Poison by ingestion, intravenous, and intraperitoneal routes. Moderately toxic by skin contact. Human systemic effects by ingestion: somnolence, convulsions, coma, and nausea or vomiting. Can cause liver and kidney injury. A skin and severe eye irritant. Human mutation data reported. Experimental reproductive effects. When heated to decomposition it emits toxic fumes of Cl^-.

DAB600
DACARBAZINE
CAS: 4342-03-4

mf: $C_6H_{10}N_6O$ mw: 182.22

SYNS: DETICENE ◇ DIC ◇ (DIMETHYLTRIAZENO)IMIDAZOLECARBOXAMIDE ◇ 4-(DIMETHYLTRIAZENO)IMIDAZOLE-5-CARBOXAMIDE ◇ 4-(3,3-DIMETHYL-1-TRIAZENO)IMIDAZOLE-5-CARBOX-AMIDE ◇ 4-(5)-(3,3-DIMETHYL-1-TRIAZENO)IMIDAZOLE-5(4)-CARBOXAMIDE ◇ 5-(DIMETHYLTRIAZENO)IMIDA-ZOLE-4-CARBOXAMIDE ◇ 5-(3,3-DIMETHYLTRIAZENO)IM-IDAZOLE-4-CARBOXAMIDE ◇ 5-(3,3-DIMETHYL-1-TRIAZENO)IMIDAZOLE-4-CARBOXAMIDE ◇ 5-(3,3-DIMETHYL-1-TRIAZENYL)-1H-IMIDAZOLE-4-CARBOXAMIDE ◇ DTIC ◇ DTIC-DOME ◇ NCI-C04717 ◇ NSC-45388

TOXICITY DATA with REFERENCE
CAR: ipr-mus TDLo: 1950 mg/kg/26W-I   RRCRBU 52,1,75
CAR: ipr-rat TDLo: 3900 mg/kg/26W-I   RRCRBU 52,1,75
CAR: orl-rat TD: 3700 mg/kg/14W-C   PAACA3 11,73,70
CAR: orl-rat TDLo: 1730 mg/kg/15W-C   JNCIAM 54,951,75
ETA: ipr-rat TDLo: 25 mg/kg (20D preg): TER   ARGEAR 50,3-06,80
MUT: mma-esc 100 μg/plate   CRNGDP 3,467,82
MUT: mma-sat 100 μg/plate   CRNGDP 3,467,82
MUT: mmo-esc 100 μg/plate   CRNGDP 3,467,82
MUT: msc-ham: lng 20 mg/L   CRNGDP 3,467,82
MUT: msc-ham: ovr 400 mg/L   CNREA8 43,577,83
MUT: par-ham LD10: 250 mg/kg   JSONAU 15,355,80
MUT: sce-ham: ovr 200 mg/L   CNREA8 43,577,83

CONSENSUS REPORTS: IARC Cancer Review: GROUP 2B IMEMDT 7,184,87; Human Limited Evidence IMEMDT 26,203,81; Animal Sufficient Evidence IMEMDT 26,203,81. NCI Carcinogenesis Studies (ipr); Clear Evidence: mouse, rat RRCRBU 52,1,75. EPA Genetic Toxicology Program.

SAFETY PROFILE: Suspected carcinogen with experimental carcinogenic, tumorigenic, and teratogenic data. Poison by intraperitoneal and parenteral routes. Moderately toxic by ingestion and intravenous routes. Human systemic effects by intravenous route: nausea or vomiting, luekopenia (reduced white blood cell count), and changes in dehydrogenase enzymatic activity. Mutation data reported. When heated to decomposition it emits toxic fumes of NO_x.

DAC000
DAUNOMYCIN
CAS: 20830-81-3

mf: $C_{27}H_{29}NO_{10}$ mw: 527.57

PROP: Thin, red needles. Mp: 190° (decomp). Isolated from cultures of a *Streptomyces* (CNREA8 32,1029,72).

SYNS: ACETYLADRIAMYCIN ◇ CERUBIDIN ◇ DAUNA-MYCIN ◇ DAUNORUBICIN ◇ DAUNORUBICINE ◇ DM ◇ FI6339 ◇ LEUKAEMOMYCIN C ◇ NCI-C04693 ◇ NSC-82151 ◇ RCRA WASTE NUMBER U059 ◇ RP 13057 ◇ 13,057 R.P. ◇ RUBIDOMYCIN ◇ RUBIDOMYCINE ◇ RUBOMYCIN C ◇ RUBOMYCIN C 1 ◇ STREPTOMYCES PEUCETIUS

TOXICITY DATA with REFERENCE
CAR: ivn-rat TD: 10 mg/kg   JJIND8 66,81,81
CAR: ivn-rat TD: 10 mg/kg   LAPPA5 38,71,78
CAR: ivn-rat TD: 13 mg/kg   EXPEAM 27,1209,71
CAR: ivn-rat TD: 40 mg/kg/4W-I   AFCPDR 34,369,82
CAR: ivn-rat TDLo: 6250 μg/kg   CNREA8 38,1444,78
CAR: scu-mus TDLo: 15 g/kg/12W-I   RRCRBU 20,73,69
NEO: ivn-rat TD: 5 mg/kg   CNREA8 32,1029,72
NEO: scu-mus TD: 15 mg/kg/12W-I   ARZNAD 17,948,67
ETA: ipr-mus TDLo: 2340 μg/kg/26W-I   CANCAR 40,1935,77
ETA: ipr-rat TDLo: 2200 μg/kg/7W-I   CANCAR 40,1935,77
ETA: ivn-rat TD: 5 mg/kg   CNREA8 36,2065,76
MUT: cyt-ham: fbr 1 mg/L   ICHUDW 6(6),26,84
MUT: dni-hmn: oth 30 nmol/L   CNREA8 44,2421,84
MUT: dns-rat: lvr 10 mg/L   CNREA8 44,5599,84
MUT: mmo-sat 1 μg/plate   ENMUDM 7,129,85
MUT: pic-sat 800 ng/plate   MUREAV 110,243,83

CONSENSUS REPORTS: IARC Cancer Review: GROUP 2B IMEMDT 7,56,87; Animal Sufficient Evidence IMEMDT 10,145,76. NCI Carcinogenesis Studies (ipr); Clear Evidence: rat CANCAR 40,1935,77; No Evidence: mouse CANCAR 40,1935,77. EPA Genetic Toxicology Program.

SAFETY PROFILE: Suspected carcinogen with experimental carcinogenic, neoplastigenic, tumorigenic, and teratogenic data. Human poison by ingestion. Experimental poison by subcutaneous, intravenous, and intraperitoneal routes. Experimental reproductive effects. Human mutation data reported. When heated to decomposition it emits toxic fumes of NO_x.

DAL600   CAS: 84-17-3
DEHYDROSTILBESTROL
mf: $C_{18}H_{18}O_2$ mw: 266.36

SYNS: 3,4-BIS(p-HYDROXYPHENYL)-2,4-HEXADIENE
◇ 3,4-BIS(4-HYDROXYPHENYL)-2,4-HEXADIENE
◇ CYCLADIENE ◇ DEHYDROSTILBOESTROL ◇ DIENES-
TROL ◇ DIENOESTROL ◇ β-DIENOESTROL ◇ DIENOL
◇ 4,4'-(1,2-DIETHYLIDENE-1,2-ETHANEDIYL)BISPHENOL
◇ p,p'-(DIETHYLIDENEETHYLENE)DIPHENOL ◇ 4,4'-(DI-
ETHYLIDENEETHYLENE)DIPHENOL ◇ DINOVEX
◇ DI(p-OXYPHENYL)-2,4-HEXADIENE ◇ DV ◇ ESTRAGARD
◇ ESTRODIENOL ◇ ESTRORAL ◇ FOLLIDIENE ◇ FOLLOR-
MON ◇ GYNEFOLLIN ◇ HORMOFEMIN ◇ 4,4'-HYDROXY-
γ,Δ-DIPHENYL-β,Δ-HEXADIENE ◇ ISODIENESTROL
◇ OESTRASID ◇ OESTRODIENE ◇ OESTRODIENOL
◇ OESTRORAL ◇ PARA-DIEN ◇ RESTROL ◇ RETALON
◇ SEXADIEN ◇ SYNESTROL ◇ TESERENE ◇ WILLNESTROL

TOXICITY DATA with REFERENCE
MUT: dns-ham:emb 3 mg/L   CNREA8 44,184,84
MUT: sce-hmn:fbr 5 nmol/L   NATUAS 281,392,79

CONSENSUS REPORTS: IARC Cancer Review: Animal Inadequate Evidence IMEMDT
21,161,79; Human Limited Evidence IMEMDT
21,161,79

SAFETY PROFILE: Suspected human carcinogen. Human mutation data reported. Experimental reproductive effects. Used as a drug for the
treatment of postmenopausal symptoms. When
heated to decomposition it emits acrid smoke
and irritating fumes.

DBD400   CAS: 9004-54-0
DEXTRAN 10

PROP: A branched, water-soluble polymer of
average molecular weight 89,400 (ARPAAQ
67,589,59).

TOXICITY DATA with REFERENCE
CAR: ipr-mus TDLo:8000 mg/kg   AMPLAO
67,589,59
CAR: ivn-rbt TDLo:8750 mg/kg/I   AMPLAO
67,589,59
CAR: scu-rat TDLo:2500 mg/kg   AMPLAO
67,589,59

CONSENSUS REPORTS: Reported in EPA
TSCA Inventory.

SAFETY PROFILE: Suspected carcinogen with
experimental carcinogenic data. When heated
to decomposition it emits acrid smoke and
fumes.

DBF200   CAS: 642-65-9
2-DIACETAMIDOFLUORENE
mf: $C_{17}H_{15}NO_2$ mw: 265.33

SYNS: N-ACETYL-N-9H-FLUOREN-2-YL-ACETAMIDE
◇ N-DIACETYL-2-AMINOFLUORENE ◇ 2-DIACETYLAMI-
NOFLUORENE ◇ N,N-DIACETYL-2-AMINOFLUORENE
◇ N,N-DIACETYL-2-FLUORENAMINE ◇ F-diAA ◇ 2-FLUOR-
ENYLDIACETAMIDE ◇ N-FLUOREN-2-YLDIACETAMIDE
◇ N-2-FLUORENYLDIACETAMIDE

TOXICITY DATA with REFERENCE
CAR: orl-ham TDLo:6174 mg/kg/49W-C
GANNA2 59,239,68
CAR: skn-rat TDLo:290 mg/kg/77W-I   JNCIAM
10,1201,50
NEO: orl-rat TDLo:970 mg/kg/23W-C   JNCIAM
10,1201,50
ETA: orl-rat TD:475 mg/kg/5W-C   AICCA6
20,1364,64
ETA: orl-rat TD:613 mg/kg/8W-I   JNCIAM
31,1407,63
ETA: orl-rat TD:945 mg/kg/9W-I   JNCIAM
34,697,65
ETA: orl-rat TD:1138 mg/kg/16W-I   JNCIAM
29,933,62
ETA: orl-rat TD:1365 mg/kg/16W-I   EJCAAH
12,137,76
ETA: orl-rat TD:1540 mg/kg/19W-I   CNREA8
28,2177,68
ETA: orl-rat TD:4000 mg/kg/23W-C   CNREA8
7,730,47

SAFETY PROFILE: Suspected carcinogen with
experimental carcinogenic, neoplastigenic, and
tumorigenic data. When heated to decomposition it emits toxic fumes of NO_x.

DBL200   CAS: 131-17-9
DIALLYL PHTHALATE
mf: $C_{14}H_{14}O_4$ mw: 246.28

PROP: Nearly colorless, oily liquid. Bp: 157°,
flash p: 330°F, d: 1.120 @ 20°/20°, vap d: 8.3.

SYNS: DAPON 35 ◇ DAPON R ◇ DI-2-PROPENYL ESTER,
1,2-BENZENEDICARBOXYLIC ACID ◇ NCI-C50657
◇ PHTHALIC ACID, DIALLYL ESTER ◇ o-PHTHALIC ACID,
DIALLYL ESTER

TOXICITY DATA with REFERENCE
CAR: orl-mus TDLo:156 g/kg/2Y-I   EVHPAZ
65,271,86
CAR: orl-rat TDLo:52 g/kg/2Y-I   EVHPAZ
65,271,86
MUT: mma-mus:lyms 67200 μg/L   SCIEAS
236,933,87   SCIEAS 236,933,87

CONSENSUS REPORTS: NTP Carcinogenesis Studies (gavage); Equivocal Evidence: rat NTPTR* NTP-TR-284,85. Reported in EPA TSCA Inventory.

SAFETY PROFILE: Suspected carcinogen with experimental carcinogenic data. Moderately toxic by ingestion, skin contact, intraperitoneal, and subcutaneous routes. An eye irritant. Mutation data reported. Combustible when exposed to heat or flame; can react with oxidizing materials. To fight fire use CO_2 or dry chemical. When heated to decomposition it emits acrid smoke and irritating fumes.

DCY200   CAS: 189-64-0
DIBENZO(b,def)CHRYSENE
mf: $C_{24}H_{14}$ mw: 302.38

SYNS: BD(a,h)P ◊ DIBENZO(a,h)PYRENE ◊ 1,2,6,7-DI-BENZOPYRENE ◊ 3,4,8,9-DIBENZOPYRENE ◊ 3,4,8,9-DI-BENZPYRENE

TOXICITY DATA with REFERENCE
CAR: skn-mus TDLo:287 mg/kg/30W-I
ZKKOBW 89,113,77
ETA: imp-rat TDLo:100 mg/kg   NEOLA4 26,23,79
ETA: scu-mus TDLo:72 mg/kg/9W-I   COREAF
246,1477,58
ETA: skn-mus TD:330 mg/kg/15W   AVBNAN
56,39,39
ETA: skn-mus TD:700 mg/kg/42W-I   PRLBA4
129,439,40
ETA: skn-mus TD:1060 mg/kg/44W-I   PRLBA4
123,343,37
MUT: mma-sat 12500 pmol/plate   CNREA8
41,2589,81
MUT: msc-ham:lng 30 μg/L   CNREA8 42,1646,82

CONSENSUS REPORTS: IARC Cancer Review: GROUP 2B IMEMDT 7,56,87; Animal Sufficient Evidence IMEMDT 32,331,83; IMEMDT 3,207,73

SAFETY PROFILE: Suspected carcinogen with experimental carcinogenic and tumorigenic data. When heated to decomposition it emits acrid smoke and irritating fumes. Mutation data reported.

DCY400   CAS: 191-30-0
DIBENZO(def,p)CHRYSENE
mf: $C_{24}H_{14}$ mw: 302.38

SYNS: BA 51-090462 ◊ DB(a,l)P ◊ DIBENZO(a,d)PYRENE ◊ DIBENZO(a,l)PYRENE ◊ 1,2:3,4-DIBENZOPYRENE ◊ 1,2,9,10-DIBENZOPYRENE ◊ 2,3:4,5-DIBENZOPYRENE ◊ 1,2,3,4-DIBENZPYRENE ◊ 4,5,6,7-DIBENZPYRENE

TOXICITY DATA with REFERENCE
ETA: scu-mus TD:72 mg/kg/9W-I   COREAF
258,3387,64
ETA: scu-mus TDLo:48 mg/kg/4W-I   NATWAY
55,43,68
ETA: skn-mus TDLo:890 mg/kg/37W-I
PRLBA4 123,343,37

CONSENSUS REPORTS: IARC Cancer Review: GROUP 2B IMEMDT 7,56,87; Animal Sufficient Evidence IMEMDT 32,343,83; Animal Limited Evidence IMEMDT 3,224,73

SAFETY PROFILE: Suspected carcinogen with experimental tumorigenic data. When heated to decomposition it emits acrid smoke and irritating fumes.

DDG800   CAS: 63-92-3
DIBENZYLINE HYDROCHLORIDE
mf: $C_{18}H_{22}ClNO•ClH$ mw: 340.32

SYNS: 688A ◊ BENSYLYT NEN ◊ 2-(N-BENZYL-2-CHLO-ROETHYLAMINO)-1-PHENOXYPROPANE HYDROCHLO-RIDE ◊ BENZYL(2-CHLOROETHYL)(1-METHYL-2-PHEN-OXYETHYL)AMINE HYDROCHLORIDE ◊ N-BENZYL-N-PHENOXYISOPROPYL-β-CHLORETHYLAMINE HYDRO-CHLORIDE ◊ BENZYLYT ◊ BLOCADREN ◊ N-(2-CHLORO-ETHYL)-N-(1-METHYL-2-PHENOXYETHYL)BENZENE-METHANAMINE HYDROCHLORIDE ◊ N-(2-CHLORO-ETHYL)-N-(1-METHYL-2-PHENOXYETHYL)BENZYLAMINE HYDROCHLORIDE ◊ DIBENZYLENE ◊ DIBENZYLIN ◊ DIBENZYRAN ◊ FENOXYBENZAMIN ◊ NCI-C01661 ◊ PHENOXYBENZAMIDE HYDROCHLORIDE ◊ N-PHENOX-YISOPROPYL-N-BENZYL-β-CHLOROETHYLAMINE HY-DROCHLORIDE ◊ N-2-PHENOXYISOPROPYL-N-BENZYL-CHLOROETHYLAMINE HYDROCHLORIDE ◊ SKF 688A

TOXICITY DATA with REFERENCE
CAR: ipr-mus TDLo:3900 mg/kg/52W-I
NCITR* NCI-CG-TR-72,78
CAR: ipr-rat TD:1560 mg/kg/1Y-I   NCITR* NCI-CG-TR-72,78
CAR: ipr-rat TDLo:780 mg/kg/1Y-I   NCITR*
NCI-CG-TR-72,78

CONSENSUS REPORTS: IARC Cancer Review: GROUP 2B IMEMDT 7,56,87; Animal Sufficient Evidence IMEMDT 24,185,80. NCI Carcinogenesis Bioassay Completed; Results Positive: mouse, rat NCITR* NCI-CG-TR-72,78.

SAFETY PROFILE: Suspected carcinogen with experimental carcinogenic and teratogenic data. Poison by intraperitoneal, intravenous, and subcutaneous routes. Moderately toxic by ingestion. Other experimental reproductive effects. A long-acting adrenergic blocker. When heated to decomposition it emits very toxic fumes of NO_x and Cl^-.

DEP800   CAS: 106-46-7
p-DICHLOROBENZENE
DOT: 1592
mf: $C_6H_4Cl_2$ mw: 147.00

PROP: White crystals, penetrating odor. Mp: 53°, bp: 173.4°, flash p: 150°F (CC), d: 1.4581 @ 20.5°/4°, vap press: 10 mm @ 54.8°, vap d: 5.08.

SYNS: p-CHLOROPHENYL CHLORIDE ◇ p-DICHLOOR-BENZEEN (DUTCH) ◇ 1,4-DICHLOORBENZEEN (DUTCH) ◇ p-DICHLORBENZOL (GERMAN) ◇ 1,4-DICHLOR-BENZOL (GERMAN) ◇ DI-CHLORICIDE ◇ 1,4-DICHLOROBENZENE (MAK) ◇ p-DICLOROBENZENE (ITALIAN) ◇ DICHLORO-BENZENE, PARA, solid (DOT) ◇ 1,4-DICLOROBENZENE (ITALIAN) ◇ p-DICHLOROBENZOL ◇ EVOLA ◇ NCI-C54955 ◇ PARACIDE ◇ PARA CRYSTALS ◇ PARADI ◇ PARADI-CHLORBENZOL (GERMAN) ◇ PARADICHLOROBENZENE ◇ PARADICHLOROBENZOL ◇ PARADOW ◇ PARAMOTH ◇ PARANUGGETS ◇ PARAZENE ◇ PDB ◇ PDCB ◇ PERSIA-PERAZOL ◇ RCRA WASTE NUMBER U070 ◇ RCRA WASTE NUMBER U071 ◇ RCRA WASTE NUMBER U072 ◇ SANTOCHLOR

TOXICITY DATA with REFERENCE
CAR: orl-mus TDLo:155 g/kg/2Y-I   NTPTR* NTP-TR-319,87
CAR: orl-rat TDLo:155 g/kg/2Y-I   NTPTR* NTP-TR-319,87
MUT: mmo-asn 200 mg/L   CJMIAZ 16,369,70

CONSENSUS REPORTS: IARC Cancer Review: GROUP 2B IMEMDT 7,192,87; Animal Inadequate Evidence IMEMDT 7,231,74; Human Inadequate Evidence IMEMDT 7,231,74; Animal Inadequate Evidence IMEMDT 29,213,82. Reported in EPA TSCA Inventory. EPA Genetic Toxicology Program. Community Right-To-Know List.

OSHA PEL: (Transitional: TWA 75 ppm) TWA 75 ppm; STEL 110 ppm   ACGIH TLV: TWA 75 ppm; STEL 110 ppm   DFG MAK: 75 ppm (450 mg/m^3)   DOT Classification: ORM-A; Label: None; IMO: Poison B; Label: St. Andrews Cross.

SAFETY PROFILE: Suspected carcinogen with experimental carcinogenic data. An experimental teratogen. A human poison by an unspecified route. Moderately toxic to humans by ingestion. Moderately toxic experimentally by ingestion, subcutaneous, and intraperitoneal routes. Mildly toxic by subcutaneous route. Other experimental reproductive effects. Human systemic effects by ingestion: unspecified changes in the eyes, lungs, thorax and respiration, and decreased motility or constipation. Can cause liver injury in humans. A human eye irritant. Mutation data reported. A fumigant. Flammable when exposed to heat, flame, or oxidizers. Dangerous; can react vigorously with oxidizing materials. To fight fire, use water, foam, CO_2, dry chemical. When heated to decomposition it emits toxic fumes of Cl^-.

DER000   CAS: 510-15-6
4,4'-DICHLOROBENZILIC ACID ETHYL ESTER
mf: $C_{16}H_{14}Cl_2O_3$ mw: 325.20

PROP: Viscous liquid, sometimes yellow, sltly sol in water. Bp: 156-158°, vap press: 2.2 × 10^{-6} mm @ 20°.

SYNS: ACAR ◇ ACARABEN 4E ◇ AKAR ◇ BENZILAN ◇ BENZ-o-CHLOR ◇ CHLORBENZILATE ◇ CHLOROBENZY-LATE ◇ COMPOUND 338 ◇ 4,4'-DICHLORBENZIL-SAEUREAETHYLESTER (GERMAN) ◇ 4,4'-DICHLO-ROBENZILATE ◇ ENT 18,596 ◇ ETHYL 4-CHLORO-α-(4-CHLOROPHENYL)-α-HYDROXYBENZENEACETATE ◇ ETHYL-p,p'-DICHLOROBENZILATE ◇ ETHYL-4,4'-DI-CHLOROBENZILATE ◇ ETHYL-4,4'-DICHLORODIPHENYL GLYCOLLATE ◇ ETHYL-4,4'-DICHLOROPHENYL GLYCOL-LATE ◇ ETHYL ESTER of 4,4'-DICHLOROBENZILIC ACID ◇ ETHYL-2-HYDROXY-2,2-BIS(4-CHLOROPHENYL)ACE-TATE ◇ FOLBEX ◇ FOLBEX SMOKE-STRIPS ◇ G 338 ◇ G 23992 ◇ GEIGY 338 ◇ KOP MITE ◇ NCI-C00408 ◇ NCI-C60413 ◇ RCRA WASTE NUMBER U038

TOXICITY DATA with REFERENCE
CAR: orl-mus TD:125 g/kg/83W-C   DIGEBW 16,308,77
CAR: orl-mus TD:210 g/kg/78W-C   NCITR* NCI-CG-TR-75,78
CAR: orl-mus TDLo:71 g/kg/82W-C   JNCIAM 42,1101,69
CAR: orl-rat TD:17520 mg/kg/2Y-C   CTOXAO 16,67,80
CAR: orl-rat TDLo:5475 mg/kg/2Y-C   CTOXAO 16,67,80
NEO: orl-rat TD:1752 mg/kg/2Y-C   CTOXAO 16,67,80
ETA: orl-rat TD:72 g/kg/78W-C   NCITR* NCI-CG-TR-75,78

CONSENSUS REPORTS: IARC Cancer Review: GROUP 3 IMEMDT 7,56,87; Animal Limited Evidence IMEMDT 30,73,83; Animal Sufficient Evidence IMEMDT 5,75,74. NCI Carcinogenesis Bioassay Completed; Results Positive: mouse (NCITR* NCI-CG-TR-75,78). NCI Carcinogenesis Bioassay Completed; Results Indefinite: rat (NCITR* NCI-CG-TR-75,78). Community Right-To-Know List. Reported in EPA TSCA Inventory.

SAFETY PROFILE: Suspected carcinogen with experimental carcinogenic, neoplastigenic, and tumorigenic data. Moderately toxic by ingestion and possibly other routes. A skin and eye irritant. A pesticide. When heated to decomposition it emits toxic fumes of Cl^-.

DFX800   CAS: 120-83-2
2,4-DICHLOROPHENOL
mf: $C_6H_4Cl_2O$ mw: 163.00

PROP: Colorless crystals. Mp: 45°, bp: 210°, flash p: 237°F, d: 1.383 @ 60°/25°, vap d: 5.62, vap press: 1 mm @ 53.0°.

SYNS: DCP ◇ 2,4-DCP ◇ NCI-C55345 ◇ RCRA WASTE NUMBER U081

TOXICITY DATA with REFERENCE
CAR: skn-mus TDLo: 16 g/kg/39W-I   CNREA8 19,413,59

CONSENSUS REPORTS: IARC Cancer Review: Human Limited Evidence IMEMDT 41,319,86. Reported in EPA TSCA Inventory. EPA Genetic Toxicology Program. Community Right-To-Know List.

SAFETY PROFILE: Suspected carcinogen with experimental carcinogenic and teratogenic data. Poison by intraperitoneal route. Moderately toxic by ingestion, skin contact, and subcutaneous routes. Combustible when exposed to heat or flame. To fight fire, use alcohol foam, foam, CO_2, dry chemical. When heated to decomposition, or on contact with acid or acid fumes it emits highly toxic fumes of Cl^-.

DGB000   CAS: 120-36-5
2-(2,4-DICHLOROPHENOXY)
PROPIONIC ACID
mf: $C_9H_8Cl_2O_3$ mw: 235.07

SYNS: ACIDE-2-(2,4-DICHLORO-PHENOXY) PROPIONIQUE (FRENCH) ◇ ACIDO-2-(2,4-DICLORO-FENOSSI)-PROPIONICO (ITALIAN) ◇ CORNOX RD ◇ CORNOX RK

◇ DESORMONE ◇ 2-(2,4-DICHLOOR-FENOXY)-PROPIONZUUR (DUTCH) ◇ α-(2,4-DICHLOROPHENOXY) PROPIONIC ACID ◇ DICHLOROPROP ◇ 2-(2,4-DICHLOR-PHENOXY)-PROPIONSAEURE (GERMAN) ◇ DICHLORPROP ◇ 2,4-DP ◇ 2-(2,4-DP) ◇ HEDONAL ◇ HEDONAL DP ◇ HORMATOX ◇ KILDIP ◇ POLYCLENE ◇ POLYMONE ◇ POLYTOX ◇ RD 406 ◇ SERITOX 50 ◇ U46 ◇ U46 DP-FLUID ◇ VISKO-RHAP ◇ WEEDONE DP ◇ WEEDONE 170

TOXICITY DATA with REFERENCE
MUT: mmo-smc 700 mg/L   ZAPOAK 9,483,69

CONSENSUS REPORTS: IARC Cancer Review: GROUP 2B IMEMDT 7,156,87; Human Limited Evidence IMEMDT 41,357,86. Reported in EPA TSCA Inventory.

SAFETY PROFILE: Suspected carcinogen. Poison by ingestion. Moderately toxic by skin contact. An experimental teratogen. Mutation data reported. A fumigant. When heated to decomposition it emits toxic fumes of Cl^-.

DHB600   CAS: 298-18-0
dl-DIEPOXYBUTANE
mf: $C_4H_6O_2$ mw: 86.10

PROP: Colorless liquid. Bp: 138°, mp: 4°, d: 1.112 @ 18°/4°.

SYNS: dl-BUTADIENE DIOXIDE ◇ 1,2:3,4-DIANHYDRO-dl-THREITOL ◇ (±)-1,2:3,4-DIEPOXYBUTANE ◇ dl-1,2:3,4-DIEPOXYBUTANE

TOXICITY DATA with REFERENCE
CAR: scu-mus TDLo: 13200 μg/kg/68W-I   CNREA8 43,159,83
CAR: skn-mus TD: 24 g/kg/68W-I   14JTAF -,275,74
CAR: skn-mus TDLo: 132 mg/kg/66W-I   CNREA8 43,159,83
ETA: skn-mus TD: 13 g/kg/11W-I   JNCIAM 31,41,63
NEO: scu-mus TD: 260 mg/kg/65W-I   JNCIAM 37,825,66
ETA: scu-rat TDLo: 335 mg/kg/67W-I   JNCIAM 37,825,66
ETA: skn-mus TD: 13 g/kg/11W-I   JNCIAM 31,41,63
ETA: skn-mus TD: 13 g/kg/11W-I   JNCIAM 31,41,63
MUT: dns-ham: lvr 1 μmol/L   ENMUDM 6,1,84
MUT: mmo-ssp 20 mmol/L   ADWMAX -,193,62

CONSENSUS REPORTS: IARC Cancer Review: GROUP 2B IMEMDT 7,56,87; Animal

Sufficient Evidence IMEMDT 11,115,76. EPA Genetic Toxicology Program.

SAFETY PROFILE: Suspected carcinogen with experimental carcinogenic, neoplastigenic, and tumorigenic data. Poison by ingestion, inhalation, and skin contact. Mutation data reported. When heated to decomposition it emits acrid smoke and irritating fumes.

DHB800   CAS: 564-00-1
meso-1,2,3,4-DIEPOXYBUTANE
mf: $C_4H_6O_2$ mw: 86.10

SYNS: (R*,S*)-2,2'-BIOXIRANE ◇ 1,2:3,4-DIANHY-DROERYTHRITOL ◇ meso-DIEPOXYBUTANE ◇ (R*,S*)-DI-EPOXYBUTANE ◇ ERYTHRITOL ANHYDRIDE

TOXICITY DATA with REFERENCE
NEO: skn-mus TDLo: 26 g/kg/22W-I   14JTAF -,275,64

ETA: skn-mus TD: 26 g/kg/22W-I   JNCIAM 31,41,63

MUT: mma-sat 3300 ng/plate   ENMUDM 6(Suppl 2),1,84

MUT: mma-sat 33300 ng/plate   ENMUDM 6(Suppl 2),1,84

MUT: mmo-esc 100 µg/plate   ENMUDM 6(Suppl 2),1,84

MUT: mmo-sat 100 µg/plate   ENMUDM 6(Suppl 2),1,84

MUT: mmo-ssp 51 mmol/L   ADWMAX -,193,62

CONSENSUS REPORTS: IARC Cancer Review: GROUP 2B IMEMDT 7,56,87; Animal Sufficient Evidence IMEMDT 11,115,76.

SAFETY PROFILE: Suspected carcinogen with experimental carcinogenic, neoplastigenic, and tumorigenic data. Poison by skin contact and intraperitoneal routes. Mutation data reported. When heated to decomposition it emits acrid smoke and irritating fumes.

DIW400   CAS: 88-10-8
DIETHYLCARBAMOYL CHLORIDE
mf: $C_5H_{10}ClNO$ mw: 135.61

PROP: Liquid. Mp: −44°, bp: 190-195°, vap d: 4.1.

SYNS: DIETHYLCARBAMIC CHLORIDE ◇ DIETHYLCAR-BAMIDOYL CHLORIDE ◇ N,N-DIETHYLCARBAMOYL CHLORIDE ◇ DIETHYLCARBAMYL CHLORIDE

TOXICITY DATA with REFERENCE
CAR: skn-mus TDLo: 43200 mg/kg/72W-I

   JACTDZ 6(4),479,87

CONSENSUS REPORTS: Reported in EPA TSCA Inventory.

DFG MAK: Suspected Carcinogen.

SAFETY PROFILE: Suspected carcinogen with experimental carcinogenic data. Moderately toxic by intraperitoneal route. Mutation data reported. Reacts with water or steam to produce toxic and corrosive fumes. When heated to decomposition it emits highly toxic fumes of Cl^- and NO_x.

DJL400   CAS: 1615-80-1
1,2-DIETHYLHYDRAZINE
mf: $C_4H_{12}N_2$ mw: 88.18

PROP: Bp: 86°, d: 0.797 @ 26°. Sol in alcohol and ether.

SYNS: 1,2-DIAETHYLHYDRAZINE (GERMAN) ◇ N-N'-DI-ETHYLHYDRAZINE ◇ sym-DIETHYLHYDRAZINE ◇ HYDRAZOETHANE ◇ HYDROAZOETHANE ◇ RCRA WASTE NUMBER U086 ◇ SDEH

TOXICITY DATA with REFERENCE
CAR: ivn-rat TDLo: 50 mg/kg (15D preg): TER

   IARCCD 4,45,73

ETA: ivn-rat TDLo: 1850 mg/kg/37W-I

   XENOBH 3,271,73

ETA: scu-rat TDLo: 700 mg/kg/28W-I   NATWAY 53,557,66

ETA: ivn-rat TD: 50 mg/kg (15D preg): TER

   FCTXAV 6,584,68

CONSENSUS REPORTS: IARC Cancer Review: GROUP 2B IMEMDT 7,56,87; Animal Sufficient Evidence IMEMDT 4,153,74.

SAFETY PROFILE: Suspected carcinogen with experimental carcinogenic, tumorigenic, and teratogenic data. It is also a transplacental carcinogenic. When heated to decomposition it emits toxic fumes of NO_x.

DKM200   CAS: 2238-07-5
DIGLYCIDYL ETHER
mf: $C_6H_{10}O_3$ mw: 130.16

PROP: Liquid.

SYNS: BIS(2,3-EPOXYPROPYL)ETHER ◇ DGE ◇ DI(2,3-EPOXYPROPYL) ETHER

TOXICITY DATA with REFERENCE
ETA: unr-mus TDLo: 1300 mg/kg   RARSAM 3,193,63

MUT: mma-sat 50 µg/plate   MUREAV 66,367,79
MUT: mmo-sat 50 µg/plate   MUREAV 66,367,79

CONSENSUS REPORTS: EPA Extremely Hazardous Substances List. Reported in EPA TSCA Inventory. EPA Genetic Toxicology Program.

OSHA PEL: (Transitional: CL 0.5 ppm) TWA 0.1 ppm   ACGIH TLV: TWA 0.1 ppm   DFG MAK: 0.1 ppm (0.6 mg/m^3); Suspected Carcinogen.   NIOSH REL: (Glycidyl Ethers) CL 1 mg/m^3/15M

SAFETY PROFILE: Suspected carcinogen with experimental tumorigenic data. Poison by ingestion, inhalation, and intravenous routes. Moderately toxic by skin contact. A severe eye and skin irritant. Mutation data reported. Chronic exposure can cause bone marrow depression. When heated to decomposition it emits acrid smoke and fumes.

DMD600   CAS: 94-58-6
DIHYDROSAFROLE
mf: $C_{10}H_{12}O_2$ mw: 164.22

PROP: An oily liquid. Bp: 228°, d: 1.0695 @ 20°.

SYNS: 1,2-(METHYLENEDIOXY)-4-PROPYLBENZENE ◇ 5-PROPYL-1,3-BENZODIOXOLE ◇ 4-PROPYL-1,2-METHYLENEDIOXYBENZENE ◇ RCRA WASTE NUMBER U090

TOXICITY DATA with REFERENCE
CAR: orl-mus TD: 101 g/kg/81W-C   DIGEBW 19,42,79
CAR: orl-mus TDLo: 101 g/kg/81W-C   FCTXAV 19,130,81
CAR: orl-mus TDLo: 163 g/kg/81W-C   JNCIAM 42,1101,69

CONSENSUS REPORTS: IARC Cancer Review: GROUP 2B IMEMDT 7,56,87; Animal Sufficient Evidence IMEMDT 10,231,76; Animal Limited Evidence IMEMDT 1,169,72. Reported in EPA TSCA Inventory. EPA Genetic Toxicology Program.

SAFETY PROFILE: Suspected carcinogen with experimental carcinogenic data. Moderately toxic by ingestion and intraperitoneal routes. A skin irritant. When heated to decomposition it emits acrid smoke and irritating fumes.

DMI400   CAS: 2373-98-0
3,3'-DIHYDROXYBENZIDINE
mf: $C_{12}H_{12}N_2O_2$ mw: 216.26

SYNS: 6,6'-DIAMINO-m,m'-BIPHENOL ◇ 4,4'-DIAMINO-3,3'-BIPHENYLDIOL ◇ 3,3'-DIOXYBENZIDINE ◇ 3,3'-DWUOKSYBENZYDYNA (POLISH)

TOXICITY DATA with REFERENCE
CAR: mul-rat TDLo: 6900 mg/kg/43W-I   VOONAW 7(2),33,61
CAR: scu-mus TDLo: 1620 g/kg/45W-I   AICCA6 7,46,50
CAR: scu-rat TDLo: 5900 mg/kg/43W-I   VOONAW 7(2),33,61
NEO: orl-rat TDLo: 9950 mg/kg/52W-I   VOONAW 7(2),33,61
ETA: orl-mus TDLo: 11 g/kg/47W-I   VOONAW 7(2),33,61
ETA: scu-mus TD: 14 g/kg/43W-I   VOONAW 7(2),33,61
ETA: skn-mus TDLo: 5040 mg/kg/52W-I   VOONAW 7(2),33,61
MUT: pic-esc 100 mmol/L   MDMIAZ 31,11,79

SAFETY PROFILE: Suspected carcinogen with experimental carcinogenic, neoplastigenic, and tumorigenic data. Mutation data reported. When heated to decomposition it emits toxic fumes of NO_x.

DNB200   CAS: 53609-64-6
DI(2-HYDROXY-n-PROPYL)AMINE
mf: $C_6H_{14}N_2O_3$ mw: 162.22

SYNS: BHP ◇ N-BIS(2-HYDROXYPROPYL)NITROSAMINE ◇ 2,2'-BISHYDROXYPROPYLNITROSAMINE ◇ DHPN ◇ 2,2'-DIHYDROXY-DI-n-PROPYLNITROSOAMINE ◇ N,N-DI-(2-HYDROXYPROPYL)NITROSAMINE ◇ DIISOPROPANOLNITROSAMINE ◇ DIPN ◇ N-NITROSOBIS(2-HYDROXYPROPYL)AMINE ◇ N-NITROSO-N,N-DI(2-HYDROXYPROPYL)AMINE ◇ N-NITROSO-1,1'-IMINODI-2-PROPANOL ◇ 1,1'-NITROSOIMINODI-2-PROPANOL

TOXICITY DATA with REFERENCE
CAR: ipr-mus TDLo: 125 mg/kg   JTSCDR 10,315,85
CAR: ipr-rat TD: 2000 mg/kg   IAPUDO 41,611,82
CAR: ipr-rat TDLo: 3000 mg/kg   CALEDQ 6,115,79
CAR: orl-ham TDLo: 1875 mg/kg/15W-I   CNREA8 41,4715,81
CAR: orl-rat TDLo: 4600 mg/kg/42W-C   CRNGDP 5,167,84
CAR: orl-rbt TDLo: 29 g/kg/25W-C   CALEDQ 5,339,78
CAR: scu-gpg TDLo: 7500 mg/kg/30W-I   JNCIAM 58,387,77
CAR: scu-ham TD: 500 mg/kg   JCREA8 102,265,82
CAR: scu-ham TD: 2750 mg/kg/34W-I   ZEKBAI 90,141,77
CAR: scu-ham TD: 4125 mg/kg/33W-I   CANCAR 36,379,75
CAR: scu-ham TD: 4250 mg/kg/17W-I   CRNGDP 3,1021,82

CAR: scu-ham TD: 5250 mg/kg/15W-I   CRNGDP 7,801,86

CAR: scu-ham TDLo: 2375 mg/kg/19W-I   CANCAR 36,379,75

CAR: scu-mus TDLo: 6049 mg/kg/23W-I   CALEDQ 9,257,80

CAR: scu-rat TD: 3000 mg/kg   IGAYAY 107,248,78

CAR: scu-rat TD: 3560 mg/kg/20W-I   JNCIAM 58,361,77

CAR: scu-rat TD: 14000 mg/kg/20W-I   NAIZAM 32,670,81

CAR: scu-rat TDLo: 1400 mg/kg/2W-I   CTRRDO 63,1181,79

CAR: scu-uns TDLo: 20 g/kg/80W-I   JJIND8 65,835,80

CAR: skn-ham TDLo: 688 mg/kg/43W-I   CALEDQ 10,365,80

NEO: ipr-rat TD: 2800 mg/kg   JJIND8 72,471,84

NEO: orl-mus TDLo: 28 g/kg/16W-I   CALEDQ 3,255,77

NEO: scu-ham TDLo: 100 mg/kg (14D post): REP,TER   ZEKBAI 90,119,77

ETA: ims-mus TDLo: 125 mg/kg   IGSBAL 109,99,84

MUT: dns-rat: lvr 5 mmol/L   MUREAV 144,197,85

MUT: mma-sat 250 µg/plate   MUREAV 111,135,83

MUT: msc-ham: lng 700 µmol/L   CNREA8 40,3463,80

MUT: otr-hmn: oth 5 mg/L   BANRDU 12,15,82

SAFETY PROFILE: Suspected carcinogen with experimental carcinogenic, neoplastigenic, tumorigenic, and teratogenic data. Moderately toxic by subcutaneous route. Experimental reproductive effects. Human mutation data reported. When heated to decomposition it emits toxic fumes of NO_x.

DNX500   CAS: 8015-19-8
DIMETHISTERONE and ETHINYL ESTRADIOL
mf: $C_{23}H_{32}O_2 \cdot C_{20}H_{24}O_2$ mw: 636.99

SYNS: ETHINYL ESTRADIOL and DIMETHISTERONE ◊ ORACON ◊ OVIN ◊ SECROVIN

TOXICITY DATA with REFERENCE
CAR: orl-wmn TDLo: 92 mg/kg/3Y-I   OBGNAS 47,639,76

CAR: orl-wmn TDLo: 244 mg/kg/8Y-I   AJOGAH 123,299,75

SAFETY PROFILE: Suspected human carcinogen producing uterine tumors. Human reproductive effects by ingestion: abnormalities of the uterus, cervix, and vagina. A steroid. When

heated to decomposition it emits acrid smoke and irritating fumes.

DOA800   CAS: 20325-40-0
3,3'-DIMETHOXYBENZIDINE DIHYDROCHLORIDE
mf: $C_{14}H_{16}N_2O_2 \cdot 2ClH$ mw: 317.24

SYNS: C.I. DISPERSE BLACK-6-DIHYDROCHLORIDE ◊ o-DIANISIDINE DIHYDROCHLORIDE ◊ 3,3-DIMETHOXY-(1,1'-BIPHENYL)-4,4'-DIAMINE DIHYDROCHLORIDE

TOXICITY DATA with REFERENCE
CAR: orl-rat TDLo: 1040 mg/kg/1Y-I   JNCIAM 41,985,68

CAR: orl-rat TD: 11 g/kg/51W-I   JNCIAM 41,985,68

ETA: orl-mus TDLo: 5760 mg/kg/2Y-I   VOONAW 25(7),43,79

ETA: scu-mus TDLo: 1152 mg/kg/2Y-I   VOONAW 25(7),43,79

MUT: mma-sat 100 nmol/plate   MUREAV 136,33,84

MUT: mmo-sat 100 nmol/plate   MUREAV 136,33,84

CONSENSUS REPORTS: Reported in EPA TSCA Inventory.

NIOSH REL: (Benzidine-Based Dye) Reduce to lowest feasible level

SAFETY PROFILE: Questionable carcinogen with experimental carcinogenic and tumorigenic data. Mutation data reported. When heated to decomposition it emits very toxic fumes of NO_x and HCl.

DOK200   CAS: 6358-53-8
1-((2,5-DIMETHOXYPHENYL)AZO)-2-NAPHTHOL
mf: $C_{18}H_{16}N_2O_3$ mw: 308.36

PROP: Mp: 156°. Sltly water-sol; mod sol in alc.

SYNS: C.I. 12156 ◊ C.I. SOLVENT RED 80 ◊ CITRUS RED NO. 2 ◊ 2,5-DIMETHOXYBENZENEAZO-β-NAPHTHOL ◊ 1-((2,5-DIMETHOXYPHENYL)AZO)-2-NAPHTHALENOL ◊ 2,5-DIMETHOXY-1-(PHENYLAZO)-2-NAPHTHOL ◊ 1-(1-(2,5-DIMETHOXYPHENYL)AZO)-2-NAPHTHOL ◊ 1-(2,5-DIMETHYLOXYPHENYLAZO)-2-NAPHTHOL

TOXICITY DATA with REFERENCE
CAR: imp-mus TDLo: 80 mg/kg   BJCAAI 22,825,68

CAR: scu-mus TDLo: 20 g/kg/80W-C   FCTXAV 4,493,66

MUT: mmo-sat 500 µg/plate   MUREAV 56,249,78

CONSENSUS REPORTS: IARC Cancer Review: GROUP 2B IMEMDT 7,56,87; Animal

Sufficient Evidence IMEMDT 8,101,75. EPA Genetic Toxicology Program.

SAFETY PROFILE: Suspected carcinogen with experimental carcinogenic data. Mutation data reported. When heated to decomposition it emits toxic fumes of NO_x.

DON400 CAS: 23435-31-6
2′,5′-DIMETHOXYSTILBENAMINE
mf: $C_{16}H_{17}NO_2$ mw: 255.34

SYNS: (trans)-2,5-DIMETHOXY-4′-AMINOSTILBENE ◇ 4-(2,5-DIMETHOXYPHENETHYL)ANILINE ◇ 4-(2-(2,5-DIMETHOXYPHENYL)ETHYL)BENZENAMINE ◇ 4-(2,5-DIMETHOXY)STILBENAMINE ◇ 2,5-DIMETHOXY-4′-STILBENAMINE

TOXICITY DATA with REFERENCE
CAR: orl-mus TDLo: 130 g/kg/78W-C JEPTDQ 2,325,78
CAR: orl-rat TD: 4725 mg/kg/78W-C JEPTDQ 2,325,78
CAR: orl-rat TDLo: 2360 mg/kg/78W-C JEPTDQ 2,325,78

SAFETY PROFILE: Suspected carcinogen with experimental carcinogenic data. When heated to decomposition it emits toxic fumes of NO_x.

DPL000 CAS: 55738-54-0
trans-2-((DIMETHYLAMINO)METHYLIMINO)-5-(2-(5-NITRO-2-FURYL)VINYL)-1,3,4-OXADIAZOLE
mf: $C_{11}H_{12}N_5O_4$ mw: 277.27

TOXICITY DATA with REFERENCE
CAR: orl-rat TD: 42 g/kg/46W-C JNCIAM 54,841,75
CAR: orl-rat TDLo: 42 g/kg/46W-I JNCIAM 51,403,73
MUT: mma-sat 100 ng/plate MUREAV 40,9,76

CONSENSUS REPORTS: IARC Cancer Review: Animal Limited Evidence IMEMDT 7,147,74. EPA Genetic Toxicology Program.

SAFETY PROFILE: Suspected carcinogen with experimental carcinogenic data. Mutation data reported. When heated to decomposition it emits toxic fumes of NO_x.

DQD400 CAS: 1596-84-5
DIMETHYLAMINOSUCCINAMIC ACID
mf: $C_6H_{12}N_2O_3$ mw: 160.20

SYNS: ALAR ◇ ALAR-85 ◇ AMINOZIDE ◇ B 995 ◇ BERNSTEINSAEURE-2,2-DIMETHYLHYDRAZID (GER-MAN) ◇ B-NINE ◇ BUTANEDIOIC ACID MONO(2,2-DIMETHYLHYDRAZIDE) ◇ DAMINOZIDE (USDA) ◇ DIMAS ◇ N-DIMETHYL AMINO-β-CARBAMYL PROPIONIC ACID ◇ N-(DIMETHYLAMINO)SUCCINAMIC ACID ◇ N-DIMETHYLAMINO-SUCCINAMIDSAEURE (GERMAN) ◇ DMASA ◇ DMSA ◇ KYLAR ◇ NCI-C03827 ◇ SADH ◇ SUCCINIC ACID-2,2-DIMETHYLHYDRAZIDE ◇ SUCCINIC-1,1-DIMETHYL HYDRAZIDE

TOXICITY DATA with REFERENCE
CAR: orl-mus TDLo: 2600 g/kg/62W-C CNREA8 37,3497,77
CAR: orl-rat TDLo: 182 g/kg/2Y-C: TER NCITR* NCI-CG-TR-83,78
ETA: orl-mus TD: 873 g/kg/2Y-C NCITR* NCI-CG-TR-83,78

CONSENSUS REPORTS: EPA Genetic Toxicology Program. NCI Carcinogenesis Bioassay (feed); Clear Evidence: mouse, rat NCITR* NCI-CG-TR-83,78.

SAFETY PROFILE: Suspected carcinogen with experimental carcinogenic, tumorigenic, and teratogenic data. Poison by intraperitoneal route. Moderately toxic by ingestion and possibly other routes. When heated to decomposition it emits toxic fumes of NO_x.

DQJ200 CAS: 57-97-6
DIMETHYLBENZANTHRACENE
mf: $C_{20}H_{16}$ mw: 256.36

SYNS: DBA ◇ DIMETHYLBENZ(a)ANTHRACENE ◇ 7,12-DIMETHYLBENZANTHRACENE ◇ 7,12-DIMETHYL-BENZ(a)ANTHRACENE ◇ 9,10-DIMETHYL-BENZANTHRACENE ◇ 9,10-DIMETHYLBENZ(a)ANTHRACENE ◇ 9,10-DIMETHYL-1,2-BENZANTHRACENE ◇ 9,10-DIMETHYL-1,2-BENZANTHRAZEN (GERMAN) ◇ DIMETHYLBENZANTHRENE ◇ 7,12-DIMETHYLBENZO(a)ANTHRACENE ◇ 1,4-DIMETHYL-2,3-BENZPHENANTHRENE ◇ DMBA ◇ 7,12-DMBA ◇ NCI-C03918 ◇ RCRA WASTE NUMBER U094

TOXICITY DATA with REFERENCE
CAR: imp-rat TD: 5 mg/kg NGGZAK 85,555,84
CAR: ims-rat TDLo: 2400 μg/kg NTIS** DOE/EV/03140-5
CAR: itr-mus TDLo: 4 mg/kg AJCAA7 35,538,39
CAR: ivg-mus TDLo: 40 mg/kg (19D preg): TER VOONAW 22(6),44,76
CAR: ivg-mus TDLo: 744 mg/kg/31W-I: TER BJCAAI 20,184,66
CAR: ivn-mus TDLo: 4800 mg/kg/24W-I APJAAG 31,799,81
CAR: orl-mus TD: 60 mg/kg/2W-I JTEHD6 10,131,82

CAR: orl-rat TD:10 mg/kg   CNREA8 45,4827,85
CAR: orl-rat TD:15 mg/kg   BCTRD6 4,129,84
CAR: orl-rat TD:150 mg/kg   IJCNAW 26,349,80
CAR: orl-rat TD:37500 μg/kg   CRNGDP 5,1539,84
CAR: orl-rat TDLo:15 mg/kg   LIFSAK 7,259,68
CAR: orl-rat TDLo:37500 μg/kg (14-20D preg):TER   CCSUDL 3,413,78
CAR: scu-ham TDLo:400 μg/kg   BJCAAI 21,184,67
CAR: scu-rat TDLo:500 μg/kg   CRNGDP 6,769,85
CAR: skn-ham TDLo:1600 μg/kg   PEXTAR 26,128,83
CAR: skn-mky TDLo:1600 mg/kg/65W-I   JNCIAM 57,1269,76
NEO: ims-ckn TDLo:125 mg/kg/2W-I   BJCAAI 41,130,80
NEO: ivn-mus TDLo:120 mg/kg (18-20D preg):TER   VOONAW 20(8),65,74
NEO: ivn-rat TD:30 mg/kg/7D-I   ACLSCP 13,289,83
NEO: ivn-rat TDLo:30 mg/kg   KIDZAK 23(Suppl 1),34,71
NEO: ivn-rbt TDLO:20 mg/kg (25D preg): TER   BEXBAN 85,369,78
NEO: mul-ham TDLo:272g/kg/18W-I   AEMBAP 91,57,77
NEO: orl-ham TDLo:80 mg/kg   PEXTAR 26,128,83
NEO: scu-mus TD:1880 μg/kg/47W-I   JNCIAM 37,825,66
NEO: scu-mus TDLo:60 mg/kg (13-17D preg):TER   LIFSAK 26,1955,80
NEO: scu-mus TDLo:833 μg/kg   BJCAAI 20,148,66
NEO: scu-rat TD:13 mg/kg   EJCAAH 6,417,70
NEO: scu-rat TD:20 mg/kg/39D-I   CNREA8 31,1951,71
ETA: imp-dog TDLo:378mg/kg/52W-C   JJIND8 65,921,80
ETA: imp-gpg TDLo:100 mg/kg   COREAF 252,1236,61
ETA: imp-mus TDLo:40mg/kg   OSOMAE 48,47,79
ETA: imp-rat TDLo:11 μg/kg:TER   NISFAY 34,1853,82
ETA: ims-grb TDLo:350 μg/kg/7W-I   CNREA8 26,844,66
ETA: ims-ham TDLo:12500 μg/kg   CMBID4 24,127,79
ETA: ipc-rat TDLo:1250 μg/kg:TER   GANNA2 62,55,71
ETA: ipr-mus TDLo:112 mg/kg (14-21D preg):TER   IJCNAW 4,219,69
ETA: ipr-rat TDLo:24 mg/kg (20D preg):TER   CCSUDL 3,413,78
ETA: ipr-rat TDLo:25 mg/kg   CNREA8 39,3968,79

ETA: itr-dog TDLo:11 mg/kg/53W-I   JTCSAQ 49,364,65
ETA: itr-ham TDLo:5200 μg/kg/13W-I   EJCAAH 10,483,74
ETA: ivn-ham TDLo:24 mg/kg/13W-I:TER   INURAQ 15,42,77
ETA: ivn-rat TDLo:15 mg/kg (21D preg):TER   JNCIAM 52,1365,74
ETA: ivn-rat TDLo:15 mg/kg (21D preg):TER   NEOLA4 23,285,76
ETA: par-dog TDLo:1235 mg/kg/52W-I   JJIND8 65,921,80
ETA: par-rbt TDLo:40 mg/kg/16W-I   AOUNAZ 102,111,83
ETA: scu-gpg TDLo:20 mg/kg/9W-I   COREAF 252,1236,61
ETA: skn-gpg TDLo:240 mg/kg/20W-I   PGTCA4 5,120,79
ETA: skn-grb TDLo:70 mg/kg/7W-I   CNREA8 26,844,66
ETA: skn-rat TDLo:60 mg/kg/30W-I   JCUPBN 7,277,80
ETA: skn-rbt TDLo:7 mg/kg/8W-I   ONCOAR 15,98,62
MUT: dnd-hmn:emb 220 nmol/L   MUREAV 89,95,81
MUT: dni-hmn:hla 44 μmol/L   MUREAV 92,427,82
MUT: dni-hmn:lvr 1 mmol/L   VOONAW 28(11),53,82
MUT: otr-mus:emb 300 μg/L   PMRSDJ 5,659,85
MUT: sce-mus:mmr 7800 nmol/L   MUREAV 147,165,85
MUT: skn-mus 64 μg MLD   CALEDQ 4,333,78

CONSENSUS REPORTS: Reported in EPA TSCA Inventory. EPA Genetic Toxicology Program.

SAFETY PROFILE: Suspected carcinogen with experimental carcinogenic, neoplastigenic, tumorigenic, and teratogenic data. A transplacental carcinogen. Poison by ingestion, intravenous, subcutaneous, intraperitoneal and intratracheal routes. Other experimental reproductive effects. Human mutation data reported. A skin irritant. When heated to decomposition it emits acrid smoke and irritating fumes.

DSF800   CAS: 306-37-6
1,2-DIMETHYLHYDRAZINE DIHYDROCHLORIDE
mf: $C_2H_8N_2 \cdot 2ClH$ mw: 133.04

SYNS: N,N'-DIMETHYLHYDRAZINE DIHYDROCHLORIDE ◇ sym-DIMETHYLHYDRAZINE DIHYDROCHLORIDE ◇ DMH

TOXICITY DATA with REFERENCE

CAR: ipr-rat TDLo: 160 mg/kg/16W-I   NUCADQ
4,146,82

CAR: orl-gpg TDLo: 2190 mg/kg/73W-I
TXAPA9 38,647,76

CAR: orl-mus TD: 284 mg/kg/40W-C   TJXMAH
27,5,80

CAR: orl-mus TD: 672 mg/kg/48W-C   VAPHDQ
384,263,79

CAR: orl-mus TD: 720 mg/kg/24W-I   VAPHDQ
384,263,79

CAR: orl-mus TDLo: 23 mg/kg/2Y-C   ANTRD4
2,365,82

CAR: orl-rat TD: 75 mg/kg/5W-I   CNREA8
43,4083,83

CAR: orl-rat TDLo: 35 mg/kg   CALEDQ 14,47,81

CAR: orl-rat TDLo: 150 mg/kg/10W-I   TXAPA9
55,417,80

CAR: scu-mus TD: 400 mg/kg/20W-I   FCTXAV
19,281,81

CAR: scu-mus TD: 480 mg/kg/16W-I   VAPHDQ
384,263,79

CAR: scu-mus TDLo: 150 mg/kg/10W-I
CALEDQ 9,111,80

CAR: scu-rat TD: 240 mg/kg/16W-I   JSGRA2
29,363,80

CAR: scu-rat TD: 400 mg/kg/22W-I   JJIND8
64,263,80

CAR: scu-rat TD: 500 mg/kg/20W-I   APLMAS
105,29,81

CAR: scu-rat TDLo: 200 mg/kg/20W-I   PSEBAA
151,237,76

NEO: olr-ham TDLo: 446 mg/kg/51W-C
CNREA8 32,804,72

ETA: ipr-mus TDLo: 212 mg/kg/8W-I   JNCIAM
42,337,69

ETA: par-mus TDLo: 133 mg/kg/6W-I   CALEDQ
8,23,79

ETA: scu-gpg TDL0: 2040 mg/kg/34W-I
TXAPA9 38,647,76

MUT: dnd-rat-orl 1700 μg/kg/2D-C   CRNGDP
4,529,83

MUT: dni-mus: oth 500 μmol/L   JJIND8 68,1015,82

MUT: dni-rat-orl 1700 μg/kg/2D-C   CRNGDP
4,529,83

MUT: dns-rat-orl 1700 μg/kg/4D-C   CRNGDP
4,529,83

MUT: otr-rat-ipr 100 mg/kg   CALEDQ 26,191,82

CONSENSUS REPORTS: Reported in EPA
TSCA Inventory. EPA Genetic Toxicology Program.

SAFETY PROFILE: Suspected carcinogen with
experimental carcinogenic, neoplastigenic, and tumorigenic data. Poison by ingestion and subcutaneous routes. Experimental reproductive effects. Mutation data reported. A rocket fuel. When heated to decomposition it emits very toxic fumes of HCl and NO_x.

DSG400   CAS: 26049-69-4
2-(2,2-DIMETHYLHYDRAZINO)-4-(5-NITRO-2-FURYL)THIAZOLE
mf: $C_9H_{10}N_4O_3S$ mw: 254.29

SYN: DMNT

TOXICITY DATA with REFERENCE

CAR: orl-mus TDLo: 15 g/kg/17W-C   CNREA8
33,1593,73

CAR: orl-rat TD: 31 g/kg/44W-C   PAACA3
10,15,69

CAR: orl-rat TDLo: 4800 mg/kg/46W-I   CNREA8
30,897,70

MUT: dnr-sat 500 nmol/well   CNREA8 34,2266,74

MUT: mma-sat 100 ng/plate   MUREAV 40,9,76

MUT: mmo-esc 300 nmol/well   CNREA8 34,2266,74

MUT: mrc-esc 500 nmol/well   CNREA8 34,2266,74

MUT: pic-esc 1 mg/L   MUREAV 26,3,74

CONSENSUS REPORTS: EPA Genetic Toxicology Program.

SAFETY PROFILE: Suspected carcinogen with
experimental carcinogenic data. Mutation data reported. When heated to decomposition it emits very toxic fumes of NO_x and SO_x.

DTA000   CAS: 1456-28-6
2,6-DIMETHYLNITROSOMORPHOLINE
mf: $C_6H_{12}N_2O_2$ mw: 144.20

SYNS: DIMETHYLNITROSOMORPHOLINE ◇ 2,6-DIMETHYL-N-NITROSOMORPHOLINE ◇ DMNM ◇ Me2NMOR ◇ NITROSO-2,6-DIMETHYLMORPHOLINE ◇ N-NITROSO-2,6-DIMETHYLMORPHOLINE

TOXICITY DATA with REFERENCE

CAR: orl-gpg TD: 400 mg/kg/23W-I   JJIND8
64,529,80

CAR: orl-gpg TDLo: 960 mg/kg/12W-I   CNREA8
40,1879,80

CAR: orl-ham TD: 937 mg/kg/51W-I   JNCIAM
58,429,77

CAR: orl-ham TDLo: 819 mg/kg/45W-I
JNCIAM 60,371,78

CAR: scu-ham TDLo: 2040 mg/kg/24W-I
JCROD7 109,183,85

CAR: scu-rat TDLo: 1684 mg/kg/18W-I
CALEDQ 13,159,81

NEO: orl-ham TD: 1073 mg/kg/29W-I   JCROD7
109,183,85

NEO: scu-ham TD: 1200 mg/kg/15W-I   PAACA3 24,62,83

NEO: scu-rat TD: 1198 mg/kg/20W-I   CALEDQ 13,159,81

ETA: orl-ham TD: 644 mg/kg/35W-I   VTPHAK 17,352,80

ETA: orl-rat TD: 300 mg/kg/30W-I   CALEDQ 10,325,80

ETA: orl-rat TD: 300 mg/kg/30W-I   CRNGDP 1,501,80

ETA: orl-rat TD: 400 mg/kg/5W-I   CALEDQ 16,281,82

ETA: orl-rat TD: 2025 mg/kg/30W-I   CNREA8 35,2123,75

ETA: orl-rat TDLo: 135 mg/kg/30W-I   ZKKOBW 92,221,78

MUT: dns-rat: lvr 1 mmol/L   MUREAV 144,197,85

MUT: mma-sat 50 nmol/plate   MUREAV 57,1,78

MUT: mmo-sat 1 mg/plate   TCMUD8 1,295,80

CONSENSUS REPORTS: EPA Genetic Toxicology Program.

SAFETY PROFILE: Suspected carcinogen with experimental carcinogenic, tumorigenic, and neoplastigenic data. Poison by ingestion and subcutaneous routes. Mutation data reported. Used as a model carcinogenic and carcinogenic metabolite. When heated to decomposition it emits toxic fumes of NO_x.

DTB200   CAS: 13256-32-1
1,3-DIMETHYLNITROSOUREA
mf: $C_3H_7N_3O_2$ mw: 117.13

SYNS: DIMETHYLNITROSOHARNSTOFF (GERMAN) ◇ N,N'-DIMETHYLNITROSOUREA ◇ 1,3-DIMETHYL-N-NITROSOUREA ◇ NITROSODIMETHYLUREA ◇ N-NITROSODIMETHYLUREA

TOXICITY DATA with REFERENCE

CAR: scu-ham TDLo: 680 mg/kg/17W-I   AMOKAG 28,333,74

CAR: scu-mus TDLo: 720 mg/kg/9W-I   GANNA2 62,135,71

NEO: scu-rat TDLo: 836 mg/kg/20W-I   AMOKAG 32,119,78

ETA: ivn-rat TDLo: 660 mg/kg/66W-I   ZEKBAI 69,103,67

ETA: orl-rat TDLo: 1300 mg/kg/65W-C   ZEKBAI 69,103,67

MUT: dni-mus-ipr 80 mg/kg   INSSDM 19,85,81

MUT: dni-mus/oth 80 mg/kg   INSSDM 19,85,81

MUT: hma-mus/sat 150 mg/kg   ARZNAD 23,746,73

MUT: mmo-omi 1 pph   ANTBAL 27,738,82

MUT: mmo-omi 500 ppm   ANTBAL 21,501,76

MUT: mmo-omi 500 ppm   ANTBAL 21,501,76

MUT: mmo-sat 1400 μmol/L/48H   MUREAV 48,131,77

CONSENSUS REPORTS: EPA Genetic Toxicology Program.

SAFETY PROFILE: Suspected carcinogen with experimental carcinogenic, neoplastigenic, tumorigenic, and teratogenic data. Poison by ingestion and intravenous routes. Experimental reproductive effects. Mutation data reported. When heated to decomposition it emits toxic fumes of NO_x.

DUQ180   CAS: 25154-54-5
DINITROBENZENE
DOT: 1597
mf: $C_6H_4N_2O_4$ mw: 168.12

SYNS: DINITROBENZENE, solution (DOT) ◇ DINITROBENZOL solid (DOT)

OSHA PEL: TWA 1 mg/m³ (skin)   ACGIH TLV: TWA 0.15 ppm (skin)   DFG MAK: 0.15 ppm (1 mg/m³); Suspected Carcinogen   DOT Classification: Poison B; Label: Poison, Solid and Solution.

SAFETY PROFILE: Suspected carcinogen. A poison. When heated to decomposition it emits toxic fumes of NO_x.

DUQ200   CAS: 99-65-0
m-DINITROBENZENE
DOT: 1597
mf: $C_6H_4N_2O_4$ mw: 168.12

PROP: Yellowish crystals. Mp: 89°, bp: 301°.

SYNS: BINITROBENZENE ◇ 1,3-DINITROBENZENE ◇ 2,4-DINITROBENZENE ◇ 1,3-DINITROBENZOL ◇ DWUNITROBENZEN (POLISH)

TOXICITY DATA with REFERENCE

MUT: mma-sat 100 nmol/plate   MUREAV 58,11,78

MUT: mmo-sat 3300 ng/plate   ENMUDM 2,531,80

CONSENSUS REPORTS: Reported in EPA TSCA Inventory. EPA Genetic Toxicology Program.

OSHA PEL: TWA 1 mg/m³ (skin)   ACGIH TLV: TWA 0.15 ppm (skin)   DFG MAK: 0.15 ppm (1 mg/m³); Suspected Carcinogen   DOT Classification: Poison B; Label: Poison.

SAFETY PROFILE: Suspected carcinogen. Human poison by ingestion. Experimental poison by ingestion, intraperitoneal and intravenous routes. Human systemic effects by skin contact: cyanosis and motor activity changes. Experi mental reproductive effects. Mutation data reported. Mixture with nitric acid is a high explosive. Mixture with tetranitromethane is a high explosive very sensitive to sparks. When heated to decomposition it emits toxic fumes of NO_x.

DUQ400   CAS: 528-29-0
o-DINITROBENZENE
DOT: 1597
mf: $C_6H_4N_2O_4$ mw: 168.12

PROP: Colorless needles or plates. Mp: 118°, bp: 319°, flash p: 302°F (CC), d: 1.571 @ 0°/4°, vap d: 5.79.

SYN: 1,2-DINITROBENZENE

OSHA PEL: TWA 1 mg/m³ (skin) ACGIH TLV: TWA 0.15 ppm (skin) DFG MAK: 0.15 ppm (1 mg/m³); Suspected Carcinogen DOT Classification: Poison B; Label: Poison.

SAFETY PROFILE: Suspected carcinogen. Poison by inhalation and ingestion. Moderately toxic by skin contact. Can cause liver, kidney, and central nervous system injury. A severe explosion hazard when shocked or exposed to heat or flame. It is used in bursting charges and to fill artillery shells. To fight fire, use water, CO_2, dry chemical. Dangerous; when heated to decomposition it emits highly toxic fumes of NO_x and explodes.

DUQ600   CAS: 100-25-4
p-DINITROBENZENE
DOT: 1597
mf: $C_6H_4N_2O_4$ mw: 168.12

PROP: White crystals. Mp: 173°, bp: 299°. Volatile with steam.

SYN: DITHANE A-4

TOXICITY DATA with REFERENCE
MUT: mma-sat 25 μg/plate CRNGDP 6,727,85
MUT: mmo-sat 5 μg/plate CRNGDP 6,727,85

CONSENSUS REPORTS: Reported in EPA TSCA Inventory.

OSHA PEL: TWA 1 mg/m³ (skin) ACGIH TLV: TWA 0.15 ppm (skin) DFG MAK: 0.15 ppm (1 mg/m³); Suspected Carcinogen DOT Classification: Poison B; Label: Poison.

SAFETY PROFILE: Suspected carcinogen. Poison by ingestion. Mutation data reported. Mixture with nitric acid is a high explosive. When heated to decomposition it emits toxic fumes of NO_x.

DVD400   CAS: 75321-20-9
1,3-DINITROPYRENE
mf: $C_{16}H_8N_2O_4$ mw: 292.26

TOXICITY DATA with REFERENCE
CAR: ipr-rat TDLo: 23 mg/kg/4W-I DTESD7 13,279,86
CAR: scu-rat TDLo: 16 mg/kg/10W-I CRNGDP 5,583,84
MUT: mmo-esc 80 ng/plate MUREAV 142,163,85
MUT: mmo-sat 1 nmol/plate SCIEAS 209,1039,80
MUT: msc-ham: lng 2500 μg/L CRNGDP 3,917,82
MUT: msc-ham: ovr 500 μg/L MUREAV 119,387,83

DFG MAK: Suspected Carcinogen.

SAFETY PROFILE: Suspected carcinogen with experimental carcinogenic data. Mutation data reported. When heated to decomposition it emits toxic fumes of NO_x.

DVD600   CAS: 42397-64-8
1,6-DINITROPYRENE
mf: $C_{16}H_8N_2O_4$ mw: 292.26

TOXICITY DATA with REFERENCE
CAR: ipl-rat TDLo: 600 μg/kg JJIND8 76,693,86
CAR: ipr-rat TDLo: 23 mg/kg/4W-I DTESD7 13,279,86
CAR: itr-ham TDLo: 104 mg/kg/26W-I JJCREP 76,457,85
CAR: scu-mus TDLo: 80 mg/kg/20W-I DTESD7 13,253,86
CAR: scu-rat TD: 16 mg/kg/10W-I CALEDQ 25,239,85
CAR: scu-rat TDLo: 9206 μg/kg/8W-I DTESD7 13,279,86
MUT: dns-hmn: lvr 80 nmol/L ENMUDM 5,488,83
MUT: dns-hmn: oth 500 nmol/L TXAPA9 79,28,85
MUT: mma-smc 2900 ng/L PCBRD2 109,249,82
MUT: mmo-esc 5 ng/plate JJIND8 73,1359,84
MUT: mmo-sat 600 pg/plate JJIND8 73,1359,84
MUT: mrc-smc 1400 ng/L PCBRD2 109,249,82

DFG MAK: Suspected Carcinogen.

SAFETY PROFILE: Suspected carcinogen with experimental carcinogenic data. Human mutation data reported. When heated to decomposition it emits toxic fumes of NO_x.

DVD800   CAS: 42397-65-9
1,8-DINITROPYRENE
mf: $C_{16}H_8N_2O_4$ mw: 292.26

TOXICITY DATA with REFERENCE
CAR: ipr-rat TDLo: 23 mg/kg/4W-I DTESD7 13,279,86

CAR: scu-mus TD:40 mg/kg/20W-I   JJIND8
79,185,87
CAR: scu-mus TDLo:40 mg/kg/20W-I   DTESD7
13,253,86
CAR: scu-rat TD:160 µg/kg/10W-I   CALEDQ
25,239,85
CAR: scu-rat TDLo:16 mg/kg/10W-I   CRNGDP
5,583,84
MUT: mma-sat 1 µg/plate   MUREAV 91,321,81
MUT: mmo-sat 1 nmol/plate   SCIEAS 209,1039,80
MUT: msc-hmn:lym 100 µg/L   ENMUDM5,457,83
MUT: msc-mus:lym 500 µg/L   EVSRBT 25,397,82

DFG MAK: Suspected Carcinogen.

SAFETY PROFILE: Suspected carcinogen with experimental carcinogenic data. Human mutation data reported. When heated to decomposition it emits toxic fumes of NO_x.

DVF200   CAS: 140-79-4
DINITROSOPIPERAZINE
mf: $C_4H_8N_4O_2$ mw: 144.16

PROP: White crystals. Mp: 158°, vap d: 4.97.

SYNS: DINITROSOPIPERAZIN (GERMAN) ◇ N,N'-DINI-
TROSOPIPERAZINE ◇ 1,4-DINITROSOPIPERAZINE
◇ DNPZ ◇ NSC 339 ◇ USAF DO-36

TOXICITY DATA with REFERENCE
CAR: orl-rat TDLo:1040 mg/kg/1Y-I   JNCIAM
41,985,68
NEO: orl-mus TD:7300 mg/kg/52W-C   CNREA8
40,2925,80
NEO: orl-mus TDLo:1568 mg/kg/28W-C
JNCIAM 46,1029,71
ETA: orl-mus TD:5280 mg/kg/44W-I   VOONAW
15(6),104,69
ETA: orl-rat TD:300 mg/kg/50W-I   CNREA8
26,619,66
ETA: orl-rat TD:560 mg/kg/10W-C   CNREA8
42,4236,82
ETA: orl-rat TD:1120 mg/kg/20W-C   CNREA8
42,4236,82
ETA: orl-rat TD:1680 mg/kg/30W-C   CNREA8
42,4236,82
ETA: orl-rat TD:1800 mg/kg/64W-C   ARZNAD
19,1077,69
ETA: orl-rat TD:2250 mg/kg/50W-I   ZKKOBW
77,257,72
ETA: scu-mus TDLo:720 mg/kg/72W-I
VOONAW 15(6),104,69
ETA: scu-rat TD:1086 mg/kg/69W-I   ZEKBAI
66,138,64

ETA: scu-rat TD:1100 mg/kg/110W-I   ARZNAD
19,1077,69
ETA: scu-rat TDLo:1070 mg/kg/53W-I   ZEKBAI
69,103,67
MUT: cyt-mus-ipr 50 mg/kg   MUREAV 46,220,77
MUT: dnd-rat-ipr 50 mg/kg   CNREA8 33,3209,73
MUT: hma-mus/sat 10 mg/kg   CNREA8 37,4572,77
MUT: mma-esc 16700 µmol/L   CNREA836,4099,76
MUT: mma-sat 50 nmol/plate   MUREAV 57,1,78
MUT: mma-smc 50 µmol/plate   MUREAV77,143,80
MUT: sce-hmn:lym 10 mmol/L   TCMUE91,129,84

CONSENSUS REPORTS: EPA Genetic Toxicology Program. Reported in EPA TSCA Inventory.

SAFETY PROFILE: Suspected carcinogen with experimental carcinogenic, neoplastigenic, tumorigenic, and teratogenic data. Poison by ingestion, subcutaneous, and intraperitoneal routes. Experimental reproductive effects. Human mutation data reported. When heated to decomposition it emits toxic fumes of NO_x.

DVH000   CAS: 121-14-2
2,4-DINITROTOLUENE
mf: $C_7H_6N_2O_4$ mw: 182.15

PROP: Yellow needles. Mp: 69.5°, bp: 300°, d: 1.521 @ 15°, vap d: 6.27, flash p: 404°F.

SYNS: 2,4-DINITROTOLUOL ◇ DNT ◇ 2,4-DNT
◇ 1-METHYL-2,4-DINITROBENZENE ◇ NCI-C01865
◇ RCRA WASTE NUMBER U105

TOXICITY DATA with REFERENCE
CAR: orl-mus TDLo:10080 mg/kg/2Y-C
JACTDZ 4(4),257,85
CAR: orl-rat TD:28 g/kg/2Y-C   NTIS** AD-A080-
146
NEO: orl-mus TDLo:8760 mg/kg/2Y-C   NTIS**
AD-A080-146
NEO: orl-rat TD:5460 mg/kg/78W-C   NCITR*
NCI-CG-TR-54,78
NEO: orl-rat TDLo:2620 mg/kg/78W-C
NCITR* NCI-CG-TR-54,78
ETA: orl-rat TD:12775 mg/kg/2Y-C   NCITR*
NCI-CG-TR-54,78
MUT: cyt-mus-orl 840 µg/kg   MUREAV 38,387,76
MUT: dlt-mus-orl 2 mg/kg   MUREAV 38,387,76
MUT: dnd-rat:lvr 3 mmol/L   SinJF# 260CT82
MUT: mma-sat 125 µg/plate   ENMUDM 7(Suppl
5),1,85
MUT: mmo-sat 10 µg/plate   NTIS** AD-A080-146
MUT: oms-rat-orl 10 mg/kg   JTEHD6 11,555,83

CONSENSUS REPORTS: NCI Carcinogenesis Bioassay (feed); No Evidence: mouse NCITR* NCI-CG-TR-54,78; Some Evidence: rat NCITR* NCI-CG-TR-54,78. Reported in EPA TSCA Inventory.

OSHA PEL: TWA 1.5 mg/m^3 (skin) ACGIH TLV: TWA 1.5 mg/m^3 (skin) NIOSH REL: (Dinitrotoluene): Reduce to lowest level

SAFETY PROFILE: Suspected carcinogen with experimental carcinogenic and neoplastigenic data. Poison by ingestion and subcutaneous routes. Experimental reproductive effects. Mutation data reported. An irritant and an allergen. Can cause anemia, methemoglobinemia, cyanosis, and liver damage. Combustible when exposed to heat or flame; can react with oxidizing materials. To fight fire, use water spray or mist, dry chemical. When heated to decomposition it emits toxic fumes of NO$_x$.

DWW700   CAS: 67730-10-3
DIPYRIDO(1,2-a:3′,2′-d)IMIDAZOL-2-AMINE
mf: C$_{10}$H$_8$N$_4$ mw: 184.22

SYNS: 2-AMINODIPYRIDO(1,2-a:3′,2′-d)-IMIDAZOLE ◇ GLU-P-2

TOXICITY DATA with REFERENCE
CAR: orl-mus TD:23232 mg/kg/69W-C
  CRNGDP 5,815,84
CAR: orl-mus TD:24024 mg/kg/66W-C
  CRNGDP 5,815,84
CAR: orl-mus TDLo:23100 mg/kg/83W-C
  EVHPAZ 67,129,86
CAR: orl-rat TD:13 g/kg/2Y-C   EVHPAZ67,129,86
CAR: orl-rat TDLo:12500 mg/kg/2Y-C
  EVHPAZ 67,129,86
MUT: dnd-mus:lvr 200 μmol/L   JJCREP76,835,85
MUT: dns-rat:lvr 1 μmol/L   CALEDQ 20,283,83
MUT: mma-sat 100 ng/plate   MUREAV 136,23,84
MUT: pic-sat 10 μg/plate   MUREAV 110,243,83
MUT: sce-hmn:lym 10 μmol/L   MUREAV
  116,137,83

CONSENSUS REPORTS: IARC Cancer Review: GROUP 2B IMEMDT 7,56,87; Animal Sufficient Evidence IMEMDT 40,235,86

SAFETY PROFILE: Suspected carcinogen with experimental carcinogenic data. Human mutation data reported. When heated to decomposition it emits toxic fumes of NO$_x$.

EBR000   CAS: 96-09-3
1,2-EPOXYETHYLBENZENE
mf: C$_8$H$_8$O   mw: 120.16

PROP: Colorless liquid. Bp: 194.2, flash p: 165°F (OC), fp: −36.7°, d: 1.0469 @ 25°/4°, vap d: 4.14.

SYNS: EPOXYETHYLBENZENE (8CI) ◇ EPOXYSTYRENE ◇ α,β-EPOXYSTYRENE ◇ NCI-C54977 ◇ PHENETHYLENE OXIDE ◇ 1-PHENYL-1,2-EPOXYETHANE ◇ PHENYLETHYLENE OXIDE ◇ PHENYLOXIRANE ◇ 1-PHENYLOXIRANE ◇ 2-PHENYLOXIRANE ◇ STYRENE EPOXIDE ◇ STYRENE OXIDE ◇ STYRENE-7,8-OXIDE ◇ STYRYL OXIDE

TOXICITY DATA with REFERENCE
CAR: orl-rat TD:200 g/kg/2Y-C   JJIND8 77,471,86
CAR: orl-rat TD:52 g/kg/52W-I   MELAAD
  70,358,79
CAR: orl-rat TDLo:10 g/kg/52W-I   MELAAD
  70,358,79
CAR: orl-mus TDLo:273 g/kg/2Y-C   JJIND8
  77,471,86
ETA: skn-mus TDLo:74 g/kg/62W-I   JNCIAM
  31,41,63
ETA: unr-mus TDLo:96 mg/kg   RARSAM3,193,63
MUT: dni-hmn:hla 4400 μmol/L   MUREAV
  93,447,82
MUT: msc-ham:lng 2080 μmol/L/2H   CBINA8
  39,57,82
MUT: msc-mus:lym 13800 μg/L   MUREAV
  97,49,82
MUT: oms-mus:fbr 1 μmol/L   CRNGDP
  6,1367,85
MUT: sce-ham:lng 100 mg/L   CNREA8 44,3270,84

CONSENSUS REPORTS: IARC Cancer Review: GROUP 2B IMEMDT 7,345,87; Animal Sufficient Evidence IMEMDT 36,245,85; Animal Inadequate Evidence IMEMDT 19,275,79; IMEMDT 11,201,76. Reported in EPA TSCA Inventory. EPA Genetic Toxicology Program.

SAFETY PROFILE: Suspected carcinogen with experimental carcinogenic, tumorigenic, and teratogenic data. Moderately toxic by ingestion, inhalation, skin contact, and intraperitoneal routes. Experimental reproductive effects. Human mutation data reported. A skin and eye irritant. Flammable when exposed to heat, flame, or oxidizers; can react with oxidizing materials. To fight fire, use foam, CO$_2$, dry chemical. When heated to decomposition it emits acrid smoke and fumes.

EBW500 CAS: 1024-57-3
EPOXYHEPTACHLOR
mf: $C_{10}H_5Cl_7O$ mw: 389.30

SYNS: ENT 25,584 ◇ HCE ◇ HEPTACHLOR EPOXIDE
(USDA) ◇ 1,4,5,6,7,8,8-HEPTACHLORO-2,3-EPOXY-2,3,-
3a,4,7,7a-HEXAHYDRO-4,7-METHANOINDENE ◇ 1,4,5,-
6,7,8,8-HEPTACHLORO-2,3-EPOXY-3a,4,7,7a-TETRAHY-
DRO-4,7-METHANOINDAN ◇ 2,3,4,5,6,7,7-HEPTACHLORO-
1a,1b,5,5a,6,6a-HEXAHYDRO-2,5-METHANO-2H-
INDENO(1,2-b)OXIRENE ◇ VELSICOL 53-CS-17

TOXICITY DATA with REFERENCE
CAR: orl-mus TD:876 mg/kg/2Y-C   ECEBDI
    45,147,77
CAR: orl-mus TDLo:580 mg/kg/69W-C
    ARTODN 38,163,77
MUT: mma-hmn:fbr 10 μmol/L   MUREAV
    42,161,77

CONSENSUS REPORTS: IARC Cancer Re-
view: Human Inadequate Evidence IMEMDT
20,129,79;   Animal   Inadequate   Evidence
IMEMDT 5,173,74; Animal Limited Evidence
IMEMDT 20,129,79. EPA Genetic Toxicology
Program.

SAFETY PROFILE: Suspected carcinogen with
experimental carcinogenic data. Poison by ingestion and intravenous routes. Human mutation
data reported. When heated to decomposition
it emits toxic fumes of Cl^-.

EDS100 CAS: 979-32-8
ESTRADIOL-17-VALERATE
mf: $C_{24}H_{32}O_3$ mw: 368.56

SYNS: ALTADIOL ◇ DELADIOL ◇ DELAHORMONE UNI-
MATIC ◇ DELESTROGEN ◇ DELESTROGEN 4X ◇ DURA-
ESTRADIOL ◇ ESTRADIOL VALERATE ◇ ESTRADIOL 17-
β-VALERATE ◇ ESTRADIOL VALERIANATE ◇ (17-β)-ES-
TRA-1,3,5(10)-TRIENE-3,17-DIOL-17-PENTANOATE (9CI)
◇ ESTRAVEL ◇ FEMOGEX ◇ NEOFOLLIN ◇ PHARLON
◇ PROGYNON ◇ PROGYNON-DEPOT ◇ PROGYNOVA

TOXICITY DATA with REFERENCE
CAR: scu-mus TDLo:400 μg/kg/W-I   AVBIB9
    22/23,359,79
CAR: scu-rat TDLo:104 mg/kg/2Y-I   CRNGDP
    5,1003,84

SAFETY PROFILE: Suspected carcinogen with
carcinogenic and teratogenic data. Experimental

reproductive effects. When heated to decomposition it emits acrid smoke and irritating fumes.

EDU500 CAS: 50-27-1
ESTRIOL
mf: $C_{18}H_{24}O_3$ mw: 288.42
PROP: Small, white crystals. D: 0.965, bp:
214.6°

SYNS: AACIFEMINE ◇ COLPOVISTER ◇ DESTRIOL
◇ DEUSLON-A ◇ ESTRA-1,3,5(10)-TRIENE-3,16-α,17-β-
TRIOL ◇ 1,3,5-ESTRATRIENE-3-β,16-α,17-β-TRIOL
◇ (16-α,17-β)-ESTRA-1,3,5(10)-TRIENE-3,16,17-TRIOL
◇ ESTRATRIOL ◇ 3,16-α,17-β-ESTRIOL ◇ 16-α,17-β-ES-
TRIOL ◇ ESTRIOLO (ITALIAN) ◇ FOLLICULAR HORMONE
HYDRATE ◇ GYNAESAN ◇ HEMOSTYPTANON ◇ HOLIN
◇ HORMOMED ◇ HORMONIN ◇ 16-α-HYDROXYESTRA-
DIOL ◇ 16-α-HYDROXYOESTRADIOL ◇ KLIMORAL
◇ NSC-12169 ◇ OE3 ◇ OESTRA-1,3,5(10)-TRIENE-3,16-α,17-
β-TRIOL ◇ 1,3,5-OESTRATRIENE-3-β-3,16-α,17-β-TRIOL
◇ (16-α,17-β)-OESTRA-1,3,5(10)-TRIENE-3,16,17-TRIOL
◇ OESTRATRIOL ◇ OESTRIOL ◇ 3,16-α,17-β-OESTRIOL
◇ 16-α,17-β-OESTRIOL ◇ ORGASTYPTIN ◇ OVESTERIN
◇ OVESTIN ◇ OVESTINON ◇ OVESTRION ◇ STIPTANON
◇ SYNAPAUSE ◇ THEELOL ◇ THULOL ◇ TRIDESTRIN
◇ 3,16-α,17-β-TRIHYDROXY-Δ-1,3,5-ESTRATRIENE
◇ 3,16-α,17-β-TRIHYDROXY-Δ-1,3,5-OESTRATRIENE
◇ 3,16-α,17-β-TRIHYDROXYESTRA-1,3,5(10)-TRIENE
◇ TRIHYDROXYESTRIN ◇ 3,16-α,17-β-TRIHYDROXYOES-
TRA-1,3,5(10)-TRIENE ◇ TRIHYDROXYOESTRIN ◇ TRIODU-
RIN ◇ TRIOVEX

TOXICITY DATA with REFERENCE
NEO: imp-mus TD:34 mg/kg   EJCAAH 11,39,75
NEO: imp-mus TDLo:26 mg/kg   EJCAAH11,39,75
ETA: imp-gpg TDLo:20 mg/kg:TER   RBBIAL
    5,1,45
ETA: imp-ham TDLo:480 mg/kg/64W-C
    NCIMAV 1,1,59
MUT: cyt-ham:ovr 50 μmol/L   TOLED5 29,201,85

CONSENSUS REPORTS: IARC Cancer Review: Animal Limited Evidence IMEMDT
21,327,79; Human Limited Evidence IMEMDT
21,327,79; Animal Inadequate Evidence IM-
EMDT 6,117,74.

SAFETY PROFILE: Suspected carcinogen with
experimental carcinogenic, neoplastigenic, tumorigenic, and teratogenic data. Mutation data
reported. A steroid drug for the treatment of
menopause. When heated to decomposition it
emits acrid smoke and irritating fumes.

EDV500 CAS: 2393-53-5
ESTRONE BENZOATE
mf: $C_{25}H_{26}O_3$ mw: 374.51

SYNS: BENZOATE d'OESTRONE (FRENCH) ◇ 3-(BENZOY-LOXY)ESTRA-1,3,5(10)-TRIEN-17-ONE ◇ 3-HYDROXYES-TRA-1,3,5(10)-TRIEN-17-ONE BENZOATE ◇ KETOHYDROX-YESTRIN BENZOATE ◇ OESTRONBENZOAT (GERMAN)

TOXICITY DATA with REFERENCE
NEO: scu-mus TDLo: 760 μg/kg/19W-I
ZEKBAI 56,482,49
ETA: par-mus TDLo: 52 mg/kg/26W-I   CRSBAW
122,183,36
ETA: scu-mus TD: 6450 μg/kg/43W-I   JPBAA7
42,169,36
ETA: scu-rat TDLo: 80 mg/kg/87W-I   CRSBAW
137,325,43

CONSENSUS REPORTS: IARC Cancer Review: Animal Limited Evidence IMEMDT 21,343,79.

SAFETY PROFILE: Suspected carcinogen with experimental carcinogenic, neoplastigenic, and tumorigenic data. A steroid. When heated to decomposition it emits acrid smoke and irritating fumes.

EEH520   CAS: 8015-12-1
ETHINYLESTRADIOL and
NORETHINDRONE ACETATE
mf: $C_{22}H_{28}O_3 \cdot C_{20}H_{24}O_2$ mw: 636.94

SYNS: ANOVLAR 21 ◇ CONTROVLAR ◇ ETHINYL OES-TRADIOL mixed with NORETHISTERONE ACETATE ◇ GYN-ANOVLAR ◇ GYNONLAR 21 ◇ MINORLAR ◇ NORLESTRIN ◇ NORETHINDRONE ACETATE and ETHI-NYLESTRADIOL ◇ NORETHISTERONE ACETATE mixed with ETHINYL OESTRADIOL ◇ MINOVLAR ◇ PRIMODOS

TOXICITY DATA with REFERENCE
CAR: orl-wmn TDLo: 23562 μg/kg/94W-I
LANCAO 1,207,78
NEO: orl-wmn TD: 41 mg/kg/2Y-I   MJAUAJ
2,223,78
NEO: orl-wmn TD: 81 mg/kg/8Y-I   BMJOAE
3,7,74
ETA: orl-mus TDLo: 69 mg/kg/69W-I   PEXTAR
11,440,69
ETA: orl-rat TD: 11087 mg/kg/1Y-C   GANNA2
71,576,80
ETA: orl-rat TD: 22174 mg/kg/1Y-C   KNZOAU
23,57,82
ETA: orl-rat TDLo: 11087 mg/kg/1Y-C
KNZOAU 23,57,82

SAFETY PROFILE: Suspected human carcinogen producing lung and liver tumors. Experimental neoplastigenic and tumorigenic data. Human and experimental teratogenic and reproductive effects. When heated to decomposition it emits acrid smoke and irritating fumes.

EEH550   CAS: 68-23-5
17-α-ETHINYL-5,10-ESTRENOLONE
mf: $C_{20}H_{26}O_2$ mw: 298.46

SYNS: 17-α-ETHINYL-Δ$^{5,10-19}$-NORTESTOSTERONE ◇ 17-ETHINYL-5(10)-ESTRAENEOLONE ◇ 17-α-ETHINYL-ESTRA(5,10)ENEOLONE ◇ 17-α-ETHYNYL-5(10)-ESTREN-17-OL-3-ONE ◇ 17-α-ETHYNYLESTR-5(10)-EN-17-β-OL-3-ONE ◇ 17-α-ETHYNYL-ESTR-5(10)-EN-3-ON-17-β-OL ◇ 17-α-ETHYNYL-17-HYDROXYESTR-5(10)-EN-3-ONE ◇ 17-α-ETHYNYL-17-HYDROXY-5(10)-ESTREN-3-ONE ◇ 17-α-ETHYNYL-17-β-HYDROXY-5(10)-ESTREN-3-ONE ◇ 17-α-ETHYNYL-17-β-HYDROXYESTR-5(10)-EN-3-ONE ◇ 17-α-ETHINYL-17-β-HYDROXY-Δ$^{5(10)}$-ESTREN-3-ONE ◇ 17-α-ETHYNYL-17-β-HYDROXY-Δ$^{-5(10)}$-ESTREN-3-ONE ◇ 17-α-ETHYNYL-17-β-HYDROXY-3-OXO-Δ$^{5(10)}$-ESTRENE ◇ 17-α-ETHYNYL-19-NOR-5(10)-ANDROSTEN-17-β-OL-3-ONE ◇ 17-HYDROXY-19-NOR-17-α-PREGN-5(10)-EN-20-YN-3-ONE ◇ (17-α)-17-HYDROXY-19-NORPREGN-5(10)-EN-20-YN-3-ONE ◇ 17-HYDROXY(17-α)-19-NORPREGN-5(10)-EN-20-YN-3-ONE ◇ 17-β-HYDROXY-17-α-ETHINYL-5(10)-ES-TREN-3-ONE ◇ LYNESTROL ◇ NORETHINODREL ◇ 19-NOR-ETHINYL-5,10-TESTOSTERONE ◇ NORETHINY-NODREL ◇ NORETHYNODRAL ◇ NORETHYNODREL ◇ 19-NORETHYNODREL ◇ NSC-15432 ◇ SC-4642

TOXICITY DATA with REFERENCE
ETA: imp-mus TDLo: 119 mg/kg/77W-C
NATUAS 212,686,66
ETA: orl-rat TDLo: 60 mg/kg/17W-C   PAACA3
21,76,80
ETA: scu-mus TDLo: 135 mg/kg/83W-C
BJCAAI 21,153,67
MUT: cyt-ctl: oth 100 μg/L   AJOGAH 120,390,74
MUT: cyt-mus: oth 10 mg/L   AJOGAH 120,390,74
MUT: dni-hmn: lyms 50 μmol/L   PSEBAA
146,401,74
MUT: dns-rat: lvr 100 μmol/L   CRNGDP 6,1201,85
MUT: oth-ctl: oth 10 mg/L   AJOGAH 120,390,74
MUT: oth-dom: oth 74100 μg/L   AJOGAH
120,390,74
MUT: oth-mus-par 16 μg/kg   AJOGAH 120,390,74

CONSENSUS REPORTS: IARC Cancer Review: Animal Limited Evidence IMEMDT 21,461,79; Animal Sufficient Evidence IMEMDT 6,191,74.

SAFETY PROFILE: Suspected carcinogen with experimental tumorigenic data. Human and experimental reproductive effects. Mutation data reported. When heated to decomposition it emits acrid smoke and irritating fumes.

EEI000   CAS: 67-21-0
dl-ETHIONINE
mf: $C_6H_{13}NO_2S$ mw: 163.26

PROP: Crystals. Decomp @ 273°.

SYNS: AETHIONIN ◇ 2-AMINO-4-(ETHYLTHIO)BUTYRIC
ACID ◇ dl-2-AMINO-4-(ETHYLTHIO)BUTYRIC ACID
◇ CN 8676 ◇ ETH ◇ ETHIONIN ◇ ETHIONINE ◇ (±)-ETHIO-
NINE ◇ S-ETHYL-HOMOCYSTEINE ◇ S-ETHYL-dl-HOMO-
CYSTEINE ◇ NSC 751 ◇ U-1434

TOXICITY DATA with REFERENCE
CAR: orl-mus TD:57 g/kg/68W-C   PAACA3
  25,78,84
CAR: orl-mus TDLo:44 g/kg/2Y-C   PAACA3
  25,78,84
CAR: orl-rat TD:28800 mg/kg/69W-C   CNREA8
  42,4364,82
CAR: orl-rat TDLo:7200 mg/kg/34W-C
  CNREA8 42,4364,82
ETA: ipr-rat TDLo:5625 mg/kg/12W-I   CNREA8
  42,4364,82
ETA: orl-mus TD:32 g/kg/30W-C   PAACA3
  25,252,84
ETA: orl-rat TD:24 g/kg/23W-C   CNREA8
  28,1703,68
MUT: dns-rat:lvr 1 μmol/L   CNREA8 42,3010,82
MUT: dns-sat 2 μg   ECEBDI 50,271,82
MUT: mmo-ssp 240 μg/L   PMRSDJ 1,424,81
MUT: otr-mus:emb 9200 μmol/L   MUREAV
  152,113,85
MUT: otr-rat:lvr 7500 μmol/L/12W-C   ITCSAF
  20,291,84

CONSENSUS REPORTS: EPA Genetic Toxicology Program. Reported in EPA TSCA Inventory.

SAFETY PROFILE: Suspected carcinogen with
experimental carcinogenic and tumorigenic
data. Moderately toxic by intraperitoneal route.
Mildly toxic by ingestion. Experimental reproductive effects. Mutation data reported. When
heated to decomposition it emits toxic fumes
of SO_x and NO_x.

EFT000   CAS: 140-88-5
ETHYL ACRYLATE
DOT: 1917
mf: $C_5H_8O_2$ mw: 100.13

PROP: Colorless liquid; acrid penetrating odor.
Bp: 99.8°, fp: <−72°: lel: 1.8%, flash p: 60°F
(OC), 48.2°F d: 0.916-0.919, vap press, 29.3
mm @ 20°, vap d: 3.45. Misc with alc, ether;
sltly sol in water.

SYNS: ACRYLATE d'ETHYLE (FRENCH) ◇ ACRYLIC
ACID ETHYL ESTER ◇ ACRYLSAEUREAETHYLESTER
(GERMAN) ◇ AETHYLACRYLAT (GERMAN) ◇ ETHOXY-
CARBONYLETHYLENE ◇ ETHYLACRYLAAT (DUTCH)
◇ ETHYLAKRYLAT (CZECH) ◇ ETHYL PROPENOATE
◇ ETHYL-2-PROPENOATE ◇ ETIL ACRILATO (ITALIAN)
◇ ETILACRILATULUI (ROMANIAN) ◇ FEMA No. 2418
◇ NCI-C50384 ◇ 2-PROPENOIC ACID, ETHYL ESTER (MAK)
◇ RCRA WASTE NUMBER U113

TOXICITY DATA with REFERENCE
CAR: orl-mus TDLo:103 g/kg/2Y-I   NTPTR*
  NTP-TR-259,86
CAR: orl-rat TDLo:51500 mg/kg/2Y-I   NTPTR*
  NTP-TR-259,86
MUT: cyt-ham:lng 9800 μg/L   GMCRDC 27,95,81
MUT: cyt-mus:lym 20 mg/L   ENMUDM 8(Suppl
  6),4,86
MUT: mma-mus:lym 20 mg/L   ENMUDM 8(Suppl
  6),4,86
MUT: mnt-mus-ipr 225 mg/kg   MUREAV135,189,84
MUT: msc-mus:lym 20 mg/L   ENMUDM 8(Suppl
  6),4,86

CONSENSUS REPORTS: IARC Cancer Review: GROUP 2B IMEMDT 7,56,87; Animal
Sufficient Evidence IMEMDT 39,81,86; Animal Inadequate Evidence IMEMDT 19,47,79;
Human Inadequate Evidence IMEMDT 19,
47,79. NTP Carcinogenesis Studies (gavage);
Clear Evidence: mouse, rat NTPTR* NTP-TR-
259,86. Reported in EPA TSCA Inventory.
Community Right-To-Know List.

OSHA PEL: (Transitional: TWA 25 mg/m³
(skin)) TWA 5 ppm; STEL 25 ppm
(skin)   ACGIH TLV: TWA 5 ppm; STEL 25
ppm (Proposed: 5 ppm; STEL 25 ppm Suspected
Human Carcinogen)   DFG MAK: 5 ppm (20
mg/m³)   DOT   Classification: Flammable
Liquid; Label: Flammable Liquid.

SAFETY PROFILE: Suspected carcinogen with
experimental carcinogenic data. Poison by ingestion and inhalation. Moderately toxic by skin
contact and intraperitoneal routes. Human systemic effects by inhalation: eye, olfactory and
pulmonary changes. A skin and eye irritant.
Flammable liquid. To fight fire, use CO_2, dry
chemical or alcohol foam. When heated to decomposition it emits acrid smoke and irritating
fumes.

ELG500   CAS: 13147-25-6
ETHYL-2-
HYDROXYETHYLNITROSAMINE
mf: $C_4H_{10}N_2O_2$ mw: 118.16

SYNS: AETHYL-AETHANOL-NITROSOAMIN (GERMAN) ◇ EENA ◇ EHEN ◇ N-ETHYL-N-HYDROXYETHYLNITROSA-MINE ◇ 2-(ETHYLNITROSAMINO)ETHANOL ◇ N-NITRO-SOAETHYLAETHANOLAMIN (GERMAN) ◇ N-NITROSOE-THYLETHANOLAMINE ◇ N-NITROSOETHYL-2-HYDROXYETHYLAMINE ◇ N-NITROSO-N-ETHYL-N-(2-HY-DROXYETHYL)AMINE

TOXICITY DATA with REFERENCE

CAR: ivn-rat TDLo:50 mg/kg/10W-I   CRNGDP 7,1313,86

CAR: orl-rat TD:700 mg/kg/2W-C   NAIZAM 31,361,80

CAR: orl-rat TD:840 mg/kg/2W-C   SAIGAK 37,1771,82

CAR: orl-rat TD:1400 mg/kg/2W-C   NAIZAM 31,361,80

CAR: orl-rat TD:5146 mg/kg/23W-C   CRNGDP 8,719,87

CAR: orl-rat TDLo:1680 mg/kg/14D-C GANNA2 70,817,79

NEO: orl-rat TD:840 mg/kg/2W-C   JJIND8 72,483,84

NEO: orl-rat TD:1400 mg/kg/2W-C   GANNA2 74,607,83

ETA: orl-rat TD:700 mg/kg/1W-C   JJIND8 70,477,83

ETA: orl-rat TD:1400 mg/kg/2W-C   CRNGDP 4,523,83

ETA: orl-rat TD:1400 mg/kg/2W-C   CRNGDP 5,525,84

ETA: orl-rat TD:1400 mg/kg/2W-C   CRNGDP 2,1299,81

MUT: mma-sat 20 μg/plate   MUREAV 66,1,79

CONSENSUS REPORTS: IARC Cancer Review: Animal Limited Evidence IMEMDT 17,83,78. EPA Genetic Toxicology Program.

SAFETY PROFILE: Suspected carcinogen with experimental carcinogenic, neoplastigenic, and tumorigenic data. Mutation data reported. Explodes when heated to 170°C. When heated to decomposition it emits toxic fumes of NO_x.

EMF500   CAS: 62-50-0
ETHYL METHANESULFONATE
mf: $C_3H_8O_3S$ mw: 124.17

SYNS: EMS ◇ ENT 26,396 ◇ ETHYL ESTER of METHANE-SULFONIC ACID ◇ ETHYL ESTER of METHYLSULFONIC ACID ◇ ETHYL ESTER of METHYLSULPHONIC ACID ◇ ETHYL METHANESULPHONATE ◇ ETHYL METHANSUL-FONATE ◇ ETHYL METHANSULPHONATE ◇ HALF-MYL-ERAN ◇ METHANESULPHONIC ACID ETHYL ESTER ◇ METHYLSULFONIC ACID, ETHYL ESTER ◇ NSC 26805 ◇ RCRA WASTE NUMBER U119

TOXICITY DATA with REFERENCE

CAR: ipr-rat TDLo:300 mg/kg   BJCAAI 29,50,74

CAR: orl-rat TD:3353 mg/kg/13W-C   CRNGDP 2,1223,81

CAR: orl-rat TDLo:1050 g/kg/12W-C   CALEDQ 7,79,79

NEO: ipr-mus TDLo:373 mg/kg   CBINA8 83,117,71

NEO: ipr-rat TD:825 mg/kg/10D-I   NATUAS 223,947,69

ETA: ipr-mus TD:400 mg/kg   BIJOAK 174,1031,78

ETA: ipr-mus TD:600 mg/kg/6W-I   BECCAN 39,77,61

ETA: ipr-rat TD:413 mg/kg/10D-I   NATUAS 223,947,69

ETA: ivn-rat TD:1650 mg/kg/30W-I   EXPTAX 16,157,78

ETA: ivn-rat TDLo:100 mg/kg (21D post) EXPTAX 16,157,78

ETA: ivn-rat TDLo:1650 mg/kg/2W-I 43XWAI-,15,78

ETA: par-rat TDLo:800 mg/kg/3W-I   RCOCB8 7,25,74

MUT: cyt-ham:ovr 1 mmol/L   CNREA8 45,1556,85

MUT: dnd-rat-ipr 33800 μg/kg   MUREAV 130,283,84

MUT: mnt-ham:lng 100 mg/L   MUREAV 130,272,84

MUT: msc-hmn:lym 50 μmol/L   MUREAV 128,221,84

MUT: oms-hmn:lym 400 μmol/L   MUREAV 155,75,85

MUT: oms-mam:lym 49 mmol/L   CBINA8 46,179,83

MUT: sce-frg-mul 300 mg/L   ENMUDM 8(Suppl 6),30,86

MUT: sln-dmg-orl 500 ppm   ENMUDM 7(Suppl 3),76,85

CONSENSUS REPORTS: IARC Cancer Review: GROUP 2B IMEMDT 7,56,87; Animal Sufficient Evidence IMEMDT 7,245,74. Reported in EPA TSCA Inventory. EPA Genetic Toxicology Program.

SAFETY PROFILE: Suspected carcinogen with experimental carcinogenic, neoplastigenic, tumorigenic, and teratogenic data. Poison by intraperitoneal route. Experimental reproductive effects. Human mutation data reported. When heated to decomposition it emits toxic fumes of SO_x.

ENV500   CAS: 139-94-6
1-ETHYL-3-(5-NITRO-2-THIAZOLYL) UREA
mf: $C_6H_8N_4O_3S$ mw: 216.24

SYNS: N-ETHYL-N′-(5-NITRO-2-THIAZOLYL)UREA
◇ HEPZIDE ◇ NCI-C03792 ◇ NITHIAZID ◇ NITHIAZIDE

TOXICITY DATA with REFERENCE
CAR: orl-mus TDLo: 395 g/kg/94W-I   NCITR*
NCI-CG-TR-146,79
CAR: orl-rat TDLo: 41 g/kg/94W-I   NCITR*
NCI-CG-TR-146,79
MUT: mma-sat 75 μg/plate   ENMUDM 5(Suppl
1),3,83
MUT: mmo-sat 75 μg/plate   ENMUDM 5(Suppl
1),3,83

CONSENSUS REPORTS: IARC Cancer Review: Animal Limited Evidence IMEMDT 31,179,83. NCI Carcinogenesis Bioassay (feed); Clear Evidence: mouse, rat NCITR* NCI-CG-TR-146,79

SAFETY PROFILE: Suspected carcinogen with experimental carcinogenic data. Moderately toxic by ingestion. Mutation data reported. When heated to decomposition it emits very toxic fumes of NO_x and PO_x.

EOK000   CAS: 50-06-6
5-ETHYL-5-PHENYLBARBITURIC ACID
mf: $C_{12}H_{12}N_2O_3$ mw: 232.26

SYNS: ACIDO-5-FENIL-5-ETILBARBITURICO (ITALIAN)
◇ ADONAL ◇ AEPHENAL ◇ AGRYPNAL ◇ AMYLOFENE
◇ APHENYLBARBIT ◇ APHENYLETTEN ◇ AUSTROMINAL
◇ BARBAPIL ◇ BARBELLON ◇ BARBENYL ◇ BARBILEHAE
(BARBILETTAE) ◇ BARBINAL ◇ BARBIPHENYL
◇ BARBITA ◇ BARBIVIS ◇ BARBONAL ◇ BARBOPHEN
◇ BARDORM ◇ BARTOL ◇ BIALMINAL ◇ BLU-PHEN
◇ CABRONAL ◇ CALMETTEN ◇ CALMINAL ◇ CARDENAL
◇ CODIBARBITA ◇ CORONALETTA ◇ CRATECIL
◇ DAMORAL ◇ DEZIBARBITUR ◇ DORMINA ◇ DORMIRAL
◇ DOSCALUN ◇ DUNERYL ◇ ENSOBARB ◇ ENSODORM
◇ EPANAL ◇ EPIDORM ◇ EPILOL ◇ EPISEDAL ◇ EPSY-
LONE ◇ ESKABARB ◇ 5-ETHYL-5-PHENYL-2,4,6--
(1H,3H,5H)PYRIMIDINETRIONE ◇ ETILFEN ◇ EUNERYL
◇ FENBITAL ◇ FENEMAL ◇ FENOBARBITAL ◇ FENOSED
◇ FENYLETTAE ◇ GARDENAL ◇ GARDEPANYL
◇ GLYSOLETTEN ◇ HAPLOPAN ◇ HAPLOS ◇ HELIONAL
◇ HENNOLETTEN ◇ HYPNALETTEN ◇ HYPNOGEN
◇ HYPNOLONE ◇ HYPNO-TABLINETTEN ◇ HYSTEPS
◇ LEFEBAR ◇ LEONAL ◇ LEPHEBAR ◇ LEPINAL
◇ LEPINALETTEN ◇ LINASEN ◇ LIQUITAL ◇ LIXOPHEN
◇ LUBERGAL ◇ LUBROKAL ◇ LUMEN ◇ LUMESETTES
◇ LUMESYN ◇ LUMINAL ◇ LUMOFRIDETTEN ◇ LUPHENIL
◇ LURAMIN ◇ MOLINAL ◇ NEUROBARB ◇ NIRVONAL
◇ NOPTIL ◇ NOVA-PHENO ◇ NUNOL ◇ PARKOTAL
◇ PHARMETTEN ◇ PHENAEMAL ◇ PHENOBAL ◇ PHENO-
BARBITAL ◇ PHENOBARBITONE ◇ PHENOBARBITURIC

ACID ◇ PHENOLURIC ◇ PHENOMET ◇ PHENONYL
◇ PHENOTURIC ◇ PHENYLETHYLBARBITURATE
◇ PHENYL-ETHYL-BARBITURIC ACID ◇ 5-PHENYL-5-
ETHYLBARBITURIC ACID ◇ PHENYLETHYLMALONYLU-
REA ◇ PHENYLETTEN ◇ PHENYRAL ◇ PHOB ◇ POLCOMI-
NAL ◇ PROMPTONAL ◇ SEDABAR ◇ SEDA-TABLINEN
◇ SEDICAT ◇ SEDIZORIN ◇ SEDLYN ◇ SEDOFEN
◇ SEDONAL ◇ SEDONETTES ◇ SEDOPHEN ◇ SEVENAL
◇ SK-PHENOBARBITAL ◇ SOLFOTON ◇ SOMBUTOL
◇ SOMNOLENS ◇ SOMNOLETTEN ◇ SOMNOSAN
◇ SOMONAL ◇ SPASEPILIN ◇ STARIFEN ◇ STARILETTAE
◇ STENTAL EXTENTABS ◇ TALPHENO ◇ TEOLAXIN
◇ THENOBARBITAL ◇ THEOLOXIN ◇ THEOMINAL
◇ TRIABARB ◇ TRIDEZIBARBITUR ◇ TRIPHENATOL
◇ VERSOMNAL ◇ ZADOLETTEN ◇ ZADONAL

TOXICITY DATA with REFERENCE
CAR: orl-rat TD: 2100 mg/kg/12W-C   IGAYAY
123,1069,82
CAR: orl-rat TD: 3990 mg/kg/19W-C   CRNGDP
4,935,83
NEO: orl-mus TD: 38 g/kg/90W-C   FCTXAV
11,433,73
NEO: orl-mus TDLo: 22 g/kg/1Y-C   JNCIAM
51,1349,73
NEO: orl-rat TD: 2520 mg/kg/12W-C   CRNGDP
4,935,83
ETA: orl-rat TD: 4200 mg/kg/20W-C   CALEDQ
5,139,78
ETA: orl-rat TDLo: 7560 mg/kg/36W-C
GANNA2 69,679,78
MUT: cyt-ham: lvr 100 mg/L   PMRSDJ 5,397,85
MUT: cyt-hmn: lym 388 mg/L   AGMGAK 21,305,72
MUT: dns-rat: lvr 100 pmol/L   CRNGDP 6,811,85
MUT: mmo-sat 100 μg/plate   MUREAV 147,255,85
MUT: mmo-smc 500 mg/L   PMRSDJ 5,271,85
MUT: otr-ham: emb 100 mg/L   PMRSDJ 5,665,85
MUT: sce-ham: ovr 15 mmol/L   PMRSDJ 5,433,85

CONSENSUS REPORTS: EPA Genetic Toxicology Program. IARC Cancer Review: GROUP 2B IMEMDT 7,313,87; Human Inadequate Evidence IMEMDT 13,157,77.

SAFETY PROFILE: Suspected carcinogen with experimental carcinogenic, neoplastigenic, tumorigenic, and teratogenic data. A human teratogen. A human poison by ingestion. An experimental poison by ingestion, intraperitoneal, subcutaneous, intravenous, and rectal routes. Human systemic effects by ingestion: somnolence, motor activity changes, pulmonary changes, allergic dermatitis and fever. Human reproductive effects by ingestion and possibly other routes: drug dependence and other postnatal measures or effects. Human teratogenic effects include developmental abnormalities of the central nervous system, body wall, musculoskeletal, respiratory, gastrointestinal and urogenital systems. Experimental reproductive effects. Human mutation data reported. Used as a drug in the treatment of epilepsy, and as an hypnotic and sedative. When heated to decomposition it emits toxic fumes of NO_x.

EQE000
ETHYLUREA and SODIUM NITRITE (2:1)

SYNS: AETHYLHARNSTOFF UND NATRIUMNITRIT (GERMAN) ◇ AETHYLHARNSTOFF UND NITRIT (GERMAN) ◇ SODIUM NITRITE and ETHYLUREA (1:2)

TOXICITY DATA with REFERENCE
CAR: orl-ham TDLo: 300 mg/kg (15D preg): TER   JNCIAM 55,1389,75
CAR: orl-rat TDLo: 1650 mg/kg (13-23D preg): TER   IARCCD 4,92,73
NEO: orl-ham TDLo: 600 mg/kg (12-15D preg): TER   ZKKOBW 85,201,76
NEO: orl-rat TDLo: 750 mg/kg (15D preg): TER   ZAPPAN 121,61,77
ETA: orl-rat TD: 25 g/kg/35D-C   ARZNAD 21,1707,71
ETA: orl-rat TD: 1650 mg/kg (13-23D preg): TER   NATWAY 57,460,70
ETA: orl-rbt TDLo: 450 mg/kg/(17-19D preg): TER   JNCIAM 59,427,77

SAFETY PROFILE: Suspected carcinogen with experimental carcinogenic, neoplastigenic, tumorigenic, and teratogenic data. Experimental reproductive effects. When heated to decomposition it emits toxic fumes of NO_x and Na_2O.

EQJ500   CAS: 297-76-7
ETHYNODIOL ACETATE
mf: $C_{24}H_{32}O_4$ mw: 384.56

SYNS: CERVICUNDIN ◇ 3-β, 17-β-DIACETOXY-17-α-ETHYNYL-4-OESTRENE ◇ 3-β,17-β-DIACETOXY-19-NOR-17-α-PREGN-4-EN-20-YNE ◇ ETHINODIOL DIACETATE ◇ ETHYNODIOL DIACETATE ◇ β-ETHYNODIOL DIACETATE ◇ 17-α-ETHYNYL-3,17-DIHYDROXY-4-ESTRENE DIACETATE ◇ 17-α-ETHYNYLESTR-4-ENE-3-β,17-β-DIOL ACETATE ◇ 17-α-ETHYNYL-4-ESTRENE-3-β,17-β-DIOL DIACETATE ◇ 17-α-ETHYNYL-4-ESTRENE-3-β,17-β-DIOL DIACETATE ◇ 17-α-ETHYNYL-19-NORANDROST-4-ENE-3-β,17-β-DIOL DIACETATE ◇ FEMULEN ◇ LUTO-METRODIOL ◇ METRODIOL ◇ METRODIOL DIACETATE ◇ (3-β,17-α)-19-NORPREGN-4-EN-20-YNE-3,17-DIOL DIACETATE ◇ OVULEN 50

TOXICITY DATA with REFERENCE
MUT: oth-mus-par 16 μg/kg   AJOGAH 120,390,74
MUT: cyt-ctl: oth 10 mg/L   AJOGAH 120,390,74

CONSENSUS REPORTS: IARC Cancer Review: Animal Limited Evidence IMEMDT 21,387,79; Animal Sufficient Evidence IMEMDT 6,173,74.

SAFETY PROFILE: Suspected carcinogen. Human reproductive effects by ingestion: menstrual cycle changes. Experimental reproductive effects. Mutation data reported. A steroid. When heated to decomposition it emits acrid smoke and irritating fumes.

FAG018   CAS: 3564-09-8
FD&C RED No. 1
mf: $C_{19}H_{16}N_2O_7S_2 \cdot 2Na$ mw: 494.47

SYNS: A.F. RED NO. 1 ◇ CERVEN KUMIDINOVA ◇ C.I. 16155 ◇ C.I. FOOD RED 6 ◇ C.I. FOOD RED 6, DISODIUM SALT ◇ DISODIUM 3-HYDROXY-4-((2,4,5-TRIMETHYLPHENYL)AZO)-2,7-NAPHTHALENEDISULFONATE ◇ DISODIUM 3-HYDROXY-4-((2,4,5-TRIMETHYLPHENYL)AZO)-2,7-NAPHTHALENEDISULFONIC ACID ◇ DISODIUM 3-HYDROXY-4-((2,4,5-TRIMETHYLPHENYL)AZO)-2,7-NAPHTHALENEDISULPHONATE ◇ DISODIUM 3-HYDROXY-4-((2,4,5-TRIMETHYLPHENYL)AZO)-2,7-NAPHTHALENEDISULPHONIC ACID ◇ DOLKWAL PONCEAU 3R ◇ EXT. D&C RED No. 15 ◇ 3-HYDROXY-4-((2,4,5-TRIMETHYLPHENYL)AZO)-2,7-NAPHTHALENEDISULPHONIC ACID, DISODIUM SALT ◇ 3-HYDROXY-4-((2,4,5-TRIMETHYLPHENYL)AZO)-2,7-NAPHTHALENEDISULFONIC ACID, DISODIUM SALT ◇ MAPLE PONCEAU 3R ◇ PONCEAU 3R ◇ SODIUM CUMENEAZO-β-NAPHTHOL DISULPHONATE ◇ USACERT RED No. 1

TOXICITY DATA with REFERENCE
CAR: imp-mus TDLo: 80 mg/kg   BJCAAI 17,127,63
CAR: orl-mus TDLo: 1640 g/kg/65W-C   TXAPA9 3,509,61
CAR: orl-rat TDLo: 730 g/kg/2Y-C   TXAPA9 5,105,63
NEO: orl-rat TD: 200 g/kg/24W-C   TXAPA9 5,105,63
ETA: orl-mus TD: 1140 g/kg/68W-C   TXAPA9 5,105,63
MUT: mma-sat 660 nmol/plate   INFIBR 23,686,79
MUT: oth-esc 300 μmol/L   SKEZAP 12,298,71

CONSENSUS REPORTS: IARC Cancer Review: GROUP 2B IMEMDT 7,56,87; Animal Sufficient Evidence IMEMDT 8,199,75

SAFETY PROFILE: Suspected carcinogen with experimental carcinogenic and tumorigenic data. Mutation data reported. When heated to decomposition it emits toxic fumes of NO_x and SO_x.

FAG120   CAS: 1694-09-3
FD&C VIOLET No. 1
mf: $C_{39}H_{41}N_3O_6S_2 \cdot Na$ mw: 734.94

SYNS: ACID VIOLET ◇ A.F. VIOLET No 1 ◇ AIZEN FOOD VIOLET No 1 ◇ BENZYL VIOLET ◇ BENZYL VIOLET 3B ◇ CALCOCID VIOLET 4BNS ◇ C.I. 42640 ◇ C.I. FOOD VIOLET 2 ◇ COOMASSIE VIOLET ◇ DISPERSED VIOLET 12197 ◇ FORMYL VIOLET S4BN ◇ PERGACID VIOLET 2B ◇ SOLAR VIOLET 5BN ◇ WOOL VIOLET

TOXICITY DATA with REFERENCE
CAR: orl-rat TDLo:498 g/kg/28W-C   JNCIAM 51,1337,73
ETA: scu-rat TDLo:9360 mg/kg/2Y-I   FEPRA7 16,367,57
MUT: mma-sat 320 µg/plate   MUREAV 89,21,81

CONSENSUS REPORTS: IARC Cancer Review: GROUP 2B IMEMDT 7,56,87; Animal Sufficient Evidence IMEMDT 16,153,78. EPA Genetic Toxicology Program. Reported in EPA TSCA Inventory.

SAFETY PROFILE: Suspected carcinogen with experimental carcinogenic and tumorigenic data. Mutation data reported. When heated to decomposition it emits very toxic fumes of NO_x, NH_3, Na_2O, and SO_x.

FBU509   CAS: 67774-32-7
FIREMASTER FF-1

PROP: 2,4,5,2′,4′,5′-hexabromobiphenyl is the predominant isomer (LANCAO 2,602,77).

SYNS: 2,4,5,2′,4′,5′-HEXABROMOBIPHENYL ◇ PBB ◇ POLYBROMINATED BIPHENYL ◇ POLYBROMINATED BIPHENYL (FF-1)

TOXICITY DATA with REFERENCE
CAR: orl-mus TDLo:1250 mg/kg/26W-I   NTPTR* NTP-TR-244,83
CAR: orl-rat TD:1250 mg/kg/26W-I   NTPTR* NTP-TR-244,83
CAR: orl-rat TDLo:375 mg/kg/26W-I   NTPTR* NTP-TR-244,83
NEO: orl-rat TD:1000 mg/kg   LANCAO 2,602,77

CONSENSUS REPORTS: IARC Cancer Review: GROUP 2B IMEMDT 7,321,87; Human Inadequate Evidence IMEMDT 41,261,86; Animal Sufficient Evidence IMEMDT 41,261,86.

NTP Carcinogenesis Studies (gavage); Clear Evidence: mouse, rat NTPTR* NTP-TR-244,83. Polybrominated biphenyl compounds are on the Community Right-To-Know List.

SAFETY PROFILE: Suspected carcinogen with experimental carcinogenic, neoplastigenic, and teratogenic data. Experimental reproductive effects. When heated to decomposition it emits very toxic fumes of Br^-.

FDI000   CAS: 153-78-6
FLUOREN-2-AMINE
mf: $C_{13}H_{11}N$ mw: 181.25

SYNS: AMINOFLUOREN (GERMAN) ◇ 2-AMINOFLUORENE ◇ 2-FLUORENAMINE ◇ 2-FLUORENEAMINE

TOXICITY DATA with REFERENCE
CAR: imp-mus TDLo:50 mg/kg   BJCAAI 12,222,58
CAR: orl-rat TDLo:3600 mg/kg/32W-C   CNREA8 15,188,55
CAR: skn-rat TDLo:240 mg/kg/73W-I   JNCIAM 10,1201,50
NEO: orl-rat TD:2420 mg/kg/23W-C   JNCIAM 10,1201,50
NEO: skn-mus TDLo:11 g/kg/34W-C   BJCAAI 14,195,60
ETA: imp-mus TD:100 mg/kg   BMBUAQ 14,147,58
ETA: orl-mus TDLo:100 mg/kg/47W-C   CNREA8 7,453,47
ETA: orl-rat TD:3200 mg/kg/58W-C   CNREA8 7,453,47
ETA: orl-rat TD:4000 mg/kg/23W-C   CNREA8 7,730,47
ETA: scu-rat TDLo:400 mg/kg/26W-I   CNREA8 7,453,47
ETA: skn-rat TD:18 g/kg/30W-I   BJEPA5 25,1,44
ETA: skn-rat TD:1080 mg/kg/30W-I   ENDOAO 76,1027,65
MUT: dns-gpg:lng 10 µmol/L   ENMUDM 7,245,85
MUT: dns-ham:lng 10 µmol/L   ENMUDM 7,245,85
MUT: mma-sat 150 ng/plate   CBINA8 54,71,85
MUT: msc-rat:lvr 50 µmol/L   MUREAV 130,53,84
MUT: pic-sat 10 µg/plate   MUREAV 110,243,83

CONSENSUS REPORTS: EPA Genetic Toxicology Program.

SAFETY PROFILE: Suspected carcinogen with experimental carcinogenic, neoplastigenic, and tumorigenic data. Poison by intraperitoneal route. Mutation data reported. When heated to decomposition it emits toxic fumes of NO_x.

FGI100
6-FLUOROBENZO(a)PYRENE
mf: $C_{20}H_{11}F$ mw: 270.31

TOXICITY DATA with REFERENCE
CAR: scu-mus TDLo:9 mg/kg   JJIND8 71,309,83
CAR: scu-rat TDLo:35 mg/kg/1W-I   JJIND8 71,309,83
NEO: skn-mus TDLo:49 mg/kg/60W-I   JJIND8 71,309,85
ETA: skn-mus TD:16 mg/kg/60W-I   JJIND8 71,309,83

SAFETY PROFILE: Suspected carcinogen with experimental carcinogenic and neoplastigenic data. When heated to decomposition it emits toxic fumes of F⁻.

FNW000   CAS: 758-17-8
N-FORMYL-N-METHYLHYDRAZINE
mf: $C_2H_6N_2O$ mw: 74.10

SYNS: FORMIC ACID, METHYLHYDRAZIDE ◇ 1-FOR-MYL-1-METHYLHYDRAZINE ◇ N-METHYL-N-FORMLYHY-DRAZINE ◇ MFH

TOXICITY DATA with REFERENCE
CAR: orl-ham TDLo:6100 mg/kg/80W-C JCROD7 93,109,79
CAR: orl-mus TD:84 mg/kg/70W-C   MYCPAH 78,11,82
CAR: orl-mus TD:158 mg/kg/79W-C   MYCPAH 78,11,82
CAR: orl-mus TD:187 mg/kg/78W-C   MYCPAH 78,11,82
CAR: orl-mus TD:3158 mg/kg/94W-C   NEOLA4 27,25,80
CAR: orl-mus TD:3360 mg/kg/2Y-C   NEOLA4 27,25,80
CAR: orl-mus TD:3920 mg/kg/2Y-C   NEOLA4 27,25,80
CAR: orl-mus TD:7840 mg/kg/70W-C MYCPAH 68,121,79
CAR: orl-mus TDLo:14 mg/kg/62W-C   JNCIAM 60,201,78
CAR: orl-rat TD:64 mg/kg/80W-C   MYCPAH 78,11,82
CAR: scu-mus TD:100 mg/kg:TER   JTEHD6 6,577,80
CAR: scu-mus TD:180 mg/kg   JTEHD6 6,577,80
CAR: scu-mus TDLo:400 mg/kg/40W-I NEOLA4 39,437,83
MUT: mma-sat 100 μmol/plate   TXCYAC26,155,83
MUT: mmo-sat 100 μmol/plate   TXCYAC26,155,83

SAFETY PROFILE: Suspected carcinogen with experimental carcinogenic and teratogenic data. Poison by ingestion and possibly other routes. Mutation data reported. When heated to decomposition it emits toxic fumes of NO_x.

FPI150   CAS: 3031-51-4
l-FURALTADONE HYDROCHLORIDE
mf: $C_{13}H_{16}N_4O_6$•ClH   mw: 360.79

PROP: Yellow crystals. Decomposes @ 206°.

SYNS: FURMETHONOL ◇ l-5-(MORPHOLINOMETHYL)-3-((5-NITROFURFURYLIDENE)AMINO)-2-OXAZOLIDINO-NEHYDROCHLORIDE

TOXICITY DATA with REFERENCE
CAR: orl-rat TDLo:25 g/kg/46W-C   JNCIAM 51,403,73
MUT: mmo-eug 10 mg/L   JPROAR 17,129,70

CONSENSUS REPORTS: IARC Cancer Review: GROUP 2B IMEMDT 7,56,87; Animal Limited Evidence IMEMDT 7,161,74.

SAFETY PROFILE: Suspected carcinogen with experimental carcinogenic data. Poison by intravenous route. Moderately toxic by ingestion. Mutation data reported. When heated to decomposition it emits very toxic fumes of HCl and NO_x.

FQN000   CAS: 3688-53-7
2-(2-FURYL)-3-(5-NITRO-2-FURYL)ACRYLAMIDE
mf: $C_{11}H_8N_2O_5$ mw: 248.21

SYNS: AF-2 (PRESERVATIVE) ◇ FF ◇ FURYLAMIDE ◇ FURYLFURAMIDE ◇ α-2-FURYL-5-NITRO-2-FURANA-CYRLAMIDE ◇ 2-(2-FURYL)-3-(5-NITRO-2-FURYL)ACRYLIC ACID AMIDE ◇ α-(FURYL)-β-(5-NITRO-2-FURYL)ACRYLIC AMIDE ◇ TOFURON

TOXICITY DATA with REFERENCE
CAR: orl-ham TD:116 g/kg/80W-C   ZKKOBW 89,61,77
CAR: orl-ham TD:127 g/kg/94W-C   FCTXAV 17,339,79
CAR: orl-ham TDLo:63 g/kg/94W-C   FCTXAV 17,339,79
CAR: orl-mus TD:158 g/kg/47W-C   CALEDQ 3,115,77
CAR: orl-mus TD:211 g/kg/63W-C   GANNA2 68,825,77
CAR: orl-mus TD:32400 mg/kg/72W-C ESKHA5 (100),80,82
CAR: orl-mus TDLo:156 g/kg/44W-C   ZKKOBW 89,61,77
CAR: orl-rat TDLo:52 g/kg/40W-C   CALEDQ 3,115,77
NEO: orl-mus TD:42 g/kg/63W-C   GANNA2 68,825,77
NEO: orl-rat TD:25 g/kg/78W-C   TOLED5 1,11,77

MUT: cyt-ham: ovr 500 μg/L   ENMUDM 7,8,85
MUT: mmo-esc 100 ng/plate   MUREAV 142,163,85
MUT: mmo-sat 4 μg/L   MUREAV 147,219,85
MUT: pic-esc 40 μg/L   MUREAV 165,57,86
MUT: sce-ham: ovr 160 μg/L   ENMUDM 7,1,85
MUT: sce-hmn: lym 500 μg/L   CNREA8 40,4775,80

CONSENSUS REPORTS: IARC Cancer Review: GROUP 2B IMEMDT 7,56,87; Human Inadequate Evidence IMEMDT 31,47,83; Animal Sufficient Evidence IMEMDT 31,47,83. EPA Genetic Toxicology Program.

SAFETY PROFILE: Suspected carcinogen with experimental carcinogenic, neoplastigenic, and teratogenic data. Poison by ingestion. Experimental reproductive effects. Human mutation data reported. When heated to decomposition it emits toxic fumes of NO_x.

GCE100
GASOLINE, UNLEADED

SYNS: UNLEADED GASOLINE ◇ UNLEADED MOTOR GASOLINE

TOXICITY DATA with REFERENCE
CAR: ihl-mus TCLo: 2056 ppm/6H/78W-I
   NTIS** PB86-209152
CAR: ihl-rat TC: 2056 ppm/6H/78W-I   NTIS**
   PB86-209152
CAR: ihl-rat TCLo: 1501 ppm/78W-C   AETODY
   7,65,84

SAFETY PROFILE: Suspected carcinogen with experimental carcinogenic data. Moderately toxic by inhalation. Pulmonary aspiration can cause severe pneumonitis. Skin irritant. Flammable liquid. When heated to decomposition it emits acrid smoke and irritating fumes.

GGI000   CAS: 38571-73-2
GLYCEROL
(TRI(CHLOROMETHYL))ETHER
mf: $C_6H_{11}Cl_3O_3$ mw: 237.52

SYN: TRIS-1,2,3-(CHLOROMETHOXY)PROPANE

TOXICITY DATA with REFERENCE
NEO: ipr-mus TDLo: 910 mg/kg/76W-I
   CNREA8 35,2553,75
NEO: scu-mus TDLo: 970 mg/kg/81W-I
   CNREA8 35,2553,75
ETA: skn-mus TDLo: 8640 mg/kg/72W-I
   CNREA8 35,2553,75

CONSENSUS REPORTS: IARC Cancer Review: GROUP 2A IMEMDT 7,56,87; Animal Sufficient Evidence IMEMDT 15,301,77.

SAFETY PROFILE: Suspected carcinogen with experimental neoplastigenic and tumorigenic data. When heated to decomposition it emits toxic fumes of Cl^-.

GGW000   CAS: 765-34-4
GLYCIDALDEHYDE
DOT: 2622
mf: $C_3H_4O_2$ mw: 72.07

PROP: Colorless liquid. Bp: 113°, d: 1.1403 @ 20°/4°.

SYNS: EPIHYDRINALDEHYDE ◇ EPIHYDRINE ALDEHYDE ◇ 2,3-EPOXYPROPANAL ◇ 2,3-EPOXY-1-PROPANAL ◇ 2,3-EPOXYPROPIONALDEHYDE ◇ GLYCIDAL ◇ GLYCIDYLALDEHDYE ◇ OXIRANE-CARBOXALDEHYDE ◇ RCRA WASTE NUMBER U126

TOXICITY DATA with REFERENCE
CAR: scu-rat TDLo: 13 g/kg/77W-I   JNCIAM
   39,1213,67
CAR: skn-mus TD: 26 g/kg/71W-I
   14JTAF -,275,65
CAR: skn-mus TDLo: 17 g/kg/48W-I   JNCIAM
   35,707,65
NEO: scu-mus TDLo: 8844 mg/kg/67W-I
   JNCIAM 37,825,66
ETA: scu-rat TDLo: 390 mg/kg/78W-I   JNCIAM
   37,825,66
ETA: skn-mus TD: 26 g/kg/22W-I   JNCIAM
   39,1217,67
MUT: mma-esc 33300 ng/plate   ENMUDM 6(Suppl
   2),1,84
MUT: mma-mus: lym 8900 μg/L   MUREAV
   97,49,82
MUT: mma-sat 3300 ng/plate   ENMUDM 6(Suppl
   2),1,84
MUT: mmo-esc 10 μg/plate   ENMUDM 6(Suppl
   2),1,84
MUT: otr-ham: emb 1 mg/L   JJIND8 67,1303,81
MUT: otr-mus: fbr 1 mg/L   JJIND8 67,1303,81

CONSENSUS REPORTS: IARC Cancer Review: GROUP 2B IMEMDT 7,56,87; Animal Sufficient Evidence IMEMDT 11,175,76. EPA Genetic Toxicology Program.

DOT Classification: Flammable or Combustible Liquid; Label: Flammable and Poison.

SAFETY PROFILE: Suspected carcinogen with experimental carcinogenic, neoplastigenic, and tumorigenic data. Poison by ingestion, skin contact, intraperitoneal, and intravenous routes. Moderately toxic by inhalation. Human systemic effects by inhalation: changes in central nervous system electrical activity, olfactory changes, and excitement. Mutation data reported. A human eye irritant. Powerful skin sensitizer and mucous membrane irritant. Flammable when exposed to heat, flame or oxidizing materials. When heated to decomposition it emits acrid smoke and irritating fumes.

GKE000
GRISOFULVIN

CAS: 126-07-8

mf: $C_{17}H_{17}ClO_6$ mw: 352.79

SYNS: AMUDANE ◇ BIOGRISIN-FP ◇ 7-CHLORO-4,6,2'-TRIMETHOXY-6'-METHYLGRIS-2'-EN-3,4'-DIONE ◇ DELMOFULVINA ◇ FULCIN ◇ FULCINE ◇ FULVICAN GRISACTIN ◇ FULVICIN ◇ FULVINA ◇ FULVISTATIN ◇ FUNGIVIN ◇ GREOSIN ◇ GRESFEED ◇ GRICIN ◇ GRIFULVIN ◇ GRISACTIN ◇ GRISCOFULVIN ◇ GRISEFULINE ◇ GRISEO ◇ (+)-GRISEOFULVIN ◇ GRISEOFULVIN-FORTE ◇ GRISEOFULVINUM ◇ GRISETIN ◇ GRISOVIN ◇ GRIS-PEG ◇ GRYSIO ◇ GUSERVIN ◇ LAMORYL ◇ LIKUDEN ◇ MURFULVIN ◇ NEO-FULCIN ◇ NSC 34533 ◇ PONCYL ◇ SPIROFULVIN ◇ SPOROSTATIN ◇ USAF SC-2

TOXICITY DATA with REFERENCE
NEO: orl-mus TD:730 g/kg/52W-C   CNREA8 26,721,66
NEO: orl-mus TDLo:440 g/kg/52W-C   CNREA8 26,721,66
NEO: orl-rat TDLo:462 g/kg/2Y-I   BJCAAI 38,237,78
NEO: scu-mus TDLo:120 mg/kg/49W-I CNREA8 27,1900,67
MUT: cyt-ham:fbr 10 mg/L   CRNGDP 3,499,82
MUT: cyt-hmn:lym 40 mg/L/3D   MUREAV 25,123,74
MUT: dni-hmn:fbr 20 mg/L/3D-C   KAMJDW 2,127,76
MUT: dni-hmn:lym 20 mg/L/3D-C   KAMJDW 2,127,76
MUT: dnr-bcs 100 μL/plate   MUREAV 97,1,82

CONSENSUS REPORTS: IARC Cancer Review: GROUP 2B IMEMDT 7,56,87; Animal Sufficient Evidence IMEMDT 10,153,76. EPA Genetic Toxicology Program.

SAFETY PROFILE: Suspected carcinogen with experimental neoplastigenic and teratogenic data. Poison by intravenous and intraperitoneal routes. Moderately toxic by subcutaneous route. Human mutation data reported. Experimental reproductive effects. Used as a antibiotic, pharmaceutical and veterinary drug. When heated to decomposition it emits toxic fumes of Cl⁻.

HAR000
HEPTACHLOR

CAS: 76-44-8

DOT: 2761

mf: $C_{10}H_5Cl_7$ mw: 373.30

PROP: Crystals. Mp: 96°. Nearly insol in water; sol in organic solvents.

SYNS: AGROCERES ◇ 3-CHLOROCHLORDENE ◇ DRINOX ◇ E 3314 ◇ ENT 15,152 ◇ EPTACLORO (ITALIAN) ◇ 1,4,5,6,7,8,8-EPTACLORO-3a,4,7,7a-TETRAIDRO-4,7-endo-METANO-INDENE (ITALIAN) ◇ GPKh ◇ H-34 ◇ HEPTACHLOOR (DUTCH) ◇ 1,4,5,6,7,8,8-HEPTACHLOOR-3a,4,7,7a-TETRAHYDRO-4,7-endo-METHANO-INDEEN (DUTCH) ◇ HEPTACHLORE (FRENCH) ◇ 3,4,5,6,7,8,8-HEPTACHLORODICYCLOPENTADIENE ◇ 3,4,5,6,7,8,8a-HEPTACHLORODICYCLOPENTADIENE ◇ 1,4,5,6,7,10,10-HEPTACHLORO-4,7,8,9,-TETRAHYDRO-4,7-ENDOMETHYLENEINDENE ◇ 1,4,5,6,7,8,8-HEPTACHLORO-3a,4,7,7a-TETRAHYDRO-4,7-ENDOMETHANOINDENE ◇ 1,4,5,6,7,8,8a-HEPTACHLORO-3a,4,7,7a-TETRAHYDRO-4,7-METHANOINDANE ◇ 1,4,5,6,7,8,8-HEPTACHLORO-3a,4,7,7a-TETRAHYDRO-4,7-METHANOINDENE ◇ 1(3a),4,5,6,7,8,8-HEPTACHLORO-3a(1),4,7,7a-TETRAHYDRO-4,7-METHANOINDENE ◇ 1,4,5,6,7,8,8-HEPTACHLORO-3a,4,7,7a-TETRAHYDRO-4,7-METHANOL-1H-INDENE ◇ 1,4,5,6,7,8,8-HEPTACHLORO-3a,4,7,7a-TETRAHYDRO-4,7-METHYLENE INDENE ◇ 1,4,5,6,7,8,8-HEPTACHLOR-3a,4,7,7,7a-TETRAHYDRO-4,7-endo-METHANO-INDEN (GERMAN) ◇ HEPTAGRAN ◇ HEPTAMUL ◇ NCI-C00180 ◇ RCRA WASTE NUMBER P059 ◇ RHODIACHLOR ◇ VELSICOL 104

TOXICITY DATA with REFERENCE
CAR: orl-mus TD:876 mg/kg/2Y-C   ECEBDI 45,147,77
CAR: orl-mus TD:930 mg/kg/80W-C   NCITR* NCI-CG-TR-9,77
CAR: orl-mus TDLo:403 mg/kg/80W-C NCITR* NCI-CG-TR-9,77
MUT: cyt-mus-ipr 5200 μg/kg   SOGEBZ 2,80,66
MUT: cyt-rat-orl 60 μg/kg   34LXAP -,555,76
MUT: dlt-rat-orl 60 μg/kg   34LXAP -,555,76
MUT: mma-hmn:fbr 100 μmol/L   MUREAV 42,161,77

CONSENSUS REPORTS: IARC Cancer Review: GROUP 3 IMEMDT 7,146,87; Human Inadequate Evidence IMEMDT 20,129,79; Animal Inadequate Evidence IMEMDT 5,173,74; Animal Sufficient Evidence IMEMDT 20,-129,79. NCI Carcinogenesis Bioassay (feed) Clear Evidence: Mouse (NCITR* NCI-CG-TR-9,77); Results negative: rat (NCITR* NCI-CG-TR-9,77). EPA Genetic Toxicology Program. Community Right-To-Know List.

OSHA PEL: TWA 0.5 mg/m³ (skin)   ACGIH TLV: TWA 0.5 mg/m³ (skin)   DFG MAK: 0.5 mg/m³, Suspected Carcinogen.   DOT Classification: ORM-E; Label; None.

SAFETY PROFILE: Suspected carcinogen with experimental carcinogenic data. A poison by ingestion, skin contact, intraperitoneal, intravenous, and possibly other routes. Human mutation data reported. Acute exposure and chronic doses have caused liver damage. When heated to decomposition it emits toxic fumes of Cl⁻.

HCD250   CAS: 87-68-3
HEXACHLORBUTADIENE
DOT: 2279
mf: C_4Cl_6 mw: 260.74

PROP: Autoign temp: 1130°F, vap d: 8.99.

SYNS: DOLEN-PUR ◇ GP-40-66:120 ◇ HCBD ◇ HEXA-CHLOR-1,3-BUTADIEN (CZECH) ◇ HEXACHLORO-1,3-BU-TADIENE (MAK) ◇ 1,1,2,3,4,4-HEXACHLORO-1,3-BUTA-DIENE ◇ PERCHLOROBUTADIENE ◇ RCRA WASTE NUMBER U128

TOXICITY DATA with REFERENCE
CAR: orl-rat TDLo:15 g/kg/2Y-C   AIHAAP 38(1),589,77
MUT: dns-ham:emb 2 mg/L   CALEDQ 23,297,84
MUT: dns-rat-orl 77 g/kg/11W   TXAPA9 60,287,81
MUT: mma-sat 320 µg/plate   CRNGDP 7,431,86
MUT: otr-ham:emb 10 mg/L   CALEDQ 23,297,84

CONSENSUS REPORTS: IARC Cancer Review: Animal Suspected IMEMDT 20,179,79. Community Right-To-Know List. Reported in EPA TSCA Inventory.

OSHA PEL: TWA 0.02 ppm   ACGIH TLV: TWA 0.02 ppm (skin); Suspected Human Carcinogen.   DFG MAK: Suspected Carcinogen.

DOT Classification: Poison B; Label: St. Andrews Cross.

SAFETY PROFILE: Suspected carcinogen with experimental carcinogenic data. Poison by ingestion, intraperitoneal, and possibly other routes. Moderately toxic by inhalation and skin contact. A skin and eye irritant. Experimental reproductive effects. Mutation data reported. Combustible when exposed to heat or flame; can react vigorously with oxidizing materials. To fight fire, use dry chemical, CO_2, alcohol foam, water spray, fog, mist. When heated to decomposition it emits very toxic fumes of Cl⁻. A solvent, heat transfer fluid, transformer, hydraulic fluid, and wash liquor.

HCF500
1,2,3,6,7,8-HEXACHLORODIBENZO-p-DIOXIN mixed with 1,2,3,7,8,9-HEXACHLORODIBENZO-p-DIOXIN

PROP: Composed of 67% of 1,2,3,7,8,9-hexachlorodibenzo-p-dioxin and 31% of 1,2,3,6,7,8-hexachlorodibenzo-p-dioxin   (NCITR* NCI-CG-TR-198,80)

SYNS: 1,2,3,7,8,9-HEXACHLORODIBENZO-p-DIOXIN mixed with 1,2,3,6,7,8-HEXACHLORODIBENZO-p-DIOXIN ◇ NCI-C03703

TOXICITY DATA with REFERENCE
CAR: orl-mus TDLo:520 µg/kg/2Y-I   NCITR* NCI-CG-TR-198,80

CONSENSUS REPORTS: NCI Carcinogenesis Bioassay (gavage); Clear Evidence: mouse, rat NCITR* NCI-CG-TR-198,80. NCI Carcinogenesis Bioassay (dermal); No Evidence: mouse NCITR* NCI-CG-TR-202,80.

SAFETY PROFILE: Suspected carcinogen with experimental carcinogenic data. A deadly poison by ingestion. When heated to decomposition it emits very toxic fumes of Cl⁻ and dioxin.

HGP500   CAS: 304-20-1
HYDRALAZINE HYDROCHLORIDE
mf: $C_8H_8N_4$•ClH   mw: 196.66

PROP: Yellow crystals. Decomp @ 273°, very sltly sol in ether.

SYNS: AISELAZINE ◇ APPRESINUM ◇ APRELAZINE ◇ APRESAZIDE ◇ APRESINE ◇ APRESOLIN ◇ APRESOLINE-ESIDRIX ◇ APRESOLINE HYDROCHLORIDE ◇ APREZOLIN ◇ BA 5968 ◇ CIBA 5968 ◇ DRALZINE ◇ HIDRALAZIN ◇ HIPOFTALIN ◇ HYDRALAZINE CHLORIDE ◇ HYDRALA-ZINE MONOHYDROCHLORIDE ◇ HYDRALLAZINE HYDRO-CHLORIDE ◇ HYDRAPRESS ◇ 1-HYDRAZINOPHTHALA-ZINE HYDROCHLORIDE ◇ 1-HYDRAZINOPHTHLAZINE MONOHYDROCHLORIDE ◇ HYPERAZIN ◇ HYPOPHTHA-LIN ◇ HYPOS ◇ IPOLINA ◇ LOPRESS ◇ NOR-PRESS 25 ◇ 1(2H)-PHTHALAZINONE HYDRAZONE HYDROCHLORIDE ◇ 1(2H)-PHTHLAZINONE, HYDRAZONE, MONOHYDRO-CHLORIDE ◇ PRAPARAT 5968 ◇ ROLAZINE ◇ SERPASIL APRESOLINE No. 2

TOXICITY DATA with REFERENCE
NEO: orl-mus TDLo:2950 mg/kg/78W-C   JJIND8 61,1363,78
MUT: dni-hmn:hla 150 µmol/L   MUREAV 92,427,82
MUT: dns-rat:lvr 100 µmol/L   RCOCB8 49,415,85

MUT: mma-sat 500 μg/plate RCOCB8 49,415,85
MUT: mmo-sat 500 μg/plate RCOCB8 49,415,85
MUT: sce-mus-ipr 83 mg/kg ENMUDM 4,605,82

CONSENSUS REPORTS: IARC Cancer Review: Animal Limited Evidence IMEMDT 24,85,80. Reported in EPA TSCA Inventory.

SAFETY PROFILE: Suspected carcinogen with experimental neoplastigenic data. A poison by ingestion, subcutaneous, intravenous, and intraperitoneal routes. Human mutation data reported. An antihypertensive agent. When heated to decomposition it emits very toxic NO_x and HCl.

HIM000 CAS: 103-90-2
4′-HYDROXYACETANILIDE
mf: $C_8H_9NO_2$ mw: 151.18

SYNS: ABENSANIL ◇ ACAMOL ◇ ACETAGESIC ◇ ACETALGIN ◇ p-ACETAMIDOPHENOL ◇ 4-ACETAMIDO-PHENOL ◇ ACETAMINOPHEN ◇ p-ACETAMINOPHENOL ◇ N-ACETYL-p-AMINOPHENOL ◇ p-ACETYLAMINOPHENOL ◇ ALGOTROPYL ◇ ALPINYL ◇ ALVEDON ◇ AMADIL ◇ ANAFLON ◇ ANELIX ◇ ANHIBA ◇ APADON ◇ APAMIDE ◇ APAP ◇ BEN-U-RON ◇ BICKIE-MOL ◇ CALPOL ◇ CETADOL ◇ CLIXODYNE ◇ DATRIL ◇ DIAL-A-GESIC ◇ DIROX ◇ DOLIPRANE ◇ DYMADON ◇ ENELFA ◇ ENERIL ◇ EXDOL ◇ FEBRILIX ◇ FEBRO-GESIC ◇ FEBROLIN ◇ FENDON ◇ FINIMAL ◇ G 1 ◇ GELOCATIL ◇ HEDEX ◇ HOMOOLAN ◇ p-HYDROXYACETANILIDE ◇ 4-HYDROXYACETANILIDE ◇ N-(4-HYDROXYPHENYL) ACETAMIDE ◇ JANUPAP ◇ KORUM ◇ LESTEMP ◇ LIQUAGESIC ◇ LONARID ◇ LYTECA SYRUP ◇ MOMENTUM ◇ MULTIN ◇ NAPA ◇ NAPRINOL ◇ NCI-C55801 ◇ NOBEDON ◇ PACEMO ◇ PANADOL ◇ PANETS ◇ PANEX ◇ PANOFEN ◇ PARACETAMOLE ◇ PARACETAMOLO (ITALIAN) ◇ PARACETANOL ◇ PARAPAN ◇ PARASPEN ◇ PARMOL ◇ PEDRIC ◇ PYRINAZINE ◇ SK-Apap ◇ TABALGIN ◇ TAPAR ◇ TEMLO ◇ TEMPANAL ◇ TEMPRA ◇ TRALGON ◇ TUSSAPAP ◇ TYLENOL ◇ VALADOL ◇ VALGESIC

TOXICITY DATA with REFERENCE
CAR: orl-mus TDLo: 135 g/kg/77W-C CRNGDP 4,363,83
CAR: orl-rat TDLo: 164 g/kg/78W-C ACPADQ 93,367,85
CAR: orl-rat TD: 329 g/kg/78W-C ACPADQ 93,367,85
ETA: orl-mus TD: 270 g/kg/77W-C CRNGDP 4,363,83
MUT: cyt-ham: fbr 60 mg/L ESKHA5 96,55,78
MUT: cyt-ham: lng 10 mg/L ARTODN (4),41,80
MUT: cyt-hmn: lym 200 mg/L NEZAAQ 37,673,82

MUT: cyt-mus-orl 50 mg/kg CYTBAI 27,27,80
MUT: oms-hmn: lym 200 mg/L NEZAAQ37,673,82

CONSENSUS REPORTS: Reported in EPA TSCA Inventory. EPA Genetic Toxicology Program.

SAFETY PROFILE: Suspected carcinogen with experimental carcinogenic and tumorigenic data. A human poison by ingestion and possibly other routes. An experimental poison by intraperitoneal route. Moderately toxic by subcutaneous, intravenous, and possibly other routes. Human systemic effects by ingestion: changes in exocrine pancreas, diarrhea, nausea, irritability, somnolence, general anesthetic, fever, hepatitis, kidney tubule damage. Experimental teratogenic and reproductive effects. Human mutation data reported. Used as an analgesic and antipyretic. When heated to decomposition it emits toxic fumes of NO_x.

HIP000 CAS: 53-95-2
N-HYDROXY-N-ACETYL-2-AMINOFLUORENE
mf: $C_{15}H_{13}NO_2$ mw: 239.29

SYNS: FLUORENYL-2-ACETHYDROXAMIC ACID ◇ N-FLUOREN-2-YL ACETOHYDROXAMIC ACID ◇ N-2-FLUORENYL ACETOHYDROXAMIC ACID ◇ N-HYDROXY-AAF ◇ N-HYDROXY-2-ACETAMIDOFLUORENE ◇ 2-(N-HYDROXYACETAMIDO)FLUORENE ◇ N-HYDROXY-2-ACETYLAMINOFLUORENE ◇ N-HYDROXY-2-FAA ◇ N-HYDROXY-N-(2-FLUORENYL)ACETAMIDE ◇ NOHFAA

TOXICITY DATA with REFERENCE
CAR: ipr-gpg TDLo: 4700 mg/kg/26W-I: TER CNREA8 24,2018,64
CAR: ipr-ham TDLo: 1250 mg/kg/26W-I CNREA8 24,2018,64
CAR: ipr-rat TD: 237 mg/kg/4W-I CNREA8 30,1485,70
CAR: ipr-rat TD: 540 mg/kg/4W-I CNREA8 27,1443,67
CAR: ipr-rat TDLo: 120 mg/kg/4W-I CNREA8 32,1554,72
CAR: ipr-rbt TDLo: 3880 mg/kg/40W-I CNREA8 27,838,67
CAR: orl-gpg TDLo: 13 g/kg/94W-C CNREA8 24,2018,64
CAR: orl-ham TDLo: 8640 mg/kg/32W-C CNREA8 24,2018,64
CAR: orl-mus TDLo: 27 g/kg/60W-C CNREA8 24,2018,64
CAR: orl-rat TD: 1075 mg/kg/16W-C ENDOAO 82,685,68

CAR: orl-rat TD: 2677 mg/kg/32W-C   FCTXAV 11,199,73

CAR: orl-rat TDLo: 1000 mg/kg   CNREA8 26,619,66

CAR: par-rat TDLo: 2991 µg/kg   CRNGDP3,233,82

CAR: scu-rat TD: 205 mg/kg/7W-I   CNREA8 25,527,65

CAR: scu-rat TD: 216 mg/kg/8W-I   CNREA8 27,1600,67

CAR: scu-rat TD: 485 mg/kg/9W-I   CNREA8 31,1645,71

CAR: scu-rat TDLo: 102 mg/kg/3W-I   CNREA8 25,527,65

NEO: imp-mus TDLo: 160 mg/kg   ANYAA9 108,924,63

NEO: imp-rat TDLo: 24 mg/kg   CNREA8 37,111,77

NEO: orl-rat TD: 806 mg/kg/12W-C   IJCNAW 2,337,67

NEO: orl-rat TD: 1344 mg/kg/20W-C   IJCNAW 2,337,67

NEO: scu-rat TD: 61 mg/kg/5W-I   CNREA8 37,1461,77

ETA: orl-rbt TDLo: 9800 mg/kg/56W-I   CNREA8 27,838,67

MUT: dnd-hmn: hla 25 µmol/L   MUREAV 89,95,81

MUT: dnd-mus: lvr 20 µmol/L   CRNGDP 5,797,84

MUT: dns-hmn: oth 1 µmol/L   JJIND8 72,847,84

MUT: mmo-sat 1 µg/plate   ENMUDM 6(Suppl 2),1,84

MUT: msc-ham: lng 25 µmol/L   MUREAV 149,265,85

CONSENSUS REPORTS: EPA Genetic Toxicology Program.

SAFETY PROFILE: Suspected carcinogen with experimental carcinogenic, neoplastigenic, and tumorigenic data. A poison by intraperitoneal route. Experimental teratogenic and other reproductive effects. Human mutation data reported. When heated to decomposition it emits toxic fumes of NO_x.

HKW500   CAS: 13743-07-2
1-(2-HYDROXYETHYL)-1-NITROSOUREA
mf: $C_3H_7N_3O_3$ mw: 133.13

SYNS: HENU ◇ HNU ◇ NITROSO-2-HYDROXYETHYLUREA ◇ N-NITROSOHYDROXYETHYLUREA ◇ 1-NITROSO-1-(2-HYDROXYETHYL)UREA

TOXICITY DATA with REFERENCE
CAR: orl-rat TD: 672 mg/kg/30W-C   CNREA8 43,214,83

CAR: orl-rat TD: 717 mg/kg/52W-I   JNCIAM 56,445,76

CAR: orl-rat TD: 738 mg/kg/28W-I   JJIND8 78,387,87

CAR: orl-rat TD: 840 mg/kg/38W-I   JJIND8 62,1523,79

CAR: orl-rat TD: 882 mg/kg/34W-I   JJIND8 78,387,87

CAR: orl-rat TD: 1400 mg/kg/25W-C   CNREA8 43,214,83

CAR: orl-rat TDLo: 520 mg/kg/37W-I   JJCREP 79,181,88

CAR: skn-mus TDLo: 479 mg/kg/45W-I   CNREA8 43,214,83

ETA: ipr-mus TDLo: 8 mg/kg   JJIND8 63,1469,79

ETA: orl-ham TD: 533 mg/kg/24W-I   IAPUDO 57,617,84

ETA: orl-ham TDLo: 533 mg/kg/22W-I   PAACA3 24,92,83

ETA: orl-rat TD: 202 mg/kg/18W-I   JCREA8 112,221,86

ETA: orl-rat TD: 399 mg/kg/51W-I   IAPUDO 57,617,84

MUT: mma-sat 2500 ng/plate   TCMUE9 1,13,84

MUT: mmo-sat 41 µmol/L/48H   MUREAV 48,131,77

MUT: spm-mus-ipr 455 mg/kg   MUREAV 108,337,83

CONSENSUS REPORTS: EPA Genetic Toxicology Program.

SAFETY PROFILE: Suspected carcinogen with experimental carcinogenic and tumorigenic data. A poison by intraperitoneal route. Experimental reproductive effects. Mutation data reported. When heated to decomposition it emits toxic fumes of NO_x.

HLX925   CAS: 78246-54-5
4-(HYDROXYMETHYL)BENZENEDIAZONIUM TETRAFLUOROBORATE
mf: $C_7H_7N_2O•BF_4$ mw: 221.97

SYNS: HMBD ◇ BENZENEDIAZONIUM, 4-(HYDROXYMETHYL)-, TETRAFLUOROBORATE(1-)

TOXICITY DATA with REFERENCE
CAR: orl-mus TDLo: 400 mg/kg   BJCAAI46,417,82

CAR: scu-mus TDLo: 1300 mg/kg/26W-I   CNREA8 41,2444,81

MUT: mma-sat 1 µmol/plate   ZLUFAR 183,85,86

MUT: mmo-sat 1 µmol/plate   ZLUFAR 183,85,86

SAFETY PROFILE: Suspected carcinogen with experimental carcinogenic data. Mutation data reported. When heated to decomposition it emits toxic fumes of NO_x, B, and F^-.

HMG000   CAS: 590-96-5
1-HYDROXYMETHYL-2-METHYLDITMIDE-2-OXIDE
mf: $C_2H_6N_2O_2$ mw: 90.10

SYNS: MAM ◇ METHYLAZOXYMETHANOL ◇ (METHYL-ONN-AZOXY)METHANOL

TOXICITY DATA with REFERENCE
ETA: ipr-gpg TD: 18 mg/kg/3W-I   25NJAN -,24,70
ETA: ipr-gpg TDLo: 10 mg/kg/9W-I
25NJAN -,24,70
ETA: ipr-rat TD: 20 mg/kg   IGKEAO 44,211,74
ETA: ipr-rat TD: 50 mg/kg/2W-I   CRNGDP
6,1529,85
ETA: ipr-rat TD: 80 mg/kg/35W-I   APAVAY
340,151,65
ETA: ipr-rat TDLo: 20 mg/kg/2W-I   JNCIAM
37,217,66
ETA: ivn-gpg TDLo: 1800 μg/kg   25NJAN -,24,70
ETA: ivn-ham TDLo: 20 mg/kg   PAACA3 10,86,69
ETA: scu-rat TDLo: 234 mg/kg/39W-I   DICRAG
16,438,73
MUT: dnd-mam: lym 1 mol/L   BIJOAK 98,20c,66
MUT: hma-mus/sat 1200 mg/kg   22XWAN -,260,70
MUT: mma-sat 10 μmol/plate   CNREA8 39,3780,79
MUT: mmo-sat 10 μmol/plate   CNREA8 39,3780,79
MUT: otr-ham: emb 2500 mg/kg   NATUAS
235,278,72
MUT: sln-dmg-orl 90 ng   PSEBAA 125,988,67

CONSENSUS REPORTS: IARC Cancer Review: GROUP 2B IMEMDT 7,56,87; Animal Sufficient Evidence IMEMDT 10,121,76. EPA Genetic Toxicology Program.

SAFETY PROFILE: Suspected carcinogen with experimental tumorigenic and teratogenic data. Other experimental reproductive effects. Mutation data reported. When heated to decomposition it emits toxic fumes of NO_x.

HNX500   CAS: 61499-28-3
1-((2-HYDROXYPROPYL)NITROSO)AMINO)ACETONE
mf: $C_6H_{12}N_2O_3$ mw: 160.20

SYNS: HPOP ◇ 1-((2-HYDROXYPROPYL)NITROSO-AMINO)-2-PROPANONE ◇ N-NITROSO(2-HYDROXYPROPYL)(2-OXOPROPYL)AMINE

TOXICITY DATA with REFERENCE
CAR: ipr-rat TDLo: 160 g/kg   JJIND8 74,209,85

CAR: orl-ham TD: 1008 mg/kg/21W-C   JJIND8
72,685,84
CAR: scu-ham TDLo: 817 mg/kg/43W-I
CNREA8 39,3828,79
CAR: skn-ham TDLo: 1900 mg/kg/50W-I
CALEDQ 10,163,80
NEO: scu-ham TD: 500 mg/kg/53W-I   CNREA8
39,3828,79
ETA: orl-ham TDLo: 961 mg/kg/27W-I   IAPUDO
57,617,84
ETA: orl-rat TDLo: 881 mg/kg/41W-I   IAPUDO
57,617,84
MUT: dnd-ham: oth 1 mg/L   CBINA8 48,59,84
MUT: dnd-rat: oth 25 mg/L   CBINA8 48,59,84
MUT: dns-rat: lvr 100 μmol/L   MUREAV 144,197,85
MUT: mma-ham: lng 400 μmol/L   CNREA8
45,5219,85
MUT: mmo-sat 2 μmol/plate   MUREAV 77,215,80

SAFETY PROFILE: Suspected carcinogen with experimental carcinogenic, neoplastigenic, and tumorigenic data. A poison by subcutaneous route. Mutation data reported. When heated to decomposition it emits toxic fumes of NO_x.

IAN000   CAS: 5034-77-5
IMIDAZOLE MUSTARD
mf: $C_8H_{12}Cl_2N_6O$ mw: 279.16

SYNS: BIC ◇ 5-(3,3-BIS(2-CHLOROETHYL)-1-TRIA-ZENO)IMIDAZOLE-4-CARBOXAMIDE ◇ NCI-C01616
◇ NSC-82196 ◇ SRI 2489 ◇ TIC MUSTARD

TOXICITY DATA with REFERENCE
NEO: ipr-mus TDLo: 1500 mg/kg/8W-I
CNREA8 33,3069,73
ETA: ipr-mus TD: 1170 mg/kg/26W-I   CANCAR
40(Suppl 4),1935,77
ETA: ipr-rat TDLo: 600 mg/kg/7W-I   CANCAR
40(Suppl 4),1935,77

CONSENSUS REPORTS: NCI Carcinogenesis Studies (ipr); Clear Evidence: mouse, rat CANCAR 40,1935,77.

SAFETY PROFILE: Suspected carcinogen with experimental neoplastigenic and tumorigenic data. Poison by ingestion and intraperitoneal routes. Experimental teratogenic and reproductive effects. Human systemic effects by intravenous route: nausea. When heated to decomposition it emits very toxic fumes of Cl^- and NO_x.

IAR000
2-IMIDAZOLIDINETHIONE mixed with SODIUM NITRITE

SYNS: ETHYLENETHIOUREA mixed with SODIUM NITRITE ◇ SODIUM NITRITE mixed with ETHYLENETHIOUREA

TOXICITY DATA with REFERENCE
MUT: dlt-mus-orl 1000 mg/kg/5D-I   MUREAV 56,335,78
MUT: hma-mus/sat 5 mg/kg   MUREAV 106,27,82
MUT: mmo-sat 1 μL/plate   MUREAV 48,225,77

SAFETY PROFILE: Suspected carcinogen. 2-Imidazolidinethione and sodium nitrite are experimental carcinogens. Experimental teratogenic and reproductive data. Sodium nitrite is a poison. Mutation data reported. When heated to decomposition it emits very toxic fumes of SO_x, Na_2O, and NO_x.

IGW000
IRON DUST

PROP: Silvery-white, tenacious, lustrous, ductile metal. Mp: 1535°, bp: 3000°, d: 7.86, vap press: 1 mm @ 1787°. Iron dust from open hearth furnace contained 52% iron (85AGAF -,480,76).

TOXICITY DATA with REFERENCE
NEO: itr-rat TDLo: 506 mg/kg/15W-I
85AGAF -,480,76

SAFETY PROFILE: Suspected carcinogen with experimental neoplastigenic data. Iron dust can cause conjunctivitis, choroiditis, retinitis, and siderosis of tissues if iron contacts and remains in these tissues. Iron ore dust can cause palpebral conjunctivitis, massive pulmonary fibrosis, and an increased incidence of lung cancer. Flammable in the form of dust when exposed to heat or flame. To fight fire, use special mixtures of dry chemical.

IHF000
IRON OXIDE FUME
mf: Fe_2O_3 mw: 159.70

SYN: ZELAZA TLENKI (POLISH)

OSHA PEL: TWA 10 mg/m³   ACGIH TLV: TWA 5 mg/m³, welding fumes.

SAFETY PROFILE: Suspected carcinogen.

IMH000   CAS: 3778-73-2
ISOPHOSPHAMIDE
mf: $C_7H_{15}Cl_2N_2O_2P$ mw: 261.11

SYNS: A 4942 ◇ ASTA Z 4942 ◇ N,N-BIS(β-CHLORO-ETHYL)-AMINO-N'-O-PROPYLENE-PHOSPHORIC ACID ESTER DIAMIDE ◇ 2,3-(N,N(1)-BIS(2-CHLOROETHYL)DIAMIDO-1,3,2-OXAZAPHOSPHORIDINOXY ◇ N,3-BIS(2-CHLOROETHYL)TETRAHYDRO-2H-1,3,2-OXAZAPHOSPHORIN-2-AMINE 2-OXIDE ◇ N-(2-CHLORAETHYL)-N'-(2 CHLORO-ETHYL)-N'-o-PROPYLEN-PHOSPHORSAUREESTER-DIAMID (GERMAN) ◇ 3-(2-CHLOROETHYL)-2-((2-CHLOROETHYL)AMINO)PERHYDRO-2H-1,3,2-OXAZAPHOSPHORINE OXIDE ◇ 3-(2-CHLOROETHYL)-2-((2-CHLOROETHYL)AMINO)TETRAHYDRO-2H-1,3,2-OXAZAPHOSPHORINE-2-OXIDE ◇ N-(2-CHLOROETHYL)-N'-(2-CHLOROETHYL)-N', O-PROPYLENEPHOSPHORIC ACID DIAMIDE ◇ N-(2-CHLOROETHYL)-N'-(2-CHLOROETHYL)-N',O-PROPYLENE-PHOSPHORIC ACID ESTER DIAMIDE ◇ CYFOS ◇ HOLOXAN ◇ IFOSFAMID ◇ IFOSFAMIDE ◇ IPHOSPHAMIDE ◇ ISOENDOXAN ◇ ISOFOSFAMIDE ◇ MITOXANA ◇ MJF 9325 ◇ NAXAMIDE ◇ NCI-C01638 ◇ NSC-109724 ◇ Z 4942

TOXICITY DATA with REFERENCE
CAR: ipr-mus TD: 3120 mg/kg/1Y-I   NCITR* NCI-TR-32,78
CAR: ipr-rat TD: 1872 mg/kg/1Y-I   NCITR* NCI-TR-32,78
CAR: ipr-rat TDLo: 940 mg/kg/1Y-I   NCITR* NCI-TR-32,78
CAR: scu-mus TDLo: 2600 mg/kg/65W-I   ARZNAD 29,483,79
NEO: ipr-mus TDLo: 450 mg/kg/8W-I   CNREA8 33,3069,73
MUT: bfa-rat/sat 2 g/kg   HIKYAJ 26,813,80
MUT: cyt-hmn: leu 130 mg/L   HUMAA7 5,321,68
MUT: cyt-hmn: lym 75 mg/L   CYTOAN 46,387,81
MUT: dnd-mam: lym 5600 μmol/L   JPMSAE 61,2009,72
MUT: mma-sat 400 μg/plate   TCMUD8 5,319,85

CONSENSUS REPORTS: IARC Cancer Review: Animal Limited Evidence IMEMDT 26,237,81. NCI Carcinogenesis Bioassay (ipr); Clear Evidence: mouse, rat NCITR* NCI-CG-TR-32,77. EPA Genetic Toxicology Program.

SAFETY PROFILE: Suspected carcinogen with experimental carcinogenic and neoplastigenic data. A poison by ingestion, intraperitoneal, subcutaneous, intravenous, and possibly other routes. Human systemic effects by ingestion and intravenous routes: nausea or vomiting; proteinuria, hematuria, inflammation, necrosis or scarring of the bladder, and other kidney, ureter, or bladder changes; changes in hair covering the skin; leukopenia (decreased white blood cell count), thrombocytopenia (decrease in the number of blood platelets); hallucinations, distorted perceptions; tumorigenic effects (active as an anti-cancer agent) data. Experimental teratogenic and reproductive effects. Human mutation data reported. When heated to decomposition it emits very toxic Cl^-, NO_x, and PO_x.

IQU000
ISOPROPYL OILS

PROP: A by-product of isopropyl alcohol manufacture composed of trimeric and tetrameric polypropylene + small amounts of benzene, toluene, alkyl benzenes, polyaromatic ring compounds, hexane, heptane, acetone, ethanol, isopropyl ether, and isopropyl alcohol (IARC** 15,225,77).

TOXICITY DATA with REFERENCE
NEO: ihl-mus TC:24 mg/m³/22W-I   AMIHBC 5,535,52
NEO: scu-mus TDLo:20 g/kg/20W-I   AMIHBC 5,535,52

CONSENSUS REPORTS: IARC Cancer Review: Animal Inadequate Evidence IMEMDT 15,223,77; Human Limited Evidence IMEMDT 15,223,77. DFG MAK: Suspected Carcinogen.

SAFETY PROFILE: Suspected carcinogen with experimental neoplastigenic data. When heated to decomposition they emit acrid smoke and fumes.

ISV000   CAS: 2835-39-4
ISOVALERIC ACID, ALLYL ESTER
mf: $C_8H_{14}O_2$ mw: 142.22

SYNS: ALLYL ISOVALERATE ◇ ALLYL ISOVALERIANATE ◇ ALLYL 3-METHYLBUTYRATE ◇ FEMA No. 2045 ◇ 3-METHYLBUTANOIC ACID, 2-PROPENYL ESTER ◇ 3-METHYLBUTYRIC ACID, ALLYL ESTER ◇ NCI-C54717 ◇ 2-PROPENYL ISOVALERATE ◇ 2-PROPENYL 3-METHYLBUTANOATE

TOXICITY DATA with REFERENCE
CAR: orl-mus TDLo:31930 mg/kg/2Y-I
   NTPTR* NTP-TR-253,83
CAR: orl-rat TDLo:31930 mg/kg/2Y-I   NTPTR* NTP-TR-253,83
ETA: orl-rat TD:15065 mg/kg/2Y-I   NTPTR* NTP-TR-253,83

CONSENSUS REPORTS: IARC Cancer Review: Animal Limited Evidence IMEMDT

36,69,85. NTP Carcinogenesis Studies (gavage); Clear Evidence: mouse, rat NTPTR* NTP-TR-253,83. Reported in EPA TSCA Inventory.

SAFETY PROFILE: Suspected carcinogen with experimental carcinogenic and tumorigenic data. A poison by ingestion. Moderately toxic by skin contact. A skin irritant. When heated to decomposition it emits acrid smoke and fumes.

LBG000   CAS: 303-34-4
LASIOCARPINE
mf: $C_{21}H_{33}NO_7$ mw: 411.55

PROP: An alkaloid isolated from *H. Lasiocarpum*.

SYNS: HELIOTRIDINE ESTER with LASIOCARPUM and ANGELIC ACID ◇ NCI-C01478 ◇ RCRA WASTE NUMBER U143

TOXICITY DATA with REFERENCE
CAR: ipr-rat TDLo:470 mg/kg/56W-I   CNREA8 32,908,72
CAR: orl-rat TD:546 mg/kg/2Y-C   NCITR* NCI-CG-TR-39,78
CAR: orl-rat TD:760 mg/kg/48W-C   BJCAAI 37,289,78
CAR: orl-rat TD:1310 mg/kg/2Y-C   NCITR* NCI-CG-TR-39,78
CAR: orl-rat TDLo:255 mg/kg/2Y-C   NCITR* NCI-CG-TR-39,78
MUT: mma-sat 200 µg/plate   MUREAV 68,211,79
MUT: msc-hmn:lym 60 µmol/L   ENMUDM 4,304,82
MUT: sln-dmg-orl 750 ppm   ENMUDM 7,349,85
MUT: sln-dmg-par 20 µmol/L   ZEVBA5 91,74,60
MUT: trn-dmg-orl 750 ppm   ENMUDM 7,349,85

CONSENSUS REPORTS: IARC Cancer Review: GROUP 2B IMEMDT 7,56,87; Animal Limited Evidence IMEMDT 10,281,76. NCI Carcinogenesis Bioassay (feed); No Evidence: mouse, rat NCITR* NCI-CG-TR-39,78. EPA Genetic Toxicology Program.

SAFETY PROFILE: Suspected carcinogen with experimental carcinogenic data. Poison by ingestion, intravenous, intraperitoneal, parenteral, and possibly other routes. Human mutation data reported. When heated to decomposition it emits toxic fumes of NO_x.

LCF000   CAS: 7439-92-1
LEAD
af: Pb   aw: 207.19

PROP: Bluish-gray, soft metal. Mp: 327.43°, bp: 1740°, d: 11.34 @ 20°/4°. vap press: 1 mm @ 973°.

SYNS: C.I. 77575 ◊ C.I. PIGMENT METAL 4 ◊ GLOVER ◊ LEAD FLAKE ◊ LEAD S2 ◊ OLOW (POLISH) ◊ OMAHA ◊ OMAHA & GRANT ◊ SI ◊ SO

TOXICITY DATA with REFERENCE
MUT: cyt-hmn-unr 50 μg/m³   MUREAV 147,301,85
MUT: cyt-mky-orl 42 mg/kg/30W   TOLED5 8,165,81
MUT: cyt-rat-ihl 23 μg/m³/16W   GTPZAB 26(10),38,82

CONSENSUS REPORTS: IARC Cancer Review: GROUP 2B IMEMDT 7,230,87; Animal Inadequate Evidence IMEMDT 23,325,80. Lead and its compounds are on the Community Right-To-Know List. Reported in EPA TSCA Inventory. EPA Genetic Toxicology Program.

OSHA PEL: TWA 0.05 mg(Pb)/m³   ACGIH TLV: TWA 0.15 mg(Pb)/m³; BEI: 50 μg(lead)/L in blood; 150 μg(lead)/g creatinine in urine. DFG MAK: 0.1 mg/m³; BAT: 70 μg(lead)/L in blood, 30 μg(lead)/L in blood of women less than 45 years old. NIOSH REL: TWA (Inorganic Lead) 0.10 mg(Pb)/m³

SAFETY PROFILE: Suspected carcinogen. Poison by ingestion. Moderately toxic by intraperitoneal route. Human systemic effects by ingestion and inhalation: loss of appetite, anemia, malaise, insomnia, headache, irritability, muscle and joint pains, tremors, flaccid paralysis without anesthesia, hallucinations and distorted perceptions, muscle weakness, gastritis and liver changes. Severe toxicity can cause sterility, abortion and neonatal mortality and morbidity. An experimental teratogen. Experimental reproductive effects. Human mutation data reported.'' Flammable in the form of dust when exposed to heat or flame. When heated to decomposition it emits highly toxic fumes of Pb.

LJE000   CAS: 8015-14-3
LYNDIOL
mf: $C_{21}H_{26}O_2 \cdot C_{20}H_{28}O$ mw:594.95

SYNS: LYNESTRENOL mixed with MESTRANOL ◊ LYNESTROL mixed with MESTRANOL ◊ LYNOESTRENOL mixed with MESTRANOL ◊ MESTRANOL mixed with LYNESTRENOL ◊ MESTRANOL mixed with LYNESTROL ◊ NORACYCLINE ◊ OVANON ◊ OVARIOSTAT (FRENCH) ◊ RESTOVAR ◊ SISTOMETRENOL

TOXICITY DATA with REFERENCE
CAR: orl-wmn TD:34 mg/kg/2Y-I:LIV
   HEGAD4 29,187,82
CAR: orl-wmn TDLo:32 mg/kg/130W-I:LIV
   MJAUAJ 2,223,78
NEO: orl-wmn TD:91 mg/kg/7Y-I:LIV
   NPMDAD 5,3014,76
NEO: orl-wmn TD:104 mg/kg/10Y-I:LIV
   MJAUAJ 2,223,78

CONSENSUS REPORTS: EPA Genetic Toxicology Program.

SAFETY PROFILE: Suspected human carcinogen producing liver tumors. An experimental teratogen. Human systemic effects by ingestion: dyspnea, nausea or vomiting, and fever. Experimental reproductive effects. Used as an oral contraceptive. When heated to decomposition it emits acrid smoke and irritating fumes.

MCA000   CAS: 71-58-9
MEDROXYPROGESTERONE ACETATE
mf: $C_{24}H_{34}O_4$ mw: 386.58

PROP: White to off-white, odorless, crystalline powder. Melting range 207-209°. Insol in water; freely sol in chloroform; sparingly sol in alc.

SYNS: 17-α-ACETOXY-6-α-METHYLPREGN-4-ENE-3,20-DIONE ◊ 17-ACETOXY-6-α-METHYLPROGESTERONE ◊ (6-α)-17-(ACETYLOXY)-6-METHYLPREG-4-ENE-3,20-DIONE ◊ DEPO-PROVERA ◊ FARLUTIN ◊ 17-α-HYDROXY-6-α-METHYLPREGN-4-ENE-3,20-DIONE ACETATE ◊ 17-HYDROXY-6-α-METHYLPREGN-4-ENE-3,20-DIONE ACETATE ◊ 17-α-HYDROXY-6-α-METHYLPROGESTERONE ACETATE ◊ 6-α-METHYL-17-α-ACETOXYPREGN-4-ENE-3,20-DIONE ◊ 6-α-METHYL-17-α-ACETOXYPROGESTERONE ◊ 6-α-METHYL-17-α-HYDROXYPROGESTERONE ACETATE ◊ 6-α-METHYL-4-PREGNENE-3,20-DION-17-α-OL ACETATE ◊ METIPREGNONE ◊ NOGEST ◊ ORAGEST ◊ PERLUTEX ◊ REPROMIX

TOXICITY DATA with REFERENCE
CAR: scu-mus TDLo:9600 mg/kg/1Y-I
   CALEDQ 33,215,86
NEO: ims-dog TDLo:30 mg/kg/26W-I
   36PYAS-,145,77
ETA: ims-dog TD:324 mg/kg/4Y-I   FESTAS 31,340,79
ETA: ims-dog TD:1240 mg/kg/4Y-I   FESTAS 31,340,79
MUT: dni-hmn:lym 50 μmol/L   PSEBAA 146,401,74

CONSENSUS REPORTS: IARC Cancer Review: Animal Limited Evidence IMEMDT

21,417,79; IMEMDT 6,157,74; Human Inadequate Evidence IMEMDT 21,417,79. Reported in EPA TSCA Inventory. EPA Genetic Toxicology Program.

SAFETY PROFILE: Suspected carcinogen with experimental carcinogenic, neoplastigenic, tumorigenic, and teratogenic data. Human systemic effects by intravenous route: increased intraocular pressure. Human teratogenic effects by an unspecified route: developmental abnormalities of the urogenital system. Human reproductive effects by multiple routes: spermatogenesis, menstrual cycle changes or disorders, postpartum effects, female fertility effects, abortion, newborn behavioral effects. Human mutation data reported. Experimental reproductive effects. A drug for the treatment of secondary amenorrhoea and dysfunctional uterine bleeding. When heated to decomposition it emits acrid smoke and irritating fumes.

MCB500   CAS: 3771-19-5
MELIPAN
mf: $C_{20}H_{22}O_3$ mw: 310.42

SYNS: 2-METHYL-2-(4-(1,2,3,4-TETRAHYDRO-1-NAPHTHALENYL)PHENOXY)PROPANOIC ACID ◇ α-METHYL-α-(p-1,2,3,4-TETRAHYDRONAPHTH-1-YLPHENOXY)PROPIONIC ACID ◇ 2-METHYL-2-(4-(1,2,3,4-TETRAHYDRO-1-NAPHTHYL)PHENOXY)PROPANOIC ACID ◇ 2-METHYL-2-(p-(1,2,3,4-TETRAHYDRO-1-NAPHTHYL)PHENOXY)PROPIONIC ACID ◇ NAFENOIC ACID ◇ NAFENOPIN ◇ SU-13437

TOXICITY DATA with REFERENCE
CAR: orl-mus TDLo:56 g/kg/81W-C   CNREA8
  36,1211,76
CAR: orl-rat TDLo:39 g/kg/92W-C   JNCIAM
  59,1645,77
ETA: orl-rat TD:33 g/kg/78W-C   CNREA8
  36,1211,76
MUT: dni-mus:oth 100 μmol/L   CNREA8 40,36,80
MUT: dns-rat:lvr 10 mg/L   CRNGDP 5,1033,84

CONSENSUS REPORTS: IARC Cancer Review: GROUP 2B IMEMDT 7,56,87; Human Limited Evidence IMEMDT 24,125,80; Animal Sufficient Evidence IMEMDT 24,125,80.

SAFETY PROFILE: Suspected carcinogen with experimental carcinogenic and tumorigenic data. Mutation data reported. A drug for the treatment of hypercholesterolemia or hypertriglyceridemia. When heated to decomposition it emits acrid smoke and irritating fumes.

MEI450   CAS: 72-43-5
METHOXYCHLOR
DOT: 2761
mf: $C_{16}H_{15}Cl_3O_2$ mw: 345.66
PROP: Crystals. Mp: 78°, vap d: 12.

SYNS: 2,2-BIS(p-ANISYL)-1,1,1-TRICHLOROETHANE ◇ 1,1-BIS(p-METHOXYPHENYL)-2,2,2-TRICHLOROETHANE ◇ 2,2-BIS(p-METHOXYPHENYL)-1,1,1-TRICHLOROETHANE ◇ CHEMFORM ◇ DIANISYLTRICHLORETHANE ◇ 2,2-DI-p-ANISYL-1,1,1-TRICHLOROETHANE ◇ p,p'-DIMETHOXYDIPHENYLTRICHLOROETHANE ◇ DIMETHOXY-DT ◇ DIMETHOXY-DDT ◇ 2,2-DI-(p-METHOXYPHENYL)-1,1,1-TRICHLOROETHANE ◇ DI(p-METHOXYPHENYL)-TRICHLOROMETHYL METHANE ◇ DMDT ◇ p,p'-DMDT ◇ ENT 1,716 ◇ MARALATE ◇ MARLATE ◇ METHOXCIDE ◇ METHOXO ◇ p,p'-METHOXYCHLOR ◇ METHOXY-DDT ◇ METOKSYCHLOR (POLISH) ◇ METOX ◇ MOXIE ◇ NCI-C00497 ◇ RCRA WASTE NUMBER U247 ◇ 1,1,1-TRICHLOR-2,2-BIS(4-METHOXY-PHENYL)-AETHAN (GERMAN) ◇ 1,1,1-TRICHLORO-2,2-BIS (p-ANISYL)ETHANE ◇ 1,1,1-TRICHLORO-2,2-BIS(p-METHOXYPHENOL)ETHANOL ◇ 1,1,1-TRICHLORO-2,2-BIS(p-METHOXYPHENYL)ETHANE ◇ 1,1,1-TRICHLORO-2,2-DI(4-METHOXYPHENYL)ETHANE ◇ 1,1'-(2,2,2-TRICHLOROETHYLIDENE)BIS(4-METHOXYBENZENE)

TOXICITY DATA with REFERENCE
CAR: orl-mus TDLo:56700 mg/kg/90W-C:
  TER   JCROD7 93,173,79
CAR: orl-rat TD:80 g/kg/2Y-C:TER   LIFSAK
  24,1367,79
CAR: orl-rat TD:72800 mg/kg/2Y-C   EVHPAZ
  36,205,80
CAR: orl-rat TD:87360 mg/kg/2Y-C   EVHPAZ
  36,205,80
CAR: orl-rat TDLo:18200 mg/kg/2Y-C:TER
  EVHPAZ 36,205,80
ETA: orl-dog TDLo:383 g/kg/3Y-C   EVHPAZ
  36,205,80
ETA: orl-mus TD:62622 mg/kg/2Y-C   EVHPAZ
  36,205,80
ETA: orl-rat TD:41 g/kg/2Y-C   TXAPA9
  11,88,67
ETA: orl-rat TD:10920 mg/kg/1Y-C   AIPTAK
  83,491,50
ETA: orl-rat TD:45500 mg/kg/1Y-C   AIPTAK
  83,491,50
MUT: cyt-ham-ipr 50 mg/kg   ARTODN 58,152,85
MUT: cyt-mus-orl 6 mg/kg/50D-I   FOMOAJ
  36,361,76
MUT: otr-mus:fbr 2 mg/L   JJIND8 67,1303,81
MUT: spm-rat-orl 28 g/kg/10W-C   PSEBAA
  176,187,84

CONSENSUS REPORTS: IARC Cancer Review: Animal No Evidence IMEMDT 20,-259,79; Animal Inadequate Evidence IMEMDT 5,193,74. NCI Carcinogenesis Bioassay (feed); No Evidence: mouse, rat NCITR* NCI-CG-TR-35,78. EPA Genetic Toxicology Program. Community Right-To-Know List.

OSHA PEL: (Transitional: TWA Total Dust: 10 mg/m^3; Respirable Fraction: 5 mg/m^3 TWA Total Dust: 10 mg/m^3; 5 mg/m^3 ACGIH TLV: TWA 10 mg/m^3 DFG MAK: 15 mg/m^3 DOT Classification: ORM-E; Label: None.

SAFETY PROFILE: Suspected carcinogen with experimental carcinogenic, tumorigenic, and teratogenic data. Moderately toxic by ingestion, intraperitoneal, and skin contact. Human systemic effects by skin contact: somnolence. Experimental reproductive effects. Mutation data reported. When heated to decomposition emits highly toxic fumes of Cl$^-$.

MFB400   CAS: 75965-74-1
7-METHOXY-2-NITRONAPHTHO(2,1-b) FURAN
mf: $C_{13}H_9NO_4$ mw: 243.23

SYNS: 2-NITRO-7-METHOXYNAPHTHO(2,1-b)FURAN ◇ R7000

TOXICITY DATA with REFERENCE
CAR: orl-rat TDLo: 210 mg/kg/91W-C   CRNGDP 7,1447,86
CAR: scu-rat TDLo: 24 mg/kg/36W-I   CALEDQ 35,59,87
CAR: skn-mus TDLo: 11967 μg/kg   JJCREP 78,565,87
ETA: scu-rat TD: 10 mg/kg/5W-I   PAACA3 25,96,84
ETA: scu-rat TD: 20 mg/kg/10W-I   PAACA3 25,96,84
ETA: scu-rat TD: 360 mg/kg/12W-I   CRNGDP 6,109,85
MUT: cyt-ham: lng 1 mg/L   MUREAV 157,53,85
MUT: dni-ckn: emb 500 μg/L   AMACCQ 23,328,83
MUT: mnt-ham: lng 100 μg/L   MUREAV 130,273,84
MUT: oms-ckn: emb 1 mg/L   AMACCQ 23,328,83
MUT: oms-ham: lng 4 mg/L   MUREAV 157,53,85
MUT: sce-ham: lng 100 μg/L   MUREAV 130,273,84

SAFETY PROFILE: Suspected carcinogen with experimental experimental carcinogenic and tumorigenic data. Mutation data reported. When heated to decomposition it emits toxic fumes of NO$_x$.

MFN275   CAS: 484-20-8
5-METHOXY PSORALEN
mf: $C_{12}H_8O_4$ mw: 216.20

PROP: Naturally occurring analog of psoralen and isomer of methoxsalen. Found in a wide variety of plants. Needles from alc. Mp: 188° (subl). Practically insol in boiling water; sltly sol in glacial acetic acid, chloroform, benzene, warm phenol. Sol in abs alc: 1 part in 60.

SYNS: BERGAPTEN ◇ 4-METHOXY-7H-FURO(3,2-g)(1)BENZOPYRAN-7-ONE ◇ PSORADERM

TOXICITY DATA with REFERENCE
MUT: dnd-esc 20 μmol/L   CBINA8 21,103,78
MUT: dnd-mam: lym 20 μmol/L   CBINA8 21,103,78
MUT: dnd-omi 20 μmol/L   CBINA8 21,103,78
MUT: dnd-omi 20 μmol/L   CBINA8 21,103,78
MUT: dnd-sal: spr 20 μmol/L   CBINA8 21,103,78

CONSENSUS REPORTS: IARC Cancer Review: GROUP 2A IMEMDT 7,242,87; Animal Inadequate Evidence IMEMDT 40,327,86; Human Inadequate Evidence IMEMDT 40,327,86.

SAFETY PROFILE: Suspected carcinogen. Mutation data reported. When heated to decomposition it emits acrid smoke and irritating fumes.

MGO500   CAS: 102-50-1
2-METHYL-p-ANISIDINE
mf: $C_8H_{11}NO$ mw: 137.20

SYNS: m-CRESIDINE ◇ 4-METHOXY-2-METHYLANILINE ◇ 4-METHOXY-2-METHYLBENZENAMINE ◇ 2-METHYL-4-METHOXYANILINE ◇ NCI-C02993

TOXICITY DATA with REFERENCE
CAR: orl-mus TDLo: 29800 mg/kg/53W-I   IARC** 27,91,82
CAR: orl-rat TD: 61600 mg/kg/77W-I   IARC** 27,91,82
CAR: orl-rat TDLo: 62 g/kg/77W-I   NCITR* NCI-CG-TR-105,78
ETA: orl-mus TD: 29 mg/kg/53W-I   NCITR* NCI-CG-TR-105,78
ETA: orl-mus TD: 14900 mg/kg/53W-I   IARC** 27,91,82
ETA: orl-rat TD: 31 g/kg/77W-I   NCITR* NCI-CG-TR-105,78
ETA: orl-rat TD: 30800 mg/kg/77W-I   IARC** 27,91,82
MUT: otr-rat: emb 51500 ng/plate   JJATDK 1,190,81

CONSENSUS REPORTS: IARC Cancer Review: Animal Inadequate Evidence IMEMDT

27,91,82. NCI Carcinogenesis Bioassay (gavage); Clear Evidence: rat NCITR* NCI-CG-
TR-105,78; (gavage); Inadequate Studies:
mouse NCITR* NCI-CG-TR-105,78. Reported
in EPA TSCA Inventory.

SAFETY PROFILE: Suspected carcinogen with
experimental carcinogenic and tumorigenic
data. Mutation data reported. When heated to
decomposition it emits toxic fumes of NO_x.

MGS750   CAS: 592-62-1
METHYL AZOXYMETHYL ACETATE
mf: $C_4H_8N_2O_3$ mw: 132.14

SYNS: MAM AC ◇ MAM ACETATE ◇ METHYLAZOXY-
METHANOL ACETATE ◇ (METHYL-ONN-AZOXY)METHA-
NOL, ACETATE (ESTER)

TOXICITY DATA with REFERENCE
CAR: ipr-mus TD: 120 mg/kg/22D-I   JJIND8
72,1181,84
CAR: ipr-mus TDLo: 60 mg/kg/11D-I   JJIND8
72,1181,84
CAR: ipr-rat LDLo: 50 mg/kg   CBINA8 17,291,77
CAR: ipr-rat TDLo: 35 mg/kg   CBINA8 17,291,77
CAR: ipr-rat TDLo: 180 mg/kg/9W-I   DIGEBW
14,311,76
CAR: ivn-rat TDLo: 35 mg/kg   CNREA8 42,1774,82
CAR: scu-mus TDLo: 200 mg/kg/10W-I
PSEBAA 161,347,79
CAR: scu-rat TDLo: 62 mg/kg/21D-I   JNCIAM
39,355,67
CAR: skn-mus TDLo: 1440 mg/kg/24W-I
GANNA2 72,886,81
NEO: scu-rat TDLo: 30 mg/kg   JJIND8 63,1089,79
ETA: ipr-mky TD: 992 mg/kg/7Y-I   JJIND8
65,177,80
ETA: ipr-mky TDLo: 776 mg/kg/5Y-I   JJIND8
65,177,80
ETA: ipr-mus TDLo: 180 mg/kg/18W-I   FEPRA7
34,827,75
ETA: ipr-rat TDLo: 35 mg/kg   CNREA8 37,4156,77
ETA: ipr-rat TDLo: 75 mg/kg/3W-I   JTSCDR
9,319,84
ETA: orl-mus TDLo: 240 mg/kg/12W-I   APJAAG
33,1197,83
ETA: orl-rat TDLo: 50 mg/kg/21D-C   JNCIAM
39,355,67
ETA: par-rat TDLo: 360 mg/kg/18W-I   CALEDQ
2,133,77
ETA: rec-mus TDLo: 360 mg/kg/18W-I   FEPRA7
34,827,75
ETA: rec-rat TDLo: 50 mg/kg/7D-C   GANNA2
64,93,73

ETA: scu-mus TD: 160 mg/kg/10W-I   CANCAR
54,18,84
ETA: scu-rat TD: 50 mg/kg/21D-I   JNCIAM
39,355,67
ETA: skn-mus TDLo: 1440 mg/kg/24W-I
GANNA2 73,358,82
MUT: dnd-gpg-scu 25 mg/kg   CALEDQ 29,293,85
MUT: dnd-hmn: fbr 7 μmol/L   PNASA6 80,7219,83
MUT: dnd-hmn: oth 1500 μmol/L/4H   PAACA3
21,69,80
MUT: dnd-rat-scu 25 mg/kg   CALEDQ 29,293,85
MUT: mma-esc 100 μg/plate   ENMUDM 6(Suppl
2),1,84
MUT: otr-hmn: fbr 7 μmol/L   PNASA6 80,7219,83

CONSENSUS REPORTS: EPA Genetic Toxicology Program.

SAFETY PROFILE: Suspected carcinogen with
experimental carcinogenic, neoplastigenic, tumorigenic, and teratogenic data. Poison by ingestion, intraperitoneal, and intravenous routes.
Experimental reproductive effects. Human mutation data reported. When heated to decomposition it emits toxic fumes of NO_x.

MHR200   CAS: 74-83-9
METHYL BROMIDE
DOT: 1062
mf: CH_3Br mw: 94.95

PROP: Colorless, transparent, volatile liquid
or gas; burning taste, chloroform-like odor. Bp:
3.56°, lel: 13.5%, uel: 14.5%, fp: −93°, flash
p: none, d: 1.732 @ 0°/0°, autoign temp: 998°F,
vap d: 3.27, vap press: 1824 mm @ 25°.

SYNS: BROM-METHAN (GERMAN) ◇ BROMO METHANE
◇ BROMO-O-GAS ◇ BROMOMETANO (ITALIAN)
◇ BROMURE de METHYLE (FRENCH) ◇ BROMURO di ME-
TILE (ITALIAN) ◇ BROOMMETHAAN (DUTCH) ◇ DAWSON
100 ◇ DOWFUME ◇ DOWFUME MC-2 SOIL FUMIGANT
◇ EDCO ◇ EMBAFUME ◇ FUMIGANT-1 (OBS.) ◇ HALON
1001 ◇ ISCOBROME ◇ KAYAFUME ◇ MB ◇ MBX
◇ MEBR ◇ METAFUME ◇ METHOGAS ◇ METHYLBROMID
(GERMAN) ◇ METYLU BROMEK (POLISH) ◇ MONOBROMO-
METHANE ◇ PESTMASTER (OBS.) ◇ PROFUME (OBS.)
◇ R 40B1 ◇ RCRA WASTE NUMBER U029 ◇ ROTOX
◇ TERABOL ◇ TERR-O-GAS 100 ◇ ZYTOX

TOXICITY DATA with REFERENCE
CAR: orl-rat TDLo: 3250 mg/kg/13W-I   TXAPA9
72,262,84
MUT: mma-sat 5 g/m³   MUREAV 116,185,83
MUT: mmo-klp 4750 mg/m³   MUREAV 155,41,85
MUT: mmo-sat 400 ppm   DHEFDK FDA-78-1046,78
MUT: msc-mus: lym 300 μg/L   MUREAV 155,41,85

MUT: sce-hmn:lym 43000 ppm   ENMUDM 7(Suppl 3),48,85

MUT: sln-dmg-ihl 150 mg/m³/6H   MUREAV 113,272,83

CONSENSUS REPORTS: IARC Cancer Review: GROUP 3 IMEMDT 7,245,87; Human Inadequate Evidence IMEMDT 41,187,86; Animal Limited Evidence IMEMDT 41,187,86. Reported in EPA TSCA Inventory. Community Right-To-Know List. EPA Extremely Hazardous Substances List.

OSHA PEL: (Transitional: CL 20 ppm (skin)) TWA 5 ppm (skin) ACGIH TLV: TWA 5 ppm (skin) DFG MAK: 5 ppm (20 mg/m³), Suspected Carcinogen. NIOSH REL: Reduce to lowest level DOT Classification: Poison A; Label: Poison Gas.

SAFETY PROFILE: Suspected carcinogen with experimental with experimental carcinogenic data. A human poison by inhalation. Human systemic effects by inhalation: anorexia, nausea or vomiting. Corrosive to skin; can produce severe burns. Human mutation data reported. A powerful fumigant gas which is one of the most toxic of the common organic halides. Mixtures of 10-15 percent with air may be ignited with difficulty. To fight fire, use foam, water, CO_2, dry chemical. When heated to decomposition it emits toxic fumes of Br^-.

MHW350   CAS: 71016-15-4
**N-3-METHYLBUTYL-N-1-METHYL
ACETONYLNITROSAMINE**
mf: $C_9H_{18}N_2O_2$ mw: 186.29

SYNS: 3-((ISOPENTYL)NITROSOAMINO)-2-BUTANONE ◇ MAMBNA

TOXICITY DATA with REFERENCE
CAR: orl-mus TDLo:8400 mg/kg/19W-C
   CCLCDY 7,329,85
CAR: orl-rat TDLo:21600 mg/kg/74W-C
   CCLCDY 7,329,85
NEO: orl-mus TD:19600 mg/kg/32W-C
   CCLCDY 7,329,85
ETA: orl-mus TD:8400 mg/kg/19W-C   CMJODS 97,311,84
ETA: orl-rat TD:27 g/kg/74W-C   CMJODS 97,311,84
MUT: mma-sat 2 g/L   CRNGDP 1,867,80
MUT: otr-ham:lng 500 mg/L   SSBSEF 25,738,82

SAFETY PROFILE: Suspected carcinogen with experimental carcinogenic, neoplastigenic, and

tumorigenic data. Mutation data reported. When heated to decomposition it emits toxic fumes of NO_x.

MIF765   CAS: 74-87-3
METHYL CHLORIDE
DOT: 1063
mf: CH_3Cl mw: 50.49

PROP: Colorless gas; ethereal odor and sweet taste. D: 0.918 @ 20°/4°, mp: −97°, bp: −23.7°, flash p: <32°F, lel: 8.1%, uel: 17%, autoign temp: 1170°F, vap d: 1.78. Sltly sol in water; miscible with chloroform, ether, glacial acetic acid, sol in alcohol.

SYNS: ARTIC ◇ CHLOOR-METHAAN (DUTCH) ◇ CHLOR-METHAN (GERMAN) ◇ CHLOROMETHANE ◇ CHLORURE de METHYLE (FRENCH) ◇ CLOROMETANO (ITALIAN) ◇ CLORURO di METILE (ITALIAN) ◇ METHYL-CHLORID (GERMAN) ◇ METYLU CHLOREK (POLISH) ◇ MONOCHLOROMETHANE ◇ RCRA WASTE NUMBER U045

TOXICITY DATA with REFERENCE
MUT: dlt-rat-ihl 3000 ppm/6H/5D-C   ENMUDM 6,392,84
MUT: dns-rat:spr 30 ppm/3H-C   ENMUDM 6,392,84
MUT: msc-hmn:lym 5 pph   MUREAV 155,75,85
MUT: oms-hmn:lym 3 pph   MUREAV 155,75,85
MUT: otr-ham:emb 6 mL/plate   EVSRBT 25,75,82
MUT: sce-hmn:lym 3 pph   MUREAV 155,75,85

CONSENSUS REPORTS: IARC Cancer Review: GROUP 3 IMEMDT 7,246,87; Human Inadequate Evidence IMEMDT 41,161,86; Animal Inadequate Evidence IMEMDT 41,161,86. Reported in EPA TSCA Inventory. EPA Genetic Toxicology Program.

OSHA PEL: (Transitional: TWA 100; CL 200 ppm; Pk 300 ppm/5M)TWA 50 ppm; STEL 100 ppm ACGIH TLV: TWA 50 ppm; STEL 100 ppm DFG MAK: 50 ppm (105 mg/m³); Suspected Carcinogen. NIOSH REL: (Monohalomethanes) TWA Reduce to lowest level.

DOT Classification: Flammable Gas; Label: Flammable Gas; IMO: Poison A; Label: Poison Gas and Flammable Gas.

SAFETY PROFILE: Suspected carcinogen. Very mildly toxic by inhalation. An experimental teratogen. Other experimental reproductive effects. Human mutation data reported. Human systemic effects by inhalation: convulsions, nausea or vomiting, and unspecified effects on the eye. Flammable gas. To fight fire, stop flow of gas and use CO_2, dry chemical or water spray. When heated to decomposition it emits highly toxic fumes of Cl^-.

MIJ750   CAS: 56-49-5
3-METHYLCHOLANTHRENE
mf: $C_{21}H_{16}$ mw: 268.37

PROP: Pale yellow needles from benzene. Mp: 176.5°, bp: 280° @ 80 mm, d: 1.28 @ 20°. Sol in benzene, xylene, toluene; sltly sol in amyl alc; insol in water.

SYNS: 1,2-DIHYDRO-3-METHYL-BENZ(j)ACEANTHRYL-ENE ◇ 3-MCA ◇ METHYLCHOLANTHRENE ◇ 20-METHYL-CHOLANTHRENE ◇ RCRA WASTE NUMBER U157

TOXICITY DATA with REFERENCE
CAR: icv-mus TDLo:46 mg/kg   AMPLAO 60,451,55
CAR: imp-mus TDLo:24 mg/kg   IJEBA6 22,195,84
CAR: imp-rat TDLo:20 mg/kg   CRNGDP 7,831,86
CAR: ims-mus TDLo:40 mg/kg   IJCAAR 19,126,82
CAR: ipl-rat TDLo:2 mg/kg   JJIND8 76,693,86
CAR: ipr-mus TDLo:5 mg/kg (17D post):TER   CRNGDP 6,1389,85
CAR: itr-dck TDLo:27 mg/kg   CNREA8 21,571,61
CAR: itr-mus TD:200 mg/kg/10W-I   PWPSA8 22,269,79
CAR: itr-mus TDLo:4 mg/kg   AJCAA7 35,538,39
CAR: ivn-mus TDLo:4 mg/kg   AJCAA7 35,538,39
CAR: orl-ham TDLo:1632 mg/kg/17W-I   PEXTAR 24,408,79
CAR: orl-mus TDLo:21 mg/kg (15-17D post): TER   TXAPA9 72,427,84
CAR: orl-mus TDLo:336 mg/kg   JJIND8 47,645,71
CAR: orl-rat TDLo:600 mg/kg (60D pre):TER   CNREA8 12,296,52
CAR: orl-rat TDLo:600 mg/kg (MGN):TER   CNREA8 12,296,52
CAR: scu-gpg TDLo:20 mg/kg/15D-I   CNREA8 22,1155,62
CAR: scu-mus TD:80 mg/kg   IJCNAW 27,501,81
CAR: scu-mus TDLo:20 mg/kg   JCREA8 102,245,82
CAR: scu-rat TDLo:8 mg/kg   HOIZAK 57,53,82
CAR: skn-mus TDLo:120 mg/kg (MGN):TER   BEXBAN 71,677,71
CAR: skn-mus TDLo:4800 µg/kg/2W-I   JTEHD6 14,115,84
CAR: skn-mus TDLo:76800 µg/kG (MGN)   BEXBAN 71,677,71
CAR: skn-rat TDLo:480 mg/kg/20W-I   GANNA2 61,367,70

NEO: imp-mus TD:2800 µg/kg   AJPAA4 16,287,40
NEO: ims-ckn TDLo:50 mg/kg/2W-I   BJCAAI 41,130,80
NEO: ipr-ckn TDLo:36 mg/kg/6W-I   GROWAH 27,199,63
NEO: ipr-mus TD:20 mg/kg   TXAPA9 72,313,84
NEO: ipr-mus TDLo:10 mg/kg   ARTODN 4,74,80
NEO: itr-rat TDLo:40 mg/kg   JJIND8 49,541,72
NEO: orl-mus TD:20 mg/kg   TXAPA9 72,313,84
NEO: orl-rat TD:1680 mg/kg/28W-I   13BYAH-,305,62
NEO: scu-mus TD:120 mg/kg/6W-I   IJCNAW 2,505,67
NEO: scu-mus TD:312 µg/kg   JJIND8 3,503,43
NEO: scu-mus TD:400 µg/kg   JJIND8 62,353,79
NEO: skn-mus TD:43 mg/kg/18W-I   CNREA8 33,832,73
ETA: ice-rat TDLo:22 mg/kg   CNREA8 29,1927,69
ETA: imp-cat TDLo:25 mg/kg   CANCAR 8,689,55
ETA: imp-dog TDLo:20 mg/kg   CANCAR 14,1127,61
ETA: imp-ham TDLo:48 mg/kg   CNREA8 19,93,59
ETA: ipl-mus TDLo:120 mg/kg   BAFEAG 27,706,38
ETA: ipl-rbt TDLo:100 mg/kg/9W-I   GANNA2 59,497,68
ETA: ipr-gpg TDLo:8 mg/kg   BJCAAI 27,445,73
ETA: irn-mus TDLo:32 mg/kg   CNREA8 22,1177,62
ETA: itr-rbt TDLo:800 mg/kg/12W-I   CNREA8 32,1209,72
ETA: itt-mus TDLo:40 mg/kg   BAFEAG 27,706,38
ETA: ivn-gpg TDLo:20 mg/kg   JJIND8 13,705,52
ETA: ivn-rat TDLo:5 mg/kg   AIHAAP 30,236,69
ETA: orl-rat TDLo:200 mg/kg   JJIND8 48,185,72
ETA: par-dog TDLo:90 mg/kg/18W-I   TIDZAH 38,317,80
ETA: par-rat TDLo:4 mg/kg   IJEBA6 9,296,71
ETA: scu-ham TDLo:4000 µg/kg   CNREA8 32,360,72
ETA: skn-ham TDLo:7700 mg/kg/40W-I   CNREA8 20,100,60
ETA: unr-mus TDLo:32 mg/kg   AOBIAR 1,325,60
MUT: cyt-ofs-ipr 10 mg/kg   CBPCBB 82,489,85
MUT: mma-mus:lym 2500 µg/L   ENMUDM 7(Suppl 3),10,85
MUT: otr-hmn:lng 500 µg/L/2W   GANNA2 74,615,83
MUT: otr-mus-skn 5000 ppm/12W-I   TUMOAB 71,1,85

CONSENSUS REPORTS: Reported in EPA TSCA Inventory. EPA Genetic Toxicology Program.

SAFETY PROFILE: Suspected carcinogen with experimental carcinogenic, neoplastigenic, and tumorigenic data. Poison by intravenous and intraperitoneal routes. Experimental teratogenic and reproductive effects. Human mutation data reported. When heated to decomposition it emits acrid smoke and irritating fumes.

MJE500   CAS: 892-17-1
11-METHYL-15,16-DIHYDRO-17-OXOCYCLOPENTA(a)PHENANTHRENE
mf: $C_{18}H_{14}O$ mw: 246.32

SYNS: 15,16-DIHYDRO-11-METHYLCYCLOPENTA(a)PHE-
NANTHREN-17-ONE ◇ 15,16-DIHYDRO-11-METHYL-17H-
CYCLOPENTA(a)PHENANTHREN-17-ONE ◇ 11-METHYL-
15,16-DIHYDRO-17H-CYCLOPENTA(a)PHENANTHREN-17-
ONE

TOXICITY DATA with REFERENCE
CAR: orl-rat TDLo: 150 mg/kg   BJCAAI 40,914,79
CAR: scu-mus TD: 400 mg/kg   CRNGDP 3,677,82
CAR: scu-mus TD: 2000 mg/kg   PEXTAR 11,69,69
CAR: scu-mus TDLo: 360 mg/kg   PEXTAR 11,69,69
CAR: skn-mus TD: 200 mg/kg/50W-I   BJCAAI 38,148,78
CAR: skn-mus TDLo: 16 mg/kg   BJCAAI 40,914,79
NEO: skn-mus TD: 16 mg/kg/4D-C   BJCAAI 38,148,78
NEO: skn-mus TD: 46 mg/kg/19W-I   CNREA8 33,832,73
NEO: skn-mus TD: 120 mg/kg/30W-I   CNREA8 43,2261,83
ETA: skn-mus TD: 125 mg/kg/52W-I   NATUAS 210,1281,66
ETA: skn-mus TD: 125 mg/kg/52W-I   NATUAS 210,1281,66
MUT: dnd-mus-ims 120 mg/kg   CNREA8 41,4115,81
MUT: dnd-mus: oth 10 μg/L   CNREA8 43,2261,83
MUT: mma-sat 1 μg/plate   CNREA8 40,882,80

CONSENSUS REPORTS: EPA Genetic Toxicology Program.

SAFETY PROFILE: Suspected carcinogen with experimental carcinogenic, neoplastigenic, and tumorigenic data. Mutation data reported. When heated to decomposition it emits acrid smoke and irritating fumes.

MJP450   CAS: 75-09-2
METHYLENE CHLORIDE
DOT: 1593
mf: CH_2Cl_2 mw: 84.93

PROP: Colorless, volatile liquid; odor of chloroform. Bp: 39.8°, lel: 15.5% in O_2, uel: 66.4% in O_2, fp: −96.7°, d: 1.326 @ 20°/4°, autoign temp: 1139°F, vap press: 380 mm @ 22°, vap d: 2.93, refr index: 1.424 @ 20L. Sol in water; misc with alcohol, acetone, chloroform, ether, carbon tetrachloride.

SYNS: AEROTHENE MM ◇ CHLORURE de METHYLENE (FRENCH) ◇ DCM ◇ DICHLOROMETHANE (MAK, DOT) ◇ FREON 30 ◇ METHANE DICHLORIDE ◇ METHYLENE BICHLORIDE ◇ METHYLENE DICHLORIDE ◇ METYLENU CHLOREK (POLISH) ◇ NCI-C50102 ◇ RCRA WASTE NUMBER U080 ◇ SOLMETHINE

TOXICITY DATA with REFERENCE
CAR: ihl-mus TCLo: 2000 ppm/5H/2Y-C   NTPTR* NTP-TR-306,86
CAR: ihl-rat TCLo: 3500 ppm/6H/2Y-I   FAATDF 4,30,84
ETA: ihl-rat TCLo: 500 ppm/6H/2Y   TXAPA9 48,A185,79
MUT: cyt-ham: ovr 5 g/L   MUREAV 116,361,83
MUT: dni-ham: lng 5000 ppm/1H-C   MUREAV 81,203,81
MUT: dni-hmn: fbr 5000 ppm/1H-C   MUREAV 81,203,81
MUT: sce-ham: lng 5000 ppm/1H-C   MUREAV 81,203,81

CONSENSUS REPORTS: IARC Cancer Review: GROUP 2B IMEMDT 7,194,87; Human Inadequate Evidence IMEMDT 41,43,86; Animal Sufficient Evidence IMEMDT 41,43,86; Animal Inadequate Evidence IMEMDT 20,-449,79. NTP Carcinogenesis Studies (inhalation); Clear Evidence: mouse, rat NTPTR* NTP-TR-306,86. Reported in EPA TSCA Inventory. EPA Genetic Toxicology Program. Community Right-To-Know List.

OSHA PEL: (Transitional: TWA 500 ppm; CL 1000 ppm; Pk 2000/5M/2H)   ACGIH TLV: TWA 50 ppm, Suspected Human Carcinogen   DFG MAK: 100 ppm (360 mg/m³); BAT: 5% CO-Hb in blood at end of shift; Suspected Carcinogen.   NIOSH REL: (Methylene Chloride) Reduce to lowest feasible level.   DOT Classification: Poison B; Label: St. Andrews Cross.

SAFETY PROFILE: Suspected carcinogen with experimental carcinogenic and tumorigenic data. Poison by intravenous route. Moderately toxic by ingestion, subcutaneous, and intraperitoneal routes. Mildly toxic by inhalation. Human systemic effects by ingestion and inhalation: paresthesia, somnolence, altered sleep time, convulsions, euphoria, and change in cardiac rate. An experimental teratogen. Experimental reproductive effects. An eye and severe skin irritant. Human mutation data reported. It is flammable in the range of 12-19 percent in air but ignition is difficult. When heated to decomposition it emits highly toxic fumes of phosgene and Cl^-.

MKN000   CAS: 60-34-4
METHYL HYDRAZINE
DOT: 1244
mf: CH_6N_2 mw: 46.09

PROP: Colorless, hydroscopic liquid; ammonia-like odor. D: 0.874 @ 25°, mp: −20.9°, bp: 87.8°, vap d: 1.6, flash p: 73.4°F, fp: −52.4°, autoign temp: 196°, lel: 2.5%, uel: 97 ±2%. Sltly sol in water, sol in alc, hydrocarbons, and ether. Misc with H_2O, hydrazine. Strong reducing agent.

SYNS: HYDRAZOMETHANE ◇ 1-METHYL HYDRAZINE ◇ METHYLHYDRAZINE (DOT) ◇ METYLOHYDRAZYNA (POLISH) ◇ MMH ◇ MONOMETHYL HYDRAZINE ◇ RCRA WASTE NUMBER P068

TOXICITY DATA with REFERENCE
CAR: ihl-mus TCLo:2 ppm/6H/1Y-I   NTIS**
  AD-A154-659
CAR: ihl-rat TCLo:20 ppb/6H/1Y-I   NTIS**
  AD-A154-659
CAR: orl-ham TDLo:3000 mg/kg/47W-C
  CNREA8 33,2744,73
NEO: ihl-ham TCLo:5 ppm/6H/1Y-I   NTIS**
  AD-A154-659
NEO: orl-mus TDLo:10 g/kg/1Y-C   IJCNAW
  9,109,72
ETA: ipr-mus TDLo:72 mg/kg/8W-I   JNCIAM
  42,337,69
MUT: dlt-rat-ipr 1075 mg/kg/5D-I   NTIS**
  AD-A041-973
MUT: dnd-hmn:fbr 116 pmol   NTIS**
  AD-A092-249
MUT: dns-ham:ovr 1 μmol/L   NTIS**
  AD-A075-605
MUT: mmo-sat 2 μmol/plate/48H   MUREAV
  54,167,78

CONSENSUS REPORTS: Community Right-To-Know List. EPA Extremely Hazardous Substances List. Reported in EPA TSCA Inventory. EPA Genetic Toxicology Program.

OSHA PEL: CL 0.2 ppm (skin))   ACGIH

TLV: CL 0.2 ppm; Suspected Human Carcinogen   NIOSH REL: CL 0.08 mg/m³/2H   DOT Classification: Flammable Liquid; Label: Flammable Liquid, Corrosive.

SAFETY PROFILE: Suspected carcinogen with experimental carcinogenic, neoplastigenic, tumorigenic, and teratogenic data. Poison by inhalation, ingestion, skin contact, intraperitoneal, subcutaneous, and intravenous routes. Experimental reproductive effects. Human mutation data reported. Corrosive to skin, eyes, and mucous membranes. May self-ignite in air. Very dangerous fire hazard when exposed to heat or flame. To fight fire, use alcohol foam, CO_2, dry chemical. Explosive in the form of vapor when exposed to heat or flame. A powerful reducing agent. It is hypergolic with many oxidants (e.g., dinitrogen tetraoxide and hydrogen peroxide). When heated to decomposition it emits toxic fumes of NO_x.

MME500   CAS: 10546-24-4
3-METHYL-2-NAPHTHYLAMINE
mf: $C_{11}H_{11}N$ mw: 157.23

TOXICITY DATA with REFERENCE
CAR: scu-ham TDLo:4440 mg/kg/94W-I
  JJIND8 67,481,81
ETA: scu-mus TDLo:4100 mg/kg/17W-I
  CUSCAM 33,45,64
ETA: scu-rat TDLo:1800 mg/kg/18W-I
  CUSCAM 33,45,64

SAFETY PROFILE: Suspected carcinogen with experimental carcinogenic and tumorigenic data. When heated to decomposition it emits toxic fumes of NO_x.

MMG000   CAS: 129-15-7
2-METHYL-1-NITROANTHRAQUINONE
mf: $C_{15}H_9NO_4$ mw: 267.25

SYNS: 2-METHYL-1-NITRO-9,10-ANTHRACENEDIONE ◇ NCI-C01923 ◇ 1-NITRO-2-METHYLANTHRAQUINONE ◇ 1-N-2-MA (RUSSIAN)

TOXICITY DATA with REFERENCE
CAR: orl-mus TD:19 g/kg/37W-C   IJCNAW
  19,117,77
CAR: orl-mus TDLo:10 g/kg/41W-C   IJCNAW
  19,117,77
CAR: orl-rat TDLo:45 g/kg/2Y-C   NCITR*
  NCI-CG-TR-29,78
NEO: orl-rat TD:19 g/kg/77W-C   TOLED5 4,71,79
NEO: orl-rat TD:20 g/kg/78W-C   NCITR*
  NCI-CG-TR-29,78

MUT: mma-sat 3 μg/plate   ENMUDM 8(Suppl 7),1,86
MUT: mmo-sat 33 μg/plate   ENMUDM 8(Suppl 7),1,86

CONSENSUS REPORTS: IARC Cancer Review: GROUP 2B IMEMDT 7,56,87; Animal Sufficient Evidence IMEMDT 27,205,82. NCI Carcinogenesis Bioassay (feed); Clear Evidence: rat NCITR* NCI-CG-TR-29,78; (feed); Clear Evidence: mouse IJCNAW 19,117, 77.

SAFETY PROFILE: Suspected carcinogen with experimental carcinogenic and neoplastigenic data. Moderately toxic by intraperitoneal route. Mutation data reported. When heated to decomposition it emits toxic fumes of NO_x.

MMP000   CAS: 70-25-7
N-METHYL-N′-NITRO-N-NITROSOGUANIDINE
mf: $C_2H_5N_5O_3$ mw: 147.12

PROP: Crystals.

SYNS: METHYLNITRONITROSOGUANIDINE ◇ 1-METHYL-3-NITRO-1-NITROSOGUANIDINE ◇ N-METHYL-N′-NITRO-N-NITROSOGUANIDINE, not exceeding 25 grams in one outside packaging (DOT) ◇ 1-METHYL-1-NITROSO-3-NITROGUANIDINE ◇ METHYLNITROSOGUANIDINE ◇ N-METHYL-N-NITROSO-N′-NITROGUANIDINE ◇ N-METHYL-N-NITROSONITROGUANIDIN (GERMAN) ◇ N-METYLO-N′-NITRO-N-NITROZOGOUANIDYNY (POLISH) ◇ MNG ◇ MNNG ◇ N′-NITRO-N-NITROSO-N-METHYLGUANIDINE ◇ N-NITROSO-N-METHYLNITROGUANIDINE ◇ NSC 9369 ◇ RCRA WASTE NUMBER U163

TOXICITY DATA with REFERENCE
CAR: orl-mus TD: 6220 mg/kg/88W-C   CCLCDY 4,161,82
CAR: orl-mus TDLo: 1984 mg/kg/70W-I   CCLCDY 4,161,82
CAR: orl-rat TD: 107 mg/kg/35W-C   JCROD7 100,1,81
CAR: orl-rat TD: 125 mg/kg/10W-I   VOONAW 26(2),62,80
CAR: orl-rat TD: 155 mg/kg/11W-I   CNREA8 35,2469,75
CAR: orl-rat TD: 250 mg/kg   GANNA2 75,362,84
CAR: orl-rat TD: 280 mg/kg/8W-C   CNREA8 43,1334,83
CAR: orl-rat TD: 438 mg/kg/25W-I   IJCNAW 32,253,83
CAR: orl-rat TD: 651 mg/kg/34W-C   VOONAW 28(9),34,82
CAR: orl-rat TD: 697 mg/kg/12W-C   CALEDQ 22,315,84

CAR: orl-rat TD: 13500 mg/kg/78W-C   JJIND8 70,1067,83
CAR: orl-rat TDLo: 500 μg/kg   GANNA2 69,805,78
CAR: par-rat TDLo: 400 μg/kg   ARTODN 45,227,80
CAR: rec-rat TDLo: 128 mg/kg/32W-I   JNCIAM 50,927,73
CAR: scu-rat TDLo: 400 μg/kg   ARTODN 45,227,80
CAR: skn-mus TDLo: 54 mg/kg/30W-I   BANRDU 12,397,82
CAR: skn-rat TDLo: 720 mg/kg/60W-I   ARGEAR 55,117,85
ETA: ivn-rat TDLo: 25 mg/kg (15D preg): TER   KFIZAO 84,23,75
ETA: ivn-rat TDLo: 60 mg/kg   EJCAAH 16,395,80
ETA: orl-dog TDLo: 725 mg/kg/45W-I   JCROD7 97,51,80
ETA: orl-ham TDLo: 592 mg/kg/27W-C   CNREA8 30,1444,70
ETA: orl-rbt TDLo: 743 mg/kg/26W-C   HGANAO 16,321,76
ETA: scu-mus TDLo: 48 mg/kg   BJCAAI 23,757,69
MUT: dnd-hmn: fbr 20 μmol/L   ENMUDM 7,267,85
MUT: dns-mus: lvr 1 μmol/L   TOPADD 12,119,84
MUT: msc-rat: lvr 50 μmol/L   ENMUDM 2,259,80
MUT: otr-ham: fbr 500 μg/L   CNREA8 42,1274,82
MUT: otr-mus: emb 300 μg/L   PMRSDJ 5,659,85
MUT: sce-hmn: hla 300 nmol/L   CRNGDP 5,593,84
MUT: sce-mus: lym 100 μg/L   JCHODP 13,1,83

CONSENSUS REPORTS: IARC Cancer Review: GROUP 2A IMEMDT 7,248,87; Animal Sufficient Evidence IMEMDT 4,183,74. Reported in EPA TSCA Inventory. EPA Genetic Toxicology Program.

DOT Classification: Flammable Solid; Label: Flammable Solid.

SAFETY PROFILE: Suspected carcinogen with experimental carcinogenic, tumorigenic, and teratogenic data. Poison by ingestion, intraperitoneal, and intravenous routes. Moderately toxic by subcutaneous route. Experimental reproductive effects. Human mutation data reported. An explosive sensitive to heat or impact. Flammable when exposed to heat or flame, can react vigorously with oxidizing materials. When heated to decomposition it emits very toxic fumes of NO_x.

MMS200   CAS: 60153-49-3
3-METHYLNITROSAMINO-PROPIONITRILE
mf: $C_4H_7N_3O$ mw: 113.14

SYNS: MNPN ◊ PROPANENITRILE, 3-(METHYLNITRO-SOAMINO)-

TOXICITY DATA with REFERENCE
CAR: scu-rat TDLo: 103 mg/kg/20W-I   CNREA8
47,467,87
ETA: scu-rat TD: 622 mg/kg   PAACA3 25,99,84

CONSENSUS REPORTS: IARC Cancer Review: GROUP 2B IMEMDT 7,56,87, Animal Sufficient Evidence IMEMDT 37,263,85

SAFETY PROFILE: Suspected carcinogen with experimental carcinogenic and tumorigenic data. When heated to decomposition it emits toxic fumes of NO_x.

MMS500 CAS: 64091-91-4
4-(N-METHYL-N-NITROSAMINO)-1-(3-PYRIDYL)-1-BUTANONE
mf: $C_{10}H_{13}N_3O_2$ mw: 207.26

SYNS: 4-(N-METHYL-N-NITROSOAMINO)-4-(3-PYRI-DYL)-1-BUTANONE ◊ N-METHYL-N-NITROSO-4-OXO-4-(3-PYRIDYL)BUTYL AMINE ◊ 4-(NITROSOAMINO-N-METHYL)-1-(3-PYRIDYL)-1-BUTANONE ◊ 4-(N-NITROSO-N-METHYLAMINO)-1-(3-PYRIDYL)-1-BUTANONE ◊ NNK

TOXICITY DATA with REFERENCE
CAR: scu-ham TDLo: 1504 mg/kg/25W-I
IAPUDO 41,309,82
CAR: scu-rat TD: 2700 mg/kg/20W-I   CNREA8
40,298,80
CAR: scu-rat TD: 2700 mg/kg/20W-I   CNREA8
40,298,80
CAR: scu-rat TD: 68396 μg/kg/20W-I   CNREA8
46,498,86
CAR: scu-rat TDLo: 68396 μg/kg/20W-I
CRNGDP 8,291,87
NEO: ipr-mus TD: 880 mg/kg/7W-I   JNCIAM
60,819,78
NEO: ipr-mus TDLo: 880 mg/kg/I   IARCCD
19,395,78
NEO: scu-ham TD: 93 mg/kg   CRNGDP 4,1287,83
MUT: dnd-rat-ipr 1200 mg/kg/12D-C   CNREA8
46,1280,86
MUT: mma-sat 1 μmol/plate   CRNGDP 4,305,83

CONSENSUS REPORTS: IARC Cancer Review: GROUP 2B IMEMDT 7,56,87; Animal Sufficient Evidence IMEMDT 37,209,85. EPA Genetic Toxicology Program.

SAFETY PROFILE: Suspected carcinogen with experimental carcinogenic and neoplastigenic data. Mutation data reported. When heated to decomposition it emits toxic fumes of NO_x.

MMW775 CAS: 25355-61-7
1-METHYL-1-NITROSO-3-(p-CHLOROPHENYL)UREA
mf: $C_8H_8ClN_3O_2$ mw: 213.64

SYNS: 1-(p-CHLOROPHENYL)-3-METHYL-3-NITRO-SOUREA ◊ 3-(p-CHLOROPHENYL)-1-METHYL-1-NITRO-SOUREA ◊ N-METHYL-N'-(p-CHLOROPHENYL)-N-NITRO-SOUREA

TOXICITY DATA with REFERENCE
CAR: orl-rat TDLo: 598 mg/kg/20W-I   ARGEAR
56,9,86
CAR: skn-mus TDLo: 634 mg/kg/7W-I   CNREA8
44,1027,84
MUT: cyt-ham: lng 10 μmol/L   IAPUDO 31,797,80
MUT: mmo-sat 66 μmol/L   CNREA8 39,5147,79
MUT: sce-ham: lng 10 μmol/L   IAPUDO 31,685,80

SAFETY PROFILE: Suspected carcinogen with experimental carcinogenic data. Mutation data reported. When heated to decomposition it emits toxic fumes of Cl^- and NO_x.

MMX250 CAS: 615-53-2
N-METHYL-N-NITROSOETHYLCARBAMATE
mf: $C_4H_8N_2O_3$ mw: 132.14

SYNS: ETHYL ESTER of METHYLNITROSO-CARBAMIC ACID ◊ N-METHYL-N-NITROSOCARBAMIC ACID, ETHYL ESTER ◊ METHYLNITROSOURETHAN (GERMAN) ◊ METHYLNITROSOURETHANE ◊ N-METHYL-N-NITROSO-URETHANE ◊ MNU ◊ NITROSOMETHYLURETHAN (GER-MAN) ◊ NITROSOMETHYLURETHANE ◊ N-NITROSO-N-METHYLURETHANE ◊ NMUM ◊ NMUT ◊ RCRA WASTE NUMBER U178

TOXICITY DATA with REFERENCE
CAR: orl-ham TDLo: 220 mg/kg/28W-I: TER
JNCIAM 37,389,66
CAR: scu-mus TDLo: 5 mg/kg (9D preg): TER
CNREA8 34,3373,74
ETA: ipc-rat TDLo: 100 mg/kg (21D preg):
TER   IARCCD 4,1,73
ETA: ipr-mus TD: 25 mg/kg   CNREA8 45,2802,85
ETA: ipr-mus TD: 176 mg/kg/22W-I   APJAAG
29,421,79
ETA: ipr-mus TDLo: 25 mg/kg   CNREA8 30,11,70
ETA: ipr-rat TD: 50 mg/kg   BJCAAI 22,316,68
ETA: ipr-rat TDLo: 35 mg/kg/13W-I   JTEHD6
8,501,81
ETA: ivn-rat TDLo: 19 mg/kg/38W-I   XENOBH
3,271,73
ETA: ivn-rat TDLo: 20 mg/kg (15D preg): TER
IARCCD 4,100,73

ETA: orl-gpg TD:920 mg/kg/92W-I   PPTCBY 2,73,72

ETA: orl-gpg TDLo:500 mg/kg/57W-I   ZEKBAI 72,167,68

ETA: orl-rat TD:70 mg/kg/20W-I   FCTOD7 21,601,83

ETA: orl-rat TD:280 mg/kg/20W-I   FCTOD7 21,601,83

ETA: orl-rat TD:1175 mg/kg/47W-I   XENOBH 3,271,73

ETA: orl-rat TD:1200 mg/kg/49W-C   ARZNAD 19,1077,69

ETA: orl-rat TDLo:23 mg/kg/4W-I   NATUAS 199,190,63

ETA: scu-gpg TDLo:130 mg/kg/47W-I   ZEKBAI 72,167,68

ETA: scu-ham TDLo:84 mg/kg/22W-I   AJPAA4 50,639,67

MUT: cyt-ham:lng 6800 μg/L   GMCRDC 27,95,81
MUT: dnd-gpg-ipr 30 mg/kg   CBINA8 20,77,78
MUT: dnd-gpg:oth 20 mmol/L   CBINA8 20,77,78
MUT: mmo-asn 3 μg/plate   MUREAV 97,293,82
MUT: pic-esc 1 mg/L   TCMUE9 1,91,84

CONSENSUS REPORTS: IARC Cancer Review: GROUP 2B IMEMDT 7,56,87; Animal Sufficient Evidence IMEMDT 4,211,74. Reported in EPA TSCA Inventory. EPA Genetic Toxicology Program.

SAFETY PROFILE: Suspected carcinogen with experimental carcinogenic, tumorigenic, and teratogenic data. Poison by ingestion, intraperitoneal, subcutaneous, and intravenous routes. Moderately toxic by inhalation. Experimental reproductive effects. Mutation data reported. Has been implicated as a transplacental brain carcinogen. Combustible when exposed to heat, sparks, open flame, and powerful oxidizers. Explodes when heated. A storage hazard. When heated to decomposition it emits toxic fumes of NO_x.

MMY500   CAS: 21561-99-9
1-METHYL-1-NITROSO-3-PHENYLUREA
mf: $C_8H_9N_3O_2$ mw: 179.20

SYNS: N-METHYL-N-NITROSO-N'-PHENYLUREA ◇ METHYLPHENYLNITROSOUREA ◇ N-METHYL-N'-PHENYL-N-NITROSOUREA ◇ MPNU ◇ NITROSOMETHYLPHENYLUREA ◇ 3-PHENYL-1-METHYL-1-NITROSOHARNSTOFF (GERMAN)

TOXICITY DATA with REFERENCE
CAR: orl-rat TDLo:750 mg/kg/32W-I   CALEDQ 4,299,78

CAR: skn-mus TDLo:532 mg/kg/7W-I   CNREA8 44,1027,84

ETA: orl-rat TD:450 mg/kg/20W-I   MVMZA8 33,128,78

ETA: orl-rat TD:650 mg/kg/26W-I   EXPTAX 17,394,79

ETA: orl-rat TD:650 mg/kg/26W-I   IAPUDO 31,685,80

ETA: orl-rat TD:650 mg/kg/W-I   ARTODN 4,25,80

ETA: scu-rat TDLo:250 mg/kg   MVMZA8 33,128,78

MUT: cyt-ham:lng 10 μmol/L   IAPUDO 31,797,80
MUT: mmo-sat 66 μmol/L   CNREA8 39,5147,79
MUT: sce-ham:lng 10 μmol/L   IAPUDO 31,797,80

SAFETY PROFILE: Suspected carcinogen with experimental carcinogenic and tumorigenic data. Mutation data reported. When heated to decomposition it emits toxic fumes of NO_x.

MNA000   CAS: 924-46-9
N-METHYL-N-NITROSO-1-PROPANAMINE
mf: $C_4H_{10}N_2O$ mw: 102.16

SYNS: METHYL-N-PROPYLNITROSAMINE ◇ METHYL-PROPYLNITROSOAMINE ◇ MPN ◇ NITROSOMETHYL-N-PROPYLAMINE ◇ NITROSOMETHYLPROPYLAMINE

TOXICITY DATA with REFERENCE
CAR: scu-ham TDLo:1250 mg/kg/24W-I   ZKKOBW 90,141,77
CAR: scu-mus TDLo:185 mg/kg/48W-I   ZKKOBW 90,253,77
NEO: scu-ham TDLo:100 mg/kg/(14D preg)   ZKKOBW 90,119,77
NEO: scu-rat TDLo:240 mg/kg/45W-I   JNCIAM 54,937,75
ETA: orl-rat TDLo:160 mg/kg/23W-I   JJIND8 70,959,83
ETA: scu-ham TD:225 mg/kg/18W-I   JNCIAM 51,287,73
MUT: hma-mus/esc 1180 μmol/L   CRNGDP 2,909,81
MUT: mma-esc 196 mmol/L   CRNGDP 2,909,81
MUT: mma-ham:lng 10 mmol/L   CNREA8 37,1044,77
MUT: mma-sat 500 nmol/plate   ZKKOBW 86,293,76
MUT: msc-ham:lng 700 μmol/L   50EYAN-,241,83
MUT: pic-esc 50 mg/L   TCMUE9 1,91,84

CONSENSUS REPORTS: EPA Genetic Toxicology Program.

SAFETY PROFILE: Suspected carcinogen with experimental carcinogenic, neoplastigenic, and tumorigenic data. Poison by subcutaneous route. Experimental reproductive effects. Mutation data reported. When heated to decomposition it emits toxic fumes of NO$_x$.

MPW500   CAS: 56-04-2
6-METHYLTHIOURACIL
mf: C$_5$H$_6$N$_2$OS   mw: 142.19

PROP: Bitter crystals or colorless liquid; odor of onions. Decomp @ 326-331°, sublimes readily. Very sltly sol in ether, cold water, alkaline hydroxides, NH$_3$; sltly sol in alc, acetone. Almost insol in benzene, chloroform.

SYNS: ALKIRON ◊ ANTIBASON ◊ BASECIL ◊ BASETHYRIN ◊ 2,3-DIHYDRO-6-METHYL-2-THIOXO-4(1H)-PYRIMIDINONE ◊ 2-MERCAPTO-4-HYDROXY-6-METHYLPYRIMIDINE ◊ 2-MERCAPTO-6-METHYLPYRIMID-4-ONE ◊ 2-MERCAPTO-6-METHYL-4-PYRIMIDONE ◊ METACIL ◊ METHIACIL ◊ METHIOCIL ◊ 6-METHYL-2-THIO-2,4-(1H3H)PYRIMIDINEDIONE ◊ METHYLTHIOURACIL ◊ 4-METHYL-2-THIOURACIL ◊ 6-METHYL-2-THIOURACIL ◊ 4-METHYLURACIL ◊ 6-METIL-TIOURACILE (ITALIAN) ◊ MTU ◊ MURACIL ◊ ORCANON ◊ PROSTRUMYL ◊ RCRA WASTE NUMBER U164 ◊ STRUMACIL ◊ THIMECIL ◊ THIOMECIL ◊ 2-THIO-6-METHYL-1,3-PYRIMIDIN-4-ONE ◊ 6-THIO-4-METHYLURACIL ◊ THIOMIDIL ◊ 2-THIO-4-OXO-6-METHYL-1,3-PYRIMIDINE ◊ THIORYL ◊ THIOTHYMIN ◊ THIOTHYRON ◊ THIURYL ◊ THYREONORM ◊ THYREOSTAT ◊ THYRIL ◊ TIOMERACIL ◊ TIORALE M ◊ TIOTIRON ◊ USAF EK-6454

TOXICITY DATA with REFERENCE
CAR: orl-rat TDLo: 9100 mg/kg/2Y-C   CNREA8 19,870,59
NEO: orl-mus TDLo: 196 g/kg/1Y-C   CANCAR 40,2188,77
NEO: orl-rat TD: 27783 mg/kg/60W-I   BJCAAI 4,223,50
ETA: orl-rat TD: 53750 mg/kg/65W-I   BJCAAI 7,181,53

CONSENSUS REPORTS: IARC Cancer Review: GROUP 2B IMEMDT 7,56,87; Animal Sufficient Evidence IMEMDT 7,53,74. Reported in EPA TSCA Inventory.

SAFETY PROFILE: Suspected carcinogen with experimental carcinogenic, neoplastigenic, tumorigenic, and teratogenic data. Poison by intraperitoneal route. Moderately toxic by ingestion. Human teratogenic and reproductive effects by an unspecified route: developmental abnormalities of the endocrine system and effects on newborn including neonatal measures or effects. Experimental reproductive effects. Used to treat hyperthyroidism. When heated to decomposition it emits very toxic fumes of NO$_x$ and SO$_x$.

MQY325   CAS: 63642-17-1
MNCO
mf: C$_7$H$_{14}$N$_4$O$_4$ mw: 218.25

SYNS: NΔ-(N-METHYL-N-NITROSOCARBAMOYL)-l-ORNITHINE ◊ N^5-(METHYLNITROSOCARBAMOYL)-l-ORNITHINE ◊ N^5-(N-METHYL-N-NITROSOCARBAMOYL)-l-ORNITHINE

TOXICITY DATA with REFERENCE
CAR: ipr-ham TD: 3924 mg/kg/6W-I   JJIND8 71,1327,83
CAR: ipr-ham TDLo: 2616 mg/kg/12W-I   JJIND8 71,1327,83
CAR: ipr-rat TDLo: 1870 mg/kg/26W-I   JEPTDQ 4(1),117,80
ETA: ipr-ham TDLo: 1308 mg/kg/6W-I   CALEDQ 8,163,79
MUT: dnd-ham: oth 218 mg/L   JJIND8 71,1327,83
MUT: dnd-rat-ipr 1 mmol/kg   CRNGDP 5,555,84
MUT: otr-ham-par 2616 mg/kg/12W-I   JJIND8 71,1327,83

SAFETY PROFILE: Suspected carcinogen with experimental carcinogenic and tumorigenic data. Mutation data reported. When heated to decomposition it emits toxic fumes of NO$_x$.

MRH000   CAS: 315-22-0
MONOCROTALINE
mf: C$_{16}$H$_{23}$NO$_6$ mw: 325.40

PROP: Prisms from absolute ethanol. Decomp @ 197-198°.

SYNS: CROTALINE ◊ 14,19-DIHYDRO-12,13-DIHYDROXY(13-α,14-α)-20-NORCROTALANAN-11,15-DIONE ◊ MONOCRATILIN ◊ NCI-C56462 ◊ NSC 28693

TOXICITY DATA with REFERENCE
CAR: scu-rat TDLo: 130 mg/kg/1Y-I   JNCIAM 56,787,76
MUT: cyt-hmn: lvr 50 mg/L   BJCAAI 14,637,60
MUT: dnd-rat-ipr 5 mg/kg   CNREA8 44,1505,84
MUT: dnr-esc 1 g/L   CRNGDP 2,189,81
MUT: dns-ham: lvr 2 μmol/L   CNREA8 45,3125,85
MUT: dns-rat: lvr 2 μmol/L   CNREA8 45,3125,85
MUT: sce-ham: lng 2500 μg/L   MUREAV 142,209,85

CONSENSUS REPORTS: IARC Cancer Review: Animal Limited Evidence IMEMDT 10,291,76. EPA Genetic Toxicology Program.

SAFETY PROFILE: Suspected carcinogen with experimental carcinogenic data. Poison by ingestion, intravenous, intraperitoneal, subcutaneous, and possibly other routes. Human mutation data reported. When heated to decomposition it emits toxic fumes of NO_x.

NAM000   CAS: 2243-62-1
1,5-NAPHTHALENEDIAMINE
mf: $C_{10}H_{10}N_2$ mw: 158.22

SYNS: 1,5-DIAMINONAPHTHALENE ◊ 1,5-NAPHTHYLENEDIAMINE ◊ NCI-C03021

TOXICITY DATA with REFERENCE
CAR: orl-mus TD:288 g/kg/2Y-C   NCITR*
    NCI-CG-TR-143,78
CAR: orl-mus TDLo:120 g/kg/2Y-C   NCITR*
    NCI-CG-TR-143,78
CAR: orl-mus TDLo:721 g/kg/1Y-C   IARC**
    27,127,82
CAR: orl-mus TDLo:1442 g/kg/1Y-C   IARC**
    27,127,82
CAR: orl-rat TDLo:721 g/kg/1Y-C   IARC**
    27,127,82
NEO: orl-rat TDLo:54 g/kg/2Y-C:TER   NCITR*
    NCI-CG-TR-143,78
ETA: orl-rat TD:18 g/kg/88W-C:TER   NCITR*
    NCI-CG-TR-143,78
ETA: orl-rat TDLo:361 g/kg/1Y-C   IARC**
    27,127,82
MUT: mma-sat 33300 ng/plate   ENMUDM 7(Suppl 5),1,85
MUT: mma-sat 33300 ng/plate   ENMUDM 7(Suppl 5),1,85
MUT: otr-rat:emb 5200 ng/plate   JJATDK 1,190,81

CONSENSUS REPORTS: IARC Cancer Review: Animal Limited Evidence IMEMDT 27,127,82. NCI Carcinogenesis Bioassay (feed); Clear Evidence: mouse, rat NCITR* NCI-CG-TR-143,78. EPA Genetic Toxicology Program.

SAFETY PROFILE: Suspected carcinogen with experimental carcinogenic, neoplastigenic, tumorigenic, and teratogenic data. Mutation data reported. When heated to decomposition it emits toxic fumes of NO_x.

NAT500   CAS: 192-65-4
NAPHTHO(1,2,3,4-def)CHRYSENE
mf: $C_{24}H_{14}$ mw: 302.38

SYNS: DB(a,e)P ◊ DIBENZO(a,e)PYRENE ◊ 1,2,4,5-DIBENZOPYRENE

TOXICITY DATA with REFERENCE
NEO: skn-mus TDLo:312 mg/kg/52W-I
    ZEKBAI 68,137,66
ETA: scu-mus TDLo:72 mg/kg/9W-I   COREAF
    259,3899,64

CONSENSUS REPORTS: IARC Cancer Review: GROUP 2B IMEMDT 7,56,87; Animal Sufficient Evidence IMEMDT 32,327,83; IMEMDT 3,201,73.

SAFETY PROFILE: Suspected carcinogen with experimental neoplastigenic and tumorigenic data. When heated to decomposition it emits acrid smoke and irritating fumes.

NCX500   CAS: 6018-89-9
NICKEL ACETATE TETRAHYDRATE
mf: $C_4H_6O_4 \cdot Ni \cdot 4H_2O$ mw: 248.89

TOXICITY DATA with REFERENCE
MUT: cyt-mus:mmr 100 μmol/L   MUREAV
    68,337,79

CONSENSUS REPORTS: Nickel and its compounds are on the Community Right-To-Know List.

OSHA PEL: (Transitional: TWA 1 mg/m³) TWA 0.1 mg (Ni)/m³ ACGIH TLV: TWA 0.1 mg(Ni)/m³; (Proposed: TWA 0.05 mg(Ni)/m³; Human Carcinogen)   NIOSH REL: (Inorganic Nickel) TWA 0.015 mg(Ni)/m³

SAFETY PROFILE: Suspected carcinogen. Poison by intraperitoneal route. Mutation data reported. When heated to decomposition it emits acrid smoke and irritating fumes.

NDA000   CAS: 7791-20-0
NICKEL(II) CHLORIDE HEXAHYDRATE (1:2:6)
mf: $Cl_2Ni \cdot 6H_2O$ mw: 237.73

PROP: A: Yellow, deliquescent scales; b: monoclinic, green crystals. A: $NiCl_2$, b: $NiCl_2 \cdot 6H_2O$; mw (a): 129.60, mw (b): 237.70, mp (a): sublimes, bp (a): 987°, d (a): 3.55, vap press: 1 mm @ 671°.

TOXICITY DATA with REFERENCE
MUT: cyt-mus:mmr 100 μmol/L   MUREAV
    68,337,79
MUT: sce-ham:fbr 32 mg/L   MUREAV 104,141,82

CONSENSUS REPORTS: Nickel and its compounds are on the Community Right-To-Know List.

OSHA PEL: (Transitional: TWA 1 mg/m^3) TWA 0.1 mg (Ni)/m^3 ACGIH TLV: TWA 0.1 mg(Ni)/m^3; (Proposed: TWA 0.05 mg(Ni)/m^3; Human Carcinogen) NIOSH REL: (Inorganic Nickel) TWA 0.015 mg(Ni)/m^3

SAFETY PROFILE: Suspected carcinogen. Poison by intraperitoneal and intravenous routes. Mutation data reported. When heated to decomposition it emits very toxic fumes of Cl$^-$.

NDB500   CAS: 557-19-7
NICKEL CYANIDE (solid)
DOT: 1653
mf: C$_2$N$_2$Ni   mw: 110.75

PROP: Apple-green plates or powder.

SYNS: NICKEL CYANIDE (DOT) ◇ RCRA WASTE NUMBER P074

CONSENSUS REPORTS: Cyanide and its compounds, as well as nickel and its compounds, are on the Community Right-To-Know List. Reported in EPA TSCA Inventory.

OSHA PEL: (Transitional: TWA 1 mg/m^3) TWA 0.1 mg (Ni)/m^3 ACGIH TLV: TWA 0.1 mg(Ni)/m^3; (Proposed: TWA 0.05 mg(Ni)/m^3; Human Carcinogen) DOT Classification: Poison B; Label: Poison.

SAFETY PROFILE: Suspected carcinogen. A poison. When heated to decomposition it emits very toxic fumes of CN$^-$.

NDC000   CAS: 14708-14-6
NICKEL(II) FLUOBORATE
mf: B$_2$F$_8$•Ni   mw: 232.33

SYN: NICKEL BOROFLUORIDE ◇ NICKEL FLUOROBORATE ◇ NICKELOUS TETRAFLUOROBORATE ◇ NICKEL(II) TETRAFLUOROBORATE ◇ TL 1091

CONSENSUS REPORTS: Nickel and its compounds are on the Community Right-To-Know List. Reported in EPA TSCA Inventory.

OSHA PEL: (Transitional: TWA 1 mg/m^3) TWA 0.1 mg (Ni)/m^3; 2.5 mg(F)/m^3 ACGIH TLV: TWA 0.1 mg(Ni)/m^3; (Proposed: TWA 0.05 mg(Ni)/m^3; Human Carcinogen) NIOSH REL: (Inorganic Nickel) TWA 0.015 mg(Ni)/m^3

SAFETY PROFILE: Suspected carcinogen. Moderately toxic by ingestion and inhalation. When heated to decomposition it emits very toxic fumes of F$^-$.

NDC500   CAS: 10028-18-9
NICKEL(II) FLUORIDE (1:2)
mf: F$_2$Ni   mw: 96.71

PROP: Green crystals. D: 4.63. Sltly water-sol; decomp by boiling water; insol in alc, ether.

SYNS: NICKEL DIFLUORIDE ◇ NICKELOUS FLUORIDE

CONSENSUS REPORTS: Nickel and its compounds are on the Community Right-To-Know List. Reported in EPA TSCA Inventory.

OSHA PEL: (Transitional: TWA 1 mg/m^3) TWA 0.1 mg (Ni)/m^3; 2.5 mg(F)/m^3 ACGIH TLV: TWA 0.1 mg(Ni)/m^3; (Proposed: TWA 0.05 mg(Ni)/m^3; Human Carcinogen) NIOSH REL: (Inorganic Nickel) TWA 0.015 mg(Ni)/m^3

SAFETY PROFILE: Suspected carcinogen. Poison by intravenous route. When heated to decomposition it emits toxic fumes of F$^-$.

NDD000   CAS: 26043-11-8
NICKEL(II) FLUOSILICATE (1:1)
mf: F$_6$Si•Ni   mw: 200.80

SYN: HEXAFLUOROSILICATE (2−), NICKEL

CONSENSUS REPORTS: Nickel and its compounds are on the Community Right-To-Know List. Reported in EPA TSCA Inventory.

OSHA PEL: (Transitional: TWA 1 mg/m^3) TWA 0.1 mg (Ni)/m^3 ACGIH TLV: TWA 1 mg(Ni)/m^3; (Proposed: TWA 0.05 mg(Ni)/m^3; Human Carcinogen) NIOSH REL: (Inorganic Nickel) TWA 0.015 mg(Ni)/m^3

SAFETY PROFILE: Suspected carcinogen. Poison by ingestion. When heated to decomposition it emits toxic fumes of F$^-$.

NDD500   CAS: 56668-59-8
NICKEL-GALLIUM ALLOY

PROP: Nickel (60%) - gallium (40%) alloy (JDREAF 29,1023,60).

SYN: GALLIUM-NICKEL ALLOY

TOXICITY DATA with REFERENCE
ETA: imp-rat TDLo:86 mg/kg/30W-C JDREAF 39,1023,60

CONSENSUS REPORTS: Nickel and its compounds are on the Community Right-To-Know List.

OSHA PEL: TWA 1 mg(Ni)/m^3 ACGIH TLV: TWA 1 mg(Ni)/m^3; (Proposed: TWA 0.05

mg(Ni)/m^3;   Human   Carcinogen)   NIOSH REL: (Inorganic Nickel) TWA 0.015 mg(Ni)/ m^3

SAFETY PROFILE: Suspected carcinogen with experimental tumorigenic data.

NDE500   CAS: 59978-65-3
NICKEL IRON SULFIDE
mf: FeNi$_4$S$_4$ mw: 418.93

SYNS: IRON NICKEL SULFIDE ◇ NICKEL-IRON SULFIDE MATTE

TOXICITY DATA with REFERENCE
CAR: ims-rat TD:400 mg/kg   IAPUDO 53,127,84
NEO: ims-rat TD:1472 mg/kg   PAACA3 17,11,76
NEO: ims-ratTDLo:147mg/kg   RCOCB814,319,76

CONSENSUS REPORTS: Nickel and its compounds are on the Community Right-To-Know List.

OSHA PEL: TWA 1 mg(Ni)/m^3 ACGIH TLV: TWA 1 mg(Ni)/m^3; (Proposed: TWA 0.05 mg(Ni)/m^3;   Human   Carcinogen)   NIOSH REL: (Inorganic Nickel) TWA 0.015 mg(Ni)/ m^3

SAFETY PROFILE: Suspected carcinogen with experimental carcinogenic and neoplastigenic data. When heated to decomposition it emits toxic fumes of SO$_x$.

NDG000   CAS: 13138-45-9
NICKEL(II) NITRATE (1:2)
DOT: 2725
mf: N$_2$O$_6$•Ni   mw: 182.73

PROP: Green, deliquescent crystals. Mp: 56.7°, bp: 136.7°, d: 2.05.

SYNS: NICKEL NITRATE (DOT) ◇ NITRIC ACID, NICKEL(II) SALT

TOXICITY DATA with REFERENCE
MUT: dlt-mus-unr 56 mg/kg   MUREAV 97,180,82

CONSENSUS REPORTS: Nickel and its compounds are on the Community Right-To-Know List. Reported in EPA TSCA Inventory.

OSHA PEL: (Transitional: TWA 1 mg/m^3) TWA 0.1 mg (Ni)/m^3 ACGIH TLV: TWA 0.1 mg(Ni)/m^3; (Proposed: TWA 0.05 mg(Ni)/ m^3; Human Carcinogen)   NIOSH REL: (Inorganic Nickel) TWA 0.015 mg(Ni)/m^3 DOT Classification: Oxidizer; Label:Oxidizer.

SAFETY PROFILE: Suspected carcinogen. Poison by intravenous route. Experimental repro-

ductive effects. Mutation data reported. A powerful oxidizer. When heated to decomposition it emits very toxic fumes of NO$_x$.

NDG500   CAS: 13478-00-7
NICKEL(II) NITRATE, HEXAHYDRATE (1:2:6)
mf: N$_2$O$_6$•Ni•6H$_2$O   mw: 290.85

PROP: Green, deliquescent crystals. Mp: 56.7°, bp: 136.7°, d: 2.05. Sol in 0.4 parts H$_2$O, alc. Keep well closed.

SYNS: NICKEL(2+) NITRATE, HEXAHYDRATE ◇ NITRIC ACID, NICKEL(2+) SALT, HEXAHYDRATE

CONSENSUS REPORTS: Nickel and its compounds are on the Community Right-To-Know List.

OSHA PEL: (Transitional: TWA 1 mg/m^3) TWA 0.1 mg (Ni)/m^3 ACGIH TLV: TWA 0.1 mg(Ni)/m^3; (Proposed: TWA 0.05 mg(Ni)/ m^3; Human Carcinogen)   NIOSH REL: (Inorganic Nickel) TWA 0.015 mg(Ni)/m^3

SAFETY PROFILE: Suspected carcinogen. Moderately toxic by ingestion. When heated to decomposition it emits toxic fumes of NO$_x$.

NDH000   CAS: 7718-54-9
NICKELOUS CHLORIDE
DOT: 9139
mf: Cl$_2$Ni   mw: 129.61

SYNS: NICKEL CHLORIDE (DOT) ◇ NICKEL(II) CHLORIDE (1:2)

TOXICITY DATA with REFERENCE
MUT: cyt-ham-ipr 10 mg/kg   BLOAAO 38,1107,83
MUT: cyt-ham:ovr 3200 nmol/L   CNREA8 45,2320,85
MUT: dnr-esc 200 mg/L   CRNGDP 2,189,81
MUT: mmo-esc 25 mg/L   MUREAV 38,3,76
MUT: mmo-omi 500 μg/L   FOMIAZ 28,17,83
MUT: mmo-smc 1 mmol/L   CPBTAL 33,1571,85
MUT: msc-ham:lng 800 μmol/L   MUREAV 68,259,79
MUT: sln-smc 1 mmol   MUTAEX 1,21,86

CONSENSUS REPORTS: Nickel and its compounds are on the Community Right-To-Know List. Reported in EPA TSCA Inventory. EPA Genetic Toxicology Program.

OSHA PEL: (Transitional: TWA 1 mg/m^3) TWA 0.1 mg (Ni)/m^3 ACGIH TLV: TWA 0.1 mg(Ni)/m^3; (Proposed: TWA 0.05 mg(Ni)/

m³; Human Carcinogen) NIOSH REL: (Inorganic Nickel) TWA 0.015 mg(Ni)/m³ DOT Classification: ORM-E; Label: None.

SAFETY PROFILE: Suspected carcinogen. Poison by ingestion, intravenous, intramuscular, and intraperitoneal routes. An experimental teratogen. Experimental reproductive effects. Mutation data reported. When heated to decomposition it emits very toxic fumes of Cl⁻.

NDH500
CAS: 1314-06-3
NICKEL PEROXIDE
mf: Ni_2O_3 mw: 165.42

PROP: Gray-black powder. Mp: $-O_2$ @ 600°, d: 4.83. Decomp about 600° into NiO and O_2. Insol in H_2O; very sltly sol in cold acid, dissolved by hot HCl evolving Cl_2; dissolved by hot H_2SO_4 or HNO_3 evolving O_2.

SYNS: DINICKEL TRIOXIDE ◇ NICKELIC OXIDE ◇ NICKEL OXIDE ◇ NICKEL OXIDE PEROXIDE ◇ NICKEL SISQUIOXIDE ◇ NICKEL TRIOXIDE

TOXICITY DATA with REFERENCE
MUT: otr-mus:emb 500 μmol/L   PAACA3
   24,100,83

CONSENSUS REPORTS: Nickel and its compounds are on the Community Right-To-Know List. Reported in EPA TSCA Inventory.

OSHA PEL: (Transitional: TWA 1 mg/m³) TWA 0.1 mg (Ni)/m³ ACGIH TLV: TWA 1 mg(Ni)/m³; (Proposed: TWA 0.05 mg(Ni)/m³; Human Carcinogen) NIOSH REL: (Inorganic Nickel) TWA 0.015 mg(Ni)/m³

SAFETY PROFILE: Suspected carcinogen. Poison by subcutaneous route. Mutation data reported.

NDI000
CAS: 14220-17-8
NICKEL POTASSIUM CYANIDE
mf: $C_4N_4Ni•2K$ mw: 240.99

SYNS: DIPOTASSIUM NICKEL TETRACYANIDE ◇ DIPOTASSIUM TETRACYANONICKELATE ◇ POTASSIUM TETRACYANONICKELATE ◇ POTASSIUM TETRACYANONICKELATE(II)

TOXICITY DATA with REFERENCE
MUT: cyt-mus:mmr 1 mmol/L/48H   MUREAV
   67,221,79

CONSENSUS REPORTS: Nickel and its compounds, as well as cyanide and its compounds, are on the Community Right-To-Know List. Reported in EPA TSCA Inventory.

OSHA PEL: (Transitional: TWA 1 mg/m³) TWA 0.1 mg (Ni)/m³ ACGIH TLV: TWA 0.1 mg(Ni)/m³; (Proposed: TWA 0.05 mg(Ni)/m³; Human Carcinogen) NIOSH REL: (Inorganic Nickel) TWA 0.015 mg(Ni)/m³

SAFETY PROFILE: Suspected carcinogen. Poison by ingestion. Mutation data reported. When heated to decomposition it emits very toxic fumes of NO_x, K_2O and CN⁻.

NDJ000
CAS: 13520-61-1
NICKEL(2+) SALT PERCHLORIC ACID HEXAHYDRATE
mf: $Cl_2O_8•Ni•6H_2O$ mw: 365.73

SYN: NICKEL(2+) PERCHLORATE, HEXAHYDRATE

CONSENSUS REPORTS: Nickel and its compounds are on the Community Right-To-Know List.

OSHA PEL: (Transitional: TWA 1 mg/m³) TWA 0.1 mg (Ni)/m³ ACGIH TLV: TWA 0.1 mg(Ni)/m³; (Proposed: TWA 0.05 mg(Ni)/m³; Human Carcinogen) NIOSH REL: TWA 15 μg(Ni)/m³

SAFETY PROFILE: Suspected carcinogen. Poison by intraperitoneal route. A powerful oxidizer. Mixtures with 2,2-dimethoxypropane explode when heated above 65°C. When heated to decomposition it emits toxic fumes of Cl⁻.

NDK000
CAS: 13770-89-3
NICKEL (II) SULFAMATE
mf: $H_4N_2NiO_6S_2$ mw: 250.89

CONSENSUS REPORTS: Nickel and its compounds are on the Community Right-To-Know List. Reported in EPA TSCA Inventory.

OSHA PEL: (Transitional: TWA 1 mg/m³) TWA 0.1 mg (Ni)/m³ ACGIH TLV: TWA 0.1 mg(Ni)/m³; (Proposed: TWA 0.05 mg(Ni)/m³; Human Carcinogen) NIOSH REL: (Inorganic Nickel) TWA 0.015 mg(Ni)/m³

SAFETY PROFILE: Suspected carcinogen. Poison by intraperitoneal route. When heated to decomposition it emits very toxic fumes of SO_x and NO_x.

NDK500
CAS: 7786-81-4
NICKEL SULFATE
DOT: 9141
mf: $O_4S•Ni$ mw: 154.77

PROP: Cubic yellow crystals. Mp: $-SO_3$ @ 840°, d: 3.68.

SYNS: NCI-C60344 ◇ NICKELOUS SULFATE ◇ NICKEL(II) SULFATE (1:1) ◇ NICKEL(II) SULFATE ◇ NICKEL SULFATE(1:1) ◇ NICKEL(2+)SULFATE(1:1) ◇ SULFURIC ACID, NICKEL(2+)SALT ◇ SULFURIC ACID, NICKEL(2+) SALT (1:1)

TOXICITY DATA with REFERENCE

ETA: imp-rat TDLo: 95 mg/kg/78W-C   PAACA3 5,50,64

MUT: dnd-ham:emb 380 μmol/L   CNREA8 39,193,79

MUT: mmo-smc 100 mmol/L   MUREAV 117,149,83

MUT: mrc-smc 100 mmol/L   MUREAV 117,149,83

MUT: otr-ham:emb 380 μmol/L   CNREA8 39,193,79

MUT: sce-hmn:leu 23 μmol/L   DMBUAE 27,40,80

CONSENSUS REPORTS: Nickel and its compounds are on the Community Right-To-Know List. Reported in EPA TSCA Inventory. EPA Genetic Toxicology Program.

OSHA PEL: (Transitional: TWA 1 mg/m^3) TWA 0.1 mg (Ni)/m^3 ACGIH TLV: TWA 0.1 mg(Ni)/m^3; (Proposed: TWA 0.05 mg(Ni)/ m^3; Human Carcinogen)   NIOSH REL: (Inorganic Nickel) TWA 0.015 mg(Ni)/m^3 DOT Classification: ORM-E; Label: None.

SAFETY PROFILE: Suspected carcinogen with experimental tumorigenic data. Poison by intravenous, intraperitoneal, and subcutaneous routes. Human mutation data reported. A human skin irritant. When heated to decomposition it emits very toxic fumes of SO$_x$.

NDL000   CAS: 10101-97-0
NICKEL(II) SULFATE HEXAHYDRATE (1:1:6)
mf: NiO$_4$S•$_6$H$_2$O   mw: 262.89

SYNS: NICKEL MONOSULFATE HEXAHYDRATE ◇ NICKEL SULFATE HEXAHYDRATE ◇ NICKEL (II) SULFATE HEXAHYDRATE ◇ NICKEL SULPHATE HEXAHYDRATE ◇ SULFURIC ACID, NICKEL(2+) SALT, HEXAHYDRATE

TOXICITY DATA with REFERENCE

MUT: cyt-ham:emb 5 mg/L   ENMUDM 3,597,81

MUT: cyt-hmn:lym 5 mg/L   ENMUDM 3,597,81

MUT: otr-ham:emb 5 mg/L   DTESD7 8,259,80

MUT: sce-ham:emb 1 mg/L   ENMUDM 3,597,81

MUT: sce-ham:fbr 50 mg/L   MUREAV 104,141,82

MUT: sce-hmn:lym 2500 μg/L   ENMUDM 3,597,81

CONSENSUS REPORTS: Nickel and its compounds are on the Community Right-To-Know List. EPA Genetic Toxicology Program.

OSHA PEL: (Transitional: TWA 1 mg/m^3) TWA 0.1 mg (Ni)/m^3 ACGIH TLV: TWA 0.1 mg(Ni)/m^3; (Proposed: TWA 0.05 mg(Ni)/ m^3; Human Carcinogen)   NIOSH REL: (Inorganic Nickel) TWA 0.015 mg(Ni)/m^3

SAFETY PROFILE: Suspected carcinogen. Poison by intravenous and subcutaneous routes. Experimental reproductive effects. Human mutation data reported. When heated to decomposition it emits toxic fumes of SO$_x$.

NDL500   CAS: 12035-39-1
NICKEL TITANIUM OXIDE
mf: NiO$_3$Ti   mw: 154.61

SYNS: NICKEL-TITANATE ◇ TITANIUM NICKEL OXIDE

TOXICITY DATA with REFERENCE

CAR: ims-rat TDLo: 210 mg/kg/91W-I   NCIUS* PH 43-69-886,DEC,68

ETA: imp-rat TDLo: 200 mg/kg   JJIND8 67,965,81

ETA: ims-rat TD: 945 mg/kg/91W-I   NCIUS* PH 43-64-886,Aug,69

CONSENSUS REPORTS: Nickel and its compounds are on the Community Right-To-Know List. Reported in EPA TSCA Inventory.

OSHA PEL: TWA 1 mg(Ni)/m^3 ACGIH TLV: TWA 0.1 mg(Ni)/m^3; (Proposed: TWA 0.05 mg(Ni)/m^3; Human Carcinogen)   NIOSH REL: (Inorganic Nickel) TWA 0.015 mg(Ni)/ m^3

SAFETY PROFILE: Suspected carcinogen with experimental carcinogenic and tumorigenic data.

NDY000   CAS: 555-84-0
NIFURADENE
mf: C$_8$H$_8$N$_4$O$_4$ mw: 224.20

PROP: Lemon-yellow solid from nitromethane. Mp: 261.5-263° (decomp).

SYNS: NF 246 ◇ 1-(((5-NITRO-2-FURANYL)MEHTY-LENE)AMINO)-2-IMIDAZOLIDINONE ◇ N-(5-NITRO-2-FUR-FURYLIDENE)-1-AMINO-2-IMIDAZOLIDONE ◇ 1-((5-NITRO-FURFURYLIDENE)AMINO)-2-IMIDAZOLIDINONE ◇ N-(5-NITRO-2-FURFURYLIDENEAMINO)-2-IMIDAZOAIDI-NONE ◇ NSC-6470 ◇ OXAFURADENE ◇ OXYFURADENE ◇ RENAFUR

TOXICITY DATA with REFERENCE

CAR: orl-rat TDLo: 34 g/kg/46W-C   JNCIAM 51,403,73

CONSENSUS REPORTS: IARC Cancer Review: Animal Limited Evidence IMEMDT 7,181,74.

SAFETY PROFILE: Suspected carcinogen with experimental carcinogenic data. Moderately toxic by ingestion and intraperitoneal routes. When heated to decomposition it emits toxic fumes of NO_x.

NDY500   CAS: 3570-75-0
NIFURTHIAZOLE
mf: $C_8H_6N_4O_4S$ mw: 254.24

PROP: Bright yellow plates. Mp: 215.5°.

SYNS: AS-17665 ◇ FNT ◇ FORMIC 2-(4-(5-NITROFURYL)-2-THIAZOLYL)HYDRAZIDE ◇ 2-(2-FORMYLHYDRAZINO)-4-(5-NITRO-2-FURYL)THIAZOLE ◇ NEFURTHIAZOLE ◇ 2-(4-(5-NITRO-2-FURANYL)-2-THIAZOLYL)-HYDRAZINE-CARBOXALDEHYDE ◇ NSC-525334

TOXICITY DATA with REFERENCE
CAR: orl-ham TDLo: 22 g/kg/48W-C   JNCIAM 51,941,73
CAR: orl-mus TD: 28 g/kg/33W-C   CNREA8 33,1593,73
CAR: orl-mus TD: 48 g/kg/29W   CNREA8 30,906,70
CAR: orl-mus TDLo: 30 g/kg/33W-C   CNREA8 38,1398,78
CAR: orl-rat TD: 41 g/kg/49W-C   CNREA8 33,2894,73
CAR: orl-rat TD: 38640 mg/kg/46W-C   CNREA8 30,2098,70
CAR: orl-rat TDLo: 31 g/kg/44W-C   PAACA3 10,15,69
NEO: orl-rat TD: 28 g/kg/46W-C   JNCIAM 47,437,71
MUT: dnr-sat 500 nmol/well   CNREA8 34,2266,74
MUT: mma-sat 100 ng/plate   MUREAV 40,9,76
MUT: mmo-esc 300 nmol/well   CNREA8 34,2266,74
MUT: mmo-sat 200 ng/plate   CNJGA8 21,319,79
MUT: mrc-esc 500 nmol/well   CNREA8 34,2266,74
MUT: pic-esc 250 μg/L   MUREAV 26,3,74
MUT: spm-mus-ipr 1575 mg/kg/5D-I   CMMUAO 5,257,78

CONSENSUS REPORTS: IARC Cancer Review: GROUP 2B IMEMDT 7,56,87; Animal Sufficient Evidence IMEMDT 7,151,74. EPA Genetic Toxicology Program.

SAFETY PROFILE: Suspected carcinogen with experimental carcinogenic and neoplastigenic data. Mutation data reported. When heated to decomposition it emits very toxic fumes of NO_x and SO_x.

NEI000   CAS: 18662-53-8
NITRILOTRIACETIC ACID TRISODIUM SALT MONOHYDRATE
mf: $C_6H_6NO_6$•3Na•H_2O mw: 275.12

SYNS: N,N-BIS(CARBOXYMETHYL)GLYCINE TRISO-DIUM SALT MONOHYDRATE ◇ NCI-C01445 ◇ NITRILO-ACETIC ACID TRISODIUM SALT MONOHYDRATE ◇ NTA SODIUM HYDRATE ◇ TRISODIUM NITRILOTRIACE-TATE MONOHYDRATE

TOXICITY DATA with REFERENCE
CAR: orl-mus TDLo: 315 g/kg/75W-C   NCITR* NCI-CG-TR-6,77
CAR: orl-rat TDLo: 830 g/kg/2Y-C   NCITR* NCI-CG-TR-6,77
ETA: orl-rat TD: 876 g/kg/2Y-C   FCTOD7 20,441,82
MUT: msc-hmn:oth 11 μmol/L   TOLED5 25,137,85

CONSENSUS REPORTS: NCI Carcinogenesis Bioassay (feed); Clear Evidence: mouse, rat NCITR* NCI-CG-TR-6,77. Cyanides and its compounds are on the Community Right-To-Know List.

SAFETY PROFILE: Suspected carcinogen with experimental carcinogenic, tumorigenic, and teratogenic data. Moderately toxic by intraperitoneal route. Human mutation data reported. When heated to decomposition it emits toxic fumes of NO_x, CN^- and Na_2O.

NEM480   CAS: 119-34-6
2-NITRO-4-AMINOPHENOL
mf: $C_6H_6N_2O_3$ mw: 154.14

SYNS: 4-AMINO-2-NITROPHENOL ◇ C.I. 76555 ◇ FOURRINE 57 ◇ FOURRINE BROWN PR ◇ FOURRINE BROWN PROPYL ◇ 4-HYDROXY-3-NITROANILINE ◇ NCI-C03963 ◇ o-NITRO-p-AMINOPHENOL ◇ OXIDATION BASE 25

TOXICITY DATA with REFERENCE
CAR: orl-rat TDLo: 108 g/kg/2Y-C   NCITR* NCI-CG-TR-94,78
MUT: mma-sat 100 μg/plate   IAPUDO 27,283,80
MUT: mmo-sat 100 μg/plate   ENMUDM 8(Suppl 5),1,85
MUT: otr-rat:emb 11 μg/plate   JJATDK 1,190,81

CONSENSUS REPORTS: IARC Cancer Review: GROUP 3 IMEMDT 7,56,87; NCI Carcinogenesis Bioassay (feed); No Evidence: mouse NCITR* NCI-CG-TR-94,78; Clear Evidence: rat NCITR* NCI-CG-TR-94,78. Reported in EPA TSCA Inventory. EPA Genetic Toxicology Program.

DFG MAK: Suspected Carcinogen.

SAFETY PROFILE: Suspected carcinogen with experimental carcinogenic data. Very poisonous by intraperitoneal route. Moderately toxic by ingestion. A severe eye irritant. Mutation data reported. When heated to decomposition it emits toxic fumes of NO_x.

NEQ500   CAS: 99-59-2
5-NITRO-o-ANISIDINE
mf: $C_7H_8N_2O_3$ mw: 168.17

PROP: Red needles from alc. D: 1.207 @ 156°, mp: 118°. Sol in hot benzene; sol in alc and acetic acid; very sltly sol in ligroin.

SYNS: 2-AMINO-1-METHOXY-4-NITROBENZENE ◇ 3-AMINO-4-METHOXYNITROBENZENE ◇ 2-AMINO-4-NITROANISOLE ◇ o-ANISIDINE NITRATE ◇ AZOAMINE SCARLET ◇ AZOGENE ECARLATE R ◇ AZOIC DIAZO COMPONENT 13, BASE ◇ C.I. AZOIC DIAZO COMPONENT 13 ◇ C.I. 37130 ◇ FAST SCARLET R ◇ 2-METHOXY-5-NITROANILINE ◇ 2-METHOXY-5-NITROBENZENAMINE ◇ NCI-C01934 ◇ 3-NITRO-6-METHOXYANILINE ◇ 5-NITRO-2-METHOXYANILINE

TOXICITY DATA with REFERENCE
CAR: orl-mus TD:3444 g/kg/78W-C   IARC** 27,133,82
CAR: orl-mus TD:4368 g/kg/78W-C   IARC** 27,133,82
CAR: orl-mus TDLo:413 g/kg/78W-C   NCITR* NCI-CG-TR-127,78
CAR: orl-rat TD:218 g/kg/78W-C   NCITR* NCI-CG-TR-127,78
CAR: orl-rat TD:2184 g/kg/78W-C   IARC** 27,133,82
CAR: orl-rat TD:4368 g/kg/78W-C   IARC** 27,133,82
CAR: orl-rat TDLo:109 g/kg/78W-C   NCITR* NCI-CG-TR-127,78
ETA: orl-mus TD:524 g/kg/78W-C   NCITR* NCI-CG-TR-127,78
MUT: mma-sat 10 μmol/plate   MUREAV 58,11,78
MUT: mmo-sat 10 μmol/plate   MUREAV 58,11,78

CONSENSUS REPORTS: IARC Cancer Review: Animal Limited Evidence IMEMDT 27,133,82. NCI Carcinogenesis Bioassay (feed); Clear Evidence: mouse, rat NCITR* NCI-CG-TR-127,78. Reported in EPA TSCA Inventory. EPA Genetic Toxicology Program. Community Right-To-Know List.

SAFETY PROFILE: Suspected carcinogen with experimental carcinogenic and tumorigenic

data. Moderately toxic by ingestion. Mutation data reported. When heated to decomposition it emits toxic fumes of NO_x.

NGE500   CAS: 59-87-0
NITROFURAZONE
mf: $C_6H_6N_4O_4$ mw: 198.16

PROP: Odorless, lemon-yellow crystals; bitter aftertaste. Darkens upon prolonged exposure to light. Decomp @ 236-240°. Very sltly sol in water; sltly sol in alc, propylene glycol; sol in alkaline solns; insol in ether.

SYNS: ALDOMYCIN ◇ ALFUCIN ◇ AMIFUR ◇ BABROCID ◇ BIOFUREA ◇ CHEMOFURAN ◇ COCAFURIN ◇ COXISTAT ◇ DERMOFURAL ◇ DYNAZONE ◇ ELDEZOL ◇ FEDACIN ◇ FLAVAZONE ◇ FRACINE ◇ FURACILLIN ◇ FURACINETTEN ◇ FURACOCCID ◇ FURACORT ◇ FURACYCLINE ◇ FURALDON ◇ FURAN-OFTENO ◇ FURAPLAST ◇ FURASEPTYL ◇ FURAZONE ◇ FURESOL ◇ FURFURIN ◇ FUVACILLIN ◇ HEMOFURAN ◇ IBIOFURAL ◇ MAMMEX ◇ MONOFURACIN ◇ NCI-C56064 ◇ NEFCO ◇ NF ◇ NIFUZON ◇ 5-NITROFURALDEHYDE SEMICARBAZIDE ◇ 6-NITROFURALDEHYDE SEMICARBAZIDE ◇ 5-NITRO-2-FURALDEHYDE SEMICARBAZONE ◇ 5-NITROFURAN-2-ALDEHYDE SEMICARBAZONE ◇ 5-NITRO-2-FURANCARBOXALDEHYDE SEMICARBAZONE ◇ 2((5-NITRO-2-FURANYL)METHYLENE)HYDRAZINECARBOXAMIDE ◇ 5-NITROFURFURAL SEMICARBAZONE ◇ (5-NITRO-2-FURFURYLIDENEAMINO)UREA ◇ NITROZONE ◇ NSC-2100 ◇ OTOFURAN ◇ SANFURAN ◇ SPRAY-DERMIS ◇ SPRAY-FORAL ◇ U-6421 ◇ USAF EA-4 ◇ VABROCID ◇ VADROCID ◇ VETERINARY NITROFURAZONE ◇ YATROCIN

TOXICITY DATA with REFERENCE
CAR: orl-mus TDLo:10094 mg/kg/2Y-C   FEPRA7 25,419,66
CAR: orl-rat TDLo:8652 mg/kg/2Y-C   NTPTR* NTP-TR-337,88
NEO: orl-rat TD:31 g/kg/45W-C   FEPRA7 25,419,66
ETA: orl-rat TD:4500 mg/kg/27D-I   CNREA8 28,924,68
ETA: scu-mus TDLo:300 mg/kg/18D-I   SEIJBO 15,234,75
MUT: cyt-ham:lng 100 mg/L/27H   MUREAV 66,277,79
MUT: cyt-ham:ovr 100 mg/L   FCTOD7 23,1091,85
MUT: dnd-esc 1 mg/L   MUREAV 107,1,83
MUT: dnd-hmn:oth 250 μmol/L   CNREA8 35,781,75
MUT: dnd-mus:lym 500 μmol/L/90M-C   BJCAAI 40,94,79
MUT: dni-ham:lng 10 μmol/L/6D-C   BJCAAI 40,94,79

MUT: dni-mus:oth 100 mg/L   ONCODU 19,183,80
MUT: dnr-bcs 10 μg/disc   KSRNAM 17,70,83

CONSENSUS REPORTS: IARC Cancer Review: Animal Inadequate Evidence IMEMDT 7,171,74. Reported in EPA TSCA Inventory. EPA Genetic Toxicology Program.

SAFETY PROFILE: Suspected carcinogen with experimental carcinogenic, neoplastigenic, tumorigenic, and teratogenic data. Poison by ingestion and intraperitoneal routes. Moderately toxic by subcutaneous route. Experimental reproductive effects. A human sensitizer. Human mutation data reported. When heated to decomposition it emits toxic fumes of NO_x.

NGI500   CAS: 712-68-5
2-(5-NITRO-2-FURYL)-5-AMINO-1,3,4-THIADIAZOLE
mf: $C_6H_4N_4O_3S$ mw: 212.20

SYNS: 2-AMINO-5-(5-NITRO-2-FURYL)-1,3,4-THIADIA-ZOLE ◇ 5-AMINO-2-(5-NITRO-2-FURYL)-1,3,4-THIADIA-ZOLE ◇ FURIDIAZINE ◇ 5-(5-NITRO-2-FURANYL)-1,3,4-THIADIAZOL-2-AMINE ◇ 5-(5-NITRO-2-FURYL)-2-AMINO-1,3,4-THIADIAZOLE

TOXICITY DATA with REFERENCE
CAR: orl-rat TDLo:6 g/kg/46W-I   JNCIAM
54,841,75
NEO: orl-rat TD:2240 mg/kg/32W-C   FEPRA7
29,817,70

CONSENSUS REPORTS: IARC Cancer Review: Animal Limited Evidence IMEMDT 7,143,74.

SAFETY PROFILE: Suspected carcinogen with experimental carcinogenic and neoplastigenic data. When heated to decomposition it emits very toxic fumes of NO_x and SO_x.

NGI800   CAS: 75198-31-1
3-(5-NITRO-2-FURYL)-IMIDAZO (1,2-a)PYRIDINE
mf: $C_{11}H_7N_3O_3$ mw: 229.21

SYN: NFIP

TOXICITY DATA with REFERENCE
CAR: orl-mus TDLo:33600 mg/kg/40W-C
TUMOAB 66,131,80
CAR: orl-rat TDLo:11200 mg/kg/20W-C
TUMOAB 66,131,80

SAFETY PROFILE: Suspected carcinogen with experimental carcinogenic data. When heated to decomposition it emits toxic fumes of NO_x.

NGM500   CAS: 24554-26-5
N-(4-(5-NITRO-2-FURYL)-2-THIAZOLYL)FORMAMIDE
mf: $C_8H_5N_3O_4S$ mw: 239.22

SYNS: FANFT ◇ 2-FORMYLAMINO-4-(5-NITRO-2-FURYL)THIAZOLE ◇ N-(4-(5-NITRO-2-FURYL)-2-THIAZO-LYL)FORMAMID (GERMAN)

TOXICITY DATA with REFERENCE
CAR: orl-ham TDLo:23 g/kg/48W-C   JNCIAM
51,941,73
CAR: orl-mus TD:27 g/kg/33W-C   CNREA8
38,1398,78
CAR: orl-mus TD:36 g/kg/46W-C   CNREA8
30,1309,70
CAR: orl-mus TDLo:1008 mg/kg/12W-C
CNREA8 41,1397,81
CAR: orl-rat TD:2 g/kg/10W-I   CALEDQ
12,355,81
CAR: orl-rat TD:320 mg/kg/16W-I   CRNGDP
1,135,80
CAR: orl-rat TD:3360 mg/kg/4W-C   CNREA8
46,6160,86
CAR: orl-rat TD:6000 mg/kg/6W-C:TER
CNREA8 39,1207,79
CAR: orl-rat TD:7040 mg/kg/30W-C   CALEDQ
18,261,83
CAR: orl-rat TD:7700 mg/kg/10W-C   CRNGDP
2,515,81
CAR: orl-rat TD:9600 mg/kg/10W-C   JJCREP
76,577,85
CAR: orl-rat TD:10080 mg/kg/12W-C   CRNGDP
5,53,84
CAR: orl-rat TDLo:14500 mg/kg/20W-C
CALEDQ 34,249,87
ETA: imp-dog TDLo:3700 mg/kg/74W-I
NATWAY 65,665,78
ETA: orl-dog TDLo:26 g/kg/2Y-C   JNCIAM
45,535,70
ETA: scu-dog TDLo:2600 mg/kg/1Y-I   INURAQ
18,24,80
MUT: bfa-rat/sat 658 mg/kg/7D-C   MUREAV
135,169,84
MUT: dns-dog:oth 10 μmol/L   CNREA842,3974,82
MUT: mma-esc 30 ng/plate   ENMUDM 6(Suppl 2),1,84
MUT: mmo-esc 3 ng/plate   ENMUDM6(Suppl2),1,84
MUT: otr-ham:emb 1 mg/L   JJIND8 67,1303,81

CONSENSUS REPORTS: EPA Genetic Toxicology Program.

SAFETY PROFILE: Suspected carcinogen with experimental carcinogenic, tumorigenic, and teratogenic data. Mutation data reported. When heated to decomposition it emits very toxic fumes of SO_x and NO_x.

NGN500   CAS: 42011-48-3
N-(4-(5-NITRO-2-FURYL)-2-THIAZOLYL)-2,2,2-TRIFLUOROACETAMIDE
mf: $C_9H_4F_3N_3O_4S$ mw: 307.22

SYNS: 2-(2,2,2-TRIFLUOROACETAMIDO)-4-(5-NITRO-2-FURYL)THIAZOLE ◇ 2,2,2-TRIFLUORO-N-(4-(5-NITRO-2-FURYL)-2-THIAZOLYL)ACETAMIDE

TOXICITY DATA with REFERENCE
CAR: orl-mus TDLo: 108 g/kg/46W-C   CNREA8 33,1593,73
CAR: orl-rat TDLo: 18 g/kg/46W-C   JNCIAM 54,841,75
MUT: dnr-sat 500 nmol/well   CNREA8 34,2266,74
MUT: mma-sat 100 ng/plate   MUREAV 48,295,77
MUT: mmo-esc 300 nmol/well   CNREA834,2266,74
MUT: mrc-esc 500 nmol/well   CNREA8 34,2266,74
MUT: pic-esc 500 μg/L   MUREAV 26,3,74

SAFETY PROFILE: Suspected carcinogen with experimental carcinogenic data. Mutation data reported. When heated to decomposition it emits very toxic fumes of F^-, NO_x, and SO_x.

NJA000   CAS: 5522-43-0
3-NITROPYRENE
mf: $C_{16}H_9NO_2$ mw: 247.26

SYN: 1-NITROPYRENE

TOXICITY DATA with REFERENCE
CAR: ipr-mus TDLo: 1575 mg/kg/6W-I   CRNGDP 5,1449,84
CAR: ipr-rat TDLo: 20 mg/kg/4W-I   DTESD7 13,279,86
CAR: orl-rat TDLo: 396 mg/kg/16W-I   CNREA8 48,4256,88
CAR: scu-rat TD: 198 mg/kg/8W-I   CNREA8 44,1158,84
CAR: scu-rat TDLo: 160 mg/kg/10W-I   CALEDQ 15,1,82
NEO: ipr-mus TD: 1780 mg/kg   PAACA3 25,122,84
ETA: scu-rat TD: 99 mg/kg/8W-I   CNREA8 44,1158,84
ETA: scu-rat TD: 160 mg/kg/10W-I   CALEDQ 25,239,85
MUT: dnd-mus: lvr 50 μmol/L   MUREAV 151,137,85
MUT: dnd-rbt: lng 8100 nmol/L   CALEDQ 19,241,83
MUT: mma-sat 500 ng/plate   MUREAV 91,321,81
MUT: mmo-esc 3 μg/plate   MUREAV 142,163,85

MUT: msc-hmn: fbr 1 μmol/L   CRNGDP 7,89,86
MUT: otr-hmn: fbr 3 μmol/L   CRNGDP 4,353,83

CONSENSUS REPORTS: IARC Cancer Review: Animal Limited Evidence IMEMDT 33,209,84. Reported in EPA TSCA Inventory.

DFG MAK: Suspected Carcinogen.

SAFETY PROFILE: Suspected carcinogen with experimental carcinogenic, neoplastigenic, and tumorigenic data. Human mutation data reported. When heated to decomposition it emits toxic fumes of NO_x.

NJF000   CAS: 56-57-5
4-NITROQUINOLINE-N-OXIDE
mf: $C_9H_6N_2O_3$ mw: 190.17

SYNS: 4-NITROCHINOLIN N-OXID (SWEDISH) ◇ 4-NITROQUINOLINE-1-OXIDE ◇ 4-NQO

TOXICITY DATA with REFERENCE
CAR: orl-mus TD: 160 mg/kg/15W-I   GANNA2 58,389,67
CAR: orl-mus TDLo: 100 mg/kg/12W-I   GANNA2 58,389,67
CAR: orl-rat TD: 2400 μg/kg/28W-C   OSOMAE 59,600,85
CAR: scu-mus TDLo: 80 mg/kg/20W-I   DTESD7 13,253,86
CAR: scu-mus TDLo: 100 mg/kg/10W-I   GANNA2 57,559,66
CAR: scu-rat TD: 5 mg/kg   CRNGDP 6,769,85
CAR: scu-rat TDLo: 50 mg/kg/10W-I   GANNA2 57,559,66
NEO: orl-mus TD: 44 mg/kg/2W-I   AMBPBZ 83,550,75
NEO: orl-mus TD: 115 mg/kg/23W-I   GANNA2 56,429,65
ETA: imp-mus TDLo: 48 mg/kg   CNREA8 33,408,73
ETA: imp-rat TDLo: 1600 μg/kg   APJAAG23,87,73
ETA: ims-bwd TDLo: 35 mg/kg/9W-I   ARZNAD 14,842,64
ETA: orl-rat TD: 120 mg/kg/18W-I   GANNA2 61,27,70
ETA: orl-rat TD: 144 mg/kg/18W-I   JJIND8 64,835,80
ETA: orl-rat TD: 210 mg/kg/30W-C   BTDCAV 22,85,81
ETA: orl-rat TD: 1980 mg/kg/33W-I   BJCAAI 47,413,83
ETA: orl-rat TDLo: 13500 μg/kg/18W-I   ACPADQ 92,437,84
ETA: scu-mus TD: 400 μg/kg   JJEMAG 40,475,70

ETA: skn-gpg TDLo: 4800 μg/kg/80W-I
BJCAAI 20,200,66
ETA: skn-ham TDLo: 580 mg/kg/14W-I
AICCA6 19,519,63
ETA: skn-mus TDLo: 84 mg/kg/14W-I GANNA2
48,129,57
MUT: dni-hmn: fbr 5 μmol/L MUREAV 81,203,81
MUT: dni-hmn: oth 1 μmol/L/30M MUREAV
125,55,84
MUT: dns-hmn: hla 3300 nmol/L MUREAV
139,155,84
MUT: sce-hmn: lym 1 nmol/L NGCJAK 15,1085,80

CONSENSUS REPORTS: EPA Genetic Toxicology Program.

SAFETY PROFILE: Suspected carcinogen with experimental carcinogenic, neoplastigenic, and tumorigenic data. Poison by intraperitoneal and subcutaneous routes. Experimental reproductive effects. Human mutation data reported. When heated to decomposition it emits toxic fumes of NO_x.

NJN000   CAS: 60599-38-4
N-NITROSOBIS(2-OXOPROPYL)AMINE
mf: $C_6H_{10}N_2O_3$ mw: 158.18

SYNS: BIS-(2-OXOPROPYL)-N-NITROSAMINE ◇ BOP ◇ DI-OXO-DI-N-PROPYLNITROSAMINE ◇ 2,2'-DIOXO-DI-N-PROPYLNITROSAMINE ◇ 2,2'-DIOXO-N-NITROSODIPRO-PYLAMINE ◇ N,N-DI(2-OXOPROPYL)NITROSAMINE ◇ 2,2'-DIOXOPROPYL-N-PROPYLNITROSAMINE ◇ DOPN ◇ N-NITROSO-N,N-DI(2-OXYPROPYL)AMINE ◇ (NITRO-SOIMINO)DIACETONE

TOXICITY DATA with REFERENCE
CAR: orl-ham TDLo: 57 mg/kg/13W-C
CALEDQ 2,323,77
CAR: orl-rat TD: 750 mg/kg/90W-I CALEDQ
19,207,83
CAR: orl-rat TDLo: 500 mg/kg/1Y-I: TER
CALEDQ 13,303,81
CAR: scu-gpg TDLo: 180 mg/kg/5W-I CALEDQ
5,31,78
CAR: scu-ham TD: 10 mg/kg CRNGDP 4,1215,83
CAR: scu-ham TD: 10 mg/kg JJIND8 71,347,83
CAR: scu-ham TD: 40 mg/kg/3D-I BJCAAI
41,996,80
CAR: scu-ham TD: 75 mg/kg/15W-I CRNGDP
3,1021,82
CAR: scu-ham TD: 105 mg/kg/42W-I JNCIAM
58,1449,77
CAR: scu-ham TDLo: 10 mg/kg JJIND8 70,141,83
CAR: scu-rat TD: 293 mg/kg/2Y-I CALEDQ
5,13,78

CAR: scu-rat TD: 460 mg/kg/46W-I CALEDQ
4,293,78
CAR: scu-rat TDLo: 20 mg/kg (18D post)
CNREA8 46,4135,86
CAR: skn-ham TDLo: 672 mg/kg/42W-I
CALEDQ 10,365,80
NEO: scu-ham TDLo: 40 mg/kg (8-14D post)
CNREA8 46,3663,86
NEO: scu-rat TD: 100 mg/kg CALEDQ 5,13,78
ETA: scu-ham TD: 10 mg/kg JJIND8 71,355,83
MUT: dnd-ham: oth 500 μg/L CBINA8 48,59,84
MUT: dns-ham: oth 100 mg/L JJIND8 71,523,83
MUT: dns-rat: lvr 1 μmol/L MUREAV 144,197,85
MUT: mma-ham: lng 20 μmol/L CNREA8
45,5219,85
MUT: mma-sat 250 μg/plate MUREAV 111,135,83
MUT: otr-hmn: oth 200 μg/L BANRDU 12,15,82

SAFETY PROFILE: Suspected carcinogen with experimental carcinogenic, neoplastigenic, tumorigenic, and teratogenic data. Poison by ingestion and subcutaneous routes. Human mutation data reported. When heated to decomposition it emits toxic fumes of NO_x.

NKC000   CAS: 17608-59-2
N-NITROSOEPHEDRINE
mf: $C_{10}H_{14}N_2O_2$ mw: 194.26

SYNS: α-(1-(N-METHYL-N-NITROSOAMINO)ETHYL)BEN-ZYL ALCOHOL ◇ 2-(N-METHYL-N-NITROSOAMINO)-1-PHE-NYL-1-PROPANOL

TOXICITY DATA with REFERENCE
CAR: ipr-mus TDLo: 600 mg/kg/7D-I CNREA8
35,1981,75
CAR: orl-rat TDLo: 17 g/kg/71W-I CALEDQ
5,103,78
MUT: mma-sat 50 μg/plate CALEDQ 21,63,83
MUT: otr-ham: kdy 80 μg/L BJCAAI 37,873,78

SAFETY PROFILE: Suspected carcinogen with experimental carcinogenic data. Poison by intraperitoneal route. Mutation data reported. When heated to decomposition it emits toxic fumes of NO_x.

NKI000   CAS: 932-83-2
N-NITROSOHEXAHYDROAZEPINE
mf: $C_6H_{12}N_2O$ mw: 128.20

SYNS: HEXAHYDRO-1-NITROSO-1H-AZEPINE ◇ N-6-MI ◇ N-NITROSOAZACYCLOHEPTANE ◇ NITROSOHEXA-METHYLENIMINE ◇ N-NITROSOHEXAMETHYLENEIMINE ◇ N-NITROSOPERHYDROAZEPINE

TOXICITY DATA with REFERENCE

CAR: orl-mus TDLo:700 mg/kg/8W-I   JJIND8 73,1215,84

CAR: orl-rat TDLo:1570 mg/kg/28W-I
CALEDQ 12,99,81

CAR: scu-ham TD:348 mg/kg/87W-I   JNCIAM 50,323,73

CAR: scu-ham TDLo:80 mg/kg (8-15D preg):
TER   ZKKOBW 86,69,76

CAR: scu-ham TDLo:80 mg/kg/8W-I   ZKKOBW 86,69,76

ETA: orl-mus TD:1600 mg/kg/8W-I   PTLGAX 2,261,70

ETA: orl-rat TD:720 mg/kg/8W-I   CNREA8 28,1217,68

ETA: orl-rat TD:1320 mg/kg/30W-I   JJIND8 62,407,79

ETA: scu-ham TD:4 mg/kg   ZKKOBW 78,78,72
ETA: scu-mus TDLo:4 mg/kg   ZKKOBW 78,78,72
MUT: mma-esc 7500 µmol/L   IAPUDO 41,543,82

MUT: mma-sat 10 µg/plate   TCMUE9 1,13,84
MUT: pic-esc 100 mg/L   TCMUE9 1,91,84

SAFETY PROFILE: Suspected carcinogen with experimental carcinogenic, tumorigenic, and teratogenic data. Poison by ingestion, intraperitoneal, and subcutaneous routes. Experimental reproductive effects. Mutation data reported. When heated to decomposition it emits toxic fumes of NO_x.

NKO400   CAS: 71752-69-7
NITROSOISOPROPANOLUREA
mf: $C_4H_9N_3O_3$ mw: 147.16

SYNS: 1-(2-HYDROXYPROPYL)-1-NITROSOUREA ◇ NITROSO-2-HYDROXY-N-PROPYLUREA ◇ N-NITROSO-2-HYDROXY-N-PROPYLUREA

TOXICITY DATA with REFERENCE

CAR: orl-rat TD:230 mg/kg/18W-I   JCREA8 112,221,86

CAR: orl-rat TD:1560 mg/kg/25W-C   CNREA8 43,214,83

CAR: orl-rat TDLo:768 mg/kg/30W-C   CNREA8 43,214,83

CAR: skn-mus TDLo:471 mg/kg/40W-I
CNREA8 43,214,83

ETA: orl-ham TDLo:662 mg/kg/36W-I   IAPUDO 57,617,84

ETA: orl-rat TD:441 mg/kg/32W-I   IAPUDO 57,617,84

MUT: dnd-mam:lym 10 mmol/L   CBINA8 48,169,84

MUT: mma-sat 1 µg/plate   TCMUE9 1,13,84
MUT: mmo-sat 1 µg/plate   MUREAV 68,1,79

SAFETY PROFILE: Suspected carcinogen with experimental carcinogenic and tumorigenic data. Mutation data reported. When heated to decomposition it emits toxic fumes of NO_x.

NKU875   CAS: 35631-27-7
NITROSO-5-METHYLOXAZOLIDONE
mf: $C_4H_8N_2O_2$ mw: 116.14

SYNS: 5-METHYL-3-NITROSO-1,3-OXAZOLIDINE ◇ NITROSO-5-METHYL-1,3-OXAZOLIDINE ◇ N-NITROSO-5-METHYL-1,3-OXAZOLIDINE

TOXICITY DATA with REFERENCE

CAR: orl-rat TDLo:250 g/kg/50W-I   CRNGDP 3,911,82

CAR: skn-mus TDLo:465 mg/kg/50W-I
CNREA8 43,214,83

ETA: orl-ham TD:929 mg/kg/35W-I   IAPUDO 57,617,84

ETA: orl-ham TDLo:960 mg/kg/24W-I
CRNGDP 5,875,84

ETA: orl-rat TD:813 mg/kg/85W-I   IAPUDO 57,617,84

ETA: orl-rat TD:1200 mg/kg/40W-C   CNREA8 43,214,83

MUT: mma-sat 5 µg/plate   TCMUE9 1,13,84
MUT: mmo-sat 1 µg/plate   TCMUE9 1,13,84
MUT: pic-esc 10 mg/L   TCMUE9 1,91,84

SAFETY PROFILE: Suspected carcinogen with experimental carcinogenic and tumorigenic data. Mutation data reported. When heated to decomposition it emits toxic fumes of NO_x.

NKV000   CAS: 55984-51-5
N-NITROSOMETHYL-2-OXOPROPYLAMINE
mf: $C_4H_8N_2O_2$ mw: 116.14

SYNS: 1-(METHYLNITROSOAMINO)2-PROPANONE ◇ MOP ◇ NMOP

TOXICITY DATA with REFERENCE

CAR: orl-ham TDLo:176 mg/kg/2ZW-I
JCREA8 109,1,85

CAR: par-rat TDLo:600 mg/kg/30W-I   JJCREP 79,309,88

CAR: scu-ham TD:68 mg/kg/39W-I   CNREA8 40,3585,80

CAR: scu-ham TD:94 mg/kg/27W-I   CNREA8 40,3585,80

CAR: scu-ham TDLo:25 mg/kg   CNREA8 40,3585,80

ETA: orl-ham TD: 290 mg/kg/20W-I   IAPUDO
57,617,84

ETA: orl-rat TD: 375 mg/kg/30W-I   CALEDQ
22,83,84

ETA: orl-rat TD: 523 mg/kg/23W-I   IAPUDO
57,617,84

ETA: orl-rat TD: 800 mg/kg/8W-I   JJIND8
70,959,83

ETA: orl-rat TDLo: 300 mg/kg/30W-I   JJIND8
70,959,83

MUT: dnd-ham-ipr 20 mg/kg   CRNGDP 5,565,84

MUT: dnd-ham: oth 10 μmol/L   PAACA3 24,73,83

MUT: dnd-rat-ipr 60 mg/kg   CRNGDP 5,565,84

MUT: dns-rat: lvr 100 μmol/L   MUREAV 144,197,85

MUT: mma-sat 250 μg/plate   MUREAV 111,135,83

MUT: msc-ham: lng 200 μmol/L   CNREA8
40,3463,80

SAFETY PROFILE: Suspected carcinogen with experimental carcinogenic and tumorigenic data. Poison by subcutaneous route. Mutation data reported. When heated to decomposition it emits toxic fumes of NO_x.

NKY000   CAS: 4549-40-0
N-NITROSOMETHYLVINYLAMINE
mf: $C_3H_6N_2O$ mw: 86.11

SYNS: N-METHYL-N-NITROSO-ETHENYLAMINE ◇ N-METHYL-N-NITROSOVINYLAMINE ◇ METHYLVINYL-NITROSAMINE ◇ METHYLVINYLNITROSAMIN (GERMAN) ◇ MVNA ◇ NMVA ◇ RCRA WASTE NUMBER P084

TOXICITY DATA with REFERENCE
ETA: ihl-rat TD: 44 mg/kg   ZEKBAI 66,1,64
ETA: ihl-rat TD: 50 mg/kg/50D   ARZNAD
19,1077,69

ETA: ihl-rat TDLo: 2700 μg/kg/30M/33W-I
ZEKBAI 69,103,67

ETA: orl-rat TDLo: 110 mg/kg/52W-C   ARZNAD
19,1077,69

CONSENSUS REPORTS: IARC Cancer Review: GROUP 2B IMEMDT 7,56,87; Animal Sufficient Evidence IMEMDT 17,257,78; Human Limited Evidence IMEMDT 17,257,78. Community Right-To-Know List. EPA Genetic Toxicology Program.

SAFETY PROFILE: Suspected carcinogen with experimental tumorigenic data. Poison by ingestion and inhalation. When heated to decomposition it emits toxic fumes of NO_x.

NLE000   CAS: 39884-52-1
N-NITROSOOXAZOLIDINE
mf: $C_3H_6N_2O_2$ mw: 102.11

SYNS: N-NITROSOOXAZOLIDIN (GERMAN) ◇ NITROSO-OXAZOLIDONE ◇ N-NITROSO-1,3-OXAZOLIDINE ◇ 3-NITROSOOXAZOLIDINE

TOXICITY DATA with REFERENCE
CAR: orl-rat TD: 219 g/kg/50W-I   CRNGDP
3,911,82

CAR: orl-rat TD: 1080 mg/kg/40W-C   CNREA8
43,214,83

CAR: orl-rat TD: 1500 mg/kg/30W-I   ZKKOBW
88,25,76

CAR: orl-rat TDLo: 790 mg/kg/36W-I   ZKKOBW
88,25,76

CAR: skn-mus TDLo: 408 mg/kg/50W-I
CNREA8 43,214,83

ETA: orl-ham TD: 1225 mg/kg/43W-I   IAPUDO
57,617,84

ETA: orl-ham TDLo: 1288 mg/kg/35W-I
CRNGDP 5,875,84

ETA: orl-rat TD: 715 mg/kg/53W-I   IAPUDO
57,617,84

MUT: mma-sat 1 μg/plate   TCMUE9 1,13,84

MUT: mmo-sat 2500 ng/plate   TCMUE9 1,13,84

MUT: pic-esc 100 mg/L   TCMUE9 1,191,84

SAFETY PROFILE: Suspected carcinogen with experimental carcinogenic and tumorigenic data. Moderately toxic by ingestion. Mutation data reported. When heated to decomposition it emits toxic fumes of NO_x.

NLO500   CAS: 816-57-9
N-NITROSO-N-PROPYLUREA
mf: $C_4H_9N_3O_2$ mw: 131.16

SYNS: NITROSOPROPYLUREA ◇ NITROSO-N-PROPYLU-REA ◇ NPU ◇ PNU ◇ N-PROPYLNITROSOHARNSTOFF (GERMAN) ◇ N-PROPYLNITROSUREA ◇ 1-PROPYL-1-NI-TROSOUREA

TOXICITY DATA with REFERENCE
CAR: orl-ham TD: 7728 mg/kg/23W-C
GANNA2 73,695,82

CAR: orl-ham TDLo: 3024 mg/kg/36W-C
GANNA2 73,695,82

CAR: skn-mus TDLo: 525 mg/kg/50W-I
JCROD7 102,13,81

NEO: orl-rat TD: 3 g/kg/10W-C   JJIND8 73,757,84

ETA: orl-rat TD: 500 mg/kg   ANYAA9 381,250,82

ETA: orl-rat TD: 689 mg/kg/25W-C   GANNA2
71,231,80

ETA: orl-rat TD: 1054 mg/kg/30W-C   GANNA2
71,231,80

ETA: orl-rat TD: 1969 mg/kg/35W-I   BIHAA2
(40),107,73

ETA: orl-rat TD:2080 mg/kg/1Y-I   PPTCBY
2,73,72

ETA: orl-rat TD:10920 mg/kg/39W-C   JJIND8
72,367,84

ETA: orl-rat TDLo:120 mg/kg (19D preg):
TER   ARGEAR 40,99,72

ETA: orl-rat TDLo:200 mg/kg   GANNA267,121,76

ETA: scu-rat TD:420 mg/kg   ANYAA9 381,250,82

ETA: scu-rat TDLo:400 mg/kg   GANNA267,121,76

ETA: skn-mus TD:525 mg/kg/50W-I   CNREA8
43,214,83

MUT: cyt-ham:fbr 125 mg/L/48H   MUREAV
48,337,77

MUT: cyt-ham:lng 68 mg/L   GMCRDC 27,95,81

MUT: dnd-mam:lym 500 μmol/L   CRNGDP
4,1455,83

MUT: mmo-sat 1 μg/plate   MUREAV 68,1,79

MUT: msc-ham:lng 1 g/L   CNREA8 44,3270,84

MUT: sce-ham:lng 1 g/L   CNREA8 44,3270,84

CONSENSUS REPORTS: EPA Genetic Toxicology Program.

SAFETY PROFILE: Suspected carcinogen with
experimental carcinogenic, neoplastigenic, tumorigenic, and teratogenic data. Moderately
toxic by ingestion. Experimental reproductive
effects. Mutation data reported. When heated
to decomposition it emits toxic fumes of NO_x.

NLY750   CAS: 88208-15-5
NITROSO-3,4,5-TRIMETHYLPIPERAZINE
mf: $C_7H_{15}N_3O$ mw: 157.25

SYNS: N-NITROSO-3,4,5-TRIMETHYLPIPERAZINE
◇ 1-NITROSO-3,4,5-TRIMETHYLPIPERAZINE

TOXICITY DATA with REFERENCE
CAR: orl-ham TDLo:2208 mg/kg/46W-I
CRNGDP 4,1165,83

CAR: orl-rat TD:660 mg/kg/30W-I   CRNGDP
4,1165,83

CAR: orl-rat TD:1430 mg/kg/26W-I   CNREA8
41,1034,81

CAR: orl-rat TDLo:270 mg/kg/30W-I   CRNGDP
4,1165,83

ETA: orl-ham TD:2202 mg/kg/59W-I   IAPUDO
57,617,84

ETA: orl-rat TD:1100 mg/kg/27W-I   IAPUDO
57,617,84

MUT: mma-sat 10 μg/plate   TCMUE9 1,13,84

SAFETY PROFILE: Suspected carcinogen with
experimental carcinogenic and tumorigenic
data. Mutation data reported. When heated to
decomposition it emits toxic fumes of NO_x.

NML000   CAS: 61-57-4
NITROTHIAZOLE
mf: $C_6H_6N_4O_3S$ mw: 214.22

SYNS: AMBILHAR ◇ BA 32644 ◇ BA 32644 CIBA
◇ CIBA 32644 ◇ CIBA 32644-BA ◇ NIRIDAZOLE ◇ NITRIDA-
ZOLE ◇ NITROTHIAMIDAZOL ◇ NITROTHIAMIDAZOLE
◇ 1-(5-NITRO-2-THIAZOLYL)IMIDAZOLIDIN-2-ONE
◇ 1-(5-NITRO-2-THIAZOLYL)-2-IMIDAZOLIDINONE
◇ 1-(5-NITRO-2-THIAZOLYL)-2-IMIDAZOLINONE
◇ 1-(5-NITRO-2-THIAZOLYL)-2-OXOTETRAHYDROIMIDA-
ZOL ◇ 1-(5-NITRO-2-THIAZOLYL)-2-OXOTETRAHYDROIMI-
DAZOLE ◇ NTOI

TOXICITY DATA with REFERENCE
CAR: orl-mus TD:16 g/kg/75W-C   JNCIAM
59,1625,77

CAR: orl-mus TDLo:15 g/kg/49W-C   CALEDQ
1,69,75

NEO: orl-ham TDLo:21 g/kg/63W-C   JNCIAM
59,1625,77

NEO: orl-mus TD:4 g/kg/19W-C   CALEDQ1,69,75

NEO: orl-rat TDLo:8 g/kg/90W-I   CALEDQ
4,305,78

MUT: bfa-hmn/sat 25 mg/kg   CMMUAO 4,171,76

MUT: dnr-bcs 20 μL/disc   MUREAV 97,1,82

MUT: dnr-esc 20 μL/disc   MUREAV 97,1,82

MUT: mma-sat 33 ng/plate   ENMUDM 7,429,85

MUT: mmo-esc 100 ng/plate   MUREAV 142,163,85

MUT: mmo-klp 500 nmol/L   MUREAV 118,153,83

MUT: mmo-sat 12500 pg/plate   MUREAV130,79,84

CONSENSUS REPORTS: IARC Cancer Re-
view: GROUP 2B IMEMDT 7,56,87; Animal
Sufficient Evidence IMEMDT 13,123,77. EPA
Genetic Toxicology Program.

SAFETY PROFILE: Suspected carcinogen with
experimental carcinogenic and neoplastigenic
data. Poison by intraperitoneal route. Moderately toxic by ingestion. Experimental reproductive effects. Human mutation data reported.
Used as an amoebicide and schistosomicidal
agent. When heated to decomposition it emits
very toxic fumes of SO_x and NO_x.

ORS000   CAS: 39603-54-8
β-OXYPROPYLPROPYLNITROSAMINE
mf: $C_6H_{12}N_2O_2$ mw: 144.20

SYNS: N-NITROSO-2-OXO-N-PROPYL-N-PROPYLAMINE
◇ 1-(NITROSOPROPYLAMINO)-2-PROPANONE ◇ 2-OXI-
PROPYL-PROPYLNITROSAMIN (GERMAN) ◇ 2-OXO-PRO-
PYL-PROPYLNITROSAMINE ◇ (2-OXOPROPYL)PROPYLNI-
TROSOAMINE

TOXICITY DATA with REFERENCE

CAR: scu-ham TDLo: 2450 mg/kg/34W-I
ZKKOBW 90(3),141,77

CAR: scu-mus TD: 2352 mg/kg/39W-I
ZKKOBW 91,189,78

CAR: scu-mus TDLo: 1688 mg/kg/56W-I
ZKKOBW 91,189,78

CAR: scu-rat TDLo: 3100 mg/kg/33W-I
ZKKOBW 81,23,74

NEO: scu-ham TDLo: 100 mg/kg/(14D preg)
ZKKOBW 90,119,77

ETA: scu-ham TD: 700 mg/kg/14W-I   JNCIAM
51,287,73

MUT: mma-sat 500 nmol/plate   ZKKOBW86,293,76

SAFETY PROFILE: Suspected carcinogen with experimental carcinogenic, neoplastigenic, and tumorigenic data. Moderately toxic by subcutaneous route. Mutation data reported. When heated to decomposition it emits toxic fumes of NO_x.

PAH800   CAS: 63449-39-8
PARAFFIN WAXES and HYDROCARBON WAXES, CHLORINATED (C12, 60% CHLORINE)

SYN: CHLORINATED PARAFFINS (C12, 60% CHLORINE)

TOXICITY DATA with REFERENCE

CAR: orl-mus TDLo: 182 g/kg/2Y-I   NTPTR*
NTP-TR-308,86

CAR: orl-rat TD: 228 g/kg/2Y-I   FAATDF9,454,87

CAR: orl-rat TDLo: 227 g/kg/2Y-I   NTPTR*
NTP-TR-308,86

NEO: orl-mus TD: 183 g/kg/2Y-I   FAATDF
9,454,87

NEO: orl-mus TD: 917 g/kg/2Y-I   NTPTR*
NTP-TR-308,86

NEO: orl-mus TD: 91250 mg/kg/2Y-I   FAATDF
9,454,87

NEO: orl-rat TD: 227 g/kg/2Y-I   NTPTR*
NTP-TR-308,86

NEO: orl-rat TD: 227 g/kg/2Y-I   NTPTR*
NTP-TR-308,86

CONSENSUS REPORTS: NTP Carcinogenesis Studies (gavage): Clear Evidence: mouse,rat NTPTR* NTP-TR-308,86. Reported in EPA TSCA Inventory.

SAFETY PROFILE: Suspected carcinogen with experimental carcinogenic and neoplastigenic data. When heated to decomposition it emits acrid smoke and irritating fumes.

PAX250   CAS: 87-86-5
PENTACHLOROPHENOL
DOT: 2020
mf: C_6HCl_5O mw: 266.32

PROP: Dark-colored flakes and sublimed needle crystals; characteristic odor. Mp: 191°, bp: 310° (decomp), d: 1.978, vap press: 40 mm @ 211.2°. Sol in ether, benzene; very sol in alc; insol in water; sltly sol in cold petr ether.

SYNS: CHEM-TOL ◇ CHLOROPHEN ◇ CRYPTOGIL OL ◇ DOWCIDE 7 ◇ DOWICIDE 7 ◇ DOWICIDE EC-7 ◇ DOWICIDE G ◇ DOW PENTACHLOROPHENOL DP-2 ANTI-MICROBIAL ◇ DUROTOX ◇ EP 30 ◇ FUNGIFEN ◇ GLAZD PENTA ◇ GRUNDIER ARBEZOL ◇ LAUXTOL ◇ LAUXTOL A ◇ LIROPREM ◇ NCI-C54933 ◇ NCI-C55378 ◇ NCI-C56655 ◇ PCP ◇ PENCHLOROL ◇ PENTA ◇ PENTACHLOORFENOL (DUTCH) ◇ PENTACHLOROFENOL ◇ PENTACHLOROPHEN-ATE ◇ 2,3,4,5,6-PENTACHLOROPHENOL ◇ PENTACHLO-ROPHENOL, DOWICIDE EC-7 ◇ PENTACHLOROPHENOL, DP-2 ◇ PENTACHLOROPHENOL (GERMAN) ◇ PENTACHLO-ROPHENOL, TECHNICAL ◇ PENTACLOROFENOLO (ITALIAN) ◇ PENTACON ◇ PENTA-KIL ◇ PENTASOL ◇ PENWAR ◇ PERATOX ◇ PERMACIDE ◇ PERMAGARD ◇ PERMASAN ◇ PERMATOX DP-2 ◇ PERMATOX PENTA ◇ PERMITE ◇ PRILTOX ◇ RCRA WASTE NUMBER U242 ◇ SANTOBRITE ◇ SANTOPHEN ◇ SANTOPHEN 20 ◇ SINITUHO ◇ TERM-I-TROL ◇ THOMPSON'S WOOD FIX ◇ WEEDONE

TOXICITY DATA with REFERENCE

ETA: scu-mus TDLo: 46 mg/kg   NTIS**
PB223-159

MUT: mma-sat 40 nmol/plate   AIDZAC 10,305,82

CONSENSUS REPORTS: IARC Cancer Review: Human Limited Evidence IMEMDT 41,319,86; Animal Inadequate Evidence IMEMDT 20,303,79. Chlorophenol compounds are on The Community Right-To-Know List. Reported in EPA TSCA Inventory. EPA Genetic Toxicology Program.

OSHA PEL: TWA 0.5 mg/m³ (skin)   ACGIH TLV: TWA 0.5 mg/m³ (skin); BEI: 2 mg(total PCP)/L in urine prior to last shift of workweek; 5 mg(free PCP)/L in plasma at end of shift.   DFG MAK: 0.05 ppm (0.5 mg/m³); BAT: 1000 µg/L in plasma/serum.   DOT Classification: ORM-E; Label: None.

SAFETY PROFILE: Suspected human carcinogen with experimental tumorigenic data. Human poison by ingestion. Poison experimentally by ingestion, skin contact, intraperitoneal, and subcutaneous routes. An experimental teratogen.

A skin irritant. Mutation data reported. Acute poisoning is marked by weakness with changes in respiration, blood pressure, and urinary output. Also causes dermatitis, convulsions, and collapse. Chronic exposure can cause liver and kidney injury. Dangerous; when heated to decomposition it emits highly toxic fumes of Cl⁻.

PCF275   CAS: 127-18-4
PERCHLOROETHYLENE
DOT: 1897
mf: C_2Cl_4 mw: 165.82

PROP: Colorless liquid; chloroform-like odor. Mp: $-23.35°$, bp: $121.20°$, d: 1.6311 @ 15°/4°, vap press: 15.8 mm @ 22°, vap d: 5.83.

SYNS: ANKILOSTIN ◇ ANTISOL 1 ◇ CARBON BICHLO-RIDE ◇ CARBON DICHLORIDE ◇ CZTEROCHLOROETYLEN (POLISH) ◇ DIDAKENE ◇ DOW-PER ◇ ENT 1,860 ◇ ETHYLENE TETRACHLORIDE ◇ FEDAL-UN ◇ NCI-C04580 ◇ NEMA ◇ PERAWIN ◇ PERCHLOORETHYLEEN, PER (DUTCH) ◇ PERCHLOR ◇ PERCHLORAETHYLEN, PER (GERMAN) ◇ PERCHLORETHYLENE ◇ PERCHLORETHY-LENE, PER (FRENCH) ◇ PERCLENE ◇ PERCLOROETILENE (ITALIAN) ◇ PERCOSOLVE ◇ PERK ◇ PERKLONE ◇ PERSEC ◇ RCRA WASTE NUMBER U210 ◇ TETLEN ◇ TETRACAP ◇ TETRACHLOORETHEEN (DUTCH) ◇ TETRACHLORAETHEN (GERMAN) ◇ TETRACHLO-ROETHENE ◇ TETRACHLOROETHYLENE (DOT) ◇ 1,1,2,2-TETRACHLOROETHYLENE ◇ TETRACLOROETENE (ITAL-IAN) ◇ TETRALENO ◇ TETRALEX ◇ TETRAVEC ◇ TETROGUER ◇ TETROPIL

TOXICITY DATA with REFERENCE
CAR: ihl-mus TCLo: 100 ppm/6H/2Y-I   NTPTR*
  NTP-TR-311,86
CAR: ihl-rat TCLo: 200 ppm/6H/2Y-I   NTPTR*
  NTP-TR-311,86
CAR: orl-mus TD: 240 g/kg/62W-I   NCITR*
  NCI-TR-13,77
CAR: orl-mus TDLo: 195 g/kg/50W-I   NCITR*
  NCI-TR-13,77
NEO: ihl-mus TC: 100 ppm/6H/2Y-I   TOLED5
  31(Suppl),16,86
NEO: ihl-rat TC: 200 ppm/6H/2Y-I   TOLED5
  31(Suppl),16,86
MUT: dns-hmn: lng 100 mg/L   NTIS**PB82-185075
MUT: mma-sat 200 μL/plate   NIOSH* 5AUG77
MUT: mmo-sat 50 μL/plate   NIOSH* 5AUG77
MUT: otr-rat: emb 97 μmol/L   ITCSAF 14,290,78

CONSENSUS REPORTS: IARC Cancer Review: Animal Limited Evidence IMEMDT 20,491,79. NCI Carcinogenesis Bioassay (gavage); Clear Evidence: mouse NCITR* NCI-CG-TR-13,77; (inhalation); Clear Evidence: mouse, rat NTPTR* NTP-TR-311,86; (gavage); Inadequate Studies: rat NCITR* NCI-CG-TR-13,77. Reported in EPA TSCA Inventory. EPA Genetic Toxicology Program. Community Right-To-Know List.

OSHA PEL: (Transitional: TWA 100 ppm; CL 200 ppm; Pk 600 ppm/5M)TWA 25 ppm   ACGIH TLV: TWA 50 ppm; STEL 200 ppm (Proposed: BEI: 7 mg/L trichloroacetic acid in urine at end of workweek.)   DFG MAK: 50 ppm (345 mg/m³); BAT: blood 100 μg/dl   NIOSH REL: (Tetrachloroethylene) Minimize workplace exposure.   DOT Classification: Poison B; Label: St. Andrews Cross; ORM-A; Label: None.

SAFETY PROFILE: Suspected carcinogen with experimental carcinogenic, neoplastigenic, and teratogenic data. Experimental poison by intravenous route. Moderately toxic to humans by inhalation with the following effects: local anesthetic, conjunctiva irritation, general anesthesia, hallucinations, distorted perceptions, coma, and pulmonary changes. Moderately experimentally toxic by ingestion, inhalation, intraperitoneal, and subcutaneous routes. Experimental reproductive effects. Human mutation data reported. An eye and severe skin irritant. When heated to decomposition it emits highly toxic fumes of Cl⁻.

PCR000   CAS: 91845-41-9
PETASITES JAPONICUS MAXIM

PROP: Dried flower stalk of *Petasites Japonicus Maxim* (GANNA2 64,527,73).

SYNS: COLTS FOOT ◇ FUKI-NO-TOH (JAPANESE)

TOXICITY DATA with REFERENCE
CAR: orl-mus TDLo: 2300 g/kg/69W-C
  TOLED5 1,291,78
CAR: orl-rat TDLo: 1060 mg/kg/69W-C
  GANNA2 64,527,73
ETA: orl-rat TD: 960 g/kg/68W-C   GANNA2
  68(6),841,77

SAFETY PROFILE: Suspected carcinogen with experimental carcinogenic and tumorigenic data. When heated to decomposition it emits acrid smoke and irritating fumes.

PEI000   CAS: 60-09-3
p-(PHENYLAZO)ANILINE
mf: $C_{12}H_{11}N_3$ mw: 197.26

PROP: Yellow crystals. Mp: 128°, bp: 360°. Sltly sol in hot water; sol in hot alc and ether.

SYNS: AAB ◇ AMINOAZOBENZENE ◇ p-AMINOAZOBEN-ZENE ◇ 4-AMINOAZOBENZENE ◇ 4-AMINO-1,1'-AZOBEN-ZENE ◇ p-AMINOAZOBENZOL ◇ 4-AMINOAZOBENZOL ◇ p-AMINODIPHENYLIMIDE ◇ ANILINE YELLOW ◇ 4-BENZENEAZOANILINE ◇ BRASILAZINA OIL YELLOW G ◇ CERES YELLOW R ◇ C.I. 11000 ◇ C.I. SOLVENT BLUE 7 ◇ C.I. SOLVENT YELLOW 1 ◇ FAST SPIRIT YELLOW AAB ◇ OIL SOLUBLE ANILINE YELLOW ◇ OIL YELLOW AAB ◇ ORGANOL YELLOW ◇ PARAPHENOLAZO ANILINE ◇ 4-(PHENYLAZO)ANILINE ◇ 4-(PHENYLAZO)BENZENA-MINE ◇ p-PHENYLAZOPHENYLAMINE ◇ SOLVENT YEL-LOW 1 ◇ SUDAN YELLOW R ◇ USAF EK-1375

TOXICITY DATA with REFERENCE
NEO: ipr-mus TD: 10 mg/kg   CNREA8 44,2540,84
NEO: ipr-mus TDLo: 3353 µg/kg   CNREA8 44,2540,84
NEO: irn-frg TDLo: 12 mg/kg   CNREA8 24,1969,64
NEO: skn-rat TDLo: 1965 mg/kg/2Y-I   CNREA8 26,2406,66
ETA: orl-rat TDLo: 89 g/kg/57W-C   JPBAA7 59,1,47
ETA: scu-mus TDLo: 296 mg/kg (15-19D post)   CALEDQ 17,321,83
MUT: dns-rat: ivr 5 µmol/L   ENMUDM 3,11,81
MUT: hma-mus/sat 125 mg/kg   JNCIAM 62,911,79
MUT: mma-sat 100 µg/plate   PNASA6 72,5135,75
MUT: mmo-sat 50 nmol/plate   CRNGDP 3,113,82
MUT: mrc-esc 700 µg/well   MUREAV 46,53,77
MUT: otr-ham: emb 32 mg/L   NCIMAV 58,243,81
MUT: otr-ham: kdy 80 µg/L   BJCAAI 37,873,78

CONSENSUS REPORTS: IARC Cancer Review: GROUP 2B IMEMDT 7,56,87; Animal Sufficient Evidence IMEMDT 8,53,75. Community Right-To-Know List. Reported in EPA TSCA Inventory.

SAFETY PROFILE: Suspected carcinogen with experimental neoplastigenic and tumorigenic data. Poison by intraperitoneal route. Experimental reproductive effects. Mutation data reported. Used as a dye for lacquer, varnish, wax products, oil stains, and styrene resins. When heated to decomposition it emits toxic fumes of NO_x.

PFH000   CAS: 122-60-1
PHENYL GLYCYDYL ETHER
mf: $C_9H_{10}O_2$ mw: 150.19

SYNS: 1,2-EPOXY-3-PHENOXYPROPANE ◇ 2,3-EPOXY-PROPYLPHENYL ETHER ◇ FENYL-GLYCIDYLETHER

(CZECH) ◇ GLYCIDYL PHENYL ETHER ◇ PGE ◇ PHENOL-GLYCIDAETHER (GERMAN) ◇ PHENOL GLYCIDYL ETHER (MAK) ◇ 3-PHENOXY-1,2-EPOXYPROPANE ◇ PHENOXY-PROPENE OXIDE ◇ PHENOXYPROPYLENE OXIDE ◇ PHENYL-2,3-EPOXYPROPYL ETHER

TOXICITY DATA with REFERENCE
CAR: ihl-rat TCLo: 12 ppm/6H/2Y-I   AJPAA4 111,140,83
MUT: hma-mus/sat 2500 mg/kg   MUREAV 67,9,79
MUT: mmo-esc 20 µmol/L   ARTODN 46,277,80
MUT: mmo-klp 100 µmol/L   MUREAV 89,269,81
MUT: mmo-sat 50 µg/plate   MUREAV 67,9,79

CONSENSUS REPORTS: Reported in EPA TSCA Inventory. EPA Genetic Toxicology Program.

OSHA PEL: (Transitional: TWA 10 ppm) TWA 1 ppm   ACGIH TLV: TWA 1 ppm   DFG MAK: 1 ppm (6 mg/m³), Suspected Carcinogen. NIOSH REL: (Glycidyl Ethers) CL 5 mg/m³/15M

SAFETY PROFILE: Suspected carcinogen with experimental carcinogenic data. Moderately toxic by ingestion, skin contact, and subcutaneous routes. A severe eye and skin irritant. Experimental reproductive effects. Mutation data reported. When heated to decomposition it emits acrid smoke and irritating fumes. Used as a chemical intermediate.

PFI000   CAS: 100-63-0
PHENYLHYDRAZINE
DOT: 2572
mf: $C_6H_8N_2$ mw: 108.16

PROP: Yellow, monoclinic crystals or oil. Mp: 19.6°, bp: 243.5° (decomp), flash p: 192°F (CC), d: 1.0978 @ 20°/4°, vap press: 1 mm @ 71.8°, vap d: 3.7. Sltly sol in hot water; misc in alc, chloroform, ether, benzene.

SYNS: FENILIDRAZINA (ITALIAN) ◇ FENYLHYDRAZINE (DUTCH) ◇ HYDRAZINE-BENZENE ◇ HYDRAZINOBENZ-ENE ◇ PHENYLHYDRAZIN (GERMAN)

TOXICITY DATA with REFERENCE
CAR: scu-rat TDLo: 5200 mg/kg/52W-I   GTPZAB 19(6),28,75
MUT: dnd-mus-ipr 350 µmol/kg   CNREA8 41,1469,81
MUT: mma-sat 1500 µg/plate   MUREAV 66,247,79
MUT: mmo-omi 150 µg/L   MUREAV 173,233,86
MUT: mmo-sat 4600 nmol/plate   CNREA8 41,1469,81

CONSENSUS REPORTS: Reported in EPA TSCA Inventory.

OSHA PEL: (Transitional: TWA 5 ppm (skin)) TWA 5 ppm (skin); STEL 10 ppm   ACGIH TLV: TWA 5 ppm (skin); STEL 10 ppm; Suspected Human Carcinogen; (Proposed: TWA 0.1 ppm (skin); Suspected Human Carcinogen)   DFG MAK: 5 ppm (22 mg/m^3), Suspected Carcinogen.   NIOSH REL: CL 0.6 mg/m^3/2H   DOT Classification: Poison B; Label: Poison.

SAFETY PROFILE: Suspected carcinogen with experimental carcinogenic data. Poison by ingestion, subcutaneous, intravenous, and possibly other routes. Experimental reproductive effects. Mutation data reported. Ingestion or subcutaneous injection can cause hemolysis of red blood cells. Flammable when exposed to heat, flame or oxidizers. To fight fire, use alcohol foam. Dangerous; when heated to decomposition it emits highly toxic fumes of NO$_x$; can react with oxidizing materials.

PFT500   CAS: 135-88-6
N-PHENYL-β-NAPHTHYLAMINE
mf: C$_{16}$H$_{13}$N   mw: 219.30

PROP: Rhombic crystals from methanol. Mp: 107-108°, bp: 395.5°. Insol in water; sol in hot benzene; very sol in hot alc, ether.

SYNS: ACETO PBN ◇ AGERITE POWDER ◇ ANILINON-APHTHALENE ◇ 2-ANILINONAPHTHALENE ◇ ANTIOXI-DANT 116 ◇ ANTIOXIDANT PBN ◇ N-(2-NAPHTHYL)ANI-LINE ◇ 2-NAPHTHYLPHENYLAMINE ◇ β-NAPHTHYLPHE-NYLAMINE ◇ NCI-C02915 ◇ NEOZONE D ◇ NILOX PBNA ◇ NONOX D ◇ PBNA ◇ PHENYL-β-NAPHTHYLAMINE ◇ PHENYL-2-NAPHTHYLAMINE ◇ N-PHENYL-β-NAPHTHYLAMINE ◇ N-PHENYL-2-NAPHTHYLAMINE ◇ STABILIZATOR AR

TOXICITY DATA with REFERENCE
CAR: orl-mus TD: 17280 mg/kg/9W-I   CNREA8 44,3098,84
CAR: orl-mus TDLo: 208 g/kg/97W-C   SYSWAE 14,129,81
NEO: orl-mus TD: 135 g/kg/78W-I   NTIS**PB223-159
NEO: scu-mus TDLo: 464 mg/kg   NTIS** PB223-159
ETA: orl-mus TD: 264 g/kg/99W-C   SYSWAE 14,129,81
ETA: orl-mus TDLo: 433 g/kg/2Y-C   NTPTR* NTP-TR-333,88

MUT: cyt-mus-orl 360 mg/kg/18D   GTPZAB 29(9),57,79
MUT: otr-hmn: oth 23100 μg/L   ITCSAF 17,719,81

CONSENSUS REPORTS: IARC Cancer Review: Human Inadequate Evidence IMEMDT 16,325,78; Animal Limited Evidence IMEMDT 16,325,78. Reported in EPA TSCA Inventory.

ACGIH TLV: Suspected Human Carcinogen.   DFG MAK: Suspected Carcinogen.

SAFETY PROFILE: Suspected carcinogen with experimental carcinogenic, neoplastigenic, and tumorigenic data. Moderately toxic by ingestion. Human mutation data reported. When heated to decomposition it emits toxic fumes of NO$_x$.

PIK250   CAS: 21416-87-5
2,6-PIPERAZINEDIONE-4,4'-
PROPYLENE DIOXOPIPERAZINE
mf: C$_{11}$H$_{16}$N$_4$O$_4$ mw: 268.31

SYNS: (±)-1,2-BIS(3,5-DIOXOPIPERAZINE-1-YL)PRO-PANE ◇ (±)-1,2-BIS(3,5-DIOXOPIPERAZINYL)PROPANE ◇ ICRF-159 ◇ 4,4'-(1-METHYL-1,2-ETHANEDIYL)BIS-2,6-PI-PERAZINEDIONE ◇ NCI-C01627 ◇ NSC-129943 ◇ RAZOXIN ◇ (±)-(3,5,3',5'-TETRAOXO)-1,2-DIPIPERAZINOPROPANE

TOXICITY DATA with REFERENCE
CAR: ipr-mus TD: 12 g/kg/Y-I   NCITR* NCI-CG-TR-78,78
CAR: ipr-rat TD: 15 g/kg/Y-I: TER   NCITR* NCI-CG-TR-78,78
CAR: ipr-rat TDLo: 7488 mg/kg/52W-I: TER   NCITR* NCI-CG-TR-78,78
ETA: ipr-mus TD: 1 g/kg/8W-I   CNREA8 33,3069,73
MUT: dni-mus: emb 20 mg/L   IJCNAW 5,47,70
MUT: msc-mus: lng 200 μg/L   MUREAV 157,199,85

CONSENSUS REPORTS: NCI Carcinogenesis Bioassay (ipr); Clear Evidence: mouse, rat NCITR* NCI-CG-TR-78,78. EPA Genetic Toxicology Program.

SAFETY PROFILE: Suspected carcinogen with experimental carcinogenic and tumorigenic data. Moderately toxic by intraperitoneal route. Experimental teratogenic and reproductive effects. Human systemic effects by ingestion: nausea, thrombocytopenia, leukopenia. Mutation data reported. When heated to decomposition it emits toxic fumes of NO$_x$.

PJD000   CAS: 15663-27-1
cis-PLATINOUS DIAMMINE DICHLORIDE
mf: Cl$_2$H$_6$N$_2$Pt   mw: 300.07

SYNS: CACP ◇ CDDP ◇ CISPLATINO (SPANISH) ◇ CISPLATYL ◇ CPDC ◇ CPDD ◇ DDP ◇ cis-DDP ◇ cis-DIAMINEDICHLOROPLATINUM ◇ cis-DICHLORO-DIAMMINE PLATINUM(II) ◇ NCI-C55776 ◇ NEOPLATIN ◇ NSC-119875 ◇ PEYRONE'S CHLORIDE ◇ PLATIBLASTIN ◇ cis-PLATIN ◇ PLATINEX ◇ PLATINOL ◇ cis-PLATINUM(II) DIAMINEDICHLORIDE

TOXICITY DATA with REFERENCE
CAR: ipr-mus TDLo: 16 mg/kg/19W-I CNREA8 39,913,79
NEO: ipr-mus TD: 16204 μg/kg/10W-I CNREA8 41,4368,81
NEO: ipr-mus TD: 32408 μg/kg/10W-I CNREA8 41,4368,81
MUT: dnd-hmn: fbr 10 μmol/L CNREA8 41,3347,81
MUT: dnd-hmn: lym 12 μmol/L CNREA8 42,897,82
MUT: dnr-bcs 1 μg/plate TAKHAA 44,96,85
MUT: dns-hmn: fbr 20 μmol/L CNREA844,1809,84
MUT: mmo-nsc 200 μmol/L MUREAV 125,43,84
MUT: mmo-sat 250 ng/plate TAKHAA 44,96,85
MUT: sce-hmn: lym 250 ng/L/96H ARTODN 46,61,80

CONSENSUS REPORTS: IARC Cancer Review: Animal Limited Evidence IMEMDT 26,151,81. Reported in EPA TSCA Inventory. EPA Genetic Toxicology Program.

OSHA PEL: TWA 0.002 mg(Pt)/m^3 ACGIH TLV: TWA 0.002 mg(Pt)/m^3

SAFETY PROFILE: Suspected carcinogen with experimental carcinogenic and tumorigenic data. Poison by ingestion, intramuscular, subcutaneous, intravenous, and intraperitoneal routes. Human systemic effects by intravenous, intradermal and possibly other routes: nausea or vomiting, change in auditory acuity, depressed renal function tests, changes in bone marrow, change in kidney tubules, hallucinations, corrosive to skin. Experimental teratogenic and reproductive effects. Human mutation data reported. When heated to decomposition it emits very toxic fumes of Cl$^-$ and NO$_x$.

PJJ750
POLONIUM
af: Po   aw: 210

PROP: A low melting, volatile, radioactive, naturally occurring metallic element. Mp: 254°, bp: 962°, d: 9.4.

SYN: RADIUM F

SAFETY PROFILE: Suspected carcinogen. Severe radiotoxicity. Very dangerous to handle. Radiation Hazard: Natural isotope ^{210}Po (radium-F, Uranium Series), $T_{0.5} = 138$ D. Decays to stable ^{206}Pb by alphas of 5.3 MeV. When heated to decomposition it emits toxic and radioactive fumes of Po.

PJK000
POLONIUM CARBONYL
mf: PoCO   mw: 237.01

SAFETY PROFILE: Suspected carcinogen. Poison by ingestion, inhalation, intravenous, and subcutaneous routes. When heated to decomposition it emits toxic and radioactive fumes of Po.

PJM000   CAS: 11104-28-2
POLYCHLORINATED BIPHENYL (AROCLOR 1221)

SYNS: AROCHLOR 1221 ◇ CHLORODIPHENYL (21% Cl)

CONSENSUS REPORTS: IARC Cancer Review: Human Limited Evidence IMEMDT 18,43,78.

NIOSH REL: TWA (Polychlorinated Biphenyls) 0.001 mg/m^3

SAFETY PROFILE: Suspected human carcinogen. Moderately toxic by ingestion and skin contact. Experimental reproductive effects. When heated to decomposition it emits toxic fumes of Cl$^-$. Used in heat transfer, hydraulic fluids, lubricants, and insecticides.

PJM250   CAS: 11141-16-5
POLYCHLORINATED BIPHENYL (AROCLOR 1232)

SYNS: AROCLOR 1232 ◇ CHLORODIPHENYL (32% Cl)

CONSENSUS REPORTS: IARC Cancer Review: Human Limited Evidence IMEMDT 18,43,78.

NIOSH REL: TWA (Polychlorinated Biphenyls) 0.001 mg/m^3

SAFETY PROFILE: Suspected human carcinogen. Moderately toxic by skin contact. Mildly toxic by ingestion. When heated to decomposition it emits toxic fumes of Cl$^-$. Used in heat transfer, hydraulic fluids, lubricants, and insecticides.

PJM500   CAS: 53469-21-9
**POLYCHLORINATED BIPHENYL
(AROCLOR 1242)**

SYNS: AROCHLOR 1242 ◇ AROCLOR 1242 ◇ CHLOR-
IERTE BIPHENYLE, CHLORGEHALT 42% (GERMAN)
◇ CHLORODIPHENYL (42% Cl) (OSHA) ◇ CLORODIFENILI,
CLORO 42% (ITALIAN) ◇ DIPHENYLE CHLORE, 42% de
CHLORE (FRENCH) ◇ GECHLOREERDEDIFENYL (DUTCH)
◇ PCB's

TOXICITY DATA with REFERENCE
MUT: EESADV 3,10,79
MUT: oms-mus:oth 25 ppm/4H

CONSENSUS REPORTS: IARC Cancer Review: Human Limited Evidence IMEMDT
18,43,78. EPA Genetic Toxicology Program.

OSHA PEL: TWA 1 mg/m³ (skin)   ACGIH
TLV: TWA 1 mg/m³ (skin)   DFG MAK: 0.1
ppm (1 mg/m³)   NIOSH REL: TWA (Polychlorinated Biphenyls) 0.001 mg/m³

SAFETY PROFILE: Suspected human carcinogen. Poison by subcutaneous route. Mildly toxic
by ingestion. Human systemic effects by inhalation: pulmonary and liver effects. Moderately
toxic by ingestion. Experimental reproductive
effects. Mutation data reported. When heated
to decomposition it emits toxic fumes of Cl⁻.
Used in heat transfer, hydraulic fluids, lubricants, and insecticides.

PJM750   CAS: 12672-29-6
**POLYCHLORINATED BIPHENYL
(AROCLOR 1248)**

SYNS: AROCLOR 1248 ◇ CHLORODIPHENYL (48% Cl)

CONSENSUS REPORTS: IARC Cancer Review: Human Limited Evidence IMEMDT
18,43,78.

NIOSH REL: TWA (Polychlorinated Biphenyls) 0.001 mg/m³

SAFETY PROFILE: Suspected human carcinogen. Moderately toxic by skin contact. Experimental teratogenic and reproductive effects.
When heated to decomposition it emits toxic
fumes of Cl⁻. Used in heat transfer, hydraulic
fluids, lubricants, and insecticides.

PJN000   CAS: 11097-69-1
**POLYCHLORINATED BIPHENYL
(AROCLOR 1254)**

PROP: Composed of 11% tetra-, 49% penta-,
34% hexa- and 6% heptachlorobiphenyls
(FCTXAV 12,63,74).

SYNS: AROCHLOR 1254 ◇ AROCLOR 1254 ◇ CHLOR-
IERTE BIPHENYLE, CHLORGEHALT 54% (GERMAN)
◇ CHLORODIPHENYL (54% Cl) (OSHA) ◇ CLORODIFENILI,
CLORO 54% (ITALIAN) ◇ DIPHENYLE CHLORE, 54% de
CHLORE (FRENCH) ◇ NCI-C02664 ◇ PCB's

TOXICITY DATA with REFERENCE
CAR: orl-rat TDLo:73500 mg/kg/2Y-C
   EVHPAZ 60,89,85
NEO: orl-mus TDLo:17 g/kg/48W-C   JNCIAM
   53,547,74
ETA: orl-rat TD:1 mg/kg/D-C   CNREA8 41,5052,81
ETA: orl-rat TD:3 mg/kg/D-C   CNREA8 41,5052,81
ETA: orl-rat TDLo:4 g/kg/2Y-I   NCITR*
   NCI-CG-TR-38,78
ETA: skn-mus TDLo:4 mg/kg   BECTA6 18,552,77
MUT: cyt-ofs-ipr 50 mg/kg   CBPCBB 82,489,85
MUT: dnd-rat-orl 1295 mg/kg   BSIBAC 57,407,81
MUT: dnd-rat:lvr 300 µmol/L   SinJF# 26OCT82
MUT: otr-rat-orl 25 ppm/2Y-C   EVHPAZ 60,89,85

CONSENSUS REPORTS: IARC Cancer Review: GROUP 2A IMEMDT 7,322,87; Animal
Sufficient Evidence IMEMDT 7,261,74; Animal Limited Evidence IMEMDT 18,43,78; Human Limited Evidence IMEMDT 18,43,78.
NCI Carcinogenesis Bioassay (feed); Some Evidence: rat NCITR* NCI-CG-TR-38,78. EPA
Genetic Toxicology Program.

OSHA PEL: TWA 0.5 mg/m³ (skin)   ACGIH
TLV: TWA 0.5 mg/m³ (skin)   NIOSH REL:
TWA (Polychlorinated Biphenyls) 0.001 mg/m³

SAFETY PROFILE: Suspected carcinogen with
experimental carcinogenic and neoplastigenic
data. Poison by intravenous route. Moderately
toxic by ingestion and intraperitoneal routes.
Experimental teratogenic and reproductive effects. Mutation data reported. When heated to
decomposition it emits toxic fumes of Cl⁻. Used
in heat transfer, hydraulic fluids, lubricants, and
insecticides.

PJN250   CAS: 11096-82-5
**POLYCHLORINATED BIPHENYL
(AROCLOR 1260)**

PROP: Composed of 12% penta-, 38% hexa-,
41% hepta-, 8% octa- and 1% nonachlorobiphe-
nyls (FCTXAV 12,63,74).

SYNS: AROCHLOR 1260 ◇ AROCLOR 1260 ◇ CHLORODI-
PHENYL (60% Cl) ◇ CLOPHEN A60 ◇ PHENOCLOR DP6

TOXICITY DATA with REFERENCE
CAR: orl-rat TD:4992 mg/kg/2Y-C   TXAPA9
   75,278,84

CAR: orl-rat TDLo:4380 mg/kg/83W-C
JNCIAM 55,1453,75
NEO: orl-rat TD:360 mg/kg/17W-C CALEDQ
39,59,88
MUT: cyt-rat-orl 1080 mg/kg/26W-C APTOD9
19,A16,80

CONSENSUS REPORTS: IARC Cancer Review: Animal Limited Evidence IMEMDT 18,43,78; Human Limited Evidence IMEMDT 18,43,78.

NIOSH REL: TWA (Polychlorinated Biphenyls) 0.001 mg/m^3

SAFETY PROFILE: Suspected carcinogen with carcinogenic and neoplastigenic data. Moderately toxic by ingestion and skin contact. Experimental reproductive effects. Mutation data reported. When heated to decomposition it emits highly toxic fumes of Cl$^-$. Used in heat transfer, hydraulic fluids, lubricants, and insecticides.

PJN500 CAS: 37324-23-5
POLYCHLORINATED BIPHENYL
(AROCLOR 1262)

SYNS: AROCLOR 1262 ◇ CHLORODIPHENYL (62% Cl)

CONSENSUS REPORTS: IARC Cancer Review: Human Limited Evidence IMEMDT 18,43,78. DFG MAK: 0.1 ppm (1 mg/m^3) NIOSH REL: TWA 0.001 mg/m^3

SAFETY PROFILE: Suspected human carcinogen. Moderately toxic by skin contact. When heated to decomposition it emits toxic fumes of Cl$^-$. Used in heat transfer, hydraulic fluids, lubricants, and insecticides.

PJN750 CAS: 11100-14-4
POLYCHLORINATED BIPHENYL
(AROCLOR 1268)

SYNS: AROCLOR 1268 ◇ CHLORODIPHENYL (68% Cl)

CONSENSUS REPORTS: IARC Cancer Review: Human Limited Evidence IMEMDT 18,43,78.

NIOSH REL: TWA 0.001 mg/m^3

SAFETY PROFILE: Suspected human carcinogen. Moderately toxic by skin contact. Used in heat transfer, hydraulic fluids, lubricants, and insecticides. When heated to decomposition it emits toxic fumes of Cl$^-$.

PJO000 CAS: 37324-24-6
POLYCHLORINATED BIPHENYL
(AROCLOR 2565)

SYN: AROCLOR 2565

CONSENSUS REPORTS: IARC Cancer Review: Human Limited Evidence IMEMDT 18,43,78.

NIOSH REL: TWA 0.001 mg/m^3

SAFETY PROFILE: Suspected human carcinogen. Moderately toxic by skin contact. Mildly toxic by ingestion. When heated to decomposition it emits toxic fumes of Cl$^-$. Used in heat transfer, hydraulic fluids, lubricants, and insecticides.

PJO250 CAS: 11120-29-9
POLYCHLORINATED BIPHENYL
(AROCLOR 4465)

SYN: AROCLOR 4465

CONSENSUS REPORTS: IARC Cancer Review: Human Limited Evidence IMEMDT 18,43,78.

NIOSH REL: TWA (Polychlorinated Biphenyls) 0.001 mg/m^3

SAFETY PROFILE: Suspected human carcinogen. Moderately toxic by skin contact. Mildly toxic by ingestion. When heated to decomposition it emits toxic fumes of Cl$^-$. Used in heat transfer, hydraulic fluids, lubricants, and insecticides.

PJO500 CAS: 37353-63-2
POLYCHLORINATED BIPHENYL
(KANECHLOR 300)

PROP: Average content: 60% trichlorobiphenyl, 23% tetrachlorobiphenyl, 17% dichlorobiphenyl, 1% pentachlorobiphenyl (IARC** 7,262,74).

SYN: KANECHLOR 300

IARC Cancer Review: Animal Limited Evidence IMEMDT 7,261,74, IMEMDT 18, 43,78; Human Limited Evidence IMEMDT 18,43,78.

NIOSH REL: TWA (Polychlorinated Biphenyls) 0.001 mg/m^3

SAFETY PROFILE: Suspected human carcinogen. Used in heat transfer, hydraulic fluids, lubricants, and insecticides. When heated to decomposition it emits toxic fumes of Cl^-.

PJO750   CAS: 12737-87-0
POLYCHLORINATED BIPHENYL
(KANECHLOR 400)

PROP: Average content: 44% tetrachlorbiphenyl, 33% trichlorobiphenyl, 16% pentachlorobiphenyl, 5% hexachlorobiphenyl, 3% dichlorobiphenyl (IARC** 7,262,74).

SYNS: KANECHLOR 400 ◇ KC-400

TOXICITY DATA with REFERENCE
NEO: orl-rat TDLo:6750 mg/kg/69W-I
 GANNA2 64,105,73

CONSENSUS REPORTS: IARC Cancer Review: Animal Limited Evidence IMEMDT 7,261,74, IMEMDT 18,43,78; Human Limited Evidence IMEMDT 18,43,78.

NIOSH REL: TWA (Polychlorinated Biphenyls) 0.001 mg/m^3

SAFETY PROFILE: Suspected carcinogen with experimental neoplastigenic data. Experimental teratogenic and reproductive effects. Human systemic effects by ingestion: dermatitis, sweating. When heated to decomposition it emits toxic fumes of Cl^-.

PJP000   CAS: 37317-41-2
POLYCHLORINATED BIPHENYL
(KANECHLOR 500)

PROP: Average content, 55% pentachlorobiphenyl, 26.5% tetrachlorobiphenyl, 12.8% hexachloro biphenyl and 5% trichlorobiphenyl (JNCIAM 51,1637,73).

SYNS: KANECHLOR 500 ◇ KC-500

TOXICITY DATA with REFERENCE
CAR: orl-mus TD:23 g/kg/32W-C   JNCIAM
 51,1637,73
CAR: orl-mus TDLo:13 g/kg/32W-C   NAIZAM
 25,635,74
ETA: orl-mus TD:13440 mg/kg/32W-C   SAIGBL
 17,54,75

CONSENSUS REPORTS: IARC Cancer Review: Human Limited Evidence IMEMDT 18,43,78; Animal Limited Evidence IMEMDT 18,43,78; Animal Sufficient Evidence IMEMDT 7,261,74.

NIOSH REL: TWA (Polychlorinated Biphenyls) 0.001 mg/m^3.

SAFETY PROFILE: Suspected carcinogen with experimental carcinogenic and tumorigenic data. Experimental teratogenic and reproductive effects. When heated to decomposition it emits toxic fumes of Cl^-. Used in heat transfer, hydraulic fluids, lubricants, and insecticides.

PKQ500   CAS: 9003-39-8
POLY(1-VINYL-2-PYRROLIDINONE)
HUEPER'S POLYMER NO. 1

PROP: Polymer of average molecular weight 20,000 (AMPLAO 67,589,59).

SYNS: NCI-C60582 ◇ PVP 1

TOXICITY DATA with REFERENCE
CAR: ipr-rat TDLo:2500 mg/kg   AMPLAO
 67,589,59
CAR: ivn-rat TDLo:750 mg/kg/I   AMPLAO
 67,589,59
CAR: scu-rat TDLo:2500 mg/kg   AMPLAO
 67,589,59

CONSENSUS REPORTS: IARC Cancer Review: Animal Limited Evidence IMEMDT 19,461,79. Reported in EPA TSCA Inventory.

SAFETY PROFILE: Suspected carcinogen with experimental carcinogenic data. When heated to decomposition it emits toxic fumes of NO_x.

PKQ750   CAS: 9003-39-8
POLY(1-VINYL-2-PYRROLIDINONE)
HUEPER'S POLYMER NO. 2

PROP: Polymer of average molecular weight 20,000 (AMPLAO 67,589,59).

SYNS: NCI-C60582 ◇ PVP 2

TOXICITY DATA with REFERENCE
NEO: ipr-rat TDLo:2500 mg/kg   AMPLAO
 67,589,59
NEO: ivn-rat TDLo:750 mg/kg/I   AMPLAO
 67,589,59
NEO: scu-rat TDLo:2500 mg/kg   AMPLAO
 67,589,59
ETA: scu-mus TDLo:8000 mg/kg   AMPLAO
 67,589,59

CONSENSUS REPORTS: IARC Cancer Review: Animal Limited Evidence IMEMDT 19,461,79. Reported in EPA TSCA Inventory.

SAFETY PROFILE: Suspected carcinogen with experimental neoplastigenic and tumorigenic data. When heated to decomposition it emits toxic fumes of NO_x.

PKR000   CAS: 9003-39-8
POLY(1-VINYL-2-PYRROLIDINONE)
HUEPER'S POLYMER NO. 3

PROP: Polymer of average molecular weight 50,000 (AMPLAO 67,589,59).

SYNS: NCI-C60582 ◇ PVP 3

TOXICITY DATA with REFERENCE
CAR: ipr-rat TDLo: 2500 mg/kg   AMPLAO
  67,589,59
CAR: ivn-rat TDLo: 750 mg/kg/I   AMPLAO
  67,589,59
CAR: scu-rat TDLo: 2500 mg/kg   AMPLAO
  67,589,59
ETA: ipr-mus TDLo: 8000 mg/kg   AMPLAO
  67,589,59

CONSENSUS REPORTS: IARC Cancer Review: Animal Limited Evidence IMEMDT 19,461,79. Reported in EPA TSCA Inventory.

SAFETY PROFILE: Suspected carcinogen with experimental carcinogenic and tumorigenic data. When heated to decomposition it emits toxic fumes of NO_x.

PKR250   CAS: 9003-39-8
POLY(1-VINYL-2-PYRROLIDINONE)
HUEPER'S POLYMER NO. 4

PROP: Polymer of average molecular weight 300,000 (AMPLAO 67,589,59).

SYNS: NCI-C60582 ◇ PVP 4

TOXICITY DATA with REFERENCE
CAR: ipr-rat TDLo: 2500 mg/kg   AMPLAO
  67,589,59
CAR: ivn-rat TDLo: 750 mg/kg/I   AMPLAO
  67,589,59
CAR: scu-rat TDLo: 2500 mg/kg   AMPLAO
  67,589,59

CONSENSUS REPORTS: IARC Cancer Review: Animal Limited Evidence IMEMDT 19,461,79. Reported in EPA TSCA Inventory.

SAFETY PROFILE: Suspected carcinogen with experimental carcinogenic data. When heated to decomposition it emits toxic fumes of NO_x.

PKR500   CAS: 9003-39-8
POLY(1-VINYL-2-PYRROLIDINONE)
HUEPER'S POLYMER NO. 5

PROP: Polymer of average molecular weight 10,000 (AMPLAO 67,589,59).

SYN: PVP 5

TOXICITY DATA with REFERENCE
CAR: ipr-rat TDLo: 2500 mg/kg   AMPLAO
  67,589,59
CAR: scu-rat TDLo: 2500 mg/kg   AMPLAO
  67,589,59
ETA: ipr-mus TDLo: 8000 mg/kg   AMPLAO
  67,589,59

CONSENSUS REPORTS: IARC Cancer Review: Animal Limited Evidence IMEMDT 19,461,79. Reported in EPA TSCA Inventory.

SAFETY PROFILE: Suspected carcinogen with experimental carcinogenic and tumorigenic data. When heated to decomposition it emits toxic fumes of NO_x.

PKR750   CAS: 9003-39-8
POLY(1-VINYL-2-PYRROLIDINONE)
HUEPER'S POLYMER NO. 6

PROP: Polymer of average molecular weight 50,000 (AMPLAO 67,589,59).

SYNS: NCI-C60582 ◇ PVP 6

TOXICITY DATA with REFERENCE
CAR: scu-rat TDLo: 1000 mg/kg   AMPLAO
  67,589,59

CONSENSUS REPORTS: IARC Cancer Review: Animal Limited Evidence IMEMDT 19,461,79. Reported in EPA TSCA Inventory.

SAFETY PROFILE: Suspected carcinogen with experimental carcinogenic data. When heated to decomposition it emits toxic fumes of NO_x.

PKS000   CAS: 9003-39-8
POLY(1-VINYL-2-PYRROLIDINONE)
HUEPER'S POLYMER NO. 7

SYNS: NCI-C60582 ◇ PVP 7

TOXICITY DATA with REFERENCE
NEO: scu-rat TDLo: 3000 mg/kg/I   AMPLAO
  67,589,59

CONSENSUS REPORTS: IARC Cancer Review: Animal Limited Evidence IMEMDT 19,461,79.

SAFETY PROFILE: Suspected carcinogen with experimental neoplastigenic data. When heated to decomposition it emits toxic fumes of NO_x.

PKY300   CAS: 7758-01-2
POTASSIUM BROMATE
DOT: 1484
mf: $BrO_3 \cdot K$ mw: 167.01

PROP: White crystals or crystalline powder. Mp: 350° (approx), decomp @ 370°, d: 3.27 @ 17.5°. Sol in water; sltly sol in alc.

SYN: BROMIC ACID, POTASSIUM SALT

TOXICITY DATA with REFERENCE
CAR: orl-rat TD:9625 mg/kg/2Y-C   ESKHA5 (100),93,82

CAR: orl-rat TD:9625 mg/kg/2Y-C   EVHPAZ 69,221,86

CAR: orl-rat TD:10500 mg/kg/39W-C   JJCREP 78,358,87

CAR: orl-rat TD:19250 mg/kg/2Y-C   GANNA2 73,335,82

CAR: orl-rat TD:19635 mg/kg/2Y-C   ESKHA5 (100),93,82

CAR: orl-rat TDLo:4200 mg/kg/13W-C   JJCREP 78,358,87

CAR: orl-rat TDLo:38500 mg/kg/2Y-C   GANNA2 73,335,82

MUT: cyt-ham:lng 85 mg/L   GMCRDC 27,95,81
MUT: cyt-rat-ipr 500 μmol/kg   MUREAV 147,274,85
MUT: cyt-rat-orl 3 mmol/kg   MUREAV 147,274,85
MUT: mma-sat 1 mg/plate   AMONDS 3,253,80

CONSENSUS REPORTS: IARC Cancer Review: GROUP 2B IMEMDT 7,56,87; Animal Sufficient Evidence IMEMDT 40,207,86. Reported in EPA TSCA Inventory.

DOT Classification: Oxidizer; Label: Oxidizer.

SAFETY PROFILE: Suspected carcinogen with experimental carcinogenic data. A poison by ingestion. A powerful oxidizer. An irritant to skin, eyes, and mucous membranes. Mutation data reported. When heated to decomposition it emits very toxic fumes of Br^- and K_2O.

RCA375   CAS: 21416-67-1
RAZOXANE
mf: $C_{11}H_{16}N_4O_4$ mw: 268.31

SYNS: ICI 59118 ◇ ICRF 159 ◇ 4,4'-PROPYLENEDI-2,6-PIPERAZINEDIONE ◇ RAZOXIN

TOXICITY DATA with REFERENCE
CAR: orl-man TD:2693 mg/kg/3Y-C   BJDEAZ 109.675,83

CAR: orl-man TDLo:693 mg/kg/77W-I   LANCAO 2,1343,81

CAR: orl-wmn TD:3650 mg/kg/2Y-I   LANCAO 2,1085,87

CAR: orl-wmn TD:4650 mg/kg/2Y-C   LANCAO 2,1343,81

MUT: cyt-ham-orl 100 mg/kg   BJCAAI 52,725,85
MUT: dni-hmn:lym 20 mg/L   INNDDK 1,283,83
MUT: mnt-mus-ipr 200 mg/kg   BJCAAI 52,725,85
MUT: oms-hmn:lym 20 mg/L   INNDDK 1,283,83

SAFETY PROFILE: Suspected human carcinogen producing leukemia and skin tumors. Moderately toxic by intraperitoneal route. Human effects: normocytic anemia and thrombocytopenia. Human mutation data reported. When heated to decomposition it emits toxic fumes of NO_x.

RDK000   CAS: 50-55-5
RESERPINE
mf: $C_{33}H_{40}N_2O_9$ mw: 608.75

PROP: White or pale buff to sltly yellow powder, odorless. Mp: 264-265° (decomp). Insol in water; very sltly sol in alc; sol in chloroform and acetic acid.

SYNS: ENT 50,146 ◇ METHYLRESERPATE 3,4,5-TRIME-THOXYBENZOIC ACID ◇ METHYL RESERPATE 3,4,5-TRI-METHOXYBENZOIC ACID ESTER ◇ NCI-C50157 ◇ RAUSER-PIN ◇ RAUWOLEAF ◇ SERPASIL ◇ SERPASIL APRESOLINE ◇ 3,4,5-TRIMETHOXYBENZOYL METHYL RESERPATE ◇ USAF CB-27 ◇ YOHIMBAN-16-CARBOXYLIC ACID DE-RIVATIVE of BENZ(G)INDOLO(2,3-A)QUINOLIZINE

TOXICITY DATA with REFERENCE
CAR: orl-mus TDLo:433 mg/kg/2Y-C   NCITR* NCI-TR-193,80

CAR: orl-rat TD:216 mg/kg/2Y-C   NCITR* NCI-TR-193,80

CAR: orl-rat TDLo:54 mg/kg/77W-C   COREAF 254,1535,62

CAR: orl-wmn TDLo:456 μg/kg/Y-C   LANCAO 2,672,74

NEO: orl-mus TD:1120 mg/kg/2Y-I   VOONAW 32(7),76,86

NEO: orl-rat TD:340 mg/kg/3Y-I   VOONAW 32(7),76,86

NEO: orl-wmn TD:16 mg/kg/3Y-C   LANCAO 2,672,74

NEO: orl-wmn TD:24 mg/kg/13Y-C   LANCAO 2,672,74

NEO: orl-wmn TD:73 mg/kg/2Y-C   LANCAO 2,672,74

NEO: scu-mus TDLo:200 mg/kg/2Y-I   VOONAW 32(7),76,86

NEO: scu-rat TDLo:132 mg/kg/2.5Y-I   VOONAW 32(7),76,86

MUT: cyt-mus-ipr 30 mg/kg/48H   PCJOAU 12,298,78

MUT: dlt-mus-ipr 300 μg/kg   PCJOAU 12,298,78

CONSENSUS REPORTS: IARC Cancer Review: Animal Inadequate Evidence IMEMDT 10,217,76; Human Limited Evidence IMEMDT 24,211,80; Animal Limited Evidence IMEMDT 24,211,80. NCI Carcinogenesis Bioassay (feed); Clear Evidence: mouse, rat NCITR* NCI-CG-TR-193,80. Reported in EPA TSCA Inventory.

SAFETY PROFILE: Suspected human carcinogen producing tumors of the skin and brain. Poison by ingestion, intravenous, subcutaneous and intraperitoneal routes. Mutation data reported. An experimental teratogen. Human reproductive and teratogenic effects by ingestion and possibly other routes: stillbirth, reduced viability, and other neonatal measures or effects. In humans, 0.014 mg/kg causes psychotropic effects. Experimental reproductive effects. A medicine with side effects. Used as an additive permitted in the feed and drinking water of animals and/or for the treatment of food-producing animals. Also permitted in food for human consumption. A sedative. When heated to decomposition it emits toxic fumes of NO_x.

REF000　　　　　　　　CAS: 101-90-6
RESORCINOL DIGLYCIDYL ETHER
mf: $C_{12}H_{14}O_4$　　mw: 222.26

SYNS: ARALDITE ERE 1359 ◇ m-BIS(2,3-EPOXYPRO-POXY)BENZENE ◇ 1,3-BIS(2,3-EPOXYPROPOXY)BENZENE ◇ m-BIS(GLYCIDYLOXY)BENZENE ◇ 1,3-DIGLYCIDYLOX-YBENZENE ◇ DIGLYCIDYL RESORCINOL ETHER ◇ ERE 1359 ◇ NCI-C54966 ◇ 2,2'-(1,3-PHENYLENEBIS (OXYMETHYLENE))BISOXIRANE ◇ RDGE ◇ RESORCINOL BIS(2,3-EPOXYPROPYL)ETHER ◇ RESOR-CINYL DIGLYCIDYL ETHER

TOXICITY DATA with REFERENCE
CAR: orl-mus TD:51500 mg/kg/2Y-I　NTPTR* NTP-TR-257,86
CAR: orl-mus TDLo:25750 mg/kg/2Y-I NTPTR* NTP-TR-257,86
CAR: orl-rat TDLo:6180 mg/kg/2Y-I　NTPTR* NTP-TR-257,86
ETA: unr-mus TDLo:6700 mg/kg　RARSAM 3,193,63
MUT: cyt-ham:ovr 8 mg/L　MUREAV 135,159,84
MUT: mmo-sat 50 µg/plate　MUREAV 135,159,84
MUT: sln-dmg-orl 5 pph　ENMUDM 7,325,85
MUT: trn-dmg-orl 5 pph　ENMUDM 7,325,85

CONSENSUS REPORTS: IARC Cancer Review: GROUP 2B IMEMDT 7,56,87; Animal Sufficient Evidence IMEMDT 36,181,85; Ani-mal Inadequate Evidence IMEMDT 11,125,76. NTP Carcinogenesis Studies (gavage); Clear Evidence: mouse, rat NTPTR* NTP-TR-257,86. Reported in EPA TSCA Inventory.

SAFETY PROFILE: Suspected carcinogen with experimental carcinogenic and tumorigenic data. Poison by intraperitoneal route. Moderately toxic by ingestion. Mutation data reported. A skin irritant. When heated to decomposition it emits acrid smoke and irritating fumes.

RKP000　　　　　　　　CAS: 13292-46-1
RIFAMYCIN AMP
mf: $C_{43}H_{58}N_4O_{12}$　　mw: 823.05

SYNS: ARCHIDYN ◇ ARFICIN ◇ DIONE 21-ACETATE ◇ L-5103 ◇ 3-(4-METHYLPIPERAZINYLIMINOMETHYL)-RI-FAMYCIN SV ◇ 8-(4-METHYLPIPERAZINYLIMINOMETHYL) RIFAMYCIN SV ◇ 8-(((4-METHYL-1-PIPERAZINYL)IMINO) METHYL)RIFAMYCIN SV ◇ NSC 113926 ◇ R/AMP ◇ RIFA ◇ RIFADINE ◇ RIFAGEN ◇ RIFALDAZINE ◇ RIFALDIN ◇ RIFAMATE ◇ RIFAMPICIN ◇ RIFAMPICINE (FRENCH) ◇ RIFAMPICINUM ◇ RIFAMPIN ◇ RIFAPRODIN ◇ RIFINAH ◇ RIFOBAC ◇ RIFOLDIN ◇ RIFORAL ◇ RIMACTAN ◇ RIMACTAZID ◇ TUBOCIN

TOXICITY DATA with REFERENCE
NEO: orl-mus TDLo:8400 mg/kg/60W-C TXAPA9 43,293,78
MUT: cyt-hmn:leu 19 µg/L　EXPEAM 29,124,73
MUT: cyt-mus-ipr 5 mg/kg　MUREAV 141,171,84
MUT: dni-hmn:hla 250 mg/L　IJEBA6 22,350,84
MUT: dnr-esc 20 µL/disc　MUREAV 97,1,82
MUT: oms-hmn:hla 250 mg/L　IJEBA6 22,350,84
MUT: pic-esc 60 ng/plate　CNREA8 43,2819,83

CONSENSUS REPORTS: IARC Cancer Review: Animal Limited Evidence IMEMDT 24,243,80; Human Inadequate Evidence IMEMDT 24,243,80.

SAFETY PROFILE: Suspected carcinogen with experimental neoplastigenic and teratogenic data. Poison by intraperitoneal and intravenous routes. Moderately toxic to humans by ingestion. Moderately experimentally toxic by ingestion and subcutaneous routes. Human systemic effects by ingestion: conjunctiva irritation, iritis (inflammation of the iris), other eye effects, and skin dermatitis. Experimental reproductive effects. Human mutation data reported. When heated to decomposition it emits toxic fumes of NO_x.

RMK020　　　　　　　　CAS: 569-61-9
p-ROSANILINE HYDROCHLORIDE
mf: $C_{19}H_{17}N_3 \cdot ClH$　　mw: 323.85

SYNS: 4-((4-AMINOPHENYL)(4-IMINO-2,5-CYCLOHEXA-DIEN-1-YLIDENE)METHYL), MONOCHLORIDE ◇ BASIC PARAFUCHSINE ◇ CALCOZINE MAGENTA N ◇ C.I. 42500 ◇ C.I. BASIC RED 9, MONOHYDROCHLORIDE ◇ p-FUCHSIN ◇ FUCHSINE DR-001 ◇ FUCHSINE SPC ◇ 4,4'-((4-IMINO-2,5-CYCLOHEXADIEN-1-YLIDENE)METHYLENE)DIANILINE MONOHYDROCHLORIDE-o-TOLUIDINE ◇ NCI-C54739 ◇ PARAFUCHSIN (GERMAN) ◇ PARA-MAGENTA ◇ PARAROSANILINE ◇ PARAROSANILINE CHLORIDE ◇ PARAROSANILINE HYDROCHLORIDE ◇ p-ROSANILINE HCL ◇ SCHULTZ-TAB NO. 779 (GERMAN) ◇ 4,4'4''-TRIAMINOTRIPHENYLMETHAN-HYDROCHLORID (GERMAN)

TOXICITY DATA with REFERENCE
CAR: orl-mus TDLo: 364 mg/kg/2Y-C   NTPTR*
    NTP-TR-285,86
CAR: orl-rat TDLo: 728 mg/kg/2Y-C   NTPTR*
    NTP-TR-285,86
ETA: scu-rat TDLo: 1714 mg/kg/43W-I
    NATWAY 43,543,56
MUT: dnd-mam: lym 10 pph   BIPMAA 11,2537,72
MUT: dnr-esc 20 mg/L   JJIND8 62,873,79
MUT: dns-ham: lvr 100 nmol/L   ENMUDM 6,1,84
MUT: dns-rat: lvr 2200 μg/L   ENMUDM 5,482,83
MUT: mma-sat 100 μg/plate   ENMUDM 6(Suppl 2),1,84
MUT: mmo-sat 100 μmol/L   AMACCQ 9,77,76
MUT: otr-mus: fbr 8 μg/L   JJIND8 67,1303,81
MUT: otr-rat: emb 1400 μg/L   JJIND8 67,1303,81

CONSENSUS REPORTS: IARC Cancer Review: GROUP 3 IMEMDT 7,238,87; Animal Limited Evidence IMEMDT 4,57,74; Human Inadequate Evidence IMEMDT 4,57,74. EPA Genetic Toxicology Program. Reported in EPA TSCA Inventory.

SAFETY PROFILE: Suspected carcinogen with experimental carcinogenic and tumorigenic data. Mildly toxic by ingestion. Mutation data reported. When heated to decomposition it emits very toxic fumes of HCl and NO_x.

RPK000   CAS: 13446-73-6
RUBIDIUM DICHROMATE
mf: $Cr_2O_7Rb_2$ mw: 386.94

PROP: Crystals. D: 3.02-3.13

CONSENSUS REPORTS: Chromium and its compounds are on the Community Right-To-Know List.

OSHA PEL: CL 0.1 mg(CrO_3)/m³   ACGIH TLV: TWA 0.05 mg(Cr)/m³   NIOSH REL: TWA 0.025 mg(Cr(VI))/m³; CL 0.05/15M

SAFETY PROFILE: Suspected carcinogen. A poison. A powerful oxidizer. When heated to decomposition it emits toxic fumes of Rb_2O.

RRP000
RUSSIAN COMFREY ROOTS

PROP: Fresh roots dried, milled, and mixed with diet (JNCIAM 61,86578).

SYNS: COMFREY, RUSSIAN ◇ SYMPHYTUM OFFICINALE L

TOXICITY DATA with REFERENCE
CAR: orl-rat TD: 91 g/kg/52W-C   JJIND8
    61(3),865,78
CAR: orl-rat TDLo: 140 g/kg/43W-I   JJIND8
    61(3),865,78

CONSENSUS REPORTS: IARC Cancer Review: Animal Limited Evidence IMEMDT 31,239,83

SAFETY PROFILE: Suspected carcinogen with experimental carcinogenic data. When heated to decomposition it emits acrid smoke and irritating fumes.

SBQ000   CAS: 144-34-3
SELENIUM DIMETHYLDITHIOCARBAMATE
mf: $C_{12}H_{24}N_4S_8 \cdot Se$ mw: 559.84

PROP: Yellow powder, crystals. D: 1.58, melting range: 140-172°.

SYNS: METHYL SELENAC ◇ TETRAKIS(DIMETHYLCARBAMODITHIOATO-S,S') SELENIUM

CONSENSUS REPORTS: IARC Cancer Review: GROUP 2B IMEMDT 7,56,87; Animal Inadequate Evidence IMEMDT 12,161,76. Selenium and its compounds are on the Community Right-To-Know List. Reported in EPA TSCA Inventory.

OSHA PEL: TWA 0.2 mg(Se)/m³   ACGIH TLV: TWA 0.2 mg(Se)/m³   DFG MAK: 0.1 mg(Se)/m³

SAFETY PROFILE: Suspected carcinogen. Selenium compounds are poisons. When heated to decomposition it emits very toxic fumes of Se, SO_x, and NO_x.

SCN500   CAS: 15191-85-2
SILICIC ACID, BERYLLIUM SALT
mf: $O_4Si \cdot 2Be$ mw: 110.11

PROP: Colorless crystals. D: 3.0.

SYNS: BERYLLIUM ORTHOSILICATE ◇ BERYLLIUM SIL-ICATE ◇ BERYLLIUM SILICIC ACID ◇ ORTHOSILICATE ◇ PHENACITE ◇ PHENAKITE ◇ PHENAZITE

TOXICITY DATA with REFERENCE
ETA: imp-rbt TDLo: 10 mg/kg   ARPAAQ 88,89,69
ETA: ivn-rbt TDLo: 500 mg/kg   AICCA6 7,171,50

CONSENSUS REPORTS: IARC Cancer Review: GROUP 2A IMEMDT 7,127,87; Animal Sufficient Evidence IMEMDT 23,143,80. Beryllium and its compounds are on the Community Right-To-Know List.

OSHA PEL: (Transitional: TWA 0.002 mg(Be)/m^3; CL 0.005; Pk 0.025/30M/8H) TWA 0.002 mg(Be)/m^3; STEL 0.005 mg(Be)/m^3/30M; CL 0.025 mg(Be)/m^3 ACGIH TLV: TWA 0.002 mg(Be)/m^3; Suspected Carcinogen NIOSH REL: CL not to exceed 0.0005 mg/(Be)/m^3

SAFETY PROFILE: Suspected carcinogen with experimental carcinogenic and tumorigenic data. When heated to decomposition it emits toxic fumes of BeO.

SJN700   CAS: 128-44-9
SODIUM SACCHARIN
mf: $C_7H_4NO_3S \cdot Na$ mw: 205.17

PROP: White crystals or crystalline powder; odorless, very sweet taste. Sol in water, alc.

SYNS: ARTIFICIAL SWEETENING SUBSTANZ GENDORF 450 ◇ CRISTALLOSE ◇ CRYSTALLOSE ◇ DAGUTAN ◇ KRISTALLOSE ◇ MADHURIN ◇ ODA ◇ SACCHARIN ◇ SACCHARIN SOLUBLE ◇ SACCHARIN, SODIUM ◇ SACCHARIN, SODIUM SALT ◇ SACCHARINE SOLUBLE ◇ SACCHARINNATRIUM ◇ SACCHAROIDUM NATRICUM ◇ SAXIN ◇ SODIUM 1,2 BENZISOTHIAZOLIN-3-ONE-1,1-DI-OXIDE ◇ SODIUM o-BENZOSULFIMIDE ◇ SODIUM BENZO-SULPHIMIDE ◇ SODIUM o-BENZOSULPHIMIDE ◇ SODIUM 2-BENZOSULPHIMIDE ◇ SODIUM SACCHARIDE ◇ SODIUM SACCHARINATE ◇ SODIUM SACCHARINE ◇ SOLUBLE GLUSIDE ◇ SOLUBLE SACCHARIN ◇ SUCCARIL ◇ SUCRA ◇ o-SULFONBENZOIC ACID IMIDE SODIUM SALT ◇ SULPHOBENZOIC IMIDE, SODIUM SALT ◇ SWEETA ◇ SYKOSE ◇ WILLOSETTEN

TOXICITY DATA with REFERENCE
CAR: orl-rat TDLo: 1092 g/kg/1Y-C   GANNA2 74,8,83
NEO: imp-mus TDLo: 176 mg/kg   SCIEAS 168,1238,70
NEO: orl-rat TD: 224 g/kg/8W-C   CNREA8 37,2943,77

NEO: orl-rat TDLo: 112 g/kg/8W-C   CNREA8 37,2943,77
ETA: orl-rat TD: 1190 g/kg/85W-C   BJCAAI 39,355,79
ETA: orl-rat TD: 1330 g/kg/95W-C   CBINA8 11,225,75
ETA: orl-rat TD: 1428 g/kg/2Y-C   BJCAAI 39,355,79
ETA: orl-rat TD: 2660 g/kg/95W-C   BJCAAI 39,355,79
MUT: cyt-ham: fbr 8 g/L/48H   MUREAV 48,337,77
MUT: cyt-hmn: leu 500 mg/L   MUREAV 32,81,75
MUT: cyt-mus-ipr 4000 mg/kg   MUREAV 54,219,78
MUT: dlt-mus-orl 6 g/kg/30D   MUREAV 32,81,75
MUT: mma-mus: lym 11 g/L/4H   MUREAV 59,61,79
MUT: mrc-smc 2 g/L   MUREAV 67,215,79
MUT: sce-hmn: leu 20 μmol/L   ENMUDM 1,177,79

CONSENSUS REPORTS: IARC Cancer Review: GROUP 2B IMEMDT 7,334,87; Animal Sufficient Evidence IMEMDT 22,111,80. EPA Genetic Toxicology Program. Reported in EPA TSCA Inventory.

SAFETY PROFILE: Suspected carcinogen with experimental carcinogenic, neoplastigenic, tumorigenic, and teratogenic data. Moderately toxic by ingestion and intraperitoneal routes. A promoter. Experimental reproductive effects. Human mutation data reported. When heated to decomposition it emits very toxic fumes of SO_x, Na_2O, and NO_x.

SLP000   CAS: 10048-13-2
STERIGMATOCYSTIN
mf: $C_{18}H_{12}O_6$ mw: 328.34

PROP: A metabolite of *Aspergillus versicolor* (BJCAAI 20,134,66).

SYN: 3a,12c-DIHYDRO-8-HYDROXY-6-METHOXY-7H-FURO(3',2':4,5)FURO(2,3-C)XANTHEN-7-ONE

TOXICITY DATA with REFERENCE
CAR: ipr-rat TDLo: 240 mg/kg/23W-I   GANNA2 69,237,78
CAR: orl-mus TD: 2759 mg/kg/55W-C   FCTOD7 20,547,82
CAR: orl-mus TD: 3227 mg/kg/55W-I   FCTOD7 20,547,82
CAR: orl-mus TDLo: 1840 mg/kg/73W-C   MAIKD3 (12),20,80
CAR: orl-rat TDLo: 175 mg/kg/52W-C   FCTXAV 8,289,70
CAR: skn-rat TDLo: 560 mg/kg/70W-I   TXAPA9 26,274,73

ETA: ipr-rat TD:60 mg/kg/16W-I   SKEZAP
14,272,73

ETA: orl-mky TDLo:1040 mg/kg/2Y-I
33IUAS -,369,74

ETA: orl-mus TD:113 mg/kg/54W-I   FCTXAV
12,491,74

ETA: orl-rat TD:60 mg/kg/4W-I   SKEZAP
14,272,73

ETA: orl-rat TD:3 mg/kg/93W-C   GANNA2
70,777,79

ETA: scu-rat TDLo:96 mg/kg/24W-I   BJCAAI
20,134,66

MUT: cyt-ckn-par 22 μg/kg   47JMAE -,137,82

MUT: cyt-rat-ipr 31200 μg/kg   MUREAV139,203,84

MUT: dnr-bcs 10 μg/disc   MUREAV 97,339,82

MUT: dns-hmn:fbr 100 mmol/L/3H   IJCNAW
16,284,75

MUT: dns-hmn:hla 1 μmol/L   CNREA8 38,2621,78

MUT: dns-mus:lvr 2 μmol/L   CNREA8 44,2918,84

MUT: dns-rat:lvr 1 μmol/L   MUREAV 173,217,86

MUT: msc-hmn:emb 100 μg/L   KIKNAJ(29),38,78

MUT: sce-ckn-par 22 μg/kg   47JMAE -,137,82

MUT: sce-mus-ipr 60 μg/kg   MUREAV 137,111,84

CONSENSUS REPORTS: IARC Cancer Review: GROUP 2B IMEMDT 7,56,87; Animal Sufficient Evidence IMEMDT 10,245,76; Animal Limited Evidence IMEMDT 1,175,72. EPA Genetic Toxicology Program.

SAFETY PROFILE: Suspected carcinogen with experimental carcinogenic and tumorigenic data. Poison by ingestion and intraperitoneal routes. Human mutation data reported. When heated to decomposition it emits acrid smoke and irritating fumes.

SMQ000   CAS: 100-42-5
STYRENE
DOT: 2055
mf: C_8H_8 mw: 104.16

PROP: Colorless, refractive, oily liquid. Mp: −31°, bp: 146°, lel: 1.1%, uel: 6.1%, flash p: 88°F, d: 0.9074 @ 20°/4°, autoign temp: 914°F, vap d: 3.6, fp: −33°, ULC: 40-50. Very sltly sol in water; misc in alc, and ether.

SYNS: CINNAMENE ◇ CINNAMENOL ◇ DIAREX HF 77 ◇ ETHENYLBENZENE ◇ NCI-C02200 ◇ PHENETHYLENE ◇ PHENYLETHENE ◇ PHENYLETHYLENE ◇ STIROLO (ITALIAN) ◇ STYREEN (DUTCH) ◇ STYREN (CZECH) ◇ STYRENE MONOMER (ACGIH) ◇ STYRENE MONOMER, inhibited (DOT) ◇ STYROL (GERMAN) ◇ STYROLE ◇ STYROLENE ◇ STYRON ◇ STYROPOR ◇ VINYLBENZEN (CZECH) ◇ VINYLBENZENE ◇ VINYLBENZOL

TOXICITY DATA with REFERENCE

MUT: cyt-hmn:lym 300 ppm/72H   MUREAV
58,277,78

MUT: dnd-mus-ipr 10 mmol/kg   CALEDQ 21,9,83

MUT: dni-hmn:hla 28 mmol/L   MUREAV93,447,82

MUT: dns-hmn:lym 100 μmol/L   CRNGDP
3,681,82

MUT: hma-mus/smc 1 g/kg   MUREAV 40,317,76

MUT: mma-sat 1 μmol/plate   MUREAV 56,147,77

MUT: mmo-smc 1 mmol/L   BSIBAC 59,233,83

MUT: mrc-smc 1 mmol/L   BSIBAC 59,233,83

MUT: sce-hmn:lym 500 μmol/L   ATSUDG
7,286,84

MUT: sce-mus-ihl 125 ppm/4D-I   APTOD9
19,A34,80

MUT: sce-mus-ihl 46400 μg/kg/4D-I   TXAPA9
55,37,80

CONSENSUS REPORTS: IARC Cancer Review: GROUP 2B IMEMDT 7,345,87; Animal Sufficient Evidence IMEMDT 19,231,79; Human Inadequate Evidence IMEMDT 19,231,79. NCI Carcinogenesis Bioassay (gavage); Inadequate Studies: mouse, rat NCITR* NCI-CG-TR-170,79; (gavage). Reported in EPA TSCA Inventory. EPA Genetic Toxicology Program. Community Right To Know List.

OSHA PEL: (Transitional: TWA 100 ppm; CL 200; Pk 600/5M/3H) TWA 50 ppm; STEL: 100 ppm   ACGIH TLV: TWA 50 ppm; STEL: 100 ppm (skin); BEI: 1 g(mandelic acid)/L in urine at end of shift; 40 ppb styrene in mixed-exhaled air prior to shift; 18 ppm styrene in mixed-exhaled air during shift; 0.55 mg/L styrene in blood end of shift; 0.02 mg/L styrene in blood prior to shift.   DFG MAK: 20 ppm (85 mg/m^3); BAT: 2g/L of mandelic acid in urine at end of shift.   NIOSH REL: (Styrene) TWA 50 ppm; CL 100 ppm   DOT Classification: Flammable Liquid; Label: Flammable Liquid; Flammable or Combustible Liquid; Label: Flammable Liquid

SAFETY PROFILE: Suspected carcinogen. Confirmed carcinogen. Experimental poison by ingestion, inhalation, and intravenous routes. Moderately toxic experimentally by intraperitoneal route. Mildly toxic to humans by inhalation. An experimental teratogen. Human systemic effects by inhalation: eye and olfactory changes. Experimental reproductive effects. Human mutation data reported. A human skin irritant. An experimental skin and eye irritant. A very dangerous fire hazard when exposed to flame, heat or oxidants. To fight fire, use foam, CO_2, dry chemical. When heated to decomposition it emits acrid smoke and irritating fumes.

TAA100   CAS: 93-76-5
2,4,5-T
DOT: 2765
mf: $C_8H_5Cl_3O_3$ mw: 255.48

PROP: Crystals; light tan solid. Mp: 151-153°. Usually has 2,3,7,8-TCDD as a minor component.

SYNS: ACIDE 2,4,5-TRICHLORO PHENOXYACETIQUE (FRENCH) ◊ ACIDO (2,4,5-TRICLORO-FENOSSI)-ACETICO (ITALIAN) ◊ AMINE 2,4,5-T FOR RICE ◊ BCF-BUSHKILLER ◊ BRUSH-OFF 445 MLD VOLATILE BRUSH KILLER ◊ BRUSH RHAP ◊ BRUSHTOX ◊ DACAMINE ◊ DEBROUS-SAILLANT CONCENTRE ◊ DECAMINE 4T ◊ DED-WEED BRUSH KILLER ◊ DED-WEED LV-6 BRUSH KIL and T-5 BRUSH KIL ◊ DINOXOL ◊ ENVERT-T ◊ ESTERCIDE T-2 and T-245 ◊ ESTERON 245 BE ◊ ESTERON BRUSH KILLER ◊ FARMCO FENCE RIDER ◊ FORRON ◊ FORST U 46 ◊ FORTEX ◊ FRUITONE A ◊ INVERTON 245 ◊ LINE RIDER ◊ PHORTOX ◊ RCRA WASTE NUMBER U232 ◊ REDDON ◊ REDDOX ◊ SPONTOX ◊ SUPER D WEEDONE ◊ TIPPON ◊ TORMONA ◊ TRANSAMINE ◊ TRIBUTON ◊ (2,4,5-TRICHLOOR-FENOXY)-AZIJNZUUR (DUTCH) ◊ 2,4,5-TRI-CHLOROPHENOXYACETIC ACID ◊ (2,4,5-TRICHLOR-PHE-NOXY)-ESSIGSAEURE (GERMAN) ◊ TRINOXOL ◊ TRIOXON ◊ TRIOXONE ◊ U 46 ◊ VEON 245 ◊ VERTON 2T ◊ VISKO RHAP LOW VOLATILE ESTER ◊ WEEDAR ◊ WEEDONE

TOXICITY DATA with REFERENCE
NEO: orl-mus TDLo:3379 mg/kg/33W-C
    BJCAAI 33,626,76
ETA: scu-mus TDLo:215 mg/kg   NTIS**
    PB223-159
MUT: cyt-dmg-orl 250 ppm   MUREAV 65,83,79
MUT: cyt-grb-ipr 250 mg/kg   MUREAV 65,83,79
MUT: dnd-mam:lym 100 μmol/L   PYTCAS
    11,3135,72
MUT: mmo-bcs 1 nmol/plate   MSERDS 5,93,81
MUT: mmo-smc 35 mg/L   ECBUDQ 27,193,78
MUT: sln-dmg-orl 1000 ppm/15D   MUREAV
    65,83,79

CONSENSUS REPORTS: IARC Cancer Review: GROUP 2B IMEMDT 7,156,87; Animal Inadequate Evidence IMEMDT 15,273,77; Human Inadequate Evidence IMEMDT 15,273,77; Human Limited Evidence IMEMDT 41,357,86. Reported in EPA TSCA Inventory. EPA Genetic Toxicology Program.

OSHA PEL: TWA 10 mg/m^3 ACGIH TLV: TWA 10 mg/m^3 DFG MAK: 10 mg/m^3 DOT Classification: ORM-A; Label: None.

SAFETY PROFILE: Suspected carcinogen with experimental neoplastigenic, tumorigenic, and teratogenic data. Poison by ingestion. Moderately toxic by unspecified route. Experimental reproductive effects. Mutation data reported. The teratogenicity is due in part to 2,3,7,8-TCDD, which is present as a contaminant (ARENAA 17,123,72). When heated to decomposition it emits toxic fumes of Cl$^-$.

TBO000   CAS: 15721-02-5
TETRACHLOROBENZIDINE
mf: $C_{12}H_8Cl_4N_2$ mw: 322.02

SYNS: 2,2',5,5'-TETRACHLOROBENZIDINE ◊ 3,3',6,6'-TETRACHLOROBENZIDINE ◊ 2,2',5,5'-TETRACHLORO-(1,1'-BIPHENYL)-4,4'-DIAMINE, (9CI) ◊ 2,2',5,5'-TETRA-CHLORO-4,4'-DIAMINODIPHENYL

TOXICITY DATA with REFERENCE
CAR: orl-mus TD:300 g/kg/43W-C   IARC**
    27,141,82
CAR: orl-mus TDLo:36 mg/kg/43W-C   JMEJAS
    25,123,78
CAR: orl-rat TD:900 g/kg/43W-C   IARC**
    27,141,82
ETA: orl-rat TDLo:54 mg/kg/43W-C   JMEJAS
    25,123,78

CONSENSUS REPORTS: IARC Cancer Review: Animal Inadequate Evidence IMEMDT 27,141,82. Reported in EPA TSCA Inventory.

SAFETY PROFILE: Suspected carcinogen with experimental carcinogenic and tumorigenic data. When heated to decomposition it emits very toxic fumes of NO$_x$ and Cl$^-$.

TBQ100   CAS: 79-34-5
1,1,2,2-TETRACHLOROETHANE
DOT: 1702
mf: $C_2H_2Cl_4$ mw: 167.84

PROP: Heavy, colorless, mobile liquid; chloroform-like odor. Mp: −43.8°, bp: 146.4°, d: 1.600 @ 20°/4°.

SYNS: ACETYLENE TETRACHLORIDE ◊ BONOFORM ◊ CELLON ◊ 1,1,2,2-CZTEROCHLOROETAN (POLISH) ◊ 1,1-DICHLORO-2,2-DICHLOROETHANE ◊ NCI-C03554 ◊ RCRA WASTE NUMBER U209 ◊ TCE ◊ TETRACHLORE-THANE ◊ 1,1,2,2-TETRACHLOORETHAAN (DUTCH) ◊ 1,1,2,2-TETRACHLORAETHAN (GERMAN) ◊ 1,1,2,2-TET

RACHLORETHANE (FRENCH) ◇ sym-TETRACHLORO-ETHANE ◇ 1,1,2,2-TETRACHLOROETHANE ◇ 1,1,2,2-TET-RACLOROETANO (ITALIAN) ◇ TETRACHLORURE D'ACE-TYLENE (FRENCH) ◇ WESTRON

TOXICITY DATA with REFERENCE

CAR: orl-mus TD:110 g/kg/78W-I   NCITR*
    NCI-TR-27,78
CAR: orl-mus TDLo:55 g/kg/78W-I   NCITR*
    NCI-TR-27,78
ETA: orl-rat TDLo:42 g/kg/78W-I   NCITR*
    NCI-TR-27,78
MUT: dnr-esc 15866 μg/plate   CNREA8 34,2576,74
MUT: mma-sat 10 μg/plate   TECSDY 15,101,87
MUT: mmo-sat 10 μg/plate   TECSDY 15,101,87
MUT: sce-ham:ovr 56 mg/L   EMMUEG 10(Suppl 10),1,87

CONSENSUS REPORTS: IARC Cancer Review: GROUP 3 IMEMDT 7,354,87; Animal Limited Evidence IMEMDT 20,477,79; NCI Carcinogenesis Bioassay (gavage); Clear Evidence: mouse NCITR* NCI-CG-TR-27,78; Some Evidence: rat NCITR* NCI-CG-TR-27,78. Reported in EPA TSCA Inventory. EPA Genetic Toxicology Program. Community Right-To-Know List.

OSHA PEL: (Transitional: TWA 5 ppm (skin)) TWA 1 ppm (skin) ACGIH TLV: TWA 1 ppm (skin) DFG MAK: 1 ppm (7 mg/m^3); Suspected Carcinogen. NIOSH REL: (1,1,2,2-Tetrachlorethane) Reduce to lowest level. DOT Classification: IMO: Poison B; Label: Poison.

SAFETY PROFILE: Suspected carcinogen with experimental with experimental carcinogenic and tumorigenic data. Poison by inhalation, ingestion, and intraperitoneal routes. Moderately toxic by several other routes. Mutation data reported. Human central nervous system effects by ingestion and inhalation: general anesthesia, somnolence, hallucinations, and distorted perceptions. When heated to decomposition it emits toxic fumes of Cl$^-$.

TBT000   CAS: 58-90-2
2,4,5,6-TETRACHLOROPHENOL
mf: C$_6$H$_2$Cl$_4$O   mw: 231.88

SYNS: DOWICIDE 6 ◇ RCRA WASTE NUMBER U212 ◇ 2,3,4,6-TETRACHLOROPHENOL

TOXICITY DATA with REFERENCE

CAR: scu-mus TDLo:100 mg/kg   NTIS**
    PB223-159

CONSENSUS REPORTS: IARC Cancer Review: Human Limited Evidence IMEMDT 41,319,86. Chlorophenol compounds are on the Community Right-To-Know List. Reported in EPA TSCA Inventory.

SAFETY PROFILE: Suspected carcinogen with experimental carcinogenic and teratogenic data. Poison by ingestion, skin contact, intraperitoneal and subcutaneous routes. May be a human carcinogen. Experimental reproductive effects. When heated to decomposition it emits toxic fumes of Cl$^-$. Used as a disinfectant and a preservative for wood, latex and leather.

TBW100   CAS: 961-11-5
TETRACHLORVINPHOS
mf: C$_{10}$H$_9$Cl$_4$O$_4$P   mw: 365.96

SYNS: 2-CHLORO-1-(2,4,5-TRICHLOROPHENYL)VINYL DIMETHYL PHOSPHATE ◇ 2-CHLORO-1-(2,4,5-TRICHLORO-PHENYL(VINYL PHOSPHORIC ACID DIMETHYL ESTER ◇ O,O-DIMETHYL-O-2-CHLOR-1-(2,4,5-TRICHLORPHE-NYL)-VINYL-PHOSPHAT (GERMAN) ◇ IPO 8 ◇ NCI C00168 ◇ PHOSPHORIC ACID, 2-CHLORO-1-(2,4,5-TRICHLOROPHE-NYL)ETHENYL DIMETHYL ESTER ◇ 2,4,5-TRICHLORO-α-(CHLOROMETHYLENE)BENZYL PHOSPHATE

TOXICITY DATA with REFERENCE

CAR: orl-mus TD:692 g/kg/2Y-C   FAATDF
    5,840,85
CAR: orl-mus TD:1057 g/kg/80W-C   NCITR*
    NCI-CG-TR-33,78
CAR: orl-mus TD:1384 g/kg/2Y-C   FAATDF
    5,840,85
CAR: orl-mus TDLo:450 g/kg/67W-C   NCITR*
    NCI-CG-TR-33,78
NEO: orl-rat TDLo:240 g/kg,80W-C   NCITR*
    NCI-CG-TR-33,78
ETA: orl-rat TD:120 g/kg/80W-C   NCITR*
    NCI-CG-TR-33,78

CONSENSUS REPORTS: NCI Carcinogenesis Bioassay (feed); Results Positive: Mouse, Rat (NCITR* NCI-CG-TR-33,78). Community Right-To-Know List.

SAFETY PROFILE: Suspected carcinogen with experimental carcinogenic, neoplastigenic, and tumorigenic data. Poison by ingestion. Experimental reproductive effects. When heated to decomposition it emits toxic fumes of Cl$^-$ and PO$_x$.

TBW250   CAS: 14323-41-2
TETRACYANONICKELATE(2-)
DIPOTASSIUM, HYDRATE
mf: C$_4$N$_4$Ni•K•H$_2$O   mw: 219.91

SYN: POTASSIUM CYANONICKELATE HYDRATE

TOXICITY DATA with REFERENCE
MUT: cyt-mus:mmr 1600 μmol/L   MUREAV
  68,337,79

CONSENSUS REPORTS: Nickel and its compounds, as well as cyanide and its compounds, are on the Community Right-To-Know List.

OSHA PEL: (Transitional: TWA 1 mg/m^3) TWA 0.1 mg (Ni)/m^3 ACGIH TLV: TWA 0.1 mg(Ni)/m^3; (Proposed: TWA 0.05 mg(Ni)/m^3; Human Carcinogen)

SAFETY PROFILE: Suspected human carcinogen. Mutation data reported. Many nickel compounds are poisons. When heated to decomposition it emits very toxic fumes of CN$^-$, K$_2$O and NO$_x$.

TFS750   CAS: 7440-29-1
THORIUM
af: Th   aw: 232.00
DOT: 2975

PROP: Silvery-white, air stable, soft, ductile metal. D: 11.72; mp: 1842 ± 30°. A radioactive material.

SYNS: THORIUM-232 ◇ THORIUM METAL, PYROPHORIC (DOT)

CONSENSUS REPORTS: Reported in EPA TSCA Inventory.

DOT Classification: Radioactive Material; Label: Radioactive and Flammable Solid.

SAFETY PROFILE: Suspected carcinogen. Taken internally as ThO$_2$, it has proven to be a carcinogenic due to its radioactivity. On an acute basis it has caused dermatitis. Flammable in the form of dust when exposed to heat or flame, or by chemical reaction with oxidizers. The powder may ignite spontaneously in air.

TFT250   CAS: 15457-87-1
THORIUM HYDRIDE
mf: H$_4$Th   mw: 236.07

PROP: Black, metallic crystals. D: 8.24, mp: decomp explosively @ red heat. Reacts with water.

SAFETY PROFILE: Suspected carcinogen. Explodes on heating in air. The powder ignites spontaneously in air.

TGM800   CAS: 91-08-7
TOLUENE-2,6-DIISOCYANATE
mf: C$_9$H$_6$N$_2$O$_2$ mw: 174.17

SYNS: 2,6-DIISOCYANATO-1-METHYLBENZENE ◇ 2,6-DIISOCYANATOTOLUENE ◇ HYLENE TM ◇ 2-METHYL-m-PHENYLENE ESTER, ISOCYANIC ACID ◇ 2-METHYL-m-PHENYLENE ISOCYANATE ◇ NIAX TDI ◇ 2,6-TDI ◇ 2,6-TOLUENE DIISOCYANATE ◇ TOLYLENE-2,6-DIISOCYANATE ◇ m-TOLYLENE DIISOCYANATE

CONSENSUS REPORTS: IARC Cancer Review: GROUP 2B IMEMDT 7,56,87; Human Inadequate Evidence IMEMDT 39,287,86; Animal Sufficient Evidence IMEMDT 39,287,86. Reported in EPA TSCA Inventory. Community Right-To-Know List. EPA Hazardous Substances List.

DFG MAK: 0.01 ppm (0.07 mg/m^3)   NIOSH REL: (Diisocyanates) TWA 0.005 ppm; CL 0.02 ppm/10M

SAFETY PROFILE: Suspected carcinogen. Poison by ingestion and inhalation. Human systemic effects by inhalation: olfactory, eye and pulmonary changes. When heated to decomposition it emits toxic fumes of NO$_x$.

TGN250   CAS: 88-19-7
o-TOLUENESULFONAMIDE
mf: C$_7$H$_9$NO$_2$S   mw: 171.23

PROP: Tetragonal prisms. Mp: 156°. Sol in water, alc.

SYNS: o-METHYLBENZENESULFONAMIDE ◇ 2-METHYLBENZENESULFONAMIDE ◇ ONCO-CARBIDE ◇ ORTHO-TOLUOL-SULFONAMID (GERMAN) ◇ OTS ◇ OXYUREA ◇ TOLUENE-2-SULFONAMIDE

TOXICITY DATA with REFERENCE
ETA: orl-rat TDLo:13 g/kg/96W-C   ZKKOBW
  91,19,78
MUT: mma-sat 70 μmol/plate   45OHAA -,170,80
MUT: sln-dmg-orl 2500 μmol/L   45OHAA -,170,80
MUT: sln-dmg-par 5 mmol/L   MUREAV 56,163,77

CONSENSUS REPORTS: IARC Cancer Review: Animal Limited Evidence IMEMDT 22,111,80. Reported in EPA TSCA Inventory. EPA Genetic Toxicology Program.

SAFETY PROFILE: Suspected carcinogen with experimental tumorigenic data. Mildly toxic by ingestion. Experimental reproductive effects. Mutation data reported. An eye irritant. When heated to decomposition it emits very toxic fumes of NO$_x$ and SO$_x$. Used as a chemical intermediate in the production of saccharin.

TGW000   CAS: 2646-17-5
1-(o-TOLYLAZO)-2-NAPHTHOL
mf: C$_{17}$H$_{14}$N$_2$O   mw: 262.33

SYNS: A.F.ORANGE No. 2 ◇ AIZEN FOOD ORANGE No. 2 ◇ ATUL OIL ORANGE T ◇ C.I. 12100 ◇ C.I. SOLVENT ORANGE 2 ◇ D&C ORANGE No. 2 ◇ DOLKWAL ORANGE SS ◇ EXTRACT D&C ORANGE No. 4 ◇ FAT ORANGE II ◇ HEXACOL OIL ORANGE SS ◇ LACQUER ORANGE V ◇ 1-((2-METHYLPHENYL)AZO)-2-NAPHTHALENOL ◇ OIL ORANGE O'PEL ◇ OIL ORANGE SS ◇ OLEAL ORANGE SS ◇ ORANGE 3R SOLUBLE IN GREASE ◇ ORGANOL ORANGE 2R ◇ TOLUENE-2-AZONAPHTHOL-2 ◇ o-TOLUENO-AZO-β-NAPHTHOL ◇ 1-(o-TOLYLAZO)-β-NAPHTHOL

TOXICITY DATA with REFERENCE

CAR: imp-mus TDLo: 50 mg/kg   BJCAAI 12,222,58

NEO: scu-mus TDLo: 6 g/kg/52W   BJCAAI 10,653,56

CONSENSUS REPORTS: IARC Cancer Review: GROUP 2B IMEMDT 7,56,87; Animal Sufficient Evidence IMEMDT 8,165,75. Reported in EPA TSCA Inventory. EPA Genetic Toxicology Program.

SAFETY PROFILE: Suspected carcinogen with experimental carcinogenic and neoplastigenic data. Poison by intravenous route. Mildly toxic by ingestion. When heated to decomposition it emits toxic fumes of NO_x. Used to color cosmetics, varnishes, oils, fats and waxes, petroleum products.

THP250   CAS: 17168-85-3
TRIAMMINEDIPEROXOCHROMIUM(IV)
mf: $CrH_9N_3O_4$ mw: 167.09

SAFETY PROFILE: Suspected carcinogen. Chromium compounds are generally poisons. May explode with heat or shock. May explode at 120°C. An oxidizer. When heated to decomposition it emits toxic fumes of NO_x.

TIN000   CAS: 79-00-5
1,1,2-TRICHLOROETHANE
mf: $C_2H_3Cl_3$ mw: 133.40

PROP: Liquid; pleasant odor. Bp: 114°, fp: −35°, d: 1.4416 @ 20°/4°, vap press: 40 mm @ 35.2°.

SYNS: ETHANE TRICHLORIDE ◇ NCI-C04579 ◇ RCRA WASTE NUMBER U227 ◇ β-T ◇ 1,1,2-TRICHLORETHANE ◇ β-TRICHLOROETHANE ◇ 1,2,2-TRICHLOROETHANE ◇ TROJCHLOROETAN(1,1,2) (POLISH) ◇ VINYL TRICHLORIDE

TOXICITY DATA with REFERENCE

CAR: orl-mus TD: 152 g/kg/78W-I   NCITR* NCI-CG-TR-74,78

CAR: orl-mus TDLo: 76 g/kg/78W-I   NCITR*

NCI-CG-TR-74,78

MUT: cyt-gpg-skn 2880 μg/kg   APTOA6 41,298,77

MUT: dnd-mam: lym 1 mmol/L   TOLED5 11,243,82

MUT: otr-mus: emb 25 mg/L   CALEDQ 28,85,85

CONSENSUS REPORTS: IARC Cancer Review: Animal Limited Evidence IMEMDT 20,533,79. NCI Carcinogenesis Bioassay (gavage); No Evidence: rat NCITR* NCI-CG-TR-74,78; (gavage); Clear Evidence: mouse NCITR* NCI-CG-TR-74,78. Community Right-To-Know List. Reported in EPA TSCA Inventory.

OSHA PEL: TWA 10 ppm (skin) ACGIH TLV: TWA 10 ppm (skin) DFG MAK: 10 ppm (55 mg/m³); Suspected Carcinogen.

SAFETY PROFILE: Suspected carcinogen with experimental carcinogenic data. Poison by ingestion, intravenous and subcutaneous routes. Moderately toxic by inhalation, skin contact, and intraperitoneal routes. Experimental reproductive effects. Mutation data reported. An eye and severe skin irritant. Has narcotic properties and acts as a local irritant to the eyes, nose and lungs. It may also be injurious to the liver and kidneys. When heated to decomposition it emits toxic fumes of Cl^-.

TIO750   CAS: 79-01-6
TRICHLOROETHYLENE
DOT: 1710
mf: C_2HCl_3 mw: 131.38

PROP: Clear, colorless, mobile liquid; characteristic sweet odor of chloroform. D: 1.4649 @ 20°/4°, bp: 86.7°, flash p: 89.6°F (but practically nonflammable), lel: 12.5%, uel: 90% @ > 30°, mp: −73°, fp: −86.8°, autoign temp: 788°F, vap press: 100 mm @ 32°, vap d: 4.53, refr index: 1.477 @ 20°. Immiscible with water; misc with alc, ether, acetone, carbon tetrachloride.

SYNS: ACETYLENE TRICHLORIDE ◇ ALGYLEN ◇ ANAMENTH ◇ BENZINOL ◇ BLACOSOLV ◇ CECOLENE ◇ 1-CHLORO-2,2-DICHLOROETHYLENE ◇ CHLORYLEA ◇ CHORYLEN ◇ CIRCOSOLV ◇ CRAWHASPOL ◇ DENSINFLUAT ◇ 1,1-DICHLORO-2-CHLOROETHYLENE ◇ DOW-TRI ◇ DUKERON ◇ ETHINYL TRICHLORIDE ◇ ETHYLENE TRICHLORIDE ◇ FLECK-FLIP ◇ FLUATE ◇ GERMALGENE ◇ LANADIN ◇ LETHURIN ◇ NARCOGEN ◇ NARKOSOID ◇ NCI-CO4546 ◇ NIALK ◇ PERM-A-CHLOR ◇ PETZINOL ◇ RCRA WASTE NUMBER U228 ◇ THRETHYLENE ◇ TRIAD ◇ TRIASOL ◈ TRICHLOORETHEEN (DUTCH) ◇ TRICHLOORETHYLEEN, TRI (DUTCH) ◇ TRICHLO-

RAETHEN (GERMAN) ◇ TRICHLORAETHYLEN, TRI (GER-
MAN) ◇ TRICHLORAN ◇ TRICHLORETHENE (FRENCH)
◇ TRICHLORETHYLENE, TRI (FRENCH) ◇ TRICHLOROETH-
ENE ◇ 1,2,2-TRICHLOROETHYLENE ◇ TRI-CLENE
◇ TRICLORETENE (ITALIAN) ◇ TRICHLOROETILENE (ITAL-
IAN) ◇ TRIELINA (ITALIAN) ◇ TRILENE ◇ TRIMAR
◇ TRI-PLUS ◇ VESTROL ◇ VITRAN ◇ WESTROSOL

TOXICITY DATA with REFERENCE

CAR: ihl-mus TC:150 ppm/7H/2Y-I INHEAO
21,243,83
CAR: ihl-mus TCLo:150 ppm/7H/2Y-I INHEAO
21,243,83
CAR: ihl-rat TCLo:150 ppm/7H/2Y-I INHEAO
21,243,83
CAR: orl-mus TD:912 g/kg/78W-I NCITR*
NCI-CG-TR-2,76
CAR: orl-mus TDLo:455 g/kg/78W-I NCITR*
NCI-CG-TR-2,76
ETA: ihl-ham TCLo:100 ppm/6H/77W-I
ARTODN 43,237,80
ETA: ihl-mus TC:500 ppm/6H/77W-I ARTODN
43,237,80
MUT: dns-rat:lvr 2800 μmol/L CRNGDP5,1629,84
MUT: mmo-asn 2500 ppm MUREAV 155,105,85
MUT: otr-ham:emb 5 mg/L CRNGDP 4,291,83
MUT: otr-mus:emb 20 mg/L CALEDQ 28,85,85
MUT: sln-asn 17500 ppm MUREAV 155,105,85

CONSENSUS REPORTS: IARC Cancer Review: GROUP 3 IMEMDT 7,364,87; Animal
Limited Evidence IMEMDT 20,545,79; Human
Inadequate Evidence IMEMDT 20,545,79; Animal Sufficient Evidence IMEMDT 11,263,76.
NCI Carcinogenesis Bioassay (gavage); No Evidence: rat NCITR* NCI-CG-TR-2,76; (gavage);
Clear Evidence: mouse NCITR* NCI-CG-TR-
2,76. Community Right-To-Know List. Reported in EPA TSCA Inventory. EPA Genetic
Toxicology Program.

OSHA PEL: (Transitional: TWA 100 ppm; CL
200 ppm; Pk 300 ppm/5M/2H)TWA 50 ppm;
STEL 200 ppm ACGIH TLV: TWA 50 ppm;
STEL 200 ppm; BEI: 320 mg(trichloroethanol)/
g creatinine in urine at end of shift; 0.5 ppm
trichloroethylene in end-exhaled air prior to shift
and end of work week. DFG MAK: Suspected
Carcinogen; 50 ppm (270 mg/m³); BAT: 500
μg/dL in blood at end of shift or work week.
NIOSH REL: (Trichloroethylene) TWA 250
ppm; (Waste Anesthetic Gases) CL 2 ppm/
1H DOT Classification: ORM-A; Label:
None; Poison B; Label: St. Andrews Cross.

SAFETY PROFILE: Suspected carcinogen with
experimental carcinogenic, tumorigenic, and
teratogenic data. Experimental poison by intravenous and subcutaneous routes. Moderately
toxic experimentally by ingestion and intraperitoneal routes. Mildly toxic to humans by ingestion and inhalation. Mildly toxic experimentally
by inhalation. Human systemic effects by ingestion and inhalation: eye effects, somnolence,
hallucinations or distorted perceptions, gastrointestinal changes and jaundice. Experimental reproductive effects. Human mutation data reported. An eye and severe skin irritant. When
heated to decomposition it emits toxic fumes
of Cl⁻.

TIV750   CAS: 95-95-4
2,4,5-TRICHLOROPHENOL
mf: $C_6H_3Cl_3O$ mw: 197.44

PROP: Colorless needles or gray flakes. Bp:
252°, fp: 57.0°, d: 1.678 @ 25/4°, vap press:
1 mm @ 72.0°, mp: 61-63°. Insol in water;
sol in CCl_4, alc, benzene, ether.

SYNS: COLLUNOSOL ◇ DOWICIDE 2 ◇ DOWICIDE B
◇ NCI-C61187 ◇ NURELLE ◇ PREVENTOL I ◇ RCRA WASTE
NUMBER U230

TOXICITY DATA with REFERENCE
NEO: skn-mus TDLo:6700 mg/kg/16W-I
CNREA8 19,413,59

CONSENSUS REPORTS: IARC Cancer Review: Human Limited Evidence IMEMDT
41,319,86; Animal Inadequate Evidence
IMEMDT 20,349,79. Chlorophenol compounds
are on the Community Right-To-Know List.
Reported in EPA TSCA Inventory.

SAFETY PROFILE: Suspected carcinogen with
experimental neoplastigenic data. Poison by intraperitoneal, intravenous and possibly other
routes. Moderately toxic by ingestion and subcutaneous routes. Experimental reproductive effects. When heated to decomposition it emits
toxic fumes of Cl⁻ and explodes.

TIX500   CAS: 93-72-1
α-(2,4,5-TRICHLOROPHENOXY)
PROPIONIC ACID
mf: $C_9H_7Cl_3O_3$ mw: 269.51

PROP: Crystals. Mp: 182°. Sltly water-sol.

SYNS: ACIDE 2-(2,4,5-TRICHLORO-PHENOXY) PROPIO-
NIQUE (FRENCH) ◇ ACIDO 2-(2,4,5-TRICLORO-FENOSSI)-
PROPIONICO (ITALIAN) ◇ AMCHEM 2,4,5-TP ◇ AQUA-VEX

◊ COLOR-SET ◊ DED-WEED ◊ DOUBLE STRENGTH ◊ FENOPROP ◊ FENORMONE ◊ FRUITONE T ◊ HERBI-CIDES, SILVEX ◊ KURAN ◊ KURON ◊ KUROSAL ◊ MILLER NU SET ◊ PROPON ◊ RCRA WASTE NUMBER U233 ◊ SILVEX (USDA) ◊ SILVI-RHAP ◊ STA-FAST ◊ 2,4,5-TC ◊ 2,4,5-TCPPA ◊ 2,4,5-TP ◊ 2-(2,4,5-TRICHLOOR-FENOXY)-PROPIONZUUR (DUTCH) ◊ 2-(2,4,5-TRICHLORO-PHENOXY)PROPIONIC ACID ◊ 2,4,5-TRICHLOROPHE-NOXY-α-PROPIONIC ACID ◊ 2-(2,4,5-TRICHLOR-PHE-NOXY)-PROPIONSAEURE (GERMAN) ◊ WEED-B-GON

CONSENSUS REPORTS: IARC Cancer Review: Human Limited Evidence IMEMDT 41,357,86.

SAFETY PROFILE: Suspected carcinogen. Moderately toxic by ingestion and possibly other routes. An experimental teratogen. Experimental reproductive effects. When heated to decomposition it emits toxic fumes of Cl^-.

TLH000   CAS: 6334-11-8
2,4,6-TRIMETHYLANILINE HYDROCHLORIDE
mf: $C_9H_{13}N \cdot ClH$ mw: 171.69

SYNS: AMINOMESITYLENE HYDROCHLORIDE ◊ 2-AMINOMESITYLENE HYDROCHLORIDE ◊ 2-AMINO-1,3-5-TRIMETHYLBENZENE HYDROCHLORIDE ◊ MESIDINE HYDROCHLORIDE ◊ MESITYLAMINE HYDROCHLORIDE ◊ 2,4,6-TRIMETHYLBENZENAMINE HYDROCHLORIDE

TOXICITY DATA with REFERENCE
CAR: orl-mus TD:43 g/kg/78W-C   JEPTDQ 2,325,78
CAR: orl-mus TD:180 g/kg/77W-C   IARC** 27,177,82
CAR: orl-mus TD:360 g/kg/77W-C   IARC** 27,177,82
CAR: orl-mus TDLo:22 g/kg/78W-C   JEPTDQ 2,325,78
CAR: orl-rat TD:79 g/kg/77W-C   IARC** 27,177,82
CAR: orl-rat TD:158 g/kg/77W-C   IARC** 27,177,82
CAR: orl-rat TDLo:9500 mg/kg/78W-C   JEPTDQ 2,325,78
NEO: orl-rat TD:4700 mg/kg/78W-C   JEPTDQ 2,325,78

CONSENSUS REPORTS: IARC Cancer Review: Animal Inadequate Evidence IMEMDT 27,177,82.

SAFETY PROFILE: Suspected carcinogen with experimental carcinogenic and neoplastigenic

data. Poison by intraperitoneal route. Moderately toxic by ingestion. When heated to decomposition it emits very toxic fumes of NO_x and HCl.

TLT750   CAS: 60597-20-8
TRIMETHYLHYDRAZINE HYDROCHLORIDE
mf: $C_3H_{10}N_2 \cdot ClH$ mw: 110.61

TOXICITY DATA with REFERENCE
CAR: orl-ham TDLo:80 g/kg/27W-C   JNCIAM 59,431,77
CAR: orl-mus TDLo:22 g/kg/37W-C   JNCIAM 57,187,76

SAFETY PROFILE: Suspected carcinogen with experimental carcinogenic data. When heated to decomposition it emits very toxic fumes of HCl and NO_x.

TMD250   CAS: 512-56-1
TRIMETHYL PHOSPHATE
mf: $C_3H_9O_4P$ mw: 140.09

PROP: Liquid. D: 1.97 @ 19.5/0°, bp: 197.2°. Sol in alc, water, ether.

SYNS: METHYL PHOSPHATE ◊ NCI-C03781 ◊ PHOSPHORIC ACID, TRIMETHYL ESTER ◊ TMP ◊ O,O,O-TRIMETHYL PHOSPHATE

TOXICITY DATA with REFERENCE
CAR: orl-mus TDLo:154 g/kg/2Y-C:TER   NCITR* NCI-CG-TR-81,78
NEO: orl-rat TDLo:31 g/kg/2Y-C   NCITR* NCI-CG-TR-81,78
ETA: orl-rat TD:16 g/kg/2Y-I   NCITR* NCI-CG-TR-81,78
ETA: orl-rat TD:77 g/kg/2Y-I   NCITR* NCI-CG-TR-81,78
MUT: cyt-hmn:lym 100 mmol/L/5H   MUREAV 65,121,79
MUT: dnd-rat:lvr 300 μmol/L   SinJF#26OCT82
MUT: sce-ckn-par 25424 μg/kg   47JMAE -,137,82
MUT: trn-mus-ipr 1 g/kg   MUREAV 157,205,85
MUT: trn-mus-orl 21728 mg/kg/8W-C   ENMUDM 7(Suppl 3),65,85

CONSENSUS REPORTS: NCI Carcinogenesis Bioassay (gavage); Clear Evidence: mouse, rat NCITR* NCI-CG-TR-81,78. Reported in EPA TSCA Inventory. EPA Genetic Toxicology Program.

DFG MAK: Suspected Carcinogen.

SAFETY PROFILE: Suspected carcinogen with experimental carcinogenic, neoplastigenic, tumorigenic, and teratogenic data. Moderately toxic by ingestion, skin contact, intraperitoneal, intravenous, and possibly other routes. Experimental reproductive effects. Human mutation data reported. Explodes when heat distilled. When heated to decomposition it emits toxic fumes of PO_x.

TMM250   CAS: 129-79-3
2,4,7-TRINITROFLUOREN-9-ONE
mf: $C_{13}H_5N_3O_7$ mw: 315.21

SYNS: 2,4,7-TRINITRO-9-FLUORENONE ◊ 2,4,7-TRINI-TROFLUORENONE (MAK)

TOXICITY DATA with REFERENCE
ETA: orl-rat TDLo:1000 mg/kg   SCIEAS 137,257,62

MUT: cyt-hmn:lym 3 mg/L   MUREAV 138,181,84
MUT: dns-rat-orl 100 mg/kg   ENMUDM 5,488,83
MUT: mma-sat 10 μL/plate   EPASR* 8EHQ-0280-0333
MUT: msc-mus:lym 1950 μg/L   MUREAV 118,167,83
MUT: sce-ham:ovr 900 μg/L   MUREAV 118,167,83
MUT: sce-hmn:lym 3 mg/L   MUREAV 138,181,84

CONSENSUS REPORTS: Reported in EPA TSCA Inventory.

DFG MAK: Suspected Carcinogen.

SAFETY PROFILE: Suspected carcinogen with experimental tumorigenic data. Mildly toxic by ingestion. Human mutation data reported. A skin and eye irritant. When heated to decomposition it emits highly toxic fumes of NO_x.

TNX275   CAS: 62450-06-0
TRYPTOPHAN P1
mf: $C_{13}H_{13}N_3$ mw: 211.29

SYNS: 3-AMINO-1,4-DIMETHYL-γ-CARBOLINE ◊ 3-AMINO-1,4-DIMETHYL-5H-PYRIDO(4,3-b)INDOLE ◊ 1,4-DIMETHYL-5H-PYRIDO(4,3-b)INDOL-3-AMINE ◊ TRP-P-1 ◊ dl-TRYPTOPHAN, pyrolyzate 1

TOXICITY DATA with REFERENCE
CAR: imp-mus TDLo:40 mg/kg   CALEDQ 17,101,82
CAR: orl-mus TDLo:9648 mg/kg/57W-C   EVHPAZ 67,129,86
CAR: orl-rat TDLo:2 g/kg/49W-C   EVHPAZ 67,129,86
CAR: scu-ham TDLo:240 mg/kg/20W-I   PPTCBY 9,159,79
CAR: scu-mus TD:50 mg/kg   CRNGDP 8,1721,87

CAR: scu-mus TDLo:50 mg/kg   PPTCBY 37,193,85
CAR: scu-rat TDLo:150 mg/kg/20W-I   PPTCBY 9,159,79
NEO: scu-mus TD:50 mg/kg   CRNGDP 8,1721,87
MUT: cyt-ham:lng 1250 μg/L   GMCRDC 27,95,81
MUT: cyt-hmn:fbr 200 μg/L   PJABDW 56,332,80
MUT: dnd-bcs 200 μg/disc   PMRSDJ 1,175,81
MUT: dnd-mam:lym 50 μmol/L   BICHAW 20,298,81
MUT: dnd-mus-ipr 10 mg/kg   JJCREP 76,835,85
MUT: dnd-mus:lvr 50 μmol/L   JJCREP 76,835,85
MUT: dni-rat:lvr 5 mg/L   CBINA8 54,317,85
MUT: dnr-bcs 1200 ng/disc   MUREAV 97,339,82
MUT: dns-hmn:fbr 20 mg/L   JRARAX 24,356,83
MUT: dns-rat:lvr 100 nmol/L   CALEDQ 20,283,83
MUT: mma-sat 250 ng/plate   JJCREP 76,835,85
MUT: msc-ham:lng 10 mg/L   MUREAV 118,91,83
MUT: oms-rat:lvr 10 mg/L   CBINA8 54,317,85
MUT: sce-hmn:fbr 200 μg/L   PJABDW 56,332,80

CONSENSUS REPORTS: IARC Cancer Review: GROUP 2B IMEMDT 7,56,87; Animal Sufficient Evidence IMEMDT 31,247,83. EPA Genetic Toxicology Program.

SAFETY PROFILE: Suspected carcinogen with experimental with experimental carcinogenic and neoplastigenic data. Poison by ingestion. Human mutation data reported. When heated to decomposition it emits toxic fumes of NO_x.

VLU200   CAS: 83768-87-0
VINTHIONINE
mf: $C_6H_{11}NO_2S$ mw: 161.24

SYNS: S-ETHENYL-dl-HOMOCYSTEINE ◊ S-VINYL-dl-HOMOCYSTEINE

TOXICITY DATA with REFERENCE
CAR: ipr-rat TDLo:5625 mg/kg/12W-I   CNREA8 42,4364,82
CAR: orl-mus TDLo:68040 mg/kg/75W-C   CNREA8 42,4364,82
CAR: orl-rat TD:36 g/kg/86W-C   CNREA8 42,4364,82
CAR: orl-rat TDLo:18 g/kg/86W-C   CNREA8 42,4364,82
MUT: mma-sat 50 nmol/plate   BBRCA9 88,395,79
MUT: mmo-sat 50 nmol/plate   BBRCA9 88,395,79

SAFETY PROFILE: Suspected carcinogen with experimental carcinogenic data. Mutation data reported. When heated to decomposition it emits toxic fumes of SO_x and NO_x.

VPK000   CAS: 75-35-4
VINYLIDENE CHLORIDE
mf: $C_2H_2Cl_2$ mw: 96.94

PROP: Colorless, volatile liquid. Bp: 31.6°, lel: 7.3%, uel: 16.0%, fp: −122°, flash p: 0°F (OC), d: 1.213 @ 20°/4°, autoign temp: 1058°F.

SYNS: CHLORURE de VINYLIDENE (FRENCH)
◇ 1-1-DCE ◇ 1,1-DICHLOROETHENE ◇ 1,1-DICHLORO-
ETHYLENE ◇ NCI-C54262 ◇ RCRA WASTE NUMBER U078
◇ SCONATEX ◇ VDC ◇ VINYLIDENE CHLORIDE (II)
◇ VINYLIDENE DICHLORIDE ◇ VINYLIDINE CHLORIDE

TOXICITY DATA with REFERENCE
CAR: ihl-mus TCLo:25 ppm/4H/52W-I
  MELAAD 68,241,77
NEO: skn-mus TDLo:4840 mg/kg   JJIND8
  63,1433,79
ETA: ihl-mus TC:55 ppm/6H/13W-I   JTEHD6
  7,909,81
ETA: ihl-mus TC:55 ppm/6H/52W-I   EVHPAZ
  21,25,77
ETA: ihl-rat TC:55 ppm/6H/28W-I   JTEHD6
  7,909,81
ETA: ihl-rat TC:55 ppm/6H/52W-I   EVHPAZ
  21,25,77
ETA: ihl-rat TC:150 ppm/4H/52W-I   EVHPAZ
  21,45,77
ETA: ihl-rat TC:150 ppm/4H/52W-I   MELAAD
  68,241,77
ETA: ihl-rat TCLo:55 ppm/6H/52W-I   JTEHD6
  4,15,78
MUT: dnd-rat-ihl 10 ppm   TXAPA9 53,357,80
MUT: dns-mus-ihl 50 ppm   TXAPA9 53,357,80
MUT: dns-mus-orl 200 mg/kg   TXCYAC 36,199,85
MUT: mma-sat 3 pph/2H   MUREAV 58,183,78
MUT: mmo-sat 5 pph   MUREAV 57,141,78

CONSENSUS REPORTS: IARC Cancer Review: GROUP 3 IMEMDT 7,376,87; Human Inadequate Evidence IMEMDT 39,195,86; Animal Sufficient Evidence IMEMDT 19,439,79; Animal Limited Evidence IMEMDT 39,195,86; Human Inadequate Evidence IMEMDT 19, 439,79. EPA Genetic Toxicology Program. Reported in EPA TSCA Inventory. Community Right-To-Know List.

OSHA PEL: TWA 1 ppm   ACGIH TLV: TWA 5 ppm; STEL 20 ppm   DFG MAK: Suspected Carcinogen.

SAFETY PROFILE: Suspected carcinogen with experimental carcinogenic, neoplastigenic, tumorigenic, and teratogenic data. Poison by inhalation, ingestion, and intravenous routes. Moderately toxic by subcutaneous route. Human systemic effects by inhalation: general anesthesia, liver and kidney changes. Experimental reproductive effects. Mutation data reported. A very dangerous fire hazard when exposed to heat or flame. Moderately explosive in the form of gas when exposed to heat or flame. It forms explosive peroxides upon exposure to air. To fight fire, use alcohol foam, CO_2, dry chemical. When heated to decomposition it emits toxic fumes of Cl^-.

VPP000   CAS: 75-38-7
VINYLIDENE FLUORIDE
DOT: 1959
mf: $C_2H_2F_2$ mw: 64.04

PROP: Colorless gas. Bp: $<-70°$, lel: 5.5%, uel: 21.3%.

SYNS: 1,1-DIFLUOROETHYLENE (DOT, MAK)
◇ HALOCARBON 1132A ◇ NCI-C60208 ◇ VDF

TOXICITY DATA with REFERENCE
NEO: orl-rat TDLo:1930 mg/kg/52W-I
  MELAAD 70,363,79
MUT: mma-sat 50 pph/24H   ARTODN 41,249,79

CONSENSUS REPORTS: IARC Cancer Review: Animal Inadequate Evidence IMEMDT 39,227,86. Reported in EPA TSCA Inventory.

DFG MAK: Suspected Carcinogen. DOT Classification: Flammable Gas; Label: Flammable Gas.

SAFETY PROFILE: Suspected carcinogen with experimental neoplastigenic data. Mildly toxic by inhalation. Mutation data reported. A very dangerous fire hazard when exposed to heat, flames or oxidizers. Explosive in the form of vapor when exposed to heat or flame. To fight fire, stop flow of gas. When heated to decomposition it emits toxic fumes of F^-.

VTF000   CAS: 595-33-5
VOLIDAN
mf: $C_{24}H_{32}O_4$ mw: 384.56

SYNS: 17-α-ACETOXY-6-DEHYDRO-6-METHYLPRO-
GESTERONE ◇ 17-ACETOXY-6-METHYLPREGNA-4,6-
DIENE-3,20-DIONE ◇ 17-α-ACETOXY-6-METHYLPREGNA-
4,6-DIENE-3,20-DIONE ◇ 17-α-ACETOXY-6-METHYL-4,6-
PREGNADIENE-3,20-DIONE ◇ BDH 1298 ◇ 6-DEHYDRO-6-
METHYL-17-α-ACETOXYPROGESTERONE ◇ DMAP
◇ 17-HYDROXY-6-METHYLPREGNA-4,6-DIENE-3,20-DIONE
ACETATE ◇ MEGACE ◇ MEGESTROL ACETATE

◇ MEGESTRYL ACETATE ◇ 6-METHYL-17-α-ACETOXY-PREGNA-4,6-DIENE-3,20-DIONE ◇ 6-METHYL-6-DEHYDRO-17-α-ACETOXYPROGESTERONE ◇ 6-METHYL-6-DEHYDRO-17-α-ACETYLPROGESTERONE ◇ 6-METHYL-17-α-HY-DROXY-Δ⁶-PROGESTERONE ACETATE ◇ 6-METHYL-Δ⁴,⁶-PREGNADIEN-17-α-OL-3,20-DIONE ACETATE ◇ NSC-71423 ◇ OVABAN ◇ SC10363

TOXICITY DATA with REFERENCE
CAR: orl-dog TDLo: 256 mg/kg/7Y-C   JTEHD6 3,167,77
ETA: orl-dog TD: 182 mg/kg/2Y-C   JAMAAP 219,1601,72
MUT: dni-mus-scu 200 mg/kg   JOENAK 60,167,74
MUT: dns-mus-scu 200 mg/kg   JOENAK 60,167,74

CONSENSUS REPORTS: IARC Cancer Review: Animal Limited Evidence IMEMDT 21,431,79.

SAFETY PROFILE: Suspected carcinogen with experimental carcinogenic and teratogenic data. Poison by intravenous route. Human reproductive effects by ingestion and implant routes: effects on ovaries and fallopian tubes, menstrual cycle changes and female fertility index changes. Mutation data reported. Experimental reproductive effects. When heated to decomposition it emits acrid smoke and irritating fumes. An FDA proprietary drug used to treat endometriosis and breast cancer. A steroid.

XMS000
2,4-XYLIDINE
CAS: 95-68-1

DOT: 1711
mf: $C_8H_{11}N$ mw: 121.20

PROP: Liquid. Bp: 214°, mp: 16°, d: 0.978 @ 19.6/4°. Very sltly sol in water.

SYNS: 1-AMINO-2,4-DIMETHYLBENZENE ◇ 4-AMINO-1,3-DIMETHYLBENZENE ◇ 4-AMINO-3-METHYLTOLUENE ◇ 4-AMINO-1,3-XYLENE ◇ 2,4-DIMETHYLANILINE ◇ 2,4-DIMETHYLBENZENAMINE ◇ 2,4-DIMETHYL-PHENYLAMINE ◇ 2-METHYL-p-TOLUIDINE ◇ 4-METHYL-o-TOLUIDINE ◇ 2,4-XYLIDENE (MAK) ◇ m-XYLIDINE (DOT) ◇ m-4-XYLIDINE

TOXICITY DATA with REFERENCE
MUT: dni-mus-orl 200 mg/kg   MUREAV 46,305,77
MUT: mma-sat 5 µmol/plate   MUREAV 77,317,80

CONSENSUS REPORTS: IARC Cancer Review: GROUP 3 IMEMDT 7,56,87; Animal Inadequate Evidence IMEMDT 16,367,78. Reported in EPA TSCA Inventory.

DFG MAK: 5 ppm (25 mg/m³); Suspected Carcinogen.   DOT Classification: Poison B; Label: Poison.

SAFETY PROFILE: Suspected carcinogen. Poison by ingestion. Mutation data reported. When heated to decomposition it emits toxic fumes of NO_x.

Class III/Questionable Carcinogens

AAD750
ACACIA VILLOSA

PROP: Aqueous extract from the root of the plant (JNCIAM 52,1579,74).

SYN: WATAPANA SHIMARON

TOXICITY DATA with REFERENCE
CAR: imp-ham TDLo: 1660 mg/kg   JNCIAM 53,1259,74

NEO: scu-rat TD: 300 g/kg/60W-I   JNCIAM 52,445,74

NEO: scu-rat TDLo: 198 mg/kg/22W-I   JNCIAM 52,1579,74

SAFETY PROFILE: Questionable carcinogen with experimental neoplastigenic and carcinogenic data. When heated to decomposition it emits smoke and acrid fumes.

AAE000   CAS: 3697-25-4
4,10-ACE-1,2-BENZANTHRACENE
mf: $C_{20}H_{14}$ mw: 254.34

SYN: 1,2-DIHYDROBENZ(e)ACEANTHRYLENE ◇ 5,6-DI-HYDROBENZENE(e)ACEANTHRYLENE

TOXICITY DATA with REFERENCE
ETA: scu-mus TD: 80 mg/kg   CNREA8 6,454,46
ETA: scu-mus TDLo: 4 mg/kg   AJCAA7 33,499,38

SAFETY PROFILE: Questionable carcinogen with experimental tumorigenic data. When heated to decomposition it emits acrid smoke and fumes.

AAF000   CAS: 5779-79-3
ACENAPHTHANTHRACENE
mf: $C_{20}H_{14}$ mw: 254.34

SYNS: BENZ(k)ACEPHENANTHRENE ◇ 4,5-DIHYDRO-BENZ(k)ACEPHENANTHRYLENE ◇ 3:4-DIMETHYLENE-1:2-BENZANTHRACENE

TOXICITY DATA with REFERENCE
ETA: skn-mus TDLo: 960 mg/kg/40W-I
PRLBA4 129,439,40

SAFETY PROFILE: Questionable carcinogen with experimental tumorigenic data. When heated to decomposition it emits acrid smoke and irritating fumes.

AAF250   CAS: 4657-93-6
5-ACENAPHTHENAMINE
mf: $C_{12}H_{11}N$ mw: 169.24

PROP: Colorless needles, sol in ethanol. Mp: 108°.

SYNS: 5-AMINOACENAPHTHENE ◇ 1,2-DIHYDRO-5-ACENAPHTHYLENAMINE

TOXICITY DATA with REFERENCE
CAR: imp-mus TDLo: 160 mg/kg
NEZAAQ 24,263,69
ETA: ipr-mus TDLo: 3744 mg/kg/78W-I
NEZAAQ 24,263,69

CONSENSUS REPORTS: IARC Cancer Review: GROUP 3 IMEMDT 7,56,87; Animal Inadequate Evidence IMEMDT 16,243,78

SAFETY PROFILE: Questionable carcinogen with experimental carcinogenic and tumorigenic data. Poison by intravenous route. When heated to decomposition it emits toxic fumes of NO_x.

AAH000   CAS: 16568-02-8
ACETALDEHYDE-N-METHYL-N-FORMYLHYDRAZONE
mf: $C_4H_8N_2O$ mw: 100.14

SYNS: ACETALDEHYDE-N-FORMYL-N-METHYLHYDRA-ZONE ◇ ETHYLIDENE GYROMITRIN ◇ GYROMITRIN ◇ N-METHYL-N-FORMYL HYDRAZONE of ACETALDEHYDE

TOXICITY DATA with REFERENCE
CAR: scu-mus TDLo: 600 mg/kg/12W-I
NEOLA4 28,559,81
ETA: orl-mus TD: 5200 mg/kg/52W-I   FEPRA7 39(3,Pt.2),884,80

CONSENSUS REPORTS: IARC Cancer Review: GROUP 3 IMEMDT 7,56,87; Animal

Limited Evidence IMEMDT 7,391,87. EPA Genetic Toxicology Program.

SAFETY PROFILE: Questionable carcinogen with experimental carcinogenic and tumorigenic data. Poison via ingestion and possibly other routes. When heated to decomposition it emits toxic fumes of NO_x.

AAH100 CAS: 17167-73-6
ACETALDEHYDE METHYLHYDRAZONE
mf: $C_3H_8N_2$ mw: 72.13

SYNS: ACETALDEHYDE, N-METHYLHYDRAZONE ◇ AMFH

TOXICITY DATA with REFERENCE
ETA: orl-mus TDLo: 208 mg/kg/1Y-I   JJIND8 67,881,81

SAFETY PROFILE: Questionable carcinogen with experimental tumorigenic data. Poison by ingestion. When heated to decomposition it emits toxic fumes of NO_x.

AAI100 CAS: 103416-59-7
ACETAMIDE, 2-(DIETHYLAMINO)-N-(1,3-DIMETHYL-4-(o-FLUOROBENZOYL)-5-PYRAZOLYL)-, MONOHYDROCHLORIDE
mf: $C_{18}H_{23}FN_4O_2 \cdot ClH$ mw: 382.91

SYN: 2-(DIETHYLAMINO)-N-(1,3-DIMETHYL-4-(o-FLUO-ROBENZOYL)-5-PYRAZOLYL)ACETAMI DE HYDROCHLO-RIDE ◇ 2-(DIETHYLAMINO)-N-(4-(2-FLUOROBENZOYL)-1,3-DIMETHYL-1H-PYRAZOL-5-YL)ACE TAMIDE HYDRO-CHLORIDE ◇ PD 109394

TOXICITY DATA with REFERENCE
ETA: orl-rat TD: 4550 mg/kg/13W-C   AJPAA4 124,392,86

MUT: mma-sat 1 μmol/plate   CRNGDP 7,2019,86

SAFETY PROFILE: Questionable carcinogen with experimental tumorigenic data. Mutation data reported. When heated to decomposition it emits toxic fumes of F^-, NO_x and HCl.

AAI125 CAS: 85723-21-3
ACETAMIDE, N-(4-(2-FLUOROBENZOYL)-1,3-DIMETHYL-1H-PYRAZOL-5-YL)-2-((3-(2-METHYL-1-PIPERIDINYL)PROPYL)AMINO)-, (Z)-2-BUTENEDIOATE (1:2)
mf: $C_{23}H_{32}FN_5O_2$ mw: 429.60

TOXICITY DATA with REFERENCE
ETA: orl-rat TD: 4550 mg/kg/13W-C   AJPAA4 124,392,86

SAFETY PROFILE: Questionable carcinogen with experimental tumorigenic data. When heated to decomposition it emits toxic fumes of NO_x.

AAK400 CAS: 19361-41-2
3-ACETAMIDOFLUORANTHENE
mf: $C_{18}H_{13}NO$ mw: 259.32

SYNS: 3-ACETYLAMINO-FLUORANTHEN ◇ 3-ACE-TYLAMINOFLUORANTHENE ◇ N-FLUORANTHEN-3-YL-ACETAMIDE ◇ N-3-FLUORANTHENYLACETAMIDE

TOXICITY DATA with REFERENCE
ETA: orl-rat TDLo: 4050 mg/kg/16W-C ONCOAR 8,233,55
MUT: mma-sat 1 μg/plate   NTIS** PB86-213733

SAFETY PROFILE: Questionable carcinogen with experimental tumorigenic data. Mutation data reported. When heated to decomposition it emits toxic fumes of NO_x.

AAL300 CAS: 55123-66-5
(S)-2-(2-ACETAMIDO-4-METHYLVALERAMIDO)-N-(1-FORMYL-4-GUANIDINOBUTYL)-4-M ETHYL-VALERAMIDE
mf: $C_{20}H_{38}N_6O_4$ mw: 426.64

SYN: VALERAMIDE, 2-(2-ACETAMIDO-4-METHYLVAL-ERAMIDO)-N-(1-FORMYL-4-GUANIDINOBUTYL)-4-METHYL-(S)-

TOXICITY DATA with REFERENCE
NEO: orl-mus TDLo: 57600 mg/kg/69W-C GANNA2 71,913,80

SAFETY PROFILE: Questionable carcinogen with experimental neoplastigenic data. When heated to decomposition it emits toxic fumes of NO_x.

AAL500 CAS: 24143-08-6
5-ACETAMIDO-3-(5-NITRO-2-FURYL)-6H-1,2,4-OXADIAZINE
mf: $C_9H_8N_4O_5$ mw: 252.21

SYN: N-(3-(5-NITRO-2-FURYL)-6H-1,2,4-OXADI-AZINYL)ACETAMIDE

TOXICITY DATA with REFERENCE
CAR: orl-rat TDLo: 21 g/kg/28W-C   CNREA8 29,2212,69
MUT: dnr-sat 500 nmol/well   CNREA8 34,2266,74
MUT: mma-sat 1 μg/plate   MUREAV 40,9,76
MUT: mmo-esc 300 nmol/well   CNREA8 34,2266,74

MUT: mrc-esc 500 nmol/well   CNREA8 34,2266,74
MUT: pic-esc 500 µg/L   MUREAV 26,3,74

SAFETY PROFILE: Questionable carcinogen with experimental carcinogenic data. When heated to decomposition it emits toxic fumes of NO_x.

AAM250   CAS: 4120-77-8
2-ACETAMIDOPHENATHRENE
mf: $C_{16}H_{13}NO$ mw: 235.30

SYNS: 2-ACETAMINOPHENANTHRENE ◇ 2-ACETYL-AMINOPHENANTHRENE ◇ 2-PHENANTHRYLACE-TAMIDE ◇ N-2-PHENANTHRYLACETAMIDE ◇ N-(2-PHENANTHRYL)ACETAMIDE

TOXICITY DATA with REFERENCE
CAR: orl-rat TDLo: 900 mg/kg/13W-C   CNREA8 19,210,59
ETA: orl-rat TD: 252 mg/kg/3W-C   CRNGDP 2,1235,81
ETA: orl-rat TD: 300 mg/kg/3D-I   ZEKBAI 72,321,69
ETA: scu-rat TDLo: 75 mg/kg/3W-I   CNREA8 26,2239,66
MUT: dnr-ham: fbr 1 µmol/L   JNCIAM 54,1287,75

SAFETY PROFILE: Questionable carcinogen with experimental carcinogenic and tumorigenic data. Mutation data reported. When heated to decomposition it emits toxic fumes of NO_x.

ABJ750   CAS: 26541-56-0
N-ACETOXY-4-ACETAMIDOBIPHENYL
mf: $C_{16}H_{15}NO_3$ mw: 269.32

SYNS: ACETIC ACID (N-ACETYL-N-(4-BIPHE-NYL)AMINO) ESTER ◇ ACETIC ACID ESTER with N-4-BI-PHENYLYLACETOHYDROXAMIC ACID ◇ N-ACETOXY-4-BIPHENYLACETAMIDE ◇ N-(4-BIPHENYLYL)ACETO-HYDROXAMIC ACETATE

TOXICITY DATA with REFERENCE
NEO: skn-mus TDLo: 4309 µg/kg   JNCIAM 54,491,75
MUT: mma-sat 1 µg/plate   CBINA8 26,11,79
MUT: mmo-sat 25 µg/plate   CBINA8 26,11,79

SAFETY PROFILE: Questionable carcinogen with experimental neoplastigenic data. Mutation data reported. When heated to decomposition it emits toxic fumes of NO_x.

ABK250   CAS: 26541-57-1
N-ACETOXY-2-
ACETAMIDOPHENANTHRENE
mf: $C_{18}H_{15}NO_3$ mw: 293.34

SYNS: ACETIC ACID (N-ACETYL-N-(2-PHENAN-THRYL)AMINO)ESTER ◇ ACETIC ACID ESTER with N-(2-PHENANTHRYL)ACETOHYDROXAMIC ACID ◇ N-ACETOXY-2-ACETYLAMINOPHENANTHRENE ◇ N-ACETOXY-4-PHENANTHRYLACETAMIDE ◇ N-(2-PHENANTHRYL)ACETOHYDROXAMIC ACETATE

TOXICITY DATA with REFERENCE
NEO: skn-mus TDLo: 584 µg/kg   JNCIAM 54,491,75
MUT: dnd-mam: lym 625 mg/L   CNREA8 35,1416,75
MUT: dns-hmn: fbr 10 mmol/L/5H   IJCNAW 16,284,75
MUT: mma-sat 50 ng/plate   CBINA8 26,11,79
MUT: mmo-bcs 14 mol   CNREA8 30,1473,70
MUT: mmo-sat 5 µg/plate   CBINA8 26,11,79
MUT: oms-bcs 10 g/L   CNREA8 30,1473,70

SAFETY PROFILE: Questionable carcinogen with experimental neoplastigenic data. Human mutation data reported. When heated to decomposition it emits toxic fumes of NO_x.

ABL000   CAS: 6098-44-8
N-ACETOXY-N-ACETYL-2-
AMINOFLUORENE
mf: $C_{17}H_{15}NO_3$ mw: 281.33

SYNS: ACETIC ACID (N-ACETYL-N-(2-FLUO-RENYL)AMINO) ESTER ◇ N-ACETOXY-2-ACETAMIDOFLU-ORENE ◇ N-ACETOXY-2-ACETYLAMINOFLUORENE ◇ N-ACETOXY-2-FLUORENYLACETAMIDE ◇ N-(FLU-OREN-2-YL)ACETOHYDROXAMIC ACETAMIDE

TOXICITY DATA with REFERENCE
NEO: scu-rat TDLo: 21 mg/kg   CNREA8 37,1461,77
ETA: imp-rat TDLo: 28 mg/kg   CNREA8 37,111,77
MUT: cyt-hmn: unk 10 µmol/L   PNASA6 76,462,79
MUT: dnd-hmn: lym 10 µmol/L   PNASA6 76,462,79
MUT: dni-hmn: hla 100 µmol/L/30M-C   JEPTDQ 2(1),65,78
MUT: dns-hmn: bmr 10 µmol/L   CRNGDP 1,547,80
MUT: dns-hmn: leu 10 µmol/L   CRNGDP 1,547,80
MUT: dns-hmn: lym 10 µmol/L   CALEDQ 2,311,77
MUT: mmo-sat 3100 ng/plate   MUREAV 130,79,84
MUT: msc-ham: emb 500 µg/L   CNREA8 44,1933,84

CONSENSUS REPORTS: EPA Genetic Toxicology Program.

SAFETY PROFILE: Questionable carcinogen with experimental tumorigenic and neoplastigenic data. Human mutation data reported. When heated to decomposition it emits toxic fumes of NO_x.

ABL250 CAS: 26488-34-6
trans-N-ACETOXY-4-ACETYL-AMINOSTILBENE
mf: $C_{18}H_{17}NO_3$ mw: 295.36

SYN: trans-N,o-DIACETYL-N-(p-STYRYLPHENYL)HY-DROXYLAMINE

TOXICITY DATA with REFERENCE
CAR: orl-rat TDLo: 180 mg/kg/20W-I ZEKBAI 74,200,70
MUT: mrc-smc 10 ppm ZEKBAI 74,412,70

CONSENSUS REPORTS: EPA Genetic Toxicology Program.

SAFETY PROFILE: Questionable carcinogen with experimental carcinogenic data. Mutation data reported. When heated to decomposition it emits toxic fumes of NO_x.

ABM000
3-β-ACETOXY-BIS NOR-Δ5-CHOLENIC ACID
mf: $C_{24}H_{36}O_4$ mw: 388.60

SYN: 3-β-ACETOXYPREGN-6-ENE-20-CARBOXYLIC ACID

TOXICITY DATA with REFERENCE
ETA: scu-mus TDLo: 200 mg/kg/90D-I NATUAS 209,1026,66

SAFETY PROFILE: Questionable carcinogen with experimental tumorigenic data. When heated to decomposition it emits acrid smoke and irritating fumes.

ABN250 CAS: 24684-58-0
11-ACETOXY-15-DIHYDROCYCLOPENTA(a)PHENANTHRACEN-17-ONE
mf: $C_{19}H_{14}O_3$ mw: 290.33

SYN: 11-HYDROXY-15,16-DIHYDROCYCLOPENTA(a)-PHENANTHRACEN-17-ONE ACETATE (ESTER)

TOXICITY DATA with REFERENCE
ETA: skn-mus TDLo: 108 mg/kg/1Y-I PEXTAR 11,69,69

SAFETY PROFILE: Questionable carcinogen with experimental tumorigenic data. When

heated to decomposition it emits acrid smoke and irritating fumes.

ABN500 CAS: 38539-23-0
1-ACETOXY-1,4-DIHYDRO-4-(HYDROXYAMINO)QUINOLINE ACETATE (ESTER)
mf: $C_{13}H_{13}N_2O_4$ mw: 261.28

SYN: O,O'-DIACETYL 4-HYDROXYAMINOQUINOLINE-1-OXIDE

TOXICITY DATA with REFERENCE
NEO: scu-mus TDLo: 30 mg/kg/4W-I PSEBAA 136,1206,71
ETA: scu-rat TDLo: 5 mg/kg/2W-I PSEBAA 136,1206,71
MUT: mmo-smc 50 mg/L IGSBAL 85,127,72

SAFETY PROFILE: Questionable carcinogen with experimental tumorigenic and neoplastigenic data. Mutation data reported. When heated to decomposition it emits toxic fumes of NO_x.

ABN725 CAS: 61691-82-5
1'-ACETOXYESTRAGOLE
mf: $C_{12}H_{14}O_3$ mw: 206.26

SYN: p-METHOXY-α-VINYLBENZYL ALCOHOL ACETATE (ESTER)

TOXICITY DATA with REFERENCE
CAR: ipr-mus TDLo: 20626 μg/kg CNREA8 47,2275,87
MUT: dnd-hmn: fbr 500 μmol/L CRNGDP 3,935,82
MUT: dns-hmn: oth 500 μmol/L CRNGDP 3,929,82

CONSENSUS REPORTS: EPA Genetic Toxicology Program.

SAFETY PROFILE: Questionable carcinogen with experimental carcinogenic data. Human mutation data reported. When heated to decomposition it emits acrid smoke and fumes.

ABO250 CAS: 38105-27-0
N-ACETOXYFLUORENYLACETAMIDE
mf: $C_{17}H_{15}NO_3$ mw: 281.33

SYNS: ACETIC ACID ESTER with N-(FLUOREN-3-YL)ACETOHYDROXAMIC ACID ◇ N-ACETOXY-3-FLUORENYLACETAMIDE ◇ N-(FLUOREN-3-YL)ACETOHYDROXAMIC ACETATE

TOXICITY DATA with REFERENCE
NEO: ipr-rat TDLo: 350 mg/kg/4W-I CNREA8 35,447,75

ETA: imp-rat TDLo: 28 mg/kg   CNREA8 37,111,77
ETA: ims-rat TDLo: 210 mg/kg/8W-I   CNREA8 35,447,75

SAFETY PROFILE: Questionable carcinogen with experimental tumorigenic and neoplastigenic data. When heated to decomposition it emits toxic fumes of NO_x.

ABO500   CAS: 55080-20-1
N-ACETOXY-4-FLUORENYLACETAMIDE
mf: $C_{17}H_{15}NO_3$ mw: 281.33

SYNS: ACETIC ACID(N-ACETYL-N-(4-FLUORENYL)AMINO)ESTER ◇ ACETIC ACID, ESTER with N-(FLUOREN-4-YL)ACETOXYHYDROXAMIC ACID ◇ N-(FLUOREN-4-YL)ACETOHYDROXAMIC ACETATE

TOXICITY DATA with REFERENCE
ETA: ipr-rat TDLo: 350 mg/kg/4W-I   CNREA8 35,447,75

SAFETY PROFILE: Questionable carcinogen with experimental tumorigenic data. When heated to decomposition it emits toxic fumes of NO_x.

ABO750   CAS: 29968-75-0
N-ACETOXY-2-FLUORENYLBENZAMIDE
mf: $C_{22}H_{17}NO_3$ mw: 343.40

SYN: N-FLUOREN-2-YL BENZOHYDROXAMIC ACID ACETATE

TOXICITY DATA with REFERENCE
ETA: orl-rat TDLo: 5200 mg/kg/21W-I   CNREA8 30,1485,70

SAFETY PROFILE: Questionable carcinogen with experimental tumorigenic data. When heated to decomposition it emits toxic fumes of NO_x.

ABP500   CAS: 2198-54-1
3′,4′-ACETOXYLIDIDE
mf: $C_{10}H_{13}NO$ mw: 163.24

SYNS: 3,4-DIMETHYLACETANILIDE ◇ 3′,4′-DIMETHYLACETANILIDE

TOXICITY DATA with REFERENCE
ETA: orl-rat TDLo: 9900 mg/kg/56W-C
   CNREA8 16,525,56

SAFETY PROFILE: Questionable carcinogen with experimental tumorigenic data. Moderately toxic by ingestion. When heated to decomposition it emits toxic fumes of NO_x.

ABQ600   CAS: 83876-62-4
4-ACETOXY-7-METHYLBENZ(c)ACRIDINE
mf: $C_{20}H_{15}NO_2$ mw: 301.36

SYN: BENZ(c)ACRIDIN-4-OL, 7-METHYL-, ACETATE (ESTER)

TOXICITY DATA with REFERENCE
ETA: scu-mus TDLo: 72 mg/kg/12W-I   JMCMAR 26,303,83

SAFETY PROFILE: Questionable carcinogen with experimental tumorigenic data. When heated to decomposition it emits toxic fumes of NO_x.

ABR125   CAS: 70715-92-3
N-(ACETOXYMETHYL)-N-ISOBUTYLNITROSAMINE
mf: $C_7H_{14}N_2O_3$ mw: 174.23

SYNS: N-ISOBUTYL-N-(ACETOXYMETHYL)NITROSAMINE ◇ N-NITROSO-N-(ACETOXYMETHYL)-N-ISOBUTYLAMINE

TOXICITY DATA with REFERENCE
CAR: scu-rat TD: 66 mg/kg/10W-I   IAPUDO 41,619,82
ETA: scu-rat TDLo: 50 mg/kg/10W-I   JCROD7 104,13,82
MUT: dnr-bcs 1 μmol/plate   GANNA2 70,663,79
MUT: mmo-esc 25 μmol/plate   GANNA2 70,663,79
MUT: mmo-sat 5 μmol/plate   GANNA2 70,663,79

SAFETY PROFILE: Questionable carcinogen with experimental carcinogenic and tumorigenic data. Mutation data reported. When heated to decomposition it emits toxic fumes of NO_x.

ABR250   CAS: 2517-98-8
7-ACETOXYMETHYL-12-METHYLBENZ(a)ANTHRACENE
mf: $C_{22}H_{18}O_2$ mw: 314.40

SYN: 12-METHYLBENZ(a)ANTHRACENE-7-METHANOL ACETATE (ESTER)

TOXICITY DATA with REFERENCE
NEO: scu-rat TDLo: 150 mg/kg/39D-I   CNREA8 31,1951,71
ETA: orl-rat TDLo: 100 mg/kg   JMCMAR 10,932,67
ETA: scu-mus TDLo: 120 mg/kg/6W-I   IJCNAW 2,500,67

SAFETY PROFILE: Questionable carcinogen with experimental tumorigenic and neoplastigenic data. When heated to decomposition it emits acrid smoke and fumes.

ABR625
ACETOXYMETHYLPHENYL NITROSAMINE
mf: $C_9H_{11}N_2O_3$ mw: 195.22

TOXICITY DATA with REFERENCE
ETA: scu-ham TD:55 mg/kg/35W-I   CALEDQ
15,289,82
ETA: scu-ham TD:64 mg/kg/41W-I   CALEDQ
15,289,82
ETA: scu-ham TD:119 mg/kg/38W-I   CALEDQ
15,289,82
ETA: scu-ham TD:182 mg/kg/58W-I   CALEDQ
15,289,82
ETA: scu-ham TDLo:42 mg/kg/27W-I   CALEDQ
15,289,82
MUT: mmo-sat 64400 pmol/plate   CALEDQ
15,289,82

SAFETY PROFILE: Questionable carcinogen with experimental tumorigenic data. Poison by subcutaneous route. Mutation data reported. When heated to decomposition it emits toxic fumes of NO_x.

ABT750   CAS: 53198-41-7
1-ACETOXY-N-NITROSODIPROPYLAMINE
mf: $C_8H_{16}N_2O_3$ mw: 188.26

SYNS: ACETIC ACID-1-(PROPYLNITROSAMINO)PROPYL ESTER ◇ N-(α-ACETOXY)PROPYL-N-N-PROPYLNITROS-AMINE ◇ 1-(PROPYLNITROSAMINO)PROPYL ACETATE

TOXICITY DATA with REFERENCE
CAR: scu-ham TDLo:410 mg/kg/33W-I
ZKKOBW 90,127,77
MUT: mmo-sat 100 nmol/plate   MUREAV49,187,78

SAFETY PROFILE: Questionable carcinogen with experimental carcinogenic data. Mutation data reported. Moderately toxic by subcutaneous route. When heated to decomposition it emits toxic fumes of NO_x.

ABW500   CAS: 26594-44-5
N-ACETOXY-N-(4-STILBENYL) ACETAMIDE
mf: $C_{18}H_{17}NO_3$ mw: 295.36

SYNS: ACETIC ACID-(N-ACETYL-N-(p-STYRYLPHE-NYL)AMINO) ESTER ◇ ACETIC ACID-ESTER with N-(p-STY-RYLPHENYL)ACETOHYDROXAMIC ACID ◇ N-ACETOXY-4-ACETAMIDOSTILBENE ◇ N,O-DIACETYL-N-(p-STYRYL-PHENYL)HYDROXYLAMINE ◇ N-(p-STYRYLPHENYL)ACE-TOHYDROXAMIC ACETATE ◇ N-(p-STYRYLPHE-NYL)ACETOHYDROXAMIC ACID ACETATE

TOXICITY DATA with REFERENCE
NEO: skn-mus TDLo:2360 μg/kg   JNCIAM
54,491,75
MUT: dnd-mam:lym 1375 mg/L   CBINA8
26,47,79
MUT: dns-hmn:fbr 10 mmol/L/5H   IJCNAW
16,284,75
MUT: dns-hmn:hla 100 nmol/L   CNREA8
38,2621,78
MUT: mma-sat 5 μg/plate   CBINA8 26,11,79

CONSENSUS REPORTS: EPA Genetic Toxicology Program.

SAFETY PROFILE: Questionable carcinogen with experimental neoplastigenic data by skin contact. Human mutation data reported. When heated to decomposition it emits highly toxic fumes of NO_x.

ABX250   CAS: 900-95-8
ACETOXYTRIPHENYLSTANNANE
mf: $C_{20}H_{18}O_2Sn$ mw: 409.07

PROP: Practically insol, crystalline solid. Mp: 120°.

SYNS: ACETATE de TRIPHENYL-ETAIN (FRENCH) ◇ ACETATO di STAGNO TRIFENILE (ITALIAN) ◇ ACETATO-TRIPHENYLSTANNANE ◇ ACETOXY-TRIPHENYL-STAN-NAN (GERMAN) ◇ ACETOXY-TRIPHENYLSTANNANE ◇ ACETOXYTRIPHENYLTIN ◇ (ACETYLOXY)TRIPHENYL-STANNANE (9CI) ◇ BATASAN ◇ BRESTAN ◇ ENT 25,208 ◇ FENOLOVO ACETATE ◇ FENTIN ACETAAT (DUTCH) ◇ FENTIN ACETAT (GERMAN) ◇ FENTIN ACETATE ◇ FENTINE ACETATE (FRENCH) ◇ FINTIN ACETATO (ITAL-IAN) ◇ GC 6936 ◇ HOE-2824 ◇ LIROMATIN ◇ LIROSTANOL ◇ PHENTIN ACETATE ◇ PHENTINOACETATE ◇ SUZU ◇ TINESTAN ◇ TINESTAN 60 WP ◇ TIN TRIPHENYL ACE-TATE ◇ TPTA ◇ TPZA ◇ TRIFENYLTINACETAAT (DUTCH) ◇ TRIPHENYLACETO STANNANE ◇ TRIPHENYLTIN ACE-TATE ◇ TRIPHENYL-ZINNACETAT (GERMAN) ◇ TUBOTIN ◇ VP 1940

TOXICITY DATA with REFERENCE
NEO: orl-mus TDLo:132 g/kg/78W-I   NTIS**
PB223-159

CONSENSUS REPORTS: EPA Extremely Hazardous Substances List. Reported in EPA TSCA Inventory.

OSHA PEL: TWA 0.1 mg(Sn)/m³ (skin) ACGIH TLV: TWA 0.1 mg(Sn)/m³ (skin) (Proposed: TWA 0.1 mg(Sn)/m³; STEL 0.2

mg(Sn)/m^3 (skin))   NIOSH REL: (Organotin Compounds) TWA 0.1 mg(Sn)/m^3

SAFETY PROFILE: Questionable carcinogen with experimental neoplastigenic and teratogenic data. Poison by ingestion, skin contact, intraperitoneal, intravenous, and subcutaneous routes. A fungicide and algicide used as a wood preservative. When heated to decomposition it emits acrid smoke and fumes.

ABY000   CAS: 28322-02-3
4-ACETYLAMINOFLUORENE
mf: $C_{15}H_{13}NO$ mw: 223.29

SYNS: 4-ACETYLAMINOFLUOREN (GERMAN) ◇ N-FLUOREN-4-YLACETAMIDE ◇ N-4-FLUORENYLACETAMIDE

TOXICITY DATA with REFERENCE
ETA: orl-rat TD:6300 mg/kg/30W-C   CRNGDP 3,103,82
ETA: orl-rat TD:5240 mg/kg/57W-C   JNCIAM 24,149,60
ETA: orl-rat TDLo:4175 mg/kg/17W-C   ONCOAR 8,233,55
MUT: dns-rat:lvr 100 μmol/L/2H   CNREA8 37,1845,77
MUT: mma-mus:lym 94 mg/L/4H   MUREAV 59,61,79
MUT: mma-sat 50 μg/plate   PMRSDJ 1,285,81
MUT: msc-mus:lym 375 mg/L/4H   MUREAV 59,61,79
MUT: otr-ham:kdy 25 mg/L   PMRSDJ 1,638,81
MUT: otr-mus:fbr 400 μg/L   JJIND8 67,1303,81

CONSENSUS REPORTS: EPA Genetic Toxicology Program.

SAFETY PROFILE: Questionable carcinogen with experimental tumorigenic data. Poison by intraperitoneal route. Mutation data reported. When heated to decomposition it emits toxic fumes of NO$_x$.

ABY150   CAS: 57229-41-1
2-ACETYLAMINO-9-FLUORENOL
mf: $C_{15}H_{13}NO_2$ mw: 239.29

SYNS: N-(9-HYDROXYFLUOREN-2-YL)ACETAMIDE ◇ 9-HYDROXY-2-FLUORENYLACETAMIDE

TOXICITY DATA with REFERENCE
ETA: orl-rat TDLo:4644 mg/kg/32W-C   CNREA8 15,188,55

SAFETY PROFILE: Questionable carcinogen with experimental tumorigenic data. When

heated to decomposition it emits toxic fumes of NO$_x$.

ABY250   CAS: 3096-50-2
2-ACETYLAMINOFLUORENONE
mf: $C_{15}H_{11}NO_2$ mw: 237.27

SYNS: 2-ACETYLAMINO-9-FLUORENONE ◇ 9-OXO-2-FLUORENYLACETAMIDE ◇ N-(9-OXO-2-FLUORENYL)ACETAMIDE

TOXICITY DATA with REFFERENCE
CAR: orl-rat TD:6075 mg/kg/65W-C   JNCIAM 24,149,60
CAR: orl-rat TDLo:4740 mg/kg/32W-C   CNREA8 15,188,55

SAFETY PROFILE: Questionable carcinogen with experimental carcinogenic data. When heated to decomposition it emits toxic fumes of NO$_x$.

ACA750   CAS: 73637-16-8
9-ACETYL-1,7,8-ANTHRACENETRIOL
mf: $C_{16}H_{11}O_4$ mw: 267.27

SYNS: 9-ACETYL-1,7,8-ANTHRACENETRIOL ◇ 10-ACETYL-1,8,9-ANTHRACENETRIOL ◇ 10-ACETYLANTHRALIN ◇ 1,8-DIHYDROXY-10-ACETYL-9-ANTHRONE

TOXICITY DATA with REFERENCE
NEO: skn-mus TDLo:32 mg/kg/53W-I   JMCMAR 21,26,78

SAFETY PROFILE: Questionable carcinogen with experimental neoplastigenic data. When heated to decomposition it emits acrid smoke and fumes.

ACB250   CAS: 460-07-1
1-ACETYLAZIRIDINE
mf: C_4H_7NO mw: 85.12

SYN: ACETYLETHYLENEIMINE

TOXICITY DATA with REFERENCE
NEO: scu-mus TDLo:180 mg/kg/33W-I   BJPCAL 9,306,54
NEO: scu-rat TDLo:78 mg/kg/26W-I   BJPCAL 9,306,54
ETA: scu-rat TD:80 mg/kg/16W-I   BJPCAL 9,306,54

CONSENSUS REPORTS: Reported in EPA TSCA Inventory. EPA Genetic Toxicology Program.

SAFETY PROFILE: Questionable carcinogen with experimental tumorigenic and neoplastigenic data. Poison by intraperitoneal route. When heated to decomposition it emits toxic fumes of NO_x.

ACC750   CAS: 63018-98-4
2-ACETYL-3:4-BENZPHENANTHRENE
mf: $C_{20}H_{14}O$ mw: 270.34

SYN: 5-ACETYL BENZO(C)PHENANTHRENE

TOXICITY DATA with REFERENCE
ETA: skn-mus TDLo:720 mg/kg/30W-I
  PRLBA4 131,170,42

SAFETY PROFILE: Questionable carcinogen with experimental tumorigenic data. When heated to decomposition it emits acrid smoke and irritating fumes.

ACD000   CAS: 4463-22-3
N-ACETYL-4-BIPHENYLHYDROXYLAMINE
mf: $C_{14}H_{13}NO_2$ mw: 227.28

SYNS: 4-BIPHENYLACETHYDROXAMIC ACID ◇ N-HYDROXY-AABP ◇ N-HYDROXY-4-ACETAMIDOBI-PHENYL ◇ N-4-(N-HYDROXYACETAMIDO)BIPHENYL ◇ N-HYDROXY-4-ACETAMIDODIPHENYL ◇ N-HYDROXY-4-ACETYLAMINOBIPHENYL ◇ N-HYDROXY-N-4-BIPHE-NYLACETAMIDE

TOXICITY DATA with REFERENCE
CAR: ipr-rat TDLo:91 mg/kg   CNREA8
  41,2450,81
ETA: imp-mus TDLo:80 mg/kg   BJCAAI
  22,825,68
ETA: ipr-rat TDLo:1430 mg/kg/21W-I   CNREA8
  21,1465,61
ETA: orl-rat TDLo:2400 mg/kg/16W-C
  CNREA8 21,1465,61
MUT: dnd-rat-ipr 25 mg/kg   COINAV 256,115,77
MUT: dns-dog:oth 1 µmol/L   CNREA8 42,3974,82
MUT: dns-hmn:oth 1 µmol/L   JJIND8 72,847,84
MUT: mnt-ham:ovr 290 µmol/L   MUREAV
  88,397,81

SAFETY PROFILE: Questionable carcinogen with experimental carcinogenic and tumorigenic data. Human mutation data reported. When heated to decomposition it emits toxic fumes of NO_x.

ACK250   CAS: 79-27-6
ACETYLENE TETRABROMIDE
DOT: 2504
mf: $C_2H_2Br_4$ mw: 345.68

PROP: Colorless to yellow liquid. Bp: 151° @ 54 mm, fp: −1°, d: 2.9638 @ 20°/4°, autoign temp: 635°F.

SYNS: MUTHMANN'S LIQUID ◇ TBE ◇ 1,1,2,2-TETRA-BROMAETHAN (GERMAN) ◇ TETRABROMOACETYLENE ◇ 1,1,2,2-TETRABROMOETANO (ITALIAN) ◇ S-TETRABRO-MOETHANE ◇ 1,1,2,2-TETRABROMOETHANE ◇ 1,1,2,2-TETRABROOMETHAAN (DUTCH)

TOXICITY DATA with REFERENCE
NEO: skn-mus TDLo:130 g/kg/74W-I   JJIND8
  63,1433,79
MUT: dnr-esc 10 µL/disc   MUREAV 41,61,76

CONSENSUS REPORTS: Reported in EPA TSCA Inventory. EPA Genetic Toxicology Program.

OSHA PEL: TWA 1 ppm   ACGIH TLV: TWA 1 ppm   DFG MAK: 1 ppm (14 mg/m^3)   DOT Classification: ORM-A; Label: None.

SAFETY PROFILE: Questionable carcinogen with experimental neoplastigenic data. Poison by inhalation and ingestion. Mutation data reported. An eye and skin irritant and a narcotic. When heated it emits highly toxic fumes of carbonyl bromide and Br⁻.

ACL000   CAS: 2597-54-8
N-ACETYL ETHYL CARBAMATE
mf: $C_6H_9NO_3$ mw: 131.15

SYN: ACETYLURETHANE

TOXICITY DATA with REFERENCE
NEO: ipr-mus TD:7300 mg/kg/10W-I   IJCNAW
  4,318,69
NEO: ipr-mus TDLo:2400 mg/kg/4W-I
  CNREA8 29,2184,69
ETA: ipr-mus TD:3650 mg/kg/5W-I   IJCNAW
  4,318,69

SAFETY PROFILE: Questionable carcinogen with experimental neoplastigenic and tumorigenic data. When heated to decomposition it emits toxic fumes of NO_x.

ACL500   CAS: 52217-47-7
N'-ACETYL ETHYLNITROSOUREA
mf: $C_5H_9N_3O_3$ mw: 159.17

TOXICITY DATA with REFERENCE
ETA: orl-rat TDLo:520 mg/kg/52W-I   PPTCBY
  2,73,72

SAFETY PROFILE: Questionable carcinogen with experimental tumorigenic data. Moderately toxic by ingestion. When heated to decomposition it emits toxic fumes of NO_x.

ACN500   CAS: 65734-38-5
N-ACETYL-N'-(p-HYDROXYMETHYL) PHENYLHYDRAZINE
mf: $C_9H_{12}N_2O_2$ mw: 180.23

TOXICITY DATA with REFERENCE
NEO: orl-mus TDLo: 74 g/kg/85W-C   CNREA8 38,177,78
ETA: scu-mus TDLo: 13 g/kg/26W-I   JTEHD6 8,1,81

SAFETY PROFILE: Questionable carcinogen with experimental neoplastigenic and tumorigenic data. When heated to decomposition it emits toxic fumes such as NO_x.

ACO250   CAS: 2466-76-4
N-ACETYLIMIDAZOLE
mf: $C_5H_6N_2O$ mw: 110.13

SYN: 1-ACETYLIMIDAZOLE

TOXICITY DATA with REFERENCE
NEO: ipr-mus TDLo: 50 mg/kg/I   JNCIAM 54,495,75

CONSENSUS REPORTS: Reported in EPA TSCA Inventory.

SAFETY PROFILE: Questionable carcinogen with experimental neoplastigenic data. Poison by intraperitoneal route. When heated to decomposition it emits toxic fumes of NO_x.

ACO750   CAS: 1078-38-2
1-ACETYL-2-ISONICOTINOYLHYDRAZINE
mf: $C_8H_9N_3O_2$ mw: 179.20

SYNS: ACETYL ISONIAZID ◇ N-ACETYLISONIAZID ◇ N-ACETYLISONICOTINYLHYDRAZIDE ◇ 4-PYRIDINE-CARBOXYLIC ACID-2-ACETYLHYDRAZIDE

TOXICITY DATA with REFERENCE
NEO: orl-mus TDLo: 380 g/kg/68W-C   EJCAAH 9,285,73
MUT: dni-mus-ipr 1 g/kg   IJEBA6 19,939,81

CONSENSUS REPORTS: EPA Genetic Toxicology Program.

SAFETY PROFILE: Questionable carcinogen with experimental neoplastigenic data. Mutation

data reported. When heated to decomposition it emits toxic fumes of NO_x.

ACR250   CAS: 28895-91-2
ACETYLMETHYLNITROSOUREA
mf: $C_4H_7N_3O_3$ mw: 145.14

SYNS: ACETYL-METHYL-NITROSO-HARNSTOFF (GERMAN) ◇ N'-ACETYL-METHYLNITROSOUREA ◇ N-METHYL-N-NITROSO-N'-ACETYLUREA ◇ 1-METHYL-1-NITROSOACETYLUREA

TOXICITY DATA with REFERENCE
ETA: orl-rat TD: 540 mg/kg/54W-I   PPTCBY 2,73,72
ETA: orl-rat TD: 740 mg/kg/74W-I   XENOBH 3,271,73
ETA: orl-rat TDLo: 468 mg/kg/47W-I   ZEKBAI 74,23,70
MUT: cyt-ham: fbr 500 mg/L/20H   MUREAV 48,337,77

SAFETY PROFILE: Questionable carcinogen with experimental tumorigenic data. Poison by ingestion. Mutation data reported. When heated to decomposition it emits toxic fumes of NO_x.

ACS000   CAS: 63224-44-2
N-ACETYL-N-MYRISTOYLOXY-2-AMINOFLUORENE
mf: $C_{29}H_{39}NO_3$ mw: 449.69

SYNS: N-ACETYL-N-TETRADECANOYLOXY-2-AMINO-FLUORENE ◇ N-(FLUOREN-2-YL)-o-TETRADECANOYL-ACETOHYDROXAMIC ACID ◇ N-MYRISTOYLOXY-AAF ◇ N-MYRISTOYLOXY-N-ACETYL-2-AMINOFLUORENE

TOXICITY DATA with REFERENCE
CAR: scu-rat TD: 115 mg/kg/6W-I   CRNGDP 2,655,81
NEO: scu-rat TDLo: 114 mg/kg/5W-I   CNREA8 37,1461,77
MUT: dns-hmn: fbr 10 μmol/L/5H   IJCNAW 16,284,75
MUT: msc-ham: lng 50 μmol/L/3H   CALEDQ 6,67,79

SAFETY PROFILE: Questionable carcinogen with experimental carcinogenic and neoplastigenic data. Human mutation data reported. When heated to decomposition it emits toxic fumes of NO_x.

ACU500   CAS: 42978-43-8
6-ACETYLOXYMETHYLBENZO(a) PYRENE
mf: $C_{23}H_{16}O_2$ mw: 324.39

SYN: 6-ACETOXY METHYL BENZO(a)PYRENE

TOXICITY DATA with REFERENCE
NEO: scu-rat TDLo: 584 µg/kg/60D-I CBINA8 29,159,80
ETA: scu-rat TD: 100 mg/kg/40D-I JMCMAR 16,714,73
MUT: dnd-mam: lym 500 mg/L CBINA8 25,35,79
MUT: dnd-rat: lym 500 mg/L CBINA8 25,35,79
MUT: mmo-sat 1 nmol/plate PAACA3 24,93,83

SAFETY PROFILE: Questionable carcinogen with experimental neoplastigenic and tumorigenic data. Mutation data reported. When heated to decomposition it emits acrid smoke and fumes.

ACV000   CAS: 34627-78-6
5-(1-ACETYLOXY-2-PROPENYL)-1,3-BENZODIOXOLE
mf: $C_{12}H_{12}O_4$ mw: 220.24
SYN: 1'-ACETOXYSAFROLE

TOXICITY DATA with REFERENCE
CAR: ipr-mus TDLo: 22 mg/kg CNREA8 47,2275,87
CAR: scu-rat TDLo: 529 mg/kg/10W-I CNREA8 43,1124,83
NEO: orl-rat TDLo: 62 g/kg/36W-C CNREA8 33,590,73
NEO: scu-rat TD: 328 mg/kg/10W-I CNREA8 33,590,73
NEO: scu-rat TD: 393 mg/kg/12W-I CNREA8 37,1883,77
MUT: dnd-hmn: fbr 500 µmol/L CRNGDP 3,935,82
MUT: dni-hmn: oth 300 µmol/L CRNGDP 3,929,82
MUT: dns-hmn: oth 500 µmol/L CRNGDP 3,929,82
MUT: mma-sat 50 µg/plate PNASA6 72,5135,75

CONSENSUS REPORTS: EPA Genetic Toxicology Program.

SAFETY PROFILE: Questionable carcinogen with experimental carcinogenic and neoplastigenic data. Human mutation data reported. When heated to decomposition it emits acrid smoke and fumes.

ACV500   CAS: 110-22-5
ACETYL PEROXIDE
mf: $C_4H_6O_4$ mw: 118.04
PROP: Solid or colorless crystals or liquid. Sltly sol in cold water, decomp. D: 1.18, mp: 30°, bp: 63° @ 21 mm.

SYN: DIACETYL PEROXIDE (MAK)

TOXICITY DATA with REFERENCE
ETA: unk-mus TDLo: 283 mg/kg RARSAM 3,193,63

CONSENSUS REPORTS: Reported in EPA TSCA Inventory.

DFG MAK: Strong Skin Effects. DOT Classification: Forbidden.

SAFETY PROFILE: Questionable carcinogen with experimental tumorigenic data. Severe skin and eye irritant. Dangerous fire hazard by spontaneous chemical reaction. A powerful oxidizing agent; can cause ignition of organic materials on contact. Severe explosion hazard when shocked or exposed to heat. It may explode spontaneously in storage and should be used as soon as prepared. To fight fire use CO_2, dry chemical.

ACX750   CAS: 114-83-0
ACETYLPHENYLHYDRAZINE
mf: $C_8H_{10}N_2O$ mw: 150.20

PROP: Mp: 130-132°. Sol in hot water and alc; sltly sol in ether.

SYNS: ACETIC ACID PHENYLHYDRAZONE ◇ β-ACETYLPHENYLHYDRAZINE ◇ 1-ACETYL-2-PHENYLHYDRAZINE ◇ APH ◇ HYDRACETIN ◇ N'-PHENYLACETHYDRAZIDE ◇ PYRODINE

TOXICITY DATA with REFERENCE
NEO: orl-mus TDLo: 31 g/kg/79W-I BJCAAI 39,584,79

CONSENSUS REPORTS: Reported in EPA TSCA Inventory.

SAFETY PROFILE: Questionable carcinogen with experimental neoplastigenic data. Poison by ingestion and intraperitoneal routes. When heated to decomposition it emits toxic fumes of NO_x.

ACY750
12-O-ACETYL-PHORBOL-13-DECA-(Δ-2)-ENOATE
mf: $C_{32}H_{45}O_8$ mw: 557.77

TOXICITY DATA with REFERENCE
NEO: skn-mus TDLo: 107 g/kg/12W-I PLMEAA 22,241,72

SAFETY PROFILE: Questionable carcinogen with experimental neoplastigenic data. A skin irritant. When heated to decomposition it emits acrid smoke and fumes.

ACZ000   CAS: 20839-15-0
12-O-ACETYL-PHORBOL-13-DECANOATE
mf: $C_{32}H_{48}O_8$ mw: 560.80

SYN: PHORBOL ACETATE, CAPRATE

TOXICITY DATA with REFERENCE
NEO: skn-mus TDLo: 26 mg/kg/32W-I
   NATWAY 54,282,67

SAFETY PROFILE: Questionable carcinogen with experimental neoplastigenic data. A skin irritant. When heated to decomposition it emits acrid smoke and irritating fumes.

ADA000   CAS: 17433-31-7
1-ACETYL-2-PICOLINOLHYDRAZINE
mf: $C_8H_{11}N_3O_2$ mw: 179.20

SYNS: N-ACETYL-N'-ISONICOTINYL HYDRAZIDE ◇ 1-ACETYL-2-PICOLINOYLHYDRAZINE ◇ AZAPICYL ◇ P-2292 ◇ NCI-C04739 ◇ NSC-68626 ◇ 2-PYRIDINECAR-BOXYLIC ACID-2-ACETYLHYDRAZIDE (9CI)

TOXICITY DATA with REFERENCE
NEO: ipr-mus TDLo: 9750 mg/kg/26W-I
   RRCRBU 52,1,75
NEO: ipr-rat TDLo: 9750 mg/kg/26W-I
   RRCRBU 52,1,75

CONSENSUS REPORTS: NCI Carcinogenesis Studies (ipr): Clear Evidence: mouse, rat RRCRBU 52,1,75

SAFETY PROFILE: Questionable carcinogen with experimental neoplastigenic data. Poison by ingestion and intravenous routes. When heated to decomposition it emits toxic fumes such as NO_x.

ADB250   CAS: 58086-32-1
o-ACETYLSTERIGMATOCYSTIN
mf: $C_{20}H_{14}O_7$ mw: 366.34

TOXICITY DATA with REFERENCE
CAR: ipr-rat TDLo: 245 mg/kg/23W-I   GANNA2
   69,237,78
MUT: dns-rat: lvr 1 μmol/L   MUREAV 173,217,86
MUT: mma-sat 1 μg/plate   CNREA8 38,536,78
MUT: mmo-sat 100 μg/plate   CNREA8 38,536,78
MUT: mrc-bcs 1 μg/disc   CNREA8 36,445,76

SAFETY PROFILE: Questionable carcinogen with experimental carcinogenic data. Poison by

intraperitoneal route. Mutation data reported. When heated to decomposition it emits acrid smoke and fumes.

ADE500   CAS: 129-17-9
ACID BLUE 1
mf: $C_{27}H_{31}N_2O_6S_2 \cdot Na$ mw: 566.71

SYNS: ANHYDRO-4,4'-BIS(DIETHYLAMINO)TRIPHE-NYLMETHANOL-2',4''-DISULPHONIC ACID, MONOSO-DIUM SALT ◇ BLUE 1084 ◇ C.I. ACID BLUE 1, SODIUM SALT ◇ COSMETIC GREEN BLUE R25396 ◇ 4,4'-DI(DI-ETHYLAMINO)-4',6'-DISULPHOTRIPHENYLMETHANOL ANHYDRIDE, SODIUM SALT ◇ FOOD BLUE 3 ◇ LEATHER BLUE G ◇ PATENTBLAU V (GERMAN) ◇ SCHULTZ Nr. 826 (GERMAN) ◇ SODIUM PATENT BLUE V ◇ XYLENE BLUE VS

TOXICITY DATA with REFERENCE
CAR: ims-rat TDLo: 2070 mg/kg/50W-I
   JNCIAM 37,845,66
NEO: scu-rat TDLo: 3000 mg/kg/33W-I   BJCAAI
   27,230,73
ETA: scu-rat TD: 4050 mg/kg/45W-I   FCTXAV
   9,463,71
MUT: mma-sat 1 mg/plate   ENMUDM 8(Suppl 7),1,86

CONSENSUS REPORTS: IARC Cancer Review: GROUP 3 IMEMDT 7,56,87; Animal Sufficient Evidence IMEMDT 16,163,78. Reported in EPA TSCA Inventory.

SAFETY PROFILE: Questionable carcinogen with experimental carcinogenic, tumorigenic, and neoplastigenic data. Deadly human poison by intravenous route: anaphylaxis. Moderately toxic by several routes. Mutation data reported. When heated to decomposition it emits very toxic fumes of NO_x, NH_3, Na_2O and SO_x.

ADF000   CAS: 3087-16-9
ACID BRILLIANT GREEN BS
mf: $C_{27}H_{26}N_2O_7S_2 \cdot Na$ mw: 577.66

SYNS: ACIDAL WOOL GREEN BS ◇ ACID LEATHER GREEN S ◇ BRILLIANTSAEURE GRUEN BS (GERMAN) ◇ C.I. 44090 ◇ C.I. ACID GREEN 50, MONOSODIUM SALT ◇ C.I. FOOD GREEN 4 ◇ GREEN 5 ◇ SCHULTZ Nr. 836 (GERMAN) ◇ WOOL GREEN S (BIOLOGICAL STAIN)

TOXICITY DATA with REFERENCE
ETA: par-rat TDLo: 470 mg/kg/2Y-I   FAONAU
   46A,57,69
MUT: mma-sat 1 mg/plate   MUREAV 89,21,81
MUT: mrc-smc 2840 μmol/L   FCTXAV 19,419,81

CONSENSUS REPORTS: Reported in EPA TSCA Inventory. EPA Genetic Toxicology Program.

SAFETY PROFILE: Questionable carcinogen with experimental tumorigenic data. Moderately toxic by ingestion. Mutation data reported. When heated to decomposition it emits very toxic fumes of SO_x and NO_x.

ADJ875   CAS: 146-59-8
ACRIDINE MUSTARD
mf: $C_{21}H_{25}Cl_2N_3O \cdot 2ClH$ mw: 479.31

SYNS: 6-CHLORO-9-(3-(ETHYL-2-CHLOROETHYL)AMI-NOPROPYLAMINO)-2-METHOXYACRIDINE DIHYDRO-CHLORIDE ◊ 9-(3-(ETHYL(2-CHLOROETHYL)AMINO)PRO-PYLAMINO)-6-CHLORO-2-METHOXYACRIDINE DIHYDROCHLORIDE ◊ ICR 170 ◊ 2-METHOXY-6-CHLORO-9-(3-(ETHYL-2-CHLOROETHYL)AMINOPROPYLAMINO)AC-RIDINE DIHYDROCHLORIDE

TOXICITY DATA with REFERENCE
NEO: ivn-mus TDLo:4800 μg/kg/28D-I
　CNREA8 36,2423,76
MUT: dnd-dmg-par 2100 μmol/L　CNREA8
　30,195,70
MUT: dni-hmn:hla 50 nmol/L/30M-C　JEPTDQ
　2(1),65,78
MUT: dnr-hmn:fbr 1 μmol/L/1H-C　36YFAG
　-,483,77
MUT: dns-hmn:fbr 1 μmol/L/1H　33AQAA
　-,103,76
MUT: mma-sat 10 μg/plate　PNASA6 72,5135,75
MUT: msc-ham:lng 1 mg/L　CNREA8 44,3270,84

CONSENSUS REPORTS: EPA Genetic Toxicology Program.

SAFETY PROFILE: Questionable carcinogen with experimental neoplastigenic data. Poison by intravenous and intraperitoneal routes. Experimental reproductive effects. Human mutation data reported. When heated to decomposition it emits toxic fumes of NO_x and HCl.

ADK000   CAS: 2465-29-4
ACRIDINE RED
mf: $C_{15}H_{14}N_2O \cdot ClH$ mw: 274.77
PROP: Sltly sol in water; sol in alc; insol in ether.

SYNS: ACRIDINE RED 3B ◊ ACRIDINE RED, HYDRO-CHLORIDE ◊ DIMETHYLDIAMINOXANTHENYL CHLORIDE

TOXICITY DATA with REFERENCE
ETA: scu-rat TDLo:1215 mg/kg/59W-I
　GANNA2 47,153,56

MUT: sln-dmg-orl 1000 ppm　AMNTA4 87,295,53

CONSENSUS REPORTS: Reported in EPA TSCA Inventory.

SAFETY PROFILE: Questionable carcinogen with experimental tumorigenic data. Mutation data reported. When heated to decomposition it emits very toxic fumes of HCl and NO_x.

ADK250   CAS: 191-27-5
ACRIDINO(2,1,9,8-klmna)ACRIDINE
mf: $C_{20}H_{10}N_2$ mw: 278.32

SYN: 6,12-DIAZAANTHANTHRENE

TOXICITY DATA with REFERENCE
ETA: imp-rat TDLo:600 mg/kg　NEOLA4
　18,591,71

SAFETY PROFILE: Questionable carcinogen with experimental tumorigenic data. When heated to decomposition it emits toxic fumes of NO_x.

ADR000   CAS: 107-02-8
ACROLEIN
DOT: 1092
mf: C_3H_4O mw: 56.07

PROP: Colorless or yellowish liquid; disagreeable, choking odor. Sol in water, alc, and ether. Mp: −87.7°, bp: 52.5°, flash p: <0°F, d: 0.841 @ 20°/4°, autoign temp: unstable (455°F), lel: 2.8%, uel: 31%, vap d: 1.94.

SYNS: ACQUINITE ◊ ACRALDEHYDE ◊ ACROLEINA (ITALIAN) ◊ ACROLEINE (DUTCH, FRENCH) ◊ ACRYLAL-DEHYD (GERMAN) ◊ ACRYLALDEHYDE ◊ ACRYLIC AL-DEHYDE ◊ ALDEIDE ACRILICA (ITALIAN) ◊ ALDEHYDE ACRYLIQUE (FRENCH) ◊ ALLYL ALDEHYDE ◊ AKROLEIN (CZECH) ◊ AKROLEINA (POLISH) ◊ AQUALINE ◊ BIOCIDE ◊ CROLEAN ◊ ETHYLENE ALDEHYDE ◊ MAGNACIDE H ◊ NSC 8819 ◊ PROPENAL (CZECH) ◊ 2-PROPENAL ◊ PROP-2-EN-1-AL ◊ 2-PROPEN-1-ONE ◊ PROPYLENE AL-DEHYDE ◊ RCRA WASTE NUMBER P003 ◊ SLIMICIDE

TOXICITY DATA with REFERENCE
MUT: dnd-esc 9 μmol/L　MUREAV 39,317,77
MUT: dni-mam:lym 80 μmol/L　FEBLAL 30,286,73
MUT: mma-sat 50 μg/plate　NTPTB* JAN 82
MUT: sce-ham:ovr 10 μmol/L　CGCGBR 26,108,80
MUT: sce-ham:ovr 10 μmol/L　CGCGBR 26,108,80
MUT: sce-hmn:lym 5 μmol/L　CNREA8 46,203,86

CONSENSUS REPORTS: IARC Cancer Review: GROUP 3 IMEMDT 7,78,87; Animal Inadequate Evidence IMEMDT 36,133,85;

IMEMDT 19,479,79; Human Inadequate Evidence IMEMDT 36,133,85. Community Right-To-Know List. EPA Extremely Hazardous Substances List. Reported in EPA TSCA Inventory.

OSHA PEL: (Transitional: TWA 0.1 ppm) TWA 0.1 ppm; STEL 0.3 ppm   ACGIH TLV: TWA 0.1 ppm; STEL 0.3 ppm   DFG MAK: 0.1 ppm (0.25 mg/m^3)   DOT Classification: Flammable Liquid; Label: Flammable Liquid and Poison.

SAFETY PROFILE: Questionable carcinogen. Human poison by inhalation and intradermal route. Poison experimentally by most routes. Severe eye and skin irritant. Human systemic irritant and pulmonary system effects by inhalation include: lacrimation, delayed hypersensitivity with multiple organ involvement, and respiratory system damage. Human mutation data reported. Experimental reproductive effects. Dangerous fire hazard when exposed to heat, flame, or oxidizers. An explosion hazard. To fight fire use CO_2, dry chemical or alcohol foam.

ADR750   CAS: 7008-42-6
ACRONYCINE
mf: $C_{20}H_{19}NO_3$ mw: 321.40

SYNS: ACROMYCINE ◇ ACRONINE ◇ COMPOUND 42339 ◇ 3,12-DIHYDRO-6-METHOXY-3,3,12-TRIMETHYL-7H-PYRANO(2,3-C)ACRIDIN-7-ONE ◇ NCI-C01536 ◇ NSC 403169

TOXICITY DATA with REFERENCE
CAR: ipr-rat TD: 1800 mg/kg/1Y-I   NCITR* NCI-CG-TR-49,78
CAR: ipr-rat TDLo: 1170 mg/kg/1Y-I   NCITR* NCI-CG-TR-49,78
NEO: ipr-rat TD: 585 mg/kg/1Y-I   NCITR* NCI-CG-TR-49,78
ETA: ipr-mus TD: 530 mg/kg/8W-I   CNREA8 33,3069,73
MUT: cyt-mus: fbr 10 mg/L/24H   ARZNAD 27,1549,77
MUT: dni-mus: leu 1 μmol/L   CNREA8 33,2310,73

CONSENSUS REPORTS: NCI Carcinogenesis Bioassay (ipr); Inadequate Studies: mouse NCITR* NCI-CG-TR-49,78; Clear Evidence: rat NCITR* NCI-CG-TR-49,78

SAFETY PROFILE: Questionable carcinogen with experimental carcinogenic, neoplastigenic, and tumorigenic data. Moderately toxic by ingestion and intraperitoneal routes. Mutation data reported. When heated to decomposition it emits toxic fumes of NO$_x$.

ADS750   CAS: 79-10-7
ACRYLIC ACID
DOT: 2218
mf: $C_3H_4O_2$ mw: 72.07

PROP: Liquid, acrid odor. Misc in water, benzene, alc, chloroform, ether, and acetone. Mp: 13°, bp: 141°, d: 1.062, vap press: 10 mm @ 39.9°, flash p: 130°F (OC), vap d: 2.45.

SYNS: ACROLEIC ACID ◇ ACRYLIC ACID, GLACIAL ◇ ACRYLIC ACID, inhibited (DOT) ◇ ETHYLENECARBOXYLIC ACID ◇ PROPENE ACID ◇ 2-PROPENOIC ACID ◇ RCRA WASTE NUMBER U008 ◇ VINYLFORMIC ACID

TOXICITY DATA with REFERENCE
CAR: skn-mus TDLo: 37440 mg/kg/78W-I
EPASR* 8EHQ-0386-0592
ETA: scu-mus TDLo: 2912 mg/kg/52W-I
CBINA8 61,189,87
ETA: skn-mus TD: 37440 mg/kg/78W-I   EPASR* 8EHQ-0386-0592

CONSENSUS REPORTS: IARC Cancer Review: Human Inadequate Evidence IMEMDT 19,47,79. Community Right-To-Know List. Reported in EPA TSCA Inventory.

OSHA PEL: TWA 10 ppm (skin)   ACGIH TLV: TWA 10 ppm (Proposed: 2 ppm (skin))   DFG MAK: 200 ppm (950 mg/m^3)   DOT Classification: IMO: Corrosive Material; Label: Corrosive, Flammable Liquid.

SAFETY PROFILE: Questionable carcinogen with experimental carcinogenic and tumorigenic data. Poison by ingestion, skin contact, intraperitoneal and possibly other routes. An experimental teratogen. Other experimental reproductive effects. A severe skin and eye irritant. Corrosive. Exothermic polymerization at room temperature may become explosive if confined. A fire hazard when exposed to heat or flame.

ADT050   CAS: 17831-71-9
ACRYLIC ACID, DIESTER with
TETRAETHYLENE GLYCOL
mf: $C_{14}H_{22}O_7$ mw: 302.36

SYNS: ACRYLIC ACID, OXYBIS(ETHYLENEOXYETHYLENE) ESTER ◇ 2-PROPENOIC ACID, OXYBIS(2,1-ETHANEDIYLOXY-2,1-ETHANEDIYL)ESTER ◇ TETRAETHYLENE GLYCOL DIACRYLATE

TOXICITY DATA with REFERENCE
ETA: skn-mus TDLo: 16 g/kg/80W-I   JTEHD6 19,149,86

CONSENSUS REPORTS: Reported in EPA TSCA Inventory.

SAFETY PROFILE: Questionable carcinogen with experimental tumorigenic data. Moderate skin and severe eye irritant. When heated to decomposition it emits acrid smoke and irritating fumes.

ADU250 CAS: 103-11-7
ACRYLIC ACID-2-ETHYLHEXYL ESTER
mf: $C_{11}H_{20}O_2$ mw: 184.31

PROP: Bp: 130° @ 50 mm, fp: −90°, flash p: 180°F (OC), d: 0.8869 @ 20°/20°, vap press: 1 mm @ 50°, vap d: 6.35.

SYNS: 2-ETHYLHEXYL ACRYLATE ◊ 2-ETHYLHEXYL-2-PROPENOATE ◊ OCTYL ACRYLATE ◊ 2-PROPENOIC ACID-2-ETHYLHEXYL ESTER

TOXICITY DATA with REFERENCE
CAR: skn-mus TDLo: 187 g/kg/78W-I JTEHD6 16,55,85
NEO: skn-mus TD: 240 g/kg/2Y-C EPASR* 8EHQ-1079-0262

CONSENSUS REPORTS: Reported in EPA TSCA Inventory.

SAFETY PROFILE: Questionable carcinogen with experimental carcinogenic and neoplastigenic data. Moderately toxic by inhalation and various other routes. A severe skin and eye irritant. Flammable. A fire hazard when exposed to heat or flame. To fight fire use alcohol foam, CO_2, dry chemical. When heated to decomposition it emits acrid smoke and irritating fumes.

ADW250 CAS: 25916-47-6
ACRYLIC ACID POLYMER, ZINC SALT
mf: $(C_3H_4O_2)_x \cdot xZn$

SYNS: 2-PROPENOIC ACID, HOMOPOLYMER, ZINC SALT ◊ ZINC POLYACRYLATE ◊ ZINC POLYCARBOXYLATE

TOXICITY DATA with REFERENCE
ETA: imp-ham TDLo: 320 mg/kg/64W-C JBMRBG 9,69,75
ETA: imp-mus TDLo: 1600 mg/kg/1Y-C JBMRBG 9,69,75

CONSENSUS REPORTS: Reported in EPA TSCA Inventory. Zinc and its compounds are on the Community Right-To-Know List.

SAFETY PROFILE: Questionable carcinogen with experimental tumorigenic data. When heated to decomposition it emits toxic fumes of ZnO, acrid fumes and CO.

ADY250 CAS: 9003-00-3
ACRYLONITRILE POLYMER with CHLOROETHYLENE
mf: $(C_3H_3N \cdot C_2H_3Cl)_n$

SYNS: ACROPOR ◊ DYNEL ◊ KANEKALON ◊ 2-PROPENENITRILE, POLYMER with CHLOROETHENE ◊ VINYON N

TOXICITY DATA with REFERENCE
ETA: imp-mus TDLo: 18 mg/kg CNREA8 15,333,55

CONSENSUS REPORTS: Reported in EPA TSCA Inventory. Cyanide and its compounds are on the Community Right-To-Know List.

SAFETY PROFILE: Questionable carcinogen with experimental tumorigenic data. When heated to decomposition it emits very toxic fumes of Cl^-, CN^- and NO_x.

AEB000 CAS: 50-76-0
ACTINOMYCIN D
mf: $C_{62}H_{86}N_{12}O_{16}$ mw: 1255.60

SYNS: ACT ◊ ACTINOMYCINDIOIC D ACID, DILACTONE ◊ ACTINOMYCIN I ◊ AD ◊ COSMEGEN ◊ DACTINOMYCIN ◊ DILACTONE ACTINOMYCINDIOIC D ACID ◊ HBF 386 ◊ LYOVAC COSMEGEN ◊ MERACTINOMYCIN ◊ NCI-C04682 ◊ NSC 3053 ◊ ONCOSTATIN K

TOXICITY DATA with REFERENCE
CAR: ipr-rat TDLo: 2600 μg/kg/17W-I CNREA8 30,2271,70
NEO: ipr-rat TD: 1700 μg/kg/26W-I RRCRBU 52,1,75
ETA: scu-mus TDLo: 280 μg/kg/18W-I APJAAG 17,495,67
MUT: cyt-ham: ovr 100 μg/L ENMUDM 2,455,80
MUT: cyt-hmn: lym 200 μg/L/2H CCPHDZ 3,143,79
MUT: cyt-rat-ivn 250 mg/kg JELJA7 22,205,73
MUT: dnd-hmn: hla 400 μg/L/15M ECREAL 103,175,76
MUT: dnd-rat-ipr 100 μg/kg CNREA8 36,4647,76
MUT: dni-hmn: oth 10 μg/L/2H-C NATUAS 250,786,74

CONSENSUS REPORTS: IARC Cancer Review: GROUP 3 IMEMDT 7,80,87. NCI Carcinogenesis Studies (ipr); Clear Evidence: rat RRCRBU 52,1,75; No Evidence: mouse RRCRBU 52,1,75

SAFETY PROFILE: Questionable carcinogen with experimental carcinogenic, neoplastigenic, tumorigenic, and teratogenic data. Poison by ingestion, intravenous, subcutaneous, intraperitoneal and possibly other routes. Experimental reproductive effects. Human mutation data reported. Human systemic effects by intravenous and possibly other routes: dermatitis, bone marrow damage, and gastrointestinal effects. A human systemic skin irritant by intravenous route. When heated to decomposition it emits toxic fumes of NO_x.

AEH250   CAS: 700-02-7
ADENINE-1-N-OXIDE
mf: $C_5H_5N_5O$ mw: 151.15

TOXICITY DATA with REFERENCE
NEO: scu-rat TDLo: 1300 mg/kg/26W-I
CNREA8 30,184,70

SAFETY PROFILE: Questionable carcinogen with experimental neoplastigenic data. When heated to decomposition it emits toxic fumes of NO_x.

AEN000   CAS: 628-94-4
ADIPAMIDE
mf: $C_6H_{12}N_2O_2$ mw: 144.20

PROP: Crystals. Mp: 220°. Sol in alc.

SYNS: ADIPIC ACID DIAMIDE ◇ ADIPIC DIAMIDE
◇ 1,4-BUTANEDICARBOXAMIDE ◇ HEXANEDIAMIDE (9CI)
◇ NCI-C02095

TOXICITY DATA with REFERENCE
CAR: orl-rat TDLo: 1270 mg/kg   JEPTDQ
3(5-6),149,80

CONSENSUS REPORTS: Reported in EPA TSCA Inventory.

SAFETY PROFILE: Questionable carcinogen with experimental carcinogenic data. Moderately toxic by ingestion. When heated to decomposition it emits toxic fumes of NO_x.

AEO000   CAS: 103-23-1
ADIPIC ACID BIS(2-ETHYLHEXYL) ESTER
mf: $C_{22}H_{42}O_4$ mw: 370.64

SYNS: ADIPOL 2EH ◇ BEHA ◇ BIS(2-ETHYLHEXYL) ADI-
PATE ◇ BISOFLEX DOA ◇ DEHA ◇ DI-2-ETHYLHEXYL ADI-
PATE ◇ DIOCTYL ADIPATE ◇ DOA ◇ EFFEMOLL DOA
◇ ERGOPLAST AdDO ◇ FLEXOL A 26 ◇ HEXANEDIOIC
ACID, BIS(2-ETHYLHEXYL) ESTER ◇ HEXANEDIOIC ACID,
DIOCTYL ESTER ◇ KODAFLEX DOA ◇ MONOPLEX DOA
◇ NCI-C54386 ◇ OCTYL ADIPATE ◇ PLASTOMOLL DOA

◇ PX-238 ◇ REOMOL DOA ◇ RUCOFLEX PLASTICIZER DOA
◇ SICOL 250 ◇ TRUFLEX DOA ◇ VESTINOL OA
◇ WICKENOL 158 ◇ WITAMOL 320

TOXICITY DATA with REFERENCE
CAR: orl-mus TD: 1048 g/kg/2Y-C   EVHPAZ
65,271,86
CAR: orl-mus TD: 2163 g/kg/2Y-C   NTPTR*
NTP-TR-212,82
CAR: orl-mus TDLo: 1038 g/kg/2Y-C   NTPTR*
NTP-TR-212,82
MUT: dlt-mus-ipr 1000 mg/kg   TXAPA9 32,566,75

CONSENSUS REPORTS: IARC Cancer Review: GROUP 3 IMEMDT 7,56,87; Animal Limited Evidence IMEMDT 29,257,82; NTP Carcinogenesis Bioassay (feed); Clear Evidence: mouse NTPTR* NTP-TR-212,82; No Evidence: rat NTPTR* NTP-TR-212,82. Community Right-To-Know List. Reported in EPA TSCA Inventory.

SAFETY PROFILE: Questionable carcinogen with experimental carcinogenic and teratogenic data. Experimental reproductive effects. Moderately toxic by intravenous route. Mildly toxic by ingestion and skin contact. Mutation data reported. An eye and skin irritant. When heated to decomposition it emits acrid smoke and irritating fumes.

AER000
ADIPIC ACID, UREA mixed with CARBOXYMETHYLCELLULOSE ACIDS

PROP: Consists of 97.3% urea, 0.6% adipic acid and 2.1% carboxymethylcellulose acids (ANYAA9 75,543,59).

TOXICITY DATA with REFERENCE
ETA: ivg-mus TDLo: 91 g/kg/76W-I   ANYAA9
75,543,59

SAFETY PROFILE: Questionable carcinogen with experimental tumorigenic data.

AEU500   CAS: 58209-98-6
AFLATOXIN B1-2,3-DICHLORIDE
mf: $C_{17}H_{12}Cl_2O_6$ mw: 383.19

TOXICITY DATA with REFERENCE
NEO: scu-rat TDLo: 197 µg/kg/10W-I   CNREA8
35,3811,75
NEO: skn-mus TDLo: 1533 µg/kg/20W-I
CNREA8 35,3811,75
MUT: dnd-hmn: fbr 4 µmol/L   CBINA8 50,59,84
MUT: mmo-sat 100 nmol/L   CSHCAL 4,605,77

MUT: sln-dmg-par 200 nmol/L   CNREA8
38,2608,78

SAFETY PROFILE: Questionable carcinogen with experimental neoplastigenic data. Human mutation data reported. When heated to decomposition it emits toxic fumes of Cl^-.

AEX850   CAS: 644-06-4
AGERATOCHROMENE
mf: $C_{13}H_{16}O_3$ mw: 220.29

SYNS: 2H-1-BENZOPYRAN, 6,7-DIMETHOXY-2,2-DI-METHYL- ◇ 6,7-DIMETHOXY-2,2-DIMETHYL-2H-BEN-ZO(b)PYRAN ◇ PRECOCENE 2 ◇ PRECOCENE II

TOXICITY DATA with REFERENCE
CAR: ipr-mus TDLo:27536 μg/kg   CNREA8
47,2275,87
MUT: dnd-rat:lvr 25 μmol/L   CALEDQ 26,311,85
MUT: dns-rat:lvr 1 μmol/L   CALEDQ 26,311,85

CONSENSUS REPORTS: Reported in EPA TSCA Inventory.

SAFETY PROFILE: Questionable carcinogen with experimental carcinogenic data. Mutation data reported. When heated to decomposition it emits acrid smoke and irritating fumes.

AEY000   CAS: 103-16-2
AGERITE
mf: $C_{13}H_{12}O_2$ mw: 200.25

SYNS: AGERITE ALBA ◇ ALBA-DOME ◇ BENOQUIN ◇ BENZOQUIN ◇ BENZYL HYDROQUINONE ◇ p-BEN-ZYLOXYPHENOL ◇ DEPIGMAN ◇ HYDROQUINONE BEN-ZYL ETHER ◇ HYDROQUINONE MONOBENZYL ETHER ◇ p-HYDROXYPHENYL BENZYL ETHER ◇ MONOBENZONE ◇ MONOBENZYL ETHER HYDROQUINONE ◇ MONOBEN-ZYL HYDROQUINONE ◇ 4-(PHENYLMETHOXY)PHENOL ◇ PIGMEX

TOXICITY DATA with REFERENCE
NEO: scu-mus TDLo:1000 mg/kg   NTIS**
PB223-159
ETA: orl-mus TDLo:163 g/kg/78W-I   NTIS**
PB223-159
MUT: skn-gpg 5%/48H MLD   JSCCA5 28,357,77

CONSENSUS REPORTS: Reported in EPA TSCA Inventory.

SAFETY PROFILE: Questionable carcinogen with experimental neoplastigenic and tumorigenic data. Mild acute toxicity by intraperitoneal route. A skin irritant. When heated to decomposition it emits acrid smoke and irritating fumes.

AFJ500   CAS: 52-01-7
ALDACTAZIDE
mf: $C_{24}H_{32}O_4S$ mw: 416.62

SYNS: 3'-(3-OXO-7-α-ACETYLTHIO-17-β-HYDROXYAN-DROST-4-EN-17-β-YL)PROPIONIC ACID LACTONE ◇ 7-α-ACETYLTHIO-3-OXO-17-α-PREGN-4-ENE-21,17-β-CARBOL-ACTONE ◇ ALDACTIDE ◇ ALDACTONE ◇ ALDACTONE A ◇ 3-(3-KETO-7-α-ACETYLTHIO-17-β-HYDROXY-4-AN-DROSTEN-17-α-YL)PROPIONIC ACID LACTONE ◇ OSIREN ◇ OSYROL ◇ 17-α-PREGN-4-ENE-21-CARBOXYLIC ACID, 1-HYDROXY-7-α-MERCAPTO-3-OXO-α-LACTONE ◇ SPIRESIS ◇ SPIRIDON ◇ SPIROCTANIE ◇ SPIROLACTONE ◇ SPIRONOLACTONE ◇ URACTONE ◇ VEROSPIRON ◇ VEROSPIRONE

CONSENSUS REPORTS: IARC Cancer Review: GROUP 3 IMEMDT 7,344,87; Animal Limited Evidence IMEMDT 24,259,80; Human Inadequate Evidence IMEMDT 24,259,80. Reported in EPA TSCA Inventory.

SAFETY PROFILE: Questionable carcinogen. Poison by intraperitoneal route. An experimental teratogen. Human reproductive effects by ingestion and possibly other routes: men, impotence and breast development; women, menstrual cycle changes or disorders, changes in the breasts and lactation. Other human systemic effects by ingestion: agranulocytosis, kidney tubule damage, increased urine volume, and changes in blood sodium and calcium levels. Other reproductive effects in experimental animals. When heated to decomposition it emits toxic fumes of SO_x. Used to treat hypertension, edema of congestive heart failure, cirrhosis and kidney failure.

AFK250   CAS: 309-00-2
ALDRIN
DOT: 2761
mf: $C_{12}H_8Cl_6$ mw: 364.90

PROP: Crystals. Mp: 104-105°. Insol in water; sol in aromatics, esters, ketones, paraffins, and halogenated solvents.

SYNS: ALDREX ◇ ALDREX 30 ◇ ALDRIN, cast solid (DOT) ◇ ALDRINE (FRENCH) ◇ ALDRITE ◇ ALDROSOL ◇ ALTOX ◇ COMPOUND 118 ◇ DRINOX ◇ ENT 15,949 ◇ HEXACHLOROHEXAHYDRO-endo-exo-DIMETHANO-NAPHTHALENE ◇ 1,2,3,4,10,10-HEXACHLORO-1,4,4a,5,8, 8a-HEXAHYDRO-1,4,5,8-DIMETHANONAPHTHALENE ◇ 1,2,3,4,10,10-HEXACHLORO-1,4,4a,5,8,8a-HEXAHYDRO-exo-1,4,-endo-5,8-DIMETHANONAPHTHALENE ◇ 1,2,3,4,-10,10-HEXACHLORO-1,4,4a,5,8,8a-HEXAHYDRO-1,4-endo-

exo-5, 8-DIMETHANONAPHTHALENE ◇ HHDN ◇ NCI-
C00044 ◇ OCTALENE ◇ RCRA WASTE NUMBER P004
◇ SEEDRIN

TOXICITY DATA with REFERENCE

CAR: orl-mus TD:540 mg/kg/80W-I   NCITR*
NCI-CG-TR-21,78

CAR: orl-mus TDLo:270 mg/kg/80W-I   NCITR*
NCI-CG-TR-21,78

NEO: orl-rat TDLo:200 mg/kg/2Y-C   FCTXAV
2,551,64

ETA: orl-rat TD:188 mg/kg/2Y-C   TXAPA9
11,88,67

MUT: cyt-hmn:leu 19125 μg/L   PHTHDT 6,147,79

MUT: cyt-hmn:lym 1900 mg/L   MUREAV
31,103,75

MUT: cyt-rat-ipr 9560 μg/kg   PHTHDT 6,147,79

CONSENSUS REPORTS: IARC Cancer Review: Human Inadequate Evidence IMEMDT 5,25,74; Animal Inadequate Evidence IMEMDT 5,25,74; NCI Carcinogenesis Bioassay (feed); Clear Evidence: mouse NCITR* NCI-CG-TR-21,78; Inadequate Studies: rat NCITR* NCI-CG-TR-21,78. EPA Genetic Toxicology Program. EPA Extremely Hazardous Substances List. Community Right-To-Know List.

OSHA PEL: TWA 0.25 mg/m^3 (skin)   ACGIH TLV: TWA 0.25 mg/m^3/ DFG MAK: 0.25 mg/m^3 NIOSH REL: (Aldrin) Reduce to lowest detectable level.   DOT Classification: Poison B; ORM-A.

SAFETY PROFILE: Questionable carcinogen with experimental carcinogenic, neoplastigenic, tumorigenic, and teratogenic data. Poison by ingestion, skin contact, intravenous, intraperitoneal and other routes. Human systemic effects by ingestion: excitement, tremors and nausea or vomiting. Experimental reproductive effects. Human mutation data reported. Continued acute exposure causes liver damage. When heated to decomposition it emits toxic fumes of Cl$^-$.

AFW750   CAS: 140-67-0
p-ALLYLANISOLE
mf: C$_{10}$H$_{12}$O   mw: 148.22

PROP: Isolated from rind of *Persea Gratissima Garth,* and from Oil of Estragon; found in oils of Russian Anise, Basil, Fennel, Turpentine, and others (FCTXAV 14,601,76). Colorless to sltly yellow liquid; anise odor. D: 0.960-0.968, refr index: 1.519-1.524, flash p: 178°F. Sol in alc; insol in water.

SYNS: 4-ALLYL-1-METHOXYBENZENE ◇ CHAVICOL METHYL ETHER ◇ ESDRAGOL ◇ ISOANETHOLE ◇ p-METHOXYALLYLBENZENE ◇ 1-METHOXY-4-(2-PRO-PENYL)BENZENE ◇ METHYL CHAVICOL ◇ NCI-C60946 ◇ TARRAGON

TOXICITY DATA with REFERENCE

CAR: ipr-mus TDLo:111 mg/kg   CNREA8
47,2275,87

CAR: scu-mus TDLo:140 mg/kg/22D-I   JNCIAM
57,1323,76

NEO: orl-mus TD:195 g/kg/1Y-C   CNREA8
43,1124,83

NEO: orl-mus TDLo:97 g/kg/1Y-C   CNREA8
43,1124,83

MUT: bfa-rat/sat 2500 mg/kg   NUCADQ 1,10,79

MUT: dnd-mus-ipr 80 mg/kg   CRNGDP 5,1613,84

MUT: mma-sat 1 μmol/plate   MUREAV 60,143,79

MUT: mmo-sat 1 μmol/plate   FCTXAV 14,603,76

MUT: skn-rbt 500 mg/24H MOD   FCTXAV
14,601,76

CONSENSUS REPORTS: Reported in EPA TSCA Inventory.

SAFETY PROFILE: Questionable carcinogen with experimental carcinogenic and neoplastigenic data. Moderate acute toxicity by many routes. A skin irritant. Mutation data reported. Combustible liquid. When heated to decomposition it emits acrid smoke and irritating fumes. A spice used in foods, liqueurs, and perfumes.

AGA750   CAS: 2114-11-6
ALLYL CARBAMATE
mf: C$_4$H$_7$NO$_2$ mw: 101.12

SYN: CARBAMIC ACID, ALLYL ESTER

TOXICITY DATA with REFERENCE

NEO: ipr-mus TDLo:279 mg/kg/4W-I   CNREA8
29,2184,69

MUT: sce-mus-ipr 100 μmol/kg   CNREA8
42,2165,82

CONSENSUS REPORTS: Reported in EPA TSCA Inventory.

SAFETY PROFILE: Questionable carcinogen with experimental neoplastigenic data. Mutation data reported. When heated to decomposition it emits toxic NO$_x$.

AGH500   CAS: 52207-83-7
ALLYLHYDRAZINE HYDROCHLORIDE
mf: C$_3$H$_8$N$_2$•ClH   mw: 108.59

TOXICITY DATA with REFERENCE
CAR: orl-mus TDLo: 9800 mg/kg/35W-C
   BJCAAI 34,90,76
ETA: orl-mus TDLo: 25 mg/kg   PAACA3 16,61,75

SAFETY PROFILE: Questionable carcinogen with experimental carcinogenic and tumorigenic data. When heated to decomposition it emits very toxic fumes of HCl and NO_x.

AGK750   CAS: 6728-21-8
ALLYL METHANESULFONATE
mf: $C_4H_8O_3S$ mw: 136.18

SYNS: ALLYL MESYLATE ◇ ALLYL METHANESULFO-
NATE ◇ METHANESULFONIC ACID, 2-PROPENYL ESTER
(9CI)

TOXICITY DATA with REFERENCE
NEO: skn-mus TDLo: 540 mg/kg/10W-I
   CNREA8 17,64,57
MUT: dns-hmn: hla 50 μmol/L   CALEDQ
20,263,83
MUT: mmo-sat 1 μmol/plate   BCPCA6 29,993,80

SAFETY PROFILE: Questionable carcinogen with experimental neoplastigenic data. Human mutation data reported. When heated to decomposition it emits toxic fumes of SO_x.

AGM125
1-(ALLYLNITROSAMINO)-2-PROPANONE
mf: $C_6H_{10}N_2O_2$ mw: 142.18

SYNS: NAOP ◇ N-NITROSOALLYL-2-OXOPROPYLAMINE

TOXICITY DATA with REFERENCE
ETA: orl-ham TDLo: 1848 mg/kg/50W-I
   IAPUDO 57,617,84
ETA: orl-rat TD: 1225 mg/kg/50W-I   CALEDQ
22,281,84
ETA: orl-rat TDLo: 995 mg/kg/74W-I   IAPUDO
57,617,84
MUT: mma-sat 10 μg/plate   TCMUE9 1,13,84

SAFETY PROFILE: Questionable carcinogen with experimental tumorigenic data. Mutation data reported. When heated to decomposition it emits toxic fumes of NO_x.

AGQ500   CAS: 1745-81-9
o-ALLYL PHENOL
mf: $C_9H_{10}O$ mw: 134.19

PROP: Mp: 10°, bp: 230°, d: 1.033 @ 18°/4°. Sol in water, alc, chloroform, and ether.

SYN: 2-ALLYL PHENOL

TOXICITY DATA with REFERENCE
CAR: skn-mus TDLo: 8400 mg/kg/30W-I
   CNREA8 19,413,59
NEO: skn-mus TD: 3360 mg/kg/12W-I   CNREA8
19,413,59

CONSENSUS REPORTS: Reported in EPA TSCA Inventory.

SAFETY PROFILE: Questionable carcinogen with experimental carcinogenic and neoplastigenic data. Poison by intraperitoneal route. When heated to decomposition it emits acrid smoke and fumes.

AHA250   CAS: 7047-84-9
ALUMINUM DEXTRAN
mf: $C_{18}H_{37}AlO_4$ mw: 344.48

PROP: Powder. A complex containing aluminum and dextran, a chain of molecular weight 2,500, corresponding to a chain of 15 anhydroglucose units.

SYN: ALUMINUM MONOSTEARATE ◇ STEARIC ACID
ALUMINUM DIHYDROXIDE SALT

TOXICITY DATA with REFERENCE
ETA: scu-mus TDLo: 112 g/kg/14W-I   JNCIAM
24,109,60

ACGIH TLV: TWA 2 mg(Al)/m^3

SAFETY PROFILE: Questionable carcinogen with experimental tumorigenic data. When heated to decomposition it emits acrid smoke and fumes.

AHE250   CAS: 1344-28-1
ALUMINUM OXIDE (2:3)
mf: Al_2O_3 mw: 101.96

PROP: White powder. Mp: 2050°, bp: 2977°, d: 3.5-4.0, vap press: 1 mm @ 2158°.

SYNS: A 1 (SORBENT) ◇ A1-0109 P ◇ ABRAREX
◇ ACTIVATED ALUMINUM OXIDE ◇ ALCOA F 1
◇ ALMITE ◇ ALON ◇ ALUMINA ◇ α-ALUMINA (OSHA)
◇ β-ALUMINA ◇ γ-ALUMINA ◇ ALUMINUM OXIDE
◇ α-ALUMINUM OXIDE ◇ β-ALUMINUM OXIDE
◇ γ-ALUMINUM OXIDE ◇ ALUMINUM SESQUIOXIDE
◇ ALUMITE ◇ ALUNDUM ◇ BROCKMANN, ALUMINUM
OXIDE ◇ CAB-O-GRIP ◇ COMPALOX ◇ DIALUMINUM TRI-
OXIDE ◇ DISPAL ◇ DOTMENT 324 ◇ FASERTON
◇ G 2 (OXIDE) ◇ KHP 2 ◇ LUCALOX ◇ MICROGRIT WCA
◇ PS 1 ◇ RC 172DBM

TOXICITY DATA with REFERENCE
NEO: imp-rat TDLo: 200 mg/kg   JJIND8 67,965,81

ETA: imp-rat TD:200 mg/kg   IARCCD 8,289,79
ETA: ipl-rat TDLo:90 mg/kg   BJCAAI 28,173,73

CONSENSUS REPORTS: Community Right-To-Know List. Reported in EPA TSCA Inventory.

OSHA PEL: Total Dust: (Transitional: TWA 5 mg/m^3) TWA 10 mg/m^3; Respirable Fraction: TWA 5 mg/m^3 ACGIH TLV: TWA (nuisance particulate) 10 mg/m^3 of total dust (when toxic impurities are not present, e.g., quartz $<$ 1%). DFG MAK: 6 mg/m^3 (fume)

SAFETY PROFILE: Questionable carcinogen with experimental neoplastigenic and tumorigenic data by implantation. Inhalation of finely divided particles may cause lung damage (Shaver's disease).

AHF500   CAS: 1302-76-7
ALUMINUM(III) SILICATE (2:1)
mf: $O_5Si\bullet 2Al$ mw: 162.05

SYNS: ALUMINUM OXIDE SILICATE $\diamond$ CERAMIC FIBRE $\diamond$ CYANITE $\diamond$ DISTHENE $\diamond$ KYANITE $\diamond$ OIL-DRI $\diamond$ SAFE-N-DRI $\diamond$ SILICIC ACID ALUMINUM SALT $\diamond$ SNOW TEX $\diamond$ VALFOR

TOXICITY DATA with REFERENCE
ETA: ipl-rat TDLo:90 mg/kg   BJCAAI 28,173,73

ACGIH TLV: TWA 2 mg(Al)/m^3

SAFETY PROFILE: Questionable carcinogen with experimental tumorigenic data by implantation.

AHR250   CAS: 613-89-8
2-AMINOACETOPHENONE
mf: C_8H_9NO mw: 135.18

PROP: Yellow, oily liquid. Bp: 251° (slt decomp); insol in water, sol in alc and ether.

SYNS: φ-AMINOACETOPHENONE $\diamond$ PHENACYLAMINE

TOXICITY DATA with REFERENCE
CAR: scu-mus TDLo:2000 mg/kg/7W-I
   PGPKA8 14,12,69
ETA: scu-ham TDLo:1600 mg/kg/10W-I
   VOONAW 25(6),81,79
ETA: scu-mus TD:1600 mg/kg/8W-I   VOONAW 22(6),47,76

SAFETY PROFILE: Questionable carcinogen with experimental carcinogenic, neoplastigenic, tumorigenic and teratogenic data. When heated to decomposition it emits toxic fumes of NO$_x$.

AIA750   CAS: 82-45-1
1-AMINOANTHRAQUINONE
mf: $C_{14}H_9NO_2$ mw: 223.24

PROP: Red needles. Mp: 256°, bp: subl. Insol in water; sol in HCl, alc, benzene, ether, and chloroform.

SYNS: 1-AMINO-9,10-ANTHRACENEDIONE $\diamond$ 1-AMINOANTHRACHINON (CZECH) $\diamond$ α-AMINOANTHRAQUINONE $\diamond$ 1-AMINO-9,10-ANTHRAQUINONE $\diamond$ α-ANTHRAQUINONYLAMINE $\diamond$ C.I. 37275 $\diamond$ DIAZO FAST RED AL

TOXICITY DATA with REFERENCE
ETA: orl-rat TD:3000 mg/kg/60W-I   TXAPA9 8,346,66
ETA: orl-rat TDLo:2400 mg/kg/60W-I   TXAPA9 8,346,66
MUT: dnd-mus-ipr 250 mg/kg   ATSUDG(5),355,82

CONSENSUS REPORTS: Reported in EPA TSCA Inventory.

SAFETY PROFILE: Questionable carcinogen with experimental tumorigenic data. Moderately toxic by intraperitoneal route. Mutation data reported. An eye irritant. When heated to decomposition it emits toxic NO$_x$.

AIC000   CAS: 3398-09-2
p-AMINO-2':3-AZOTOLUENE
mf: $C_{14}H_{15}N_3$ mw: 225.32

SYN: 4'-AMINO-3,2'-AZOTOLUENE

TOXICITY DATA with REFERENCE
ETA: orl-mus TDLo:30 g/kg/57W-C   BJCAAI 3,387,49

SAFETY PROFILE: Questionable carcinogen with experimental tumorigenic data. When heated to decomposition it emits toxic fumes of NO$_x$.

AIC500   CAS: 3963-79-9
4'-AMINO-4,2'-AZOTOLUENE
mf: $C_{14}H_{15}N_3$ mw: 225.32

SYN: 4-(p-TOLYLAZO)-m-TOLUIDINE

TOXICITY DATA with REFERENCE
CAR: orl-mus TDLo:30 g/kg/57W-C   BJCAAI 3,387,49

SAFETY PROFILE: Questionable carcinogen with experimental carcinogenic data. When heated to decomposition it emits toxic fumes of NO$_x$.

AIC750   CAS: 18936-75-9
10-AMINOBENZ(a)ACRIDINE
mf: $C_{17}H_{12}N_2$ mw: 244.31

SYN: BENZ(a)ACRIDIN-10-AMINE

TOXICITY DATA with REFERENCE
ETA: scu-mus TDLo:72 mg/kg/9W-I CHDDAT
267,981,68

SAFETY PROFILE: Questionable carcinogen
with experimental tumorigenic data. When
heated to decomposition it emits toxic fumes
of NO_x.

AIV750 CAS: 4363-03-5
4-AMINO-3-BIPHENYLOL
mf: $C_{12}H_{11}NO$ mw: 185.24
SYN: 4-AMINO-3-HYDROXYBIPHENYL

TOXICITY DATA with REFERENCE
CAR: scu-mus TDLo:216 mg/kg/3D JNCIAM
41,403,68

SAFETY PROFILE: Questionable carcinogen
with experimental carcinogenic data. When
heated to decomposition it emits toxic fumes
of NO_x.

AIW000 CAS: 1204-79-1
4'-AMINO-4-BIPHENYLOL
mf: $C_{12}H_{11}NO$ mw: 185.24
SYN: 4-AMINO-4'-HYDROXYBIPHENOL

TOXICITY DATA with REFERENCE
CAR: scu-mus TDLo:216 mg/kg/3D JNCIAM
41,403,68

SAFETY PROFILE: Questionable carcinogen
with experimental carcinogenic data. When
heated to decomposition it emits toxic fumes
of NO_x.

AIW250 CAS: 1204-59-7
3-AMINO-4-BIPHENYLOL
HYDROCHLORIDE
mf: $C_{12}H_{11}NO \cdot ClH$ mw: 221.70
SYNS: 3-AMINO-4-HYDROXYDIPHENYL HYDROCHLO-
RIDE ◇ 4-HYDROXY-3-AMINODIPHENYL HYDROCHLO-
RIDE

TOXICITY DATA with REFERENCE
CAR: imp-mus TDLo:50 mg/kg BJCAAI 12,222,58

SAFETY PROFILE: Questionable carcinogen
with experimental carcinogenic data by implantation. When heated to decomposition it emits
very toxic fumes of HCl and NO_x.

AJA000 CAS: 5003-71-4
1-AMINO-3-BROMOPROPANE
HYDROBROMIDE
mf: $C_3H_6BrN \cdot BrH$ mw: 216.93

SYNS: 3-BROMO-1-PROPANAMINE HYDROBROMIDE
◇ 3-BROMOPROPYLAMINE HYDROBROMIDE

TOXICITY DATA with REFERENCE
ETA: ipr-mus TDLo:1150 mg/kg/8W-I CNREA8
39,391,79

CONSENSUS REPORTS: Reported in EPA
TSCA Inventory.

SAFETY PROFILE: Questionable carcinogen
with experimental tumorigenic data. When
heated to decomposition it emits very toxic
fumes of HBr and NO_x.

AJL250 CAS: 63041-30-5
9-AMINO-1,2,5,6-DIBENZANTHRACENE
mf: $C_{22}H_{15}N$ mw: 293.38
SYN: 7-AMINODIBENZ(a,h)ANTHRACENE

TOXICITY DATA with REFERENCE
ETA: skn-mus TDLo:1250 mg/kg/52W-I
PRLBA4 117,318,35

SAFETY PROFILE: Questionable carcinogen
with experimental tumorigenic data. When
heated to decomposition it emits toxic fumes
of NO_x.

AJM000 CAS: 133-90-4
3-AMINO-2,5-DICHLOROBENZOIC ACID
mf: $C_7H_5Cl_2NO_2$ mw: 206.03

SYNS: ACP-M-728 ◇ AMBIBEN ◇ AMOBEN ◇ CHLORAM-
BEN ◇ 2,5-DICHLORO-3-AMINOBENZOIC ACID ◇ NCI-
C00055 ◇ ORNAMENTAL WEED ◇ VEGABEN

TOXICITY DATA with REFERENCE
CAR: orl-mus TD :1344 g/kg/80W-C NCITR*
NCI-CG-TR-25,77
CAR: orl-mus TDLo:672 g/kg/80W-C NCITR*
NCI-CG-TR-25,77
MUT: cyt-mus-ipr 58500 μg/kg CARYAB
33,527,80
MUT: cyt-mus-orl 234 mg/kg CARYAB 33,527,80
MUT: mma-sat 1 mg/plate NTPTB* JAN 82
MUT: mmo-sat 10 mg/plate ENMUDM 5(Suppl
1),3,83

CONSENSUS REPORTS: NCI Carcinogen-
esis Bioassay Completed; Results Positive:
mouse (NCITR* NCI-CG-TR-25,77); Results
Negative: rat (NCITR* NCI-CG-TR-25,77).
Community Right-To-Know List. Reported in
EPA TSCA Inventory.

SAFETY PROFILE: Questionable carcinogen
with experimental carcinogenic data. Moder-

ately toxic by ingestion. Mutation data reported. When heated to decomposition it emits highly toxic fumes such as Cl^- and NO_x.

AJQ500   CAS: 21554-20-1
4-AMINO-3',5'-DIMETHYL-4'-HYDROXYAZOBENZENE
mf: $C_{14}H_{15}N_3O$ mw: 241.32

TOXICITY DATA with REFERENCE
ETA: orl-rat TDLo: 40 g/kg/2Y-C   AABIAV
52,33,63

SAFETY PROFILE: Questionable carcinogen with experimental tumorigenic data. Poison by intraperitoneal route. When heated to decomposition it emits toxic fumes of NO_x.

AJQ600   CAS: 77094-11-2
2-AMINO-3,4-DIMETHYLIMIDAZO(4,5-f)QUINOLINE
mf: $C_{12}H_{12}N_4$ mw: 212.28

SYN: 3,4-DIMETHYL-3H-IMIDAZO(4,5-f)QUINOLIN-2-AMINE

TOXICITY DATA with REFERENCE
CAR: orl-mus TD: 22120 mg/kg/81W-C
CRNGDP 7,1889,86
CAR: orl-mus TD: 27888 mg/kg/83W-C
PJABDW 61,99,85
CAR: orl-mus TDLo: 7476 mg/kg/89W-C
CRNGDP 7,1889,86
MUT: dnd-mus: leu 100 μmol/L   MUREAV
144,57,85
MUT: dns-gpg: lng 10 μmol/L   ENMUDM 7,245,85
MUT: dns-ham: lng 3 μmol/L   ENMUDM 7,245,85
MUT: dns-rat: lng 3 μmol/L   ENMUDM 7,245,85
MUT: mma-sat 100 ng/plate   CRNGDP 7,273,86
MUT: msc-ham: lng 25 mg/L   MUREAV 118,91,83
MUT: slt-dmg-orl 100 ng/kg   JJCREP 76,468,85

CONSENSUS REPORTS: IARC Cancer Review: Animal Inadequate Evidence IMEMDT 40,275,86

SAFETY PROFILE: Questionable carcinogen with experimental carcinogenic data. Mutation data reported. When heated to decomposition it emits toxic fumes of NO_x.

AJR400   CAS: 31272-21-6
5-AMINO-1,3-DIMETHYL-4-PYRAZOLYL o-FLUOROPHENYL KETONE
mf: $C_{12}H_{12}FN_3O$ mw: 233.27

SYNS: (5-AMINO-1,3-DIMETHYL-1H-PYRAZOL-4-YL)(2-FLUOROPHENYL)METHANONE ◇ KETONE, 5-AMINO-1,3-

DIMETHYLPYRAZOL-4-YL o-FLUOROPHENYL ◇ METHA-NONE, (5-AMINO-1,3-DIMETHYL-1H-PYRAZOL-4-YL)(2-FLUOROPHENYL)- ◇ PD 71627

TOXICITY DATA with REFERENCE
ETA: orl-rat TD: 2366 mg/kg/13W-C   AJPAA4
124,392,86
MUT: mma-sat 10 nmol/plate   CRNGDP 7,2019,86

SAFETY PROFILE: Questionable carcinogen with experimental tumorigenic data. Mutation data reported. When heated to decomposition it emits toxic fumes of F^- and NO_x.

AJS225
2-AMINODIPYRIDO(1,2-a:3',2'-d)IMIDAZOLE HYDROCHLORIDE
mf: $C_{10}H_8N_4 \cdot ClH$ mw: 220.68

SYN: DIPYRIDO(1,2-a:3',2'-d)IMIDAZOLE, 2-AMINO-, HY-DROCHLORIDE

TOXICITY DATA with REFERENCE
CAR: orl-rat TDLo: 4116 mg/kg/24W-C
GANNA2 75,207,84
MUT: slt-dmg-orl 100 ng/kg   JJCREP 76,468,85

SAFETY PROFILE: Questionable carcinogen with experimental carcinogenic data. Mutation data reported. When heated to decomposition it emits toxic fumes of NO_x and HCl.

AJT750   CAS: 17026-81-2
3-AMINO-4-ETHOXYACETANILIDE
mf: $C_{10}H_{14}N_2O_2$ mw: 194.26

SYNS: 2-AMINO-4-ACETAMINIFENETOL (CZECH) ◇ NCI-C01887

TOXICITY DATA with REFERENCE
CAR: orl-mus TDLo: 524 mg/kg/78W-C
NCITR* NCI-CG-TR-112,78
ETA: orl-mus TD: 260 g/kg/78W-C   NCITR*
NCI-CG-TR-112,78
ETA: orl-rat TDLo: 130 g/kg/78W-C   NCITR*
NCI-CG-TR-112,78
MUT: mma-esc 333 μg/plate   ENMUDM 7(Suppl 5),1,85
MUT: mma-sat 33300 ng/plate   ENMUDM 7(Suppl 5),1,85
MUT: mmo-sat 1 mg/plate   ENMUDM 7(Suppl 5),1,85

CONSENSUS REPORTS: NTP Carcinogenesis Bioassay (feed): Clear Evidence: mouse NCITR* NCI-TR-112,78; Inadequate Studies: rat NCITR* NCI-TR-112,78. Reported in EPA TSCA Inventory.

SAFETY PROFILE: Questionable carcinogen with experimental carcinogenic and tumorigenic data. Moderately toxic by ingestion. An eye irritant. Mutation data reported. When heated to decomposition it emits toxic fumes of NO_x.

AKB250 CAS: 13073-35-3
2-AMINO-4-(ETHYLTHIO)BUTYRIC ACID
mf: $C_6H_{13}NO_2S$ mw: 163.26

SYNS: l-2-AMINO-4-(ETHYLTHIO)BUTYRIC ACID ◇ ETHIONINE ◇ l-ETHIONINE ◇ S-ETHYL-l-HOMOCYS-TEINE

TOXICITY DATA with REFERENCE
CAR: orl-mus TDLo:44100 mg/kg/2Y-C
  CRNGDP 7,1143,86
MUT: dni-esc 2 g/L CYTOAN 50,387,85
MUT: dni-hmn:lym 2 mmol/L BBACAQ
  520,139,79
MUT: otr-ham:emb 5 mg/L CRNGDP 4,291,83

CONSENSUS REPORTS: Reported in EPA TSCA Inventory. EPA Genetic Toxicology Program.

SAFETY PROFILE: Questionable carcinogen with experimental carcinogenic data. Human mutation data reported. When heated to decomposition it emits very toxic fumes of NO_x and SO_x.

AKC000 CAS: 63019-67-0
2-AMINO-N-FLUOREN-2-YLACETAMIDE
mf: $C_{15}H_{14}N_2O$ mw: 238.31

SYN: 2-GLYCYLAMINOFLUORENE

TOXICITY DATA with REFERENCE
ETA: orl-rat TDLo:1200 mg/kg/20W-I NATUAS
  184,2018,59

SAFETY PROFILE: Questionable carcinogen with experimental tumorigenic data. When heated to decomposition it emits toxic fumes of NO_x.

AKC500 CAS: 324-93-6
4-AMINO-4'-FLUORODIPHENYL
mf: $C_{12}H_{10}FN$ mw: 187.23

SYNS: 4'-FLUORO-4-AMINODIPHENYL ◇ 4'-FLUORO-4-BIPHENYLAMINE

TOXICITY DATA with REFERENCE
CAR: orl-rat TDLo:300 mg/kg CNREA8
  26,619,66
NEO: orl-mus TDLo:520 mg/kg/26W-I BJCAAI
  19,297,65

ETA: scu-rat TD:1990 mg/kg/20W-I NATUAS
  175,1131,55
ETA: scu-rat TD:2000 mg/kg/W-I BMBUAQ
  14,141,58

CONSENSUS REPORTS: EPA Genetic Toxicology Program.

SAFETY PROFILE: Questionable carcinogen with experimental carcinogenic, neoplastigenic, and tumorigenic data. Poison by ingestion. When heated to decomposition it emits very toxic fumes of F^- and NO_x.

AKE000 CAS: 4502-10-7
2-AMINO-3-HYDROXYACETOPHENONE
mf: $C_8H_9NO_2$ mw: 151.18

SYN: 2-AMINO-3-HYDROXYPHENYL METHYL KETONE

TOXICITY DATA with REFERENCE
NEO: imp-mus TDLo:80 mg/kg BJCAAI
  11,212,57

SAFETY PROFILE: Questionable carcinogen with experimental neoplastigenic data. When heated to decomposition it emits toxic fumes of NO_x.

AKE500 CAS: 103-18-4
4-AMINO-4'-HYDROXYAZOBENZENE
mf: $C_{12}H_{11}N_3O$ mw: 213.26

TOXICITY DATA with REFERENCE
ETA: orl-rat TDLo:28 g/kg/2Y-C AABIAV
  52,33,63

CONSENSUS REPORTS: Reported in EPA TSCA Inventory.

SAFETY PROFILE: Questionable carcinogen with experimental tumorigenic data. Poison by intraperitoneal route. Moderately toxic by ingestion. When heated to decomposition it emits toxic fumes of NO_x.

AKE750 CAS: 548-93-6
2-AMINO-3-HYDROXYBENZOIC ACID
mf: $C_7H_7NO_3$ mw: 153.15

SYNS: 3-HYDROXYANTHRANILIC ACID ◇ 3-HYDROXY-ANTHRANILSAEURE (GERMAN) ◇ 3-OHAA ◇ 3-OXYAN-THRANILIC ACID

TOXICITY DATA with REFERENCE
CAR: scu-mus TD:2000 mg/kg/7W-I PGPKA8
  14,12,69
CAR: scu-mus TDLo:1600 mg/kg/8W-I
  VOONAW 22(6),47,76

NEO: imp-mus TD:80 mg/kg   BJCAAI 11,212,57
ETA: scu-dog TDLo:500 mg/kg/20W-I
VOONAW 26(3),93,80
ETA: scu-mus TD:121 mg/kg/21D-I   JCREA8
96,163,80
ETA: scu-mus TD:2040 mg/kg/59W-C
VOONAW 20(8),75,74
ETA: scu-mus TD:8000 mg/kg/19W-I   KLWOAZ
37,1053,59
ETA: scu-mus TDLo:185 mg/kg (13-17D post)
JCREA8 96,163,80
MUT: cyt-hmn:emb 30 mg/L   BEXBAN 67,200,69
MUT: cyt-hmn:leu 100 mg/L   TSITAQ 15,1505,73

SAFETY PROFILE: Questionable carcinogen with experimental carcinogenic, neoplastigenic, and tumorigenic data. Human mutation data reported. When heated to decomposition it emits toxic fumes such as NO_x.

AKF250   CAS: 73728-82-2
4-AMINO-3-HYDROXYBIPHENYL SULFATE
mf: $C_{12}H_{11}NO \cdot H_2O_4S$ mw: 283.32

SYNS: 4-AMINO-3-BIPHENYLOL HYDROGEN SULFATE
◇ 3-HYDROXY-4-AMINODIPHENYL SULPHATE

TOXICITY DATA with REFERENCE
CAR: imp-mus TDLo:100 mg/kg   BJCAAI
10,539,56

SAFETY PROFILE: Questionable carcinogen with experimental carcinogenic data. When heated to decomposition it emits very toxic fumes of SO_x and NO_x.

AKI500   CAS: 63019-81-8
4-AMINO-3-HYDROXY-4'-NITRODIPHENYLHYDROCHLORIDE
mf: $C_{12}H_{10}N_2O_3 \cdot ClH$ mw: 266.70

SYNS: 4-AMINO-4'-NITRO-3-BIPHENYLOL HYDROCHLO-
RIDE ◇ 4'-NITRO-4-AMINO-3-HYDROXYDIPHENYL HY-
DROCHLORIDE ◇ 4'-NITRO-4-AMINO-3-HYDROXYDIPHE-
NYL HYDROGEN CHLORIDE

TOXICITY DATA with REFERENCE
ETA: imp-mus TDLo:100 mg/kg   BJCAAI
10,539,56

SAFETY PROFILE: Questionable carcinogen with experimental tumorigenic data. When heated to decomposition it emits very toxic fumes of HCl and NO_x.

AKK250   CAS: 360-97-4
5-AMINOIMIDAZOLE-4-CARBOXAMIDE
mf: $C_4H_6N_4O$ mw: 126.14

SYN: DIAZOL-C

TOXICITY DATA with REFERENCE
ETA: orl-rat TDLo:6390 mg/kg/21W-C
JNCIAM 54,951,75
MUT: mma-sat 10 µg/plate   JTEHD6 2,1095,77
MUT: mmo-klp 5 mmol/L/20H   MUREAV
66,297,79

CONSENSUS REPORTS: Reported in EPA TSCA Inventory.

SAFETY PROFILE: Questionable carcinogen with experimental tumorigenic data. Mutation data reported. When heated to decomposition it emits toxic fumes of NO_x.

AKN250   CAS: 63040-25-5
4-AMINO-4'-METHOXY-3-BIPHENYLOLHYDROCHLORIDE
mf: $C_{13}H_{13}NO_2 \cdot ClH$ mw: 251.73

SYN: 3-HYDROXY-4'-METHOXY-4-AMINODIPHENYL HY-
DROCHLORIDE

TOXICITY DATA with REFERENCE
ETA: imp-mus TDLo:80 mg/kg   BJCAAI
17,127,63

SAFETY PROFILE: Questionable carcinogen with experimental tumorigenic data. When heated to decomposition it emits very toxic fumes of HCl and NO_x.

AKN500   CAS: 951-39-3
2-AMINO-3-METHOXYDIPHENYLENE OXIDE
mf: $C_{13}H_{11}NO_2$ mw: 213.25

SYN: 3-METHOXY-2-AMINODIPHENYLENE OXIDE

TOXICITY DATA with REFERENCE
CAR: orl-rat TDLo:15 g/kg/70W-I   ZEKBAI
61,45,56
ETA: orl-rat TD:21 g/kg/76W-C   JNCIAM
39,1069,67

SAFETY PROFILE: Questionable carcinogen with experimental carcinogenic and tumorigenic data. When heated to decomposition it emits toxic fumes of NO_x.

AKS275
2-AMINO-6-METHYLDIPYRIDO(1,2-a:3',2'-d)IMIDAZOLE HYDROCHLORIDE
mf: $C_{11}H_{10}N_4 \cdot ClH$ mw: 234.71

SYN: DIPYRIDO(1,2-a:3',2'-d)IMIDAZOLE, 2-AMINO-6-
METHYL-, HYDROCHLORIDE

TOXICITY DATA with REFERENCE
CAR: orl-rat TDLo: 3612 mg/kg/24W-C

GANNA2 75,207,84

MUT: slt-dmg-orl 100 ng/kg   JJCREP 76,468,85

SAFETY PROFILE: Questionable carcinogen with experimental carcinogenic data. Mutation data reported. When heated to decomposition it emits toxic fumes of NO_x and HCl.

AKT620
2-AMINO-3-METHYLIMIDAZO(4,5-f) QUINOLINE DIHYDROCHLORIDE
mf: $C_{11}H_{10}N_4 \cdot 2ClH$ mw: 271.17

SYN: IQ DIHYDROCHLORIDE

TOXICITY DATA with REFERENCE
CAR: orl-rat TDLo: 4081 mg/kg/31W-I   JJCREP 76,570,85

SAFETY PROFILE: Questionable carcinogen with experimental carcinogenic data. When heated to decomposition it emits toxic fumes of NO_x.

ALE750
CAS: 72254-58-1
3-AMINO-1-METHYL-5H-PYRIDO(4,3-b) INDOLE ACETATE
mf: $C_{12}H_{11}N_3 \cdot C_2H_4O_2$ mw: 257.32

SYNS: 5H-PYRIDO(4,3-b)INDOL-3-AMINE, 1-METHYL-1, MONOACETATE ◇ TRP-P-2(ACETATE)

TOXICITY DATA with REFERENCE
CAR: orl-mus TDLo: 14 g/kg/89W-C   SCIEAS 213,346,81

MUT: mma-sat 1 μg/plate   CPBTAL 26,611,78
MUT: slt-dmg-orl 400 ppm   MUREAV 122,315,83

SAFETY PROFILE: Questionable carcinogen with experimental carcinogenic data. Mutation data reported. When heated to decomposition it emits toxic fumes of NO_x.

ALI300
CAS: 86-60-2
7-AMINO-1-NAPHTHALENESULFONIC ACID
mf: $C_{10}H_9NO_3S$ mw: 223.26

SYNS: BADEN ACID ◇ BADISCHE ACID ◇ 2-NAPH-THYLAMINE-8-SULFONIC ACID

TOXICITY DATA with REFERENCE
NEO: ipr-mus TDLo: 18 g/kg/8W-I   JJIND8 67,1299,81

SAFETY PROFILE: Questionable carcinogen with experimental neoplastigenic data. When

heated to decomposition it emits toxic fumes of NO_x and SO_x.

ALJ250
CAS: 42884-33-3
2-AMINO-1-NAPHTHOL
mf: $C_{10}H_9NO$ mw: 159.20

PROP: Mp; 255° (decomp). Sol in alc.

SYN: AMINONAPHTHALENOL

TOXICITY DATA with REFERENCE
CAR: imp-mus TDLo: 56 mg/kg   SAIGBL 24,186,82

ETA: ipr-rat TDLo: 39 mg/kg/13W-I   CNREA8 28,535,68

SAFETY PROFILE: Questionable carcinogen with experimental carcinogenic and tumorigenic data. When heated to decomposition it emits toxic fumes of NO_x.

ALK000
CAS: 1198-27-2
1-AMINO-2-NAPHTHOL HYDROCHLORIDE
mf: $C_{10}H_9NO \cdot ClH$ mw: 195.66

PROP: Needles from alc. Mp: 201°; sltly sol in water; sol in alc and ether.

SYN: 2-HYDROXY-1-NAPHTHYLAMINE HYDROCHLORIDE

TOXICITY DATA with REFERENCE
CAR: imp-mus TDLo: 100 mg/kg   BJCAAI 10,539,56

MUT: dnr-esc 500 μg/well/16H   CBINA8 15,219,76

CONSENSUS REPORTS: Reported in EPA TSCA Inventory. EPA Genetic Toxicology Program.

SAFETY PROFILE: Questionable carcinogen with experimental carcinogenic data. Mutation data reported. When heated to decomposition it emits very toxic fumes of HCl and NO_x.

ALK250
CAS: 41772-23-0
2-AMINO-1-NAPHTHOL HYDROCHLORIDE
mf: $C_{10}H_9NO \cdot ClH$ mw: 195.66

PROP: Needles. Mp: 255° (decomp); sol in alc.

SYN: 1-HYDROXY-2-NAPHTHYLAMINE HYDROCHLORIDE

TOXICITY DATA with REFERENCE
CAR: imp-mus TD: 100 mg/kg   BJCAAI 10,539,56
CAR: imp-mus TDLo: 80 mg/kg   BJCAAI
17,127,63
ETA: imp-mus TD: 40 mg/kg   BJCAAI 6,412,52
ETA: imp-mus TD: 120 mg/kg   LANCAO 2,286,51
ETA: scu-mus TDLo: 1100 mg/kg/45W-I
BJCAAI 6,412,52
ETA: scu-rat TDLo: 1100 mg/kg/45W-I   BJCAAI
6,412,52

CONSENSUS REPORTS: Reported in EPA
TSCA Inventory.

SAFETY PROFILE: Questionable carcinogen
with experimental carcinogenic and tumorigenic
data. When heated to decomposition it emits
very toxic fumes of NO_x and HCl.

ALK500   CAS: 5959-56-8
4-AMINO-1-NAPHTHOL
HYDROCHLORIDE
mf: $C_{10}H_9NO \cdot ClH$ mw: 195.66

SYN: 1-AMINO-4-NAPHTHOL HYDROCHLORIDE

TOXICITY DATA with REFERENCE
NEO: imp-mus TDLo: 50 mg/kg   BJCAAI
12,222,58

CONSENSUS REPORTS: Reported in EPA
TSCA Inventory.

SAFETY PROFILE: Questionable carcinogen
with experimental neoplastigenic data. When
heated to decomposition it emits very toxic
fumes of NO_x and HCl.

ALK750   CAS: 605-92-5
2-AMINO-1-NAPHTHYL ESTER
SULFURIC ACID
mf: $C_{10}H_9NO_4S$ mw: 239.26

PROP: Sltly sol in water.

SYNS: 2-AMINO-1-NAPHTHYL HYDROGEN SULFATE
◇ 2-AMINO-1-NAPHTHYL HYDROGEN SULPHATE

TOXICITY DATA with REFERENCE
NEO: imp-mus TDLo: 50 mg/kg   BJCAAI
12,222,58

SAFETY PROFILE: Questionable carcinogen
with experimental neoplastigenic data. When
heated to decomposition it emits very toxic
fumes of NO_x and SO_x.

ALL000   CAS: 63976-07-8
2-AMINO-1-
NAPHTHYLGLUCOSIDURONIC ACID
mf: $C_{16}H_{17}NO_7$ mw: 335.34

SYN: 2-NAPHTHYLAMINE-1-d-GLUCOSIDURONIC ACID

TOXICITY DATA with REFERENCE
NEO: imp-mus TDLo: 80 mg/kg   BJCAAI
11,212,57

SAFETY PROFILE: Questionable carcinogen
with experimental neoplastigenic data. When
heated to decomposition it emits toxic fumes
of NO_x.

ALM000   CAS: 1211-40-1
4-AMINO-4'-NITROBIPHENYL
mf: $C_{12}H_{10}N_2O_2$ mw: 214.24

SYN: 4'-NITRO-4-BIPHENYLAMINE

TOXICITY DATA with REFERENCE
ETA: orl-rat TDLo: 1440 mg/kg/73W-I   TXAPA9
14,661,69

SAFETY PROFILE: Questionable carcinogen
with experimental tumorigenic data. When
heated to decomposition it emits toxic fumes
of NO_x.

ALM250   CAS: 3775-55-1
2-AMINO-5-(5-NITRO-2-FURYL)-1,3,4-
OXADIAZOLE
mf: $C_8H_7N_4O_4$ mw: 223.19

TOXICITY DATA with REFERENCE
CAR: orl-rat TDLo: 20 g/kg/46W-C   JNCIAM
54,841,75

SAFETY PROFILE: Questionable carcinogen
with experimental carcinogenic data. When
heated to decomposition it emits toxic fumes
of NO_x.

ALM500   CAS: 38514-71-5
2-AMINO-4-(5-NITRO-2-FURYL)
THIAZOLE
mf: $C_7H_5N_3O_3S$ mw: 211.21

SYN: ANFT

TOXICITY DATA with REFERENCE
CAR: orl-rat TDLo: 30212 mg/kg/Y-C   CRNGDP
3,275,82
NEO: orl-mus TDLo: 68 g/kg/46W-C   CNREA8
33,1593,73
ETA: orl-rat TD: 40894 mg/kg/46W-C   PAACA3
21,75,80
MUT: dnd-esc 10 μmol/L   CBINA8 31,133,80
MUT: dnd-mam: lym 50 μmol/L   CRNGDP
3,1339,82
MUT: dnr-esc 670 nmol/L   MUREAV 67,133,79

MUT: dnr-sat 500 nmol/well   CNREA8 34,2266,74
MUT: dns-dog:oth 1 μmol/L   CNREA8 42,3974,82
MUT: mma-sat 100 ng/plate   MUREAV 40,9,76
MUT: mmo-esc 300 nmol/well   CNREA8 34,2266,74
MUT: mrc-esc 500 nmol/well   CNREA8 34,2266,74
MUT: oms-omi 50 μmol/L   CRNGDP 3,1339,82

CONSENSUS REPORTS: EPA Genetic Toxicology Program.

SAFETY PROFILE: Questionable carcinogen with experimental carcinogenic, neoplastigenic, and tumorigenic data. Mutation data reported. When heated to decomposition it emits very toxic fumes of NO_x and SO_x.

ALO000   CAS: 121-88-0
2-AMINO-5-NITROPHENOL
mf: $C_6H_6N_2O_3$ mw: 154.14

SYN: C.I. 76535 ◇ NCI C55970 ◇ URSOL YELLOW BROWN A

TOXICITY DATA with REFERENCE
ETA: orl-rat TDLo: 51500 mg/kg/2Y-C   NTPTR* NTP-TR-334,88
MUT: cyt-ham:lng 1 mg/L   ATSUDG (4),41,80
MUT: mma-sat 1 μmol/plate   MUREAV 58,11,78
MUT: mmo-sat 20 μg/plate   PNASA6 72,2423,75

CONSENSUS REPORTS: NTP Carcinogenesis Studies (gavage): Some Evidence: rat NTPTR* NTP-TR-334,88. Reported in EPA TSCA Inventory. EPA Genetic Toxicology Program.

SAFETY PROFILE: Questionable carcinogen with experimental tumorigenic data. Mutation data reported. When heated to decomposition it emits toxic fumes of NO_x.

ALO750   CAS: 2871-01-4
2-((4-AMINO-2-NITROPHENYL) AMINO)ETHANOL
mf: $C_8H_{11}N_3O_3$ mw: 197.22

SYNS: HC RED NO. 3 ◇ NCI-C54922

TOXICITY DATA with REFERENCE
CAR: orl-mus TDLo: 182 g/kg/2Y-C   NTPTR* NTP-TR-281,86
MUT: mma-sat 3300 ng/plate   NTPTR* NTP-TR-281,86
MUT: mmo-sat 100 μg/plate   NTPTR* NTP-TR-281,86

CONSENSUS REPORTS: NTP Carcinogenesis Studies (gavage); Equivocal Evidence: mouse NTPTR* NTP-TR-281,86; No Evidence: rat NTPTR* NTP-TR-281,86. Reported in EPA TSCA Inventory.

SAFETY PROFILE: Questionable carcinogen with experimental carcinogenic data. Mutation data reported. When heated to decomposition it emits toxic fumes of NO_x.

ALP000   CAS: 2104-09-8
2-AMINO-4-(p-NITROPHENYL)THIAZOLE
mf: $C_9H_7N_3O_2S$ mw: 221.25

TOXICITY DATA with REFERENCE
CAR: orl-rat TDLo: 2150 mg/kg/13W-C   JNCIAM 54,841,75
ETA: orl-mus TDLo: 9600 mg/kg/46W-C   CNREA8 33,1593,73

SAFETY PROFILE: Questionable carcinogen with experimental carcinogenic data. When heated to decomposition it emits toxic NO_x and SO_x.

ALQ000   CAS: 121-66-4
2-AMINO-5-NITROTHIAZOLE
mf: $C_3H_3N_3O_2S$ mw: 145.15

SYNS: AMINONITROTHIAZOLE ◇ AMINONITROTHIAZOLUM ◇ AMINZOL SOLUBLE ◇ ENHEPTIN ◇ ENTRAMIN ◇ NCI-C03065 ◇ NITRAMIN ◇ NITRAMINE ◇ 5-NITRO-2-AMINOTHIAZOLE ◇ NITROMIN IDO ◇ 5-NITRO-2-THIAZOLYLAMINE ◇ USAF EK-6561

TOXICITY DATA with REFERENCE
CAR: orl-rat TDLo: 28 g/kg/2Y-C   NCITR* NCI-CG-TR-53,78
NEO: orl-rat TD: 23 g/kg/46W-C   JNCIAM 54,841,75
ETA: orl-rat TD: 12 g/kg/2Y-C   NCITR* NCI-CG-TR-53,78
MUT: mma-esc 800 μg/plate   ENMUDM 7(Suppl 5),1,85
MUT: mma-sat 666 μg/plate   ENMUDM 7(Suppl 5),1,85
MUT: mmo-esc 50 μmol/L   MUREAV 118,153,83
MUT: mmo-klp 200 μmol/L   MUREAV 118,153,83
MUT: mmo-sat 500 μg/plate   WTMOA3 69,19,82

CONSENSUS REPORTS: IARC Cancer Review: GROUP 3 IMEMDT 7,56,87; Animal Limited Evidence IMEMDT 31,71,83. NCI Carcinogenesis Bioassay (feed); No Evidence: mouse NCITR* NCI-CG-TR-53,78; Clear Evidence: rat NCITR* NCI-CG-TR-53,78. Reported in EPA TSCA Inventory.

SAFETY PROFILE: Questionable carcinogen with experimental carcinogenic, tumorigenic, and neoplastigenic data. Poison by intraperitoneal route. Experimental reproductive effects. Mutation data reported. When heated to decomposition it emits very toxic fumes of NO_x and SO_x. An antiprotozoal agent.

ALS000   CAS: 4176-53-8
1-AMINOPHENANTHRENE
mf: $C_{14}H_{11}N$ mw: 193.26

TOXICITY DATA with REFERENCE
ETA: orl-rat TDLo: 250 mg/kg   ZEKBAI 72,321,69
MUT: mma-sat ng/plate   ENMUDM 6,497,84

SAFETY PROFILE: Questionable carcinogen with experimental tumorigenic data. Mutation data reported. When heated to decomposition it emits toxic fumes of NO_x.

AMA250   CAS: 616-30-8
3-AMINO-1,3-PROPANEDIOL
mf: $C_3H_9NO_2$ mw: 91.13

SYNS: 1-AMINOGLYCEROL ◇ 2,3-DIHYDROXYPRO-PYLAMINE

TOXICITY DATA with REFERENCE
CAR: orl-ham TDLo: 784 mg/kg/41W-I   JCROD7 109,1,85

CONSENSUS REPORTS: Reported in EPA TSCA Inventory.

SAFETY PROFILE: Questionable carcinogen with experimental carcinogenic data. Poison by intraperitoneal route. Moderately toxic by ingestion. When heated to decomposition it emits toxic fumes of NO_x.

AMA500   CAS: 78-96-6
1-AMINOPROPAN-2-OL
mf: C_3H_9NO mw: 75.13

PROP: Liquid, slt ammonia odor, sol in water. D: 0.969, mp: 1.4°, flash p: 171°F, vap d: 2.6.

SYNS: α-AMINOISOPROPYL ALCOHOL ◇ 1-AMINO-2-PROPANOL ◇ 2-HYDROXYPROPYLAMINE ◇ ISOPROPA-NOLAMINE ◇ MONO-ISO-PROPANOLAMINE ◇ THREA-MINE

TOXICITY DATA with REFERENCE
CAR: orl-ham TDLo: 168 mg/kg/21W-I   JCROD7 109,1,85

CONSENSUS REPORTS: Reported in EPA TSCA Inventory.

SAFETY PROFILE: Questionable carcinogen with experimental carcinogenic data. Poison by intraperitoneal route. Moderately toxic by ingestion and skin contact. A skin and severe eye irritant. Moderately flammable by heat, flame, sparks, powerful oxidizers. To fight fire, use alcohol foam. When heated to decomposition it emits toxic fumes of NO_x.

AMG750   CAS: 54-62-6
AMINOPTERIDINE
mf: $C_{19}H_{20}N_8O_5$ mw: 440.47

PROP: Yellow needles, sol in sodium hydroxide soln.

SYNS: 4-AMINO-4-DEOXYPTEROYLGLUTAMATE ◇ 4-AMINO-PGA ◇ AMINOPTERIN ◇ 4-AMINOPTEROYL-GLUTAMIC ACID ◇ APGA ◇ ENT 26,079 ◇ FOLIC ACID, 4-AMINO- ◇ NSC 739

TOXICITY DATA with REFERENCE
ETA: ims-rat TDLo: 1200 μg/kg/17W-C
    AMUK** 38,248,62
MUT: spm-mus-ipr 2 mg/kg/5D   PNASA6 78,4425,78

CONSENSUS REPORTS: EPA Extremely Hazardous Substances List.

SAFETY PROFILE: Questionable carcinogen with experimental tumorigenic data. Poison by ingestion and intraperitoneal routes. Human and experimental teratogenic data. Mutation data reported. Human systemic effects by ingestion: gastrointestinal. When heated to decomposition it emits toxic fumes of NO_x.

AMK500   CAS: 68-89-3
AMINOPYRINE SODIUM SULFONATE
mf: $C_{13}H_{17}N_3O_4S•Na$ mw: 334.38
SYNS:
(ANTIPYRINYLMETHYLAMINO)METHANESULFONIC ACID SODIUM SALT ◇ METHYLAMINOANTIPYRINE SODIUM METHANESULFONATE ◇ 4-METHYLAMINO-1,5-DIMETH-YL-2-PHENYL-3-PYRAZOLONE SODIUM METHANESULFO-NATE ◇ METHYLAMINOPHENYLDIMETHYL-PYRAZOLONE METHANESULFONATE SODIUM ◇ 1-PHE-NYL-2,3-DIMETHYL-5-PYRAZOLONE-4-METHYLAMINO-METHANESULFONATE SODIUM ◇ 1-PHENYL-2,3-DI-METHYLPYRAZOLONE-(5)-4-METHYLAMINOMETHANE-SULFONIC ACID SODIUM ◇ PHENYL DIMETHYL PYRAZOLON METHYL AMINOMETHANE SODIUM SULFONATE ◇ 4-SODIUM METHANESULFONATE METH-YLAMINE-ANTIPYRINE ◇ SODIUM METHYLAMINOANTI-

PYRINE METHANESULFONATE ◇ SODIUM-4-METHYL-
AMINO-1,5-DIMETHYL-2-PHENYL-3-PYRAZOLONE 4-
METHANESULFONATE ◇ SODIUM NORAMIDOPYRINE
METHANESULFONATE ◇ SODIUM-1-PHENYL-2,3-DI-
METHYL-4-METHYLAMINOPYRAZOLON-N-METHANE-
SULFONATE ◇ SODIUM-1-PHENYL-2,3-DIMETHYL-5-
PYRAZOLONE-4-METHYLAMINO METHANESULFONATE
◇ SODIUM PHENYLDIMETHYLPYRAZOLONMETH-
YLAMINOMETHANE SULFONATE

TOXICITY DATA with REFERENCE
NEO: orl-mus TD:792 mg/kg/78W-C   JJIND8
71,1295,83
NEO: orl-mus TDLo:536 mg/kg/78W-C   JJIND8
71,1295,83
MUT: cyt-hmn:lym 250 mg/L   SOGEBZ 11,528,75
MUT: mma-sat:1 mg/plate   AMONDS 3,253,80

SAFETY PROFILE: Questionable carcinogen
with experimental neoplastigenic data. Poison
by subcutaneous route. Moderately toxic by several other routes. An experimental teratogen.
Human mutation data reported. When heated
to decomposition it emits very toxic fumes of
NO_x, Na_2O and SO_x.

AMO000   CAS: 4309-66-4
trans-4-AMINOSTILBENE
mf: $C_{14}H_{13}N$ mw: 195.28

SYNS: 4-(2-PHENYLETHENYL)BENZENAMINE,(E)
◇ trans-4-STILBENE ◇ trans-4-N-STILBENAMINE

TOXICITY DATA with REFERENCE
CAR: orl-rat TDLo:200 mg/kg/13W-C   CNREA8
24,128,64
CAR: scu-rat TDLo:26 mg/kg/4W-I   CNREA8
24,128,64
ETA: scu-rat TD:63 mg/kg/6W-I   PTRMAD
241,147,48
ETA: scu-rat TD:200 mg/kg/7W-I   PTRMAD
241,147,48
MUT: mma-sat 10 µg/plate   PNASA6 70,2281,73

SAFETY PROFILE: Questionable carcinogen
with experimental carcinogenic and tumorigenic data. Mutation data reported. When
heated to decomposition it emits toxic fumes
of NO_x.

AMO250   CAS: 3432-10-8
2-(p-AMINOSTYRYL)-6-(p-ACETYLAMINOBENZOYLAMINO) QUINOLINE METHOACETATE
mf: $C_{27}H_{25}N_4O_2 \cdot C_2H_3O_2$ mw: 496.61

SYN: STYRYL 430

TOXICITY DATA with REFERENCE
ETA: scu-mus TD:350 mg/kg   JPBAA7 47,155,38
ETA: scu-mus TDLo:268 mg/kg   JPBAA7
42,155,36
MUT: mmo-esc 1 pph   CRSBAW 142,453,48

SAFETY PROFILE: Questionable carcinogen
with experimental tumorigenic data. Mutation
data reported. When heated to decomposition
it emits toxic fumes of NO_x.

AMW000   CAS: 2432-99-7
11-AMINOUNDECANOIC ACID
mf: $C_{11}H_{23}NO_2$ mw: 201.35

SYNS: AMINOUNDECANOIC ACID ◇ 11-AMINOUNDE-
CYLIC ACID ◇ NCI-C50613

TOXICITY DATA with REFERENCE
CAR: orl-rat TDLo:655 g/kg/2Y-C   NTPTR*
NTP-TR-216,82
NEO: orl-rat TD:328 g/kg/2Y-C   NTPTR* NTP-
TR-216,82
MUT: otr-ham:emb 2500 mmol/L   ENMUDM
8,515,86
MUT: sce-ham:ovr 500 mg/L   EMMUEG 10(Suppl
10),1,87

CONSENSUS REPORTS: IARC Cancer Re-
view: GROUP 3 IMEMDT 7,56,87; Animal
Limited Evidence IMEMDT 39,239,86. NTP
Carcinogenesis Bioassay (feed): Clear Evi-
dence: mouse, rat NTPTR* NTP-TR-216,82.
Reported in EPA TSCA Inventory.

SAFETY PROFILE: Questionable carcinogen
with experimental carcinogenic and neoplastigenic data. Mutation data reported. When heated
to decomposition it emits toxic fumes of NO_x.

AMW750   CAS: 6623-41-2
2-AMINO-4,5-XYLENOL
mf: $C_8H_{11}NO$ mw: 137.20

SYN: 2-AMINO-4,5-DIMETHYLPHENOL

TOXICITY DATA with REFERENCE
CAR: imp-mus TDLo:80 mg/kg   BJCAAI
11,212,57

CONSENSUS REPORTS: Reported in EPA
TSCA Inventory.

SAFETY PROFILE: Questionable carcinogen
with experimental carcinogenic data. When
heated to decomposition it emits toxic fumes
of NO_x.

ANT250   CAS: 64046-00-0
AMMONIUM POTASSIUM SELENIDE mixed with AMMONIUM POTASSIUM SULFIDE
mf: $H_4KNSe + NH_4KS$ mw: 136.11 + 89.21 = 225.32

SYN: AMMONIUM POTASSIUM SULFIDE mixed with AMMONIUM POTASSIUM SELENIDE

TOXICITY DATA with REFERENCE
ETA: orl-rat TDLo:450 mg/kg/2Y-C   CNREA8 3,230,43

CONSENSUS REPORTS: Selenium and its compounds are on the Community Right-To-Know List.

ACGIH TLV: TWA 0.2 mg(Se)/m^3

OSHA PEL: TWA 0.2 mg(Se)/m^3

SAFETY PROFILE: Questionable carcinogen with experimental tumorigenic data. When heated to decomposition it emits very toxic fumes of NO_x, NH_3, SO_x, and Se.

AOE000
AMYL ALCOHOL
mf: $C_5H_{12}O$ mw: 88.1

PROP: Clear liquid. Mp: −79°, bp: 137.8°, flash p: 91°F (CC), d: 0.8168 @ 20°/20°, ulc: 40, lel: 1.2%, uel: 10% @ 212°F, vap press: 1 mm @ 13.6°, 10 mm @ 44.9°, vap d: 3.04, sol in water; misc in alc and ether.

SYNS: ALCOOL AMYLIQUE (FRENCH) ◇ N-AMYL ALCOHOL ◇ AMYL ALCOHOL, NORMAL ◇ N-AMYLALKOHOL (CZECH) ◇ N-BUTYLCARBINOL ◇ PENTANOL-1 ◇ N-PENTANOL ◇ PENTAN-1-OL ◇ PENTASOL ◇ PENTYL ALCOHOL ◇ PRIMARY AMYL ALCOHOL

TOXICITY DATA with REFERENCE
ETA: ipr-mus TDLo:1200 mg/kg/8W-I   CNREA8 33,3069,73

CONSENSUS REPORTS: Reported in EPA TSCA Inventory.

SAFETY PROFILE: Questionable carcinogen with experimental tumorigenic data. Moderately toxic by ingestion and skin contact. An eye and upper respiratory irritant by inhalation. A severe skin and eye irritant. Ingestion can cause headache, nausea, vomiting, delirium, and methemoglobin formation. Extremely flammable if exposed to heat, flame or powerful oxidizers. To fight fire use alcohol foam, dry chemical. Moderately explosive when exposed to flame.

AOE750   CAS: 63018-99-5
5-n-AMYL-1:2-BENZANTHRACENE
mf: $C_{23}H_{22}$ mw: 298.45

SYN: 8-PENTYLBENZ(a)ANTHRACENE

TOXICITY DATA with REFERENCE
ETA: skn-mus TDLo:790 mg/kg/33W-I   PRLBA4 129,439,40

SAFETY PROFILE: Questionable carcinogen with experimental tumorigenic data. When heated to decomposition it emits acrid smoke and irritating fumes.

AOL750   CAS: 64005-62-5
n-AMYL-N-NITROSOURETHANE
mf: $C_8H_{16}N_2O_3$ mw: 188.26

SYN: N-NITROSO-N-PENTYLCARBAMIC ACID-ETHYL ESTER

TOXICITY DATA with REFERENCE
CAR: orl-rat TD:4200 mg/kg/40W-C   GANNA2 73,48,82
CAR: orl-rat TD:7350 mg/kg/35W-C   GANNA2 73,48,82
CAR: orl-rat TDLo:2625 mg/kg/50W-C   GANNA2 73,48,82
ETA: orl-rat TDLo:5880 mg/kg/24W-C   GANNA2 70,653,79
MUT: cyt-ham:fbr 63 mg/L/48H   MUREAV 48,337,77

SAFETY PROFILE: Questionable carcinogen with experimental carcinogenic and tumorigenic data. Mutation data reported. When heated to decomposition it emits toxic fumes of NO_x.

AOM150   CAS: 9047-13-6
AMYLOPECTINE SULPHATE

SYNS: AMYLOPECTIN, HYDROGEN SULFATE ◇ AMYLOPECTIN SULFATE ◇ AMYLOPECTIN SULFATE (SN-263) ◇ SULFATED AMYLOPECTIN

TOXICITY DATA with REFERENCE
CAR: orl-rat TDLo:621 g/kg/24W-C   JUIZAG 32,479,86

SAFETY PROFILE: Questionable carcinogen with experimental carcinogenic data. Poison by subcutaneous and intraperitoneal route. When heated to decomposition it emits toxic fumes of NO_x and SO_x.

AOM250   CAS: 14938-35-3
4-n-AMYLPHENOL
mf: $C_{11}H_{16}O$ mw: 164.27

PROP: Liquid. Bp: 342°, vap d: 5.66, flash p: 219°F (OC), d: 0.966.

SYN: p-PENTYLPHENOL

TOXICITY DATA with REFERENCE
NEO: skn-mus TDLo:4100 mg/kg/12W-I
CNREA8 19,413,59

CONSENSUS REPORTS: Reported in EPA TSCA Inventory.

SAFETY PROFILE: Questionable carcinogen with experimental neoplastigenic data. Moderately flammable. To fight fire, use foam, CO_2, dry chemical. When heated to decomposition it emits acrid smoke and irritating fumes.

AOM500
2-sec-AMYLPHENOL
mf: $C_{11}H_{16}O$ mw: 164.27

PROP: Clear, straw-colored liquid; very sltly sol in water, sol in oils and organic solvents. D: 0.955-0.971 @ 30°/30°, bp: 235-250°, flash p: 200°F.

SYN: o-(sec-PENTYL) PHENOL

TOXICITY DATA with REFERENCE
NEO: skn-mus TDLo:4100 mg/kg/12W-I
CNREA8 19,413,59

SAFETY PROFILE: Questionable carcinogen with experimental neoplastigenic data by skin contact. Poison by intravenous route. Moderately flammable when exposed to heat or flame. To fight fire, use foam, fog, dry chemical, water mist or spray, multi-purpose dry chemical. When heated to decomposition it emits acrid smoke and irritating fumes.

AOM750   CAS: 25735-67-5
4-sec-AMYLPHENOL
mf: $C_{11}H_{16}O$ mw: 164.27

PROP: D: <1.0, bp: 482°-516°F, flash p: 270°F.

SYN: p-(sec-PENTYL) PHENOL

TOXICITY DATA with REFERENCE
ETA: skn-mus TDLo:4080 mg/kg/12W-I
CNREA8 19,413,59

SAFETY PROFILE: Questionable carcinogen with experimental tumorigenic data. Combustible when exposed to heat or flame. To fight fire, use dry chemical, water mist, CO_2. When

heated to decomposition it emits acrid smoke and fumes.

AOO000
ANAGESTONE ACETATE mixed with MESTRANOL (10:1)
mf: $C_{24}H_{36}O_3$ mw: 372.60

SYNS: ANATROPIN mixed with MESTRANOL (10:1)
◇ MESTRANOL mixed with ANAGESTONE ACETATE (1:10)

TOXICITY DATA with REFERENCE
ETA: orl-dog TD:333 mg/kg/3Y-I   JNCIAM
59,933,77
ETA: orl-dog TD:554 mg/kg/5Y-I   JTEHD6
3,179,77
ETA: orl-dog TD:601 mg/kg/2Y-I   JJIND8
65,137,80
ETA: orl-dog TDLo:259 mg/kg/2Y-I   JJIND8
65,137,80

SAFETY PROFILE: Questionable carcinogen with experimental tumorigenic data. When heated to decomposition it emits acrid smoke and irritating fumes.

AOO425   CAS: 63-05-8
ANDROSTENEDIONE
mf: $C_{19}H_{26}O_2$ mw: 286.45

PROP: Dimorphous: Needles from acetone. Mp: 142-144°. Crystals from hexane, mp: 173-174°.

SYNS: Δ-(4)-ANDROSTEN-3,17-DIONE ◇ Δ(4)-ANDRO-STENE-3,17-DIONE ◇ Δ-4-ANDROSTENEDIONE ◇ 4-AN-DROSTENE-3,17-DIONE ◇ ANDROTEX ◇ SKF 2170

TOXICITY DATA with REFERENCE
ETA: scu-mus TDLo:600 mg/kg/72W-I
JNCIAM 19,977,57

SAFETY PROFILE: Questionable carcinogen with experimental tumorigenic data. Experimental reproductive effects. An experimental teratogen. When heated to decomposition it emits acrid smoke and irritating fumes.

AOO450   CAS: 53-43-0
ANDROSTENOLONE
mf: $C_{19}H_{28}O_2$ mw: 288.47

PROP: Dimorphous: Needles. Mp: 140-141°. Leaflets. mp: 152-153°. Sol in benzene, alcohol, ether; sparingly sol in chloroform and petr ether.

SYNS: 17-CHETOVIS ◇ trans-DEHYDROANDROSTERONE ◇ DEHYDROEPIANDROSTERONE ◇ 5-DEHYDROEPIAN-DROSTERONE ◇ DEHYDROISOANDROSTERONE

◇ 5,6-DEHYDROISOANDROSTERONE ◇ DHA ◇ DIANDRON ◇ DIANDRONE ◇ 5,6-DIDEHYDROISOANDROSTERONE ◇ 17-HORMOFORIN ◇ 3-β-HYDROXY-5-ANDROSTEN-17-ONE ◇ PRASTERONE ◇ PSICOSTERONE

TOXICITY DATA with REFERENCE
NEO: imp-mus TDLo:400 mg/kg/50D-C
CNREA8 48,2788,88
NEO: orl-mus TDLo:25 g/kg/52D-C   CNREA8 48,2788,88

SAFETY PROFILE: Questionable carcinogen with experimental neoplastigenic data. An experimental teratogen. Experimental reproductive effects. When heated to decomposition it emits acrid smoke and irritating fumes.

AOR500   CAS: 548-62-9
ANILINE VIOLET
mf: $C_{25}H_{30}N_3 \cdot Cl$ mw: 408.03

SYNS: AIZEN CRYSTAL VIOLET EXTRA PURE ◇ GENTIAN VIOLET ◇ HEXAMETHYL-p-ROSANILINE HYDROCHLORIDE ◇ HEXAMETHYL VIOLET ◇ METHYL-ROSANILINE CHLORIDE ◇ NCI-C55969

TOXICITY DATA with REFERENCE
CAR: orl-mus TDLo:25750 mg/kg/2Y-C
FAATDF 5,902,85
MUT: cyt-ham:ovr 500 μg/L   MUREAV 58,269,78
MUT: cyt-hmn:hla 500 μg/L   MUREAV 58,269,78
MUT: cyt-hmn:lym 500 μg/L   MUREAV 58,269,78
MUT: mmo-sat 100 ng/plate   MUREAV 89,21,81

CONSENSUS REPORTS: Reported in EPA TSCA Inventory.

SAFETY PROFILE: Questionable carcinogen with experimental carcinogenic data. Poison by ingestion, intravenous, intraperitoneal, and intraduodenal routes. Experimental reproductive effects. A human skin irritant. Human mutation data reported. When heated to decomposition it emits very toxic fumes of NO_x and Cl^-.

AOV250   CAS: 7466-54-8
o-ANISIC ACID, HYDRAZIDE
mf: $C_8H_{10}N_2O_2$ mw: 166.20

SYNS: o-METHOXYBENZOHYDRAZIDE ◇ o-METHOXYBENZOIC ACID HYDRAZIDE ◇ 2-METHOXYBENZOIC ACID HYDRAZIDE ◇ o-METHOXYBENZOYLHYDRAZIDE ◇ 2-METHOXYBENZOYL HYDRAZIDE ◇ 2-METHOXYBENZOYLHYDRAZINE

TOXICITY DATA with REFERENCE
NEO: orl-mus TDLo:6000 mg/kg/22W-I
34ZRA9 -,869,66

SAFETY PROFILE: Questionable carcinogen with experimental neoplastigenic data. When heated to decomposition it emits toxic fumes of NO_x.

AOV500   CAS: 3290-99-1
p-ANISIC ACID, HYDRAZIDE
mf: $C_8H_{10}N_2O_2$ mw: 166.20

SYNS: ANISIC ACID HYDRAZIDE ◇ ANISIC HYDRAZIDE ◇ ANISOYLHYDRAZINE ◇ p-ANISOYLHYDRAZINE ◇ p-METHOXYBENZOIC ACID HYDRAZIDE ◇ 4-METHOXYBENZOIC ACID HYDRAZIDE ◇ p-METHOXYBENZOIC HYDRAZIDE ◇ 4-METHOXYBENZOYL HYDRAZIDE ◇ (p-METHOXYBENZOYL)HYDRAZINE ◇ 4-METHOXYBENZOYLHYDRAZINE

TOXICITY DATA with REFERENCE
NEO: orl-mus TDLo:12 g/kg/22W-I
34ZRA9 -,869,66

SAFETY PROFILE: Questionable carcinogen with experimental neoplastigenic data. Poison by intravenous route. When heated to decomposition it emits toxic fumes of NO_x.

AOX500   CAS: 20265-97-8
p-ANISIDINE HYDROCHLORIDE
mf: $C_7H_9NO \cdot ClH$ mw: 159.63

SYN: NCI-C03758

TOXICITY DATA with REFERENCE
CAR: orl-rat TDLo:2163 g/kg/1Y-C   IMEMDT 27,63,82
ETA: orl-rat TDLo:116 g/kg/92W-C   NCITR* NCI-CG-TR-116,78

CONSENSUS REPORTS: IARC Cancer Review: Animal Inadequate Evidence IMEMDT 27,63,82; NCI Carcinogenesis Bioassay (feed); No Evidence: mouse NCITR* NCI-CG-TR-116,78; Inadequate Studies: rat NCITR* NCI-CG-TR-116,78. Reported in EPA TSCA Inventory.

SAFETY PROFILE: Questionable carcinogen with experimental carcinogenic and tumorigenic data. When heated to decomposition it emits very toxic fumes of NO_x and HCl.

APE750   CAS: 191-26-4
ANTHANTHRENE
mf: $C_{22}H_{12}$ mw: 276.34

SYNS: ANTHANTHREN (GERMAN) ◇ ANTHRANTHRENE ◇ DIBENZO-(drf,mno)CHRYSENE ◇ DIBENZO(cd,mk)PYRENE

TOXICITY DATA with REFERENCE
CAR: imp-rat TDLo: 4150 µg/kg   JJIND8 71,539,83
CAR: skn-mus TDLo: 263 mg/kg/30W-I
  ZKKOBW 89,113,77
ETA: imp-rat TD: 5 mg/kg   50NNAZ 7,571,83
ETA: skn-mus TD: 2100 mg/kg/88W-I   PRLBA4
129,439,40
MUT: mma-sat 1 µg/plate   MUREAV 51,311,78

CONSENSUS REPORTS: IARC Cancer Review: GROUP 3 IMEMDT 7,56,87; Animal Limited Evidence IMEMDT 32,95,83

SAFETY PROFILE: Questionable carcinogen with experimental carcinogenic and tumorigenic data. Mutation data reported. A polycyclic hydrocarbon found in polluted air. When heated to decomposition it emits acrid fumes.

APF750   CAS: 189-58-2
ANTHRA(9,1,2-cde)BENZO(h)
CINNOLINE
mf: $C_{22}H_{12}N_2$ mw: 304.36

SYN: 1,2-DIAZA-3,4:9,10-DIBENZPYRENE

TOXICITY DATA with REFERENCE
ETA: scu-mus TDLo: 80 mg/kg   IJMRAQ 53,638,65

SAFETY PROFILE: Questionable carcinogen with experimental tumorigenic data. When heated to decomposition it emits toxic fumes of NO_x.

APG250   CAS: 610-49-1
1-ANTHRACENAMINE
mf: $C_{14}H_{11}N$ mw: 193.26

PROP: Yellow needles from alc. Mp: 130°. Insol HCl, sol in alc.

SYNS: α-AMINOANTHRACENE ◊ 1-AMINOANTHRACENE ◊ 1-ANTHRACYLAMINE ◊ 1-ANTHRAMINE

TOXICITY DATA with REFERENCE
ETA: orl-rat TDLo: 7200 mg/kg/27D-I   CNREA8
28,924,68
MUT: dnr-esc 100 mg/L   JNCIAM 62,873,79
MUT: mma-sat 20 µg/plate   PNASA6 72,5135,75
MUT: mrc-smc 5 pph   JNCIAM 62,901,79

SAFETY PROFILE: Questionable carcinogen with experimental tumorigenic data. Mutation data reported. When heated to decomposition it emits toxic fumes of NO_x.

APG500   CAS: 120-12-7
ANTHRACENE
mf: $C_{14}H_{10}$ mw: 178.24

PROP: Colorless crystals, violet fluorescence. Mp: 217°, lel: 0.6%, flash p: 250°F (CC), d: 1.24 @ 27°/4°, autoign temp: 1004°F, vap press: 1 mm @ 145.0°, (sublimes), vap d: 6.15, bp: 339.9°. Insol in water. Solubility in alc @ 1.9/100 @ 20°; in ether 12.2/100 @ 20°.

SYNS: ANTHRACEN (GERMAN) ◊ ANTHRACIN ◊ GREEN OIL ◊ PARANAPHTHALENE ◊ TETRA OLIVE N2G

TOXICITY DATA with REFERENCE
NEO: scu-rat TDLo: 3300 mg/kg/33W-I
  NATWAY 42,159,55
ETA: orl-rat TDLo: 20 g/kg/79W-I   ZEKBAI
60,697,55
ETA: scu-rat TD: 660 mg/kg/33W-I   ZEKBAI
60,697,55
MUT: dnd-mam: lym 100 µmol   BIPMAA 9,689,70
MUT: dns-hmn: fbr 10 mg/L   CNREA8 38,2091,78
MUT: hma-mus/sat 125 mg/kg   JNCIAM 62,911,79
MUT: mma-sat 100 µg/plate   ABCHA6 43,1433,79
MUT: skn-mus 118 µg MLD   CALEDQ 4,333,78

CONSENSUS REPORTS: Reported in EPA TSCA Inventory. Community Right-To-Know List. IARC Cancer Review: Animal No Evidence IMEMDT 32,105,83

OSHA PEL: TWA 0.2 mg/m³

SAFETY PROFILE: Questionable carcinogen with experimental neoplastigenic and tumorigenic data. A skin irritant and allergen. Mutation data reported. Combustible when exposed to heat, flame, or oxidizing materials. Moderately explosive when exposed to flame; $Ca(OCl)_2$; chromic acid. To fight fire, use water, foam, CO_2, water spray or mist, dry chemical. Explodes on contact with fluorine.

APH250   CAS: 480-22-8
1,8,9-ANTHRACENETRIOL
mf: $C_{14}H_{10}O_3$ mw: 226.24

PROP: Yellow powder. Mp: 178-180°. Insol in water; sol in fat, hot alc, benzene and dilute alkalies.

SYNS: ANTHRALIN ◊ 1,8,9-ANTHRATRIOL ◊ DIHYDROXYANTHRANOL ◊ 1,8-DIHYDROXYANTHRANOL ◊ 1,8-DIHYDROXY-9-ANTHRANOL ◊ 1,8-DIHYDROXY-9-ANTHRONE ◊ DIOXYANTHRANOL ◊ 1,8,9-TRIHYDROXYANTHRACENE

TOXICITY DATA with REFERENCE
NEO: skn-mus TDLo: 509 mg/kg/53W-I
  JMCMAR 21,26,78

ETA: skn-mus TD: 240 mg/kg/50W-I   JPETAB
229,255,84

ETA: skn-mus TD: 73 mg/kg/11W-I   GANNA2
59,187,68

MUT: dnr-esc 250 μg/plate   JNCIAM 62,873,79

MUT: mma-sat 100 μg/plate   BCSTB5 5,1489,77

MUT: mmo-sat 100 μg/plate   BCSTB5 5,1489,77

MUT: mmo-smc 165 nmol/L   ADVEA4 51,45,71

CONSENSUS REPORTS: IARC Cancer Review: GROUP 3 IMEMDT 7,56,87; Animal Limited Evidence IMEMDT 13,75,77

SAFETY PROFILE: Questionable carcinogen with experimental neoplastigenic and tumorigenic data. Mutation data reported. Skin contact can cause folliculitis. Absorption can cause kidney damage and intestinal disturbances. Combustible when heated. When heated to decomposition it emits acrid smoke and irritating fumes.

API500   CAS: 118-92-3
ANTHRANILIC ACID
mf: $C_7H_7NO_2$ mw: 137.15

PROP: Needle-like crystals. Mp: 146°, bp: subl, d: 1.412 @ 20°. Solubility: in water = 0.35/100 @ 14°, in 90% alc = 10.7/100 @ 10°, in ether = 16/100 @ 70°.

SYNS: o-AMINOBENZOIC ACID ◇ 2-AMINOBENZOIC ACID ◇ 1-AMINO-2-CARBOXYBENZENE ◇ CARBOXYANILINE ◇ o-CARBOXYANILINE ◇ 2-CARBOXYANILINE ◇ NCI-C01730 ◇ o-AMIDOBENZOIC ACID ◇ VITAMIN L

TOXICITY DATA with REFERENCE
ETA: orl-rat TDLo: 16 g/kg/25W-C   APMIAL
26,447,49

ETA: scu-mus TDLo: 1345 mg/kg/21D-I
JCROD7 96,163,80

CONSENSUS REPORTS: IARC Cancer Review: Animal Inadequate Evidence IMEMDT 16,265,78. NTP Carcinogenesis Bioassay (feed): No Evidence: mouse, rat NCITR* NCI-TR-36,78. Reported in EPA TSCA Inventory.

SAFETY PROFILE: Questionable carcinogen with experimental tumorigenic data. Experimental reproductive effects. Moderately toxic by intraperitoneal route. Combustible. When heated to decomposition it emits toxic fumes of NO_x.

APM750   CAS: 1715-81-7
9-ANTHRONOL
mf: $C_{14}H_{10}O_2$ mw: 210.24

TOXICITY DATA with REFERENCE
NEO: skn-mus TDLo: 700 mg/kg/73W-I
JMCMAR 21,26,78

SAFETY PROFILE: Questionable carcinogen with experimental neoplastigenic data. When heated to decomposition it emits acrid smoke and irritating fumes.

AQB750   CAS: 7440-36-0
ANTIMONY
DOT: 2871
af: Sb   aw: 121.75

PROP: Silvery or gray, lustrous metal. Mp: 630°, bp: 1635°, d: 6.684 @ 25°, vap press: 1 mm @ 886°. Insol in water; sol in hot concentrated H_2SO_4.

SYNS: ANTIMONY BLACK ◇ ANTIMONY REGULUS ◇ ANTYMON (POLISH) ◇ C.I. 77050 ◇ STIBIUM

TOXICITY DATA with REFERENCE
CAR: ihl-rat TCLo: 50 mg/m³/7H/52W-I
JTEHD6 18,607,86

CONSENSUS REPORTS: Antimony and its compounds are on the Community Right-To-Know List. Reported in EPA TSCA Inventory.

OSHA PEL: TWA 0.5 mg(Sb)/m³ ACGIH TLV: TWA 0.5 mg(Sb)/m³ DFG MAK: 0.5 mg(Sb)/m³ NIOSH REL: TWA 0.5 mg(Sb)/m³ DOT Classification: Poison B; LABEL: St. Andrews Cross.

SAFETY PROFILE: Questionable carcinogen with experimental carcinogenic data. An experimental poison by intraperitoneal route. Moderate fire and explosion hazard in the forms of dust and vapor, when exposed to heat or flame. When heated or on contact with acid, emits toxic fumes of SbH_3.

AQN000   CAS: 60-80-0
ANTIPYRINE
mf: $C_{11}H_{12}N_2O$ mw: 188.23

PROP: Fine, white crystals. Mp: 113°, bp: 319° @ 174 mm, d: 1.19. Very sol in water and alc; sltly sol in ether.

SYNS: DIMETHYLOXYQUINAZINE ◇ 2,3-DIMETHYL-1-PHENYL-3-PYRAZOLIN-5-ONE ◇ 2,3-DIMETHYL-1-PHENYL-5-PYRAZOLONE ◇ OXYDIMETHYLQUINAZINE ◇ PHENAZONE (PHARMACEUTICAL) ◇ 1-PHENYL-2,3-DIMETHYLPYRAZOLE-5-ONE ◇ 1-PHENYL-2,3-DIMETHYL-5-PYRAZOLONE

TOXICITY DATA with REFERENCE
ETA: orl-rat TDLo: 361 g/kg/92W-C   IJCNAW
27,521,81

CONSENSUS REPORTS: Reported in EPA TSCA Inventory.

SAFETY PROFILE: Questionable carcinogen with experimental tumorigenic data. A human poison by an unspecified route. Moderately toxic via ingestion, subcutaneous, and intravenous routes. When heated to decomposition it emits toxic fumes of NO_x.

AQN635   CAS: 86-88-4
ANTU
DOT: 1651
mf: $C_{11}H_{10}N_2S$ mw: 202.29

PROP: Crystals; bitter taste. Mp: 198°. Sltly sol in hot alc.

SYNS: ALPHANAPHTHYL THIOUREA ◇ ALPHA-NAPHTYL THIOUREE (FRENCH) ◇ ALRATO ◇ ANTURAT ◇ CHEMICAL 109 ◇ DIRAX ◇ KILL KANTZ ◇ KRYSID ◇ 1-NAFTIL-TIOUREA (ITALIAN) ◇ 1-NAFTYLTHIOUREUM (DUTCH) ◇ 1-NAPHTHALENYLTHIOUREA ◇ α-NAPHTHAL-THIOHARNSTOFF (GERMAN) ◇ α-NAPHTHOTHIOUREA ◇ α-NAPHTHYLTHIOCARBAMIDE ◇ 1-NAPHTHYL-THIO-HARNSTOFF (GERMAN) ◇ 1-NAPHTHYL THIOUREA (MAK) ◇ α-NAPHTHYLTHIOUREA ◇ 1-(1-NAPHTHYL)-2-THIOUREA ◇ N-(1-NAPHTHYL)-2-THIOUREA ◇ α-NAPH-THYLTHIOUREA (DOT) ◇ 1-NAPHTHYL-THIOUREE (FRENCH) ◇ NAPHTOX ◇ RATTRACK ◇ RCRA WASTE NUMBER P072 ◇ SMEESANA ◇ U-5227 ◇ USAF EK-P-5976

TOXICITY DATA with REFERENCE
ETA: scu-mus TDLo: 5 mg/kg   NTIS**
PB223-159
MUT: mma-sat 500 µmol/L   ENMUDM 3,11,81
MUT: otr-ham:emb 1600 µg/L   NCIMAV 58,243,81

CONSENSUS REPORTS: IARC Cancer Review: Animal Inadequate Evidence IMEMDT 30,347,83. Reported in EPA TSCA Inventory. EPA Extremely Hazardous Substances List. EPA Genetic Toxicology Program.

OSHA PEL: TWA 0.3 mg/m^3 ACGIH TLV: TWA 0.3 mg/m^3 DFG MAK: 0.3 mg/m^3 DOT Classification: Poison B; Label: Poison.

SAFETY PROFILE: Questionable carcinogen with experimental tumorigenic data. Poison by ingestion and intraperitoneal routes. Moderately toxic to humans by an unspecified route. Mutagenic data. A rodenticide used extensively.

Death is caused by pulmonary edema. Chronic toxicity has been known to cause dermatitis and a decrease in the white blood cells. When heated to decomposition it emits toxic fumes of NO_x and SO_x.

AQO500   CAS: 641-81-6
APOCHOLIC ACID
mf: $C_{24}H_{38}O_4$ mw: 390.62

SYN: 3-α,12-α-DIHYDROXY-5-β-CHOL-8(14)-EN-24-OIC ACID

TOXICITY DATA with REFERENCE
ETA: scu-mus TDLo: 200 mg/kg/13W-I
NATUAS 190,1007,61

SAFETY PROFILE: Questionable carcinogen with experimental tumorigenic data. When heated to decomposition it emits acrid smoke and irritating fumes.

AQQ750   CAS: 147-94-4
ARABINOCYTIDINE
mf: $C_9H_{13}N_3O_5$ mw: 243.25

SYNS: 4-AMINO-1-ARABINOFURANOSYL-2-OXO-1,2-DIHYDROPYRIMIDINE ◇ 4-AMINO-1-β-d-ARABINOFURA-NOSYL-2(1H)-PYRIMIDINONE (9CI) ◇ 1-β-d-ARABINOFURA-NOSYL-4-AMINO-2(1H)PYRIMIDINONE ◇ 1-ARABINOFU-RANOSYLCYTOSINE ◇ 1-β-ARABINOFURANOSYLCYTO-SINE ◇ 1-(β-d-ARABINOFURANOSYL)CYTOSINE ◇ β-d-ARABINOSYLCYTOSINE ◇ CYTOSINE-β-ARABINOSIDE ◇ CYTOSINE β-d-ARABINOSIDE ◇ NCI-C04728 ◇ NSC 63878

TOXICITY DATA with REFERENCE
ETA: ipr-mus TDLo: 4836 mg/kg/26W-I
CANCAR 40,1935,77
ETA: ipr-rat TDLo: 2500 mg/kg/7W-I   CANCAR
40,1935,77
MUT: cyt-ham: fbr 100 mg/L   CNREA8 30,2477,70
MUT: cyt-hmn: leu 50 µmol/L/6H   ECREAL
46,276,67
MUT: cyt-hmn: lym 3 mg/L/4H   SOGEBZ
12,1552,76
MUT: cyt-mus-scu 315 mg/kg   MUREAV 58,67,78

CONSENSUS REPORTS: NCI Carcinogenesis Studies (ipr); No Evidence: mouse, rat CANCAR 40,1935,77

SAFETY PROFILE: Questionable carcinogen with experimental tumorigenic data. An experimental teratogen. Human systemic effects: peripheral nerve fasciculations, degenerative brain changes, allergic dermatitis (after systemic exposure), blood changes, hearing acuity change, ataxia, spleen changes, central nervous system effects. A human skin and eye irritant. Human mutagenic data. When heated to decomposition it emits toxic fumes of NO_x.

AQT500   CAS: 39300-45-3
ARATHANE
mf: $C_{18}H_{24}N_2O_6$ mw: 364.44

PROP: Liquid.

SYNS: CAPRYLDINITROPHENYL CROTONATE ◇ 2-CAPRYL-4,6-DINITROPHENYL CROTONATE ◇ CROTONATE de 2,4-DINITRO 6-(1-METHYL-HEPTYL)-PHENYLE (FRENCH) ◇ 4,6-DINITRO-2-CAPRYLPHENYL CROTONATE ◇ 4,6-DINITRO-2-(2-CAPRYL)PHENYL CROTONATE ◇ DINITRO(1-METHYLHEPTYL)PHENYL CROTONATE ◇ 2,4-DINITRO-6-(1-METHYLHEPTYL)PHENYL CROTONATE ◇ 2,4-DINITRO-6-(2-OCTYL)PHENYL CROTONATE ◇ ENT 24,727 ◇ (6-(1-METHYL-HEPTYL)-2,4-DINITRO-FENYL)-CROTONAAT (DUTCH) ◇ (6-(1-METHYL-HEPTYL)-2,3-DINITRO-PHENYL)-CROTONAT (GERMAN) ◇ 2-(1-METHYL-HEPTYL)-4,6-DINITROPHENYL CROTONATE ◇ (6-(1-METI-L-EPITL)-2,4-DINITRO-FENIL)-CROTONATO (ITALIAN)

TOXICITY DATA with REFERENCE
NEO: scu-mus TDLo: 10 mg/kg   NTIS**
     PB223-159

SAFETY PROFILE: Questionable carcinogen with experimental neoplastigenic data. Poison by ingestion and intravenous routes. When heated to decomposition it emits toxic fumes of NO_x.

AQT650
ARECA NUT

PROP: From the Areca palm tree, a native to South Asia. Orange-yellow in color when ripe. The seed, the size of a small egg, is separated from the fibrous pericarp and used fresh, after sun drying, or curing. It is chewed either alone or as a component of mixtures including Betel leaf and/or tobacco. Also known as Betel nut and supari. The nut contains several alkaloids, primarily arecoline, arecaidine, arecolidine, guvacoline, and guvacine.

SYNS: BETEL NUT ◇ SUPARI (INDIA)

SAFETY PROFILE: 3-(methylnitrosamino)propionaldehyde is a questionable experimental carcinogen. Arecoline is one of the agents responsible for betel quid addiction. It mimics the action

of acetylcholine and acts as a stimulant. It is a poison by intraperitoneal route. Reactions in the mouth and during processing can produce from these alkaloids several nitrosamines: N-nitrosoguvacoline, 3-(methylnitrosamino)propionitrile, 3-(methylnitrosamino)propionaldehyde and N-nitrosoguvacine. N-nitrosoguvacoline and N-nitrosoguvacine have been found in the mouths of betel quid users. Areca nut extracts are experimental carcinogens and mutagens.

AQT750   CAS: 63-75-2
ARECOLINE
mf: $C_8H_{13}NO_2$ mw: 155.22

PROP: Oily liquid. Bp: 209°.

SYNS: ARECAIDINE METHYL ESTER ◇ ARECOLINE BASE ◇ METHYL-1,2,5,6-TETRAHYDRO-1-METHYLNICOTINATE ◇ N-METHYL-Δ-TETRAHYDRONICOTINIC ACID METHYL ESTER ◇ N-METHYLTETRAHYDROPYRIDINE-β-CARBOXYLIC ACID METHYL ESTER ◇ 1,2,5,6-TETRAHYDRO-1-METHYLNICOTINIC ACID, METHYL ESTER

TOXICITY DATA with REFERENCE
NEO: skn-ham TDLo: 2698 mg/kg/65W-I
     JNCIAM 53,1259,74

CONSENSUS REPORTS: IARC Cancer Review: Animal Inadequate Evidence IMEMDT 37,141,85

SAFETY PROFILE: Questionable carcinogen with experimental neoplastigenic data. Poison by inhalation, ingestion, and subcutaneous routes. It mimics the action of acetylcholine a neuro transmitter, and is a parasympathetic nervous system stimulant. Its action on the central nervous system can cause tremors. A mutagen. It is easily nitrosated to several nitrosamines. It is the major alkaloid found in betel quid. Combustible, can react with oxidizing materials. When heated to decomposition it emits highly toxic fumes of NO_x.

AQU250   CAS: 61-94-9
ARECOLINE HYDROCHLORIDE
mf: $C_8H_{13}NO_2 \cdot ClH$ mw: 191.68

SYNS: NICOTINIC ACID-1,2,5,6-TETRAHYDRO-1-METHYL-, METHYL ESTER, HYDROCHLORIDE ◇ 3-PYRIDINECARBOXYLIC ACID-1,2,5,6-TETRAHYDRO-1-METHYL ESTER, HYDROCHLORIDE

TOXICITY DATA with REFERENCE
CAR: orl-mus TDLo: 10400 mg/kg/1Y-I
     JCREA8 107,169,84

MUT: dni-mus-ipr 60 mg/kg   IJEBA6 17,1141,79
MUT: oth-mus-ipr 60 mg/kg   IJEBA6 17,1141,79

SAFETY PROFILE: Questionable carcinogen with experimental carcinogenic data. Poison by intraperitoneal and intravenous routes. When heated to decomposition it emits very toxic fumes of NO_x and HCl.

AQY125
ARISTOLOCHIC ACID SODIUM SALT
mf: $C_{17}H_{10}NO_7 \cdot Na$ mw: 363.27

SYN: 8-METHOXY-6-NITROPHENANTHRO(3,4-d)-1,3-DI-OXOLE-5-CARBOXYLIC ACID SODIUM SALT

TOXICITY DATA with REFERENCE
CAR: orl-rat TD:90 mg/kg/12W-C   ARTODN
51,107,82
CAR: orl-rat TD:90 mg/kg/13W-C   ARTODN
51,107,82
CAR: orl-rat TD:900 mg/kg/13W-C   ARTODN
52,209,83
CAR: orl-rat TDLo:37 mg/kg/1Y-C   ARTODN
51,107,82

SAFETY PROFILE: Questionable carcinogen with experimental carcinogenic data. When heated to decomposition it emits toxic fumes of NO_x and Na_2O.

ARE500
ARSENICAL DUST   CAS: 8028-73-7
DOT: 1562

SYNS: ARSENICAL FLUE DUST ◇ FLUE DUST, ARSENIC containing

TOXICITY DATA with REFERENCE
ETA: itr-rat TDLo:120 mg/kg/15W-I   EVHPAZ
19,191,77

CONSENSUS REPORTS: Reported in EPA TSCA Inventory. Arsenic and its compounds are on the Community Right-To-Know List.

OSHA PEL: TWA 0.5 mg(As)/m^3 ACGIH TLV: TWA 0.2 mg(As)/m^3 NIOSH REL: CL 2 μg(As)/m^3/15M   DOT Classification: Poison B; Label: Poison.

SAFETY PROFILE: Questionable carcinogen with experimental tumorigenic data. A poison.

ARM500   CAS: 512-85-6
ASCARIDOLE
mf: $C_{10}H_{16}O_2$ mw: 168.26
PROP: Colorless unstable liquid. Mp: 3.3°, bp: 40° @ 2 mm; 115° @ 15 mm, d: 1.011 @ 13°/15°.

SYNS: ASCARISIN ◇ 1,4-PEROXIDO-p-MENTHENE-2

TOXICITY DATA with REFERENCE
NEO: skn-mus TDLo:25 g/kg/42W-I   JNCIAM
35,707,65
ETA: skn-mus TD:38 g/kg/63W-I   14JTAF-,275,64

DOT Classification: Forbidden.

SAFETY PROFILE: Questionable carcinogen with experimental neoplastigenic and tumorigenic data. Poison by ingestion. Flammable by spontaneous chemical reaction. An oxidizer.

ARN500   CAS: 16830-15-2
ASIATICOSIDE

PROP: A glycoside terpene from the plant *Centella asiatica* (CNREA8 32,1463,72)

SYNS: BLASTOESTIMULINA ◇ CENTELASE ◇ DERMATOLOGICO ◇ MADECASSOL

TOXICITY DATA with REFERENCE
ETA: skn-mus TDLo:400 mg/kg/52W-I
CNREA8 32,1463,72

SAFETY PROFILE: Questionable carcinogen with experimental tumorigenic data. When heated to decomposition it emits acrid smoke and fumes. Promotes healing of wounds.

ARN800   CAS: 9015-68-3
l-ASPARAGINASE

SYNS: ASPARAGINASE ◇ l-ASPARAGINASE X ◇ l-ASPARAGINASI (ITALIAN) ◇ l-ASPARAGINE AMIDOHYDROLASE ◇ LEUCOGEN ◇ NSC-109229

TOXICITY DATA with REFERENCE
NEO: ipr-mus TDLo:10 iu/kg/4D   BSIBAC
47,418,71

SAFETY PROFILE: Questionable carcinogen with experimental neoplastigenic data. Human (child) systemic effects by intramuscular route.

ARP250   CAS: 8003-03-0
ASPIRIN, PHENACETIN and CAFFEINE
mf: $C_{10}H_{13}NO_2 \cdot C_9H_8O_4 \cdot C_8H_{10}N_4O_2$ mw: 553.63

PROP: Composed of 50% aspirin, 46% phenacetin, and 4% caffeine (NCIMR* NIH-71-E-2144)

SYNS: 2-(ACETYLOXY)BENZOIC ACID, mixed with 3,7-DIHYDRO-1,3,7-TRIMETHYL-1H-PURINE-2,6-DIONE and N-(4-ETHOXYPHENYL)ACETAMIDE ◇ APC (pharmaceutical) ◇ ASCOPHEN ◇ CITRAMON ◇ EMPIRIN COMPOUND ◇ NCI-C02697 ◇ OSCOPHEN ◇ THOMAPYRIN

TOXICITY DATA with REFERENCE
ETA: orl-rat TDLo: 382 g/kg/78W-C   NCITR*
NCI-CG-TR-67,78

CONSENSUS REPORTS: NCI Carcinogenesis Bioassay (feed); Inadequate Studies: mouse, rat NCITR* NCI-CG-TR-67,78

SAFETY PROFILE: Questionable carcinogen with experimental tumorigenic data. Moderately toxic by ingestion. When heated to decomposition it emits toxic fumes of NO_x.

ARP500
ASSAM TEA

PROP: Tannin containing fraction of leaf used (JNCIAM 57,207,76).

SYN: CAMELLIA SINENSIS

TOXICITY DATA with REFERENCE
NEO: scu-rat TDLo: 1850 mg/kg/58W-I
JNCIAM 57,207,76

SAFETY PROFILE: Questionable carcinogen with experimental neoplastigenic data. When heated to decomposition it emits acrid smoke and irritating fumes.

ARQ725   CAS: 1912-24-9
ATRAZINE
mf: $C_8H_{14}ClN_5$ mw: 215.72

PROP: Crystals. Mp: 171-174°. Solubility at 25°: in water, 70 ppm; ether, 12,000 ppm; chloroform, 52,000 ppm; methanol, 18,000 ppm.

SYNS: A 361 ◇ AATREX ◇ AATREX 4L ◇ AATREX NINE-O ◇ AATREX 80W ◇ 2-AETHYLAMINO-4-CHLOR-6-ISOPROPYLAMINO-1,3,5-TRIAZIN (GERMAN) ◇ 2-AETHYLAMINO-4-ISOPROPYLAMINO-6-CHLOR-1,3,5-TRIAZIN (GERMAN) ◇ AKTIKON ◇ AKTIKON PK ◇ AKTINIT A ◇ AKTINIT PK ◇ ARGEZIN ◇ ATAZINAX ◇ ATRANEX ◇ ATRASINE ◇ ATRATOL A ◇ ATRAZIN ◇ ATRED ◇ ATREX ◇ CANDEX ◇ CEKUZINA-T ◇ 2-CHLORO-4-ETHYLAMINE-ISOPROPYLAMINE-s-TRIAZINE ◇ 1-CHLORO-3-ETHYL-AMINO-5-ISOPROPYLAMINO-s-TRIAZINE ◇ 1-CHLORO-3-ETHYLAMINO-5-ISOPROPYLAMINO-2,4,6-TRIAZINE ◇ 2-CHLORO-4-ETHYLAMINO-6-ISOPROPYLAMINO-s-TRIAZINE ◇ 2-CHLORO-4-ETHYLAMINO-6-ISOPROPYL-AMINO-1,3,5-TRIAZINE ◇ 6-CHLORO-N-ETHYL-N'-(1-METHYLETHYL)-1,3,5-TRIAZINE-2,4-DIAMINE (9CI) ◇ 2-CHLORO-4-(2-PROPYLAMINO)-6-ETHYLAMINO-s-TRIAZINE ◇ CRISATRINA ◇ CRISAZINE ◇ CYAZIN ◇ FARMCO ATRAZINE ◇ FENAMIN ◇ FENAMINE ◇ FENATROL ◇ G 30027 ◇ GEIGY 30,027 ◇ GESAPRIM ◇ GESOPRIM

◇ GRIFFEX ◇ HUNGAZIN ◇ HUNGAZIN PK ◇ INAKOR ◇ OLEOGESAPRIM ◇ PRIMATOL ◇ PRIMAZE ◇ RADAZIN ◇ RADIZINE ◇ SHELL ATRAZINE HERBICIDE ◇ STRAZINE ◇ TRIAZINE A 1294 ◇ VECTAL ◇ VECTAL SC ◇ WEEDEX A ◇ WONUK ◇ ZEAZIN ◇ ZEAZINE

TOXICITY DATA with REFERENCE
ETA: orl-mus TDLo: 9000 mg/kg/78W-I
NTIS** PB223-159
MUT: dns-hmn: fbr 3 mmol/L   MUREAV 74,77,80
MUT: mma-ham: lng 3 mmol/L   MUREAV 74,77,80

CONSENSUS REPORTS: EPA Genetic Toxicology Program. Reported in EPA TSCA Inventory.

OSHA PEL: TWA 5 mg/m³   ACGIH TLV: TWA 5 mg/m³   DFG MAK: 2 mg/m³

SAFETY PROFILE: Questionable carcinogen with experimental tumorigenic data. Poison by intraperitoneal route. Moderately toxic by ingestion. Mildly toxic by inhalation and skin contact. Human mutation data reported. Experimental reproductive effects. A skin and severe eye irritant. When heated to decomposition it emits toxic fumes of Cl^- and NO_x.

ARQ750   CAS: 637-07-0
ATROMID S
mf: $C_{12}H_{15}ClO_3$ mw: 242.72

SYNS: AMOTRIL ◇ ANGIOKAPSUL ◇ ANPARTON ◇ ANTILIPID ◇ APOLAN ◇ ARTERIOFLEXIN ◇ ARTEROSOL ◇ ARTES ◇ ARTEVIL ◇ ATECULON ◇ ATERIOSAN ◇ ATHEBRATE ◇ ATHEROMIDE ◇ ATHEROPRONT ◇ ATHRANID-WIRKSTOFF ◇ ATROLEN ◇ ATROMID ◇ ATROMIDIN ◇ ATROVIS ◇ AY 61123 ◇ AZIONYL ◇ BIOSCLERAN ◇ BRESIT ◇ CARTAGYL ◇ α-p-CHLORO-PHENOXYISOBUTYRYL ETHYL ESTER ◇ 2-(4-CHLOROPHE-NOXY)-2-METHYLPROPANOIC ACID ETHYL ESTER ◇ 2-(p-CHLOROPHENOXY)-2-METHYLPROPIONIC ACID ETHYL ESTER ◇ CINNARIZIN ◇ CITIFLUS ◇ CLARIPEX ◇ CLOBERAT ◇ CLOBRAT ◇ CLOBREN-SF ◇ CLOFAR ◇ CLOFIBRAM ◇ CLOFIBRAT ◇ CLOFIBRATO (SPANISH) ◇ CLOFINIT ◇ CLOFIPRONT ◇ CPIB ◇ DELIVA ◇ DURA CLOFIBRAT ◇ ELPI ◇ EPIB ◇ ETHYL CHLOROPHENOXY-ISOBUTYRATE ◇ ETHYL-p-CHLOROPHENOXYISOBUTY-RATE ◇ ETHYL-α-p-CHLOROPHENOXYISOBUTYRATE ◇ ETHYL-α-(4-CHLOROPHENOXY)ISOBUTYRATE ◇ ETHYL-2-(p-CHLOROPHENOXY)ISOBUTYRATE ◇ ETHYL-α-(p-CHLOROPHENOXY)-α-METHYLPROPION-ATE ◇ ETHYL-α-(4-CHLOROPHENOXY)-α-METHYLPRO-PIONATE ◇ ETHYL 2-(p-CHLOROPHENOXY)-2-METHYL-PROPIONATE ◇ ETHYL 2-(4-CHLOROPHENOXY)-2-

METHYLPROPIONATE ◇ ETHYL CLOFIBRATE ◇ FIBRA-LEM ◇ GERASTOP ◇ HYCLORATE ◇ ICI 28257 ◇ KLOFIRAN ◇ LEVATROM ◇ LIPAMID ◇ LIPAVIL ◇ LIPAVLON ◇ LIPIDE 500 ◇ LIPIDSENKER ◇ LIPOFACTON ◇ LIPOMID ◇ LIPONORM ◇ LIPOREDUCT ◇ LIPORIL ◇ LIPOSID ◇ LIPRIN ◇ LIPRINAL ◇ LOBETRIN ◇ MISCLERON ◇ NEGALIP ◇ NEO-ATOMID ◇ NORMALIP ◇ NORMAT ◇ NORMOLIPOL ◇ NSC-79389 ◇ OXAN 600 ◇ PERSANTINAT ◇ RECOLIP ◇ REGARDIN ◇ REGELAN ◇ ROBIGRAM ◇ SCROBIN ◇ SEROFINEX ◇ SEROTINEX ◇ SKEROLIP ◇ SKLEROMEX ◇ SKLEROMEXE ◇ SKLERO-TABLINEN ◇ SKLERO-TABULS ◇ TICLOBRAN ◇ VINCAMIN COMPOSI-TUM ◇ XYDURIL ◇ YOCLO

TOXICITY DATA with REFERENCE
ETA: orl-rat TDLo: 100 g/kg/72W-C   CNREA8 39,3419,79
MUT: dni-mus: oth 40 μmol/L   CNREA8 49,36,80
MUT: dns-rat: lvr 100 pmol/L   CRNGDP 5,1547,84
MUT: sce-ham: ovr 100 μmol/L/1H   CRNGDP 5,703,84

CONSENSUS REPORTS: IARC Cancer Review: GROUP 3 IMEMDT 7,171,87; Animal Limited Evidence IMEMDT 24,39,80; Human Inadequate Evidence IMEMDT 24,39,80

SAFETY PROFILE: Questionable carcinogen with experimental tumorigenic and teratogenic data. Poison by intravenous route. Moderately toxic by ingestion and other routes. Other experimental reproductive effects. Reduces plasma lipid levels. Human systemic effects by ingestion: muscle weakness, muscle spasms, and fever. When heated to decomposition it emits toxic fumes of Cl^-.

ARY000   CAS: 320-67-2
AZACYTIDINE
mf: $C_8H_{12}N_4O_5$ mw: 244.24

SYNS: 5-AC ◇ 5-ACZ ◇ 4-AMINO-1-β-d-RIBOFURA-NOSYL-d-TRIAZIN-2(1H)-ONE ◇ 4-AMINO-1-β-d-RIBOFURA-NOSYL-1,3,5-TRIAZIN-2(1H)-ONE ◇ ANTIBIOTIC U 18496 ◇ AZACITIDINE ◇ 5-AZACYTIDINE ◇ 5'-AZACYTIDINE ◇ LADAKAMYCIN ◇ MYLOSAR ◇ NCI-C01569 ◇ NSC-102816 ◇ U 18496

TOXICITY DATA with REFERENCE
CAR: ipr-mus TDLo: 100 mg/kg/50W-I   CALEDQ 37,51,87
CAR: unr-mus TDLo: 1 mg/kg (16D post)   TJADAB 32,33A,85
NEO: ipr-mus TD: 90 mg/kg/8W-I   CNREA8 33,3069,73
NEO: ipr-mus TD: 100 mg/kg/50W-I   CALEDQ 37,51,87

NEO: ipr-mus TD: 284 mg/kg/43W-I   NCITR* NCI-TR-42,78
ETA: ipr-rat TDLo: 190 mg/kg/38W-I   CRNGDP 5,1583,84
MUT: cyt-ham: emb 5 mg/L   CNREA8 37,2202,77
MUT: dnd-hmn: fbr 1 μmol/L   PNASA6 79,2352,82
MUT: dni-hmn: leu 3 μmol/L   CNREA8 43,763,83
MUT: msc-hmn: lym 100 nmol/L   MUREAV 160,249,86
MUT: otr-mus: emb 250 μg/L   CNREA8 37,2202,77
MUT: sce-ham: fbr 2500 μg/L   CNREA8 39,797,79
MUT: slt-dmg-orl 1 mmol/L   MUREAV 143,195,85

CONSENSUS REPORTS: IARC Cancer Review: GROUP 3 IMEMDT 7,56,87; Animal Limited Evidence IMEMDT 26,37,81; NCI Carcinogenesis Bioassay (ipr); Inadequate Studies: rat NCITR* NCI-CG-TR-42,78; Clear Evidence: mouse NCITR* NCI-CG-TR-42,78. EPA Genetic Toxicology Program.

SAFETY PROFILE: Questionable carcinogen with experimental carcinogenic, neoplastigenic, tumorigenic, and teratogenic data. Poison by ingestion, intravenous, and intraperitoneal routes. Human systemic effects by intravenous route: nausea, vomiting and diarrhea, reduction in white cell count (luekopenia and agranulocytosis). Human mutation data reported. A skin irritant. When heated to decomposition it emits toxic fumes of NO_x.

ARY500   CAS: 63907-29-9
2-AZAHYPOXANTHINE
mf: $C_4H_3N_5O$ mw: 137.12

SYN: 4-OXO-4H-IMIDAZO(4,5-D)-v-TRIAZINE

TOXICITY DATA with REFERENCE
ETA: orl-rat TDLo: 3005 mg/kg/21W-C   JNCIAM 54,951,75

SAFETY PROFILE: Questionable carcinogen with experimental tumorigenic data. When heated to decomposition it emits toxic fumes of NO_x.

ASH500   CAS: 86-50-0
AZINPHOS METHYL
mf: $C_{10}H_{12}N_3O_3PS_2$ mw: 317.34

PROP: Crystals or brown, waxy solid. D: 1.44, mp: 74°. Sltly sol in water; sol in organic solvents.
DOT: 2783

SYNS: AZINFOS-METHYL (DUTCH) ◇ AZINPHOS-METILE (ITALIAN) ◇ AZINPHOS METHYL, liquid (DOT) ◇ BAY 9027

◇ BAYER 17147 ◇ BENZOTRIAZINEDITHIOPHOSPHORIC ACID DIMETHOXY ESTER ◇ BENZOTRIAZINE derivative of a METHYL DITHIOPHOSPHATE ◇ CARFENE ◇ COTNION METHYL ◇ CRYSTHION 2L ◇ CRYSTHYON ◇ DBD ◇ S-(3,4-DIHYDRO-4-OXO-BENZO(α)(1,2,3)TRIAZIN-3-YL-METHYL)-O,O-DIMETHYL PHOSPHORODITHIOATE ◇ S-(3,4-DIHYDRO-4-OXO-1,2,3-BENZOTRIAZIN-3-YL-METHYL)- O,O-DIMETHYL PHOSPHORODITHIOATE ◇ O,O-DIMETHYL-S-(BENZAZIMINOMETHYL) DITHIO-PHOSPHATE ◇ O,O-DIMETHYL-S-(1,2,3-BENZOTRIAZINYL-4-KETO)METHYL PHOSPHORODITHIOATE ◇ O,O-DI-METHYL-S-(3,4-DIHYDRO-4-KETO-1,2,3-BENZOTRIAZIN-YL-3-METHYL) DITHIOPHOSPHATE ◇ DIMETHYLDITHIO-PHOSPHORIC-ACID N-METHYLBENZAZIMIDE ESTER ◇ O,O-DIMETHYL-S-(4-OXO-3H-1,2,3-BENZOTRIZIANE-3-METHYL)PHOSPHORODITHIOATE ◇ O,O-DIMETHYL-S-(4-OXOBENZOTRIAZINO-3-METHYL)PHOSPHORODITHIOATE ◇ O,O-DIMETHYL-S-(4-OXO-1,2,3-BENZOTRIAZINO(3)-METHYL) THIOTHIONOPHOSPHATE ◇ O,O-DIMETHYL-S-((4-OXO-3H-1,2,3-BENZOTRIAZIN-3-YL)-METHYL)-DI-THIOFOSFAAT (DUTCH) ◇ O,O-DIMETHYL-S-((4-OXO-3H-1,2,3-BENZOTRIAZIN-3-YL)-METHYL)-DITHIOPHOS-PHAT (GERMAN) ◇ O,O-DIMETHYL-S-4-OXO-1,2,3-BEN-ZOTRIAZIN-3(4H)-YLMETHYL PHOSPHORODITHIOATE ◇ O,O-DIMETIL-S-((4-OXO-3H-1,2,3-BENZOTRIA-ZIN-3-IL)-METIL)-DITIOFOSFATO (ITALIAN) ◇ ENT 23,233 ◇ GOTHNION ◇ GUSATHION ◇ GUTHION (DOT) ◇ GU-THION, liquid (DOT) ◇ 3-(MERCAPTOMETHYL)-1,2,3-BENZOTRIAZIN-4(3H)-ONE-O,O-DIMETHYL PHOSPHORO-DITHIOATE ◇ 3-(MERCAPTOMETHYL)-1,2,3-BENZO-TRIAZIN-4(3H)-ONE-O,O-DIMETHYL PHOSPHORO-DITHIOATE-S-ESTER ◇ METHYLAZINPHOS ◇ N-METHYL-BENZAZIMIDE, DIMETHYLDITHIOPHOSPHORIC ACID ESTER ◇ METHYL GUTHION ◇ METILTRIAZOTION ◇ NCI-C00066

TOXICITY DATA with REFERENCE
ETA: orl-rat TD:121 g/kg/78W-C   JEPTDQ 1(6),829,78
ETA: orl-rat TDLo:5110mg/kg/78W-C   NCITR* NCI-CG-TR-69,78
MUT: cyt-hmn:lng 120 mg/L   CNJGA8 17,455,75
MUT: cyt-hmn:oth 120 mg/L   CNJGA8 17,455,75
MUT: mmo-ssp 25 mmol/L   MUREAV 117,139,83

CONSENSUS REPORTS: NCI Carcinogenesis Bioassay (feed); Inadequate Studies: rat NCITR* NCI-CG-TR-69,78; No Evidence: mouse NCITR* NCI-CG-TR-69,78. EPA Genetic Toxicology Program. EPA Extremely Hazardous Substances List.

OSHA PEL: TWA 0.2 mg/m^3 (skin)   ACGIH TLV: TWA 0.2 mg/m^3 (skin)   DFG MAK: 0.2 mg/m^3 DOT Classification: Poison B; Label: Poison, liquid mixture.

SAFETY PROFILE: Questionable carcinogen with experimental tumorigenic and teratogenic data. Poison by inhalation, ingestion, skin contact, intravenous, intraperitoneal, and possibly other routes. Other experimental reproductive effects. Human mutation data reported. When heated to decomposition it emits very toxic fumes of PO_x, SO_x, and NO_x.

ASI000   CAS: 1072-52-2
1-AZIRIDINE ETHANOL
mf: C_4H_9NO mw: 87.14

SYNS: 2-(1-AZIRIDINYL)ETHANOL ◇ β-HYDROXY-1-ETHYLAZIRIDINE ◇ 2-HYDROXY-1-ETHYLAZIRIDINE ◇ N-(β-HYDROXYETHYL)AZIRIDINE ◇ N-(2-HYDROXY-ETHYL)AZIRIDINE ◇ N-HYDROXYETHYL ETHYLENE IMINE ◇ N-(2-HYDROXYETHYL)ETHYLENIMINE ◇ 1-(2-HYDROXYETHYL)ETHYLENIMINE

TOXICITY DATA with REFERENCE
NEO: scu-mus TDLo:900 mg/kg/75W-I
    JNCIAM 46,143,71

CONSENSUS REPORTS: IARC Cancer Review: GROUP 3 IMEMDT 7,56,87; Animal Limited Evidence IMEMDT 9,47,75. Reported in EPA TSCA Inventory.

SAFETY PROFILE: Questionable carcinogen with experimental neoplastigenic data. Poison by ingestion, skin contact, and intravenous routes. A skin and eye irritant. When heated to decomposition it emits toxic fumes of NO_x.

ASL250   CAS: 103-33-3
AZOBENZENE
mf: $C_{12}H_{10}N_2$ mw: 182.23

PROP: Orange, monoclinic crystals. Mp: 68°, bp: 297°, d: 1.203 @ 20°/4°, vap press: 1 mm @ 103.5°. Insol in water. Solubility in alc = 4.2/100 @ 20° in ether (ligroin) = 12/100 @ 20°.

SYNS: AZOBENZEEN (DUTCH) ◇ AZOBENZIDE ◇ AZOBENZOL ◇ AZOBISBENZENE ◇ AZODIBENZENE ◇ AZODIBENZENEAZOFUME ◇ BENZENEAZOBENZENE ◇ DIAZOBENZENE ◇ DIPHENYLDIAZENE ◇ 1,2-DIPHENYL-DIAZENE ◇ DIPHENYLDIIMIDE ◇ ENT 14,611 ◇ NCI-C02926 ◇ USAF EK-704

TOXICITY DATA with REFERENCE
CAR: orl-rat TD:15 g/kg/2Y-C   NCITR* NCI-CG-TR-154,79

CAR: orl-rat TDLo: 7350 mg/kg/2Y-C NCITR*
NCI-CG-TR-154,79
NEO: orl-mus TDLo: 300 mg/kg/8W-I TXAPA9
82,19,86
NEO: orl-rat TD: 7280 mg/kg/2Y-C FCTOD7
25,619,87
ETA: scu-rat TDLo: 17 g/kg/2Y-I CANCAR
3,789,50
MUT: mma-sat 40 μg/plate PNASA6 72,5135,75

CONSENSUS REPORTS: IARC Cancer Review: GROUP 3 IMEMDT 7,56,87; Animal Limited Evidence IMEMDT 8,75,75; NCI Carcinogenesis Bioassay (feed); Clear Evidence: rat NCITR* NCI-CG-TR-154,79; No Evidence: mouse NCITR* NCI-CG-TR-154,79. Reported in EPA TSCA Inventory.

SAFETY PROFILE: Questionable carcinogen with experimental carcinogenic, neoplastigenic, and tumorigenic data. Moderately toxic by ingestion and possibly other routes. When heated to decomposition it emits toxic fumes of NO_x.

ASN250   CAS: 821-14-7
AZO ETHANE
mf: $C_4H_{10}N_2$ mw: 86.16

SYN: AZOAETHAN (GERMAN)

TOXICITY DATA with REFERENCE
CAR: ihl-rat TCLo: 37 mg/kg/1H (22D post)
IARCCD 4,45,73
ETA: ihl-rat TC: 300 mg/kg/1H (15D post)
EXPEAM 24,561,68
ETA: ihl-rat TC: 4000 ppm/1H (15D post)
FCTXAV 6,584,68
ETA: scu-rat TDLo: 1250 mg/kg/26W-I ZEKBAI
67,31,65

SAFETY PROFILE: Questionable carcinogen with experimental carcinogenic and tumorigenic data. Moderate acute toxicity. An experimental teratogen. When heated to decomposition it emits toxic fumes of NO_x.

ASN500   CAS: 487-10-5
1,1'-AZONAPHTHALENE
mf: $C_{20}H_{14}N_2$ mw: 282.35

PROP: Red needles from acetic acid. Mp: 190°; bp: subl > 190°; Insol in water, sol in acetic acid, very sltly sol in alc, very sol in benzene.

TOXICITY DATA with REFERENCE
ETA: scu-mus TDLo: 6300 mg/kg/63W-I
AJCAA7 40,62,40

SAFETY PROFILE: Questionable carcinogen with experimental tumorigenic data. When heated to decomposition it emits toxic fumes of NO_x.

ASN750   CAS: 582-08-1
2,2'-AZONAPHTHALENE
mf: $C_{20}H_{14}N_2$ mw: 282.35

PROP: Red prisms from chloroform. Mp: 204°; bp: subl @ 210°; Insol in water, sltly sol in alc, sol in benzene.

SYN: DI-β-NAPHTHYLDIIMIDE

TOXICITY DATA with REFERENCE
ETA: orl-mus TDLo: 8400 mg/kg/42W-I
AJCAA7 40,62,40

SAFETY PROFILE: Questionable carcinogen with experimental tumorigenic data. When heated to decomposition it emits toxic fumes of NO_x.

ASP000   CAS: 16301-26-1
AZOXYETHANE
mf: $C_4H_{10}N_2O$ mw: 102.16

SYNS: AZOXYAETHAN (GERMAN) ◇ DIETHYLDIAZENE-1-OXIDE

TOXICITY DATA with REFERENCE
CAR: ivn-rat TDLo: 50 mg/kg (15D post)
IARCCD 4,45,73
ETA: ivn-rat TD: 50 mg/kg (15D post) XENOBH
3,271,73
ETA: orl-ham TDLo: 400 mg/kg/20W-I
CNREA8 47,3968,87
ETA: orl-rat TDLo: 500 mg/kg/20W-I CNREA8
47,3968,87
ETA: scu-rat TD: 250 mg/kg ZEKBAI 67,31,65
ETA: scu-rat TDLo: 30 mg/kg (11D post)
NATWAY 60,555,73
ETA: scu-rat TDLo: 240 mg/kg/24W-I XENOBH
3,271,73

SAFETY PROFILE: Questionable carcinogen with experimental carcinogenic and tumorigenic data. An experimental transplacental teratogen. Poison by subcutaneous and intravenous routes. When heated to decomposition it emits toxic fumes of NO_x.

ASP500   CAS: 17697-55-1
1-AZOXYPROPANE
mf: $C_6H_{14}N_2O$ mw: 130.22

SYNS: 1,1'-AZOXYPROPANE ◇ DIPROPYLDIAZENE 1-OXIDE

TOXICITY DATA with REFERENCE
CAR: orl-rat TDLo: 773 mg/kg/26W-I   CRNGDP
   8,1947,87

SAFETY PROFILE: Questionable carcinogen with experimental carcinogenic data. When heated to decomposition it emits toxic fumes of NO_x.

ASP510
2-AZOXYPROPANE
mf: $C_6H_{14}N_2O$ mw: 130.22

SYNS: AZOXYISOPROPANE ◇ BIS(1-METHYLETHYL) DIAZENE 1-OXIDE

TOXICITY DATA with REFERENCE
CAR: orl-rat TDLo: 773 mg/kg/26W I   CRNGDP
   8,1947,87

SAFETY PROFILE: Questionable carcinogen with experimental carcinogenic data. When heated to decomposition it emits toxic fumes of NO_x.

ASP750   CAS: 6580-41-2
AZULENO(5,6,7-cd)PHENALENE
mf: $C_{20}H_{12}$ mw: 252.32

TOXICITY DATA with REFERENCE
ETA: scu-mus TDLo: 80 mg/kg/4W-I   PAACA3
   10,12,69

SAFETY PROFILE: Questionable carcinogen with experimental tumorigenic data. When heated to decomposition it emits acrid smoke and irritating fumes.

BAD000   CAS: 64550-80-7
BA-10,11-DIOL-8,9-EPOXIDE-1
mf: $C_{18}H_{14}O_3$ mw: 278.32

SYN: 8,9,10,11-TETRAHYDRO-10,11-DIHYDROXY-8-α,9-α-EPOXYBENZ(a)ANTHRACENE

TOXICITY DATA with REFERENCE
ETA: skn-mus TDLo: 22 mg/kg   CNREA8
   38,1699,78

SAFETY PROFILE: Questionable carcinogen with experimental tumorigenic data. When heated to decomposition it emits acrid smoke and irritating fumes.

BAP000   CAS: 7727-43-7
BARIUM SULFATE
mf: $O_4S \cdot Ba$ mw: 233.40

PROP: White, heavy, odorless powder. D: 4.50 @ 15°, mp: 1580°. Insol in water or dilute acids.

SYNS: ACTYBARYTE ◇ ARTIFICIAL BARITE ◇ ARTIFICIAL HEAVY SPAR ◇ BAKONTAL ◇ BARIDOL ◇ BARITE ◇ BARITOP ◇ BAROSPERSE ◇ BAROTRAST ◇ BARYTA WHITE ◇ BARYTES ◇ BAYRITES ◇ BLANC FIXE ◇ C.I. 77120 ◇ C.I. PIGMENT WHITE 21 ◇ CITOBARYUM ◇ COLONATRAST ◇ ENAMEL WHITE ◇ ESOPHOTRAST ◇ EWEISS ◇ E-Z-PAQUE ◇ FINEMEAL ◇ LACTOBARYT ◇ LIQUIBARINE ◇ MACROPAQUE ◇ NEOBAR ◇ ORATRAST ◇ PERMANENT WHITE ◇ PRECIPITATED BARIUM SULPHATE ◇ RAYBAR ◇ REDI-FLOW ◇ SOLBAR ◇ SULFURIC ACID, BARIUM SALT (1:1) ◇ SUPRAMIKE ◇ TRAVAD ◇ UNIBARYT

TOXICITY DATA with REFERENCE
ETA: ipl-rat TDLo: 200 mg/kg   BJCAAI 28,173,73

CONSENSUS REPORTS: Reported in EPA TSCA Inventory. Barium and its compounds are on the Community Right-To-Know List.

OSHA PEL: (Transitional: Total Dust: TWA 15 mg/m³; Respirable Fraction: 5 mg/m³) Total Dust: TWA 10 mg/m³; Respirable Fraction: 5 mg/m³   ACGIH TLV: TWA (nuisance particulate) 10 mg/m³ of total dust (when toxic impurities are not present, e.g., quartz < 1%).

SAFETY PROFILE: Questionable carcinogen with experimental tumorigenic data. A relatively insoluble salt used as an opaque medium in radiography. When heated to decomposition it emits toxic fumes of SO_x.

BAR500
BASORA CORRA

PROP: Aqueous extract from the root of the plant (JNCIAM 52,445,74).

SYN: MELOCHIA TOMENTOSA

TOXICITY DATA with REFERENCE
NEO: scu-rat TDLo: 300 g/kg/60W-I   JNCIAM
   52,445,74

SAFETY PROFILE: Questionable carcinogen with experimental neoplastigenic data.

BAV500
BENLATE and SODIUM NITRITE

SYNS: 1-(BUTYLCARBAMOYL)-2-BENZIMIDAZOLECARBAMIC ACID METHYL ESTER and SODIUM NITRITE (1:6) ◇ SODIUM NITRITE and BENLATE

TOXICITY DATA with REFERENCE
CAR: orl-mus TDLo: 31 g/kg/26W-I   NEOLA4
   24,119,77

SAFETY PROFILE: Questionable carcinogen with experimental carcinogenic data. When heated to decomposition it emits toxic fumes of Na_2O and NO_x.

BAV750   CAS: 1302-78-9
BENTONITE

PROP: A clay containing appreciable amounts of the clay mineral montmorillonite; light yellow or green, cream, pink, gray to black solid. Insol in water and common organic solvents.

SYNS: ALBAGEL PREMIUM USP 4444 ◇ BENTONITE 2073 ◇ BENTONITE MAGMA ◇ HI-JEL ◇ IMVITE I.G.B.A. ◇ MAGBOND ◇ MONTMORILLONITE ◇ PANTHER CREEK BENTONITE ◇ SOUTHERN BENTONITE ◇ TIXOTON ◇ VOLCLAY ◇ VOLCLAY BENTONITE BC ◇ WILKINITE

TOXICITY DATA with REFERENCE
ETA: orl-mus TDLo: 12000 g/kg/28W-C
ANYAA9 57,678,54

CONSENSUS REPORTS: Reported in EPA TSCA Inventory.

SAFETY PROFILE: Questionable carcinogen with experimental tumorigenic data. Poison by intravenous route causing blood clotting.

BAW000   CAS: 7093-10-9
BENZ(1)ACEANTHRENE
mf: $C_{20}H_{14}$ mw: 254.34

SYNS: 8:9-ACE-1:2-BENZANTHRACENE ◇ 1,2-DIHYDROBENZ(1)ACEANTHRYLENE ◇ 8:9-DIMETHYLENE-1:2-BENZANTHRACENE

TOXICITY DATA with REFERENCE
ETA: scu-mus TDLo: 800 mg/kg/13W-I
AJCAA7 28,334,36

SAFETY PROFILE: Questionable carcinogen with experimental tumorigenic data. When heated to decomposition it emits acrid smoke and fumes.

BAW750   CAS: 225-51-4
BENZ(c)ACRIDINE
mf: $C_{17}H_{11}N$ mw: 229.29

PROP: Mp: 108°.

SYNS: 12-AZABENZ(a)ANTHRACENE ◇ B(c)AC ◇ 3,4-BENZACRIDINE ◇ 7,8-BENZACRIDINE (FRENCH) ◇ 3,4-BENZOACRIDINE ◇ α-CHRYSIDINE ◇ α-NAPHTHACRIDINE ◇ RCRA WASTE NUMBER U016

TOXICITY DATA with REFERENCE
NEO: ipr-mus TDLo: 9630 mg/kg/3D-I   CNREA8 44,5161,84

ETA: skn-mus TDLo: 2400 mg/kg/67W-I
IJCAAR-5,183,68
MUT: mma-sat 1 nmol/plate   GANNA2 70,749,79
MUT: sce-ham: lng 1 μmol/L   MUREAV 118,103,83
MUT: sce-ham: ovr 10 μmol/L   MUREAV 118,103,83

CONSENSUS REPORTS: IARC Cancer Review: GROUP 3 IMEMDT 7,56,87; Animal Sufficient Evidence IMEMDT 3,241,73; Animal Limited Evidence IMEMDT 32,129,83

SAFETY PROFILE: Questionable carcinogen with experimental neoplastigenic and tumorigenic data. Mutation data reported. When heated to decomposition it emits toxic fumes of NO_x.

BAX000   CAS: 3123-27-1
BENZ(c)ACRIDINE-7-CARBONITRILE
mf: $C_{18}H_{10}N_2$ mw: 254.30

SYNS: 7-CYANOBENZ(c)ACRIDINE ◇ 7-CYANOBENZO-(c)ACRIDINE

TOXICITY DATA with REFERENCE
ETA: scu-mus TDLo: 120 mg/kg/9W-I   CHDDAT 267,981,68

CONSENSUS REPORTS: Cyanide and its compounds are on the Community Right-To-Know List.

SAFETY PROFILE: Questionable carcinogen with experimental tumorigenic data. When heated to decomposition it emits toxic fumes of NO_x and CN^-.

BAX250   CAS: 3301-75-5
BENZ(c)ACRIDINE-7-CARBOXALDEHYDE
mf: $C_{18}H_{11}NO$ mw: 257.30

SYNS: 3,4-BENZACRIDINE-9-ALDEHYDE ◇ 7-FORMYL-BENZ(c)ACRIDINE ◇ 7-FORMYLBENZO(c)ACRIDINE

TOXICITY DATA with REFERENCE
ETA: scu-mus TDLo: 200 mg/kg   VOONAW 1,52,55
MUT: mma-sat 10 μg/plate   CRNGDP 7,23,86

SAFETY PROFILE: Questionable carcinogen with experimental tumorigenic data. Mutation data reported. When heated to decomposition it emits toxic fumes of NO_x.

BAY250   CAS: 63019-50-1
α-(BENZ(c)ACRIDIN-7-YL)-N-(p-(DIMETHYLAMINO)PHENYL)NITRONE
mf: $C_{26}H_{21}N_3O$ mw: 391.50

SYN: α-(9-(3,4-BENZACRIDYL)-N-(p-DIMETHYLAMINO-
PHENYL)-NITRONE

TOXICITY DATA with REFERENCE
ETA: scu-mus TDLo: 200 mg/kg   VOONAW
  1,52,55

SAFETY PROFILE: Questionable carcinogen
with experimental tumorigenic data. When
heated to decomposition it emits toxic fumes
of NO_x.

BBB500   CAS: 63018-69-9
BENZ(a)ANTHRACEN-7-ACETONITRILE
mf: $C_{20}H_{13}N$ mw: 267.34

SYN: 10-CYANOMETHYL-1,2-BENZANTHRACENE

TOXICITY DATA with REFERENCE
ETA: scu-mus TDLo: 600 mg/kg   JNCIAM 1,303,40

CONSENSUS REPORTS: Cyanide and its
compounds are on the Community Right-To-
Know List.

SAFETY PROFILE: Questionable carcinogen
with experimental tumorigenic data. When
heated to decomposition it emits toxic fumes
of NO_x and CN^-.

BBB750   CAS: 2381-18-2
BENZ(a)ANTHRACEN-7-AMINE
mf: $C_{18}H_{13}N$ mw: 243.32

SYN: 10-AMINO-1,2-BENZANTHRACENE

TOXICITY DATA with REFERENCE
ETA: scu-mus TDLo: 1500 mg/kg/23W-I
  PRLBA4 129,439,40

SAFETY PROFILE: Questionable carcinogen
with experimental tumorigenic data. When
heated to decomposition it emits toxic fumes
of NO_x.

BBC000   CAS: 56961-60-5
BENZ(a)ANTHRACEN-8-AMINE
mf: $C_{18}H_{13}N$ mw: 243.32

SYN: 5-AMINO-1:2-BENZANTHRACENE

TOXICITY DATA with REFERENCE
ETA: scu-mus TDLo: 400 mg/kg/3W-I   PRLBA4
  131,170,42

SAFETY PROFILE: Questionable carcinogen
with experimental tumorigenic data. When
heated to decomposition it emits toxic fumes
of NO_x.

BBC500   CAS: 63018-40-6
1,2-BENZANTHRACENE-10-ACETIC
ACID, METHYL ESTER
mf: $C_{21}H_{16}O_2$ mw: 300.37

SYN: BENZ(a)ANTHRACEN-7-ACETIC ACID, METHYL ES-
TER

TOXICITY DATA with REFERENCE
ETA: scu-mus TDLo: 600 mg/kg   JNCIAM 1,303,40

SAFETY PROFILE: Questionable carcinogen
with experimental tumorigenic data. When
heated to decomposition it emits acrid smoke
and fumes.

BBC750   CAS: 7505-62-6
BENZ(a)ANTHRACENE-7-
CARBOXALDEHYDE
mf: $C_{19}H_{12}O$ mw: 256.31

SYN: 1,2-BENZANTHRACENE-10-ALDEHYDE

TOXICITY DATA with REFERENCE
ETA: scu-mus TDLo: 280 mg/kg   JNCIAM 1,303,40

SAFETY PROFILE: Questionable carcinogen
with experimental tumorigenic data. When
heated to decomposition it emits acrid smoke
and fumes.

BBD000   CAS: 19926-22-8
BENZ(a)ANTHRACENE-7,12-
DICARBOXALDEHYDE
mf: $C_{20}H_{12}O_2$ mw: 284.32

SYN: 7,12-DIFORMYLBENZ(a)ANTHRACENE

TOXICITY DATA with REFERENCE
NEO: skn-mus TDLo: 8000 mg/kg   JJIND8
  61,135,78
MUT: dnd-omi 2 mg/L   PNASA6 74,1378,77

SAFETY PROFILE: Questionable carcinogen
with experimental neoplastigenic data by skin
contact. Mutation data reported. When heated
to decomposition it emits acrid smoke and irritating fumes.

BBD250   CAS: 60967-88-6
BENZ(a)ANTHRACENE-1,2-
DIHYDRODIOL
mf: $C_{18}H_{14}O_2$ mw: 262.32

SYNS: BA-1,2-DIHYDRODIOL ◇ trans-1,2-DIHYDROXY-
1,2-DIHYDROBENZ(a)ANTHRACENE

TOXICITY DATA with REFERENCE
ETA: skn-mus TD: 10 mg/kg   PNASA6 74,3176,77

ETA: skn-mus TDLo:2100 µg/kg   CNREA8 38,1699,78

MUT: mma-sat 10 µmol/L   CNREA8 42,1620,82

MUT: msc-ham:lng 1200 µg/L/3H   BJCAAI 39,540,79

CONSENSUS REPORTS: EPA Genetic Toxicology Program.

SAFETY PROFILE: Questionable carcinogen with experimental tumorigenic data by skin contact. Mutation data reported. When heated to decomposition it emits acrid smoke and irritating fumes.

BBD500   CAS: 60967-89-7
BENZ(a)ANTHRACENE-3,4-DIHYDRODIOL
mf: $C_{18}H_{14}O_2$ mw: 262.32

SYNS: BA-3,4-DIHYDRODIOL ◇ trans-3,4-DIHYDRO-3,4-DIHYDROXYBENZO(a)ANTHRACENE ◇ trans-3,4-DIHYDROXY-3,4-DIHYDROBENZ(a)ANTHRACENE

TOXICITY DATA with REFERENCE

NEO: skn-mus TD:4200 µg/kg   CNREA8 38,1705,78

NEO: skn-mus TD:4200 µg/kg   PNASA6 74,3176,77

NEO: skn-mus TDLo:2100 µg/kg   CNREA8 38,1699,79

MUT: mma-sat 25 µmol/L   BBRCA9 72,680,76

MUT: msc-ham:lng 2500 µg/L/3H   BJCAAI 39,540,79

CONSENSUS REPORTS: EPA Genetic Toxicology Program.

SAFETY PROFILE: Questionable carcinogen with experimental neoplastigenic data by skin contact. Mutation data reported. When heated to decomposition it emits acrid smoke and irritating fumes.

BBD750   CAS: 67335-43-7
(+)-(3S,4S)trans-BENZ(a)ANTHRACENE-3,4-DIHYDRODIOL
mf: $C_{18}H_{10}O_3$ mw: 274.28

SYNS: (+)-(3S,4S)-trans-3,4-DIHYDRO-3,4-DIHYDROXY-BENZ(a)ANTHRACENE ◇ (+)-(3S,4S)-trans-3,4-DIHYDRO-3,4-DIHYDROXYBENZO(a)ANTHRACENE

TOXICITY DATA with REFERENCE

ETA: skn-mus TDLo:4390 µg/kg   CNREA8 38,1705,78

SAFETY PROFILE: Questionable carcinogen with experimental tumorigenic data by skin con-

tact. When heated to decomposition it emits acrid smoke and irritating fumes.

BBE250   CAS: 3719-37-7
BENZ(a)ANTHRACENE-5,6-DIHYDRODIOL
mf: $C_{18}H_{14}O_2$ mw: 262.32

SYNS: BA-5,6-DIHYDRODIOL ◇ BA-5,6-trans-DIHYDRODIOL ◇ BENZ(a)ANTHRACENE-5,6-trans-DIHYDRODIOL ◇ trans-5,6-DIHYDROXY-5,6-DIHYDROBENZ(a)ANTHRACENE

TOXICITY DATA with REFERENCE

NEO: skn-mus TDLo:21 mg/kg   PNASA6 74,3176,77

ETA: skn-mus TD:2100 µg/kg   CNREA8 38,1699,78

MUT: otr-ham:emb 4 mg/L   CNREA8 32,1391,72

CONSENSUS REPORTS: EPA Genetic Toxicology Program.

SAFETY PROFILE: Questionable carcinogen with experimental tumorigenic and neoplastigenic data by skin contact. Mutation data reported. When heated to decomposition it emits acrid smoke and irritating fumes.

BBE750   CAS: 34501-24-1
trans-BENZ(a)ANTHRACENE-8,9-DIHYDRODIOL
mf: $C_{18}H_{14}O_2$ mw: 262.32

SYNS: BA-8,9-DIHYDRODIOL ◇ trans-8,9-DIHYDROXY-8,9-DIHYDROBENZ(a)ANTHRACENE

TOXICITY DATA with REFERENCE

NEO: skn-mus TDLo:2100 µg/kg   CNREA8 38,1699,78

ETA: skn-mus TD:4200 µg/kg   PNASA6 74,3176,77

MUT: mma-sat 25 µmol/L   BBRCA9 72,680,76

CONSENSUS REPORTS: EPA Genetic Toxicology Program.

SAFETY PROFILE: Questionable carcinogen with experimental tumorigenic and neoplastigenic data by skin contact. Mutation data reported. When heated to decomposition it emits acrid smoke and irritating fumes.

BBF000   CAS: 60967-90-0
BENZ(a)ANTHRACENE-10,11-DIHYDRODIOL
mf: $C_{18}H_{14}O_2$ mw: 262.32

SYNS: BA-10,11-DIHYDRODIOL ◊ trans-10,11-DIHY-
DROXY-10,11-DIHYDROBENZ(a)ANTHRACENE

TOXICITY DATA with REFERENCE
ETA: skn-mus TD:4200 µg/kg   CNREA8
   38,1699,78
ETA: skn-mus TDLo:2100 µg/kg   PNASA6
   74,3176,77
MUT: mma-sat 100 µmol/L   CNREA8 42,1620,82

CONSENSUS REPORTS: EPA Genetic Toxicology Program.

SAFETY PROFILE: Questionable carcinogen
with experimental tumorigenic data by skin contact. When heated to decomposition it emits
acrid smoke and irritating fumes.

BBF500   CAS: 2564-65-0
BENZ(a)ANTHRACENE-7,12-
DIMETHANOL
mf: $C_{20}H_{16}O_2$ mw: 288.36

SYNS: 9:10-BISHYDROXYMETHYL-1:2-BENZANTHRA-
CENE ◊ 7:12-DIHYDROXYMETHYLBENZ(a)ANTHRACENE

TOXICITY DATA with REFERENCE
ETA: scu-mus TDLo:2600 mg/kg/40W-I
   PRLBA4 129,439,40
MUT: mma-sat 20 nmol/plate   46OJAN -,675,81
MUT: mmo-esc 1 g/L/2H   GENTAE 39,141,54

CONSENSUS REPORTS: EPA Genetic Toxicology Program.

SAFETY PROFILE: Questionable carcinogen
with experimental tumorigenic data. Mutation
data reported. When heated to decomposition
it emits acrid smoke and irritating fumes.

BBF750   CAS: 63018-62-2
BENZ(a)ANTHRACENE-7,12-
DIMETHANOLDIACETATE
mf: $C_{24}H_{20}O_4$ mw: 372.44

SYNS: ACETIC ACID, BENZ(a)ANTHRACENE-7,12-DI-
METHANOL DIESTER ◊ 9,10-BISACETOXYMETHYL-1,2-
BENZANTHRACENE

TOXICITY DATA with REFERENCE
ETA: scu-mus TDLo:3000 mg/kg/45W-I
   PRLBA4 129,439,40
ETA: skn-mus TDLo:1700 mg/kg/71W-I
   PRLBA4 129,439,40

SAFETY PROFILE: Questionable carcinogen
with experimental tumorigenic data. When

heated to decomposition it emits acrid smoke
and irritating fumes.

BBG000   CAS: 67335-42-6
(−)(3R,4R)-trans-
BENZ(a)ANTHRACENE-3,4-DIOL
mf: $C_{18}H_{10}O_3$ mw: 274.28

SYNS: (−)(3R,4R)-trans-3,4-DIHYDRO-3,4-DIHYDROXY-
BENZ(a)ANTHRACENE ◊ (−)(3R,4R)trans-3,4-DIHYDRO-3,4-
DIHYDROXYBENZO(a)ANTHRACENE

TOXICITY DATA with REFERENCE
NEO: skn-mus TDLo:1100 µg/kg   CNREA8
   38,1705,78

SAFETY PROFILE: Questionable carcinogen
with experimental neoplastigenic data by skin
contact. When heated to decomposition it emits
acrid smoke and irritating fumes.

BBG500   CAS: 63020-45-1
BENZ(a)ANTHRACENE-7-ETHANOL
mf: $C_{20}H_{16}O$ mw: 272.36

SYN: 10-β-HYDROXYETHYL-1:2-BENZANTHRACENE

TOXICITY DATA with REFERENCE
ETA: scu-mus TDLo:1700 mg/kg/26W-I
   PRLBA4 129,439,40
ETA: skn-mus TDLo:1220 mg/kg/51W-I
   PRLBA4 131,170,42

SAFETY PROFILE: Questionable carcinogen
with experimental tumorigenic data. When
heated to decomposition it emits acrid smoke
and irritating fumes.

BBG750   CAS: 17012-91-8
BENZ(a)ANTHRACENE-7-
METHANEDIOLDIACETATE (ester)
mf: $C_{23}H_{18}O_4$ mw: 358.41

SYN: 7-DIACETOXYMETHYLBENZ(a)ANTHRACENE

TOXICITY DATA with REFERENCE
CAR: scu-mus TDLo:120 mg/kg/6W-I   IJCNAW
   2,500,67

SAFETY PROFILE: Questionable carcinogen
with experimental carcinogenic data. When
heated to decomposition it emits acrid smoke
and irritating fumes.

BBH000   CAS: 63018-59-7
BENZ(a)ANTHRACENE-7-
METHANETHIOL
mf: $C_{19}H_{14}S$ mw: 274.39

SYN: 1,2-BENZANTHRYL-10-METHYLMERCAPTAN

TOXICITY DATA with REFERENCE
ETA: scu-mus TDLo: 80 mg/kg   CNREA8 6,454,46

SAFETY PROFILE: Questionable carcinogen with experimental tumorigenic data. When heated to decomposition it emits toxic fumes of SO_x.

BBH250   CAS: 16110-13-7
BENZ(a)ANTHRACENE-7-METHANOL
mf: $C_{19}H_{14}O$ mw: 258.33

SYNS: 7-HMBA ◇ 7-HYDROXYMETHYLBENZ(a)AN-THRACENE ◇ 10-HYDROXYMETHYL-1,2-BENZANTHRA-CENE

TOXICITY DATA with REFERENCE
ETA: scu-mus TDLo: 1000 mg/kg/16W-I
    PRLBA4 129,439,40
ETA: skn-mus TDLo: 56 mg/kg/60W-I   CNREA8
    43,2034,83
ETA: skn-mus TDLo: 700 mg/kg/29W-I
    PRLBA4 129,439,40
MUT: dnd-mam: lym 30 μmol/L   CBINA8 31,51,80
MUT: dnd-mus: emb 800 μg/L   CNREA8
    33,2386,73
MUT: dnd-omi 30 μmol/L   CBINA8 31,51,80
MUT: otr-mus: oth 100 μg/L   IJCNAW 13,304,74

CONSENSUS REPORTS: EPA Genetic Toxicology Program.

SAFETY PROFILE: Questionable carcinogen with experimental tumorigenic data. Mutation data reported. When heated to decomposition it emits acrid smoke and irritating fumes.

BBH500   CAS: 17526-24-8
BENZ(a)ANTHRACENE-7-METHANOL ACETATE
mf: $C_{21}H_{16}O_2$ mw: 300.37

SYNS: ACETIC ACID, BENZ(a)ANTHRACENE-7-METHA-NOL ESTER ◇ 10-ACETOXYMETHYL-1,2-BENZANTHRA-CENE

TOXICITY DATA with REFERENCE
ETA: scu-mus TDLo: 1200 mg/kg/17W-I
    PRLBA4 129,439,40
ETA: skn-mus TD: 744 mg/kg/31W-I   PRLBA4
    129,439,40
ETA: skn-mus TDLo: 16 mg/kg/17W-I
    VOONAW 21(10),50,75

SAFETY PROFILE: Questionable carcinogen with experimental tumorigenic data. When heated to decomposition it emits acrid smoke and irritating fumes.

BBH750   CAS: 63018-57-5
BENZ(a)ANTHRACENE-7-THIOL
mf: $C_{18}H_{12}S$ mw: 260.36

SYNS: 1,2-BENZANTHRYL-10-MERCAPTAN ◇ 7-MER-CAPTOBENZ(a)ANTHRACENE

TOXICITY DATA with REFERENCE
ETA: scu-mus TDLo: 80 mg/kg   CNREA8 6,454,46

SAFETY PROFILE: Questionable carcinogen with experimental tumorigenic data. When heated to decomposition it emits toxic fumes of SO_x.

BBI000   CAS: 960-92-9
BENZ(a)ANTHRACEN-5-OL
mf: $C_{18}H_{12}O$ mw: 244.30

SYNS: 3-HYDROXY-1,2-BENZANTHRACENE ◇ 5-HY-DROXYBENZ(a)ANTHRACENE

TOXICITY DATA with REFERENCE
ETA: scu-mus TDLo: 1240 mg/kg   JNCIAM
    1,303,40
MUT: dnd-ham: kdy 5 mg/L   BCPCA6 20,1297,71
MUT: dnd-ham: lng 1 mg/L   CBINA8 4,389,71/72
MUT: dnd-mus: oth 1 mg/L   CBINA8 4,389,71/72
MUT: oms-ham: lng 1 mg/L   CBINA8 4,389,71/72
MUT: oms-mus: oth 1 mg/L   CBINA8 4,389,71/72

CONSENSUS REPORTS: EPA Genetic Toxicology Program.

SAFETY PROFILE: Questionable carcinogen with experimental tumorigenic data. Mutation data reported. When heated to decomposition it emits acrid smoke and irritating fumes.

BBI750   CAS: 63018-49-5
1,2-BENZANTHRYL-3-CARBAMIDOACETIC ACID
mf: $C_{21}H_{16}N_2O_3$ mw: 344.39

SYN: N-(BENZ(a)ANTHRACEN-5-YLCARBAMOYL)GLY-CINE

TOXICITY DATA with REFERENCE
ETA: scu-mus TDLo: 120 mg/kg   CNREA8
    6,454,46

SAFETY PROFILE: Questionable carcinogen with experimental tumorigenic data. When heated to decomposition it emits toxic fumes such as NO_x.

BBJ000   CAS: 63018-50-8
1,2-BENZANTHRYL-10-CARBAMIDOACETIC ACID
mf: $C_{21}H_{16}N_2O_3$ mw: 344.39

SYN: N-(BENZ(a)ANTHRACEN-7-YLCARBAMOYL)GLY-CINE

TOXICITY DATA with REFERENCE
ETA: scu-mus TDLo:160 mg/kg   CNREA8
  6,454,46

SAFETY PROFILE: Questionable carcinogen with experimental tumorigenic data. When heated to decomposition it emits toxic fumes of NO_x.

BBJ250   CAS: 63018-56-4
1,2-BENZANTHRYL-10-ISOCYANATE
mf: $C_{19}H_{11}NO$ mw: 269.31

SYN: ISOCYANIC ACID, BENZ(a)ANTHRACEN-7-YL ESTER

TOXICITY DATA with REFERENCE
ETA: scu-mus TDLo:40 mg/kg   CNREA8 6,454,46

SAFETY PROFILE: Questionable carcinogen with experimental tumorigenic data. When heated to decomposition it emits toxic fumes of NO_x.

BBM250   CAS: 2227-79-4
BENZENECARBOTHIOAMIDE
mf: C_7H_7NS mw: 137.21

SYNS: BENZOTHIAMIDE ◊ BENZOTHIOAMIDE ◊ THIOBENZAMIDE ◊ TIOBENZAMIDE (ITALIAN)

TOXICITY DATA with REFERENCE
ETA: orl-rat TD:13 g/kg/38W-C   ARTODN
  55,34,84
ETA: orl-rat TD:13 g/kg/38W-C   ARTODN
  55,34,84
ETA: orl-rat TD:13300 mg/kg/38W-C   ARTODN
  55,34,84
ETA: orl-rat TDLo:6300 mg/kg/15W-C   BSIBAC
  54,1027,78
MUT: mnt-mus-orl 180 μmol/kg   MUREAV
  192,141,87

CONSENSUS REPORTS: Reported in EPA TSCA Inventory.

SAFETY PROFILE: Questionable carcinogen with experimental tumorigenic data. Poison by ingestion. Moderately toxic by intraperitoneal route. Mutation data reported. When heated to decomposition it emits very toxic fumes of NO_x and SO_x.

BBM500   CAS: 63021-32-9
BENZENECARBOXALDEHYDE
mf: $C_{19}H_{15}N$ mw: 257.35

SYNS: BENZALDEHYDE FFC ◊ 7-ETHYLBENZ(c)ACRIDINE ◊ 9-ETHYL-3,4-BENZACRIDINE ◊ PHENYLMETHANAL

TOXICITY DATA with REFERENCE
ETA: scu-mus TDLo:200 mg/kg   VOONAW
  1,52,55

SAFETY PROFILE: Questionable carcinogen with experimental tumorigenic data. When heated to decomposition it emits toxic fumes of NO_x.

BBO325   CAS: 369-57-3
BENZENEDIAZONIUM TETRAFLUOROBORATE
mf: $C_6H_5N_2•BF_4$ mw: 191.94

SYNS: BENZENEDIAZONIUM FLUOBORATE ◊ BENZENEDIAZONIUM FLUOROBORATE ◊ PHENYLDIAZONIUM FLUOROBORATE (SALT) ◊ PHENYLDIAZONIUM TETRAFLUOROBORATE

TOXICITY DATA with REFERENCE
ETA: scu-ham TD:157 mg/kg/66W-I   CALEDQ
  15,289,82
ETA: scu-ham TD:200 mg/kg/84W-I   CALEDQ
  15,289,82
ETA: scu-ham TD:100 mg/kg/84W-I   CALEDQ
  15,289,82
ETA: scu-ham TD:119 mg/kg/50W-I   CALEDQ
  15,289,82
ETA: scu-ham TDLo:85 mg/kg/71W-I   CALEDQ
  15,289,82
MUT: mmo-sat 10 μmol/L   CNREA8 42,1446,82

SAFETY PROFILE: Questionable carcinogen with experimental tumorigenic data. Poison by ingestion and subcutaneous routes. Mutation data reported. When heated to decomposition it emits toxic fumes of NO_x and F^-.

BBR750   CAS: 1678-25-7
BENZENESULFONANILIDE
mf: $C_{12}H_{11}NO_2S$ mw: 233.30
SYN: BENZENESULFANILIDE

TOXICITY DATA with REFERENCE
ETA: ipr-rat TDLo:593 mg/kg/4W-I   CNREA8
  30,1485,70

SAFETY PROFILE: Questionable carcinogen with experimental tumorigenic data. When heated to decomposition it emits very toxic fumes of SO_x and NO_x.

BBV250   CAS: 613-94-5
BENZHYDRAZIDE
mf: $C_7H_8N_2O$ mw: 136.17

SYNS: BENZOHYDRAZIDE ◇ BENZOHYDRAZINE ◇ BENZOIC HYDRAZIDE ◇ BENZOYL HYDRAZIDE

TOXICITY DATA with REFERENCE
CAR: orl-mus TDLo: 15 g/kg/77W-C   EJCAAH 8,341,72
NEO: orl-mus TD: 13 g/kg/30W-I   34ZRA9 -,869,65

CONSENSUS REPORTS: Reported in EPA TSCA Inventory.

SAFETY PROFILE: Questionable carcinogen with experimental carcinogenic and neoplastigenic data. Poison by subcutaneous and intraperitoneal routes. When heated to decomposition it emits toxic fumes of NO_x.

BBX250   CAS: 16993-94-5
3,3'-BENZIDINE DICARBOXYLIC ACID, DISODIUM SALT
mf: $C_{14}H_{10}N_2O_4 \cdot 2Na$ mw: 316.24

SYN: 4,4'-DIAMINO-3,3'-BIPHENYLDICARBOXYLIC ACID DISODIUM SALT

TOXICITY DATA with REFERENCE
ETA: scu-mus TDLo: 9 g/kg/43W-I   VOONAW 15(5),60,69
ETA: scu-rat TDLo: 7 g/kg/77W-I   VOONAW 15(5),60,69

SAFETY PROFILE: Questionable carcinogen with experimental tumorigenic data. When heated to decomposition it emits toxic fumes of NO_x and Na_2O.

BBY250   CAS: 2051-89-0
BENZIDINE-3-SULFURIC ACID
mf: $C_{12}H_{12}N_2O_3S$ mw: 264.32

SYNS: BENZIDINE-3-SULPHURIC ACID ◇ 4,4'-DIAMINO-3-BIPHENYL-3-SULFONIC ACID ◇ 4:4'-DIAMINO-3-DIPHE-NYLYL HYDROGEN SULFATE ◇ 3-SULFOBENZIDINE

TOXICITY DATA with REFERENCE
ETA: imp-mus TDLo: 80 mg/kg   BJCAAI 17,127,63

CONSENSUS REPORTS: Reported in EPA TSCA Inventory.

SAFETY PROFILE: Questionable carcinogen with experimental tumorigenic data. When heated to decomposition it emits very toxic fumes of NO_x and SO_x.

BBY500   CAS: 3365-94-4
BENZIDIN-3-YL ESTER SULFURIC ACID
mf: $C_{12}H_{12}N_2O_4S$ mw: 280.32

SYNS: BENZIDIN-3-YL HYDROGEN SULFATE ◇ 4,4'-DIAMINO-3-DIPHENYLYL HYDROGEN SULFATE

TOXICITY DATA with REFERENCE
ETA: imp-mus TDLo: 80 mg/kg   BJCAAI 17,127,63

SAFETY PROFILE: Questionable carcinogen with experimental tumorigenic data. When heated to decomposition it emits very toxic fumes of NO_x and SO_x.

BCC250   CAS: 6898-43-7
BENZIMIDAZOLE METHYLENE MUSTARD
mf: $C_{14}H_{19}Cl_2N_3 \cdot ClH$ mw: 336.72

SYNS: BENZIMIDAZOLE MUSTARD ◇ 2-(BIS(2-CHLORO-ETHYL)AMINOMETHYL)-5,5-DIMETHYLBENZIMIDAZOLE HYDROCHLORIDE ◇ 2-(DI-2-CHLOROETHYL)AMINO-METHYL-5,6-DIMETHYLBENZIMIDAZOLE ◇ NSC-23892

TOXICITY DATA with REFERENCE
CAR: ipr-mus TDLo: 12 mg/kg/4W   JNCIAM 36,915,66

SAFETY PROFILE: Questionable carcinogen with experimental carcinogenic data. When heated to decomposition it emits very toxic fumes HCl and NO_x.

BCE000   CAS: 208-07-1
BENZ(e)INDENO(1,2-b)INDOLE
mf: $C_{19}H_{11}N$ mw: 253.31

SYN: 4,5-BENZO-2,3-1',2'-INDENOINDOLE (FRENCH)

TOXICITY DATA with REFERENCE
ETA: scu-mus TDLo: 120 mg/kg/9W-I   BAFEAG 42,3,55

SAFETY PROFILE: Questionable carcinogen with experimental tumorigenic data. Poison by subcutaneous route. When heated to decomposition it emits toxic fumes of NO_x.

BCF500   CAS: 1491-10-7
BENZO(f)(1)BENZOTHIENO(3,2-b) QUINOLINE
mf: $C_{19}H_{11}NS$ mw: 285.37

SYN: NAPHTHO(1,2-e)THIANAPHTHENO(3,2-b)PYRIDINE

TOXICITY DATA with REFERENCE
ETA: scu-mus TDLo: 72 mg/kg/9W-I   EJCAAH 4,123,68

SAFETY PROFILE: Questionable carcinogen with experimental tumorigenic data. When heated to decomposition it emits very toxic fumes of SO_x and NO_x.

BCF750   CAS: 1491-09-4
BENZO(h)(1)BENZOTHIENO(3,2-b) QUINOLINE
mf: $C_{19}H_{11}NS$ mw: 285.37

SYN: NAPHTHO(2,1-e)THIANAPHTHENO(3,2-b)PYRIDINE

TOXICITY DATA with REFERENCE
ETA: scu-mus TDLo:72 mg/kg/9W-I   EJCAAH
   4,123,68

SAFETY PROFILE: Questionable carcinogen with experimental tumorigenic data. When heated to decomposition it emits very toxic fumes of SO_x and NO_x.

BCG000   CAS: 846-35-5
BENZO(e)(1)BENZOTHIOPYRANO (4,3-b)INDOLE
mf: $C_{19}H_{11}NS$ mw: 285.37

TOXICITY DATA with REFERENCE
NEO: scu-mus TDLo:360 mg/kg/25W-I
   JNCIAM 46,1257,71

SAFETY PROFILE: Questionable carcinogen with experimental neoplastigenic data. When heated to decomposition it emits very toxic fumes of SO_x and NO_x.

BCG250   CAS: 239-01-0
11H-BENZO(a)CARBAZOLE
mf: $C_{16}H_{11}N$ mw: 217.28

SYN: 1,2-BENZCARBAZOLE

TOXICITY DATA with REFERENCE
ETA: skn-mus TDLo:840 mg/kg/21W-I
   HSZPAZ 236,79,35

SAFETY PROFILE: Questionable carcinogen with experimental tumorigenic data. When heated to decomposition it emits toxic fumes such as NO_x.

BCG500   CAS: 214-17-5
BENZO(b)CHRYSENE
mf: $C_{22}H_{14}$ mw: 278.36

SYNS: 2,3-BENZOCHRYSENE ◇ 3,4-BENZOTETRACENE ◇ 3,4-BENZOTETRAPHENE ◇ BENZO(c)TETRAPHENE ◇ 1,2:6,7-DIBENZOPHENANTHRENE ◇ 2,3:7,8-DIBENZO-PHENANTHRENE ◇ DIBENZO-2,3,7,8-PHENANTHRENE

TOXICITY DATA with REFERENCE
NEO: skn-mus TDLo:28 mg/kg   JNCIAM
   50,1717,73
MUT: mma-sat 50 μg/plate   MUREAV 174,247,86

SAFETY PROFILE: Questionable carcinogen with experimental neoplastigenic data by skin contact. Mutation data reported. When heated to decomposition it emits acrid smoke and irritating fumes.

BCG750   CAS: 194-69-4
BENZO(c)CHRYSENE
mf: $C_{22}H_{14}$ mw: 278.36

SYN: 1,2,5,6-DIBENZPHENANTHRENE

TOXICITY DATA with REFERENCE
ETA: scu-mus TDLo:2400 mg/kg/36W-I
   PRLBA4 129,439,40
ETA: skn-mus TDLo:1630 mg/kg/68W-I
   PRLBA4 129,439,40

SAFETY PROFILE: Questionable carcinogen with experimental tumorigenic data. When heated to decomposition it emits acrid smoke and irritating fumes.

BCH000   CAS: 196-78-1
BENZO(g)CHRYSENE
mf: $C_{22}H_{14}$ mw: 278.36

SYNS: 1,2,3,4-DIBENZOPHENANTHRENE ◇ 1,2,3,4-DI-BENZPHENANTHRENE

TOXICITY DATA with REFERENCE
ETA: orl-mus TDLo:15 g/kg/74W-I   PRLBA4
   129,439,40
ETA: scu-mus TDLo:1400 mg/kg/21W-I
   PRLBA4 129,439,40
ETA: skn-mus TDLo:720 mg/kg/30W-I
   PRLBA4 129,439,40

SAFETY PROFILE: Questionable carcinogen with experimental tumorigenic data. When heated to decomposition it emits acrid smoke and irritating fumes.

BCH250   CAS: 5096-19-5
N-6-(3,4-BENZOCOUMARINYL) ACETAMIDE
mf: $C_{15}H_{10}NO_3$ mw: 252.26

SYN: N-(6-OXO-6H-DIBENZO(b,d)PYRAN-1-YL)ACET-AMIDE

TOXICITY DATA with REFERENCE
CAR: orl-rat TDLo:5000 mg/kg   CNREA8
   26,619,66
ETA: orl-rat TD:9000 mg/kg/27D-I   CNREA8
   28,924,68

SAFETY PROFILE: Questionable carcinogen with experimental carcinogenic and tumorigenic data. When heated to decomposition it emits very toxic fumes of NO_x.

BCI000
CAS: 198-46-9
BENZO(de)CYCLOPENT(a) ANTHRACENE

mf: $C_{20}H_{12}$　　mw: 252.32

SYN: Δ^3-DEHYDRO-3,4-TRIMETHYLENE-ISOBENZAN-THRENE-2

TOXICITY DATA with REFERENCE
ETA: imp-mus TDLo:600 mg/kg/40W-I
JNCIAM 2,241,41

SAFETY PROFILE: Questionable carcinogen with experimental tumorigenic data. When heated to decomposition it emits acrid smoke and irritating fumes.

BCI250
CAS: 240-44-8
1H-BENZO(a)CYCLOPENT(b) ANTHRACENE

mf: $C_{21}H_{16}$　　mw: 268.37

SYN: 6,7-CYCLOPENTENO-1,2-BENZANTHRACENE

TOXICITY DATA with REFERENCE
ETA: skn-mus TDLo:820 mg/kg/34W-I
PRLBA4 117,318,35

SAFETY PROFILE: Questionable carcinogen with experimental tumorigenic data. When heated to decomposition it emits acrid smoke and irritating fumes.

BCL100
CAS: 42242-58-0
p-(7-BENZOFURYLAZO)-N,N-DIMETHYLANILINE

mf: $C_{16}H_{15}N_3O$　　mw: 265.34

SYNS: ANILINE, p-(7-BENZOFURYLAZO)-N,N-DI-METHYL- ◇ N,N-DIMETHYL-p-(7-BENZOFURYLAZO) ANILINE

TOXICITY DATA with REFERENCE
ETA: orl-rat TDLo:1620 mg/kg/13W-C
JMCMAR 16,717,73

SAFETY PROFILE: Questionable carcinogen with experimental tumorigenic data. When heated to decomposition it emits toxic fumes of NO_x.

BCP750
CAS: 192-70-1
BENZO(a)NAPHTHO(8,1,2-cde) NAPHTHACENE

mf: $C_{28}H_{16}$　　mw: 352.44

SYN: NAPHTO(1,2-c-d-e)NAPHTACENE (FRENCH)

TOXICITY DATA with REFERENCE
ETA: scu-mus TDLo:72 mg/kg/9W-I　CHDDAT
266,301,68

SAFETY PROFILE: Questionable carcinogen with experimental tumorigenic data. When heated to decomposition it emits acrid smoke and irritating fumes.

BCQ000
CAS: 196-79-2
BENZO(h)NAPHTHO(1,2-f,s-3) QUINOLINE

mf: $C_{21}H_{13}N$　　mw: 279.35

SYN: PYRIDO(3',2':5,6)CHRYSENE

TOXICITY DATA with REFERENCE
ETA: scu-mus TDLo:72 mg/kg/9W-I　COREAF
252,1711,61

SAFETY PROFILE: Questionable carcinogen with experimental tumorigenic data. When heated to decomposition it emits toxic fumes such as NO_x.

BCQ750
CAS: 63040-53-9
BENZO(rst)PENTAPHENE-5-CARBOXALDEHYDE

mf: $C_{25}H_{14}O$　　mw: 330.39

SYN: 5-FORMYL-3,4:9,10-DIBENZOPYRENE

TOXICITY DATA with REFERENCE
ETA: scu-mus TDLo:72 mg/kg/9W-I　COREAF
252,1236,61

SAFETY PROFILE: Questionable carcinogen with experimental tumorigenic data. When heated to decomposition it emits acrid smoke and irritating fumes.

BCR000
CAS: 191-24-2
BENZO(ghi)PERYLENE

mf: $C_{22}H_{12}$　　mw: 276.34

SYNS: 1,12-BENZPERYLENE ◇ 1,12-BENZOPERYLENE

TOXICITY DATA with REFERENCE
MUT: mma-sat 2 μg/plate/48H　FCTXAV 17,141,79

CONSENSUS REPORTS: IARC Cancer Review: GROUP 3 IMEMDT 7,56,87, Animal Inadequate Evidence IMEMDT 32,195,83. EPA Genetic Toxicology Program.

SAFETY PROFILE: Questionable carcinogen. Mutation data reported. When heated to decomposition it emits acrid smoke and irritating fumes.

BCR250   CAS: 190-07-8
BENZO(a)PHENALENO(1,9-hi)ACRIDINE
mf: $C_{27}H_{15}N$ mw: 353.43

SYN: BENZO(c)PHENALENO(1,9-I,j)ACRIDINE

TOXICITY DATA with REFERENCE
ETA: scu-mus TDLo: 72 mg/kg/9W-I   BAFEAG
52,49,65

SAFETY PROFILE: Questionable carcinogen with experimental tumorigenic data. When heated to decomposition it emits toxic fumes such as NO_x.

BCR500   CAS: 190-03-4
BENZO(a)PHENALENO(1,9-i,j)ACRIDINE
mf: $C_{27}H_{15}N$ mw: 353.43

SYN: BENZO(h)PHENALENO(1,9-bc)ACRIDINE

TOXICITY DATA with REFERENCE
ETA: scu-mus TDLo: 72 mg/kg/9W-I   BAFEAG
52,49,65

SAFETY PROFILE: Questionable carcinogen with experimental tumorigenic data. When heated to decomposition it emits toxic fumes of NO_x.

BCR750   CAS: 195-19-7
BENZO(c)PHENANTHRENE
mf: $C_{18}H_{12}$ mw: 228.30

SYNS: 3,4-BENZOPHENANTHRENE ◇ 3,4-BENZPHENAN-THRENE ◇ TETRAHELICENE

TOXICITY DATA with REFERENCE
ETA: skn-mus TD: 1220 mg/kg/51W-I   PRLBA4
129,439,40
ETA: skn-mus TD: 1270 mg/kg/53W-I   PRLBA4
123,343,37
ETA: skn-mus TDLo: 940 mg/kg/39W-I
PRLBA4 117,318,35
MUT: mma-sat 25 nmol/plate   CNREA8 40,2876,80

CONSENSUS REPORTS: IARC Cancer Review: Animal Inadequate Evidence IMEMDT 32,205,83

SAFETY PROFILE: Questionable carcinogen with experimental tumorigenic data. Mutation data reported. When heated to decomposition it emits acrid and irritating fumes.

BCS000   CAS: 4466-76-6
BENZO(c)PHENATHRENE-8-CARBOXALDEHYDE
mf: $C_{19}H_{12}O$ mw: 256.31

SYN: 2-FORMYL-3:4-BENZPHENANTHRENE

TOXICITY DATA with REFERENCE
ETA: scu-mus TDLo: 5200 mg/kg/52W-I
PRLBA4 131,170,42

SAFETY PROFILE: Questionable carcinogen with tumorigenic data. When heated to decomposition it emits acrid smoke and irritating fumes.

BCS100
(±)-BENZO(c)PHENANTHRENE-3,4-DIHYDRODIOL
mf: $C_{18}H_{14}O_2$ mw: 262.32

TOXICITY DATA with REFERENCE
NEO: ipr-mus TDLo: 11 mg/kg/15D-I   CNREA8
46,2257,86

SAFETY PROFILE: Questionable carcinogen with experimental neoplastigenic data. When heated to decomposition it emits toxic and irritating fumes.

BCS103
(+)-BENZO(c)PHENANTHRENE-3,4-DIOL-1,2-EPOXIDE-1
mf: $C_{18}H_{14}O_3$ mw: 278.32

SYNS: BENZO(c)PHENANTHRENE-3,4-DIOL, 1,2,3,4-TET-RAHYDRO-1,2-EPOXY-, (Z)-(+)-(1R,2S,3R,4S)- ◇ cis-1-β,2-β-EPOXY-1,2,3,4-TETRAHYDROBENZO(c)PHENANTHRENE-3-α-4-β-DIOL

TOXICITY DATA with REFERENCE
NEO: ipr-mus TDLo: 12 mg/kg/15D-I   CNREA8
46,2257,86
NEO: skn-mus TDLo: 111 μg/kg   CNREA8
46,2257,86

SAFETY PROFILE: Questionable carcinogen with experimental neoplastigenic data. When heated to decomposition it emits toxic and irritating fumes.

BCS105
(+)-BENZO(c)PHENANTHRENE-3,4-DIOL-1,2-EPOXIDE-2
mf: $C_{18}H_{14}O_3$ mw: 278.32

SYNS: BENZO(c)PHENANTHRENE-3,4-DIOL, 1,2,3,4-TET-RAHYDRO-1,2-EPOXY-1, (E)-(+)-(1S,2R,3R,4S)- ◇ trans-1-α-2-α-EPOXY-1,2,3,4-TETRAHYDROBENZO(c)PHENAN-THRENE-3-α,4-β-DIOL

TOXICITY DATA with REFERENCE
NEO: ipr-mus TDLo: 12 mg/kg/15D-I   CNREA8
46,2257,86
NEO: skn-mus TDLo: 278 μg/kg   CNREA8
46,2257,86

SAFETY PROFILE: Questionable carcinogen with experimental neoplastigenic data. When heated to decomposition it emits toxic and irritating fumes.

BCS110
(−)-BENZO(c)PHENANTHRENE-3,4-DIOL-1,2-EPOXIDE-2
mf: $C_{18}H_{14}O_3$ mw: 278.32

SYNS: BENZO(c)PHENANTHRENE-3,4-DIOL, 1,2,3,4-TET-RAHYDRO-1,2-EPOXY-, (E)-(−)-(1R,2S,3S,4R)- ◊ trans-1-β,2-β-EPOXY-1,2,3,4-TETRAHYDROBENZO(c)PHENAN-THRENE-3-β, 4-α-DIOL

TOXICITY DATA with REFERENCE
NEO: ipr-mus TDLo:12 mg/kg/15D-I   CNREA8 46,2257,86
NEO: skn-mus TDLo:111 μg/kg   CNREA8 46,2257,86

SAFETY PROFILE: Questionable carcinogen with experimental neoplastigenic data. When heated to decomposition it emits toxic and irritating fumes.

BCT000   CAS: 192-97-2
BENZO(e)PYRENE
mf: $C_{20}H_{12}$ mw: 252.32

SYNS: 1,2-BENZOPYRENE ◊ 4,5-BENZOPYRENE ◊ 1,2-BENZPYRENE ◊ B(e)P

TOXICITY DATA with REFERENCE
ETA: orl-mus TDLo:360 mg/kg/43W-I   VRRAAT 20,276,38
ETA: scu-gpg TDLo:140 mg/kg/37W-I   AJCAA7 27,474,36
ETA: scu-mus TDLo:160 mg/kg   AJCAA7 27,474,36
ETA: skn-mus TD:516 mg/kg/43W-I   CANCAR 12,1079,59
ETA: skn-mus TDLo:240 mg/kg/30W-I   CALEDQ 7,51,79
MUT: dnd-ham:lng 100 μmol/L/4H   BBRCA9 72,732,76
MUT: dnd-mus-skn 192 μmol/kg   CRNGDP 5,231,84
MUT: dns-hmn:fbr 1 mg/L   CNREA8 38,2091,78
MUT: dns-hmn:hla 1 μmol/L   CNREA8 38,2621,78
MUT: dns-rat:lvr 79 nmol/L   CNREA8 42,3010,82
MUT: mma-mus:lym 10 mg/L   MUREAV 59,61,79
MUT: mma-sat 50 μg/plate   JNCIAM 62,893,79
MUT: mma-sat 1 μg/plate   ENMUDM 6(Suppl 2),1,84
MUT: mmo-sat 1 nmol/plate   CNREA8 40,1985,80

MUT: msc-hmn:oth 12 μmol/L   MUREAV 130,127,84
MUT: otr-ham:emb 10 mg/L   JNCIAM 42,867,69
MUT: otr-ham:kdy 25 μg/L   TOLED5 7,143,80
MUT: sce-ham-ipr 900 mg/kg/24H   MUREAV 66,65,79
MUT: sce-ham:ovr 1 μmol/L   MUREAV 53,284,78

CONSENSUS REPORTS: IARC Cancer Review: GROUP 3 IMEMDT 7,56,87; Animal Inadequate Evidence IMEMDT 32,225,83; Animal Limited Evidence IMEMDT 3,137,73. EPA Genetic Toxicology Program.

SAFETY PROFILE: Questionable carcinogen with experimental tumorigenic and teratogenic data. Other experimental reproductive effects. Human mutation data reported. When heated to decomposition it emits acrid smoke and irritating fumes.

BCT250   CAS: 13312-42-0
BENZO(a)PYRENE-6-CARBOXYALDEHYDE
mf: $C_{21}H_{12}O$ mw: 280.33

SYNS: 3,4-BENZPYRENE-5-ALDEHYDE ◊ 6-FORMYL-BENZO(a)PYRENE

TOXICITY DATA with REFERENCE
NEO: scu-mus TDLo:40 mg/kg   BJCAAI 26,506,72
NEO: scu-rat TDLo:17 mg/kg/60D-I   CBINA8 29,159,80
NEO: skn-mus TDLo:180 mg/kg/20W-I   CBINA8 22(1),53,78
ETA: scu-mus TD:200 mg/kg   COREAF 245,876,57
ETA: scu-rat TD:100 mg/kg/40D-I   JMCMAR 16,714,73
ETA: skn-mus TD:32 mg/kg/20W-I   BEXBAN 87,474,79
ETA: skn-mus TD:179 mg/kg/20W-I   PAACA3 18,59,77
ETA: unk-mus TDLo:80 mg/kg/8D-I   BEBMAE 88(11),592,79

SAFETY PROFILE: Questionable carcinogen with experimental tumorigenic and neoplastigenic data. When heated to decomposition it emits acrid smoke and fumes.

BCT500   CAS: 64048-70-0
BENZO(a)PYRENE-6-CARBOXALDEHYDE THIOSEMICARBAZONE
mf: $C_{22}H_{15}N_3S$ mw: 353.46

SYN: 3,4-BENZPYRENE-5-ALDEHYDE THIOSEMICARBAZONE

TOXICITY DATA with REFERENCE
ETA: scu-mus TDLo: 200 mg/kg   COREAF 245,876,57

SAFETY PROFILE: Questionable carcinogen with experimental tumorigenic data. When heated to decomposition it emits very toxic fumes of SO_x and NO_x.

BCT750   CAS: 13345-25-0
BENZO(a)PYRENE-7,8-DIHYDRODIOL
mf: $O_2C_{20}H_{14}$ mw: 286.34

SYN: BP-7,8-DIHYDRODIOL

TOXICITY DATA with REFERENCE
NEO: skn-mus TDLo: 4580 µg/kg   CCSUDL 3,371,78
ETA: par-mus TDLo: 4 mg/kg   BJCAAI 37,657,78
ETA: skn-mus TD: 2290 µg/kg   CALEDQ 2,115,76
MUT: dnd-ham: emb 250 mg/L   NATUAS 252,326,74
MUT: dnd-hmn: fbr 30 µmol/L   CBINA8 41,155,82
MUT: dnd-rat: lvr 30 µmol/L   CBINA8 20,311,78
MUT: dnd-sal: spr 215 mg/L   NATUAS 252,326,74
MUT: mma-sat 8 µmol/L   CALEDQ 24,281,84
MUT: msc-ham: fbr 100 µg/L   NATUAS 264,360,76

CONSENSUS REPORTS: EPA Genetic Toxicology Program.

SAFETY PROFILE: Questionable carcinogen with experimental neoplastigenic and tumorigenic data. Human mutation data reported. When heated to decomposition it emits acrid smoke and irritating fumes.

BCU000   CAS: 60268-85-1
anti-BENZO(a)PYRENE-7,8-DIHYDRODIOL-9,10-OXIDE
mf: $C_{20}H_{14}O_3$ mw: 302.34

SYNS: BENZO(a)PYRENE-7,8-DIHYDRODIOL-9,10-EPOXIDE (anti) ◇ BP-7,8-DIHYDRODIOL-9,10-EPOXIDE (anti) ◇ anti-BP-7,8-DIHYDRODIOL-9,10-OXIDE

TOXICITY DATA with REFERENCE
ETA: skn-mus TD: 4840 µg/kg   CALEDQ 3,23,77
ETA: skn-mus TDLo: 2400 µg/kg   CALEDQ 2,115,76
MUT: dnd-hmn: lym 800 µg/L   CRNGDP 3,1107,82
MUT: dns-hmn: lym 100 µg/L   CRNGDP 3,1107,82

MUT: msc-ham: lng 100 µg/L   IJCNAW 24,203,79
MUT: msc-mus: fbr 200 nmol/L   CNREA8 42,1866,82
MUT: otr-mus: fbr 200 nmol/L   CNREA8 42,1866,82

SAFETY PROFILE: Questionable carcinogen with experimental tumorigenic data by skin contact. Human mutation data reported. When heated to decomposition it emits acrid smoke and irritating fumes.

BCU500   CAS: 3067-13-8
BENZO(a)PYRENE-1,6-DIONE
mf: $C_{20}H_{10}O_2$ mw: 282.30

SYNS: 1,6-BENZO(a)PYRENEDIONE ◇ BENZO(a)PYRENE-1,6-QUINONE ◇ PB-1,6-QUINONE

TOXICITY DATA with REFERENCE
NEO: skn-mus TDLo: 4520 µg/kg   CCSUDL 3,371,78
MUT: msc-ham: lng 2 mg/L   CNREA8 36,3350,76

CONSENSUS REPORTS: EPA Genetic Toxicology Program.

SAFETY PROFILE: Questionable carcinogen with experimental neoplastigenic data by skin contact. Mutation data reported. When heated to decomposition it emits acrid smoke and irritating fumes.

BCU750   CAS: 3067-14-9
BENZO(a)PYRENE-3,6-DIONE
mf: $C_{20}H_{10}O_2$ mw: 282.30

SYNS: 3,6-BENZO(a)PYRENEDIONE ◇ BENZO(a)PYRENE-3,6-QUINONE ◇ BP-3,6-QUINONE

TOXICITY DATA with REFERENCE
NEO: skn-mus TDLo: 4520 µg/kg   CCSUDL 3,371,78
MUT: dnd-hmn: fbr 1 µmol/L   TOLED5 28,37,85
MUT: mma-sat 5 µg/plate   ENMUDM 7,839,85
MUT: msc-ham: lng 2 mg/L   CNREA8 36,3350,76

CONSENSUS REPORTS: EPA Genetic Toxicology Program.

SAFETY PROFILE: Questionable carcinogen with experimental neoplastigenic data by skin contact. Human mutation data reported. When heated to decomposition it emits acrid smoke and irritating fumes.

BCV000   CAS: 3067-12-7
BENZO(a)PYRENE-6,12-DIONE
mf: $C_{20}H_{10}O_2$ mw: 282.30

SYNS: 6,12-BENZO(a)PYRENEDIONE ◇ BENZO(a)PY-
RENE-6,12-QUINONE ◇ 6,12-BENZOPYRENE QUINONE
◇ BP-6,12-QUINONE

TOXICITY DATA with REFERENCE
NEO: skn-mus TDLo:4520 µg/kg   CCSUDL
3,371,78
MUT: msc-ham:lng 4 mg/L   CNREA8 36,3350,76

CONSENSUS REPORTS: EPA Genetic Toxicology Program.

SAFETY PROFILE: Questionable carcinogen
with experimental neoplastigenic data. Mutation
data reported. When heated to decomposition
it emits acrid smoke and irritating fumes.

BCV500   CAS: 37574-47-3
BENZO(a)PYRENE-4,5-OXIDE
mf: $C_{20}H_{12}O$ mw: 268.32

SYNS: BENZO(1,2)PYRENO(4,5-b)OXIRENE-3b,4b-DIHY-
DRO ◇ BENZ(a)PYRENE 4,5-OXIDE ◇ BENZO(a)PYRENE-4,5-
EPOXIDE ◇ BP-4,5-EPOXIDE ◇ BP 4,5-OXIDE

TOXICITY DATA with REFERENCE
NEO: skn-mus TDLo:2144 µg/kg   CCSUDL
3,371,78
ETA: scu-rat TDLo:40 mg/kg/50D-I   IJCNAW
18,351,76
ETA: skn-mus TD:32 mg/kg/60W-I   PNASA6
73,243,76
ETA: skn-mus TD:2160 µg/kg   CALEDQ 2,115,76
ETA: skn-mus TD:2160 µg/kg   CNREA8
37,4130,77
MUT: dnd-mam:lym 800 nmol   CRNGDP 3,267,82
MUT: dnr-bcs 1- µg/plate   CNREA8 45,2600,85
MUT: mma-sat 1 µg/plate   ENMUDM 7,839,85
MUT: mmo-esc 1 µg/plate   TCMUD8 5,339,85
MUT: mmo-sat 250 ng/plate   ENMUDM 7,839,85

CONSENSUS REPORTS: EPA Genetic Toxicology Program.

SAFETY PROFILE: Questionable carcinogen
with experimental tumorigenic and neoplastigenic data. Mutation data reported. When heated
to decomposition it emits acrid and irritating
fumes.

BCV750   CAS: 36504-65-1
BENZO(a)PYRENE-7,8-OXIDE
mf: $C_{20}H_{12}O$ mw: 268.32

SYNS: BENZO(10,11)CHRYSENO(1,2-b)OXIRENE-6-β,7-α-
DIHYDRO ◇ BENZO(a)PYRENE-7,8-DIHYDRO-7,8-EPOXY
◇ BENZO(a)PYRENE-7,8-EPOXIDE ◇ 6-β,7-α-
DIHYDROBENZO(10,11)CHRYSENO(1,2-b)OXIRENE

◇ BP 7,8-EPOXIDE ◇ BP 7,8-OXIDE ◇ 7,8-EPOXY-7,8-DIHY-
DROBENZO(a)PYRENE

TOXICITY DATA with REFERENCE
CAR: skn-mus TDLo:32 mg/kg/60W-I   PNASA6
73,243,76
NEO: skn-mus TD:99 mg/kg   PNASA6 73,243,76
NEO: skn-mus TD:2144 µg/kg   CCSUDL 3,371,78
ETA: scu-mus TDLo:10 mg/kg   JJIND8 64,617,80
ETA: skn-mus TD:68 mg/kg/42W-I   PNASA6
73,3867,76
ETA: skn-mus TD:2160 µg/kg   CALEDQ 2,115,76
ETA: skn-mus TD:2160 µg/kg   CNREA8
37,4130,77
MUT: mma-sat 25 µmol/L   JBCHA3 251,4882,76
MUT: mmo-sat 250 ng/plate   CNREA8 36,3350,76

CONSENSUS REPORTS: EPA Genetic Toxicology Program.

SAFETY PROFILE: Questionable carcinogen
with experimental carcinogenic, neoplastigenic,
and tumorigenic data. Mutation data reported.
When heated to decomposition it emits irritating
fumes.

BCW000   CAS: 36504-66-2
BENZO(a)PYRENE-9,10-OXIDE
mf: $C_{20}H_{12}O$ mw: 268.32

SYN: BP-9,10-OXIDE

TOXICITY DATA with REFERENCE
ETA: skn-mus TD:2160 µg/kg   CNREA8
37,4130,77
ETA: skn-mus TDLo:2140 µg/kg   CCSUDL
3,371,78
MUT: mmo-sat 250 ng/plate   CNREA8 36,3350,76

CONSENSUS REPORTS: EPA Genetic Toxicology Program.

SAFETY PROFILE: Questionable carcinogen
with experimental tumorigenic data by skin contact. Mutation data reported. When heated to
decomposition it emits acrid smoke and irritating
fumes.

BCW250   CAS: 60448-19-3
BENZO(a)PYRENE-11,12-OXIDE
mf: $C_{20}H_{12}O$ mw: 268.32

SYN: BP-11,12-OXIDE

TOXICITY DATA with REFERENCE
NEO: skn-mus TDLo:2140 µg/kg   CCSUDL
3,371,78
ETA: skn-mus TD:2160 µg/kg   CNREA8
37,4130,77

MUT: mmo-sat 1 µg/plate   CNREA8 36,3350,76
MUT: msc-ham:lng 5 mg/L   CNREA8 36,3350,76

CONSENSUS REPORTS: EPA Genetic Toxicology Program.

SAFETY PROFILE: Questionable carcinogen with experimental tumorigenic and neoplastigenic data by skin contact. Mutation data reported. When heated to decomposition it emits acrid smoke and irritating fumes.

BCX000   CAS: 56892-30-9
BENZO(a)PYREN-2-OL
mf: $C_{20}H_{12}O$ mw: 268.32

SYN: 2-HYDROXYBENZO(a)PYRENE

TOXICITY DATA with REFERENCE
NEO: skn-mus TDLo: 69 mg/kg/32W-I   CNREA8 37,2608,77
ETA: scu-mus TDLo: 10 mg/kg   JJIND8 64,617,80
MUT: dnd-hmn:fbr 30 µmol/L   CBINA8 41,155,82
MUT: mma-ham:lng 25 nmol/plate   CNREA8 39,2660,79
MUT: mma-sat 2 nmol/plate   CNREA8 39,2660,79
MUT: mmo-sat 8500 pmol/L   RRBCAD 18,291,81
MUT: msc-ham:lng 10 mg/L   CNREA8 36,3350,76

CONSENSUS REPORTS: EPA Genetic Toxicology Program.

SAFETY PROFILE: Questionable carcinogen with experimental tumorigenic and neoplastigenic data. Human mutation data reported. When heated to decomposition it emits acrid smoke and irritating fumes.

BCX250   CAS: 13345-21-6
BENZO(a)PYREN-3-OL
mf: $C_{20}H_{12}O$ mw: 268.32

SYNS: BP-3-HYDROXY ◇ 3-HYDROXYBENZO(a)PYRENE ◇ 8-HYDROXY-3,4-BENZPYRENE

TOXICITY DATA with REFERENCE
NEO: skn-mus TD: 4280 µg/kg   CCSUDL 3,371,78
NEO: skn-mus TDLo: 117 µg/kg   CNREA8 38,678,78
ETA: scu-mus TDLo: 160 mg/kg/21W-I   BJCAAI 6,400,52
ETA: skn-mus TD: 2760 mg/kg/69W-I   BJCAAI 6,400,52
ETA: skn-mus TD: 4300 µg/kg   CALEDQ 3,23,77
MUT: cyt-ham:emb 10 mg/L/48H-C   IJCNAW 9,435,72

MUT: cyt-mus:leu 10 mg/L/48H-C   IJCNAW 9,435,72
MUT: dnd-hmn:fbr 30 µmol/L   CBINA8 41,155,82
MUT: dnd-rat:lvr 30 µmol/L   CBINA8 20,311,78
MUT: dnr-esc 250 mg/L   JNCIAM 62,873,79
MUT: mma-sat 2500 ng/plate   BCPCA6 28,1615,79
MUT: mmo-sat 5 µg/plate   JJIND8 62,893,79
MUT: msc-ham:lng 12 µmol/L   PNASA6 73,607,76
MUT: otr-ham:emb 30 µg/L/7D-C   IJCNAW 9,435,72

CONSENSUS REPORTS: EPA Genetic Toxicology Program.

SAFETY PROFILE: Questionable carcinogen with experimental tumorigenic and neoplastigenic data by skin contact. Human mutation data reported. When heated to decomposition it emits acrid smoke and irritating fumes.

BCX500   CAS: 24027-84-7
BENZO(a)PYREN-5-OL
mf: $C_{20}H_{12}O$ mw: 268.32

SYN: 5-HYDROXYBENZO(a)PYRENE

TOXICITY DATA with REFERENCE
ETA: skn-mus TD: 4290 µg/kg   CNREA8 38,678,78
ETA: skn-mus TDLo: 4280 µg/kg   CCSUDL 3,371,78

CONSENSUS REPORTS: EPA Genetic Toxicology Program.

SAFETY PROFILE: Questionable carcinogen with experimental tumorigenic data by skin contact. When heated to decomposition it emits acrid smoke and irritating fumes.

BCX750   CAS: 33953-73-0
BENZO(a)PYREN-6-OL
mf: $C_{20}H_{12}O$ mw: 268.32

SYN: 6-HYDROXYBENZO(a)PYRENE

TOXICITY DATA with REFERENCE
NEO: scu-mus TDLo: 12 mg/kg   GANNA2 62,419,71
NEO: skn-mus TD: 4290 µg/kg   CNREA8 38,678,78
NEO: skn-mus TDLo: 4280 µg/kg   CCSUDL 3,371,78
ETA: idr-mus TDLo: 2400 µg/kg   GANNA2 62,419,71

MUT: mma-ham:lng 3700 nmol/L   PNASA6 73,607,76

MUT: mma-sat 25 μmol/L   JBCHA3 251,4882,76

MUT: mmo-sat 7 μg/plate   ENMUDM 7,839,85

MUT: msc-ham:lng 5 mg/L   CNREA8 36,3350,76

CONSENSUS REPORTS: EPA Genetic Toxicology Program.

SAFETY PROFILE: Questionable carcinogen with experimental neoplastigenic and tumorigenic data. Mutation data reported. When heated to decomposition it emits acrid smoke and fumes.

BCY000   CAS: 37994-82-4
BENZO(a)PYREN-7-OL
mf: $C_{20}H_{12}O$ mw: 268.32

SYN: 7-HYDROXYBENZO(a)PYRENE

TOXICITY DATA with REFERENCE
NEO: skn-mus TDLo:4280 μg/kg   CCSUDL 3,371,78

ETA: skn-mus TD:4290 μg/kg   CNREA8 38,678,78

MUT: dnd-hmn:fbr 30 μmol/L   CBINA8 41,155,82

MUT: dni-omi 200 μg/L   PNASA6 74,1378,77

MUT: mma-sat 7 μg/plate   ENMUDM 7,839,85

MUT: mmo-sat 16 μg/plate   MUREAV 36,379,76

MUT: msc-ham:lng 12 μmol/L   PNASA6 73,607,76

CONSENSUS REPORTS: EPA Genetic Toxicology Program.

SAFETY PROFILE: Questionable carcinogen with experimental tumorigenic and neoplastigenic data by skin contact. Human mutation data reported. When heated to decomposition it emits acrid smoke and fumes.

BCY250   CAS: 17573-21-6
BENZO(a)PYREN-9-OL
mf: $C_{20}H_{12}O$ mw: 268.32

SYN: 9-HYDROXYBENZO(a)PYRENE

TOXICITY DATA with REFERENCE
NEO: skn-mus TD:4290 μg/kg   CNREA8 38,678,78
NEO: skn-mus TDLo:4280 μg/kg   CCSUDL 3,371,78

MUT: dnd-esc 10 μmol/L   IJCNAW 18,339,76

MUT: dnd-hmn:fbr 30 μmol/L   CBINA8 41,155,82

MUT: dnd-mam:lym 447 nmol   CRNGDP 3,267,82

MUT: dnd-rat:lvr 30 μmol/L   CBINA8 20,311,78

MUT: mma-sat 7 μg/plate   ENMUDM 7,839,85

MUT: mmo-sat 16 μg/plate   MUREAV 36,379,76

MUT: msc-ham:lng 37 μmol/L   PNASA6 73,607,76

CONSENSUS REPORTS: EPA Genetic Toxicology Program.

SAFETY PROFILE: Questionable carcinogen with experimental neoplastigenic data by skin contact. Human mutation data reported. When heated to decomposition it emits acrid smoke and irritating fumes.

BCY500   CAS: 56892-31-0
BENZO(a)PYREN-10-OL
mf: $C_{20}H_{12}O$ mw: 268.32

SYN: 10-HYDROXYBENZO(a)PYRENE

TOXICITY DATA with REFERENCE
ETA: skn-mus TD:4290 μg/kg   CNREA8 38,678,78

ETA: skn-mus TDLo:4280 μg/kg   CCSUDL 3,371,78

MUT: mmo-sat 18600 pmol/L   RRBCAD 18,291,81

CONSENSUS REPORTS: EPA Genetic Toxicology Program.

SAFETY PROFILE: Questionable carcinogen with experimental tumorigenic data by skin contact. Mutation data reported. When heated to decomposition it emits acrid smoke and irritating fumes.

BCY750   CAS: 56892-32-1
BENZO(a)PYREN-11-OL
mf: $C_{20}H_{12}O$ mw: 268.32

SYN: 11-HYDROXYBENZO(a)PYRENE

TOXICITY DATA with REFERENCE
ETA: skn-mus TDLo:82 mg/kg/38W-I   CNREA8 37,2608,77

MUT: dnd-hmn:fbr 30 μmol/L   CBINA8 41,155,82

CONSENSUS REPORTS: EPA Genetic Toxicology Program.

SAFETY PROFILE: Questionable carcinogen with experimental tumorigenic data by skin contact. Human mutation data reported. When heated to decomposition it emits acrid smoke and irritating fumes.

BCZ000   CAS: 56892-33-2
BENZO(a)PYREN-12-OL
mf: $C_{20}H_{12}O$ mw: 268.32

SYN: 12-HYDROXYBENZO(a)PYRENE

TOXICITY DATA with REFERENCE
NEO: skn-mus TD:4290 µg/kg   CNREA8 38,678,78
NEO: skn-mus TDLo:4280 µg/kg   CCSUDL 3,371,78
MUT: mma-sat 7 µg/plate   ENMUDM 7,839,85
MUT: mmo-sat 1 µg/plate   CNREA8 36,3350,76
MUT: msc-ham:lng 15 mg/L   CNREA8 36,3350,76

CONSENSUS REPORTS: EPA Genetic Toxicology Program.

SAFETY PROFILE: Questionable carcinogen with experimental neoplastigenic data by skin contact. Mutation data reported. When heated to decomposition it emits acrid smoke and irritating fumes.

BDA000   CAS: 207-89-6
7H-BENZO(a)PYRIDO(3,2-g) CARBAZOLE
mf: $C_{19}H_{12}N_2$ mw: 268.33

SYN: 1,2-BENZOPYRIDO(3',2':5,6)CARBAZOLE

TOXICITY DATA with REFERENCE
ETA: scu-mus TDLo:72 mg/kg/9W-I   NATUAS 191,1005,61

SAFETY PROFILE: Questionable carcinogen with experimental tumorigenic data. When heated to decomposition it emits toxic fumes such as NO_x.

BDA250   CAS: 194-62-7
7H-BENZO(c)PYRIDO(2,3-g) CARBAZOLE
mf: $C_{19}H_{12}N_2$ mw: 268.33

SYN: 5,6-BENZOPYRIDO(3',2':3,4)CARBAZOLE

TOXICITY DATA with REFERENCE
ETA: scu-mus TDLo:72 mg/kg/9W-I   COREAF 257,818,63

SAFETY PROFILE: Questionable carcinogen with experimental tumorigenic data. When heated to decomposition it emits toxic fumes such as NO_x.

BDA500   CAS: 194-60-5
7H-BENZO(c)PYRIDO(3,2-g) CARBAZOLE
mf: $C_{19}H_{12}N_2$ mw: 268.33

SYN: 3,4-BENZOPYRIDO(3',2':5,6)CARBAZOLE

TOXICITY DATA with REFERENCE
ETA: scu-mus TDLo:72 mg/kg/9W-I   NATUAS 191,1005,61

SAFETY PROFILE: Questionable carcinogen with experimental tumorigenic data. When heated to decomposition it emits toxic fumes such as NO_x.

BDA750   CAS: 239-67-8
13H-BENZO(a)PYRIDO(3,2-i) CARBAZOLE
mf: $C_{19}H_{12}N_2$ mw: 268.33

SYN: 7,8-BENZOPYRIDO(2',3':1,2)CARBAZOLE

TOXICITY DATA with REFERENCE
ETA: scu-mus TDLo:72 mg/kg/9W-I   COREAF 257,818,63

SAFETY PROFILE: Questionable carcinogen with experimental tumorigenic data. When heated to decomposition it emits toxic fumes such as NO_x.

BDB000   CAS: 207-88-5
13H-BENZO(g)PYRIDO(2,3-a) CARBAZOLE
mf: $C_{19}H_{12}N_2$ mw: 268.33

SYN: 5,6-BENZOPYRIDO(2',3':1,2)CARBAZOLE

TOXICITY DATA with REFERENCE
ETA: orl-mus TDLo:2880 mg/kg/24W-I   COREAF 257,818,63
ETA: scu-mus TDLo:72 mg/kg/9W-I   NATUAS 191,1005,61

SAFETY PROFILE: Questionable carcinogen with experimental tumorigenic data. When heated to decomposition it emits toxic fumes as NO_x.

BDB250   CAS: 207-85-2
13H-BENZO(g)PYRIDO(3,2-a) CARBAZOLE
mf: $C_{19}H_{12}N_2$ mw: 268.33

SYN: 5,6-BENZOPYRIDO(3',2':1,2)CARBAZOLE

TOXICITY DATA with REFERENCE
ETA: orl-mus TDLo:3720 mg/kg/31W-I   COREAF 257,818,63
ETA: scu-mus TDLo:72 mg/kg/9W-I   NATUAS 191,1005,61

SAFETY PROFILE: Questionable carcinogen with experimental tumorigenic data. When

heated to decomposition it emits toxic fumes such as NO_x.

BDB500   CAS: 318-03-6
11H-BENZO(g)PYRIDO(4,3-b)INDOLE
mf: $C_{15}H_{10}N_2$ mw: 218.27

SYN: 8,9-BENZO-γ-CARBOLINE

TOXICITY DATA with REFERENCE
NEO: scu-mus TDLo: 72 mg/kg/9W-I   CHDDAT
271,1474,70

SAFETY PROFILE: Questionable carcinogen with experimental neoplastigenic data. When heated to decomposition it emits toxic fumes such as NO_x.

BDC750   CAS: 800-24-8
BENZOQUINONE AZIRIDINE
mf: $C_{16}H_{22}N_2O_6$ mw: 338.40

SYNS: A-139 ◇ AZIRIDYL BENZOQUINONE ◇ BAYER A 139 ◇ BAYER R39 SOLUBLE ◇ 2,5-BIS(1-AZIRIDINYL)-3,6-BIS(2-METHOXYETHOXY)-p-BENZOQUINONE ◇ 2,5-BIS(1-AZIRIDINYL)-3,6-BIS(2-METHOXYETHOXY)-2,5-CYCLOHEXADIENE-1,4-DIONE ◇ 2,5-BISMETHOXY-ETHOXY-3,6-BISETHYLENEIMINO-1,4-BENZOQUINONE ◇ 3,6-BIS(β-METHOXYETHOXY)-2,5-BIS(ETHYLENIMINO)-p-BENZOQUINONE ◇ 3,6-BIS (β-METHOXYETHOXY)-2,5-BIS(ETHYLENEIMINO)-p-BENZOQUINONE ◇ E 39 SOLUBLE ◇ NSC-17262

TOXICITY DATA with REFERENCE
CAR: ipr-mus TDLo: 4 mg/kg/4W   JNCIAM
36,915,66
MUT: dlt-dmg-orl 1 μmol/L   MUREAV 14,250,72

CONSENSUS REPORTS: IARC Cancer Review: GROUP 3 IMEMDT 7,56,87; Animal Limited Evidence IMEMDT 9,51,75. EPA Genetic Toxicology Program.

SAFETY PROFILE: Questionable carcinogen with experimental carcinogenic data. Deadly poison by intravenous route. Mutation data reported. When heated to decomposition it emits toxic fumes of NO_x.

BDE750   CAS: 120-78-5
BENZOTHIAZOLE DISULFIDE
mf: $C_{14}H_8N_2S_4$ mw: 332.48

PROP: Cream to light yellow powder; mp: 175°, d: 1.5.

SYNS: ALTAX ◇ BENZOTHIAZOLYL DISULFIDE ◇ 2-BENZOTHIAZOLYL DISULFIDE ◇ BIS(BENZOTHIA-ZOLYL)DISULFIDE ◇ BIS(2-BENZOTHIAZYL) DISULFIDE ◇ DI-2-BENZOTHIAZOLYLDISULFIDE ◇ DIBENZOTHIAZYL DISULFIDE ◇ 2,2'-DIBENZOTHIAZYLDISULFIDE ◇ DIBENZOYLTHIAZYL DISULFIDE ◇ DIBENZTHIAZYL DISULFIDE ◇ 2,2'-DITHIOBIS(BENZOTHIAZOLE) ◇ DWUSI-ARCZEK DWUBENZOTIAZYLU (POLISH) ◇ MBTS ◇ MBTS RUBBER ACCELERATOR ◇ 2-MERCAPTOBEN-ZOTHIAZOLEDISULFIDE ◇ 2-MERCAPTOBENZOTHIA-ZYLDISULFIDE ◇ ROYAL MBTS ◇ THIOFIDE ◇ USAF B-33 ◇ USAF CY-5 ◇ USAF EK-5432 ◇ VULKACIT DM ◇ VULKACIT DM/MGC

TOXICITY DATA with REFERENCE
ETA: orl-mus TDLo: 172 g/kg/78W-I   NTIS**
PB223-159
MUT: mma-mus: lym 15 mg/L   ENMUDM 5,193,83

CONSENSUS REPORTS: Reported in EPA TSCA Inventory.

SAFETY PROFILE: Questionable carcinogen with experimental tumorigenic and teratogenic data. Poison by intravenous and intraperitoneal routes. Mildly toxic by ingestion. Other experimental reproductive effects. Mutation data reported. When heated to decomposition it emits very toxic fumes of SO_x and NO_x.

BDG000   CAS: 102-77-2
2-BENZOTHIAZOLYL-N-MORPHOLINOSULFIDE
mf: $C_{11}H_{12}N_2OS_2$ mw: 252.37

SYNS: AMAX ◇ 2-BENZOTHIAZOLYLSULFENYL MOR-PHOLINE ◇ 4-(2-BENZOTHIAZOLYLTHIO)MORPHOLINE ◇ 2-(MORPHOLINOTHIO)BENZOTHIAZOLE ◇ MORPHO-LINYLMERCAPTOBENZOTHIAZOLE ◇ 2-(4-MORPHO-LINYLTHIO)BENZOTHIAZOLE ◇ N-(OXYDIETHYLENE) BENZOTHIAZOLE-2-SULFENAMIDE ◇ SANTOCURE MOR ◇ SULFENAMIDE M ◇ USAF CY-7 ◇ VULCAFOR BSM

TOXICITY DATA with REFERENCE
NEO: scu-mus TDLo: 464 mg/kg   NTIS**
PB223-159
MUT: dnr-esc 10 μg/tube   ENMUDM 5,193,83
MUT: mma-mus: lym 15 mg/L   ENMUDM 5,193,83
MUT: msc-mus: lym 10 mg/L   ENMUDM 5,193,83
MUT: otr-mus: emb 200 μg/L   ENMUDM 5,193,83

CONSENSUS REPORTS: Reported in EPA TSCA Inventory.

SAFETY PROFILE: Questionable carcinogen with experimental neoplastigenic and teratogenic data. Poison by intraperitoneal route.

Moderately toxic by ingestion. Mutation data reported. When heated to decomposition it emits very toxic fumes of NO_x and SO_x.

BDH250   CAS: 95-14-7
1H-BENZOTRIAZOLE
mf: $C_6H_5N_3$ mw: 119.14

PROP: Needle-like crystals. Mp: 100°, bp: 204° @ 15 mm.

SYNS: 1,2,-AMINOZOPHENYLENE ◇ AZIMIDOBENZENE ◇ AZIMINOBENZENE ◇ BENZENE AZIMIDE ◇ BENZISO-TRIAZOLE ◇ 1,2,3-BENZOTRIAZOLE ◇ COBRATEC #99 ◇ 2,3-DIAZAINDOLE ◇ NCI-C03521 ◇ NSC-3058 ◇ 1,2,3-TRIAZAINDENE ◇ U-6233

TOXICITY DATA with REFERENCE
ETA: orl-mus TDLo:770 g/kg/78W-I   NCITR* NCI-CG-TR-88,78
ETA: orl-rat TDLo:220 g/kg/78W-I   NCITR* NCI-CG-TR-88,78
MUT: mma-esc 33300 ng/plate   ENMUDM 7(Suppl 5),1,85
MUT: mma-sat 100 µg/plate   IARCCD 27,283,80
MUT: mmo-esc 333 µg/plate   ENMUDM 7(Suppl 5),1,85
MUT: otr-rat:emb 94 µg/plate   JJATDK 1,190,81

CONSENSUS REPORTS: NCI Carcinogenesis Bioassay (feed); Inadequate Studies: mouse, rat NCITR* NCI-CG-TR-88,78. Reported in EPA TSCA Inventory.

SAFETY PROFILE: Questionable carcinogen with experimental tumorigenic data. Poison by intravenous route. Moderately toxic by ingestion and intraperitoneal routes. Mutation data reported. May detonate at 220°C or during vacuum distillation. When heated to decomposition it emits toxic fumes of NO_x.

BDH750   CAS: 215-58-7
BENZO(b)TRIPHENYLENE
mf: $C_{22}H_{14}$ mw: 278.36

PROP: Clear plates or leaflets. Mp: 267°.

SYNS: DB(a,c)A ◇ DIBENZ(a,c)ANTHRACENE ◇ 1,2:3,4-DIBENZANTHRACENE ◇ DIBENZO(a,c)ANTHRACENE ◇ 1,2:3,4-DIBENZOANTHRACENE

TOXICITY DATA with REFERENCE
ETA: scu-mus TDLo:12 mg/kg   IJCNAW 32,765,83
ETA: skn-mus TD:22 mg/kg   CNREA8 40,1981,80

ETA: skn-mus TD:40 mg/kg   JNCIAM 44,1167,70
ETA: skn-mus TDLo:440 mg/kg/65W-I   JNCIAM 44,641,70
MUT: dnd-esc 10 µmol/L   MUREAV 89,95,81
MUT: dnd-hmn:emb 360 nmol/L   CBINA8 22,257,78
MUT: dnd-hmn:hla 10 nmol/L   MUREAV 89,95,81
MUT: dnd-mam:lym 100 µmol   BIPMAA 9,689,70
MUT: dnd-mus-skn 1 g/L   CNREA8 27,1678,67
MUT: dnd-mus:ast 10 µmol/L   MUREAV 89,95,81
MUT: dnd-mus:lvr 6 µmol/L   JNCIAM 62,947,79
MUT: dns-hmn:hla 100 nmol/L   CNREA8 38,2625,78
MUT: mma-ham:lng 40200 nmol/L   MUREAV 46,27,77
MUT: mma-sat 10 µg/plate   PNASA6 72,5135,75
MUT: msc-ham:fbr 1 mg/L   DTESD7 8,121,80
MUT: msc-ham:lng 1 mg/L   PNASA6 73,188,76

CONSENSUS REPORTS: EPA Genetic Toxicology Program. IARC Cancer Review: GROUP 3 IMEMDT 7,56,87; Animal Limited Evidence IMEMDT 32,289,83

SAFETY PROFILE: Questionable carcinogen with experimental tumorigenic data. Human mutation data reported. When heated to decomposition it emits acrid smoke and irritating fumes.

BDM500   CAS: 98-88-4
BENZOYL CHLORIDE
DOT: 1736
mf: C_7H_5ClO mw: 140.57

PROP: Colorless, fuming, pungent liquid; decomposes in water. Mp: −0.5°, bp: 197°, flash p: 162°F (CC), d: 1.2187 @ 15°/15°, vap press: 1 mm @ 32.1°, vap d: 4.88.

SYNS: BENZENECARBONYL CHLORIDE ◇ BENZOIC ACID, CHLORIDE ◇ BENZOYL CHLORIDE (DOT) ◇ α-CHLOROBENZALDEHYDE

TOXICITY DATA with REFERENCE
ETA: skn-mus TD:17600 mg/kg/42W-I   GANNA2 72,655,81
ETA: skn-mus TD:35200 mg/kg/42W-I   GANNA2 72,655,81
ETA: skn-mus TDLo:9200 mg/kg/50W-I   GANNA2 72,655,81
MUT: mmo-sat 1 µmol/plate   MUREAV 58,11,78

CONSENSUS REPORTS: IARC Cancer Review: Human Inadequate Evidence IMEMDT

29,83,82; Animal Inadequate Evidence IMEMDT 29,83,82. Community Right-To-Know List. Reported in EPA TSCA Inventory. EPA Genetic Toxicology Program.

DOT Classification: Corrosive Material; Label: Corrosive.

SAFETY PROFILE: Questionable carcinogen with experimental tumorigenic data by skin contact. Human systemic effects by inhalation: unspecified effects on olfaction, and respiratory systems. Corrosive effects on the skin, eyes, and mucous membranes by inhalation. Flammable when exposed to heat or flame. To fight fire, use alcohol foam, CO_2, dry chemical. When heated to decomposition it emits toxic fumes of Cl^-.

BDO199 CAS: 55398-24-8
N-BENZOYLOXY-N-ETHYL-4-AMINOAZOBENZENE
mf: $C_{21}H_{19}N_3O_2$ mw: 345.43

TOXICITY DATA with REFERENCE
NEO: scu-rat TDLo: 262 mg/kg/8W-I   CNREA8 35,880,75

SAFETY PROFILE: Questionable carcinogen with experimental neoplastigenic data. When heated to decomposition it emits toxic fumes of NO_x.

BDO500 CAS: 55398-26-0
N-BENZOYLOXY-4'-ETHYL-N-METHYL-4-AMINOAZOBENZENE
mf: $C_{22}H_{21}N_3O_2$ mw: 359.46

TOXICITY DATA with REFERENCE
NEO: scu-rat TDLo: 272 mg/kg/8W-I   CNREA8 35,880,75

SAFETY PROFILE: Questionable carcinogen with experimental neoplastigenic data. When heated to decomposition it emits toxic fumes such as NO_x.

BDP000 CAS: 6098-46-0
N-BENZOYLOXY-N-METHYL-4-AMINOAZOBENZENE
mf: $C_{20}H_{17}N_3O_2$ mw: 331.40

SYNS: o-BENZOYL-N-METHYL-N-(p-(PHENYLAZO) PHENYL)HYDROXYLAMINE ◇ N-(BENZOYLOXY)-N-METHYL-4-(PHENYLAZO)-BENZENAMINE

TOXICITY DATA with REFERENCE
NEO: scu-rat TD: 318 mg/kg/12W-I   CNREA8 39,3441,79

NEO: scu-rat TD: 375 mg/kg/12W-I   CNREA8 27,1600,67
MUT: dnd-esc 60 mmol/L   CNREA8 40,2493,80
MUT: dnd-mam: lym 50 mmol/L   CBINA8 31,1,80
MUT: dnd-mus-ipr 120 mg/kg   CNREA8 40,2493,80
MUT: dnd-rat: lvr 50 mmol/L   CBINA8 31,1,80
MUT: mma-sat 10 nmol/plate   CALEDQ 1,91,75
MUT: mmo-sat 100 nmol/plate   CALEDQ 1,91,75
MUT: sln-dmg-par 10 mmol/L   IJCNAW 10,194,72
MUT: slt-dmg-par 10 mmol/L   MUREAV 9,239,70

CONSENSUS REPORTS: EPA Genetic Toxicology Program.

SAFETY PROFILE: Questionable carcinogen with experimental neoplastigenic data. Mutation data reported. When heated to decomposition it emits toxic fumes of NO_x.

BDP500 CAS: 42978-42-7
6-BENZOYLOXYMETHYLBENZO(a)PYRENE
mf: $C_{28}H_{18}O_2$ mw: 386.46

TOXICITY DATA with REFERENCE
CAR: scu-rat TDLo: 100 mg/kg/40D-I   JMCMAR 16,714,73
NEO: scu-rat TD: 2898 μg/kg/60D-I   CBINA8 29,159,80

SAFETY PROFILE: Questionable carcinogen with experimental carcinogenic and neoplastigenic data. When heated to decomposition it emits acrid smoke and irritating fumes.

BDQ000 CAS: 55398-25-9
N-BENZOYLOXY-4'-METHYL-N-METHYL-4-AMINOAZOBENZENE
mf: $C_{21}H_{19}N_3O_2$ mw: 345.43

TOXICITY DATA with REFERENCE
NEO: scu-rat TDLo: 262 mg/kg/8W-I   CNREA8 35,880,75

SAFETY PROFILE: Questionable carcinogen with experimental neoplastigenic data. When heated to decomposition it emits toxic fumes of NO_x.

BDQ250 CAS: 31012-29-0
7-BENZOYLOXYMETHYL-12-METHYLBENZ(a)ANTHRACENE
mf: $C_{27}H_{20}O_2$ mw: 376.47

SYN: 12-METHYLBENZ(a)ANTHRACENE-7-METHANOL BENZOATE (ESTER)

TOXICITY DATA with REFERENCE
NEO: scu-rat TDLo:20 mg/kg/39D-I   CNREA8
31,1951,71

SAFETY PROFILE: Questionable carcinogen with experimental neoplastigenic data. When heated to decomposition it emits very acrid smoke and irritating fumes.

BDS000   CAS: 94-36-0
BENZOYL PEROXIDE
DOT: 2085
mf: $C_{14}H_{10}O_4$ mw: 242.24

PROP: White, granular, tasteless, odorless powder. Mp: 103-106° (decomp), bp: decomposes explosively, autoign temp: 176°F. Sol in benzene, acetone, chloroform; sltly sol in alc; insol in water.

SYNS: ACETOXYL ◇ ACNEGEL ◇ AZTEC BPO ◇ BENOXYL ◇ BENZAC ◇ BENZAKNEW ◇ BENZOIC ACID, PEROXIDE ◇ BENZOPEROXIDE ◇ BENZOYL ◇ BENZOYL-PEROXID (GERMAN) ◇ BENZOYLPEROXYDE (DUTCH) ◇ BENZOYL SUPEROXIDE ◇ BZF-60 ◇ CADET ◇ CADOX ◇ CLEARASIL BENZOYL PEROXIDE LOTION ◇ CLEARASIL BP ACNE TREATMENT ◇ CUTICURA ACNE CREAM ◇ DEBROXIDE ◇ DIBENZOYLPEROXID (GERMAN) ◇ DIBENZOYL PEROXIDE (MAK) ◇ DIBENZOYLPEROXYDE (DUTCH) ◇ DIPHENYLGLYOXAL PEROXIDE ◇ DRY AND CLEAR ◇ EPI-CLEAR ◇ FOSTEX ◇ GAROX ◇ INCIDOL ◇ LOROXIDE ◇ LUCIDOL ◇ LUPERCO ◇ LUPEROX FL ◇ NAYPER B and BO ◇ NOROX BZP-250 ◇ NOVADELOX ◇ OXY-5 ◇ OXY-10 ◇ OXYLITE ◇ OXY WASH ◇ PANOXYL ◇ PEROSSIDO di BENZOILE(ITALIAN) ◇ PEROXYDE de BEN-ZOYLE (FRENCH) ◇ PERSADOX ◇ QUINOLOR COMPOUND ◇ SULFOXYL ◇ SUPEROX ◇ THERADERM ◇ TOPEX ◇ VANOXIDE ◇ XERAC

TOXICITY DATA with REFERENCE
ETA: skn-mus TDLo:24 g/kg/30W-I   SCIEAS
213,1023,81
MUT: dnd-hmn:oth 100 μmol/L   CNREA8
45,2522,85
MUT: dnd-mus:oth 1 μmol/L   PAACA3 24,108,83
MUT: dni-ham:oth 56 μmol/L   CNREA8
45,2522,85
MUT: dns-rat:lvr 100 pmol/L   CRNGDP 5,1547,84
MUT: oms-hmn:oth 56 μmol/L   CNREA8
45,2522,85

CONSENSUS REPORTS: IARC Cancer Review: Animal Inadequate Evidence IMEMDT 36,267,85; Human Inadequate Evidence IMEMDT 36,267,85. Reported in EPA TSCA Inventory. EPA Genetic Toxicology Program. Community Right-To-Know List.

OSHA PEL: TWA 5 mg/m³ ACGIH TLV: TWA 5 mg/m³ DFG MAK: 5 mg/m³ NIOSH REL: TWA 5 mg/m³ DOT Classification: Organic Peroxide; Label: Organic Peroxide.

SAFETY PROFILE: Questionable carcinogen with experimental tumorigenic data. Poison by ingestion and intraperitoneal routes. Can cause dermatitis, asthmatic effects, testicular atrophy, and vasodilation. An allergen and eye irritant. Human mutation data reported. Moderate fire hazard by spontaneous chemical reaction in contact with reducing agents.

BDV750   CAS: 5929-01-1
1:2-BENZPYRENE PICRATE
mf: $C_{20}H_{12} \cdot C_6H_3N_3O_7$ mw: 481.44

SYN: BENZO(a)PYRENE MONOPICRATE

TOXICITY DATA with REFERENCE
ETA: skn-mus TDLo:1200 mg/kg/50W-I
PRLBA4 117,318,35

SAFETY PROFILE: Questionable carcinogen with experimental tumorigenic data by skin contact. When heated to decomposition it emits toxic fumes of NO_x.

BDX000   CAS: 140-11-4
BENZYL ACETATE
mf: $C_9H_{10}O_2$ mw: 150.19

PROP: Colorless liquid; sweet, floral fruity odor. Mp: −51.5°, bp: 213.5°, flash p: 216°F (CC), d: 1.06, autoign temp: 862°F, vap press: 1 mm @ 45°, vap d: 5.1, refr index: 1.501. Sol in alc, most fixed oils, propylene glycol; insol in glycerin and water @ 214°.

SYNS: ACETIC ACID BENZYL ESTER ◇ ACETIC ACID PHENYLMETHYL ESTER ◇ α-ACETOXYTOLUENE ◇ BENZYL ETHANOATE ◇ FEMA No. 2135 ◇ NCI-C06508

TOXICITY DATA with REFERENCE
NEO: orl-mus TDLo:258 g/kg/2Y-I   NTPTR*
NTP-TR-250,86
NEO: orl-rat TDLo:258 g/kg/2Y-I   NTPTR*NTP-TR-250,86
MUT: dnr-bcs 21 mg/disc   OIGZDE 34,267,85
MUT: mma-hmn:lyms 1500 mg/L   MUREAV
196,61,88
MUT: mma-mus:lyms 500 mg/L   MUREAV
196,61,88
MUT: msc-mus:lyms 700 mg/L   SCIEAS
236,933,87

CONSENSUS REPORTS: IARC Cancer Review: GROUP 3 IMEMDT 7,56,87; Animal

Limited Evidence IMEMDT 40,109,86. NTP Carcinogenesis Studies (gavage); Some Evidence: mouse, rat NTPTR* NTP-TR-250,86. Reported in EPA TSCA Inventory.

SAFETY PROFILE: Questionable carcinogen with experimental tumorigenic data. A poison by inhalation. Moderately toxic by ingestion and subcutaneous routes. Human systemic effects by inhalation: an antipsychotic, unspecified respiratory and urinary system effects. Combustible liquid. To fight fire, use alcohol foam, CO_2. When heated to decomposition it emits irritating fumes.

BDY669   CAS: 61-33-6
BENZYL-6-AMINOPENICILLINIC ACID
mf: $C_{16}H_{18}N_2O_4S$ mw: 334.42

SYNS: ABBOCILLIN ◊ (5R,6R)-BENXYLPENICILLIN ◊ BENZOPENICILLIN ◊ BENZYLPENICILLIN ◊ BENZYL-PENICILLIN G ◊ BENZYLPENICILLINIC ACID ◊ CILLORAL ◊ CILOPEN ◊ COMPOCILLIN G ◊ COSMOPEN ◊ DROPCILLIN ◊ FREE BENZYLPENICILLIN ◊ PENICILLIN G ◊ GALOFAK ◊ GELACILLIN ◊ LIQUACILLIN ◊ PHENYL-ACETAMIDOPENICILLANIC ACID ◊ (PHENYLMETHYL) PENICILLINIC ACID ◊ PRADUPEN ◊ SPECILLINE G

TOXICITY DATA with REFERENCE
ETA: scu-rat TDLo:2600 mg/kg/65W-I
  LANCAO 1,394,86
MUT: dnr-bcs 100 µL/plate   MUREAV 97,1,82
MUT: dnr-esc 20 µL/disc   MUREAV 97,1,82
MUT: mmo-omi 12 µg/L   ARMKA7 81,1,72
MUT: oms-omi 20 µg/L   AMACCQ 17,572,80

CONSENSUS REPORTS: EPA Genetic Toxicology Program.

SAFETY PROFILE: Questionable carcinogen with experimental tumorigenic data. Poison by ingestion, intravenous, intracerebral, intraspinal, subcutaneous and possibly other routes. Human (child) systemic effects by parenteral route: changes in cochlear (inner ear) structure or function, convulsions, and dyspnea. Mutation data reported. When heated to decomposition it emits very toxic fumes of NO_x and SO_x.

BEC500   CAS: 85-68-7
BENZYL BUTYL PHTHALATE
mf: $C_{19}H_{20}O_4$ mw: 312.39

PROP: Clear, oily liquid. Mp: <−35°, bp: 370°, flash p: 390°F, d: 1.116 @ 25°/25°, vap d: 10.8.

SYNS: BBP ◊ 1,2-BENZENEDICARBOXYLIC ACID, BUTYL PHENYLMETHYL ESTER ◊ BUTYL BENZYL PHTHALATE ◊ n-BUTYL BENZYL PHTHALATE ◊ NCI-C54375 ◊ PALATINOL BB ◊ SANTICIZER 160 ◊ SICOL 160 ◊ UNIMOLL BB

TOXICITY DATA with REFERENCE
CAR: orl-rat TD:437 g/kg/2Y-C   EVHPAZ 65,271,86
CAR: orl-rat TDLo:433 g/kg/2Y-C   NTPTR* NTP-TR-213,82

CONSENSUS REPORTS: IARC Cancer Review: Animal Inadequate Evidence IMEMDT 29,193,82; NTP Carcinogenesis Bioassay (feed); No Evidence: mouse NTPTR* NTP-TR-213,82; Clear Evidence: rat NTPTR* NTP-TR-213,82. Reported in EPA TSCA Inventory. Community Right-To-Know List.

SAFETY PROFILE: Questionable carcinogen with experimental carcinogenic data. Moderately toxic by ingestion and intraperitoneal routes. Experimental reproductive effects. Combustible when exposed to heat or flame; can react with oxidizers. To fight fire, use spray or mist, CO_2, dry chemical. When heated to decomposition it emits acrid smoke and irritating fumes.

BED750   CAS: 14504-15-5
3-BENZYL-4-CARBAMOYLMETHYLSYDNONE
mf: $C_{11}H_{11}N_3O_3$ mw: 233.25

SYN: 3-BENZYLSYDNONE-4-ACETAMIDE

TOXICITY DATA with REFERENCE
NEO: orl-rat TDLo:23 mg/kg/13W-I   GANNA2 65,273,74

SAFETY PROFILE: Questionable carcinogen with experimental neoplastigenic data. Mildly toxic by ingestion. When heated to decomposition it emits toxic fumes of NO_x.

BEN000   CAS: 121-54-0
BENZYLDIMETHYL(2-(2-(p-(1,1,3,3-TETRAMETHYLBUTYL)PHENOXY)ETHOXY)ETHYL) AMMONIUM CHLORIDE
mf: $C_{27}H_{42}NO_2 \cdot Cl$ mw: 448.15

PROP: Colorless crystals. Sol in water.

SYNS: ANTI-GERM 77 ◊ ANTISEPTOL ◊ BENZETHONIUM CHLORIDE ◊ BENZETONIUM CHLORIDE ◊ BENZYL-DIMETHYL-p-(1,1,3,3-TETRAMETHYLBUTYL)PHENOXY-ETHOXY-ETHYLAMMONIUM CHLORIDE ◊ BZT ◊ DIAPP

◇ DIISOBUTYLPHENOXYETHOXYETHYLDIMETHYL BEN-
ZYL AMMONIUM CHLORIDE ◇ DISILYN ◇ HYAMINE
◇ HYAMINE 1622 ◇ NCI-C61494 ◇ p-tert-OCTYLPHEN-
OXYETHOXYETHYLDIMETHYLBENZYL AMMONIUM
CHLORIDE ◇ PHEMERIDE ◇ PHEMEROL CHLORIDE
◇ PHEMITHYN ◇ POLYMINE D ◇ QUATRACHLOR
◇ SOLAMINE

TOXICITY DATA with REFERENCE
NEO: scu-rat TDLo: 104 mg/kg/1Y-I   CTOXAO
4,185,71

CONSENSUS REPORTS: Reported in EPA
TSCA Inventory.

SAFETY PROFILE: Questionable carcinogen
with experimental neoplastigenic data. Poison
by ingestion, subcutaneous, intraperitoneal, and
intravenous routes. A severe eye irritant. When
heated to decomposition it emits very toxic
fumes of Cl^-, NH_3 and NO_x. A topical anti-
infective agent.

BEQ250   CAS: 20570-96-1
BENZYLHYDRAZINE
DIHYDROCHLORIDE
mf: $C_7H_{10}N_2$•2ClH   mw: 195.11

TOXICITY DATA with REFERENCE
NEO: orl-mus TDLo: 10 g/kg/29W-C   ZEKBAI
87,267,76

SAFETY PROFILE: Questionable carcinogen
with experimental neoplastigenic data. Poison
by intraperitoneal route. When heated to decomposition it emits very toxic fumes of HCl and
NO_x.

BFD250   CAS: 69-57-8
BENZYL PENICILLINIC ACID SODIUM
SALT
mf: $C_{16}H_{17}N_2O_4S$•Na   mw: 356.40

SYNS: AMERICAN PENICILLIN ◇ BENZYLPENICILLIN
SODIUM ◇ CRYSTAPEN ◇ MYCOFARM ◇ NOVOCILLIN
◇ PEN-A-BRASIVE ◇ PENICILLIN-G, MONOSODIUM SALT
◇ PENICILLIN G, SODIUM ◇ PENICILLIN G, SODIUM SALT
◇ PENILARYN ◇ PENZYLPENICILLIN SODIUM SALT
◇ SODIUM BENZYLPENICILLIN ◇ SODIUM BENZYLPENI-
CILLIN G ◇ SODIUM BENZYLPENICILLINATE ◇ SODIUM
PENICILLIN ◇ SODIUM PENICILLIN G ◇ SODIUM PENICIL-
LIN II ◇ VETICILLIN

TOXICITY DATA with REFERENCE
ETA: scu-rat TDLo: 1840 mg/kg/46W-I   BJCAAI
15,85,61

CONSENSUS REPORTS: EPA Genetic Toxicology Program.

SAFETY PROFILE: Questionable carcinogen
with experimental tumorigenic and teratogenic
data. Poison by intracerebral, parenteral, and
intramuscular routes. Moderately toxic via intravenous route. Mildly toxic by ingestion.
Other experimental reproductive effects. When
heated to decomposition it emits very toxic
fumes of NO_x, Na_2O, and SO_x. An antibiotic.

BFV975
BETEL LEAVES

TOXICITY DATA with REFERENCE
ETA: orl-rat TDLo: 3000 g/kg/43W-C   EXPEAM
35,384,79

CONSENSUS REPORTS: IARC Cancer Review: Animal Inadequate Evidence IMEMDT
37,141,85

SAFETY PROFILE: Questionable carcinogen
with experimental tumorigenic data. When
heated to decomposition it emits toxic and irritating fumes.

BFW050
BETEL NUT TANNIN

SYN: TANNIN from BETEL NUT

TOXICITY DATA with REFERENCE
ETA: orl-mus TDLo: 27740 mg/kg/1Y-I   IJEBA6
24,229,86
MUT: sce-mus-ipr 1500 mg/kg/15D-C   CRNGDP
7,37,86

SAFETY PROFILE: Questionable carcinogen
with experimental tumorigenic data. Mutation
data reported. When heated to decomposition
it emits toxic and irritating fumes.

BFW750   CAS: 128-37-0
BHT (food grade)
mf: $C_{15}H_{24}O$ mw: 220.39

PROP: White, crystalline solid; faint characteristic odor. Bp: 265°, fp: 68°, flash p: 260°F
(TOC), d: 1.048 @ 20°/4°, vap d: 7.6. Sol in
alc; insol in water and propylene glycol.

SYNS: ADVASTAB 401 ◇ AGIDOL ◇ ANTIOXIDANT DBPC
◇ ANTIOXIDANT 29 ◇ AO 29 ◇ AO 4K ◇ 2,6-BIS(1,1-DI-
METHYLETHYL)-4-METHYLPHENOL ◇ BUKS ◇ BUTYL-
ATED HYDROXYTOLUENE ◇ BUTYLHYDROXYTOLUENE
◇ CAO 1 ◇ CAO 3 ◇ CATALIN CAO-3 ◇ CHEMANOX 11
◇ DBMP ◇ DBPC (technical grade) ◇ DIBUTYLATED HY-
DROXYTOLUENE ◇ 2,6-DI-tert-BUTYL-p-CRESOL (OSHA,
ACGIH) ◇ 2,6-DI-tert-BUTYL-1-HYDROXY-4-METHYLBEN

ZENE ◇ 3,5-DI-tert-BUTYL-4-HYDROXYTOLUENE ◇ 2,6-DI-terc. BUTYL-p-KRESOL (CZECH) ◇ 2,6-DI-tert-BU-TYL-p-METHYLPHENOL ◇ 2,6-DI-tert-BUTYL-4-METHYL-PHENOL ◇ FEMA No. 2184 ◇ 4-HYDROXY-3,5-DI-tert-BU-TYLTOLUENE ◇ IMPRUVOL ◇ IONOL ◇ IONOL (antioxidant) ◇ 4-METHYL-2,6-DI-terc. BUTYLFENOL (CZECH) ◇ METHYL DI-tert-BUTYLPHENOL ◇ 4-METHYL-2,6-DI-tert-BUTYLPHENOL ◇ NCI-C03598 ◇ NONOX TBC ◇ PARABAR 441 ◇ SUSTANE ◇ TENOX BHT ◇ TOPANOL ◇ VANLUBE PCX

TOXICITY DATA with REFERENCE
CAR: orl-mus TDLo: 435 mg/kg/69W-C
FCTXAV 12,367,74
CAR: orl-rat TD: 247 g/kg FCTOD7 24,1121,86
CAR: orl-rat TD: 247 g/kg/3Y-C: CAR FCTOD7 24,1,86
CAR: orl-rat TD: 247 g/kg/3Y-C: NEO FCTOD7 24,1,86
CAR: orl-rat TD: 963 g/kg FCTOD7 24,1071,86
CAR: orl-rat TDLo: 134 g/kg/32W-C CRNGDP 4,895,83
NEO: orl-mus TD: 1423 mg/kg/43W-C TXCYAC 38,151,86
MUT: dni-hmn: lym 20 μmol/L BBRCA9 80,963,78
MUT: dns-rat: lvr 100 pmol/L CRNGDP 5,1547,84
MUT: spm-mus-ipr 350 mg/kg/5D-I CMMUAO 5,257,78

CONSENSUS REPORTS: IARC Cancer Review: GROUP 3 IMEMDT 7,56,87; Animal Limited Evidence IMEDT 40,161,86. NCI Carcinogenesis Bioassay Completed; (feed): No Evidence: mouse, rat (NCITR* NCI-CG-TR-150,79). Reported in EPA TSCA Inventory. EPA Genetic Toxicology Program.

OSHA PEL: TLV 10 mg/m^3 ACGIH TLV: TLV 10 mg/m^3

SAFETY PROFILE: Questionable carcinogen with experimental carcinogenic and neoplastigenic data. Poison by intraperitoneal and intravenous routes. Moderately toxic by ingestion. Experimental reproductive effects. A human skin irritant. A skin and eye irritant in experimental animals. Combustible when exposed to heat or flame. To fight fire, use CO_2, dry chemical. When heated to decomposition it emits acrid smoke and fumes.

BFX250   CAS: 2130-56-5
5,5'-BIANTHRANILIC ACID
mf: $C_{14}H_{12}N_2O_4$ mw: 272.28

SYNS: 3,3'-BENZIDINEDICARBOXYLIC ACID ◇ 4,4'-DIAMINO-3,3'-BIPHENYLDICARBOXYLIC ACID ◇ 4,4'-DIAMINOBIPHENYL-3,3'-DICARBOXYLIC ACID ◇ 3,3'-DI-CARBOXYBENZIDINE ◇ KWAS BENZYDYNODWUKARO-KSYLOWY (POLISH)

TOXICITY DATA with REFERENCE
ETA: orl-mus TDLo: 22 g/kg/45W-I VOONAW 15(5),60,69
ETA: scu-mus TDLo: 12 g/kg/60W-I VOONAW 15(5),60,69
ETA: scu-rat TDLo: 7 g/kg/77W-I VOONAW 15(5),60,69
MUT: pic-esc 100 mmol/L MDMIAZ 31,11,79

CONSENSUS REPORTS: Reported in EPA TSCA Inventory.

SAFETY PROFILE: Questionable carcinogen with experimental tumorigenic data. Mutation data reported. When heated to decomposition it emits toxic fumes of NO_x.

BGB750   CAS: 4488-22-6
(1,1'-BINAPHTHALENE)-2,2'-DIAMINE
mf: $C_{20}H_{16}N_2$ mw: 284.38

SYN: 2,2'-DIAMINO-1,1'-DINAPHTHYL

TOXICITY DATA with REFERENCE
ETA: scu-mus TDLo: 2700 mg/kg/27W-I AJCAA7 40,62,40
ETA: skn-mus TDLo: 590 mg/kg/25W-I AJCAA7 40,62,40

SAFETY PROFILE: Questionable carcinogen with experimental tumorigenic data. When heated to decomposition it emits toxic fumes of NO_x.

BGC000   CAS: 795-95-9
(1,2'-BINAPHTHALENE)-1,2'-DIAMINE
mf: $C_{20}H_{16}N_2$ mw: 284.38

SYN: 1:2'-DIAMINO-1':2-DINAPHTHYL

TOXICITY DATA with REFERENCE
ETA: skn-mus TDLo: 2880 mg/kg/60W-I PRLBA4 131,170,72

SAFETY PROFILE: Questionable carcinogen with experimental tumorigenic data by skin contact. When heated to decomposition it emits toxic fumes of NO_x.

BGE000   CAS: 92-52-4
BIPHENYL
mf: $C_{12}H_{10}$ mw: 154.22

PROP: White scales, pleasant odor. Mp: 70°, bp: 255°, flash p: 235°F (CC), d: 0.991 @ 75°/4°, autoign temp: 1004°F, vap d: 5.31, lel: 0.6% @ 232°, uel: 5.8% @ 331°F.

SYNS: BIBENZENE ◇ 1,1'-BIPHENYL ◇ DIPHENYL ◇ LEMONENE ◇ PHENADOR-X ◇ PHENYLBENZENE ◇ PHPH ◇ XENENE

TOXICITY DATA with REFERENCE
NEO: scu-mus TDLo: 46 mg/kg   NTIS** PB223-159
ETA: orl-mus TDLo: 56 g/kg   NTIS** PB223-159
MUT: sce-ham: fbr 100 μmol/L   JNCIAM 58,1635,77

CONSENSUS REPORTS: EPA Genetic Toxicology Program. Reported in EPA TSCA Inventory. Community Right-To-Know List.

OSHA PEL: TWA 0.2 ppm   ACGIH TLV: TWA 0.2 ppm   DFG MAK: 0.2 ppm (1 mg/m^3)

SAFETY PROFILE: Questionable carcinogen with experimental tumorigenic and neoplastigenic data. Poison by intravenous route. Moderately toxic by ingestion. A powerful irritant by inhalation in humans. Human systemic effects by inhalation of very small amounts: flaccid paralysis, nausea or vomiting, and other unspecified gastrointestinal effects. Mutation data reported. Combustible when exposed to heat or flame; can react with oxidizing materials. To fight fire, use CO_2, dry chemical, water spray, mist, fog. When heated to decomposition it emits acrid smoke and fumes.

BGE300
4-BIPHENYLAMINE, DIHYDROCHLORIDE
mf: $C_{12}H_{11}N \cdot 2ClH$ mw: 242.16

SYN: 4-AMINOBIPHENYL DIHYDROCHLORIDE

TOXICITY DATA with REFERENCE
CAR: orl-rat TDLo: 2238 mg/kg/31W-I   JJCREP 76,570,85

SAFETY PROFILE: Questionable carcinogen with experimental carcinogenic data. When heated to decomposition it emits toxic fumes of NO_x and HCl.

BGE325
2-BIPHENYLAMINE, HYDROCHLORIDE
CAS: 2185-92-4
mf: $C_{12}H_{11}N \cdot ClH$ mw: 205.70

SYN: NCI-C50282

TOXICITY DATA with REFERENCE
CAR: orl-mus TD: 262 g/kg/2Y-C   FAATDF 2,201,82
CAR: orl-mus TDLo: 260 g/kg/2Y-C   NTPTR* NTP-TR-233,82
MUT: cyt-ham: ovr 200 mg/L   SCIEAS 236,933,87
MUT: mma-mus: lyms 110 mg/L   EMMUEG 12,85,88
MUT: mma-sat 10 μg/plate   SCIEAS 236,933,87

CONSENSUS REPORTS: NCI Carcinogenesis Studies (feed): Clear Evidence: mouse NTPTR* NTP-TR-233,82; No Evidence: rat NTPTR* NTP-TR-233,82

SAFETY PROFILE: Questionable carcinogen with experimental carcinogenic data. Mutation data reported. When heated to decomposition it emits toxic fumes of NO_x and HCl.

BGF000
N-4-BIPHENYLBENZAMIDE
CAS: 20743-57-1
mf: $C_{19}H_{15}NO$ mw: 273.35

SYNS: N-4-BIPHENYLYLBENZAMIDE ◇ 4'-PHENYL-BENZANILIDE

TOXICITY DATA with REFERENCE
ETA: ipr-rat TDLo: 508 mg/kg/4W-I   CNREA8 30,1485,70

SAFETY PROFILE: Questionable carcinogen with experimental tumorigenic data. When heated to decomposition it emits toxic fumes of NO_x.

BGF109
2,4'-BIPHENYLDIAMINE
CAS: 492-17-1
mf: $C_{12}H_{12}N_2$ mw: 184.26

PROP: Needles, very sltly sol in alcohol and ether. Mp: 54.4°, bp: 363°.

SYNS: o,p'-BIANILINE ◇ (1,1'-BIPHENYL)-2,4'-DIAMINE ◇ o,p'-DIAMINOBIPHENYL ◇ 2,4'-DIAMINODIPHENYL ◇ o,p'-DIANILINE ◇ DIFENYLIN ◇ 2,4'-DIPHENYLDIAMINE ◇ DIPHENYLINE

TOXICITY DATA with REFERENCE
ETA: orl-dog TDLo: 7020 mg/kg/5Y-I   NEOLA4 15,3,68
MUT: mma-sat 100 μg/plate   MUREAV 149,9,85

CONSENSUS REPORTS: IARC Cancer Review: GROUP 3 IMEMDT 7,56,87; Animal Inadequate Evidence IMEMDT 16,313,78

SAFETY PROFILE: Questionable carcinogen with experimental tumorigenic data. A poison by ingestion. Mutation data reported. When heated to decomposition it emits toxic fumes of NO_x.

BGF899　　　　　　　　　　　CAS: 1137-79-7
4-BIPHENYLDIMETHYLAMINE
mf: $C_{14}H_{15}N$　　mw: 197.30

SYN: 4-DIMETHYLAMINOBIPHENYL

TOXICITY DATA with REFERENCE
CAR: orl-rat TDLo:19 g/kg/43W-C　CNREA8 16,525,56

SAFETY PROFILE: Questionable carcinogen with experimental carcinogenic data. When heated to decomposition it emits toxic fumes of NO_x.

BGI250　　　　　　　　　　　CAS: 6810-26-0
4-BIPHENYLHYDROXYLAMINE
mf: $C_{12}H_{11}NO$　　mw: 185.24

SYNS: N-4-BIPHENYLYLHYDROXYLAMINE ◇ 4-HYDROXYLAMINOBIPHENYL

TOXICITY DATA with REFERENCE
CAR: scu-mus TDLo:216 mg/kg/3D　JNCIAM 41,403,68
MUT: dns-hmn:oth 1 μmol/L　JJIND8 72,847,84
MUT: dns-rat:lvr 5 μmol/L　ENMUDM 3,11,81
MUT: dns-rbt:oth 10 μmol/L　CNREA8 45,221,85
MUT: mmo-esc 2500 nmol/L　MUREAV 151,201,85
MUT: mmo-sat 5 μg/plate　MUREAV 151,201,85

CONSENSUS REPORTS: EPA Genetic Toxicology Program.

SAFETY PROFILE: Questionable carcinogen with experimental carcinogenic data. Human mutation data reported. When heated to decomposition it emits highly toxic fumes of NO_x.

BGJ250　　　　　　　　　　　CAS: 90-43-7
2-BIPHENYLOL
mf: $C_{12}H_{10}O$　　mw: 170.22

SYNS: o-BIPHENYLOL ◇ (1,1'-BIPHENYL)-2-OL ◇ o-DIPHENYLOL ◇ DOWCIDE 1 ◇ DOWCIDE 1 ANTIMICROBIAL ◇ 2-HYDROXYBIFENYL (CZECH) ◇ o-HYDROXYBIPHENYL ◇ 2-HYDROXYBIPHENYL ◇ o-HYDROXYDIPHENYL ◇ 2-HYDROXYDIPHENYL ◇ KIWI LUSTR 277 ◇ NCI-C50351 ◇ OPP ◇ ORTHOHYDROXYDIPHENYL ◇ ORTHOPHENYLPHENOL ◇ ORTHOXENOL ◇ o-PHENYLPHENOL ◇ 2-PHENYLPHENOL ◇ PREVENTOL O EXTRA ◇ REMOL TRF ◇ TETROSIN OE ◇ TORSITE ◇ TUMESCAL OPE ◇ USAF EK-2219 ◇ o-XENOL

TOXICITY DATA with REFERENCE
CAR: orl-rat TD:478 g/kg/91W-C　FCTOD7 22,865,84
CAR: orl-rat TDLo:478 g/kg/91W-C　FCTOD7 22,865,84
NEO: orl-rat TD:135 g/kg/26W-C　FCTOD7 25,359,87
MUT: cyt-ham:ovr 100 mg/L　MUREAV 141,95,84
MUT: cyt-hmn:fbr 200 μg/L　MUREAV 54,255,78
MUT: mmo-sat 60 μg/plate　ENMUDM 5(Suppl 1),3,83
MUT: msc-hmn:emb 20 mg/L　MUREAV 156,123,85
MUT: msc-hmn:oth 15 mg/L　TRENAF 35,399,84

CONSENSUS REPORTS: IARC Cancer Review: Animal Inadequate Evidence IMEMDT 30,329,83; NTP Carcinogenesis Studies (dermal); No Evidence: mouse NTPTR* NTP-TR-301,86. Reported in EPA TSCA Inventory. On Community Right-To-Know List.

SAFETY PROFILE: Questionable carcinogen with experimental carcinogenic data. A poison by intraperitoneal route. Moderately toxic by ingestion and possibly other routes. An experimental teratogen. Other experimental reproductive effects. Human mutation data reported. Severe eye and moderate skin irritant. When heated to decomposition it emits acrid smoke and irritating fumes.

BGJ500　　　　　　　　　　　CAS: 92-69-3
4-BIPHENYLOL
mf: $C_{12}H_{10}O$　　mw: 170.22

SYNS: p-HYDROXYBIPHENYL ◇ 4-HYDROXYBIPHENYL ◇ p-HYDROXYDIPHENYL ◇ 4-HYDROXYDIPHENYL ◇ PARAXENOL ◇ p-PHENYLPHENOL ◇ 4-PHENYLPHENOL

TOXICITY DATA with REFERENCE
CAR: scu-mus TDLo:1000 mg/kg　NTIS** PB223-159
ETA: orl-mus TDLo:153 g/kg/78W-I　NTIS** PB223-159

CONSENSUS REPORTS: Reported in EPA TSCA Inventory.

SAFETY PROFILE: Questionable carcinogen with experimental carcinogenic and tumorigenic data. Acute poison by intraperitoneal route. When heated to decomposition it emits acrid, irritating fumes.

BGK500　　　　　　　　　　　CAS: 91-95-2
3,3',4,4'-BIPHENYLTETRAMINE
mf: $C_{12}H_{14}N_4$　　mw: 214.30

SYNS: 3,3'-DIAMINOBENZIDENE ◊ 3,3',4,4'-DIPHE-
NYLTETRAMINE ◊ 3,3',4,4'-TETRAAMINOBIPHENYL

TOXICITY DATA with REFERENCE
ETA: orl-rat TDLo: 9000 mg/kg/27D-I   CNREA8
28,924,68

MUT: dnd-esc 20 μmol/L   MUREAV 89,95,81
MUT: dns-rat: lvr 500 μmol/L   ENMUDM 3,11,81
MUT: mma-sat 100 μg/plate   BJCAAI 37,873,78
MUT: mmo-smc 140 μmol/L   MGGEAE
174,39, 79

CONSENSUS REPORTS: Reported in EPA
TSCA Inventory.

SAFETY PROFILE: Questionable carcinogen
with experimental tumorigenic data. Moderately
toxic by ingestion. Mutation data reported.
When heated to decomposition it emits toxic
fumes of NO_x.

BGK750   CAS: 7411-49-6
3,3',4,4'-BIPHENYLTETRAMINE
TETRAHYDROCHLORIDE
mf: $C_{12}H_{14}N_4 \cdot 4ClH$ mw: 360.14

SYNS: 3,3'-DIAMINOBENZIDINE TETRAHYDROCHLO-
RIDE ◊ 3,3',4,4'-TETRAAMINOBIPHENYL TETRAHYDRO-
CHLORIDE

TOXICITY DATA with REFERENCE
NEO: orl-mus TD: 520 g/kg/78W-C   JEPTDQ
2,325,78
NEO: orl-mus TDLo: 260 g/kg/78W-C   JEPTDQ
2,325,78
ETA: orl-rat TDLo: 260 g/kg/78W-C   JEPTDQ
2,325,78

CONSENSUS REPORTS: Reported in EPA
TSCA Inventory.

SAFETY PROFILE: Questionable carcinogen
with experimental neoplastigenic and tumorigenic data. Poison by intraperitoneal route.
When heated to decomposition it emits very
toxic fumes of HCl and NO_x.

BGL000   CAS: 13607-48-2
N-4-BIPHENYLYLBENZENE-
SULFONAMIDE
mf: $C_{18}H_{15}NO_2S$ mw: 309.40

SYN: N-4-BIPHENYLYL BENZENESULFONAMIDE

TOXICITY DATA with REFERENCE
ETA: ipr-rat TDLo: 634 mg/kg/4W-I   CNREA8
30,1485,70

SAFETY PROFILE: Questionable carcinogen
with experimental tumorigenic data. When

heated to decomposition it emits very toxic
fumes of SO_x and NO_x.

BGN000   CAS: 29968-68-1
N-4-BIPHENYLYL-N-
HYDROXYBENZENESULFONAMIDE
mf: $C_{18}H_{15}NO_3S$ mw: 325.40

SYN: HYDROXY-4-BIPHENYLYLBENZENESULFON-
AMIDE

TOXICITY DATA with REFERENCE
NEO: ipr-rat TDLo: 618 mg/kg/4W-I   CNREA8
30,1485,70

SAFETY PROFILE: Questionable carcinogen
with experimental neoplastigenic data. When
heated to decomposition it emits very toxic
fumes of SO_x and NO_x.

BGO500   CAS: 366-18-7
2,2'-BIPYRIDINE
mf: $C_{10}H_8N_2$ mw: 156.20

PROP: White crystals. Sol in 2200 parts water;
very sol in alc, ether, benzene, chloroform, and
petroleum ether. Mp: 69.7°, bp: 272°-273°.

SYNS: 2,2'-BYPYRIDIN ◊ BIPYRIDINE ◊ α,α'-BIPYRI-
DINE ◊ α,α'-BIPYRIDYL ◊ 2,2'-BIPYRIDYL ◊ CI-588
◊ α,α'-DIPYRIDYL ◊ 2,2'-DIPYRIDYL

TOXICITY DATA with REFERENCE
ETA: scu-mus TDLo: 8000 mg/kg/40W-I
JNCIAM 24,109,60

MUT: mma-sat 20 μg/plate   ABCHA6 45,327,81
MUT: mmo-sat 20 μg/plate   ABCHA6 45,327,81

CONSENSUS REPORTS: Reported in EPA
TSCA Inventory.

SAFETY PROFILE: Questionable carcinogen
with experimental tumorigenic data. Experimental teratogenic data. Poison by ingestion,
subcutaneous, and intraperitoneal route. Mutation data reported. When heated to decomposition it emits toxic fumes of NO_x.

BGP500   CAS: 63981-20-4
BIS-4-ACETAMINO PHENYL
SELENIUMDIHYDROXIDE
mf: $C_8H_{11}NO_3 \cdot Se$ mw: 248.16

TOXICITY DATA with REFERENCE
ETA: orl-rat TDLo: 2890 mg/kg/15W-C   SCIEAS
103,762,46

CONSENSUS REPORTS: Selenium and its
compounds are on the Community Right-To-
Know List

OSHA PEL: TWA 0.2 mg(Se)/m^3 ACGIH TLV: TWA 0.2 mg(Se)m^3

SAFETY PROFILE: Questionable carcinogen with experimental tumorigenic data. When heated to decomposition it emits very toxic fumes of NO$_x$ and Se.

BGQ750   CAS: 14024-64-7
BIS(ACETYLACETONATO) TITANIUM OXIDE
mf: C$_{10}$H$_{14}$O$_5$Ti   mw: 262.14

SYNS: BIS(2,4-PENTANEDIONATO)TITANIUM OXIDE ◇ TITANIUM ACETONYL ACETONATE ◇ TITANIUM OXIDE BIS(ACETYLACETONATE) ◇ TITANIUM, OXOBIS(2,4-PENTANEDIONATO-O,O') ◇ TITANYL BIS(ACETYLACETONATE)

TOXICITY DATA with REFERENCE
ETA: ims-rat TD: 2025 mg/kg/34W-I   NCIUS*
   PH 43-64-886,DEC,68
ETA: ims-rat TDLo: 360 mg/kg/69W-I   NCIUS*
   PH 43-64-886,AUG,69

SAFETY PROFILE: Questionable carcinogen with experimental tumorigenic data. Moderate toxic by intraperitoneal route. When heated to decomposition it emits acrid smoke and irritating fumes.

BGR250   CAS: 22750-65-8
2,5-BIS(ACETYLAMINO)FLUORENE
mf: C$_{17}$H$_{16}$N$_2$O$_2$ mw: 280.35

SYNS: N,N'-FLUOREN-2,5-YLENEBISACETAMIDE ◇ 2,5-FLUORENYLENEBISACETAMIDE

TOXICITY DATA with REFERENCE
CAR: orl-rat TDLo: 4550 mg/kg/26W-C
   CNREA8 22,1002,62

SAFETY PROFILE: Questionable carcinogen with experimental carcinogenic data. When heated to decomposition it emits toxic fumes of NO$_x$.

BGT250   CAS: 314-13-6
4,4'-BIS(1-AMINO-8-HYDROXY-2,4-DISULFO-7-NAPHTHYLAZO)-3,3'-BITOLYL, TETRASODIUM SALT
mf: C$_{34}$H$_{24}$N$_6$O$_{14}$S$_4$•4Na   mw: 960.84

SYNS: 4,4'-BIS(7-(1-AMINO-8-HYDROXY-2,4-DISULFO) NAPHTHYLAZO)-3,3'-BITOLYL, TETRASODIUM SALT ◇ 4,4'-BIS(1-AMINO-8-HYDROXY-2,4-DISULPHO-7-NAPHTHYLAZO)-3,3'-BITOLYL, TETRASODIUM SALT ◇ BLEKIT EVANSA (POLISH) ◇ CHLORAZOL SKY BLUE

FF ◇ C.I. 23860 ◇ C.I. DIRECT BLUE 53 ◇ DIAMINE SKY BLUE FF ◇ DIAZOBLEU ◇ DIAZOL PURE BLUE FF ◇ DYE EVANS BLUE ◇ EB ◇ EVABLIN ◇ EVANS BLUE DYE ◇ GEIGY-BLAU 536 ◇ T 1824

TOXICITY DATA with REFERENCE
ETA: ipr-rat TDLo: 850 mg/kg/34W-I   APHGBP
   33,1,53
MUT: dnd-mus-skn 192 µmol/kg   CRNGDP
   5,231,84
MUT: dns-ham: lvr 10 µmol/L   MUREAV
   136,255,84
MUT: dns-rat-orl 200 mg/kg   ENMUDM 7,101,85
MUT: dns-rat: lvr 100 µmol/L   MUREAV
   136,255,84
MUT: mma-sat 33 µg/plate   CRNGDP 3,21,82
MUT: pic-esc 100 mmol/L   MDMIAZ 31,11,79

CONSENSUS REPORTS: IARC Cancer Review: GROUP 3 IMEMDT 7,56,87, Animal Limited Evidence IMEMDT 8,151,75. Reported in EPA TSCA Inventory. EPA Genetic Toxicology Program.

SAFETY PROFILE: Questionable carcinogen with experimental tumorigenic data. An experimental teratogen and tumorigenic. Poison by intraperitoneal route. Moderately toxic by intravenous route. Other experimental reproductive effects. Mutation data reported. When heated to decomposition it emits very toxic fumes of SO$_x$, Na$_2$O and NO$_x$.

BGU000   CAS: 63077-09-8
BIS(2-AMINO-1-NAPHTHYL)SODIUM PHOSPHATE
mf: C$_{20}$H$_{17}$N$_2$O$_4$P•Na   mw: 403.35

SYN: 2-AMINO-1-NAPHTHOL PHOSPHATE (ESTER) SODIUM SALT

TOXICITY DATA with REFERENCE
CAR: imp-mus TDLo: 80 mg/kg   BJCAAI
   17,127,63

SAFETY PROFILE: Questionable carcinogen with experimental carcinogenic data. When heated to decomposition it emits very toxic fumes of PO$_x$, NO$_x$, and Na$_2$O.

BHA750   CAS: 155-04-4
BIS(2-BENZOTHIAZOLYLTHIO)ZINC
mf: C$_{14}$H$_8$N$_2$S$_4$•Zn   mw: 397.85

SYNS: 2-BENZOTHIAZOLETHIOL, ZINC SALT (2:1) ◇ BIS(MERCAPTOBENZOTHIAZOLATO)ZINC ◇ HERMAT Zn-MBT ◇ 2-MERCAPTOBENZOTHIAZOLE ZINC SALT

◇ OXAF ◇ PENNAC ZT ◇ TISPERSE MB-58 ◇ USAF GY-7 ◇ VULKACIT ZM ◇ ZENITE ◇ ZENITE SPECIAL ◇ ZETAX ◇ ZINC-2-BENZOTHIAZOLETHIOLATE ◇ ZINC BENZOTHIAZOLYL MERCAPTIDE ◇ ZINC BENZO-THIAZOL-2-YLTHIOLATE ◇ ZINC BENZOTHIAZYL-2-MER-CAPTIDE ◇ ZINC MERCAPTOBENZOTHIAZOLATE ◇ ZINC-2-MERCAPTOBENZOTHIAZOLE ◇ ZINC MERCAP-TOBENZOTHIAZOLE SALT ◇ ZMBT ◇ ZnMB

TOXICITY DATA with REFERENCE
CAR: scu-mus TDLo: 1000 mg/kg   NTIS** PB223-159

CONSENSUS REPORTS: Reported in EPA TSCA Inventory. Zinc compounds are on the Community Right-To-Know List.

SAFETY PROFILE: Questionable carcinogen with experimental carcinogenic data. Poison by intraperitoneal route. Moderately toxic by inges-tion and subcutaneous routes. When heated to decomposition it emits very toxic fumes of SO_x, NO_x, and ZnO.

BHB750   CAS: 4420-79-5
2,5-BIS(BIS-(2-CHLOROETHYL) AMINOMETHYL)HYDROQUINONE
mf: $C_{16}H_{24}Cl_4N_2O_2$ mw: 418.22

SYNS: HYDROQUINONE MUSTARD ◇ NSC 18321 ◇ WEATHERBEE MUSTARD

TOXICITY DATA with REFERENCE
CAR: ipr-mus TDLo: 28 mg/kg/4W   JNCIAM 36,915,66
MUT: ipr-rat LD10: 4700 μg/kg   CNCRA6 17,1,62

SAFETY PROFILE: Questionable carcinogen with experimental carcinogenic data. Deadly poison by intravenous and intraperitoneal routes. A powerful irritant. When heated to de-composition it emits highly toxic fumes of NO_x and Cl^-.

BHV250   CAS: 3223-07-2
l-3-(p-(BIS(2-CHLOROETHYL)AMINO) PHENYL)ALANINE MONOHYDROCHLORIDE
mf: $C_{13}H_{18}Cl_2N_2O_2 \cdot ClH$ mw: 341.69

SYNS: ALANINE NITROGEN MUSTARD ◇ CB 3025 ◇ MELPHALAN HYDROCHLORIDE ◇ NSC-8806 ◇ l-PHE-NYLALANINE MUSTARD HYDROCHLORIDE ◇ l-SARCOLY-SINE HYDROCHLORIDE

TOXICITY DATA with REFERENCE
CAR: ipr-mus TDLo: 1300 μg/kg/4W   JNCIAM 36,915,66

SAFETY PROFILE: Questionable carcinogen with experimental carcinogenic data. Deadly poison by intravenous route. Human systemic effects by ingestion: nausea and vomiting. When heated to decomposition it emits very toxic fumes of Cl^-, NO_x, and HCl.

BIC600   CAS: 4213-41-6
N,N-BIS(2-CHLOROETHYL)-2,3-DIMETHOXYANILINE
mf: $C_{12}H_{17}Cl_2NO_2$ mw: 278.20

SYNS: ANILINE, N,N-BIS(2-CHLOROETHYL)-2,3-DI-METHOXY- ◇ 2,3-DIMETHOXYANILINE MUSTARD ◇ NSC-18439

TOXICITY DATA with REFERENCE
CAR: ipr-mus TDLo: 27 mg/kg/4W   JNCIAM 36,915,66

SAFETY PROFILE: Questionable carcinogen with experimental carcinogenic data. When heated to decomposition it emits toxic fumes of NO_x.

BID000   CAS: 6986-48-7
BIS(α-CHLOROETHYL) ETHER
mf: $C_4H_8Cl_2O$ mw: 143.02

SYN: 1,1'-OXYBIS(1-CHLOROETHANE)

TOXICITY DATA with REFERENCE
ETA: scu-mus TDLo: 648 mg/kg/54W-I   JNCIAM 48,1431,72

SAFETY PROFILE: Questionable carcinogen with experimental tumorigenic data. When heated to decomposition it emits toxic fumes of Cl^-.

BIF500   CAS: 67856-68-2
BIS(2-CHLOROETHYL)NITROSOAMINE
mf: $C_4H_8Cl_2N_2O$ mw: 171.04

SYNS: NITROSOBIS(2-CHLOROETHYL)AMINE ◇ N-NITROSO-2,2'-DICHLORODIETHYLAMINE

TOXICITY DATA with REFERENCE
ETA: orl-rat TDLo: 345 mg/kg/30W-I   CNREA8 38,2391,78
MUT: mma-sat 10 μg/plate   MUREAV 66,1,79
MUT: mmo-sat-10 μg/plate   MUREAV 66,1,79

SAFETY PROFILE: Questionable carcinogen with experimental tumorigenic data. Mutation data reported. When heated to decomposition it emits toxic fumes of Cl^- and NO_x.

BII250 CAS: 108-60-1
BIS(2-CHLOROISOPROPYL) ETHER
DOT: 2490
mf: $C_6H_{12}Cl_2O$ mw: 171.08

PROP: Colorless liquid. Bp: 187.8°, fp: >−20°, flash p: 185°F (OC), d: 1.11 @ 25°/25°, vap d: 6.0, vap press: 0.10 mm @ 20°.

SYNS: BIS(2-CHLORO-1-METHYLETHYL) ETHER ◇ (2-CHLORO-1-METHYLETHYL) ETHER ◇ DICHLORODI-ISOPROPYL ETHER ◇ DICHLOROISOPROPYL ETHER (DOT) ◇ 2,2′-DICHLOROISOPROPYL ETHER ◇ NCI-C50044 ◇ RCRA WASTE NUMBER U027

TOXICITY DATA with REFERENCE
MUT: mma-sat 333 μg/plate ENMUDM 8(Suppl 7),1,86
MUT: mmo-sat 1 mL/plate/3H DHEFDK FDA-78-1046,78

CONSENSUS REPORTS: IARC Cancer Review: GROUP 3 IMEMDT 7,56,87, Animal Limited Evidence IMEMDT 41,149,86. NCI Carcinogenesis Bioassay (gavage); No Evidence: rat NCITR* NCI-CG-TR-191,79. Community Right-To-Know List. Reported in EPA TSCA Inventory.

DOT Classification: Corrosive Material; Label: Corrosive; IMO: Poison B; Label: Poison.

SAFETY PROFILE: Questionable carcinogen. Poison by ingestion. Moderately toxic by skin contact and inhalation. An eye irritant. Mutation data reported. A corrosive material. Moderate fire hazard when exposed to heat, flame, or powerful oxidizers. Incompatible with oxidizing materials. To fight fire, use water to blanket fire; foam, CO_2, dry chemical. When heated to decomposition it emits highly toxic fumes of Cl^-.

BIJ250 CAS: 13483-18-6
BIS-1,2-(CHLOROMETHOXY)ETHANE
mf: $C_4H_8Cl_2O_2$ mw: 159.02

PROP: Viscous liquid. Bp: 99°-100° @ 22 mm, d: 1.2879 @ 14°/15°.

SYN: ETHYLENE GLYCOL BIS(CHLOROMETHYL)ETHER

TOXICITY DATA with REFERENCE
NEO: ipr-mus TDLo:940 mg/kg/78W-I
CNREA8 35,2553,75
NEO: scu-mus TDLo:970 mg/kg/81W-I
CNREA8 35,2553,75
NEO: skn-mus TDLo:8640 mg/kg/72W-I
CNREA8 35,2553,75

CONSENSUS REPORTS: IARC Cancer Review: GROUP 3 IMEMDT 7,56,87; Animal Sufficient Evidence IMEMDT 15,31,77. Reported in EPA TSCA Inventory. Glycol ethers are on the Community Right-To-Know List.

SAFETY PROFILE: Questionable carcinogen with experimental neoplastigenic data. When heated to decomposition it emits toxic fumes of Cl^-.

BIJ500 CAS: 56894-91-8
1,4-BIS(CHLOROMETHOXYMETHYL) BENZENE
mf: $C_{10}H_{12}Cl_2O_2$ mw: 235.12

SYN: BIS-1,4-(CHLOROMETHOXY)-p-XYLENE

TOXICITY DATA with REFERENCE
NEO: scu-mus TDLo:970 mg/kg/81W-I
CNREA8 35,2553,75
NEO: skn-mus TDLo:2590 mg/kg/72W-I
CNREA8 35,2553,75
ETA: ipr-mus TDLo:310 mg/kg/78W-I CNREA8 35,2553,75

CONSENSUS REPORTS: IARC Cancer Review: GROUP 3 IMEMDT 7,56,87; Animal Sufficient Evidence IMEMDT 15,37,77

SAFETY PROFILE: Questionable carcinogen with experimental neoplastigenic and tumorigenic data. When heated to decomposition it emits toxic fumes of Cl^-.

BIJ750 CAS: 10387-13-0
9,10-BIS(CHLOROMETHYL) ANTHRACENE
mf: $C_{16}H_{12}Cl_2$ mw: 275.18

SYNS: 9,10-DI(CHLOROMETHYL)ANTHRACENE ◇ ICR-450

TOXICITY DATA with REFERENCE
NEO: ivn-mus TDLo:1100 μg/kg CNREA8 36,2423,76
MUT: mma-sat 100 ng/plate PNASA6 72,5135,75

CONSENSUS REPORTS: Reported in EPA TSCA Inventory. EPA Genetic Toxicology Program.

SAFETY PROFILE: Questionable carcinogen with experimental neoplastigenic data. Poison by intravenous route. Mutation data reported. When heated to decomposition it emits toxic fumes of Cl^-.

BIK100
BIS(2-CHLORO-1-METHYLETHYL) ETHER mixed with 2-CHLORO-1-METHYLETHYL-(2-CHLOROPROPYL) ETHER

mf: $C_6H_{12}Cl_2O$ mw: 171.08

SYN: ETHER, BIS(2-CHLORO-1-METHYLETHYL), mixed with 2-CHLORO-1-METHYLETHYL-(2-CHLOROPRO-PYL)ETHER (7:3)

TOXICITY DATA with REFERENCE
CAR: orl-mus TD:103 g/kg/2Y-I   NTPTR*
  NTP-TR-239,82
CAR: orl-mus TDLo:51500 mg/kg/2Y-I
  NTPTR* NTP-TR-239,82

CONSENSUS REPORTS: NTP CARCINO-GENESIS BIOASSAY (gavage); Clear Evidence: mouse NTPTR* NTP-TR-239,83

SAFETY PROFILE: Questionable carcinogen with experimental carcinogenic data. When heated to decomposition it emits toxic fumes of Cl⁻.

BIL250   CAS: 14579-91-0
1,3-BIS(CHLOROMETHYL)-1,1,3,3-TETRAMETHYLDISILAZANE

mf: $C_6H_{17}Cl_2N-Si_2$ mw: 230.32

SYN: 1-(CHLOROMETHYL)-N-((CHLOROMETHYL)DI-METHYLSILYL)-1,1-DIMETHYL-SILANAMINE

TOXICITY DATA with REFERENCE
NEO: ipr-mus TDLo:40 mg/kg/I   JNCIAM
  54,495,75

CONSENSUS REPORTS: Reported in EPA TSCA Inventory.

SAFETY PROFILE: Questionable carcinogen with experimental neoplastigenic data. Poison by intraperitoneal route. When heated to decomposition it emits very toxic fumes of Cl⁻ and NO_x.

BIO750   CAS: 115-32-2
1,1-BIS(p-CHLOROPHENYL)-2,2,2-TRICHLOROETHANOL

DOT: 2761
mf: $C_{14}H_9Cl_5O$ mw: 370.48

PROP: Material used in cancer bioassay was 40-60% pure (NCITR* NCI-CG-TR-90,78).

SYNS: ACARIN ◇ 1,1-BIS(CHLOROPHENYL)-2,2,2-TRI-CHLOROETHANOL ◇ 1,1-BIS(4-CHLOROPHENYL)-2,2,2-TRICHLOROETHANOL ◇ CARBAX ◇ CEKUDIFOL

◇ 4-CHLORO-α-(4-CHLOROPHENYL)-α-(TRICHLOROMETHYL)BENZENEMETHANOL ◇ CPCA ◇ DECOFOL ◇ DICHLOROKELTHANE ◇ DI-(p-CHLOROPHENYL)TRICHLOROMETHYLCARBINOL ◇ 4,4'-DICHLORO-α-(TRICHLOROMETHYL)BENZHYDROL ◇ DICOFOL ◇ DTMC ◇ ENT 23,648 ◇ FW 293 ◇ HIFOL ◇ KELTANE ◇ p,p'-KELTHANE ◇ KELTHANE (DOT) ◇ KELTHANE DUST BASE ◇ KELTHANETHANOL ◇ MILBOL ◇ MITIGAN ◇ NCI-C00486 ◇ 2,2,2-TRICHLOOR-1,1-BIS(4-CHLOOR FENYL)-ETHANOL (DUTCH) ◇ 1,1,1-TRICHLOR-2,2-BIS(4-CHLORPHENYL)-AETHANOL (GER-MAN) ◇ 2,2,2-TRICHLOR-1,1-BIS(4-CHLOR-PHENYL)-AETHANOL (GERMAN) ◇ 2,2,2-TRICHLORO-1,1-BIS(4-CHLOROPHENYL)-ETHANOL (FRENCH) ◇ 2,2,2-TRICHLO-RO-1,1-BIS(4-CLORO-FENIL)-ETANOLO (ITALIAN) ◇ 2,2,2-TRICHLORO-1,1-DI-(4-CHLOROPHENYL)ETHANOL

TOXICITY DATA with REFERENCE
CAR: orl-mus TD:35 g/kg/78W-C   NCITR*
  NCI-CG-TR-90,78
CAR: orl-mus TDLo:17 g/kg/78W-C   NCITR*
  NCI-CG-TR-90,78
MUT: sce-hmn:lym 1 μmol/L   ARTODN 52,221,83

CONSENSUS REPORTS: IARC Cancer Review: GROUP 3 IMEMDT 7,56,87; Animal Limited Evidence IMEMDT 30,87,83. NCI Carcinogenesis Bioassay (feed); Clear Evidence: mouse NCITR* NCI-CG-TR-90,78; No Evidence: rat NCITR* NCI-CG-TR-90,78. Community Right-To-Know List.

DOT Classification: ORM-E; Label: None.

SAFETY PROFILE: Questionable carcinogen with experimental carcinogenic data. Poison by ingestion and skin contact. Moderately toxic by intraperitoneal route. Human mutation data reported. When heated to decomposition it emits toxic fumes of Cl⁻.

BIR529   CAS: 1277-43-6
BIS(CYCLOPENTADIENYL)COBALT

mf: $C_{10}H_{10}Co$ mw: 189.13

SYNS: COBALTOCENE ◇ DICYCLOPENTADIENYLCO-BALT

TOXICITY DATA with REFERENCE
ETA: ims-rat TDLo:200 mg/kg/60W-I   NCIUS*
  PH 42-64-886,SEPT,71

CONSENSUS REPORTS: Reported in EPA TSCA Inventory. Cobalt and its compounds are on the Community Right-To-Know List.

SAFETY PROFILE: Questionable carcinogen with experimental tumorigenic data. Poison by intraperitoneal route. When heated to decomposition it emits acrid smoke and fumes.

BIS250 CAS: 38780-36-8
cis-BIS(CYCLOPENTYLAMMINE) PLATINUM(II)
mf: $C_{10}H_{22}Cl_2N_2Pt$ mw: 436.33

SYNS: cis-DICHLOROBIS(CYCLOPENTYLAMMINE) PLATINUM(II) ◇ cis-DICYCLOPENTYLAMMINEDICHLORO-PLATINUM(II)

TOXICITY DATA with REFERENCE
CAR: ipr-mus TDLo: 189 mg/kg/10W-I CNREA8 39,913,79
CAR: scu-rat TDLo: 109 mg/kg/6W-I CNREA8 39,913,79
MUT: cyt-ham: ovr 46 mg/L CBINA8 14,217,76
MUT: dni-ham: ovr 26 mg/L CBINA8 14,217,76
MUT: mma-sat 10 μg/plate MUREAV 95,79,82
MUT: mmo-sat 1 μmol/plate CBINA8 26,179,79

SAFETY PROFILE: Questionable carcinogen with experimental carcinogenic data. Moderately toxic by intraperitoneal and possibly other routes. Mutation data reported. When heated to decomposition it emits very toxic fumes of Cl^- and NO_x.

BIT000 CAS: 5684-13-9
BISDEHYDROISYNOLIC ACID METHYL ESTER
mf: $C_{19}H_{22}O_3$ mw: 298.41

SYNS: DEHYDROFOLLICULINIC ACID ◇ DOISYNOES-TROL ◇ 1-ETHYL-2-METHYL-7-METHOXY-1,2,3,4-TETRA-HYDROPHENANTHRYL-2-CARBOXYLIC ACID ◇ FENO-CYCLIN ◇ FENOCYCLINE ◇ 7-METHYLBISDEHYDRO-DOISYNOLIC ACID ◇ METILESTER DEL ACIDO BISDEHI-DROISYNOLICO (SPANISH) ◇ 16,17-SECO-13-α-ESTRA-1,3,5,6,7,9-PENTAEN-17-OIC ACID, METHYL ESTER ◇ SURESTRINE ◇ SURESTRYL ◇ TETRADEHYDRODO-ISYNOLIC ACID METHYL ETHER

TOXICITY DATA with REFERENCE
ETA: imp-gpg TDLo: 3952 μg/kg BSBSAS 8,142,51
ETA: imp-ham TDLo: 437 mg/kg CNREA8 12,274,52

SAFETY PROFILE: Questionable carcinogen with experimental tumorigenic data. Experimental reproductive effects. When heated to decomposition it emits acrid smoke and irritating fumes.

BIT030
BISDEHYDRODOISYNOLIC ACID 7-METHYL ETHER
mf: $C_{19}H_{22}O_3$ mw: 298.41

SYNS: 7-METILETER del ACIDO BISDEHIDRODOISYNOL-ICO ◇ 16,17-SECOESTRA-1,3,5(10),6,8-PENTAEN-17-OIC ACID, 3-METHOXY-

TOXICITY DATA with REFERENCE
ETA: imp-gpg TDLo: 21 mg/kg BSBSAS 8,142,51

SAFETY PROFILE: Questionable carcinogen with experimental tumorigenic data. When heated to decomposition it emits toxic fumes of NO_x.

BIW750 CAS: 13927-77-0
BIS(DIBUTYLDITHIOCARBAMATO) NICKEL
mf: $C_{18}H_{36}N_2S_4•Ni$ mw: 467.51

SYNS: DIBUTYLDITHIOCARBAMIC ACID, NICKEL SALT ◇ NICKEL DIBUTYLDITHIOCARBAMATE ◇ UV CHEK AM 104 ◇ VANGUARD N

TOXICITY DATA with REFERENCE
ETA: orl-mus TDLo: 22 mg/kg/78W-I NTIS** PB223-159
ETA: scu-mus TDLo: 1000 mg/kg NTIS** PB223-159

CONSENSUS REPORTS: Reported in EPA TSCA Inventory. Nickel and its compounds are on The Community Right-To-Know List.

NIOSH REL: TWA 0.015 mg(Ni)/m³

SAFETY PROFILE: Questionable carcinogen with experimental tumorigenic data. When heated to decomposition it emits very toxic fumes of SO_x and NO_x.

BIX000 CAS: 136-23-2
BIS(DIBUTYLDITHIOCARBAMATO)ZINC
mf: $C_{18}H_{38}N_2S_4Zn$ mw: 476.19

PROP: White powder. Mp: 104-108°; d: 1.24 @ 20°/20°.

SYNS: ACETO ZDBD ◇ BUTAZATE ◇ BUTAZATE 50-D ◇ BUTYL ZIMATE ◇ BUTYL ZIRAM ◇ DIBUTYLDITHIO-CARBAMIC ACID ZINC COMPLEX ◇ DIBUTYLDITHIOCAR-BAMIC ACID ZINC SALT ◇ USAF GY-5 ◇ VULCACURE ◇ VULKACIT LDB/C ◇ ZINC-BIBUTYLDITHIOCARBAMATE ◇ ZINC-DIBUTYLDITHIOCARBAMATE ◇ ZINC-N,N-DIBU-TYLDITHIOCARBAMATE

TOXICITY DATA with REFERENCE
ETA: orl-mus TDLo: 290 g/kg/78W-I NTIS** PB223-159

ETA: scu-mus TDLo:1000 mg/kg   NTIS**
PB223-159

CONSENSUS REPORTS: Reported in EPA TSCA Inventory. Zinc and its compounds are on the Community Right-To-Know List.

SAFETY PROFILE: Questionable carcinogen with experimental tumorigenic data. Poison by intraperitoneal route. When heated to decomposition it emits very toxic fumes of NO_x, ZnO and SO_x.

BJC000   CAS: 14324-55-1
BIS(DIETHYLDITHIOCARBAMATO)ZINC
mf: $C_{10}H_{22}N_2S_4 \cdot Zn$ mw: 363.95

PROP: White powder. D: 1.47 @ 20°/20°.

SYNS: DIETHYLDITHIOCARBAMIC ACID ZINC SALT ◇ ETHAZATE ◇ ETHYL CYMATE ◇ ETHYL ZIMATE ◇ ETHYL ZIRUM ◇ VULCACURE ◇ VULKACIT LDA ◇ ZINC DIETHYLDITHIOCARBAMATE ◇ ZINC-N,N-DI-ETHYLDITHIOCARBAMATE

TOXICITY DATA with REFERENCE
CAR: scu-mus TDLo:464 mg/kg   NTIS**
PB223-159
ETA: orl-mus TDLo:28 g/kg/78W-I   NTIS**
PB223-159
MUT: mma-sat 25 µg/plate   MUREAV 68,313,79
MUT: mmo-sat 25 µg/plate   MUREAV 68,313,79

CONSENSUS REPORTS: Reported in EPA TSCA Inventory. Zinc and its compounds are on the Community Right-To-Know List.

SAFETY PROFILE: Questionable carcinogen with experimental carcinogenic and tumorigenic data. Poison by intraperitoneal route. Moderately toxic by ingestion and subcutaneous routes. Mutation data reported. Severe irritant to eyes, nose, and throat. When heated to decomposition it emits very toxic fumes of NO_x and SO_x.

BJF000   CAS: 494-38-2
3,6-BIS(DIMETHYLAMINO)ACRIDINE
mf: $C_{17}H_{19}N_3$ mw: 265.39

SYNS: ACRIDINE ORANGE ◇ ACRIDINE ORANGE FREE BASE ◇ BASIC ORANGE 3RN ◇ 2,8-BISDIMETHYLAMINO-ACRIDINE ◇ BRILLIANT ACRIDINE ORANGE E ◇ C.I. 46005 ◇ C.I. NO. 46005:1 ◇ C.I. BASIC ORANGE 14 ◇ C.I. SOLVENT ORANGE 15 ◇ 3,6-DI(DIMETHYLAMINO)ACRI-DINE ◇ EUCHRYSINE ◇ RHODULINE ORANGE ◇ SOLVENT ORANGE 15 ◇ N,N,N'-TETRAMETHYL-3,6-ACRIDINEDIAMINE ◇ WAXOLINE ORANGE A

TOXICITY DATA with REFERENCE
ETA: scu-mus TDLo:657 mg/kg/63W-I   BJCAAI
23,587,69
ETA: skn-mus TDLo:6630 mg/kg   BJCAAI
23,587,69
MUT: cyt-ckn-par 1695 µg/kg   47JMAE
-,137,82
MUT: cyt-ham:ovr 20 µmol/L/5H-C   ENMUDM
1,27,79
MUT: dnd-esc 5 µmol/L   MUREAV 89,95,81
MUT: dns-rat:lvr 1 mmol/L   ENMUDM 3,11,81
MUT: mmo-omi 10 µg/L   MIBLAO 49,223,80
MUT: msc-ham:ovr 1 mg/L   MUREAV 94,449,82
MUT: otr-ham:emb 1 µg/L   NCIMAV 58,243,81

CONSENSUS REPORTS: IARC Cancer Review: GROUP 3 IMEMDT 7,56,87; Animal Inadequate Evidence IMEMDT 16,145,78

SAFETY PROFILE: Questionable carcinogen with experimental tumorigenic and carcinogenic data. Poison by subcutaneous route. Mutation data reported. When heated to decomposition it emits toxic fumes of NO_x.

BJK500   CAS: 137-30-4
BIS(DIMETHYLDITHIOCARBAMATO) ZINC
mf: $C_6H_{12}N_2S_4 \cdot Zn$ mw: 305.81

PROP: White powder. Mp: 248-250°; d: 1.65 @ 20°/20°.

SYNS: AAPROTECT ◇ AAVOLEX ◇ AAZIRA ◇ ACCELER-ATOR L ◇ ACETO ZDED ◇ ACETO ZDMD ◇ ALCOBAM ZM ◇ AMYL ZIMATE ◇ ANTENE ◇ BIS(DIMETHYLCAR-BAMODITHIOATO-S,S')ZINC ◇ BIS(DIMETHYLDITHIOCAR-BAMATE de ZINC) (FRENCH) ◇ BIS(N,N-DIMETIL-DITIO-CARBAMMATO) DI ZINCO (ITALIAN) ◇ CARBAMIC ACID, DIMETHYLDITHIO-, ZINC SALT (2:) ◇ CARBAZINC ◇ CIRAM ◇ CORONA COROZATE ◇ COROZATE ◇ CUMAN ◇ CUMAN L ◇ CYMATE ◇ DIMETHYLCARBAM-ODITHIOIC ACID, ZINC COMPLEX ◇ DIMETHYLCARBAMO-DITHIOIC ACID, ZINC SALT ◇ DIMETHYLDITHIOCAR-BAMATE ZINC SALT ◇ DIMETHYLDITHIOCARBAMIC ACID, ZINC SALT ◇ DRUPINA 90 ◇ EPTAC 1 ◇ ENT 988 ◇ FUCLASIN ◇ FUCLASIN ULTRA ◇ FUKLASIN ◇ FUNGOSTOP ◇ HERMAT ZDM ◇ HEXAZIR ◇ KARBAM WHITE ◇ METHASAN ◇ METHAZATE ◇ METHYL ZIMATE ◇ METHYL ZINEB ◇ METHYL ZIRAM ◇ MEXENE ◇ MEZENE ◇ MILBAM ◇ MILBAN ◇ MOLURAME ◇ MYCRONIL ◇ NCI-C50442 ◇ ORCHARD BRAND ZIRAM ◇ POMARSOL Z FORTE ◇ PRODARAM ◇ RHODIACID ◇ SOXINAL PZ ◇ SOXINOL PZ ◇ TRICARBAMIX Z ◇ TSIMAT ◇ TSIRAM (RUSSIAN) ◇ USAF P-2 ◇ VANCIDE MZ-96 ◇ VULCACURE ◇ VULKACITE L ◇ Z 75 ◇ ZARLATE

◇ Z-C SPRAY ◇ ZERLATE ◇ ZIMATE ◇ ZIMATE METHYL ◇ ZINC BIS(DIMETHYLDITHIOCARBAMATE) ◇ ZINC BIS(DIMETHYLDITHIOCARBAMOYL)DISULPHIDE ◇ ZINC BIS(DIMETHYLTHIOCARBAMOYL)DISULFIDE ◇ ZINC DIMETHYLDITHIOCARBAMATE ◇ ZINC N,N-DI-METHYLDITHIOCARBAMATE ◇ ZINCMATE ◇ ZINK-BIS (N,N-DIMETHYL-DITHIOCARBAMAAT) (DUTCH) ◇ ZINK-BIS(N,N-DIMETHYL-DITHIOCARBAMAT) (GER-MAN) ◇ ZINKCARBAMATE ◇ ZINK-(N,N-DIMETHYL-DI-THIOCARBAMAT) (GERMAN) ◇ ZIRAM ◇ ZIRAM TECHNI-CAL ◇ ZIRAMVIS ◇ ZIRASAN ◇ ZIRBERK ◇ ZIREX 90 ◇ ZIRIDE ◇ ZIRTHANE ◇ ZITOX

TOXICITY DATA with REFERENCE

CAR: orl-rat TD:13160 mg/kg/94W-I   VPITAR 29,71,70

CAR: orl-rat TD:25956 mg/kg/2Y-I   NTPTR* NTP-TR-238,82

CAR: orl-rat TDLo:12978 mg/kg/2Y-I   NTPTR* NTP-TR-238,82

ETA: imp-rat TDLo:60 mg/kg   VPITAR 29,71,70

ETA: orl-mus TDLo:840 mg/kg/13W-I   GISAAA 37(9),25,72

MUT: cyt-hmn:lym 10 nmol/L   TXCYAC 4,331,75

MUT: dnd-esc 1 μmol/L   ARTODN 46,277,80

MUT: mma-sat 5 μg/plate   MUREAV 68,313,79

MUT: mmo-sat 5 μg/plate   MUREAV 68,313,79

MUT: mrc-bcs 600 ng/disc/24H   MUREAV 40,19,76

CONSENSUS REPORTS: IARC Cancer Review: Animal Inadequate Evidence IMEMDT 12,259,76; NTP Carcinogenesis Bioassay (feed); Clear Evidence: mouse, rat NTPTR* NTP-TR-238,83. EPA Genetic Toxicology Program. Reported in EPA TSCA Inventory. Zinc and its compounds are on the Community Right-To-Know List.

SAFETY PROFILE: Questionable carcinogen with experimental carcinogenic and tumorigenic data. Poison by ingestion, intraperitoneal, and intravenous routes. Moderately toxic by inhalation. Mutation data reported. Severe irritant to eyes, nose, and throat. When heated to decomposition it emits very toxic fumes of NO_x and SO_x.

BJL600   CAS: 97-74-5
BIS(DIMETHYLTHIOCARBAMOYL) SULFIDE

mf: $C_6H_{12}N_2S_3$ mw: 208.38

SYNS: ACETO TMTM ◇ BIS(DIMETHYLTHIOCARBAM-YL) MONOSULFIDE ◇ CARBAMIC ACID, DIMETHYLDI-THIO-, ANHYDROSULFIDE ◇ MONEX ◇ MONO-THIURAD ◇ MONOTHIURAM ◇ PENNAC MS ◇ TETRAMETHYLTHI-URAMMONIUM SULFIDE ◇ TETRAMETHYLTHIURAM MONOSULFIDE ◇ TETRAMETHYLTHIURAMONOSUL-FIDE ◇ TETRAMETHYLTHIURAM SULFIDE ◇ TETRA-METHYLTRITHIO CARBAMIC ANHYDRIDE ◇ 1,1'-THIO-BIS(N,N-DIMETHYLTHIO)FORMAMIDE ◇ THIONEX ◇ THIONEX RUBBER ACCELERATOR ◇ TMTM ◇ TMTMS ◇ UNADS ◇ USAF B-32 ◇ USAF EK-P-6255 ◇ VULKACIT THIURAM MS/C

TOXICITY DATA with REFERENCE

ETA: scu-mus TDLo:100 mg/kg   NTIS** PB223-159

MUT: mma-sat 5 μg/plate   MUREAV 68,313,79

MUT: mmo-sat 100 μg/plate   MUREAV 68,313,79

MUT: mnt-ham-ipr 250 mg/kg   SWEHDO 9(Suppl 2),27,83

MUT: sce-ham:ovr 100 nmol/L   SWEHDO 9(Suppl 2),27,83

CONSENSUS REPORTS: Reported in EPA TSCA Inventory.

SAFETY PROFILE: Questionable carcinogen with experimental tumorigenic data. Poison by ingestion and intraperitoneal routes. Mutation data reported. Experimental reproductive effects. When heated to decomposition it emits very toxic fumes of NO_x and SO_x.

BJN250   CAS: 2386-90-5
BIS(2,3-EPOXYCYCLOPENTYL) ETHER

mf: $C_{10}H_{14}O_3$ mw: 182.24

SYNS: EP-205 ◇ ERR 4205 ◇ 2,2'-OXYBIS-6-OXABICY-CLO-(3.1.0)HEXANE

TOXICITY DATA with REFERENCE

CAR: skn-mus TDLo:156 g/kg/2Y-I   NTIS** ORNL-5375

NEO: skn-mus TD:312 g/kg/2Y-I   CNREA8 39,1718,79

ETA: skn-mus TD:395 g/kg/132W-I   NTIS** ORNL-5762

MUT: mma-sat 5700 μg/plate   CIHPDR 6,210,84

MUT: mmo-sat 5700 μg/plate   CIHPDR 6,210,84

MUT: mnt-mus-orl 1 g/kg   CIHPDR 6,210,84

MUT: sce-hmn:lym 50 mg/L   CIHPDR 6,210,84

CONSENSUS REPORTS: EPA Genetic Toxicology Program. Reported in EPA TSCA Inventory.

SAFETY PROFILE: Questionable carcinogen with experimental carcinogenic and neoplastigenic data. A systemic irritant by skin contact and ingestion. When heated to decomposition it emits acrid smoke and irritating fumes.

BJN850   CAS: 63951-08-6
N,N-BIS(2-(2,3-EPOXYPROPOXY)ETHOXY)ANILINE
mf: $C_{16}H_{23}NO_6$ mw: 325.40

SYNS: ANILINE, N,N-BIS(2-(2,3-EPOXYPROPOXY) ETHOXY)- ◇ DIGLYCIDYL ETHER of N,N-BIS(2-HYDROXY-ETHOXYETHYL)ANILINE

TOXICITY DATA with REFERENCE
ETA: scu-mus TDLo: 5600 mg/kg/60W-I
FCTXAV 4,365,66

SAFETY PROFILE: Questionable carcinogen with experimental tumorigenic data. When heated to decomposition it emits toxic fumes of NO_x.

BJN875   CAS: 7329-29-5
N,N-BIS(2-(2,3-EPOXYPROPOXY)ETHYL)ANILINE
mf: $C_{16}H_{23}NO_4$ mw: 293.40

SYNS: ANILINE, N,N-BIS(2-(2,3-EPOXYPROPOXY) ETHYL)- ◇ DIGLYCIDYL ETHER of PHENYLDIETHANOL-AMINE

TOXICITY DATA with REFERENCE
ETA: scu-mus TD: 22 g/kg/39W-I   FCTXAV 4,365,66
ETA: scu-rat TDLo: 2820 mg/kg/43W-I
BECCAN 42,37,64

SAFETY PROFILE: Questionable carcinogen with experimental tumorigenic data. When heated to decomposition it emits toxic fumes of NO_x.

BJO250   CAS: 67856-66-0
BIS(2-ETHOXYETHYL)NITROSOAMINE
mf: $C_8H_{18}N_2O$ mw: 158.28

SYN: N-NITROSOBIS(2-ETHOXYETHYL)AMINE

TOXICITY DATA with REFERENCE
ETA: orl-rat TDLo: 3250 mg/kg/50W-I   CNREA8 38,2391,78
MUT: mma-sat 50 μg/plate   MUREAV 66,1,79

SAFETY PROFILE: Questionable carcinogen with experimental tumorigenic data. Mutation data reported. When heated to decomposition it emits highly toxic fumes of NO_x.

BJP000   CAS: 122-34-9
2,4-BIS(ETHYLAMINO)-6-CHLORO-s-TRIAZINE
mf: $C_7H_{12}ClN_5$ mw: 201.69

SYNS: A 2079 ◇ AKTINIT S ◇ AQUAZINE ◇ BATAZINA ◇ 2,4-BIS(AETHYLAMINO)-6-CHLOR-1,3,5-TRIAZIN (GERMAN) ◇ BITEMOL ◇ BITEMOL S 50 ◇ CAT (HERBICIDE) ◇ CDT ◇ CEKUSAN ◇ CEKUZINA-S ◇ CET ◇ 1-CHLORO-3,5-BISETHYLAMINO-2,4,6-TRIAZINE ◇ 2-CHLORO-4,6-BIS(ETHYLAMINO)-s-TRIAZINE ◇ 2-CHLORO-4,6-BIS (ETHYLAMINO)-1,3,5-TRIAZINE ◇ FRAMED ◇ G 27692 ◇ GEIGY 27,692 ◇ GESARAN ◇ GESATOP ◇ GESATOP 50 ◇ H 1803 ◇ HERBAZIN ◇ HERBAZIN 50 ◇ HERBEX ◇ HERBOXY ◇ HUNGAZIN DT ◇ PREMAZINE ◇ PRIMATOL S ◇ PRINCEP ◇ PRINTOP ◇ RADOCON ◇ RADOKOR ◇ SIMADEX ◇ SIMANEX ◇ SIMAZIN ◇ SIMAZINE (USDA) ◇ SIMAZINE 80W ◇ SYMAZINE ◇ TAFAZINE ◇ TAFAZINE 50-W ◇ TAPHAZINE ◇ TRIAZINE A 384 ◇ W 6658 ◇ ZEAPUR

TOXICITY DATA with REFERENCE
ETA: scu-mus TDLo: 35 g/kg/87W-I   VOONAW 16(1),82,70
ETA: scu-rat TDLo: 16 g/kg/61W-I   VOONAW 16(1),82,70
MUT: dlt-dmg-orl 6000 ppm   JTEHD6 3,691,77
MUT: dlt-dmg-par 396 μmol/L   JTEHD6 3,691,77
MUT: msc-mus: lym 400 mg/L   NTIS** PB84-138973
MUT: sln-dmg-orl 2000 ppm   JPFCD2 15,867,80
MUT: sln-dmg-par 396 μmol/L   JTEHD6 3,691,77

CONSENSUS REPORTS: EPA Genetic Toxicology Program. Reported in EPA TSCA Inventory.

SAFETY PROFILE: Questionable carcinogen with experimental tumorigenic data. Poison by intravenous route. Mutation data reported. A skin and eye irritant. When heated to decomposition it emits very toxic fumes of Cl^- and NO_x.

BJP899   CAS: 19218-16-7
1,3-BIS(ETHYLENIMINOSULFONYL)PROPANE
mf: $C_7H_{14}N_2O_4S_2$ mw: 254.35

SYNS: BEP ◇ omega,omega'-BIS-(ETHYLENEIMINOSUL-PHONYL)PROPANE ◇ 1,3,-DI(ETHYLENESULPHAMOYL)PROPANE

TOXICITY DATA with REFERENCE
NEO: scu-rat TDLo: 80 mg/kg/I   ANYAA9 68,750,58
MUT: cyt-rat-ipr 4 mg/kg   BJPCAL 6,357,51
MUT: oms-rat-ipr 4 mg/kg   BJPCAL 6,357,51

SAFETY PROFILE: Questionable carcinogen with experimental neoplastigenic data. When heated to decomposition it emits very toxic fumes of SO_x and NO_x.

BJT750 CAS: 76-20-0
2,2-BIS(ETHYLSULFONYL)BUTANE
mf: $C_8H_{18}O_4S_2$ mw: 242.38

SYNS: DIETHYLSULFONMETHYLETHYLMETHANE
◇ ETHYLSULFONAL ◇ METHYLSULFONAL ◇ METHYL-
SULPHONAL ◇ SULFONETHYLMETHANE ◇ TIONAL
◇ TRIONAL

TOXICITY DATA with REFERENCE
ETA: skn-mus TDLo: 1900 mg/kg/1W-I BJCAAI
9,177,55

SAFETY PROFILE: Questionable carcinogen
with experimental tumorigenic data. When
heated to decomposition it emits toxic fumes
of SO_x.

BJW250 CAS: 20929-99-1
**1,1-BIS(4-FLUOROPHENYL)-2-
PROPYNYL-N-
CYCLOHEPTYLCARBAMATE**
mf: $C_{23}H_{23}F_2NO_2$ mw: 383.47

SYN: CYCLOHEPTANECARBAMIC ACID-1,1-BIS(p-FLUO-
ROPHENYL)-2-PROPYNYL ESTER

TOXICITY DATA with REFERENCE
CAR: orl-rat TDLo: 620 mg/kg/13W-C CNREA8
30,2881,70

SAFETY PROFILE: Questionable carcinogen
with experimental carcinogenic data. Poison by
ingestion and intraperitoneal routes. When
heated to decomposition it emits very toxic
fumes of F^- and NO_x.

BJW500 CAS: 20930-00-1
**1,1-BIS(4-FLUOROPHENYL)-2-
PROPYNYL-N-CYCLOOCTYL
CARBAMATE**
mf: $C_{24}H_{25}F_2NO_2$ mw: 397.50

SYN: CYCLOOCTANECARBAMIC ACID-1,1-BIS(p-FLUO-
ROPHENYL)-2-PROPYNYL ESTER

TOXICITY DATA with REFERENCE
CAR: orl-rat TDLo: 1900 mg/kg/66D-C
CNREA8 30,2881,70·

SAFETY PROFILE: Questionable carcinogen
with experimental carcinogenic data. Moderately toxic by intraperitoneal route. When heated
to decomposition it emits very toxic fumes of
F^- and NO_x.

BKB750 CAS: 5055-20-9
**4-BIS(2-HYDROXYETHYL)AMINO-2-(5-
NITRO-2-FURYL)QUINAZOLINE**
mf: $C_{16}H_{16}N_4O_5$ mw: 344.36

TOXICITY DATA with REFERENCE
CAR: orl-rat TDLo: 8437 mg/kg/22W-C
JNCIAM 57,277,76

SAFETY PROFILE: Questionable carcinogen
with experimental carcinogenic data. When
heated to decomposition it emits toxic fumes
of NO_x.

BKC250 CAS: 33372-39-3
**4-BIS(2-HYDROXYETHYL)AMINO-2-(5-
NITRO-2-THIENYL)QUINAZOLINE**
mf: $C_{16}H_{16}N_4O_4S$ mw: 360.42

TOXICITY DATA with REFERENCE
CAR: orl-rat TDLo: 3800 mg/kg/15W-C
JNCIAM 57,277,76
MUT: mma-sat 1250 μg/plate CNREA8
35,3611,75

CONSENSUS REPORTS: EPA Genetic Toxicology Program.

SAFETY PROFILE: Questionable carcinogen
with experimental carcinogenic data. Mutation
data reported. When heated to decomposition
it emits very toxic fumes of NO_x and SO_x.

BKM500 CAS: 1187-00-4
**BIS(METHANE SULFONYL)-d-
MANNITOL**
mf: $C_8H_{18}O_{10}S_2$ mw: 338.38

SYNS: 1,6-BIS-o-METHYLSULFONYL-d-MANNITOL
◇ CB 2511 ◇ 1,6-DIMESYL-d-MANNITOL ◇ 1,6-DIMETH-
ANESULFONATE-d-MANNITOL ◇ 1,6-DIMETHANE-SULFO-
NOXY-d-MANNITOL ◇ 1,6-DIMETHANESULPHONOXY-1,6-
DIDEOXY-d-MANNITOL ◇ DMM ◇ d-MANNITOL BUSUL-
FAN ◇ MANNITOL MYLERAN ◇ MANNOGRANOL
◇ MM ◇ NSC-37538

TOXICITY DATA with REFERENCE
NEO: ipr-mus TDLo: 1000 mg/kg/4W JNCIAM
36,915,66
MUT: sln-dmg-unk 160 mmol/L ANYAA9
160,228,69

CONSENSUS REPORTS: EPA Genetic Toxicology Program.

SAFETY PROFILE: Questionable carcinogen
with experimental neoplastigenic data. Poison
by intravenous route. Moderately toxic by intraperitoneal route. Mildly toxic by ingestion. Mutation data reported. When heated to decomposition it emits toxic fumes of SO_x.

BKM750 CAS: 7306-46-9
3,4-BIS(METHOXY)BENZYL CHLORIDE
mf: $C_9H_{11}ClO_2$ mw: 186.65

SYNS: 3,4-DIMETHOXYBENZYL CHLORIDE ◇ VERA-
TRYL CHLORID (GERMAN) ◇ VERATRYL CHLORIDE

TOXICITY DATA with REFERENCE
ETA: scu-rat TDLo: 2100 mg/kg/42W-I   ZEKBAI
74,241,70

SAFETY PROFILE: Questionable carcinogen
with experimental tumorigenic data. Moderately
toxic by subcutaneous route. Mildly toxic by
ingestion. When heated to decomposition it
emits toxic fumes of Cl^-.

BKO000   CAS: 67856-65-9
**BIS(2-METHOXYETHYL)
NITROSOAMINE**
mf: $C_6H_{14}N_2O_3$ mw: 162.22

SYN: N-NITROSOBIS(2-METHOXYETHYL)AMINE

TOXICITY DATA with REFERENCE
ETA: orl-rat TDLo: 2750 mg/kg/50W-I   CNREA8
38,2391,78

SAFETY PROFILE: Questionable carcinogen
with experimental tumorigenic data. When
heated to decomposition it emits toxic fumes
of NO_x.

BKW000   CAS: 21260-46-8
**BISMUTH DIMETHYL
DITHIOCARBAMATE**
mf: $C_9H_{18}N_3S_6 \cdot Bi$ mw: 569.64

SYNS: BISMATE ◇ TRIS(DIMETHYLDITHIOCAR-
BAMATO)BISMUTH

TOXICITY DATA with REFERENCE
ETA: scu-mus TDLo: 1000 mg/kg   NTIS**
PB223-159

CONSENSUS REPORTS: Reported in EPA
TSCA Inventory.

SAFETY PROFILE: Questionable carcinogen
with experimental tumorigenic data. When
heated to decomposition it emits very toxic
fumes of SO_x and NO_x.

BLC250   CAS: 10380-28-6
BIS(8-OXYQUINOLINE)COPPER
mf: $C_{18}H_{12}CuN_2O_2$ mw: 351.86

PROP: Yellow-green powder.

SYNS: BIOQUIN ◇ BIOQUIN 1 ◇ BIS(8-QUINOLINATO)
COPPER ◇ BIS(8-QUINOLINOLATO)COPPER ◇ BIS(8-QUI-
NOLINOLATO-N(¹),O(⁸))-COPPER ◇ CELLU-QUIN

◇ COPPER-8 ◇ COPPER HYDROXYQUINOLATE ◇ COPPER-
8-HYDROXYQUINOLATE ◇ COPPER-8-HYDROXYQUINOLI-
NATE ◇ COPPER-8-HYDROXYQUINOLINE ◇ COPPER OXI-
NATE ◇ COPPER (2+) OXINATE ◇ COPPER OXINE
◇ COPPER OXYQUINOLATE ◇ COPPER OXYQUINOLINE
◇ COPPER QUINOLATE ◇ COPPER-8-QUINOLATE
◇ COPPER-8-QUINOLINOL ◇ COPPER QUINOLINOLATE
◇ COPPER-8-QUINOLINOLATE ◇ CUNILATE ◇ CUNILATE
2472 ◇ CUPRIC-8-HYDROXYQUINOLATE ◇ CUPRIC-8-QUI-
NOLINOLATE ◇ DOKIRIN ◇ FRUITDO ◇ 8-HYDROXYQUI-
NOLINE COPPER COMPLEX ◇ MILMER ◇ OXIME COPPER
◇ OXINE COPPER ◇ OXINE CUIVRE ◇ OXYQUINOLINO-
LEATE de CUIVRE (FRENCH) ◇ QUINONDO

TOXICITY DATA with REFERENCE
ETA: scu-mus TDLo: 156 mg/kg/39W-I
JNCIAM 24,109,60
MUT: mma-sat 5 μg/plate   MUREAV
116,185,83

CONSENSUS REPORTS: IARC Cancer Review: Animal Inadequate Evidence IMEMDT
15,103,77. Reported in EPA TSCA Inventory.
Copper and its compounds are on the Community Right-To-Know List.

SAFETY PROFILE: Questionable carcinogen
with experimental tumorigenic data. Poison by
intraperitoneal route. Mutation data reported.
When heated to decomposition it emits toxic
fumes of NO_x.

BLD750   CAS: 1675-54-3
BISPHENOL A DIGLYCIDYL ETHER
mf: $C_{21}H_{24}O_4$ mw: 340.45

SYNS: 2,2-BIS(4-(2,3-EPOXYPROPYLOXY)PHENYL)PRO-
PANE ◇ BIS(4-GLYCIDYLOXYPHENYL)DIMETHYAMETH-
ANE ◇ 2,2-BIS(p-GLYCIDYLOXYPHENYL)PROPANE ◇ BIS
(4-HYDROXYPHENYL)DIMETHYLMETHANE DIGLYCIDYL
ETHER ◇ 2,2-BIS(4-HYDROXYPHENYL)PROPANE,
DIGLYCIDYL ETHER ◇ 2,2-BIS(p-HYDROXYPHENYL)PRO-
PANE, DIGLYCIDYL ETHER ◇ D.E.R. 332 ◇ DIGLYC-
IDYL BISPHENOL A ETHER ◇ DIGLYCIDYL ETHER of
2,2-BIS(p-HYDROXYPHENYL)PROPANE ◇ DIGLYCIDYL
ETHER of 2,2-BIS(4-HYDROXYPHENYL)PROPANE ◇ DI-
GLYCIDYL ETHER of BISPHENOL A ◇ DIGLYCIDYL
ETHER of 4,4'-ISOPROPYLIDENEDIPHENOL ◇ 4,4'-
DIHYDROXYDIPHENYLDIMETHYLMETHANE DIGLYCI-
DYL ETHER ◇ p,p'-DIHYDROXYDIPHENYLDIMETHYL-
METHANE DIGLYCIDYL ETHER ◇ EPI-REZ 508 ◇ EPI-
REZ 510 ◇ EPON 828 ◇ EPOXIDE A ◇ ERL-2774 ◇ 4,4'-
ISOPROPYLIDENEDIPHENOL DIGLYCIDYL ETHER
◇ 2,2'-((1-METHYLETHYLIDENE)BIS(4,1-
PHENYLENEOXYMETHYLENE))BISOXIRANE

TOXICITY DATA with REFERENCE
CAR: skn-mus TD:312 g/kg/2Y-I CNREA8
   39,1718,79
CAR: skn-mus TDLo:312 g/kg/2Y-I NTIS**
   ORNL-5375
ETA: skn-mus TD:16480 mg/kg/2Y-I FCTOD7
   23,1081,85
MUT: dnd-esc 1 μmol/L ARTODN 46,277,80
MUT: mma-sat 50 μg/plate MUREAV 66,367,79
MUT: mmo-esc 20 μmol/L ARTODN 46,277,80
MUT: mmo-sat 50 μg/plate MUREAV 66,367,79

CONSENSUS REPORTS: EPA Genetic Toxicology Program. Reported in EPA TSCA Inventory.

SAFETY PROFILE: Questionable carcinogen with experimental carcinogenic and tumorigenic data. Poison by skin contact. Mildly toxic by ingestion. Mutation data reported. A skin and severe eye irritant. When heated to decomposition it emits acrid and irritating fumes.

BLE000
BISPHENOL DIGLYCIDYL ETHER, MODIFIED

TOXICITY DATA with REFERENCE
ETA: skn-mus TD:1200 g/kg/2Y-I AIHAAP
   24,305,63
ETA: skn-mus TDLo:470 g/kg/39W-I AIHAAP
   24,305,63

SAFETY PROFILE: Questionable carcinogen with experimental tumorigenic data.

BLE500   CAS: 74-31-7
1,4-BIS(PHENYL AMINO)BENZENE
mf: $C_{18}H_{16}N_2$ mw: 260.36

PROP: A solid. D: 1.20, vap d: 9.0.

SYNS: AGERITE ◇ AGERITEDPPD ◇ N,N′-DIFENYL-p-FENYLENDIAMIN (CZECH) ◇ N,N′-DIPHENYL-p-PHENYLENEDIAMINE ◇ DIPHENYL-p-PHENYLENEDIAMINE ◇ DPPD ◇ FLEXAMINE G ◇ JZF ◇ NONOX DPPD ◇ p-PHENYLAMINODIPHENYLAMINE ◇ 4-PHENYLAMINODIPHENYLAMINE ◇ USAF GY-2

TOXICITY DATA with REFERENCE
ETA: scu-mus TDLo:1000 mg/kg NTIS**
   PB223-159
MUT: mma-sat 10 μg/plate PCBRD2 141,407,84
MUT: msc-ham:lng 30 mg/L SWEHDO 9(Suppl 2),27,83

CONSENSUS REPORTS: Reported in EPA TSCA Inventory.

SAFETY PROFILE: Questionable carcinogen with experimental tumorigenic and teratogenic data. Poison by intraperitoneal route. Moderately toxic by ingestion. A weak allergen. Other experimental reproductive effects. Mutation data reported. An eye irritant. Combustible when exposed to heat or flame; can react with oxidizing materials. When heated to decomposition it emits toxic fumes of NO_x.

BLJ250   CAS: 142-46-1
BIS(THIOUREA)
mf: $C_2H_6N_4S_2$ mw: 150.24

SYNS: BISTHIOCARBAMYL HYDRAZINE ◇ 2,5-DITHIOBIUREA ◇ 1,2-HYDRAZINEDICARBOTHIOAMIDE ◇ NCI-C03009 ◇ USAF B-44 ◇ USAF EK-P-6281

TOXICITY DATA with REFERENCE
ETA: orl-mus TD:1310 g/kg/78W-C NCITR*
   NCI-CG-TR-132,79
ETA: orl-mus TDLo:655 g/kg/78W-C NCITR*
   NCI-CG-TR-132,79

CONSENSUS REPORTS: NCI Carcinogenesis Bioassay (feed); No Evidence: mouse, rat NCITR* NCI-CG-TR-132,79. Reported in EPA TSCA Inventory.

SAFETY PROFILE: Questionable carcinogen with experimental tumorigenic data. Poison by intraperitoneal route. When heated to decomposition it emits very toxic fumes of NO_x and SO_x.

BLQ600
2,3-BISTRIMETHYLACETOXYMETHYL-1-METHYLPYRROLE
mf: $C_{17}H_{27}NO_4$ mw: 309.45

TOXICITY DATA with REFERENCE
CAR: skn-mus TDLo:291 mg/kg/47W-I CALEDQ 17,61,82

SAFETY PROFILE: Questionable carcinogen with experimental carcinogenic data. When heated to decomposition it emits toxic fumes of NO_x.

BLY780   CAS: 9041-93-4
BLEOMYCIN SULFATE

SYNS: BLENOXANE ◇ BLEXANE

TOXICITY DATA with REFERENCE
CAR: par-rat TD:36 mg/kg/52W-I PAACA3
   24,96,83

CAR: par-rat TDLo: 18 mg/kg/52W-I   PAACA3 24,96,83

CAR: scu-rat TDLo: 14 mg/kg/68W-I   ONCOBS 41,114,84

MUT: cyt-ham: ovr 10 mg/L   MUREAV 93,149,82

MUT: dlt-oin-orl 110 ppm   MUREAV 149,375,85

MUT: dnd-ham: ovr 10 mg/L   MUREAV 93,149,82

MUT: dnr-esc 20 μmol/L   MUREAV 164,19,86

MUT: hma-mus/esc 10 mg/kg   MUREAV 164,19,86

CONSENSUS REPORTS: IARC Cancer Review: Human Inadequate Evidence IMEMDT 26,97,81. EPA Genetic Toxicology Program.

SAFETY PROFILE: Questionable carcinogen with experimental carcinogenic data. Poison by subcutaneous and intraperitoneal routes. Mutation data reported. When heated to decomposition it emits toxic fumes of SO_x.

BMK500   CAS: 774-64-1
BOVOLIDE
mf: $C_{11}H_{16}O_2$ mw: 180.27

TOXICITY DATA with REFERENCE

NEO: scu-rat TDLo: 2600 mg/kg/65W-I   BJCAAI 19,392,65

SAFETY PROFILE: Questionable carcinogen with experimental neoplastigenic data. It is found in butter made from cow's milk and many other places. When heated to decomposition it emits acrid smoke and irritating fumes.

BMK620   CAS: 63323-31-9
(+)-BP-7-β,8-α-DIOL-9-α,10-α-EPOXIDE 2
mf: $C_{20}H_{14}O_3$ mw: 302.34

SYNS: (+)-trans-7-β,8-α-DIHYDROXY-9-α,10-α-EPOXY-7,8,9,10-TETRAHDYROBENZO(a)PYRENE ◇ (+)-E-7,8,9,10-TETRAHYDRO-7-α,8-β-DIHYDROXY-9-β,19-β-EPOXY-BENZO(a)PYRENE

TOXICITY DATA with REFERENCE

NEO: skn-mus TDLo: 1200 μg/kg   CNREA8 39,67,79

MUT: mmo-sat 100 pmol/plate   BBRCA977,1389,77

MUT: msc-ham: lng 300 nmol/L   BBRCA9 77,1389,77

SAFETY PROFILE: Questionable carcinogen with experimental neoplastigenic data by skin contact. Mutation data reported. When heated to decomposition it emits acrid smoke and fumes.

BMK630
B(a)P EPOXIDE II
mf: $C_{20}H_{14}O_3$ mw: 302.34

SYN: anti-(±)-7-β,8-α-DIHYDROXY-9-α,10-α-EPOXY-7,-8,9,10-TETRAHYDROBENZO(a)PYRENE

TOXICITY DATA with REFERENCE

NEO: skn-mus TDLo: 4830 μg/kg   CCSUDL 3,371,78

ETA: scu-mus TDLo: 11 mg/kg   JJIND8 64,617,80

MUT: dnd-hmn: fbr 1500 nmol/L/15M-C   CBINA8 38,261,82

MUT: dnd-hmn: lng 2700 nmol/L   CNREA8 38,2118,78

MUT: dnd-hmn: lym 5 μmol/L   PAACA3 24,70,83

MUT: dnd-mus: emb 1800 μg/L   SCIEAS 209,297,80

MUT: dnd-rat: lvr 50 μg/L   CRNGDP 4,189,83

MUT: dni-hmn: lng 2700 nmol/L   CNREA8 38,2118,78

MUT: dni-mky: kdy 166 nmol/L   CRNGDP 3,473,82

MUT: dnr-hmn: fbr 1 μmol/L   CBINA8 20,279,78

MUT: dns-hmn: oth 10 μmol/L   JJIND8 69,557,82

MUT: msc-hmn: fbr 50 nmol/L   MUREAV 94,435,82

MUT: msc-mus: fbr 1200 μg/L   CRNGDP 1,215,80

MUT: otr-mus: fbr 1200 μg/L   CRNGDP 1,215,80

CONSENSUS REPORTS: EPA Genetic Toxicology Program.

SAFETY PROFILE: Questionable carcinogen with experimental neoplastigenic and tumorigenic data by skin contact. Human mutation data reported. When heated to decomposition it emits acrid smoke and fumes.

BMK634   CAS: 75410-89-8
B(c)PH DIOL EPOXIDE-1
mf: $C_{18}H_{14}O_3$ mw: 278.32

SYNS: (±)-BENZO(c)PHENANTHRENE-3,4-DIOL-1,2-EPOXIDE-1 ◇ BENZO(c)PHENANTHRENE-3-α-4-β-DIOL,1,2,3,4-TETRAHYDRO-1-β,2-β-EPOXY-, (±)- ◇ (±)-3-α-4-β-DIHYDROXY-1-β,2-β-EPOXY-1,2,3,4-TETRAHYDROBENZO(c)PHENANTHRENE

TOXICITY DATA with REFERENCE

NEO: skn-mus TDLo: 278 μg/kg   CNREA8 46,2257,86

MUT: mmo-sat 100 pmol/plate   CNREA8 40,2876,80

MUT: msc-ham: lng 200 nmol/L   CNREA8 40,2876,80

SAFETY PROFILE: Questionable carcinogen with experimental neoplastigenic data. Mutation data reported. When heated to decomposition it emits toxic and irritating fumes.

BMK635
B(c)PH DIOL EPOXIDE-2
mf: $C_{18}H_{14}O_3$ mw: 278.32

SYN: (±)-3-α,4-β-DIHYDROXY-1-α,2-α-EPOXY-1,2,3,4-TETRAHYDROBENZ(c)PHENANTHRACENE

TOXICITY DATA with REFERENCE
NEO: ipr-mus TDLo:12 mg/kg/15D-I   CNREA8
46,2257,86
NEO: skn-mus TDLo:278 μg/kg   CNREA8
46,2257,86
MUT: mma-sat 300 pmol/plate   CRNGDP
4,1631,83
MUT: mmo-sat 100 pmol/plate   CNREA8
40,2876,80
MUT: msc-ham:lng 200 nmol/L   CNREA8
40,2876,80

SAFETY PROFILE: Questionable carcinogen with experimental neoplastigenic data. Mutation data reported. When heated to decomposition it emits toxic fumes of NO_x.

BMK750
BRACKEN FERN, CHLOROFORM FRACTION

PROP: Chloroform fraction of tannin isolated from Bracken Fern (*Pteridium aquilinum*).

TOXICITY DATA with REFERENCE
CAR: orl-rat TDLo:1000 g/kg/56W-C   JJIND8
65,131,80

SAFETY PROFILE: Questionable carcinogen with experimental carcinogenic data. Mutation data reported.

BML250
BRACKEN FERN TANNIN

SYNS: PTERIDIUM AQUILINUM TANNIN ◇ TANNIN from BRACKEN FERN

TOXICITY DATA with REFERENCE
NEO: imp-mus TDLo:50 mg/kg/1Y-C   JNCIAM
56,33,76
NEO: scu-rat TDLo:1595 mg/kg/38W-I   JJIND8
65,131,80
MUT: bfa-rat/sat 2000 g/kg/56W-C   JJIND8
65,131,80

SAFETY PROFILE: Questionable carcinogen with experimental neoplastigenic data. Poison by intraperitoneal route. Mutation data reported.

BMM500   CAS: 2580-78-1
BRILLIANT BLUE R
mf: $C_{22}H_{16}N_2O_{11}S_3 \cdot 2Na$ mw: 626.56

SYNS: CAVALITE BRILLIANT BLUE R ◇ C.I. 61200 ◇ C.I. REACTIVE BLUE 19 ◇ C.I. REACTIVE BLUE 19, DISODIUM SALT ◇ REACTIVE BLUE 19 ◇ REMALAN BRILLIANT BLUE R ◇ REMAZOL BRILLIANT BLUE R

TOXICITY DATA with REFERENCE
ETA: orl-rat TDLo:87 g/kg/2Y-I   TKORAS
3,53,67
ETA: scu-mus TDLo:47 g/kg/39W-I   TKORAS
3,53,67

CONSENSUS REPORTS: Reported in EPA TSCA Inventory.

SAFETY PROFILE: Questionable carcinogen with experimental tumorigenic data. When heated to decomposition it emits very toxic fumes of Na_2O, NO_x and SO_x.

BMO250   CAS: 15086-94-9
BROMEOSIN
mf: $C_{20}H_8Br_4O_5$ mw: 647.92

SYNS: BROMOEOSIN ◇ BROMOFLUORESCEIC ACID ◇ C.I. 45380:2 ◇ C.I. SOLVENT RED 43 ◇ D&C RED NO. 21 ◇ EOSIN ◇ EOSINE ◇ 2,4,5,7-TETRABROMO-3,6-FLUORANDIOL ◇ TETRABROMOFLUORESCEIN ◇ 2′,4′,5′,7′-TETRABROMOFLUORESCEIN

TOXICITY DATA with REFERENCE
MUT: dnr-bcs 2 mg/disc   TRENAF 27,153,76

CONSENSUS REPORTS: IARC Cancer Review: GROUP 3 IMEMDT 7,56,87, Animal Inadequate Evidence IMEMDT 15,183,77. Reported in EPA TSCA Inventory.

SAFETY PROFILE: Questionable carcinogen. Moderately toxic by subcutaneous route. Mutation data reported. Incompatible with reducing agents. When heated to decomposition it emits very toxic fumes of Br^-.

BMT300
3′-BROMO-trans-ANETHOLE
mf: $C_{10}H_{11}BrO$ mw: 227.12

SYNS: ANISOLE, p-(3-BROMOPROPENYL)-, (E)- ◇ (E)-p-(3-BROMOPROPENYL)ANISOLE

TOXICITY DATA with REFERENCE
CAR: ipr-mus TDLo:69600 μg/kg/4D-I
CNREA8 47,2275,87
MUT: mmo-sat 2 μmol/plate   CRNGDP 7,2089,86

SAFETY PROFILE: Questionable carcinogen with experimental carcinogenic data. Mutation

data reported. When heated to decomposition it emits toxic fumes of Br⁻.

BMT750   CAS: 32795-84-9
10-BROMO-1,2-BENZANTHRACENE
mf: $C_{18}H_{11}Br$ mw: 307.20

SYN: 10-BROM-1,2-BENZANTHRACEN (GERMAN)

TOXICITY DATA with REFERENCE
ETA: scu-rat TDLo: 25 mg/kg   SCPHA4 22,224,54

SAFETY PROFILE: Questionable carcinogen with experimental tumorigenic data. When heated to decomposition it emits toxic fumes of Br⁻.

BMU500   CAS: 21248-00-0
6-BROMOBENZO(a)PYRENE
mf: $C_{20}H_{11}Br$ mw: 331.22

TOXICITY DATA with REFERENCE
ETA: scu-mus TDLo: 40 mg/kg   BJCAAI
26,506,72

SAFETY PROFILE: Questionable carcinogen with experimental tumorigenic data. When heated to decomposition it emits toxic fumes of HBr.

BMX000   CAS: 60883-74-1
α-BROMO-β,β-BIS
(p-ETHOXYPHENYL)STYRENE
mf: $C_{24}H_{23}BrO_2$ mw: 423.38

SYN: α,α-DI(p-ETHOXYPHENYL)-β-BROMO-β-PHENYL-ETHYLENE

TOXICITY DATA with REFERENCE
CAR: scu-mus TDLo: 94 mg/kg/26W-I   MMJJAI
11,95,61

SAFETY PROFILE: Questionable carcinogen with experimental carcinogenic data. When heated to decomposition it emits toxic fumes of Br⁻.

BMX250   CAS: 34346-98-0
4-BROMO-7-
BROMOMETHYLBENZ(a)ANTHRACENE
mf: $C_{19}H_{12}Br_2$ mw: 400.13

TOXICITY DATA with REFERENCE
ETA: skn-mus TDLo: 16 mg/kg   EJCAAH 7,473,71

SAFETY PROFILE: Questionable carcinogen with experimental tumorigenic data. When heated to decomposition it emits toxic fumes of Br⁻.

BMX750   CAS: 78-76-2
2-BROMOBUTANE
DOT: 2339
mf: C_4H_9Br mw: 137.04

PROP: Colorless liquid, fp: $<-50°$, bp: 91.4°, flash p: 70°F, d: 1.257 @ 25°/25°.

SYNS: sec-BUTYL BROMIDE ◇ METHYLETHYLBROMO-METHANE

TOXICITY DATA with REFERENCE
NEO: ipr-mus TDLo: 3000 mg/kg/8W-I
CNREA8 35,1411,75

CONSENSUS REPORTS: EPA Genetic Toxicology Program. Reported in EPA TSCA Inventory.

DOT Classification: Flammable Liquid; Label: Flammable Liquid.

SAFETY PROFILE: Questionable carcinogen with experimental neoplastigenic data. Narcotic in high concentrations. Dangerous fire hazard when exposed to heat or flame. When heated to decomposition it emits toxic fumes of Br⁻; can react with oxidizing materials. To fight fire, use water, spray or mist, foam, CO_2, dry chemical.

BMY800   CAS: 83463-62-1
BROMOCHLOROACETONITRILE
mf: $C_2HBrClN$ mw: 154.40

SYN: BROMOCHLOROMETHYL CYANIDE

TOXICITY DATA with REFERENCE
CAR: skn-mus TDLo: 2400 mg/kg/2W-I
FAATDF 5,1065,85
MUT: dnd-hmn: lyms 2 μmol/L   NTIS**
PB84-246230
MUT: mma-sat 170 nmol/plate   FAATDF
5,1065,85
MUT: mmo-sat 1 nmol/plate   ENMUDM 5,447,83
MUT: sce-ham: ovr 4200 nmol/L   FAATDF
5,1065,85

SAFETY PROFILE: Questionable carcinogen with experimental carcinogenic data. Experimental reproductive data. Mutation data reported. When heated to decomposition it emits toxic fumes of Br⁻, Cl⁻, and NO_x.

BNB250   CAS: 25614-03-3
BROMOCRIPTINE
mf: $C_{32}H_{40}BrN_5O_5$ mw: 654.68

SYNS: BROMOCRIPTIN ◇ α-BROMOERGOCRIPTINE
◇ BROMOERGOCRYPTINE ◇ 2-BROMOERGOCRYPTINE

◇ 2-BROMO-α-ERGOKRYPTIN ◇ 2-BROMO-12'-HYDROXY-2'-(1-METHYLETHYL)-5'-α-(2-METHYLPROPYL)ERGOTAMIN-3',6',18-TRIONE ◇ CB-154

TOXICITY DATA with REFERENCE
ETA: orl-rat TDLo: 7 g/kg/2Y-C   BMJOAE
2,1605,77
MUT: dna-rat-ipr 4 mg/kg   CNREA8 36,2223,76
MUT: oms-hmn: lym 100 µmol/L   MUREAV
117,163,83

CONSENSUS REPORTS: EPA Genetic Toxicology Program.

SAFETY PROFILE: Questionable carcinogen with experimental tumorigenic data. Poison by intravenous and possibly other routes. Human teratogenic effects by an unspecified route: developmental abnormalities of the respiratory system, musculoskeletal system, urogenital system, craniofacial area and body wall. Human systemic effects by ingestion including: olfaction changes. Experimental reproductive effects. Human mutation data reported. When heated to decomposition it emits very toxic fumes such as Br⁻ and NO$_x$.

BNE600   CAS: 17576-88-4
3'-BROMO-4-DIMETHYLAMINOAZOBENZENE
mf: $C_{14}H_{14}BrN_3$ mw: 304.22

SYNS: ANILINE, p-(m-BROMOPHENYLAZO)-N,N-DIMETHYL- ◇ BENZENAMINE, 4-((3-BROMOPHENYL)AZO)-N,N-DIMETHYL-(9CI) ◇ p-(m-BROMOPHENYLAZO)-N,N-DIMETHYLANILINE

TOXICITY DATA with REFERENCE
CAR: orl-rat TDLo: 7980 mg/kg/25W-C
CBINA8 53,107,85

SAFETY PROFILE: Questionable carcinogen with experimental carcinogenic data. Low oral toxicity. When heated to decomposition it emits toxic fumes of Br⁻ and NO$_x$.

BNF300
3-BROMO-7,12-DIMETHYLBENZ(a)ANTHRACENE
mf: $C_{20}H_{15}Br$ mw: 335.26

SYN: 3-BROMO-DMBA

TOXICITY DATA with REFERENCE
ETA: skn-mus TDLo: 520 mg/kg/50W-I
CRNGDP 4,1221,83
MUT: mma-sat 5 µg/plate   CRNGDP 4,1221,83

SAFETY PROFILE: Questionable carcinogen with experimental tumorigenic data. Mutation data reported. When heated to decomposition it emits toxic fumes of Br⁻.

BNF310
4-BROMO-7,12-DIMETHYLBENZ(a)ANTHRACENE
mf: $C_{20}H_{15}Br$ mw: 335.26

SYN: 4-BROMO-DMBA

TOXICITY DATA with REFERENCE
CAR: skn-mus TDLo: 520 mg/kg/50W-I
CRNGDP 4,1221,83
MUT: mma-sat 10 µg/plate   CRNGDP 4,1221,83

SAFETY PROFILE: Questionable carcinogen with experimental carcinogenic data. Mutation data reported. When heated to decomposition it emits toxic fumes of Br⁻.

BNF315   CAS: 63018-63-3
5-BROMO-9,10-DIMETHYL-1,2-BENZANTHRACENE
mf: $C_{20}H_{15}Br$ mw: 335.26

SYN: BENZ(a)ANTHRACENE, 8-BROMO-7,12-DIMETHYL-

TOXICITY DATA with REFERENCE
ETA: scu-mus TDLo: 80 mg/kg   CNREA8
6,454,46

SAFETY PROFILE: Questionable carcinogen with experimental tumorigenic data. When heated to decomposition it emits toxic fumes of Br⁻.

BNH500   CAS: 17372-87-1
BROMOEOSINE
mf: $C_{20}H_8Br_4O_5 \cdot 2Na$ mw: 693.90

SYNS: AIZEN EOSINE GH ◇ BROMO ACID ◇ BROMOFLUORESCEIC ACID ◇ BROMO FLUORESCEIN ◇ BRONZE BROMO ◇ CERTIQUAL EOSINE ◇ C.I. 45380 ◇ D&C RED NO. 22 ◇ DISODIUM EOSIN ◇ EOSINE ◇ EOSINE SODIUM SALT ◇ EOSINE YELLOWISH ◇ EOSIN GELBLICH (GERMAN) ◇ FENAZO EOSINE XG ◇ HIDACID DIBROMO FLUORESCEIN ◇ IRGALITE BRONZE RED CL ◇ PHLOXINE TONER B ◇ PHLOX RED TONER X-1354 ◇ PURE EOSINE YY ◇ 11445 RED ◇ SODIUM EOSINATE ◇ SYMULER EOSIN TONER ◇ 2,4,5,7-TETRABROMO-9-o-CARBOXYPHENYL-6-HYDROXY-3-ISOXANTHONE, DISODIUM SALT ◇ 2,4,5,7-TETRABROMO-3,6-FLUORANDIOL ◇ TETRABROMOFLUORESCEIN ◇ 2',4',5',7'-TETRABROMOFLUORESCEIN DISODIUM SALT ◇ TETRABROMOFLUORESCEIN S ◇ TETRABROMOFLUORESCEIN SOLUBLE ◇ 2-(2,4,5,7-TET-

RABROMO-6-HYDROXY-3-OXO-3H-XANTHENE-9-YL)BEN-
ZOIC ACID, DISODIUM SALT ◇ TOYO EOSINE G
◇ 1903 YELLOW PINK

TOXICITY DATA with REFERENCE
ETA: scu-rat TDLo: 13 g/kg/1Y-I   GANNA2
47,51,56

MUT: dnr-bcs 2 mg/disc   TRENAF 27,153,76

CONSENSUS REPORTS: IARC Cancer Review: Animal Inadequate Evidence IMEMDT
15,183,77. EPA Genetic Toxicology Program.
Reported in EPA TSCA Inventory.

SAFETY PROFILE: Questionable carcinogen
with experimental tumorigenic data. Poison by
intravenous route. Moderately toxic by ingestion, subcutaneous and intraperitoneal routes.
When heated to decomposition it emits very
toxic fumes of Br^- and Na_2O.

BNI500   CAS: 540-51-2
2-BROMO ETHANOL
mf: C_2H_5BrO mw: 124.98

SYNS: BE ◇ BROMOETHANOL ◇ ETHYLENEBROMO-
HYDRIN ◇ GLYCOL BROMOHYDRIN

TOXICITY DATA with REFERENCE
NEO: ipr-mus TDLo: 150 mg/kg/8W-I   CNREA8
39,391,79

ETA: orl-mus TDLo: 43 g/kg/80W-C   JACTDZ
2(2),246,83

MUT: dnr-bcs 20 µL/disc   AEMIDF 43,177,82
MUT: dnr-esc 10 µmol/plate   EVHPAZ 21,79,77
MUT: mma-sat 10 µL/plate   EVHPAZ 21,79,77
MUT: mmo-klp 15 mmol/L   EXPEAM 25,85,69
MUT: mmo-sat 10 µL/plate   EVHPAZ 21,79,77

CONSENSUS REPORTS: EPA Genetic Toxicology Program. Reported in EPA TSCA Inventory.

SAFETY PROFILE: Questionable carcinogen
with experimental neoplastigenic and tumorigenic data. Poison by intraperitoneal route. Mutation data reported. When heated to decomposition it emits toxic fumes of Br^-.

BNK100
4'-BROMO-3'-ETHYL-4-
DIMETHYLAMINOAZOBENZENE
mf: $C_{16}H_{18}BrN_3$ mw: 332.28

SYNS: ANILINE, p-((4-BROMO-3-ETHYLPHENYL)AZO)-
N,N-DIMETHYL- ◇ BENZENAMINE, N,N-DIMETHYL-4'-
BROMO-3'-ETHYL-4-(PHENYLAZO)- ◇ p-((4-BROMO-3-
ETHYLPHENYL)AZO)-N,N-DIMETHYLANILINE

TOXICITY DATA with REFERENCE
CAR: orl-rat TDLo: 14414 mg/kg/52W-C
CBINA8 53,107,85

SAFETY PROFILE: Questionable carcinogen
with experimental carcinogenic data. When
heated to decomposition it emits toxic fumes
of Br^- and NO_x.

BNK275
p-((3-BROMO-4-ETHYLPHENYL)AZO)-
N,N-DIMETHYLANILINE
mf: $C_{16}H_{18}BrN_3$ mw: 332.28

SYNS: ANILINE, p-((3-BROMO-4-ETHYLPHENYL)AZO)-
N,N-DIMETHYL- ◇ BENZENAMINE, N,N-DIMETHYL-3'-
BROMO-4'-ETHYL-4-(PHENYLAZO)- ◇ 3'-BROMO-4'-
ETHYL-4-DIMETHYLAMINOAZOBENZENE

TOXICITY DATA with REFERENCE
CAR: orl-rat TDLo: 6930 mg/kg/25W-C
CBINA8 53,107,85

SAFETY PROFILE: Questionable carcinogen
with experimental carcinogenic data. When
heated to decomposition it emits toxic fumes
of Br^- and NO_x.

BNK700   CAS: 548-26-5
BROMOFLUORESCEIC ACID
mf: $C_{20}H_8Br_4O_5 \cdot 2Na$ mw: 693.90

SYNS: AIZEN EOSINE GH ◇ BROMO ACID ◇ BROMO B
◇ BROMOEOSINE ◇ BROMO FLUORESCEIN ◇ BRONZE
BROMO ◇ CERTIQUAL EOSINE ◇ C.I. 45380 ◇ C.I. ACID
RED 87 ◇ EOSIN ◇ EOSINE B ◇ EOSINE FA ◇ EOSINE
LAKE RED Y ◇ FENAZO EOSINE XG ◇ FLUORESCEIN, 2',
4',5',7'-TETRABROMO-, DISODIUM SALT ◇ HIDACID
BROMO ACID REGULAR ◇ HIDACID DIBROMO FLUORES-
CEIN ◇ IRGALITE BRONZE RED CL ◇ PHLOXINE RED 20-
7600

TOXICITY DATA with REFERENCE
ETA: scu-rat TDLo: 13 g/kg/1Y-I   GANNA2
47,51,56

SAFETY PROFILE: Questionable carcinogen
with experimental tumorigenic data. Moderately
toxic by subcutaneous and intravenous routes.
When heated to decomposition it emits toxic
fumes of Br^-.

BNL000   CAS: 75-25-2
BROMOFORM
DOT: 2515
mf: $CHBr_3$ mw: 252.75

PROP: Colorless liquid or hexagonal crystals.
Mp: 6-7°, bp: 149.5°, flash p: none, d: 2.890
@ 20°/4°.

SYNS: BROMOFORME (FRENCH) ◇ BROMOFORMIO (ITALIAN) ◇ METHENYL TRIBROMIDE ◇ NCI-C55130 ◇ RCRA WASTE NUMBER U225 ◇ TRIBROMMETHAAN (DUTCH) ◇ TRIBROMMETHAN (GERMAN) ◇ TRIBROMO-METAN (ITALIAN) ◇ TRIBROMOMETHANE

TOXICITY DATA with REFERENCE
NEO: ipr-mus TDLo:1100 mg/kg/8W-I
CNREA8 37,2717,77
MUT: cyt-ham:ovr 110 µg/L ENMUDM 7,1,85
MUT: mmo-sat 50 µl/plate DHEFDK FDA-78-1046,78
MUT: sce-ham:ovr 290 µg/L ENMUDM 7,1,85
MUT: sce-hmn:lym 80 µmol/L ENVRAL 32,72,83
MUT: sce-mus-orl 100 mg/kg/4D-I ENVRAL 32,72,83
MUT: sln-dmg-orl 3000 ppm ENMUDM 7,677,85

CONSENSUS REPORTS: Reported in EPA TSCA Inventory. Community Right-To-Know List.

OSHA PEL: TWA 0.5 ppm (skin) ACGIH TLV: TWA 0.5 ppm (skin) DOT Classification: Poison B; Label: St. Andrews Cross.

SAFETY PROFILE: Questionable carcinogen with experimental neoplastigenic data. A human poison by ingestion. Moderately toxic via intraperitoneal and subcutaneous routes. Human mutation data reported. A lachrymator. Inhalation of small amounts causes irritation, provoking the flow of tears and saliva, and reddening of the face. Abuse can lead to addiction and serious consequences. When heated to decomposition it emits highly toxic fumes of Br^-.

BNO500 CAS: 2417-77-8
9-BROMOMETHYLANTHRACENE
mf: $C_{15}H_{11}Br$ mw: 271.17

SYN: ICR 506

TOXICITY DATA with REFERENCE
NEO: ivn-mus TDLo:1350 µg/kg CNREA8 36,2423,76
MUT: mma-sat 10 µg/plate PNASA6 72,5135,75

CONSENSUS REPORTS: EPA Genetic Toxicology Program.

SAFETY PROFILE: Questionable carcinogen with experimental neoplastigenic data. Deadly poison by intravenous route. Mutation data reported. When heated to decomposition it emits toxic fumes of Br^-.

BNO750 CAS: 24961-39-5
7-BROMO METHYL BENZ(a)ANTHRACENE
mf: $C_{19}H_{13}Br$ mw: 321.23

SYNS: 7-BMBA ◇ ICR 498

TOXICITY DATA with REFERENCE
CAR: scu-rat TD:80 mg/kg CRNGDP 2,103,81
CAR: scu-rat TDLo:27 mg/kg CRNGDP 2,103,81
NEO: ivn-mus TDLo:800 µg/kg CNREA8 36,2423,76
ETA: skn-mus TD:10 mg/kg/40W-I CNREA8 43,2034,83
ETA: skn-mus TD:31 mg/kg/40W-I CNREA8 43,2034,83
MUT: dnd-ham:ovr 100 nmol/L SCMGDN 10,183,84
MUT: dnr-esc 1 mg/L PNASA6 79,534,82
MUT: dnr-ham:ovr 800 nmol/L PNASA6 79,534,82
MUT: dns-hmn:fbr 1 µmol/L NARHAD 7,1343,79
MUT: msc-ham:ovr 50 nmol/L PNASA6 79,534,82
MUT: sce-ham:ovr 400 nmol/L PNASA6 79,534,82

CONSENSUS REPORTS: EPA Genetic Toxicology Program.

SAFETY PROFILE: Questionable carcinogen with experimental carcinogenic, neoplastigenic, and tumorigenic data. A deadly poison by intravenous route. Human mutation data reported. When heated to decomposition it emits toxic fumes of Br^-.

BNP000 CAS: 49852-85-9
6-BROMOMETHYLBENZO(a)PYRENE
mf: $C_{21}H_{13}Br$ mw: 345.25

TOXICITY DATA with REFERENCE
ETA: scu-rat TDLo:100 mg/kg/40D-I JMCMAR 16,714,73
MUT: dnd-mam:lum 100 mg/L CBINA8 47,111,83

SAFETY PROFILE: Questionable carcinogen with experimental tumorigenic data. Mutation data reported. When heated to decomposition it emits toxic fumes of Br^-.

BNP850 CAS: 25855-92-9
9-(BROMOMETHYL)-10-CHLOROANTHRACENE
mf: $C_{15}H_{10}BrCl$ mw: 305.61

SYN: 10-BROMOMETHYL-9-CHLOROANTHRACENE

TOXICITY DATA with REFERENCE
NEO: ivn-mus TDLo: 3066 µg/kg   CNREA8
    40,782,80

SAFETY PROFILE: Questionable carcinogen
with experimental neoplastigenic data. When
heated to decomposition it emits toxic fumes
of Br⁻ and Cl⁻.

BNQ000   CAS: 34346-99-1
7-BROMOMETHYL-4-CHLOROBENZ(a)ANTHRACENE
mf: $C_{19}H_{12}BrCl$ mw: 355.67

SYN: 4-CHLORO-7-BROMOMETHYLBENZ(a)ANTHRA-
CENE

TOXICITY DATA with REFERENCE
ETA: skn-mus TDLo: 14 mg/kg   EJCAAH 7,473,71

SAFETY PROFILE: Questionable carcinogen
with experimental tumorigenic data by skin contact. When heated to decomposition it emits
very toxic fumes of Br⁻ and Cl⁻.

BNQ100
3′-BROMO-4′-METHYL-4-DIMETHYLAMINOAZOBENZENE
mf: $C_{15}H_{16}BrN_3$ mw: 318.25

SYNS: ANILINE, p-((3-BROMO-p-TOLYL)AZO)-N,N-DI-
THYL- ◇ BENZENAMINE, N,N-DIMETHYL-3′-BROMO-
4′-METHYL-4-(PHENYLAZO)- ◇ p-((3-BROMO-p-TO-
LYL)AZO)-N,N-DIMETHYLANILINE

TOXICITY DATA with REFERENCE
CAR: orl-rat TDLo: 13977 mg/kg/52W-C
    CBINA8 53,107,85

SAFETY PROFILE: Questionable carcinogen
with experimental carcinogenic data. When
heated to decomposition it emits toxic fumes
of Br⁻ and NO_x.

BNQ110
4′-BROMO-3′-METHYL-4-DIMETHYLAMINOAZOBENZENE
mf: $C_{15}H_{16}BrN_3$ mw: 318.25

SYNS: ANILINE, p-((4-BROMO-m-TOLYL)AZO)-N,N-DI-
METHYL- ◇ BENZENAMINE, N,N-DIMETHYL-4′-BROMO-3′-
METHYL-4-(PHENYLAZO)- ◇ p-((4-BROMO-m-TOLYL)AZO)-
N,N-DIMETHYLANILINE

TOXICITY DATA with REFERENCE
CAR: orl-rat TDLo: 9677 mg/kg/36W-C
    CBINA8 53,107,85

SAFETY PROFILE: Questionable carcinogen

with experimental carcinogenic data. When
heated to decomposition it emits toxic fumes
of Br⁻ and NO_x.

BNQ250   CAS: 34346-97-9
7-BROMOMETHYL-6-FLUOROBENZ(a)ANTHRACENE
mf: $C_{19}H_{12}BrF$ mw: 339.22

SYN: 6-FLUORO-7-BROMOMETHYLBENZ(a)ANTHRA-
CENE

TOXICITY DATA with REFERENCE
ETA: skn-mus TDLo: 14 mg/kg   EJCAAH 7,473,71

SAFETY PROFILE: Questionable carcinogen
with experimental tumorigenic data by skin contact. When heated to decomposition it emits
very toxic fumes of Br⁻ and F⁻.

BNQ750   CAS: 34346-96-8
7-BROMOMETHYL-1-METHYLBENZ(a)ANTHRACENE
mf: $C_{20}H_{15}Br$ mw: 335.26

SYN: 1-METHYL-7-BROMOMETHYLBENZ(a)ANTHRA-
CENE

TOXICITY DATA with REFERENCE
ETA: skn-mus TDLo: 13 mg/kg   EJCAAH 7,473,71

SAFETY PROFILE: Questionable carcinogen
with experimental tumorigenic data by skin contact. When heated to decomposition it emits
toxic fumes of Br⁻.

BNR000   CAS: 16238-56-5
7-BROMO METHYL-12-METHYLBENZ(a)ANTHRACENE
mf: $C_{20}H_{15}Br$ mw: 335.26

SYN: ICR 502

TOXICITY DATA with REFERENCE
CAR: scu-rat TD: 188 mg/kg   CRNGDP 2,103,81
CAR: scu-rat TDLo: 6 mg/kg   CRNGDP 2,103,81
NEO: ivn-mus TDLo: 1700 µg/kg   CNREA8
    36,2423,76
NEO: scu-rat TD: 13 mg/kg   EJCAAH 6,417,70
NEO: scu-rat TD: 20 mg/kg/39D-I   CNREA8
    31,1951,71
NEO: skn-mus TDLo: 8040 mg/kg   JJIND8
    61,135,78
MUT: dnd-mus: emb 500 nmol/L   CALEDQ
    7,103,79
MUT: mmo-esc 1 µg/plate   ENMUDM
    6(Suppl 2),1,84

MUT: mmo-sat 300 ng/plate   ENMUDM 6(Suppl 2),1,84

MUT: otr-mus:fbr 16 μg/L   JJIND8 67,1303,81

MUT: otr-rat:emb 270 μg/L   JJIND8 67,1303,81

CONSENSUS REPORTS: EPA Genetic Toxicology Program.

SAFETY PROFILE: Questionable carcinogen with experimental carcinogenic and neoplastigenic data. Mutation data reported. When heated to decomposition it emits toxic fumes of Br⁻.

BNR250   CAS: 59230-81-8
12-BROMOMETHYL-7-METHYLBENZ(a)ANTHRACENE
mf: $C_{20}F_{15}Br$ mw: 605.11

TOXICITY DATA with REFERENCE
NEO: skn-mus TDLo:8040 mg/kg   JJIND8 61,135,78

SAFETY PROFILE: Questionable carcinogen with experimental neoplastigenic data. When heated to decomposition it emits very toxic fumes of F⁻ and Br⁻.

BNR750   CAS: 78-77-3
1-BROMO-2-METHYL PROPANE
DOT: 2342
mf: C_4H_9Br mw: 137.04
PROP: Flash p: 22°C.
SYNS: 1-BUTYL BROMIDE ◇ i-BUTYL BROMIDE ◇ ISOBUTYL BROMIDE

TOXICITY DATA with REFERENCE
NEO: ipr-mus TDLo:3000 mg/kg/8W-I   CNREA8 35,1411,75

CONSENSUS REPORTS: EPA Genetic Toxicology Program. Reported in EPA TSCA Inventory.

DOT Classification: IMO: Flammable or Combustible Liquid; Label: Flammable Liquid.

SAFETY PROFILE: Questionable carcinogen with experimental neoplastigenic data. Moderately toxic by intraperitoneal route. A dangerous fire hazard when exposed to heat or flame. When heated to decomposition it emits toxic fumes of Br⁻.

BNT500   CAS: 14173-58-1
3-BROMO-4-NITROQUINOLINE-1-OXIDE
mf: $C_9H_5BrN_2O_3$ mw: 269.07

TOXICITY DATA with REFERENCE
ETA: scu-mus TD:120 mg/kg/50D-I   BCPCA6 16,631,67

ETA: scu-mus TDLo:60 mg/kg/I   CPBTAL 17,544,69

MUT: cyt-omi 37 μmol   GANNA2 60,155,69

SAFETY PROFILE: Questionable carcinogen with experimental tumorigenic data. Mutation data reported. When heated to decomposition it emits very toxic fumes of Br⁻ and NO$_x$.

BNU750   CAS: 106-41-2
4-BROMOPHENOL
mf: C_6H_5BrO mw: 173.02

SYN: p-BROMOPHENOL

TOXICITY DATA with REFERENCE
ETA: skn-mus TDLo:7200 mg/kg/18W-I   CNREA8 19,413,59

CONSENSUS REPORTS: Reported in EPA TSCA Inventory.

SAFETY PROFILE: Questionable carcinogen with experimental tumorigenic data. Moderately toxic by ingestion and intraperitoneal routes. When heated to decomposition it emits toxic fumes of Br⁻.

BNX125   CAS: 23139-02-8
3-(p-BROMOPHENYL)-1-METHYL-1-NITROSOUREA
mf: $C_8H_8BrN_3O_2$ mw: 258.10

SYNS: 1-METHYL-3-(p-BROMPHENYL)-1-NITROSO-HARNSTOFF (GERMAN) ◇ 1-METHYL-3-(p-BROMOPHE-NYL)-1-NITROSOUREA ◇ 1-METHYL-1-NITROSO-3-(p-BRO-MOPHENYL)UREA

TOXICITY DATA with REFERENCE
CAR: orl-rat TDLo:774 mg/kg/88W-I   ARGEAR 53,329,83

ETA: orl-rat TD:1080 mg/kg/30W-I   IAPUDO 31,685,80

MUT: cyt-ham:lng 10 μmol/L   IAPUDO 31,797,80

MUT: sce-ham:lng 10 μmol/L   IAPUDO 31,797,80

SAFETY PROFILE: Questionable carcinogen with experimental carcinogenic and tumorigenic data. Mutation data reported. When heated to decomposition it emits toxic fumes of Br⁻ and NO$_x$.

BOA750   CAS: 42461-89-2
5-(3-BROMO-1-PROPENYL)-1,3-BENZODIOXOLE
mf: $C_{10}H_9BrO_2$ mw: 241.10

SYNS: 3'-BROMOISOSAFROLE ◇ 1,2-(METHYLENEDI-OXY)-4-(3-BROMO-1-PROPENYL)BENZENE

TOXICITY DATA with REFERENCE
ETA: scu-rat TDLo: 359 mg/kg/10W-   CNREA8
33,590,73

SAFETY PROFILE: Questionable carcinogen with experimental tumorigenic data. When heated to decomposition it emits toxic fumes such as Br^-.

BOB250   CAS: 590-92-1
3-BROMOPROPIONIC ACID
mf: $C_3H_5BrO_2$ mw: 152.99

SYN: β-BROMOPROPIONIC ACID

TOXICITY DATA with REFERENCE
ETA: ipr-mus TDLo: 580 mg/kg/8W-I   CNREA8
39,391,79

MUT: mmo-sat 25 μg/plate   DHEFDK
FDA-78-1046,78

CONSENSUS REPORTS: Reported in EPA TSCA Inventory.

SAFETY PROFILE: Questionable carcinogen with experimental tumorigenic data. Moderately toxic by intraperitoneal route. Mutation data reported. When heated to decomposition it emits toxic fumes of Br^-.

BOI250   CAS: 63041-00-9
3-BROMOTRICYCLOQUINAZOLINE
mf: $C_{21}H_{11}BrN_4$ mw: 399.27

TOXICITY DATA with REFERENCE
NEO: skn-mus TDLo: 1240 mg/kg/1Y-I   BJCAAI
16,275,62

SAFETY PROFILE: Questionable carcinogen with experimental neoplastigenic data. When heated to decomposition it emits very toxic fumes of Br^- and NO_x.

BOV000   CAS: 96-48-0
4-BUTANOLIDE
mf: $C_4H_6O_2$ mw: 86.10

PROP: Colorless liquid; mild caramel odor. Mp: −44°, bp: 206°, flash p: 209°F (OC), d: 1.124 @ 25°/4°, refr index: 1.434-1.454 @ 25°, vap d: 3.0.

SYNS: γ-6480 ◇ γ-BL ◇ BLO ◇ BLON ◇ BUTYRIC ACID LACTONE ◇ γ-BUTYROLACTONE (FCC) ◇ α-BUTYROLAC-TONE ◇ BUTYRYL LACTONE ◇ 4-DEOXYTETRONIC ACID ◇ DIHYDRO-2(3H)-FURANONE ◇ FEMA No. 3291 ◇ 4-HYDROXYBUTANOIC ACID LACTONE ◇ γ-HYDROXY-BUTYRIC ACID CYCLIC ESTER ◇ 4-HYDROXYBUTYRIC

ACID γ-LACTONE ◇ γ-HYDROXYBUTYROLACTONE ◇ NCI-C55878 ◇ TETRAHYDRO-2-FURANONE

TOXICITY DATA with REFERENCE
ETA: skn-mus TDLo: 50 g/kg/42W-I   JNCIAM
31,41,63
MUT: dnd-bcs 20 μL/disc   PMRSDJ 1,175,81
MUT: otr-ham: kdy 25 mg/L   PMRSDJ 1,638,81

CONSENSUS REPORTS: IARC Cancer Review: GROUP 3 IMEMDT 7,56,87; Animal No Evidence IMEMDT 11,231,76. EPA Genetic Toxicology Program. Reported in EPA TSCA Inventory.

SAFETY PROFILE: Questionable carcinogen with experimental tumorigenic data by skin contact. Moderately toxic by ingestion, intravenous and intraperitoneal routes. Experimental reproductive effects. Mutation data reported. Less acutely toxic than β-propiolactone. Combustible when exposed to heat or flame; can react with oxidizing materials. To fight fire, use foam, alcohol foam, CO_2, dry chemical. When heated to decomposition it emits acrid and irritating fumes.

BOX750   CAS: 106-88-7
1-BUTENE OXIDE
mf: C_4H_8O mw: 72.12

PROP: Colorless liquid, sol in water, miscible with most organic solvents. D: 0.8312 @ 20°/20°, bp: 63°, flash p: 5°F, lel: 1.5%, uel: 18.3%.

SYNS: 1,2-BUTENE OXIDE ◇ 1,2-BUTYLENE OXIDE ◇ 1,2-EPOXYBUTANE ◇ NCI-C55527 ◇ PROPYL OXIRANE

TOXICITY DATA with REFERENCE
CAR: ihl-rat TCLo: 400 ppm/6H/5D/2Y-C
NTPTR* NTP-TR-329,88
MUT: dnd-esc 1 μmol/L   ARTODN 46,277,80
MUT: dnd-mam: lym 100 mmol/L   CBINA8
9,97,74
MUT: mma-ssp 1600 μmol/L   TCMUD8 3,75,83
MUT: mmo-klp mmol/L   MUREAV 89,269,81
MUT: mmo-ssp 3200 μmol/L   TCMUD8 3,75,83
MUT: otr-ham: emb 50 μg/L   JJIND8 67,1303,81
MUT: otr-rat: emb 700 mg/L   JJIND8 67,1303,81
MUT: sln-dmg-orl 5 pph   ENMUDM 7,349,85
MUT: trn-dmg-orl 5 pph   ENMUDM 7,349,85

CONSENSUS REPORTS: NTP CARCINO-GENESIS STUDIES (inhalation); Clear Evidence: rat; No Evidence: mouse NTPTR* NTP-TR-329,88. Community Right-To-Know List. EPA Genetic Toxicology Program. Reported in EPA TSCA Inventory.

SAFETY PROFILE: Questionable carcinogen with experimental carcinogenic data. Moderately toxic by ingestion and skin contact. Mildly toxic by inhalation. Experimental reproductive effects. Mutation data reported. Dangerous fire hazard when exposed to heat, flame, or powerful oxidizers. To fight fire, use dry chemical, water spray, mist or fog, alcohol foam. When heated to decomposition it emits acrid smoke and fumes.

BPC600
3-(3-BUTENYLNITROSAMINO)-1-PROPANOL
mf: $C_7H_{14}N_2O_2$ mw: 158.23

SYN: BUTENYL(3-HYDROXYPROPYL)NITROSAMINE

TOXICITY DATA with REFERENCE
CAR: scu-ham TDLo: 22800 mg/kg/76W-I
CDPRD4 4,79,81

SAFETY PROFILE: Questionable carcinogen with experimental carcinogenic data. When heated to decomposition it emits toxic fumes of NO_x.

BPD000   CAS: 54746-50-8
3-BUTENYL-(2-PROPENYL)-N-NITROSAMINE
mf: $C_7H_{12}N_2O$ mw: 140.21

SYN: N-ALLYL-N-NITROSO-3-BUTENYLAMINE

TOXICITY DATA with REFERENCE
CAR: scu-ham TDLo: 15300 mg/kg/51W-I
CDPRD4 4,79,81
MUT: mmo-sat 250 μg/plate   MUREAV 68,195,79

SAFETY PROFILE: Questionable carcinogen with experimental carcinogenic data. Mutation data reported. When heated to decomposition it emits acrid smoke and irritating fumes.

BPI300   CAS: 832-06-4
2-BUTOXYCARBONYLMETHYLENE-4-OXOTHIAZOLIDONE
mf: $C_9H_{13}NO_3S$ mw: 215.29

SYNS: ACETIC ACID, (4-OXO-2-THIAZOLIDINYLIDENE)-, BUTYL ESTER (9CI) ◇ 2-(n-BUTYLOXYCARBONYLMETH-YLENE)THIAZOLID-4-ONE ◇ ICI 43823

TOXICITY DATA with REFERENCE
ETA: orl-rat TDLo: 193 g/kg/2Y-C   EXMDA4
(145),289,68

SAFETY PROFILE: Questionable carcinogen with experimental tumorigenic data. When heated to decomposition it emits toxic fumes of NO_x and SO_x.

BPV325   CAS: 56986-35-7
N-BUTYL-N-(1-ACETOXYBUTYL)NITROSAMINE
mf: $C_{10}H_{20}N_2O_3$ mw: 216.32

SYNS: ACETIC ACID-1-(BUTYLNITROSOAMINO)BUTYL ESTER ◇ N-(α-ACETOXY)BUTYL-N-BUTYLNITROSAMINE ◇ 1-ACETOXY-N-NITROSODIBUTYLAMINE ◇ BABN ◇ 1-(BUTYLNITROSOAMINO)BUTYL ACETATE

TOXICITY DATA with REFERENCE
CAR: scu-rat TDLo: 82 mg/kg/10W-I   IAPUDO 41,619,82
ETA: scu-rat TD: 70500 μg/kg/10W-I   GANNA2 73,687,82
MUT: cyt-ham: fbr 125 mg/L/48H   MUREAV 48,337,77
MUT: cyt-ham: lng 32 mg/L   GMCRDC 27,95,81
MUT: dnr-bcs 500 nmol/plate   CNREA8 40,162,80
MUT: dns-rat: oth 10 μmol/L   CBINA8 53,99,85
MUT: mmo-esc 500 nmol/plate   CNREA8 40,162,80
MUT: mmo-sat 50 nmol/plate   CNREA8 40,162,80

CONSENSUS REPORTS: EPA Genetic Toxicology Program.

SAFETY PROFILE: Questionable carcinogen with experimental carcinogenic and tumorigenic data. Mutation data reported. When heated to decomposition it emits toxic fumes of NO_x.

BPX750   CAS: 109-73-9
n-BUTYLAMINE
DOT: 1125
mf: $C_4H_{11}N$ mw: 73.16

PROP: Liquid, ammonia-like odor. Mp: −50°, bp: 77°, flash p: 10°F (OC), 10°F (CC), d: 0.74-0.76 @ 20°/20°, autoign temp: 594°F, vap d: 2.52, lel: 1.7%, uel: 9.8%.

SYNS: 1-AMINO-BUTAAN (DUTCH) ◇ 1-AMINOBUTAN (GERMAN) ◇ 1-AMINOBUTANE ◇ 1-BUTANAMINE ◇ n-BUTILAMINA (ITALIAN) ◇ n-BUTYLAMIN (GERMAN) ◇ MONO-n-BUTYLAMINE ◇ NORVALAMINE

TOXICITY DATA with REFERENCE
ETA: ipr-mus TDLo: 800 mg/kg   BCPCA62,168,59
MUT: cyt-rat-orl 110 mg/kg   ZKKOBW 86,47,76

CONSENSUS REPORTS: Reported in EPA TSCA Inventory.

OSHA PEL: CL 5 ppm (skin)   ACGIH TLV: CL 5 ppm   DFG MAK: 5 ppm (15 mg/m^3) DOT Classification: Flammable Liquid; Label: Flammable Liquid.

SAFETY PROFILE: Questionable carcinogen with experimental tumorigenic data. Poison by ingestion, skin contact, and intravenous routes. Moderately toxic by inhalation, intraperitoneal, parenteral, and possibly other routes. A severe skin irritant. Mutation data reported. Dangerous fire hazard when exposed to heat, flame or oxidizing materials. To fight fire, use alcohol foam, CO_2, dry chemical. Explodes on contact with perchloryl fluoride. When heated to decomposition it emits toxic fumes of NO_x.

BQF750   CAS: 86166-58-7
1-(tert-BUTYLAMINO)3-(3-METHYL-2-NITROPHENOXY)-2-PROPANOL
mf: $C_{13}H_{22}N_2O_4$ mw: 282.38

SYNS: dl-1-(2-NITRO-3-EMTHYLPHENOXY)-3-tert-BU-TYLAMINO-PROPAN-2-OL ◇ ZAMI 1305 ◇ dl-ZAMI 1305

TOXICITY DATA with REFERENCE
CAR: orl-rat TD: 18 g/kg/26W-C   JJIND8 68,669,82
CAR: orl-rat TDLo: 9 g/kg/26W-C   JJIND8 68,669,82
MUT: dni-rat-ipr 100 mg/kg   TOPADD 13,18,85
MUT: dni-rat: lvr 14 mmol/L   CBINA8 50,77,84
MUT: oms-rat-ipr 300 mg/kg/6D   CBINA8 52,203,84
MUT: oms-rat: lvr 28 mmol/L   CBINA8 50,77,84

SAFETY PROFILE: Questionable carcinogen with experimental carcinogenic data. Mutation data reported. When heated to decomposition it emits toxic fumes of NO_x.

BQI010   CAS: 88-32-4
3-tert-BUTYLATED HYDROXYANISOLE
mf: $C_{11}H_{16}O_2$ mw: 180.27

SYNS: 3-tert-BHA ◇ 3-tert-BUTYL-4-METHOXYPHENOL

TOXICITY DATA with REFERENCE
ETA: orl-ham TDLo: 27 g/kg/3W-C   JJIND8 76,143,86

SAFETY PROFILE: Questionable carcinogen with experimental tumorigenic data. When heated to decomposition it emits acrid and irritating fumes.

BQI500   CAS: 63018-64-4
5-n-BUTYL-1,2-BENZANTHRACENE
mf: $C_{22}H_{20}$ mw: 284.42

SYN: 8-BUTYLBENZ(a)ANTHRACENE

TOXICITY DATA with REFERENCE
ETA: skn-mus TDLo: 860 mg/kg/36W-I
   PRLBA4 129,439,40

SAFETY PROFILE: Questionable carcinogen with experimental tumorigenic data. When heated to decomposition it emits acrid smoke and irritating fumes.

BQM250   CAS: 507-19-7
tert-BUTYL BROMIDE
DOT: 2342
mf: C_4H_9Br mw: 137.04

PROP: Colorless liquid. Mp: $-20°$, bp: 73.3°, fp: $-18°$, d: 1.215 @ 25°/25°.

SYNS: 2-BROMOISOBUTANE ◇ 2-BROMO-2-METHYL-PROPANE (DOT) ◇ TRIMETHYLBROMOMETHANE

TOXICITY DATA with REFERENCE
NEO: ipr-mus TDLo: 3000 mg/kg/8W-I
   CNREA8 35,1411,75

CONSENSUS REPORTS: EPA Genetic Toxicology Program. Reported in EPA TSCA Inventory.

DOT Classification: Flammable or Combustible Liquid; Label: Flammable Liquid.

SAFETY PROFILE: Questionable carcinogen with experimental neoplastigenic data. Moderately toxic by intraperitoneal route. When heated to decomposition it emits toxic fumes of Br^-.

BQP250   CAS: 592-35-8
BUTYL CARBAMATE
mf: $C_5H_{11}NO_2$ mw: 117.17

SYNS: CARBAMIC ACID, BUTYL ESTER ◇ USAF EL-101 ◇ USAF FO-1

TOXICITY DATA with REFERENCE
NEO: ipr-mus TDLo: 1980 mg/kg/6D-C
   PSEBAA 132,422,69
MUT: mmo-esc 5000 ppm/3H   AMNTA4 85,119,51

CONSENSUS REPORTS: Reported in EPA TSCA Inventory.

SAFETY PROFILE: Questionable carcinogen with experimental neoplastigenic and teratogenic data. A poison via intraperitoneal route. Moderately toxic via subcutaneous route. Mutation data reported. When heated to decomposition it emits toxic fumes of NO_x.

BQR000 CAS: 507-20-0
tert-BUTYL CHLORIDE
mf: C_4H_9Cl mw: 92.58

PROP: Flash p: 32°F, d: 0.87, vap d: 3.2, bp: 51°.

SYNS: 2-CHLOROISOBUTANE ◇ 2-CHLORO-2-METHYL-PROPANE ◇ TRIMETHYLCHLOROMETHANE

TOXICITY DATA with REFERENCE
NEO: ipr-mus TDLo:3000 mg/kg/8W-I
CNREA8 35,1411,75

CONSENSUS REPORTS: Reported in EPA TSCA Inventory.

SAFETY PROFILE: Questionable carcinogen with experimental neoplastigenic data. Dangerous fire hazard when exposed to heat, flame (sparks), and oxidizers. To fight fire, use water, spray, fog, alcohol foam, dry chemical. When heated to decomposition it emits toxic fumes of Cl^-.

BQU750 CAS: 67195-50-0
tert-20-BUTYLCHOLANTHRENE
mf: $C_{24}H_{22}$ mw: 310.46

SYN: 3-tert-BUTYLCHOLANTHRENE

TOXICITY DATA with REFERENCE
ETA: scu-mus TDLo:600 mg/kg/39W-I
JNCIAM 2,99,41

SAFETY PROFILE: Questionable carcinogen with experimental tumorigenic data. When heated to decomposition it emits acrid smoke and irritating fumes.

BQV750 CAS: 2409-55-4
2-tert-BUTYL-p-CRESOL
mf: $C_{11}H_{16}O$ mw: 164.27

PROP: Clear liquid, sol in organic solvents and aqueous potassium hydroxide. Fp: 23.1°, bp: 244°, d: 0.922, flash p: 116°F.

SYNS: 2-tert-BUTYL-p-KRESOL (CZECH) ◇ 2-tert-BUTYL-4-METHYLPHENOL

TOXICITY DATA with REFERENCE
NEO: orl-ham TDLo:84 g/kg/20W-C CRNGDP
7,1285,86
MUT: dni-hmn:lyms 25 μmol/L RCOCB8
54,133,86

CONSENSUS REPORTS: Reported in EPA TSCA Inventory.

SAFETY PROFILE: Questionable carcinogen with experimental neoplastigenic data. A poison by intraperitoneal and intravenous routes. Moderately toxic by ingestion and skin contact. Mutation data reported. A severe skin and eye irritant. Flammable when exposed to heat, flame, or oxidizers. To fight fire, use alcohol foam, foam, water spray, fog, dry chemical. When heated to decomposition it emits acrid and irritating fumes.

BQY000 CAS: 10457-58-6
14-n-BUTYL DIBENZ(a,h)ACRIDINE
mf: $C_{25}H_{21}N$ mw: 335.47

SYN: 10-n-BUTYL-1,2,5,6-DIBENZACRIDINE (FRENCH)

TOXICITY DATA with REFERENCE
ETA: scu-mus TD:60 mg/kg/9W-I ACRSAJ
4,315,56
ETA: scu-mus TDLo:60 mg/kg/9W-I BAFEAG
42,186,55

SAFETY PROFILE: Questionable carcinogen with experimental tumorigenic data. When heated to decomposition it emits toxic fumes of NO_x.

BQZ000 CAS: 94-80-4
BUTYL DICHLOROPHENOXYACETATE
mf: $C_{12}H_{14}Cl_2O_3$ mw: 277.16

SYNS: BUTYL 2,4-D ◇ BUTYL (2,4-DICHLOROPHE-NOXY)ACETATE ◇ 2,4-D BUTYL ESTER ◇ BUTYL ESTER-2,4-D ◇ (2,4-DICHLOROPHENOXY)ACETIC ACID, BUTYL ESTER ◇ ESSO HERBICIDE 10 ◇ FERNESTA ◇ LIRONOX ◇ SHELL 40

CONSENSUS REPORTS: IARC Cancer Review: Animal Inadequate Evidence IMEMDT 15,111,77

SAFETY PROFILE: Questionable carcinogen. Poison by an unspecified route. Moderately toxic by ingestion and possibly other routes. An experimental teratogen. Experimental reproductive effects. An herbicide. When heated to decomposition it emits toxic fumes of Cl^-.

BRB450 CAS: 24596-39-2
4'-n-BUTYL-4-DIMETHYLAMINOAZOBENZENE
mf: $C_{18}H_{23}N_3$ mw: 281.44

SYNS: ANILINE, p-((p-BUTYLPHENYL)AZO)-N,N-DI-METHYL- ◇ p-((p-BUTYLPHENYL)AZO)-N,N-DIMETHYL-ANILINE

TOXICITY DATA with REFERENCE
ETA: orl-rat TDLo: 13 mg/kg/Y-C   JNCIAM
27,663,61

SAFETY PROFILE: Questionable carcinogen
with experimental tumorigenic data. When
heated to decomposition it emits toxic fumes
of NO_x.

BRB460   CAS: 24596-41-6
4'-tert-BUTYL-4-DIMETHYLAMINOAZOBENZENE
mf: $C_{18}H_{23}N_3$ mw: 281.44

SYNS: ANILINE, p-((p-(tert-BUTYL)PHENYL)AZO)-N,N-DI-
METHYL- ◇ p-((p-tert-BUTYLPHENYL)AZO)-N,N-DIMETH-
YLANILINE

TOXICITY DATA with REFERENCE
ETA: orl-rat TDLo: 12852 mg/kg/Y-C   JNCIAM
27,663,61

SAFETY PROFILE: Questionable carcinogen
with experimental tumorigenic data. When
heated to decomposition it emits toxic fumes
of NO_x.

BRE000   CAS: 56654-53-6
1-BUTYL-3,3-DIMETHYL-1-NITROSOUREA
mf: $C_7H_{15}N_3O_2$ mw: 173.25

TOXICITY DATA with REFERENCE
ETA: orl-rat TDLo: 3140 mg/kg/45W-C
JNCIAM 56,1177,76

SAFETY PROFILE: Questionable carcinogen
with experimental tumorigenic data. When
heated to decomposition it emits toxic fumes
of NO_x.

BRE500   CAS: 88-85-7
2-sec-BUTYL-4,6-DINITROPHENOL
mf: $C_{10}H_{12}N_2O_5$ mw: 240.24

PROP: Crystals. Vap d: 7.73.

SYNS: ARETIT ◇ BASANITE ◇ BNP 30 ◇ BUTAPHENE
◇ CALDON ◇ CHEMOX GENERAL ◇ CHEMOX P.E.
◇ DINITRO ◇ DINITRO-3 ◇ 4,6-DINITRO-2-sec.BUTYL-
FENOL (CZECH) ◇ 2,4-DINITRO-6-sec-BUTYLPHENOL
◇ 4,6-DINITRO-o-sec-BUTYLPHENOL ◇ 4,6-DINITRO-2-sec-
BUTYLPHENOL ◇ DINITROBUTYLPHENOL ◇ 4,6-DINITRO-
2-(1-METHYL-N-PROPYL)PHENOL ◇ 2,4-DINITRO-6-(1-
METHYL-PROPYL)PHENOL (FRENCH) ◇ DINOSEB ◇ DI-
NOSEBE (FRENCH) ◇ DN 289 ◇ DNBP ◇ DNOSBP
◇ DNSBP ◇ DOW GENERAL ◇ DOW GENERAL WEED

KILLER ◇ DOW SELECTIVE WEED KILLER ◇ ELGETOL
◇ ELGETOL 318 ◇ ENT 1,122 ◇ GEBUTOX ◇ HEL-FIRE
◇ KILOSEB ◇ 6-(1-METHYL-PROPYL)-2,4-DINITROFE-
NOL (DUTCH) ◇ 2-(1-METHYLPROPYL)-4,6-DINITROPHE-
NOL ◇ 6-(1-METIL-PROPIL)-2,4-DINITRO-FENOLO (ITAL-
IAN) ◇ NITROPONE C ◇ PHENOTAN ◇ PREMERGE
◇ PREMERGE 3 ◇ RCRA WASTE NUMBER P020 ◇ SINOX
GENERAL ◇ SPARIC ◇ SPURGE ◇ SUBITEX ◇ UNICROP
DNBP ◇ VERTAC DINITRO WEED KILLER ◇ VERTAC GEN-
ERAL WEED KILLER ◇ VERTAC SELECTIVE WEED KILLER

TOXICITY DATA with REFERENCE
ETA: orl-mus TDLo: 764 mg/kg/78W-I   NTIS**
PB223-159
MUT: mrc-smc 185 ppm   MUREAV 21,83,73
MUT: orl-rat 25 mg/kg   TXAPA9 7,353,65

CONSENSUS REPORTS: EPA Genetic Toxicology Program. EPA Extremely Hazardous
Substances List.

SAFETY PROFILE: Questionable carcinogen
with experimental tumorigenic and teratogenic
data. A poison by ingestion, inhalation, skin
contact, subcutaneous, intraperitoneal, and possibly other routes. Experimental reproductive
effects. Mutation data reported. A severe eye
irritant. An herbicide. When heated to decomposition it emits toxic fumes of NO_x.

BRG000   CAS: 110-57-6
2-BUTYLENE DICHLORIDE
mf: $C_4H_6Cl_2$ mw: 125.00

PROP: Colorless liquid. Mp: 1-3°, bp: 156°,
d: 1.183 @ 25°/4°.

SYNS: 1,4-DICHLOROBUTENE-2 (trans) ◇ 1,4-DICHLORO-
2-BUTENE

TOXICITY DATA with REFERENCE
NEO: scu-mus TDLo: 150 mg/kg/77W-I
CNREA8 35,2553,75
ETA: ipr-mus TDLo: 150 mg/kg/77W-I   CNREA8
35,2553,75

CONSENSUS REPORTS: IARC Cancer Review: GROUP 3 IMEMDT 7,56,87; Animal
Inadequate Evidence IMEMDT 15,149,77. Reported in EPA TSCA Inventory. EPA Extremely
Hazardous Substances List.

SAFETY PROFILE: Questionable carcinogen
with experimental neoplastigenic and tumorigenic data. A poison by inhalation. When heated
to decomposition it emits toxic fumes of Cl^-

BRH250   CAS: 106-83-2
BUTYL-9,10-EPOXYSTEARATE
mf: $C_{22}H_{42}O_3$ mw: 354.64

SYN: 9,10-EPOXYOCTADECANOIC ACID BUTYL ESTER

TOXICITY DATA with REFERENCE
ETA: unr-mus TDLo:24 g/kg   RARSAM 3,193,63
CONSENSUS REPORTS: Reported in EPA
TSCA Inventory.
SAFETY PROFILE: Questionable carcinogen
with experimental tumorigenic data. When
heated to decomposition it emits acrid smoke
and irritating fumes.

BRK100   CAS: 16120-70-0
N-n-BUTYL-N-FORMYLHYDRAZINE
mf: $C_5H_{12}N_2O$ mw: 116.19

SYNS: BFH ◊ FORMIC ACID, 1-BUTYLHYDRAZIDE

TOXICITY DATA with REFERENCE
CAR: orl-mus TDLo:70 g/kg/84W-C   CRNGDP
1,589,80

SAFETY PROFILE: Questionable carcinogen
with experimental carcinogenic data. When
heated to decomposition it emits toxic fumes
of NO_x.

BRL500   CAS: 56795-65-4
n-BUTYLHYDRAZINE HYDROCHLORIDE
mf: $C_4H_{12}N_2 \cdot ClH$ mw: 124.64

TOXICITY DATA with REFERENCE
NEO: orl-mus TDLo:14/g/kg/8W-C   EJCAAH
11,473,75

SAFETY PROFILE: Questionable carcinogen
with experimental neoplastigenic data. When
heated to decomposition it emits very toxic
fumes of NO_x and HCl.

BRM750   CAS: 21070-33-7
6-BUTYL-4-HYDROXYAMINOQUINOLINE-1-OXIDE
mf: $C_{13}H_{16}N_2O_2$ mw: 232.31

TOXICITY DATA with REFERENCE
ETA: scu-mus TDLo:60 mg/kg/I   CPBTAL
17,544,69

SAFETY PROFILE: Questionable carcinogen
with experimental tumorigenic data. When
heated to decomposition it emits toxic fumes
of NO_x.

BRN000   CAS: 121-00-6
3-tert-BUTYL-4-HYDROXYANISOLE
mf: $C_{11}H_{16}O_2$ mw: 180.27

SYNS: 2-tert-BUTYL-4-METHOXYPHENOL ◊ 4-METH-
OXY-2-tert-BUTYLPHENOL

TOXICITY DATA with REFERENCE
NEO: orl-ham TDLo:168 g/kg/20W-C   CRNGDP
7,1285,86

CONSENSUS REPORTS: Reported in EPA
TSCA Inventory.

SAFETY PROFILE: Questionable carcinogen
with experimental neoplastigenic data. Poison
by intraperitoneal route. Moderately toxic by
ingestion. When heated to decomposition it
emits acrid smoke and irritating fumes.

BRO000   CAS: 51938-14-8
BUTYL(2-HYDROXYETHYL)NITROSOAMINE
mf: $C_6H_{14}N_2O_2$ mw: 146.22

SYNS: BHEN ◊ 2-(BUTYLNITROSAMINO)ETHANOL

TOXICITY DATA with REFERENCE
ETA: orl-rat TDLo:4800 mg/kg/20W-C
GANNA2 65,13,74
MUT: mma-sat 5 μmol/plate   CNREA8 37,399,77
MUT: mmo-sat 100 μg/plate   MUREAV 56,219,78

CONSENSUS REPORTS: EPA Genetic Toxicology Program.

SAFETY PROFILE: Questionable carcinogen
with experimental tumorigenic data. Mutation
data reported. When heated to decomposition
it emits toxic fumes of NO_x.

BRQ250   CAS: 542-69-8
n-BUTYL IODIDE
mf: C_4H_9I mw: 184.03

SYN: 1-IODOBUTANE

TOXICITY DATA with REFERENCE
NEO: ipr-mus TDLo:480 mg/kg/8W-I   CNREA8
35,1411,75

CONSENSUS REPORTS: EPA Genetic Toxicology Program. Reported in EPA TSCA Inventory.

SAFETY PROFILE: Questionable carcinogen
with experimental neoplastigenic data. A poison
by intraperitoneal route. Moderately toxic by
inhalation. When heated to decomposition it
emits toxic fumes of I^-.

BRW750   CAS: 21070-32-6
6-BUTYL-4-NITROQUINOLINE-1-OXIDE
mf: $C_{13}H_{14}N_2O_3$ mw: 246.29

TOXICITY DATA with REFERENCE
ETA: scu-mus TDLo:60 mg/kg/I   CPBTAL
17,544,69

MUT: dnd-mus:fbr 100 μmol/L   CNREA8
35,521,75
MUT: dns-ham:oth 4 μmol/L   NATUAS
229,416,71

CONSENSUS REPORTS: EPA Genetic Toxicology Program.

SAFETY PROFILE: Questionable carcinogen with experimental tumorigenic data. Mutation data reported. When heated to decomposition it emits toxic fumes of NO_x.

BRX500   CAS: 56986-36-8
BUTYLNITROSOAMINOMETHYL ACETATE
mf: $C_7H_{14}N_2O_3$ mw: 174.23

SYNS: ACETOXYMETHYLBUTYLNITROSAMINE ◇ N-(ACETOXY)METHYL-N,N-BUTYLNITROSAMINE ◇ BAMN ◇ BUTYL ACETOXYMETHYLNITROSAMINE ◇ N-BUTYL-N-(ACETOXYMETHYL)NITROSAMINE ◇ N-NITROSO-N-(1-ACETOXYMETHYL)BUTYLAMINE

TOXICITY DATA with REFERENCE
CAR: scu-rat TD:66 mg/kg/10W-I   IAPUDO
41,619,82
CAR: scu-rat TDLo:50 mg/kg/10W-I   JCROD7
104,13,82
ETA: orl-rat TDLo:555 mg/kg/90D-I   ZKKOBW
91,317,78
MUT: cyt-ham:fbr 16 mg/L/24H   MUREAV
48,337,77
MUT: dnd-mus:fbr 260 nmol/L   GANNA2
73,565,82
MUT: dnr-bcs 500 nmol/plate   GANNA2 66,457,75
MUT: dns-rat:oth 10 μmol/L   CBINA8 53,99,85
MUT: mmo-esc 1 μmol/plate   GANNA2 71,124,80
MUT: mmo-sat 1 μmol/plate   MUREAV 49,187,78
MUT: msc-ham:lng 100 μmol/L   GANNA2
75,531,81

CONSENSUS REPORTS: EPA Genetic Toxicology Program.

SAFETY PROFILE: Questionable carcinogen with experimental carcinogenic and tumorigenic data. Moderately toxic by ingestion. Mutation data reported. When heated to decomposition it emits toxic fumes of NO_x.

BRY000   CAS: 51938-15-9
1-(BUTYLNITROSOAMINO)-2-PROPANONE
mf: $C_7H_{14}N_2O_2$ mw: 158.23

SYNS: BUTYL(2-OXOPROPYL)NITROSOAMINE ◇ N-NITROSO-1-BUTYLAMINO-2-PROPANONE ◇ N-NITROSO-(2-OXOPROPYL)-N-BUTYLAMINE

TOXICITY DATA with REFERENCE
ETA: orl-rat TDLo:2000 mg/kg/13W-C
GANNA2 65,13,74
MUT: mma-sat 4 μmol/plate   CNREA8 37,399,77
MUT: mmo-sat 31 μmol/plate   CNREA8 37,399,77

CONSENSUS REPORTS: EPA Genetic Toxicology Program.

SAFETY PROFILE: Questionable carcinogen with experimental tumorigenic data. Mutation data reported. When heated to decomposition it emits toxic fumes of NO_x.

BRY250   CAS: 16339-05-2
N-BUTYL-N-NITROSO AMYL AMINE
mf: $C_9H_{20}N_2O$ mw: 172.31

SYNS: BUTYLAMYLNITROSAMIN (GERMAN) ◇ N-BUTYL-N-NITROSOPENTYLAMINE ◇ N-BUTYL-N-PENTYLINITROSAMINE ◇ N-NITROSO-N-BUTYLPENTYLAMINE ◇ N-NITROSO-N-BUTYL-N-PENTYLAMINE

TOXICITY DATA with REFERENCE
ETA: scu-mus TDLo:17 g/kg/21W-I   ZEKBAI
69,103,67

SAFETY PROFILE: Questionable carcinogen with experimental tumorigenic data. Moderately toxic by subcutaneous route. When heated to decomposition it emits toxic fumes of NO_x.

BRZ000   CAS: 6558-78-7
N-BUTYL-N-NITROSO ETHYL CARBAMATE
mf: $C_7H_{14}N_2O_3$ mw: 174.23

SYNS: N-BUTYL-N-NITROSOURETHAN ◇ 1-BUTYL-1-NITROSOURETHAN ◇ TL 478

TOXICITY DATA with REFERENCE
NEO: orl-mus TDLo:5300 mg/kg/20W-C
GANNA2 67,231,76
ETA: orl-mam TD:5 g/kg/16W-C   AMBNAS
28,85,81
ETA: orl-rat TD:5 g/kg/16W-C   AMBNAS
28,85,81
ETA: orl-rat TD:5040 mg/kg/18W-C   NIPAA4
78,157,81
ETA: orl-rat TDLo:2240 mg/kg/8W-C   GANNA2
65,227,74
MUT: cyt-ham:fbr 120 mg/L/48H   MUREAV
48,337,77
MUT: cyt-ham:lng 35 mg/L   GMCRDC 27,95,81
MUT: dnr-bcs 5 g/L   MUREAV 42,19,77
MUT: mmo-bcs 5 g/L   MUREAV 42,19,77
MUT: sce-ham:fbr 100 μmol/L   JNCIAM
58,1635,77

CONSENSUS REPORTS: EPA Genetic Toxicology Program.

SAFETY PROFILE: Questionable carcinogen with experimental neoplastigenic, tumorigenic, and teratogenic data. A poison by inhalation. Moderately toxic by ingestion. Mutation data reported. When heated to decomposition it emits toxic fumes of NO_x.

BRZ200　　　　　CAS: 17721-94-7
4-tert-BUTYL-1-NITROSOPIPERIDINE
mf: $C_9H_{18}N_2O$　　mw: 170.29

SYN: N-NITROSO-4-tert-BUTYLPIPERIDINE

TOXICITY DATA with REFERENCE
CAR: orl-rat TDLo: 4500 mg/kg/2Y-I　CRNGDP 2,1045,81

MUT: mma-sat 250 μg/plate　MUREAV 111,135,83

SAFETY PROFILE: Questionable carcinogen with experimental carcinogenic data. Mutation data reported. When heated to decomposition it emits toxic fumes of NO_x.

BSB500　　　　　CAS: 61734-89-2
N-BUTYL-N-(2-OXOBUTYL) NITROSAMINE
mf: $C_8H_{16}N_2O_2$　　mw: 172.26

SYN: N-NITROSO-N-(2-OXOBUTYL)BUTYLAMINE

TOXICITY DATA with REFERENCE
ETA: orl-rat TDLo: 69 g/kg/20W-C　GANNA2 67,825,76

MUT: mma-sat 4 μmol/plate　CNREA8 37,399,77

CONSENSUS REPORTS: EPA Genetic Toxicology Program.

SAFETY PROFILE: Questionable carcinogen with experimental tumorigenic data. Mutation data reported. When heated to decomposition it emits toxic fumes of NO_x.

BSB750　　　　　CAS: 61734-90-5
N-BUTYL-N-(3-OXOBUTYL) NITROSAMINE
mf: $C_8H_{16}N_2O_2$　　mw: 172.26

SYN: N-NITROSO-N-(3-OXOBUTYL)BUTYLAMINE

TOXICITY DATA with REFERENCE
ETA: orl-rat TDLo: 69 g/kg/20W-C　GANNA2 67,825,76

MUT: mma-sat 4 μmol/plate　CNREA8 37,399,77

CONSENSUS REPORTS: EPA Genetic Toxicology Program.

SAFETY PROFILE: Questionable carcinogen with experimental tumorigenic data. Mutation data reported. When heated to decomposition it emits toxic fumes of NO_x.

BSC500　　　　　CAS: 614-45-9
tert-BUTYL PERBENZOATE
DOT: 2097
mf: $C_{11}H_{14}O_3$　　mw: 194.25

PROP: Colorless to slight yellow liquid, mild aromatic odor. Bp: 112° (decomp), flash p: 19°, fp: 8°, vap press: 0.33 mm @ 50°, d: 1.0. Insol in water; sol in organic solvents.

SYNS: tert-BUTYLPERBENZOAN (CZECH) ◇ tert-BUTYL PEROXY BENZOATE ◇ tert-BUTYL PEROXYBENZOATE, technical pure or in concentration of more than 75% (DOT) ◇ ESPEROX 10 ◇ NOVOX ◇ PERBENZOATE de BUTYLE TERTIAIRE (FRENCH) ◇ TRIGONOX C

TOXICITY DATA with REFERENCE
ETA: unr-mus TDLo: 311 mg/kg　RARSAM 3,193,63

MUT: mma-sat 67 μg/plate　ENMUDM 8(Suppl 7),52,72

CONSENSUS REPORTS: Reported in EPA TSCA Inventory.

DOT Classification: Organic Peroxide; Label: Organic Peroxide.

SAFETY PROFILE: Questionable carcinogen with experimental tumorigenic data. Moderately toxic by ingestion. A skin and eye irritant. Mutation data reported. Potentially explosive when heated above 115°C. When heated to decomposition it emits acrid smoke and fumes.

BSC750　　　　　CAS: 110-05-4
tert-BUTYL PEROXIDE
DOT: 2102
mf: $C_8H_{18}O_2$　　mw: 146.26

PROP: Clear, water white liquid. Mp: −40°, bp: 80° @ 284 mm, flash p: 65°F (OC), d: 0.79, vap press: 19.51 mm @ 20°, vap d: 5.03.

SYNS: CADOX ◇ DI-tert-BUTYLPEROXID (GERMAN) ◇ DI-tert-BUTYL PEROXIDE (MAK) ◇ DI-tert-BUTYL PEROXYDE (DUTCH) ◇ DTBP ◇ PEROSSIDO di BUTILE TERZIARIO (ITALIAN) ◇ PEROXYDE de BUTYLE TERTIAIRE (FRENCH) ◇ (TRIBUTYL)PEROXIDE

TOXICITY DATA with REFERENCE
ETA: unr-mus TDLo: 585 mg/kg　RARSAM 3,193,63

CONSENSUS REPORTS: Reported in EPA ISCA Inventory

DFG MAK: Mild skin irritant.   DOT Classification: Organic Peroxide; Label: Organic Peroxide, Flammable Liquid.

SAFETY PROFILE: Questionable carcinogen with experimental tumorigenic data. Moderately toxic by intraperitoneal route. A powerful irritant by ingestion and inhalation. A mild skin and eye irritant. Warning: Water may not work to fight fire. When heated to decomposition it emits acrid smoke and fumes.

BSD500   CAS: 3180-09-4
2-n-BUTYLPHENOL
DOT: 2228/2229
mf: $C_{10}H_{14}O$ mw: 150.24

SYNS: o-BUTYLPHENOL, liquid (DOT) ◇ o-BUTYLPHE-NOL, solid (DOT)

TOXICITY DATA with REFERENCE
NEO: skn-mus TDLo: 3800 mg/kg/12W-I
   CNREA8 19,413,59

DOT Classification: Poison B; Label: St. Andrews Cross.

SAFETY PROFILE: Questionable carcinogen with experimental neoplastigenic data. When heated to decomposition it emits acrid smoke and irritating fumes.

BSD750   CAS: 1638-22-8
4-n-BUTYLPHENOL
DOT: 2228/2229
mf: $C_{10}H_{14}O$ mw: 150.24

TOXICITY DATA with REFERENCE
ETA: skn-mus TDLo: 3840 mg/kg/12W-I
   CNREA8 19,413,59

CONSENSUS REPORTS: Reported in EPA TSCA Inventory.

DOT Classification: Poison B; Label: St. Andrews Cross.

SAFETY PROFILE: Questionable carcinogen with experimental tumorigenic data. A poison. When heated to decomposition it emits acrid smoke and irritating fumes.

BSE500   CAS: 98-54-4
4-tert-BUTYLPHENOL
mf: $C_{10}H_{14}O$ mw: 150.24

PROP: Crystals or practically white flakes. Bp: 238°, fp: 97°, d: 0.9081 @ 114°/4°, vap press: 1 mm @ 70.0°, vap d: 5.1.

SYNS: p-tert-BUTYLFENOL (CZECH) ◇ BUTYLPHEN ◇ p-tert-BUTYLPHENOL (MAK) ◇ 4-(1,1-DIMETHYL-ETHYL)PHENOL ◇ 1-HYDROXY-4-tert-BUTYLBENZENE ◇ UCAR BUTYLPHENOL 4-T

TOXICITY DATA with REFERENCE
NEO: orl-ham TDLo: 252 g/kg/20W-C   CRNGDP 7,1285,86

CONSENSUS REPORTS: Reported in EPA TSCA Inventory.

DFG MAK: 0.08 ppm (0.5 mg/m³)

SAFETY PROFILE: Questionable carcinogen with experimental neoplastigenic data. Poison by intraperitoneal route. Moderately toxic by skin contact and ingestion. A skin and severe eye irritant. Combustible when exposed to heat or flame; can react with oxidizing materials. To fight fire, use foam, CO_2, dry chemical. When heated to decomposition it emits acrid and irritating fumes.

BSR500   CAS: 313-94-0
3-tert-BUTYLTRICYCLOQUINAZOLINE
mf: $C_{25}H_{21}N_4$ mw: 377.50

TOXICITY DATA with REFERENCE
CAR: skn-mus TDLo: 1200 mg/kg/50W-I
   BCPCA6 14,323,65

SAFETY PROFILE: Questionable carcinogen with experimental carcinogenic data. When heated to decomposition it emits toxic fumes of NO_x.

BSX500   CAS: 67557-56-6
N-(1-BUTYROXYMETHYL)METHYLNITROSAMINE
mf: $C_6H_{12}N_2O_3$ mw: 160.20

SYNS: N-(1-BUTYROXYMETHYL)-N-NITROSOMETHYL-AMINE ◇ N-NITROSO-N-(1-BUTYROXYMETHYL)METHYL AMINE

TOXICITY DATA with REFERENCE
ETA: orl-rat TDLo: 60 mg/kg/90D-I   ZKKOBW 91,317,78
MUT: mma-sat 200 nmol/plate   ARTODN 39,51,77
MUT: mmo-sat 1 μmol/plate   ARTODN 39,51,77

SAFETY PROFILE: Questionable carcinogen with experimental tumorigenic data. Moderately toxic by ingestion. Mutation data reported. When heated to decomposition it emits toxic fumes of NO_x.

BSX750
CAS: 37415-56-8

12-o-BUTYROYL-PHORBOLDODECANOATE

mf: $C_{36}H_{57}O_8$ mw: 617.93

SYN: PHORBOL-12-o-BUTYROYL-13-DODECANOATE

TOXICITY DATA with REFERENCE
ETA: skn-mus TDLo: 12 mg/kg/12W-I   85CVA2 5,213,70

SAFETY PROFILE: Questionable carcinogen with experimental tumorigenic data. A skin irritant. When heated to decomposition it emits acrid smoke and irritating fumes.

BSY000
CAS: 10431-86-4

1-n-BUTYRYLAZIRIDINE

mf: $C_6H_{11}NO$ mw: 113.18

SYNS: 1-BUTYRYLAZIRIDINE ◇ BUTYRYLETHYLENEI-MINE ◇ BUTYRYLETHYLENIMINE ◇ 1-(1-OXOBUTYL)-AZIRIDINE

TOXICITY DATA with REFERENCE
ETA: scu-mus TDLo: 488 mg/kg/20W-I   BJPCAL 9,306,54
ETA: scu-rat TD: 488 mg/kg/20W-I   BJPCAL 9,306,54
ETA: scu-rat TDLo: 225 mg/kg/26W-I   BJPCAL 9,306,54
MUT: cyt-rat-ipr 50 mg/kg   BJPCAL 9,306,54

SAFETY PROFILE: Questionable carcinogen with experimental tumorigenic data. Moderately toxic by intraperitoneal route. Mutation data reported. When heated to decomposition it emits toxic fumes of NO_x.

CAC500

CADIA DEL PERRO

PROP: Aqueous extract from the dried leaves of the plant (JNCIAM 46,1131,71).

SYNS: K. IXINA ◇ KRAMERIA IXINA

TOXICITY DATA with REFERENCE
CAR: skn-ham TDLo: 53950 mg/kg/65W-I   JNCIAM 53,1259,74
NEO: scu-rat TD: 990 mg/kg/55W-I   JNCIAM 52,1579,74
NEO: scu-rat TDLo: 300 mg/kg/1Y-I   JNCIAM 46,1131,71
ETA: ims-rat TDLo: 45 g/kg/1Y-I   JNCIAM 46,1131,71

SAFETY PROFILE: Questionable carcinogen with experimental carcinogenic, tumorigenic,

and neoplastigenic data. When heated to decomposition it emits acrid smoke and fumes.

CAK500
CAS: 58-08-2

CAFFEINE

mf: $C_8H_{10}N_4O_2$ mw: 194.22

PROP: White, fleecy masses; odorless with bitter taste. Mp: 236.8°. Sol in water, alc, chloroform, ether.

SYNS: CAFFEIN ◇ COFFEIN (GERMAN) ◇ COFFEINE ◇ 3,7-DIHYDRO-1,3,7-TRIMETHYL-1H-PURINE-2,6-DIONE ◇ ELDIATRIC C ◇ FEMA No. 2224 ◇ GUARANINE ◇ KOFFEIN (GERMAN) ◇ METHYLTHEOBROMIDE ◇ 1-METHYLTHEOBROMINE ◇ 7-METHYLTHEOPHYLLINE ◇ NCI-C02733 ◇ NO-DOZ ◇ ORGANEX ◇ THEIN ◇ THEINE ◇ 1,3,7-TRIMETHYL-2,6-DIOXOPURINE ◇ 1,3,7-TRIMETHYLXANTHINE

TOXICITY DATA with REFERENCE
CAR: orl-mus TDLo: 30800 mg/kg/44W-C   CNREA8 48,2078,88
MUT: cyt-hmn: fbr 2600 μmol/L/24H   MUREAV 46,297,77
MUT: cyt-hmn: lym 100 μg/L/24H   MUREAV 46,205,77
MUT: dni-hmn: oth 4 mmol/L   BIOJAU 35,665,81
MUT: dns-hmn: oth 1 mmol/L   BIOJAU 35,665,81
MUT: sce-hmn: lym 1 mmol/L   RBPMB2 10,60,77

CONSENSUS REPORTS: Reported in EPA TSCA Inventory. EPA Genetic Toxicology Program.

SAFETY PROFILE: Questionable carcinogen with experimental carcinogenic data. A human poison by ingestion. An experimental poison by ingestion, subcutaneous, intraperitoneal, intramuscular, rectal, and intravenous routes. Human systemic effects by ingestion, intravenous and intramuscular routes include: ataxia, blood pressure elevation, convulsions or effect on seizure threshold, diarrhea, distorted perceptions, hallucinations, hypermotility, muscle contraction or spasticity, somnolence (general depressed activity), nausea or vomiting, toxic psychosis, tremors. A human teratogen causing developmental abnormalities of the craniofacial and musculoskeletal systems, pregnancy termination (abortion) and stillbirth. Human maternal effects include an unspecified effect on labor or childbirth. Human mutation data reported. An experimental teratogen. Large doses (above 1.0 gram) cause palpitation, excitement, insomnia, dizziness, headache, and vomiting. Continued excessive use of caffeine in tea or coffee may lead to digestive disturbances, constipation, palpitations, shortness of breath, and depressed mental states. It is also implicated in cardiac disorders under those conditions. When heated to decomposition it emits toxic fumes of NO_x.

CAO750   CAS: 10043-52-4
CALCIUM CHLORIDE
mf: $CaCl_2$ mw: 110.98

PROP: Cubic, colorless, deliquescent crystals. Mp: 772°, bp: >1600°, d: 2.512 @ 25°. Sol in water and alc.

SYNS: CALCIUM CHLORIDE, ANHYDROUS ◇ CALPLUS ◇ CALTAC ◇ DOWFLAKE ◇ LIQUIDOW ◇ PELADOW ◇ SNOMELT ◇ SUPERFLAKE ANHYDROUS

TOXICITY DATA with REFERENCE
ETA: orl-rat TDLo: 112 g/kg/20W-C   AJCAA7 23,550,35
MUT: cyt-rat: ast 3500 mg/kg   GANNA2 7,165,87
MUT: dns-rat-ipr 2500 μmol/kg   JOENAK 65,45,75

CONSENSUS REPORTS: Reported in EPA TSCA Inventory. EPA Genetic Toxicology Program.

SAFETY PROFILE: Questionable carcinogen with experimental tumorigenic data. Moderately toxic by ingestion. Poison by intravenous, intramuscular, intraperitoneal, and subcutaneous routes. Mutation data reported. When heated to decomposition it emits toxic fumes of Cl^-.

CAQ250   CAS: 156-62-7
CALCIUM CYANAMIDE
mf: $CN_2 \cdot Ca$ mw: 80.11
DOT: 1403

PROP: Hexagonal, rhombohedral, colorless crystals. Mp: 1300°, subl > 1500°. Compound not hydrated; compound contains more than 0.1% calcium (FEREAC 41,15972,76).

SYNS: AERO-CYANAMID ◇ AERO CYANAMID GRANULAR ◇ AERO CYANAMID SPECIAL GRADE ◇ ALZODEF ◇ CALCIUM CARBIMIDE ◇ CALCIUM CYANAMID ◇ CCC ◇ CYANAMIDE ◇ CYANAMIDE, CALCIUM SALT (1:1) ◇ CYANAMIDE CALCIQUE (FRENCH) ◇ CYANAMID GRANULAR ◇ CYANAMID SPECIAL GRADE ◇ CY-L 500 ◇ LIME-NITROGEN (DOT) ◇ NCI-C02937 ◇ NITROGEN LIME ◇ NITROLIME ◇ USAF CY-2

TOXICITY DATA with REFERENCE
ETA: orl-mus TDLo: 170 g/kg/2Y-C   NCITR* NCI-CG-TR-163,79

MUT: mma-sat 100 μg/plate   ENMUDM 5(Suppl 1),3,83
MUT: mmo-sat 1 mg/plate   ENMUDM 5(Suppl 1),3,83

CONSENSUS REPORTS: NCI Carcinogenesis Bioassay (feed); No Evidence: mouse, rat NCITR*   NCI-CG-TR-163,79.   Community Right-To-Know List. Reported in EPA TSCA Inventory.

OSHA PEL: TWA 0.5 mg/m³   ACGIH TLV: TWA 0.5 mg/m³   DFG MAK: 1 mg/m³   DOT Classification: ORM-C; Label: None; IMO: Flammable Solid; Label: Dangerous When Wet.

SAFETY PROFILE: Questionable carcinogen with experimental tumorigenic data. Poison by ingestion, inhalation, skin contact, intravenous, and intraperitoneal routes. Moderately toxic to humans by ingestion. Mutation data reported. Calcium cyanamide is not believed to have a cumulative action. Flammable. Reaction with water forms the explosive acetylene gas. When heated to decomposition it emits toxic fumes of NO_x and CN^-.

CAR000   CAS: 139-06-0
CALCIUM CYCLOHEXYLSULPHAMATE
mf: $C_{12}H_{24}N_2O_6S_2 \cdot Ca$ mw: 396.58

PROP: White, crystalline powder; almost odorless; freely sol in water; practically insol in alc, benzene, chloroform, and ether.

SYNS: CALCIUM CYCLAMATE ◇ CALCIUM CYCLOHEXANESULFAMATE ◇ CALCIUM CYCLOHEXANE SULPHAMATE ◇ CALCIUM CYCLOHEXYLSULFAMATE ◇ CYCLAMATE CALCIUM ◇ CYCLAMATE, CALCIUM SALT ◇ CYCLAN ◇ CYCLOHEXANESULFAMIC ACID, CALCIUM SALT ◇ CYCLOHEXYLSULPHAMIC ACID, CALCIUM SALT ◇ CYLAN ◇ DIETIL ◇ KALZIUMZYKLAMATE (GERMAN) ◇ SUCARYL CALCIUM

TOXICITY DATA with REFERENCE
NEO: orl-rat TDLo: 3465 g/kg/88W-C   JNCIAM 49,751,72
ETA: scu-rat TDLo: 45 g/kg/66W-I   FCTXAV 9,463,71
MUT: cyt-grb-ipr 150 mg/kg   CNJGA8 13,189,71
MUT: cyt-ham: fbr 10 mg/L   MUREAV 39,1,76
MUT: cyt-ham: lng 100 mg/L   HEREAY 70,271,72
MUT: cyt-hmn: leu 250 mg/L   SCIEAS 164,568,69
MUT: dni-hmn: lng 100 mg/L   JCLBA3 47,30a,70
MUT: sln-dmg-orl 5 mmol/L   DRISAA 46,114,71

CONSENSUS REPORTS: IARC Cancer Review: GROUP 3 IMEMDT 7,178,87; Animal

Limited Evidence IMEMDT 22,55,80. Reported in EPA TSCA Inventory. EPA Genetic Toxicology Program.

SAFETY PROFILE: Questionable carcinogen with experimental tumorigenic and neoplastigenic data. Poison by ingestion and intravenous routes. Experimental reproductive effects. Human mutation data reported. When heated to decomposition it emits very toxic fumes of SO_x and NO_x.

CAX260   CAS: 23209-59-8
CALCIUM SODIUM METAPHOSPHATE
mf: $HO_3P•Ca•Na$ mw: 143.05

SYN: METAPHOSPHORIC ACID, CALCIUM SODIUM SALT

TOXICITY DATA with REFERENCE
ETA: ipl-rat TDLo:200 mg/kg/2Y-C   EPASR*
  8EHQ-0386-0619

CONSENSUS REPORTS: Reported in EPA TSCA Inventory.

SAFETY PROFILE: Questionable carcinogen with experimental tumorigenic data. When heated to decomposition it emits toxic fumes of PO_x.

CAX750   CAS: 10101-41-4
CALCIUM(II) SULFATE DIHYDRATE
(1:1:2)
mf: $O_4S•Ca•2H_2O$ mw: 172.18

PROP: Colorless crystals. D: 2.32, mp: 128° (loses $1.5H_2O$), bp: 163° (loses $2H_2O$).

SYNS: ALABASTER ◇ ANNALINE ◇ C.I. 77231 ◇ C.I. PIGMENT WHITE 25 ◇ GYPSUM ◇ GYPSUM STONE ◇ LAND PLASTER ◇ LIGHT SPAR ◇ MAGNESIA WHITE ◇ MINERAL WHITE ◇ NATIVE CALCIUM SULFATE ◇ PRECIPITATED CALCIUM SULFATE ◇ SATINITE ◇ SATIN SPAR ◇ SULFURIC ACID, CALCIUM(2+) SALT, DIHYDRATE ◇ TERRA ALBA

TOXICITY DATA with REFERENCE
CAR: ipr-rat TDLo:450 mg/kg/3W-I   ZHPMAT
  162,467,76

OSHA PEL: Total Dust: 15 mg/m^3; Respirable Fraction: 5 mg/m^3 ACGIH TLV: TWA (nuisance particulate) 10 mg/m^3 of total dust (when toxic impurities are not present, e.g., quartz < 1%)

SAFETY PROFILE: Questionable carcinogen with experimental carcinogenic data. Human systemic effects by inhalation: fibrosing alveolitis (growth of fibrous tissue in the lung); unspecified respiratory system effects and unspecified effects on the nose. Long considered a nuisance dust (depending on silica content). When heated to decomposition it emits toxic fumes of SO_x.

CAZ000
CALOMEL and MAGNESIUM SULFATE
(5:8)

SYN: MAGNESIUM SULFATE and CALOMEL (8:5)

TOXICITY DATA with REFERENCE
ETA: orl-mus TDLo:44 g/kg/69W-I   CNREA8
  28,2272,68

CONSENSUS REPORTS: Mercury and its compounds are on the Community Right-To-Know List.

SAFETY PROFILE: Questionable carcinogen with experimental tumorigenic data. When heated to decomposition it emits very toxic fumes of Hg, Cl$^-$ and SO_x.

CBD760
CANNABIS SMOKE RESIDUE

SYN: MARIJUANA, SMOKE RESIDUE

TOXICITY DATA with REFERENCE
ETA: scu-rat TDLo:11640 mg/kg/18D-I
  VHTODE 21(Suppl),148,79
MUT: dnd-esc 10 ppm   MUREAV 89,95,81

SAFETY PROFILE: Questionable carcinogen with experimental tumorigenic data. Mutation data reported. When heated to decomposition it emits acrid smoke and irritating fumes.

CBE750   CAS: 56-25-7
CANTHARIDINE
mf: $C_{10}H_{12}O_4$ mw: 196.22

SYNS: CANTHARIDES CAMPHOR ◇ CANTHARIDIN ◇ CANTHARONE ◇ exo-1,2-cis-DIMETHYL-3,6-EPOXY-HEXAHYDROPHTHALIC ANHYDRIDE ◇ 2,3-DIMETHYL-7-OXABICYCLO(2.2.1)HEPTANE-2,3-DICARBOXYLIC ANHYDRIDE ◇ HEXAHYDRO-3A,7A-DIMETHYL-4,7-EPOXYISO-BENZOFURAN-1,3-DIONE

TOXICITY DATA with REFERENCE
NEO: skn-mus TDLo:25 mg/kg/14W-I   BJCAAI
  9,177,55
ETA: skn-mus TD:70 mg/kg/52W-I   CNREA8
  32,1463,72

CONSENSUS REPORTS: IARC Cancer Review: GROUP 3 IMEMDT 7,56,87; Animal

Limited Evidence IMEMDT 10,79,76. EPA Extremely Hazardous Substances List. Reported in EPA TSCA Inventory.

SAFETY PROFILE: Questionable carcinogen with experimental tumorigenic and neoplastigenic data. A suspected animal carcinogenic. A deadly human poison by ingestion. An experimental poison by ingestion and subcutaneous routes. When heated to decomposition it emits acrid and irritating fumes.

CBF700   CAS: 105-60-2
CAPROLACTAM
mf: $C_6H_{11}NO$ mw: 113.18

PROP: White crystals. Mp: 69°, vap press: 6 mm @ 120°.

SYNS: AMINOCAPROIC LACTAM ◇ 6-AMINOHEXANOIC ACID CYCLIC LACTAM ◇ 2-AZACYCLOHEPTANONE ◇ CAPROLACTAM ◇ 6-CAPROLACTAM ◇ omega-CAPROLACTAM (MAK) ◇ CAPROLATTAME (FRENCH) ◇ CYCLOHEXANONE ISO-OXIME ◇ EPSYLON KAPROLAKTAM (POLISH) ◇ HEXAHYDRO-2-AZEPINONE ◇ HEXAHYDRO-2H-AZEPIN-2-ONE ◇ 6-HEXANELACTAM ◇ HEXANONE ISOXIME ◇ HEXANONISOXIM (GERMAN) ◇ 1,6-HEXOLACTAM ◇ e-KAPROLAKTAM (CZECH) ◇ 2-KETOHEXAMETHYLENIMINE ◇ NCI-C50646 ◇ 2-OXOHEXAMETHYLENIMINE ◇ 2-PERHYDROAZEPINONE

TOXICITY DATA with REFERENCE
MUT: cyt-hmn:lym 270 mg/L   PMRSDJ 5,457,85
MUT: mma-smc 100 mg/L   PMRSDJ 5,257,85
MUT: mmo-smc 100 mg/L   PMRSDJ 5,271,85
MUT: otr-mus:emb 2500 mg/L   PMRSDJ 5,639,85
MUT: slt-dmg-orl 5 mmol/L   PMRSDJ 5,313,85

CONSENSUS REPORTS: IARC Cancer Review: GROUP 4 IMEMDT 7,56,87; Animal No Evidence IMEMDT 39,247,86. Reported in EPA TSCA Inventory.

OSHA PEL: Dust: 1 mg/m³; STEL 3 mg/m³; Vapor: 5 ppm; STEL 10 ppm   ACGIH TLV: Dust: 1 mg/m³; STEL 3 mg/m³; Vapor: 5 ppm; STEL 10 ppm; (Proposed: TWA Dust: 1 mg/m³; 5 ppm (vapor and aerosol)   DFG MAK: 25 mg/m³

SAFETY PROFILE: No evidence of carcinogenicity. Moderately toxic by ingestion, skin contact, intraperitoneal, and subcutaneous routes. Human systemic effects by inhalation: cough. Experimental reproductive effects. Human mutation data reported. A skin and eye irritant. When heated to decomposition it emits toxic fumes of NO_x.

CBF800   CAS: 2425-06-1
CAPTAFOL
mf: $C_{10}H_9Cl_4NO_2S$ mw: 349.06

SYNS: CAPTOFOL ◇ DIFOLATAN ◇ DIFOSAN ◇ FOLCID ◇ ORTHO 5865 ◇ SANSPOR ◇ SULFONIMIDE ◇ SULPHEIMIDE ◇ N-(1,1,2,2-TETRACHLORAETHYLTHIO) CYCLOHEX-4-EN-1,4-DIACARBOXIMID (GERMAN) ◇ N-(1,1,2,2-TETRACHLORAETHYLTHIO) TETRAHYDROPHTHALAMID (GERMAN) ◇ N-1,1,2,2-TETRACHLOROETHYLMERCAPTO-4-CYCLOHEXENE-1,2-CARBOXIMIDE ◇ N-((1,1,2,2-TETRACHLOROETHYL)SULFENYL)-cis-4-CYCLOHEXENE-1,2-DICARBOXIMIDE ◇ N-(1,1,2,2-TETRACHLOROETHYLTHIO)-4-CYCLOHEXENE-1,2-DICARBOXIMIDE

TOXICITY DATA with REFERENCE
CAR: orl-mus TDLo:60480 mg/kg/96W-C
    GANNA2 75,853,84
MUT: cyt-ham:lng 10 μmol/L   MUREAV 78,177,80
MUT: dlt-rat-ipr 25 mg/kg/5D   FCTXAV 10,353,72
MUT: mma-esc 50 μg/plate   MUREAV 116,185,83
MUT: mmo-esc 50 μg/plate   MUREAV 40,19,76
MUT: mrc-bcs 100 ng/disc/24H   MUREAV 40,19,76
MUT: sce-ham:lng 2 μmol/L   MUREAV 78,177,80

CONSENSUS REPORTS: EPA Genetic Toxicology Program.

OSHA PEL: TWA 0.1 mg/m³   ACGIH TLV: TWA 0.1 mg/m³

SAFETY PROFILE: Questionable carcinogen with experimental carcinogenic and teratogenic data. Poison by intraperitoneal route. Moderately toxic by ingestion. Other experimental reproductive effects. Mutation data reported. A fungicide. When heated to decomposition it emits very toxic fumes of Cl^-, NO_x and SO_x.

CBG000   CAS: 133-06-2
CAPTAN
DOT: 9099
mf: $C_9H_8Cl_3NO_2S$ mw: 300.59

PROP: Odorless crystals. Insol in water; sol in benzene and chloroform.

SYNS: AACAPTAN ◇ AGROSOL S ◇ AGROX 2-WAY and 3-WAY ◇ AMERCIDE ◇ BANGTON ◇ BEAN SEED PROTECTANT ◇ CAPTAF ◇ CAPTANCAPTENEET 26,538 ◇ CAPTANE ◇ CAPTAN-STREPTOMYCIN 7.5-0.1 POTATO SEED PIECE PROTECTANT ◇ CAPTEX ◇ ENT 26,538 ◇ ESSO FUNGICIDE 406 ◇ FLIT 406 ◇ FUNGUS BAN TYPE II ◇ GLYODEX 3722 ◇ GRANOX PPM ◇ GUSTAFSON CAPTAN 30-DD ◇ HEXACAP ◇ KAPTAN ◇ LE CAPTANE (FRENCH) ◇ MALIPUR ◇ MERPAN ◇ MICRO-CHECK 12 ◇ NCI-CO0077

◇ NERACID ◇ ORTHOCIDE ◇ OSOCIDE ◇ SR406 ◇ STAUFFER CAPTAN ◇ 3a,4,7,7a-TETRAHYDRO-N-(TRICHLOROMETHANESULPHENYL)PHTHALIMIDE ◇ 3a,4,7,7a-TETRAHYDRO-2-((TRICHLOROMETHYL)THIO)-1H-ISOINDOLE-1,3(2H)-DIONE ◇ 1,2,3,6-TETRAHYDRO-N-(TRICHLOROMETHYLTHIO)PHTHALIMIDE ◇ N-(TRICHLOR-METHYLTHIO)-PHTHALIMID (GERMAN) ◇ N-TRICHLOROMETHYLMERCAPTO-4-CYCLOHEXENE-1,2-DICARBOXIMIDE ◇ N-(TRICHLOROMETHYLMER-CAPTO)-Δ⁴-TETRAHYDROPHTHALIMIDE ◇ N-TRICHLORO-METHYLTHIOCYCLOHEX-4-ENE-1,2-DICARBOXIMIDE ◇ N-TRICHLOROMETHYLTHIO-cis-Δ⁴-CYCLOHEXENE-1,2-DICARBOXIMIDE ◇ N-((TRICHLOROMETHYL)THIO)-4-CYCLOHEXENE-1,2-DICARBOXIMIDE ◇ TRICHLORO-METHYLTHIO-1,2,5,6-TETRAHYDROPHTHALAMIDE ◇ N-((TRICHLOROMETHYL)THIO)TETRAHYDROPHTHALI-MIDE ◇ N-TRICHLOROMETHYLTHIO-3A,4,7,7A-TETRA-HYDROPHTHALIMIDE ◇ VANCIDE 89 ◇ VANGARD K ◇ VANICIDE ◇ VONDCAPTAN

TOXICITY DATA with REFERENCE
ETA: orl-mus TD:540 g/kg/80W-C NCITR* NCI-TR-15,77

NEO: orl-mus TDLo:1075 g/kg/80W-C NCITR* NCI-TR-15,77

MUT: cyt-hmn:lng 10 mg/L ANYAA9 160,344,69

MUT: dns-hmn:fbr 1 μmol/L MUREAV 42,161,77

MUT: mmo-sat 310 ng/plate MUREAV 130,79,84

MUT: oms-ctl:lvr 1 mmol/L CBINA8 56,289,85

MUT: oms-hmn:lym 1 mg/L CYGEDX 17(1),29,82

MUT: sce-hmn:lym 30 μmol/L MUREAV 79,53,80

CONSENSUS REPORTS: IARC Cancer Review: GROUP 3 IMEMDT 7,56,87; Animal Limited Evidence IMEMDT 30,295,83. NCI Carcinogenesis Bioassay (feed); Clear Evidence: mouse NCITR* NCI-CG-TR-15,77; No Evidence: rat NCITR* NCI-CG-TR-15,77. EPA Genetic Toxicology Program. Community Right-To-Know List. Reported in EPA TSCA Inventory.

OSHA PEL: TWA 5 mg/m³ ACGIH TLV: TWA 5 mg/m³ DOT Classification: ORM-E; Label; None.

SAFETY PROFILE: Questionable carcinogen with experimental tumorigenic, neoplastigenic, and teratogenic data. Moderately toxic to humans by ingestion. Moderately toxic experimentally by ingestion, inhalation, and intraperitoneal routes. Experimental reproductive effects. Human mutation data reported. When heated to decomposition it emits toxic fumes of Cl⁻, SO_x, and NO_x.

CBJ000   CAS: 121-59-5
N-CARBAMOYLARSANILIC ACID
mf: $C_7H_9AsN_2O_4$ mw: 260.10

PROP: White, nearly odorless powder; slt acid taste; sol in alc and water. Mp: 174°.

SYNS: AMABEVAN ◇ AMEBAN ◇ AMEBARSONE ◇ AMIBIARSON ◇ AMINARSON ◇ AMINARSONE ◇ AMINOARSON ◇ (4-((AMINOCARBONYL)AMINO)PHE-NYL)ARSONIC ACID ◇ ARSAMBIDE ◇ p-ARSONOPHE-NYLUREA ◇ p-CARBAMIDOBENZENEARSONIC ACID ◇ p-CARBAMINO PHENYL ARSONIC ACID ◇ CARBAMINO-PHENYL-p-ARSONIC ACID ◇ 4-CARBAMYLAMINOPHE-NYLARSONIC ACID ◇ N-CARBAMYL ARSANILIC ACID ◇ CARBARSONE (USDA) ◇ CARBASONE ◇ FEN-ARSONE ◇ HISTOCARB ◇ LEUCARSONE ◇ p-UREIDOBEN-ZENEARSONIC ACID ◇ 4-UREIDO-1-PHENYLARSONIC ACID

TOXICITY DATA with REFERENCE
ETA: orl-rat TDLo:5000 mg/kg CNREA8 26,619,66

CONSENSUS REPORTS: Arsenic and its compounds are on the Community Right-To-Know List.

OSHA PEL: TWA 10 μmg/m³ ACGIH TLV: TWA 0.2 mg(As)/m³

SAFETY PROFILE: Questionable carcinogen with experimental tumorigenic data. Poison by ingestion. Moderately toxic by intraperitoneal route. When heated to decomposition it emits very toxic fumes of As and NO_x.

CBK000   CAS: 817-99-2
N-(CARBAMOYLMETHYL)-2-DIAZOACETAMIDE
mf: $C_4H_6N_4O_2$ mw: 142.14

SYNS: N-(2-AMINO-2-OXOETHYL)-2-DIAZOACETAMIDE ◇ N-DIAZOACETILGLICINA-AMIDE (ITALIAN) ◇ DIAZO-ACETYLGLYCINAMIDE ◇ N-(DIAZOACETYL)GLYCINAM-IDE ◇ DIAZOACETYLGLYCINE AMIDE ◇ N-DIAZOACETYL-GLYCINE AMIDE

TOXICITY DATA with REFERENCE
CAR: ipr-mus TDLo:720 mg/kg/4D-I BSIBAC 45,227,69

MUT: dnd-mus:fbr 620 μmol/L TOLED5 1,115,77

MUT: dnd-rat-ipr 3700 μg/kg BSIBAC 57,414,81

MUT: dni-mus/ast 1500 mg/kg BCPCA6 23,289,74

MUT: mma-sat 10 μg/plate PNASA6 72,5135,75

MUT: mmo-sat 10 μg/plate AMACCQ 6,655,74

CONSENSUS REPORTS: EPA Genetic Toxicology Program.

SAFETY PROFILE: Questionable carcinogen with experimental carcinogenic data. Moderately toxic by intraperitoneal route. Mutation data reported. When heated to decomposition it emits toxic fumes of NO_x.

CBL000   CAS: 103-03-7
1-CARBAMYL-2-PHENYL HYDRAZINE
mf: $C_7H_9N_3O$ mw: 151.19

PROP: Crystals. Mp: 172°.

SYNS: 1-CARBAMYL-2-PHENYLHYDRAZINE ◇ CPH ◇ CRYOGENINE ◇ KRYOGENIN ◇ 2-PHENYLDIAZENECARBOXAMIDE ◇ 2-PHENYLHYDRAZIDE, CARBAMIC ACID ◇ 1-PHENYLHYDRAZINE CARBOXAMIDE ◇ 2-PHENYLHYDRAZINECARBOXAMIDE ◇ PHENYLSEMICARBAZIDE ◇ 1-PHENYLSEMICARBAZIDE

TOXICITY DATA with REFERENCE
NEO: orl-mus TDLo:394 mg/kg/62W-C
    JNCIAM 52,241,74
MUT: dnd-esc 250 µg/well   MUREAV 133,161,84

CONSENSUS REPORTS: IARC Cancer Review: GROUP 3 IMEMDT 7,56,87; Animal Limited Evidence IMEMDT 12,177,76. Reported in EPA TSCA Inventory.

SAFETY PROFILE: Questionable carcinogen with experimental carcinogenic and neoplastigenic data. Poison by intraperitoneal route. Mutation data reported. When heated to decomposition it emits toxic fumes of NO_x.

CBL750   CAS: 101-99-5
CARBANILIC ACID ETHYL ESTER
mf: $C_9H_{11}NO_2$ mw: 165.21

PROP: Crystals. Mp: 53°, bp: 238° (slt decomp), d: 1.106.

SYNS: EPC (the plant regulator) ◇ ETHYL CARBANILATE ◇ ETHYL-N-PHENYLCARBAMATE ◇ EUPHORIN ◇ KEIMSTOP ◇ PHENYLETHYL CARBAMATE ◇ PHENYLURETHAN ◇ PHENYLURETHAN(E) ◇ N-PHENYLURETHANE

TOXICITY DATA with REFERENCE
NEO: skn-mus TD:72 g/kg/15W-I   BJCAAI
    10,363,56
NEO: skn-mus TDLo:20 g/kg/2W-I   BJCAAI
    9,177,55
MUT: cyt-smc 12 mmol/tube   HEREAY 33,457,47

CONSENSUS REPORTS: Reported in EPA TSCA Inventory.

SAFETY PROFILE: Questionable carcinogen with experimental neoplastigenic data. Poison by intraperitoneal and intravenous routes. Moderately toxic by subcutaneous, and possibly other routes. Mutation data reported. When heated to decomposition it emits toxic fumes of NO_x.

CBM000   CAS: 122-42-9
CARBANILIC ACID ISOPROPYL ESTER
mf: $C_{10}H_{13}NO_2$ mw: 179.24

PROP: A white, crystalline solid; sol in acetone and benzene. Mp: 90°.

SYNS: BAN-HOE ◇ BEET-KLEEN ◇ CHEM-HOE ◇ IFC ◇ IPPC ◇ ISOPROPIL-N-FENIL-CARBAMMATO (ITALIAN) ◇ ISOPROPYL CARBANILATE ◇ ISOPROPYL CARBANILIC ACID ESTER ◇ ISOPROPYL-N-FENYL-CARBAMAAT (DUTCH) ◇ ISOPROPYL-N-PHENYL-CARBAMAT (GERMAN) ◇ ISOPROPYL PHENYLCARBAMATE ◇ ISOPROPYL-N-PHENYLCARBAMATE ◇ o-ISOPROPYL-N-PHENYL CARBAMATE ◇ ISOPROPYL-N-PHENYLURETHAN (GERMAN) ◇ ORTHO GRASS KILLER ◇ N-PHENYLCARBAMATE D'ISOPROPYLE (FRENCH) ◇ PHENYLCARBAMIC ACID-1-METHYLETHEL ESTER ◇ N-PHENYL ISOPROPYL CARBAMATE ◇ PREMALOX ◇ PROFAM ◇ PROPHAM ◇ TRIHERBIDE ◇ TRIHERBIDE-IPC ◇ TUBERIT ◇ TUBERITE ◇ USAF D-9 ◇ Y 2

TOXICITY DATA with REFERENCE
NEO: orl-mus TDLo:6 g/kg/10W-I   BJCAAI
    12,355,58
MUT: cyt-omi 550 µmol/L   JCLBA3 63,84,74
MUT: sce-hmn:lym 2 mg/L   MUREAV 147,296,85

CONSENSUS REPORTS: IARC Cancer Review: Animal Inadequate Evidence IMEMDT 12,189,76. Reported in EPA TSCA Inventory. EPA Genetic Toxicology Program.

SAFETY PROFILE: Questionable carcinogen with experimental neoplastigenic and teratogenic data. Poison by intraperitoneal route. Moderately toxic to humans by ingestion. Moderately toxic experimentally by ingestion and possibly other routes. Human mutation data reported. An herbicide. When heated to decomposition it emits toxic fumes of NO_x.

CBM750   CAS: 63-25-2
CARBARYL
mf: $C_{12}H_{11}NO_2$ mw: 201.24

PROP: White crystals. Mp: 142°, d: 1.232 @ 20°/20°.

SYNS: CARBATOX-60 ◇ CRAG SEVIN ◇ ENT 23,969 ◇ EXPERIMENTAL INSECTICIDE 7744 ◇ KARBARYL (POLISH) ◇ N-METHYLCARBAMATE de 1-NAPHTYLE (FRENCH)

◇ METHYLCARBAMATE-1-NAPHTHALENOL ◇ METHYL-CARBAMATE-1-NAPHTHOL ◇ METHYLCARBAMIC ACID-1-NAPHTHYL ESTER ◇ N-METHYL-1-NAFTYL-CARBA-MAAT (DUTCH) ◇ N-METHYL-1-NAPHTHYL-CARBAMAT (GERMAN) ◇ N-METHYL-α-NAPHTHYLCARBAMATE ◇ N-METHYL-1-NAPHTHYL CARBAMATE ◇ N-METHYL-α-NAPHTHYLURETHAN ◇ N-METIL-1-NAFTIL-CARBAM-MATO (ITALIAN) ◇ α-NAFTYL-N-METHYLKARBAMAT (CZECH) ◇ 1-NAPHTHOL-N-METHYLCARBAMATE ◇ 1-NAPHTHYL METHYLCARBAMATE ◇ α-NAPHTHYL N-METHYLCARBAMATE ◇ 1-NAPHTHYL-N-METHYLCARBA-MATE ◇ SEVIN

TOXICITY DATA with REFERENCE

ETA: orl-rat TDLo: 5640 mg/kg/94W-I VPITAR 29,71,70

CAR: imp-rat TDLo: 80 mg/kg VPITAR 29,71,70

MUT: cyt-ham: fbr 30 mg/L/48H MUREAV 48,337,77

MUT: cyt-hmn: emb 40 μg/kg ZDVKAP20(4),14,77

MUT: dns-hmn: fbr 1 μmol/L MUREAV 42,161,77

MUT: mma-hmn: fbr 1 μmol/L MUREAV 42,161,77

MUT: mma-sat 100 μmol/L ARTODN 39,159,77

MUT: mmo-sat 250 μg/plate RPZHAW 30,81,79

MUT: sln-dmg-orl 1 pph/24H SOGEBZ 8,151,72

MUT: spm-mus-ipr 1 mmol/L BSRSA6 45,46,76

MUT: spm-mus-orl 1 mmol/L BSRSA6 45,46,76

CONSENSUS REPORTS: IARC Cancer Review: Animal Inadequate Evidence IMEMDT 12,37,76. Community Right-To-Know List.

OSHA PEL: TWA 5 mg/m³ ACGIH TLV: TWA 5 mg/m³ DFG MAK: 5 mg/m³ NIOSH REL: TWA 5 mg/m³ DOT Classification: ORM-A; Label: None.

SAFETY PROFILE: Questionable carcinogen with experimental carcinogenic, tumorigenic, and teratogenic data. Poison by ingestion, intravenous, intraperitoneal, and possibly other routes. Human systemic effects by ingestion: sensory change involving peripheral nerve, muscle weakness. Human mutation data reported. Experimental reproductive effects. An eye and severe skin irritant. Absorbed by all routes, although skin absorption is slow. No accumulation in tissue. Symptoms include blurred vision, headache, stomach ache, vomiting. Symptoms similar to but less severe than those due to parathion. A reversible cholinesterase inhibitor. When heated to decomposition it emits toxic fumes of NO_x.

CBN000 CAS: 86-74-8
CARBAZOLE
mf: $C_{12}H_9N$ mw: 167.22

PROP: White crystals. Mp: 244.8°, bp: 354.8°, d: 1.10 @ 18°/4°, vap press: 400 mm @ 323.0°.

SYNS: 9-AZAFLUORENE ◇ 9H-CARBAZOLE ◇ DIBENZO-PYRROLE ◇ DIBENZO(b,d)PYRROLE ◇ DIPHENYLENEI-MINE ◇ DIPHENYLENIMIDE ◇ DIPHENYLENIMINE ◇ USAF EK-600

CONSENSUS REPORTS: IARC Cancer Review: GROUP 3 IMEMDT 7,56,87; Animal Limited Evidence IMEMDT 32,239,83. Reported in EPA TSCA Inventory.

SAFETY PROFILE: Questionable carcinogen. Poison by intraperitoneal route. Moderately toxic by ingestion. A pesticide. When heated to decomposition it emits toxic fumes of NO_x.

CBP250 CAS: 21600-51-1
1(4-CARBETHOXYPHENYL)-3,3-DIMETHYLTRIAZENE
mf: $C_{11}H_{15}N_3O_2$ mw: 221.29

SYNS: 1-(p-CARBOXYAETHYLPHENYL)-3,3-DIMETHYL-TRIAZEN (GERMAN) ◇ 1-(p-ETHYLCARBOXYPHENYL)-3,3-DIMETHYLTRIAZENE

TOXICITY DATA with REFERENCE

CAR: ivn-rat TDLo: 805 mg/kg/23W-I ARZNAD 23,800,73

CAR: scu-rat TDLo: 760 mg/kg/19W-I ARZNAD 23,800,73

ETA: scu-mus TDLo: 760 mg/kg/19W-I ARZNAD 23,800,73

MUT: hma-mus/smc 1 mmol/L CBINA8 9,365,74

MUT: mrc-smc 10 mmol/L CBINA8 9,365,74

MUT: sln-dmg-orl 1 mmol/L CBINA8 9,365,74

CONSENSUS REPORTS: EPA Genetic Toxicology Program.

SAFETY PROFILE: Questionable carcinogen with experimental carcinogenic and tumorigenic data. Poison by intravenous route. Moderately toxic by subcutaneous route. Mutation data reported. When heated to decomposition it emits toxic fumes of NO_x.

CBT750 CAS: 1333-86-4
CARBON BLACK

PROP: A generic term applied to a family of high-purity colloidal carbons commercially produced by carefully controlled pyrolysis of gaseous or liquid hydrocarbons. Carbon blacks, including commercial colloidal carbons such as furnace blacks, lamp blacks and acetylene blacks, usually contain less than several tenths percent of extractable organic matter and less than one percent ash.

SYNS: ACETYLENE BLACK ◊ CHANNEL BLACK ◊ FURNACE BLACK ◊ LAMP BLACK

CONSENSUS REPORTS: IARC Cancer Review: GROUP 3 IMEMDT 7,142,87; Human Inadequate Evidence IMEMDT 33,35,84; Animal Inadequate Evidence IMEMDT 33,35,84

OSHA PEL: TWA 3.5 mg/m^3 ACGIH TLV: TWA 3.5 mg/m^3 NIOSH REL: TWA 3.5 mg/m^3

SAFETY PROFILE: Questionable carcinogen. Mildly toxic by ingestion, inhalation, and skin contact. A nuisance dust in high concentrations. While it is true that the tiny particulates of carbon black contain some molecules of carcinogenic materials, the carcinogens are apparently held tightly and are not eluted by hot or cold water, gastric juices, or blood plasma.

CCE500   CAS: 493-52-7
2-CARBOXY-4′-(DIMETHYLAMINO) AZOBENZENE
mf: $C_{15}H_{15}N_3O_2$ mw: 269.33

PROP: Shiny violet crystals.

SYNS: C.I. 13020 ◊ C.I. ACID RED 2 ◊ p-(DIMETHYL-AMINO)AZOBENZENE-o-CARBOXYLIC ACID ◊ 4′-DI-METHYLAMINOAZOBENZENE-2-CARBOXYLIC ACID ◊ o-((p-(DIMETHYLAMINO)PHENYL)AZO)BENZOIC ACID ◊ 2-((4-DIMETHYLAMINO)PHENYLAZO)BENZOIC ACID ◊ METHYL RED

TOXICITY DATA with REFERENCE
ETA: orl-rat TDLo: 12 g/kg/57W-C   BJCAAI 9,310,55
MUT: dnr-bcs 2 mg/disc   TRENAF 27,153,76
MUT: dns-rat: lvr 10 μmol/L   CNREA8 46,1654,86
MUT: mma-sat 50 μg/plate   MUREAV 56,249,78

CONSENSUS REPORTS: IARC Cancer Review: Animal Inadequate Evidence IMEMDT 8,161,75. Reported in EPA TSCA Inventory. EPA Genetic Toxicology Program.

SAFETY PROFILE: Questionable carcinogen with experimental tumorigenic data. Mutation data reported. When heated to decomposition it emits toxic fumes of NO$_x$.

CCE750   CAS: 20691-84-3
3′-CARBOXY-4-DIMETHYLAMINOAZOBENZENE
mf: $C_{15}H_{15}N_3O_2$ mw: 269.33

SYN: 3-((p-(DIMETHYLAMINO)PHENYL)AZO)BENZOIC ACID

TOXICITY DATA with REFERENCE
ETA: orl-rat TDLo: 12 g/kg/57W-C   BJCAAI 9,310,55
MUT: dns-rat: lvr 10 μmol/L   CNREA8 46,1654,86
MUT: mma-sat 1 μmol/plate   CRNGDP 1,121,80

SAFETY PROFILE: Questionable carcinogen with experimental tumorigenic data. Moderately toxic by ingestion. Mutation data reported. When heated to decomposition it emits toxic fumes of NO$_x$.

CCF250   CAS: 4033-46-9
3-((2-CARBOXYETHYL)THIO)ALANINE
mf: $C_6H_{11}NO_4S$ mw: 193.24

SYN: S-2-CARBOXYETHYL-1-CYSTEINE

TOXICITY DATA with REFERENCE
ETA: scu-rat TDLo: 520 mg/kg/52W-I   BJCAAI 15,85,61

SAFETY PROFILE: Questionable carcinogen with experimental tumorigenic data. When heated to decomposition it emits very toxic fumes of SO$_x$ and NO$_x$.

CCF750   CAS: 13442-14-3
6-CARBOXYL-4-HYDROXYLAMINOQUINOLINE-1-OXIDE
mf: $C_{10}H_8N_2O_4$ mw: 220.20

SYN: 4-(HYDROXYAMINO)-6-QUINOLINECARBOXYLIC ACID-1-OXIDE

TOXICITY DATA with REFERENCE
ETA: scu-mus TDLo: 120 mg/kg/50D-I   BCPCA6 16,631,67

SAFETY PROFILE: Questionable carcinogen with experimental tumorigenic data. When heated to decomposition it emits toxic fumes of NO$_x$.

CCG000   CAS: 1425-67-8
6-CARBOXYL-4-NITROQUINOLINE-1-OXIDE
mf: $C_{10}H_6N_2O_5$ mw: 234.18

SYNS: 6-CARBOXY-4-NITROQUINOLINE-1-OXIDE ◊ 4-NITROQUINOLINE-6-CARBOXYLIC ACID-1-OXIDE ◊ 4-NITRO-6-QUINOLINECARBOXYLIC ACID-1-OXIDE

TOXICITY DATA with REFERENCE
ETA: scu-mus TDLo: 120 mg/kg/50D-I   BCPCA6 16,631,67
ETA: scu-rat TDLo: 90 mg/kg/20W-I   GANNA2 58,397,67

MUT: dnd-mam:lym 5 mg   BIPMAA 4,409,66
MUT: dnd-mus:fbr 100 μmol/L   CNREA8 35,521,75
MUT: dns-ham:oth 4 μmol/L   NATUAS 229,416,71
MUT: mmo-esc 500 μg/plate   CNREA8 32,2369,72
MUT: mmo-smc 100 mg/L   IGSBAL 85,127,72
MUT: mrc-esc 500 μg/well   CNREA8 32,2369,72

CONSENSUS REPORTS: EPA Genetic Toxicology Program.

SAFETY PROFILE: Questionable carcinogen with experimental tumorigenic data. Mutation data reported. When heated to decomposition it emits toxic fumes of NO$_x$.

CCH000   CAS: 9086-60-6
CARBOXYMETHYLCELLULOSE NORDIC

SYNS: AMMONIUM CARBOXYMETHYL CELLULOSE ◇ CARBOXYMETHYL CELLULOSE, AMMONIUM SALT

TOXICITY DATA with REFERENCE
NEO: scu-rat TDLo: 6600 mg/kg/73W-I   RCBIAS 20,701,61

CONSENSUS REPORTS: Reported in EPA TSCA Inventory.

SAFETY PROFILE: Questionable carcinogen with experimental neoplastigenic data. When heated to decomposition it emits toxic fumes of NO$_x$ and NH$_3$.

CCH500
CARBOXYMETHYLNITROSOUREA
mf: C$_3$H$_5$N$_3$O$_4$ mw: 147.11

TOXICITY DATA with REFERENCE
NEO: orl-rat TDLo: 4 g/kg/74W-I   JJIND8 62,1523,79

SAFETY PROFILE: Questionable carcinogen with experimental neoplastigenic data. Poison by intraperitoneal route. When heated to decomposition it emits toxic fumes of NO$_x$.

CCJ375
3-CARBOXYPROPYL(2-PROPENYL) NITROSAMINE
mf: C$_7$H$_{12}$N$_2$O$_3$ mw: 172.21

SYN: 4-(ALLYLNITROSOAMINO)BUTRIC ACID

TOXICITY DATA with REFERENCE
CAR: scu-ham TDLo: 23100 mg/kg/77W-I
    CDPRD4 4,79,81

SAFETY PROFILE: Questionable carcinogen with experimental carcinogenic data. When heated to decomposition it emits toxic fumes of NO$_x$.

CCJ500   CAS: 19477-24-8
CARCINOLIPIN
mf: C$_{44}$H$_{78}$O$_2$ mw: 639.22

SYNS: CHOLESTERYL-14-METHYLHEXADECANOATE ◇ 3-β-14-METHYLHEXADECANOATE-CHOLEST-5-EN-3-OL

TOXICITY DATA with REFERENCE
ETA: scu-mus TDLo: 720 mg/kg/(14-21D preg)   NEOLA4 20,347,73

SAFETY PROFILE: Questionable carcinogen with experimental tumorigenic data. When heated to decomposition it emits acrid smoke and irritating fumes.

CCL250   CAS: 9000-07-1
CARRAGEEN

PROP: A sulfated polysaccharide. Dried plant of seaweed *Chondrus crispus, Chondrus ocellatus, Eucheuma cottonil, Eucheuma spinosum, Gigartina acicularis, Gigartina pistillata, Gigartina radula, Gigartina stellata.* Yellow-white when powdered. Sol in water @ 80°; insol in organic solvents. Dried, bleached *Chondrus crispus* containing salts of sulfated polygalactose esters.

SYNS: 3,6-ANHYDRO-d-GALACTAN ◇ AUBYGEL GS ◇ AUBYGUM DM ◇ BURTONITE-V-40-E ◇ CARASTAY ◇ CARASTAY G ◇ CARRAGEENAN (FCC) ◇ CARRAGEENAN GUM ◇ CARRAGHEANIN ◇ CARRAGHEEN ◇ CARRAGHEENAN ◇ CHONDRUS ◇ CHONDRUS EXTRACT ◇ COLLOID 775 ◇ COREINE ◇ EUCHEUMA SPINOSUM GUM ◇ FLANOGEN ELA ◇ GALOZONE ◇ GELCARIN ◇ GELCARIN HMR ◇ GELOZONE ◇ GENU ◇ GENUGEL ◇ GENUGEL CJ ◇ GENUGOL RLV ◇ GENUVISCO J ◇ GUM CARRAGEENAN ◇ GUM CHON 2 ◇ GUM CHROND ◇ IRISH GUM ◇ IRISH MOSS EXTRACT ◇ IRISH MOSS GELOSE ◇ KILLEEN ◇ LYGOMME CDS ◇ PEARLPUSS ◇ PELLUGEL ◇ PENCOGEL ◇ PIG-WRACK ◇ SATIAGEL GS350 ◇ SATIAGUM 3 ◇ SATIAGUM STANDARD ◇ SEAKEM CARRAGEENIN ◇ SEATREM ◇ SELF ROCK MOSS ◇ VISCARIN

TOXICITY DATA with REFERENCE
NEO: scu-rat TDLo: 525 mg/kg/21W-I   13BYAH -,83,62
ETA: orl-rat TDLo: 2100 g/kg/40W-C   CNREA8 38,4427,78

ETA: par-rat TDLo: 430 mg/kg   BJCAAI 15,607,61
ETA: par-rat TD: 320 mg/kg   OYYAA2 32,711,86

CONSENSUS REPORTS: IARC Cancer Review: GROUP 3 IMEMDT 7,56,87; Animal Limited Evidence IMEMDT 10,181,76. Reported in EPA TSCA Inventory.

SAFETY PROFILE: Questionable carcinogen with experimental neoplastigenic and tumorigenic data. Poison by intravenous route. When heated to decomposition it emits acrid smoke and fumes.

CCL350   CAS: 11114-20-8
kappa-CARRAGEENAN

SYNS: kappa-CARRAGEEN ◇ kappa-CARRAGEENIN ◇ SATIAGEL GS 350

TOXICITY DATA with REFERENCE
ETA: par-rat TDLo: 320 mg/kg   OYYAA2 32,711,86

SAFETY PROFILE: Questionable carcinogen with experimental tumorigenic data. Poison by ingestion. When heated to decomposition it emits acrid smoke and irritating fumes.

CCP850   CAS: 120-80-9
CATECHOL
mf: $C_6H_6O_2$ mw: 110.12

PROP: Colorless crystals. Mp: 105°, bp: 246°, flash p: 261°F (CC), d: 1.341 @ 15°, vap press: 10 mm @ 118.3°, vap d: 3.79. Sol in water, chloroform, and benzene; very sol in alc and ether.

SYNS: o-BENZENEDIOL ◇ 1,2-BENZENEDIOL ◇ CATECHIN ◇ C.I. 76500 ◇ C.I. OXIDATION BASE 26 ◇ o-DIHYDROXYBENZENE ◇ 1,2-DIHYDROXYBENZENE ◇ o-DIOXYBENZENE ◇ o-DIPHENOL ◇ DURAFUR DEVELOPER C ◇ FOURAMINE PCH ◇ FOURRINE 68 ◇ o-HYDROQUINONE ◇ o-HYDROXYPHENOL ◇ 2-HYDROXYPHENOL ◇ NCI-C55856 ◇ OXYPHENIC ACID ◇ PELAGOL GREY C ◇ o-PHENYLENEDIOL ◇ PYROCATECHIN ◇ PYROCATECHINIC ACID ◇ PYROCATECHOL ◇ PYROCATECHUIC ACID

TOXICITY DATA with REFERENCE
MUT: dni-hmn: hla 200 μmol/L   MUREAV 92,427,82
MUT: dns-rat-orl 1 g/kg   JJIND8 74,1283,85
MUT: mma-sat 4 μg/plate   ABCHA6 45,327,81
MUT: mrc-smc 300 mg/L   MUREAV 135,109,84
MUT: oms-rbt: bmr 2 mmol/L   AJIMD8 7,485,85

CONSENSUS REPORTS: IARC Cancer Review: GROUP 3 IMEMDT 7,56,87; Animal

Inadequate Evidence IMEMDT 15,155,77. EPA Extremely Hazardous Substances List. Reported in EPA TSCA Inventory. EPA Genetic Toxicology Program.

OSHA PEL: TWA 5 ppm (skin)   ACGIH TLV: TWA 5 ppm

SAFETY PROFILE: Questionable carcinogen. Poison by ingestion, subcutaneous, intraperitoneal, intravenous, parenteral and possibly other routes. Moderately toxic by skin contact. Human mutation data reported. Experimental reproductive effects. Can cause dermatitis on skin contact. An allergen. Combustible when exposed to heat or flame; can react vigorously with oxidizing materials. To fight fire, use water, CO_2, dry chemical. When heated to decomposition it emits acrid smoke and irritating fumes.

CCT250   CAS: 9005-81-6
CELLOPHANE
mf: $(C_6H_{10}O_5)_n$

SYN: VISKING CELLOPHANE

TOXICITY DATA with REFERENCE
ETA: imp-mus TDLo: 720 mg/kg   CNREA8 15,333,55
ETA: imp-rat TD: 4200 mg/kg   PSEBAA 67,33,48
ETA: imp-rat TDLo: 18 mg/kg   CNREA8 15,333,55

CONSENSUS REPORTS: Reported in EPA TSCA Inventory.

SAFETY PROFILE: Questionable carcinogen with experimental tumorigenic data by implant. When heated to decomposition it emits acrid smoke and irritating fumes.

CDL325   CAS: 474-25-9
CHENODESOXYCHOLIC ACID
mf: $C_{24}H_{40}O_4$ mw: 392.64

PROP: Needles from ethyl acetate + heptane. Mp: 119°. Freely sol in methanol, alc, acetone, acetic acid; more sol in ether and ethyl acetate than deoxycholic acid. Practically insol in water, petr ether, benzene. Forms beautiful crystalline salts of Na, K and Ba. While the acid is tasteless, the Na salt tastes slightly sweet at first, then bitter.

SYNS: ANTHROPODEOXYCHOLIC ACID ◇ ANTHROPODESOXYCHOLIC ACID ◇ ANTHROPODODESOXYCHOLIC ACID ◇ CDC ◇ CDCA ◇ CHENDAL ◇ CHENDOL ◇ CHENIC ACID ◇ CHENIX ◇ CHENOCEDON ◇ CHENODE-

OXYCHOLIC ACID ◇ CHENODESOXYCHOLSAEURE (GER-MAN) ◇ CHENODEX ◇ CHENODIOL ◇ CHENOFALK ◇ CHENOSAURE ◇ CHENOSSIL ◇ CHOLANORM ◇ 3-α,7-α-DIHYDROXYCHOLANIC ACID ◇ 3-α,7-α-DIHY-DROXY-5-β-CHOLAN-24-OIC ACID ◇ FLUIBIL ◇ GALLO-DESOXYCHOLIC ACID ◇ HEKBILIN ◇ KEBILIS ◇ ULMEN-IDE

TOXICITY DATA with REFERENCE
CAR: orl-wmn TDLo:24 g/kg/5Y-C   CLONEA 7,245,81
MUT: mmo-sat 20 mg/L   MUREAV 158,45,85
MUT: sln-smc 100 mg/L   CRNGDP 5,447,84

SAFETY PROFILE: Questionable human carcinogen producing liver tumors. Poison by intravenous and intraperitoneal routes. Moderately toxic by ingestion. An experimental teratogen. Experimental reproductive effects. Mutation data reported. When heated to decomposition it emits acrid smoke and fumes.

CDL750
CHERRY BARK OAK

PROP: Tannin containing fraction of bark used (JNCIAM 57,207,76)

SYNS: QUERCUS FALCATA PAGODAEFOLIA ◇ TANNIN from CHERRY BARK OAK

TOXICITY DATA with REFERENCE
NEO: scu-rat TDLo:720 mg/kg/45W-I   JNCIAM 57,207,76

SAFETY PROFILE: Questionable carcinogen with experimental neoplastigenic data. When heated to decomposition it emits acrid and irritating fumes.

CDM250   CAS: 1401-55-4
CHESTNUT TANNIN

SYNS: CASTANEA SATIVA MILL TANNIN ◇ TANNIN from CHESTNUT

TOXICITY DATA with REFERENCE
ETA: scu-mus TDLo:750 mg/kg/12W-I   BJCAAI 14,147,60

SAFETY PROFILE: Questionable carcinogen with experimental tumorigenic data. Poison by subcutaneous, intramuscular, intravenous and intraperitoneal routes. When heated to decomposition it emits acrid and irritating fumes.

CDN000   CAS: 53-19-0
CHLODITHANE
mf: $C_{14}H_{10}Cl_4$ mw: 320.04

SYNS: CHLODITAN ◇ 1-CHLORO-2-(2,2-DICHLORO-1-(4-CHLOROPHENYL)ETHYL)BENZENE ◇ 2-(o-CHLOROPHE-NYL)-2-(p-CHLOROPHENYL)-1,1-DICHLOROETHANE ◇ o,p′-DDD ◇ 2,4′-DDD ◇ 1,1-DICHLORO-2,2-BIS(2,4′-DI-CHLOROPHENYL)ETHANE ◇ 1,1-DICHLORO-2-(o-CHLORO-PHENYL)-2-(p-CHLOROPHENYL)ETHANE ◇ o,p′-DICHLORODIPHENYLDICHLOROETHANE ◇ 2,4′-DICHLO-ROPHENYLDICHLOROETHANE ◇ MITOTANE ◇ NCI-C04933 ◇ NSC 38721 ◇ o,p-TDE ◇ o,p′-TDE

TOXICITY DATA with REFERENCE
ETA: ipr-rat TDLo:2500 mg/kg/7W-I:TER
    CANCAR 40(Suppl 4),1935,77
ETA: ipr-mus TDLo:9750 mg/kg/26W-I
    CANCAR 40(Suppl 4),1935,77
ETA: orl-rat TDLo:10 g/kg/52W-C   BAFEAG 52,89,65
MUT: cyt-rat:oth 10 μg/L   34LXAP -,555,76

CONSENSUS REPORTS: NCI Carcinogenesis Studies (ipr); Equivocal Evidence: mouse, rat CANCAR 40,1935,77. EPA Genetic Toxicology Program.

SAFETY PROFILE: Questionable carcinogen with experimental carcinogenic, tumorigenic, and teratogenic data. Human systemic effects by ingestion: somnolence, blood pressure depression, diarrhea, nausea or vomiting, normocytic anemia (decrease in the number of red blood cells), and pigmented or nucleated red blood cells. Other experimental reproductive effects. Mutation data reported. When heated to decomposition it emits toxic fumes of Cl⁻.

CDN500   CAS: 107-14-2
CHLORACETONITRILE
DOT: 2668
mf: C_2H_2ClN mw: 75.50

SYNS: CHLOROACETONITRILE (DOT) ◇ α-CHLOROACE-TONITRILE ◇ 2-CHLOROACETONITRILE ◇ CHLOROME-THYL CYANIDE ◇ MONOCHLOROACETONITRILE ◇ MONOCHLOROMETHYL CYANIDE ◇ USAF KF-5

TOXICITY DATA with REFERENCE
CAR: skn-mus TDLo:4800 mg/kg/2W-I
    FAATDF 5,1065,85
MUT: dnd-hmn:lym 50 μmol/L   AIHAAP 23,95,62
MUT: sce-ham:ovr 79100 nmol/L   FAATDF 5,1065,85

CONSENSUS REPORTS: Reported in EPA TSCA Inventory. Cyanide and its compounds are on the Community Right-To-Know List.

DOT Classification: Poison B; Label: Flammable Liquid and Poison.

SAFETY PROFILE: Questionable carcinogen with experimental tumorigenic data. Poison by ingestion, skin contact, and intraperitoneal route. Moderately toxic by inhalation. A skin irritant. Human mutation data reported. When heated to decomposition it emits very toxic fumes of Cl^-, NO_x, and CN^-.

CDO000   CAS: 302-17-0
CHLORAL HYDRATE
mf: $C_2HCl_3O \cdot H_2O$ mw: 165.40

PROP: Transparent, colorless crystals; aromatic, penetrating, sltly acrid odor and sltly bitter, caustic taste. Mp: 52°, bp: 97.5°, d: 1.9.

SYNS: AQUACHLORAL ◇ Bi 3411 ◇ CHLORALDURAT ◇ DORMAL ◇ FELSULES ◇ HYDRAL ◇ HYDRAL de CHLO-RAL ◇ KESSODRATE ◇ LORINAL ◇ NOCTEC ◇ NORTEC ◇ NYCOTON ◇ PHALDRONE ◇ RECTULES ◇ SK-CHORAL HYDRATE ◇ SOMNI SED ◇ SOMNOS ◇ SONTEC ◇ TOSYL ◇ TRAWOTOX ◇ TRICHLORACETALDEHYD-HYDRAT (GERMAN) ◇ TRICHLOROACETALDEHYDE HY-DRATE ◇ TRICHLOROACETALDEHYDE MONOHYDRATE ◇ 2,2,2-TRICHLORO-1,1-ETHANEDIOL

TOXICITY DATA with REFERENCE
CAR: orl-mus TDLo: 10 mg/kg   CDPRD4 9,279,86
ETA: skn-mus TDLo: 960 mg/kg/1W-I   BJCAAI 9,177,55
MUT: mma-sat 1 mg/plate   ENMUDM 5(Suppl 1),3,83
MUT: mmo-asn 5 mg/plate   CBINA8 30,9,80
MUT: mmo-sat 1 mg/plate   ENMUDM 5(Suppl 1),3,83
MUT: mrc-smc 15 mmol/L   MUREAV 141,19,84
MUT: sce-hmn: lym 54 mg/L   AGTQAH 24,105,81
MUT: sln-asn 5 mmol/L   MUREAV 155,105,85

CONSENSUS REPORTS: Reported in EPA TSCA Inventory. EPA Genetic Toxicology Program.

SAFETY PROFILE: Questionable carcinogen with experimental carcinogenic and tumorigenic data by skin contact. A human poison by ingestion and possibly other routes. Poison experimentally by ingestion, intravenous, and rectal routes. Moderately toxic by subcutaneous, parenteral, and intraperitoneal routes. Human systemic effects by ingestion: general anesthetic; cardiac arrythmias, blood pressure depression. Human mutation data reported. A sedative, anesthetic, and narcotic. Combustible when exposed to heat or flame. When heated to decomposition it emits toxic fumes of Cl^-.

CDT750   CAS: 96-24-2
CHLORHYDRIN
DOT: 2689
mf: $C_3H_7ClO_2$ mw: 110.55

PROP: Colorless liquid. Bp: 213° decomp, d: 1.326.

SYNS: α-CHLORHYDRIN ◇ CHLORODEOXYGLYCEROL ◇ 1-CHLORO-2,3-DIHYDROXYPROPANE ◇ 3-CHLORO-1,2-DIHYDROXYPROPANE ◇ α-CHLOROHYDRIN ◇ 1-CHLORO-PROPANE-2,3-DIOL ◇ 1-CHLORO-2,3-PROPANEDIOL ◇ 3-CHLOROPROPANE-1,2-DIOL ◇ 3-CHLORO-1,2-PRO-PANEDIOL ◇ 3-CHLOROPROPYLENE GYLCOL ◇ β,β'-DIHY-DROXYISOPROPYL CHLORIDE ◇ 2,3-DIHYDROXYPROPYL CHLORIDE ◇ EPIBLOC ◇ GLYCERIN-α-MONOCHLORHY-DRIN ◇ GLYCEROL CHLOROHYDRIN ◇ GLYCEROL-α-CHLOROHYDRIN ◇ GLYCEROL-α-MONOCHLOROHYDRIN (DOT) ◇ GLYCERYL-α-CHLOROHYDRIN ◇ MONOCHLO-RHYDRIN ◇ MONOCHLOROHYDRIN ◇ α-MONOCHLORO-HYDRIN ◇ U-5897

TOXICITY DATA with REFERENCE
ETA: orl-rat TDLo: 34580 mg/kg/72W-C   JJIND8 67,75,81
MUT: mma-ssp 300 mmol/L   MUREAV 118,213,83
MUT: mmo-ssp 100 mmol/L   MUREAV 118,213,83
MUT: msc-mus: lym 10 mmol/L   PAACA3 21,74,80
MUT: spm-rat-orl 600 mg/kg/24D-C   CUSCAM 44,193,75

CONSENSUS REPORTS: Reported in EPA TSCA Inventory. EPA Genetic Toxicology Program.

DOT Classification: Poison B; Label: St. Andrews Cross.

SAFETY PROFILE: Questionable carcinogen with experimental tumorigenic data. Poison by ingestion and intraperitoneal routes. Moderately toxic by inhalation. Experimental reproductive effects. Mutation data reported. An eye irritant. A chemosterilant for rodents. Combustible when exposed to heat or flame. When heated to decomposition it emits toxic fumes of Cl^-.

CDV575
CHLORINATED NAPHTHALENES

SAFETY PROFILE: Questionable carcinogens which can cause tumors of the liver. Severe irritants by ingestion, inhalation and skin contact. The action of the chlorinated naphthalenes on the body is quite similar to that of the chlorinated biphenyls. The chief effects being the production of chloracne of the skin, and systemically an acute yellow atrophy of the liver. When heated to decomposition they emit toxic fumes of Cl^-.

CEA000   CAS: 79-11-8
CHLOROACETIC ACID
mf: $C_2H_3ClO_2$ mw: 94.50
DOT: 1750/1751

PROP: Colorless crystals. Mp: (α) 63°, (β) 56°, (τ) 50°, bp: 189°, flash p: 259°F, d: 1.58 @ 20°/20°, vap d: 3.26.

SYNS: ACIDE CHLORACETIQUE (FRENCH) ◇ ACIDE MONOCHLORACETIQUE (FRENCH) ◇ ACIDOMONOCLORO-ACETICO (ITALIAN) ◇ CHLORACETIC ACID ◇ α-CHLORO-ACETIC ACID ◇ CHLOROACETIC ACID, LIQUID (DOT) ◇ CHLOROACETIC ACID, SOLID (DOT) ◇ CHLOROETHA-NOIC ACID ◇ MCA ◇ MONOCHLOORAZIJNZUUR (DUTCH) ◇ MONOCHLORACETIC ACID ◇ MONOCHLORESSIG-SAEURE (GERMAN) ◇ MONOCHLOROACETIC ACID ◇ MONOCHLOROETHANOIC ACID ◇ NCI-C60231

TOXICITY DATA with REFERENCE
ETA: scu-mus TD: 1300 mg/kg/65W-I   JNCIAM 53,695,74
ETA: scu-mus TDLo: 100 mg/kg   NTIS** PB223-159
MUT: mma-mus: lym 548 mg/L   MUREAV 97,49,82

CONSENSUS REPORTS: Reported in EPA TSCA Inventory. EPA Genetic Toxicology Program. EPA Extremely Hazardous Substances List. Community Right-To-Know List.

DOT Classification: Corrosive Material; Label: Corrosive, liquid, solution or solid.

SAFETY PROFILE: Questionable carcinogen with experimental tumorigenic data. Poison by ingestion, inhalation, subcutaneous, and intravenous route. A corrosive skin, eye, and mucous membrane irritant. Mutation data reported. Combustible liquid when exposed to heat or flame. To fight fire, use water spray, fog, mist, dry chemical, foam. When heated to decomposition it emits toxic fumes of Cl^-.

CEA750   CAS: 532-27-4
α-CHLOROACETOPHENONE
DOT: 1697
mf: C_8H_7ClO mw: 154.60

SYNS: CAF ◇ CAP ◇ CHEMICAL MACE ◇ 1-CHLOROACE-TOPHENONE ◇ omega-CHLOROACETOPHENONE ◇ CHLOROACETOPHENONE, gas, liquid or solid (DOT) ◇ CHLOROMETHYL PHENYL KETONE ◇ 2-CHLORO-1-PHE-NYLETHANONE ◇ CN ◇ MACE (lacrimator) ◇ NCI-C55107 ◇ PHENACYL CHLORIDE ◇ PHENYLCHLOROMETHYLKE-TONE

TOXICITY DATA with REFERENCE
NEO: skn-mus TDLo: 2400 mg/kg/27W-I
BJCAAI 7,482,53

CONSENSUS REPORTS: Reported in EPA TSCA Inventory. Community Right-To-Know List.

OSHA PEL: TWA 0.05 ppm   ACGIH TLV: TWA 0.05 ppm   DOT Classification: Irritating Material; Label: Irritant; Poison B; Label: Poison.

SAFETY PROFILE: Questionable carcinogen with experimental neoplastigenic data by skin contact. A human poison by inhalation. An experimental poison by ingestion, inhalation, intraperitoneal, and intravenous routes. Human systemic effects by inhalation: lacrimation, conjunctiva irritation, and unspecified eye effects, cough, and dyspnea. A severe eye and moderate skin irritant. A riot control agent. When heated to decomposition it emits toxic fumes of Cl^-.

CEG625   CAS: 6219-71-2
3-CHLORO-4-AMINOANILINE SULFATE
mf: $C_6H_5ClN_2 \cdot H_2O_4S$ mw: 238.66

SYNS: 2-CHLORO-1,4-BENZENEDIAMINE SULFATE ◇ 2-CHLORO-p-PHENYLENEDIAMINE SULFATE ◇ C.I. 76066 ◇ C.I. OXIDATION BASE 13A ◇ 2-Cl-P-PD ◇ FOURRINE 81 ◇ FOURRINE SO ◇ NCI-C03316 ◇ RENAL SO

TOXICITY DATA with REFERENCE
ETA: orl-mus TD: 12150 g/kg/96W-C   CRNGDP 1,495,80
ETA: orl-mus TDLo: 194 g/kg/77W-C   CRNGDP 1,495,80
ETA: orl-rat TDLo: 41 g/kg/77W-C   CRNGDP 1,495,80
MUT: mma-sat 100 µg/plate   ENMUDM 5(Suppl 1),3,83
MUT: mmo-sat 333 µg/plate   ENMUDM 5(Suppl 1),3,83

CONSENSUS REPORTS: NCI Carcinogenesis Bioassay (Feed); Results Negative: mouse, rat (NCITR* NCI-CG-TR-113,78)

SAFETY PROFILE: Questionable carcinogen with experimental tumorigenic data. Mutation data reported. When heated to decomposition it emits toxic fumes of Cl^-, SO_x and NO_x.

CEH000   CAS: 5730-85-8
3-CHLORO-4-AMINODIPHENYL
mf: $C_{12}H_{10}ClN$ mw: 203.68

SYN: 3-CHLOROBIPHENYLAMINE

TOXICITY DATA with REFERENCE
ETA: scu-rat TDLo: 7000 mg/kg/W-I   BMBUAQ
14,141,58

SAFETY PROFILE: Questionable carcinogen
with experimental tumorigenic data. When
heated to decomposition it emits very toxic
fumes of Cl^- and NO_x.

CEH125   CAS: 101-79-1
4-CHLORO-4'-AMINODIPHENYL ETHER
mf: $C_{12}H_{10}ClNO$ mw: 219.68

SYNS: 4'-CHLORO-4-AMINOBIPHENYL ETHER
◇ p-(p-CHLOROPHENOXY)ANILINE ◇ 4-(4-CHLOROPHEN-
OXY)ANILINE ◇ 4-(4-CHLOROPHENOXY)-BENZENAMINE
(9CI)

TOXICITY DATA with REFERENCE
CAR: orl-rat TDLo: 38 g/kg/78W-C   JEPTDQ
2(2),325,78
NEO: orl-mus TDLo: 150 g/kg/78W-C   JEPTDQ
2(2),325,78
ETA: orl-mus TD: 302 g/kg/78W-C   JEPTDQ
2(2),325,78
MUT: mma-sat 100 μg/plate   CBINA8 44,133,83

CONSENSUS REPORTS: Reported in EPA
TSCA Inventory.

SAFETY PROFILE: Questionable carcinogen
with experimental carcinogenic, neoplastigenic,
and tumorigenic data. Mutation data reported.
When heated to decomposition it emits toxic
fumes of Cl^- and NO_x.

CEH680   CAS: 106-47-8
4-CHLOROANILINE
DOT: 2018/2019
mf: C_6H_6ClN mw: 127.58

PROP: Orthorhombic crystals from alcohol or
petr ether. Mp: 72.5°, bp: 232°, d: 1.169. Sol
in hot water; freely sol in alc, ether, acetone,
carbon disulfide.

SYNS: 1-AMINO-4-CHLOROBENZENE ◇ 4-CHLORANILIN
(CZECH) ◇ p-CHLORANILINE ◇ p-CHLOROANILINE
◇ p-CHLOROANILINE, liquid (DOT) ◇ p-CHLOROANILINE,
solid (DOT) ◇ 4-CHLOROBENZENAMINE ◇ 4-CHLORO BEN-
ZENEAMINE ◇ 4-CHLOROPHENYLAMINE ◇ NCI-C02039
◇ RCRA WASTE NUMBER P024

TOXICITY DATA with REFERENCE
NEO: orl-rat TDLo: 18200 mg/kg/2Y-C
FCTOD7 25,619,87
ETA: orl-mus TDLo: 328 g/kg/78W-C   NCITR*
NCI-CG-TR-189,79
ETA: orl-rat TDLo: 14 g/kg/78W-C   NCITR*
NCI-CG-TR-189,79
MUT: dnr-esc 5 mg/L   JJIND8 62,873,79
MUT: dns-rat: lvr 5 mg/L   MUREAV 97,359,82
MUT: ihl-mus LC12: 250 mg/m^3/6H   85GMAT
-,34,82
MUT: mma-sat 100 μg/plate   ENMUDM 7(Suppl
5),1,85
MUT: mmo-asn 200 mg/L   CJMIAZ 16,369,70
MUT: otr-ham: emb 10 μg/L   NCIMAV 58,243,81
MUT: otr-rat: emb 14500 ng/plate   JJATDK
1,190,81

CONSENSUS REPORTS: EPA Genetic Toxicology Program. Reported in EPA TSCA Inventory.

DOT Classification: Poison B; Label: Poison.

SAFETY PROFILE: Questionable carcinogen
with experimental neoplastigenic and tumorigenic data. Poison by ingestion, inhalation, skin
contact, subcutaneous and intravenous routes.
Moderately toxic by inhalation and intraperitoneal routes. A skin and severe eye irritant. Mutation data reported. When heated to decomposition it emits toxic fumes of Cl^- and NO_x.

CEJ000   CAS: 20268-52-4
10-CHLORO-1,2-BENZANTHRACENE
mf: $C_{18}H_{11}Cl$ mw: 262.74

SYN: 7-CHLOROBENZ(a)ANTHRACENE

TOXICITY DATA with REFERENCE
ETA: skn-mus TDLo: 530 mg/kg/22W-I
COREAF 226,1852,48
MUT: mma-sat 20 μg/plate   MUREAV 155,91,85

SAFETY PROFILE: Questionable carcinogen
with experimental tumorigenic data. Mutation
data reported. When heated to decomposition
it emits toxic fumes of Cl^-.

CEK425   CAS: 106-54-7
4-CHLOROBENZENETHIOL
mf: C_6H_5ClS mw: 144.62

SYNS: p-CHLORO-PHENYL MERCAPTAN ◇ p-CHLORO-
THIOPHENOL ◇ 4-CHLOROTHIOPHENOL ◇ p-CHLOR-
THIOFENOL (CZECH)

TOXICITY DATA with REFERENCE
ETA: skn-mus TDLo: 8000 mg/kg/20W-I
CNREA8 19,413,59

CONSENSUS REPORTS: Chlorophenol compounds are on the Community Right-To-Know List. Reported in EPA TSCA Inventory.

SAFETY PROFILE: Questionable carcinogen with experimental tumorigenic data by skin contact. Poison by intraperitoneal route. Moderately toxic by ingestion. A severe eye and moderate skin irritant. When heated to decomposition it emits toxic fumes of Cl$^-$ and SO$_x$.

CEK500 CAS: 21248-01-1
6-CHLOROBENZENO(a)PYRENE
mf: $C_{20}H_{11}Cl$ mw: 286.69

TOXICITY DATA with REFERENCE
ETA: unk-mus TDLo: 80 mg/kg/8D-I BEBMAE 88(11),592,79

SAFETY PROFILE: Questionable carcinogen with experimental tumorigenic data. When heated to decomposition it emits toxic fumes of Cl$^-$.

CEL000 CAS: 32226-65-6
2-CHLOROBENZO(e) (1)BENZOTHIOPYRANO(4,3-b) INDOLE
mf: $C_{19}H_{10}ClNS$ mw: 319.81

TOXICITY DATA with REFERENCE
NEO: scu-mus TDLo: 378 mg/kg/27W-I
JNCIAM 46,1257,71

SAFETY PROFILE: Questionable carcinogen with experimental neoplastigenic data. When heated to decomposition it emits very toxic fumes of Cl$^-$, NO$_x$ and SO$_x$.

CEU250 CAS: 78-86-4
2-CHLOROBUTANE
mf: C_4H_9Cl mw: 92.58

PROP: Flash p: 14°F, d: 0.87, vap d: 3.2, bp: 68.50.

SYN: sec-BUTYL CHLORIDE

TOXICITY DATA with REFERENCE
NEO: ipr-mus TDLo: 3240 mg/kg/8W-I
CNREA8 35,1411,75

CONSENSUS REPORTS: Reported in EPA TSCA Inventory.

DOT Classification: Flammable Liquid; Label: Flammable Liquid.

SAFETY PROFILE: Questionable carcinogen with experimental neoplastigenic data. Mildly toxic by ingestion, inhalation, and skin contact. Dangerous fire hazard when exposed to heat, open flame (sparks), or oxidizers. To fight fire, use water, water spray, fog, mist, dry chemical, alcohol foam. When heated to decomposition it emits toxic fumes of Cl$^-$.

CEU500 CAS: 928-51-8
4-CHLORO-1-BUTANOL
mf: C_4H_9ClO mw: 108.58

SYNS: 4-CHLORBUTAN-1-OL (GERMAN) ◇ 4-CHLORO-1-BUTANE-OL ◇ 4-CHLOROBUTANOL ◇ TETRAMETHYLENE CHLOROHYDRIN

TOXICITY DATA with REFERENCE
NEO: ipr-mus TDLo: 3650 mg/kg/8W-I
CNREA8 39,391,79
MUT: mmo-sat 20 μmol/plate MUREAV 90,91,81

CONSENSUS REPORTS: Reported in EPA TSCA Inventory.

SAFETY PROFILE: Questionable carcinogen with experimental neoplastigenic data. Moderately toxic by ingestion. Mutation data reported. When heated to decomposition it emits toxic fumes of Cl$^-$.

CEW000 CAS: 1951-12-8
β-CHLOROBUTYRIC ACID
mf: $C_4H_7ClO_2$ mw: 122.56

SYNS: 3-CHLOROBUTANOIC ACID ◇ 3-CHLOROBUTYRIC ACID

TOXICITY DATA with REFERENCE
ETA: ipr-mus TDLo: 1180 mg/kg/8W-I CNREA8 39,391,79

CONSENSUS REPORTS: Reported in EPA TSCA Inventory.

SAFETY PROFILE: Questionable carcinogen with experimental tumorigenic data. When heated to decomposition it emits toxic fumes of Cl$^-$.

CFA250
6-CHLORO-9-(3-(2-CHLOROETHYL) MERCAPTOPROPYLAMINO)-2-METHOXYACRIDINE HYDROCHLORIDE
mf: $C_{19}H_{20}Cl_2N_2OS•ClH$ mw: 431.83

SYNS: ICR 342 ◇ 2-METHOXY-6-CHLORO-9-(3-(2-CHLOROETHYL) MERCAPTO PROPYLAMINO) ACRIDINE HYDROCHLORIDE

TOXICITY DATA with REFERENCE
NEO: ivn-mus TDLo: 6500 μg/kg CNREA8 36,2423,76

SAFETY PROFILE: Questionable carcinogen with experimental neoplastigenic data. Poison by intravenous route. When heated to decomposition it emits very toxic fumes of Cl⁻, SO$_x$, and NO$_x$.

CFA500   CAS: 126-85-2
2-CHLORO-N-(2-CHLOROETHYL)-N-METHYL ETHANAMINE-N-OXIDE
mf: $C_5H_{11}Cl_2NO$ mw: 172.07

SYNS: 2,2′-DICHLORO-N-METHYLDIETHYLAMINE-N-OXIDE ◇ MECHLORETHAMINE OXIDE ◇ METHYLBIS(β-CHLOROETHYL)AMINE-N-OXIDE ◇ N-METHYL-DI-2-CHLOROETHYLAMINE-N-OXIDE ◇ NITROGEN MUSTARD AMINE OXIDE ◇ NITROGEN MUSTARD-N-OXIDE ◇ N-OXYD-LOST (GERMAN) ◇ N-OXYD-MUSTARD (GERMAN) ◇ NSC 10107

TOXICITY DATA with REFERENCE
CAR: ivn-rat TDLo:218 mg/kg/1Y-I   ARZNAD 20,1461,70
ETA: skn-mus TDLo:204 g/kg/17W-I   GANNA2 57,295,66
MUT: dlt-mus-ipr-20 mg/kg   MUREAV 26,285,74
MUT: mmo-esc 50 μg/plate   TAKHAA 44,96,85

SAFETY PROFILE: Questionable carcinogen with experimental carcinogenic and tumorigenic data. Poison by ingestion, intravenous, intraperitoneal, and subcutaneous routes. Experimental reproductive effects. Mutation data reported. When heated to decomposition it emits toxic fumes of Cl⁻ and NO$_x$.

CFB500   CAS: 19996-03-3
9-CHLORO-10-CHLOROMETHYL ANTHRACENE
mf: $C_{15}H_{10}Cl_2$ mw: 261.15

SYNS: 10-CHLOROMETHYL-9-CHLOROANTHRACENE ◇ ICR 486

TOXICITY DATA with REFERENCE
NEO: ivn-mus TD:2612 μg/kg   CNREA8 40M782,80
NEO: ivn-mus TDLo:2600 μg/kg   CNREA8 36,2423,76
MUT: mma-sat 1 μg/plate   PNASA6 72,5135,75
MUT: pic-esc 50 ng/plate   CNREA8 43,2819,83

CONSENSUS REPORTS: EPA Genetic Toxicology Program.

SAFETY PROFILE: Questionable carcinogen with experimental neoplastigenic data. Mutation data reported. When heated to decomposition it emits toxic fumes of Cl⁻.

CFX500   CAS: 75-45-6
CHLORODIFLUOROMETHANE
DOT: 1018
mf: $CHClF_2$ mw: 86.47

PROP: Gas. D: 3.87 air @ 0°, mp: −146°, bp: −40.8°, autoign temp: 1170°F.

SYNS: ALGOFRENE TYPE 6 ◇ ARCTON 4 ◇ DIFLUORO-CHLOROMETHANE ◇ DIFLUOROMONOCHLOROMETHANE ◇ ELECTRO-CF 22 ◇ ESKIMON 22 ◇ F 22 ◇ FLUOROCARBON-22 ◇ FREON ◇ FREON 22 ◇ FRIGEN ◇ GENETRON 22 ◇ ISCEON 22 ◇ ISOTRON 22 ◇ MONOCHLORODIFLUOROMETHANE ◇ PROPELLANT 22 ◇ R 22 (DOT) ◇ REFRIGERANT 22 ◇ UCON 22/HALOCARBON 22

TOXICITY DATA with REFERENCE
MUT: mma-sat 33 pph/24H-C   TOLED5 2,1,78
MUT: mmo-sat 33 pph/24H-C   TOLED5 2,1,78

CONSENSUS REPORTS: IARC Cancer Review: GROUP 3 IMEMDT 7,149,87; Human Inadequate Evidence IMEMDT 41,237,86; Animal Limited Evidence IMEMDT 41,237,86. Reported in EPA TSCA Inventory. EPA Genetic Toxicology Program.

OSHA PEL: TWA 1000 ppm   ACGIH TLV: TWA 1000 ppm   DFG MAK: 500 ppm (1800 mg/m³)   DOT Classification: Nonflammable Gas; Label: Nonflammable Gas.

SAFETY PROFILE: Questionable carcinogen. Mildly toxic by inhalation. Experimental reproductive effects. Mutation data reported. An asphyxiant in high concentrations. At elevated pressures, 50% mixtures with air are combustible although ignition is difficult. When heated to decomposition it emits toxic fumes of F⁻ and Cl⁻.

CFZ000   CAS: 604-75-1
7-CHLORO-1,3-DIHYDRO-3-HYDROXY-5-PHENYL-2H-1,4-BENZODIAZEPINE-2-ONE
mf: $C_{15}H_{11}ClN_2O_2$ mw: 286.73

SYNS: ADUMBRAN ◇ ANSIOLISINA ◇ ANSIOXACEPAM ◇ ANXIOLIT ◇ APLAKIL ◇ ASTRESS ◇ BONARE ◇ 7-CHLORO-3-HYDROXY-5-PHENYL-1,3-DIHYDRO-2H-1,4-BENZODIAZEPIN-2-ONE ◇ ENIDREL ◇ HILONG ◇ ISODIN ◇ LIMBIAL ◇ NESONTIL ◇ NOCTAZEPAM ◇ NOTARAL ◇ OX ◇ OXAZEPAM ◇ PACIENX ◇ PRAXITEN ◇ PROPAX ◇ PSICOPAX ◇ QUEN ◇ QUILIBREX ◇ RO 5-6789 ◇ RONDAR ◇ SERAX ◇ SERENAL ◇ SERENID ◇ SERENID-D ◇ SEREPAX ◇ SERESTA ◇ SERPAX ◇ SIGACALM ◇ SOBRIL ◇ TAZEPAM ◇ TRANQUO-BUSCOPAN-WIRKSTOFF ◇ VABEN ◇ WY-3498 ◇ Z10-TR

TOXICITY DATA with REFERENCE
NEO: orl-mus TDLo: 65 g/kg/52W-C   RCOCB8
8,481,74
MUT: mma-sat 5200 pmol/plate   CNREA8
38,4478,78

CONSENSUS REPORTS: IARC Cancer Review: GROUP 3 IMEMDT 7,56,87; Animal Limited Evidence IMEMDT 13,57,77

SAFETY PROFILE: Questionable carcinogen with experimental neoplastigenic data. Moderately toxic by ingestion and intraperitoneal routes. Human (child) systemic effects by ingestion: somnolence, changes in REM sleep, and loss of muscle control (ataxia). Experimental reproductive effects. Mutation data reported. Used to treat anxiety and tension. When heated to decomposition it emits very toxic fumes of NO_x and HCl.

CGD250   CAS: 2491-76-1
p-CHLORO
DIMETHYLAMINOAZOBENZENE
mf: $C_{14}H_{14}ClN_3$ mw: 259.76

SYNS: 4'-CHLORO-4-DIMETHYLAMINOAZOBENZENE ◊ N,N-DIMETHYL-p-((p-CHLOROPHENYL)AZO)ANILINE

TOXICITY DATA with REFERENCE
NEO: orl-rat TDLo: 6100 mg/kg/21W-C
JEMEAV 87,139,48

SAFETY PROFILE: Questionable carcinogen with experimental neoplastigenic and teratogenic data. Moderately toxic by subcutaneous route. When heated to decomposition it emits very toxic fumes of Cl^- and NO_x.

CGH250   CAS: 63019-52-3
9-CHLORO-8,12-DIMETHYLBENZ(a)
ACRIDINE
mf: $C_{19}H_{14}ClN$ mw: 291.79

SYNS: 2-CHLORO-1,10-DIMETHYL-5,6-BENZACRIDINE (FRENCH) ◊ 1,10-DIMETHYL-2-CHLORO-5,6-BENZACRIDINE ◊ 8,12-DIMETHYL-9-CHLOROBENZ(a)ACRIDINE

TOXICITY DATA with REFERENCE
ETA: skn-mus TD : 540 mg/kg/45W-I   ACRSAJ
4,315,56
ETA: skn-mus TDLo: 500 mg/kg/41W-I
AICCA6 11,736,55

SAFETY PROFILE: Questionable carcinogen with experimental tumorigenic data by skin con-

tact. When heated to decomposition it emits very toxic fumes of NO_x and Cl^-.

CGH500   CAS: 64050-23-3
10-CHLORO-6,9-DIMETHYL-5,10-
DIHYDRO-3,4-BENZOPHENARSAZINE
mf: $C_{18}H_{15}AsClN$ mw: 355.71

SYN: 12-CHLORO-7,12-DIHYDRO-8,11-DIMETHYLBENZO (a)PHENARSAZINE

TOXICITY DATA with REFERENCE
ETA: skn-mus TDLo: 380 mg/kg/16W-I
CRSBAW 145,1451,51

CONSENSUS REPORTS: Arsenic and its compounds are on the Community Right-To-Know List.

OSHA PEL: TWA 0.5 mg(As)/m^3

SAFETY PROFILE: Questionable carcinogen with experimental tumorigenic data by skin contact. When heated to decomposition it emits very toxic fumes of As, Cl^- and NO_x.

CGJ250   CAS: 24358-29-0
2-CHLORO-5-(3,5-
DIMETHYLPIPERIDINO
SULPHONYL)BENZOIC ACID
mf: $C_{14}H_{18}ClNO_4S$ mw: 331.84

SYN: TIBRIC ACID

TOXICITY DATA with REFERENCE
CAR: orl-rat TDLo: 39 g/kg/71W-C   NATUAS
283,397,80
MUT: dni-mus: oth 500 μmol/L   CNREA8 40,36,80

SAFETY PROFILE: Questionable carcinogen with experimental carcinogenic data. Mutation data reported. When heated to decomposition it emits very toxic fumes of SO_x, NO_x and Cl^-.

CGK500   CAS: 63020-91-7
2'-CHLORO-N,N-DIMETHYL-4-
STILBENAMINE
mf: $C_{16}H_{16}ClN$ mw: 257.78

SYNS: 2'-CHLORO-4-DIMETHYLAMINOSTILBENE ◊ 2'-CHLORO-4-STILBENYL-N,N-DIMETHYLAMINE

TOXICITY DATA with REFERENCE
CAR: ipr-rat TDLo: 300 mg/kg/8W-I   BJCAAI
10,123,56
ETA: ipr-rat TD : 420 mg/kg/9W-I   BJCAAI
6,392,52
ETA: orl-rat TDLo: 625 mg/kg/60W-C   ABMGAJ
9,87,62

SAFETY PROFILE: Questionable carcinogen with experimental carcinogenic and tumorigenic data. When heated to decomposition it emits very toxic fumes of Cl⁻ and NO$_x$.

CGK750   CAS: 63040-27-7
3'-CHLORO-N,N-DIMETHYL-4-STILBENAMINE
mf: $C_{16}H_{16}ClN$ mw: 257.78

SYNS: 3'-CHLORO-N,N-DIMETHYLAMINOSTIBEN (GERMAN) ◇ 3'-CHLORO-4-DIMETHYLAMINOSTILBENE ◇ 3'-CHLORO-4-STILBENYL-N,N-DIMETHYLAMINE

TOXICITY DATA with REFERENCE
ETA: orl-rat TDLo: 440 mg/kg/42W-C   ABMGAJ 9,87,62

SAFETY PROFILE: Questionable carcinogen with experimental tumorigenic data. When heated to decomposition it emits very toxic fumes of Cl⁻ and NO$_x$.

CGL000   CAS: 7378-50-9
4'-CHLORO-N,N-DIMETHYL-4-STILBENAMINE
mf: $C_{16}H_{16}ClN$ mw: 257.78

SYNS: 4'-CHLORO-N,N-DIMETHYLAMINOSTIBEN (GERMAN) ◇ 4'-CHLORO-4-DIMETHYLAMINOSTILBENE ◇ 4'-CHLORO-4-STILBENYL-N,N-DIMETHYLAMINE

TOXICITY DATA with REFERENCE
ETA: orl-rat TDLo: 625 mg/kg/59W-C   ABMGAJ 9,87,62

SAFETY PROFILE: Questionable carcinogen with experimental tumorigenic data. When heated to decomposition it emits very toxic fumes of Cl⁻ and NO$_x$.

CGW100
3'-CHLORO-4'-ETHYL-4-DIMETHYLAMINOAZOBENZENE
mf: $C_{16}H_{18}ClN_3$ mw: 287.82

SYNS: BENZENAMINE, N,N-DIMETHYL-3'-CHLORO-4'-ETHYL-4-(PHENYLAZO)- ◇ p-((3-CHLORO-4-ETHYLPHENYL)AZO)-N,N-DIMETHYLANILINE

TOXICITY DATA with REFERENCE
CAR: orl-rat TDLo: 4515 mg/kg/25W-C
   CBINA8 53,107,85

SAFETY PROFILE: Questionable carcinogen with experimental carcinogenic data. When heated to decomposition it emits toxic fumes of Cl⁻ and NO$_x$.

CGW105
4'-CHLORO-3'-ETHYL-4-DIMETHYLAMINOAZOBENZENE
mf: $C_{16}H_{18}ClN_3$ mw: 287.82

SYNS: BENZENAMINE, N,N-DIMETHYL-4'-CHLORO-3'-ETHYL-4-(PHENYLAZO)- ◇ p-((4-CHLORO-3-ETHYLPHENYL)AZO)-N,N-DIMETHYLANILINE

TOXICITY DATA with REFERENCE
CAR: orl-rat TDLo: 15725 mg/kg/52W-C
   CBINA8 53,107,85

SAFETY PROFILE: Questionable carcinogen with experimental carcinogenic data. When heated to decomposition it emits toxic fumes of Cl⁻ and NO$_x$.

CGW750   CAS: 63019-51-2
4-CHLORO-6-ETHYLENEIMINO-2-PHENYLPYRIMIDINE
mf: $C_{12}H_{10}ClN_3$ mw: 231.70

SYN: 6-(1-AZIRIDINYL)-4-CHLORO-2-PHENYLPYRIMIDINE

TOXICITY DATA with REFERENCE
NEO: scu-rat TDLo: 960 mg/kg/16W-I   BJPCAL 9,306,54

SAFETY PROFILE: Questionable carcinogen with experimental neoplastigenic data. When heated to decomposition it emits very toxic fumes of Cl⁻ and NO$_x$.

CGX000   CAS: 7763-77-1
CHLOROETHYLENE OXIDE
mf: C_2H_3ClO mw: 78.50

SYNS: CHLOROEPOXYETHANE ◇ CHLOROOXIRANE ◇ MONOCHLOROETHYLENE OXIDE

TOXICITY DATA with REFERENCE
NEO: scu-mus TDLo: 128 mg/kg/42W-I
   CNREA8 40,352,80
MUT: dns-rat-ivn 5 g/kg   CBINA8 17,239,77
MUT: mma-sat 400 μmol/L   MUREAV 58,217,78
MUT: mmo-esc 500 μmol/L   MUREAV 152,147,85
MUT: mrc-smc 1 mmol/L   TOERD9 3,131,81
MUT: msc-ham: lng 6 μmol/L   IJCNAW 16,639,75

CONSENSUS REPORTS: EPA Genetic Toxicology Program.

SAFETY PROFILE: Questionable carcinogen with experimental neoplastigenic data. Mutation data reported. When heated to decomposition it emits very toxic fumes of Cl⁻.

CHB750 CAS: 60784-46-5
1-(2-CHLOROETHYL)-3-(2-HYDROXYETHYL)-1-NITROSOUREA
mf: $C_5H_{10}ClN_3O_3$ mw: 195.63

SYNS: CNU-ETHANOL ◇ HECNU ◇ 1-(2-HYDROXY-ETHYL)-3-(2-CHLOROETHYL)-3-NITROSOUREA ◇ HY-DROXYETHYL CNU ◇ NSC 294895

TOXICITY DATA with REFERENCE
ETA: ivn-rat TD:64 mg/kg/60W-I   DTESD7
  8,273,80
ETA: ivn-rat TD:96 mg/kg/60W-I   DTESD7
  8,273,80
ETA: ivn-rat TDLo:16 mg/kg/60W-I   DTESD7
  8,273,80
MUT: cyt-mus:lng 1 mg/L/1H   MUREAV 44,87,77
MUT: dnd-rat-ipr 100 μmol/kg   CNREA8 44,514,84
MUT: mrc-smc 1 mmol/L/16H   MUREAV 42,45,77
MUT: sln-dmg-orl 5 mmol/L   DRISAA 52,20,77
MUT: sln-dmg-par 5 mmol/L   DRISAA 52,20,77

CONSENSUS REPORTS: EPA Genetic Toxicology Program.

SAFETY PROFILE: Questionable carcinogen with experimental tumorigenic data. Poison by intraperitoneal route. Mutation data reported. Many N-nitroso compounds are carcinogens. When heated to decomposition it emits very toxic fumes of Cl⁻ and NO_x.

CHF500 CAS: 6296-45-3
2-CHLOROETHYL-N-NITROSOURETHANE
mf: $C_5H_9ClN_2O_3$ mw: 180.61

SYNS: N-(2-CHLOROETHYL)-N-NITROSOETHYLCARBA-MATE ◇ N-(β-CHLOROETHYL)-N-NITROSOURETHAN ◇ ETHYL-N-(β-CHLOROETHYL)-N-NITROSOCARBAMATE ◇ TL 154

TOXICITY DATA with REFERENCE
ETA: orl-rat TDLo:6 mg/kg   CNREA8 31,573,71
MUT: dnd-mus:leu 500 nmol/L   CNREA8 43,175,83
MUT: mmo-sat 1 nmol/plate   CNREA8 43,175,83

SAFETY PROFILE: Questionable carcinogen with experimental tumorigenic data. Poison by inhalation, ingestion, and intraperitoneal routes. Mutation data reported. Many N-nitroso compounds are carcinogens. When heated to decomposition it emits very toxic fumes of Cl⁻ and NO_x.

CHH000 CAS: 38915-59-2
7-(3-(2-CHLOROETHYL-n-PROPYLAMINO)PROPYLAMINO)BENZO(b)(1,10)-PHENATHROLINE HYDROCHLORIDE
mf: $C_{24}H_{27}ClN_4 \cdot 3ClH$ mw: 516.38

SYN: ICR 394

TOXICITY DATA with REFERENCE
NEO: ivn-mus TDLo:1550 μg/kg   CNREA8
  36,2423,76
MUT: ipr-mus LD20:1 mg/kg   JMCMAR 15,739,72
MUT: mmo-sat 5 μg/plate   JMCMAR 15,739,72

SAFETY PROFILE: Questionable carcinogen with experimental neoplastigenic data. Poison by intraperitoneal route. Mutation data reported. When heated to decomposition it emits very toxic fumes of Cl⁻ and NO_x.

CHI750
CHLOROETHYNYL NORGESTREL mixed with MESTRANOL (20:1)

SYNS: MESTRANOL mixed with CHLOROETHYNYL NOR-GESTREL (1:20) ◇ WY-4355 mixed with MESTRANOL (20:1)

TOXICITY DATA with REFERENCE
CAR: orl-dog TDLo:463 mg/kg/90W-I   JJIND8
  65,137,80
ETA: orl-dog TD:383 mg/kg/4Y-I   JNCIAM
  59,933,77
ETA: orl-dog TD:423 mg/kg/4Y-I   JTEHD6
  3,179,77

SAFETY PROFILE: Questionable carcinogen with experimental carcinogenic and tumorigenic data. When heated to decomposition it emits very toxic fumes of Cl⁻ and NO_x.

CHI825 CAS: 5096-17-3
N-(7-CHLORO-2-FLUORENYL)ACETAMIDE
mf: $C_{15}H_{11}ClNO$ mw: 256.72

SYN: N-2-(7-CHLORO)FLUORENYLACETAMIDE

TOXICITY DATA with REFERENCE
ETA: orl-rat TD:5000 mg/kg   CNREA8 26,619,66
ETA: orl-rat TDLo:1265 mg/kg/11W-C
  JNCIAM 24,149,60

SAFETY PROFILE: Questionable carcinogen with experimental tumorigenic data. Mildly toxic by ingestion. When heated to decomposition it emits toxic fumes of Cl⁻ and NO_x.

CHL500   CAS: 18979-94-7
4-CHLORO-2-HEXYLPHENOL
mf: $C_{12}H_{17}ClO$ mw: 212.74

SYN: 2-HEXYL-4-CHLOROPHENOL

TOXICITY DATA with REFERENCE
NEO: skn-mus TDLo: 8400 mg/kg/21W-I
    CNREA8 19,413,59

CONSENSUS REPORTS: Chlorophenol compounds are on the Community Right-To-Know List.

SAFETY PROFILE: Questionable carcinogen with experimental neoplastigenic data by skin contact. When heated to decomposition it emits toxic fumes of Cl^- and NO_x.

CHM500   CAS: 13442-11-0
5-CHLORO-4-(HYDROXYAMINO) QUINOLINE-1-OXIDE
mf: $C_9H_7ClN_2O_2$ mw: 210.63

TOXICITY DATA with REFERENCE
ETA: scu-mus TDLo: 120 mg/kg/50D-I   BCPCA6
    16,631,67

SAFETY PROFILE: Questionable carcinogen with experimental tumorigenic data. When heated to decomposition it emits very toxic fumes of Cl^- and NO_x.

CHM750   CAS: 14076-05-2
6-CHLORO-4-(HYDROXYAMINO) QUINOLINE-1-OXIDE
mf: $C_9H_7ClN_2O_2$ mw: 210.63

TOXICITY DATA with REFERENCE
ETA: scu-mus TDLo: 120 mg/kg/50D-I   BCPCA6
    16,631,67

SAFETY PROFILE: Questionable carcinogen with experimental tumorigenic data. When heated to decomposition it emits very toxic fumes of Cl^- and NO_x.

CHN000   CAS: 13442-12-1
7-CHLORO-4-(HYDROXYAMINO) QUINOLINE-1-OXIDE
mf: $C_9H_7ClN_2O_2$ mw: 210.63

TOXICITY DATA with REFERENCE
ETA: scu-mus TDLo: 120 mg/kg/50D-I   BCPCA6
    16,631,67

SAFETY PROFILE: Questionable carcinogen with experimental tumorigenic data. When heated to decomposition it emits very toxic fumes of Cl^- and NO_x.

CHP250   CAS: 303-47-9
(−)-N-((5-CHLORO-8-HYDROXY-3-METHYL-1-OXO-7-ISOCHROMANYL) CARBONYL)-3-PHENYLALANINE
mf: $C_{29}H_{18}ClNO_6$ mw: 403.84

PROP: Crystals. Mp: 169°.

SYNS: (R)N-((5-CHLORO-3,4-DIHYDRO-8-HYDROXY-3-METHYL-1-OXO-1H-2-BENZOPYRAN-7-YL)PHENYLALANINE ◇ NCI-C56586 ◇ OCHRATOXIN A

TOXICITY DATA with REFERENCE
CAR: orl-mus TD: 3504 mg/kg/2Y-C   JJIND8
    75,733,85
CAR: orl-mus TDLo: 2216 mg/kg/44W-C
    GANNA2 69,599,78
NEO: orl-mus TD: 1478 mg/kg/44W-C   MAIKD3
    (18),15,83
ETA: orl-mus TD: 2 g/kg/30W-C   TOLED5
    31(Suppl),206,86
ETA: orl-mus TD: 1478 mg/kg/44W-C   GANRAE
    30,1445,84
MUT: cyt-mky: kdy 20 mg/L   TXAPA9
    32,198,75

CONSENSUS REPORTS: IARC Cancer Review: GROUP 3 IMEMDT 7,271,87; Animal Limited Evidence IMEMDT 31,191,83; Animal Inadequate Evidence IMEMDT 10,191,76; Human Inadequate Evidence IMEMDT 31,191,83.

SAFETY PROFILE: Questionable carcinogen with experimental carcinogenic, neoplastigenic, tumorigenic, and teratogenic data. Poison by ingestion, intraperitoneal, intravenous, and subcutaneous routes. Experimental reproductive effects. Mutation data reported. When heated to decomposition it emits very toxic fumes of Cl^- and NO_x.

CHP500   CAS: 5160-02-1
5-CHLORO-2-((2-HYDROXY-1-NAPHTHYL)AZO)-p-TOLUENE SULFONIC ACID, BARIUM SALT
mf: $C_{17}H_{12}ClN_2O_4S \cdot 1/2Ba$ mw: 444.49

SYNS: BRIGHT RED ◇ BRILLIANT RED ◇ BRILLIANT SCARLET ◇ BRILLIANT TONER Z ◇ BRONZE RED RO ◇ BRONZE SCARLET ◇ 5-CHLORO-2-((2-HYDROXY-1-NAPHTHALENYL)AZO)-4-METHYLBENZENE SULFONIC

ACID, BARIUM SALT (2:1) ◇ 5-CHLORO-2-((2-HYDROXYI-
NAPHTHALENYL)AZO)-4-METHYLBENZENE SULPHONIC
ACID, BARIUM SALT ◇ 1-(4-CHLORO-o-SULFO-5-TOLY-
LAZO)-2-NAPHTHOL,BARIUM SALT ◇ C.I. PIGMENT RED
◇ COSMETIC CORAL RED KO BLUISH ◇ DAINICHI LAKE
RED C ◇ D&C RED No. 9 ◇ DESERT RED ◇ ELJON LAKE
RED C ◇ HAMILTON RED ◇ HELIO RED TONER LCLL
◇ IRGALITE RED CBN ◇ ISOL LAKE RED LCS 12527
◇ LAKE RED C ◇ LATEXOL SCARLET R ◇ LD RUBBER
RED 16913 ◇ LUTETIA RED CLN ◇ MICROTEX LAKE RED
CR ◇ MOHICAN RED A-8008 ◇ NCI-C53792 ◇ No. 3 CONC.
SCARLET ◇ PARIDINE RED LCL ◇ PIGMENT RED CD
◇ POTOMAC RED ◇ RECOLITE RED LAKE C ◇ 1860 RED
◇ RED SCARLET ◇ SANYO LAKE RED C ◇ SEGNALE RED
LC ◇ SICO LAKE RED 2L ◇ SUPEROL RED C RT-265
◇ SYMULER LAKE RED C ◇ TERMOSOLIDO RED LCG
◇ TEXAN RED TONER D ◇ TONER LAKE RED C
◇ TRANSPARENT BRONZE SCARLET ◇ VULCAFIX SCAR-
LET R ◇ VULCAN RED LC ◇ VULCOL FAST RED L
◇ WAYNE RED X-2486

TOXICITY DATA with REFERENCE
CAR: orl-rat TDLo: 130 g/kg/2Y-C   NTPTR*
NTP-TR-225,82
NEO: orl-rat TD: 109 g/kg/2Y-C   FCTOD7
25,619,87
MUT: mmo-sat 1 mg/plate   SCIEAS 236,933,87

CONSENSUS REPORTS: IARC Cancer Re-
view: Animal Inadequate Evidence IMEMDT
8,107,75; NTP Carcinogenesis Bioassay (feed);
Clear Evidence: rat NTPTR* NTP-TR-225,82;
No Evidence: mouse NTPTR* NTP-TR-225,82.
Reported in EPA TSCA Inventory.

SAFETY PROFILE: Questionable carcinogen
with experimental carcinogenic and tumorigenic
data. Mutation data reported. When heated to
decomposition it emits very toxic fumes of SO_x,
NO_x, and Cl^-.

CHP750   CAS: 3124-93-4
21-CHLORO-17-HYDROXY-19-NOR-17-
α-PREGNA-4,9-DIEN-20-YN-3-ONE
mf: $C_{20}H_{23}ClO_2$ mw: 330.88

SYNS: 17-α-CHLOROETHINYL-17-β-HYDROXYESTRA-
4,9-DIEN-3-ONE ◇ 17-α-CHLOROETHYNYL-17-β-HY-
DROXY-19-NOR-4,9-ANDROSTADIEN-3-ONE ◇ 17-α-CHLO-
ROETHYNLY-19-NOR-4,9-ANDROSTADIEN-17-β-OL-3-ONE
◇ ETHYNERONE ◇ MK 665

TOXICITY DATA with REFERENCE
ETA: orl-dog TDLo: 1008 mg/kg/4Y-I   JTEHD6
3,179,77

SAFETY PROFILE: Questionable carcinogen
with experimental tumorigenic data. When
heated to decomposition it emits toxic fumes
of Cl^-.

CHT500   CAS: 20794-96-1
β-CHLORO-N-ISOPROPYL-2-
NAPHTHALENEETHYLAMINE
HYDROCHLORIDE
mf: $C_{15}H_{18}ClN \cdot ClH$ mw: 284.25

SYNS: 2-(α-CHLORO-β-ISOPROPYLAMINE)ETHYL-
NAPHTHALENE HYDROCHLORIDE ◇ ICI 42464

TOXICITY DATA with REFERENCE
CAR: orl-rat TDLo: 19800 mg/kg/38W-C
PSDTAP 10,183,69
ETA: orl-mus TDLo: 18 g/kg/11W-C   NATUAS
207,594,65

CONSENSUS REPORTS: EPA Genetic Toxicology Program.

SAFETY PROFILE: Questionable carcinogen
with experimental carcinogenic and tumorigenic
data. When heated to decomposition it emits
very toxic fumes of Cl^- and NO_x.

CIG000   CAS: 63018-67-7
5-CHLORO-10-METHYL-1,2-
BENZANTHRACENE
mf: $C_{19}H_{13}Cl$ mw: 276.77

SYN: 8-CHLORO-7-METHYLBENZ(a)ANTHRACENE

TOXICITY DATA with REFERENCE
ETA: scu-mus TDLo: 80 mg/kg   JNCIAM 1,303,40

SAFETY PROFILE: Questionable carcinogen
with experimental tumorigenic data. When
heated to decomposition it emits toxic fumes
of Cl^-.

CIG250   CAS: 6325-54-8
7-CHLOROMETHYL BENZ(a)
ANTHRACENE
mf: $C_{19}H_{13}Cl$ mw: 276.77

SYN: ICR 451

TOXICITY DATA with REFERENCE
NEO: ivn-mus TDLo: 700 μg/kg   CNREA8
36,2423,76
MUT: mma-sat 1 μg/plate   PNASA6 72,5135,75

SAFETY PROFILE: Questionable carcinogen
with experimental neoplastigenic data. Poison
by intravenous route. Mutation data reported.

When heated to decomposition it emits toxic Cl⁻.

CIG500   CAS: 6366-24-1
7-CHLORO-10-METHYL-1,2-BENZANTHRACENE
mf: $C_{19}H_{13}Cl$ mw: 276.77

SYN: 10-CHLORO-7-METHYLBENZ(a)ANTHRACENE

TOXICITY DATA with REFERENCE
ETA: scu-mus TDLo:80 mg/kg   JNCIAM 1,303,40

SAFETY PROFILE: Questionable carcinogen with experimental tumorigenic data. When heated to decomposition it emits toxic fumes of Cl⁻.

CIH000   CAS: 49852-84-8
6-CHLOROMETHYL BENZO(a)PYRENE
mf: $C_{21}H_{13}Cl$ mw: 300.79

TOXICITY DATA with REFERENCE
CAR: scu-rat TDLo:100 mg/kg/40D-I   JMCMAR 16,714,73
NEO: scu-rat TD:2256 mg/kg/60D-I   CBINA8 29,159,80
MUT: mmo-sat 750 ng/plate   CBINA8 56,101,85

SAFETY PROFILE: Questionable carcinogen with experimental carcinogenic and neoplastigenic data. Mutation data reported. When heated to decomposition it emits very toxic fumes of Cl⁻.

CIL700   CAS: 63951-11-1
3'-CHLORO-4'-METHYL-4-DIMETHYLAMINOAZOBENZENE
mf: $C_{15}H_{16}ClN_3$ mw: 273.79

SYNS: p-((3-CHLORO-p-TOLYL)AZO)-N,N-DIMETHYL-ANILINE ◇ N,N-DIMETHYL-3'-CHLORO-4'-METHYL-4-(PHENYLAZO)-BENZENAMINE

TOXICITY DATA with REFERENCE
CAR: orl-rat TDLo:14062 mg/kg/36W-C
   CBINA8 53,107,85
ETA: orl-rat TD:9774 mg/kg/34W-I   CNREA8 30,1520,70
MUT: dns-rat:lvr 10 μmol/L   CNREA8 46,1654,86
MUT: mma-sat 250 nmol/plate   CNREA846,1654,86

SAFETY PROFILE: Questionable carcinogen with experimental carcinogenic and tumorigenic data. Mutation data reported. When heated to decomposition it emits toxic fumes of Cl⁻ and NOₓ.

CIL710   CAS: 17010-59-2
4'-CHLORO-3'-METHYL-4-DIMETHYLAMINOAZOBENZENE
mf: $C_{15}H_{16}ClN_3$ mw: 273.79

SYNS: ANILINE, N,N-DIMETHYL-p-(4'-CHLORO-3'-ME-THYLPHENYLAZO)- ◇ p-((4-CHLORO-m-TOLYL)AZO)-N,N-DIMETHYLANILINE ◇ N,N-DIMETHYL-p-((4-CHLORO-m-TOLYL)AZO)ANILINE

TOXICITY DATA with REFERENCE
CAR: orl-rat TDLo:3927 mg/kg/17W-C
   CBINA8 53,107,85
ETA: orl-rat TD:1027 mg/kg/50D-I   CNREA8 30,1520,70

SAFETY PROFILE: Questionable carcinogen with experimental carcinogenic and tumorigenic data. When heated to decomposition it emits toxic fumes of Cl⁻ and NOₓ.

CIN500   CAS: 25148-26-9
10-CHLOROMETHYL-9-METHYLANTHRACENE
mf: $C_{16}H_{13}Cl$ mw: 240.74

SYN: ICR 433

TOXICITY DATA with REFERENCE
NEO: ivn-mus TD:2407 μg/kg   CNREA840,782,80
NEO: ivn-mus TDLo:2400 μg/kg   CNREA8 36,2423,76
MUT: mma-sat 5 μg/plate   PNASA6 72,5135,75

SAFETY PROFILE: Questionable carcinogen with experimental neoplastigenic data. Mutation data reported. When heated to decomposition it emits toxic fumes of Cl⁻.

CIN750   CAS: 13345-62-5
7-CHLOROMETHYL-12-METHYL BENZ(a)ANTHRACENE
mf: $C_{20}H_{15}Cl$ mw: 290.80

SYN: IRC 453

TOXICITY DATA with REFERENCE
NEO: ivn-mus TDLo:1150 μg/kg   CNREA8 36,2423,76
NEO: scu-rat TDLo:150 mg/kg/39D-I   CNREA8 31,1951,71
MUT: mma-sat 1 μg/plate   PNASA6 72,5135,75

CONSENSUS REPORTS: EPA Genetic Toxicology Program.

SAFETY PROFILE: Questionable carcinogen with experimental neoplastigenic data. Poison by intravenous route. Mutation data reported. When heated to decomposition it emits toxic Cl⁻.

CIQ500 CAS: 16339-16-5
2-CHLORO-N-METHYL-N-NITROSOETHYLAMINE
mf: $C_3H_7ClN_2O$ mw: 122.57

SYNS: 2-CHLORO-2-METHYL-N-NITROSOETHANAMINE ◇ METHYL-2-CHLORAETHYLNITROSAMIN (GERMAN) ◇ METHYL(2-CHLOROETHYL)NITROSAMINE ◇ N-NITRO-SOMETHYL-2-CHLOROETHYLAMINE

TOXICITY DATA with REFERENCE
ETA: orl-rat TDLo: 111 mg/kg/53W-C ZEKBAI 69,103,67

SAFETY PROFILE: Questionable carcinogen with experimental tumorigenic data. Poison by ingestion, intravenous and possibly other routes. Many nitrosamine compounds are carcinogens. When heated to decomposition it emits very toxic fumes of Cl⁻ and NO_x.

CJB750 CAS: 88-73-3
CHLORO-o-NITROBENZENE
DOT: 1578
mf: $C_6H_4ClNO_2$ mw: 157.56

PROP: Yellow crystals. Mp: 32-33°, bp: 245-246°, d: 1.348, flash p: 123°.

SYNS: o-CHLORONITROBENZENE ◇ o-CHLORONITRO-BENZENE (DOT) ◇ 1-CHLORO-2-NITROBENZENE ◇ 2-CHLORONITROBENZENE ◇ 2-CHLORO-1-NITROBEN-ZENE ◇ o-NITROCHLOROBENZENE ◇ o-NITROCHLORO-BENZENE LIQUID (DOT) ◇ ONCB

TOXICITY DATA with REFERENCE
CAR: orl-mus TD: 280 g/kg/78W-C JEPTDQ 2(2),325,78
CAR: orl-mus TDLo: 140 g/kg/78W-C JEPTDQ 2(2),325,78
NEO: orl-rat TDLo: 22 g/kg/78W-C JEPTDQ 2(2),325,78
MUT: mma-sat 100 μg/plate ENMUDM 5(Suppl 1),3,83
MUT: mmo-sat 205 μg/plate MUREAV 116,217,83

CONSENSUS REPORTS: Reported in EPA TSCA Inventory.

DOT Classification: Poison B; Label: Poison.

SAFETY PROFILE: Questionable carcinogen with experimental carcinogenic and neoplastigenic data. Poison by ingestion and probably

inhalation. Combustible when exposed to heat or flame. To fight fire, use water, foam. When heated to decomposition it emits toxic fumes of Cl⁻, NO_x, and phosgene.

CJE500 CAS: 14100-52-8
3-CHLORO-4-NITROQUINOLINE-1-OXIDE
mf: $C_9H_5ClN_2O_3$ mw: 224.61

TOXICITY DATA with REFERENCE
ETA: scu-mus TDLo: 347 mg/kg/I CPBTAL 17,544,59
MUT: cyt-omi 36 μmol/L GANNA2 60,155,69

SAFETY PROFILE: Questionable carcinogen with experimental tumorigenic data. Mutation data reported. When heated to decomposition it emits very toxic fumes of Cl⁻ and NO_x.

CJE750 CAS: 14076-19-8
5-CHLORO-4-NITROQUINOLINE-1-OXIDE
mf: $C_9H_5ClN_2O_3$ mw: 224.61

TOXICITY DATA with REFERENCE
ETA: scu-mus TDLo: 120 mg/kg/50D-I BCPCA6 16,631,67

SAFETY PROFILE: Questionable carcinogen with experimental tumorigenic data. When heated to decomposition it emits very toxic fumes of Cl⁻ and NO_x.

CJF000 CAS: 3741-12-6
6-CHLORO-4-NITROQUINOLINE-1-OXIDE
mf: $C_9H_5ClN_2O_3$ mw: 224.61

TOXICITY DATA with REFERENCE
ETA: scu-mus TDLo: 120 mg/kg/50D-I BCPCA6 16,631,67
ETA: skn-mus TDLo: 43 mg/kg/7W-I GANNA2 49,33,58
ETA: skn-rat TDLo: 38 mg/kg/17W-I GANNA2 53,167,62
MUT: cyt-hmn: lvr 5260 nmol/L JNCIAM 47,367,71
MUT: dnd-mam: lym 5 mg BIPMAA 4,409,66
MUT: dnd-mus: fbr 10 μmol/L CNREA8 35,521,75
MUT: dns-ham: oth 500 μmol/L NATUAS 229,416,71
MUT: otr-ham: emb 4 μmol/L PJACAW 42,1211,66

CONSENSUS REPORTS: EPA Genetic Toxicology Program.

SAFETY PROFILE: Questionable carcinogen with experimental tumorigenic data by skin contact and other routes. Mutation data reported. When heated to decomposition it emits very toxic fumes of Cl^- and NO_x.

CJF250   CAS: 14753-14-1
7-CHLORO-4-NITROQUINOLINE-1-OXIDE
mf: $C_9H_5ClN_2O_3$ mw: 224.61

TOXICITY DATA with REFERENCE
ETA: scu-mus TDLo: 120 mg/kg/50D-I   BCPCA6 16,631,67
MUT: cyt-omi 44 μmol/L   GANNA2 60,155,69
MUT: mmo-smc 2 mg/L   IGSBAL 85,127,72
MUT: pic-esc 94 mg/L   EXPEAM 24,1245,68

SAFETY PROFILE: Questionable carcinogen with experimental tumorigenic data. Mutation data reported. When heated to decomposition it emits very toxic fumes of Cl^- and NO_x.

CJG375   CAS: 65445-60-5
3-CHLORONITROSOPIPERIDINE
mf: $C_5H_9ClN_2O$ mw: 148.61

SYNS: 3-CHLORO-1-NITROSOPIPERIDINE ◇ N-NITROSO-3-CHLOROPIPERIDINE

TOXICITY DATA with REFERENCE
ETA: orl-rat TDLo: 300 mg/kg/30W-C   CNREA8 40,3325,80
MUT: mma-sat 1 μg/plate   MUREAV 56,131,77
MUT: sln-dmg-orl 5 mmol/L/24H   MUREAV 67,27,79

SAFETY PROFILE: Questionable carcinogen with experimental tumorigenic data. Mutation data reported. Many N-nitroso compounds are carcinogens. When heated to decomposition it emits toxic fumes of Cl^- and NO_x.

CJG500   CAS: 65445-61-6
4-CHLORONITROSOPIPERIDINE
mf: $C_5H_9ClN_2O$ mw: 148.61

SYNS: 4-CHLORO-1-NITROSOPIPERIDINE ◇ N-NITROSO-4-CHLOROPIPERIDINE

TOXICITY DATA with REFERENCE
ETA: orl-rat TDLo: 300 mg/kg/30W-C   CNREA8 40,3325,80
ETA: orl-rat TDLo: 540 mg/kg/27W-I   ZKKOBW 92,217,78
MUT: mma-sat 1 μmol/plate   MUREAV 56,131,77
MUT: sce-hmn: lym 1 mmol/L   TCMUE9 1,129,84
MUT: sln-dmg-orl 5 mmol/L/24H   MUREAV 67,27,79

CONSENSUS REPORTS: EPA Genetic Toxicology Program.

SAFETY PROFILE: Questionable carcinogen with experimental tumorigenic data. Human mutation data reported. Many N-nitroso compounds are carcinogens. When heated to decomposition it emits very toxic fumes of Cl^- and NO_x.

CJI000
CHLOROPARAFFIN XP-470

SYN: XP-470

TOXICITY DATA with REFERENCE
CAR: scu-rat TDLo: 90 g/kg/52W-I   GISAAA 44(7),68,79

SAFETY PROFILE: Questionable carcinogen with experimental carcinogenic data. When heated to decomposition it emits toxic fumes of Cl^-.

CJI100   CAS: 7203-90-9
CHLORO-PDMT
mf: $C_8H_{10}ClN_3$ mw: 183.66

SYNS: 1-p-CHLORFENYL-3,3-DIMETHYLTRIAZEN (CZECH) ◇ 1-(p-CHLOROPHENYL)-3,3-DIMETHYL-TRI-AZENE ◇ 1-(4-CHLOROPHENYL)-3,3-DIMETHYLTRIAZENE ◇ 1-(p-CHLOR-PHENYL)-3,3-DIMETHYL-TRIAZEN (GERMAN)

TOXICITY DATA with REFERENCE
CAR: scu-rat TDLo: 3200 mg/kg/70W-I   ZKKOBW 81,285,74
NEO: scu-rat TD: 300 mg/kg   ZKKOBW 81,285,74
MUT: mma-sat 5 mmol/L   MUREAV 36,1,76
MUT: mnt-mus-ipr 50 mg/kg/24H   MUREAV 56,319,78
MUT: sln-dmg-orl 100 μmol/L   CBINA8 9,365,74

CONSENSUS REPORTS: EPA Genetic Toxicology Program.

SAFETY PROFILE: Questionable carcinogen with experimental carcinogenic and neoplastigenic data. Poison by ingestion and subcutaneous routes. Mutation data reported. When heated to decomposition it emits toxic fumes of Cl^- and NO_x.

CJI750   CAS: 937-14-4
3-CHLOROPEROXYBENZOIC ACID
mf: $C_7H_5ClO_3$ mw: 172.57

PROP: Mp: 94°.

SYNS: 3-CHLORO-BENZENECARBOPEROXOIC ACID
(9CI) ◇ m-CHLOROBENZOYL HYDROPEROXIDE ◇ m-CHLO-
ROPERBENZOIC ACID ◇ 3-CHLOROPERBENZOIC ACID
◇ m-CHLOROPEROXYBENZOIC ACID

TOXICITY DATA with REFERENCE
ETA: skn-mus TDLo:21 g/kg/52W-I   JNCIAM
    55,1359,75

CONSENSUS REPORTS: Reported in EPA
TSCA Inventory.

SAFETY PROFILE: Questionable carcinogen
with experimental tumorigenic data. When
heated to decomposition it emits toxic fumes
of Cl⁻.

CJJ250   CAS: 6164-98-3
CHLOROPHENAMIDINE
mf: $C_{10}H_{13}ClN_2$ mw: 196.70

SYNS: ACARON ◇ BERMAT ◇ C 8514 ◇ CARZOL
◇ CDM ◇ CHLORDIMEFORM ◇ CHLORFENAMIDINE
◇ N'-(4-CHLORO-2-METHYLPHENYL)-N,N-DIMETHYL-
METHANIMIDAMIDE ◇ CHLOROPHENAMADIN
◇ N'-(4-CHLORO-o-TOLYL)-N,N-DIMETHYLFORMAMIDINE
◇ CHLORPHENAMIDINE ◇ N'-(4-CHLOR-o-TOLYL)-N,N-
DIMETHYLFORMAMIDIN (GERMAN) ◇ CIBA 8514
◇ N,N-DIMETHYL-N'-(2-METHYL-4-CHLOROPHE-
NYL)-FORMAMIDINE ◇ N,N-DIMETHYL-N'-(2-METHYL-4-
CHLORPHENYL)-FORMADIN (GERMAN) ◇ ENT 27,335
◇ ENT 27,567 ◇ EP-333 ◇ FUNDAL ◇ FUNDAL 500
◇ FUNDEX ◇ GALECRON ◇ N'-(2-METHYL-4-
CHLOROPHENYL)-N,N-DIMETHYLFORMAMIDINE
◇ N'-(2-METHYL-4-CHLORPHENYL)-FORMAMIDIN-HY-
DROCHLORID (GERMAN) ◇ NSC 190935 ◇ RS 141
◇ SCHERING 36268 ◇ SN 36268 ◇ SPANON ◇ SPANONE

TOXICITY DATA with REFERENCE
CAR: orl-mus TDLo:6552 mg/kg/78W-C
    CHYCDW 19,154,85
MUT: dni-hmn:hla 1 mmol/L   BECTA6 11,184,74
MUT: mmo-smc 5 ppm   RSTUDV 6,161,76
MUT: oms-hmn:hla 1 mmol/L   BECTA6 11,184,74

CONSENSUS REPORTS: EPA Genetic Toxicology Program.

SAFETY PROFILE: Questionable carcinogen
with experimental carcinogenic data. Poison by
ingestion, skin contact, and intraperitoneal
routes. Experimental reproductive effects. Human mutation data reported. An eye and skin
irritant. When heated to decomposition it emits
very toxic fumes of NO_x and Cl⁻.

CJK250   CAS: 95-57-8
2-CHLOROPHENOL
DOT: 2020/2021
mf: C_6H_5ClO mw: 128.56

PROP: Light amber liquid. Bp: 174.5°, fp: 7°,
d: 1.256 @ 25°/25°, flash p: 147°F, vap press:
1 mm @ 12.1°. Sltly water-sol; very sol in
alc, ether, alkali.

SYNS: o-CHLOROPHENOL ◇ o-CHLOROPHENOL, LIQUID
(DOT) ◇ o-CHLOROPHENOL, SOLID (DOT) ◇ o-CHLORPHE-
NOL (GERMAN) ◇ RCRA WASTE NUMBER U048

TOXICITY DATA with REFERENCE
ETA: skn-mus TDLo:4800 mg/kg/12W-I
    CNREA8 19,413,59

CONSENSUS REPORTS: Reported in EPA
TSCA Inventory. Chlorophenol compounds are
on the Community Right-To-Know List.

DOT Classification: Poison B; Label: St. Andrews Cross.

SAFETY PROFILE: Questionable carcinogen
with experimental tumorigenic data. Poison by
ingestion, intraperitoneal, intravenous, and subcutaneous routes. Experimental reproductive effects. Flammable when exposed to heat, flame,
or oxidizers. To fight fire, use alcohol foam.
When heated to decomposition it emits toxic
fumes of Cl⁻.

CJK500   CAS: 108-43-0
3-CHLOROPHENOL
DOT: 2020/2021
mf: C_6H_5ClO mw: 128.56

PROP: Crystals. Mp: 33.5°, bp: 214°, d: 1.245
@ 45°/4°, vap press: 1 mm @ 44.2°, flash p:
>112°.

SYNS: m-CHLOROPHENOL ◇ m-CHLOROPHENOL, LIQ-
UID (DOT) ◇ m-CHLOROPHENOL, SOLID (DOT)

TOXICITY DATA with REFERENCE
ETA: skn-mus TDLo:6000 mg/kg/15W-I
    CNREA8 19,413,59

CONSENSUS REPORTS: Reported in EPA
TSCA Inventory. Chlorophenol compounds are
on the Community Right-To-Know List.

DOT Classification: Poison B; Label: St. Andrews Cross.

SAFETY PROFILE: Questionable carcinogen
with experimental tumorigenic data by skin contact. Poison by intraperitoneal route. Moderately

toxic by ingestion and subcutaneous routes. When heated to decomposition it emits toxic fumes of Cl⁻.

CJR250   CAS: 3647-19-6
N-(3-CHLOROPHENYL)-1-AZIRIDINECARBOXAMIDE
mf: $C_9H_9ClN_2O$ mw: 196.65

SYNS: 1-(1-AZIRIDINYL)-N-(m-CHLOROPHENYL)FORMAMIDE ◇ 3-CHLOROPHENYL-N-CARBAMOYLAZIRIDINE

TOXICITY DATA with REFERENCE
NEO: ipr-mus TDLo: 120 mg/kg/4W-I   CNREA8 29,2184,69

SAFETY PROFILE: Questionable carcinogen with experimental neoplastigenic data. Poison by intravenous route. When heated to decomposition it emits very toxic fumes of Cl⁻ and NO_x.

CJT750   CAS: 80-33-1
4-CHLOROPHENYL-4-CHLOROBENZENESULFONATE
mf: $C_{12}H_8Cl_2O_3S$ mw: 303.16

SYNS: ACARICYDOL E 20 ◇ C-854 ◇ C 1,006 ◇ CCS ◇ CHLOORFENSON (DUTCH) ◇ (4-CHLOOR-FENYL)-4-CHLOOR-BENZEEN-SULFONAAT (DUTCH) ◇ CHLOREFENIZON (FRENCH) ◇ CHLORFENSON ◇ CHLORFENSONE ◇ 4-CHLOROBENZENESULFONATE de 4-CHLOROPHENYLE (FRENCH) ◇ p-CHLOROBENZENESULFONIC ACID-p-CHLOROPHENYL ESTER ◇ CHLOROFENIZON ◇ p-CHLOROPHENYL-p-CHLOROBENZENE SULFONATE ◇ 4-CHLOROPHENYL-4-CHLOROBENZENESULPHONATE ◇ 4-CHLORPHENYL-4'-CHLORBENZOLSULFONAT (GERMAN) ◇ (4-CHLOR-PHENYL)-4-CHLOR-BENZOL-SULFONATE (GERMAN) ◇ (4-CLORO-FENIL)-4-CLORO-VENZOL-SOLFONATO (ITALIAN) ◇ COROTRAN ◇ CPCBS ◇ D 854 ◇ DIFENSON ◇ ENT 16,358 ◇ EPHIRSULPHONATE ◇ ESTER SULFONATE ◇ ESTONMITE ◇ ETHERSULFONATE ◇ GENITE 883 ◇ K 6451 ◇ LETHALAIRE G-58 ◇ MITICIDE K-101 ◇ NIAGARATRAN ◇ ONEX ◇ ORTHOTRAN ◇ OTRACID ◇ OVATRAN ◇ OVEX ◇ OVOCHLOR ◇ OVOTOX ◇ OVOTRAN ◇ PCPCBS ◇ SAPPILAN ◇ SAPPIRAN ◇ TRICHLORFENSON (OBS.)

TOXICITY DATA with REFERENCE
ETA: orl-mus TDLo: 115 g/kg/78W-I   NTIS** PB223-159

SAFETY PROFILE: Questionable carcinogen with experimental tumorigenic data. Moderately toxic by ingestion and possibly other routes. A pesticide. When heated to decomposition it emits very toxic fumes of Cl⁻ and SO_x.

CJU250   CAS: 120-32-1
4-CHLORO-α-PHENYL-o-CRESOL
mf: $C_{13}H_{11}ClO$ mw: 218.69

PROP: Nearly colorless flakes. Mp: 49°, bp: 175° @ 5 mm, d: 1.2 @ 55°/25°.

SYNS: o-BENZYL-p-CHLOROPHENOL ◇ 2-BENZYL-4-CHLOROPHENOL ◇ BIO-CLAVE ◇ 5-CHLORO-2-HYDROXYDIPHENYLMETHANE ◇ CHLOROPHENE ◇ 4-CHLORO-2-(PHENYLMETHYL)PHENOL ◇ CLOROPHENE ◇ KETOLIN-H ◇ NCI-C61201 ◇ NEOSABENYL ◇ SANTOPHEN ◇ SANTOPHEN I GERMICIDE ◇ SENTIPHENE

TOXICITY DATA with REFERENCE
ETA: skn-mus TDLo: 14 g/kg/34W-I   CNREA8 19,413,59

CONSENSUS REPORTS: Reported in EPA TSCA Inventory. Chlorophenol compounds are on the Community Right-To-Know List.

SAFETY PROFILE: Questionable carcinogen with experimental tumorigenic data. Moderately toxic by ingestion. When heated to decomposition it emits toxic fumes of Cl⁻.

CJX750   CAS: 150-68-5
3-(p-CHLOROPHENYL)-1,1-DIMETHYLUREA
mf: $C_9H_{11}ClN_2O$ mw: 198.67

PROP: Crystals, nearly water-insol, slight odor. Mp: 171°, vap press: 0.002 mm @ 100°.

SYNS: 3-(4-CHLOOR-FENYL)-1,1-DIMETHYLUREUM (DUTCH) ◇ CHLORFENIDIM ◇ N-(p-CHLOROPHENYL)-N',N'-DIMETHYLUREA ◇ N'-(4-CHLOROPHENYL)-N,N-DIMETHYLUREA ◇ 1-(p-CHLOROPHENYL)-3,3-DIMETHYLUREA ◇ 3-(4-CHLOROPHENYL)-1,1-DIMETHYLUREA ◇ 1-(4-CHLORO PHENYL)-3,3-DIMETHYLUREE (FRENCH) ◇ 3-(4-CHLOR-PHENYL)-1,1-DIMETHYL-HARNSTOFF (GERMAN) ◇ 3-(4-CLORO-FENIL)-1,1-DIMETIL-UREA (ITALIAN) ◇ CMU ◇ N,N-DIMETHYL-N'-(4-CHLOROPHENYL)UREA ◇ 1,1-DIMETHYL-3-(p-CHLOROPHENYL)UREA ◇ HERBICIDES, MONURON ◇ KARMEX MONURON HERBICIDE ◇ KARMEX W. MONURON HERBICIDE ◇ LIROBETAREX ◇ MONUREX ◇ MONURON ◇ MONUROX ◇ MONURUON ◇ MONUURON ◇ NCI-C02846 ◇ TELVAR ◇ TELVAR MONURON WEEDKILLER ◇ USAF P-8 ◇ USAF XR-41

TOXICITY DATA with REFERENCE
CAR: orl-mus TDLo: 4320 mg/kg/16W-I   VOONAW 16(10),51,70
CAR: orl-rat TDLo: 58 g/kg/18W-C   VOONAW 16(10),51,70
MUT: dni-mus-orl 200 mg/kg   MUREAV 58,353,78

MUT: mma-sat 1 μg/plate MUREAV 58,353,78
MUT: otr-ham:emb 5 mg/L CRNGDP 4,291,83

CONSENSUS REPORTS: IARC Cancer Review: GROUP 3 IMEMDT 7,56,87; Animal Sufficient Evidence IMEMDT 12,167,76. Reported in EPA TSCA Inventory. EPA Genetic Toxicology Program.

SAFETY PROFILE: Questionable carcinogen with experimental carcinogenic and teratogenic data. Moderately toxic by ingestion, intraperitoneal, and possibly other routes. Other experimental reproductive effects. Mutation data reported. An herbicide. When heated to decomposition it emits very toxic fumes of NO_x and Cl^-.

CKC000   CAS: 101-21-3
N-3-CHLOROPHENYLISOPROPYL CARBAMATE
mf: $C_{10}H_{12}ClNO_2$ mw: 213.68

PROP: Light brown, crystalline solid; faint characteristic odor. Mp: 41°, bp: 247° (decomp).

SYNS: BEET-KLEEN ◇ BUD-NIP ◇ N-(3-CHLOOR-FENYL)-ISOPROPYL CARBAMAAT (DUTCH) ◇ CHLOR-IFC ◇ CHLOR-IPC ◇ m-CHLOROCARBANILIC ACID, ISOPROPYL ESTER ◇ 3-CHLOROCARBANILIC ACID, ISOPROPYL ESTER ◇ N-(3-CHLORO PHENYL) CARBAMATE D'ISOPROPYLE (FRENCH) ◇ N-(3-CHLOROPHENYL)CARBAMIC ACID, ISO-PROPYL ESTER ◇ (3-CHLOROPHENYL)CARBAMIC ACID, 1-METHYLETHYL ESTER ◇ CHLOROPROPHAM ◇ N-(3-CHLOR-PHENYL)-ISOPROPYL-CARBAMAT (GERMAN) ◇ CHLORPROPHAM ◇ CHLORPROPHAME (FRENCH) ◇ CICP ◇ CI-IPC ◇ CIPC ◇ N-(3-CLORO-FENIL)-ISOPROPIL-CARBAMMATO (ITALIAN) ◇ ELBANIL ◇ ENT 18,060 ◇ FASCO WY-HOE ◇ FURLOE ◇ FURLOE 4EC ◇ ISOPRO-PYL-m-CHLOROCARBANILATE ◇ ISOPROPYL-3-CHLORO-CARBANILATE ◇ ISOPROPYL-3-CHLOROPHENYLCARBA-MATE ◇ ISOPROPYL-N-(3-CHLOROPHENYL)CARBAMATE ◇ o-ISOPROPYL-N-(3-CHLOROPHENYL)CARBAMATE ◇ ISOPROPYL-N-(3-CHLORPHENYL)-CARBAMAT (GER-MAN) ◇ JACK WILSON CHLORO 51 (oil) ◇ LIRO CIPC ◇ METOXON ◇ NEXOVAL ◇ PREVENOL ◇ PREVENOL 56 ◇ PREVENTOL ◇ PREVENTOL 56 ◇ PREWEED ◇ SPROUT NIP ◇ SPROUT-NIP EC ◇ SPUD-NIC ◇ SPUD-NIE ◇ STOPGERME-S ◇ TATERPEX ◇ TRIHERBICIDE CIPC ◇ UNICROP CIPC ◇ Y 3

TOXICITY DATA with REFERENCE
NEO: orl-mus TDLo:600 mg/kg BJCAAI 12,355,58
MUT: cyt-mus:fbr 100 μmol/L ECREAL 116,229,78
MUT: dns-hmn:fbr 4 mg/L PMRSDJ 1,528,81

MUT: mmo-smc 100 mg/L PMRSDJ 1,414,81
MUT: msc-mus:lym 31500 μg/L PMRSDJ 1,580,81
MUT: otr-ham:kdy 2500 μg/L PMRSDJ 1,638,81
MUT: sln-smc 25 mg/L PMRSDJ 1,468,81

CONSENSUS REPORTS: IARC Cancer Review: Animal Inadequate Evidence IMEMDT 12,55,76. EPA Genetic Toxicology Program.

SAFETY PROFILE: Questionable carcinogen with experimental neoplastigenic and teratogenic data. Moderately toxic by ingestion, intraperitoneal, and possibly other routes. Human mutation data reported. An herbicide. When heated to decomposition it emits highly toxic fumes of Cl^-, NO_x, and phosgene.

CKI250
1-(p-CHLOROPHENYL)-1-PHENYL-2-PROPYN-1-OL CARBAMATE
mf: $C_{16}H_{12}ClNO_2$ mw: 285.74

SYNS: 4-CHLORO-α-ETHYNYL-α-PHENYLBENZENE-METHANOL CARBAMATE ◇ 1-(4-CHLOROPHENYL)-1-PHENYL-2-PROPYNYL ESTER CARBAMIC ACID

TOXICITY DATA with REFERENCE
CAR: orl-rat TDLo:4040 mg/kg/42W-C TXAPA9 21,414,72
ETA: orl-rat TD:14 g/kg/77W-C JJIND8 71,211,83

SAFETY PROFILE: Questionable carcinogen with experimental carcinogenic and tumorigenic data. Poison by intraperitoneal route. When heated to decomposition it emits toxic fumes of Cl^- and NO_x.

CKI500   CAS: 10473-70-8
1-(4-CHLOROPHENYL)-1-PHENYL-2-PROPYNYL CARBAMATE
mf: $C_{16}H_{12}ClNO_2$ mw: 285.74

SYNS: CARBAMIC ACID, 1-(4-CHLOROPHENYL)-1-PHE-NYL-2-PROPYNYL ESTER ◇ 4-CHLORO-α-ETHYNYL-α-PHE-NYLBENZENEMETHANOL CARBAMATE

TOXICITY DATA with REFERENCE
CAR: orl-rat TDLo:4040 mg/kg/42W-C TXAPA9 21,414,72
ETA: orl-rat TD:14 g/kg/77W-C JJIND8 71,211,83

SAFETY PROFILE: Questionable carcinogen with experimental carcinogenic and tumorigenic data. When heated to decomposition it emits very toxic fumes of Cl^- and NO_x.

CKN500   CAS: 76-06-2
CHLOROPICRIN
DOT: 1580/1583
mf: CCl_3NO_2 mw: 164.37

PROP: Sltly oily, colorless liquid. D: 1.651
@ 22.8°/4°, mp: −64°, bp: 112.3 @ 766 mm,
vap press: 40 mm @ 33.80, vap d: 6.69. Sol
in water, alc, and ether.

SYNS: ACQUINITE ◇ CHLOORPIKRINE (DUTCH)
◇ CHLOR-O-PIC ◇ CHLOROPICRIN ◇ CHLOROPICRIN, AB-
SORBED (DOT) ◇ CHLOROPICRIN, LIQUID (DOT)
◇ CHLOROPICRINE (FRENCH) ◇ CHLORPIKRIN (GERMAN)
◇ CLOROPICRINA (ITALIAN) ◇ DOJYOPICRIN ◇ DOLO-
CHLOR ◇ LARVACIDE ◇ MICROLYSIN ◇ NCI-C00533
◇ NITROCHLOROFORM ◇ NITROTRICHLOROMETHANE
◇ PIC-CLOR ◇ PICFUME ◇ PICRIDE ◇ PROFUME A
◇ PS ◇ TRICHLOORNITROMETHAAN (DUTCH) ◇ TRI-
CHLORNITROMETHAN (GERMAN) ◇ TRICHLORONITRO-
METHANE ◇ TRI-CLOR ◇ TRICLORO-NITRO-METANO
(ITALIAN)

TOXICITY DATA with REFERENCE
ETA: orl-mus TDLo:26 g/kg/78W-I   NCITR*
NCI-CG-TR-65,78

MUT: mma-sat 50 μg/plate   MUREAV 116,185,83

CONSENSUS REPORTS: NCI Carcinogen-
esis Bioassay (gavage); No Evidence: mouse
NCITR* NCI-GC-TR-65,78. Reported in EPA
TSCA Inventory.

OSHA PEL: TWA 0.1 ppm   ACGIH TLV:
TWA 0.1 ppm   DFG MAK: 0.1 ppm (0.7 mg/
m³)   DOT Classification: Poison B; Label: Poison, Liquid and Absorbed.

SAFETY PROFILE: Questionable carcinogen
with experimental tumorigenic data. Poison by
ingestion, intravenous and intraperitoneal
routes. Moderately toxic by inhalation. Human
systemic effects by inhalation: lacrimation, conjunctiva irritation, and pulmonary changes. Mutation data reported. A powerful irritant that
affects all body surfaces. It causes lachrymation,
vomiting, bronchitis, pulmonary edema, irritation to gastrointestinal and respiratory tracts.
Industrially it is used as a warning agent in
commercial fumigants. Used for insect and rodent control in grain elevators and bins and as
a soil fumigant and fungicide.

CKR100   CAS: 683-50-1
2-CHLOROPROPANAL
mf: C_3H_5ClO mw: 92.53

SYNS: α-CHLOROPROPANAL ◇ 3-CHLOROPROPANAL
◇ α-CHLOROPROPIONALDEHYDE ◇ 2-CHLOROPROPION-
ALDEHYDE ◇ α-CHLOROPROPYLALDEHYDE ◇ PROPA-
NAL, 2-CHLORO-(9CI)

TOXICITY DATA with REFERENCE
NEO: orl-mus TDLo:3560 mg/kg/89W-I
JJIND8 63,1433,79
NEO: scu-mus TDLo:3560 mg/kg/89W-I
JJIND8 63,1433,79

SAFETY PROFILE: Questionable carcinogen
with experimental neoplastigenic data. When
heated to decomposition it emits toxic fumes
of Cl⁻.

CKS099   CAS: 21947-75-1
cis-1-CHLOROPROPENE OXIDE
mf: C_3H_3ClO mw: 90.51

SYNS: cis-1-CHLORO-1,2-EPOXYPROPANE ◇ cis-2-
CHLORO-3-METHYLOXIRANE ◇ cis-CPO ◇ OXIRANE, 2-
CHLORO-3-METHYL-, cis-(9CI) ◇ PROPANE, 1-CHLORO-1,2-
EPOXY-, (Z)-

TOXICITY DATA with REFERENCE
CAR: scu-mus TDLo:40 mg/kg/69W-I   CNREA8
43,159,83
CAR: skn-mus TDLo:400 mg/kg/62W-I
CNREA8 43,159,83
MUT: dnr-esc 110 μmol/L   MUREAV 101,115,82
MUT: mmo-esc 1130 μmol/L   MUREAV 101,115,82
MUT: mmo-sat 550 μmol/L   MUREAV 101,115,82
MUT: otr-ham:emb 110 μmol/L   JJIND8 69,531,82

SAFETY PROFILE: Questionable carcinogen
with experimental carcinogenic data. Mutation
data reported. When heated to decomposition
it emits toxic fumes of Cl⁻.

CKS100   CAS: 21947-76-2
trans-1-CHLOROPROPENE OXIDE
mf: C_3H_5ClO mw: 92.53

SYNS: trans-1-CHLORO-1,2-EPOXYPROPANE ◇ trans-2-
CHLORO-3-METHYLOXIRANE ◇ trans-CPO ◇ OXIRANE, 2-
CHLORO-3-METHYL-, trans-(9CI) ◇ PROPANE, 1-CHLORO-
1,2-EPOXY-, (E)-

TOXICITY DATA with REFERENCE
CAR: scu-mus TDLo:40 mg/kg/60W-I   CNREA8
43,159,83
CAR: skn-mus TDLo:400 mg/kg/73W-I
CNREA8 43,159,83
MUT: dnr-esc 110 μmol/L   MUREAV 101,115,82
MUT: mmo-esc 2250 μmol/L   MUREAV 101,115,82
MUT: mmo-sat 550 μmol/L   MUREAV 101,115,82
MUT: otr-ham:emb 550 μmol/L   JJIND8 69,531,82

SAFETY PROFILE: Questionable carcinogen
with experimental carcinogenic data. Mutation

data reported. When heated to decomposition it emits toxic fumes of Cl^-.

CKS500 CAS: 107-94-8
3-CHLOROPROPIONIC ACID
mf: $C_3H_5ClO_2$ mw: 108.53

SYNS: β-CHLOROPROPIONIC ACID ◇ β-MONOCHLORO-PROPIONIC ACID

TOXICITY DATA with REFERENCE
NEO: ipr-mus TDLo: 730 mg/kg/4W-I   CNREA8 39,391,79

CONSENSUS REPORTS: Reported in EPA TSCA Inventory.

SAFETY PROFILE: Questionable carcinogen with experimental neoplastigenic data. Moderately toxic by skin contact. Mutation data reported. When heated to decomposition it emits toxic fumes of Cl^-.

CLD000 CAS: 54-05-7
CHLOROQUINE
mf: $C_{18}H_{26}ClN_3$ mw: 319.92

SYNS: AMOKIN ◇ ARALEN ◇ ARTHROCHIN ◇ AVLO-CLOR ◇ BEMACO ◇ BEMAPHATE ◇ BEMASULPH ◇ CHEMOCHIN ◇ CHINGAMIN ◇ CHLORAQUINE ◇ CHLOROCHIN ◇ 7-CHLORO-4-(4-DIETHYLAMINO-1-METHYLBUTYLAMINO)QUINOLINE ◇ CHLOROQUINIUM ◇ N^4-(7-CHLORO-4-QUINOLINYL)-N^1,N^1-DIETHYL-1,4-PEN-TANEDIAMINE ◇ CIDANCHIN ◇ CLOROCHINA ◇ COCAR-TRIT ◇ DELAGIL ◇ DICHINALEX ◇ ELESTOL ◇ GONTO-CHIN ◇ HELIOPAR ◇ IMAGON ◇ IROQUINE ◇ KLOROKIN ◇ LAPAQUIN ◇ MALAQUIN ◇ MALAREN ◇ MALAREX ◇ MESYLITH ◇ NEOCHIN ◇ NIVACHINE ◇ NIVAQUINE B ◇ QUINACHLOR ◇ QUINAGAMINE ◇ QUINERCYL ◇ QUINILON ◇ QUINOSCAN ◇ RESOCHIN ◇ RESOQUINA ◇ RESOQUINE ◇ REUMACHLOR ◇ REUMAQUIN ◇ ROQUINE ◇ RP 3377 ◇ SANOQUIN ◇ SENAQUIN ◇ SILBESAN ◇ SIRAGAN ◇ SN 6718 ◇ SN 7618 ◇ SOLPRINA ◇ SOPAQUIN ◇ TANAKAN ◇ TRESOCHIN ◇ TROCHIN ◇ W 7618 ◇ WIN 244

TOXICITY DATA with REFERENCE
MUT: cyt-hmn: lym 100 mg/L   BEXBAN82,1095,76
MUT: dnr-esc 250 μg/disc   MUREAV 41,61,76
MUT: mmo-sat 100 μmol/L   AMACCQ 9,77,76

CONSENSUS REPORTS: IARC Cancer Review: GROUP 3 IMEMDT 7,56,87; Animal Inadequate Evidence IMEMDT 13,47,77. EPA Genetic Toxicology Program.

SAFETY PROFILE: Questionable carcinogen. Poison by ingestion, intraperitoneal, intrave-

nous, intramuscular, and subcutaneous routes. Human systemic effects by ingestion: visual field changes, gastrointestinal changes, and weight loss. Human reproductive effects by an unspecified route: terminates pregnancy. Human teratogenic effects by an unspecified route include developmental abnormalities of the urogenital system, eyes and ears, other unspecified areas, and postnatal effects. Human mutation data reported. An antimalarial agent. When heated to decomposition it emits very toxic fumes of Cl^- and NO_x.

CLD500 CAS: 4213-44-9
CHLOROQUINE MUSTARD
mf: $C_{18}H_{24}Cl_3N_3 \cdot 2ClH$ mw: 461.72

SYNS: 4-((4-(BIS(2-CHLOROETHYL)AMINO)-1-METHYL-BUTYL)AMINO-7-CHLOROQUINOLINE, DIHYDROCHLO-RIDE ◇ ICR-25A ◇ NSC-17118

TOXICITY DATA with REFERENCE
CAR: ipr-mus TDLo: 8 mg/kg/4W   JNCIAM 36,915,66
MUT: dnd-mus: lvr 70 μmol/L   CNREA8 21,1124,61
MUT: dnd-mus: oth 70 μmol/L   CNREA8 21,1124,61
MUT: ipr-rat LD10: 1100 μg/kg   CCROBU 17,63,62

SAFETY PROFILE: Questionable carcinogen with experimental carcinogenic data. A deadly poison by intraperitoneal and intravenous routes. Mutation data reported. When heated to decomposition it emits very toxic fumes of Cl^- and NO_x.

CLE500 CAS: 73928-01-5
3-CHLORO-4-STILBENAMINE
mf: $C_{12}H_{12}ClN$ mw: 205.70

SYN: 3-CHLORO-4-AMINOSTILBENE

TOXICITY DATA with REFERENCE
ETA: scu-rat TDLo: 200 mg/kg/W-I   BMBUAQ 14,141,58

SAFETY PROFILE: Questionable carcinogen with experimental tumorigenic data. When heated to decomposition it emits very toxic fumes of Cl^- and NO_x.

CLX000 CAS: 54749-90-5
CHLOROZOTOCIN
mf: $C_9H_{16}ClN_3O_7$ mw: 313.73

SYNS: 1-(2-CHLOROETHYL)-3-(d-GLUCOPYRANOS-2-YL)-1-NITROSOUREA ◇ 2-((((2-CHLOROETHYL)

NITROSOAMINO)CARBONYL)AMINO)-2-DEOXY-d-
GLUCOPYRANOSE ◇ 2-((((2-CHLOROETHYL)NITRO-
SOAMINO)CARBONYL)AMINO)-2-DEOXY-d-GLUCOSE
◇ 2-(3-(2-CHLOROETHYL)-3-NITROSOUREIDO)-2-DEOXY-
d-GLUCOSOPYRANOSE ◇ 2-(3-(2-CHLOROETHYL)-3-
NITROSOUREIDO)-d-GLUCO-PYRANOSE ◇ CHLZ
◇ CZT ◇ DCNU ◇ NSC 178248 ◇ NSC D 254157

TOXICITY DATA with REFERENCE
CAR: ipr-rat TDLo:34 mg/kg/85W-I   CALEDQ
8,133,79
ETA: ivn-rat TD:64 mg/kg/60W-I   DTESD7
8,273,80
ETA: ivn-rat TDLo:16 mg/kg/60W-I   DTESD7
8,273,80
MUT: dnd-mam:lym 10 mmol/L   CNREA8
44,1887,84
MUT: dnd-rat-ipr 100 μmol/kg   CNREA8 44,514,84
MUT: ivn-mus LD10:15 mg/kg   GANNA2
71,686,80
MUT: mma-sat 100 mg/L/1H   MUREAV 40,281,76
MUT: mmo-sat 100 nmol/plate   JJIND8 65,149,80
MUT: sce-rat:oth 1 μmol/L   CNREA8 43,473,83

CONSENSUS REPORTS: EPA Genetic Toxicology Program.

SAFETY PROFILE: Questionable carcinogen
with experimental carcinogenic and tumorigenic
data. Poison by subcutaneous, intravenous, and
intraperitoneal routes. Human systemic effects
by intravenous route: anorexia, nausea or vomiting, and thrombocytopenia (decrease in the
number of blood platelets). Mutation data reported. When heated to decomposition it emits
very toxic fumes of Cl^- and NO_x.

CLY500   CAS: 52-86-8
γ-(4-(p-CHLORPHENYL)-4-
HYDROXPIPERIDINO)-p-
FLUORBUTYROPHENONE
mf: $C_{21}H_{23}ClFNO_2$ mw: 375.90

SYNS: ALDO ◇ ALOPERIDIN ◇ ALOPERIDOLO
◇ BROTOPON ◇ 4-(4-(4-CHLOROPHENYL)-4-HYDROXY-1-
PIPERIDINYL)-1-(4-FLUOROPHENYL)-1-BUTANONE
◇ EINALON S ◇ EUKYSTOL ◇ 1-(3-p-FLUOROBENZOYL-
PROPYL)-4-p-CHLOROPHENYL-4-HYDROXYPIPERIDINE
◇ 4'-FLUORO-4-(4-HYDROXY-4-(4'-
CHLOROPHENYL)PIPERIDINO)BUTYROPHENONE
◇ GALOPERIDOL ◇ HALDOL ◇ HALOPERIDOL ◇ HALOS-
TEN ◇ 4-(4-(HYDROXY-4'-CHLORO-4-PHENYLPIPERIDINO)-
4'-FLUOROBUTYROPHENONE ◇ KESELAN ◇ LEALGIN
COMPOSITUM ◇ LINTON ◇ PELUCES ◇ PERNOX
◇ R 1625 ◇ SERENACE ◇ SERNAS ◇ SERNEL ◇ ULCOLIND
◇ ULIOLIND ◇ VESALIUM

TOXICITY DATA with REFERENCE
CAR: ipr-mus TD:50 mg/kg/10D-C   CRNGDP
3,223,82
CAR: ipr-mus TDLo:25 mg/kg/5D-C   CRNGDP
3,223,82
MUT: cyt-hmn:fbr 10 g/L   AMBUCH 6,42,79
MUT: mma-sat 100 nmol/plate   CRNGDP 3,223,82
MUT: sln-dmg-orl 200 mg   SOGEBZ 7,1042,71

CONSENSUS REPORTS: EPA Genetic Toxicology Program.

SAFETY PROFILE: Questionable carcinogen
with experimental carcinogenic data. Poison by
ingestion, intraperitoneal, intravenous, subcutaneous, and possibly other routes. Human systemic effects by ingestion and possibly other
routes: somnolence, cardiac arrythmias, body
temperature decrease, change in motor activity,
muscle weakness, muscle contraction or spasticity, tremors, and ataxia (loss of muscle coordination). A human teratogen by ingestion which
causes developmental abnormalites of the mus-
culosketal and cardiovascular (circulatory) systems, and abnormal conditions of newborn at
birth. Human mutation data reported. An experimental teratogen. Experimental reproductive effects. A tranquilizer used in the treatment of
schizophrenia and agitated psychoses. When
heated to decomposition it emits very toxic
fumes of F^-, Cl^-, and NO_x.

CMC000   CAS: 479-23-2
CHOLANTHRENE
mf: $C_{20}H_{14}$ mw: 254.34

SYNS: BENZ(j)ACEANTHRYLENE ◇ 1,2-DIHYDRO-
BENZ(j)ACEANTHRYLENE ◇ 7,8-DIMETHYLENE-
BENZ(a)ANTHRACENE

TOXICITY DATA with REFERENCE
CAR: scu-mus TDLo:40 mg/kg   CNREA8 1,695,41
ETA: scu-mus TD:200 mg/kg   CNREA8 1,685,41
ETA: skn-mus TDLo:170 mg/kg/7W-I   PRLBA4
123,343,37
MUT: mma-sat 3 μg/plate   MUREAV 119,259,83
MUT: msc-ham:lng 10 mg/L   CNREA8 44,4993,84

SAFETY PROFILE: Questionable carcinogen
with experimental carcinogenic and tumorigenic
data. Mutation data reported. When heated to
decomposition it emits acrid smoke and irritating
fumes.

CMD000   CAS: 80-99-9
5-α-CHOLEST-7-EN-3-β-OL
mf: $C_{27}H_{46}O$ mw: 386.73

SYNS: Δ⁷-CHOLESTENOL ◇ 7-CHOLESTEN-3-β-OL ◇ CHOLESTERIN (GERMAN) ◇ LATHOSTEROL

TOXICITY DATA with REFERENCE
ETA: scu-mus TDLo:800 mg/kg/4W-I
  NATWAY 60,525,73

SAFETY PROFILE: Questionable carcinogen with experimental tumorigenic data. When heated to decomposition it emits acrid smoke and irritating fumes.

CMD250   CAS: 3328-25-4
CHOLEST-6-EN-3-β-OL-5-α-HYDROPEROXIDE
mf: $C_{27}H_{46}O_3$ mw: 418.73

SYNS: Δ⁶-CHOLESTEN-3-β-OL-5-α-HYDROPEROXIDE ◇ Δ⁶-CHOLESTEN-3-β-OL-5-α-HYDROPEROXYD (GERMAN) ◇ CHOLESTEROL-5-α-HYDROPEROXIDE

TOXICITY DATA with REFERENCE
NEO: ipr-mus TDLo:200 mg/kg   STRAAA
  124,626,64

SAFETY PROFILE: Questionable carcinogen with experimental neoplastigenic data. When heated to decomposition it emits acrid smoke and irritating fumes.

CMD500   CAS: 601-54-7
CHOLEST-5-EN-3-ONE
mf: $C_{27}H_{44}O$ mw: 384.71

SYNS: CHOLESTENONE ◇ Δ(⁵)-CHOLESTENONE ◇ 5-CHOLESTEN-3-ONE ◇ CHOLESTERONE

TOXICITY DATA with REFERENCE
CAR: scu-mus TDLo:760 mg/kg/16W   CNREA8
  6,403,46

SAFETY PROFILE: Questionable carcinogen with experimental carcinogenic data. When heated to decomposition it emits acrid smoke and irritating fumes.

CMD750   CAS: 57-88-5
CHOLESTEROL
mf: $C_{27}H_{46}O$ mw: 386.73

PROP: White or faint yellow, pearly leaflets. Mp: 148.5°, bp: 360° decomp.

SYNS: CHOLEST-5-EN-3-β-OL ◇ Δ⁵-CHOLESTEN-3-β-OL ◇ 5-CHOLESTEN-3-β-OL ◇ 5:6-CHOLESTEN-3-β-OL ◇ CHOLESTERIN ◇ CHOLESTEROL BASE H ◇ CHOLESTERYL ALCOHOL ◇ CHOLESTRIN ◇ CHOLESTROL ◇ CORDULAN ◇ DUSOLINE ◇ DUSORAN ◇ DYTHOL ◇ HYDROCERIN ◇ 3-β-HYDROXYCHOLEST-5-ENE

◇ KATHRO ◇ LANOL ◇ NIMCO CHOLESTEROL BASE H ◇ PROVITAMIN D ◇ SUPER HARTOLAN ◇ TEGOLAN

TOXICITY DATA with REFERENCE
CAR: scu-mus TDLo:15 g/kg/47W-I   NATUAS
  160,270,47
ETA: imp-mus TDLo:800 mg/kg   SCIEAS
  167,996,70
ETA: ipr-rat TDLo:800 mg/kg/43W-I   EMSUA8
  3,95,45
ETA: scu-mus TDLo:600 mg/kg/72W-I
  JNCIAM 19,977,57
MUT: dnd-mus:oth 1 μmol/L   CJBBDU 62,94,84
MUT: mmo-sat 500 μg/plate   FCTOD7 20,35,82

CONSENSUS REPORTS: IARC Cancer Review: Human Inadequate Evidence IMEMDT 31,95,83; Animal Inadequate Evidence IMEMDT 10,99,76. Reported in EPA TSCA Inventory. EPA Genetic Toxicology Program.

SAFETY PROFILE: Questionable carcinogen with experimental carcinogenic, tumorigenic, and teratogenic data. Other experimental reproductive effects. Mutation data reported. Used in pharmaceutical and dermal preparations as an emulsifying agent. When heated to decomposition it emits acrid smoke and irritating fumes.

CME000   CAS: 63019-46-5
CHOLESTEROL ISOHEPTYLATE
mf: $C_{34}H_{58}O_2$ mw: 498.92

SYN: CHOLESTEROL-5-METHYL-1-HEXANOATE

TOXICITY DATA with REFERENCE
CAR: scu-mus TDLo:600 mg/kg/72W-I
  JNCIAM 19,977,57

SAFETY PROFILE: Questionable carcinogen with experimental carcinogenic data. When heated to decomposition it emits acrid smoke and irritating fumes.

CME400   CAS: 11041-12-6
CHOLESTYRAMINE

SYNS: CHOLESTYRAMINE CHLORIDE ◇ CHOLESTYRAMINE RESIN ◇ COLESTYRAMIN ◇ CUEMID ◇ QUANTALAN ◇ QUESTRAN

TOXICITY DATA with REFERENCE
CAR: orl-man TDLo:112 g/kg/W-C   NEJMAG
  301,1007,79

CONSENSUS REPORTS: Reported in EPA TSCA Inventory.

SAFETY PROFILE: Questionable human carcinogen producing colon tumors. Experimental reproductive data. Toxic effects by ingestion: acidosis and nose bleeds. When heated to decomposition it emits acrid smoke and irritating fumes.

CMF400   CAS: 999-81-5
CHOLINE DICHLORIDE
mf: $C_5H_{13}ClN \cdot Cl$ mw: 158.09

SYNS: ANTYWYLEGACZ ◇ CCC PLANT GROWTH REGU-LANT ◇ CE CE CE ◇ 2-CHLORAETHYL-TRIMETHYLAM-MONIUMCHLORID ◇ CHLORCHOLINCHLORID ◇ CHLOR-CHOLINE CHLORIDE ◇ CHLORMEQUAT ◇ CHLORMEQUAT CHLORIDE ◇ CHLOROCHOLINE CHLORIDE ◇ (β-CHLORO-ETHYL)TRIMETHYLAMMONIUM CHLORIDE ◇ (2-CHLORO-ETHYL)TRIMETHYLAMMONIUM CHLORIDE ◇ 2-CHLORO-N,N,N-TRIMETHYLETHANAMINIUM CHLORIDE ◇ 60-CS-16 ◇ CYCLOCEL ◇ CYCOCEL ◇ CYCOCEL-EXTRA ◇ CYCO-GAN ◇ CYCOGAN EXTRA ◇ CYCOEL ◇ EI 38,555 ◇ ETHANAMINIUM, 2-CHLORO-N,N,N-TRIMETHYL-, CHLORIDE (9CI) ◇ HICO CCC ◇ HORMOCEL-2CCC ◇ INCRECEL ◇ LIHOCIN ◇ NCI-C02960 ◇ RETACEL ◇ STABILAN ◇ TRIMETHYL-β-CHLORETHYLAMMONIUM-CHLORID ◇ TUR

TOXICITY DATA with REFERENCE
NEO: orl-mus TDLo:7100 mg/kg/78W-I
    NTIS** PB223-159
MUT: dni-mus-ivg 5 pph   JIDEAE 62,378,74
MUT: mmo-esc 500 mmol/L/30M   MUREAV 40,229,76

CONSENSUS REPORTS: NTP Carcinogenesis Bioassay (feed): No Evidence: mouse, rat NCITR* NCI-TR-158,79. Reported in EPA TSCA Inventory.

SAFETY PROFILE: Questionable carcinogen with experimental neoplastigenic data. Human poison by ingestion and intravenous routes. Moderately toxic by skin contact. Human systemic effects: respiratory depression. Mutation data reported. When heated to decomposition it emits toxic fumes of Cl^-.

CMG850   CAS: 7788-99-0
CHROME ALUM (DODECAHYDRATE)
mf: $CrKO_8S_2 \cdot 12H_2O$ mw: 499.41

SYNS: CHROME ALUM ◇ POTASSIUM CHROMIUM ALUM ◇ SULFURIC ACID, CHROMIUM(3+)POTASSIUM SALT(2:1:1), DODECAHYDRATE

TOXICITY DATA with REFERENCE
ETA: scu-rat TDLo:135 mg/kg   PBPHAW 14,47,78
MUT: dnr-esc 125 μg/well   MUREAV 133,161,84

OSHA PEL: CL 0.5 mg(Cr)/m³   ACGIH TLV: TWA 0.5 mg(Cr)/m³

SAFETY PROFILE: Questionable carcinogen with experimental tumorigenic data. Poison by intravenous route. Mutation data reported. When heated to decomposition it emits toxic fumes of Cr^-.

CMH000   CAS: 1066-30-4
CHROMIC ACETATE
DOT: 9101
mf: $C_6H_9O_6 \cdot Cr$ mw: 229.15

PROP: Gray, green powder or bluish-green pasty mass.

SYNS: CHROMIC ACETATE(III) ◇ CHROMIUM ACETATE ◇ CHROMIUM(III) ACETATE ◇ CHROMIUM TRIACETATE

TOXICITY DATA with REFERENCE
ETA: imp-rat TDLo:1000 mg/kg/56W-I
    AEHLAU 5,445,62
MUT: cyt-ham:ovr 150 mg/L   TXCYAC 17,219,80
MUT: cyt-hmn:leu 16 μmol/L   MUREAV 58,175,78
MUT: mmo-esc 16 mmol/L   MUREAV 58,175,78
MUT: mrc-bcs 160 mmol/L   MUREAV 58,175,78
MUT: msc-ham:ovr 200 μmol/L   MUREAV 117,279,83

CONSENSUS REPORTS: IARC Cancer Review: Animal Inadequate Evidence IMEMDT 2,100,73; IMEMDT 23,205,80. Chromium and its compounds are on the Community Right-To-Know List. Reported in EPA TSCA Inventory.

OSHA PEL: TWA 0.5 mg(Cr)/m³   ACGIH TLV: TWA 0.5 mg(Cr)/m³   DOT Classification: ORM-E; Label: None.

SAFETY PROFILE: Questionable carcinogen with experimental tumorigenic data. Moderately toxic by intravenous route. Human mutation data reported. When heated to decomposition it emits acrid smoke and irritating fumes.

CMJ900   CAS: 12018-40-5
CHROMIUM OXIDE, aerosols
mf: Cr_5O_{12} mw: 452.00

TOXICITY DATA with REFERENCE
ETA: ihl-rat TCLo:143 μg/m³/78W-I   TXCYAC 42,219,86

SAFETY PROFILE: Questionable carcinogen with experimental tumorigenic data. When heated to decomposition it emits toxic fumes of Cr^-.

CML800   CAS: 2642-98-0
6-CHRYSENAMINE
mf: $C_{18}H_{13}N$ mw: 243.32

PROP: Leaflets from alc. Mp: 210-211°. Sltly sol in alc, benzene, ethyl acetate.

SYNS: 6-AMC ◇ 6-AMINOCHRYSENE ◇ CHRYSENEX ◇ CHRYSONEX

TOXICITY DATA with REFERENCE
CAR: skn-mus TDLo:1100 g/kg/39W-I
EJCAAH 11,327,75
MUT: dnr-bcs 20 uL/disc   MUREAV 97,1,82
MUT: dns-rat:lvr 500 nmol/L   ENMUDM 3,11,81
MUT: mma-sat 500 ng/plate   MUREAV 155,7,85
MUT: mmo-sat 2500 ng/plate   CNREA8 44,3408,84
MUT: msc-ham:ovr 50 mg/L   JTEHD6 13,531,84

CONSENSUS REPORTS: EPA Genetic Toxicology Program.

SAFETY PROFILE: Questionable carcinogen with experimental carcinogenic data by skin contact. Mutation data reported. When heated to decomposition it emits toxic fumes of NO_x.

CML815   CAS: 15131-84-7
CHRYSENE-5,6-EPOXIDE
mf: $C_{18}H_{12}O$ mw: 244.30

SYNS: CHRYSENE-K-REGION EPOXIDE ◇ CHRYSENE-5,6-OXIDE ◇ 5,6-EPOXY-5,6-DIHYDROCHRYSENE

TOXICITY DATA with REFERENCE
ETA: scu-mus TDLo:400 mg/kg/10W-I
IJCNAW 2,500,67
MUT: dnr-esc 100 μmol/L   ZKKOBW 92,157,78
MUT: dns-esc 100 μmol/L   ZKKOBW 92,157,78
MUT: mma-sat 50 μg/plate   PNASA6 72,5135,75

CONSENSUS REPORTS: EPA Genetic Toxicology Program.

SAFETY PROFILE: Questionable carcinogen with experimental tumorigenic data. Mutation data reported. When heated to decomposition it emits acrid smoke and fumes.

CMP000   CAS: 2586-60-9
C.I. DIRECT VIOLET 1, DISODIUM SALT
mf: $C_{32}H_{22}N_6O_8S_2 \cdot 2Na$ mw: 728.70

SYNS: AIREDALE VIOLET ND ◇ AMANIL FAST VIOLET N ◇ ATLANTIC VIOLET N ◇ ATUL DIRECT VIOLET N ◇ AZOCARD VIOLET N ◇ BENCIDAL FAST VIOLET N ◇ BENZANIL VIOLET N ◇ BENZO VIOLET N ◇ BRASILAMINA VIOLET 3R ◇ CALCOMINE VIOLET N ◇ CHLORAZOL

VIOLET N ◇ C.I. 22570 ◇ COTTON VIOLET R ◇ DIAMINE VIOLET N ◇ DIAPHTAMINE VIOLET N ◇ DIAZINE VIOLET N ◇ DIAZOL VIOLET N ◇ DIRECT FAST VIOLET N ◇ DIRECT VIOLET C ◇ ERIE VIOLET 3R ◇ FIXANOL VIOLET N ◇ HISPAMIN VIOLET 3R ◇ JAPANOL VIOLET J ◇ NAPHTAMINE VIOLET N ◇ PARAMINE FAST VIOLET N ◇ PHENO VIOLET N ◇ PONTAMINE VIOLET N ◇ TERTRODIRECT VIOLET N ◇ TRISULFON VIOLET N

TOXICITY DATA with REFERENCE
ETA: orl-rat TDLo:1125 g/kg/71W-C   VOONAW 23(7),72,77
ETA: unk-rat TDLo:125 g/kg/71W-C   GTPZAB 22(10),22,78

SAFETY PROFILE: Questionable carcinogen with experimental tumorigenic data. When heated to decomposition it emits very toxic fumes of NO_x, Na_2O, and SO_x.

CMS210   CAS: 52214-84-3
CIPROFIBRATE
mf: $C_{13}H_{14}Cl_2O_3$ mw: 289.17

SYNS: 2-(p-(2,2-DICHLOROCYCLOPROPYL)PHENOXY)-2-METHYL PROPIONIC ACID ◇ PROPANOIC ACID, 2-(4-(2,2-DICHLOROCYCLOPROPYL)PHENOXY)-2-METHYL- ◇ WIN 35833

TOXICITY DATA with REFERENCE
ETA: orl-rat TD:6720 mg/kg/64W-C   CALEDQ 32,33,86
ETA: orl-rat TDLo:6390 mg/kg/60W-C   CALEDQ 38,65,87
MUT: otr-rat Oral 3650 mg/kg/1Y-C   CNREA8 46,4601,86

SAFETY PROFILE: Questionable carcinogen with experimental tumorigenic data. Experimental reproductive data. Mutation data reported. When heated to decomposition it emits toxic fumes of Cl^-.

CMS775   CAS: 518-75-2
CITRININ
mf: $C_{13}H_{14}O_5$ mw: 250.27

SYNS: ANTIMYCIN ◇ 3H-2-BENZOPYRAN-7-CARBOXYLIC ACID, 4,6-DIHYDRO-8-HYDROXY-3,4,5-TRIMETHYL-6-OXO-, (3R-trans)- ◇ (3R,4S)-4,6-DIHYDROXY-3,4,5-TRIMETHYL-6-OXO-3H-2-BENZOPYRAN-7-CARBOXYLIC ACID

TOXICITY DATA with REFERENCE
ETA: orl-rat TD:13 g/kg/32W-C   FGIGDO 5,77,81
NEO: orl-rat TDLo:25200 mg/kg/60W-C
CALEDQ 17,281,83

MUT: dnd-esc 100 mg/L   AEMIDF 52,1273,86
MUT: dnr-bcs 20 µg/disc   CNREA8 36,445,76
MUT: pic-esc 300 mg/L   AEMIDF 52,1273,86

CONSENSUS REPORTS: IARC Cancer Review: GROUP 3 IMEMDT 7,56,87, Animal Limited Evidence IMEMDT 40,67,86

SAFETY PROFILE: Questionable carcinogen with experimental neoplastigenic and tumorigenic data. Poison by ingestion and other routes. Experimental reproductive data. A severe skin irritant. Mutation data reported. When heated to decomposition it emits acrid smoke and irritating fumes.

CMV000   CAS: 149-29-1
CLAVACIN
mf: $C_7H_6O_4$ mw: 154.13

PROP: Colorless crystals. Mp: 111°.

SYNS: CLAIRFORMIN ◇ 2,4-DIHYDROXY-2H-PYRAN-Δ-3(6H),α-ACETIC ACID-3,4-LACTONE ◇ (2,4-DIHYDROXY-2H-PYRAN-3(6H)-YLIDENE)ACETIC ACID-3,4-LACTONE ◇ EXPANSIN ◇ GIGANTIN ◇ 4-HYDROXY-4H-FURO(3,2-C)PYRAN-2(6H)-ONE ◇ LEUCOPIN ◇ MYCOIN ◇ PATULIN ◇ PENATIN ◇ PENICIDIN ◇ TERCININ ◇ TERININ

TOXICITY DATA with REFERENCE
NEO: scu-rat TDLo: 232 mg/kg/58W-I   BJCAAI 15,85,61
MUT: dni-hmn: hla 3200 mg/L   FCTOD7 20,893,82
MUT: dni-hmn: lym 50 mg/L   FCTOD7 20,893,82
MUT: oms-hmn: hla 3200 mg/L   FCTOD7 20,893,82
MUT: sce-hmn: lym 100 µg/L   FCTOD7 20,893,82
MUT: sln-dmg-orl 3200 nmol/L   CBTOE2 1,133,85

CONSENSUS REPORTS: IARC Cancer Review: Animal Limited Evidence IMEMDT 10,205,76; Animal Inadequate Evidence IMEMDT 40,83,86. EPA Genetic Toxicology Program.

SAFETY PROFILE: Questionable carcinogen with experimental neoplastigenic and teratogenic data. Poison by ingestion, subcutaneous, intracerebral, intraperitoneal, intravenous, and possibly other routes. Other experimental reproductive effects. Human mutation data reported. An antimicrobial agent. When heated to decomposition it emits acrid smoke and irritating fumes.

CMV475   CAS: 1532-19-0
CLEP
mf: $C_7H_7Cl_2N \cdot ClH$ mw: 212.51

SYNS: 2-(α,β-DICHLORETHYL)PYRIDINE HYDROCHLORIDE ◇ 2-(1,2-DICHLOROETHYL)PYRIDINE HYDROCHLORIDE

TOXICITY DATA with REFERENCE
CAR: orl-rat TDLo: 5940 mg/kg/84W-C   GANMAX 3,51,66
NEO: mul-mus TDLo: 2640 mg/kg/37W-I   GANMAX 3,51,66
ETA: orl-rat TD: 8580 mg/kg/89W-C   PAACA3 9,28,68
ETA: skn-mus TDLo: 19 g/kg/37W-I   PAACA3 9,28,68

SAFETY PROFILE: Questionable carcinogen with experimental carcinogenic, neoplastigenic, and tumorigenic data. When heated to decomposition it emits very toxic fumes of Cl^- and NO_x.

CMV850   CAS: 12173-10-3
CLINOPTILOLITE
SYN: KLINOSORB

TOXICITY DATA with REFERENCE
ETA: ipl-rat TDLo: 240 mg/kg/13W-I   GTPZAB 30(5),29,86

SAFETY PROFILE: Questionable carcinogen with experimental tumorigenic data. When heated to decomposition it emits acrid smoke and irritating fumes.

CMV950   CAS: 33979-15-6
CLIVORINE
mf: $C_{21}H_{28}NO_7$ mw: 406.50

SYN: SENECIONANIUM, 12-(ACETYLOXY)-14,15,20,21-TETRADEHYDRO-15,20-DIHYDRO-8-HYDROXY-4-METHYL-11,16-DIOXO-, (8-xi,12-β,14-Z)-

TOXICITY DATA with REFERENCE
CAR: orl-rat TDLo: 1700 mg/kg/49W-C   CALEDQ 10,117,80
MUT: dns-ham: lvr 2 µmol/L   CNREA8 45,3125,85
MUT: dns-rat: lvr 2 µmol/L   CNREA8 45,3125,85
MUT: mma-sat 1 mg/plate   MUREAV 68,211,79
MUT: slt-slw-par 10 µg   KIKNAJ (30),70,79

SAFETY PROFILE: Questionable carcinogen with experimental carcinogenic data. Mutation data reported. When heated to decomposition it emits toxic fumes of NO_x.

CMX500   CAS: 911-45-5
CLOMIPHENE
mf: $C_{26}H_{28}ClNO$ mw: 406.00

SYNS: CHLOMAPHENE ◇ CHLORAMIFENE ◇ CHLORA-
MIPHENE ◇ 2-(4-(2-CHLORO-1,2-DIPHENYLETHENYL)PHE-
NOXY)-N,N-DIETHYLETHANAMINE ◇ 2-(p-(β-CHLORO-α-
PHENYLSTYRYL)PHENOXY)-TRIETHYLAMINE ◇ CISCLO-
MIPHENE ◇ CLOMEPHENE B ◇ CLOMIFENE ◇ 1-(p-(β-DI-
ETHYLAMINOETHOXY)PHENYL)-1,2-DIPHENYLCHLORO-
ETHYLENE

TOXICITY DATA with REFERENCE
CAR: orl-wmn TDLo: 15 mg/kg/13W-I:
  SPN,SKN   LANCAO 2,1176,77
ETA: orl-mus TDLo: 552 mg/kg/69W-I   PEXTAR
  11,440,69

SAFETY PROFILE: Questionable human carcinogen producing spinal cord and skin tumors.
Experimental teratogenic data. Poison by intraperitoneal route. Moderately toxic by ingestion.
Human systemic effects by ingestion: dermatitis.
Human reproductive effects by unspecified
routes: death of fetus, stillbirth, and poor viability. Human teratogenic effects by unspecified
routes include developmental abnormalities of
the central nervous system, cardiovascular system, gastrointestinal system, and urogenital system. Other experimental teratogenic and reproductive effects. When heated to decomposition
it emits very toxic fumes of Cl^- and NO_x.

CMX700   CAS: 50-41-9
racemic-CLOMIPHENE CITRATE
mf: $C_{26}H_{28}ClNO \cdot C_6H_8O_7$ mw: 598.14

SYNS: CHLORAMIPHENE ◇ CHLORAMIPHENE CITRATE
◇ 2-CHLORO-1-(p-(β-DIETHYLAMINOETHOXY)PHENYL)-
1,2-DIPHENYLETHYLENE ◇ 2-(p-(2-CHLORO-1,2-DIPHENYL
VINYL)PHENOXY)TRIETHYLAMINE CITRATE (1:1)
◇ CLOMID ◇ CLOMIFEN CITRATE ◇ CLOMIFENO
◇ CLOMIPHENE CITRATE ◇ CLOMIPHENE DIHYDROGEN
CITRATE ◇ CLOMIPHENE-R ◇ CLOMIPHINE ◇ CLOMIVID
◇ CLOMPHID ◇ 1-(p-(β-DIETHYLAMINO ETHOXY)PHE-
NYL)-1,2-DIPHENYL-2-CHLOROETHYLENE CITRATE
◇ DYNERIC ◇ GENOZYM ◇ IKACLOMIN ◇ MER-41
◇ MRL 41 ◇ NSC 35770 ◇ OMIFIN

TOXICITY DATA with REFERENCE
ETA: par-rat TD: 50 mg/kg   SCIEAS 197,164,77
ETA: par-rat TDLo: 2 mg/kg   OGSUA8 35,12,80
ETA: scu-rat TDLo: 2500 μg/kg   JSTBBK 12,47,80
MUT: dnd-esc 25 mg/L   MUREAV 165,57,86
MUT: dni-esc 50 mg/L   MUREAV 165,57,86

CONSENSUS REPORTS: IARC Cancer Review: Human Inadequate Evidence IMEMDT
21,551,79; Animal Inadequate Evidence
IMEMDT 21,551,79. EPA Genetic Toxicology
Program.

SAFETY PROFILE: Questionable carcinogen
with experimental tumorigenic and teratogenic
data. Moderately toxic by ingestion and intraperitoneal routes. Human reproductive effects by
ingestion: changes in spermatogenesis and effects on testes, epididymis and sperm duct. Human teratogenic effects by an unspecified route:
developmental abnormalities of the eye and ear.
Experimental reproductive effects. Used as a
drug to induce ovulation and for the treatment
of oligospermia. When heated to decomposition
it emits very toxic fumes of Cl^- and NO_x.

CMX845   CAS: 55600-34-5
CLOPHEN A-30

TOXICITY DATA with REFERENCE
NEO: orl-rat TDLo: 4992 mg/kg/2Y-C   TXAPA9
  75,278,84

SAFETY PROFILE: Questionable carcinogen
with experimental neoplastigenic data. When
heated to decomposition it emits acrid smoke
and irritating fumes.

CMY635
COAL DUST
DOT: 1361

PROP: Black powder or dust.

SYN: ANTHRACITE PARTICLES ◇ COAL FACINGS
◇ COAL, GROUND BITUMINOUS (DOT) ◇ COAL-MILLED
◇ COAL SLAG-MILLED ◇ SEA COAL

TOXICITY DATA with REFERENCE
ETA: ihl-rat TC: 14900 μg/m³/6H/86W-I
  AIHAAP 42,382,81
ETA: ihl-rat TCLo: 6600 μg/m³/6H/86W-I
  AIHAAP 42,382,81

OSHA PEL: (Transitional: Respirable Quartz
Fraction less than 5% SiO_2: TWA 2.4 mg/m³;
Respirable Quartz Fraction greater than or equal
to 5% SiO_2: 10 mg/m³) Respirable Quartz Fraction less than 5% SiO_2: TWA 2 mg/m³; Respirable Quartz Fraction greater than or equal to
5% SiO_2: 0.1 mg/m³   ACGIH TLV: TWA 2
mg/m³   DOT Classification: Flammable Solid;
Label: Flammable Solid.

SAFETY PROFILE: Questionable carcinogen
with experimental tumorigenic data. Variable
toxicity depending upon SiO_2 content. Moderately flammable when exposed to heat, flame,
or chemical reaction with oxidizers.

CMY805   CAS: 8007-45-2
COAL TAR, AEROSOL

TOXICITY DATA with REFERENCE
CAR: ihl-mus TCLo: 22 g/m³/55W-I   JNCIAM
39,175,67

OSHA PEL: TWA 0.2 mg/m³   NIOSH REL:
TWA 0.1 mg/m³ CHE fraction

CONSENSUS REPORTS: Reported in EPA
TSCA Inventory.

SAFETY PROFILE: Questionable carcinogen
with experimental carcinogenic data. When
heated to decomposition it emits acrid smoke
and irritating fumes.

CNB599   CAS: 7646-79-9
COBALT(II) CHLORIDE
mf: Cl_2Co mw: 129.83

PROP: Blue powder. Mp: 724°, bp: 1049°, d:
3.348.

SYNS: COBALT DICHLORIDE ◇ COBALT MURIATE
◇ COBALTOUS CHLORIDE ◇ COBALTOUS DICHLORIDE
◇ KOBALT CHLORID (GERMAN)

TOXICITY DATA with REFERENCE
CAR: scu-rat TDLo: 400 mg/kg   LBANAX 11,43,77
MUT: dni-hmn: hla 1 mmol/L   MUREAV 92,427,82
MUT: dns-ham: emb 200 μmol/L   MUREAV
131,173,84
MUT: mmo-smc 100 mmol/L   CPBTAL 33,1571,85
MUT: mrc-bcs 50 mmol/L   MUREAV 77,109,80
MUT: mrc-smc: 3 g/L   MUREAV 155,117,85
MUT: msc-ham: lng 200 μmol/L   MUREAV
68,259,79

CONSENSUS REPORTS: Reported in EPA
TSCA Inventory. EPA Genetic Toxicology Program. Cobalt and its compounds are on the Community Right-To-Know List.

SAFETY PROFILE: Questionable carcinogen
with experimental carcinogenic and teratogenic
data. Poison experimentally by ingestion, skin
contact, intraperitoneal, intravenous, and subcutaneous routes. Moderately toxic to humans by
ingestion. Human systemic effects by ingestion:
anorexia, goiter (increased thyroid size), and
weight loss. Experimental reproductive effects.
Human mutation data reported. When heated
to decomposition it emits toxic fumes of Cl^-.

CNC500   CAS: 10141-05-6
COBALT(II) NITRATE
mf: CoN_2O_6 mw: 182.95

PROP: Mp: 55°, d: 1.87.

SYNS: COBALT DINITRATE ◇ COBALTOUS NITRATE
◇ NITRIC ACID, COBALT (2+) SALT

TOXICITY DATA with REFERENCE
ETA: scu-rbt TDLo: 4530 μg/kg/5D-C   COREAF
236,1387,53

CONSENSUS REPORTS: Reported in EPA
TSCA Inventory. Cobalt and its compounds are
on the Community Right-To-Know List.

SAFETY PROFILE: Questionable carcinogen
with experimental tumorigenic data. Poison by
ingestion, intramuscular, and subcutaneous
routes. Experimental reproductive effects. Used
in animal feed. When heated to decomposition
it emits toxic fumes of NO_x.

CND125   CAS: 1307-96-6
COBALT(II) OXIDE
mf: CoO   mw: 74.93

PROP: Powder, or cubic or hexagonal crystals.
Color varies from olive green to red, depending
on the particle size, but the commercial material
is usually dark grey and contains about 76%
Co. Mp: about 1935°, d: 5.7 to 6.7. Practically
insol in water; sol in acids or alkalies. Easily
reduced to Co by C or CO.

SYNS: C.I. 77322 ◇ C.I. PIGMENT BLACK 13 ◇ COBALT
BLACK ◇ COBALT MONOOXIDE ◇ COBALT MONOXIDE
◇ COBALTOUS OXIDE ◇ COBALT OXIDE ◇ COBALT(2+)
OXIDE ◇ MONOCOBALT OXIDE ◇ ZAFFRE

TOXICITY DATA with REFERENCE
CAR: ims-rat TDLo: 135 mg/kg   CNREA8 22,152,62
ETA: ims-rat TD: 90 mg/kg   CNREA8 22,158,62

CONSENSUS REPORTS: Cobalt and its compounds are on the Community Right-To-Know
List. Reported in EPA TSCA Inventory.

SAFETY PROFILE: Questionable carcinogen
with experimental carcinogenic and tumorigenic
data. Poison by ingestion, subcutaneous, and
intratracheal routes. Moderately toxic by intramuscular route. Note: The commercial oxides
are usually not definite chemical compounds
but mixtures of the cobalt oxides.

CNE200   CAS: 1317-42-6
COBALT(II) SULFIDE
mf: CoS   mw: 90.99

PROP: Exists in two forms. α-CoS: black,
amorphous powder. Sol in HCl. β-CoS: grey

powder or reddish-silver octahedral crystals. Mp: above 1100°, d: 5.45. Practically insol in water; sol in acids.

SYNS: COBALT MONOSULFIDE ◇ COBALTOUS SULFIDE ◇ COBALT SULFIDE ◇ COBALT SULFIDE (AMORPHOUS)

TOXICITY DATA with REFERENCE
ETA: ims-rat TDLo: 180 mg/kg   CNREA8 22,158,62
MUT: dnd-ham: ovr 10 mg/L   CRNGDP 3,657,82
MUT: otr-ham: emb 1 mg/L   CNREA8 42,2757,82

CONSENSUS REPORTS: Reported in EPA TSCA Inventory. Cobalt and its compounds are on the Community Right-To-Know List.

SAFETY PROFILE: Questionable carcinogen with experimental tumorigenic data. Mutation data reported. If dried at 300°C it ignites spontaneously in air.

CNH250
COLTSFOOT

PROP: It is an herb of the tribe *Senecione* and from the family *Compositae* (GANNA2 67,-125,76).

SYNS: KAN-TO-KA (JAPANESE) ◇ TUSSILAGO FAR-FARA L

TOXICITY DATA with REFERENCE
CAR: orl-rat TDLo: 4800 g/kg/77W-C   GANNA2 67,125,76

SAFETY PROFILE: Questionable carcinogen with experimental carcinogenic data.

CNI000   CAS: 7440-50-8
COPPER
af: Cu   aw: 63.54

PROP: A metal with a distinct reddish color. Mp: 1083°, bp: 2324°, d: 8.92, vap press: 1 mm @ 1628°.

SYNS: ALLBRI NATURAL COPPER ◇ ANAC 110 ◇ ARWOOD COPPER ◇ BRONZE POWDER ◇ CDA 101 ◇ CDA 102 ◇ CDA 110 ◇ CDA 122 ◇ C.I. 77400 ◇ C.I. PIGMENT METAL 2 ◇ COPPER-AIRBORNE ◇ COPPER BRONZE ◇ COPPER-MILLED ◇ COPPER SLAG-AIRBORNE ◇ COPPER SLAG-MILLED ◇ 1721 GOLD ◇ GOLD BRONZE ◇ KAFAR COPPER ◇ M1 (COPPER) ◇ M2 (COPPER) ◇ OFHC Cu ◇ RANEY COPPER

TOXICITY DATA with REFERENCE
ETA: ipl-rat TDLo: 100 mg/kg   AIHAAP 41,836,80

CONSENSUS REPORTS: Reported in EPA TSCA Inventory. Copper and its compounds are on the Community Right-To-Know List.

OSHA PEL: TWA (dust, mist) 1 mg(Cu)/m^3; (fume) 0.1 mg/m^3 ACGIH TLV: TWA (dust, mist) 1 mg(Cu)/m^3; (fume) 0.2 mg/m^3 DFG MAK: (dust) 1 mg/m^3; (fume) 0.1 mg/m^3

SAFETY PROFILE: Questionable carcinogen with experimental tumorigenic data. Experimental teratogenic and reproductive effects. Human systemic effects by ingestion: nausea and vomiting. Liquid copper explodes on contact with water.

CNP250   CAS: 7758-98-7
COPPER(II) SULFATE (1:1)
DOT: 9109
mf: O$_4$S•Cu   mw: 159.60

PROP: Blue crystals or blue, crystalline granules or powder. D: 2.284.

SYNS: BCS COPPER FUNGICIDE ◇ BLUE COPPER ◇ BLUE STONE ◇ BLUE VITRIOL ◇ COPPER MONOSULFATE ◇ COPPER SULFATE ◇ CP BASIC SULFATE ◇ CUPRIC SULFATE ◇ KUPPERSULFAT (GERMAN) ◇ ROMAN VITRIOL ◇ SULFATE de CUIVRE (FRENCH) ◇ SULFURIC ACID, COPPER(2+) SALT (1:1) ◇ TNCS 53 ◇ TRINAGLE

TOXICITY DATA with REFERENCE
ETA: par-ckn TDLo: 10 mg/kg   BEXBAN 9,519,40
MUT: dnd-ham: emb 2200 μmol/L   CNREA8 39,193,79
MUT: dnd-rat: lvr 1 mmol/L   SinJF# 26OCT82
MUT: dni-mus-ipr 20 g/kg   ARGEAR 51,605,81
MUT: dns-ham: emb 200 μmol/L   MUREAV 131,173,84
MUT: mmo-bcs 400 μmol/L   AMAHA5 21,297,74
MUT: otr-ham: emb 80 μmol/L   CNREA8 39,193,79

CONSENSUS REPORTS: Copper and its compounds are on the Community Right-To-Know List. Reported in EPA TSCA Inventory. EPA Genetic Toxicology Program.

DOT Classification: ORM-E; label: None.

SAFETY PROFILE: Questionable carcinogen with experimental tumorigenic data. A human poison by ingestion. An experimental poison by ingestion, subcutaneous, parenteral, intravenous, and intraperitoneal routes. Human systemic effects by ingestion: gastritis, diarrhea, nausea or vomiting, damage to kidney tubules, and hemolysis. Mutation data reported. When heated to decomposition it emits toxic fumes of SO$_x$.

CNS250
CORONENE
CAS: 191-07-1

mf: $C_{24}H_{12}$ mw: 300.36

SYN: HEXABENZOBENZENE

TOXICITY DATA with REFERENCE
ETA: skn-mus TDLo: 20 mg/kg/W-I NCIMAV 28,173,68
MUT: dnd-mam: lym 20 mg BIPMAA 4,409,66
MUT: mma-sat 1 μg/plate/48H FCTXAV 17,141,79

CONSENSUS REPORTS: IARC Cancer Review: Animal Inadequate Evidence IMEMDT 32,263,83.

SAFETY PROFILE: Questionable carcinogen with experimental tumorigenic data. Mutation data reported. A polycyclic hydrocarbon air pollutant. When heated to decomposition it emits acrid smoke and irritating fumes.

CNS825
CORTISONE-21-ACETATE
CAS: 50-04-4

mf: $C_{23}H_{30}O_6$ mw: 402.53

SYNS: ACETATE CORTISONE ◇ 21-ACETOXY-17,α-HYDROXYPREGN-4-ENE-3,11,20-TRIONE ◇ 21-ACETOXY-17,α-HYDROXY-3,11,20-TRIKETOPREGNENE-4 ◇ 21-(ACETYLOXY)-17-HYDROXY-PREGN-4-ENE-3,11,20-TRIONE (9CI) ◇ ADRESON ◇ ARTRIONA ◇ BIOCORT ACETATE ◇ COMPOUND E ACETATE ◇ CORTADREN ◇ CORTELAN ◇ CORTISAL ◇ CORTISATE ◇ CORTISONE ACETATE ◇ CORTISONE MONOACETATE ◇ CORTISTAB ◇ CORTISYL ◇ CORTIVITE ◇ CORTOGEN ◇ CORTOGEN ACETATE ◇ CORTONE ◇ CORTONE ACETATE ◇ 11-DEHYDRO-17-HYDROXYCORTICOSTERONE ACETATE ◇ 11-DEHYDRO-17-HYDROXYCORTICOSTERONE-21-ACETATE ◇ 17,21-DI-HYDROXYPREGN-4-ENE-3,11,20-TRIONE ACETATE ◇ 17,21-DIHYDROXY-PREGN-4-ENE-3,11,20-TRIONE 21-ACETATE ◇ INCORTIN ◇ IRISONE ACETATE ◇ 4-PREGNENE-17,α,21-DIOL-3,11,20-TRIONE 21-ACETATE ◇ RICORTEX ◇ SCHEROSON

TOXICITY DATA with REFERENCE
ETA: ipr-mus TDLo: 35 mg/kg EXPEAM 33,1640,77
MUT: dnr-bcs 5 g/L MUREAV 42,19,77
MUT: mmo-bcs 5 g/L MUREAV 42,19,77

SAFETY PROFILE: Questionable carcinogen with experimental tumorigenic data. An experimental teratogen. Experimental reproductive effects. Mutation data reported. When heated to decomposition it emits acrid smoke and fumes.

CNU000
COTTONSEED OIL (UNHYDROGENATED)
CAS: 8001-29-4

PROP: Oily, pale yellow, nearly odorless liquid from seeds of species of *Gossypium hirsutum*. Flash p: 486°F (CC), fp: 0° to 5°, d: 0.915-0.921 @ 25°/25°, autoign temp: 650°F.

SYNS: DEODORIZED WINTERIZED COTTONSEED OIL ◇ NCI-C50168

TOXICITY DATA with REFERENCE
ETA: orl-mus TDLo: 2940 g/kg/35W-C LPDSAP 17,115,82

SAFETY PROFILE: Questionable carcinogen with experimental tumorigenic and teratogenic data. An allergen. Combustible liquid when exposed to heat or flame. To fight fire, use CO_2, dry chemical.

CNV000
COUMARIN
CAS: 91-64-5

mf: $C_9H_6O_2$ mw: 146.15

PROP: Crystals; fragrant, pleasant odor; burning taste. Mp: 70°, bp: 291.0°, vap press: 1 mm @ 106.0°.

SYNS: 2H-1-BENZOPYRAN-2-ONE ◇ 1,2-BENZOPYRONE ◇ cis-o-COUMARINIC ACID LACTONE ◇ COUMARINIC ANHYDRIDE ◇ o-HYDROXYCINNAMIC ACID LACTONE ◇ o-HYDROXYZIMTSAURE-LACTON (GERMAN) ◇ NCI-C60297 ◇ 2-OXO-1,2-BENZOPYRAN ◇ RATTEX ◇ TONKA BEAN CAMPHOR

TOXICITY DATA with REFERENCE
ETA: orl-rat TD: 200 g/kg/2Y-C TXCYAC 1,93,73
MUT: dnd-mam: Lym 20 mmol/L PNASA6 48,686,62
MUT: mma-sat 1 mg/plate ENMUDM 5(Suppl 1),3,83

CONSENSUS REPORTS: IARC Cancer Review: GROUP 3 IMEMDT 7,56,87; Animal Limited Evidence IMEMDT 10,113,76. EPA Genetic Toxicology Program. Reported in EPA TSCA Inventory.

SAFETY PROFILE: Questionable carcinogen with experimental tumorigenic and teratogenic data. Poison by ingestion, intraperitoneal, and subcutaneous routes. Mutation data reported. Combustible when exposed to heat or flame. When heated to decomposition it emits acrid smoke and fumes.

CNV750   CAS: 8065-91-6
C-QUENS

SYNS: ACONCEN ◇ CHLORMADINONE ACETATE mixed
with MESTRANOL ◇ 6-CHLORO-6-DEHYDRO-17-α-ACE-
TOXYPROGESTERONE mixed with MESTRENOL ◇ LUTES-
TRAL (FRENCH) ◇ MESTRANOL mixed with CHLORMADI-
NONE ACETATE ◇ MESTRANOL mixed with 6-CHLORO-6-
DEHYDRO-17-α-ACETOXYPROGESTERONE ◇ MESTRENOL
mixed with 6-CHLORO-6-DEHYDRO-17-α-ACETOXYPRO-
GESTERONE

TOXICITY DATA with REFERENCE
NEO: orl-wmn TDLo:60480 μg/kg/6Y-I
    SURGAZ 77,137,75

SAFETY PROFILE: Questionable human carcinogen producing liver tumors. Human reproductive effects by ingestion: changes in the
uterus, cervix, vagina, and fertility. Other experimental reproductive effects. Mildly toxic by
subcutaneous and intraperitoneal routes. A steroid. When heated to decomposition it emits
toxic fumes of Cl⁻.

CNW750   CAS: 108-39-4
m-CRESOL
DOT: 2076
mf: C_7H_8O mw: 108.15

PROP: Colorless to yellowish liquid, phenolic
odor. Mp: 10.9° bp: 202.8°, lel: 1.1% @ 302°F,
flash p: 202°F, d: 1.034 @ 20°/4°, autoign temp:
1038°F, vap press: 1 mm @ 52.0°, vap d: 3.72.

SYNS: 3-CRESOL ◇ m-CRESYLIC ACID ◇ 1-HYDROXY-
3-METHYLBENZENE ◇ m-HYDROXYTOLUENE ◇ m-KRE-
SOL ◇ m-METHYLPHENOL ◇ 3-METHYLPHENOL
◇ m-OXYTOLUENE ◇ RCRA WASTE NUMBER U052
◇ m-TOLUOL

TOXICITY DATA with REFERENCE
NEO: skn-mus TDLo:2280 mg/kg/20W-I
    CNREA8 19,413,59
MUT: dni-hmn:hla 10 μmol/L/4H   BECTA6
    32,220,84

CONSENSUS REPORTS: Community Right-
To-Know List. Reported in EPA TSCA Inventory. EPA Genetic Toxicology Program.

OSHA PEL: TWA 5 ppm (skin)   ACGIH TLV:
TWA 5 ppm NIOSH REL: TWA 10 mg/
m³ DOT Classification: Poison B; Label: Poison.

SAFETY PROFILE: Questionable carcinogen
with experimental neoplastigenic data. Poison

by ingestion, intravenous, intraperitoneal, and
subcutaneous routes. Moderately toxic by skin
contact. Severe eye and skin irritant. Human
mutation data reported. Flammable when exposed to heat or flame. Moderately explosive
in the form of vapor when exposed to heat or
flame.

CNX000   CAS: 95-48-7
o-CRESOL
DOT: 2076
mf: C_7H_8O mw: 108.15

PROP: Crystals or liquid darkening with exposure to air and light. Mp: 30.8°, bp: 190.8°,
flash p: 178°F, d: 1.047 @ 20°/4°, autoign temp:
1110°F, vap press: 1 mm @ 38.2°, vap d: 3.72,
lel: 1.4% @ 300°F.

SYNS: 2-CRESOL ◇ o-CRESYLIC ACID ◇ 1-HYDROXY-
2-METHYLBENZENE ◇ o-HYDROXYTOLUENE ◇ o-KRESOL
(GERMAN) ◇ o-METHYLPHENOL ◇ 2-METHYLPHENOL
◇ ORTHOCRESOL ◇ o-OXYTOLUENE ◇ RCRA WASTE
NUMBER U052 ◇ o-TOLUOL

TOXICITY DATA with REFERENCE
NEO: skn-mus TDLo:4800 mg/kg/12W-I
    CNREA8 19,413,59
MUT: sce-hmn:fbr 8 mmol/L   MUREAV 137,51,84

CONSENSUS REPORTS: EPA Extremely
Hazardous Substances List. Community Right
To Know Lit. EPA Genetic Toxicology Pro-
gram. Reported in EPA TSCA Inventory.

OSHA PEL: TWA 5 ppm (skin)   ACGIH TLV:
TWA 5 ppm NIOSH REL: TWA 10 mg/
m³ DOT Classification: Poison B; Label: Poison.

SAFETY PROFILE: Questionable carcinogen
with experimental neoplastigenic data. Poison
by ingestion, inhalation, subcutaneous, intravenous, and intraperitoneal routes. Moderately
toxic by skin contact. A severe eye and skin
irritant. Human mutation data reported. Flammable when exposed to heat, flame, or oxidants.
To fight fire, water may be used to blanket
fire; foam, fog, mist, dry chemical.

CNX250   CAS: 106-44-5
p-CRESOL
DOT: 2076
mf: C_7H_8O mw: 108.15

PROP: Found in a score of essential oils, including ylang-ylang and oil of jasmine (FCTXAV

12,385,74) Crystals, phenolic odor. Mp: 35.5°, bp: 201.8°, lel: 1.1% @ 302°F, flash p: 202°F, d: 1.0341 @ 20°/4°, autoign temp: 1038°F, vap press 1 mm @ 53.0°, vap d: 3.72.

SYNS: 4-CRESOL ◇ p-CRESYLIC ACID ◇ 1-HYDROXY-4-METHYLBENZENE ◇ p-HYDROXYTOLUENE ◇ 4-HYDROXYTOLUENE ◇ p-KRESOL ◇ 1-METHYL-4-HYDROXYBENZENE ◇ p-METHYLPHENOL ◇ 4-METHYLPHENOL ◇ p-OXYTOLUENE ◇ PARAMETHYL PHENOL ◇ RCRA WASTE NUMBER U052 ◇ p-TOLUOL ◇ p-TOLYL ALCOHOL

TOXICITY DATA with REFERENCE
NEO: skn-mus TDLo: 2280 mg/kg/20W-I
   CNREA8 19,413,59

CONSENSUS REPORTS: Community Right-To-Know List. Reported in EPA TSCA Inventory. EPA Genetic Toxicology Program.

OSHA PEL: TWA 5 ppm (skin)   ACGIH TLV: TWA 5 ppm NIOSH REL: TWA 10 mg/m³ DOT Classification: Poison B; Label: Poison.

SAFETY PROFILE: Questionable carcinogen with experimental neoplastigenic data by itself and with 7,12-dimethyl benz(a)anthracene. Poison by ingestion, skin contact, subcutaneous, intravenous, and intraperitoneal routes. A severe skin and eye irritant. Combustible when exposed to heat or flame. Moderately explosive in the form of vapor when exposed to heat or flame. To fight fire, use CO_2, dry chemical, alcohol foam.

COC250   CAS: 8001-28-3
CROTON OIL

PROP: Oil from the seeds of *Croton tiglium* (BJCAAI 10,72,56). Brownish-yellow, viscid oil; slt offensive odor. Composition: croton resin, glycerides of fatty acids and crotin. D: 0.935 @ 25°/25°.

SYNS: CROTONOEL (GERMAN) ◇ CROTON RESIN ◇ CROTON TIGLIUM L. OIL ◇ OLEUM TIGLII ◇ OLIO DI CROTON (ITALIAN)

TOXICITY DATA with REFERENCE
NEO: skn-mus TD: 150 mg/kg/15W-I   CNREA8
   19,413,59
NEO: skn-mus TDLo: 2 mg/kg/27W-I   BJCAAI
   7,482,53
ETA: skn-mus TD: 75 mg/kg/25W-I   JNCIAM
   39,1217,67
ETA: skn-mus TD: 120 mg/kg/3W-C   ZEKBAI
   65,325,63

ETA: skn-mus TD: 160 mg/kg/8W-I   GANNA2
   59,187,68
ETA: skn-mus TD: 285 mg/kg/42W-I   BJCAAI
   10,72,56
ETA: skn-mus TD: 340 µg/kg/17W-I   CNREA8
   28,653,68
ETA: skn-mus TD: 540 mg/kg/45W-I   IJCNAW
   1,491,66
ETA: skn-mus TD: 850 mg/kg/18W-I   BJCAAI
   7,472,53
ETA: skn-mus TD: 5714 mg/kg/14W-I   BJCAAI
   11,206,57
MUT: dni-hmn: fbr 10 ppm   CNREA8 35,1392,75
MUT: dni-hmn: lym 50 ppm   BBRCA9 45,630,71
MUT: mma-sat 2500 µg/plate   BJCAAI 37,873,78

CONSENSUS REPORTS: Reported in EPA TSCA Inventory.

SAFETY PROFILE: Questionable carcinogen with experimental neoplastigenic and tumorigenic data by skin contact. Poison by parenteral, intraperitoneal, and possibly other routes. A skin and eye irritant. An allergen. Human mutation data reported. When heated to decomposition it emits toxic fumes.

COD725
CRUDE OIL, synthetic

TOXICITY DATA with REFERENCE
CAR: skn-mus TDLo: 339 g/kg/2Y-I   FAATDF
   7,228,86

SAFETY PROFILE: Questionable carcinogen with experimental carcinogenic data. When heated to decomposition it emits acrid smoke and irritating fumes.

COG250   CAS: 29929-77-9
CURETARD
mf: $(C_{12}H_{14}N_2O)_n$

SYNS: N-NITROSO-2,2,4-TRIMETHYL-1,2-DIHYDRO-QUINOLINE,POLYMER ◇ 1-NITROSO-2,2,4-TRIMETHYL-1,2,-DIHYDRO-QUINOLINE (POLYMER) ◇ 1-NITROSO-2,2,4-TRIMETHYL-1(2H)QUINOLINE, POLYMER

TOXICITY DATA with REFERENCE
CAR: scu-rat TDLo: 2500 mg/kg/20W-I   BJCAAI
   23,408,69
NEO: ipr-rat TDLo: 2600 mg/kg/26W-I   EJCAAH
   4,233,68
ETA: ipr-rat TD: 2500 mg/kg/20W-I   BJCAAI
   23,408,69

SAFETY PROFILE: Questionable carcinogen with experimental carcinogenic, tumorigenic, and neoplastigenic data. When heated to decomposition it emits toxic fumes of NO_x.

COJ750   CAS: 6629-04-5
N-CYANOACETYL ETHYL CARBAMATE
mf: $C_6H_8N_2O_3$ mw: 156.16

TOXICITY DATA with REFERENCE
NEO: ipr-mus TDLo: 2400 mg/kg/4W-I

  CNREA8 29,2184,69

CONSENSUS REPORTS: Cyanide and its compounds are on the Community Right-To-Know List.

SAFETY PROFILE: Questionable carcinogen with experimental neoplastigenic data. When heated to decomposition it emits toxic fumes of NO_x.

COK500   CAS: 7476-08-6
10-CYANO-1,2-BENZANTHRACENE
mf: $C_{19}H_{11}N$ mw: 253.31

SYN: 7-CYANOBENZ(a) ANTHRACENE

TOXICITY DATA with REFERENCE
ETA: scu-mus TDLo: 2400 mg/kg/36W-I

  PRLBA4 129,439,40

ETA: skn-mus TDLo: 1370 mg/kg/57W-I

  PRLBA4 131,170,42

CONSENSUS REPORTS: Cyanide and its compounds are on the Community Right-To-Know List.

SAFETY PROFILE: Questionable carcinogen with experimental tumorigenic data. When heated to decomposition it emits toxic fumes of NO_x and CN^-.

COM000   CAS: 63018-68-8
5-CYANO-9,10-DIMETHYL-1,2-BENZANTHRACENE
mf: $C_{21}H_{15}N$ mw: 281.37

SYN: 7,12-DIMETHYLBENZ(a)ANTHRACENE-8-CARBONI-TRILE

TOXICITY DATA with REFERENCE
ETA: scu-mus TDLo: 80 mg/kg   CNREA8 6,454,46

CONSENSUS REPORTS: Cyanide and its compounds are on the Community Right-To-Know List.

SAFETY PROFILE: Questionable carcinogen with experimental tumorigenic data. When

heated to decomposition it emits toxic fumes of NO_x and CN^-.

COP765   CAS: 88254-07-3
CYANOMORPHOLINOADRIAMYCIN
mf: $C_{32}H_{34}N_2O_{12}$ mw: 638.68

SYNS: 3'-DEAMINO-3'-(3-CYANO-4-MORPHOLINYL) DOXORUBICIN ◇ MRA-CN ◇ 5,12-NAPHTHACENEDIONE, 7,8,9,10-TETRAHYDRO-10-((3-(3-CYANOMORPHOLINO)-2,3,6-TRIDEOXY-α-L-lyxo-HEXOPYRANOSYL)OXY)-8-(HY-DROXYACETYL)-1-METHOXY-6,8,11-TRIHYDR OXY-, (8s-cis)-

TOXICITY DATA with REFERENCE
CAR: ivn-rat TDLo: 10 μg/kg   CBTOE2 3,17,87
MUT: cyt-mus: leu 200 ng/L   CBTOE2 1,87,85
MUT: dnd-hmn: leu 10 nmol/L   CNREA846,4041,86
MUT: dni-hmn: leu 2200 pmol/L   CNREA8
  46,4041,86
MUT: dni-mus: leu 3 nmol/L   PAACA3 24,252,83
MUT: dns-rat: lvr 200 μg/L   CNREA8 44,5599,84
MUT: mma-sat 500 ng/plate   CNREA8 44,5599,84
MUT: msc-ham: lng 30 ng/L   CNREA8 44,5599,84
MUT: oth-hmn: leu 2800 pmol/L   CNREA8
  46,4041,86
MUT: oth-mus: leu 530 pmol/L   PAACA3 24,252,83
MUT: otr-mus: fbr 30 ng/L   CBTOE2 3,17,87

SAFETY PROFILE: Questionable carcinogen with experimental carcinogenic data. Mutation data reported. When heated to decomposition it emits toxic fumes of NO_x.

COS750   CAS: 41427-34-3
2-CYANO-4-STILBENAMINE
mf: $C_{15}H_{12}N_2$ mw: 220.29

SYNS: 4-AMINO-2-STILBENECARBONITRILE ◇ 2-CYANO-4-AMINOSTILBENE

TOXICITY DATA with REFERENCE
NEO: scu-rat TDLo: 2700 mg/kg/30W-I

  TXAPA9 5,344,63

CONSENSUS REPORTS: Cyanide and its compounds are on the Community Right-To-Know List.

SAFETY PROFILE: Questionable carcinogen with experimental neoplastigenic data. When heated to decomposition it emits toxic fumes of NO_x and CN^-.

COT500
CYCAD HUSK

PROP: The active substance in the cycad meal is aglycone of Cycasin, a methylazoxymethanol (JNCIAM 41,605,68).

SYN: CYCAS CIRCINALIS HUSK

TOXICITY DATA with REFERENCE
ETA: orl-rat TDLo:28 g/kg/10D-C   JNCIAM
41,605,68

SAFETY PROFILE: Questionable carcinogen with experimental tumorigenic data. When heated to decomposition it emits toxic and irritating fumes.

COT750
CYCAD MEAL

PROP: Obtained from the nut of *Cycas circinalis L.* (FEPRA7 23,1384,64).

SYN: CYCAD NUT, aqueous extract

TOXICITY DATA with REFERENCE
CAR: orl-rat TDLo:21 g/kg/3W-C   FEPRA7
23,1383,64
NEO: orl-gpg TDLo:30 g/kg/44W-I   FEPRA7
23,1384,64
ETA: skn-mus TDLo:68 g/kg/6D-C   FEPRA7
23,1383,64

SAFETY PROFILE: Questionable carcinogen with experimental carcinogenic, neoplastigenic, and tumorigenic data. When heated to decomposition it emits acrid smoke and fumes.

COV750   CAS: 3741-38-6
CYCLIC ETHYLENE SULFITE
mf: $C_2H_4O_3S$ mw: 108.12

SYNS: 1,3,2-DIOXATHIOLANE-2-OXIDE (9CI) ◇ ETHYLENE SULFITE ◇ 1,2-ETHYLENE SULFITE ◇ GLYCOL SULFITE

TOXICITY DATA with REFERENCE
ETA: ipr-mus TDLo:768 mg/kg/64W-I   JNCIAM
53,695,74

CONSENSUS REPORTS: Reported in EPA TSCA Inventory.

SAFETY PROFILE: Questionable carcinogen with experimental tumorigenic data. Poison by intraperitoneal route. When heated to decomposition it emits toxic fumes of SO_x.

COW750   CAS: 12663-46-6
CYCLOCHLOROTINE
mf: $C_{24}H_{30}Cl_2N_5O_7$ mw: 571.49

PROP: White needles. Mp: 251°, decomp. Chlorine containing peptide produced by *P. islandicum* (85CVA2 5,177,70).

SYN: ISLANDITOXIN

TOXICITY DATA with REFERENCE
ETA: orl-mus TDLo:362 mg/kg/32W-C
FCTXAV 10,193,72

CONSENSUS REPORTS: IARC Cancer Review: GROUP 3 IMEMDT 7,56,87; Animal Limited Evidence IMEMDT 10,139,76.

SAFETY PROFILE: Questionable carcinogen with experimental tumorigenic data. A deadly poison by ingestion, subcutaneous, intraperitoneal, and intravenous routes. When heated to decomposition it emits very toxic fumes of Cl^- and NO_x.

COX250   CAS: 64058-30-6
p-N-CYCLO
ETHYLENEUREIDOAZOBENZENE
mf: $C_{15}H_{14}N_4O$ mw: 266.33

SYNS: 4-N-CYCLOETHYLENEUREIDOAZOBENZENE
◇ AZOBENZEN (CZECH)

TOXICITY DATA with REFERENCE
ETA: scu-rat TDLo:1140 mg/kg/15W-I   BJPCAL
9,306,54

SAFETY PROFILE: Questionable carcinogen with experimental tumorigenic data. When heated to decomposition it emits toxic fumes of NO_x.

CPD000   CAS: 286-20-4
CYCLOHEXENE OXIDE
mf: $C_6H_{10}O$ mw: 98.16

PROP: Clear liquid. Bp: 129.5°, flash p: 81°F, d: 0.9678 @ 25°/4°, vap d: 3.5.

SYNS: CCHO ◇ CYCLOHEXANE OXIDE ◇ CYCLOHEXENE EPOXIDE ◇ CYCLOHEXENE-1-OXIDE ◇ 1,2-CYCLOHEXENE OXIDE ◇ CYCLOHEXYLENE OXIDE ◇ 1,2-EPOXYCYCLOHEXANE ◇ 7-OXABICYCLO(4.1.0)HEPTANE ◇ TETRAMETHYLENEOXIRANE

TOXICITY DATA with REFERENCE
ETA: unk-mus TDLo:79 mg/kg   RARSAM3,193,63
MUT: mma-sat 1 mg/plate   MUREAV 58,217,78
MUT: mmo-klp 5 mmol/L   MUREAV 89,269,81
MUT: mmo-sat 10 μmol/plate   BCPCA6 29,1068,80
MUT: msc-ham:lng 5 mmol/L   CBINA8 51,77,84

CONSENSUS REPORTS: Reported in EPA TSCA Inventory. EPA Genetic Toxicology Program.

SAFETY PROFILE: Questionable carcinogen with experimental tumorigenic data. Moderately

toxic by ingestion, skin contact, intraperitoneal, and intramuscular routes. Mildly toxic by inhalation. Mutation data reported. A dangerous fire hazard when exposed to heat or flame. When heated to decomposition it emits acrid smoke and irritant fumes.

CPD750   CAS: 100-40-3
CYCLOHEXENYLETHYLENE
mf: C_8H_{12} mw: 108.20

PROP: Liquid. Bp: 128°, fp: −109°, flash p: 60°F (TOC), d: 0.832 @ 20°/4°, autoign temp: 517°F, vap press: 25.8 mm @ 38°, vap d: 3.76.

SYNS: BUTADIENE DIMER ◇ 4-ETHENYL-1-CYCLOHEX-ENE ◇ NCI-C54999 ◇ 1,2,3,4-TETRAHYDROSTYRENE ◇ 1-VINYLCYCLOHEXENE-3 ◇ 1-VINYLCYCLOHEX-3-ENE ◇ 4-VINYLCYCLOHEXENE-1 ◇ 4-VINYL-1-CYCLOHEXENE

TOXICITY DATA with REFERENCE
CAR: orl-mus TD: 206 g/kg/2Y-I   NTPTR* NTP-TR-303,86

CAR: orl-mus TDLo: 103 g/kg/2Y-I   JTEHD6 21,507,87

NEO: orl-mus TD: 103 g/kg/2Y-I   NTPTR* NTP-TR-303,86

ETA: skn-mus TDLo: 16 g/kg/54W-I   JNCIAM 31,41,63

CONSENSUS REPORTS: IARC Cancer Review: GROUP 3 IMEMDT 7,56,87; Animal Inadequate Evidence IMEMDT 11,277,76; Animal Limited Evidence IMEMDT 39,181,86. NTP Carcinogenesis Studies (gavage); Clear Evidence: mouse NTPTR* NTP-TR-303,86; Inadequate Studies: rat NTPTR* NTP-TR-303,86. Reported in EPA TSCA Inventory.

SAFETY PROFILE: Questionable carcinogen with experimental carcinogenic, neoplastigenic, and tumorigenic data. Moderately toxic by ingestion and inhalation. Mildly toxic by skin contact. Dangerous fire hazard when exposed to heat, flame or oxidizers. Can react with oxidizers. To fight fire, use foam, CO_2, dry chemical.

CPF500   CAS: 108-91-8
CYCLOHEXYLAMINE
DOT: 2357
mf: $C_6H_{13}N$ mw: 99.20

PROP: Liquid; strong, fishy odor. Mp: −17.7°, bp: 134.5°, flash p: 69.8°F, d: 0.865 @ 25°/25°, autoign temp: 560°F, vap d. 3.42.

SYNS: AMINOCYCLOHEXANE ◇ AMINOHEXAHYDRO-BENZENE ◇ CHA ◇ CYCLOHEXANAMINE ◇ HEXAHY-DROANILINE ◇ HEXAHYDROBENZENAMINE

TOXICITY DATA with REFERENCE
MUT: cyt-ham:fbr 10 mg/L   MUREAV 39,1,76
MUT: cyt-hmn:leu 10 μmol/L/5H   MUREAV 39,1,76
MUT: cyt-rat-unk 50 mg/kg   MUREAV 26,199,74
MUT: dni-hmn:hla 100 μg/L   INHEAO 9,188,71
MUT: hma-mus/leu 450 mg/kg/3D   MUREAV 31,5,75

CONSENSUS REPORTS: IARC Cancer Review: GROUP 3 IMEMDT 7,178,87; Animal No Evidence IMEMDT 22,55,80. EPA Extremely Hazardous Substances List. EPA Genetic Toxicology Program. Reported in EPA TSCA Inventory.

OSHA PEL: TWA 10 ppm   ACGIH TLV: TWA 10 ppm   DFG MAK: 10 ppm (40 mg/m³) DOT Classification: Flammable Liquid; Label: Flammable Liquid, Corrosive; Flammable or Combustible Liquid; Label: Flammable, Corrosive.

SAFETY PROFILE: Questionable carcinogen. A poison by ingestion, skin contact, and intraperitoneal routes. Moderately toxic by subcutaneous and parenteral routes. An experimental teratogen. Other experimental reproductive effects. Severe human skin irritant. Can cause dermatitis; convulsions. Human mutation data reported. Flammable liquid. Dangerous fire hazard when exposed to heat, flame, or oxidizers. To fight fire, use alcohol foam, CO_2, dry chemical. When heated to decomposition it emits toxic fumes of NO_x.

CPF750   CAS: 19834-02-7
CYCLOHEXYLAMINE SULFATE
mf: $C_6H_{13}N \cdot H_2O_4S$ mw: 197.28

SYNS: CHA-SULFATE ◇ CHS ◇ CYCLOHEXAMINE SULFATE

TOXICITY DATA with REFERENCE
ETA: orl-rat TDLo: 11 g/kg/2Y-C   SCIEAS 167,1131,70

SAFETY PROFILE: Questionable carcinogen with experimental tumorigenic and teratogen data. Other experimental reproductive effects. When heated to decomposition it emits very toxic fumes of SO_x and NO_x.

CPI000   CAS: 13311-57-4
N-CYCLOHEXYL-1-AZIRIDINECARBOXAMIDE
mf: $C_9H_{16}N_2O$ mw: 168.27

SYNS: CYCLOHEXYL-N-CARBAMOYLAZIRIDINE ◇ N-CYCLOHEXYL-N-CARBAMOYLAZIRIDINE

TOXICITY DATA with REFERENCE
NEO: ipr-mus TDLo: 240 mg/kg/4W-I CNREA8 29,2184,69

SAFETY PROFILE: Questionable carcinogen with experimental neoplastigenic data. When heated to decomposition it emits toxic fumes of NO_x.

CPI250   CAS: 95-33-0
N-CYCLOHEXYL-2-BENZOTHIAZOLESULFENAMIDE
mf: $C_{13}H_{16}N_2S_2$ mw: 264.43

PROP: Light tan or buff powder. Mp: 94°, d: 1.27 @ 25°.

SYNS: DURAX ◇ PENNAC CBS ◇ SANTOCURE ◇ SULFENAMIDE TS

TOXICITY DATA with REFERENCE
ETA: orl-mus TDLo: 76 g/kg/78W-I NTIS** PB223-159

CONSENSUS REPORTS: Reported in EPA TSCA Inventory.

SAFETY PROFILE: Questionable carcinogen with experimental tumorigenic and teratogenic data. A poison by intravenous route. When heated to decomposition it emits toxic fumes of SO_x and NO_x.

CPU000   CAS: 202-98-2
4H-CYCLOPENTA(def)CHRYSENE
mf: $C_{19}H_{12}$ mw: 240.31

SYN: 4,5-METHYLENECHRYSENE

TOXICITY DATA with REFERENCE
ETA: scu-mus TDLo: 80 mg/kg CNREA8 3,606,43

SAFETY PROFILE: Questionable carcinogen with experimental tumorigenic data. When heated to decomposition it emits acrid smoke and irritating fumes.

CPX250   CAS: 203-64-5
4H-CYCLOPENTA(def)PHENANTHRENE
mf: $C_{15}H_{10}$ mw: 190.25

SYN: CYCLOPENTAPHENANTHRENE

TOXICITY DATA with REFERENCE
ETA: orl-rat TDLo: 3000 mg/kg CNREA8 26,619,66

SAFETY PROFILE: Questionable carcinogen with experimental tumorigenic data. When heated to decomposition it emits acrid smoke and irritating fumes.

CPX500   CAS: 27208-37-3
CYCLOPENTA(cd)PYRENE
mf: $C_{18}H_{10}$ mw: 226.28

SYNS: ACEPYRENE ◇ ACEPYRYLENE ◇ CYCLOPENTENO(c,d)PYRENE

TOXICITY DATA with REFERENCE
NEO: skn-mus TDLo: 9051 µg/kg CNREA8 40,642,80
ETA: scu-mus TDLo: 260 mg/kg HLSCAE 9,32,72
MUT: mma-hmn: lym 4 mg/L JJIND8 63,309,79
MUT: msc-ham: lng 300 µg/L CRNGDP 3,763,82
MUT: msc-hmn: lym 50 nmol/L MUREAV 128,221,84
MUT: msc-mus: lym 1200 µg/L CNREA8 40,4482,80
MUT: otr-mus: emb 300 µg/L EVSRBT 22,445,81
MUT: otr-mus: fbr 300 µg/L CNREA8 40,4482,80

CONSENSUS REPORTS: IARC Cancer Review: GROUP 3 IMEMDT 7,56,87; Animal Limited Evidence IMEMDT 32,269,83. EPA Genetic Toxicology Program.

SAFETY PROFILE: Questionable carcinogen with experimental neoplastigenic and tumorigenic data. Human mutation data reported. When heated to decomposition it emits acrid smoke and irritating fumes.

CPY500   CAS: 7129-91-1
1,2-CYCLOPENTENO-5,10-ACEANTHRENE
mf: $C_{19}H_{16}$ mw: 244.35

SYN: 2,7,8,9-TETRAHYDRO-1H-CYCLOPENT(j)ACEANTHRYLENE

TOXICITY DATA with REFERENCE
NEO: scu-mus TDLo: 160 mg/kg/43W-I JNCIAM 2,99,41

SAFETY PROFILE: Questionable carcinogen with experimental neoplastigenic data. When heated to decomposition it emits acrid smoke and irritating fumes.

CPY750   CAS: 7099-43-6
5:6-CYCLOPENTENO-1:2-BENZANTHRACENE
mf: $C_{21}H_{18}$ mw: 270.39

SYN: 2,3-DIHYDRO-1H-BENZO(a)CYCLOPENT(b)AN-THRACENE

TOXICITY DATA with REFERENCE
ETA: skn-mus TDLo:480 mg/kg/20W-I

PRLBA4 111,485,32

SAFETY PROFILE: Questionable carcinogen with experimental tumorigenic data. When heated to decomposition it emits acrid smoke and irritating fumes.

CQD250   CAS: 39071-30-2
5H-CYCLOPROPA(3,4)BENZ(1,2-e) AZULEN-5-ONE,1,1a-α,1b-β,4,4a,7a-α,7b,8,9,9a-DECAHYDRO-4a-α,7b-α,9a-α-TRIHYDROXY-3-HYDROXYMETHYL-1,6,8-α-TRIMETHYL-1-ACETOXY METHYL-,9a-(2-METHYLBUT-2-ENOATE)
mf: $C_{27}H_{36}O_8$ mw: 488.63

TOXICITY DATA with REFERENCE
ETA: skn-mus TDLo:225 mg/kg/36W-I

85CVA2 5,213,70

SAFETY PROFILE: Questionable carcinogen with experimental tumorigenic data. A skin irritant. When heated to decomposition it emits acrid smoke and irritating fumes.

CQH100   CAS: 59865-13-3
CYCLOSPORIN A
mf: $C_{62}H_{111}N_{11}O_{12}$ mw: 1202.84

SYNS: ANTIBIOTIC S 7481F1 ◇ CICLOSPORIN ◇ CYCLOSPORIN ◇ CYCLOSPORINE ◇ CYCLOSPORINE A ◇ OL 27-400 ◇ S 7481F1 ◇ SANDIMMUN ◇ SANDIMMUNE

TOXICITY DATA with REFERENCE
CAR: orl-man TDLo:259 mg/kg/2W-C

CEDEDE 8,159,83

MUT: sce-hmn:lyms 1 mg/L   IGAYAY 134,403,85

SAFETY PROFILE: Questionable human carcinogen producing Hodgkin's disease. Experimental carcinogenic data. Experimental reproductive effects. Poison by intraperitoneal and intravenous routes. Moderately toxic by ingestion. Human systemic effects by ingestion: increased body temperature, cyanosis. Mutation data reported. When heated to decomposition it emits toxic fumes of NO_x.

CQJ500   CAS: 427-51-0
CYPROSTERONE ACETATE
mf: $C_{24}H_{29}ClO_4$ mw: 416.98

SYNS: 17-α-ACETOXY-6-CHLORO-1-α,2-α-METHYLENE-PREGNA-4,6-DIENE-3,20-DIONE ◇ 6-CHLORO-1,2-α-METHYLENE-6-DEHYDRO-17-α-HYDROXYPROGESTER-ONE ACETATE ◇ 6-CHLORO-Δ⁶-1,2-α-METHYLENE-17-α-HYDROXYPROGESTERONE ACETATE ◇ 6-CHLORO-1,2-α-METHYLENE-17-α-HYDROXY-Δ⁶-PROGESTERONE ACE-TATE ◇ CPA ◇ CYPROTERONE ACETATE ◇ CYPRO-TERON-R ACETATE ◇ 1,2-α-METHYLENE-6-CHLORO-Δ⁶-17-α-HYDROXYPROGESTERONE ACETATE ◇ 1,2-α-METH-YLENE-6-CHLORO-PREGNA-4,6-DIENE-3,20-DIONE 17-α-ACETATE ◇ 1,2-α-METHYLENE-6-CHLORO-Δ⁻⁴,⁶-PREG-NADIENE-17-α-OL-3,20-DIONE 17-α-ACETATE ◇ 1,2-α-METHYLENE-6-CHLORO-Δ⁻⁴,⁶-PREGNADIENE-17-α-OL-3,20-DIONE ACETATE ◇ NSC-81430 ◇ PREGNA-4,6-DIENE-3,20-DIONE, 6-CHLORO-17-HYDROXY-1-α,2-α-METHYLENE-, ACETATE ◇ SH 714

TOXICITY DATA with REFERENCE
ETA: orl-rat TLDo:27 g/kg/78W   LANCAO
2,688,76
MUT: dns-rat-orl 40 mg/kg   CBINA8 31,287,80

CONSENSUS REPORTS: EPA Genetic Toxicology Program.

SAFETY PROFILE: Questionable carcinogen with experimental tumorigenic and teratogenic data. Moderately toxic by intraperitoneal route. Human reproductive effects by ingestion and possibly other routes: abnormal spermatogenesis, changes in the testes, epididymis, and sperm duct, impotence, and other paternal effects. Experimental reproductive effects. Mutation data reported. Used as a drug to arrest precocious puberty in children and hirsutism in women. A steroid. When heated to decomposition it emits toxic fumes of Cl^-.

CQM750   CAS: 3543-75-7
CYTOSTASAN
mf: $C_{16}H_{21}Cl_2N_3O_2 \cdot ClH$ mw: 394.76

SYNS: IMET 3393 ◇ γ(1-METHYL-5-BIS(β-CHLORA-ETHYL)AMINOBENZIMIDAZOLYL)BUTTERSAEUREHY-DROCHLORID(GERMAN) ◇ γ-(1-METHYL-5-BIS(β-CHLORO-AETHYL)AMINOBENZIMIDAZOYL) BUTTERSAUERHY-DROCHLORID(GERMAN)

TOXICITY DATA with REFERENCE
CAR: ipr-mus TDLo:50 mg/kg/4D-I   ARGEAR
43,16,74
CAR: orl-mus TDLo:250 mg/kg/4D-I   ARGEAR
43,16,74

SAFETY PROFILE: Questionable carcinogen with experimental carcinogenic and teratogenic data. A poison by ingestion, intravenous and intraperitoneal routes. When heated to decomposition it emits very toxic fumes of HCl and NO_x.

DAB020   CAS: 2307-55-3
2,4-D AMMONIUM SALT
mf: $C_8H_6Cl_2O_3 \cdot H_3N$ mw: 238.08

TOXICITY DATA with REFERENCE
ETA: skn-mus TDLo:1300 mg/kg/86W-I
   VPITAR 33(5),83,74

CONSENSUS REPORTS: IARC Cancer Review: Animal Inadequate Evidence IMEMDT 15,111,77

SAFETY PROFILE: Questionable carcinogen with experimental tumorigenic data. A poison by intraperitoneal route. When heated to decomposition it emits very toxic fumes of Cl^-, NO_x, and NH_3.

DAB830   CAS: 17230-88-5
DANOCRINE
mf: $C_{22}H_{27}NO_2$ mw: 337.50

PROP: Crystals from acetone. Mp: 224.4-226.8°.

SYNS: CHRONOGYN ◇ CYCLOMEN ◇ DANAZOL ◇ DANOL ◇ LADOGAL ◇ 17-α-2,4-PREGNADIEN-20-YNO(2,3-d)ISOXAZOL-17-OL ◇ 17-α-PREGNA-2,4-DIEN-20-YNO(2,3-d)ISOXAZOL-17-OL ◇ 17-α-PREGN-4-EN-20-YNO(2,3-d)ISOXAZOL-17-OL ◇ WIN 17757 ◇ WINOBANIN

TOXICITY DATA with REFERENCE
CAR: orl-wmn TDLo:2920 mg/kg/2Y-C
   JSONAU 28,114,85

SAFETY PROFILE: Questionable human carcinogen producing liver tumors. Human systemic effects by ingestion: allergic dermatitis. Human male reproductive effects by ingestion: changes in spermatogenesis, impotence, and other unspecified effects. Human female reproductive effects by ingestion: menstrual cycle changes or disorders, changes in fertility, and other unspecified effects. When heated to decomposition it emits toxic fumes of NO_x.

DAB845   CAS: 7261-97-4
DANTROLENE
mf: $C_{14}H_{10}N_4O_5$ mw: 314.28

SYN: HYDANTOIN, 1-((5-(p-NITROPHENYL)FURFURYLI-DENE)AMINO)-

TOXICITY DATA with REFERENCE
CAR: unr-man TDLo:9386 mg/kg/3Y-C
   PGMJAO 56,261,80

SAFETY PROFILE: Questionable human carcinogen producing Hodgkin's disease. When heated to decomposition it emits toxic fumes of NO_x.

DAC450   CAS: 12011-76-6
DAWSONITE
mf: $CH_2AlO_5 \cdot Na$ mw: 144.00

SYN: CRYSTALLINE DEHYDROXY SODIUM ALUMINUM, CARBONATE

TOXICITY DATA with REFERENCE
NEO: imp-rat TDLo:200 mg/kg   JJIND8 67,965,81

SAFETY PROFILE: Questionable carcinogen with experimental neoplastigenic data.

DAC800   CAS: 33857-26-0
DCDD
mf: $C_{12}H_6Cl_2O_2$ mw: 253.08

PROP: Colorless crystals. Mp: 210°.

SYNS: 2,7-DICHLORODIBENZO(b,e)(1,4)DIOXIN ◇ 2,7-DICHLORODIBENZO-p-DIOXIN ◇ 2,7-DICHLORODI-BENZODIOXIN ◇ NCI-C03667

TOXICITY DATA with REFERENCE
ETA: orl-mus TD:756 g/kg/90W-C   NCITR*
   NCI-CG-TR-123,79
ETA: orl-mus TDLo:378 g/kg/90W-C   NCITR*
   NCI-CG-TR-123,79

CONSENSUS REPORTS: IARC Cancer Review: Animal Inadequate Evidence IMEMDT 15,41,77. NCI Carcinogenesis Bioassay (feed); Clear Evidence: mouse NCITR* NCI-CG-TR-123,79; No Evidence: rat NCITR* NCI-CG-TR-123,79.

SAFETY PROFILE: Questionable carcinogen with experimental tumorigenic and teratogenic data. An eye irritant. When heated to decomposition it emits toxic fumes of Cl^-.

DAC975   CAS: 66826-72-0
cis-DCPO
mf: $C_3H_4Cl_2O$ mw: 126.97

SYNS: cis-2-CHLORO-3-(CHLOROMETHYL)OXIRANE ◇ cis-1,3-DICHLORO-1,2-EPOXYPROPANE ◇ cis-1,3-DI-CHLOROPROPENE OXIDE

TOXICITY DATA with REFERENCE
CAR: scu-mus TDLo:20 mg/kg/71W-I   CNREA8
   43,159,83

CAR: skn-mus TDLo:400 mg/kg/53W-I
CNREA8 43,159,83
MUT: otr-ham:emb 5 μmol/L JJIND8 69,531,82

SAFETY PROFILE: Questionable carcinogen with experimental carcinogenic data. Mutation data reported. When heated to decomposition it emits toxic fumes of Cl⁻.

DAD040 CAS: 61848-70-2
cis-DDCP
mf: $C_6H_4Cl_2N_2Pt$ mw: 370.11

SYNS: 1,2-DIAMINOCYCLOHEXANEPLATINUM(II) CHLORIDE ◊ DICHLORO(1,2-CYCLOHEXANEDIAMINE) PLATINUM ◊ DICHLORO(1,2-DIAMINOCYCLOHEXANE) PLATINUM ◊ DICHLORO(1,2-DIAMINOCYCLOHEXANE) PLATINUM(II) ◊ cis-DICHLORO-1,2-DIAMINOCYCLOHEX-ANE PLATINUM(II) ◊ NSC 194814 ◊ PT 155

TOXICITY DATA with REFERENCE
NEO: ipr-mus TD:41060 μg/kg/10W-I CNREA8 41,4368,81
NEO: ipr-mus TDLo:20530 μg/kg/10W-I CNREA8 41,4368,81
MUT: dnd-sat 10 mg/L/20H-C CNREA8 41,4368,81
MUT: mmo-sat 20 nmol/plate CNREA8 41,4368,81
MUT: oms-bcs 9900 nmol/L/3H-C CNREA8 41,4368,81

SAFETY PROFILE: Questionable carcinogen with experimental neoplastigenic data. Poison by intraperitoneal route. Mutation data reported. When heated to decomposition it emits toxic fumes of Cl⁻ and NO_x.

DAD050
trans(+)-DDCP
mf: $C_6H_{14}Cl_2N_2Pt$ mw: 380.176

SYNS: (SP-4-2)-trans(+)-DICHLORO(1,2-CYCLOHEXANE-DIAMINE-N,N')- (9CI) ◊ XX 212

TOXICITY DATA with REFERENCE
NEO: ipr-mus TD:41060 μg/kg/10W-I CNREA8 41,4368,81
NEO: ipr-mus TDLo:20530 μg/kg/10W-I CNREA8 41,4368,81
MUT: dnd-sat 10 mg/L/20H-C CNREA8 41,4368,81
MUT: mmo-sat 20 nmol/plate CNREA8 41,4368,81
MUT: oms-bcs 20 μmol/L/3H-C CNREA8 41,4368,81

SAFETY PROFILE: Questionable carcinogen with experimental neoplastigenic data. Mutation data reported. When heated to decomposition it emits toxic fumes of Cl⁻ and NO_x.

DAD075 CAS: 61848-66-6
trans(−)-DDCP
mf: $C_6H_{14}Cl_2N_2Pt$ mw: 380.21

SYN: trans(−)-DICHLORO-1,2-DIAMINOCYCLOHEXANE-PLATINUM(II)

TOXICITY DATA with REFERENCE
NEO: ipr-mus TD:41060 μg/kg/10W-I CNREA8 41,4368,81
NEO: ipr-mus TDLo:20530 μg/kg/10W-I CNREA8 41,4368,81
MUT: dnd-sat 10 mg/L/20H-C CNREA8 41,4368,81
MUT: mmo-sat 20 nmol/plate CNREA8 41,4368,81
MUT: oms-bcs 13 μmol/L/3H-C CNREA8 41,4368,81

SAFETY PROFILE: Questionable carcinogen with experimental neoplastigenic data. Mutation data reported. When heated to decomposition it emits toxic fumes of Cl⁻ and NO_x.

DAE800 CAS: 91-17-8
DECAHYDRONAPHTHALENE
DOT: 1147
mf: $C_{10}H_{18}$ mw: 138.28

PROP: Water-white liquid. Mp (cis): −43.3°, mp (trans): −30.7°, bp: (cis): 195.6°, bp: (trans) 187.3°, flash p: 136°F, (CC), autoign temp: 482°F, vap press: (cis) 1 mm @ 22.5°, (trans) 10 mm @ 47.2°, d: (cis) 0.8963 @ 20°/4°, vap d: 4.76, lel: 0.7% @ 212°F, uel: 4.9% @ 212°F.

SYNS: BICYCLO(4.4.0)DECANE ◊ DEC ◊ DECALIN ◊ DECALIN (DOT) ◊ DECALIN SOLVENT ◊ DE-KALIN ◊ DEKALINA (POLISH) ◊ NAPHTHALANE ◊ NAPHTHANE ◊ PERHYDRONAPHTHALENE

TOXICITY DATA with REFERENCE
CAR: ihl-mus TCLo:50 ppm/24H/90D-C FAATDF 5,785,85
NEO: ihl-rat TCLo:5 ppm/24H/90D-C FAATDF 5,785,85

CONSENSUS REPORTS: Reported in EPA TSCA Inventory.

DOT Classification: Combustible Liquid; Label: None; Flammable or Combustible Liquid; Label: Flammable Liquid.

SAFETY PROFILE: Questionable carcinogen with experimental carcinogenic and neoplastigenic data. Moderately toxic by inhalation and ingestion. Mildly toxic by skin contact. Human systemic effects by inhalation: conjuctiva irritation, unspecified olfactory and pulmonary system changes. Can cause kidney damage. Mutation data reported. A skin and eye irritant. Flammable when exposed to heat or flame, can react with oxidizing materials. To fight fire, use foam, CO_2, dry chemical. When heated to decomposition it emits acrid smoke and fumes.

DAG400   CAS: 124-18-5
DECANE
DOT: 2247
mf: $C_{10}H_{22}$ mw: 142.29

PROP: Liquid. Mp: −29.7°, bp: 174.1°, lel: 0.8%, uel: 5.4%, flash p: 115°F (CC), d: 0.730 @ 20°/4°, autoign temp: 410°F, vap press: 1 mm @ 16.5°, vap d: 4.90.

SYN: n-DECANE (DOT)

TOXICITY DATA with REFERENCE
ETA: skn-mus TDLo:25 g/kg/52W-I   TXAPA9 9,70,66

CONSENSUS REPORTS: Reported in EPA TSCA Inventory.

DOT Classification: Flammable or Combustible Liquid; Label: Flammable Liquid.

SAFETY PROFILE: Questionable carcinogen with experimental tumorigenic data. A simple asphyxiant. Narcotic in high concentrations. Flammable when exposed to heat or flame. Moderately explosive in its vapor form. To fight fire, use foam, CO_2, dry chemical.

DAI600   CAS: 112-30-1
DECYL ALCOHOL
mf: $C_{10}H_{22}O$ mw: 158.32

PROP: Found in sweet orange and a few other essential oils (FCTXAV 11,95,73). Colorless, viscous, refractive liquid; floral fruity odor. Mp: 7°, bp: 232.9°, flash p: 180°F (OC), d: 0.8297 @ 20°/4°, refr index: 1.435-1.439, vap press: 1 mm @ 69.5°, vap d: 5.3. Sol in alc, ether, mineral oil, propylene glycol, fixed oils; insol in glycerin water @ 233°.

SYNS: AGENT 504 ◇ ALCOHOL C-10 ◇ ANTAK ◇ C 10 ALCOHOL ◇ CAPRIC ALCOHOL ◇ CAPRINIC ALCOHOL ◇ DECANAL DIMETHYL ACETAL ◇ DECANOL ◇ n-DECANOL ◇ 1-DECANOL (FCC) ◇ n-DECATYL ALCOHOL ◇ n-DECYL ALCOHOL ◇ DECYLIC ALCOHOL ◇ DYTOL S-91 ◇ EPAL 10 ◇ FEMA No. 2365 ◇ LOROL 22 ◇ NONYLCARBINOL ◇ PRIMARY DECYL ALCOHOL ◇ ROYALTAC ◇ SIPOL L10

TOXICITY DATA with REFERENCE
ETA: skn-mus TDLo:12 g/kg/25W-I   TXAPA9 9,70,66

CONSENSUS REPORTS: Reported in EPA TSCA Inventory.

SAFETY PROFILE: Questionable carcinogen with experimental tumorigenic data. Moderately toxic by skin contact. Mildly toxic by ingestion, inhalation, and possibly other routes. A severe human skin and eye irritant. Combustible when exposed to heat or flame; can react with oxidizing materials. To fight fire, use foam, CO_2, dry chemical. When heated to decomposition it emits acrid smoke and irritating fumes.

DAK600   CAS: 434-16-2
7-DEHYDROCHOLESTEROL
mf: $C_{27}H_{44}O$ mw: 384.71

SYNS: (3-β)CHOLESTA-5,7-DIEN-3-OL ◇ 5,7-CHOLESTA-DIEN-3-β-OL ◇ Δ⁷-CHOLESTEROL ◇ Δ⁵,⁷-CHOLESTEROL ◇ DEHYDROCHOLESTERIN (GERMAN) ◇ 7-DEHYDROCHOLESTERIN ◇ DEHYDROCHOLESTEROL ◇ 7,8-DIDEHYDRO-CHOLESTEROL ◇ PROVITAMIN D₃

TOXICITY DATA with REFERENCE
ETA: scu-mus TDLo:800 mg/kg/4W-I   NATWAY 60,525,73

CONSENSUS REPORTS: Reported in EPA TSCA Inventory.

SAFETY PROFILE: Questionable carcinogen with experimental tumorigenic data. When heated to decomposition it emits acrid smoke and irritating fumes.

DAK800   CAS: 1059-86-5
7-DEHYDROCHOLESTEROL ACETATE
mf: $C_{29}H_{46}O_2$ mw: 426.75

SYNS: CHOLESTA-5,7-DIEN-3-β-OL ACETATE ◇ 7-DEHYDROCHOLESTERYL ACETATE

TOXICITY DATA with REFERENCE
ETA: scu-mus TDLo:200 mg/kg/90D-I   NATUAS 209,1026,66

SAFETY PROFILE: Questionable carcinogen with experimental tumorigenic data. When heated to decomposition it emits acrid smoke and irritating fumes.

DAL200   CAS: 3343-10-0
1,2-DEHYDRO-3-METHYLCHOLANTHRENE
mf: $C_{21}H_{14}$ mw: 266.35

SYNS: DEHYDRO-3-METHYLCHOLANTHRENE ◇ 3-METHYLBENZ(j)ACEANTHRYLENE ◇ 3-METHYLCHO-LANTHRYLENE ◇ 20-METHYLCHOLANTHRYLENE

TOXICITY DATA with REFERENCE

CAR: skn-mus TDLo: 85 mg/kg/20W-I CBINA8 22,69,78

NEO: scu-mus TDLo: 120 mg/kg/6W-I IJCNAW 2,505,67

SAFETY PROFILE: Questionable carcinogen with experimental carcinogenic and neoplastigenic data. When heated to decomposition it emits acrid smoke and irritating fumes.

DAL300   CAS: 72-63-9
1-DEHYDRO-17-α-
METHYLTESTOSTERONE

mf: $C_{20}H_{28}O_2$ mw: 300.42

PROP: Crystals from acetone + ether. Mp: 163-164°.

SYNS: ABIROL ◇ ANABOLIN ◇ CIBA 17309 BA ◇ COMPOUND 17309 ◇ CREIN ◇ DANABOL ◇ DEHYDRO-METHYLTESTERONE ◇ A1-DEHYDROMETHYLTESTERONE ◇ DIANABOL ◇ DIANABOLE ◇ GEABOL ◇ 17-β-HYDROXY-17-α-METHYLANDROSTRA-1,4-DIEN-3-ONE ◇ MA ◇ METANABOL ◇ METANDIENON ◇ METANDIENONE ◇ METANDIENONUM ◇ METANDROSTENOLON ◇ METANDROSTENOLONE ◇ METASTENOL ◇ METHAN-DIENONE ◇ METHANDROLONE ◇ METHANDROSTENO-LONE ◇ 17-α-METHYL-17-β-HYDROXY-1,4-ANDROSTA-DIEN-3-ONE ◇ Δ′-17-METHYLTESTOSTERONE ◇ Δ(^{1})-17-α-METHYLTESTOSTERONE ◇ NEROBOL ◇ NEROBOLETTES ◇ NSC-42722 ◇ PROTOBOLIN ◇ STENOLON ◇ STENOLONE

TOXICITY DATA with REFERENCE

CAR: orl-man TDLo: 561 mg/kg/7Y-C LANCAO 2,1273,72

MUT: dlt-mus-orl 200 mg/kg/10D-I VPITAR 38(4),63,80

CONSENSUS REPORTS: EPA Genetic Toxicology Program.

SAFETY PROFILE: Questionable human carcinogen producing liver tumors. Human reproductive effects by ingestion route: changes in spermatogenesis. Mutation data reported. When heated to decomposition it emits acrid smoke and irritating fumes.

DAL350   CAS: 23291-96-5
DEHYDROMONOCROTALINE

mf: $C_{16}H_{21}NO_6$ mw: 323.38

SYNS: MONOCROTALINE, 3,8-DIDEHYDRO- ◇ 20-NOR-CROTALANAN-11,15-DIONE, 3,8-DIDEHYDRO-14,19-DIHY-DRO-12,13-DIHYDROXY-, (13-α-14-α)-

TOXICITY DATA with REFERENCE

ETA: skn-mus TDLo: 1504 mg/kg/47W-I CALEDQ 17,61,82

SAFETY PROFILE: Questionable carcinogen with experimental tumorigenic data. Poison by intraperitoneal route. When heated to decomposition it emits toxic fumes of NO_x.

DAP700   CAS: 2955-38-6
DEMETRIN

mf: $C_{19}H_{17}ClN_2O$ mw: 324.83

PROP: Crystals from methanol. Mp: 145-146°.

SYNS: CENTRAX ◇ 7-CHLORO-1-(CYCLOPROPYL-METHYL)-1,3-DIHYDRO-5-PHENYL-2H-1,4-BENZODIAZE-PIN-2-ONE ◇ 7-CHLORO-1-CYCLOPROPYLMETHYL-5-PHE-NYL-1H-1,4-BENZODIAZEPIN-2(3H)-ONE ◇ K-373 ◇ LYSANXIA ◇ PRAZEPAM ◇ SEDAPRAN ◇ SETTIMA ◇ TREPIDAN ◇ VERSTRAN

TOXICITY DATA with REFERENCE

ETA: orl-mus TDLo: 14 g/kg/80W-C TXAPA9 57,39,81

ETA: orl-rat TDLo: 5284 mg/kg/2Y-C TXAPA9 57,39,81

MUT: orl-rat TD: 55 g/kg/2Y-C TXAPA9 57,39,81

SAFETY PROFILE: Questionable carcinogen with experimental tumorigenic and teratogenic data. Moderately toxic by ingestion and intraperitoneal routes. Experimental reproductive effects. Note: This is a controlled substance (depressant) listed in the U.S. Code of Federal Regulations, Title 21 Part 1308.14 (1985). A tranquilizer and muscle relaxant. When heated to decomposition it emits toxic fumes of Cl^- and NO_x.

DAQ400   CAS: 83-44-3
DEOXYCHOLATIC ACID

mf: $C_{24}H_{40}O_4$ mw: 392.64

PROP: A white crystalline powder. Mp: 178°. Sol in alc, acetone; sltly sol in ether, and chloroform; insol in water.

SYNS: CHOLEIC ACID ◇ CHOLEREBIC ◇ CHOLOREBIC ◇ DEGALOL ◇ DEOXYCHOLIC ACID (FCC) ◇ 7-α-DEOXY-CHOLIC ACID ◇ DESOXYCHOLIC ACID ◇ DESOXYCHOL-SAEURE (GERMAN) ◇ 3,12-DIHYDROXYCHOLANIC ACID ◇ 3-α,12-α-DIHYDROXYCHOLANIC ACID ◇ 3-α,12-α-DIHY-DROXY-5-β-CHOLAN-24-OIC ACID ◇ 3-α,12-α-DIHY-DROXY-5-β-CHOLANOIC ACID ◇ 3-α,12-α-DIHYDROXY-CHOLANSAEURE (GERMAN) ◇ DROXOLAN ◇ 17-β-(1-METHYL-3-CARBOXYPROPYL)-ETIOCHOLANE-3-α,12-α-DIOL ◇ PYROCHOL ◇ SEPTOCHOL

TOXICITY DATA with REFERENCE
ETA: scu-mus TD: 1400 mg/kg/22W-I   PRLBA4
129,439,40
ETA: scu-mus TDLo: 1120 mg/kg/22W-I
NATUAS 145,627,40
ETA: skn-mus TDLo: 2700 mg/kg/10W-I
BJCAAI 10,363,56
MUT: mmo-sat 20 mg/L   MUREAV 158,45,85
MUT: otr-ham: emb 7250 μg/L   TOLED5 9,177,81
MUT: sln-smc 100 mg/L   CRNGDP 5,447,84

CONSENSUS REPORTS: Reported in EPA
TSCA Inventory.

SAFETY PROFILE: Questionable carcinogen
with experimental tumorigenic data. Poison by
intraperitoneal route. Moderately toxic by ingestion and intravenous routes. Mutation data reported. When heated to decomposition it emits
acrid smoke and irritating fumes.

DAQ800   CAS: 56-47-3
**11-DEOXYCORTICOSTERONE
ACETATE**
mf: $C_{23}H_{32}O_4$ mw: 372.55

SYNS: 21-ACETOXY-3,20-DIKETOPREGN-4-ENE
◇ CORTACET ◇ CORTATE ◇ CORTENIL ◇ CORTESAN
◇ CORTEXONE ACETATE ◇ CORTIFAR ◇ CORTIGEN
◇ CORTINAQ ◇ CORTIRON ◇ CORTIVIS ◇ CORTIXYL
◇ DCA ◇ DECORTIN ◇ DECORTON ◇ DECOSTERONE
◇ DECOSTRATE ◇ 11-DEOXYCORTICOSTERONE-21-ACE-
TATE ◇ DEOXYCORTONE ACETATE ◇ DESCORTERONE
◇ DESCOTONE ◇ DESOXYCORTICOSTERONE ACETATE
◇ DESOXYCORTONE ACETATE ◇ DOCA ◇ DOCA ACETATE
◇ DOC-AC ◇ DOC ACETATE ◇ DORCOSTRIN ◇ DOXO
◇ 21-HYDROXYPREGN-4-ENE-3,20-DIONE-21-ACETATE
◇ KRINOCORTS ◇ OCRITEN ◇ ORGANON'S DOCA ACE-
TATE ◇ PERCORTEN ◇ PERCOTOL ◇ 4-PREGNENE-3,20-
DIONE-21-OL ACETATE ◇ PRIMOCORT ◇ PRIMOCORTAN
◇ SINCORTEX ◇ STERAQ ◇ SYNCORT ◇ SYNCORTA
◇ SYNCORTYL ◇ UNIDOCAN

TOXICITY DATA with REFERENCE
ETA: scu-mus TDLo: 520 mg/kg/13W-I
PSEBAA 83,14,53

SAFETY PROFILE: Questionable carcinogen
with experimental tumorigenic data. Experimental reproductive effects. A steroid. When
heated to decomposition it emits acrid smoke
and irritating fumes.

DAS000   CAS: 54-42-2
2'-DEOXY-5-IODOURIDINE
mf: $C_9H_{11}IN_2O_5$ mw: 354.12

SYNS: ALLERGAN 211 ◇ DENDRID ◇ 1-(2-DEOXY-β-d-
RIBOFURANOSYL)-5-IODOURACIL ◇ 1-β-d-2'-DEOXYRIBO-
FURANOSYL-5-IODOURACIL ◇ EMANIL ◇ HERPESIL
◇ HERPIDU ◇ HERPLEX ◇ HERPLEX LIQUIFILM
◇ IDEXUR ◇ IDOXENE ◇ IDOXURIDIN ◇ IDOXURIDINE
◇ IDU ◇ IDUCHER ◇ IDULEA ◇ IDUOCULOS ◇ IDUR
◇ IDURIDIN ◇ 5-IODODEOXYURIDINE ◇ 5-IODO-2'-DE-
OXYURIDINE ◇ 5-IODOURACIL DEOXYRIBOSIDE
◇ IUDR ◇ 5-IUDR ◇ JODDEOXIURIDIN ◇ KERECID
◇ NSC 39661 ◇ OPHTHALMADINE ◇ SK&F 14287
◇ STOXIL ◇ SYNMIOL

TOXICITY DATA with REFERENCE
CAR: ipr-mus TDLo: 100 mg/kg/8W-I   EXPEAM
29,1132,73
MUT: dni-rbt: kdy 1 mg/L   JMCMAR 24,390,81
MUT: msc-ham: lng 1 mg/L   CRNGDP 6,1207,85
MUT: msc-hmn: lym 100 μmol/L   LIFSAK
19,563,76
MUT: sce-hmn: fbr 50 mg/L   BMJOAE 283,817,81
MUT: sce-hmn: lym 50 mg/L   BMJOAE 283,817,81

CONSENSUS REPORTS: Reported in EPA
TSCA Inventory. EPA Genetic Toxicology Program.

SAFETY PROFILE: Questionable carcinogen
with experimental carcinogenic and teratogenic
data. Moderately toxic by intraperitoneal route.
Experimental reproductive effects. Human mutation data reported. When heated to decomposition it emits very toxic fumes of I^- and NO_x.

DAS400   CAS: 10356-92-0
**1-DEOXY-1-(N-
NITROSOMETHYLAMINO)-d-GLUCITOL**
mf: $C_7H_{16}N_2O_6$ mw: 224.25

SYNS: 1-DEOXY-1-(METHYLNITROSAMINO)-d-GLUCI-
TOL ◇ 1-(N-METHYL-N-NITROSOAMINO)-1-DEOXY-d-GLU-
CITOL ◇ 1-N-METHYL-N-NITROSOAMINO-1-DEOXY-d-GLU-
CITOLE ◇ 1-N-METHYL-N-NITROSOAMINO-1-DESOXY-d-
GLUCIT (GERMAN)

TOXICITY DATA with REFERENCE
ETA: orl-rat TDLo: 2500 mg/kg/25W-I   ZEKBAI
75,296,71

SAFETY PROFILE: Questionable carcinogen
with experimental tumorigenic data. Many N-
nitroso compounds are carcinogens. When
heated to decomposition it emits toxic fumes
of NO_x.

DAU200   CAS: 65700-59-6
**12-DEOXYPHORBOL-13-ANGELATE-20-
ACETATE**
mf: $C_{27}H_{36}O_7$ mw: 472.63

TOXICITY DATA with REFERENCE
ETA: skn-mus TDLo: 180 mg/kg/24W-I
EXPEAM 30,1438,74

SAFETY PROFILE: Questionable carcinogen with experimental tumorigenic data. A skin irritant. When heated to decomposition it emits acrid smoke and irritating fumes.

DBA500
DESGLUCODIGITONIN

TOXICITY DATA with REFERENCE
ETA: ipr-mus LD10: 20 mg/kg   PCJOAU 11,749,77

SAFETY PROFILE: Questionable carcinogen with experimental tumorigenic data. When heated to decomposition it emits acrid smoke and irritating fumes.

DBC800   CAS: 9004-54-0
DEXTRAN 1

PROP: A linear water-sol polymer of average molecular weight 200,000 (ARPAAQ 67, 589,59).

TOXICITY DATA with REFERENCE
ETA: ipr-mus TDLo: 8000 mg/kg   AMPLAO
67,589,59
ETA: scu-mus TDLo: 8000 mg/kg   AMPLAO
67,589,59

CONSENSUS REPORTS: Reported in EPA TSCA Inventory.

SAFETY PROFILE: Questionable carcinogen with experimental neoplastigenic, tumorigenic, and teratogenic data. When heated to decomposition it emits acrid smoke and fumes.

DBD000   CAS: 9004-54-0
DEXTRAN 2

PROP: A linear, water-sol polymer of average molecular weight 100,000 (ARPAAQ 67, 589,59).

TOXICITY DATA with REFERENCE
NEO: ipr-mus TDLo: 8000 mg/kg   AMPLAO
67,589,59
NEO: ipr-rat TDLo: 2500 mg/kg   AMPLAO
67,589,59
NEO: scu-rat TDLo: 2500 mg/kg   AMPLAO
67,589,59

CONSENSUS REPORTS: Reported in EPA TSCA Inventory.

SAFETY PROFILE: Questionable carcinogen with experimental neoplastigenic data. When

heated to decomposition it emits acrid smoke and fumes.

DBD200   CAS: 9004-54-0
DEXTRAN 5

PROP: A highly branched, water-sol polymer (ARPAAQ 67,589,59).

TOXICITY DATA with REFERENCE
NEO: scu-mus TDLo: 8000 mg/kg   AMPLAO
67,589,59

CONSENSUS REPORTS: Reported in EPA TSCA Inventory.

SAFETY PROFILE: Questionable carcinogen with experimental neoplastigenic data. When heated to decomposition it emits acrid smoke and fumes.

DBD600   CAS: 9004-54-0
DEXTRAN 11

PROP: A highly branched, water-sol polymer of average molecular weight 71,400 (ARPAAQ 67,589,59).

TOXICITY DATA with REFERENCE
NEO: ipr-rat TDLo: 2500 mg/kg   AMPLAO
67,589,59
ETA: ivn-rbt TDLo: 8750 mg/kg   AMPLAO
67,589,59
ETA: scu-mus TDLo: 8000 mg/kg   AMPLAO
67,589,59

CONSENSUS REPORTS: Reported in EPA TSCA Inventory.

SAFETY PROFILE: Questionable carcinogen with experimental neoplastigenic and tumorigenic data. When heated to decomposition it emits acrid smoke and fumes.

DBD750   CAS: 9011-18-1
DEXTRAN SULFATE SODIUM

PROP: White powder from alcohol + ether. Freely sol in water.

SYNS: ASURO ◇ COLYONAL ◇ DEXTRARINE ◇ DEXULATE ◇ DS-M-1 ◇ MDS

TOXICITY DATA with REFERENCE
CAR: orl-rat TD: 335 g/kg/19W-C   JJIND8
66,579,81
CAR: orl-rat TD: 600 g/kg/69W-C   CALEDQ
18,29,83
CAR: orl-rat TDLo: 330 g/kg/94W-C   CRNGDP
3,353,82

SAFETY PROFILE: Questionable carcinogen with experimental carcinogenic data. Moderately toxic by intravenous route. When heated to decomposition it emits toxic fumes of SO_x and Na_2O.

DBF000   CAS: 63019-65-8
N-1-DIACETAMIDOFLUORENE
mf: $C_{17}H_{15}NO_2$ mw: 265.33

SYNS: N-FLUOREN-1-YLDIACETAMIDE ◇ N-1-FLUORE-NYLDIACETAMIDE

TOXICITY DATA with REFERENCE
ETA: orl-rat TDLo:5200 mg/kg/52W-C
  JNCIAM 24,149,60

SAFETY PROFILE: Questionable carcinogen with experimental tumorigenic data. When heated to decomposition it emits toxic fumes of NO_x.

DBF400   CAS: 51325-35-0
2,4-DIACETAMIDO-6-(5-NITRO-2-FURYL)-s-TRIAZINE
mf: $C_{11}H_{10}N_6O_5$ mw: 306.27

SYN: N,N'-(6-(5-NITRO-2-FURYL)-s-TRIAZINE-2,4-DIYL) BISACETAMIDE

TOXICITY DATA with REFERENCE
CAR: orl-rat TDLo:57 g/kg/46W-C   JNCIAM
  51,403,73
MUT: mma-sat 100 ng/plate   MUREAV 48,295,77

CONSENSUS REPORTS: EPA Genetic Toxicology Program.

SAFETY PROFILE: Questionable carcinogen with experimental carcinogenic data. Mutation data reported. When heated to decomposition it emits toxic fumes of NO_x.

DBG200   CAS: 73785-34-9
trans-7,8-DIACETOXY-7,8-DIHYDROBENZO(a)PYRENE
mf: $C_{24}H_{16}O_4$ mw: 368.40

SYN: trans-BP-7,8-DIHYDRODIOL DIACETATE

TOXICITY DATA with REFERENCE
NEO: scu-mus TDLo:13 mg/kg   JJIND8 64,617,80

SAFETY PROFILE: Questionable carcinogen with experimental neoplastigenic data. When heated to decomposition it emits acrid smoke and irritating fumes.

DBI200   CAS: 2303-16-4
DIALLATE
mf: $C_{10}H_{17}Cl_2NOS$ mw: 270.24

PROP: Brown liquid, sltly sol in water, sol in organic solvents. Bp: 150° @ 9 mm, mp: 25-30°.

SYNS: AVADEX ◇ CP 15,336 ◇ DATC ◇ 2,3-DCDT ◇ DIALLAAT (DUTCH) ◇ DIALLAT (GERMAN) ◇ S-(2,3-DICHLORO-ALLIL)-N,N-DIISOPROPIL-MONOTIOCARBAM-MATO (ITALIAN) ◇ S-(2,3-DICHLOR-ALLYL)-N,N-DIISO-PROPYL-MONOTHIOCARBAMAAT (DUTCH) ◇ 2,3-DICHLO-RALLYL-N,N-(DIISOPROPYL)-THIOCARBAMAT (GERMAN) ◇ DICHLOROALLYL DIISOPROPYLTHIOCARBAMATE ◇ S-2,3-DICHLOROALLYL DIISOPROPYLTHIOCARBAMATE ◇ 2,3-DICHLOROALLYL-N,N-DIISOPROPYLTHIOLCARBA-MATE ◇ 2,3-DICHLORO-2-PROPENE-1-THIOL DIISOPRO-PYLCARBAMATE ◇ S-(2,3-DICHLORO-2-PROPENYL)ES-TER, BIS(1-METHYLETHYL) CARBAMOTHIOIC ACID ◇ DI-ISOPROPYLTHIOLOCARBAMATE de S-(2,3-DICHLO-ROALLYLE) (FRENCH) ◇ PYRADEX ◇ RCRA WASTE NUM-BER U062

TOXICITY DATA with REFERENCE
CAR: orl-mus TDLo:68 g/kg/84W-C   JNCIAM
  42,1101,69
ETA: orl-rat TDLo:4095 mg/kg/78W-C   JJIND8
  67,75,81
ETA: unr-mus TDLo:1 mg/kg   JPFCD2 15,929,80
MUT: cyt-ham:ovr 200 μmol/L   MUREAV85,45,81
MUT: dnd-ham:ovr 200 μmol/L   MUREAV
  85,45,81
MUT: mmo-sat 500 μg/plate   MUREAV 85,45,81
MUT: sce-ham:ovr 20 μmol/L   MUREAV85,45,81

CONSENSUS REPORTS: IARC Cancer Review: GROUP 3 IMEMDT 7,56,87; Animal Limited Evidence IMEMDT 30,235,83; Animal Sufficient Evidence IMEMDT 12,69,76. EPA Genetic Toxicology Program. Community Right-To-Know List.

SAFETY PROFILE: Questionable carcinogen with experimental carcinogenic and tumorigenic data. Poison by ingestion and possibly other routes. Moderately toxic by skin contact. Mutation data reported. When heated to decomposition it emits very toxic fumes of Cl^-, NO_x and SO_x.

DBK100   CAS: 5164-11-4
1,1-DIALLYLHYDRAZINE
mf: $C_6H_{12}N_2$ mw: 112.20

SYNS: 1,1-DAH ◇ DIALLYLHYDRAZINE ◇ HYDRAZINE, 1,1-DI-2-PROPENYL-(9CI)

TOXICITY DATA with REFERENCE
CAR: orl-mus TD:59220 mg/kg/90W-C
  ANTRD4 1,259,81

CAR: orl-mus TDLo:56000 mg/kg/2Y-C

ANTRD4 1,259,81

SAFETY PROFILE: Questionable carcinogen with experimental carcinogenic data. When heated to decomposition it emits toxic fumes of NO_x.

DBK120 CAS: 26072-78-6
1,2-DIALLYLHYDRAZINE DIHYDROCHLORIDE
mf: $C_6H_{12}N_2 \cdot 2ClH$ mw: 185.12

SYN: 1,2-DAH HYDROCHLORIDE

TOXICITY DATA with REFERENCE
CAR: orl-mus TD:89152 mg/kg/80W-C

ONCOBS 39,104,82

CAR: orl-mus TDLo:78176 mg/kg/80W-C

ONCOBS 39,104,82

SAFETY PROFILE: Questionable carcinogen with experimental carcinogenic data. When heated to decomposition it emits toxic fumes of NO_x.

DBK800 CAS: 3382-99-8
2,6-DIALLYLPHENOL
mf: $C_{12}H_{10}O$ mw: 170.22

TOXICITY DATA with REFERENCE
NEO: skn-mus TDLo:4600 mg/kg/12W-I

CNREA8 19,413,59

SAFETY PROFILE: Questionable carcinogen with experimental neoplastigenic data by skin contact. When heated to decomposition it emits acrid smoke and irritating fumes.

DBM800 CAS: 59-33-6
DIAMINIDE MALEATE
mf: $C_{17}H_{23}N_3O \cdot C_4H_4O_4$ mw: 401.51

SYNS: AH ◇ ANISOPYRADAMINE ◇ ANTHISAN MALEATE ◇ ANTIHIST ◇ N-DIMETHYLAMINOETHYL-N-p-METHOXY-α-AMINOPYRIDINE MALEATE ◇ 2-((2-(DIMETHYLAMINO)ETHYL)(p-METHOXYBENZYL)AMINO)PYRIDINE BIMALEATE ◇ 2-((2-(DIMETHYLAMINO)ETHYL) (p-METHOXYBENZYL)AMINO)PYRIDINE MALEATE ◇ N,N-DIMETHYL-N′-(4-METHOXYBENZYL)-N′-(2-PYRIDYL)ETHYLENEDIAMINE MALEATE ◇ HISTATEX ◇ MEPYRAMINE MALEATE ◇ N-p-METHOXYBENZYL-N′-N′-DIMETHYL-N-α-PYRIDYLETHYLENEDIAMINE MALEATE ◇ MINIHIST ◇ NEOANTERGAN MALEATE ◇ PARAMAL ◇ PARAMINYL MALEATE ◇ PYMAFED ◇ PYRA MALEATE ◇ PYRANILAMINE MALEATE ◇ PYRANINYL ◇ PYRANISAMINE MALEATE

◇ PYRILAMINE MALEATE ◇ RENSTAMIN ◇ 2786 R.P. MALEATE ◇ STANGEN MALEATE ◇ STATOMIN MALEATE ◇ THYLOGEN MALEATE

TOXICITY DATA with REFERENCE
ETA: orl-rat TDLo:77 g/kg/2Y-C FCTOD7

22,27,84

MUT: dns-rat:lvr 5 μmol/L ENMUDM 3,11,81

CONSENSUS REPORTS: Reported in EPA TSCA Inventory.

SAFETY PROFILE: Questionable carcinogen with experimental tumorigenic data. A human poison by ingestion. An experimental poison by ingestion, subcutaneous, intravenous, and intraperitoneal routes. Experimental reproductive effects. Mutation data reported. An antihistamine. When heated to decomposition it emits toxic fumes of NO_x.

DBN200
3,6-DIAMINOACRIDINE HYDROCHLORIDE HEMIHYDRATE
mf: $Cl_3H_{11}N_3 \cdot ClH \cdot 1/2H_2O$ mw: 254.74

SYNS: NCI-C04137 ◇ PROFLAVINE MONOHYDROCHLORIDE HEMIHYDRATE

TOXICITY DATA with REFERENCE
ETA: orl-mus TDLo:35 g/kg/104W-C NCITR*

NCI-CG-TR-5,77

ETA: orl-rat TDLo:27 g/kg/109W-C NCITR*

NCI-CG-TR-5,77

CONSENSUS REPORTS: IARC Cancer Review: Animal Inadequate Evidence IMEMDT 24,195,80. NCI Carcinogenesis Bioassay (feed); Inadequate Studies: mouse NCITR* NCI-CG-TR-5,77; Clear Evidence: rat NCITR* NCI-CG-TR-5,77.

SAFETY PROFILE: Questionable carcinogen with experimental tumorigenic data. When heated to decomposition it emits very toxic fumes of NO_x and Cl^-.

DBN600 CAS: 92-62-6
3,6-DIAMINOACRIDINIUM
mf: $C_{13}H_{11}N_3$ mw: 209.27

SYNS: 3,6-ACRIDINEDIAMINE ◇ 3,6-DIAMINOACRIDINE ◇ 2,8-DIAMINOACRIDINE (EUROPEAN) ◇ 2,8-DIAMINOACRIDINIUM ◇ 3,7-DIAMINO-5-AZAANTHRACENE ◇ ISOFLAV BASE ◇ PROFLAVIN ◇ PROFLAVINE ◇ PROFOLIOL ◇ PROFORMIPHEN ◇ PROFUNDOL ◇ PROFURA ◇ PROGARMED ◇ PRO-GEN ◇ PROGESIC

TOXICITY DATA with REFERENCE
MUT: dnd-esc 10 mg/L   MUREAV 107,1,83
MUT: dni-mus:emb 1 μmol/L   MOPMA3 21,739,82
MUT: oms-mus:emb 1 μmol/L   MOPMA3 21,739,82
MUT: otr-mus:emb 1 μmol/L   MOPMA3 21,739,82
MUT: sce-ham:ovr 20 μg/L   ENMUDM 4,65,82

CONSENSUS REPORTS: IARC Cancer Review: Animal Inadequate Evidence IMEMDT 24,195,80. Reported in EPA TSCA Inventory. EPA Genetic Toxicology Program.

SAFETY PROFILE: Questionable carcinogen. Poison by intravenous and subcutaneous routes. Mutation data reported. When heated to decomposition it emits toxic fumes of NO_x.

DBR400   CAS: 609-20-1
1,4-DIAMINO-2,6-DICHLOROBENZENE
mf: $C_6H_6Cl_2N_2$ mw: 177.04

SYNS: C.I. 37020 ◇ 2,6-DICHLORO-p-PHENYLENEDIA-MINE ◇ NCI-C50260

TOXICITY DATA with REFERENCE
CAR: orl-mus TD:260 g/kg/2Y-C   NTPTR* NTP-TR-219,82
CAR: orl-mus TDLo:87 g/kg/2Y-C   NTPTR* NTP-TR-219,82
MUT: mma-sat 1 mg/plate   ENMUDM 8(Suppl 7),1,86

CONSENSUS REPORTS: IARC Cancer Review: GROUP 3 IMEMDT 7,56,87; Animal Limited Evidence IMEMDT 39,325,86. NTP Carcinogenesis Bioassay (feed); Clear Evidence: mouse NTPTR* NTP-TR-219,82; No Evidence: rat NTPTR* NTP-TR-219,82. Reported in EPA TSCA Inventory.

SAFETY PROFILE: Questionable carcinogen with experimental carcinogenic data. Moderately toxic by ingestion. Mutation data reported. When heated to decomposition it emits very toxic fumes of Cl^- and NO_x.

DBX400   CAS: 8048-52-0
3,6-DIAMINO-10-METHYLACRIDINIUM CHLORIDE with 3,6-ACRIDINEDIAMINE
mf: $C_{14}H_{14}N_3 \cdot Cl \cdot C_{13}H_{11}N_3$ mw: 469.03

SYNS: ACRIFLAVIN ◇ ACRIFLAVINE mixture with PRO-FLAVINE ◇ ACRIFLAVINIUM CHLORIDE ◇ ACRIFLAVI-NIUM CHLORIDUM ◇ ACRIFLAVON ◇ ANGIFLAN ◇ ASSIFLAVINE ◇ AVLON ◇ BIALFLAVINA ◇ BIOACRIDIN ◇ BOVOFLAVIN ◇ BURNOL ◇ BUROFLAVIN ◇ CHOLIFLA-VIN ◇ CHROMOFLAVINE ◇ DIACRID ◇ 3,6-DIAMINOACRI-DINE mixture with 3,6-DIAMINO-10-METHYLACRIDINIUM CHLORIDE ◇ 2,8-DIAMINO-10-METHYLACRIDINIUM CHLORIDE mixture with 2,8-DIAMINOACRIDINE ◇ EUFLA-VINE ◇ FLAVACRIDINUM HYDROCHLORICUM ◇ FLAVINE ◇ FLAVIOFORM ◇ FLAVIPIN ◇ FLAVISEPT ◇ GLYCO-FLA-VINE ◇ GONACRINE ◇ ISRAVIN ◇ MEDIFLAVIN ◇ NEUTRAL ACRIFLAVINE ◇ PANFLAVIN ◇ PANTONSI-LETTEN ◇ TRACHOSEPT ◇ TRIPLA-ETILO ◇ TRYPAFLA-VINE ◇ VETAFLAVIN ◇ XANTHACRIDINUM ◇ ZORIFLA-VIN

TOXICITY DATA with REFERENCE
ETA: scu-rat TDLo:160 mg/kg/60W-I   SEMEAS 159,778,52
MUT: dni-hmn:hla 10 μmol/L   RAREAE 37,334,69
MUT: dns-rat:lvr 5 μmol/L   ENMUDM 3,11,81
MUT: mmo-esc 5 μg/plate   MUREAV 131,193,84
MUT: mmo-sat 40 μmol/L   ENMUDM 3,11,81
MUT: msc-mus:lym 500 μg/L   MUREAV 125,291,84
MUT: otr-ham:kdy 25 mg/L   TXCYAC 19,55,81
MUT: sln-dmg-mul 5000 ppm   MUREAV 138,169,84

CONSENSUS REPORTS: IARC Cancer Review: Animal Inadequate Evidence IMEMDT 13,31,77. EPA Genetic Toxicology Program.

SAFETY PROFILE: Questionable carcinogen with experimental tumorigenic data. Poison by subcutaneous route. Human mutation data reported. A topical antiseptic used in the treatment of gonorrhea. When heated to decomposition it emits very toxic fumes of NO_x and Cl^-.

DBY700   CAS: 82-33-7
1,4-DIAMINO-5-NITRO ANTHRAQUINONE
mf: $C_{14}H_9N_3O_4$ mw: 283.26

SYN: 9,10-ANTHRACENEDIONE, 1,4-DIAMINO-5-NITRO (9CI)

TOXICITY DATA with REFERENCE
ETA: skn-rat TD:25600 mg/kg/65W-I   VINIT* #1684-81
ETA: skn-rat TDLo:22500 mg/kg/65W-I   VINIT* #1684-81
MUT: mma-sat 50 μg/plate   MUREAV 40,203,76

CONSENSUS REPORTS: Reported in EPA TSCA Inventory.

SAFETY PROFILE: Questionable carcinogen with experimental tumorigenic data. Poison by intravenous route. Mutation data reported. When heated to decomposition it emits toxic fumes of NO_x.

DBY800 CAS: 720-69-4
4,6-DIAMINO-2-(5-NITRO-2-FURYL)-S-TRIAZINE
mf: $C_7H_6N_6O_3$ mw: 222.19

TOXICITY DATA with REFERENCE
CAR: orl-rat TDLo:13 g/kg/46W-C   JNCIAM 51,403,73
MUT: dnr-sat 500 nmol/well   CNREA8 34,2266,74
MUT: mma-sat 100 ng/plate   MUREAV 40,9,76
MUT: mmo-esc 300 nmol/well   CNREA8 34,2266,74
MUT: mrc-esc 500 nmol/well   CNREA8 34,2266,74

CONSENSUS REPORTS: EPA Genetic Toxicology Program.

SAFETY PROFILE: Questionable carcinogen with experimental carcinogenic data. Mutation data reported. When heated to decomposition it emits toxic fumes of NO_x.

DCE000 CAS: 636-23-7
2,4-DIAMINOTOLUENE DIHYDROCHLORIDE
mf: $C_7H_{10}N_2 \cdot 2ClH$ mw: 195.11

SYNS: METATOLYLENEDIAMINE DIHYDROCHLORIDE ◇ 2,4-TOLUENEDIAMINE DIHYDROCHLORIDE

TOXICITY DATA with REFERENCE
NEO: orl-mus TD:65 g/kg/78W-C   JEPTDQ 2,325,78
NEO: orl-mus TDLo:32 g/kg/78W-C   JEPTDQ 2,325,78
NEO: orl-rat TD:20 g/kg/78W-C   JEPTDQ 2,325,78
NEO: orl-rat TDLo:9900 mg/kg/78W-C   JEPTDQ 2,325,78

CONSENSUS REPORTS: Reported in EPA TSCA Inventory.

SAFETY PROFILE: Questionable carcinogen with experimental neoplastigenic data. Poison by intraperitoneal route. Moderately toxic by ingestion. When heated to decomposition it emits very toxic fumes of NO_x and HCl.

DCE600 CAS: 615-50-9
2,5-DIAMINOTOLUENE SULFATE
mf: $C_7H_{10}N_2 \cdot H_2O_4S$ mw: 220.27

SYNS: C.I. 76043 ◇ p-DIAMINOTOLUENE SULFATE ◇ 2,5-DIAMINOTOLUENE SULPHATE ◇ 2-METHYL-1,4-BENZENEDIAMINE SULFATE ◇ 2-METHYL-p-PHENYLENE-DIAMINE SULPHATE ◇ NCI-C01832 ◇ p-TOLUENEDIAMINE SULFATE ◇ 2,5-TOLUENEDIAMINE SULFATE ◇ TOLUENE-2,5-DIAMINE, SULFATE (1:1) (8CI) ◇ TOLUENE-2,5-DIAMINE SULPHATE ◇ p-TOLUENEDIAMINE SULPHATE

◇ TOLUYLENE-2,5-DIAMINE SULPHATE ◇ p-TOLUYLENE-DIAMINE SULPHATE ◇ p-TOLYLENEDIAMINE SULPHATE

TOXICITY DATA with REFERENCE
ETA: orl-mus TDLo:66 g/kg/78W-C   NCITR* NCI-CG-TR-126,78

CONSENSUS REPORTS: IARC Cancer Review: Animal Indefinite Evidence IMEMDT 16,97,78. NCI Carcinogenesis Bioassay Completed; Results Indefinite: mouse, rat (NCITR* NCI-CG-TR-126,78). Reported in EPA TSCA Inventory.

SAFETY PROFILE: Questionable carcinogen with experimental tumorigenic data. Poison by ingestion and intraperitoneal routes. When heated to decomposition it emits very toxic fumes of NO_x and SO_x.

DCF200 CAS: 1455-77-2
3,5-DIAMINO-s-TRIAZOLE
mf: $C_2H_5N_5$ mw: 99.12

SYNS: GUANAZOLE ◇ NCI-C04819 ◇ NSC 1895

TOXICITY DATA with REFERENCE
ETA: ipr-mus TDLo:9750 mg/kg/26W-I   CANCAR 40(Suppl 4),1935,77
ETA: ipr-rat TDLo:2500 mg/kg/7W-I   CANCAR 40(Suppl 4),1935,77
MUT: oms-hmn:oth 500 µg/L   CNREA8 32,2661,72

CONSENSUS REPORTS: NCI Carcinogenesis Studies (ipr); Equivocal Evidence: rat CANCAR 40,1935,77; No Evidence: mouse CANCAR 40,1935,77. Reported in EPA TSCA Inventory.

SAFETY PROFILE: Questionable carcinogen with experimental tumorigenic data. Human systemic effects by intravenous route: leukopenia (reduced white blood cell count) and thrombocytopenia (reduced blood platelet count). Human mutation data reported. When heated to decomposition it emits toxic fumes of NO_x.

DCH600 CAS: 13256-06-9
DI-n-AMYLNITROSAMINE
mf: $C_{10}H_{22}N_2O$ mw: 186.34

SYNS: DIAMYLNITROSAMIN (GERMAN) ◇ DIPENTYLNITROSAMINE ◇ DI-n-PENTYLNITROSAMINE ◇ N-NITROSO-DIPENTYLAMINE ◇ N-NITROSODI-n-PENTYLAMINE

TOXICITY DATA with REFERENCE
CAR: orl-rat TDLo:7733 mg/kg/8W-C   IJCNAW 27,249,81

ETA: orl-rat TD:48 g/kg/51W-C   ZEKBAI
69,103,67

ETA: scu-mus TDLo:11 g/kg/17W-I   BEXBAN
83,83,77

ETA: scu-rat TD:12 g/kg/49W-C   ZEKBAI
69,103,67

ETA: scu-rat TDLo:11 g/kg/25W-I   NATWAY
49,111,62

MUT: mma-ham:lng 500 μmol/L   IAPUDO
27,179,80

MUT: mma-sat 465 μg/plate   PNASA6 72,5135,75

CONSENSUS REPORTS: EPA Genetic Toxicology Program.

SAFETY PROFILE: Questionable carcinogen with experimental carcinogenic and tumorigenic data. Moderately toxic by ingestion and subcutaneous routes. Mutation data reported. When heated to decomposition it emits toxic fumes of NO_x.

DCJ400   CAS: 91-93-0
DIANISIDINE DIISOCYANATE
mf: $C_{16}H_{12}N_2O_4$ mw: 296.30

SYNS: 4,4'-DIISOCYANATO-3,3'-DIMETHOXY-1,1'-BI-PHENYL ◇ 3,3'-DIMETHOXYBENZIDINE-4,4'-DIISOCYA-NATE ◇ 3,3'-DIMETHOXY-4,4'-BIPHENYLENE DIISOCYA-NATE ◇ NCI-C02175

TOXICITY DATA with REFERENCE
CAR: orl-rat TD:1200 g/kg/78W-I   NCITR* NCI-CG-TR-128,79
CAR: orl-rat TDLo:565 g/kg/78W-I   NCITR* NCI-CG-TR-128,79
MUT: mma-sat 3 μg/plate   ENMUDM 7(Suppl 5),1,85
MUT: mmo-sat 3300 ng/plate   ENMUDM 7(Suppl 5),1,85
MUT: otr-rat:emb 81 μg/plate   JJATDK 1,190,81

CONSENSUS REPORTS: IARC Cancer Review: GROUP 3 IMEMDT 7,56,87; Animal Limited Evidence IMEMDT 39,279,86. NCI Carcinogenesis Bioassay (feed); No Evidence: mouse NCITR* NCI-CG-TR-128,79; Clear Evidence: rat NCITR* NCI-CG-TR-128,79.

NIOSH REL: (Diisocyanates) TWA 0.005 ppm; CL 0.02 ppm/10M

SAFETY PROFILE: Questionable carcinogen with experimental carcinogenic data. Poison by intravenous route. When heated to decomposition it emits toxic fumes of NO_x.

DCK200   CAS: 34494-09-2
6,12-DIAZAANTHANTHRENE SULFATE
mf: $C_{20}H_{10}N_2 \cdot H_2O_4S$ mw: 376.40

SYNS: ACRIDINO(2,1,9,8-klmna)ACRIDINE SULFATE ◇ 6,12-DIAZAANTHANTHRENE SULPHATE

TOXICITY DATA with REFERENCE
ETA: imp-rat TDLo:600 mg/kg   NEOLA418,591,71

SAFETY PROFILE: Questionable carcinogen with experimental tumorigenic data. When heated to decomposition it emits very toxic fumes of NO_x and SO_x.

DCK759   CAS: 439-14-5
DIAZEPAM
mf: $C_{16}H_{13}ClN_2O$ mw: 284.76

PROP: Plates. Mp: 125-126°.

SYNS: ALBORAL ◇ ALISEUM ◇ AMIPROL ◇ ANSIOLIN ◇ ANSIOLISINA ◇ APAURIN ◇ APOZEPAM ◇ ASSIVAL ◇ ATENSINE ◇ ATILEN ◇ BIALZEPAM ◇ CALMOCITENE ◇ CALMPOSE ◇ CERCINE ◇ CEREGULART ◇ 7-CHLORO-1,3-DIHYDRO-1-METHYL-5-PHENYL-2H-1,4-BENZODIAZE-PIN-2-ONE ◇ 7-CHLORO-1-METHYL-5-3H-1,4-BENZODIAZE-PIN-2(1H)-ONE ◇ 7-CHLORO-1-METHYL-2-OXO-5-PHENYL-3H-1,4-BENZODIAZEPINE ◇ 7-CHLORO-1-METHYL-5-PHE-NYL-2H-1,4-BENZODIAZEPIN-2-ONE ◇ 7-CHLORO-1-METHYL-5-PHENYL-3H-1,4-BENZODIAZEPIN-2(1H)-ONE ◇ 7-CHLORO-1-METHYL-5-PHENYL-1,3-DIHYDRO-2H-1,4-BENZODIAZEPIN-2-ONE ◇ CONDITION ◇ DAP ◇ DIACEPAN ◇ DIAPAM ◇ DIAZETARD ◇ DIENPAX ◇ DIPAM ◇ DIPEZONA ◇ DOMALIUM ◇ DUKSEN ◇ DUXEN ◇ E-PAM ◇ ERIDAN ◇ FAUSTAN ◇ FREUDAL ◇ FRUSTAN ◇ GIHITAN ◇ HORIZON ◇ KIATRIUM ◇ LA-III ◇ LEMBROL ◇ LEVIUM ◇ LIBERETAS ◇ METHYL DIAZEPINONE ◇ 1-METHYL-5-PHENYL-7-CHLORO-1,3-DIHYDRO-2H-1,4-BENZODIAZEPIN-2-ONE ◇ MOROSAN ◇ NOAN ◇ NSC-77518 ◇ PACITRAN ◇ PARANTEN ◇ PAXATE ◇ PAXEL ◇ PLIDAN ◇ QUETINIL ◇ QUIATRIL ◇ QUIEVITA ◇ RELAMINAL ◇ RELANIUM ◇ RELAX ◇ RENBORIN ◇ RO 5-2807 ◇ S.A. R.L. ◇ SAROMET ◇ SEDIPAM ◇ SEDUKSEN ◇ SEDUXEN ◇ SERENACK ◇ SERENAMIN ◇ SERENZIN ◇ SETONIL ◇ SIBAZON ◇ SONACON ◇ STESOLID ◇ STESOLIN ◇ TENSOPAM ◇ TRANIMUL ◇ TRANQDYN ◇ TRANQUIRIT ◇ UMBRIUM ◇ UNISEDIL ◇ USEMPAX AP ◇ VALEO ◇ VALITRAN ◇ VALIUM ◇ VATRAN ◇ VELIUM ◇ VIVAL ◇ VIVOL ◇ WY-3467 ◇ ZIPAN

TOXICITY DATA with REFERENCE
ETA: orl-mus TDLo:42 g/kg/80W-C   TXAPA9 57,39,81
MUT: bfa-mus/sat 200 mg/kg   CNREA8 38,4478,78
MUT: cyt-ham:fbr 100 mg/L   MUREAV 122,201,83
MUT: cyt-hmn:leu 10 mg/L   AJOGAH 103,836,69
MUT: cyt-wmn-unr 328 mg/kg/78W   AJOGAH 107,456,70

MUT: mma-sat 958 nmol/plate CNREA8 38,4478,78
MUT: spm-mus-orl 300 mg/kg/15D-C CYTBAI
36,45,83

CONSENSUS REPORTS: Reported in EPA TSCA Inventory. EPA Genetic Toxicology Program.

SAFETY PROFILE: Questionable carcinogen with experimental tumorigenic data. Poison by ingestion, parenteral, subcutaneous, intravenous, or intraperitoneal routes data. Moderately toxic by skin contact. Human systemic effects by ingestion, intramuscular, and intravenous routes: dermatitis, effect on inflammation or mediation of inflammation, change in cardiac rate, somnolence, respiratory depression, and other respiratory changes, visual field changes, diplopia (double vision), change in motor activity, muscle contraction or spasticity, ataxia (loss of muscle coordination), an antipsychotic and general anesthetic. A human teratogen by ingestion and intravenous routes which causes developmental abnormalities of the fetal cardiovascular (circulatory) system and postnatal effects. An experimental teratogen. Experimental reproductive effects. Human mutation data reported. An allergen. A drug for the treatment of anxiety. When heated to decomposition it emits very toxic fumes of Cl^- and NO_x.

DCN800   CAS: 623-73-4
DIAZOACETIC ESTER
mf: $C_4H_6N_2O_2$ mw: 114.12

SYNS: DAAE ◇ DIAZOACETIC ACID, ETHYL ESTER ◇ DIAZOESSIGSAEURE-AETHYLESTER (GERMAN) ◇ EDA ◇ ETHOXYCARBONYLDIAZOMETHANE ◇ ETHYL DIAZOACETATE

TOXICITY DATA with REFERENCE
CAR: ipr-rat TDLo: 30 mg/kg/20W-I ARGEAR
55,117,85
CAR: ivn-rat TD: 100 mg/kg CRNGDP 3,785,82
CAR: ivn-rat TDLo: 75 mg/kg/30W-I ARGEAR
55,117,85
CAR: skn-rat TDLo: 4167 mg/kg/48W-I
ARGEAR 55,117,85
ETA: ivn-rat TD: 1000 mg/kg/40W-I PSEBAA
135,219,70
ETA: ivn-rat TD: 1330 mg/kg/53W-I BTPGAZ
146,33,72
ETA: ivn-rat TD: 2150 mg/kg 86W-I ADRCAC
19,51,65
ETA: ivn-rat TD: 2850 mg/kg/57W-I XENOBH
3,271,73

ETA: ivn-rat TD: 4300 mg/kg/86W-I ADRCAC
19,51,65
ETA: orl-rat TD: 2400 mg/kg/68W-C NATWAY
50,99,63
ETA: orl-rat TDLo: 2025 mg/kg/81W-I
XENOBH 3,271,73

SAFETY PROFILE: Questionable carcinogen with experimental carcinogenic and tumorigenic data. Poison by ingestion and intravenous routes. Can explode. Explodes on contact with tris(dimethylamino) antimony. When heated to decomposition it emits toxic fumes of NO_x.

DCO800   CAS: 820-75-7
N-(DIAZOACETYL)GLYCINE
HYDRAZINE
mf: $C_4H_7N_5O_2$ mw: 157.16

SYNS: N-DIAZOACETILGLICINA-IDRAZIDE (ITALIAN) ◇ DIAZOACETYLGLYCINE HYDRAZIDE ◇ N-DIAZOACETYL GLYCYLHYDRAZIDE ◇ NSC-58404

TOXICITY DATA with REFERENCE
CAR: ipr-mus TDLo: 1200 mg/kg/4D-I BSIBAC
45,227,69
NEO: ipr-mus TD: 720 mg/kg/4D-I BSIBAC
45,227,69
MUT: dns-mus: fbr 2500 μmol/L JCROD7 94,7,79
MUT: mma-sat 10 μg/plate PNASA6 72,5135,75
MUT: mmo-sat 10 μg/plate AMACCQ 6,655,74

CONSENSUS REPORTS: EPA Genetic Toxicology Program.

SAFETY PROFILE: Questionable carcinogen with experimental carcinogenic and neoplastigenic data. Poison by intravenous route. Moderately toxic by ingestion, intraperitoneal and subcutaneous routes. Mutation data reported. When heated to decomposition it emits toxic fumes including NO_x.

DCP400   CAS: 7008-85-7
5-DIAZOIMIDAZOLE-4-CARBOXAMIDE
mf: $C_4H_3N_5O$ mw: 137.12

SYNS: DIAZO-ICA ◇ DIAZOIMIDAZOLE-4-CARBOXAMIDE ◇ NSC 22420

TOXICITY DATA with REFERENCE
ETA: orl-rat TDLo: 2175 mg/kg/14W-C
JNCIAM 54,951,75
MUT: dni-esc 10 μg/L BCPCA6 18,1463,69
MUT: dni-rat: lvr 100 μmol/L CNREA8 2827,76
MUT: oms-esc 500 μg/L BCPCA6 18,1463,69

SAFETY PROFILE: Questionable carcinogen with experimental tumorigenic data. A deadly poison by intraperitoneal route. Mutation data reported. When heated to decomposition it emits toxic fumes of NO_x.

DCP600   CAS: 64038-55-7
5-DIAZOIMIDAZOLE-4-CARBOXAMIDE HYDROCHLORIDE
mf: $C_4H_3N_5O \cdot HCl$ mw: 137.12

TOXICITY DATA with REFERENCE
ETA: orl-rat TDLo: 105 mg/kg/10W-C   JNCIAM 54,951,75

SAFETY PROFILE: Questionable carcinogen with experimental tumorigenic data. When heated to decomposition it emits very toxic fumes of NO_x and HCl.

DCQ575
3-DIAZOTYRAMINE HYDROCHLORIDE
PROP: A nitrosated product of TYRAMINE
mf: $C_8H_9N_3O$ mw: 163.20

SYNS: 4-(2-AMINOETHYL)-6-DIAZO-2,4-CYCLOHEXA-DIENONE HYDROCHLORIDE ◇ TYRAMINE, 3-DIAZO-, HYDROCHLORIDE

TOXICITY DATA with REFERENCE
CAR: orl-rat TDLo: 77700 mg/kg/2Y-C
CRNGDP 8,527,87

SAFETY PROFILE: Questionable carcinogen with experimental carcinogenic data. When heated to decomposition it emits toxic fumes of NO_x.

DCQ650   CAS: 94362-44-4
DIAZO V
SYN: DIAZO RESIN V

TOXICITY DATA with REFERENCE
NEO: scu-rat TDLo: 900 mg/kg/26W-I   VINIT* #5689-83

SAFETY PROFILE: Questionable carcinogen with experimental neoplastigenic data. When heated to decomposition it emits acrid smoke and irritating fumes.

DCR300   CAS: 5385-75-1
DIBENZ(a,e)ACEANTHRYLENE
mf: $C_{24}H_{14}$ mw: 302.38

SYNS: DIBENZO(a,e)FLUORANTHENE ◇ 2,3,5,6-DIBENZOFLUORANTHENE

TOXICITY DATA with REFERENCE
CAR: skn-mus TDLo: 2880 μg/kg/15W-I
CRNGDP 8,461,87
MUT: dns-mus: emb 1 μmol/L   CRNGDP 5,379,84
MUT: mma-sat 500 nmol/L   CRNGDP 5,1263,84

CONSENSUS REPORTS: IARC Cancer Review: GROUP 3 IMEMDT 7,56,87; Animal Limited Evidence IMEMDT 32,321,83

SAFETY PROFILE: Questionable carcinogen with experimental carcinogenic data. Mutation data reported. When heated to decomposition it emits acrid smoke and fumes.

DCR400   CAS: 203-20-3
DIBENZ(a,j)ACEANTHRYLENE
mf: $C_{24}H_{14}$ mw: 302.38

SYN: 15,16-BENZDEHYDROCHOLANTHRENE

TOXICITY DATA with REFERENCE
ETA: ivn-mus TDLo: 20 mg/kg   JNCIAM 1,225,40
ETA: scu-mus TDLo: 800 mg/kg/9W-I   AJCAA7 28,334,36

SAFETY PROFILE: Questionable carcinogen with experimental tumorigenic data. Poison by intravenous route. When heated to decomposition it emits acrid smoke and irritating fumes.

DCR600   CAS: 201-42-3
13H-DIBENZ(bc,j)ACEANTHRYLENE
mf: $C_{23}H_{14}$ mw: 290.37

SYNS: 13H-ACENAPHTHO(1,8-ab)PHENANTHRENE ◇ 1',9-METHYLENE-1,2:5,6-DIBENZANTHRACENE

TOXICITY DATA with REFERENCE
ETA: scu-mus TDLo: 400 mg/kg   AJCAA7 28,334,36

SAFETY PROFILE: Questionable carcinogen with experimental tumorigenic data. When heated to decomposition it emits acrid smoke and irritating fumes.

DCR800   CAS: 517-85-1
4H-DIBENZ(f,g,j)ACEANTHRYLENE, 5,5a,6,7-TETRAHYDRO-
mf: $C_{23}H_{18}$ mw: 294.41

SYNS: ANG.-STERANTHREN (GERMAN) ◇ ANG-STERANTHRENE

TOXICITY DATA with REFERENCE
ETA: scu-mus TDLo: 40 mg/kg   ZEKBAI 62,217,57
ETA: skn-mus TDLo: 1120 mg/kg/35W-I
ZEKBAI 62,217,57

SAFETY PROFILE: Questionable carcinogen with experimental tumorigenic data. When heated to decomposition it emits acrid smoke and irritating fumes.

DCS800 CAS: 224-53-3
DIBENZ(c,h)ACRIDINE
mf: $C_{21}H_{13}N$ mw: 279.35

SYNS: 14-AZADIBENZ(a,j)ANTHRACENE ◇ 3,4:5,6-DI-BENZACRIDINE ◇ 1,2,7,8-DIBENZACRIDINE (FRENCH)

TOXICITY DATA with REFERENCE
ETA: scu-mus TDLo:4400 mg/kg/65W-I
PRLBA4 129,439,40
ETA: skn-mus TD:300 mg/kg/25W-I ACRSAJ
4,315,56
ETA: skn-mus TDLo:2040 mg/kg/85W-I
PRLBA4 129,439,40
MUT: mma-sat 4 µg/plate BJCAAI 37,873,78

SAFETY PROFILE: Questionable carcinogen with experimental tumorigenic data. Mutation data reported. When heated to decomposition it emits toxic fumes of NO_x.

DCT000 CAS: 63918-83-2
DIBENZ(a,j)ACRIDINE METHOSULFATE
mf: $C_{21}H_{13}N \cdot C_2H_6O_4S$ mw: 405.49

SYN: 3,4:5,6-DIBENZACRIDINE METHOSULFATE

TOXICITY DATA with REFERENCE
ETA: scu-mus TDLo:3750 mg/kg/56W-I
PRLBA4 129,439,40

SAFETY PROFILE: Questionable carcinogen with experimental tumorigenic data. When heated to decomposition it emits very toxic fumes of SO_x and NO_x.

DCT600 CAS: 224-41-9
DIBENZ(a,j)ANTHRACENE
mf: $C_{22}H_{14}$ mw: 278.36

SYN: 1,2:7,8-DIBENZANTHRACENE

TOXICITY DATA with REFERENCE
ETA: scu-mus TD:4 mg/kg JNCIAM 1,45,40
ETA: scu-mus TD:16 mg/kg JNCIAM 44,641,70
ETA: scu-mus TDLo:4 mg/kg JNCIAM 1,45,40
ETA: skn-mus TD:1250 mg/kg/52W-I PRLBA4
117,318,35
ETA: skn-mus TDLo:252 mg/kg/81W-I
JNCIAM 44,641,70
MUT: mma-sat 1 µg/plate MUREAV 51,311,78

CONSENSUS REPORTS: IARC Cancer Review: GROUP 3 IMEMDT 7,56,87; Animal Limited Evidence IMEMDT 32,309,83.

SAFETY PROFILE: Questionable carcinogen with experimental tumorigenic data. Mutation data reported. When heated to decomposition it emits acrid smoke and irritating fumes.

DCT800
1,2,5,6-DIBENZANTHRACENECHOLEIC ACID
mf: $C_{96}H_{160}O_{16} \cdot C_{22}H_{14}$ mw: 1848.92

SYN: 3-α-12-α-DIHYDROXY-5-β-CHOLAN-24-OIC ACID with DIBENZ(a,h)ANTHRACENE

TOXICITY DATA with REFERENCE
ETA: scu-mus TDLo:800 mg/kg/9W-I JNCIAM
2,99,41

SAFETY PROFILE: Questionable carcinogen with experimental tumorigenic data. When heated to decomposition it emits acrid smoke and irritating fumes.

DCU200 CAS: 4665-48-9
1,2:5,6-DIBENZANTHRACENE-9,10-ENDO-α,β-SUCCINIC ACID
mf: $C_{26}H_{18}O_4$ mw: 394.44

SYN: 7,14-DIHYDRO-7,14-ETHANODIBENZ(a,b)ANTHRACENE-15,16-DICARBOXYLIC ACID

TOXICITY DATA with REFERENCE
CAR: scu-rat TDLo:665 mg/kg/50D-I
85DLAB -,-,75
MUT: mmo-esc 2040 mg/L/4H GENTAE 39,141,54

SAFETY PROFILE: Questionable carcinogen with experimental carcinogenic data. Mutation data reported. When heated to decomposition it emits acrid smoke and irritating fumes.

DCU600 CAS: 63041-44-1
DIBENZANTHRANYL GLYCINE COMPLEX
mf: $C_{25}H_{18}N_2O_3$ mw: 394.45

SYNS: 1:2:5:6-DIBENZANTHRACENE-9-CARBAMIDO-ACETIC ACID ◇ N-(DIBENZ(a,h)ANTHRACEN-7-YLCARBAMOYL)GLYCINE

TOXICITY DATA with REFERENCE
ETA: scu-mus TDLo:80 mg/kg/12W-I AJCAA7
35,203,39

SAFETY PROFILE: Questionable carcinogen with experimental tumorigenic data. When heated to decomposition it emits toxic fumes of NO_x.

DCX000 CAS: 201-65-0
1,2,3,4-DIBENZFLUORENE
mf: $C_{21}H_{14}$ mw: 266.35

SYN: 13H-INDENO(1,2-1)PHENANTHRENE

TOXICITY DATA with REFERENCE
ETA: skn-mus TDLo: 1040 mg/kg/43W-I
   PRLBA4 129,439,40

SAFETY PROFILE: Questionable carcinogen with experimental tumorigenic data. When heated to decomposition it emits acrid smoke and irritating fumes.

DCX400   CAS: 193-40-8
DIBENZ(c,f)INDENO(1,2,3-ij)(2,7) NAPHTHYRIDINE
mf: $C_{22}H_{12}N_2$ mw: 304.36

TOXICITY DATA with REFERENCE
NEO: skn-mus TDLo: 1200 mg/kg/52W-I
   BJCAAI 17,266,63

SAFETY PROFILE: Questionable carcinogen with experimental neoplastigenic data. When heated to decomposition it emits toxic fumes of NO_x.

DCX600   CAS: 207-84-1
7H-DIBENZO(a,g)CARBAZOLE
mf: $C_{20}H_{13}N$ mw: 267.34

SYN: 1,2,5,6-DIBENZCARBAZOLE

TOXICITY DATA with REFERENCE
ETA: skn-mus TD: 900 mg/kg/38W-I   PRLBA4
   131,170,72
ETA: skn-mus TDLo: 275 mg/kg/23W-I
   PRLBA4 122,429,37

SAFETY PROFILE: Questionable carcinogen with experimental tumorigenic data. When heated to decomposition it emits toxic fumes of NO_x.

DCX800   CAS: 239-64-5
7H-DIBENZO(a,i)CARBAZOLE
mf: $C_{20}H_{13}N$ mw: 267.34

SYN: 1,2,7,8-DIBENZCARBAZOLE

TOXICITY DATA with REFERENCE
ETA: skn-mus TDLo: 515 mg/kg/43W-I
   PRLBA4 122,429,37

SAFETY PROFILE: Questionable carcinogen with experimental tumorigenic data. When heated to decomposition it emits toxic fumes of NO_x.

DCY600   CAS: 63040-54-0
DIBENZO(b,def)CHRYSENE-7-CARBOXALDEHYDE
mf: $C_{25}H_{14}O$ mw: 330.39

SYN: 5-FORMYL-3,4:8,9-DIBENZOPYRENE

TOXICITY DATA with REFERENCE
ETA: scu-mus TDLo: 72 mg/kg/9W-I   COREAF
   252,1711,61

SAFETY PROFILE: Questionable carcinogen with experimental tumorigenic data. When heated to decomposition it emits acrid smoke and irritating fumes.

DCY800   CAS: 2869-59-2
DIBENZO(def,p)CHRYSENE-10-CARBOXALDEHYDE
mf: $C_{25}H_{14}O$ mw: 330.39

SYN: 5-FORMYL-1,2:3,4-DIBENZOPYRENE

TOXICITY DATA with REFERENCE
ETA: scu-mus TDLo: 72 mg/kg/9W-I   COREAF
   259,3899,64

SAFETY PROFILE: Questionable carcinogen with experimental tumorigenic data. When heated to decomposition it emits acrid smoke and irritating fumes.

DCZ000   CAS: 128-66-5
DIBENZO(b,def)CHRYSENE-7,14-DIONE
mf: $C_{24}H_{12}O_2$ mw: 332.36

PROP: C.I. vat yellow 4 tested in NCITR* NCI-CG-TR-134,79 consists of 18.2% dibenzo(b,def)chrysene-7,14-dione, 30.8% sorbitol, 5.5% lomar twc, 2.7% glycerin and 42.8% water (NCITR* NCI-CG-TR-134,79).

SYNS: AHCOVAT PRINTING GOLDEN YELLOW ◇ AMANTHRENE GOLDEN YELLOW ◇ ANTHRAVAT GOLDEN YELLOW ◇ ARLANTHRENE GOLDEN YELLOW ◇ BENZADONE GOLDEN YELLOW ◇ CALCOLOID GOLDEN YELLOW ◇ CALEDON GOLDEN YELLOW ◇ CALEDON PRINTING YELLOW ◇ CARBANTHRENE GOLDEN YELLOW ◇ C.I. 59100 ◇ CIBANONE GOLDEN YELLOW ◇ C.I. VAT YELLOW ◇ DIBENZO(a,b)PYRENE-7,14-DIONE ◇ 2,3,7,8-DIBENZOPYRENE-1,6-QUINONE ◇ 1',2',6',7'-DIBENZPYRENE-7,14-QUINONE ◇ FEMANTHREN GOLDEN YELLOW ◇ GOLDEN YELLOW ◇ HELANTHRENE YELLOW ◇ HOSTAVAT GOLDEN YELLOW ◇ INDANTHRENE GOLDEN YELLOW ◇ LEUCOSOL GOLDEN YELLOW ◇ MAYVAT GOLDEN YELLOW ◇ MIKETHRENE GOLD YELLOW ◇ NCI-C03565 ◇ NIHONTHRENE GOLDEN YELLOW ◇ NYANTHRENE GOLDEN YELLOW ◇ PALANTHRENE GOLDEN YELLOW ◇ PARADONE GOLDEN YELLOW ◇ PHARMANTHRENE GOLDEN YELLOW ◇ ROMANTRENE GOLDEN YELLOW ◇ SANDOTHRENE PRINTING YELLOW

◇ SOLANTHRENE BRILLIANT YELLOW ◇ TINON GOLDEN YELLOW ◇ TYRION YELLOW ◇ VAT GOLDEN YELLOW ◇ YELLOW

TOXICITY DATA with REFERENCE
CAR: orl-mus TDLo: 7420 g/kg/2Y-C   NCITR*
NCI-CG-TR-134,79

ETA: orl-mus TD: 2225 g/kg/106W-C   NCITR*
NCI-CG-TR-134,79

CONSENSUS REPORTS: NCI Carcinogenesis Bioassay Completed; Results Positive: Mouse (NCITR* NCI-CG-TR-134,79); Negative: Rat (NCITR* NCI-CG-TR-134,79). Reported in EPA TSCA Inventory. Community Right-To-Know List.

SAFETY PROFILE: Questionable carcinogen with experimental carcinogenic and tumorigenic data. When heated to decomposition it emits acrid smoke and irritating fumes.

DDA800   CAS: 262-12-4
DIBENZO-p-DIOXIN
mf: $C_{12}H_8O_2$ mw: 184.20

PROP: Crystals. Mp: 123°.

SYNS: DIBENZODIOXIN ◇ DIBENZO(1,4)DIOXIN ◇ DIBENZO(b.e)(1,4)DIOXIN ◇ DIPHENYLENE DIOXIDE ◇ NCI-C03656 ◇ OXANTHRENE ◇ PHENODIOXIN

TOXICITY DATA with REFERENCE
ETA: skn-mus TDLo: 110 g/kg/58W-I   EVHPAZ
5,163,73

CONSENSUS REPORTS: IARC Cancer Review: Animal Inadequate Evidence IMEMDT 15,41,77. NCI Carcinogenesis Bioassay Completed; Results Negative (NCITR* NCI-CG-TR-122,79).

SAFETY PROFILE: Questionable carcinogen with experimental tumorigenic data. When heated to decomposition it emits acrid smoke and irritating fumes.

DDB000   CAS: 207-83-0
13H-DIBENZO(a,g)FLUORENE
mf: $C_{21}H_{14}$ mw: 266.35

SYN: 1,2,5,6-DIBENZOFLUORENE

TOXICITY DATA with REFERENCE
ETA: skn-mus TD: 240 mg/kg/37W-I   CNREA8
11,892,51
ETA: skn-mus TD: 1220 mg/kg/51W-I   PRLBA4
123,343,37

ETA: skn-mus TDLo: 48 mg/kg/15W-I   CNREA8
11,301,51

SAFETY PROFILE: Questionable carcinogen with experimental tumorigenic data. When heated to decomposition it emits acrid smoke and irritating fumes.

DDB200   CAS: 239-60-1
13H-DIBENZO(a,i)FLUORENE
mf: $C_{21}H_{14}$ mw: 266.35

SYN: 1,2,7,8-DIBENZFLUORENE

TOXICITY DATA with REFERENCE
ETA: skn-mus TDLo: 1340 mg/kg/56W-I
PRLBA4 129,439,40

SAFETY PROFILE: Questionable carcinogen with experimental tumorigenic data. When heated to decomposition it emits acrid smoke and irritating fumes.

DDB600   CAS: 3693-22-9
2-DIBENZOFURANAMINE
mf: $C_{12}H_9NO$ mw: 183.22

SYNS: 2-ADO ◇ 3-AMINODIBENZOFURAN ◇ 2-AMINODIPHENYLENE OXIDE

TOXICITY DATA with REFERENCE
CAR: orl-rat TDLo: 168 mg/kg/90W-I   ZEKBAI
61,45,56
ETA: orl-mus TDLo: 22 g/kg/52W-C   BECCAN
46,271,68
MUT: dns-mus-orl 80 mg/kg   BIJOAK 111,12P,69

SAFETY PROFILE: Questionable carcinogen with experimental carcinogenic and tumorigenic data. Mutation data reported. When heated to decomposition it emits toxic fumes of NO_x.

DDB800   CAS: 4106-66-5
3-DIBENZOFURANAMINE
mf: $C_{12}H_9NO$ mw: 183.22

SYNS: 2-AMINODIPHENYLENOXYD (GERMAN) ◇ DIBENZOFURANYLAMINE

TOXICITY DATA with REFERENCE
CAR: orl-rat TDLo: 1400 mg/kg/66W-C
ZEKBAI 61,45,56

SAFETY PROFILE: Questionable carcinogen with experimental carcinogenic data. When heated to decomposition it emits toxic fumes of NO_x.

DDC000   CAS: 5834-25-3
N-3-DIBENZOFURANYLACETAMIDE
mf: $C_{14}H_{11}NO_2$ mw: 225.26

SYNS: 3-ACETAMIDODIBENZFURANE ◇ 3-ACETAMIDO-
DIBENZOFURAN ◇ 3-ACETYLAMINODIBENZOFURAN
◇ 3-DIBENZOFURANYLACETAMIDE

TOXICITY DATA with REFERENCE
ETA: orl-rat TDLo: 4496 mg/kg/35W-C
    CNREA8 9,504,49

SAFETY PROFILE: Questionable carcinogen
with experimental tumorigenic data. When
heated to decomposition it emits toxic fumes
of NO$_x$.

DDC200   CAS: 192-47-2
DIBENZO(h,rst)PENTAPHENE
mf: C$_{28}$H$_{16}$ mw: 352.44

PROP: Pale yellow needles. Mp: 321°.

SYNS: TRIBENZO(a,e,i)PYRENE ◇ (1,2,4,5,7,8)TRI-
BENZOPYRENE ◇ (1,2,4,5,8,9)TRIBENZOPYRENE
◇ 1,2:4,5:8,9-TRIBENZOPYRENE

TOXICITY DATA with REFERENCE
ETA: scu-mus TDLo: 72 mg/kg/9W-I   COREAF
    259,3899,64

CONSENSUS REPORTS: IARC Cancer Review: GROUP 3 IMEMDT 7,56,87; Animal
Limited Evidence IMEMDT 3,197,73

SAFETY PROFILE: Questionable carcinogen
with experimental tumorigenic data. When
heated to decomposition it emits acrid smoke
and irritating fumes.

DDC400   CAS: 188-96-5
DIBENZO(cd,lm)PERYLENE
mf: C$_{26}$H$_{14}$ mw: 326.40

SYN: PEROPYRENE

TOXICITY DATA with REFERENCE
ETA: scu-mus TDLo: 72 mg/kg/9W-I   CHDDAT
    266,301,68

SAFETY PROFILE: Questionable carcinogen
with experimental tumorigenic data. When
heated to decomposition it emits acrid smoke
and irritating fumes.

DDC600   CAS: 215-64-5
DIBENZO(a,c)PHENAZINE
mf: C$_{20}$H$_{12}$N$_2$ mw: 280.34

SYN: 1,2,3,4-DIBENZPHENAZINE

TOXICITY DATA with REFERENCE
ETA: imp-rat TDLo: 7 mg/kg   COREAF 240,1738,55

SAFETY PROFILE: Questionable carcinogen
with experimental tumorigenic data. When
heated to decomposition it emits toxic fumes
of NO$_x$.

DDC800   CAS: 226-47-1
DIBENZO(a,h)PHENAZINE
mf: C$_{20}$H$_{12}$N$_2$ mw: 280.34

SYNS: 7,14-DIAZADIBENZ(a,h)ANTHRACENE ◇ DI-
BENZ(a,h)PHENAZINE ◇ 1,2:5,6-DIBENZPHENAZINE

TOXICITY DATA with REFERENCE
ETA: imp-rat TD: 100 mg/kg   NEOLA4 25,641,78
ETA: imp-rat TDLo: 7 mg/kg   COREAF 240,1738,55

CONSENSUS REPORTS: EPA Genetic Toxicology Program.

SAFETY PROFILE: Questionable carcinogen
with experimental tumorigenic data. When
heated to decomposition it emits toxic fumes
of NO$_x$.

DDD400   CAS: 54818-88-1
N-2-DIBENZOTHIENYLACETAMIDE
mf: C$_{14}$H$_{11}$NOS   mw: 241.32

SYN: 2-ACETYLAMINODIBENZOTHIOPHENE

TOXICITY DATA with REFERENCE
CAR: orl-rat TDLo: 4680 mg/kg/32W-C
    CNREA8 15,188,55

SAFETY PROFILE: Questionable carcinogen
with experimental carcinogenic data. When
heated to decomposition it emits very toxic
fumes of SO$_x$ and NO$_x$.

DDD600   CAS: 64057-52-9
N-3-DIBENZOTHIENYLACETAMIDE
mf: C$_{14}$H$_{11}$NOS   mw: 241.32

SYNS: 3-ACETAMIDODIBENZTHIOPHENE ◇ 3-ACETAMI-
NODIBENZOTHIOPHENE ◇ 3-ACETYLAMINODIBENZO-
THIOPHENE

TOXICITY DATA with REFERENCE
ETA: orl-rat TDLo: 4739 mg/kg/35W-C
    CNREA8 9,504,49

SAFETY PROFILE: Questionable carcinogen
with experimental tumorigenic data. Moderately
toxic by ingestion. When heated to decomposition it emits very toxic fumes of NO$_x$ and SO$_x$.

DDD800   CAS: 63020-21-3
N-3-DIBENZOTHIENYLACETAMIDE-5-
OXIDE
mf: C$_{14}$H$_{11}$NO$_2$S   mw: 257.32

SYNS: 3-ACETAMIDODIBENZTHIOPHENE OXIDE ◇ 3-ACETYLAMINODIBENZOTHIOPHENE-5-OXIDE

TOXICITY DATA with REFERENCE
ETA: orl-rat TDLo: 5103 mg/kg/35W-C
CNREA8 9,504,49

SAFETY PROFILE: Questionable carcinogen with experimental tumorigenic data. When heated to decomposition it emits very toxic fumes of SO_x and NO_x.

DDE200   CAS: 257-07-8
DIBENZ(b,f)(1,4)OXAZEPINE
mf: $C_{13}H_9NO$ mw: 195.23

SYNS: CR ◇ EA 3547

TOXICITY DATA with REFERENCE
CAR: ihl-mus TCLo: 236 mg/m³/18W-I
TOLED5 17,13,83
ETA: ihl-mus TC: 204 mg/m³/18W-I   TOLED5 17,13,83

CONSENSUS REPORTS: Reported in EPA TSCA Inventory.

SAFETY PROFILE: Questionable carcinogen with experimental carcinogenic, tumorigenic, and teratogenic data. Poison by intraperitoneal and intravenous routes. Moderately toxic by ingestion and inhalation. Experimental reproductive effects. A human skin and eye irritant. When heated to decomposition it emits toxic fumes of NO_x.

DDF400   CAS: 59766-02-8
7,14-DIBENZYLDIBENZ(a,h) ANTHRACENE
mf: $C_{36}H_{26}$ mw: 458.62

SYN: 9,10-DIBENZYL-1,2,5,6-DIBENZANTHRACENE

TOXICITY DATA with REFERENCE
ETA: skn-mus TDLo: 1250 mg/kg/52W-I
PRLBA4,111,485,32

SAFETY PROFILE: Questionable carcinogen with experimental tumorigenic data. When heated to decomposition it emits acrid smoke and irritating fumes.

DDJ000   CAS: 10318-26-0
DIBROMDULCITOL
mf: $C_6H_{12}Br_2O_4$ mw: 308.00

SYNS: DBD ◇ DIBROMODULCITOL ◇ 1,6-DIBROMODI-DEOXYDULCITOL ◇ 1,6-DIBROMO-1,6-DIDEOXYDULCI-TOL ◇ 1,6-DIBROMO-1,6-DIDEOXYGALACTITOL

◇ 1,6-DIBROMO-1,6-DIDEOXY-d-GALACTITOL ◇ 1,6-DI-BROMODULCITOL ◇ ELOBROMOL ◇ GALACTICOL ◇ MITOLAC ◇ MITOLACTOL ◇ NCI-C04795 ◇ NSC-104800

TOXICITY DATA with REFERENCE
NEO: ipr-mus TDLo: 3500 mg/kg/26W-I
RRCRBU 52,1,75
NEO: ipr-rat TDLo: 5850 mg/kg/26W-I
RRCRBU 52,1,75
MUT: bfa rat/sat 450 mg/kg   CRNGDP 3,333,82
MUT: dnd-mam: lym 150 mmol/L   CBINA8 47,133,83
MUT: dnd-rat-ipr 110 mg/kg   CBINA8 47,133,83
MUT: mmo-sat 100 µg/plate   CRNGDP 3,333,82
MUT: sce-ham: oth 5500 ng/L   CNREA8 43,4530,83

CONSENSUS REPORTS: NCI Carcinogenesis Bioassay Completed; Results Positive: mouse, rat (RRCRBU 52,1,75).

SAFETY PROFILE: Questionable carcinogen with experimental carcinogenic, neoplastigenic, and tumorigenic data. Poison by ingestion. Moderately toxic by intraperitoneal and possibly other routes. Human mutation data reported. An anti-cancer agent taken orally. When heated to decomposition it emits very toxic fumes of Br^-.

DDJ400   CAS: 3252-43-5
DIBROMOACETONITRILE
mf: C_2HBr_2N mw: 198.86

TOXICITY DATA with REFERENCE
CAR: skn-mus TDLo: 2400 mg/kg/2W-I
FAATDF 5,1065,85
MUT: dnd-hmn: lym 50 µmol/L   FAATDF 6,447,86
MUT: mma-sat 16 µg/plate   ENMUDM 8(Suppl 7),1,86

CONSENSUS REPORTS: Cyanide and its compounds are on the Community Right-To-Know List. Reported in EPA TSCA Inventory.

SAFETY PROFILE: Questionable carcinogen with experimental carcinogenic data. Poison by intravenous route. Human mutation data reported. When heated to decomposition it emits very toxic fumes of NO_x, Br^- and CN^-.

DDP600   CAS: 488-41-5
1,6-DIBROMOMANNITOL
mf: $C_6H_{12}Br_2O_4$ mw: 308.00

SYNS: DBM ◇ DIBROMANNIT ◇ DIBROMANNITOL ◇ d-DIBROMANNITOL ◇ 1,6-DIBROMO-1,6-DIDEOXY-d-MANNITOL ◇ 1,6-DIBROMO-1,6-d-DIDESOXYMANNITOL

◇ MIEOBROMOL ◇ MITOBRONITOL ◇ MYEBROL
◇ MYELOBROMOL ◇ NCI-C04762 ◇ NSC-94100 ◇ R 54

TOXICITY DATA with REFERENCE
NEO: ipr-mus TDLo: 7000 mg/kg/26W-I
    RRCRBU 52,1,75
NEO: ipr-rat TDLo: 9750 mg/kg/26W-I
    RRCRBU 52,1,75
MUT: cyt-mus-ivn 90 mg/kg   MUREAV 60,329,79
MUT: mma-sat 667 μg/plate   ENMUDM 8(Suppl
    7),1,86
MUT: mmo-sat 1 mg/plate   CNREA8 43,4530,83
MUT: sce-ham: oth 1300 ng/L   CNREA8 43,4530,83
MUT: sce-hmn: lym 10 nmol/L   NGCJAK
    15,1085,80

CONSENSUS REPORTS: NCI Carcinogenesis Bioassay Completed; Results Positive:
mouse, rat (RRCRBU 52,1,75).

SAFETY PROFILE: Questionable carcinogen
with experimental carcinogenic, neoplastigenic,
and teratogenic data. Moderately toxic by ingestion, intravenous, intraperitoneal, and subcutaneous routes. Other experimental reproductive
effects. Human mutation data reported. When
heated to decomposition it emits toxic fumes
of Br^-.

DDQ800   CAS: 57541-73-8
3,4-DIBROMONITROSOPIPERIDINE
mf: $C_5H_8Br_2N_2O$ mw: 271.97

SYN: N-NITROSO-3,4-DIBROMOPIPERIDINE

TOXICITY DATA with REFERENCE
ETA: orl-rat TDLo: 1090 mg/kg/27W-C
    CNREA8 35,3209,75
MUT: mma-sat 1 μmol/plate   MUREAV 56,131,77
MUT: mmo-sat 200 μg/plate   MUREAV 56,131,77
MUT: pic-esc 10 mg/L   TCMUE9 1,91,84
MUT: sln-dmg-orl 1 mmol/L/24H   MUREAV
    67,27,79

CONSENSUS REPORTS: EPA Genetic Toxicology Program.

SAFETY PROFILE: Questionable carcinogen
with experimental tumorigenic data. Mutation
data reported. Many N-nitroso compounds are
carcinogens. When heated to decomposition it
emits very toxic fumes of Br^- and NO_x.

DDX200   CAS: 63041-48-5
9,10-DI-n-BUTYL-1,2,5,6-
DIBENZANTHRACENE
mf: $C_{30}H_{30}$ mw: 390.60

TOXICITY DATA with REFERENCE
ETA: skn-mus TDLo: 1250 mg/kg/52W-I
    PRLBA4 117,318,35

SAFETY PROFILE: Questionable carcinogen
with experimental tumorigenic data. When
heated to decomposition it emits acrid smoke
and irritating fumes.

DEC000   CAS: 625-22-9
DIBUTYL ESTER SULFURIC ACID
mf: $C_8H_{18}O_4S$ mw: 210.32

SYNS: DIBUTYL SULFATE ◇ DI-n-BUTYLSULFAT (GER-
MAN)

TOXICITY DATA with REFERENCE
ETA: orl-rat TDLo: 12 g/kg/24W-I   ZEKBAI
    74,241,70
ETA: scu-rat TDLo: 9500 mg/kg/19W-I   ZEKBAI
    74,241,70

SAFETY PROFILE: Questionable carcinogen
with experimental tumorigenic data. Poison by
ingestion. Mildly toxic by subcutaneous route.
When heated to decomposition it emits toxic
fumes of SO_x.

DEC725   CAS: 7422-80-2
1,1-DIBUTYLHYDRAZINE
mf: $C_8H_{20}N_2$ mw: 144.30

SYNS: 1,1-DBH ◇ N,N-DIBUTYLHYDRAZINE ◇ 1,1-DI-
n-BUTYLHYDRAZINE

TOXICITY DATA with REFERENCE
CAR: orl-mus TDLo: 49280 mg/kg/2Y-C
    CRNGDP 2,651,81

SAFETY PROFILE: Questionable carcinogen
with experimental carcinogenic data. When
heated to decomposition it emits toxic fumes
of NO_x.

DEC775   CAS: 78776-28-0
1,2-DI-n-BUTYLHYDRAZINE
DIHYDROCHLORIDE
mf: $C_8H_{20}N_2 \cdot 2ClH$ mw: 217.22

TOXICITY DATA with REFERENCE
CAR: orl-mus TD: 142 g/kg/90W-C   EXPEAM
    37,773,81
CAR: orl-mus TDLo: 92 g/kg/90W-C   EXPEAM
    37,773,81

SAFETY PROFILE: Questionable carcinogen
with experimental carcinogenic data. When

heated to decomposition it emits toxic fumes of NO_x and HCl.

DEK000　　　　　　CAS: 56455-90-4
DICARBOXIDINE HYDROCHLORIDE
mf: $C_{20}H_{24}N_2O_6 \cdot 2ClH$　　mw: 461.38

SYNS: 4,4'-((4,4'-DIAMINO-(1,1'-BIPHENYL)-3,3'-DIYL) BIS(OXY)BISBUTANOIC ACID, DIHYDROCHLORIDE ◊ HYDROCHLORIC ACID DICARBOXIDE

TOXICITY DATA with REFERENCE
ETA: scu-rat TD: 37500 mg/kg/2Y-I　　VOONAW 25(7),43,79
ETA: scu-rat TDLo: 21250 mg/kg/2Y-I　　JJIND8 62,301,79

SAFETY PROFILE: Questionable carcinogen with experimental tumorigenic data. When heated to decomposition it emits very toxic fumes of NO_x and HCl.

DEK400　　　　　　CAS: 73758-56-2
DICARBOXYDINE
mf: $C_{20}H_{24}N_2O_6$　　mw: 388.46

SYNS: γ,γ'-,3,3'-BENZIDINE DIOXYDIBUTYRIC ACID ◊ 3,3'-BENZIDINE-γ,γ'-DIOXYDIBUTYRIC ACID ◊ 4,4'-(3,3'-DIAMINO-p,p'-BIPHENYLENEDIOXY)DIBUTYRIC ACID

TOXICITY DATA with REFERENCE
ETA: scu-rat TDLo: 19 g/kg/2Y-I　　JJIND8 62,301,79

SAFETY PROFILE: Questionable carcinogen with experimental tumorigenic data. When heated to decomposition it emits toxic fumes of NO_x.

DEL000　　　　　　CAS: 79-43-6
DICHLORACETIC ACID
DOT: 1764
mf: $C_2H_2Cl_2O_2$　　mw: 128.94

PROP: Colorless, corrosive liquid; pungent odor. Mp (a): 10°, (b): −4°, bp: 194°, d: 1.5634 @ 20°/4°, vap press: 1 mm @ 44.0°, vap d: 4.45.

SYNS: BICHLORACETIC ACID ◊ DCA ◊ DICHLORETHANOIC ACID ◊ 2,2-DICHLOROACETIC ACID ◊ DICHLOROETHANOIC ACID ◊ URNER'S LIQUID

TOXICITY DATA with REFERENCE
CAR: orl-mus TDLo: 427 g/kg/61W-C　　TXAPA9 90,183,87

CONSENSUS REPORTS: Reported in EPA TSCA Inventory.

DOT Classification: Corrosive Material; Label: Corrosive.

SAFETY PROFILE: Questionable carcinogen with experimental tumorigenic data. Moderately toxic by skin contact and ingestion. It is corrosive to the skin, eyes, and mucous membranes. Will react with water or steam to produce toxic and corrosive fumes. When heated to decomposition it emits toxic fumes of Cl^-.

DEN400　　　　　　CAS: 79-36-7
DICHLOROACETYL CHLORIDE
DOT: 1765
mf: C_2HCl_3O　　mw: 147.38

PROP: Fuming liquid, acrid odor, misc in ether. D: 1.5315 @ 16°/4°, bp: 108°, flash p: 151°F, vap d: 5.8.

SYNS: CHLORURE de DICHLORACETYLE (FRENCH) ◊ DICHLORACETYL CHLORIDE ◊ α,α-DICHLOROACETYL CHLORIDE ◊ 2,2-DICHLOROACETYL CHLORIDE ◊ DICHLOROACETYL CHLORIDE (DOT) ◊ DICHLOROETHANOYL CHLORIDE

TOXICITY DATA with REFERENCE
ETA: scu-mus TDLo: 2 mg/kg/80W-I　　CNREA8 43,159,83

CONSENSUS REPORTS: Reported in EPA TSCA Inventory.

DOT Classification: Corrosive Material; Label: Corrosive.

SAFETY PROFILE: Questionable carcinogen with experimental tumorigenic data. Moderately toxic by ingestion, inhalation, and skin contact. Corrosive to the skin, eyes, and mucous membranes. Flammable when exposed to heat or flame. When heated to decomposition it emits toxic fumes of Cl^-.

DEP600　　　　　　CAS: 95-50-1
o-DICHLOROBENZENE
DOT: 1591
mf: $C_6H_4Cl_2$　　mw: 147.00

PROP: Clear liquid. Mp: −17.5°, bp: 180-183°, fp: −22°, flash p: 151°F, d: 1.307 @ 20°/20°, vap d: 5.05, autoign temp: 1198°F, lel: 2.2%, uel: 9.2%.

SYNS: CHLOROBEN ◊ CHLORODEN ◊ CLOROBEN ◊ DCB ◊ o-DICHLORBENZENE ◊ o-DICHLOR BENZOL ◊ 1,2-DICHLOROBENZENE (MAK) ◊ DICHLOROBENZENE, ORTHO, liquid (DOT) ◊ DILANTIN DB ◊ DILATIN DB

◇ DIZENE ◇ DOWTHERM E ◇ NCI-C54944 ◇ ODB ◇ ODCB ◇ ORTHODICHLOROBENZENE ◇ ORTHODICHLO-ROBENZOL ◇ RCRA WASTE NUMBER U070 ◇ SPECIAL TERMITE FLUID ◇ TERMITKIL

TOXICITY DATA with REFERENCE

MUT: spm-rat-ipr 250 mg/kg   JACTDZ 4(2),224,85

CONSENSUS REPORTS: IARC Cancer Review: GROUP 3 IMEMDT 7,192,87; Animal Inadequate Evidence IMEMDT 7,231,74, IMEMDT 29,213,82; Human Inadequate Evidence IMEMDT 7,231,74, IMEMDT 29,-213,82. Reported in EPA TSCA Inventory. Community Right-To-Know List.

OSHA PEL: CL 50 ppm   ACGIH TLV: CL 50 ppm   DFG MAK: 50 ppm (300 mg/m^3) DOT Classification: ORM-A; Label: None; IMO: Poison B; Label: St. Andrews Cross.

SAFETY PROFILE: Questionable carcinogen. An experimental teratogen. Poison by ingestion and intravenous routes. Moderately toxic by inhalation and intraperitoneal routes. An eye, skin, and mucous membrane irritant. Causes liver and kidney injury. Experimental reproductive effects. Mutation data reported. A pesticide. Flammable when exposed to heat or flame. To fight fire, use water, foam, CO_2 dry chemical. When heated to decomposition it emits toxic fumes of Cl^-.

DER800   CAS: 1194-65-6
2,6-DICHLOROBENZONITRILE
DOT: 2769
mf: $C_7H_3Cl_2N$ mw: 172.01

PROP: White solid. Mp: 144°. Almost insol in water; sol in organic solvents.

SYNS: CARSORON ◇ CASORON 133 ◇ CODE H 133 ◇ 2,6-DBN ◇ DBN (THE HERBICIDE) ◇ DCB ◇ DECABANE ◇ DICHLOBENIL (DOT) ◇ 2,6-DICHLORBENZONITRIL (GERMAN) ◇ DU-SPREX ◇ H 133 ◇ H 1313 ◇ NIA 5996 ◇ NIAGARA 5006 ◇ NIAGARA 5,996

TOXICITY DATA with REFERENCE

ETA: ipr-mus TDLo: 260 μg/kg/39D-I   AAATAP 122,107,79
ETA: scu-mus TDLo: 260 μg/kg/39D-I   AAATAP 122,107,79

CONSENSUS REPORTS: Cyanide and its compounds are on the Community Right-To-Know List. EPA Genetic Toxicology Program.

DOT Classification: ORM-E; Label: None.

SAFETY PROFILE: Questionable carcinogen with experimental tumorigenic data. Moderately toxic by ingestion, skin contact, and possibly other routes. Does not hydrolyze to HCN in body. Less toxic than most aliphatic nitriles. When heated to decomposition it emits toxic fumes of Cl^-, CN^-, and NO_x.

DEU200   CAS: 38780-42-6
cis-DICHLOROBIS(PYRROLIDINE) PLATINUM(II)
mf: $C_8H_{18}Cl_2N_2Pt$ mw: 408.27

SYN: cis-DIPYRROLIDINEDICHLOROPLATINUM(II)

TOXICITY DATA with REFERENCE
ETA: scu-rat TDLo: 91 mg/kg/6W-I   CNREA8 39,913,79
MUT: mmo-sat 100 nmol/plate   CNREA8 39,913,79

SAFETY PROFILE: Questionable carcinogen with experimental tumorigenic data. Poison by intraperitoneal route. Mutation data reported. When heated to decomposition it emits very toxic fumes of Cl^- and NO_x.

DEX000   CAS: 14913-33-8
trans-DICHLORODIAMMINEPLATINUM(II)
mf: $C_{12}H_6N_2Pt$ mw: 300.07

SYNS: trans-DIAMMINEDICHLOROPLATINUM(II) ◇ trans-PLATINUM(II)DIAMMINEDICHLORIDE

TOXICITY DATA with REFERENCE
ETA: ipr-mus TDLo: 32408 μg/kg/10W-I CNREA8 41,4368,81
MUT: dnd-hmn: fbr 50 μmol/L/4H   CNREA8 42,145,82
MUT: dnd-hmn: lng 100 μmol/L   CBINA8 36,345,81
MUT: dnd-hmn: oth 20 mg/L   CNREA8 45,6232,85
MUT: mma-sat 2 μg/plate   MUREAV 77,45,80
MUT: msc-ham: lng 100 mg/L   CNREA8 44,3270,84

CONSENSUS REPORTS: EPA Genetic Toxicology Program.

SAFETY PROFILE: Questionable carcinogen with experimental tumorigenic data. Poison by intraperitoneal route. Human mutation data reported. When heated to decomposition it emits toxic fumes of NO_x and Cl^-.

DFD400   CAS: 17010-61-6
3′,4′-DICHLORO-4-DIMETHYLAMINOAZOBENZENE
mf: $C_{14}H_{13}Cl_2N_3$ mw: 294.20

SYNS: BENZENAMINE, 4-((3,4-DICHLOROPHENYL)AZO)-N,N-DIMETHYL-(9CI) ◊ 3′,4′-Cl2-DAB ◊ p-((3,4-DICHLORO-PHENYL)AZO)-N,N-DIMETHYLANILINE

TOXICITY DATA with REFERENCE
CAR: orl-rat TDLo: 15120 mg/kg/36W-C
CBINA8 53,107,85
ETA: orl-rat TD: 11 g/kg/17W-I CNREA8 30,1520,70

SAFETY PROFILE: Questionable carcinogen with experimental carcinogenic and tumorigenic data. When heated to decomposition it emits toxic fumes of Cl^- and NO_x.

DFE600   CAS: 3883-43-0
trans-2,3-DICHLORO-1,4-DIOXANE
mf: $C_4H_6Cl_2O_2$ mw: 157.00

SYN: trans-2,3-DICHLORO-p-DIOXANE

TOXICITY DATA with REFERENCE
NEO: scu-mus TDLo: 1260 mg/kg/63W-I
JNCIAM 53,695,74

SAFETY PROFILE: Questionable carcinogen with experimental neoplastigenic and tumorigenic data. Moderately toxic by ingestion and skin contact. When heated to decomposition it emits toxic fumes of Cl^-.

DFF809   CAS: 75-34-3
1,1-DICHLOROETHANE
DOT: 2362
mf: $C_2H_4Cl_2$ mw: 98.96

PROP: Colorless liquid; aromatic, ethereal odor; hot, saccharine taste. Mp: −97.7°, lel: 5.6%, bp: 57.3°, flash p: 22°F (TOC), d: 1.174 @ 20°/4°, vap press: 230 mm @ 25°, vap d: 3.44, autoign temp: 856°F.

SYNS: AETHYLIDENCHLORID (GERMAN) ◊ CHLORINATED HYDROCHLORIC ETHER ◊ CHLORURE d′ETHYLIDENE (FRENCH) ◊ CLORURO di ETILIDENE (ITALIAN) ◊ 1,1-DICHLOORETHAAN (DUTCH) ◊ 1,1-DICHLORAETHAN (GERMAN) ◊ 1,1-DICLOROETANO (ITALIAN) ◊ ETHYLIDENE CHLORIDE ◊ ETHYLIDENE DICHLORIDE ◊ NCI-C04535 ◊ RCRA WASTE NUMBER U076

TOXICITY DATA with REFERENCE
ETA: orl-mus TD: 1300 g/kg/78W-I: TER
NCITR* NCI-CG-TR-66,78
ETA: orl-mus TDLo: 185 g/kg/78W-I: TER
NCITR* NCI-CG-TR-66,78

CONSENSUS REPORTS: NCI Carcinogenesis Bioassay (gavage); Inadequate Studies: mouse, rat NCITR* NCI-CG-TR-66,78. Reported in EPA TSCA Inventory.

OSHA PEL: TWA 100 ppm ACGIH TLV: TWA 200 ppm; STEL 250 ppm DFG MAK: 100 ppm (400 mg/m³) DOT Classification: Flammable Liquid; Label: Flammable Liquid.

SAFETY PROFILE: Questionable carcinogen with experimental tumorigenic and teratogenic data. Moderately toxic by ingestion. Experimental reproductive effects. Liver damage reported in experimental animals. A very dangerous fire hazard and moderate explosion hazard when exposed to heat or flame; can react vigorously with oxidizing materials. To fight fire, use alcohol foam, water, foam, CO_2, dry chemical. When heated to decomposition it emits highly toxic fumes of phosgene and Cl^-.

DFH000   CAS: 10072-25-0
9-(2-(DI(2-CHLOROETHYL)AMINO) ETHYLAMINO)-6-CHLORO-2-METHOXYACRIDINE
mf: $C_{20}H_{22}Cl_3N_3O \cdot 2ClH \cdot H_2O$ mw: 517.74

SYNS: 9-(2-(BIS(2-CHLOROETHYL)AMINO)ETHYLAMINO)-6-CHLORO-2-METHOXYACRIDINE DIHYDROCHLORIDE ◊ ICR-48b ◊ NSC-34372 ◊ QUINACRINE ETHYL MUSTARD

TOXICITY DATA with REFERENCE
CAR: ipr-mus TDLo: 16 mg/kg/4W JNCIAM 36,915,66

SAFETY PROFILE: Questionable carcinogen with experimental carcinogenic data. When heated to decomposition it emits very toxic fumes of Cl^- and NO_x.

DFI800   CAS: 3967-55-3
1,2-DICHLOROETHYLENE CARBONATE
mf: $C_3H_2Cl_2O_3$ mw: 156.95

SYN: 4,5-DICHLORO-2-OXO-1,3-DIOXOLANE

TOXICITY DATA with REFERENCE
ETA: scu-mus TDLo: 648 mg/kg/54W-I
JNCIAM 48,1431,72

SAFETY PROFILE: Questionable carcinogen with experimental tumorigenic data. When heated to decomposition it emits toxic fumes of Cl^-.

DFJ050   CAS: 111-44-4
DICHLOROETHYL ETHER
DOT: 1916
mf: $C_4H_8Cl_2O$ mw: 143.02

PROP: Colorless, stable liquid. Bp: 178.5°, fp: −51.9°, flash p: 131°F (CC), d: 1.2220 @ 20°/

20°, autoign temp: 696°F, vap press: 0.7 mm @ 20°, vap d: 4.93.

SYNS: BIS(2-CHLOROETHYL) ETHER ◇ BIS(β-CHLORO-ETHYL) ETHER ◇ CHLOREX ◇ 1-CHLORO-2-(β-CHLORO-ETHOXY)ETHANE ◇ CHLOROETHYL ETHER ◇ CLOREX ◇ DCEE ◇ 2,2'-DICHLOOORETHYLETHER (DUTCH) ◇ 2,2'-DICHLOR-DIAETHYLAETHER (GERMAN) ◇ 2,2'-DI-CHLORETHYL ETHER ◇ β,β-DICHLORODIETHYL ETHER ◇ DICHLOROETHER ◇ DI(β-CHLOROETHYL)ETHER ◇ β,β'-DICHLOROETHYL ETHER (MAK) ◇ sym-DICHLORO-ETHYL ETHER ◇ 2,2'-DICHLOROETHYL ETHER ◇ DICHLO-ROETHYL OXIDE ◇ 2,2'-DICLOROETILETERE (ITALIAN) ◇ DWUCHLORODWUETYLOWY ETER (POLISH) ◇ ENT 4,504 ◇ ETHER DICHLORE (FRENCH) ◇ 1,1'-OXYBIS(2-CHLORO)ETHANE ◇ OXYDE de CHLORETHYLE (FRENCH) ◇ RCRA WASTE NUMBER U025

TOXICITY DATA with REFERENCE
CAR: orl-mus TDLo:33 g/kg/79W-C   JNCIAM 42,1101,69
ETA: scu-mus TDLo:2400 mg/kg/60W-I
JNCIAM 48,1431,72
MUT: mma-sat 1 mg/plate   ENMUDM 8 (Suppl 7),1,86
MUT: mmo-sat 1 mL/plate/2H   DHEFDK FDA-78-1046,78

CONSENSUS REPORTS: IARC Cancer Review: GROUP 3 IMEMDT 7,56,87; Animal Sufficient Evidence IMEMDT 9,117,75. Reported in EPA TSCA Inventory. On Community Right-To-Know List. On EPA Extremely Hazardous Substances List.

OSHA PEL: (Transitional: CL 15 ppm (skin)) TWA 5 ppm; STEL 10 ppm (skin) ACGIH TLV: TWA 5 ppm; STEL 10 ppm (skin) DFG MAK: 10 ppm (60 mg/m^3) DOT Classification: IMO: Poison B; Label: Poison.

SAFETY PROFILE: Questionable carcinogen with experimental carcinogenic and tumorigenic data. A poison by ingestion, skin contact and inhalation. A skin, eye, and mucous membrane irritant. Mutation data reported. Flammable when exposed to heat, flame or oxidants. Reacts with water or steam to evolve toxic and corrosive fumes. To fight fire, use water, foam, mist, fog, spray, dry chemical. When heated to decomposition it emits toxic fumes of Cl^-.

DFM200   CAS: 13442-13-2
6,7-DICHLORO-4-(HYDROXYAMINO) QUINOLINE-1-OXIDE
mf: $C_9H_6Cl_2N_2O_2$ mw: 245.07

TOXICITY DATA with REFERENCE
ETA: scu-mus TDLo:120 mg/kg/50D-I   BCPCA6 16,631,67

SAFETY PROFILE: Questionable carcinogen with experimental tumorigenic data. When heated to decomposition it emits very toxic fumes of Cl^- and NO_x.

DFO000   CAS: 528-74-5
3'5'-DICHLOROMETHOTREXATE
mf: $C_{20}H_{20}Cl_2N_8O_5$ mw: 523.38

SYNS: DCM ◇ DICHLOROAMETHOPTERIN ◇ 3',5'-DI-CHLOROAMETHOPTERIN ◇ 3',5'-DICHLORO-4-AMINO-4-DEOXY-N$_{10}$-METHYLPTEROGLUTAMIC ACID ◇ N-(3,5-DI-CHLORO-4-((2,4-DIAMINO-6-PTERIDINYL METHYL)METHYLAMINO)BENZOYL)GLUTAMIC ACID ◇ DICHLOROMETHOTREXATE ◇ NCI-C04875 ◇ NSC-29630

TOXICITY DATA with REFERENCE
ETA: ipr-mus TDLo:5850 mg/kg/26W-I
CANCAR 40(Suppl 4),1935,77
ETA: ipr-rat TDLo:75 mg/kg/7W-I   CANCAR 40(Suppl 4),1935,77

CONSENSUS REPORTS: NCI Carcinogenesis Studies (ipr): Equivocal Evidence: rat; No Evidence: mouse CANCAR 40,1935,77

SAFETY PROFILE: Questionable carcinogen with experimental tumorigenic data. Moderately toxic by intraperitoneal and intravenous routes. When heated to decomposition it emits very toxic fumes of NO_x and Cl^-.

DFQ000   CAS: 4885-02-3
α,α-DICHLOROMETHYL METHYL ETHER
mf: $C_2H_4Cl_2O$ mw: 114.96

SYNS: BIS(CHLOROPHENYL) ETHER ◇ α,α-DICHLORO-METHYL ETHER

TOXICITY DATA with REFERENCE
ETA: skn-mus TDLo:40 mg/kg   ANYAA9 163,633,69

CONSENSUS REPORTS: Reported in EPA TSCA Inventory.

SAFETY PROFILE: Questionable carcinogen with experimental tumorigenic data. When heated to decomposition it emits toxic fumes of Cl^-.

DFT000   CAS: 117-80-6
2,3-DICHLORO-1,4-NAPHTHOQUINONE
DOT: 2761
mf: $C_{10}H_4Cl_2O_2$ mw: 227.04

PROP: Golden-yellow crystals. Mp: 193°, vap d: 7.8. Insol in water, moderately sol in organic solvents.

SYNS: ALGISTAT ◇ COMPOUND 604 ◇ DICHLONE (DOT) ◇ 2,3-DICHLOR-1,4-NAPHTHOCHINON (GERMAN) ◇ 2,3-DICHLORO-1,4-NAPHTHALENEDIONE ◇ 2,3-DI-CHLORO-1,4-NAPHTHAQUINONE ◇ DICHLORONAPHTHO-QUINONE ◇ 2,3-DICHLORONAPHTHOQUINONE ◇ 2,3-DI-CHLORO-α-NAPHTHOQUINONE ◇ 2,3-DICHLORONAPH-THOQUINONE-1,4 ◇ ENT 3,776 ◇ PHYGON ◇ PHYGON PASTE ◇ PHYGON SEED PROTECTANT ◇ PHYGON XL ◇ QUINTAR ◇ QUINTAR 540F ◇ SANQUINON ◇ UNIROYAL ◇ USR 604 ◇ U.S. RUBBER 604

TOXICITY DATA with REFERENCE
CAR: scu-mus TDLo: 22 mg/kg
    NTIS** PB223-159
NEO: orl-mus TDLo: 3300 mg/kg/78W-I
    NTIS** PB223-159

CONSENSUS REPORTS: Reported in EPA TSCA Inventory.

DOT Classification: ORM-E; Label: None.

SAFETY PROFILE: Questionable carcinogen with experimental carcinogenic and neoplastigenic data. Poison by ingestion and intraperitoneal routes. Mildly toxic by skin contact. A skin, eye, and mucous membrane irritant. Large doses can cause central nervous system depression. A fungicide and algaecide. When heated to decomposition it emits toxic fumes of Cl^-.

DFU400   CAS: 6240-55-7
1,2-DICHLORO-3-NITRONAPHTHALENE
mf: $C_{10}H_5Cl_2NO_2$ mw: 242.06

TOXICITY DATA with REFERENCE
ETA: orl-rat TDLo: 13 g/kg/52W-I   JNCIAM
    41,985,68

SAFETY PROFILE: Questionable carcinogen with experimental tumorigenic data. When heated to decomposition it emits very toxic fumes of Cl^- and NO_x.

DFV200   CAS: 14094-48-5
6,7-DICHLORO-4-NITROQUINOLINE-1-OXIDE
mf: $C_9H_4Cl_2N_2O_3$ mw: 259.05

TOXICITY DATA with REFERENCE
ETA: scu-mus TDLo: 120 mg/kg/50D-I   BCPCA6
    16,631,67

SAFETY PROFILE: Questionable carcinogen with experimental tumorigenic data. When heated to decomposition it emits very toxic fumes of Cl^- and NO_x.

DFW000   CAS: 69112-96-5
2,2'-DICHLORO-N-NITROSODIPROPYLAMINE
mf: $C_6H_{12}Cl_2N_2O$ mw: 199.10

SYN: NITROSOBIS(2-CHLOROPROPYL)AMINE

TOXICITY DATA with REFERENCE
ETA: orl-rat TDLo: 1360 mg/kg/20W-I   EESADV
    2,421,78
MUT: mma-sat 10 μg/plate   MUREAV 66,1,79
MUT: mmo-sat 10 μg/plate   MUREAV 66,1,79

SAFETY PROFILE: Questionable carcinogen with experimental tumorigenic data. Many N-nitroso compounds are carcinogens. Mutation data reported. When heated to decomposition it emits very toxic fumes of Cl^- and NO_x.

DFW200   CAS: 57541-72-7
3,4-DICHLORONITROSOPIPERIDINE
mf: $C_5H_8Cl_2N_2O$ mw: 183.05

SYN: N-NITROSO-3,4-DICHLOROPIPERIDINE

TOXICITY DATA with REFERENCE
ETA: orl-rat TD: 260 mg/kg/21W-C   CNREA8
    40,3325,80
ETA: orl-rat TD: 366 mg/kg/15W-C   CNREA8
    35,3209,75
ETA: orl-rat TDLo: 169 mg/kg/30W-I   ZKKOBW
    92,221,78
MUT: mma-sat 10 nmol/plate   MUREAV 57,85,78
MUT: mmo-sat 200 μg/plate   MUREAV 56,131,77
MUT: sce-hmn: lym 100 μmol/L   TCMUE9
    1,129,84
MUT: sln-dmg-orl 200 μmol/L/24H   MUREAV
    67,27,79

CONSENSUS REPORTS: EPA Genetic Toxicology Program.

SAFETY PROFILE: Questionable carcinogen with experimental tumorigenic data. Human mutation data reported. Many N-nitroso compounds are carcinogens. When heated to decomposition it emits very toxic fumes of Cl^- and NO_x.

DFW600   CAS: 59863-59-1
3,4-DICHLORO-N-NITROSOPYRROLIDINE
mf: $C_4H_6Cl_2N_2O$ mw: 169.02

TOXICITY DATA with REFERENCE
ETA: orl-rat TDLo: 1550 mg/kg/31W-I   CNREA8
36,1988,76

MUT: mma-sat 250 μg/plate   MUREAV 89,35,81

SAFETY PROFILE: Questionable carcinogen
with experimental tumorigenic data. Mutation
data reported. Many N-nitroso compounds are
carcinogens. When heated to decomposition it
emits very toxic fumes of Cl⁻ and NO$_x$.

DFY400   CAS: 97-16-5
2,4-DICHLOROPHENOL
BENZENESULFONATE
mf: $C_{12}H_8Cl_2O_3S$ mw: 303.16

SYNS: COMPOUND 923 ◇ 2,4-DICHLOROPHENYL BEN-
ZENESULFONATE ◇ 2,4-DICHLOROPHENYL BENZENESUL-
PHONATE ◇ 2,4-DICHLOROPHENYL ESTER of BENZENE-
SULFONIC ACID ◇ 2,4-DICHLOROPHENYL ESTER
BENZENESULPHONIC ACID ◇ DPBS ◇ EM 923 ◇ GENITE
◇ GENITOL

TOXICITY DATA with REFERENCE
CAR: scu-mus TDLo: 1000 mg/kg
NTIS** PB223-159
ETA: orl-mus TDLo: 260 g/kg/78W-I
NTIS** PB223-159

CONSENSUS REPORTS: Chlorophenol compounds are on the Community Right-To-Know
List.

SAFETY PROFILE: Questionable carcinogen
with experimental carcinogenic and tumorigenic
data. Poison by intravenous route. Moderately
toxic by ingestion and possibly other routes.
An irritant. A pesticide. When heated to decomposition it emits very toxic fumes of Cl⁻ and
SO$_x$.

DGB200   CAS: 6965-71-5
2-(2,5-DICHLOROPHENOXY)PROPIONIC
ACID
mf: $C_9H_8Cl_2O_3$ mw: 235.07

SYN: α-(2,5-DICHLOROPHENOXY)PROPIONIC ACID

TOXICITY DATA with REFERENCE
ETA: scu-mus TDLo: 100 mg/kg
NTIS** PB223-159

SAFETY PROFILE: Questionable carcinogen
with experimental tumorigenic data. When
heated to decomposition it emits toxic fumes
of Cl⁻.

DGB800   CAS: 15460-48-7
N-(3,4-DICHLOROPHENYL)-1-
AZIRIDINECARBOXAMIDE
mf: $C_9H_8Cl_2N_2O$ mw: 231.09

SYN: 3,4-DICHLOROPHENYL-N-CARBAMOYLAZIRIDINE

TOXICITY DATA with REFERENCE
NEO: ipr-mus TDLo: 20 mg/kg/4W-I   CNREA8
29,2184,69

SAFETY PROFILE: Questionable carcinogen
with experimental neoplastigenic data. When
heated to decomposition it emits very toxic
fumes of Cl⁻ and NO$_x$.

DGF000   CAS: 24096-53-5
N-(3,5-DICHLOROPHENYL)
SUCCINIMIDE
mf: $C_{10}H_7Cl_2NO_2$ mw: 244.08

SYNS: 1-(3,5-DICHLOROPHENYL)-2,5-PYRROLIDINE-
DIONE ◇ DIMETHACHLON ◇ OHRIC

TOXICITY DATA with REFERENCE
ETA: orl-rat TDLo: 17 g/kg/8W-C   GANNA2
67,147,76

SAFETY PROFILE: Questionable carcinogen
with experimental tumorigenic data. Moderately
toxic by ingestion. When heated to decomposition it emits very toxic fumes of Cl⁻ and NO$_x$.

DGH500   CAS: 66826-73-1
trans-1,3-DICHLOROPROPENE OXIDE
mf: $C_3H_4Cl_2O$ mw: 126.97

SYNS: trans-2-CHLORO-3-(CHLOROMETHYL)OXIRANE
◇ trans-DCPO ◇ trans-1,3-DICHLORO-1,2-EPOXYPROPANE

TOXICITY DATA with REFERENCE
CAR: scu-mus TDLo: 20 mg/kg/71W-I   CNREA8
43,159,83
CAR: skn-mus TDLo: 400 mg/kg/73W-I
CNREA8 43,159,83
MUT: otr-ham: emb 10 μmol/L   JJIND8 69,531,82

SAFETY PROFILE: Questionable carcinogen
with experimental carcinogenic data. Mutation
data reported. When heated to decomposition
it emits toxic fumes of Cl⁻.

DGK400   CAS: 73926-91-7
2,2′-DICHLORO-4,4′-STILBENEDIAMINE
mf: $C_{14}H_{12}Cl_2N_2$ mw: 279.18

SYNS: 4:4′-DIAMINO-2:2′-DICHLOROSTILBENE
◇ 2,2′-DICHLORO-4,4′-STILBENAMINE

TOXICITY DATA with REFERENCE
ETA: scu-rat TDLo:1400 mg/kg/W-I   BMBUAQ
   14,141,58

SAFETY PROFILE: Questionable carcinogen with experimental tumorigenic data. When heated to decomposition it emits very toxic fumes of Cl^- and NO_x.

DGK600   CAS: 73926-92-8
3,3'-DICHLORO-4,4'-STILBENEDIAMINE
mf: $C_{14}H_{12}Cl_2N_2$ mw: 279.18

SYN: 4:4'-DIAMINO-3:3'-DICHLOROSTILBENE

TOXICITY DATA with REFERENCE
ETA: scu-rat TDLo:200 mg/kg/W-I   BMBUAQ
   14,141,58

SAFETY PROFILE: Questionable carcinogen with experimental tumorigenic data. When heated to decomposition it emits very toxic fumes of Cl^- and NO_x.

DGL800   CAS: 3511-19-1
2,3-DICHLOROTETRAHYDROFURAN
mf: $C_4H_6Cl_2O$ mw: 141.00

TOXICITY DATA with REFERENCE
ETA: scu-mus TDLo:888 mg/kg/74W-I
   JNCIAM 48,1431,72

SAFETY PROFILE: Questionable carcinogen with experimental tumorigenic data. When heated to decomposition it emits toxic fumes of Cl^-.

DGT600   CAS: 101-83-7
N,N-DICYCLOHEXYLAMINE
DOT: 2565
mf: $C_{12}H_{23}N$ mw: 181.36

PROP: Liquid, fishy odor. Mp: $-1°$, bp: $256°$, flash p: $>210°F$ (OC), d: 0.910, vap d: 6.27.

SYNS: CDHA ◇ N-CYCLOHEXYLCYCLOHEXANAMINE ◇ DICYCLOHEXYLAMINE (DOT) ◇ DICYKLOHEXYLAMIN (CZECH) ◇ DODECAHYDRODIPHENYLAMINE

TOXICITY DATA with REFERENCE
ETA: orl-rat TDLo:40 g/kg/52W-I   VOONAW
   4,659,58
ETA: scu-mus TDLo:2404 mg/kg/48W-I
   VOONAW 4,659,58
MUT: cyt-hmn:leu 200 μg/L   INHEAO 9,188,71

CONSENSUS REPORTS: IARC Cancer Review: Animal Inadequate Evidence IMEMDT 22,55,80. Reported in EPA TSCA Inventory.

DOT Classification: Corrosive Material; Label: Corrosive.

SAFETY PROFILE: Questionable carcinogen with experimental tumorigenic data. Poison by ingestion and subcutaneous routes. Human mutation data reported. Corrosive. A severe skin and eye irritant. Combustible when exposed to heat or flame; can react with oxidizing materials. To fight fire, use alcohol foam, CO_2, dry chemical. When heated to decomposition it emits toxic fumes of NO_x.

DGU200   CAS: 3129-91-7
DICYCLOHEXYLAMINE NITRITE
mf: $C_{12}H_{23}N \cdot HNO_2$ mw: 228.38

SYNS: DECHAN ◇ DICHAN (CZECH) ◇ DICYCLOHEXY-LAMINONITRITE ◇ DICYCLOHEXYLAMMONIUM NITRITE ◇ DICYKLOHEXYLAMIN NITRIT (CZECH) ◇ DICYNIT (CZECH) ◇ DODECAHYDROPHENYLAMINE NITRITE ◇ DUSITAN DICYKLOHEXYLAMINU (CZECH)

TOXICITY DATA with REFERENCE
ETA: scu-mus TDLo:2040 mg/kg/52W-I
   VOONAW 4,659,58
ETA: scu-rat TDLo:2400 mg/kg/48W-I
   VOONAW 4,659,58

CONSENSUS REPORTS: Reported in EPA TSCA Inventory.

SAFETY PROFILE: Questionable carcinogen with experimental tumorigenic data. Poison by ingestion and subcutaneous routes. When heated to decomposition it emits very toxic fumes of HNO_2 and NO_x.

DGW200   CAS: 1271-19-8
DICYCLOPENTADIENYLDICHLORO-TITANIUM
mf: $C_{10}H_{10}Cl_2Ti$ mw: 249.00

SYNS: DICHLOROBIS(ETA^5-2,4-CYCLOPENTADIEN-1-YL-TITANIUM (9CI) ◇ DICHLORODICYCLOPENTADIENYL-TITANIUM ◇ DICHLORODI-pi-CYCLOPENTADIENYLTI-TANIUM ◇ DICHLOROTITANOCENE ◇ DICYCLOPENTA-DIENYLTITANIUMDICHLORIDE ◇ NCI-C04502 ◇ TI-TANIUM FERROCENE ◇ TITANOCENE ◇ TITANO-CENE, DICHLORIDE

TOXICITY DATA with REFERENCE
NEO: ims-mus TDLo:75 mg/kg   NCIUS* PH
   43-64-886,JUL,68
NEO: ims-rat TD:900 mg/kg/2Y-I   PWPSA8
   14,68,71

NEO: ims-rat TDLo: 720 mg/kg/2Y-I
NCIUS* PH 43-64-886,JUL,68

ETA: ims-rat TD: 430 mg/kg/81W-I
NCIUS* PH 43-64-886,AUG,69

MUT: mma-sat 1 mg/plate   ENMUDM 5(Suppl 1),3,83

MUT: mmo-sat 100 μg/plate   ENMUDM 5(Suppl 1),3,83

MUT: otr-ham: emb 100 μg/L   JJIND8 67,1303,81

MUT: otr-mus: fbr 800 μg/L   JJIND8 67,1303,81

MUT: otr-rat: emb 2960 μg/L   JJIND8 67,1303,81

CONSENSUS REPORTS: Reported in EPA TSCA Inventory. EPA Genetic Toxicology Program.

SAFETY PROFILE: Questionable carcinogen with experimental neoplastigenic, tumorigenic, and teratogenic data. Poison by intravenous and intraperitoneal routes. Mutation data reported. When heated to decomposition it emits toxic fumes of Cl^-.

DGW300
DICYCLOPENTA(c,lmn)PHENANTHREN-1(9H)-ONE, 2,3-DIHYDRO-
mf: $C_{18}H_{12}O$ mw: 244.30

SYNS: 2,3-DIHYDRODICYCLOPEN-TA(c,lmn)PHENANTHREN-1(9H)-ONE ◇ 15,16-DIHYDRO-1,11-METHANOCYCLOPENTA(a)PHENANTHREN-17-ONE

TOXICITY DATA with REFERENCE
CAR: skn-mus TDLo: 16 mg/kg   CRNGDP
5,1485,84

SAFETY PROFILE: Questionable carcinogen with experimental carcinogenic data. When heated to decomposition it emits acrid smoke and irritating fumes.

DHA425   CAS: 53866-33-4
2,4-DIDEUTERIOESTRADIOL
mf: $C_{18}H_{22}D_2O_2$ mw: 274.42

SYN: ESTRA-1,3,5(10)-TRIENE-2,4-D2-3,17-DIOL, (17-β)-

TOXICITY DATA with REFERENCE
CAR: imp-ham TDLo: 360 mg/kg/15W-I
MOPMA3 23,278,83

SAFETY PROFILE: Questionable carcinogen with experimental carcinogenic data. When heated to decomposition it emits acrid smoke and irritating fumes.

DHB400   CAS: 60-57-1
DIELDRIN
DOT: 2761
mf: $C_{12}H_8Cl_6O$ mw: 380.90

PROP: White crystals; odorless. Mp: 150°, vap d: 13.2. Insol in water, sol in common organic solvents.

SYNS: ALVIT ◇ COMPOUND 497 ◇ DIELDREX ◇ DIELDRINE (FRENCH) ◇ DIELDRITE ◇ ENT 16,225 ◇ HEOD ◇ HEXACHLOROEPOXYOCTAHYDRO-ENDO,EXO-DIMETHANONAPHTHALENE ◇ 3,4,5,6,9,9-HEXACHLORO-1a,2,2a,3,6,6a,7,7a-OCTAHYDRO-2,7:3,6-DIMETHANO-NAPHTH(2,3-b)OXIRENE ◇ ILLOXOL ◇ INSECTI-CIDE No. 497 ◇ NCI-C00124 ◇ OCTALOX ◇ PANO-RAM D-31 ◇ QUINTOX ◇ RCRA WASTE NUMBER P037

TOXICITY DATA with REFERENCE
CAR: orl-mus TD: 714 mg/kg/85W-C   LAINAW
44,392,81

CAR: orl-mus TD: 4550 mg/kg/65W-C   CNREA8
41,3615,81

CAR: orl-mus TDLo: 546 mg/kg/65W-C
ARTODN Suppl.2,197,79

NEO: orl-mus TD: 11 g/kg/3Y-C   FCTXAV
11,415,73

NEO: orl-mus TD: 610 mg/kg/73W-C   FCTXAV
11,433,73

ETA: orl-mus TD: 8 mg/kg/2Y-C   CRNGDP
3,941,82

ETA: orl-rat TDLo: 200 mg/kg/2Y-C   FCTXAV
2,551,64

MUT: dni-hmn: hla 400 μmol/L   MUREAV
92,427,82

MUT: dns-hmn: fbr 1 μmol/L   MUREAV 42,161,77

MUT: mma-hmn: fbr 1 μmol/L   MUREAV 42,161,77

MUT: mmo-sat 1 mg/L   JOHEA8 68,184,77

MUT: otr-rat-orl 5 mg/kg   CNREA8 40,1157,80

CONSENSUS REPORTS: IARC Cancer Review: GROUP 3 IMEMDT 7,196,87; Human Inadequate Evidence IMEMDT 5,125,74; Animal Sufficient Evidence IMEMDT 5,125,74. NCI Carcinogenesis Bioassay (feed); Clear Evidence: mouse NCITR* NCI-CG-TR-21,78; No Evidence: rat NCITR* NCI-CG-TR-22,78; Inadequate Studies: rat NCITR* NCI-CG-TR-21,78.

OSHA PEL: TWA 0.25 mg/m^3 (skin)   ACGIH TLV: TWA 0.25 mg/m^3 (skin)   DFG MAK: 0.25 mg/m^3 NIOSH REL: Lowest reliable detectable level.   DOT Classification: ORM-A; Label: None.

SAFETY PROFILE: Questionable carcinogen with experimental carcinogenic, neoplastigenic, tumorigenic, and teratogenic data. A human poison by ingestion and possibly other routes. Poison experimentally by inhalation, ingestion, skin contact, intravenous, intraperitoneal and possibly other routes. Experimental reproductive effects. Absorbed readily through the skin and by other routes. It is a central nervous system stimulant. Human mutation data reported. An insecticide. Dieldrin is considerably more toxic than DDT by ingestion and skin contact. Dieldrin or its derivatives may accumulate in the body from chronic low dosages. When heated to decomposition it emits toxic fumes of Cl^-.

DHB550   CAS: 13029-44-2
(E,E)-DIENESTROL
mf: $C_{18}H_{18}O_2$ mw: 266.36

SYNS: α-DIENESTROLPHENOL, 4,4′-(DIETHYLIDENEE-THYLENE)DI-, trans-, (E,E)- ◇ PHENOL, 4,4′-(1,2-DIETHYLI-DENE-1,2-ETHANEDIYL)BIS-, (E,E)-(9CI)

TOXICITY DATA with REFERENCE
ETA: imp-ham TDLo:640 mg/kg/38W-I
CNREA8 43,5200,83
MUT: mnt-ham:emb 10 mg/L   TOLED5
31(Suppl),204,86

SAFETY PROFILE: Questionable carcinogen with experimental tumorigenic data. Mutation data reported. When heated to decomposition it emits acrid smoke and irritating fumes.

DHC000   CAS: 24854-67-9
1,2,9,10-DIEPOXYDECANE
mf: $C_{10}H_{18}O_2$ mw: 170.28

TOXICITY DATA with REFERENCE
ETA: unk-mus TDLo:510 mg/kg   RARSAM
3,193,63

SAFETY PROFILE: Questionable carcinogen with experimental tumorigenic data. When heated to decomposition it emits acrid smoke and irritating fumes.

DHC200   CAS: 63869-17-0
DIEPOXYDIHYDROMYRCENE
mf: $C_{10}H_{18}O_2$ mw: 170.28

SYN: DIEPOXYDIHYDRO-7-METHYL-3-METHYLENE-1,6-OCTADIENE

TOXICITY DATA with REFERENCE
ETA: unk-mus TDLo:5100 mg/kg   RARSAM
3,193,63

SAFETY PROFILE: Questionable carcinogen with experimental tumorigenic data. When

heated to decomposition it emits acrid smoke and irritating fumes.

DHC600   CAS: 4247-19-2
1,2,6,7-DIEPOXYHEPTANE
mf: $C_7H_{12}O_2$ mw: 128.19

TOXICITY DATA with REFERENCE
NEO: skn-mus TD:7560 mg/kg/63W-I
14JTAF -,275,64
NEO: skn-mus TDLo:2400 mg/kg/20W-I
JNCIAM 35,707,65

SAFETY PROFILE: Questionable carcinogen with experimental neoplastigenic data. When heated to decomposition it emits acrid smoke.

DHC800   CAS: 1888-89-7
1,2:5,6-DIEPOXYHEXANE
mf: $C_6H_{10}O_2$ mw: 114.16

TOXICITY DATA with REFERENCE
NEO: scu-mus TDLo:2068 mg/kg/47W-I
JNCIAM 37,825,66
ETA: skn-mus TD:28 g/kg/46W-I   14JTAF-,275,64
ETA: skn-mus TDLo:6960 mg/kg/29W-I
JNCIAM 39,1217,67
ETA: unk-mus TDLo:4600 mg/kg   RARSAM
3,193,63
MUT: mmo-ssp 116 mmol/L   ADWMAX -,193,62

CONSENSUS REPORTS: EPA Genetic Toxicology Program.

SAFETY PROFILE: Questionable carcinogen with experimental neoplastigenic and tumorigenic data. Mutation data reported. When heated to decomposition it emits acrid smoke and irritating fumes.

DHD200   CAS: 6341-85-1
1,2,3,4-DIEPOXY-2-METHYLBUTANE
mf: $C_5H_8O_2$ mw: 100.13

SYN: 2-METHYL-2,2′-BIOXIRANE (9CI)

TOXICITY DATA with REFERENCE
ETA: unk-mus TDLo:800 mg/kg   RARSAM
3,193,63
MUT: mmo-sat 7500 μmol/L   MUREAV 156,77,85

SAFETY PROFILE: Questionable carcinogen with experimental tumorigenic data. Mutation data reported. When heated to decomposition it emits acrid smoke and irritating fumes.

DHD400   CAS: 24829-11-6
1,2:8,9-DIEPOXYNONANE
mf: $C_9H_{16}O_2$ mw: 156.25

TOXICITY DATA with REFERENCE
ETA: unr-mus TDLo: 3750 mg/kg   RARSAM
   3,193,63

SAFETY PROFILE: Questionable carcinogen with experimental tumorigenic data. When heated to decomposition it emits acrid smoke and irritating fumes.

DHD600   CAS: 3012-69-9
9,10:12,13-DIEPOXYOCTADECANOIC ACID
mf: $C_{18}H_{32}O_4$ mw: 312.50

SYN: 9,10:12,13-DIEPOXYSTEARIC ACID

TOXICITY DATA with REFERENCE
ETA: skn-mus TDLo: 3360 mg/kg/28W-I
   JNCIAM 31,41,63

SAFETY PROFILE: Questionable carcinogen with experimental tumorigenic data. When heated to decomposition it emits acrid smoke and irritating fumes.

DHD800   CAS: 2426-07-5
1,2,7,8-DIEPOXYOCTANE
mf: $C_8H_{14}O_2$ mw: 142.22

SYN: 1,2-EPOXY-7,8-EPOXYOCTANE

TOXICITY DATA with REFERENCE
ETA: skn-mus TDLo: 6600 mg/kg/55W-I
   JNCIAM 39,1217,67
MUT: cyt-ham: lng 6 μmol/L   JEPTDQ 2(2),587,79
MUT: mma-sat 990 μg/plate   PNASA6 72,5135,75
MUT: mmo-klp 500 μmol/L   MUREAV 89,269,81
MUT: mmo-nsc 75 mmol/L   CNREA8 32,1890,72
MUT: msc-ham: lng 6 μmol/L   JEPTDQ 2(2),587,79

CONSENSUS REPORTS: EPA Genetic Toxicology Program.

SAFETY PROFILE: Questionable carcinogen with experimental tumorigenic data. Poison by skin contact. Moderately toxic by ingestion. Mutation data reported. A skin irritant. When heated to decomposition it emits acrid and irritating fumes.

DHE000   CAS: 4051-27-8
1,2,4,5-DIEPOXYPENTANE
mf: $C_5H_8O_2$ mw: 100.13

SYNS: 2,2'-METHYLENEBIS OXIRANE (9CI) ◇ 1:4-PEN-TADIENE DIOXIDE

TOXICITY DATA with REFERENCE
CAR: skn-mus TDLo: 70 g/kg/58W-I   JNCIAM
   35,707,65

NEO: skn-mus TD: 76 g/kg/63W-I
   14JTAF -,275,64
MUT: cyt-rat-ipr 2500 mg/kg   BJPCAL 6,235,51
MUT: mmo-nsc 75 mmol/L   CNREA8 32,1890,72

SAFETY PROFILE: Questionable carcinogen with experimental carcinogenic and neoplastigenic data. Mutation data reported. When heated to decomposition it emits acrid smoke and irritating fumes.

DHE485
DIESEL EXHAUST

TOXICITY DATA with REFERENCE
CAR: ihl-rat TC: 7 mg/m^3/7H/2Y-I   FAATDF
   9,208,87
CAR: ihl-rat TCLo: 4900 μg/m^3/8H/2Y-C
   DTESD7 13,349,86

SAFETY PROFILE: Questionable carcinogen with experimental carcinogenic data. When heated to decomposition it emits acrid smoke and irritating fumes.

DHE700
DIESEL EXHAUST PARTICLES

PROP: Particulate samples collected from the exhaust of a 1979 2.3 L diesel powered automobile running on No. 2 diesel fuel   TXAPA9 56,110,80

TOXICITY DATA with REFERENCE
NEO: ihl-rat TCLo: 2200 μg/m^3/16H/2Y-I
   DTESD7 13,471,86
ETA: ihl-rat TC: 7 mg/m^3/7H/2Y-I   ACGHD2
   13,3,85
ETA: ihl-rat TC: 8300 μg/kg/6H/86W-I   AIHAAP
   42,382,81
ETA: ihl-rat TC: 8300 μg/m^3/6H/86W-I
   AIHAAP 42,382,81
MUT: mma-sat 200 μg/plate   TXAPA9 56,110,80
MUT: mmo-sat 200 μg/plate   TXAPA9 56,110,80
MUT: msc-hmn: lyms 100 mg/L   DTESD7 10,277,82
MUT: sce-mus-uns 300 mg/kg   DTESD7 10,265,82

NIOSH REL: TWA reduce to lowest feasible level

SAFETY PROFILE: Questionable carcinogen with experimental neoplastigenic and tumorigenic data. Human mutation data reported. When heated to decomposition it emits acrid smoke and irritating fumes.

DHF200   CAS: 5716-15-4
DIETHANOLAMMONIUM MALEIC HYDRAZIDE
mf: $C_4H_{11}NO_2 \cdot C_4H_4N_2O_2$ mw: 217.26

SYNS: 6-HYDROXY-3-(2H)-PYRIDAZINONE DIETHA-
NOLAMINE ◇ 2,2′-IMINODI-ETHANOL with 1,2-DIHYDRO-
3,6-PYRIDAZINEDIONE (1:1) ◇ MALEIC HYDRAZIDE
DIETHANOLAMINE SALT ◇ MH-30 ◇ NCI-C54660

TOXICITY DATA with REFERENCE
ETA: scu-rat TD:1350 mg/kg/60W-I   NATUAS
180,62,57
ETA: scu-rat TDLo:1300 mg/kg/65W-I
TXCYAC 1,301,73
MUT: cyt-ham:lng 20 g/L   MUREAV 67,249,79
MUT: mma-sat 50 μL/plate   MUREAV 66,247,79

CONSENSUS REPORTS: Reported in EPA
TSCA Inventory.

SAFETY PROFILE: Questionable carcinogen
with experimental tumorigenic data. Moderately
toxic by ingestion. Mutation data reported.
When heated to decomposition it emits toxic
fumes of NO_x and NH_3.

DHI200   CAS: 685-91-6
N,N-DIETHYLACETAMIDE
mf: $C_6H_{13}NO$ mw: 115.20

PROP: Liquid. Mp: <65°, bp: 180°, flash p:
170°F, d: 0.92, vap d: 4.0.

TOXICITY DATA with REFERENCE
ETA: orl-rat TDLo:910 mg/kg/73W-I   JNCIAM
35,949,65

CONSENSUS REPORTS: Reported in EPA
TSCA Inventory.

SAFETY PROFILE: Questionable carcinogen
with experimental tumorigenic data. Moderately
toxic by ingestion, intravenous, and intraperitoneal routes. Flammable when exposed to heat
or flame. To fight fire, use foam, mist, CO_2,
dry chemical. When heated to decomposition
it emits toxic fumes of NO_x.

DHI800   CAS: 63019-57-8
1-DIETHYLACETYLAZIRIDINE
mf: $C_8H_{15}NO$ mw: 141.24

SYN: DIETHYLACETYLETHYLENEIMINE

TOXICITY DATA with REFERENCE
NEO: scu-mus TDLo:488 mg/kg/20W-I
BJPCAL 9,306,54
NEO: scu-rat TD:420 mg/kg/28W-I   BJPCAL
9,306,54
NEO: scu-rat TDLo:400 mg/kg/35W-I   BJPCAL
9,306,54
MUT: cyt-rat-ipr 50 mg/kg   BJPCAL 9,306,54

SAFETY PROFILE: Questionable carcinogen
with experimental neoplastigenic data. Mutation
data reported. When heated to decomposition
it emits toxic fumes of NO_x.

DHM500   CAS: 2869-83-2
3-(DIETHYLAMINO)-7-
((p-(DIMETHYLAMINO)PHENYL)AZO)-5-
PHENYLPHENAZINIUM CHLORIDE
mf: $C_{30}H_{31}N_6$•Cl   mw: 511.12

SYNS: C.I. 11050 ◇ JANUS GREEN B ◇ JANUS
GREEN V

TOXICITY DATA with REFERENCE
ETA: scu-rat TDLo:960 mg/kg/13W-I   GANNA2
44,293,53
MUT: cyt-ham:ovr 20 μmol/L/5H-C   ENMUDM
1,27,79

CONSENSUS REPORTS: Reported in EPA
TSCA Inventory.

SAFETY PROFILE: Questionable carcinogen
with experimental tumorigenic data. Mutation
data reported. When heated to decomposition
it emits toxic fumes of NO_x.

DHS000   CAS: 67-98-1
(p-2-DIETHYLAMINOETHOXYPHENYL)-
1-PHENYL-2-p-ANISYLETHANOL
mf: $C_{27}H_{33}NO_3$ mw: 419.61

SYNS: 1-(p-2-DIETHYLAMINOETHOXYPHENYL)-1-PHE-
NYL-2-p-ANISYLETHANOL ◇ 1-(4-(2-DIETHYLAMINO-
ETHOXY)PHENYL)-1-PHENYL-2-(p-ANISYL)ETHANOL
◇ 1-(p-(2-(DIETHYLAMINO)ETHOXY)PHENYL)-1-PHENYL-
2-(p-METHOXYPHENYL)ETHANOL ◇ ETHAMOXYTRIPHE-
TOL ◇ ETHANOXYTRIPHETOL ◇ MER 25

TOXICITY DATA with REFERENCE
ETA: scu-mus TDLo:30 mg/kg/5D-I   IRLCDZ
4,379,76
ETA: scu-mus TDLo:120 mg/kg (12-15D
preg):TER   IRLCDZ 4,379,76

SAFETY PROFILE: Questionable carcinogen
with experimental tumorigenic and teratogenic
data. Moderately toxic by ingestion. Experimental reproductive effects. When heated to decomposition it emits toxic fumes of NO_x.

DHW600   CAS: 9015-73-0
DIETHYLAMINOETHYL-DEXTRAN

SYNS: DEAE-D ◇ DIETHYLAMINOETHYLDEXTRAN
POLYMER

TOXICITY DATA with REFERENCE
NEO: scu-mus TDLo:1200 mg/kg/30W-I
    JNCIAM 50,387,73

SAFETY PROFILE: Questionable carcinogen with experimental neoplastigenic data. When heated to decomposition it emits toxic fumes of NO_x.

DIP000   CAS: 7347-49-1
4-((4-(DIETHYLAMINO)PHENYL)AZO) PYRIDINE-1-OXIDE
mf: $C_{15}H_{18}N_4O$ mw: 270.37

SYN: N,N-DIETHYL-4-(4′-(PYRIDYL-1′-OXIDE)AZO)ANILINE

TOXICITY DATA with REFERENCE
NEO: orl-rat TDLo:6426 mg/kg/52W-C
    JNCIAM 37,365,66

SAFETY PROFILE: Questionable carcinogen with experimental neoplastigenic data. When heated to decomposition it emits toxic fumes of NO_x.

DIT400   CAS: 36911-94-1
6,8-DIETHYLBENZ(a)ANTHRACENE
mf: $C_{22}H_{20}$ mw: 284.42

TOXICITY DATA with REFERENCE
ETA: ims-rat TDLo:50 mg/kg   JMCMAR 15,905,72

SAFETY PROFILE: Questionable carcinogen with experimental tumorigenic data. When heated to decomposition it emits acrid smoke and irritating fumes.

DIT600   CAS: 36911-95-2
8,12-DIETHYLBENZ(a)ANTHRACENE
mf: $C_{22}H_{20}$ mw: 284.42

TOXICITY DATA with REFERENCE
ETA: ims-rat TDLo:50 mg/kg   JMCMAR 15,905,72

SAFETY PROFILE: Questionable carcinogen with experimental tumorigenic data. When heated to decomposition it emits acrid smoke and irritating fumes.

DIT800   CAS: 16354-52-2
9,10-DIETHYL-1,2-BENZANTHRACENE
mf: $C_{22}H_{20}$ mw: 284.42

SYN: 7,12-DIETHYLBENZ(a)ANTHRACENE

TOXICITY DATA with REFERENCE
ETA: skn-mus TDLo:380 mg/kg/16W-I
    PRLBA4 129,439,40

SAFETY PROFILE: Questionable carcinogen with experimental tumorigenic data. When heated to decomposition it emits acrid smoke and irritating fumes.

DIX200   CAS: 105-58-8
DIETHYL CARBONATE
DOT: 2366
mf: $C_5H_{10}O_3$ mw: 118.15

PROP: Colorless liquid, mild odor. Mp: 43°, bp: 125.8°, flash p: 77°F (OC), d: 0.975 @ 20°/4°, vap press: 10 mm @ 23.8°, vap d: 4.07.

SYNS: DEC ◇ DIAETHYLCARBONAT (GERMAN) ◇ DIETHYL CARBONATE (DOT) ◇ ETHOXYFORMIC ANHYDRIDE ◇ ETHYL CARBONATE ◇ EUFIN ◇ NCI-C60899

TOXICITY DATA with REFERENCE
ETA: ipr-mus TDLo:456 mg/kg   BCPCA62,168,59
ETA: orl-mus TDLo:500 mg/kg   BCPCA62,168,59

CONSENSUS REPORTS: Reported in EPA TSCA Inventory.

DOT Classification: IMO: Flammable or Combustible Liquid; Label: Flammable Liquid.

SAFETY PROFILE: Questionable carcinogen with experimental tumorigenic and teratogenic data. Mildly toxic by subcutaneous route. A dangerous fire hazard when exposed to heat or flame; can react with oxidizing materials. To fight fire, use foam, CO_2, dry chemical. When heated to decomposition it emits acrid smoke and fumes.

DJB200   CAS: 7773-34-4
α,α′-DIETHYL-4,4′-DIMETHOXYSTILBENE
mf: $C_{20}H_{24}O_2$ mw: 296.44

SYNS: 3,4-BIS(p-METHOXYPHENYL)-3-HEXENE ◇ DEPOT-OESTROMENINE ◇ DEPOT-OESTROMON ◇ trans-α,α′-DIETHYL-4,4′-DIMETHOXYSTILBENE ◇ 3,4-DIANISYL-3-HEXENE ◇ (E)-1,1′-(1,2-DIETHYL-1,2-ETHENE-DIYL)BIS(4-METHOXYBENZENE) ◇ DIETHYLSTILBESTROL DIMETHYL ETHER ◇ DIMESTROL ◇ 4,4′-DIMETHOXY-α,β-DIETHYLSTILBENE ◇ STILBESTROL DIMETHYL ETHER ◇ SYNTHILA

TOXICITY DATA with REFERENCE
ETA: scu-ham TDLo:560 g/kg/35W-I   CNREA8
    31,1251,71

SAFETY PROFILE: Questionable carcinogen with experimental tumorigenic data. When

heated to decomposition it emits acrid and irritating fumes.

DJB400　CAS: 17010-64-9
3',4'-DIETHYL-4-DIMETHYLAMINOAZOBENZENE
mf: $C_{18}H_{23}N_3$　mw: 281.44

SYNS: BENZENAMINE, 4-((3,4-DIETHYLPHENYL)AZO)-N,N-DIMETHYL-(9CI) ◇ p-((3,4-DIETHYLPHENYL)AZO)-N,N-DIMETHYLANILINE ◇ N,N-DIMETHYL-p-((3,4-DIETHYLPHENYL)AZO)ANILINE ◇ 3',4'-Et2-DAB

TOXICITY DATA with REFERENCE
CAR: orl-rat TDLo: 8467 mg/kg/36W-C
　CBINA8 53,107,85
ETA: orl-rat TD: 2511 mg/kg/17W-I　CNREA8 30,1520,70

SAFETY PROFILE: Questionable carcinogen with experimental carcinogenic and tumorigenic data. When heated to decomposition it emits toxic fumes of NO_x.

DJB800　CAS: 7346-14-7
N,N'-DIETHYL-N,N'-DINITROSOETHYLENEDIAMINE
mf: $C_6H_{14}N_4O_2$　mw: 174.24

SYNS: N,N'-DINITROSO-N,N'-DIETHYLETHYLENEDIAMINE ◇ NSC 62579

TOXICITY DATA with REFERENCE
CAR: orl-rat TD: 34 mg/kg/50W-I　JNCIAM 41,985,68
CAR: orl-rat TDLo: 12 mg/kg/1Y-I　JNCIAM 41,985,68

SAFETY PROFILE: Questionable carcinogen with experimental carcinogenic data. When heated to decomposition it emits toxic fumes of NO_x.

DJC000　CAS: 72-56-0
DIETHYLDIPHENYL DICHLOROETHANE
mf: $C_{18}H_{20}Cl_2$　mw: 307.28

SYNS: 1,1-BIS(p-ETHYLPHENYL)-2,2-DICHLOROETHANE ◇ 2,2-BIS(p-ETHYLPHENYL)-1,1-DICHLOROETHANE ◇ 1,1-DICHLORO-2,2-BIS(p-ETHYLPHENYL)ETHANE ◇ 1,1-DICHLORO-2,2-BIS(4-ETHYLPHENYL)ETHANE ◇ 2,2-DICHLORO-1,1-BIS(p-ETHYLPHENYL)ETHANE ◇ α,α-DICHLORO-2,2-BIS(p-ETHYLPHENYL)ETHANE ◇ DI(p-ETHYLPHENYL)DICHLOROETHANE ◇ ETHYLAN ◇ p,p-ETHYL DDD ◇ p,p'-ETHYL-DDD ◇ NCI-C02868 ◇ PERTHANE ◇ Q-137

TOXICITY DATA with REFERENCE
CAR: orl-mus TDLo: 210 g/kg/2Y-C　TUMOAB 66,277,80

ETA: orl-mus TD: 547 g/kg/2Y-C
　NCITR* NCI-CG-TR-156,79
MUT: mma-sat 333 μg/plate　NTPTB* APR 82

NCI Carcinogenesis Bioassay (feed); Clear Evidence: mouse NCITR* NCI-CG-TR-156,79; No Evidence: rat NCITR* NCI-CG-TR-156,79.

SAFETY PROFILE: Questionable carcinogen with experimental carcinogenic, tumorigenic, and teratogenic data. Poison by intravenous route. Mildly toxic by ingestion. Experimental reproductive effects. Mutation data reported. A pesticide. When heated to decomposition it emits toxic fumes of Cl^-.

DJD600　CAS: 111-46-6
DIETHYLENE GLYCOL
mf: $C_4H_{10}O_3$　mw: 106.14

PROP: Clear, colorless, practically odorless, syrupy liquid. Bp: 245.8°, fp: −8°, flash p: 255°F, d: 1.1184 @ 20°/20°, autoign temp: 444°F, vap press: 1 mm @ 91.8°, vap d: 3.66.

SYNS: BIS(2-HYDROXYETHYL) ETHER ◇ BRECOLANE NDG ◇ CARBITOL ◇ DEACTIVATOR E ◇ DEACTIVATOR H ◇ DEG ◇ DICOL ◇ DIGLYCOL ◇ DIHYDROXYDIETHYL ETHER ◇ β,β'-DIHYDROXYDIETHYL ETHER ◇ 2,2'-DIHYDROXYETHYL ETHER ◇ DISSOLVANT APV ◇ ETHYLENE DIGLYCOL ◇ GLYCOL ETHER ◇ GLYCOL ETHYL ETHER ◇ 3-OXAPENTANE-1,5-DIOL ◇ 3-OXA-1,5-PENTANEDIOL ◇ 2,2'-OXYBISETHANOL ◇ 2,2'-OXYDIETHANOL ◇ TL4N

TOXICITY DATA with REFERENCE
CAR: orl-rat TDLo: 890 g/kg/53W-C　JIHTAB 28,40,46
ETA: orl-rat TD: 584 g/kg/2Y-C　FEPRA7 4,149,45
ETA: orl-rat TD: 1752 g/kg/2Y-C　IMSUAI 36,55,67

CONSENSUS REPORTS: Reported in EPA TSCA Inventory. Glycol ether compounds are on the Community Right-To-Know List.

SAFETY PROFILE: Questionable carcinogen with experimental carcinogenic, tumorigenic, and teratogenic data. Moderately toxic to humans by ingestion. Poison by experimentally inhalation; moderately toxic by ingestion and intravenous routes. An eye and human skin irritant. Combustible when exposed to heat or flame; can react with oxidizing materials. To fight fire, use alcohol foam, water, CO_2, dry chemical. When heated to decomposition it emits acrid smoke and irritating fumes.

DJD700   CAS: 13988-26-6
DIETHYLENE GLYCOL BISPHTHALATE
mf: $C_{12}H_{12}O_5$ mw: 236.24

SYNS: 2,5,8-BENZOTRIOXACYCLOUNDECIN-1,9-DIONE,
3,4,6,7-TETRAHYDRO-(9CI) ◇ HOWFLEX GBP

TOXICITY DATA with REFERENCE
ETA: orl-rat TDLo:45 g/kg/13W-C   EJCAAH
5,415,69

CONSENSUS REPORTS: Reported in EPA
TSCA Inventory.

SAFETY PROFILE: Questionable carcinogen
with experimental tumorigenic data. When
heated to decomposition it emits acrid smoke
and irritating fumes.

DJH200   CAS: 7316-37-2
**DIETHYL-β,γ-
EPOXYPROPYLPHOSPHONATE**
mf: $C_7H_{15}O_4P$ mw: 194.19

TOXICITY DATA with REFERENCE
NEO: scu-mus TDLo:13 g/kg/63W-I   JNCIAM
53,695,74
ETA: ipr-mus TDLo:13 g/kg/64W-I   JNCIAM
53,695,74

SAFETY PROFILE: Questionable carcinogen
with experimental neoplastigenic and tumorigenic data. When heated to decomposition it
emits toxic fumes of PO_x.

DJL600   CAS: 7699-31-2
**1,2-DIETHYLHYDRAZINE
DIHYDROCHLORIDE**
mf: $C_4H_{12}N_2 \cdot 2ClH$ mw: 161.10

TOXICITY DATA with REFERENCE
ETA: ivn-rat TDLo:50 mg/kg (15D preg)
EXPEAM 24,561,68

SAFETY PROFILE: Questionable carcinogen
with experimental tumorigenic and teratogenic
data. When heated to decomposition it emits
very toxic fumes of HCl and NO_x.

DJP600   CAS: 50285-72-8
**1,1-DIETHYL-3-METHYL-3-
NITROSOUREA**
mf: $C_6H_{13}N_3O_2$ mw: 159.22

SYNS: NITROSO-1,1-DIETHYL-3-METHYLUREA
◇ NITROSOMETHYLDIAETHYLHARNSTOFF ◇ NITROSO-
METHYLDIETHYLUREA ◇ 1-NITROSO-1-METHYL-3,3-DI-
ETHYLUREA

TOXICITY DATA with REFERENCE
CAR: scu-ham TD:623 mg/kg/22W-I   CALEDQ
23,177,84
ETA: orl-gpg TDLo:1200 mg/kg/32W-I
CNREA8 40,1879,80
ETA: orl-ham TD:1592 mg/kg/29W-I   IAPUDO
57,617,84
ETA: orl-ham TD:1592 mg/kg/W-I   PAACA3
24,92,83
ETA: orl-ham TDLo:1592 mg/kg/W-I   PAACA3
24,92,83
ETA: orl-rat TD:1911 mg/kg/32W-I   IAPUDO
57,617,84
ETA: orl-rat TD:2475 mg/kg/33W-C   JJIND8
65,451,80
ETA: orl-rat TDLo:1400 mg/kg/50W-I
ZKKOBW 83,315,75
ETA: scu-ham TDLo:585 mg/kg/24W-I
EXPADD 20,153,81
MUT: mma-sat 250 μg/plate   JJIND8 67,1117,81
MUT: sce-ham:lng 500 μmol/L   MUREAV
126,259,84

SAFETY PROFILE: Questionable carcinogen
with experimental carcinogenic and tumorigenic
data. Poison by subcutaneous route. Mutation
data reported. When heated to decomposition
it emits toxic fumes of NO_x.

DJS500   CAS: 7119-92-8
DIETHYLNITRAMINE
mf: $C_4H_{10}N_2O_2$ mw: 118.16

SYNS: N-ETHYL-N-NITROETHANAMINE (9CI) ◇ N-NI-
TRODIETHYLAMINE

TOXICITY DATA with REFERENCE
ETA: orl-rat TDLo:18200 mg/kg/2Y-C
ARGEAR 52,629,82
MUT: hma-rat/sat 200 mg/kg   CNREA8 41,3205,81
MUT: mmo-esc 20 μmol/plate   IAPUDO 57,485,84

SAFETY PROFILE: Questionable carcinogen
with experimental tumorigenic data. Moderately
toxic by intraperitoneal route. Mutation data
reported. When heated to decomposition it emits
toxic fumes of NO_x.

DJY000   CAS: 21600-43-1
3,3-DIETHYL-1-(m-PYRIDYL)TRIAZENE
mf: $C_9H_{14}N_4$ mw: 178.27

SYNS: PYDT ◇ 1-(PYRIDYL-3-)-3,3-DIAETHYL-TRIAZEN
(GERMAN) ◇ 1-PYRIDYL-3,3-DIETHYLTRIAZENE
◇ 1-(PYRIDYL-3)-3,3-DIETHYLTRIAZENE ◇ m-PYRIDYL-DI-
ETHYL-TRIAZENE ◇ 1-(3-PYRIDYL)-3,3-DIETHYLTRIA-
ZENE

TOXICITY DATA with REFERENCE
CAR: ivn-rat TDLo: 55 mg/kg (15D preg): TER
IARCCD 4,45,73
NEO: scu-rat TDLo: 500 mg/kg/50W-I
ZKKOBW 81,285,74
ETA: orl-rat TDLo: 660 mg/kg/73W-I   ZKKOBW
77,217,72
ETA: scu-rat TD: 50 mg/kg   ZKKOBW 81,285,74
MUT: cyt-ham: lng 10 mg/L   MUREAV 88,197,81
MUT: cyt-hmn: leu 25 μmol/L   MUREAV 21,123,73
MUT: hma-mus/smc 1600 μmol/kg   MUREAV
21,123,73
MUT: mrc-smc 21 mmol/L   MUREAV 21,123,73
MUT: sln-dmg-orl 2 mmol/L/3D-I   ARTODN
43,201,80

SAFETY PROFILE: Questionable carcinogen
with experimental carcinogenic, neoplastigenic,
tumorigenic, and teratogenic data. Poison by
ingestion and subcutaneous routes. Human mutation data reported. A transplacental carcinogen. When heated to decomposition it emits
toxic fumes of NO_x.

DJY050
DIETHYL PYROCARBONATE mixed with AMMONIA
mf: $C_6H_{10}O_5 \cdot 2H_3N$ mw: 196.24

SYN: DEPC and AMMONIA

TOXICITY DATA with REFERENCE
ETA: orl-mus TDLo: 1936 mg/kg/4W-I   JCREA8
97,205,80

SAFETY PROFILE: Questionable carcinogen
with experimental tumorigenic data. When
heated to decomposition it emits toxic fumes
of ammonia.

DKA000   CAS: 40193-47-3
N,N-DIETHYL-4-STILBENAMINE
mf: $C_{18}H_{21}N$ mw: 251.40

SYNS: DIETHYLAMINO STILBENE ◊ 4-STILBENYL-N,N-
DIETHYLAMINE

TOXICITY DATA with REFERENCE
NEO: scu-rat TDLo: 160 mg/kg/9W-I   XPHPAW
149,328,57
ETA: scu-rat TD: 180 mg/kg/8W-I   PTRMAD
241,147,48

SAFETY PROFILE: Questionable carcinogen
with experimental neoplastigenic and tumorigenic data. When heated to decomposition it
emits toxic fumes of NO_x.

DKA400   CAS: 63528-82-5
α,α'-DIETHYL-4,4'-STILBENEDIOL DISODIUM SALT
mf: $C_{18}H_{18}O_2 \cdot 2Na$ mw: 312.34

SYNS: DES DISODIUM SALT ◊ DIETHYLSTILBESTROL
DISODIUM SALT

TOXICITY DATA with REFERENCE
NEO: scu-mus TDLo: 10 mg/kg/(15D preg):
TER   CNREA8 37,1099,77

SAFETY PROFILE: Questionable carcinogen
with experimental neoplastigenic and teratogenic data. Other experimental reproductive effects. When heated to decomposition it emits
toxic fumes of Na_2O.

DKA800   CAS: 63019-08-9
DIETHYLSTILBESTROL DIPALMITATE
mf: $C_{50}H_{80}O_4$ mw: 745.30

SYNS: α,α'-DIETHYL-4,4'-STILBENEDIOL DIPALMITATE
◊ 4,4'-DIHYDROXY-α,β-DIETHYLSTILBENE PALMITATE

TOXICITY DATA with REFERENCE
ETA: ims-rbt TDLo: 38 mg/kg/45W-I: TER
CANCAR 10,500,57

SAFETY PROFILE: Questionable carcinogen
with experimental tumorigenic and teratogenic
data. Other experimental reproductive effects.
When heated to decomposition it emits acrid
smoke and irritating fumes.

DKB100   CAS: 6052-82-0
DIETHYLSTILBOESTROL-3,4-OXIDE
mf: $C_{18}H_{20}O_3$ mw: 284.38

SYNS: DES-α,β-OXIDE ◊ DES-3,4-OXIDE ◊ α,α'-DI-
ETHYL-α,α'-EPOXYBIBENZYL-4,4'-DIOL ◊ DIETHYLSTIL-
BOESTROL-α,β-OXIDE

TOXICITY DATA with REFERENCE
ETA: imp-ham TDLo: 640 mg/kg/38W-I
CNREA8 43,5200,83
MUT: dnd-hmn: leu 300 μmol/L   BCPCA6
34,3251,85
MUT: sce-hmn: fbr 40 nmol/L   NATUAS 281,392,79

SAFETY PROFILE: Questionable carcinogen
with experimental tumorigenic data. Human
mutation data reported. When heated to decomposition it emits acrid smoke and fumes.

DKC400   CAS: 105-55-5
1,3-DIETHYLTHIOUREA
mf: $C_5H_{12}N_2S$ mw: 132.25

SYNS: N,N'-DIETHYLTHIOCARBAMIDE ◇ N,N'-DI-
ETHYLTHIOUREA ◇ 1,3-DIETHYL-2-THIOUREA ◇ NCI-
C03816 ◇ PENNZONE E ◇ THIATE H ◇ U 15030 ◇ USAF
EK-1803

TOXICITY DATA with REFERENCE
CAR: orl-rat TDLo: 11 g/kg/2Y-C
　　NCITR* NCI-CG-TR-149,79

CONSENSUS REPORTS: NCI Carcinogenesis Bioassay (feed); Clear Evidence: rat
NCITR* NCI-CG-TR-149,79; No Evidence:
mouse NCITR* NCI-CG-TR-149,79. Reported
in EPA TSCA Inventory. EPA Genetic Toxicology Program.

SAFETY PROFILE: Questionable carcinogen
with experimental carcinogenic data. Poison by
ingestion. Moderately toxic by intraperitoneal
route. When heated to decomposition it emits
very toxic fumes of NO_x and SO_x.

DKD200   CAS: 63980-20-1
DIETHYL TRIAZENE
mf: $C_4H_{11}N_3$ mw: 101.18

TOXICITY DATA with REFERENCE
CAR: orl-rat TDLo: 400 mg/kg/20W-I   CALEDQ
　　35,129,87
ETA: scu-rat TDLo: 110 mg/kg (15D post)
　　XENOBH 3,271,73

SAFETY PROFILE: Questionable carcinogen
with experimental carcinogenic and tumorigenic
data. An experimental teratogen. When heated
to decomposition it emits toxic fumes of NO_x.

DKG400   CAS: 61735-78-2
**2,10-
DIFLUOROBENZO(rst)PENTAPHENE**
mf: $C_{24}H_{12}F_2$ mw: 338.36

SYN: 2,10-DIFLUORODIBENZO(a,i)PYRENE

TOXICITY DATA with REFERENCE
ETA: scu-mus TDLo: 20 mg/kg   PAACA3 13,37,72
MUT: mma-sat 12500 pmol/plate   CNREA8
　　41,2589,81

SAFETY PROFILE: Questionable carcinogen
with experimental tumorigenic data. Mutation
data reported. When heated to decomposition
it emits toxic fumes of F^-.

DKG980   CAS: 351-63-3
**2',4'-DIFLUORO-4-
DIMETHYLAMINOAZOBENZENE**
mf: $C_{14}H_{13}F_2N_3$ mw: 261.30

TOXICITY DATA with REFERENCE
ETA: orl-rat TD: 3400 mg/kg/12W-C   CNREA8
　　13,93,53
ETA: orl-rat TDLo: 2727 mg/kg/14W-I   CNREA8
　　18,469,58

SAFETY PROFILE: Questionable carcinogen
with experimental tumorigenic data. When
heated to decomposition it emits toxic fumes
of F^- and NO_x.

DKH000   CAS: 349-37-1
**2',5'-DIFLUORO-4-
DIMETHYLAMINOAZOBENZENE**
mf: $C_{14}H_{13}F_2N_3$ mw: 261.30

SYN: N,N-DIMETHYL-p-(2,5-DIFLUOROPHENYLAZO)ANI-
LINE

TOXICITY DATA with REFERENCE
ETA: orl-rat TDLo: 3400 mg/kg/12W-C
　　CNREA8 13,93,53

SAFETY PROFILE: Questionable carcinogen
with experimental tumorigenic data. When
heated to decomposition it emits very toxic
fumes of F^- and NO_x.

DKH100   CAS: 350-87-8
**3',5'-DIFLUORO-4-
DIMETHYLAMINOAZOBENZENE**
mf: $C_{14}H_{13}F_2N_3$ mw: 261.30

SYNS: ANILINE, N,N-DIMETHYL-p-(3,5-DIFLUOROPHE-
NYLAZO)- ◇ p-((3,5-DIFLUOROPHENYL)AZO)-N,N-DI-
METHYLANILINE ◇ N,N-DIMETHYL-p-(3,5-DIFLUOROPHE-
NYLAZO)ANILINE

TOXICITY DATA with REFERENCE
ETA: orl-rat TDLo: 3400 mg/kg/12W-C
　　CNREA8 13,93,53

SAFETY PROFILE: Questionable carcinogen
with experimental tumorigenic data. When
heated to decomposition it emits toxic fumes
of F^- and NO_x.

DKJ200   CAS: 314-04-5
3,8-DIFLUOROTRICYCLOQUINAZOLINE
mf: $C_{21}H_{10}F_2N_4$ mw: 356.35

TOXICITY DATA with REFERENCE
NEO: skn-mus TDLo: 1200 mg/kg/50W-I
　　BCPCA6 14,323,65

SAFETY PROFILE: Questionable carcinogen
with experimental neoplastigenic data. When

heated to decomposition it emits very toxic fumes of F^- and NO_x.

DKJ600 CAS: 628-36-4
1,2-DIFORMYLHYDRAZINE
mf: $C_2H_4N_2O_2$ mw: 88.08

SYNS: 1,2-DIFORMYLHYDRAZIN (GERMAN) ◇ HYDRA-ZODIFORMIC ACID

TOXICITY DATA with REFERENCE
CAR: orl-mus TDLo: 5800 mg/kg/66W-C

ZKKOBW 92,11,78

CONSENSUS REPORTS: Reported in EPA TSCA Inventory.

SAFETY PROFILE: Questionable carcinogen with experimental carcinogenic data. When heated to decomposition it emits toxic fumes of NO_x.

DKM130 CAS: 15336-81-9
N,N'-DIGLYCIDYL-5,5-DIMETHYLHYDANTOIN
mf: $C_{11}H_{16}N_2O_4$ mw: 240.29

SYNS: 1,3-BIS(2,3-EPOXYPROPYL)-5,5-DIMETHYLHY-DANTOIN ◇ 5,5-DIMETHYL-1,3-BIS(OXIRANYLMETHYL)-2,4-IMIDAZOLIDINEDIONE ◇ 5,5-DIMETHYL-1,3-BIS(OXI-RANYLMETHYL)-2,4-IMIDAZOLIDINEDIONE (9CI)
◇ XB 2793

TOXICITY DATA with REFERENCE
ETA: skn-mus TD: 12 g/kg/77W-I NTIS**ORNL-5762
ETA: skn-mus TD: 13 g/kg/85W-I NTIS**ORNL-5762
ETA: skn-mus TD: 3792 mg/kg/2Y-I
  NTIS** ORNL-5762
ETA: skn-mus TD: 5263 mg/kg/84W-I
  NTIS** ORNL-5762
ETA: skn-mus TD: 6903 mg/kg/92W-I
  NTIS** ORNL-5762
ETA: skn-mus TDLo: 3513 mg/kg/93W-I
  NTIS** ORNL-5762

CONSENSUS REPORTS: Reported in EPA TSCA Inventory.

SAFETY PROFILE: Questionable carcinogen with experimental tumorigenic data by skin contact. When heated to decomposition it emits toxic fumes of NO_x.

DKM400 CAS: 63041-01-0
DIGLYCIDYL ETHER of N,N-BIS(2-HYDROXYPROPYL)-tert-BUTYLAMINE
mf: $C_{16}H_{31}NO_4$ mw: 301.48

SYN: 2,2'-BIS(2,3-EPOXYPROPOXY)-N-tert-BUTYLDIPRO-PYLAMINE

TOXICITY DATA with REFERENCE
ETA: scu-mus TDLo: 3600 mg/kg/9W-I
  FCTXAV 4,365,66

SAFETY PROFILE: Questionable carcinogen with experimental tumorigenic data. When heated to decomposition it emits toxic fumes of NO_x.

DKM800 CAS: 63040-98-2
N,N-DIGLYCIDYL-p-TOLUENESULPHONAMIDE
mf: $C_{13}H_{17}NO_4S$ mw: 283.37

SYNS: N,N-BIS(2,3-EPOXYPROPYL)-p-TOLUENESUL-FONAMIDE ◇ N,N-DIGLYCIDYL-p-TOLUENESULFON-AMIDE

TOXICITY DATA with REFERENCE
ETA: scu-mus TDLo: 17 g/kg/43W-I FCTXAV 4,365,66

SAFETY PROFILE: Questionable carcinogen with experimental tumorigenic data. When heated to decomposition it emits very toxic fumes of NO_x and SO_x.

DKS400 CAS: 60968-08-3
1,2-DIHYDROBENZO(a)ANTHRACENE
mf: $C_{18}H_{14}$ mw: 230.32

SYN: 1,2-DIHYDROBENZ(a)ANTHRACENE

TOXICITY DATA with REFERENCE
NEO: skn-mus TDLo: 18 mg/kg CNREA8 38,1705,78

SAFETY PROFILE: Questionable carcinogen with experimental neoplastigenic data by skin contact. When heated to decomposition it emits acrid smoke and irritating fumes.

DKS600 CAS: 60968-01-6
3,4-DIHYDROBENZO(a)ANTHRACENE
mf: $C_{18}H_{14}$ mw: 230.32

SYN: 3,4-DIHYDROBENZ(a)ANTHRACENE

TOXICITY DATA with REFERENCE
NEO: skn-mus TDLo: 3700 µg/kg CNREA8 38,1705,78

SAFETY PROFILE: Questionable carcinogen with experimental neoplastigenic data by skin contact. When heated to decomposition it emits acrid smoke and irritating fumes.

DKS800   CAS: 10023-25-3
**6,13-DIHYDROBENZO(e)
(1)BENZOTHIOPYRANO(4,3-b)INDOLE**
mf: $C_{19}H_{13}NS$ mw: 287.39

TOXICITY DATA with REFERENCE
NEO: scu-mus TD: 270 mg/kg/20W-I   JNCIAM
46,1257,71
NEO: scu-mus TDLo: 72 mg/kg/9W-I   MUREAV
66,307,79
MUT: mma-sat 100 μg/plate   MUREAV 66,307,79

SAFETY PROFILE: Questionable carcinogen
with experimental neoplastigenic data. Mutation
data reported. When heated to decomposition
it emits very toxic fumes of SO_x and NO_x.

DKT400   CAS: 100466-04-4
2,3-DIHYDRO-1H-BENZO(h,i)CHRYSENE
mf: $C_{21}H_{16}$ mw: 268.37

SYNS: 5 : 10-TRIMETHYLENE-1 : 2-BENZANTHRACENE
◇ 1 : 12-TRIMETHYLENECHRYSENE

TOXICITY DATA with REFERENCE
ETA: scu-mus TDLo: 240 mg/kg/20D-I
AKBNAE 62(2),30,41
ETA: skn-mus TDLo: 3000 mg/kg/43W-I
AKBNAE 62(2),30,41

SAFETY PROFILE: Questionable carcinogen
with experimental tumorigenic data. When
heated to decomposition it emits acrid smoke
and fumes.

DKU000   CAS: 17573-23-8
7,8-DIHYDROBENZO(a)PYRENE
mf: $C_{20}H_{14}$ mw: 254.34

TOXICITY DATA with REFERENCE
NEO: scu-mus TDLo: 9 mg/kg   JJIND8 64,617,80
MUT: mma-sat 10 μg/plate   PNASA6 72,5135,75

CONSENSUS REPORTS: EPA Genetic Toxicology Program.

SAFETY PROFILE: Questionable carcinogen
with experimental neoplastigenic data. Mutation
data reported. When heated to decomposition
it emits acrid smoke and irritating fumes.

DKU400   CAS: 66788-01-0
9,10-DIHYDROBENZO(e)PYRENE
mf: $C_{20}H_{14}$ mw: 254.34

SYN: 9,10-H2 B(e)P

TOXICITY DATA with REFERENCE
NEO: skn-mus TDLo: 25 mg/kg   CNREA8
40,203,80

ETA: scu-mus TDLo: 9 mg/kg   JJIND8 64,617,80
MUT: mma-sat 10 nmol/plate   JBCHA3 254,4408,79
MUT: mmo-sat nmol/plate   CNREA8 40,1985,80

SAFETY PROFILE: Questionable carcinogen
with experimental neoplastigenic and tumorigenic data. Mutation data reported. When heated
to decomposition it emits acrid smoke and irritating fumes.

DKV800   CAS: 63041-49-6
meso-DIHYDROCHOLANTHRENE
mf: $C_{20}H_{16}$ mw: 256.36

SYN: 6,12,b-DIHYDROCHOLANTHRENE

TOXICITY DATA with REFERENCE
ETA: scu-mus TD: 100 mg/kg   CNREA8 1,685,41
ETA: scu-mus TDLo: 40 mg/kg   CNREA8 1,695,41

SAFETY PROFILE: Questionable carcinogen
with experimental tumorigenic data. A cho-
linergic agent. When heated to decomposition
it emits acrid smoke and irritating fumes.

DKW000   CAS: 360-68-9
DIHYDROCHOLESTEROL
mf: $C_{27}H_{48}O$ mw: 388.75

SYNS: (3-β,5-β)-CHOLESTAN-3-OL ◇ 3-β-CHOLESTANOL
◇ COPROSTANOL ◇ COPROSTAN-3-β-OL ◇ COPROSTEROL
◇ 3-β-HYDROXYCHOLESTANE ◇ KOPROSTERIN (GER-
MAN) ◇ STERCORIN ◇ XYMOSTANOL

TOXICITY DATA with REFERENCE
NEO: scu-mus TDLo: 800 mg/kg/4W-I
NATWAY 60,525,73

SAFETY PROFILE: Questionable carcinogen
with experimental neoplastigenic data. When
heated to decomposition it emits acrid smoke
and irritating fumes.

DKW200   CAS: 41593-31-1
1,2-DIHYDROCHRYSENE
mf: $C_{18}H_{14}$ mw: 230.32

SYN: DIHYDROCHRYSENE

TOXICITY DATA with REFERENCE
CAR: ipr-mus TDLo: 59 mg/kg/15D-I   CNREA8
39,5063,79

SAFETY PROFILE: Questionable carcinogen
with experimental carcinogenic data. When
heated to decomposition it emits acrid smoke
and irritating fumes.

DKW400   CAS: 71435-43-3
3,4-DIHYDROCHRYSENE
mf: $C_{18}H_{14}$ mw: 230.32

TOXICITY DATA with REFERENCE
ETA: ipr-mus TDLo:59 mg/kg/15D-I   CNREA8
  39,5063,79

SAFETY PROFILE: Questionable carcinogen with experimental tumorigenic data. When heated to decomposition it emits acrid smoke and irritating fumes.

DKX875   CAS: 74339-98-3
trans-1,2-DIHYDRODIBENZ(a,e) ACEANTHRYLENE-1,2-DIOL
mf: $C_{24}H_{16}O_2$ mw: 336.40

SYN: trans-12,13-DIHYDRO-12,13-DIHYDROXYDI-BENZO(a,e)FLUORANTHENE

TOXICITY DATA with REFERENCE
ETA: skn-mus TDLo:1200 µg/kg   CRNGDP
  8,461,87

SAFETY PROFILE: Questionable carcinogen with experimental tumorigenic data. When heated to decomposition it emits acrid smoke and irritating fumes.

DKX900   CAS: 74340-04-8
trans-10,11-DIHYDRODIBENZ(a,e) ACEANTHRYLENE-10,11-DIOL
mf: $C_{24}H_{16}O_2$ mw: 336.40

SYN: trans-3,4-DIHYDRO-3,4-DIHYDROXYDI-BENZO(a,e)FLUORANTHENE

TOXICITY DATA with REFERENCE
ETA: skn-mus TDLo:1200 µg/kg   CRNGDP
  8,461,87
MUT: dnd-man:lyms 208 nmol   CRNGDP 4,27,83
MUT: mma-sat 1200 nmol/L   CRNGDP 5,1263,84

SAFETY PROFILE: Questionable carcinogen with experimental tumorigenic data. Mutation data reported. When heated to decomposition it emits acrid smoke and irritating fumes.

DKY000   CAS: 153-34-4
5,6-DIHYDRODIBENZ(a,h)ANTHRACENE
mf: $C_{22}H_{16}$ mw: 280.38

TOXICITY DATA with REFERENCE
NEO: skn-mus TDLo:130 mg/kg/44W-I
  JNCIAM 34,1,65
ETA: scu-mus TDLo:16 mg/kg   JNCIAM 44,641,70
MUT: mma-sat 1 µg/plate   MUREAV 51,311,78

SAFETY PROFILE: Questionable carcinogen with experimental neoplastigenic and tumorigenic data. Mutation data reported. When heated

to decomposition it emits acrid smoke and irritating fumes.

DKY200   CAS: 16361-01-6
5,6-DIHYDRODIBENZ(a,j)ANTHRACENE
mf: $C_{22}H_{16}$ mw: 280.38

TOXICITY DATA with REFERENCE
ETA: skn-mus TDLo:268 mg/kg/85W-I
  JNCIAM 44,641,70
MUT: mma-sat 1 µg/plate   MUREAV 51,311,78

SAFETY PROFILE: Questionable carcinogen with experimental tumorigenic data. Mutation data reported. When heated to decomposition it emits acrid smoke and irritating fumes.

DKY400   CAS: 57816-08-7
7,14-DIHYDRODIBENZ(a,h)ANTHRACENE
mf: $C_{22}H_{16}$ mw: 280.38

SYN: 9,10-DIHYDRO-1,2,5,6-DIBENZANTHRACENE

TOXICITY DATA with REFERENCE
ETA: skn-mus TD:1250 mg/kg/52W-I   PRLBA4
  117,318,35
ETA: skn-mus TDLo:1150 mg/kg/48W-I
  PRLBA4 129,439,40
MUT: mma-sat 1 µg/plate   MUREAV 51,311,78

CONSENSUS REPORTS: EPA Genetic Toxicology Program.

SAFETY PROFILE: Questionable carcinogen with experimental tumorigenic data. Mutation data reported. When heated to decomposition it emits acrid smoke and irritating fumes.

DLA000   CAS: 63077-00-9
3,4-DIHYDRO-1,2,5,6-DIBENZCARBAZOLE
mf: $C_{20}H_{15}N$ mw: 269.36

SYN: 12,13-DIHYDRO-7H-DIBENZO(a,g)CARBAZOLE

TOXICITY DATA with REFERENCE
ETA: scu-mus TDLo:120 mg/kg/9W-I   BAFEAG
  42,3,55

SAFETY PROFILE: Questionable carcinogen with experimental tumorigenic data. When heated to decomposition it emits toxic fumes of NO_x.

DLA100
5,8-DIHYDRODIBENZO(a,def) CHRYSENE
mf: $C_{24}H_{16}$ mw: 304.40

SYN: 5,8-DIHYDRO-3,4:9,10-DIBENZOPYRENE

TOXICITY DATA with REFERENCE
ETA: scu-mus TDLo:72 mg/kg/9W-I COREAF
251,1322,60

SAFETY PROFILE: Questionable carcinogen with experimental tumorigenic data. When heated to decomposition it emits acrid smoke and irritating fumes.

DLA120   CAS: 7350-86-9
7,14-DIHYDRODIBENZO(b,def) CHRYSENE
mf: $C_{24}H_{16}$ mw: 304.40

SYN: 5,10-DIHYDRO-3,4:8,9-DIBENZOPYRENE

TOXICITY DATA with REFERENCE
ETA: scu-mus TDLo:72 mg/kg/9W-I COREAF
251,1322,60

SAFETY PROFILE: Questionable carcinogen with experimental tumorigenic data. When heated to decomposition it emits acrid smoke and irritating fumes.

DLB400   CAS: 84-16-2
DIHYDRODIETHYLSTILBESTROL
mf: $C_{18}H_{22}O_2$ mw: 270.40

PROP: Needles from benzene, thin plates from dil alc. Mp: 185-188°. Freely sol in ether; sol in acetone, alc, methanol; sltly sol in benzene, chloroform. Sol in dil solns of alkali hydroxides. Practically insol in water and in dil mineral acids.

SYNS: meso-3,4-BIS(p-HYDROXYPHENYL)-n-HEXANE ◇ 3,4-BIS(p-HYDROXYPHENYL)HEXANE ◇ CYCLOESTROL ◇ 4,4'-(1,2-DIETHYLETHYLENE)DIPHENOL ◇ DIHYDRO-STILBESTROL ◇ 4,4'-DIHYDROXY-α,β-DIETHYLDIPHE-NYLETHANE ◇ 4,4'-DIHYDROXY-γ,Δ-DIPHENYLHEXANE ◇ γ,Δ-DI(p-HYDROXYPHENYL)-HEXANE ◇ meso-3,4-DI(p-HYDROXYPHENYL)-n-HEXANE ◇ EXTRA-PLEX ◇ HEXA-NOESTROL ◇ HEXESTROL ◇ meso-HEXESTROL ◇ HEXOES-TROL ◇ HORMOESTROL ◇ SINESTROL ◇ SYNESTROL ◇ SYNTHOVO ◇ SYNTROGENE ◇ VITESTROL

TOXICITY DATA with REFERENCE
CAR: scu-mus TDLo:74 mg/kg/56W-I VRDEA5
(6),46,62
NEO: ivg-mus TDLo:18 mg/kg/17W-I
VOONAW 22(3),68,76
NEO: scu-gpg TDLo:74 mg/kg/69W-I VRDEA5
(6),46,62
ETA: imp-gpg TDLo:540 μg/kg BSBSAS8,142,51

ETA: imp-ham TDLo:640 mg/kg/38W-I
CNREA8 43,5200,83
ETA: scu-ham TDLo:360 mg/kg CBINA8
55,157,85
MUT: dns-ham:emb 1 mg/L CNREA8 44,184,84

SAFETY PROFILE: Questionable carcinogen with experimental carcinogenic, neoplastigenic, and tumorigenic data. Poison by intraperitoneal route. Moderately toxic by ingestion and subcutaneous routes. Experimental reproductive effects. Mutation data reported.

DLB800   CAS: 28622-84-6
4,5-DIHYDRO-4,5-DIHYDROXYBENZO (a)PYRENE
mf: $C_{20}H_{14}O_2$ mw: 286.34

SYNS: BENZO(a)PYRENE, 4,5-DIHYDROXY-4,5-DIHY-DRO- ◇ BP-4,5-DIHYDRODIOL

TOXICITY DATA with REFERENCE
NEO: skn-mus TDLo:4580 μg/kg CRNGDP
3,371,78
MUT: dnd-hmn:fbr 30 μmol/L CBINA8 41,155,82

SAFETY PROFILE: Questionable carcinogen with experimental neoplastigenic data. Mutation data reported. When heated to decomposition it emits acrid smoke and irritating fumes.

DLC000   CAS: 24909-09-9
9,10-DIHYDRO-9,10-DIHYDROXYBENZO (a)PYRENE
mf: $C_{20}H_{14}O_2$ mw: 286.34

SYN: 9,10-DIHYDROBENZO(a)PYRENE-9,10-DIOL

TOXICITY DATA with REFERENCE
NEO: skn-mus TD:4580 μg/kg CNREA8
40,1981,80
NEO: skn-mus TDLo:1 mg/kg BJCAAI 34,523,76
ETA: skn-mus TD:4580 μg/kg CCSUDL 3,371,78
MUT: dnd-hmn:fbr 30 μmol/L CBINA8 41,155,82

CONSENSUS REPORTS: EPA Genetic Toxicology Program.

SAFETY PROFILE: Questionable carcinogen with experimental neoplastigenic and tumorigenic data by skin contact. Human mutation data reported. When heated to decomposition it emits acrid smoke and irritating fumes.

DLC400   CAS: 58030-91-4
(±)-trans-9,10-DIHYDRO-9,10-DIHYDROXYBENZO(a)PYRENE
mf: $C_{20}H_{14}O_2$ mw: 286.34

SYN: BP-9,10-DIHYDRODIOL

TOXICITY DATA with REFERENCE
ETA: skn-mus TDLo: 4600 μg/kg   CALEDQ
3,23,77
MUT: mma-sat 50 μg/plate   CNREA8 41,270,81

SAFETY PROFILE: Questionable carcinogen with experimental tumorigenic data. Mutation data reported. When heated to decomposition it emits acrid smoke and irritating fumes.

DLC600   CAS: 37571-88-3
trans-4,5-DIHYDRO-4,5-DIHYDROXYBENZO(a)PYRENE
mf: $C_{20}H_{14}O_2$ mw: 286.34

SYNS: (E)-BENZO(a)PYRENE-4,5-DIHYDRODIOL ◇ trans-4,5-DIHYDROBENZO(a)PYRENE-4,5-DIOL ◇ trans-4,5-DIHYDROXY-4,5-DIHYDROBENZO(a)PYRENE

TOXICITY DATA with REFERENCE
NEO: skn-mus TDLo: 1 mg/kg   BJCAAI 34,523,76
MUT: dni-omi 2 mg/L   PNASA6 74,1378,77
MUT: mma-sat 30 mg/L   ENMUDM 7,839,85
MUT: msc-ham: lng 25 mg/L   CNREA8 36,3350,76
MUT: otr-ham: emb 1 mg/L   IJCNAW 19,814,77
MUT: sce-ham: ovr 8 mg/L   MUREAV 50,367,78

CONSENSUS REPORTS: EPA Genetic Toxicology Program.

SAFETY PROFILE: Questionable carcinogen with experimental neoplastigenic data by skin contact. Mutation data reported. When heated to decomposition it emits acrid smoke and irritating fumes.

DLD200   CAS: 64920-31-6
trans-1,2-DIHYDRO-1,2-DIHYDROXYCHRYSENE
mf: $C_{18}H_{14}O_2$ mw: 262.32

SYNS: (E)-1,2-DIHYDRO-1,2-CHYRSENEDIOL ◇ trans-1,2-DIHYDROCHRYSENE-1,2-DIOL ◇ trans-1,2-DIHYDROXY-1,2-DIHYDROCHRYSENE

TOXICITY DATA with REFERENCE
NEO: ipr-mus TDLo: 67 mg/kg/15D-I   CNREA8
39,5063,79
MUT: mma-sat 37500 pmol/plate   BBRCA9
78,847,77
MUT: mmo-sat 5 μg/plate   CNREA8 44,3408,84

SAFETY PROFILE: Questionable carcinogen with neoplastigenic data. Mutation data reported. When heated to decomposition it emits acrid smoke and irritating fumes.

DLD400   CAS: 66267-19-4
trans-3,4-DIHYDRO-3,4-DIHYDROXYDIBENZ(a,h)ANTHRACENE
mf: $C_{22}H_{16}O_2$ mw: 312.38

SYNS: trans-DBA-3,4-DIHYDRODIOL ◇ trans-3,4-DIHYDRO-3,4-DIHYDROXYDIBENZO(a,h)ANTHRACENE

TOXICITY DATA with REFERENCE
NEO: skn-mus TDLo: 500 μg/kg   CNREA8
39,1310,79

SAFETY PROFILE: Questionable carcinogen with experimental neoplastigenic data by skin contact. When heated to decomposition it emits acrid smoke and irritating fumes.

DLD600   CAS: 68162-13-0
trans-3,4-DIHYDRO-3,4-DIHYDROXY-7,12-DIMETHYLBENZ(a)ANTHRACENE
mf: $C_{20}H_{18}O_2$ mw: 290.38

SYN: trans-3,4-DIHYDRO-3,4-DIHYDROXY DMBA

TOXICITY DATA with REFERENCE
NEO: skn-mus TDLo: 105 μg/kg   CNREA8
39,1934,79
ETA: skn-mus TD: 34846 ng/kg   CNREA8
40,3661,80
MUT: mma-sat 5 μmol/L   BBRCA9 83,1468,78
MUT: mma-sat 2500 nmol/L   CBINA8 32,257,80
MUT: msc-ham: lng 120 μg/L/3H   BJCAAI
39,540,79
MUT: otr-mus: fbr 120 μg/L   BBRCA9 85,357,78
MUT: sce-ham: ovr 2 mg/L   CALEDQ 7,45,79

SAFETY PROFILE: Questionable carcinogen with experimental neoplastigenic and tumorigenic data by skin contact. Mutation data reported. When heated to decomposition it emits acrid smoke and irritating fumes.

DLD800   CAS: 65763-32-8
trans-8,9-DIHYDRO-8,9-DIHYDROXY-7,12-DIMETHYLBENZ(a)ANTHRACENE
mf: $C_{20}H_{18}O_2$ mw: 290.38

SYNS: (E)-8,9-DIHYDRO-8,9-DIHYDROXY-7,12-DIMETHYLBENZ(a)ANTHRACENE ◇ trans-8,9-DIHYDRO-8,9-DIHYDROXY DMBA

TOXICITY DATA with REFERENCE
ETA: skn-mus TDLo: 1050 μg/kg   CNREA8
39,1934,79
MUT: mma-sat 5 μmol/L   BBRCA9 83,1468,78
MUT: msc-ham: lng 250 μg/L/3H   BJCAAI
39,540,79

MUT: otr-mus:fbr 250 mg/L   BBRCA9 85,357,78
MUT: sce-ham:ovr 8 mg/L   CALEDQ 7,45,79

SAFETY PROFILE: Questionable carcinogen with experimental tumorigenic data by skin contact. Mutation data reported. When heated to decomposition it emits acrid smoke and irritating fumes.

DLE000   CAS: 64598-80-7
(±)-(1R,2S,3R,4R)-3,4-DIHYDRO-3,4-DIHYDROXY-1,2-EPOXYBENZ(a)ANTHRACENE
mf: $C_{18}H_{14}O_3$ mw: 278.32

SYNS: BA 3,4-DIOL-1,2-EPOXIDE 1 ◊ BA 3,4-DIOL-1,2-EPOXIDE-2 ◊ BENZ(a)ANTHRACENE 3,4-DIOL-1,2-EPOXIDE-2 ◊ (E)-1,2,3,4-TETRAHYDRO-3-α,4-β-DIHYDROXY-1-α,2-α-EPOXYBENZ(a)ANTHRACENE ◊ (±)-3-α,4-β-DIHYDROXY-1-α,2-α-EPOXY-1,2,3,4-TETRAHYDROBENZ(a)ANTHRACENE

TOXICITY DATA with REFERENCE
ETA: skn-mus TDLo:22 mg/kg   CNREA8 38,1699,78
MUT: mma-sat 150 pmol/plate   CRNGDP4,1631,83
MUT: mmo-sat 100 pmol/plate   CNREA843,1656,83
MUT: msc-ham:lng 20 μmol/L   CNREA8 43,1656,83

CONSENSUS REPORTS: EPA Genetic Toxicology Program.

SAFETY PROFILE: Questionable carcinogen with experimental tumorigenic data by skin contact. Mutation data reported. When heated to decomposition it emits acrid smoke and irritating fumes.

DLE200   CAS: 64598-81-8
(±)-(1S,2R,3R,4R)-3,4-DIHYDRO-3,4-DIHYDROXY-1,2-EPOXYBENZ(a)ANTHRACENE
mf: $C_{18}H_{14}O_3$ mw: 278.32

SYN: BA 3,4-DIOL-1,2-EPOXIDE 1

TOXICITY DATA with REFERENCE
NEO: ipr-mus TDLo:3100 μg/kg/15D-I   JJIND8 63,201,79

SAFETY PROFILE: Questionable carcinogen with experimental neoplastigenic data. When heated to decomposition it emits acrid smoke and irritating fumes.

DLE400   CAS: 102420-56-4
trans-1,2-DIHYDRO-1,2-DIHYDROXYINDENO(1,2,3-cd)PYRENE
mf: $C_{22}H_{14}O_2$ mw: 310.36

SYN: IP-1,2-DIOL

TOXICITY DATA with REFERENCE
ETA: skn-mus TDLo:40 mg/kg/20D-I   CRNGDP 7,1761,86

SAFETY PROFILE: Questionable carcinogen with experimental tumorigenic data. When heated to decomposition it emits acrid smoke and irritating fumes.

DLE500   CAS: 83876-50-0
cis-5,6-DIHYDRO-5,6-DIHYDROXY-12-METHYLBENZ(a)ACRIDINE
mf: $C_{18}H_{15}NO_2$ mw: 277.34

SYN: BENZ(a)ACRIDINE-5,6-DIOL, 5,6-DIHYDRO-12-METHYL-, (Z)-

TOXICITY DATA with REFERENCE
ETA: scu-mus TDLo:72 mg/kg/12W-I   JMCMAR 26,303,83

SAFETY PROFILE: Questionable carcinogen with experimental tumorigenic data. When heated to decomposition it emits toxic fumes of NO_x.

DLF200   CAS: 64521-15-9
trans-8,9-DIHYDRO-8,9-DIHYDROXY-7-METHYLBENZ(a)ANTHRACENE
mf: $C_{18}H_{16}O_2$ mw: 264.34

TOXICITY DATA with REFERENCE
ETA: skn-mus TDLo:1000 μg/kg   CALEDQ 3,247,77
MUT: mma-sat 30 μg/L   BBRCA9 75,427,77
MUT: msc-ham:lng 1 mg/L   IJCNAW 19,828,77
MUT: otr-mus:fbr 1 mg/L   IJCNAW 19,828,77
MUT: sce-ham:ovr 8 mg/L   MUREAV 50,367,78

CONSENSUS REPORTS: EPA Genetic Toxicology Program.

SAFETY PROFILE: Questionable carcinogen with experimental tumorigenic data by skin contact. Mutation data reported. When heated to decomposition it emits acrid smoke and irritating fumes.

DLF400   CAS: 67411-81-8
1,2-DIHYDRO-1,2-DIHYDROXY-5-METHYLCHRYSENE
mf: $C_{19}H_{16}O_2$ mw: 276.35

SYN: 1,2-DIHYDRO-5-METHYL-1,2-CHRYSENEDIOL

TOXICITY DATA with REFERENCE
CAR: skn-mus TDLo:36 μg/kg   CNREA8 45,6406,79

NEO: skn-mus TDLo:1200 µg/kg/18D-I
CNREA8 40,1396,80

MUT: mma-sat 7200 pmol/plate CNREA8
38,2191,78

SAFETY PROFILE: Questionable carcinogen with experimental carcinogenic and neoplastigenic data. Mutation data reported. When heated to decomposition it emits acrid smoke and irritating fumes.

DLF600 CAS: 67523-22-2
7,8-DIHYDRO-7,8-DIHYDROXY-5-METHYLCHRYSENE
mf: $C_{19}H_{16}O_2$ mw: 276.35

SYN: 7,8-DIHYDRO-5-METHYL-7,8-CHRYSENEDIOL

TOXICITY DATA with REFERENCE
NEO: skn-mus TDLo:1200 µg/kg/18D-I
CNREA8 40,1396,80

MUT: mma-sat 2700 pmol/plate CNREA8
38,2191,78

SAFETY PROFILE: Questionable carcinogen with experimental neoplastigenic data by skin contact. Mutation data reported. When heated to decomposition it emits acrid and irritating fumes.

DLH800 CAS: 35281-29-9
5,6-DIHYDRO-7,12-DIMETHYLBENZ(a) ANTHRACENE
mf: $C_{20}H_{18}$ mw: 258.38

TOXICITY DATA with REFERENCE
CAR: skn-mus TDLo:128 mg/kg/50W-I
ZKKOBW 77,226,72

SAFETY PROFILE: Questionable carcinogen with experimental carcinogenic data by skin contact. When heated to decomposition it emits acrid smoke and irritating fumes.

DLI000 CAS: 52171-93-4
3,4-DIHYDRO-1,11-DIMETHYLCHRYSENE
mf: $C_{20}H_{18}$ mw: 258.38

TOXICITY DATA with REFERENCE
NEO: skn-mus TDLo:120 mg/kg/50W-I
CNREA8 34,1315,74

MUT: mma-sat 20 µg/plate CNREA8 36,4525,76

CONSENSUS REPORTS: EPA Genetic Toxicology Program.

SAFETY PROFILE: Questionable carcinogen with experimental neoplastigenic data by skin

contact. Mutation data reported. When heated to decomposition it emits acrid smoke and irritating fumes.

DLI200 CAS: 5831-16-3
16,17-DIHYDRO-11,17-DIMETHYLCYCLOPENTA(a) PHENANTHRENE
mf: $C_{19}H_{17}$ mw: 245.36

SYN: 11,17-DIMETHYL-16,17-DIHYDRO-15H-CYCLO-PENTA(a)PHENANTHRENE

TOXICITY DATA with REFERENCE
ETA: skn-mus TDLo:108 mg/kg/1Y-I PEXTAR
11,69,69

CONSENSUS REPORTS: EPA Genetic Toxicology Program.

SAFETY PROFILE: Questionable carcinogen with experimental tumorigenic data by skin contact. When heated to decomposition it emits acrid smoke and irritating fumes.

DLI300 CAS: 85616-56-4
15,16-DIHYDRO-7,11-DIMETHYL-17H-CYCLOPENTA(a)PHENANTHREN-17-ONE
mf: $C_{19}H_{16}O$ mw: 260.35

SYN: 7,11-DIMETHYL-15,16-DIHYDROCYCLOPENTA (a)PHENANTHREN-17-ONE

TOXICITY DATA with REFERENCE
CAR: skn-mus TDLo:40 mg/kg/10W-I CNREA8
46,1817,86

SAFETY PROFILE: Questionable carcinogen with experimental carcinogenic data. When heated to decomposition it emits acrid smoke and irritating fumes.

DLI400 CAS: 894-52-0
15,16-DIHYDRO-11,12-DIMETHYLCYCLOPENTA(a) PHENANTHREN-17-ONE
mf: $C_{19}H_{16}O$ mw: 260.35

TOXICITY DATA with REFERENCE
CAR: scu-mus TDLo:360 mg/kg PEXTAR
11,69,69

CAR: skn-mus TDLo:108 mg/kg/1Y-I PEXTAR
11,69,69

MUT: mma-sat 50 µg/plate CNREA8 36,4525,76

CONSENSUS REPORTS: EPA Genetic Toxicology Program.

SAFETY PROFILE: Questionable carcinogen with experimental carcinogenic data. Mutation data reported. When heated to decomposition it emits acrid smoke and irritating fumes.

DLJ500   CAS: 66289-74-5
endo,endo-DIHYDRODI (NORBORNADIENE)
mf: $C_{14}H_{18}$ mw: 186.32

SYNS: 4,7-METHANO-2,3,8-METHENOCYCLOPENT(a)IN-DENE, DODECAHYDRO-, stereoisomer ◇ RJ 5 ◇ SHELLOYNE H

TOXICITY DATA with REFERENCE
ETA: ihl-rat TC: 150 mg/m³/6H/1Y-I   AETODY 7,133,84
ETA: ihl-rat TCLo: 150 mg/m³/6H/1Y-I   NTIS** AD-A134-150

SAFETY PROFILE: Questionable carcinogen with experimental tumorigenic data. Poison by ingestion. When heated to decomposition it emits acrid smoke and irritating fumes.

DLK600   CAS: 63041-56-5
7,14-DIHYDRO-7,14-DIPROPYLDIBENZ (a,h)ANTHRACENE-7,14-DIOL
mf: $C_{28}H_{28}O_2$ mw: 396.56

SYNS: 9,10-DIHYDRO-9,10-DIHYDROXY-9,10-DI-n-PRO-PYL-1,2:5,6-DIBENZANTHRACENE ◇ 9,10-DIHYDROXY-9,10-DI-n-PROPYL-9,10-DIHYDRO-1,2:5,6-DIBENZANTHRA-CENE ◇ 9,10-DI-n-PROPYL-9-10-DIHYDROXY-9,10-DIHY-DRO-1,2,5,6-DIBENZANTHRACENE

TOXICITY DATA with REFERENCE
ETA: scu-rat TDLo: 8 mg/kg   JOCEAH 2,175,37

SAFETY PROFILE: Questionable carcinogen with experimental tumorigenic data. When heated to decomposition it emits acrid smoke and irritating fumes.

DLK750
1,2-DIHYDRO-1,2-EPOXYINDENO(1,2,3-cd)PYRENE
mf: $C_{22}H_{12}O$ mw: 292.34

SYN: INDENO(1,2,3-cd)PYRENE-1,2-OXIDE

TOXICITY DATA with REFERENCE
ETA: skn-mus TDLo: 40 mg/kg/20D-I   CRNGDP 7,1761,86
MUT: mmo-sat 1 µg/plate   CNREA8 45,5421,85

THR: Questionable carcinogen with experimental tumorigenic data. Mutation data reported.

When heated to decomposition it emits acrid smoke and irritating fumes.

DLM000   CAS: 42028-27-3
15,16-DIHYDRO-11-ETHYLCYCLOPENTA(a)PHENANTHREN-17-ONE
mf: $C_{19}H_{16}O$ mw: 260.35

TOXICITY DATA with REFERENCE
NEO: skn-mus TDLo: 120 mg/kg/50W-I   CNREA8 33,832,73
MUT: mma-sat 50 µg/plate   CNREA8 36,4525,76

CONSENSUS REPORTS: EPA Genetic Toxicology Program.

SAFETY PROFILE: Questionable carcinogen with experimental neoplastigenic data. Mutation data reported. When heated to decomposition it emits acrid smoke and irritating fumes.

DLM600   CAS: 5096-24-2
2,3-DIHYDRO-3-ETHYL-6-METHYL-1H-CYCLOPENTA(a)ANTHRACENE
mf: $C_{20}H_{20}$ mw: 260.40

SYN: 3-ETHYL-2,3-DIHYDRO-6-METHYL-1H-CYCLOPEN-T(a)ANTHRACENE

TOXICITY DATA with REFERENCE
ETA: orl-rat TDLo: 1000 mg/kg   CNREA8 26,619,66

SAFETY PROFILE: Questionable carcinogen with experimental tumorigenic data. Moderately toxic by ingestion. When heated to decomposition it emits acrid smoke and irritating fumes.

DLN000   CAS: 52831-41-1
6,13-DIHYDRO-2-FLUOROBENZO(g)(1)BENZOTHIOPYRANO(4,3-b)INDOLE
mf: $C_{19}H_{12}FNS$ mw: 305.38

TOXICITY DATA with REFERENCE
NEO: scu-mus TDLo: 78 mg/kg/9W-I   MUREAV 66,307,79
MUT: mma-sat 30 µg/plate   MUREAV 66,307,79

SAFETY PROFILE: Questionable carcinogen with experimental neoplastigenic data. Mutation data reported. When heated to decomposition it emits very toxic fumes of F^-, NO_x, and SO_x.

DLN200   CAS: 52831-55-7
6,13-DIHYDRO-3-FLUOROBENZO(e)(1)BENZOTHIOPYRANO(4,3-b)INDOLE
mf: $C_{19}H_{12}FNS$ mw: 305.38

TOXICITY DATA with REFERENCE

NEO: scu-mus TDLo:72 mg/kg/9W-I   MUREAV
66,307,79

MUT: mma-sat 30 µg/plate   MUREAV 66,307,79

SAFETY PROFILE: Questionable carcinogen with experimental neoplastigenic data. Mutation data reported. When heated to decomposition it emits very toxic fumes of F^-, NO_x, and SO_x.

DLN400   CAS: 52831-67-1
6,13-DIHYDRO-4-FLUOROBENZO(e)(1) BENZOTHIOPYRANO(4,3-b)INDOLE
mf: $C_{19}H_{12}FNS$ mw: 305.38

TOXICITY DATA with REFERENCE

NEO: scu-mus TDLo:72 mg/kg/9W-I   MUREAV
66,307,79

MUT: mma-sat 30 µg/plate   MUREAV 66,307,79

SAFETY PROFILE: Questionable carcinogen with experimental neoplastigenic data. Mutation data reported. When heated to decomposition it emits very toxic fumes of F^-, NO_x, and SO_x.

DLO000   CAS: 22298-04-0
6,11-DIHYDRO-2-FLUORO(1) BENZOTHIOPYRANO(4,3-b)INDOLE
mf: $C_{15}H_{10}FNS$ mw: 255.32

SYN: 6,11-DIHYDRO-2-FLUORO-THIOPYRANO(4,3-b) BENZ(e)INDOLE

TOXICITY DATA with REFERENCE

NEO: scu-mus TDLo:72 mg/kg/9W-I   MUREAV
66,307,79

MUT: mma-sat 100 µg/plate   MUREAV 66,307,79

SAFETY PROFILE: Questionable carcinogen with experimental neoplastigenic data. Mutation data reported. When heated to decomposition it emits very toxic fumes of F^-, SO_x, and NO_x.

DLO200   CAS: 21243-26-5
6,11-DIHYDRO-4-FLUORO(1) BENZOTHIOPYRANO(4,3-b)INDOLE
mf: $C_{15}H_{10}FNS$ mw: 255.32

TOXICITY DATA with REFERENCE

NEO: scu-mus TDLo:78 mg/kg/9W-I   MUREAV
66,307,79

MUT: mma-sat 90 µg/plate   MUREAV 66,307,79

SAFETY PROFILE: Questionable carcinogen with experimental neoplastigenic data. Mutation data reported. When heated to decomposition it emits very toxic fumes of F^-, SO_x, and NO_x.

DLO950   CAS: 83053-63-8
15,16-DIHYDRO-11-HYDROXYCYCLOPENTA(a) PHENANTHREN-17-ONE
mf: $C_{17}H_{12}O_2$ mw: 248.29

TOXICITY DATA with REFERENCE

ETA: skn-mus TDLo:400 mg/kg   CRNGDP
3,677,82

SAFETY PROFILE: Questionable carcinogen with experimental tumorigenic data. When heated to decomposition it emits acrid smoke and irritating fumes.

DLP200   CAS: 55651-36-0
15,16-DIHYDRO-11-HYDROXYMETHYL-17H-CYCLOPENTA(a)PHENANTHREN-17-ONE

TOXICITY DATA with REFERENCE

ETA: skn-mus TDLo:16 mg/kg   CNREA840,882,80

MUT: mma-sat 1 µg/plate   CNREA8 40,882,80

SAFETY PROFILE: Questionable carcinogen with experimental tumorigenic data. Mutation data reported. When heated to decomposition it emits acrid smoke and fumes.

DLP400   CAS: 55651-31-5
15,16-DIHYDRO-15-HYDROXY-11-METHYL-17H-CYCLOPENTA(a) PHENANTHREN-17-ONE

TOXICITY DATA with REFERENCE

ETA: skn-mus TDLo:16 mg/kg   CNREA840,882,80

MUT: mma-sat 1 µg/plate   CNREA8 40,882,80

SAFETY PROFILE: Questionable carcinogen with experimental tumorigenic data. Mutation data reported. When heated to decomposition it emits acrid smoke and fumes.

DLP600   CAS: 24684-56-8
15,16-DIHYDRO-16-HYDROXY-11-METHYLCYCLOPENTA(a) PHENANTHREN-17-ONE
mf: $C_{18}H_{14}O_2$ mw: 262.32

SYN: 15,16-DIHYDRO-16-HYDROXY-11-METHYL-17H-CYCLOPENTA(a)PHENANTHREN-17-ONE

TOXICITY DATA with REFERENCE

NEO: skn-mus TDLo:115 mg/kg/48W-I
CNREA8 33,832,73

MUT: mma-sat 1 µg/plate   CNREA8 40,882,80

CONSENSUS REPORTS: EPA Genetic Toxicology Program.

SAFETY PROFILE: Questionable carcinogen with experimental neoplastigenic data. Mutation data reported. When heated to decomposition it emits acrid smoke and irritating fumes.

DLR200   CAS: 5836-85-1
15,16-DIHYDRO-11-METHOXYCYCLOPENTA(a)PHENANTHREN-17-ONE
mf: $C_{18}H_{14}O_2$ mw: 262.32

SYN: 11-METHOXY-15,16-DIHDYROCYCLOPENTA(a)PHENANTHREN-17-ONE

TOXICITY DATA with REFERENCE
CAR: skn-mus TDLo: 108 mg/kg/1Y-I   PEXTAR 11,69,69

ETA: skn-mus TD: 1600 µg/kg   CRNGDP 3,677,82

SAFETY PROFILE: Questionable carcinogen with experimental carcinogenic and tumorigenic data. When heated to decomposition it emits acrid smoke and irritating fumes.

DLR600   CAS: 30835-61-1
15,16-DIHYDRO-11-METHOXY-7-METHYLCYCLOPENTA(a)PHENANTHREN-17-ONE
mf: $C_{19}H_{16}O_2$ mw: 276.35

SYN: 15,16-DIHYDRO-11-METHOXY-7-METHYL-17H-CYCLOPENTA(a)PHENANTHREN-17-ONE

TOXICITY DATA with REFERENCE
NEO: skn-mus TDLo: 96 mg/kg/40W-I   CNREA8 33,832,73

MUT: mma-sat 20 µg/plate   CNREA8 36,4525,76

CONSENSUS REPORTS: EPA Genetic Toxicology Program.

SAFETY PROFILE: Questionable carcinogen with experimental neoplastigenic data. Mutation data reported. When heated to decomposition it emits acrid smoke and irritating fumes.

DLT000   CAS: 7499-32-3
9,10-DIHYDRO-7-METHYLBENZO(a)PYRENE
mf: $C_{21}H_{16}$ mw: 268.37

SYN: 1':2'-DIHYDRO-4'-METHYL-3:4-BENZPYRENE

TOXICITY DATA with REFERENCE
ETA: imp-mus TDLo: 520 mg/kg/10W-I

AJCAA7 36,211,39

SAFETY PROFILE: Questionable carcinogen with experimental tumorigenic data. When heated to decomposition it emits acrid smoke and irritating fumes.

DLT200   CAS: 63041-50-9
meso-DIHYDRO-3-METHYLCHOLANTHRENE
mf: $C_{21}H_{18}$ mw: 270.39

SYN: 6,12b-DIHYDRO-3-METHYLCHOLANTHRENE

TOXICITY DATA with REFERENCE
ETA: scu-mus TD: 200 mg/kg   CNREA8 1,685,41
ETA: scu-mus TDLo: 40 mg/kg   CNREA8 1,695,41

SAFETY PROFILE: Questionable carcinogen with experimental tumorigenic data. When heated to decomposition it emits acrid smoke and irritating fumes.

DLT400   CAS: 25486-92-4
11,12-DIHYDRO-3-METHYLCHOLANTHRENE
mf: $C_{21}H_{18}$ mw: 270.39

TOXICITY DATA with REFERENCE
ETA: skn-mus TDLo: 168 mg/kg/57W-I

JNCIAM 44,641,70

MUT: mma-sat 1 µg/plate   MUREAV 51,311,78

SAFETY PROFILE: Questionable carcinogen with experimental tumorigenic data. Mutation data reported. When heated to decomposition it emits acrid smoke and irritating fumes.

DLT600
9,10-DIHYDRO-3-METHYLCHOLANTHRENE-1,9,10-TRIOL
mf: $C_{21}H_{18}O_3$ mw: 318.39

SYNS: (E)-1-HYDROXY-MC-9,10-DIHYDRODIOL
◇ (E)-1-HYDROXY-3-METHYLCHOLANTHRENE 9,10-DIHYDRODIOL

TOXICITY DATA with REFERENCE
NEO: skn-mus TDLo: 127 µg/kg   CNREA8 39,3549,79

SAFETY PROFILE: Questionable carcinogen with experimental neoplastigenic data. When heated to decomposition it emits acrid smoke and irritating fumes.

DLT800   CAS: 40951-13-1
15,16-DIHYDRO-11-METHYL-17H-CYCLOPENTA(a)PHENANTHREN-17-OL
mf: $C_{18}H_{16}O$ mw: 248.34

TOXICITY DATA with REFERENCE
NEO: skn-mus TDLo: 91 mg/kg/38W-I   CNREA8
33,832,73

SAFETY PROFILE: Questionable carcinogen
with experimental neoplastigenic data. When
heated to decomposition it emits acrid smoke
and irritating fumes.

DLU200   CAS: 24684-42-2
16,17-DIHYDRO-11-
METHYLCYCLOPENTA(a)
PHENANTHREN-15-ONE
mf: $C_{18}H_{14}O$ mw: 246.32

TOXICITY DATA with REFERENCE
ETA: skn-mus TDLo: 120 mg/kg/50W-I
CNREA8 33,832,73
MUT: mma-sat 50 μg/plate   CNREA8 36,4525,76

CONSENSUS REPORTS: EPA Genetic Toxicology Program.

SAFETY PROFILE: Questionable carcinogen
with experimental tumorigenic data. Mutation
data reported. When heated to decomposition
it emits acrid smoke and irritating fumes.

DLU400   CAS: 30835-65-5
15,16-DIHYDRO-7-
METHYLCYCLOPENTA(a)
PHENANTHREN-17-ONE
mf: $C_{18}H_{14}O$ mw: 246.32

SYN: 15,16-DIHYDRO-7-METHYL-17H-CYCLOPENTA
(a)PHENANTHREN-17-ONE

TOXICITY DATA with REFERENCE
ETA: skn-mus TDLo: 72 mg/kg/30W-I   CNREA8
33,832,73

CONSENSUS REPORTS: EPA Genetic Toxicology Program.

SAFETY PROFILE: Questionable carcinogen
with experimental tumorigenic data. When
heated to decomposition it emits acrid smoke
and irritating fumes.

DLU600   CAS: 5837-17-2
16,17-DIHYDRO-17-METHYLENE-15H-
CYCLOPENTA(a)PHENANTHRENE
mf: $C_{18}H_{14}$ mw: 230.32

TOXICITY DATA with REFERENCE
ETA: skn-mus TDLo: 125 mg/kg/52W-I
NATUAS 210,1281,66

SAFETY PROFILE: Questionable carcinogen
with experimental tumorigenic data. When
heated to decomposition it emits acrid smoke
and irritating fumes.

DLU700   CAS: 83053-62-7
15,16-DIHYDRO-11-METHYL-15-
METHOXYCYCLOPENTA(a)
PHENANTHREN-17-ONE
mf: $C_{19}H_{16}O_2$ mw: 276.35

TOXICITY DATA with REFERENCE
ETA: skn-mus TDLo: 1600 μg/kg   CRNGDP
3,677,82

SAFETY PROFILE: Questionable carcinogen
with experimental tumorigenic data. When
heated to decomposition it emits acrid smoke
and irritating fumes.

DLU800   CAS: 29676-95-7
1,4-DIHYDRO-1-METHYL-7-(2-(5-NITRO-
2-FURYL)VINYL)-4-OXO-1,8-
NAPHTHYRIDINE-3-CARBOXYLIC ACID,
POTASSIUM SALT
mf: $C_{16}H_{10}N_3O_6 \cdot K$ mw: 379.39

SYN: NFN

TOXICITY DATA with REFERENCE
CAR: orl-mus TD: 3276 mg/kg/26W-C   CIGZAF
50,249,74
CAR: orl-mus TDLo: 1411 mg/kg/14W-C
JJIND8 69,1317,82
CAR: orl-mus TDLo: 3150 mg/kg/25W-C
CIZAAZ 50,249,74

SAFETY PROFILE: Questionable carcinogen
with experimental carcinogenic data. When
heated to decomposition it emits toxic fumes
of NO_x and K_2O.

DLX800   CAS: 17247-77-7
1,2-DIHYDRO-2-(5'-NITROFURYL)-4-
HYDROXYQUINAZOLINE-3-OXIDE
mf: $C_{12}H_9N_3O_5$ mw: 275.24

SYN: 1,2-DIHYDRO-2-(5'-NITROFURYL)-4-HYDROXY-
CHINAZOLIN-3-OXID (GERMAN)

TOXICITY DATA with REFERENCE
ETA: orl-rat TDLo: 40 g/kg/26W-C   ZKKOBW
79,165,73

SAFETY PROFILE: Questionable carcinogen
with experimental tumorigenic data. When
heated to decomposition it emits toxic fumes
of NO_x.

DLY200   CAS: 33389-33-2
1,2-DIHYDRO-2-(5-NITRO-2-THIENYL)
QUINAZOLIN-4(3H)-ONE
mf: $C_{12}H_9N_3O_3S$ mw: 275.30

SYN: 1,2-DIHYDRO-2-(5-NITRO-2-THIENYL)-4(3H)-
QUINAZOLINONE

TOXICITY DATA with REFERENCE
CAR: orl-rat TDLo: 13 g/kg/49W-C   JNCIAM
57,277,76

CONSENSUS REPORTS: EPA Genetic Toxicology Program.

SAFETY PROFILE: Questionable carcinogen with experimental carcinogenic data. When heated to decomposition it emits very toxic fumes of SO_x and NO_x.

DLY800   CAS: 7374-66-5
5,13-DIHYDRO-5-OXOBENZO(e)(2)
BENZOPYRANO(4,3-b)INDOLE
mf: $C_{19}H_{11}NO_2$ mw: 285.31

SYNS: 5-OXO-5H-BENZO(E)ISOCHROMENO(4,3-b)IN-
DOLE ◇ 5-OXO-5,13-
DIHYDROBENZO(E)(2)BENZOPYRANO(4,3-b)INDOLE

TOXICITY DATA with REFERENCE
ETA: scu-mus TDLo: 72 mg/kg/9W-I   SCIEAS
158,387,67

SAFETY PROFILE: Questionable carcinogen with experimental tumorigenic data. When heated to decomposition it emits toxic fumes of NO_x.

DLZ000   CAS: 56179-83-0
1,2-DIHYDROPHENANTHRENE
mf: $C_{14}H_{12}$ mw: 180.26

TOXICITY DATA with REFERENCE
ETA: skn-mus TDLo: 72 mg/kg   CNREA8
39,4069,79

SAFETY PROFILE: Questionable carcinogen with experimental tumorigenic data. When heated to decomposition it emits acrid smoke and irritating fumes.

DMA000   CAS: 28622-66-4
1,2-DIHYDRO-1,2-PHENANTHRENEDIOL
mf: $C_{14}H_{12}O_2$ mw: 212.26

SYN: PHENANTHRENE-1,2-DIHYDRODIOL

TOXICITY DATA with REFERENCE
ETA: skn-mus TDLo: 85 mg/kg   CNREA8
39,4069,79

SAFETY PROFILE: Questionable carcinogen with experimental tumorigenic data. When heated to decomposition it emits acrid smoke and irritating fumes.

DMA400   CAS: 18264-88-5
N-(9,10-DIHYDRO-2-PHENANTHRYL)
ACETAMIDE
mf: $C_{16}H_{15}NO$ mw: 237.32

SYN: 2-ACETYLAMINO-9,10-DIHYDROPHENANTHRENE

TOXICITY DATA with REFERENCE
CAR: orl-rat TDLo: 4608 mg/kg/32W-C
CNREA8 15,188,55

SAFETY PROFILE: Questionable carcinogen with experimental carcinogenic data. When heated to decomposition it emits toxic fumes of NO_x.

DMB200   CAS: 66731-42-8
2,3-DIHYDROPHORBOL MYRISTATE
ACETATE
mf: $C_{36}H_{58}O_8$ mw: 618.94

SYNS: 2,3-DIHYDROPHORBOL ACETATE MYRISTATE
◇ DPMA

TOXICITY DATA with REFERENCE
NEO: skn-mus TDLo: 37 mg/kg/31W-I   CNREA8
38,921,78

SAFETY PROFILE: Questionable carcinogen with experimental neoplastigenic data. When heated to decomposition it emits acrid smoke and irritating fumes.

DMC600   CAS: 123-33-1
1,2-DIHYDROPYRIDAZINE-3,6-DIONE
mf: $C_4H_4N_2O_2$ mw: 112.10

PROP: Crystals. Mp: > 300°. Sol in water and alc.

SYNS: 1,2-DIHYDRO-3,6-PYRIDAZINEDIONE ◇ ENT
18,870 ◇ 6-HYDROXY-3(2H)-PYRIDAZINONE ◇ MALEIC
ACID HYDRAZIDE ◇ MALEIC HYDRAZIDE ◇ N,N-MA-
LEOYLHYDRAZINE ◇ 1,2,3,6-TETRAHYDRO-3,6-DIOXOPY-
RIDAZINE

TOXICITY DATA with REFERENCE
ETA: scu-rat TDLo: 2600 mg/kg/65W-I   BJCAAI
19,392,65
MUT: cyt-grh-orl 5 mg   CYTOAN 37,345,72
MUT: cyt-mus-ipr 5000 ppm   CISCB7 20,28,76
MUT: dns-esc 30 μmol/L   ZKKOBW 92,177,78
MUT: mma-sat 50 μL/plate   MUREAV 66,247,79

MUT: sln-dmg-orl 4000 ppm MUREAV 55,15,78
MUT: sln-dmg-par 4000 ppm NATUAS 207,439,65

CONSENSUS REPORTS: IARC Cancer Review: Animal Inadequate Evidence IMEMDT 4,173,74. Reported in EPA TSCA Inventory.

SAFETY PROFILE: Questionable carcinogen with experimental tumorigenic data. Moderately toxic by ingestion. Mutation data reported. Can cause chronic liver damage and acute central nervous system effects. When heated to decomposition emits highly toxic fumes of NO_x.

DMF600   CAS: 5831-17-4
16,17-DIHYDRO-11,12,17-TRIMETHYLCYCLOPENTA(a)PHENANTHRENE
mf: $C_{20}H_{19}$ mw: 259.39

SYN: 11,12,17-TRIMETHYL-16,17-DIHYDRO-15H-CYCLO-PENTA(a)PHENANTHRENE

TOXICITY DATA with REFERENCE
CAR: skn-mus TDLo: 108 mg/kg/1Y-I PEXTAR 11,69,69

SAFETY PROFILE: Questionable carcinogen with experimental carcinogenic data. When heated to decomposition it emits acrid smoke and irritating fumes.

DMH400   CAS: 117-10-2
1,8-DIHYDROXYANTHRAQUINONE
mf: $C_{14}H_8O_4$ mw: 240.22

PROP: Crystals. Mp: 193°, vap d: 8.3.

SYNS: ALTAN ◇ ANTRAPUROL ◇ CHRYSAZIN ◇ DANTHRON ◇ DANTRON ◇ DIAQUONE ◇ 1,8-DIHYDROXY-9,10-ANTHRACENEDIONE ◇ 1,8-DIHYDROXYAN-THRACHINON (CZECH) ◇ DIONONE ◇ DORBANE ◇ DORBANEX ◇ DUOLAX ◇ ISTIN ◇ LAXANORM ◇ LAXANTHREEN ◇ LAXIPUR ◇ LAXIPURIN ◇ LTAN ◇ MODANE ◇ USAF ND-59 ◇ ZWITSALAX

TOXICITY DATA with REFERENCE
CAR: orl-mus TDLo: 129 g/kg/77W-C JJCREP 77,871,86
CAR: orl-rat TDLo: 292 g/kg/70W-C BJCAAI 52,781,85
NEO: orl-mus TD: 130 g/kg/77W-C TOLED5 31(Suppl),206,86
MUT: dni-hmn: fbr 100 μmol/L CNREA8 35,1392,75
MUT: dns-mus: lvr 20 μmol/L CNREA8 44,2918,84
MUT: mma-sat 100 μg/plate MUREAV 40,203,76

MUT: mmo-sat 100 μg/plate MUREAV 40,203,76
MUT: mmo-smc 5000 ppm/2D ADVEA4 51,45,71

CONSENSUS REPORTS: Reported in EPA TSCA Inventory.

SAFETY PROFILE: Questionable carcinogen with experimental carcinogenic and neoplastigenic data. Moderately toxic by intraperitoneal route. Human mutation data reported. An eye irritant. A laxative. When heated to decomposition it emits acrid smoke and irritating fumes.

DMJ600   CAS: 2892-51-5
3,4-DIHYDROXY-3-CYCLOBUTENE-1,2-DIONE
mf: $C_4H_2O_4$ mw: 114.06

SYNS: DIHYDROXYCYCLOBUTENEDIONE ◇ 3,4-DIHY-DROXYCYCLOBUTENE-1,2-DIONE ◇ QUADRATIC ACID ◇ SQUARIC ACID

TOXICITY DATA with REFERENCE
ETA: scu-mus TDLo: 368 mg/kg/92W-I JNCIAM 46,143,71

CONSENSUS REPORTS: Reported in EPA TSCA Inventory.

SAFETY PROFILE: Questionable carcinogen with experimental tumorigenic data. When heated to decomposition it emits acrid smoke and fumes.

DMK200   CAS: 66267-18-3
trans-1,2-DIHYDROXY-1,2-DIHYDROBENZO(a,h)ANTHRACENE
mf: $C_{22}H_{16}O_2$ mw: 312.38

SYNS: DBA-1,2-DIHYDRODIOL ◇ (E)-1,2-DIHYDRO-1,2-DIHYDROXYDIBENZ(a,h)ANTHRACENE ◇ trans-1,2-DIHY-DROXY-1,2-DIHYDROBENZ(a,h)ANTHRACENE

TOXICITY DATA with REFERENCE
ETA: skn-mus TDLo: 2000 μg/kg CNREA8 39,1310,79

SAFETY PROFILE: Questionable carcinogen with experimental tumorigenic data. When heated to decomposition it emits acrid smoke and irritating fumes.

DMK400   CAS: 24961-49-7
trans-4,5-DIHYDROXY-4,5-DIHYDROBENZO(e)PYRENE
mf: $C_{20}H_{14}O_2$ mw: 286.34

SYNS: BENZO(e)PYRENE-4,5-DIHDYRODIOL ◇ 4,5-DIHY-DRO-4,5-DIHYDROXYBENZO(e)PYRENE ◇ B(e)P-4,5-DIHY-DRODIOL

TOXICITY DATA with REFERENCE

ETA: ipr-mus TDLo: 32 mg/kg/15D-I   CNREA8
40,203,80

MUT: mma-sat 10 nmol/plate   JBCHA3 254,4408,79

SAFETY PROFILE: Questionable carcinogen with experimental tumorigenic data. Mutation data reported. When heated to decomposition it emits acrid smoke and irritating fumes.

DMK600   CAS: 66788-06-5
trans-9,10-DIHYDROXY-9,10-DIHYDROBENZO(e)PYRENE
mf: $C_{20}H_{14}O_2$ mw: 286.34

SYN: B(E)P 9,10-DIHYDRODIOL

TOXICITY DATA with REFERENCE

NEO: ipr-mus TDLo: 32 mg/kg/15D-I   CNREA8
40,203,80

MUT: mma-sat 10 nmol/plate   JBCHA3 254,4408,79

SAFETY PROFILE: Questionable carcinogen with experimental neoplastigenic data. Mutation data reported. When heated to decomposition it emits acrid smoke and fumes.

DML000   CAS: 61443-57-0
(+,−)-trans-7,8-DIHYDROXY-7,8-DIHYDROBENZO(a)PYRENE
mf: $C_{20}H_{14}O_2$ mw: 286.34

SYN: BP-7,8-DIHYDRODIOL

TOXICITY DATA with REFERENCE

CAR: orl-mus TDLo: 206 mg/kg/6W-I   JJIND8
62,1103,79

NEO: scu-mus TDLo: 10 mg/kg   JJIND8 64,617,80

NEO: skn-mus TDLo: 34 mg/kg/60W-I   CNREA8
37,3356,77

ETA: skn-mus TD: 22 mg/kg/25W-I   PNASA6
73,3867,76

ETA: skn-mus TD: 2160 μg/kg   CNREA8
37,4130,77

MUT: cyt-mus: fbr 5 μmol/L   CNREA8 42,1866,82

MUT: dnd-mam: lym 5 μmol/L   CRNGDP 3,697,82

MUT: dnd-rat: lvr 20 μmol/L   CRNGDP 3,861,82

MUT: msc-mus: fbr 200 nmol/L   CNREA8
42,1866,82

MUT: otr-mus: fbr 600 nmol/L   CNREA8 42,1866,82

MUT: sce-mus: fbr 10 μmol/L   CNREA8 42,1866,82

CONSENSUS REPORTS: EPA Genetic Toxicology Program.

SAFETY PROFILE: Questionable carcinogen with experimental carcinogenic, neoplastigenic,

and tumorigenic data by skin contact. Mutation data reported. When heated to decomposition it emits toxic fumes of NO_x.

DML200   CAS: 60864-95-1
(−)-trans-7,8-DIHYDROXY-7,8-DIHYDROBENZO(a)PYRENE
mf: $C_{20}H_{14}O_2$ mw: 286.34

SYN: BP-7,8-DIHYDRODIOL

TOXICITY DATA with REFERENCE

NEO: skn-mus TD: 1 mg/kg   BJCAAI 34,523,76

NEO: skn-mus TD: 1144 μg/kg   CCSUDL 3,371,78

NEO: skn-mus TDLo: 573 μg/kg   CNREA8
37,2721,77

MUT: cyt-rat: lvr 10 mg/L   CNREA8 40,1281,80

MUT: mma-sat 6 μg/plate   MUREAV 58,361,78

MUT: mmo-sat 8 μg/plate   MUREAV 58,361,78

MUT: msc-ham: lng 40 nmol/L/2D   CALEDQ
4,35,77

MUT: otr-rat: lvr 10 mg/L   CNREA8 40,1281,80

CONSENSUS REPORTS: EPA Genetic Toxicology Program.

SAFETY PROFILE: Questionable carcinogen with experimental neoplastigenic data. Mutation data reported. When heated to decomposition it emits acrid smoke and fumes.

DML400   CAS: 62314-67-4
(+)-trans-7,8-DIHYDROXY-7,8-DIHYDROBENZO(a)PYRENE
mf: $C_{20}H_{14}O_2$ mw: 286.34

TOXICITY DATA with REFERENCE

NEO: skn-mus TD: 1144 μg/kg   CCSUDL 3,371,78

NEO: skn-mus TDLo: 573 μg/kg   CNREA8
37,2721,77

MUT: mma-sat 4 μg/plate   MUREAV 58,361,78

MUT: msc-ham: lng 1200 nmol/L/2D   CALEDQ
4,35,77

MUT: otr-rat: lvr 10 mg/L   CNREA8 40,1281,80

CONSENSUS REPORTS: EPA Genetic Toxicology Program.

SAFETY PROFILE: Questionable carcinogen with experimental neoplastigenic data. Mutation data reported. When heated to decomposition it emits acrid smoke and fumes.

DML775   CAS: 69260-85-1
trans-3,4-DIHYDROXY-3,4-DIHYDRO-7,12-DIHYDROXYMETHYLBENZ(a) ANTHRACENE
mf: $C_{20}H_{18}O_4$ mw: 322.38

SYN: (E)-3,4-DIHYDROXY-3,4-DIHYDROBENZ(a)AN-
THRACENE-7,12-DIMETHANOL

TOXICITY DATA with REFERENCE
ETA: skn-mus TDLo: 116 µg/kg   CNREA8
40,3661,80

MUT: mma-sat 50 nmol/plate   CNREA8 40,3661,80

SAFETY PROFILE: Questionable carcinogen with experimental tumorigenic data. Mutation data reported. When heated to decomposition it emits acrid smoke and irritating fumes.

DML800   CAS: 3343-12-2
11,12-DIHYDROXY-11,12-DIHYDRO-3-METHYLCHOLANTHRENE (E)
mf: $C_{21}H_{18}O_2$ mw: 302.39

SYNS: trans-11,12-DIHYDRO-11,12-DIHYDROXY-3-
METHYLCHOLANTHRENE ◇ (E)-MC 11,12-DIHYDRODIOL
◇ (E)-11,12-DIHYDRO-3-METHYLCHOLANTHRENE-11,12-
DIOL ◇ (E)-3-METHYLCHOLANTHRENE-11,12-DIHYDRO-
DIOL ◇ trans-3-METHYL-11,12-DIHYDROCHOLANTHRENE-
11,12-DIOL

TOXICITY DATA with REFERENCE
ETA: skn-mus TDLo: 121 µg/kg   CNREA8
39,3549,79

MUT: mma-sat 20 µmol/L   BBRCA9 85,1568,78
MUT: msc-ham: lng 1 mg/L   BBRCA9 85,1568,78
MUT: sce-ham: ovr 1 mg/L   CALEDQ 7,45,79

CONSENSUS REPORTS: EPA Genetic Toxicology Program.

SAFETY PROFILE: Questionable carcinogen with experimental tumorigenic data. Mutation data reported. When heated to decomposition it emits acrid smoke and fumes.

DMO500   CAS: 64551-89-9
(±)-cis-3,4-DIHYDROXY-1,2-EPOXY-1,2,3,4-TETRAHYDROBENZ(a)ANTHRACENE
mf: $C_{18}H_{10}O_3$ mw: 274.28

SYNS: BENZ(a)ANTHRACENE, 3,4-DIHYDROXY-1,2-
EPOXY-1,2,3,4-TETRAHYDRO-, (Z), (+)- ◇ (±)-cis-3,4-DIHY-
DROXY-1,2-EPOXY-1,2,3,4-TETRAHYDROBENZO(a)AN-
THRACENE ◇ DIOL-EPOXIDE-1

TOXICITY DATA with REFERENCE
NEO: skn-mus TDLo: 4400 µg/kg   CNREA8
38,1705,78

SAFETY PROFILE: Questionable carcinogen with experimental neoplastigenic data. When

heated to decomposition it emits acrid smoke and irritating fumes.

DMO600   CAS: 64598-83-0
(±)-trans-8-β,9-α-DIHYDROXY-10-α,11-α-EPOXY-8,9,10,11-TETRAHYDROBENZ(a)ANTHRACENE
mf: $C_{18}H_{14}O_3$ mw: 278.32

SYNS: BA 8,9-DIOL-10,11-EPOXIDE 1 ◇ (E)-8,9,10,11-TET-
RAHYDRO-8-β,9-α-DIHYDROXY-10-α,11-α-BENZ(a)AN-
THRACENE

TOXICITY DATA with REFERENCE
ETA: skn-mus TDLo: 22 mg/kg   CNREA8
38,1699,78

CONSENSUS REPORTS: EPA Genetic Toxicology Program.

SAFETY PROFILE: Questionable carcinogen with experimental tumorigenic data. When heated to decomposition it emits acrid smoke and fumes.

DMO800   CAS: 63438-26-6
(+)-trans-3,4-DIHYDROXY-1,2-EPOXY-1,2,3,4-TETRAHYDROBENZ(a) ANTHRACENE
mf: $C_{18}H_{10}O_3$ mw: 274.28

SYNS: (E)-(+)-3,4-DIHYDROXY-1,2-EPOXY-1,2,3,4-TET-
RAHYDROBENZ(a)ANTHRACENE ◇ (+)-trans-3,4-DIHY-
DROXY-1,2-EPOXY-1,2,3,4-TETRAHYDROBENZO(a)AN-
THRACENE ◇ DIOL-EPOXIDE 2

TOXICITY DATA with REFERENCE
NEO: skn-mus TD: 4390 µg/kg   CNREA8
40,1981,80
NEO: skn-mus TDLo: 4400 µg/kg   CNREA8
38,1705,78

SAFETY PROFILE: Questionable carcinogen with experimental neoplastigenic data. When heated to decomposition it emits acrid smoke and fumes.

DMP000   CAS: 64838-75-1
(±)-trans-1,β,2,α-DIHYDROXY-3,α,4,α-EPOXY-1,2,3,4-TETRAHYDROBENZ(a)ANTHRACENE
mf: $C_{18}H_{14}O_3$ mw: 278.32

SYN: BA 1,2-DIOL-3,4-EPOXIDE 1

TOXICITY DATA with REFERENCE
ETA: skn-mus TDLo: 22 mg/kg   CNREA8
38,1699,78

SAFETY PROFILE: Questionable carcinogen with experimental tumorigenic data. When heated to decomposition it emits acrid smoke and fumes.

DMP200   CAS: 64598-82-9
(±)-trans-8-β,9-α-DIHYDROXY-10-β,11-β-EPOXY-8,9,10,11-TETRAHYDRO-BENZ(a)ANTHRACENE
mf: $C_{18}H_{14}O_3$ mw: 278.32

SYN: (E)-(±)-8,9,10,11-TETRAHYDRO-8-β,9-α-DIHY-DROXY-10-β,11-β-EPOXYBENZ(a)ANTHRACENE

TOXICITY DATA with REFERENCE
ETA: skn-mus TDLo: 22 mg/kg   CNREA8
38,1699,78

CONSENSUS REPORTS: EPA Genetic Toxicology Program.

SAFETY PROFILE: Questionable carcinogen with experimental tumorigenic data. When heated to decomposition it emits acrid smoke and fumes.

DMP600   CAS: 63323-29-5
(+)cis-7,α,8,β-DIHYDROXY-9,α,10,α-EPOXY-7,8,9,10-TETRAHYDRO-BENZO(a)PYRENE
mf: $C_{20}H_{14}O_3$ mw: 302.34

SYNS: (+)-BP-7,α,8-β-DIOL-9,α,10,α-EPOXIDE 1
◇ (+)-Z-7,8,9,10-TETRAHYDRO-7-α,8-β-DIHDYROXY-9-α,10-α-EPOXYBENZO(a)PYRENE ◇ (+)-cis-7,8,9,10-TET-RAHYDRO-7-β,8-α-DIHYDROXY-9-β,10-β-EPOXY-BENZO(a)PYRENE

TOXICITY DATA with REFERENCE
ETA: skn-mus TDLo: 1200 μg/kg   CNREA8
39,67,79
MUT: mmo-sat 100 pmol/plate   BBRCA977,1389,77

SAFETY PROFILE: Questionable carcinogen with experimental tumorigenic data. Mutation data reported. When heated to decomposition it emits acrid smoke and fumes.

DMP800   CAS: 63357-09-5
(−)-cis-7,β,8,α-DIHYDROXY-9,β,10,β-EPOXY-7,8,9,10-TETRAHYDRO-BENZO(a)PYRENE
mf: $C_{20}H_{14}O_3$ mw: 302.34

SYNS: (−)BP-7,β,8,α-DIOL-9,β,10,β-EPOXIDE 1
◇ (−)-Z-7,8,9,10-TETRAHYDRO-7-α,8-β-DIHDYROXY-9-α,10-α-EPOXYBENZO(a)PYRENE ◇ (−)-Z-7,8,9,10-TETRA-HYDRO-7-β,8-α-DIHYDROXY-9-β,10-β-EPOXYBENZO(a)PY-RENE

TOXICITY DATA with REFERENCE
ETA: skn-mus TDLo: 1200 μg/kg   CNREA8
39,67,79
MUT: dnd-mus-skn 8 μmol/kg   CNREA844,1081,84
MUT: mmo-sat 100 pmol/plate   BBRCA977,1389,77
MUT: msc-ham: lng 1 μmol/L   MUREAV44,313,77

SAFETY PROFILE: Questionable carcinogen with experimental tumorigenic data. Mutation data reported. When heated to decomposition it emits acrid smoke and irritating fumes.

DMP900   CAS: 58917-67-2
(±)-(E)-7,8-DIHYDROXY-9,10-EPOXY-7,8,9,10-TETRAHYDRO-BENZO(a)PYRENE
mf: $C_{20}H_{14}O_3$ mw: 302.34
SYN: BP 7,8-DIOL-9,10-EPOXIDE 2

TOXICITY DATA with REFERENCE
ETA: skn-mus TDLo: 2400 μg/kg   CNREA8
39,67,79

SAFETY PROFILE: Questionable carcinogen with experimental tumorigenic data. When heated to decomposition it emits acrid smoke and irritating fumes.

DMR000   CAS: 58917-91-2
(±)-7,β,8,α-DIHYDROXY-9,β,10,β-EPOXY-7,8,9,10-TETRAHYDRO-BENZO(a)PYRENE
mf: $C_{20}H_{14}O_3$ mw: 302.34

SYNS: BPDE-syn ◇ B(a)P EPOXIDE I ◇ (±)-7-α,8-β-DIHYDROXY-9-α,10-α-EPOXY-7,8,9,10-TETRAHYDROBEN-ZO(a)PYRENE ◇ (±)-7,8,8a,9a-TETRAHYDRO-BENZO(10,11)CHYRSENO(3,4-b)OXIRENE-7,8-DIOL
◇ (±)-7,8,9,10-TETRAHYDRO-7-α,8-β-DIHYDROXY-9-α,10-α-EPOXYBENZO(a)PYRENE

TOXICITY DATA with REFERENCE
ETA: skn-mus TD: 89 mg/kg/37W-I   CNREA8
37,3356,77
ETA: skn-mus TDLo: 2420 μg/kg   CCSUDL
3,371,78
MUT: dnd-mam: lym 600 nmol   CRNGDP3,267,82
MUT: dnd-mus-skn 20 μmol/kg   CRNGDP
3,1135,82
MUT: dnr-hmn: fbr 1 μmol/L   CBINA8 20,279,78

MUT: mma-sat 300 pmol/plate CNREA8 36,3358,76
MUT: mmo-sat 300 pmol/plate CNREA8 36,3358,76
MUT: oms-mus-skn 20 μmol/kg CRNGDP
3,1135,82

SAFETY PROFILE: Questionable carcinogen with experimental tumorigenic data. Human mutation data reported. When heated to decomposition it emits acrid smoke and fumes.

DMR150
(±)-9-α-10-β-DIHYDROXY-11-β,12-β-EPOXY-9,10,11,12-TETRAHYDRO-BENZO(e)PYRENE
mf: $C_{20}H_{14}O_3$ mw: 302.34

SYNS: BENZO(e)PYRENE, 9,10-DIOL-11,12-EPOXIDE 1 (cis) ◇ B(e)P DIOL EPOXIDE-1 ◇ B(e)P 9,10-DIOL-11,12-EPOX-IDE-1

TOXICITY DATA with REFERENCE
CAR: ipr-mus TDLo:476 mg/kg CNREA8
41,915,81

SAFETY PROFILE: Questionable carcinogen with experimental carcinogenic data. When heated to decomposition it emits acrid smoke and irritating fumes.

DMR200
(±)-9,β,10,α-DIHYDROXY-11,α,12,α-EPOXY-9,10,11,12-TETRAHYDRO-BENZO(e)PYRENE
mf: $C_{20}H_{14}O_3$ mw: 302.3

SYN: B(E)P DIOL EPOXIDE-2

TOXICITY DATA with REFERENCE
CAR: ipr-mus TDLo:476 mg/kg CNREA8
41,915,81

MUT: mma-sat 1 nmol/plate CNREA8 40,1985,80
MUT: mmo-sat 1 nmol/plate CNREA8 40,1985,80
MUT: msc-ham:lng 1 nmol/L CNREA8 40,1985,80

SAFETY PROFILE: Questionable carcinogen with experimental carcinogenic data. Mutation data reported. When heated to decomposition it emits acrid smoke and fumes.

DMS000
trans-1,2-DIHYDROXY-anti-3,4-EPOXY-1,2,3,4-TETRAHYDROCHRYSENE
mf: $C_{18}H_{14}O$ mw: 278.32

SYN: (+)-(E)-3,4-EPOXY-1,2,3,4-TETRAHYDRO-CHRYS-ENEDIOL

TOXICITY DATA with REFERENCE
NEO: skn-mus TDLo:20 mg/kg CNREA8
40,1981,80

SAFETY PROFILE: Questionable carcinogen with experimental neoplastigenic data. When heated to decomposition it emits acrid smoke and fumes.

DMS200   CAS: 72074-67-0
(±)-1,β,2,α-DIHYDROXY-3,α,4,α-EPOXY-1,2,3,4-TETRAHYDROCHRYSENE
mf: $C_{18}H_{14}O_3$ mw: 278.32

SYN: (±)-1,2,3,4-TETRAHYDRO-3,α,4,α-EPOXY-1,β,2,α-CHRYSENEDIOL

TOXICITY DATA with REFERENCE
CAR: ipr-mus TDLo:72 mg/kg/15D-I CNREA8
39,5063,79
MUT: mma-sat 1 nmol/plate CNREA8 39,4069,79
MUT: mmo-sat 1 nmol/L CRNGDP 6,237,85

SAFETY PROFILE: Questionable carcinogen with experimental carcinogenic data. Mutation data reported. When heated to decomposition it emits acrid smoke and fumes.

DMS400   CAS: 72074-66-9
(±)-1,β,2,α-DIHYDROXY-3,β,4,β-EPOXY-1,2,3,4-TETRAHYDROCHRYSENE
mf: $C_{18}H_{14}O_3$ mw: 278.32

SYN: (±)-1,2,3,4-TETRAHYDRO-3,β,4,β-EPOXY-1-β,2-α-CHRYSENEDIOL

TOXICITY DATA with REFERENCE
ETA: ipr-mus TDLo:72 mg/kg/15D-I CNREA8
39,5063,79
MUT: mma-sat 1 nmol/plate CNREA8 39,4069,79
MUT: msc-ham:lng 1 nmol/plate CNREA8
39,4069,79

SAFETY PROFILE: Questionable carcinogen with experimental tumorigenic data. Mutation data reported. When heated to decomposition it emits acrid smoke and fumes.

DMX000   CAS: 69260-83-9
(E)-3,4-DIHYDROXY-7-METHYL-3,4-DIHYDROBENZ(a)ANTHRACENE-12-METHANOL
mf: $C_{20}H_{18}O_3$ mw: 306.38

SYNS: trans-3,4-DIHYDRO-12-(HYDROXYMETHYL)-7-METHYLBENZ(a)ANTHRACENE-3,4-DIOL ◇ trans-3,4-DIHY-DROXY-3,4-DIHYDRO-7-METHYL-12-HYDROXYMETHYL-BENZ(a)ANTHRACENE

TOXICITY DATA with REFERENCE
ETA: skn-mus TDLo:110 μg/kg CNREA8
40,3661,80

MUT: mma-ham:lng 400 nmol/L   PNASA6
76,862,79

MUT: mma-sat 35 nmol/plate   CNREA8 40,3661,80

SAFETY PROFILE: Questionable carcinogen with experimental tumorigenic data. Mutation data reported. When heated to decomposition it emits acrid smoke and fumes.

DMX200   CAS: 2318-18-5
2,12-DIHYDROXY-4-METHYL-11,16-DIOXOSENECIONANIUM
mf: $C_{19}H_{28}NO_6$ mw: 366.48

SYNS: trans-15-ETHYLIDENE-12-β-HYDROXY-4,12-α,13-β-TRIMETHYL 8-OXO-4,8 SECOSENEC-1-ENINE ◇ 12-HYDROXY-4-METHYL-4,8-SECOSENECIONAN-8,11,16-TRIONE ◇ NSC-89945 ◇ RENARDIN ◇ RENARDINE ◇ SENKIRKIN ◇ SENKIRKINE

TOXICITY DATA with REFERENCE
NEO: ipr-rat TDLo: 1320 mg/kg/56W-I   JJIND8
63,469,79

MUT: dns-ham:lvr 2 μmol/L   CNREA8 45,3125,85
MUT: dns-mus:lvr 20 μmol/L   CNREA8 45,3125,85
MUT: dns-rat:lvr 2 μmol/L   CNREA8 45,3125,85
MUT: mma-sat 1 mg/plate   MUREAV 68,211,79
MUT: sce-ham:lng 60 μg/L   MUREAV 142,209,85
MUT: sln-dmg-orl 10 μmol/L/3D-I   FCTOD7
22,223,84

CONSENSUS REPORTS: IARC Cancer Review: GROUP 3 IMEMDT 7,56,87; Animal Limited Evidence IMEMDT 31,231,83; Animal Inadequate Evidence IMEMDT 10,327,76.

SAFETY PROFILE: Questionable carcinogen with experimental neoplastigenic data. Poison by ingestion and intraperitoneal routes. Mutation data reported. When heated to decomposition it emits toxic fumes of NO_x.

DNA200   CAS: 59-92-7
l-DIHYDROXYPHENYL-l-ALANINE
mf: $C_9H_{11}NO_4$ mw: 197.21

SYNS: 2-AMINO-3-(3,4-DIHYDROXYPHENYL)PROPANOIC ACID ◇ BENDOPA ◇ BIODOPA ◇ BROCADOPA ◇ CEREPAP ◇ CIDANDOPA ◇ DA ◇ DEADOPA ◇ DIHYDROXY-l-PHENYLALANINE ◇ (−)-3-(3,4-DIHYDROXYPHENYL)-l-ALANINE ◇ β-(3,4-DIHYDROXYPHENYL)-α-ALANINE ◇ l-α-DIHYDROXYPHENYLALANINE ◇ l-β-(3,4-DIHYDROXYPHENYL)ALANINE ◇ l-3,4-DIHYDROXYPHENYL-α-ALANINE ◇ β-(3,4-DIHYDROXYPHENYL)-l-ALANINE ◇ 3-(3,4-DIHYDROXYPHENYL)-l-ALANINE ◇ 3,4-DIHYDROXYPHENYLALANINE ◇ (−)-3,4-DIHYDROXY-

PHENYLALANINE ◇ 3,4-DIHYDROXYPHENYL-l-ALANINE ◇ 3,4-DIHYDROXY-l-PHENYLALANINE ◇ l-3,4-DIHYDROXYPHENYLALANINE ◇ (−)-DOPA ◇ l-DOPA ◇ DOPAFLEX ◇ DOPAL ◇ DOPARKINE ◇ DOPASOL ◇ DOPRIN ◇ ELDOPAL ◇ EURODOPA ◇ HELFO DOPA ◇ l-o-HYDROXYTYROSINE ◇ 3-HYDROXY-l-TYROSINE ◇ INSULAMINA ◇ LARODOPA ◇ MAIPEDOPA ◇ PARDA ◇ RO 4-6316 ◇ SOBIODOPA ◇ VELDOPA

TOXICITY DATA with REFERENCE
CAR: orl-man TDLo: 87520 mg/kg/1.5Y-C: SKN   NEURAI 24,340,74
MUT: dnd-hmn:fbr 3 mmol/L   CNREA8 42,3783,82
MUT: dnd-rat:lng 25 μmol/L   ABCHA6 39,795,75
MUT: dni-hmn:fbr 3 mmol/L   CNREA8 42,3783,82
MUT: dni-rat:lng 25 μmol/L   ABCHA6 39,795,75
MUT: dnr-bcs 500 μg/disc   MUREAV 137,17,84

CONSENSUS REPORTS: Reported in EPA TSCA Inventory.

SAFETY PROFILE: Questionable human carcinogen producing skin tumors. Experimental teratogenic data. Poison by ingestion. Moderately toxic by intravenous, intraperitoneal, and possibly other routes. Human systemic effects by ingestion: somnolence, hallucinations and distorted perceptions, toxic psychosis, motor activity changes, ataxia, dyspnea. Experimental reproductive effects. Human mutation data reported. An anticholinergic agent used as an antiparkinsonian drug. When heated to decomposition it emits toxic fumes of NO_x.

DNB600   CAS: 33372-40-6
4-(2,3-DIHYDROXYPROPYLAMINO)-2-(5-NITRO-2-THIENYL)QUINAZOLINE
mf: $C_{15}H_{14}N_4O_4S$ mw: 346.39

TOXICITY DATA with REFERENCE
CAR: orl-rat TDLo: 8313 mg/kg/47W-C   JNCIAM 57,277,76
MUT: mma-sat 1250 μg/plate   CNREA8 35,3611,75

SAFETY PROFILE: Questionable carcinogen with experimental carcinogenic data. Mutation data reported. When heated to decomposition it emits very toxic fumes of NO_x and SO_x.

DNC200   CAS: 59-00-7
4,8-DIHYDROXYQUINALDIC ACID
mf: $C_{10}H_7NO_4$ mw: 205.18

PROP: Sulfur-yellow crystals. Mp: 286°. Insol in water; sol in aqueous alkali, hydroxides, and hot dil HCl.

SYNS: 4,8-DIHYDROXYQUINALDINIC ACID ◇ 4,8-DIHY-DROXYQUINOLINE-2-CARBOXYLIC ACID ◇ XANTHU-RENIC ACID

TOXICITY DATA with REFERENCE
NEO: imp-mus TDLo:160 mg/kg   ANYAA9
108,924,63

SAFETY PROFILE: Questionable carcinogen with experimental neoplastigenic data. When heated to decomposition it emits toxic fumes of NO_x.

DNC400   CAS: 66788-03-2
trans-9,10-DIHYDROXY-9,10,11,12-TETRAHYDROBENZO(e)PYRENE
mf: $C_{20}H_{16}O_2$ mw: 288.36

SYN: B(E)P H4-9,10-DIOL

TOXICITY DATA with REFERENCE
ETA: skn-mus TDLo:69 mg/kg   CNREA840,203,80
MUT: mma-sat 10 nmol/plate   JBCHA3 254,4408,79

SAFETY PROFILE: Questionable carcinogen with experimental tumorigenic data. Mutation data reported. When heated to decomposition it emits acrid smoke and fumes.

DNC600   CAS: 73771-79-6
trans-1,2-DIHYDROXY-1,2,3,4-TETRAHYDROCHRYSENE
mf: $C_{18}H_{16}O_2$ mw: 264.34

SYN: trans-1,2,3,4-TETRAHYDROCHRYSENE-1,2,-DIOL

TOXICITY DATA with REFERENCE
NEO: skn-mus TDLo:42 mg/kg   CNREA8
38,1831,78

SAFETY PROFILE: Questionable carcinogen with experimental neoplastigenic data. When heated to decomposition it emits acrid smoke and irritating fumes.

DNC800   CAS: 70443-38-8
trans-3,4-DIHYDROXY-1,2,3,4-TETRAHYDRODIBENZ(a,h)ANTHRACENE
mf: $C_{22}H_{18}O_2$ mw: 314.40

SYN: trans-3,4-DIHYDROXY-1,2,3,4-TETRAHYDRODI-BENZO(a,h)ANTHRACENE

TOXICITY DATA with REFERENCE
ETA: skn-mus TDLo:2010 mg/kg   CNREA8
39,1310,79
MUT: mma-sat 60 μg/plate   MUREAV 96,1,82

SAFETY PROFILE: Questionable carcinogen with experimental tumorigenic data. Mutation data reported. When heated to decomposition it emits acrid smoke and fumes.

DNE400   CAS: 3468-11-9
1,3-DIIMINOISOINDOLINE
mf: $C_8H_7N_3$ mw: 145.18

SYNS: AFASTOGEN BLUE 5040 ◇ 1,3-DIIMINOISOINDO-LIN (CZECH) ◇ FASTOGEN BLUE FP-3100 ◇ FASTOGEN BLUE SH-100 ◇ MODR FRALOSTANOVA 3G (CZECH) ◇ PHTHALIMIDIMIDE ◇ PHTHALOCYANINE BLUE 01206 ◇ PHTHALOGEN

TOXICITY DATA with REFERENCE
CAR: scu-mus TDLo:140 mg/kg/51W-I
VOONAW 21(11),75,75
ETA: scu-rat TDLo:990 mg/kg/44W-I
VOONAW 21(11),75,75

CONSENSUS REPORTS: Reported in EPA TSCA Inventory.

SAFETY PROFILE: Questionable carcinogen with experimental carcinogenic and tumorigenic data. Poison by ingestion. A severe eye and skin irritant. When heated to decomposition it emits toxic fumes of NO_x.

DNO900   CAS: 2973-10-6
DIISOPROPYL ESTER SULFURIC ACID
mf: $C_6H_{14}O_4S$ mw: 182.26

SYNS: DI-ISOPROPYLSULFAT (GERMAN) ◇ DI-ISOPRO-PYLSULFATE ◇ ISOPROPYL SULFATE

TOXICITY DATA with REFERENCE
ETA: scu-rat TDLo:300 mg/kg   ZKKOBW
79,135,73

SAFETY PROFILE: Questionable carcinogen with experimental tumorigenic data. Moderately toxic by ingestion and skin contact. When heated to decomposition it emits toxic fumes of SO_x.

DNP600   CAS: 20652-39-5
N,N-DIISOPROPYL ETHYL CARBAMATE
mf: $C_9H_{19}NO_2$ mw: 173.29

SYNS: DIISOPROPYLCARBAMIC ACID, ETHYL ESTER ◇ DIISOPROPYL ETHYL CARBAMATE

TOXICITY DATA with REFERENCE
ETA: ipr-mus TDLo:6500 mg/kg/13W-I
JNCIAM 9,35,48

SAFETY PROFILE: Questionable carcinogen with experimental tumorigenic data. When heated to decomposition it emits toxic fumes of NO_x.

DNS000   CAS: 26762-93-6
DIISOPROPYLPHENYLHYDROPEROX-IDE (SOLUTION)
DOT: 2171
mf: $C_{12}H_{19}O_2$ mw: 195.31

PROP: Colorless to pale yellow liquid.

SYN: DIISOPROPYLBENZENE HYDROPEROXIDE, not more than 72% in solution (DOT)

TOXICITY DATA with REFERENCE
ETA: unr-mus TDLo:391 mg/kg   RARSAM 3,193,63

CONSENSUS REPORTS: Reported in EPA TSCA Inventory.

DOT Classification: Organic Peroxide; Label: Organic Peroxide.

SAFETY PROFILE: Questionable carcinogen with experimental tumorigenic data. A powerful oxidizer. When heated to decomposition it emits acrid smoke and fumes.

DNW800   CAS: 2303-47-1
cis-1,4-DIMETHANE SULFONOXY-2-BUTENE
mf: $C_6H_{12}O_6S_2$ mw: 244.30

TOXICITY DATA with REFERENCE
NEO: skn-mus TDLo:480 mg/kg/10W-I
   CNREA8 17,64,57
MUT: sln-dmg-par 10 mmol/L   JOGNAU 54,146,56

SAFETY PROFILE: Questionable carcinogen with experimental neoplastigenic data. Mutation data reported. When heated to decomposition it emits toxic fumes of SO_x.

DNX000   CAS: 1953-56-6
trans-1,4-DIMETHANE SULFONOXY-2-BUTENE
mf: $C_6H_{12}O_6S_2$ mw: 244.30

SYNS: CB 2095 ◊ 2-BUTENE-1,4-DIOL, DIMETHANESUL-FONATE, (E)-

TOXICITY DATA with REFERENCE
NEO: skn-mus TDLo:480 mg/kg/10W-I
   CNREA8 17,64,57
MUT: sln-dmg-par 10 mmol/L   JOGNAU 54,146,56

SAFETY PROFILE: Questionable carcinogen with experimental neoplastigenic data. Mutation data reported. When heated to decomposition it emits toxic fumes of SO_x.

DNX200   CAS: 2917-96-6
1,4-DIMETHANESULFONOXY-2-BUTYNE
mf: $C_6H_{10}O_6S_2$ mw: 242.28

SYN: CB2058

TOXICITY DATA with REFERENCE
NEO: skn-mus TDLo:320 mg/kg/5W-I   CNREA8 17,64,57
MUT: sln-dmg-par 10 mmol/L   JOGNAU 54,146,56
MUT: sln-dmg-unk 10 mmol/L   ANYAA9 160,228,69

SAFETY PROFILE: Questionable carcinogen with experimental neoplastigenic data by skin contact. Mutation data reported. When heated to decomposition it emits toxic fumes of SO_x.

DNY400   CAS: 17210-48-9
3,4'-DIMETHOXY-4-AMINOAZOBENZENE
mf: $C_{14}H_{15}N_3O_2$ mw: 257.32

SYN: 4-((p-METHOXYPHENYL)AZO)-o-ANISIDINE

TOXICITY DATA with REFERENCE
ETA: orl-rat TDLo:10 g/kg/24W-C   GANNA2 59,131,68

CONSENSUS REPORTS: IARC Cancer Review: Human Inadequate Evidence IMEMDT 27,39,82; Animal Inadequate Evidence IMEMDT 27,39,82.

SAFETY PROFILE: Questionable carcinogen with experimental tumorigenic data. Human systemic effects by ingestion: methemoglobine-mia-carboxhemoglobinemia, and changes in porphyrin metabolism. When heated to decomposition it emits toxic fumes of NO_x.

DOA000   CAS: 16354-53-3
7,12-DIMETHOXYBENZ(a)ANTHRACENE
mf: $C_{20}H_{16}O_2$ mw: 288.36

TOXICITY DATA with REFERENCE
NEO: ims-rat TD:50 mg/kg   PNASA6 58,2253,67
NEO: ims-rat TDLO:50 mg/kg   CNREA8 29,506,69

SAFETY PROFILE: Questionable carcinogen with experimental neoplastigenic data. When heated to decomposition it emits acrid smoke and irritating fumes.

DOB600 CAS: 63040-49-3
5,6-DIMETHOXYDIBENZ(a,h) ANTHRACENE
mf: $C_{24}H_{18}O_2$ mw: 338.42

SYNS: 3,4-DIMETHOXY-DBA ◇ 3,4-DIMETHOXY-1,2:5,6-DIBENZANTHRACENE

TOXICITY DATA with REFERENCE
NEO: skn-mus TDLo:600 mg/kg/60W-I
CNREA8 22,78,62
ETA: scu-mus TDLo:80 mg/kg/4W-I CNREA8 22,78,62

SAFETY PROFILE: Questionable carcinogen with experimental neoplastigenic and tumorigenic data. When heated to decomposition it emits acrid smoke and irritating fumes.

DOO400 CAS: 6483-64-3
3,3'-DIMETHOXYTRIPHENYLMETHANE-4,4'-BIS(1''-AZO-2''-NAPHTHOL)
mf: $C_{41}H_{32}N_4O_4$ mw: 644.77

SYN: 1,1'-(BENZYLIDENEBIS((2-METHOXY-p-PHENYLENE)(AZO))DI-2-NAPHTHOL

TOXICITY DATA with REFERENCE
ETA: orl-rat TDLo:40 g/kg/83W-C ZEKBAI 57,530,51

CONSENSUS REPORTS: Reported in EPA TSCA Inventory.

SAFETY PROFILE: Questionable carcinogen with experimental tumorigenic data. When heated to decomposition it emits toxic fumes of NO_x.

DOR600 CAS: 506-59-2
DIMETHYLAMINE HYDROCHLORIDE
mf: $C_2H_7N \cdot ClH$ mw: 81.56

SYNS: DIMETHYLAMMONIUM CHLORIDE ◇ HYDROCHLORIC ACID DIMETHYLAMINE ◇ N-METHYLMETHANAMINE HYDROCHLORIDE

TOXICITY DATA with REFERENCE
NEO: orl-mus TDLo:12 g/kg/Y-C GISAAA 44(8),15,79

CONSENSUS REPORTS: Reported in EPA TSCA Inventory. EPA Genetic Toxicology Program.

SAFETY PROFILE: Questionable carcinogen with experimental neoplastigenic data. Moderately toxic by ingestion, intravenous, subcutaneous, and intraperitoneal routes. When heated to decomposition it emits very toxic fumes of NO_x, NH_3 and HCl.

DOS000 CAS: 315-18-4
4-(DIMETHYLAMINE)-3,5-XYLYL-N-METHYLCARBAMATE
DOT: 2757
mf: $C_{12}H_{18}N_2O_2$ mw: 222.32

PROP: Crystals. Mp: 85°, vap press: <0.1 mm @ 139°.

SYNS: 4-(DIMETHYLAMINO)-3,5-DIMETHYLPHENOL METHYLCARBAMATE (ESTER) ◇ 4-(DIMETHYLAMINO)-3,5-DIMETHYLPHENYL ESTER, METHYLCARBAMIC ACID ◇ 4-(DIMETHYLAMINO)-3,5-DIMETHYLPHENYL-N-METHYLCARBAMATE ◇ 4-(DIMETHYLAMINO)-3,5-XYLENOL METHYLCARBAMATE (ESTER) ◇ 4-(DIMETHYLAMINO)-3,5-XYLYL ESTER METHYLCARBAMIC ACID ◇ 4-DIMETHYLAMINO-3,5-XYLYL METHYLCARBAMATE ◇ 4-DIMETHYLAMINO-3,5-XYLYL-N-METHYLCARBAMATE ◇ 4-(N,N-DIMETHYLAMINO)-3,5-XYLYL N-METHYLCARBAMATE ◇ DOWCO 139 ◇ ENT 25,766 ◇ METHYL-4-DIMETHYLAMINO-3,5-XYLYL CARBAMATE ◇ METHYL-4-DIMETHYLAMINO-3,5-XYLYL ESTER of CARBAMIC ACID ◇ MEXACARBATE (DOT) ◇ NCI-C00544 ◇ OMS-47 ◇ ZACTRAN ◇ ZECTANE ◇ ZECTRAN ◇ ZEXTRAN

TOXICITY DATA with REFERENCE
NEO: orl-mus TDLo:1200 mg/kg/78W-I
NTIS** PB223-159

CONSENSUS REPORTS: IARC Cancer Review: Animal Inadequate Evidence IMEMDT 12,237,76. NCI Carcinogenesis Bioassay (feed); No Evidence: mouse, rat NCITR* NCI-CG-TR-147,78. EPA Extremely Hazardous Substances List.

DOT Classification: Poison B; Label: Poison.

SAFETY PROFILE: Questionable carcinogen with experimental neoplastigenic and teratogenic data. Poison by ingestion, intraperitoneal, and possibly other routes. Moderately toxic by skin contact. Experimental reproductive effects. When heated to decomposition it emits toxic fumes of NO_x.

DOT000 CAS: 58-15-1
DIMETHYLAMINOANTIPYRINE
mf: $C_{13}H_{17}N_3O$ mw: 231.33

PROP: Colorless leaflets, somewhat water-sol. Mp: 107-109°.

SYNS: AMIDAZOPHEN ◇ AMIDOFEBRIN ◇ AMIDOPHEN ◇ AMIDOPHENAZONE ◇ AMIDOPYRAZOLINE ◇ AMIDOPYRIN ◇ AMINOFENAZONE (ITALIAN) ◇ AMINOPHENAZONE ◇ AMINOPYRINE ◇ ANAFEBRINA ◇ BRUFANEUXOL

◇ DAP ◇ DEREUMA ◇ DIMAPYRIN ◇ DIMETHYLAMINO-ANALGESINE ◇ 4-(DIMETHYLAMINO)ANTIPYRINE ◇ DIMETHYLAMINOAZOPHENE ◇ 4-(DIMETHYLAMINO)-1,2-DIHYDRO-1,5-DIMETHYL-2-PHENYL-3H-PYRAZOL-3-ONE ◇ 4-DIMETHYLAMINO-2,3-DIMETHYL-1-PHENYL-3-PYRAZOLIN-5-ONE ◇ 4-DIMETHYLAMINO-2,3-DIMETHYL-1-PHENYL-5-PYRAZOLONE ◇ DIMETHYLAMINOPHENA-ZON (GERMAN) ◇ DIMETHYLAMINOPHENAZONE ◇ 4-DIMETHYLAMINOPHENAZONE ◇ DIMETHYLAMINO-PHENYLDIMETHYLPYRAZOLIN ◇ 4-DIMETHYL-AMINO-1-PHENYL-2,3-DIMETHYLPYRAZOLONE ◇ 3-keto-1,5-DIMETHYL-4-DIMETHYLAMINO-2-PHENYL-2,3-DIHYDROPYRAZOLE ◇ 1,5-DIMETHYL-4-DI-METHYLAMINO-2-PHENYL-3-PYRAZOLONE ◇ 2,3-DI-METHYL-4-DIMETHYLAMINO-1-PHENYL-5-PYRAZO-LONE ◇ DIPIRIN ◇ DIPYRIN ◇ FEBRININA ◇ FEBRON ◇ ITAMIDONE ◇ MAMALLET-A ◇ NETSUSARIN ◇ NOVAMIDON ◇ 1-PHENYL-2,3-DIMETHYL-4-DIMETH-YLAMINOPYRAZOL-5-ONE ◇ 1-PHENYL-2,3-DIMETHYL-4-DIMETHYLAMINOPYRAZOLONE-5 ◇ PIRAMIDON ◇ PIRIDOL ◇ PIROMIDINA ◇ POLINALIN ◇ PYRADONE ◇ PYRAMIDON ◇ PYRAMIDONE

TOXICITY DATA with REFERENCE

MUT: cyt-ham:fbr 3 mmol/L   HDSKEK 10,63,85
MUT: dni-mus:oth 100 mg/L   ONCODU 19,183,80
MUT: mma-sat 31 μmol/plate   MUREAV 66,33,79
MUT: msc-ham-orl 100 mg/kg   IAPUDO 41,585,82
MUT: otr-ham-orl 100 mg/kg   IAPUDO 41,585,82

CONSENSUS REPORTS: Reported in EPA TSCA Inventory. EPA Genetic Toxicology Program.

SAFETY PROFILE: Mixed with $NaNO_2$ (1:1) it is a questionable carcinogen. Human poison by unspecified route. Experimental poison by ingestion, subcutaneous, intramuscular, intravenous, intraperitoneal and possibly other routes. Moderately toxic by parenteral route. An experimental teratogen. Experimental reproductive effects. Mutation data reported. Can cause bone marrow depression resulting in leucopenia. Has been implicated in development of aplastic anemia. A tranquilizer. When heated to decomposition it emits toxic fumes of NO_x.

DOT200
4-(DIMETHYLAMINO)ANTIPYRINE mixed with SODIUM NITRITE (1:1)
mf: $C_{13}H_{17}N_3O \cdot NNaO_2$ mw: 300.33

SYNS: AMINOPHENAZONE mixed with SODIUM NITRITE (1:1) ◇ AMINOPYRINE mixed with SODIUM NITRITE (1:1) ◇ SODIUM NITRITE mixed with AMINOPYRINE (1:1)

◇ SODIUM NITRITE mixed with 4-(DIMETHYLAMINO)ANTI-PYRINE (1:1)

TOXICITY DATA with REFERENCE
CAR: orl-rat TD: 10 g/kg/40W-I   IARCCD 14,461,76
CAR: orl-rat TD: 8000 mg/kg/40W-I   IARCCD 14,461,76
CAR: orl-rat TDLo: 3438 mg/kg/50W-I   NATUAS 244,176,73
MUT: cyt-rat-orl 600 mg/kg   MFEPDX 1,225,79
MUT: hma-mus/esc 10 mg/kg   CBINA8 35,199,81
MUT: hma-mus/sat 2 mmol/L/kg   ATSUDG (4),49,80
MUT: mma-sat 1 mg/plate   TOLED5 12,281,82
MUT: mmo-sat 1 mg/plate   TOLED5 12,281,82

SAFETY PROFILE: Questionable carcinogen with experimental carcinogenic data. Mutation data reported. When heated to decomposition it emits toxic fumes of NO_x and Na_2O.

DOT600   CAS: 443-30-1
1-(4-DIMETHYLAMINOBENZAL)INDENE
mf: $C_{18}H_{17}N$ mw: 247.36

SYNS: DABI ◇ (4-DIMETHYLAMINOBENZYLIDENE) INDENE ◇ N,N-DIMETHYL-α-INDOLYLIDENE-p-TOLUI-DINE ◇ 4-(1H-INDEN-1-YLIDENEMETHYL)-N,N-DIMETHYL-BENZENAMINE ◇ NSC-80087

TOXICITY DATA with REFERENCE
ETA: orl-mus TDLo: 4000 mg/kg/26W-C   PTEUA6 7,229,72
ETA: orl-rat TDLo: 270 mg/kg/15D-I: TER   NATUAS 222,383,69

SAFETY PROFILE: Questionable carcinogen with experimental tumorigenic and teratogenic data. Moderately toxic by intraperitoneal route. When heated to decomposition it emits toxic fumes of NO_x.

DOU600   CAS: 140-56-7
p-DIMETHYLAMINOBENZENEDIAZO-SODIUM SULPHONATE
mf: $C_8H_{10}N_3O_3S \cdot Na$ mw: 251.26

PROP: Yellow-brown crystals.

SYNS: BAYER 5072 ◇ DAPA ◇ DAS ◇ DEKSONAL ◇ DEXON ◇ p-DIMETHYLAMINOBENZENE DIAZO SODIUM SULFONATE ◇ p-(DIMETHYLAMINO)BENZENEDIAZO-SULFONATE ◇ p-DIMETHYLAMINOBENZENEDIAZO-SULFONIC ACID, SODIUM SALT ◇ 4-DIMETHYL-AMINOBENZENEDIAZOSULFONIC ACID, SODIUM SALT ◇ p-(DIMETHYLAMINO)BENZENEDIAZOSULPHONATE

◇ p-(DIMETHYLAMINO)BENZENEDIAZOSULPHONIC ACID, SODIUM SALT ◇ 4-DIMETHYLAMINOBENZENEDIAZO-SULPHONIC ACID, SODIUM SALT ◇ p-DIMETHYL-AMINOBENZOLDIAZOSULFONAT (NATRIUMSALZ) (GERMAN) ◇ (4-(DIMETHYLAMINO)PHENYL)DIAZENE-SULFONIC ACID, SODIUM SALT ◇ 4-((DIMETHYLAMINO)PHENYL)DIAZENESULFONIC ACID, SODIUM SALT ◇ p-(DIMETHYLAMINO)-PHENYLDIAZO-NATRIUM-SULFONAT (GERMAN) ◇ N,N-DIMETHYL-p-ANILINE-DIAZOSULFONIC ACID SODIUM SALT ◇ FENAMINO-SULF ◇ GOLD ORANGE MP ◇ LESAN ◇ NCI-C03010 ◇ SODIUM-p-(DIMETHYLAMINO)BENZENEDIAZOSUL-FONATE ◇ SODIUM-4-(DIMETHYLAMINO)BENZENE-DIAZOSULFONATE ◇ SODIUM-p-(DIMETHYLAMINO)BENZENEDIAZOSULPHONATE ◇ SODIUM-4-(DIMETHYL-AMINO)BENZENEDIAZOSULPHONATE ◇ SODIUM-(4-(DIMETHYLAMINO)PHENYL)DIAZENESULFONATE ◇ TROPAEOLIN D

TOXICITY DATA with REFERENCE

MUT: cyt-ham: lng 50 μmol/L   MUREAV 78,177,80
MUT: dnr-bcs 1 μg/disc   MUREAV 97,339,82
MUT: mmo-esc 25 μg/plate   YACHDS 13,4923,85
MUT: mmo-sat 25 μg/plate   YACHDS 13,4923,85
MUT: sce-hmn: lym 25 μmol/L   MUREAV 79,53,80

CONSENSUS REPORTS: IARC Cancer Review: GROUP 3 IMEMDT 7,56,87; Animal Inadequate Evidence IMEMDT 8,147,75. NCI Carcinogenesis Bioassay (feed); No Evidence: mouse, rat NCITR* NCI-CG-TR-101,78. EPA Genetic Toxicology Program.

SAFETY PROFILE: Questionable carcinogen. Poison by ingestion, intravenous, intraperitoneal, and possibly other routes. An experimental teratogen. Experimental reproductive effects. Human mutation data reported. A fungicide. When heated to decomposition it emits very toxic fumes of NO_x, Na_2O and SO_x.

DOV000   CAS: 63918-82-1
p-DIMETHYLAMINOBENZYLIDENE-3,4,5,6-DIBENZ-9-METHYLACRIDINE
mf: $C_{31}H_{24}N_2$ mw: 424.57

SYN: 14-(p-(DIMETHYLAMINO)STYRYL)DI-BENZ(a,j)ACRIDINE

TOXICITY DATA with REFERENCE
ETA: scu-mus TDLo: 200 mg/kg   VOONAW 1,52,55

SAFETY PROFILE: Questionable carcinogen with experimental tumorigenic data. When

heated to decomposition it emits toxic fumes of NO_x.

DOV200   CAS: 13629-82-8
3,3′-DIMETHYL-4-AMINOBIPHENYL
mf: $C_{14}H_{15}N$ mw: 197.30

SYNS: 3,3′-DIMETHYL-4-AMINODIPHENYL ◇ 3,3′-DI-METHYL-4-BIPHENYLAMINE

TOXICITY DATA with REFERENCE
CAR: scu-rat TDLo: 960 mg/kg/21W-I   ANZJA7 29,38,59
ETA: scu-rat TD: 2400 mg/kg/W-I   BMBUAQ 14,141,58

SAFETY PROFILE: Questionable carcinogen with experimental carcinogenic and tumorigenic data. When heated to decomposition it emits toxic fumes of NO_x.

DOV400   CAS: 63019-93-2
4-(DIMETHYLAMINO)-3-BIPHENYLOL
mf: $C_{14}H_{15}NO$ mw: 213.30

SYN: 4-DIMETHYLAMINO-3-HYDROXYDIPHENYL

TOXICITY DATA with REFERENCE
ETA: imp-mus TDLo: 80 mg/kg   BJCAAI 11,212,57

SAFETY PROFILE: Questionable carcinogen with experimental tumorigenic data. When heated to decomposition it emits toxic fumes of NO_x.

DPJ400   CAS: 135-23-9
2-((2-(DIMETHYLAMINO)ETHYL)-2-THENYL-AMINO)PYRIDINE HYDROCHLORIDE
mf: $C_{14}H_{19}N_3S \cdot ClH$ mw: 297.88

SYNS: BARHIST ◇ CAPATHYN ◇ CORYZOL ◇ N,N-DI-METHYL-N′-2-PYRIDINYL-N′-(2-THIENYLMEHTYL)-1,2-ETHANEDIAMINE MONOHYDROCHLORIDE ◇ N,N-DIME-THYL-N′-(2-PYRIDYL)-N′-THENYLETHYLENEDIAMINE HYDROCHLORIDE ◇ N,N-DIMETHYL-N′-(2-THENYL)-N′-(2-PYRIDYL-ETHYLENE-DIAMINE HYDROCHLORIDE) ◇ DOZAR ◇ HISTADYL HYDROCHLORIDE ◇ HISTAFED ◇ HISTIDYL ◇ LULLAMIN ◇ METHACON ◇ METHAPYRI-LENE HYDROCHLORIDE ◇ METHAPYRILENE HYDRO-CHLORIDE (L.A.) ◇ METHAPYRILENE HYDROCHLORIDE (S.A.) ◇ METHOXYLENE ◇ PYRATHYN ◇ N-(2-PYRI-DYL)-N-(2-THIENYL)-N,N′-DIMETHYL-ETHYLENEDIA-MINE HYDROCHLORIDE ◇ SEMIKON ◇ SEMIKON HYDROCHLORIDE ◇ SOMNICAPS ◇ TEM-HISTINE ◇ TERALIN ◇ THENYLENE ◇ THENYLENE HYDRO-CHLORIDE ◇ THENYLPYRAMINE HYDROCHLORIDE

◇ W-53 HYDROCHLORIDE ◇ WIN 2848 HYDROCHLO-
RIDE SALT

TOXICITY DATA with REFERENCE

CAR: orl-rat TD:22 g/kg/64W-C   SCIEAS
209,817,80

CAR: orl-rat TD:9625 mg/kg/2Y-C   FCTOD7
22,27,84

CAR: orl-rat TD:18200 mg/kg/26W-C   TXAPA9
66,252,82

CAR: orl-rat TDLo:9100 mg/kg/26/W-C
TXAPA9 66,252,82

ETA: orl-rat TD:4813 mg/kg/2Y-C   FCTOD7
22,27,84

ETA: orl-rat TD:10080 mg/kg/24W-C   TXAPA9
74,63,84

MUT: dns-rat:lvr 1 μmol/L   CNREA8 42,3010,82

MUT: mmo-smc 500 mg/L   IAPUDO 57,721,84

MUT: mrc-smc 1250 mg/L   IAPUDO 57,721,84

MUT: oms-rat:lvr 100 μmol/L   MUREAV
135,131,84

CONSENSUS REPORTS: NCI Carcinogen-
esis Studies (feed): Clear Evidence: rat FCTOD7
22,27,84; Clear Evidence: rat SCIEAS 209,
817,80; (gavage); No Evidence: guinea pig, ham
JTEHD6 12,653,83. Reported in EPA TSCA
Inventory.

SAFETY PROFILE: Questionable carcinogen
with experimental carcinogenic and tumorigenic
data. Poison by ingestion, intravenous, and subcutaneous routes. Human systemic effects by
ingestion: gastritis. Mutation data reported. An
antihistamine. When heated to decomposition
it emits very toxic fumes of Cl^-, SO_x, and NO_x.

DPJ600   CAS: 13261-62-6
2-DIMETHYLAMINOFLUORENE
mf: $C_{15}H_{15}N$ mw: 209.31

SYNS: 2-DIMETHYLAMINO-FLUOREN (GERMAN)
◇ N,N-DIMETHYL-2-AMINOFLUORENE ◇ 2-FLUORENYL-
DIMETHYLAMINE

TOXICITY DATA with REFERENCE

ETA: orl-rat TD:3960 mg/kg/13W-C   ONCOAR
8,233,55

ETA: orl-rat TD:4250 mg/kg/47W-I   JBCHA3
221,845,56

ETA: orl-rat TDLo:1370 mg/kg/47W-I   BJCAAI
6,89,52

SAFETY PROFILE: Questionable carcinogen
with experimental tumorigenic data. When
heated to decomposition it emits toxic fumes
of NO_x.

DPN400   CAS: 6632-68-4
1,3-DIMETHYL-4-AMINO-5-
NITROSOURACIL
mf: $C_6H_8N_4O_3$ mw: 184.18

SYN: DANU

TOXICITY DATA with REFERENCE
ETA: scu-rat TDLo:16 g/kg/34W-I   ZKKOBW
80,297,73

CONSENSUS REPORTS: Reported in EPA
TSCA Inventory.

SAFETY PROFILE: Questionable carcinogen
with experimental tumorigenic data. Moderately
toxic by intraperitoneal route. When heated to
decomposition it emits toxic fumes of NO_x.

DPO400   CAS: 18463-85-9
6-((p-(DIMETHYLAMINO)PHENYL)AZO)
BENZOTHIAZOLE
mf: $C_{15}H_{14}N_4S$ mw: 282.39

SYNS: 6-DIMETHYLAMINOPHENYLAZOBENZO-
THIAZOLE ◇ 6-DIMETHYLAMINOPHENYLAZO-
BENZTHIAZOLE ◇ N,N-DIMETHYL-p-(6-BENZTHIAZOLY-
LAZO)ANILINE ◇ N,N-DIMETHYL-4-(6'-BENZTHIAZOLY-
LAZO)ANILINE

TOXICITY DATA with REFERENCE
ETA: orl-rat TD:600 mg/kg/60D-C   CALEDQ
21,69,83

ETA: orl-rat TDLo:540 mg/kg/4W-C   JMCMAR
11,1074,68

MUT: dns-rat-orl 10 mg/kg   MUREAV 156,1,85

MUT: dns-rat-unr 10 mg/kg   CRNGDP 6,611,85

MUT: dns-rat:lvr 100 nmol/L   MUREAV 156,1,85

MUT: mma-sat 800 ng/plate   MUREAV 116,271,83

SAFETY PROFILE: Questionable carcinogen
with experimental tumorigenic data. Mutation
data reported. When heated to decomposition
it emits very toxic fumes of SO_x and NO_x.

DPO600   CAS: 18559-92-7
7-((p-(DIMETHYLAMINO)PHENYL)AZO)
BENZOTHIAZOLE
mf: $C_{15}H_{14}N_4S$ mw: 282.39

SYNS: N,N-DIMETHYL-p-(7-BENZTHIAZOLYLAZO)ANI-
LINE ◇ N,N-DIMETHYL-4-(7'-BENZTHIAZOLYLAZO)ANI-
LINE

TOXICITY DATA with REFERENCE
ETA: orl-rat TDLo:1620 mg/kg/13W-C
JMCMAR 11,1074,68

MUT: mma-sat 4 μg/plate   MUREAV 93,67,82

SAFETY PROFILE: Questionable carcinogen with experimental tumorigenic data. Mutation data reported. When heated to decomposition it emits very toxic fumes of NO_x and SO_x.

DPO800   CAS: 63040-63-1
4-((p-(DIMETHYLAMINO)PHENYL)AZO) ISOQUINOLINE
mf: $C_{17}H_{16}N_4$ mw: 276.37

SYN: N,N-DIMETHYL-4-(4'-ISOQUINOLINYLAZO)ANI-LINE

TOXICITY DATA with REFERENCE
ETA: orl-ratTDLo:3276mg/kg/26W-C   AICCA6 19,531,63

SAFETY PROFILE: Questionable carcinogen with experimental tumorigenic data. When heated to decomposition it emits toxic fumes of NO_x.

DPP000   CAS: 63040-64-2
5-((p-(DIMETHYLAMINO)PHENYL)AZO) ISOQUINOLINE
mf: $C_{17}H_{16}N_4$ mw: 276.37

SYN: N,N'-DIMETHYL-4-(5'-ISOQUINOLINYLAZO)ANI-LINE

TOXICITY DATA with REFERENCE
ETA: orl-rat TD:2196 mg/kg/17W-C   AICCA6 19,531,63
ETA: orl-ratTDLo:1092mg/kg/26W-C   AICCA6 19,531,63

SAFETY PROFILE: Questionable carcinogen with experimental tumorigenic data. When heated to decomposition it emits toxic fumes of NO_x.

DPP200   CAS: 63040-65-3
7-(p-(DIMETHYLAMINO)PHENYL)AZO) ISOQUINOLINE
mf: $C_{17}H_{16}N_4$ mw: 276.37

SYN: N,N-DIMETHYL-4-(7'-ISOQUINOLINYLAZO)ANI-LINE

TOXICITY DATA with REFERENCE
ETA: orl-ratTDLo:3276mg/kg/26W-C   AICCA6 19,531,63

SAFETY PROFILE: Questionable carcinogen with experimental tumorigenic data. When heated to decomposition it emits toxic fumes of NO_x.

DPP400   CAS: 10318-23-7
5-((p-(DIMETHYLAMINO)PHENYL)AZO) ISOQUINOLINE-2-OXIDE
mf: $C_{17}H_{16}N_4O$ mw: 292.37

SYN: N,N-DIMETHYL-4-(5'-ISOQUINOLYL-2'-OX-IDE)AZOANILINE

TOXICITY DATA with REFERENCE
ETA: orl-rat TDLo:720 mg/kg/17W-C   AICCA6 19,531,66

SAFETY PROFILE: Questionable carcinogen with experimental tumorigenic data. When heated to decomposition it emits toxic fumes of NO_x.

DPP600   CAS: 19471-27-3
4-((p-(DIMETHYLAMINO)PHENYL)AZO)-2,5-LUTIDINE 1-OXIDE
mf: $C_{15}H_{18}N_4O$ mw: 270.37

SYN: N,N-DIMETHYL-4-(4'-(2',5'-DIMETHYLPYRIDYL-1'-OXIDE)AZO)ANILINE

TOXICITY DATA with REFERENCE
ETA: orl-rat TDLo:2646 mg/kg/21W-C   JNCIAM 41,855,68

SAFETY PROFILE: Questionable carcinogen with experimental tumorigenic data. When heated to decomposition it emits toxic fumes of NO_x.

DPP709   CAS: 19456-77-0
4-((p-(DIMETHYLAMINO)PHENYL)AZO)-3,5-LUTIDINE-1-OXIDE
mf: $C_{15}H_{18}N_4O$ mw: 270.37

SYNS: N,N-DIMETHYL-4-(4'-(3',5'-DIMETHYLPYRIDYL-1'-OXIDE)AZO)ANILINE ◇ N,N-DIMETHYL-4-(3',5'-LUTI-DYL-1'-OXIDE)AZO)ANILINE

TOXICITY DATA with REFERENCE
ETA: orl-rat TDLo:5292 mg/kg/21W-C   JNCIAM 41,855,68

SAFETY PROFILE: Questionable carcinogen with experimental tumorigenic data. When heated to decomposition it emits toxic fumes of NO_x.

DPP800   CAS: 7349-99-7
4-((4-(DIMETHYLAMINO)PHENYL)AZO)-2,6-LUTIDINE-1-OXIDE
mf: $C_{15}H_{18}N_4O$ mw: 270.37

SYNS: N,N-DIMETHYL-4-(4'-(2',6'-DIMETHYLPYRIDYL-1'-OXIDE)AZO)ANILINE ◇ 2,6-DIMETHYLPYRIDINE-1-OX-IDE-4-AZO-p-DIMETHYLANILINE

TOXICITY DATA with REFERENCE
NEO: orl-rat TDLo: 714 mg/kg/17W-C   JNCIAM
37,365,66
ETA: orl-rat TD: 4300 mg/kg/17W-C   CNREA8
14,715,54

SAFETY PROFILE: Questionable carcinogen with experimental neoplastigenic and tumorigenic data. When heated to decomposition it emits toxic fumes of NO_x.

DPQ200   CAS: 33804-48-7
4-((p-(DIMETHYLAMINO)PHENYL)AZO)-N-METHYLACETANILIDE
mf: $C_{17}H_{20}N_4O$ mw: 296.41

SYNS: N'-ACETYL-N'-METHYL-4'-AMINO-N,N-DI-METHYL-4-AMINOAZOBENZENE ◇ 4-(N-ACETYL-N-METHYL)AMINO-4'-(N',N'-DIMETHYLAMINO)AZOBEN-ZENE ◇ N',N'-DIMETHYL-4'-AMINO-N-ACETYL-N-MONO-METHYL-4-AMINOAZOBENZENE ◇ N-(4-((4-(DIMETHYL-AMINO)PHENYL)AZO)PHENYL)-N-METHYLACETAMIDE

TOXICITY DATA with REFERENCE
ETA: orl-rat TDLo: 1630 mg/kg/21W-C
CNREA8 34,2274,74
MUT: dns-rat: lvr 1 μmol/L   CNREA8 46,1654,86
MUT: mma-sat 250 nmol/plate   CNREA846,1654,86

SAFETY PROFILE: Questionable carcinogen with experimental tumorigenic data. Poison by intraperitoneal route. Mutation data reported. When heated to decomposition it emits toxic fumes of NO_x.

DPQ400   CAS: 17400-65-6
5-((p-(DIMETHYLAMINO)PHENYL)AZO)-7-METHYLQUINOLINE
mf: $C_{18}H_{18}N_4$ mw: 290.40

SYNS: N,N-DIMETHYL-4-(5'-(7'-METHYLQUINO-LYL)AZO)ANILINE ◇ 7'-METHYL-5'-(p-DIMETHYLAMI-NOPHENYLAZO)QUINOLINE

TOXICITY DATA with REFERENCE
CAR: orl-rat TDLo: 540 mg/kg/30D-C   JNCIAM
40,891,68

SAFETY PROFILE: Questionable carcinogen with experimental carcinogenic data. When heated to decomposition it emits toxic fumes of NO_x.

DPQ600   CAS: 17416-18-1
5-((p-(DIMETHYLAMINO)PHENYL)AZO)QUINALDINE
mf: $C_{18}H_{18}N_4$ mw: 290.40

SYN: 2'-METHYL-5'-(p-DIMETHYLAMINOPHE-NYLAZO)QUINOLINE

TOXICITY DATA with REFERENCE
CAR: orl-rat TDLo: 540 mg/kg/30D-C   JNCIAM
40,891,68

SAFETY PROFILE: Questionable carcinogen with experimental carcinogenic data. When heated to decomposition it emits toxic fumes of NO_x.

DPQ800   CAS: 17416-17-0
5-((p-(DIMETHYLAMINO)PHENYL)AZO)QUINOLINE
mf: $C_{17}H_{16}N_4$ mw: 276.37

SYNS: N,N-DIMETHYL-p-(5'-QUINOLYLAZO)ANILINE ◇ N,N-DIMETHYL-4-(5'-QUINOLYLAZO)ANILINE

TOXICITY DATA with REFERENCE
CAR: orl-rat TDLo: 714 mg/kg/17W-C   JNCIAM
40,891,68
ETA: orl-rat TD: 714 mg/kg/17W-C   JNCIAM
26,1461,61
ETA: orl-rat TD: 720 mg/kg/17W-C   AICCA6
19,531,63

SAFETY PROFILE: Questionable carcinogen with experimental carcinogenic and tumorigenic data. When heated to decomposition it emits toxic fumes of NO_x.

DPR000   CAS: 30041-69-1
6-((p-(DIMETHYLAMINO)PHENYL)AZO)QUINOLINE
mf: $C_{17}H_{16}N_4$ mw: 276.37

SYNS: N,N-DIMETHYL-4-(6'-QUINOLYLAZO)ANILINE ◇ QUINOLINE-6-AZO-p-DIMETHYLANILINE

TOXICITY DATA with REFERENCE
ETA: orl-rat TDLo: 714 mg/kg/17W-C   AICCA6
19,531,63
MUT: dns-rat-orl 40 mg/kg   CALEDQ 27,115,85

CONSENSUS REPORTS: EPA Genetic Toxicology Program.

SAFETY PROFILE: Questionable carcinogen with experimental tumorigenic data. Mutation data reported. When heated to decomposition it emits toxic fumes of NO_x.

DPR200   CAS: 22750-85-2
5-((p-(DIMETHYLAMINO)PHENYL)AZO)QUINOLINE-1-OXIDE
mf: $C_{17}H_{16}N_4O$ mw: 292.37

SYN: N,N-DIMETHYL-4-((5'-QUINOLYL-1'-OX-IDE)AZO)ANILINE

TOXICITY DATA with REFERENCE
ETA: orl-rat TDLo: 714 mg/kg/17W-C AICCA6
19,531,63

SAFETY PROFILE: Questionable carcinogen with experimental tumorigenic data. When heated to decomposition it emits toxic fumes of NO_x.

DPR400 CAS: 22750-86-3
6-((p-(DIMETHYLAMINO)PHENYL)AZO) QUINOLINE-1-OXIDE
mf: $C_{17}H_{16}N_4O$ mw: 292.37

SYN: N,N'-DIMETHYL-4-((6'-QUINOLYL-1'-OX-IDE)AZO)ANILINE

TOXICITY DATA with REFERENCE
ETA: orl-rat TDLo: 714 mg/kg/17W-C AICCA6
19,531,63

SAFETY PROFILE: Questionable carcinogen with experimental tumorigenic data. When heated to decomposition it emits toxic fumes of NO_x.

DQC000 CAS: 63019-60-3
7-(p-(DIMETHYLAMINO)STYRYL)BENZ (c)ACRIDINE
mf: $C_{27}H_{22}N_2$ mw: 374.51

SYN: p-DIMETHYLAMINOBENZYLIDEN-3,4-BENZ-9-METHYLACRIDINE

TOXICITY DATA with REFERENCE
ETA: scu-mus TDLo: 200 mg/kg VOONAW
1,52,55

SAFETY PROFILE: Questionable carcinogen with experimental tumorigenic data. When heated to decomposition it emits toxic fumes of NO_x.

DQC200 CAS: 63019-59-0
12-(p-DIMETHYLAMINO)STYRYL-BENZ(a)ACRIDINE
mf: $C_{27}H_{22}N_2$ mw: 374.51

SYN: p-DIMETHYLAMINOBENZYLIDEN-1,2-BENZ-9-METHYL-ACRIDINE

TOXICITY DATA with REFERENCE
ETA: scu-mus TDLo: 200 mg/kg VOONAW
1,52,55

SAFETY PROFILE: Questionable carcinogen with experimental tumorigenic data. When heated to decomposition it emits toxic fumes of NO_x.

DQC400 CAS: 1628-58-6
2-(p-(DIMETHYLAMINO)STYRYL) BENZOTHIAZOLE
mf: $C_{17}H_{16}N_2S$ mw: 280.41

SYN: 2-(4-DIMETHYLAMINOSTYRYL)BENZOTHIAZOLE

TOXICITY DATA with REFERENCE
NEO: orl-rat TDLo: 35 g/kg/1Y-I: TER JNCIAM
41,985,68

CONSENSUS REPORTS: Reported in EPA TSCA Inventory.

SAFETY PROFILE: Questionable carcinogen with experimental neoplastigenic and terato-genic data. When heated to decomposition it emits very toxic fumes of NO_x and SO_x.

DQC600 CAS: 19716-21-3
4-(p-(DIMETHYLAMINO)STYRYL)-6,8-DIMETHYLQUINOLINE
mf: $C_{21}H_{22}N_2$ mw: 302.45

SYN: 6,8-DIMETHYL-(4-p-(DIMETHYLAMINO)STY-RYL)QUINOLINE

TOXICITY DATA with REFERENCE
ETA: orl-rat TDLo: 38 mg/kg/51W-I JNCIAM
41,985,68

SAFETY PROFILE: Questionable carcinogen with experimental tumorigenic data. When heated to decomposition it emits toxic fumes of NO_x.

DQD000 CAS: 897-55-2
4-(4-DIMETHYLAMINOSTYRYL) QUINOLINE
mf: $C_{19}H_{18}N_2$ mw: 274.39

SYNS: 2-(4-N,N-DIMETHYLAMINOSTYRYL)QUINOLINE
◇ 4-(p-(DIMETHYLAMINO)STYRYL)QUINOLINE

TOXICITY DATA with REFERENCE
NEO: ivn-mus TDLo: 100 mg/kg CNREA8
25,938,65

CONSENSUS REPORTS: Reported in EPA TSCA Inventory.

SAFETY PROFILE: Questionable carcinogen with experimental neoplastigenic data. Poison by intravenous route. When heated to decomposition it emits toxic fumes of NO_x.

DQD200   CAS: 21970-53-6
4-(p-(DIMETHYLAMINO)STYRYL)
QUINOLINE MONOHYDROCHLORIDE
mf: $C_{19}H_{18}N_2 \cdot ClH$ mw: 310.85

SYN: NSC 63346

TOXICITY DATA with REFERENCE
NEO: orl-rat TDLo: 115 mg/kg/1Y-I   JNCIAM
41,985,68

SAFETY PROFILE: Questionable carcinogen with experimental neoplastigenic data. When heated to decomposition it emits very toxic fumes of NO_x and HCl.

DQD600   CAS: 7347-47-9
4-((4-(DIMETHYLAMINO)-m-TOLYL)
AZO)-2-PICOLINE-1-OXIDE
mf: $C_{14}H_{16}N_4O$ mw: 256.34

SYN: N,N-DIMETHYL-2-METHYL-4-(4'-(2'-METHYLPYRI-DYL-1'-OXIDE)AZO)ANILINE

TOXICITY DATA with REFERENCE
NEO: orl-rat TDLo: 2142 mg/kg/17W-C
JNCIAM 37,365,66

SAFETY PROFILE: Questionable carcinogen with experimental neoplastigenic data. When heated to decomposition it emits toxic fumes of NO_x.

DQD800   CAS: 7347-48-0
4-((4-(DIMETHYLAMINO)-o-TOLYL)
AZO)-2-PICOLINE-1-OXIDE
mf: $C_{15}H_{18}N_4O$ mw: 270.37

SYNS: N,N'DIMETHYL-3-METHYL-4-(4'-(2'-METHYL-PYRIDYL-1'OXIDE)AZO)ANILINE ◇ N,N'-DIMETHYL-4-(4'-(2'-METHYLPYRIDYL-1-OXIDE)AZO)-o-TOLUIDINE

TOXICITY DATA with REFERENCE
NEO: orl-rat TDLo: 2142 mg/kg/17W-C
JNCIAM 37,365,66

SAFETY PROFILE: Questionable carcinogen with experimental neoplastigenic data. When heated to decomposition it emits toxic fumes of NO_x.

DQE000   CAS: 19456-74-7
4-((4-(DIMETHYLAMINO)-m-TOLYL)
AZO)-3-PICOLINE-1-OXIDE
mf: $C_{15}H_{18}N_4O$ mw: 270.37

SYN: N,N,2-TRIMETHYL-4-(4'-(3'-METHYLPYRIDYL-1'-OXIDE)AZO)ANILINE

TOXICITY DATA with REFERENCE
ETA: orl-rat TDLo: 4284 mg/kg/17W-C
JNCIAM 41,85,68

SAFETY PROFILE: Questionable carcinogen with experimental tumorigenic data. When heated to decomposition it emits toxic fumes of NO_x.

DQE200   CAS: 19471-28-4
4-((4-(DIMETHYLAMINO)-o-TOLYL)
AZO)-3-PICOLINE-1-OXIDE
mf: $C_{15}H_{18}N_4O$ mw: 270.37

SYN: N,N,3-TRIMETHYL-4-(4'-(3'-METHYLPYRIDYL-1'-OXIDE)AZO)ANILINE

TOXICITY DATA with REFERENCE
ETA: orl-rat TDLo: 4284 mg/kg/17W-C
JNCIAM 41,855,68

SAFETY PROFILE: Questionable carcinogen with experimental tumorigenic data. When heated to decomposition it emits toxic fumes of NO_x.

DQE400   CAS: 17400-68-9
5-((4-(DIMETHYLAMINO)-m-TOLYL)
AZO)QUINOLINE
mf: $C_{18}H_{18}N_4$ mw: 290.40

SYNS: N,N-DIMETHYL-4-(5'-QUINOLYLAZO)-m-TOLUI-DINE ◇ 3-METHYL-5'-(p-DIMETHYLAMINOPHENYL-AZO)QUINOLINE

TOXICITY DATA with REFERENCE
CAR: orl-rat TDLo: 2142 mg/kg/17W-C
JNCIAM 40,891,68

SAFETY PROFILE: Questionable carcinogen with experimental carcinogenic data. When heated to decomposition it emits toxic fumes of NO_x.

DQE600   CAS: 17416-21-6
5-((4-(DIMETHYLAMINO)-o-TOLYL)
AZO)QUINOLINE
mf: $C_{18}H_{18}N_4$ mw: 290.40

SYN: 2-METHYL-5'-(p-DIMETHYLAMINOPHENYL-AZO)QUINOLINE

TOXICITY DATA with REFERENCE
CAR: orl-rat TDLo: 2142 mg/kg/17W-C
JNCIAM 40,891,68

SAFETY PROFILE: Questionable carcinogen with experimental carcinogenic data. When heated to decomposition it emits toxic fumes of NO$_x$.

DQF000   CAS: 6120-10-1
4-DIMETHYLAMINO-3,5-XYLENOL
mf: C$_{10}$H$_{15}$NO   mw: 165.26

TOXICITY DATA with REFERENCE
ETA: orl-mus TDLo:33 g/kg/78W-I

NTIS** PB223-159

SAFETY PROFILE: Questionable carcinogen with experimental tumorigenic data. When heated to decomposition it emits toxic fumes of NO$_x$.

DQF200   CAS: 19456-73-6
4-((4-(DIMETHYLAMINO)-2,3-XYLYL) AZO)PYRIDINE-1-OXIDE
mf: C$_{15}$H$_{18}$N$_4$O   mw: 270.37

SYN: N,N,2,3-TETRAMETHYL-4-(4'-(PYRIDYL-1'-OX-IDE)AZO)ANILINE

TOXICITY DATA with REFERENCE
ETA: orl-rat TDLo:6552 mg/kg/26W-C

JNCIAM 41,855,68

SAFETY PROFILE: Questionable carcinogen with experimental tumorigenic data. When heated to decomposition it emits toxic fumes of NO$_x$.

DQF400   CAS: 19456-75-8
4-((4-(DIMETHYLAMINO)-2,5-XYLYL) AZO)PYRIDINE-1-OXIDE
mf: C$_{15}$H$_{18}$N$_4$O   mw: 270.37

SYN: N,N,2,5-TETRAMETHYL-4-(4'-(PYRIDYL-1'-OX-IDE)AZO)ANILINE

TOXICITY DATA with REFERENCE
ETA: orl-rat TDLo:3276 mg/kg/26W-C

JNCIAM 41,855,68

SAFETY PROFILE: Questionable carcinogen with experimental tumorigenic data. When heated to decomposition it emits toxic fumes of NO$_x$.

DQF600   CAS: 19595-66-5
4-((4-(DIMETHYLAMINO)-3,5-XYLYL) AZO)PYRIDINE-1-OXIDE
mf: C$_{15}$H$_{18}$N$_4$O   mw: 270.37

SYN: N,N,2,6-TETRAMETHYL-4-(4'-(PYRIDYL-1'-OX-IDE)AZO)ANILINE

TOXICITY DATA with REFERENCE
ETA: orl-rat TDLo:6552 mg/kg/26W-C

JNCIAM 41,855,68

SAFETY PROFILE: Questionable carcinogen with experimental tumorigenic data. When heated to decomposition it emits toxic fumes of NO$_x$.

DQF700   CAS: 4063-41-6
4,5'-DIMETHYL ANGELICIN
mf: C$_{13}$H$_{10}$O$_3$ mw: 214.23

SYN: 4,8-DIMETHYL-2H-FURO(2,3-h)-1-BENZOPYRAN-2-ONE

TOXICITY DATA with REFERENCE
MUT: dnd-esc 20 μmol/L   CBINA8 21,103,78
MUT: dnd-mam:lym 20 μmol/L   CBINA8 21,103,78
MUT: dnd-omi 20 μmol/L   CBINA8 21,103,78
MUT: dnd-omi 20 μmol/L   CBINA8 21,103,78
MUT: dnd-sal:spr 20 μmol/L   CBINA8 21,103,78

CONSENSUS REPORTS: IARC Cancer Review: Animal Inadequate Evidence IMEMDT 40,291,86.

SAFETY PROFILE: Questionable carcinogen. Mutation data reported. When heated to decomposition it emits acrid smoke and fumes.

DQG000   CAS: 41217-05-4
6,12-DIMETHYLANTHANTHRENE
mf: C$_{24}$H$_{16}$ mw: 304.40

SYN: 6,12-DIMETHYL-BIBENZO(def,mno)CHRYSENE

TOXICITY DATA with REFERENCE
ETA: scu-mus TDLo:72 mg/kg/9W-I   COREAF 246,1477,58
MUT: dnd-mam:lym 30 μmol/L   CBINA847,87,83

SAFETY PROFILE: Questionable carcinogen with experimental tumorigenic data. Mutation data reported. When heated to decomposition it emits acrid smoke and irritating fumes.

DQG200   CAS: 781-43-1
9,10-DIMETHYLANTHRACENE
mf: C$_{16}$H$_{14}$ mw: 206.30

TOXICITY DATA with REFERENCE
CAR: skn-mus TDLo:40 mg/kg/20D-I   CRNGDP 6,1483,85
ETA: skn-mus TDLo:1100 mg/kg/46W-I   CNREA8 2,157,42
MUT: dnr-esc 500 mg/L   PMRSDJ 1,195,81
MUT: mma-esc 10 μg/plate   PMRSDJ 1,387,81
MUT: mmo-sat 20 μg/plate   CRNGDP 6,1483,85

MUT: mrc-smc 200 ppm   PMRSDJ 1,481,81
MUT: sln-dmg-par 5 mmol/L   MUREAV 125,243,84

CONSENSUS REPORTS: EPA Genetic Toxicology Program.

SAFETY PROFILE: Questionable carcinogen with experimental carcinogenic and tumorigenic data. Mutation data reported. When heated to decomposition it emits acrid smoke and irritating fumes.

DQH000   CAS: 28842-05-9
3,6'-DIMETHYLAZOBENZENE
mf: $C_{14}H_{14}N_2$ mw: 210.30

SYNS: 2:3'-AZOTOLUENE ◇ 2,3'-DIMETHYLAZOBENZENE

TOXICITY DATA with REFERENCE
NEO: orl-rat TDLo: 26 g/kg/36W-C   JPBAA7 58,275,46
ETA: mul-mus TDLo: 400 mg/kg/I   CNREA8 1,397,41
ETA: orl-rat TD: 321 g/kg/36W-C   JPBAA7 58,275,46

SAFETY PROFILE: Questionable carcinogen with experimental neoplastigenic and tumorigenic data. When heated to decomposition it emits toxic fumes of NO_x.

DQH200   CAS: 35077-51-1
N,N'-DIMETHYL-4,4'-AZODIACETANILIDE
mf: $C_{18}H_{20}N_4O_2$ mw: 324.42

SYNS: N'-ACETYL-N'-MONOMETHYL-4'-AMINO-N-ACETYL-N-MONOMETHYL-4-AMINOAZOBENZENE ◇ N,N'-(AZODI-4,1-PHENYLENE)BIS(N-METHYLACETAMIDE) ◇ 4,4'-BIS(N-ACETYL-N-METHYLAMINO)AZOBENZENE

TOXICITY DATA with REFERENCE
ETA: orl-rat TDLo: 2200 mg/kg/13W-C   CNREA8 34,2274,74
MUT: dns-rat: lvr 1 μmol/L   CNREA8 46,1654,86

SAFETY PROFILE: Questionable carcinogen with experimental tumorigenic data. Moderately toxic by intraperitoneal route. Mutation data reported. When heated to decomposition it emits toxic fumes of NO_x.

DQH550
1,3-DIMETHYLBENZ(e)ACEPHENANTHRYLENE
mf: $C_{22}H_{18}$ mw: 282.40

SYN: 1,3-DIMETHYLBENZO(b)FLUORANTHENE

TOXICITY DATA with REFERENCE
ETA: skn-mus TDLo: 452 μg/kg/20D-I   CRNGDP 6,1023,85
MUT: mma-sat 63 nmol/plate   CRNGDP 6,1023,85

SAFETY PROFILE: Questionable carcinogen with experimental tumorigenic data. Mutation data reported. When heated to decomposition it emits acrid smoke and irritating fumes.

DQH600   CAS: 3518-05-6
1,10-DIMETHYL-5,6-BENZACRIDINE
mf: $C_{19}H_{15}N$ mw: 257.35

SYN: 8,12-DIMETHYLBENZ(a)ACRIDINE

TOXICITY DATA with REFERENCE
ETA: scu-mus TDLo: 200 mg/kg/4W-I   ACRSAJ 4,315,56
ETA: scu-mus TDLo: 250 mg/kg/10D-I   BAFEAG 34,22,47

SAFETY PROFILE: Questionable carcinogen with experimental tumorigenic data. When heated to decomposition it emits toxic fumes of NO_x.

DQH800   CAS: 17401-48-8
2,10-DIMETHYL-5,6-BENZACRIDINE
mf: $C_{19}H_{15}N$ mw: 257.35

SYN: 9,12-DIMETHYLBENZ(a)ACRIDINE

TOXICITY DATA with REFERENCE
ETA: skn-mus TDLo: 540 mg/kg/45W-I   ACRSAJ 4,315,56

SAFETY PROFILE: Questionable carcinogen with experimental tumorigenic data. When heated to decomposition it emits toxic fumes of NO_x.

DQI200   CAS: 963-89-3
7,9-DIMETHYLBENZ(c)ACRIDINE
mf: $C_{19}H_{15}N$ mw: 257.35

SYN: 3,10-DIMETHYL-7,8-BENZACRIDINE (FRENCH)

TOXICITY DATA with REFERENCE
ETA: scu-mus TD: 250 mg/kg/10D-I   BAFEAG 34,22,47
ETA: scu-mus TDLo: 200 mg/kg/4W-I   ACRSAJ 4,315,56
ETA: skn-mus TDLo: 180 mg/kg/15W-I   ACRSAJ 4,315,56
MUT: dnr-esc 250 mg/L   JJIND8 67,873,79

MUT: mma-sat 10 μg/plate   ENMUDM 6(Suppl 2),1,84

MUT: otr-ham:emb 100 μg/L   JJIND8 67,1303,81

MUT: otr-ham:kdy 80 μg/L   BJCAAI 37,873,78

MUT: otr-rat:emb 40800 μg/L   JJIND8 67,1303,81

CONSENSUS REPORTS: EPA Genetic Toxicology Program.

SAFETY PROFILE: Questionable carcinogen with experimental tumorigenic data. Mutation data reported. When heated to decompositions it emits toxic fumes of NO_x.

DQI400   CAS: 32740-01-5
7,11-DIMETHYLBENZ(c)ACRIDINE
mf: $C_{19}H_{15}N$ mw: 257.35

SYN: 1,10-DIMETHYL-7,8-BENZACRIDINE (FRENCH)

TOXICITY DATA with REFERENCE

ETA: scu-mus TD:250 mg/kg/10D-I   BAFEAG 34,22,47

ETA: scu-mus TDLo:200 mg/kg/4W-I   ACRSAJ 4,315,56

ETA: skn-mus TDLo:360 mg/kg/30W-I   ACRSAJ 4,315,56

MUT: mma-sat 1 nmol/plate   GANNA2 70,749,79

SAFETY PROFILE: Questionable carcinogen with experimental tumorigenic data. Mutation data reported. When heated to decomposition it emits toxic fumes of NO_x.

DQI800   CAS: 2381-40-0
6,9-DIMETHYL-1,2-BENZACRIDINE
mf: $C_{19}H_{15}N$ mw: 257.35

SYNS: 7,10-DIMETHYLBENZ(c)ACRIDINE ◊ 2,10-DIMETHYL-7,8-BENZACRIDINE (FRENCH)

TOXICITY DATA with REFERENCE

ETA: scu-mus TD:250 mg/kg/10D-I   BAFEAG 34,22,47

ETA: scu-mus TDLo:200 mg/kg/4W-I   ACRSAJ 4,315,56

ETA: skn-mus TDLo:190 mg/kg/16W-I   ACRSAJ 4,315,56

MUT: mma-sat 50 μg/plate   PNASA6 72,5135,75

MUT: otr-ham:emb 2 mg/L   EJCAAH 17,179,81

MUT: otr-ham:kdy 80 μg/L   BJCAAI 37,873,78

CONSENSUS REPORTS: EPA Genetic Toxicology Program.

SAFETY PROFILE: Questionable carcinogen with experimental tumorigenic data. Mutation data reported. When heated to decomposition it emits toxic fumes of NO_x.

DQJ400   CAS: 313-74-6
1,12-DIMETHYLBENZ(a)ANTHRACENE
mf: $C_{20}H_{16}$ mw: 256.36

SYN: 1',9-DIMETHYL-1,2-BENZANTHRACENE

TOXICITY DATA with REFERENCE

ETA: scu-mus TDLo:72 mg/kg/9W-I   BAFEAG 49,312,62

SAFETY PROFILE: Questionable carcinogen with experimental tumorigenic data. When heated to decomposition it emits acrid smoke and irritating fumes.

DQJ600   CAS: 18429-70-4
4,5-DIMETHYLBENZ(a)ANTHRACENE
mf: $C_{20}H_{16}$ mw: 256.36

SYN: 3,4'-DIMETHYL-1,2-BENZANTHRACENE

TOXICITY DATA with REFERENCE

ETA: scu-rat TDLo:18 mg/kg   PSEBAA 128,720,68

SAFETY PROFILE: Questionable carcinogen with experimental tumorigenic data. When heated to decomposition it emits acrid smoke and irritating fumes.

DQJ800   CAS: 20627-28-5
6,7-DIMETHYLBENZ(a)ANTHRACENE
mf: $C_{20}H_{16}$ mw: 256.36

SYN: 4,10-DIMETHYL-1,2-BENZANTHRACENE

TOXICITY DATA with REFERENCE

ETA: scu-mus TDLo:40 mg/kg   JNCIAM 1,303,40

SAFETY PROFILE: Questionable carcinogen with experimental tumorigenic data. When heated to decomposition it emits acrid smoke and fumes.

DQK000   CAS: 317-64-6
6,8-DIMETHYLBENZ(a)ANTHRACENE
mf: $C_{20}H_{16}$ mw: 256.36

SYN: 6,8-DIMETHYL-1,2-BENZANTHRACENE

TOXICITY DATA with REFERENCE

NEO: ims-rat TDLo:50 mg/kg   CNREA8 29,506,69

ETA: skn-mus TDLo:240 mg/kg/37W-I   CNREA8 11,892,51

SAFETY PROFILE: Questionable carcinogen with experimental neoplastigenic and tumorigenic data. When heated to decomposition it emits acrid smoke and irritating fumes.

DQK200   CAS: 568-81-0
6,12-DIMETHYLBENZ(a)ANTHRACENE
mf: $C_{20}H_{16}$ mw: 256.36

SYN: 4,9-DIMETHYL-1,2-BENZANTHRACENE

TOXICITY DATA with REFERENCE
ETA: imp-mus TDLo: 80 mg/kg   JNCIAM 2,241,41

SAFETY PROFILE: Questionable carcinogen with experimental tumorigenic data. When heated to decomposition it emits acrid smoke and irritating fumes.

DQK400   CAS: 35187-28-1
7,11-DIMETHYLBENZ(a)ANTHRACENE
mf: $C_{20}H_{16}$ mw: 256.36

SYN: 8,10-DIMETHYL-1,2-BENZANTHRACENE

TOXICITY DATA with REFERENCE
ETA: scu-mus TDLo: 40 mg/kg   CNREA8 6,454,46

SAFETY PROFILE: Questionable carcinogen with experimental tumorigenic data. When heated to decomposition it emits acrid smoke and irritating fumes.

DQK600   CAS: 58430-00-5
5,6-DIMETHYL-1,2-BENZANTHRACENE
mf: $C_{20}H_{16}$ mw: 256.36

SYN: 8,9-DIMETHYLBENZ(a)ANTHRACENE

TOXICITY DATA with REFERENCE
ETA: skn-mus TDLo: 500 mg/kg/21W-I
     PRLBA4 117,318,35

SAFETY PROFILE: Questionable carcinogen with experimental tumorigenic data. When heated to decomposition it emits acrid smoke and irritating fumes.

DQK800   CAS: 20627-31-0
5,9-DIMETHYL-1,2-BENZANTHRACENE
mf: $C_{20}H_{16}$ mw: 256.36

SYNS: 5:9-DIMETHYL-1:2-BENZANTHRACENE
◇ 8,12-DIMETHYLBENZ(a)ANTHRACENE

TOXICITY DATA with REFERENCE
ETA: scu-mus TDLo: 40 mg/kg   AJCAA7 33,499,38

SAFETY PROFILE: Questionable carcinogen with experimental tumorigenic data. When heated to decomposition it emits acrid smoke and irritating fumes.

DQK900   CAS: 71964-72-2
7,12-DIMETHYLBENZ(a)ANTHRACENE-3,4-DIOL
mf: $C_{20}H_{16}O_2$ mw: 288.36

TOXICITY DATA with REFERENCE
ETA: skn-mus TDLo: 35 µg/kg   CNREA8
     40,3661,80
MUT: mma-sat 10 nmol/plate   46OJAN-,675,81

SAFETY PROFILE: Questionable carcinogen with experimental tumorigenic data. Mutation data reported. When heated to decomposition it emits acrid smoke and irritating fumes.

DQL000   CAS: 604-81-9
5,10-DIMETHYL-1,2-BENZANTHRACENE
mf: $C_{20}H_{16}$ mw: 256.36

SYN: 7,8-DIMETHYLBENZ(a)ANTHRACENE

TOXICITY DATA with REFERENCE
ETA: scu-mus TD: 400 mg/kg   JACSAT 58,2376,36
ETA: scu-mus TDLo: 40 mg/kg   AJCAA7 33,499,38

SAFETY PROFILE: Questionable carcinogen with experimental tumorigenic data. When heated to decomposition it emits acrid smoke and irritating fumes.

DQL200   CAS: 58429-99-5
6,7-DIMETHYL-1,2-BENZANTHRACENE
mf: $C_{20}H_{16}$ mw: 256.36

SYN: 9,10-DIMETHYLBENZ(a)ANTHRACENE

TOXICITY DATA with REFERENCE
ETA: skn-mus TDLo: 1250 mg/kg/52W-I
     PRLBA4 117,318,35
MUT: dnd-mus-skn 110 mg/L   CNREA8 32,643,72
MUT: dni-mus-ipr 100 mg/kg   MUREAV 46,305,77
MUT: dns-rat: lvr 50 µmol/L   ENMUDM 3,11,81
MUT: mma-sat 2500 µg/plate   BJCAAI 37,873,78
MUT: otr-ham: kdy 80 µg/L   BJCAAI 37,873,78

SAFETY PROFILE: Questionable carcinogen with experimental tumorigenic data. Mutation data reported. When heated to decomposition it emits acrid smoke and irritating fumes.

DQL400   CAS: 32976-87-7
7,12-DIMETHYLBENZ(a)ANTHRACENE, DEUTERATED
mf: $C_{20}D_{16}$ mw: 272.36

SYN: 7,12-DIMETHYLBENZ(a)ANTHRACENE-D16

TOXICITY DATA with REFERENCE
ETA: scu-mus TDLo: 60 mg/kg/9W-I   NATWAY
     58,371,71

SAFETY PROFILE: Questionable carcinogen with experimental tumorigenic data. When heated to decomposition it emits acrid smoke and irritating fumes.

DQL800   CAS: 63019-25-0
9:10-DIMETHYL-1:2-BENZANTHRACENE-9:10-OXIDE
mf: $C_{20}H_{16}O$ mw: 272.36

SYN: 9:10-DIMETHYL-9-10-DIHYDRO-1,2-BENZANTHRACENE-9,10-OXIDE

TOXICITY DATA with REFERENCE
ETA: skn-mus TDLo:860 mg/kg/36W-I
   PRLBA4, 129,439,40

SAFETY PROFILE: Questionable carcinogen with experimental tumorigenic data. When heated to decomposition it emits acrid smoke and irritating fumes.

DQM200   CAS: 18463-86-0
N,N-DIMETHYL-p-(4-BENZIMIDAZOLYAZO)ANILINE
mf: $C_{15}H_{15}N_5$ mw: 265.35

SYNS:
4-((p-(DIMETHYLAMINO)PHENYL)AZO)BENZIMIDAZOLE
◇ N,N-DIMETHYL-4(4'-BENZIMIDAZOLYLAZO)ANILINE

TOXICITY DATA with REFERENCE
ETA: orl-rat TDLo:1080 mg/kg/9W-C   JMCMAR
   11,1074,68

SAFETY PROFILE: Questionable carcinogen with experimental tumorigenic data. When heated to decomposition it emits toxic fumes of NO_x.

DQM400   CAS: 4699-26-7
6,12-DIMETHYLBENZO(1,2-b:5,4-b')BIS(1)BENZOTHIOPHENE
mf: $C_{20}H_{14}S_2$ mw: 318.46

TOXICITY DATA with REFERENCE
ETA: scu-mus TDLo:80 mg/kg   JNCIAM
   18,555,57

SAFETY PROFILE: Questionable carcinogen with experimental tumorigenic data. When heated to decomposition it emits toxic fumes of SO_x.

DQM800   CAS: 37750-86-0
6,12-DIMETHYLBENZO(1,2-b:4,5-b') DITHIONAPHTHENE
mf: $C_{20}H_{14}S_2$ mw: 318.46

TOXICITY DATA with REFERENCE
ETA: scu-mus TDLo:80 mg/kg   JNCIAM 18,555,57
MUT: cyt-mus:fbr 1500 µg/L   NULSAK 6,17,63
MUT: mnt-mus:fbr 1500 µg/L   NULSAK 6,17,63

SAFETY PROFILE: Questionable carcinogen with experimental tumorigenic data. Mutation data reported. When heated to decomposition it emits toxic fumes of SO_x.

DQN000   CAS: 16757-85-0
1,2-DIMETHYLBENZO(a)PYRENE
mf: $C_{22}H_{16}$ mw: 280.38

TOXICITY DATA with REFERENCE
ETA: scu-mus TDLo:72 mg/kg/13W-I   IJCNAW
   3,238,68
MUT: cyt-ckn:leu 1 pph/30M   BBRCA9 93,954,80

SAFETY PROFILE: Questionable carcinogen with experimental tumorigenic data. Mutation data reported. When heated to decomposition it emits acrid smoke and irritating fumes.

DQN200   CAS: 16757-86-1
1,3-DIMETHYLBENZO(a)PYRENE
mf: $C_{22}H_{16}$ mw: 280.38

TOXICITY DATA with REFERENCE
ETA: scu-mus TDLo:72 mg/kg/13W-I   IJCNAW
   3,238,68

SAFETY PROFILE: Questionable carcinogen with experimental tumorigenic data. When heated to decomposition it emits acrid smoke and irritating fumes.

DQN400   CAS: 16757-88-3
1,4-DIMETHYLBENZO(a)PYRENE
mf: $C_{22}H_{16}$ mw: 280.38

TOXICITY DATA with REFERENCE
ETA: scu-mus TDLo:72 mg/kg/13W-I   IJCNAW
   3,238,68

SAFETY PROFILE: Questionable carcinogen with experimental tumorigenic data. When heated to decomposition it emits acrid smoke and irritating fumes.

DQN600   CAS: 16757-90-7
1,6-DIMETHYLBENZO(a)PYRENE
mf: $C_{22}H_{16}$ mw: 280.38

TOXICITY DATA with REFERENCE
ETA: scu-mus TDLo:72 mg/kg/13W-I   IJCNAW
   3,238,68

SAFETY PROFILE: Questionable carcinogen with experimental tumorigenic data. When heated to decomposition it emits acrid smoke and irritating fumes.

DQN800   CAS: 16757-87-2
2,3-DIMETHYLBENZO(a)PYRENE
mf: $C_{22}H_{16}$ mw: 280.38

TOXICITY DATA with REFERENCE
ETA: scu-mus TDLo: 72 mg/kg/13W-I   IJCNAW
3,238,68

SAFETY PROFILE: Questionable carcinogen with experimental tumorigenic data. When heated to decomposition it emits acrid smoke and irritating fumes.

DQO000   CAS: 16757-91-8
3,6-DIMETHYLBENZO(a)PYRENE
mf: $C_{22}H_{16}$ mw: 280.38

TOXICITY DATA with REFERENCE
ETA: scu-mus TDLo: 72 mg/kg/13W-I   IJCNAW
3,238,68

SAFETY PROFILE: Questionable carcinogen with experimental tumorigenic data. When heated to decomposition it emits acrid smoke and irritating fumes.

DQO200   CAS: 16757-84-9
3,12-DIMETHYLBENZO(a)PYRENE
mf: $C_{22}H_{16}$ mw: 280.38

TOXICITY DATA with REFERENCE
ETA: scu-mus TDLo: 72 mg/kg/13W-I   IJCNAW
3,238,68

SAFETY PROFILE: Questionable carcinogen with experimental tumorigenic data. When heated to decomposition it emits acrid smoke and irritating fumes.

DQO400   CAS: 16757-89-4
4,5-DIMETHYLBENZO(a)PYRENE
mf: $C_{22}H_{16}$ mw: 280.38

TOXICITY DATA with REFERENCE
ETA: scu-mus TDLo: 72 mg/kg/13W-I   IJCNAW
3,238,68

SAFETY PROFILE: Questionable carcinogen with experimental tumorigenic data. When heated to decomposition it emits acrid smoke and irritating fumes.

DQP400   CAS: 32362-68-8
4,9-DIMETHYL-2,3-BENZTHIOPHANTHRENE
mf: $C_{18}H_{14}S$ mw: 262.38

TOXICITY DATA with REFERENCE
ETA: skn-mus TDLo: 440 mg/kg/11W-I
XPHPAW 149,477,51

SAFETY PROFILE: Questionable carcinogen with experimental tumorigenic data. When

heated to decomposition it emits toxic fumes of SO_x.

DRB800   CAS: 64038-38-6
7,11-DIMETHYL-10-CHLOROBENZ(c) ACRIDINE
mf: $C_{19}H_{14}ClN$ mw: 291.79

SYNS: 2-CHLORO-1,10-DIMETHYL-7,8-BENZACRIDINE (FRENCH) ◇ 1,10-DIMETHYL-2-CHLORO-7,8-BENZACRIDINE (FRENCH)

TOXICITY DATA with REFERENCE
ETA: skn-mus TD: 380 mg/kg/31W-I   AICCA6
11,736,55
ETA: skn-mus TDLo: 250 mg/kg/21W-I
ACRSAJ 4,315,56

SAFETY PROFILE: Questionable carcinogen with experimental tumorigenic data. When heated to decomposition it emits very toxic fumes of NO_x and Cl^-.

DRC000   CAS: 4584-46-7
DIMETHYL(2-CHLOROETHYL)AMINE HYDROCHLORIDE
mf: $C_4H_{10}ClN \cdot ClH$ mw: 144.06

SYNS: 2-CHLORO-N,N-DIMETHYLETHYLAMINE HYDROCHLORIDE ◇ DIMETHYL-β-CHLOROETHYLAMINE HYDROCHLORIDE

TOXICITY DATA with REFERENCE
NEO: ipr-mus TDLo: 720 mg/kg/8W-I   CNREA8
39,391,79
MUT: dns-rat: lvr 5 μmol/L   ENMUDM 3,33,81
MUT: mmo-esc 1 μmol/L   JPPMAB 31,67P,79
MUT: mmo-sat 1 mg/L   ENMUDM 3,33,81
MUT: sln-dmg-orl 1700 mmol/L   MUREAV
95,237,82

CONSENSUS REPORTS: Reported in EPA TSCA Inventory.

SAFETY PROFILE: Questionable carcinogen with experimental neoplastigenic data. Poison by intraperitoneal and subcutaneous routes. Mutation data reported. When heated to decomposition it emits very toxic fumes of Cl^- and NO_x.

DRC800   CAS: 3789-77-3
N,N-DIMETHYL-p-((m-CHLOROPHENYL)AZO)ANILINE
mf: $C_{14}H_{14}ClN_3$ mw: 259.76

SYN: 3'-CHLORO-4-DIMETHYLAMINOAZOBENZENE

TOXICITY DATA with REFERENCE
NEO: orl-rat TDLo:4900 mg/kg/17W-C
    JEMEAV 87,139,48

SAFETY PROFILE: Questionable carcinogen with experimental neoplastigenic data. When heated to decomposition it emits very toxic fumes of Cl^- and NO_x.

DRD000 CAS: 3010-47-7
N,N-DIMETHYL-p-((o-CHLOROPHENYL) AZO)ANILINE
mf: $C_{14}H_{14}ClN_3$ mw: 259.76

SYN: 2'-CHLORO-4-DIMETHYLAMINOAZOBENZENE

TOXICITY DATA with REFERENCE
NEO: orl-rat TDLo:4900 mg/kg/17W-C
    JEMEAV 87,139,48

SAFETY PROFILE: Questionable carcinogen with experimental neoplastigenic data. When heated to decomposition it emits very toxic fumes of Cl^- and NO_x.

DRD800 CAS: 63041-62-3
2,3-DIMETHYLCHOLANTHRENE
mf: $C_{22}H_{18}$ mw: 282.40

SYN: 16:20-DIMETHYLCHOLANTHRENE

TOXICITY DATA with REFERENCE
ETA: scu-mus TDLo:400 mg/kg AJCAA7
    28,334,36

SAFETY PROFILE: Questionable carcinogen with experimental tumorigenic data. When heated to decomposition it emits acrid smoke and irritating fumes.

DRD850 CAS: 85923-37-1
3,6-DIMETHYLCHOLANTHRENE
mf: $C_{22}H_{18}$ mw: 282.40

SYN: BENZ(j)ACEANTHRYLENE, 1,2-DIHYDRO-3,6-DI-METHYL-(9CI)

TOXICITY DATA with REFERENCE
ETA: skn-mus TDLo:706 ng/kg CALEDQ
    28,223,85
MUT: mma-ham:lng 50 µg/L CALEDQ 28,223,85
MUT: msc-ham:lng 100 µg/L PAACA3 24,94,83

SAFETY PROFILE: Questionable carcinogen with experimental tumorigenic data. Mutation data reported. When heated to decomposition it emits acrid smoke and irritating fumes.

DRE000 CAS: 63041-61-2
15,20-DIMETHYLCHOLANTHRENE
mf: $C_{22}H_{18}$ mw: 282.40

SYN: 1,3-DIMETHYLCHOLANTHRENE

TOXICITY DATA with REFERENCE
ETA: scu-mus TDLo:200 µg/kg JNCIAM 2,99,41

SAFETY PROFILE: Questionable carcinogen with experimental tumorigenic data. When heated to decomposition it emits acrid smoke and irritating fumes.

DRE200 CAS: 15914-23-5
1,2-DIMETHYLCHRYSENE
mf: $C_{20}H_{16}$ mw: 256.36

TOXICITY DATA with REFERENCE
ETA: scu-mus TDLo:3200 mg/kg/48W-I
    PRLBA4 129,439,40
ETA: skn-mus TDLo:800 mg/kg/33W-I
    PRLBA4 129,439,40

SAFETY PROFILE: Questionable carcinogen with experimental tumorigenic. When heated to decomposition it emits acrid smoke and irritating fumes.

DRE400 CAS: 52171-92-3
1,11-DIMETHYLCHRYSENE
mf: $C_{20}H_{16}$ mw: 256.36

SYN: 5,7-DIMETHYLCHRYSENE

TOXICITY DATA with REFERENCE
NEO: skn-mus TDLo:120 mg/kg/50W-I
    CNREA8 34,1315,74
MUT: mma-sat 20 µg/plate CNREA8 36,4525,76

CONSENSUS REPORTS: EPA Genetic Toxicology Program.

SAFETY PROFILE: Questionable carcinogen with experimental neoplastigenic data. Poison by intraperitoneal and intravenous routes. Mutation data reported. When heated to decomposition it emits acrid smoke and irritating fumes.

DRE600 CAS: 63019-23-8
4,5-DIMETHYLCHRYSENE
mf: $C_{20}H_{16}$ mw: 256.36

TOXICITY DATA with REFERENCE
ETA: scu-mus TDLo:80 mg/kg CNREA8 3,606,43

SAFETY PROFILE: Questionable carcinogen with experimental tumorigenic data. When heated to decomposition it emits acrid smoke and irritating fumes.

DRE800 CAS: 3697-27-6
5,6-DIMETHYLCHRYSENE
mf: $C_{20}H_{16}$ mw: 256.36

TOXICITY DATA with REFERENCE
ETA: scu-mus TDLo: 80 mg/kg   CNREA8 3,606,43

SAFETY PROFILE: Questionable carcinogen with experimental tumorigenic data. When heated to decomposition it emits acrid smoke and irritating fumes.

DRF000   CAS: 14207-78-4
5,11-DIMETHYLCHRYSENE
mf: $C_{20}H_{16}$ mw: 256.36

TOXICITY DATA with REFERENCE
ETA: skn-mus TDLo: 400 μg/kg/20D-I
    CALEDQ 8,65,79

SAFETY PROFILE: Questionable carcinogen with experimental tumorigenic data. When heated to decomposition it emits acrid smoke and irritating fumes.

DRH200   CAS: 5831-10-7
11,17-DIMETHYL-15H-CYCLOPENTA(a)PHENANTHRENE
mf: $C_{19}H_{16}$ mw: 244.35

TOXICITY DATA with REFERENCE
CAR: skn-mus TDLo: 108 mg/kg/1Y-I   PEXTAR
11,69,69
MUT: mma-sat 50 μg/plate   CNREA8 36,4525,76

CONSENSUS REPORTS: EPA Genetic Toxicology Program.

SAFETY PROFILE: Questionable carcinogen with experimental carcinogenic data. Mutation data reported. When heated to decomposition it emits acrid smoke and irritating fumes.

DRH400   CAS: 5831-09-4
12,17-DIMETHYL-15H-CYCLOPENTA(a)PHENANTHRENE
mf: $C_{19}H_{16}$ mw: 244.35

TOXICITY DATA with REFERENCE
ETA: skn-mus TDLo: 108 mg/kg/1Y-I   PEXTAR
11,69,69
MUT: mma-sat 50 μg/plate   CNREA8 36,4525,76

CONSENSUS REPORTS: EPA Genetic Toxicology Program.

SAFETY PROFILE: Questionable carcinogen with experimental tumorigenic data. Mutation data reported. When heated to decomposition it emits acrid smoke and irritating fumes.

DRH800   CAS: 63020-69-9
3,4-DIMETHYL-1,2-CYCLOPENTENOPHENANTHRENE
mf: $C_{19}H_{18}$ mw: 246.37

SYN: 16,17-DIHYDRO-11,12-DIMETHYL-15H-CYCLO-PENTA(a)PHENANTHRENE

TOXICITY DATA with REFERENCE
ETA: skn-mus TDLo: 1260 mg/kg/39W-I
    ARGEAR 6,1,53

SAFETY PROFILE: Questionable carcinogen with experimental tumorigenic data. When heated to decomposition it emits acrid smoke and irritating fumes.

DRI400   CAS: 3546-11-0
3,3'-DIMETHYL-N,N'-DIACETYLBENZIDINE
mf: $C_{18}H_{20}N_2O_2$ mw: 296.40

SYNS: N,N'-DIACETYL-3,3'-DIMETHYLBENZIDINE
◇ 3',3'''-DIMETHYL-4',4'''-BIACETANILIDE

TOXICITY DATA with REFERENCE
CAR: orl-rat TDLo: 7900 mg/kg/43W-C
    CNREA8 16,525,56
MUT: mma-sat 10 μg/plate   SAIGBL 23,168,81

SAFETY PROFILE: Questionable carcinogen with experimental carcinogenic data. Mutation data reported. When heated to decomposition it emits toxic fumes of NO_x.

DRI800   CAS: 35335-07-0
9,10-DIMETHYL-1,2,5,6-DIBENZANTHRACENE
mf: $C_{24}H_{18}$ mw: 306.42

SYNS: 9,10-DIMETHYL-DBA ◇ 7,14-DIMETHYLDIBEN-Z(a,h)ANTHRACENE

TOXICITY DATA with REFERENCE
NEO: skn-mus TDLo: 200 mg/kg/20W-I
    CNREA8 22,78,62
ETA: scu-mus TDLo: 20 mg/kg   CNREA8 22,78,62
MUT: msc-ham: lng 25 μg/L   MUREAV 136,65,84

SAFETY PROFILE: Questionable carcinogen with experimental neoplastigenic and tumorigenic data. Mutation data reported. When heated to decomposition it emits acrid smoke and irritating fumes.

DRJ000   CAS: 63042-50-2
4,9-DIMETHYL-2,3,5,6-DIBENZOTHIOPHENTHRENE
mf: $C_{22}H_{16}S$ mw: 312.44

SYN: 7,13-DIMETHYLBENZO(b)PHENANTHRO(3,2-d)THIOPHENE

TOXICITY DATA with REFERENCE
ETA: scu-mus TDLo: 80 mg/kg   JNCIAM 18,555,57

SAFETY PROFILE: Questionable carcinogen with experimental tumorigenic data. When heated to decomposition it emits toxic fumes of SO_x.

DRK400   CAS: 42149-31-5
2,5-DIMETHYL-1,2,5,6-DIEPOXYHEX-3-YNE
mf: $C_8H_{10}O_2$ mw: 138.18

TOXICITY DATA with REFERENCE
NEO: scu-mus TDLo:1040 mg/kg/26W-I
JNCIAM 53,695,74

SAFETY PROFILE: Questionable carcinogen with experimental neoplastigenic data. When heated to decomposition it emits acrid smoke and irritating fumes.

DRK500   CAS: 34983-45-4
trans-4,4'-DIMETHYL-α-α'-DIETHYLSTILBENE
mf: $C_{20}H_{24}$ mw: 264.44

SYNS: STILBENE, α-α'-DIETHYL-4,4'-DIMETHYL-, (E)- ◇ DMES

TOXICITY DATA with REFERENCE
ETA: orl-dog TDLo:6 g/kg/30D-C   TXAPA9 21,582,72

SAFETY PROFILE: Questionable carcinogen with experimental tumorigenic data. When heated to decomposition it emits acrid smoke and irritating fumes.

DRK800   CAS: 578-32-5
N,N-DIMETHYL-2,5-DIFLUORO-p-(2,5-DIFLUOROPHENYLAZO)ANILINE
mf: $C_{14}H_{11}F_4N_3$ mw: 297.28

SYN: 2,5,2',5'-TETRAFLUORO-4-DIMETHYLAMINOAZOBENZENE

TOXICITY DATA with REFERENCE
NEO: orl-rat TDLo:6400 mg/kg/21W-C
CNREA8 17,387,57

SAFETY PROFILE: Questionable carcinogen with experimental neoplastigenic data. When heated to decomposition it emits very toxic fumes of F^- and NO_x.

DRL000   CAS: 351-65-5
N,N-DIMETHYL-p-(3,4-DIFLUOROPHENYLAZO)ANILINE
mf: $C_{14}H_{13}F_2N_3$ mw: 261.30

SYNS: 3',4'-DIFLUORO-4-DIMETHYLAMINOAZOBENZENE ◇ N,N-DIMETHYL-3',4'-DIFLUORO-4-(PHENYLAZO)BENZENEAMINE

TOXICITY DATA with REFERENCE
CAR: orl-rat TDLo:2356 mg/kg/17W-C
CBINA8 53,107,85
NEO: orl-rat TD:3400 mg/kg/13W-C   CNREA8 17,387,57

SAFETY PROFILE: Questionable carcinogen with experimental carcinogenic and neoplastigenic data. When heated to decomposition it emits very toxic fumes of F^- and NO_x.

DRL400   CAS: 35653-70-4
2,4'-DIMETHYL-4-DIMETHYLAMINOAZOBENZENE
mf: $C_{16}H_{19}N_3$ mw: 253.38

TOXICITY DATA with REFERENCE
ETA: orl-rat TDLo:8940 mg/kg/35W-C
ARZNAD 12,270,62

SAFETY PROFILE: Questionable carcinogen with experimental tumorigenic data. When heated to decomposition it emits toxic fumes of NO_x.

DRN400   CAS: 3844-60-8
1,6-DIMETHYL-1,6-DINITROSOBIUREA
mf: $C_4H_8N_6O_4$ mw: 204.18

SYNS: N,N'-DIMETHYL-N,N'-DINITROSO-1,2-HYDRAZINEDICARBOXAMIDE ◇ HYDRAZODICARBONSAEUREABIS(METHYLNITROSAMID) (GERMAN) ◇ HYDRAZODICARBOXYLIC ACID BIS(METHYLNITROSAMIDE) ◇ HYDROAZODICARBOXYBIS(METHYLNITROSAMIDE) ◇ NSC 409425 ◇ SRI 1666

TOXICITY DATA with REFERENCE
ETA: scu-rat TDLo:420 mg/kg/28W-I   ZEKBAI 69,103,67

SAFETY PROFILE: Questionable carcinogen with experimental tumorigenic data. Poison by subcutaneous and intraperitoneal routes. Many N-nitroso compounds are carcinogens. When heated to decomposition it emits toxic fumes of NO_x.

DRN800   CAS: 55556-88-2
2,5-DIMETHYLDINITROSOPIPERAZINE
mf: $C_6H_{14}N_4O_2$ mw: 174.24

PROP: Mixture approximately 25% cis and 75% trans conformers (CNREA8 35,1270,75)

SYNS: 2,5-DIMETHYL-1,4-DINITROSOPIPERAZINE ◇ 2,5-DIMETHYL-DNPZ ◇ DINITROSO-2,5-DIMETHYLPI-PERAZINE

TOXICITY DATA with REFERENCE
ETA: orl-rat TDLo: 2740 mg/kg/50W-I   CNREA8 35,1270,75
MUT: mma-sat 25 μg/plate   TCMUE9 1,13,84
MUT: mma-smc 50 μmol/plate   MUREAV77,143,80

CONSENSUS REPORTS: EPA Genetic Toxicology Program.

SAFETY PROFILE: Questionable carcinogen with experimental tumorigenic data. Mutation data reported. Many N-nitroso compounds are carcinogens. When heated to decomposition it emits toxic fumes of NO_x.

DRO000   CAS: 55380-34-2
2,6-DIMETHYLDINITROSOPIPERAZINE
mf: $C_6H_{14}N_4O_2$ mw: 174.24

SYNS: 2,6-DIMETHYL-DNPZ ◇ DINITROSO-2,6-DI-METHYLPIPERAZINE ◇ N,N′-DINITROSO-2,6-DIMETH-YLPIPERAZINE ◇ 1,4-DINITROSO-2,6-DIMETHYLPIPER-AZINE ◇ DNDMP

TOXICITY DATA with REFERENCE
CAR: orl-rat TD: 1200 mg/kg/20W-I   CRNGDP 4,1165,83
CAR: orl-rat TDLo: 240 mg/kg/20W-I   CRNGDP 4,1165,83
NEO: orl-ham TDLo: 1960 mg/kg35W-I   CRNGDP 4,1165,83
ETA: orl-gpg TDLo: 4800 mg/kg/50W-I   CNREA8 40,1879,80
ETA: orl-ham TD: 2091 mg/kg/67W-I   IAPUDO 57,617,84
ETA: orl-rat TD: 63 mg/kg/25W-I   FCTOD7 21,601,83
ETA: orl-rat TD: 958 mg/kg/27W-I   IAPUDO 57,617,84
ETA: orl-rat TD: 1800 mg/kg/33W-I   CNREA8 35,1270,75
MUT: mma-sat 50 μg/plate   MUREAV 77,143,80
MUT: mma-smc 50 μmol/plate   TCMUE9 1,13,84

CONSENSUS REPORTS: EPA Genetic Toxicology Program.

SAFETY PROFILE: Questionable carcinogen with experimental carcinogenic, neoplastigenic, and tumorigenic data. Mutation data reported. A model carcinogen and carcinogenic metabolite. When heated to decomposition it emits toxic fumes of NO_x.

DRO200   CAS: 6972-76-5
N,N′-DIMETHYL-N,N′-DINITROSO-1,3-PROPANEDIAMINE
mf: $C_5H_{12}N_4O_2$ mw: 160.21

SYNS: DINITROSODIMETHYLPROPANEDIAMINE ◇ N,N′-DINITROSO-N,N′-DIMETHYL-1,3-PROPANEDI-AMINE ◇ NSC 62580

TOXICITY DATA with REFERENCE
NEO: orl-rat TD: 640 mg/kg/32W-I   JNCIAM 41,985,68
NEO: orl-rat TDLo: 360 mg/kg/48W-I   JNCIAM 41,985,68

SAFETY PROFILE: Questionable carcinogen with experimental neoplastigenic data. Many N-nitroso compounds are carcinogens. When heated to decomposition it emits toxic fumes of NO_x.

DRQ000   CAS: 13865-57-1
N,N-DIMETHYL-4-(DIPHENYLMETHYL)ANILINE
mf: $C_{21}H_{21}N$ mw: 287.43

SYNS: 4-DIMETHYLAMINOTRIPHENYLMETHANE ◇ 4-DIMETHYLAMINOTRIPHENYLMETHAN (GERMAN)

TOXICITY DATA with REFERENCE
ETA: scu-rat TDLo: 1620 mg/kg/12W-I   NATWAY 42,215,55

SAFETY PROFILE: Questionable carcinogen with experimental tumorigenic data. When heated to decomposition it emits toxic fumes of NO_x.

DRQ200   CAS: 997-95-5
2,2′-DIMETHYLDIPROPYLINITROSO AMINE
mf: $C_8H_{18}N_2O$ mw: 158.28

SYNS: DI-ISO-BUTYLNITROSAMINE ◇ DMDPN ◇ NITROSODIISOBUTYLAMINE ◇ N-NITROSODIISOBU-TYLAMINE ◇ N-NITROSODI-ISO-BUTYLAMINE ◇ N-NI-TROSO-2,2′-DIMETHYLDI-n-PROPYLAMINE

TOXICITY DATA with REFERENCE
ETA: orl-rat TD: 11 g/kg/50W-C   CALEDQ 14,297,81
ETA: orl-rat TDLo: 1750 mg/kg/30W-I   JJIND8 62,407,79
ETA: scu-ham TDLo: 3063 mg/kg/49W-I   JNCIAM 55,1209,75
MUT: mma-sat 25 μg/plate   TCMUE9 1,13,84

SAFETY PROFILE: Questionable carcinogen with experimental neoplastigenic and tumorigenic data. Mildly toxic by subcutaneous route. Mutation data reported. Many nitrosamines compounds are carcinogens. When heated to decomposition it emits toxic fumes of NO_x.

DRQ600   CAS: 598-64-1
DIMETHYLDITHIOCARBAMIC ACID with DIMETHYLAMINE (1:1)
mf: $C_5H_{12}N_2S_2$ mw: 164.31

SYNS: DIMETHYLDITHIOCARBAMIC ACID DIMETHYL AMINE SALT ◇ DIMETHYLDITHIOCARBAMIC ACID DI-METHYLAMMONIUM SALT

TOXICITY DATA with REFERENCE
ETA: orl-mus TDLo:29 g/kg/78W-I
NTIS** PB223-159
ETA: scu-mus TDLo:464 mg/kg
NTIS** PB223-159

CONSENSUS REPORTS: Reported in EPA TSCA Inventory.

SAFETY PROFILE: Questionable carcinogen with experimental tumorigenic data. When heated to decomposition it emits very toxic fumes of NO_x, NH_3 and SO_x.

DRT000
7,14-DIMETHYL-7,14-ETHANODIBENZ(a,b)ANTHRACENE-15,16-DICARBOXYLIC ACID
mf: $C_{24}H_{20}O_4$ mw: 372.44

SYN: 7,12-DIMETHYLBENZANTHRACENE-7,12-endo-α,β-SUCCINIC ACID

TOXICITY DATA with REFERENCE
CAR: scu-rat TDLo:600 mg/kg/50D-I:TER
85DLAB -,-,75

SAFETY PROFILE: Questionable carcinogen with experimental carcinogenic and teratogenic data. Poison by intraperitoneal route. When heated to decomposition it emits acrid smoke and irritating fumes.

DRT200   CAS: 79-64-1
6-α,21-DIMETHYLETHISTERONE
mf: $C_{23}H_{32}O_2$ mw: 340.55

SYNS: DIMETHESTERONE ◇ DIMETHISTERON ◇ DIMETHISTERONE ◇ 6-α,21-DIMETHYL-17-β-HYDROXY-17-α-PREG-4-EN-20-YN-3-ONE ◇ 6-α,21-DIMETHYL-17-β-HYDROXY-17-α-PREGN-4-EN-20-YN-3-ONE ◇ 17-α-ETHY-NYL-6-α,21-DIMETHYLTESTOSTERONE ◇ 17-α-ETHYNYL-17-HYDROXY-6-α,21-DIMETHYLANDROST-4-EN-3-ONE

◇ (6-α,17-β)-17-HYDROXY-6-METHYL-17-(1-PROPYNYL)-ANDROST-4-EN-3-ONE ◇ 17-β-HYDROXY-6-α-METHYL-17-(1-PROPYNYL)ANDROST-4-EN-3-ONE ◇ LUTOGAN ◇ LUTOSAN ◇ 6-α-METHYL-17-α-PROPYNYLTESTOSTER-ONE ◇ 6-α-METHYL-17-(1-PROPYNYL)TESTOSTERONE ◇ P-5048 ◇ SECROSTERON

CONSENSUS REPORTS: IARC Cancer Review: Animal Inadequate Evidence IMEMDT 21,377,79.

SAFETY PROFILE: Questionable carcinogen. Mildly toxic by ingestion. An experimental teratogen. Experimental reproductive effects. A steroid used as a progestin and in the treatment of menstrual disorders. When heated to decomposition it emits acrid smoke and irritating fumes.

DRU000   CAS: 3837-54-5
N,N-DIMETHYL-p-((3-ETHOXYPHENYL)AZO)ANILINE
mf: $C_{16}H_{19}N_3O$ mw: 269.38

SYN: 3'-ETHOXY-4-DIMETHYLAMINOAZOBENZENE

TOXICITY DATA with REFERENCE
NEO: orl-rat TDLo:9202 mg/kg/30W-C
JEMEAV 87,139,48

SAFETY PROFILE: Questionable carcinogen with experimental neoplastigenic data. When heated to decomposition it emits toxic fumes of NO_x.

DRU600   CAS: 63021-00-1
DIMETHYL ETHYL ALLENOLIC ACID METHYL ETHER
mf: $C_{16}H_{18}O_3$ mw: 258.34

SYNS: ACIDE DIMETHYL-ETHYL-ALLENOLIQUE ETHER METHYLIQUE (FRENCH) ◇ α,α-DIMETHYL-2-(6-METHOXY-NAPHTHYL)PROPIONIC ACID

TOXICITY DATA with REFERENCE
ETA: orl-mus TDLo:139 mg/kg/24W-I
CRSBAW 146,916,52

SAFETY PROFILE: Questionable carcinogen with experimental tumorigenic data. When heated to decomposition it emits acrid smoke and irritating fumes.

DRV600   CAS: 50285-71-7
1,1-DIMETHYL-3-ETHYL-3-NITROSOUREA
mf: $C_5H_{11}N_3O_2$ mw: 145.19

SYNS: NITROSOAETHYLDIMETHYLHARNSTOFF ◇ NITROSO-1,1-DIMETHYL-3-ETHYLUREA ◇ NITROSO-

ETHYLDIMETHYLUREA ◇ 1-NITROSO-1-ETHYL-3,3-DI-
METHYLUREA

TOXICITY DATA with REFERENCE
ETA: orl-rat TDLo: 1230 mg/kg/50W-I
    ZKKOBW 83,315,75
MUT: mma-sat 250 μg/plate   JJIND8 67,1117,81

SAFETY PROFILE: Questionable carcinogen
with experimental tumorigenic data. Mutation
data reported. Many N-nitroso compounds are
carcinogens. When heated to decomposition it
emits toxic fumes of NO_x.

DRX600   CAS: 23339-04-0
2,3-DIMETHYLFLUORANTHENE
mf: $C_{18}H_{14}$ mw: 230.32

TOXICITY DATA with REFERENCE
NEO: skn-mus TDLo: 40 mg/kg/20D   JNCIAM
    49,1165,72

CONSENSUS REPORTS: IARC Cancer Review: Animal No Evidence IMEMDT 32,
355,83.

SAFETY PROFILE: Questionable carcinogen
with experimental neoplastigenic data. When
heated to decomposition it emits acrid smoke
and irritating fumes.

DRX800   CAS: 38048-87-2
7,8-DIMETHYLFLUORANTHENE
mf: $C_{18}H_{14}$ mw: 230.32

TOXICITY DATA with REFERENCE
NEO: skn-mus TDLo: 40 mg/kg/20D   JNCIAM
    49,1165,72

SAFETY PROFILE: Questionable carcinogen
with experimental neoplastigenic data. An initiator. When heated to decomposition it emits
acrid smoke and irritating fumes.

DRY000   CAS: 25889-63-8
8,9-DIMETHYLFLUORANTHENE
mf: $C_{18}H_{14}$ mw: 230.32

TOXICITY DATA with REFERENCE
ETA: skn-mus TDLo: 40 mg/kg/20D-I   JNCIAM
    49,1165,72

SAFETY PROFILE: Questionable carcinogen
with experimental tumorigenic data. An initiator. When heated to decomposition it emits acrid
smoke and irritating fumes.

DRY100   CAS: 17057-98-6
1,9-DIMETHYLFLUORENE
mf: $C_{15}H_{14}$ mw: 194.29

SYN: 9H-FLUORENE, 1,9-DIMETHYL-

TOXICITY DATA with REFERENCE
NEO: ipr-mus TDLo: 42 mg/kg/3D-I   JTEHD6
    21,525,87
MUT: mma-sat 10 μg/plate   MUREAV 91,167,81

SAFETY PROFILE: Questionable carcinogen
with experimental neoplastigenic data. Mutation
data reported. When heated to decomposition
it emits acrid smoke and irritating fumes.

DRY400   CAS: 737-22-4
7,12-DIMETHYL-4-FLUOROBENZ(a)
ANTHRACENE
mf: $C_{20}H_{15}F$ mw: 274.35

SYN: 4-FLUORO-7,12-DIMETHYLBENZ(a)ANTHRACENE

TOXICITY DATA with REFERENCE
NEO: ims-rat TDLo: 10 mg/kg   NATUAS273,566,78

SAFETY PROFILE: Questionable carcinogen
with experimental neoplastigenic data. When
heated to decomposition it emits toxic fumes
of F^-.

DRY600   CAS: 794-00-3
7,12-DIMETHYL-5-FLUOROBENZ(a)
ANTHRACENE
mf: $C_{20}H_{15}F$ mw: 274.35

SYN: 5-FLUORO-7,12-DIMETHYLBENZ(a)ANTHRACENE

TOXICITY DATA with REFERENCE
ETA: scu-rat TDLo: 823 mg/kg/10W-I   JMCMAR
    21,1076,78
ETA: skn-mus TDLo: 110 μg/kg   CNREA8
    39,411,79
MUT: dni-hmn: hla 70 μmol/L   MUREAV92,427,82

CONSENSUS REPORTS: EPA Genetic Toxicology Program.

SAFETY PROFILE: Questionable carcinogen
with experimental tumorigenic data. Human
mutation data reported. An initiator. When
heated to decomposition it emits toxic fumes
of F^-.

DRY800   CAS: 2023-60-1
7,12-DIMETHYL-8-FLUOROBENZ(a)
ANTHRACENE
mf: $C_{20}H_{15}F$ mw: 274.35

SYN: 8-FLUORO-7,12-DIMETHYLBENZ(a)ANTHRACENE

TOXICITY DATA with REFERENCE
NEO: ims-rat TDLo: 10 mg/kg   NATUAS273,566,78

SAFETY PROFILE: Questionable carcinogen
with experimental neoplastigenic data. When

heated to decomposition it emits toxic fumes of F⁻.

DRZ000   CAS: 2023-61-2
7,12-DIMETHYL-11-FLUOROBENZ(a) ANTHRACENE

mf: $C_{20}H_{15}F$ mw: 274.35

SYN: 11-FLUORO-7,12-DIMETHYLBENZ(a)ANTHRACENE

TOXICITY DATA with REFERENCE
NEO: ims-rat TDLo: 10 mg/kg   NATUAS 273,566,78
ETA: skn-mus TDLo: 110 μg/kg   CNREA8 39,411,79

CONSENSUS REPORTS: EPA Genetic Toxicology Program.

SAFETY PROFILE: Questionable carcinogen with experimental neoplastigenic and tumorigenic data. An initiator. When heated to decomposition it emits toxic fumes of F⁻.

DSA000   CAS: 150-74-3
N,N-DIMETHYL-p-((p-FLUOROPHENYL) AZO)ANILINE

mf: $C_{14}H_{14}FN_3$ mw: 243.31

SYNS: 4-(DIMETHYLAMINO)-4'-FLUOROAZOBENZENE
◇ 4'-FLUORO-N,N-DIMETHYL-4-AMINOAZOBENZENE
◇ 4'-FLUORO-p-DIMETHYLAMINOAZOBENZENE
◇ 4'-FLUORO-4-DIMETHYLAMINOAZOBENZENE
◇ 4'-FLUORO-N,N-DIMETHYL-p-PHENYLAZOANILINE
◇ p-((p-FLUOROPHENYL)AZO)-N,N-DIMETHYLANILINE
◇ 4-((4-FLUOROPHENYL)AZO)-N,N-DIMETHYLBENZEN-AMINE

TOXICITY DATA with REFERENCE
ETA: orl-rat TD: 3150 mg/kg/13W-C   CNREA8 9,652,49
ETA: orl-rat TD: 3200 mg/kg/12W-C   CNREA8 13,93,53
ETA: orl-rat TD: 4730 mg/kg/19W-C   ARZNAD 12,270,62
ETA: orl-rat TDLo: 2720 mg/kg/14W-I   CNREA8 18,469,58
MUT: dns-rat-orl 2520 mg/kg/12W-I   CNREA8 29,2039,69

SAFETY PROFILE: Questionable carcinogen with experimental tumorigenic and teratogenic data. Experimental reproductive effects. Mutation data reported. When heated to decomposition it emits very toxic fumes of F⁻ and NO$_x$.

DSG000   CAS: 593-82-8
1,1-DIMETHYLHYDRAZINE HYDROCHLORIDE

mf: $C_2H_8N_2 \cdot ClH$ mw: 96.58

TOXICITY DATA with REFERENCE
ETA: orl-rat TDLo: 35 g/kg/73W-C   ZEKBAI 69,103,67

NIOSH REL: (Hydrazines) CL 0.15 mg/m³/2H

SAFETY PROFILE: Questionable carcinogen with experimental tumorigenic data. Poison by ingestion, intraperitoneal and intravenous routes. When heated to decomposition it emits very toxic fumes of HCl and NO$_x$.

DSG200   CAS: 56400-60-3
1,2-DIMETHYLHYDRAZINE HYDROCHLORIDE

mf: $C_2H_8N_2 \cdot ClH$ mw: 96.58

SYNS: sym-DIMETHYLHYDRAZINE HYDROCHLORIDE
◇ DMH

TOXICITY DATA with REFERENCE
CAR: scu-rat TDLo: 300 mg/kg/20W-I   CANCAR 40,2502,77
NEO: orl-rat TDLo: 150 mg/kg/5W-I   JJIND8 63,1089,79
ETA: orl-rat TD: 150 mg/kg/3W-I   CALEDQ 25,311,85
ETA: scu-rat TD: 20 mg/kg   CNREA8 41,1240,81
ETA: scu-rat TD: 80 mg/kg/4W-I   CNREA8 41,1240,81
ETA: scu-rat TD: 160 mg/kg/8W-I   CNREA8 41,1240,81
ETA: scu-rat TD: 320 mg/kg/16W-I   CNREA8 41,1240,81
ETA: scu-rat TD: 532 mg/kg/20W-I   LAINAW 30,505,74
ETA: scu-rat TDLo: 120 mg/kg/6W-I   CNREA8 33,940,73
MUT: dns-mus-orl 20 mg/kg   FEPRA7 33,596,74

SAFETY PROFILE: Questionable carcinogen with experimental carcinogenic, neoplastigenic, and tumorigenic data. Poison by ingestion, intraperitoneal, subcutaneous, and intravenous routes. Mutation data reported. When heated to decomposition it emits very toxic fumes of HCl and NO$_x$.

DSG600   CAS: 868-85-9
DIMETHYLHYDROGENPHOSPHITE

mf: $C_2H_7O_3P$ mw: 110.06

SYNS: DIMETHYLESTER KYSELINY FOSFORITE (CZECH)
◇ NCI-C54773 ◇ PHOSPHONIC ACID, DIMETHYL ESTER

TOXICITY DATA with REFERENCE
CAR: orl-rat TDLo: 103 g/kg/2Y-I
NTPTR* NTP-TR-287,85

MUT: mma-sat 7500 µg/plate   ENMUDM 8(Suppl 7),1,86

CONSENSUS REPORTS: Reported in EPA TSCA Inventory. NTP Carcinogenesis Studies (gavage); No Evidence: mouse NTPTR* NTP-TR-287,85; Clear Evidence: rat NTPTR* NTP-TR-287,85.

SAFETY PROFILE: Questionable carcinogen with experimental carcinogenic data. Moderately toxic by ingestion and skin contact. Mutation data reported. A skin and eye irritant. When heated to decomposition it emits toxic fumes of PO_x.

DSI800   CAS: 17309-87-4
N,N-DIMETHYL-p-(6-INDAZYLAZO) ANILINE
mf: $C_{15}H_{15}N_5$ mw: 265.35

SYNS: 6-((p-(DIMETHYLAMINO)PHENYL)AZO)-1H-INDA-ZOLE ◊ N,N-DIMETHYL-4-(6'-1H-INDAZYLAZO)ANILINE

TOXICITY DATA with REFERENCE
CAR: orl-rat TDLo: 2700 mg/kg/21W-C
  JMCMAR 12,1113,69
MUT: mma-sat 20 µg/plate   MUREAV 93,67,82

SAFETY PROFILE: Questionable carcinogen with experimental carcinogenic data. Mutation data reported. When heated to decomposition it emits toxic fumes of NO_x.

DSK200   CAS: 119-38-0
DIMETHYL-5-(1-ISOPROPYL-3-METHYLPYRAZOLYL)CARBAMATE
mf: $C_{10}H_{17}N_3O_2$ mw: 211.30

SYNS: DIMETHYLCARBAMATE-d'1-ISOPROPYL-3-METHYL-5-PYRAZOLYLE (FRENCH) ◊ DIMETHYLCAR-BAMIC ACID 3-METHYL-1-(1-METHYLETHYL)-1H-PYRA-ZOL-5-YL ESTER ◊ ENT 19,060 ◊ GEIGY G-23611 ◊ ISOLAN ◊ ISOLANE (FRENCH) ◊ (1-ISOPROPIL-3-METIL-1H-PIRAZOL-5-IL)-N,N-DIMETIL-CARBAMMATO (ITALIAN) ◊ (1-ISOPROPYL-3-METHYL-1H-PYRAZOL-5-YL)-N,N-DI-METHYLCARBAMAAT (DUTCH) ◊ (1-ISOPROPYL-3-METHYL-1H-PYRAZOL-5-YL)-N,N-DIMETHYL-CARBAMAT (GERMAN) ◊ ISOPROPYLMETHYLPYRAZOLYL DI-METHYLCARBAMATE ◊ 1-ISOPROPYL-3-METHYL-5-PYRAZOLYL DIMETHYLCARBAMATE ◊ 1-ISOPROPYL-3-METHYLPYRAZOLYL-(5)-DIMETHYLCARBAMATE ◊ 5-METHYL-2-ISOPROPYL-3-PYRAZOLYL DIMETHYL-CARBAMATE ◊ PRIMIN ◊ SAOLAN

TOXICITY DATA with REFERENCE
ETA: orl-mus TDLo: 6600 mg/kg/78W-I
  NTIS** PB223-159

MUT: mmo-smc 5 ppm   RSTUDV 6,161,76

CONSENSUS REPORTS: EPA Extremely Hazardous Substances List.

SAFETY PROFILE: Questionable carcinogen with experimental tumorigenic data. Poison by ingestion, skin contact, intraperitoneal, and possibly other routes. Mutation data reported. An insecticide. When heated to decomposition it emits toxic fumes of NO_x.

DSM000   CAS: 766-39-2
α,β-DIMETHYLMALEIC ANHYDRIDE
mf: $C_6H_6O_3$ mw: 126.12

SYN: DIMETHYLMALEIC ANHYDRIDE

TOXICITY DATA with REFERENCE
ETA: scu-rat TDLo: 2600 mg/kg/65W-I   BJCAAI 19,392,65

CONSENSUS REPORTS: Reported in EPA TSCA Inventory.

SAFETY PROFILE: Questionable carcinogen with experimental tumorigenic data. When heated to decomposition it emits acrid smoke and irritating fumes.

DSN000   CAS: 3009-55-0
N,N-DIMETHYL-p-(2-METHOXYPHENYLAZO)ANILINE
mf: $C_{15}H_{17}N_3O$ mw: 255.35

SYN: 2'-METHOXY-4-DIMETHYLAMINOAZOBENZENE

TOXICITY DATA with REFERENCE
NEO: orl-rat TDLo: 6600 mg/kg/26W-C
  CNREA8 17,387,57

SAFETY PROFILE: Questionable carcinogen with experimental neoplastigenic data. When heated to decomposition it emits toxic fumes of NO_x.

DSN200   CAS: 20691-83-2
N,N-DIMETHYL-p-(3-METHOXYPHENYLAZO)ANILINE
mf: $C_{15}H_{17}N_3O$ mw: 255.35

SYN: 3'-METHOXY-4-DIMETHYLAMINOAZOBENZENE

TOXICITY DATA with REFERENCE
NEO: orl-rat TDLo: 2800 mg/kg/13W-C
  CNREA8 17,387,57

SAFETY PROFILE: Questionable carcinogen with experimental neoplastigenic data. When

heated to decomposition it emits toxic fumes of NO_x.

DSN400 CAS: 3009-50-5
N,N-DIMETHYL-p-(4-METHOXYPHENYLAZO)ANILINE
mf: $C_{15}H_{17}N_3O$ mw: 255.35

SYN: 4'-METHOXY-4-DIMETHYLAMINOAZOBENZENE

TOXICITY DATA with REFERENCE
NEO: orl-rat TDLo: 6600 mg/kg/26W-C

CNREA8 17,387,57

ETA: orl-rat TD: 10204 mg/kg/48W-C ARZNAD 12,270,62

SAFETY PROFILE: Questionable carcinogen with experimental neoplastigenic and tumorigenic data. When heated to decomposition it emits toxic fumes of NO_x.

DSN600 CAS: 7203-92-1
3,3-DIMETHYL-1-p-METHOXYPHENYLTRIAZENE
mf: $C_9H_{13}N_3O$ mw: 179.25

SYNS: 1-p-METHOXYFENYL-3,3-DIMETHYLTRIAZEN (CZECH) ◇ 1-(p-METHOXYPHENYL)-3,3-DIMETHYLTRI-AZENE ◇ 1-(4-METHYLOXYPHENYL)-3,3-DIMETHYLTRI-AZINE

TOXICITY DATA with REFERENCE
CAR: scu-rat TDLo: 1700 mg/kg/45W-I

ZKKOBW 81,285,74

MUT: hma-mus/smc 10 mmol/L CBINA8 9,365,74
MUT: mrc-smc 1 mmol/L/1H CBINA8 9,365,74
MUT: sln-dmg-orl 1 mmol/L CBINA8 9,365,74

CONSENSUS REPORTS: EPA Genetic Toxicology Program.

SAFETY PROFILE: Questionable carcinogen with experimental carcinogenic data. Poison by ingestion. Moderately toxic by subcutaneous route. Mutation data reported. When heated to decomposition it emits toxic fumes of NO_x.

DSP400 CAS: 60-51-5
O,O-DIMETHYL METHYLCARBAMOYLMETHYL PHOSPHORODITHIOATE
mf: $C_5H_{12}NO_3PS_2$ mw: 229.27

SYNS: AC-12682 ◇ AMERICAN CYANAMID 12880 ◇ BI-58 ◇ CEKUTHOATE ◇ CL 12880 ◇ CYGON ◇ CYGON INSECTICIDE ◇ DAPHENE ◇ DE-FEND ◇ DEMOS-L40 ◇ DEVIGON ◇ DIMATE 267 ◇ DIMETATE ◇ DIMETHOAAT (DUTCH) ◇ DIMETHOATE (USDA) ◇ DIMETHOAT (GER-MAN) ◇ DIMETHOAT TECHNISCH 95% ◇ DIMETHOGEN ◇ O,O-DIMETHYLDITHIOPHOSPHORYLACETIC ACID-N-MONOMETHYLAMIDE SALT ◇ O,O-DIMETHYL-DITHIO-PHOSPHORYLESSIGSAEURE MONOMETHYLAMID (GER-MAN) ◇ O,O-DIMETHYL-S-(2-(METHYLAMINO)-2-OXO-ETHYL) PHOSPHORODITHIOATE ◇ O,O-DIMETHYL-S-(N-METHYL-CARBAMOYL)-METHYL-DITHIOFOSFAAT (DUTCH) ◇ (O,O-DIMETHYL-S-(N-METHYL-CARBAMOYL-METHYL)-DITHIOPHOSPHAT) (GERMAN) ◇ O,O-DI-METHYL-S-(N-METHYLCARBAMOYLMETHYL) DITHIO-PHOSPHATE ◇ O,O-DIMETHYL-S-(N-METHYLCARBA-MOYLMETHYL) PHOSPHORODITHIOATE ◇ O,O-DI-METHYL-S-(N-METHYLCARBAMYLMETHYL) THIOTHIO-NOPHOSPHATE ◇ O,O-DIMETHYL-S-(N-MONOMETHYL)-CARBAMYL METHYLDITHIOPHOSPHATE ◇ O,O-DI-METHYL-S-(2-OXO-3-AZA-BUTYL)-DITHIOPHOSPHAT (GERMAN) ◇ O,O-DIMETIL-S-(N-METIL-CARBAMOIL-METIL)-DITIOFOSFATO (ITALIAN) ◇ DIMETON ◇ DIMEVUR ◇ DITHIOPHOSPHATE de O,O-DIMETHYLE et de S(-N-METHYLCARBAMOYL-METHYLE) (FRENCH) ◇ EI-12880 ◇ ENT 24,650 ◇ EXPERIMENTAL INSECTI-CIDE 12,880 ◇ FERKETHION ◇ FORTION NM ◇ FOSFAMID ◇ FOSFOTOX ◇ FOSTION MM ◇ L-395 ◇ LURGO ◇ S-METHYLCARBAMOYLMETHYL-O,O-DIMETHYL PHOSPHORODITHIOATE ◇ N-MONOMETHYLAMIDE of O,O-DIMETHYLDITHIOPHOSPHORYLACETIC ACID ◇ NC-262 ◇ NCI-C00135 ◇ PERFECTHION ◇ PHOSPHAMID ◇ PHOSPHORODITHIOIC ACID-O,O-DIMETHYL-S-(2-(METHYLAMINO)-2-OXOETHYL) ESTER ◇ RACUSAN ◇ RCRA WASTE NUMBER P044 ◇ REBELATE ◇ ROGODIAL ◇ ROGOR ◇ ROXION U.A. ◇ SINORATOX ◇ TRIMETION

TOXICITY DATA with REFERENCE
CAR: ims-rat TDLo: 176 mg/kg/6W-I ARGEAR 41,311,73
CAR: orl-rat TDLo: 256 mg/kg/4W-I ARGEAR 41,311,73
MUT: cyt-ham-ipr 16 mg/kg ARTODN 58,152,85
MUT: mma-hmn: fbr 100 μmol/L MUREAV 42,161,77
MUT: mma-sat 500 μg/plate JTEHD6 16,403,85
MUT: mmo-omi 100 mg/L TGANAK 15(3),68,81
MUT: sce-hmn: lym 20 mg/L MUREAV 88,307,81

CONSENSUS REPORTS: NCI Carcinogenesis Bioassay (feed); No Evidence: mouse, rat NCITR* NCI-CG-TR-4,77. Reported in EPA TSCA Inventory. EPA Genetic Toxicology Program. EPA Extremely Hazardous Substances List.

SAFETY PROFILE: Questionable carcinogen with experimental carcinogenic and teratogenic data. Poison by ingestion, skin contact, intraper itoneal, subcutaneous, and possibly other routes. Moderately toxic by intravenous route. Experimental reproductive effects. Human mutation data reported. When heated to decomposition it emits very toxic fumes of NO_x, PO_x, and SO_x.

DSR200   CAS: 20241-03-6
3,3-DIMETHYL-1-(m-METHYLPHENYL) TRIAZENE
mf: $C_9H_{13}N_3$ mw: 163.25

SYNS: 3,3-DIMETHYL-1-(m-TOLYL)TRIAZENE ◇ 1-(m-METHYLPHENYL)-3,3-DIMETHYLTRIAZENE ◇ 1-(3-METHYLPHENYL)-3,3-DIMETHYLTRIAZENE

TOXICITY DATA with REFERENCE
CAR: orl-rat TDLo: 250 mg/kg   ZKKOBW 81,285,74
CAR: scu-rat TD: 2700 mg/kg/56W-I   ZKKOBW 81,285,74
CAR: scu-rat TDLo: 500 mg/kg   ZKKOBW 81,285,74
MUT: mma-sat 400 nmol/L   JMCMAR 22,473,79

SAFETY PROFILE: Questionable carcinogen with experimental carcinogenic data. Poison by ingestion and intraperitoneal routes. Moderately toxic by subcutaneous route. Mutation data reported. When heated to decomposition it emits toxic fumes of NO_x.

DSS200   CAS: 7347-46-8
N,N-DIMETHYL-4-(2-METHYL-4-PYRIDYLAZO)ANILINE-N-OXIDE
mf: $C_{14}H_{16}N_4O$ mw: 256.34

SYNS: 4-((4-(DIMETHYLAMINO)PHENYL)AZO)-2-PICOLINE-1-OXIDE ◇ N,N-DIMETHYL-4-((2-METHYL-4-PYRIDINYL)AZO)BENZENAMINE-N-OXIDE ◇ N,N-DIMETHYL-4-(4'-(2'-METHYLPYRIDYL-1'-OXIDE)AZO)ANILINE ◇ 2'-MePO4' ◇ 2-METHYLPYRIDINE-1-OXIDE-4-AZO-p-DIMETHYLANILINE

TOXICITY DATA with REFERENCE
NEO: orl-rat TDLo: 714 mg/kg/17W-C   JNCIAM 37,365,66
ETA: orl-rat TD: 2142 mg/kg/17W-C   JNCIAM 41,855,68

SAFETY PROFILE: Questionable carcinogen with experimental neoplastigenic and tumorigenic data. When heated to decomposition it emits toxic fumes of NO_x.

DST800   CAS: 597-25-1
DIMETHYLMORPHOLINO-PHOSPHONATE
mf: $C_6H_{14}NO_4P$ mw: 195.18

SYNS: DIMETHYL MORPHOLINOPHOSPHORAMIDATE ◇ DMMPA ◇ MORPHOLINOPHOSPHONIC ACID DIMETHYL ESTER ◇ 4-MORPHOLINYLPHOSPHONIC ACID DIMETHYL ESTER ◇ NCI-C54740

TOXICITY DATA with REFERENCE
CAR: orl-rat TDLo: 309 g/kg/2Y-I   NTPTR* NTP-TR-298,86
MUT: cyt-ham: ovr 3 g/L   NTPTR* NTP-TR-298,86
MUT: msc-mus: lym 2200 mg/L   NTPTR* NTP-TR-298,86
MUT: sce-ham: ovr 3 g/L   NTPTR* NTP-TR-298,86

CONSENSUS REPORTS: NTP Carcinogenesis Studies (gavage); Some Evidence: rat NTPTR* NTP-TR-298,86; No Evidence: mouse NTPTR* NTP-TR-298,86.

SAFETY PROFILE: Questionable carcinogen with experimental carcinogenic data. Poison by intravenous route. Moderately toxic by ingestion and intraperitoneal routes. Mutation data reported. When heated to decomposition it emits very toxic fumes of NO_x and PO_x. See also ESTERS.

DSU600   CAS: 607-59-0
N,N-DIMETHYL-p-(1-NAPHTHYLAZO) ANILINE
mf: $C_{18}H_{17}N_3$ mw: 275.38

SYNS: DAN ◇ p-DIMETHYLAMINOBENZENEAZO-1-NAPHTHALENE ◇ p-DIMETHYLAMINOBENZENE-1-AZO-1-NAPHTHALENE

TOXICITY DATA with REFERENCE
CAR: scu-rat TDLo: 90 mg/kg/2W-I   JNCIAM 18,843,57
ETA: orl-rat TDLo: 25 g/kg/79W-C   JNCIAM 13,57,52
MUT: dns-ham: lvr 10 μmol/L   MUREAV 136,255,84
MUT: dns-rat-orl 100 mg/kg   ENMUDM 7,101,85
MUT: dns-rat: lvr 100 μmol/L   MUREAV 136,255,84

SAFETY PROFILE: Questionable carcinogen with experimental carcinogenic and tumorigenic data. Mutation data reported. When heated to decomposition it emits toxic fumes of NO_x.

DSU800   CAS: 613-65-0
N,N-DIMETHYL-4(2'-NAPHTHYLAZO) ANILINE
mf: $C_{18}H_{17}N_2$ mw: 261.37

SYNS: DA-2-N ◇ p-DIMETHYLAMINOBENZENE-1-AZO-2-NAPHTHALENE ◇ 2-(4-DIMETHYLAMINOPHENYLAZO) NAPHTHALENE

TOXICITY DATA with REFERENCE
CAR: orl-rat TDLo:8630 mg/kg/230D-C
JNCIAM 14,571,53
ETA: skn-mus TDLo:4800 mg/kg   JNCIAM
13,1259,53
MUT: dns-ham:lvr 2 μmol/L   MUREAV 136,255,84
MUT: dns-rat-orl 100 mg/kg   ENMUDM 7,101,85
MUT: dns-rat:lvr 10 μmol/L   MUREAV 136,255,84

SAFETY PROFILE: Questionable carcinogen with experimental carcinogenic and tumorigenic data. Mutation data reported. When heated to decomposition it emits toxic fumes of NO_x.

DSV000   CAS: 63019-14-7
N,N-DIMETHYL-p-(2-(1-NAPHTHYL) VINYL)ANILINE
mf: $C_{20}H_{19}N$ mw: 273.40

SYN: 1-(4'-DIMETHYLAMINOPHENYL)-2-(1'-NAPHTHYL) ETHYLENE

TOXICITY DATA with REFERENCE
ETA: scu-mus TDLo:320 mg/kg/W-I   PTRMAD
241,147,48
ETA: scu-rat TDLo:215 mg/kg/W-I   PTRMAD
241,147,48

SAFETY PROFILE: Questionable carcinogen with experimental tumorigenic data. When heated to decomposition it emits toxic fumes of NO_x.

DSV200   CAS: 4164-28-7
DIMETHYLNITRAMINE
mf: $C_2H_6N_2O_2$ mw: 90.10

SYNS: DIMETHYLNITRAMIN (GERMAN) ◇ DIMETHYL-NITROAMINE ◇ DMNM ◇ DMNO ◇ N-NITRODIMETHYL-AMINE ◇ N-NITRO-DMA

TOXICITY DATA with REFERENCE
ETA: orl-rat TD:34 g/kg/82W-C   ZEKBAI
69,103,67
ETA: orl-rat TD:40 g/kg/D   NATWAY 48,134,61
ETA: orl-rat TDLo:20 g/kg/1Y-C   JJIND8
64,1435,80
MUT: hma-rat/sat 200 mg/kg   CNREA8 41,3205,81
MUT: mma-sat 250 μmol/plate   CRNGDP 5,809,84

SAFETY PROFILE: Questionable carcinogen with experimental tumorigenic data. Poison by intraperitoneal route. Moderately toxic by ingestion. Mutation data reported. When heated to decomposition it emits toxic fumes of NO_x.

DSV400   CAS: 59-35-8
4,6-DIMETHYL-2-(5-NITRO-2-FURYL) PYRIMIDINE
mf: $C_{10}H_9N_3O_3$ mw: 219.22

TOXICITY DATA with REFERENCE
CAR: orl-rat TDLo:8988 mg/kg/49W-C
JNCIAM 57,277,76

SAFETY PROFILE: Questionable carcinogen with experimental carcinogenic data. When heated to decomposition it emits toxic fumes of NO_x.

DSV800   CAS: 551-92-8
1,2-DIMETHYL-5-NITROIMIDAZOLE
mf: $C_5H_7N_3O_2$ mw: 141.15

SYNS: 1,2-DIMETHYL-5-NITRO-1H-IMIDAZOLE
◇ DIMETRIDAZOLE ◇ EMTRYL ◇ EMTRYLVET
◇ EMTRYMIX ◇ 8595 R.P.

TOXICITY DATA with REFERENCE
NEO: orl-rat TDLo:50 g/kg/46W-C   JNCIAM
51,403,73
MUT: bfa-rat/sat 800 mg/kg   MUREAV 97,171,82
MUT: mma-sat 50 μg/plate   PNASA6 72,5135,75
MUT: mmo-esc 100 μmol/L   MUREAV 26,483,74
MUT: mmo-klp 20 μmol/L/20H   MUREAV
66,207,79
MUT: mmo-sat 25 μg/plate   MUREAV 38,203,76
MUT: mmo-smc 500 ppm   MUREAV 86,243,81

CONSENSUS REPORTS: EPA Genetic Toxicology Program.

SAFETY PROFILE: Questionable carcinogen with experimental neoplastigenic data. Mutation data reported. When heated to decomposition it emits toxic fumes of NO_x.

DSW600   CAS: 3837-55-6
N,N-DIMETHYL-p-((m-NITROPHENYL) AZO)ANILINE
mf: $C_{14}H_{14}N_4O_2$ mw: 270.32

SYN: 3'-NITRO-4-DIMETHYLAMINOAZOBENZENE

TOXICITY DATA with REFERENCE
NEO: orl-rat TDLo:5184 mg/kg/17W-C
JEMEAV 87,139,48

SAFETY PROFILE: Questionable carcinogen with experimental neoplastigenic data. When heated to decomposition it emits toxic fumes of NO_x.

DSW800   CAS: 3010-38-6
N,N-DIMETHYL-p-((o-NITROPHENYL) AZO)ANILINE
mf: $C_{14}H_{14}N_4O_2$ mw: 270.32

SYN: 2'-NITRO-4-DIMETHYLAMINOAZOBENZENE

TOXICITY DATA with REFERENCE
NEO: orl-rat TDLo:5184 mg/kg/17W-C
   JEMEAV 87,139,48

SAFETY PROFILE: Questionable carcinogen
with experimental neoplastigenic data. When
heated to decomposition it emits toxic fumes
of NO_x.

DSX400   CAS: 7227-92-1
3,3-DIMETHYL-1-(p-NITROPHENYL) TRIAZENE
mf: $C_8H_{10}N_4O_2$ mw: 194.22

SYNS: 1-p-NITROFENYL-3,3-DIMETHYLTRIAZEN
(CZECH) ◇ 1-(p-NITROPHENYL-3,3-DIMETHYL-TRIAZEN
(GERMAN) ◇ 1-(p-NITROPHENYL)-3,3-DIMETHYL-TRI-
AZENE ◇ 1-(4-NITROPHENYL)-3,3-DIMETHYLTRIAZENE

TOXICITY DATA with REFERENCE
NEO: scu-rat TDLo:3250 mg/kg/72W-I
   ZKKOBW 81,285,74
ETA: scu-rat TD:330 mg/kg   ZKKOBW 81,285,74

SAFETY PROFILE: Questionable carcinogen
with experimental neoplastigenic and tumorigenic data. Poison by subcutaneous route. Moderately toxic by ingestion. When heated to decomposition it emits toxic fumes of NO_x.

DSX800   CAS: 37699-43-7
2,3-DIMETHYL-4-NITROPYRIDINE-1-OXIDE
mf: $C_7H_8N_2O_3$ mw: 168.17

TOXICITY DATA with REFERENCE
ETA: scu-mus TDLo:1760 mg/kg/15W-I
   GANNA2 70,799,79
MUT: dnd-mus:fbr 500 μmol/L   CNREA8
   35,521,75
MUT: dnr-esc 500 μg/well   CNREA8 32,2369,72
MUT: mmo-esc 500 μmol/L   GANNA2 70,799,79
MUT: mmo-sat 100 nmol/plate   GANNA2 70,799,79
MUT: mmo-smc 500 μg/well   CNREA8 32,2369,72
MUT: mrc-esc 500 μg/well   CNREA8 32,2369,72

SAFETY PROFILE: Questionable carcinogen
with experimental tumorigenic data. Mutation
data reported. When heated to decomposition
it emits toxic fumes of NO_x.

DSY000   CAS: 21816-42-2
2,5-DIMETHYL-4-NITROPYRIDINE-1-OXIDE
mf: $C_7H_8N_2O_3$ mw: 168.17

TOXICITY DATA with REFERENCE
ETA: scu-mus TDLo:1800 mg/kg/15W-I
   GANNA2 70,799,79
MUT: dnd-mus:fbr 500 μmol/L   CNREA8
   35,521,75
MUT: mmo-esc 500 μmol/L   GANNA2
   70,799,79
MUT: mmo-sat 100 nmol/plate   GANNA2 70,799,79

SAFETY PROFILE: Questionable carcinogen
with experimental tumorigenic data. Mutation
data reported. When heated to decomposition
it emits toxic fumes of NO_x.

DSY600   CAS: 138-89-6
N,N-DIMETHYL-p-NITROSOANILINE
DOT: 1369
mf: $C_8H_{10}N_2O$ mw: 150.20

SYNS: ACCELERINE ◇ p-(DIMETHYLAMINO)NITROSO-
BENZENE ◇ 4-(DIMETHYLAMINO)NITROSOBENZENE
◇ DIMETHYL-p-NITROSOANILINE (DOT) ◇ N,N-DI-
METHYL-4-NITROSOBENZENAMINE ◇ DIMETHYL(p-NI-
TROSOPHENYL)AMINE ◇ NCI-C01821 ◇ NDMA ◇ p-NI-
TROSO-N,N-DIMETHYLANILINE ◇ 4-NITROSODIMETHY-
LANILINE ◇ p-NITROSODIMETHYLANILINE (DOT)
◇ PARANITROSODIMETHYLANILIDE ◇ ULTRA BRILLIANT
BLUE P

TOXICITY DATA with REFERENCE
ETA: orl-rat TDLo:7300 mg/kg/1Y-C   PUOMA5
   46,68,68
MUT: mma-sat 33 μg/plate   ENMUDM 8(Suppl
   7),1,86
MUT: mmo-sat 10 μg/plate   ENMUDM 8(Suppl
   7),1,86

CONSENSUS REPORTS: Reported in EPA
TSCA Inventory.

DOT Classification: Flammable Solid; Label:
Spontaneously Combustible.

SAFETY PROFILE: Questionable carcinogen
with experimental tumorigenic data. Poison by
ingestion. Mutation data reported. Flammable
when exposed to heat, flame or oxidizers. When
heated to decomposition it emits toxic fumes
of NO_x.

DSY800   CAS: 70786-64-0
3,2'-DIMETHYL-4-NITROSOBIPHENYL
mf: $C_{14}H_{13}NO$ mw: 211.28

TOXICITY DATA with REFERENCE
CAR: scu-ham TDLo:1173 mg/kg/37W-I
   CALEDQ 22,981,79

MUT: mma-sat 80 nmol/plate   JMCMAR 22,981,79
MUT: mmo-sat 120 μmol/plate   JMCMAR22,981,79

SAFETY PROFILE: Questionable carcinogen with experimental carcinogenic data. Mutation data reported. When heated to decomposition it emits toxic fumes of NO_x.

DSZ000   CAS: 16339-12-1
N,O-DIMETHYL-N-NITROSOHYDROXYLAMINE
mf: $C_2H_6N_2O_2$ mw: 90.10

SYNS: N-METHOXY-N-NITROSOMETHYLAMINE ◇ N-NITROSOMETHOXYMETHYLAMINE ◇ N-NITROSO-METHYLMETHOXYAMINE ◇ N-NITROSO-N-METHYL-o-METHYLHYDROXYLAMIN (GERMAN) ◇ N-NITROSO-N-METHYL-o-METHYL-HYDROXYLAMINE

TOXICITY DATA with REFERENCE
ETA: orl-rat TDLo:6000 mg/kg/50W-I
    ZKKOBW 89,31,77
MUT: mma-sat 1 μg/plate   MUREAV 51,319,78
MUT: mmo-omi 1 pph/72H-C   SOGEBZ 10,522,74
MUT: mmo-sat 1 μg/plate   MUREAV 51,319,78

SAFETY PROFILE: Questionable carcinogen with experimental tumorigenic data. Poison by intravenous route. Mutation data reported. Many N-nitroso compounds are carcinogens. When heated to decomposition it emits toxic fumes of NO_x.

DTA050
2,6-DIMETHYL-4-NITROSOMOR-PHOLINE cis and trans mixture (2:1)
mf: $C_6H_{12}N_2O_2$ mw: 144.20

TOXICITY DATA with REFERENCE
CAR: orl-rat TD:138 g/kg/50W-I   CRNGDP
    3,911,82
CAR: orl-rat TDLo:75 g/kg/50W-I   CRNGDP
    3,911,82

SAFETY PROFILE: Questionable carcinogen with experimental carcinogenic data. When heated to decomposition it emits toxic fumes of NO_x.

DTA400   CAS: 17721-95-8
2,6-DIMETHYLNITROSOPIPERIDINE
mf: $C_7H_{14}N_2O$ mw: 142.23

SYN: N-NITROSO-2,6-DIMETHYLPIPERIDINE

TOXICITY DATA with REFERENCE
ETA: orl-rat TDLo:2813 mg/kg/50W-I   IJCNAW
    16,318,75

CONSENSUS REPORTS: EPA Genetic Toxicology Program.

SAFETY PROFILE: Questionable carcinogen with experimental tumorigenic data. Many N-nitroso compounds are carcinogens. When heated to decomposition it emits toxic fumes of NO_x.

DTA600   CAS: 65445-59-2
3,5-DIMETHYLNITROSOPIPERIDINE
mf: $C_7H_{14}N_2O$ mw: 142.23

SYNS: 3,5-DIMETHYL-1-NITROSOPIPERIDINE ◇ N-NITROSO-3,5-DIMETHYLPIPERIDINE

TOXICITY DATA with REFERENCE
ETA: orl-rat TDLo:3100 mg/kg/50W-I   JJIND8
    68,989,82
MUT: mma-sat 1 μg/plate   MUREAV 56,131,77
MUT: mma-smc 50 mmol/L/24H   MUREAV
    57,155,78
MUT: sln-dmg-orl 5 mmol/L/24H   MUREAV
    67,27,79

CONSENSUS REPORTS: EPA Genetic Toxicology Program.

SAFETY PROFILE: Questionable carcinogen with experimental tumorigenic data. Mutation data reported. Many N-nitroso compounds are carcinogens. When heated to decomposition it emits toxic fumes of NO_x.

DTA700   CAS: 78338-32-6
trans-3,5-DIMETHYL-1-NITROSOPIPERIDINE
mf: $C_7H_{14}N_2O$ mw: 142.23

SYNS: NITROSO-3,5-DIMETHYLPIPERIDINE trans-isomer ◇ PIPERIDINE, 3,5-DIMETHYL-1-NITROSO-, (E)-

TOXICITY DATA with REFERENCE
ETA: orl-rat TDLo:500 mg/kg/50W-I   JJIND8
    68,989,82
MUT: mma-sat 50 μg/plate   TCMUE9 1,129,84

SAFETY PROFILE: Questionable carcinogen with experimental tumorigenic data. Mutation data reported. When heated to decomposition it emits toxic fumes of NO_x.

DTA690   CAS: 78338-31-5
cis-3,5-DIMETHYL-1-NITROSOPIPERIDINE
mf: $C_7H_{14}N_2O$ mw: 142.23

SYNS: NITROSO-3,5-DIMETHYLPIPERIDINE cis-isomer ◇ PIPERIDINE, 3,5-DIMETHYL-1-NITROSO-, (Z)-

TOXICITY DATA with REFERENCE
ETA: orl-rat TDLo: 2550 mg/kg/50W-I   JJIND8 68,989,82
MUT: mma-sat 100 μg/plate   TCMUD8 1,295,80

SAFETY PROFILE: Questionable carcinogen with experimental tumorigenic data. Mutation data reported. When heated to decomposition it emits toxic fumes of NO_x.

DTA800   CAS: 55556-86-0
2,5-DIMETHYL-N-NITROSOPYRROLIDINE
mf: $C_6H_{12}N_2O$ mw: 128.20

TOXICITY DATA with REFERENCE
ETA: orl-rat TDLo: 5625 mg/kg/50W-I   CNREA8 36,1988,76

SAFETY PROFILE: Questionable carcinogen with experimental tumorigenic data. Many N-nitroso compounds are carcinogens. When heated to decomposition it emits toxic fumes of NO_x.

DTH000   CAS: 1955-45-9
3,3-DIMETHYL-2-OXETHANONE
mf: $C_5H_8O_2$ mw: 100.13

SYNS: 3,3-DIMETHYL-2-OXETANONE ◇ DIMETHYL PROPIOLACTONE ◇ 3,3-DIMETHYL-β-PROPIOLACTONE ◇ NCI-C04126 ◇ PIVALIC ACID LACTONE ◇ PIVALOLACTONE

TOXICITY DATA with REFERENCE
CAR: orl-rat TDLo: 216 g/kg/2Y-I
NCITR* NCI-CG-TR-140,78
ETA: orl-rat TD: 72 g/kg/69W
NCITR* NCI-CG-TR-140,78
MUT: mma-esc 333 μg/plate   ENMUDM 7(Suppl 5),1,85
MUT: mma-sat 333 μg/plate   ENMUDM 7(Suppl 5),1,85
MUT: mmo-esc 333 μg/plate   ENMUDM 7(Suppl 5),1,85
MUT: mmo-sat 33300 ng/plate   ENMUDM 7(Suppl 5),1,85
MUT: mmo-srm 25 mg/L   ATXKA8 30,67,72

CONSENSUS REPORTS: NCI Carcinogenesis Bioassay (gavage); No Evidence: mouse NCITR* NCI-CG-TR-140,78; Clear Evidence: rat NCITR* NCI-CG-TR-140,78. Reported in EPA TSCA Inventory.

SAFETY PROFILE: Questionable carcinogen with experimental carcinogenic and tumorigenic data. Poison by ingestion. Mutation data reported. When heated to decomposition it emits acrid smoke and irritating fumes.

DTJ200   CAS: 22349-59-3
1,4-DIMETHYLPHENANTHRENE
mf: $C_{16}H_{14}$ mw: 206.30

TOXICITY DATA with REFERENCE
CAR: skn-mus TDLo: 40 mg/kg/20D-I   CNREA8 41,3441,81
MUT: mma-sat 50 μg/plate   MUREAV 116,91,83

CONSENSUS REPORTS: IARC Cancer Review: Animal Inadequate Evidence IMEMDT 32,349,83

SAFETY PROFILE: Questionable carcinogen with experimental carcinogenic data. Mutation data reported. When heated to decomposition it emits acrid smoke and irritating fumes.

DTK600   CAS: 2747-31-1
N,N-DIMETHYL-p-PHENYLAZOANILINE-N-OXIDE
mf: $C_{14}H_{15}N_3O$ mw: 241.32

SYNS: DAB-N-OXIDE ◇ 4-DIMETHYLAMINOAZOBENZENE AMINE-N-OXIDE ◇ N,N-DIMETHYLAMINOAZOBENZENE-N-OXIDE

TOXICITY DATA with REFERENCE
ETA: orl-mus TDLo: 11 g/kg/26W-C   GANNA2 54,455,63
ETA: orl-rat TDLo: 6300 mg/kg/30W-C   GANNA2 54,455,63
ETA: scu-rat TDLo: 278 mg/kg/12W-I   CNREA8 27,1600,67

SAFETY PROFILE: Questionable carcinogen with experimental tumorigenic data. Poison by intraperitoneal route. Moderately toxic by ingestion. When heated to decomposition it emits toxic fumes of NO_x.

DTK800   CAS: 2438-49-5
N,N-DIMETHYL-4-PHENYLAZO-o-ANISIDINE
mf: $C_{15}H_{17}N_3O$ mw: 255.35

SYN: 3-METHOXY-4-DIMETHYLAMINOAZOBENZENE

TOXICITY DATA with REFERENCE
ETA: orl-rat TDLo: 9800 mg/kg/34W-C   CNREA8 21,1068,61
ETA: skn-rat TDLo: 640 mg/kg/40W-I   CNREA8 25,1784,65

SAFETY PROFILE: Questionable carcinogen with experimental tumorigenic data. When heated to decomposition it emits toxic fumes of NO_x.

DTL000 CAS: 36576-23-5
2,3-DIMETHYL-4-(PHENYLAZO) BENZENAMINE
mf: $C_{14}H_{15}N_3$ mw: 225.32

SYN: 2,3-DIMETHYL-4-PHENYLAZOANILINE

TOXICITY DATA with REFERENCE
NEO: orl-mus TDLo: 6000 mg/kg/26W-C
FCTXAV 11,415,73

SAFETY PROFILE: Questionable carcinogen with experimental neoplastigenic data. When heated to decomposition it emits toxic fumes of NO_x.

DTN875 CAS: 72586-68-6
1,3-DIMETHYL-3-PHENYL-1-NITROSOUREA
mf: $C_9H_{11}N_3O_2$ mw: 193.23

SYN: N,N'-DIMETHYL-N-NITROSO-N'-PHENYLUREA

TOXICITY DATA with REFERENCE
ETA: orl-rat TDLo: 58 mg/kg/20W-I CRNGDP 8,237,87
MUT: cyt-ham: lng 5 μmol/L CRNGDP 4,409,83
MUT: mma-sat 1 μmol/plate CRNGDP 4,409,83
MUT: mmo-sat 1 μmol/plate CRNGDP 4,409,83
MUT: msc-ham: lng 500 mmol/L CRNGDP 4,409,83
MUT: sce-ham: lng 1 μmol/L CRNGDP 4,409,83
MUT: sce-ham: lng 100 nmol/L MUREAV 126,259,84

SAFETY PROFILE: Questionable carcinogen with experimental tumorigenic data. Mutation data reported. Many N-nitroso compounds are carcinogens. When heated to decomposition it emits toxic fumes of NO_x.

DTP000 CAS: 7227-91-0
3,3-DIMETHYL-1-PHENYLTRIAZENE
mf: $C_8H_{11}N_3$ mw: 149.22

SYNS: 3,3-DIMETHYL-1-PHENYL-1-TRIAZENE
◊ DMPT ◊ 1-FENYL-3,3-DIMETHYLTRIAZIN ◊ NSC 3094
◊ PDMT ◊ PDT ◊ 1-PHENYL-3,3-DIMETHYLTRIAZENE
◊ PHENYLDIMETHYLTRIAZINE ◊ X 119

TOXICITY DATA with REFERENCE
CAR: orl-rat TD: 1600 mg/kg/79W-C ZKKOBW 81,285,74

CAR: orl-rat TDLo: 310 mg/kg ZKKOBW 81,285,74
CAR: scu-rat TDLo: 75 mg/kg (23D preg) IARCCD 4,45,73
CAR: scu-rat TDLo: 1250 mg/kg/59W-I ZKKOBW 81,285,74
ETA: ivn-rat TDLo: 10 mg/kg (22D preg) ZAPPAN 115,8,72
ETA: ivn-rat TDLo: 30500 μg/kg/16W-I ZAPPAN 115,8,72
ETA: orl-rat TD: 1650 mg/kg/33W-I XENOBH 3,271,73
ETA: orl-rat TD: 2040 mg/kg/47W-I FCTXAV 6,579,68
ETA: scu-rat TD: 1166 mg/kg/47W-I FCTXAV 6,579,68
ETA: scu-rat TD: 1250 mg/kg/59W-I NATWAY 54,171,67
MUT: cyt-ham: lng 10 mg/L MUREAV 88,197,81
MUT: cyt-hmn: leu 25 μmol/L MUREAV 77,123,73
MUT: mmo-sat 1 μg/plate JNCIAM 62,873,79
MUT: mrc-smc 900 ppm JNCIAM 62,901,79
MUT: otr-ham: emb 100 μg/L NCIMAV 58,243,81

CONSENSUS REPORTS: EPA Genetic Toxicology Program.

SAFETY PROFILE: Questionable carcinogen with experimental carcinogenic, tumorigenic, and teratogenic data. Poison by ingestion and intraperitoneal routes. Experimental reproductive effects. Human mutation data reported. Decomposes explosively on attempted distillation at atmospheric pressure. When heated to decomposition it emits toxic fumes of NO_x.

DTT400 CAS: 24690-46-8
N,N-DIMETHYL-p-((p-PROPYLPHENYL) AZO)ANILINE
mf: $C_{17}H_{21}N_3$ mw: 267.41

SYN: 4'-N-PROPYL-4-DIMETHYLAMINOAZOBENZENE

TOXICITY DATA with REFERENCE
ETA: orl-rat TDLo: 4284 mg/kg/17W-C
JNCIAM 27,663,61

SAFETY PROFILE: Questionable carcinogen with experimental tumorigenic data. When heated to decomposition it emits toxic fumes of NO_x.

DTT600 CAS: 23950-58-5
N-(1,1-DIMETHYLPROPYNYL)-3,5-DICHLOROBENZAMIDE
mf: $C_{12}H_{11}Cl_2NO$ mw: 256.14

SYNS: 3,5-DICHLORO-N-(1,1-DIMETHYL-2-PRO-PYNYL)BENZAMIDE ◊ KERB ◊ PROMAMIDE ◊ PRONAM-

IDE ◇ PROPYZAMIDE ◇ RCRA WASTE NUMBER U192
◇ RH 315

TOXICITY DATA with REFERENCE
CAR: orl-mus TDLo: 65520 mg/kg/78W-C
    ENVRAL 23,1,80
ETA: orl-rat TDLo: 1092 mg/kg/2Y-C   ENVRAL
    23,1,80

SAFETY PROFILE: Questionable carcinogen
with experimental carcinogenic and tumorigenic
data. Mildly toxic by ingestion. An herbicide.
When heated to decomposition it emits very
toxic fumes of Cl$^-$ and NO$_x$.

DTV200   CAS: 21600-42-0
(3,3-DIMETHYL-1-(m-PYRIDYL-N-
OXIDE))TRIAZENE
mf: C$_7$H$_{10}$N$_4$O   mw: 166.21

SYNS: 3-(3′,3′-DIMETHYLTRIAZENO)-PYRIDIN-N-OXID
(GERMAN) ◇ 3-(3′,3′-DIMETHYLTRIAZENO)PYRIDINE-N-
OXIDE ◇ PYNDT ◇ 1-(PYRIDYL-3-N-OXID)-3,3-DIMETHYL-
TRIAZEN (GERMAN) ◇ 1-(PYRIDYL-3-N-OXIDE)-3,3-DI-
METHYLTRIAZENE

TOXICITY DATA with REFERENCE
CAR: ivn-rat TDLo: 490 mg/kg/38W-I   ZKKOBW
    81,285,74
ETA: ivn-rat TD: 540 mg/kg/36W-I   XENOBH
    3,271,73
MUT: cyt-hmn: leu 25 μmol/L   MUREAV 77,123,73
MUT: hma-mus/smc 400 μmol/L/Kg   AGACBH
    3,99,73
MUT: sln-dmg-orl 700 μmol/L   CBINA8 9,365,74

CONSENSUS REPORTS: EPA Genetic Toxicology Program.

SAFETY PROFILE: Questionable carcinogen
with experimental carcinogenic and tumorigenic
data. Poison by intravenous and subcutaneous
routes. Human mutation data reported. When
heated to decomposition it emits toxic fumes
of NO$_x$.

DTY200   CAS: 17025-30-8
N,N-DIMETHYL-4-(4′-QUINOLYLAZO)
ANILINE
mf: C$_{17}$H$_{16}$N$_4$ mw: 276.37

SYN: 4-((p-(DIMETHYLAMINO)PHENYL)AZO)QUINOLINE

TOXICITY DATA with REFERENCE
ETA: orl-rat TDLo: 2142 mg/kg/17W-C
    JNCIAM 26,1461,61

SAFETY PROFILE: Questionable carcinogen

with experimental tumorigenic data. When
heated to decomposition it emits toxic fumes
of NO$_x$.

DTY400   CAS: 63042-68-2
N,N-DIMETHYL-4-((4′-QUINOLYL-1′-
OXIDE)AZO)ANILINE
mf: C$_{17}$H$_{16}$N$_4$O   mw: 292.37

SYN:
4-((p-(DIMETHYLAMINO)PHENYL)AZO)QUINOLINE-1-OX-
IDE

TOXICITY DATA with REFERENCE
ETA: orl-rat TDLo: 2142 mg/kg/17W-C
    JNCIAM 26,1461,61

SAFETY PROFILE: Questionable carcinogen
with experimental tumorigenic data. When
heated to decomposition it emits toxic fumes
of NO$_x$.

DUA200   CAS: 23521-13-3
N,N-DIMETHYL-p-(5-QUINOXALYLAZO)
ANILINE
mf: C$_{16}$H$_{15}$N$_5$ mw: 277.36

SYN:
5-((p-(DIMETHYLAMINO)PHENYL)AZO)QUINOXALINE

TOXICITY DATA with REFERENCE
CAR: orl-rat TDLo: 2200 mg/kg/17W-C
    JMCMAR 12,1113,69

SAFETY PROFILE: Questionable carcinogen
with experimental carcinogenic data. When
heated to decomposition it emits toxic fumes
of NO$_x$.

DUA400   CAS: 23521-14-4
N,N-DIMETHYL-p-(6-QUINOXALYAZO)
ANILINE
mf: C$_{16}$H$_{15}$N$_5$ mw: 277.36

SYNS:
6-((p-(DIMETHYLAMINO)PHENYL)AZO)QUINOXALINE
◇ N,N-DIMETHYL-p-(6-QUINOXALINYLAZO)ANILINE

TOXICITY DATA with REFERENCE
CAR: orl-rat TDLo: 1100 mg/kg/60D-C
    JMCMAR 12,1113,69

SAFETY PROFILE: Questionable carcinogen
with experimental carcinogenic data. When
heated to decomposition it emits toxic fumes
of NO$_x$.

DUB600   CAS: 63148-62-9
DIMETHYL SILOXANE

PROP: Viscosity 100 at 25 degrees (ISMJAV 22,15,63).

SYN: DOW-CORNING 200 FLUID-LOT NO. AA-4163

TOXICITY DATA with REFERENCE
ETA: scu-mus TDLo:120 g/kg   ISMJAV 22,15,63
CONSENSUS REPORTS: Reported in EPA TSCA Inventory.

SAFETY PROFILE: Questionable carcinogen with experimental tumorigenic data.

DUB800   CAS: 1145-73-9
N,N-DIMETHYL-4-STILBENAMINE
mf: $C_{16}H_{17}N$ mw: 223.34

SYNS: 4-DIMETHYLAMINOSTILBEN (GERMAN) ◇ N,N-DIMETHYL-4-AMINOSTILBENE ◇ N,N-DIMETHYL-p-STYRYLANILINE ◇ STILBENYL-N,N-DIMETHYLAMINE

TOXICITY DATA with REFERENCE
CAR: orl-rat TD:4200 mg/kg/20W-C   GANNA2 61,367,70
CAR: orl-rat TDLo:50 mg/kg   CNREA8 26,619,66
ETA: ipr-rat TDLo:180 mg/kg/9W-I   BJCAAI 6,392,52
ETA: orl-rat TD:305 mg/kg/43W-C   ZEKBAI 61,230,56
ETA: orl-rat TD:370 mg/kg/26W-C   ZEKBAI 65,272,63
ETA: orl-rat TD:383 mg/kg/46W-C   ZEKBAI 67,135,65
ETA: orl-rat TD:520 mg/kg/49W-C   ABMGAJ 9,87,62
MUT: dnr-bcs 5 g/L   MUREAV 42,19,77
MUT: mma-sat 10 µg/plate   JJIND8 71,293,83
MUT: mmo-bcs 5 g/L   MUREAV 42,19,77

SAFETY PROFILE: Questionable carcinogen with experimental carcinogenic and tumorigenic data. Poison by ingestion and intraperitoneal routes. Mutation data reported. When heated to decomposition it emits toxic fumes of NO_x.

DUC000   CAS: 838-95-9
(E)-N,N-DIMETHYL-4-STILBENAMINE
mf: $C_{16}H_{17}N$ mw: 223.34

SYNS: trans-p-(DIMETHYLAMINO)STILBENE ◇ trans-4-DIMETHYLAMINOSTILBENE ◇ (E)-N,N,-DIMETHYL-4-(2-PHENYLETHENYL)BENZENAMINE ◇ 4-DIMETHYLAMINO-trans-STILBENE ◇ trans-N,N-DIMETHYL-4-STILBENAMINE

TOXICITY DATA with REFERENCE
CAR: orl-rat TDLo:240 mg/kg/20W-I   ZEKBAI 74,200,70

ETA: orl-rat TD:275 mg/kg/26W-I   PTRMAD 241,147,48
ETA: orl-rat TD:305 mg/kg/44W-C   EXPEAM 12,185,56
ETA: orl-rat TD:550 mg/kg/26W-C   EXPEAM 12,185,56
ETA: orl-rat TD:580 mg/kg/32W-C   BJCAAI 22,133,68
ETA: scu-rat TD:180 mg/kg/8W-I   PTRMAD 241,147,48
ETA: scu-rat TDLo:135 mg/kg/W-I   PTRMAD 241,147,48
MUT: dns-rat-orl 40 mg/kg   ENMUDM 7,101,85
MUT: dns-rat:lvr 1 µmol/L   ENMUDM 7,101,85
MUT: mma-sat 10 µg/plate   PNASA6 72,5135,75
MUT: oms-rat-orl 25 µmol/kg   CBINA8 24,355,79
MUT: sln-dmg-orl 1500 µmol/L   BIZNAT 102,271,83

CONSENSUS REPORTS: EPA Genetic Toxicology Program.

SAFETY PROFILE: Questionable carcinogen with experimental carcinogenic and tumorigenic data. Poison by ingestion and subcutaneous routes. Mutation data reported. When heated to decomposition it emits toxic fumes of NO_x.

DUC200   CAS: 14301-11-2
(Z)-N,N-DIMETHYL-4-STILBENAMINE
mf: $C_{16}H_{17}N$ mw: 223.34

SYNS: cis-4-DIMETHYLAMINOSTILBENE ◇ cis-N,N-DIMETHYL-4-STILBENAMINE

TOXICITY DATA with REFERENCE
NEO: orl-rat TDLo:310 mg/kg/20W-I   ZEKBAI 74,200,70

SAFETY PROFILE: Questionable carcinogen with experimental neoplastigenic data. When heated to decomposition it emits toxic fumes of NO_x.

DUD800   CAS: 67-68-5
DIMETHYL SULFOXIDE
mf: C_2H_6OS mw: 78.14

PROP: Clear, water-white, hygroscopic liquid. Mp: 18.5°, bp: 189°, flash p: 203°F (OC), d: 1.100 @ 20°, vap press: 0.37 mm @ 20°, lel: 2.6%, uel: 28.5%, autoign temp: 419°F.

SYNS: A 10846 ◇ DELTAN ◇ DEMASORB ◇ DEMAVET ◇ DEMESO ◇ DEMSODROX ◇ DERMASORB ◇ DIMETHYL SULPHOXIDE ◇ DIMEXIDE ◇ DIPIRARTRIL-TROPICO ◇ DMS-70 ◇ DMS-90 ◇ DMSO ◇ DOLICUR ◇ DOLIGUR

◇ DOMOSO ◇ DROMISOL ◇ DURASORB ◇ GAMASOL 90
◇ HYADUR ◇ INFILTRINA ◇ M 176 ◇ METHYLSULFINYL-
METHANE ◇ METHYL SULFOXIDE ◇ NSC-763 ◇ RIMSO-
50 ◇ SOMIPRONT ◇ SQ 9453 ◇ SULFINYLBIS(METHANE)
◇ SYNTEXAN ◇ TOPSYM

TOXICITY DATA with REFERENCE
ETA: orl-mus TDLo:65340 mg/kg/66W-I
  GTPZAB 28(5),39,84
ETA: orl-rat TDLo:59 g/kg/81W-I GTPZAB
  28(5),39,84
ETA: scu-mus TDLo:66 g/kg/66W-I GTPZAB
  28(5),39,84
ETA: scu-rat TDLo:220 g/kg/82W-I GTPZAB
  28(5),39,84
MUT: cyt-ham:ovr 19 pph MUREAV 88,397,81
MUT: mmo-esc 551 g/L MUREAV 130,97,84
MUT: mmo-omi 111 mL/L HEREAY 99,209,83
MUT: oms-hmn:lym 140 mmol/L PNASA6
  79,1171,82

CONSENSUS REPORTS: Reported in EPA
TSCA Inventory. EPA Genetic Toxicology Program.

SAFETY PROFILE: Questionable carcinogen
with experimental tumorigenic and teratogenic
data. Poison by ingestion. Moderately toxic by
intravenous and intraperitoneal routes. Mildly
toxic by subcutaneous route. Human systemic
effects by intravenous route: nausea or vomiting
and jaundice. Experimental reproductive effects. A skin and eye irritant. Human mutation
data reported. It freely penetrates the skin and
may carry dissolved chemicals with it into the
body. Combustible when exposed to heat or
flame; can react with oxidizing materials. To
fight fire, use foam, alcohol foam, CO_2, dry
chemical. When heated to decomposition it
emits toxic fumes of SO_x.

DUE000   CAS: 120-61-6
DIMETHYL TEREPHTHALATE
mf: $C_{10}H_{10}O_4$ mw: 194.20

SYNS: 1,4-BENZENE DICARBOXYLIC ACID DIMETHYL
ESTER (9CI) ◇ DIMETHYL-1,4-BENZENE DICARBOXYLATE
◇ METHYL-4-CARBOMETHOXY BENZOATE ◇ NCI-C50055
◇ TEREPHTHALIC ACID METHYL ESTER

TOXICITY DATA with REFERENCE
CAR: orl-mus TD:433 g/kg/103W-C
  NCITR* NCI-CG-TR-121,79
CAR: orl-mus TDLo:216 g/kg/103W-C
  NCITR* NCI-CG-TR-121,79

CONSENSUS REPORTS: NCI Carcinogenesis Bioassay (feed): Clear Evidence: mouse
(NCITR* NCI-CG-TR-121,79); No Evidence:
rat (NCITR(NCI-CG-TR-121,79). Reported in
EPA TSCA Inventory.

SAFETY PROFILE: Questionable carcinogen
with experimental carcinogenic data. Moderately toxic by intraperitoneal route. Mildly toxic
by ingestion. An eye irritant. When heated to
decomposition it emits acrid smoke and irritating
fumes.

DUF000   CAS: 25486-91-3
**7,12-DIMETHYL-8,9,10,11-
TETRAHYDROBENZ(a)ANTHRACENE**
mf: $C_{20}H_{20}$ mw: 260.40

SYN: 8,9,10,11-TETRAHYDRO-7,12-DIMETHYLBENZ(a)
ANTHRACENE

TOXICITY DATA with REFERENCE
ETA: skn-mus TDLo:212 mg/kg/65W-I
  JNCIAM 44,641,70

SAFETY PROFILE: Questionable carcinogen
with experimental tumorigenic data. When
heated to decomposition it emits acrid smoke
and irritating fumes.

DUF200   CAS: 52171-94-5
**1,11-DIMETHYL-1,2,3,4-
TETRAHYDROCHRYSENE**
mf: $C_{20}H_{20}$ mw: 260.40

TOXICITY DATA with REFERENCE
ETA: skn-mus TDLo:120 mg/kg/50W-I
  CNREA8 34,1315,74
MUT: mma-sat 20 μg/plate CNREA8 36,4525,76

CONSENSUS REPORTS: EPA Genetic Toxicology Program.

SAFETY PROFILE: Questionable carcinogen
with experimental tumorigenic data. Mutation
data reported. When heated to decomposition
it emits acrid smoke and irritating fumes.

DUH400   CAS: 3010-57-9
**N,N-DIMETHYL-4-(p-TOLYLAZO)
ANILINE**
mf: $C_{15}H_{17}N_3$ mw: 239.35

SYNS: N,N-DIMETHYL-4-((4-METHYLPHENYL)AZO)
BENZENAMINE ◇ p'-METHYL-p-DIMETHYLAMINOAZO-
BENZENE ◇ 4'-METHYL-4-DIMETHYLAMINOAZOBEN-
ZENE

TOXICITY DATA with REFERENCE
ETA: orl-rat TDLo:7776 mg/kg/35W-C
  CNREA8 5,227,45

MUT: dns-rat:lvr 10 μmol/L CNREA8 46,1654,86
MUT: mma-sat 500 nmol/plate MUREAV 121,95,83

CONSENSUS REPORTS: EPA Genetic Toxicology Program.

SAFETY PROFILE: Questionable carcinogen with experimental tumorigenic and teratogenic data. Experimental reproductive effects. Mutation data reported. When heated to decomposition it emits toxic fumes of NO_x.

DUH600   CAS: 55-80-1
N,N-DIMETHYL-p-(m-TOLYLAZO) ANILINE
mf: $C_{15}H_{17}N_3$ mw: 239.35

SYNS: 4-(N,N-DIMETHYLAMINO)-3'-METHYLAZOBEN-ZENE ◇ N,N-DIMETHYL-p-(3'-METHYLPHENYLAZO)ANI-LINE ◇ N,N-DIMETHYL-4-((3-METHYLPHENYL)AZO) BENZENAMINE ◇ MDAB ◇ 3'-MDAB ◇ 3'-METHYLBUT-TERGELB (GERMAN) ◇ 3'-METHYL-DAB ◇ 3'-METHYL-4-DIMETHYLAMINOAZOBENZEN (CZECH) ◇ M'-METHYL-p-DIMETHYLAMINOAZOBENZENE ◇ 3'-METHYL-4-DIME-THYLAMINOAZOBENZENE ◇ 3'-METHYL-N,N-DIMETHYL-4-AMINOAZOBENZENE ◇ 3'-METHYLDIMETHYLAMINO-AZOBENZOL (GERMAN)

TOXICITY DATA with REFERENCE
CAR: orl-rat TD:2419 mg/kg/12W-C CBINA8 53,107,85
CAR: orl-rat TDLo:1800 mg/kg/7W-C JJIND8 71,855,83
CAR: orl-rat TDLo:2229 mg/kg/12W-C AJPAA4 87,189,77
ETA: imp-rat TDLo:2000 mg/kg/9W-C EXPEAM 34,788,78
ETA: orl-ham TDLo:12 g/kg/38W-C ARPAAQ 71,566,61
ETA: orl-rat TD:1656 mg/kg/8W-I CNREA8 33,1119,73
ETA: orl-rat TD:1890 mg/kg/9W-C CALEDQ 9,299,80
ETA: orl-rat TD:2142 mg/kg/17W-C JNCIAM 26,1461,61
ETA: orl-rat TD:2160 mg/kg/17W-C JMCMAR 11,1074,68
ETA: orl-rat TD:2520 mg/kg/6W-C BBRCA9 92,591,80
ETA: orl-rat TD:2520 mg/kg/12W-C GANNA2 63,31,72
ETA: orl-rat TD:2600 mg/kg/13W-C CNREA8 17,387,57
ETA: scu-rat TDLo:2750 mg/kg/1Y-I CNREA8 35,3798,75
MUT: dns-ham:lvr 1 μmol/L ENMUDM 5,1,83

MUT: dns-rat-orl 10 mg/kg CALEDQ 27,115,85
MUT: dns-rat:lvr 1 μmol/L CNREA8 46,1654,86
MUT: mmo-sat 1 μmol/plate CRNGDP 4,1487,83
MUT: msc-rat:lvr 10 μmol/L MUREAV 130,53,84
MUT: otr-rat:lvr 240 μmol/L AMOKAG 39,231,85

CONSENSUS REPORTS: Reported in EPA TSCA Inventory. EPA Genetic Toxicology Program.

SAFETY PROFILE: Questionable carcinogen with experimental carcinogenic, neoplastigenic, tumorigenic, and teratogenic data. Moderately toxic by ingestion. Mutation data reported. When heated to decomposition it emits toxic fumes of NO_x.

DUH800   CAS: 3731-39-3
N,N-DIMETHYL-p-((o-TOLYL)AZO) ANILINE
mf: $C_{15}H_{17}N_3$ mw: 239.35

SYNS: N,N-DIMETHYL-p-(2'-METHYLPHENYLAZO)ANI-LINE ◇ N,N-DIMETHYL-4-((2-METHYLPHENYL)AZO) BENZENAMINE ◇ o'-METHYL-p-DIMETHYLAMINOAZO-BENZENE ◇ 2'-METHYL-4-DIMETHYLAMINOAZOBEN-ZENE ◇ 2-METHYL-N,N-DIMETHYL-4-AMINOAZOBEN-ZENE

TOXICITY DATA with REFERENCE
CAR: orl-rat TDLo:14414 mg/kg/52W-C CBINA8 53,107,85
ETA: orl-rat TD: 5856 mg/kg/26W-C CNREA8 5,227,45
MUT: dns-rat:lvr 10 μmol/L CNREA8 46,1654,86
MUT: mma-sat 100 nmol/plate CALEDQ 1,91,75

SAFETY PROFILE: Questionable carcinogen with experimental carcinogenic and tumorigenic data. Mutation data reported. When heated to decomposition it emits toxic fumes of NO_x.

DUK200   CAS: 343-75-9
N,N-DIMETHYL-p-(2,4,6-TRIFLUOROPHENYLAZO)ANILINE
mf: $C_{14}H_{12}F_3N_3$ mw: 279.29

SYN: 2',4',6'-TRIFLUORO-4-DIMETHYLAMINOAZOBEN-ZENE

TOXICITY DATA with REFERENCE
ETA: orl-rat TDLo:2700 mg/kg/13W-C CNREA8 13,93,53

SAFETY PROFILE: Questionable carcinogen with experimental tumorigenic data. When

heated to decomposition it emits very toxic fumes of F^- and NO_x.

DUK800   CAS: 2164-17-2
1,1-DIMETHYL-3-(α,α,α-TRIFLUORO-m-TOLYL) UREA
mf: $C_{10}H_{11}F_3N_2O$ mw: 232.23

SYNS: C 2059 ◇ CIBA 2059 ◇ COTORAN ◇ COTORAN MULTI 50WP ◇ COTTONEX ◇ 1,1-DIMETHYL-3-(3-TRIFLUO-ROMETHYLPHENYL)UREA ◇ N,N-DIMETHYL-N'-(3-TRI-FLUOROMETHYLPHENYL)UREA ◇ FLUOMETURON ◇ HERBICIDE C-2059 ◇ LANEX ◇ NCI-C08695 ◇ PAKHTARAN ◇ 3-(5-TRIFLUORMETHYLPHE-NYL)-,1-DIMETHYLHARNSTOFF (GERMAN) ◇ N-(m-TRI-FLUOROMETHYLPHENYL)-N',N'-DIMETHYLUREA ◇ N-(3-TRIFLUOROMETHYLPHENYL)-N'-N'-DIMETHYLUREA ◇ 3-(m-TRIFLUOROMETHYLPHE-NYL)-1,1-DIMETHYLUREA

TOXICITY DATA with REFERENCE
CAR: orl-mus TDLo:87 g/kg/2Y-C
   NCITR* NCI-CG-TR-195,80
MUT: dni-mus-orl 1 g/kg   MUREAV 58,353,78
MUT: mma-sat 1 μg/plate   MUREAV 58,353,78
MUT: otr-rat:emb 56 μg/plate   JJATDK 1,190,81

CONSENSUS REPORTS: EPA Genetic Toxicology Program. IARC Cancer Review: Animal Inadequate Evidence IMEMDT 30,245,83. NCI Carcinogenesis Bioassay (feed); No Evidence: rat NCITR* NCI-CG-TR-195,80; Equivocal Evidence: mouse NCITR* NCI-CG-TR-195,80. Reported in EPA TSCA Inventory.

SAFETY PROFILE: Questionable carcinogen with experimental carcinogenic data. Moderately toxic by ingestion, intraperitoneal, and possibly other routes. Mutation data reported. When heated to decomposition it emits very toxic fumes of F^- and NO_x.

DUL200   CAS: 2223-82-7
2,2-DIMETHYLTRIMETHYLENE ACRYLATE
mf: $C_{11}H_{16}O_4$ mw: 212.27

SYNS: DIMETHYLOLPROPANE DIACRYLATE ◇ 2,2-DI-METHYL-1,3-PROPANEDIOL DIACRYLATE ◇ 2,2-DI-METHYLTRIMETHYLENE ESTER ACRYLIC ACID ◇ NEOPENTYL GLYCOL DIACRYLATE ◇ 2-PROPENOIC ACID-2,2-DIMETHYL-1,3-PROPANEDIYL ESTER ◇ SR 247

TOXICITY DATA with REFERENCE
CAR: skn-mus TDLo:46800 mg/kg/28W-I
   JTEHD6 16,55,85

CONSENSUS REPORTS: Reported in EPA TSCA Inventory.

SAFETY PROFILE: Questionable carcinogen with experimental carcinogenic data. Poison by skin contact. Mildly toxic by ingestion. A severe skin irritant. When heated to decomposition it emits acrid smoke and irritating fumes.

DUL400   CAS: 34522-40-2
N,N-DIMETHYL-4-(3,4,5-TRIMETHYLPHENYL)AZOANILINE
mf: $C_{17}H_{21}N_3$ mw: 267.41

SYNS: N,N-DIMETHYL-4-((3,4,5-TRIMETHYLPHENYL)AZO)BENZENAMINE ◇ N,N-3',4',5'-PENTAMETHYLAMI-NOAZOBENZENE

TOXICITY DATA with REFERENCE
ETA: orl-rat TDLo:4320 mg/kg/17W-C
   JMCMAR 15,212,72

SAFETY PROFILE: Questionable carcinogen with experimental tumorigenic data. When heated to decomposition it emits toxic fumes of NO_x.

DUM400
DIMETHYLUREA and SODIUM NITRITE

SYNS: DIMETHYLHARNSTOFF and NATRIUMNITRIT (GERMAN) ◇ SODIUM NITRITE and DIMETHYLUREA

TOXICITY DATA with REFERENCE
ETA: orl-rat TDLo:14 g/kg/56D-C   ARZNAD 21,1707,71

SAFETY PROFILE: Questionable carcinogen with experimental tumorigenic data. When heated to decomposition it emits toxic fumes of NO_x and Na_2O.

DUM600   CAS: 63019-76-1
p-N,N-DIMETHYLUREIDOAZOBENZENE
mf: $C_{15}H_{16}N_4O$ mw: 268.35

TOXICITY DATA with REFERENCE
NEO: scu-rat TDLo:2600 mg/kg/83D-I   BJPCAL 9,306,54

SAFETY PROFILE: Questionable carcinogen with experimental neoplastigenic data. When heated to decomposition it emits toxic fumes of NO_x.

DUN800   CAS: 18997-62-1
N,N-DIMETHYL-p-(2,3,XYLYLAZO)ANILINE
mf: $C_{16}H_{19}N_3$ mw: 253.38

SYNS: 2′,3′-DIMETHYL-4-DIMETHYLAMINOAZOBEN-ZENE ◇ N,N-DIMETHYL-p-(2′,3′-DIMETHYLPHENYL-AZO)ANILINE

TOXICITY DATA with REFERENCE
CAR: orl-rat TDLo: 1075 mg/kg/8W-C   CBINA8 53,107,85
ETA: orl-rat TDLo: 1080 mg/kg/30D-I   JMCMAR 11,1234,68
MUT: mma-sat 4 μg/plate   MUREAV 93,67,82

SAFETY PROFILE: Questionable carcinogen with experimental carcinogenic and tumorigenic data. Mutation data reported. When heated to decomposition it emits toxic fumes of NO_x.

DUO000   CAS: 3025-73-8
N,N-DIMETHYL-p-(3,4-XYLYLAZO) ANILINE
mf: $C_{16}H_{19}N_3$ mw: 253.38

SYNS: 3′,4′-DIMETHYL-4-DIMETHYLAMINOZOBEN-ZENE ◇ N,N-DIMETHYL-p-(3′,4′-DIMETHYLPHENYL-AZO)ANILINE

TOXICITY DATA with REFERENCE
CAR: orl-rat TDLo: 9030 mg/kg/25W-C
   CBINA8 53,107,85
NEO: orl-rat TD: 6480 mg/kg/26W-C   JMCMAR 15,212,72
ETA: orl-rat TD: 4523 mg/kg/17W-I   CNREA8 30,1520,70
ETA: orl-rat TD: 6600 mg/kg/26W-C   CNREA8 17,387,57

SAFETY PROFILE: Questionable carcinogen with experimental carcinogenic, neoplastigenic, and tumorigenic data. When heated to decomposition it emits toxic fumes of NO_x.

DUP000   CAS: 258-76-4
DINAPHTHAZINE
mf: $C_{20}H_{12}N_2$ mw: 280.34

SYN: DINAPHTAZIN (GERMAN)

TOXICITY DATA with REFERENCE
ETA: scu-mus TDLo: 200 mg/kg   ZEKBAI58,56,51

SAFETY PROFILE: Questionable carcinogen with experimental tumorigenic data. When heated to decomposition it emits toxic fumes of NO_x.

DUS000   CAS: 1528-74-1
4,4′-DINITROBIPHENYL
mf: $C_{12}H_8N_2O_4$ mw: 244.22

SYN: 4,4′-DINITROBIFENYL (CZECH)

TOXICITY DATA with REFERENCE
ETA: orl-rat TDLo: 950 mg/kg/W-I   TXAPA9 6,352,64
MUT: mma-sat 5 μg/plate   MUREAV 91,321,81
MUT: mmo-sat 2500 μg/plate   MUREAV 91,321,81

CONSENSUS REPORTS: Reported in EPA TSCA Inventory.

SAFETY PROFILE: Questionable carcinogen with experimental tumorigenic data. Mildly toxic by ingestion. Mutation data reported. An eye irritant. When heated to decomposition it emits toxic fumes of NO_x.

DUS500   CAS: 29110-68-7
2,4-DINITRO-6-tert-BUTYLPHENYL METHANESULFONATE
mf: $C_{11}H_{14}N_2O_7S$ mw: 304.29

SYNS: HE 166 ◇ PREPARATION HE 166

TOXICITY DATA with REFERENCE
ETA: orl-rat TD: 1120 mg/kg/32W-C   JTSCDR 9,161,84
ETA: orl-rat TDLo: 280 mg/kg/32W-C   JTSCDR 9,161,84

SAFETY PROFILE: Questionable carcinogen with experimental tumorigenic data. Experimental reproductive effects. An herbicide. When heated to decomposition it emits toxic fumes of SO_x and NO_x.

DUS600   CAS: 2401-85-6
2,4-DINITRO-1-CHLORO-NAPHTHALENE
mf: $C_{10}H_5ClN_2O_4$ mw: 252.62

SYN: 1-CHLORO-2,4-DINITRONAPHTHALENE

TOXICITY DATA with REFERENCE
CAR: orl-rat TDLo: 5000 mg/kg   CNREA8 26,619,66
NEO: orl-rat TD: 5000 mg/kg   CNREA8 28,924,68

CONSENSUS REPORTS: Reported in EPA TSCA Inventory.

SAFETY PROFILE: Questionable carcinogen with experimental carcinogenic and neoplastigenic data. Poison by unspecified route. When heated to decomposition it emits very toxic fumes of Cl^- and NO_x.

DUV600   CAS: 1582-09-8
2,6-DINITRO-N,N-DIPROPYL-4-(TRIFLUOROMETHYL)BENZENAMINE
mf: $C_{13}H_{16}F_3N_3O_4$ mw: 335.32

PROP: Technical product contains 84-88 ppm diproplynitrosoamine (NCITR* NCI-CG-TR-34,78).

SYNS: AGREFLAN ◇ AGRIFLAN 24 ◇ CRISALIN ◇ DIGERMIN ◇ 2,6-DINITRO-N,N-DI-N-PROPYL-α,α,α-TRI-FLURO-p-TOLUIDINE ◇ 2,6-DINITRO-4-TRIFLUORMETHYL-N,N-DIPROPYLANILIN (GERMAN) ◇ 4-(DI-N-PROPYL-AMINO)-3,5-DINITRO-1-TRIFLUOROMETHYLBENZENE ◇ N,N-DI-N-PROPYL-2,6-DINITRO-4-TRIFLUOROMETH-YLANILINE ◇ N,N-DIPROPYL-4-TRIFLUOROMETHYL-2,6-DINITROANILINE ◇ ELANCOLAN ◇ L-36352 ◇ LILLY 36,352 ◇ NCI-C00442 ◇ NITRAN ◇ OLITREF ◇ SU SEGURO CARPI-DOR ◇ TREFANOCIDE ◇ TREFICON ◇ TREFLAM ◇ TREFLAN ◇ TREFLANOCIDE ELANCOLAN ◇ TRIFLUO-RALIN (USDA) ◇ TRIFLURALIN ◇ TRIFLURALINE ◇ α,α,α-TRIFLUORO-2,6-DINITRO-N,N-DIPROPYL-p-TOLUI-DINE ◇ TRIFUREX ◇ TRIKEPIN ◇ TRIM

TOXICITY DATA with REFERENCE
CAR: orl-mus TD: 340 g/kg/78W-C
  NCITR* NCI-CG-TR-34,78
CAR: orl-mus TDLo: 180 g/kg/78W-C
  NCITR* NCI-CG-TR-34,78
ETA: ipr-mus TDLo: 2600 µg/kg/39D-I
  PATHAB 73,707,81
ETA: scu-mus TDLo: 2600 µg/kg/39D-I
  PATHAB 73,707,81
MUT: cyt-hmn: lym 2 ppm   PATHAB 73,707,81
MUT: cyt-mus-ipr 200 mg/kg   EESADV 4,263,80
MUT: mma-sat 1 mg/plate   ENMUDM 8(Suppl 7),1,86
MUT: mrc-asn 100 µg/plate   AISSAW 18,123,82
MUT: sce-hmn: lym 1 mg/L   BSIBAC 60,2149,84

CONSENSUS REPORTS: NCI Carcinogenesis Bioassay (feed); Clear Evidence: mouse NCITR* NCI-CG-TR-34,78; No Evidence: rat NCITR* NCI-CG-TR-34,78. EPA Genetic Toxicology Program. Community Right-To-Know List.

SAFETY PROFILE: Questionable carcinogen with experimental carcinogenic, tumorigenic, and teratogenic data. Moderately toxic by ingestion and intraperitoneal routes. Experimental reproductive effects. Human mutation data reported. When heated to decomposition it emits very toxic fumes of F⁻ and NO$_x$.

DUW100   CAS: 105735-71-5
3,7-DINITROFLUORANTHENE
mf: $C_{16}H_8N_2O_4$ mw: 292.26

TOXICITY DATA with REFERENCE
CAR: scu-rat TDLo: 5 mg/kg/10W-I   CRNGDP
  8,1919,87

MUT: dnr-bcs 10 ng/disc   MUREAV 191,85,87
MUT: mma-sat 1 µg/plate   MUREAV 191,85,87
MUT: mmo-sat 250 pg/plate   MUREAV 191,85,87

SAFETY PROFILE: Questionable carcinogen with experimental carcinogenic data. Mutation data reported. When heated to decomposition it emits toxic fumes of NO$_x$.

DUW120   CAS: 22506-53-2
3,9-DINITROFLUORANTHENE
mf: $C_{16}H_8N_2O_4$ mw: 292.26

SYN: 4,12-DINITROFLUORANTHENE

TOXICITY DATA with REFERENCE
CAR: scu-rat TDLo: 5 mg/kg/10W-I   CRNGDP
  8,1919,87
MUT: dnr-bcs 10 ng/disc   MUREAV 191,85,87
MUT: mma-sat 1 µg/plate   MUREAV 191,85,87
MUT: mmo-sat 250 pg/plate   MUREAV 191,85,87

SAFETY PROFILE: Questionable carcinogen with experimental carcinogenic data. Mutation data reported. When heated to decomposition it emits toxic fumes of NO$_x$.

DVE000   CAS: 1596-52-7
4,6-DINITROQUINOLINE-1-OXIDE
mf: $C_9H_5N_3O_5$ mw: 235.17

TOXICITY DATA with REFERENCE
ETA: scu-mus TDLo: 560 mg/kg/I   CPBTAL
  17,544,69
MUT: cyt-hmn: lvr 5260 nmol/L   JNCIAM
  47,367,71
MUT: cyt-omi 170 µmol/L   GANNA2 60,155,69
MUT: mmo-smc 100 mg/L   IGSBAL 85,127,72

SAFETY PROFILE: Questionable carcinogen with experimental carcinogenic data. Human mutation data reported. When heated to decomposition it emits toxic fumes of NO$_x$.

DVE200   CAS: 13442-17-6
4,7-DINITROQUINOLINE-1-OXIDE
mf: $C_9H_5N_3O_5$ mw: 235.17

TOXICITY DATA with REFERENCE
NEO: skn-mus TDLo: 300 mg/kg/25W-I
  GANNA2 60,523,69

SAFETY PROFILE: Questionable carcinogen with experimental neoplastigenic data. When heated to decomposition it emits toxic fumes of NO$_x$.

DVE400   CAS: 13256-12-7
N,N'-DINITROSO-N,N'-DIMETHYLETHYLENEDIAMINE
mf: $C_4H_{10}N_4O_2$ mw: 146.18

SYNS: DIMETHYL-DI-NITROSO-AETHYLENDIAMIN (GERMAN) ◇ DIMETHYLDINITROSOETHYLENEDIAMINE ◇ N,N'-DIMETHYL-N,N'-DINITROSOETHYLENEDIAMINE

TOXICITY DATA with REFERENCE
ETA: orl-rat TDLo: 570 mg/kg/43W-C   ARZNAD 19,1077,69
MUT: mmo-omi 5000 ppm/24H-C   SOGEBZ 10,522,74

SAFETY PROFILE: Questionable carcinogen with experimental tumorigenic data. Poison by ingestion. Mutation data reported. Many N-nitroso compounds are carcinogens. When heated to decomposition it emits toxic fumes of NO_x.

DVE600   CAS: 55557-00-1
DINITROSOHOMOPIPERAZINE
mf: $C_5H_{10}N_4O_2$ mw: 158.19

SYN: HEXAHYDRO-1,4-DINITROSO-1H-1,4-DIAZEPINE

TOXICITY DATA with REFERENCE
CAR: orl-rat TD: 105 mg/kg/30W-I   EESADV 6,513,82
CAR: orl-rat TDLo: 65 mg/kg/2Y-I   EESADV 6,513,82
ETA: orl-rat TD: 1530 mg/kg/31W-I   CNREA8 35,1270,75
MUT: mma-esc 16700 μmol/L   CNREA8 36,4099,76
MUT: mma-sat 1 μg/plate   MUREAV 51,319,78
MUT: mmo-sat 1 μg/plate   MUREAV 51,319,78
MUT: msc-ham: ovr 5 μmol/L   TCMUE9 1,129,84

CONSENSUS REPORTS: EPA Genetic Toxicology Program.

SAFETY PROFILE: Questionable carcinogen with experimental carcinogenic and tumorigenic data. Mutation data reported. When heated to decomposition it emits toxic fumes of NO_x.

DVF000   CAS: 15973-99-6
DI(N-NITROSO)-PERHYDROPYRIMIDINE
mf: $C_4H_8N_4O_2$ mw: 144.16

TOXICITY DATA with REFERENCE
CAR: ipr-rat TDLo: 13 mg/kg/66W-I   JCROD7 105,191,83
NEO: ipr-rat TDLo: 525 mg/kg/35W-I   CALEDQ 6,57,79

SAFETY PROFILE: Questionable carcinogen with experimental carcinogenic and neoplastigenic data. Poison by intraperitoneal route. When heated to decomposition it emits toxic fumes of NO_x.

DVF400   CAS: 101-25-7
3,7-DINITROSO-1,3,5,7-TETRAAZABICYCLO[3.3.1]NONANE
mf: $C_5H_{10}N_6O_2$ mw: 186.18

SYNS: ACETO DNPT 40 ◇ ACETO DNPT 80 ◇ ACETO DNPT 100 ◇ CHKHZ 18 ◇ DINITROSOPENTAMETHYLENE-TETRAMINE ◇ N,N-DINITROSOPENTAMETHYLENE-TETRAMINE ◇ N^1,N^3-DINITROSOPENTAMETHYLENE-TETRAMINE ◇ 3,4-DI-N-NITROSOPENTAMETHYLENETE-TRAMINE ◇ 3,7-DI-N-NITROSOPENTAMETHYLENETE-TRAMINE ◇ DNPMT ◇ DNPT ◇ 1,5-METHYLENE-3,7-DINITROSO-1,3,5,7-TETRAAZACYCLOOCTAINE ◇ 1,5-METHYLENE-3,7-DINITROSO-1,3,5,7-TETRA-AZACYCLOOCTANE ◇ POROFOR CHKHC-18 ◇ POROPHOR B ◇ UNICEL-ND ◇ UNICEL NDX ◇ VULCACEL B-40 ◇ VULCACEL BN

TOXICITY DATA with REFERENCE
MUT: dnd-bcs 2 mg/disc   PMRSDJ 1,175,81
MUT: mmo-sat 500 μg/plate   PMRSDJ 1,302,81
MUT: otr-ham: kdy 73500 μg/L   PMRSDJ 1,626,81
MUT: pic-esc 100 mg/L   PMRSDJ 1,224,81
MUT: sce-ham: ovr 80 mg/L   PMRSDJ 1,538,81

CONSENSUS REPORTS: IARC Cancer Review: GROUP 3 IMEMDT 7,56,87; Animal No Evidence IMEMDT 11,241,76. Reported in EPA TSCA Inventory. EPA Genetic Toxicology Program.

SAFETY PROFILE: Questionable carcinogen. Poison by intravenous, intraperitoneal, and subcutaneous routes. Moderately toxic by ingestion. Mutation data reported. Can ignite when handled and burns very rapidly. A blowing agent. When heated to decomposition it emits toxic fumes of NO_x.

DVH400   CAS: 606-20-2
2,6-DINITROTOLUENE
mf: $C_7H_6N_2O_4$ mw: 182.15

SYNS: 2,6-DNT ◇ 2-METHYL-1,3-DINITROBENZENE ◇ RCRA WASTE NUMBER U106

TOXICITY DATA with REFERENCE
ETA: orl-rat TD: 2555 mg/kg/Y-C   PAACA3 24,91,83
ETA: orl-rat TDLo: 5110 mg/kg/Y-C   PAACA3 24,91,83

MUT: dnd-rat-orl 10 mg/kg   JTEHD6 11,555,83
MUT: dnd-rat:lvr 3 mmol/L   SinJF# 26OCT82
MUT: dns-rat-orl 5 mg/kg   CRNGDP 3,241,82
MUT: mmo-sat 100 μg/plate   DTESD7 2,249,77
MUT: oms-rat-orl 10 mg/kg   JTEHD6 11,555,83

CONSENSUS REPORTS: Reported in EPA TSCA Inventory.

OSHA PEL: TWA 1500 μg/m³ (skin)   NIOSH REL: (Dinitrotoluene): Reduce to lowest level

SAFETY PROFILE: Questionable carcinogen with experimental tumorigenic data. Poison by ingestion. A skin irritant. Mutation data reported. When heated to decomposition it emits toxic fumes of NO_x.

DVI600   CAS: 6379-46-0
4,6-DINITRO-1,2,3-TRICHLOROBENZENE
mf: $C_6HCl_3N_2O_4$ mw: 271.44

SYNS: 1,2,3-TRICHLORO-4,6-DINITROBENZENE ◇ VANCIDE PB

TOXICITY DATA with REFERENCE
CAR: orl-mus TDLo:13 g/kg/78W-I
    NTIS** PB223-159
CAR: scu-mus TDLo:10 mg/kg
    NTIS** PB223-159

SAFETY PROFILE: Questionable carcinogen with experimental carcinogenic data. When heated to decomposition it emits very toxic fumes of NO_x and Cl^-.

DVO175   CAS: 63323-30-8
anti-DIOLEPOXIDE
mf: $C_{20}H_{12}O_3$ mw: 300.32

SYNS: (−)-7-α,8-β-DIHYDROXY-9-β,10-β-EPOXY-7,8,9,10-TETRAHYDROBENZO(a)PYRENE ◇ (−)-BP 7-α,8-β-DIOL-9-β,10-β-EPOXIDE 2 ◇ (−)-7,8,9,10-TETRAHYDRO-7-β,8-α-DIHYDROXY-9-α,10-α-EPOXY-BENZO(a)PYRENE

TOXICITY DATA with REFERENCE
ETA: skn-mus TDLo:2400 μg/kg   CNREA8 39,67,79
MUT: cyt-ham:lng 300 μg/L   IJCNAW 24,485,79
MUT: mmo-sat 100 pmol/plate   BBRCA977,1389,77
MUT: msc-ham:lng 10 μmol   CRNGDP 3,1223,82
MUT: sce-ham:lng 600 μg/L   IJCNAW 24,485,79

SAFETY PROFILE: Questionable carcinogen with experimental tumorigenic data by skin contact. Mutation data reported. When heated to decomposition it emits toxic fumes of NO_x.

DVR200   CAS: 105-11-3
DIOXIME-p-BENZOQUINONE
mf: $C_6H_6N_2O_2$ mw: 138.14

SYNS: ACTOR Q ◇ 1,4-BENZOQUINONE DIOXINE ◇ 2,5-CYCLOHEXADIENE-1,4-DIONE DIOXIME ◇ DIBENZO PQD ◇ DIOXIME-1,4-CYCLOHEXADIENEDIONE ◇ DIOXIME-2,5-CYCLOHEXADIENE-1,4-DIONE ◇ G-M-F ◇ NCI-C03850 ◇ PQD ◇ QDO ◇ QUINONE DIOXIME ◇ p-QUINONE DIOXIME ◇ p-QUINONE OXIME

TOXICITY DATA with REFERENCE
NEO: orl-rat TDLo:14 g/kg/2Y-C
    NCITR* NCI-CG-TR-179,79
ETA: orl-mus TDLo:131 g/kg/104W-C
    NCITR* NCI-CG-TR-179,79
MUT: dnr-bcs 1 mg/disc   SAIGBL 26,147,84
MUT: mma-sat 10 μg/plate   ENMUDM 7(Suppl 5),1,85
MUT: mmo-sat 3300 ng/plate   ENMUDM 7(Suppl 5),1,85

CONSENSUS REPORTS: IARC Cancer Review: GROUP 3 IMEMDT 7,56,87; Animal Limited Evidence IMEMDT 29,185,82. NCI Carcinogenesis Bioassay (feed); Clear Evidence: rat NCITR* NCI-CG-TR-179,79; No Evidence: mouse NCITR* NCI-CG-TR-179,79. Reported in EPA TSCA Inventory.

SAFETY PROFILE: Questionable carcinogen with experimental neoplastigenic and tumorigenic data. Moderately toxic by ingestion. Mutation data reported. When heated to decomposition it emits toxic fumes of NO_x.

DVX200   CAS: 86-29-3
DIPHENYLACETONITRILE
mf: $C_{14}H_{11}N$ mw: 193.26

SYNS: BENZYHYDRYLCYANIDE ◇ α-CYANODIPHENYL-METHANE ◇ DIPAN ◇ DIPHENATRILE ◇ DIPHENYL-α-CYANOMETHANE ◇ DIPHENYLMETHYLCYANIDE ◇ α-PHENYLBENZYLCYANIDE ◇ α-PHENYLPHENYLACE-TONITRILE ◇ USAF KF-13

TOXICITY DATA with REFERENCE
CAR: scu-mus TDLo:464 mg/kg
    NTIS** PB223-159
ETA: orl-mus TDLo:61 g/kg/78W-I
    NTIS** PB223-159

CONSENSUS REPORTS: Reported in EPA TSCA Inventory. Cyanide and its compounds are on the Community Right-To-Know List.

SAFETY PROFILE: Questionable carcinogen with experimental carcinogenic and tumorigenic data. Poison by ingestion, intraperitoneal, and intravenous routes. Moderately toxic by subcutaneous and possibly other routes. When heated to decomposition it emits toxic fumes of NO_x and CN^-.

DVY900   CAS: 20930-10-3
1,1-DIPHENYL-2-BUTYNYL-N-CYCLOHEXYLCARBAMATE
mf: $C_{23}H_{25}NO_2$ mw: 347.49

SYN: CYCLOHEXANECARBAMIC ACID, 1,1-DIPHENYL-2-BUTYNYL ESTER

TOXICITY DATA with REFERENCE
ETA: orl-rat TD: 15500 mg/kg/54W-C   JJIND8 71,211,83
ETA: orl-rat TDLo: 14800 mg/kg/73W-C
JJIND8 71,211,83

SAFETY PROFILE: Questionable carcinogen with experimental tumorigenic data. When heated to decomposition it emits toxic fumes of NO_x.

DVZ000   CAS: 102-09-0
DIPHENYL CARBONATE
mf: $C_{13}H_{10}O_3$ mw: 214.23

SYNS: CARBONIC ACID, DIPHENYL ESTER ◊ PHENYL CARBONATE

TOXICITY DATA with REFERENCE
NEO: scu-mus TDLo: 1000 mg/kg
NTIS** PB223-159
ETA: orl-mus TDLo: 28 g/kg/78W-I
NTIS** PB223-159

CONSENSUS REPORTS: Reported in EPA TSCA Inventory.

SAFETY PROFILE: Questionable carcinogen with experimental neoplastigenic and tumorigenic data. When heated to decomposition it emits acrid smoke and irritating fumes.

DWA700   CAS: 56767-15-8
3,3-DIPHENYL-3-DIMETHYLCARBAMOYL-1-PROPYNE
mf: $C_{18}H_{17}NO$ mw: 263.36

SYN: N,N-DIMETHYL-α-ETHYNYL-α-PHENYLBEN-ZENEACETAMIDE

TOXICITY DATA with REFERENCE
CAR: orl-rat TDLo: 780 mg/kg/21W-I   CNREA8 35,2469,75

SAFETY PROFILE: Questionable carcinogen with experimental carcinogenic data. When heated to decomposition it emits toxic fumes of NO_x.

DWI000   CAS: 86-30-6
DIPHENYLNITROSAMINE
mf: $C_{12}H_{10}N_2O$ mw: 198.24
PROP: Green crystals. Mp: 144°.

SYNS: CURETARD A ◊ DELAC J ◊ DIPHENYLNITROSAMIN (GERMAN) ◊ DIPHENYL N-NITROSOAMINE ◊ N,N-DIPHENYLNITROSAMINE ◊ NAUGARD TJB ◊ NCI-C02880 ◊ NDPA ◊ NDPhA ◊ N-NITROSODIFENYLAMIN (CZECH) ◊ NITROSODIPHENYLAMINE ◊ N-NITROSODIPHENYLAMINE ◊ N-NITROSO-N-PHENYLANILINE ◊ NITROUS DIPHENYLAMIDE ◊ REDAX ◊ RETARDER J ◊ TJB ◊ VULCALENT A ◊ VULCATARD ◊ VULKALENT A (CZECH) ◊ VULTROL

TOXICITY DATA with REFERENCE
CAR: orl-rat TD: 146 g/kg/2Y-C   EESADV 3,29,79
CAR: orl-rat TD: 170 g/kg/2Y-C
NCITR* NCI-CG-TR-164,79
CAR: orl-rat TD: 2800 g/kg/2Y-C   IARC** 27,213,82
CAR: orl-rat TDLo: 140 g/kg/2Y-C
NCITR* NCI-CG-TR-164,79
ETA: ipr-rat TD: 7700 mg/kg/77W-I   IARC** 27,213,82
ETA: orl-mus TD: 1750 g/kg/2Y-I   IARC** 27,213,82
ETA: skn-mus TD: 800 mg/kg/20W-I   IARC** 27,213,82
ETA: skn-mus TDLo: 800 mg/kg/20W-I
EJCAAH 16,695,80
MUT: dnd-hmn: fbr 3 mmol/L   ENMUDM 7,267,85
MUT: dns-rat: lvr 500 nmol/L   CNREA8 42,3010,82
MUT: mma-sat 50 μg/plate   CANCAR 49,1970,82
MUT: otr-ham: emb 6300 μg/L   NCIMAV 58,243,81

CONSENSUS REPORTS: IARC Cancer Review: GROUP 3 IMEMDT 7,56,87; Animal Limited Evidence IMEMDT 27,213,82. NCI Carcinogenesis Bioassay (feed); Clear Evidence: rat NCITR* NCI-CG-TR-164,79; No Evidence: mouse NCITR* NCI-CG-TR-164,79. Reported in EPA TSCA Inventory. EPA Genetic Toxicology Program. Community Right-To-Know List.

SAFETY PROFILE: Questionable carcinogen with experimental carcinogenic and tumorigenic data. Moderately toxic by ingestion and possibly other routes. Human mutation data reported. An eye irritant. Dangerous fire hazard when exposed to heat, flame, or oxidizing materials. When heated to decomposition it emits highly toxic fumes of NO_x.

DWI400   CAS: 16230-71-0
3,3-DIPHENYL-2-OXETANONE
mf: $C_{15}H_{12}O_2$ mw: 224.27

SYNS: 2,2-DIPHENYL-3-HYDROXYPROPIONIC ACID LACTONE ◇ α,α-DIPHENYL-β-PROPIOLACTONE

TOXICITY DATA with REFERENCE
ETA: scu-rat TDLo: 380 mg/kg/19W-I   BJCAAI 15,85,61

SAFETY PROFILE: Questionable carcinogen with experimental tumorigenic data. When heated to decomposition it emits acrid smoke and irritating fumes.

DWL400   CAS: 10087-89-5
1,1-DIPHENYL-2-PROPYNYL-N-CYCLOHEXYLCARBAMATE
mf: $C_{22}H_{23}NO_2$ mw: 333.46

SYNS: 1,1-DIPHENYL-2-PROPYN-1-OL CYCLOHEXANE-CARBAMATE ◇ 1,1-DIPHENYL-2-PROPYNYL ESTER CY-CLOHEXANECARBAMIC ACID ◇ ENPROMATE

TOXICITY DATA with REFERENCE
ETA: orl-rat TD: 13600 mg/kg/40W-C   JJIND8 71,211,83
ETA: orl-rat TDLo: 1690 mg/kg/27W-C
   PAACA3 10,35,69
ETA: scu-rat TDLo: 1925 mg/kg/11W-C
   PAACA3 10,35,69
ETA: skn-rat TDLo: 31500 mg/kg/67W-C
   JJIND8 71,211,83
MUT: dns-rat: lvr 10 µmol/L   ENMUDM 3,11,81
MUT: mma-sat 100 µg/plate   PNASA6 72,5135,75

CONSENSUS REPORTS: EPA Genetic Toxicology Program.

SAFETY PROFILE: Questionable carcinogen with experimental tumorigenic data. Poison by intraperitoneal route. Moderately toxic by ingestion. Mutation data reported. When heated to decomposition it emits toxic fumes of NO_x.

DWL500   CAS: 10473-64-0
1,1-DIPHENYL-2-PROPYNYL-N-ETHYLCARBAMATE
mf: $C_{18}H_{17}NO_2$ mw: 279.36

SYN: ETHYLCARBAMIC ACID 1,1-DIPHENYL-2-PRO-PYNYL ESTER

TOXICITY DATA with REFERENCE
ETA: orl-rat TDLo: 8800 mg/kg/28W-C   JJIND8 71,211,83

SAFETY PROFILE: Questionable carcinogen with experimental tumorigenic data. When heated to decomposition it emits toxic fumes of NO_x.

DWL525   CAS: 10473-98-0
1,1-DIPHENYL-2-PROPYNYL 1-PYRROLIDINECARBOXYLATE
mf: $C_{20}H_{19}NO_2$ mw: 305.40

SYN: 3,3-DIPHENYL-3-(PYRROLIDINE-CARBONYL-OXY)-1-PROPYNE

TOXICITY DATA with REFERENCE
ETA: orl-rat TDLo: 2 g/kg/35W-C   JJIND8 71,211,83

SAFETY PROFILE: Questionable carcinogen with experimental tumorigenic data. When heated to decomposition it emits toxic fumes of NO_x.

DWN600   CAS: 21083-47-6
5,5-DIPHENYL-2-THIOHYDANTOIN
mf: $C_{15}H_{12}N_2OS$ mw: 268.35

TOXICITY DATA with REFERENCE
ETA: orl-rat TDLo: 3500 mg/kg   CNREA8 28,924,68

CONSENSUS REPORTS: Reported in EPA TSCA Inventory.

SAFETY PROFILE: Questionable carcinogen with experimental tumorigenic data. When heated to decomposition it emits very toxic fumes of NO_x and SO_x.

DWO800   CAS: 136-35-6
1,3-DIPHENYLTRIAZENE
mf: $C_{12}H_{11}N_3$ mw: 197.26

PROP: Golden yellow crystals. Mp: 98-99°, bp: explodes, vap d: 6.8.

SYNS: CELLOFOR (CZECH) ◇ DAAB ◇ DIAZOAMINO-BENZEN (CZECH) ◇ DIAZOAMINOBENZENE ◇ p-DIAZO-AMINOBENZENE ◇ DIAZOAMINOBENZOL (GERMAN) ◇ N-(PHENYLAZO)ANILINE

TOXICITY DATA with REFERENCE
ETA: orl-mus TDLo: 1480 mg/kg/59D-C
   GANNA2 29,209,35
ETA: skn-mus TDLo: 30 g/kg/46W-I   BJCAAI 2,290,48

CONSENSUS REPORTS: EPA Genetic Toxicology Program. Reported in EPA TSCA Inventory.

SAFETY PROFILE: Questionable carcinogen with experimental tumorigenic data. Poison by ingestion. Strongly explosive when shocked or heated to 98°C. Mixture with acetic anhydride explodes when warmed. When heated to decomposition it emits toxic fumes of NO_x.

DWT400 CAS: 6976-50-7
N,N-DI-n-PROPYL ETHYL CARBAMATE
mf: $C_9H_{19}NO_2$ mw: 173.29

SYN: DIPROPYLCARBAMIC ACID ETHYL ESTER

TOXICITY DATA with REFERENCE
ETA: ipr-mus TDLo:6500 mg/kg/13W-I
JNCIAM 9,35,48

SAFETY PROFILE: Questionable carcinogen with experimental tumorigenic data. When heated to decomposition it emits toxic fumes of NO_x.

DWU800 CAS: 53230-00-5
α-DIPROPYLNITROSAMINE METHYL ETHER

SYNS: 1-METHOXY-N-NITROSO-N-PROPYLPROPYL-AMINE ◇ 1-METHOXYPROPYLPROPYLNITROSAMIN (GERMAN) ◇ 1-METHOXYPROPYLPROPYLNITROSAMINE ◇ 1-MPPN

TOXICITY DATA with REFERENCE
NEO: scu-ham TDLo:555 mg/kg/37W-I
ZKKOBW 90,215,77

SAFETY PROFILE: Questionable carcinogen with experimental neoplastigenic data. Moderately toxic by subcutaneous route. Many nitrosamines are carcinogens. When heated to decomposition it emits toxic fumes of NO_x.

DXG000 CAS: 13410-01-0
DISODIUM SELENATE
mf: $O_4Se \cdot 2Na$ mw: 188.94

PROP: Colorless, rhombic crystals. D: 3.098.

SYNS: NATRIUMSELENIAT (GERMAN) ◇ P-40 ◇ SEL-TOX SSO2 and SS-20 ◇ SODIUM SELENATE

TOXICITY DATA with REFERENCE
CAR: orl-rat TDLo:128 mg/kg/2Y-C JONUAI 101,1531,71
MUT: dnr-sat 10 μg/plate CALEDQ 10,75,80

MUT: dns-rat:lvr 100 μmol/L CALEDQ 10,75,80
MUT: mma-sat 2 μmol/plate MUREAV 66,175,79
MUT: mmo-sat 40 μmol/L ENVRAL 36,379,85
MUT: mrc-bcs 50 μmol/plate MUREAV 66,175,79

CONSENSUS REPORTS: IARC Cancer Review: GROUP 3 IMEMDT 7,56,87. Selenium and its compounds are on the Community Right-To-Know List. EPA Genetic Toxicology Program. Reported in EPA TSCA Inventory.

OSHA PEL: TWA 0.2 mg(Se)/m^3 ACGIH TLV: TWA 0.2 mg(Se)/m^3 DFG MAK: 0.1 mg(Se)/m^3

SAFETY PROFILE: Questionable carcinogen with experimental carcinogenic and teratogenic data. Poison by ingestion, intravenous, subcutaneous, and intraperitoneal routes. Human systemic effects by ingestion: EKG changes, hypermotility, diarrhea and liver impairment. Experimental reproductive effects. Effects similar to arsenic. Mutation data reported. A pesticide. When heated to decomposition it emits toxic fumes of Se and Na_2O.

DXH250 CAS: 97-77-8
DISULFIRAM
mf: $C_{10}H_{20}N_2S_4$ mw: 296.56

PROP: Yellow-white crystals; mp: 72°.

SYNS: ABSTENSIL ◇ ABSTINYL ◇ ALCOPHOBIN ◇ ALK-AUBS ◇ ANTABUS ◇ ANTABUSE ◇ ANTADIX ◇ ANTAENYL ◇ ANTAETHAN ◇ ANTAETHYL ◇ ANTAETIL ◇ ANTALCOL ◇ ANTETAN ◇ ANTETHYL ◇ ANTETIL ◇ ANTEYL ◇ ANTIAETHAN ◇ ANTIETANOL ◇ ANTIETHYL ◇ ANTIETIL ◇ ANTIKOL ◇ ANTIVITIUM ◇ AVERSAN ◇ AVERZAN ◇ BIS(DIETHYLAMINO)THIOXOMETHYL)DISULPHIDE ◇ BIS(N,N-DIETHYL-THIOCARBAMOYL) DISULFIDE ◇ BIS(DIETHYL-THIOCARBAMOYL) DISULFIDE ◇ BIS(N,N-DIETHYL-THIOCARBAMOYL)DISULPHIDE ◇ BONIBAL ◇ CONTRALIN ◇ CONTRAPOT ◇ CRONETAL ◇ DICUPRAL ◇ DISETIL ◇ DISULFAN ◇ DISULFURAM ◇ DISULPHURAM ◇ 1,1'-DITHIOBIS(N,N-DIETHYLTHIOFORMAMIDE) ◇ EKAGOM TEDS ◇ EPHORRAN ◇ ESPENAL ◇ ESPERAL ◇ ETABUS ◇ ETHYLDITHIOURAME ◇ ETHYLDITHIURAME ◇ ETHYL THIRAM ◇ ETHYL THIUDAD ◇ ETHYL THIURAD ◇ ETHYL TUADS ◇ ETHYL TUEX ◇ EXHORAN ◇ EXHORRAN ◇ HOCA ◇ KROTENAL ◇ NCI-C02959 ◇ NOCBIN ◇ NOXAL ◇ REFUSAL ◇ RO-SULFIRAM ◇ STOPAETHYL ◇ STOPETHYL ◇ STOPETYL ◇ TATD ◇ TENURID ◇ TENUTEX ◇ TETD ◇ TETIDIS ◇ TETRADIN ◇ TETRADINE ◇ TETRAETHYLTHIOPEROXYDICARBONIC DIAMIDE ◇ TETRAETHYLTHIRAM DISULPHIDE ◇ TETRAETHYLTHIURAM ◇ TETRAETHYLTHIURAM DISULFIDE ◇ TETRA-

ETHYLTHIURAM DISULPHIDE ◇ N,N,N′,N′-TETRAETHYL-THIURAM DISULPHIDE ◇ TETRAETIL ◇ TETURAM ◇ TETURAMIN ◇ THIOSAN ◇ THIOSCABIN ◇ THIRERANIDE ◇ THIURAM E ◇ THIURANIDE ◇ TILLRAM ◇ TIURAM ◇ TTD ◇ TTS ◇ USAF B-33

TOXICITY DATA with REFERENCE

NEO: orl-mus TDLo:35 g/kg/78W-I

NTIS** PB223-159

NEO: scu-mus TDLo:1000 mg/kg

NTIS** PB223-159

MUT: dni-ckn:emb 120 nmol/L   BBACAQ
519,65,78

MUT: mma-sat 20 μg/plate   PCBRD2 141,407,84

MUT: mmo-sat 25 μg/plate   CBINA8 49,329,84

MUT: oms-ckn:emb 120 nmol/L   BBACAQ
519,65,78

MUT: sce-ham:ovr 5 μmol/L   SWEHDO 9(Suppl 2),27,83

CONSENSUS REPORTS: IARC Cancer Review: Animal Inadequate Evidence IMEMDT 12,85,76. NCI Carcinogenesis Bioassay (feed); No Evidence: mouse, rat NCITR* NCI-CG-TR-16,79. Reported in EPA TSCA Inventory.

OSHA PEL: TWA 2 mg/m^3 ACGIH TLV: TWA 2 mg/m^3 DFG MAK: 2 mg/m^3

SAFETY PROFILE: Questionable carcinogen with experimental neoplastigenic data. A human poison by ingestion. An experimental poison by intraperitoneal route. Toxic symptoms when accompanied by ingestion of alcohol. Dangerous.

DXP000   CAS: 27755-15-3
DITOLYLETHANE

mf: C$_{16}$H$_{18}$ mw: 210.34

TOXICITY DATA with REFERENCE

ETA: orl-mus TDLo:9200 mg/kg/73W-C

GTPZAB 15(5),49,71

SAFETY PROFILE: Questionable carcinogen with experimental tumorigenic data. Moderately toxic by ingestion. When heated to decomposition it emits acrid smoke and irritating fumes.

DXQ500   CAS: 330-54-1
DIURON
DOT: 2767

mf: C$_9$H$_{10}$Cl$_2$N$_2$O   mw: 233.11

PROP: Crystals. Mp: 159°. Sltly sol in water and hydrocarbon solvents.

SYNS: AF 101 ◇ CEKIURON ◇ CRISURON ◇ DAILON ◇ DCMU ◇ DIATER ◇ 3-(3,4-DICHLOOR-FENYL)-1,1-DI-

METHYLUREUM (DUTCH) ◇ DICHLORFENIDIM ◇ 3-(3,4-DICHLOROPHENOL)-1,1-DIMETHYLUREA ◇ N′-(3,4-DI-CHLOROPHENYL)-N,N-DIMETHYLUREA ◇ 1-(3,4-DICHLO-ROPHENYL)-3,3-DIMETHYLUREE (FRENCH) ◇ 3-(3,4-DI-CHLOR-PHENYL)-1,1-DIMETHYL-HARNSTOFF (GERMAN) ◇ 3-(3,4-DICLORO-FENYL)-1,1-DIMETIL-UREA (ITALIAN) ◇ 1,1-DIMETHYL-3-(3,4-DICHLOROPHENYL)UREA ◇ DI-ON ◇ DIREX 4L ◇ DIUREX ◇ DIUROL ◇ DIURON 4L ◇ DMU ◇ DREXEL ◇ DREXEL DIURON 4L ◇ DURAN ◇ DYNEX ◇ FARMCO DIURON ◇ HERBATOX ◇ HW 920 ◇ KARMEX ◇ KARMEX DIURON HERBICIDE ◇ KARMEX DW ◇ MARMER ◇ SUP'R FLO ◇ TELVAR ◇ TELVAR DIURON WEED KILLER ◇ UNIDRON ◇ USAF P-7 ◇ USAF XR-42 ◇ VONDURON

TOXICITY DATA with REFERENCE

ETA: orl-mus TDLo:153 g/kg/78W-I

NTIS** PB223-159

MUT: dni-mus-orl 1 g/kg   MUREAV 58,353,78

MUT: mma-sat 3 μg/plate   MUREAV 58,353,78

CONSENSUS REPORTS: Reported in EPA TSCA Inventory. EPA Genetic Toxicology Program. Chlorophenol compounds are on The Community Right-To-Know List.

OSHA PEL: TWA 10 mg/m^3 ACGIH TLV: TWA 10 mg/m^3 DOT Classification: ORM-E; Label: None.

SAFETY PROFILE: Questionable carcinogen with experimental tumorigenic and teratogenic data. Moderately toxic by ingestion, intraperitoneal, and possibly other routes. Mutation data reported. When heated to decomposition it emits highly toxic fumes of Cl$^-$ and NO$_x$.

DXT200   CAS: 112-40-3
DODECANE

mf: C$_{12}$H$_{26}$ mw: 170.38

SYNS: ADAKANE 12 ◇ BIHEXYL ◇ DIHEXYL ◇ n-DODECAN (GERMAN) ◇ DUODECANE

TOXICITY DATA with REFERENCE

ETA: skn-mus TDLo:11 g/kg/22W-I   TXAPA9
9,70,66

CONSENSUS REPORTS: Reported In EPA TSCA Inventory.

SAFETY PROFILE: Questionable carcinogen with experimental tumorigenic data. When heated to decomposition it emits acrid smoke and irritating fumes.

DXU400   CAS: 2855-19-8
DODECENE EPOXIDE

mf: C$_{12}$H$_{24}$O   mw: 184.36

SYN: 1,2-EPOXYDODECANE

TOXICITY DATA with REFERENCE
ETA: unr-mus TDLo: 147 mg/kg RARSAM
3,193,63

CONSENSUS REPORTS: Reported in EPA
TSCA Inventory.

SAFETY PROFILE: Questionable carcinogen
with experimental tumorigenic data. When
heated to decomposition it emits acrid smoke
and irritating fumes.

DXV600   CAS: 112-53-8
DODECYL ALCOHOL
mf: $C_{12}H_{26}O$ mw: 186.38

PROP: Colorless solid, liquid above 21°; floral
odor. D: 0.830-0.836, refr index: 1.440-1.444,
mp: 24°, bp: 259°, flash p: 260°F, autoign temp:
527°F. Sol in 2 parts of 70% alc, fixed oils,
propylene glycol; insol in water and glycerin.

SYNS: ALCOHOL C-12 ◇ ALFOL 12 ◇ CACHALOT L-50
◇ CO 12 ◇ CO-1214 ◇ n-DODECANOL ◇ 1-DODECANOL
◇ n-DODECYL ALCOHOL ◇ DUODECYL ALCOHOL
◇ DYTOL J-68 ◇ EPAL 12 ◇ FEMA No. 2617 ◇ LAURIC
ALCOHOL ◇ LAURINIC ALCOHOL ◇ LAURYL 24
◇ LAURYL ALCOHOL (FCC) ◇ n-LAURYL ALCOHOL, PRI-
MARY ◇ LOROL ◇ MA-1214 ◇ SIPOL L12

TOXICITY DATA with REFERENCE
ETA: skn-mus TDLo: 19 g/kg/39W-I TXAPA9
9,70,66

CONSENSUS REPORTS: Reported in EPA
TSCA Inventory.

SAFETY PROFILE: Questionable carcinogen
with experimental tumorigenic data. Moderately
toxic by intraperitoneal route. Mildly toxic by
ingestion. A severe human skin irritant. Combustible when exposed to heat or flame; can
react with oxidizing materials. To fight fire,
use dry chemical, CO_2. When heated to decomposition it emits acrid smoke and irritating
fumes.

DXX400   CAS: 2439-10-3
N-DODECYLGUANIDINE ACETATE
mf: $C_{13}H_{29}N_3 \cdot C_2H_4O_2$ mw: 287.51

PROP: Crystals, sol in hot water and alc. Mp:
136°.

SYNS: AC 5223 ◇ AMERICAN CYANAMID 5223
◇ APADODINE ◇ CARPENE ◇ CURITAN ◇ CYPREX
◇ CYPREX 65W ◇ N-DODECYLGUANIDINACETAT (GER-

MAN) ◇ DODECYLGUANIDINE ACETATE ◇ DODINE
◇ DODINE ACETATE ◇ DODINE, mixture with GLYODIN
◇ DODGUADINE ◇ DOGQUADINE ◇ ENT 16,436
◇ EXPERIMENTAL FUNGICIDE 5223 ◇ LAURYLGUANIDINE
ACETATE ◇ MELPREX ◇ MILPREX ◇ SYLLIT ◇ TSITREX
◇ VENTUROL ◇ VONDODINE

TOXICITY DATA with REFERENCE
ETA: scu-mus TDLo: 1000 mg/kg
NTIS** PB223-159

CONSENSUS REPORTS: Reported in EPA
TSCA Inventory. EPA Genetic Toxicology Program.

SAFETY PROFILE: Questionable carcinogen
with experimental tumorigenic data. Poison by
ingestion. Moderately toxic by skin contact and
possibly other routes. A severe eye irritant. A
pesticide. When heated to decomposition it
emits very toxic fumes of NO_x.

DXX600
DODECYLGUANIDINE ACETATE with
SODIUM NITRITE (3:5)
SYNS: DODINE with SODIUM NITRITE (3:5) ◇ SODIUM
NITRITE with DODECYL GUANIDINE ACETATE (5:3)

TOXICITY DATA with REFERENCE
CAR: orl-mus TDLo: 112 mg/kg/6D-I CALEDQ
5,107,78

SAFETY PROFILE: Questionable carcinogen
with experimental carcinogenic data. Experimental reproductive effects. When heated to decomposition it emits very toxic fumes of NO_x
and Na_2O.

DYB000   CAS: 482-49-5
DOISYNOLIC ACID
mf: $C_{18}H_{24}O_3$ mw: 288.42

SYNS: ACIDO DOISYNOLICO (SPANISH) ◇ 1-ETHYL-7-
HYDROXY-2-METHYL-1,2,3,4,4a,9,10,10a-OCTAHYDRO-
PHENANTHRENE-2-CARBOXYLIC ACID ◇ 1-ETHYL-1,2,3,
4,4a,9,10,10a-OCTAHYDRO-7-HYDROXY-2-METHYL-2-
PHENANTHRENECARBOXYLIC ACID ◇ 3-HYDROXY-16,7-
SECOESTRA-1,3,5(10)-TRIEN-17-OIC ACID

TOXICITY DATA with REFERENCE
ETA: orl-gpg TDLo: 72 mg/kg/12W-I RSABAC
25,215,49

SAFETY PROFILE: Questionable carcinogen
with experimental tumorigenic data. When
heated to decomposition it emits acrid smoke
and irritating fumes.

EAE500   CAS: 5036-03-3
EDROFURADENE
mf: $C_{10}H_{12}N_4O_5$ mw: 268.26

SYNS: 1-(2-HYDROXYETHYL)-3-((5-NITROFURFURYLI-
DENE)AMINO)-2-IMIDAZOLIDINONE ◇ NF 1010 ◇ NIFUR-
DAZIL

TOXICITY DATA with REFERENCE
CAR: orl-rat TDLo: 27 g/kg/46W-C JNCIAM
51,403,73
MUT: mma-sat 100 ng/plate   MUREAV 48,295,77

CONSENSUS REPORTS: EPA Genetic Toxicology Program.

SAFETY PROFILE: Questionable carcinogen
with experimental carcinogenic data. Mutation
data reported. When heated to decomposition
it emits toxic fumes of NO_x.

EAF000   CAS: 506-30-9
EICOSANOIC ACID
mf: $C_{20}H_{40}O_2$ mw: 312.60

PROP: White leaflets. Mp: 77°, bp: 328° slt
decomp in water, very sol in hot absolute alc
and very sol in ether.

SYNS: ARACHIC ACID ◇ ARACHIDIC ACID

TOXICITY DATA with REFERENCE
NEO: imp-mus TDLo: 1000 mg/kg   CNREA8
26,105,66

CONSENSUS REPORTS: Reported in EPA
TSCA Inventory.

SAFETY PROFILE: Questionable carcinogen
with experimental neoplastigenic data by implant route. When heated to decomposition it
emits acrid smoke and fumes.

EAG000   CAS: 23315-05-1
ELAIOMYCIN
mf: $C_{13}H_{26}N_2O_3$ mw: 258.41

PROP: Metabolite of *Streptomyces hepaticus*
(NATUAS 221,765,69).

SYN: d-threo-METHOXY-3-(1-OCTENYL-ONN-AZOXY)-2-
BUTANOL

TOXICITY DATA with REFERENCE
ETA: orl-rat TD: 35 mg/kg   29QKAZ 2,781,72
ETA: orl-rat TDLo: 35 mg/kg   NATUAS 221,765,69

SAFETY PROFILE: Questionable carcinogen
with experimental tumorigenic data. Causes tu-

mors of the brain. Poison by intravenous and
subcutaneous routes. When heated to decomposition it emits toxic fumes of NO_x.

EAG500   CAS: 50814-62-5
ELASIOMYCIN

TOXICITY DATA with REFERENCE
ETA: ivn-rat TDLo: 50 mg/kg (18D preg): TER
IARCCD 4,100,73

SAFETY PROFILE: Questionable carcinogen
with experimental tumorigenic and teratogenic
data. When heated to decomposition it emits
acrid smoke and fumes.

EAJ500   CAS: 19526-81-9
EMAZOL RED B
mf: $C_{18}H_{16}N_2O_{10}S_3 \cdot 2Na$ mw: 562.52

TOXICITY DATA with REFERENCE
ETA: orl-mus TDLo: 20 g/kg/17W-I   TKORAS
3,53,67
ETA: orl-rat TDLo: 78 g/kg/86W-I   TKORAS
3,53,67
ETA: scu-mus TDLo: 135 g/kg/56W-I   TKORAS
3,53,67
ETA: scu-rat TDLo: 10 g/kg/17W-I   TKORAS
3,53,67

CONSENSUS REPORTS: Reported in EPA
TSCA Inventory.

SAFETY PROFILE: Questionable carcinogen
with experimental tumorigenic data. When
heated to decomposition it emits very toxic
fumes of NO_x, Na_2O, and SO_x.

EAL100   CAS: 1302-74-5
EMERY
mf: Al_2O_3 mw: 101.96

PROP: A varicolored mineral. D: 3.95-4.10.

SYNS: ALUMINUM OXIDE ◇ CORUNDUM ◇ ELECTRO-
CORUNDUM ◇ EN 237 ◇ KER 710 ◇ KO 7 ◇ KORUND
◇ KU 5-3 ◇ MP 1 (REFRACTORY)

TOXICITY DATA with REFERENCE
CAR: ipr-rat TDLo: 225 mg/kg/1W-I   ZHPMAT
162,467,76

OSHA PEL: (Transitional: TWA Total Dust:
15 mg/m^3; Respirable Fraction: 5 mg/m^3) TWA
Total Dust: 10 mg/m^3; Respirable Fraction: 5
mg/m^3 ACGIH TLV: TWA (nuisance particulate) 10 mg/m^3 of total dust (when toxic impurities are not present, e.g., quartz < 1%).

SAFETY PROFILE: Questionable carcinogen with experimental carcinogenic data. May cause a pneumoconiosis. It is mainly a nuisance dust.

EAQ000
ENCEPHALARTOS HILDEBRANDTII

PROP: Flour made from the starchy kernels of *Ecephalartos hildebrandtii* (BJCAAI 22, 563,68).

TOXICITY DATA with REFERENCE
CAR: orl-rat TDLo:450 g/kg/26W-C   BJCAAI
22,563,68

SAFETY PROFILE: Questionable carcinogen with experimental carcinogenic data. When heated to decomposition it emits acrid smoke and fumes.

EAQ750   CAS: 115-29-7
ENDOSULFAN
DOT: 2761
mf: $C_9H_6Cl_6O_3S$ mw: 406.91

PROP: A mixture of 2 isomers, brown crystals, nearly insol in water; sol in most organic solvents. Mp (α): 106°, mp (β): 212°, d: 1.745 @ 20°/20°.

SYNS: BENZOEPIN ◇ BEOSIT ◇ BIO 5,462 ◇ CHLORTHIE-
PIN ◇ CRISULFAN ◇ CYCLODAN ◇ DEVISULPHAN
◇ ENDOCEL ◇ ENDOSOL ◇ ENDOSULPHAN ◇ ENSURE
◇ ENT 23,979 ◇ FMC 5462 ◇ 1,2,3,4,7,7-HEXACHLOROBI-
CYCLO(2.2.1)HEPTEN-5,6-BIOXYMETHYLENESULFITE
◇ α,β-1,2,3,4,7,7-HEXACHLOROBICYCLO(2.2.1)-2-HEP-
TENE-5,6-BISOXYMETHYLENE SULFITE ◇ HEXACHLO-
ROHEXAHYDROMETHANO 2,4,3-BENZODIOXATHIEPIN-3-
OXIDE ◇ 6,7,8,9,10,10-HEXACHLORO-1,5,5a,6,9,9a-HEXA-
HYDRO-6,9-METHANO-2,4,3-BENZODIOXATHIEPIN-3-OX-
IDE ◇ 1,4,5,6,7,7-HEXACHLORO-5-NORBORNENE-2,
3-DIMETHANOL CYCLIC SULFITE ◇ HILDAN ◇ HOE 2,671
◇ INSECTOPHENE ◇ KOP-THIODAN ◇ MALIX
◇ NCI-C00566 ◇ NIA 5462 ◇ NIAGARA 5,462 ◇ OMS 570
◇ RCRA WASTE NUMBER P050 ◇ SULFUROUS ACID,
cyclic ester with 1,4,5,6,7,7-HEXACHLORO-5-NORBORNENE-
2,3-DIMETHANOL ◇ THIFOR ◇ THIMUL ◇ THIODAN
◇ THIOFOR ◇ THIOMUL ◇ THIONEX ◇ THIOSULFAN
◇ THIOSULFAN TIONEL ◇ TIOVEL

TOXICITY DATA with REFERENCE
ETA: scu-mus TDLo:2 mg/kg
     NTIS** PB223-159
MUT: cyt-ham-ipr 8 mg/kg   ARTODN 58,152,85
MUT: cyt-mus-unr 1 mg/kg   TGANAK 16(1),45,82
MUT: mmo-smc 100 mg/L   TGANAK 18,455,84
MUT: sce-hmn:lym 1 μmol/L   ARTODN 52,221,83

MUT: sln-dmg-orl 200 ppm/48H   MUREAV
136,115,84
NEO: orl-mus TDLo:330 mg/kg/78W-I
     NTIS** PB223-159

CONSENSUS REPORTS: EPA Extremely Hazardous Substances List. NCI Carcinogenesis Bioassay (feed); No Evidence: mouse, rat NCITR* NCI-CG-TR-62,77.

OSHA PEL: TWA 0.1 mg/m^3 (skin)   ACGIH TLV: TWA 0.1 mg/m^3 (skin)   DOT Classification: Poison B; Label: Poison.

SAFETY PROFILE: Questionable carcinogen with experimental tumorigenic, neoplastigenic, and teratogenic data. Poison by ingestion, inhalation, skin contact, intraperitoneal, subcutaneous, and possibly other routes. Other experimental reproductive effects. Human mutation data reported. A central nervous system stimulant producing convulsions. A highly toxic organochlorine pesticide which does not accumulate significantly in human tissue. Absorption is normally slow, but is increased by alcohols, oil, emulsifiers. When heated to decomposition it emits toxic fumes of Cl$^-$ and SO$_x$.

EAT500   CAS: 72-20-8
ENDRIN
DOT: 2761
mf: $C_{12}H_8Cl_6O$ mw: 380.90

PROP: White crystals. Mp: decomp @ 200°.

SYNS: COMPOUND 269 ◇ ENDREX ◇ ENDRINE (FRENCH)
◇ ENT 17,251 ◇ HEXACHLOROEPOXYOCTAHYDRO-
endo,endo-DIMETHANONAPHTHALENE ◇ 3,4,5,6,9,9-HEXA-
CHLORO-1a,2,2a,3,6,6a,7,7a-OCTAHYDRO-2,7:3,6-
DIMETHANONAPHTH(2,3-b)OXIRENE ◇ HEXADRIN
◇ MENDRIN ◇ NCI-C00157 ◇ NENDRIN ◇ RCRA WASTE
NUMBER P051

TOXICITY DATA with REFERENCE
MUT: cyt-rat-par 1 mg/kg   BECTA6 9,65,73
MUT: sce-ofs-mul 54 pmol/L   MUREAV 118,61,83

CONSENSUS REPORTS: IARC Cancer Review: GROUP 3 IMEMDT 7,56,87; Animal Inadequate Evidence IMEMDT 5,157,74; Human Inadequate Evidence IMEMDT 5,157,74. NCI Carcinogenesis Bioassay (feed); No Evidence: mouse, rat NCITR* NCI-CG-TR-12,79. EPA Genetic Toxicology Program. EPA Extremely Hazardous Substances List.

OSHA PEL: TWA 0.1 mg/m^3 (skin)   ACGIH TLV: TWA 0.1 mg/m^3 (skin)   DFG MAK: 0.1

mg/m^3 DOT Classification: Poison B; Label: Poison; Poison B; Label: Poison, liquid.

SAFETY PROFILE: Questionable carcinogen. Poison by ingestion, skin contact, intravenous and possibly other routes. An experimental teratogen. Experimental reproductive effects. Mutation data reported. A central nervous system stimulant. Highly toxic to birds, fish and humans. A dangerous fire hazard.

EAT900   CAS: 13838-16-9
ENFLURANE
mf: C$_3$H$_2$ClF$_5$O   mw: 184.50

SYNS: ANESTHETIC COMPOUND NO. 347 ◇ 2-CHLORO-1-(DIFLUOROMETHOXY)-1,1,2-TRIFLUOROETHANE ◇ 2-CHLORO-1,1,2-TRIFLUOROETHYL DIFLUOROMETHYL ETHER ◇ COMPOUND 347 ◇ ETHRANE ◇ METHYLFLURETHER ◇ NSC-115944 ◇ OHIO 347

TOXICITY DATA with REFERENCE
CAR: ihl-mus TCLo:3000 ppm/4H/78W-I
    ANESAV 56,9,82
MUT: cyt-hmn:lyms 1000 ppm   ENVRAL12,366,76
MUT: cyt-mus:fbr 1000 ppm   ENVRAL 12,366,76

CONSENSUS REPORTS: Reported in EPA TSCA Inventory.

ACGIH TLV: TWA 75 ppm   NIOSH REL: (Waste Anesthetic Gases and Vapors) CL 2 ppm/1H

SAFETY PROFILE: Questionable carcinogen with experimental carcinogenic data. Experimental reproductive data by inhalation. Mildly toxic by inhalation, ingestion, and subcutaneous routes. Human systemic effects by inhalation: decreased urine volume or anuria. Experimental reproductive effects. Human mutation data reported. An eye irritant. An anesthetic. When heated to decomposition it emits very toxic fumes of F$^-$ and Cl$^-$.

EBH850
(E)-1-α-2-α-EPOXYBENZ(c)ACRIDINE-3-α-4-β-DIOL
mf: C$_{17}$H$_9$NO$_3$ mw: 275.27

SYN: BENZ(c)ACRIDINE 3,4-DIOL-1,2-EPOXIDE-2

TOXICITY DATA with REFERENCE
NEO: ipr-mus TDLo:5505 μg/kg/3D-I   CNREA8 44,5161,84

SAFETY PROFILE: Questionable carcinogen with experimental neoplastigenic data. When

heated to decomposition it emits toxic fumes of NO$_x$.

EBH875
(Z)-1-β,2-β-EPOXYBENZ(c)ACRIDINE-3-α-4-β-DIOL
mf: C$_{17}$H$_9$NO$_3$ mw: 275.27

SYN: BENZ(c)ACRIDINE 3,4-DIOL-1,2-EPOXIDE-1

TOXICITY DATA with REFERENCE
NEO: ipr-mus TDLo:11561 μg/kg/3D-I
    CNREA8 44,5161,84

SAFETY PROFILE: Questionable carcinogen with experimental neoplastigenic data. When heated to decomposition it emits toxic fumes of NO$_x$.

EBJ500   CAS: 930-22-3
3,4-EPOXY-1-BUTENE
mf: C$_4$H$_6$O   mw: 70.10

PROP: Liquid. Mp: −135°, bp: 67°, flash p: <−58°F (CC), d: 0.869, autoign temp: 806°F, vap d: 2.41.

SYNS: BUTADIENE MONOXIDE ◇ 1,2-EPOXYBUTENE-3

TOXICITY DATA with REFERENCE
ETA: skn-mus TDLo:492 g/kg/41W-I   JNCIAM 31,41,63
MUT: dnd-esc 1 μmol/L   ARTODN 46,277,80
MUT: mma-sat 100 μmol/plate   MUREAV97,204,82
MUT: mmo-esc 20 μmol/L   ARTODN 46,277,80
MUT: mmo-klp 1 μmol/L   MUREAV 89,269,81
MUT: mmo-sat 1 μmol/plate   BBRCA9 80,298,78

CONSENSUS REPORTS: Reported in EPA TSCA Inventory.

SAFETY PROFILE: Questionable carcinogen with experimental tumorigenic data. A poison by intraperitoneal route. Mutation data reported. A very dangerous fire hazard when exposed to heat or flame; can react with oxidizing materials. To fight fire, use CO$_2$, dry chemical, water spray. When heated to decomposition it emits acrid smoke and fumes.

EBK500   CAS: 6509-08-6
1,2-EPOXYBUTYRONITRILE
mf: C$_4$H$_5$NO   mw: 83.10

SYN: 3,4-EPOXYBUTYRONITRILE

TOXICITY DATA with REFERENCE
ETA: scu-mus TDLo:324 mg/kg/81W-I
    JNCIAM 46,143,71

CONSENSUS REPORTS: Cyanide and its compounds are on the Community Right-To-Know List.

SAFETY PROFILE: Questionable carcinogen with experimental tumorigenic data. When heated to decomposition it emits toxic fumes of NO_x and CN^-.

EBM000 CAS: 1250-95-9
EPOXYCHOLESTEROL
mf: $C_{27}H_{46}O_2$ mw: 402.73

SYNS: CHOLESTEROL-α-EPOXIDE ◊ CHOLESTEROL-5-α,6-α-EPOXIDE ◊ CHOLESTEROL OXIDE ◊ CHOLESTEROL-α-OXIDE ◊ 5-α,6-α-EPOXYCHOLESTANOL ◊ 5,6-α-EPOXY-5-α-CHOLESTAN-3-β-OL

TOXICITY DATA with REFERENCE
CAR: scu-mus TDLo:600 mg/kg/72W-I
  JNCIAM 19,977,57
MUT: cyt-hmn:fbr 500 μg/L/4H AJEBAK
  56,287,78
MUT: dns-hmn:fbr 10 mg/L/4H AJEBAK
  56,287,78
MUT: otr-ham:emb 625 μg/L CALEDQ 6,143,79

CONSENSUS REPORTS: EPA Genetic Toxicology Program.

SAFETY PROFILE: Questionable carcinogen with experimental carcinogenic data. Human mutation data reported. When heated to decomposition it emits acrid smoke and fumes.

EBP000 CAS: 962-32-3
5,6-EPOXY-5,6-DIHYDROBENZ(a) ANTHRACENE
mf: $C_{18}H_{12}O$ mw: 244.30

SYNS: BENZ(a)ANTHRACENE-5,6-OXIDE ◊ BENZ(a)ANTHRA-5,6-OXIDE ◊ BENZO(a)ANTHRACENE-5,6-OXIDE ◊ 1a,11b-DIHYDROBENZ(3,4)ANTHRA(1,2-b)OXIRENE ◊ 3,4-DIHYDRO-3,4-EPOXY-1,2-BENZANTHRACENE

TOXICITY DATA with REFERENCE
CAR: scu-mus TDLo:400 mg/kg/10W-I
  IJCNAW 2,500,67
MUT: dni-omi 200 μg/L PNASA6 74,1378,77
MUT: dns-hmn:fbr 10 μmol/L/3H IJCNAW
  16,284,75
MUT: mma-sat 450 nmol/L BBRCA9 66,693,75
MUT: mmo-sat 3 μg/plate IJCNAW 16,787,75
MUT: otr-mus:fbr 500 μg/L CNREA8 32,716,73
MUT: sln-dmg-par 5 mmol/L CNREA8 33,2354,73

CONSENSUS REPORTS: EPA Genetic Toxicology Program.

SAFETY PROFILE: Questionable carcinogen with experimental carcinogenic data. Human mutation data reported. When heated to decomposition it emits acrid smoke and fumes.

EBP500 CAS: 1421-85-8
5,6-EPOXY-5,6-DIHYDRODIBENZ(a,h) ANTHRACENE
mf: $C_{22}H_{14}O$ mw: 294.36

SYNS: DBA-5,6-EPOXIDE ◊ DIBENZ(a,h)ANTHRACENE-5,6-OXIDE ◊ 5,6-DIHYDRO-5,6-EPOXYDIBENZ(a,h)ANTHRACENE

TOXICITY DATA with REFERENCE
CAR: scu-mus TDLo:400 mg/kg/10W-I
  IJCNAW 2,500,67
MUT: dnd-ham:lng 1 mg/L CBINA8 4,389,71/72
MUT: dns-hmn:hla 1 μmol/L CNREA8 38,2621,78
MUT: mma-sat 5 μg/plate PNASA6 72,5135,75
MUT: mmo-sat 300 ng/plate IJCNAW 16,787,75
MUT: otr-mus:fbr 500 μg/L CNREA8 32,716,72

CONSENSUS REPORTS: EPA Genetic Toxicology Program.

SAFETY PROFILE: Questionable carcinogen with experimental carcinogenic data. Human mutation data reported. When heated to decomposition it emits acrid smoke and fumes.

EBQ500 CAS: 6921-35-3
1,3-EPOXY-2,2-DIMETHYLPROPANE
mf: $C_5H_{10}O$ mw: 86.15

SYNS: 3,3-DIMETHYLOXETANE ◊ β,β-DIMETHYLTRIMETHYLENE OXIDE ◊ 3,3-DIMETHYLTRIMETHYLENE OXIDE

TOXICITY DATA with REFERENCE
ETA: scu-rat TDLo:1020 mg/kg/61W-I BJCAAI
  17,100,63

SAFETY PROFILE: Questionable carcinogen with experimental tumorigenic data. Moderately toxic by intraperitoneal route. When heated to decomposition it emits acrid smoke and fumes.

EBX500 CAS: 7320-37-8
1,2-EPOXYHEXADECANE
mf: $C_{16}H_{32}O$ mw: 240.48

SYNS: HEXADECENE EPOXIDE ◊ NCI-C55538

TOXICITY DATA with REFERENCE
ETA: skn-mus TDLo:53 g/kg/44W-I JNCIAM
  39,1217,67
ETA: unr-mus TDLo:240 mg/kg RARSAM
  3,193,63

CONSENSUS REPORTS: Reported in EPA TSCA Inventory.

SAFETY PROFILE: Questionable carcinogen with experimental tumorigenic data. A suspected carcinogenic. When heated to decomposition it emits acrid smoke and fumes.

ECA000   CAS: 4247-30-7
4,5-EPOXY-3-HYDROXYVALERIC ACID-β-LACTONE
mf: $C_5H_6O_3$ mw: 114.11

TOXICITY DATA with REFERENCE
NEO: skn-mus TD:88 g/kg/73W-I
14JTAF -,275,64
NEO: skn-mus TDLo:76 g/kg/63W-I   JNCIAM
35,707,65

SAFETY PROFILE: Questionable carcinogen with experimental neoplastigenic data. When heated to decomposition it emits acrid smoke and fumes.

ECA500   CAS: 67195-51-1
11,12-EPOXY-3-METHYLCHOLANTHRENE
mf: $C_{21}H_{14}O$ mw: 282.35

SYNS: MCA-11,12-EPOXIDE ◇ MCA-11,12-OXIDE ◇ 3-METHYLCHOLANTHRENE-11,12-EPOXIDE ◇ 3-METHYL-11,12-EPOXYCHOLANTHRENE

TOXICITY DATA with REFERENCE
ETA: skn-mus TDLo:226 µg/kg   JNCIAM
58,1051,77
MUT: mmo-sat 50 µg/plate   CNREA8 45,2600,85
MUT: msc-ham:lng 5 mmol/L   PNASA6 68,3195,71
MUT: otr-mus:fbr 750 µg/L   CNREA8 32,716,72
MUT: pic-omi 23400 nmol/L   NNBYA7
234,186,71

SAFETY PROFILE: Questionable carcinogen with experimental tumorigenic data. Mutation data reported. When heated to decomposition it emits acrid smoke and fumes.

ECB000   CAS: 141-37-7
3,4-EPOXY-6-METHYLCYCLOHEXYLMETHYL-3',4'-EPOXY-6'-METHYLCYCLOHEXANE CARBOXYLATE
mf: $C_{16}H_{24}O_4$ mw: 280.40

SYNS: CHISSONOX 201 ◇ EP 201 ◇ EPOXIDE-201 ◇ 3,4-EPOXY-6-METHYLCYCLOHEXENECARBOXYLIC ACID (3,4-EPOXY-6-METHYLCYCLOHEXYLMETHYL) ES-TER ◇ 3,4-EPOXY-6-METHYLCYCLOHEXYLMETHYL-3,4-EPOXY-6-METHYLCYCLOHEXANECARBOXYLATE ◇ 4,5-EPOXY-2-METHYLCYCLOHEXYLMETHYL-4,5-EPOXY-2-METHYLCYCLOHEXANECARBOXYLATE ◇ 6-METHYL-3,4-EPOXYCYCLOHEXYLMETHYL-6-METHYL-3,4-EPOXYCYCLOHEXANE CARBOXYLATE ◇ UNOX 201 ◇ UNOX EPOXIDE 201

TOXICITY DATA with REFERENCE
ETA: skn-mus TD:516 g/kg/43W-I   AIHAAP
24,305,63
ETA: skn-mus TDLo:67 g/kg/56W-I   JNCIAM
39,1217,67

CONSENSUS REPORTS: IARC Cancer Review: GROUP 3 IMEMDT 7,56,87; Animal Sufficient Evidence IMEMDT 11,147,76.

SAFETY PROFILE: Questionable carcinogen with experimental tumorigenic data. Mildly toxic by ingestion. A skin irritant. When heated to decomposition it emits acrid smoke and fumes.

ECD500   CAS: 2443-39-2
cis-9,10-EPOXYOCTADECANOIC ACID
mf: $C_{18}H_{34}O_3$ mw: 298.52

SYNS: cis-9,10-EPOXYOCTADECANOATE ◇ EPOXY-OLEIC ACID ◇ 9,10-EPOXYSTEARIC ACID ◇ cis-9,10-EPOXYSTEARIC ACID ◇ cis-3-OCTYL-OXIRANE-OCTANOIC ACID

TOXICITY DATA with REFERENCE
ETA: scu-mus TDLo:164 mg/kg/41W-I
CNREA8 30,1037,70
ETA: skn-mus TDLo:2880 mg/kg/24W-I
JNCIAM 31,41,63

CONSENSUS REPORTS: IARC Cancer Review: Animal Inadequate Evidence IMEMDT 11,153,76.

SAFETY PROFILE: Questionable carcinogen with experimental tumorigenic data. When heated to decomposition it emits acrid smoke and fumes.

ECE000   CAS: 2984-50-1
1,2-EPOXYOCTANE
mf: $C_8H_{16}O$ mw: 128.24

SYN: OCTYLENE EPOXIDE

TOXICITY DATA with REFERENCE
ETA: unr-mus TDLo:103 mg/kg   RARSAM
3,193,63

SAFETY PROFILE: Questionable carcinogen with experimental tumorigenic data. When heated to decomposition it emits acrid smoke and fumes.

ECG500 CAS: 63991-57-1
p-(2,3-EPOXYPROPOXY)-N-PHENYLBENZYLAMINE
mf: $C_{16}H_{17}NO_2$ mw: 255.34

SYN: N-(4-(2,3-EPOXYPROPOXY)PHENYL)BENZYL-AMINE

TOXICITY DATA with REFERENCE
ETA: scu-rat TDLo: 4750 mg/kg/18W-I
ANYAA9 68,750,58

SAFETY PROFILE: Questionable carcinogen with experimental tumorigenic data. When heated to decomposition it emits toxic fumes of NO_x.

ECJ000 CAS: 5431-33-4
2,3-EPOXYPROPYL OLEATE
mf: $C_{21}H_{38}O_3$ mw: 338.59

SYNS: 2,3-EPOXY-1-PROPANOL OLEATE ◇ 2,3-EPOXY-PROPYL ESTER of OLEIC ACID ◇ GLYCIDOL OLEATE ◇ GLYCIDYL OCTADECENOATE ◇ GLYCIDYL OLEATE ◇ OLEIC ACID GLYCIDYL ESTER ◇ OXIRANYLMETHYL ESTER of 9-OCTADECENOIC ACID

TOXICITY DATA with REFERENCE
ETA: scu-mus TDLo: 1040 mg/kg/52W-I
CNREA8 30,1037,70
MUT: cyt-rat-ipr 10 mg/kg BJPCAL 6,235,51

CONSENSUS REPORTS: IARC Cancer Review: Animal Inadequate Evidence IMEMDT 11,183,76.

SAFETY PROFILE: Questionable carcinogen with experimental tumorigenic data. Poison by intravenous route. Moderately toxic by ingestion and subcutaneous routes. Mildly toxic by skin contact. Mutation data reported. When heated to decomposition it emits acrid smoke and fumes.

ECP000 CAS: 4509-11-9
3,4-EPOXYSULFOLANE
mf: $C_4H_6O_3S$ mw: 134.16

SYNS: 2,3-EPOXYTETRAMETHYLENE SULFONE ◇ 6-OXA-3-THIABICYCLO(3.1.0)HEXANE-3,3-DIOXIDE ◇ TETRAHYDRO-3,4-EPOXYTHIOPHENE-1,1-DIOXIDE

TOXICITY DATA with REFERENCE
ETA: scu-mus TDLo: 88 mg/kg/22W-I JNCIAM
46,143,71

SAFETY PROFILE: Questionable carcinogen with experimental tumorigenic data. Mildly toxic by intraperitoneal route. When heated to decomposition it emits toxic fumes of SO_x.

ECQ100 CAS: 36504-68-4
9,10-EPOXY-7,8,9,10-TETRAHYDROBENZO(a)PYRENE
mf: $C_{20}H_{14}O$ mw: 270.34

SYNS: 7,8,9,10-TETRAHYDRO-BENZO(a)PYRENE-9,10-EPOXIDE ◇ 7,8,9,10-TETRAHYDRO-BENZO(a)PYRENE-9,10-EPOXYIDE ◇ 7,8,9,10-TETRAHYDRO-9,10-EPOXY-BENZO(a)PYRENE

TOXICITY DATA with REFERENCE
ETA: skn-mus TDLo: 519 mg/kg/60W-I
CNREA8 37,3356,77
MUT: dnd-mam: lym 10 nmol/L CRNGDP3,247,82
MUT: dni-omi 200 μg/L PNASA6 74,1378,77'
MUT: mma-sat 300 pmol/plate CNREA836,3358,76
MUT: mmo-sat 100 pmol/plate CNREA840,642,80
MUT: msc-ham: lng 60 nmol/L CNREA8
36,3358,76

CONSENSUS REPORTS: EPA Genetic Toxicology Program.

SAFETY PROFILE: Questionable carcinogen with experimental tumorigenic data by skin contact. Mutation data reported. When heated to decomposition it emits toxic fumes of NO_x.

ECQ150 CAS: 66788-11-2
9,10-EPOXY-9,10,11,12-TETRAHYDROBENZO(e)PYRENE
mf: $C_{20}H_{14}O$ mw: 270.34

SYNS: 9,10,11,12-TETRAHYDRO-9,10-EPOXY-BENZO(e)PYRENE ◇ B(e)P H4-9,10-EPOXIDE

TOXICITY DATA with REFERENCE
ETA: scu-mus TDLo: 10 mg/kg JJIND8 64,617,80
MUT: dnd-mam: lym 10 μmol/L CRNGDP
3,247,82
MUT: mma-sat 13 pmol/plate JBCHA3 254,4408,79
MUT: mmo-sat 1 nmol/plate CNREA8 40,1985,80
MUT: msc-ham: lng 1100 nmol/L CNREA8
40,1985,80

SAFETY PROFILE: Questionable carcinogen with experimental tumorigenic data. Mutation data reported. When heated to decomposition it emits acrid smoke and fumes.

ECQ200 CAS: 67694-88-6
3,4-EPOXY-1,2,3,4-TETRAHYDROCHRYSENE
mf: $C_{18}H_{14}O$ mw: 246.32

TOXICITY DATA with REFERENCE

NEO: ipr-mus TDLo:63 mg/kg/15D-I   CNREA8
39,5063,79

MUT: mma-sat 1 nmol/plate   CNREA8 39,4069,79

MUT: msc-ham:lng 1 nmol/plate   CNREA8
39,4069,79

SAFETY PROFILE: Questionable carcinogen with experimental neoplastigenic data. Mutation data reported. When heated to decomposition it emits acrid smoke and fumes.

ECR259   CAS: 56179-80-7
1,2-EPOXY-1,2,3,4-TETRAHYDROPHENANTHRENE
mf: $C_{14}H_{12}O$ mw: 196.26

TOXICITY DATA with REFERENCE

NEO: ipr-mus TDLo:50 mg/kg/15D-I   CNREA8
39,5063,79

MUT: mma-sat 1 nmol/plate   CNREA8 39,4069,79

MUT: msc-ham:lng 1 nmol/plate   CNREA8
39,4069,79

SAFETY PROFILE: Questionable carcinogen with experimental neoplastigenic data. Mutation data reported. When heated to decomposition it emits acrid smoke and fumes.

ECR500   CAS: 66997-69-1
3,4-EPOXY-1,2,3,4-TETRAHYDROPHENANTHRENE
mf: $C_{14}H_{12}O$ mw: 196.26

SYN: PHENANTHRENETETRAHYDRO-3,4-EPOXIDE

TOXICITY DATA with REFERENCE

NEO: skn-mus TDLo:16 mg/kg   VOONAW
15(8),54,69

MUT: mma-sat 1 nmol/plate   CNREA8 39,4069,79

MUT: msc-ham:lng 1 nmol/plate   CNREA8
39,4069,79

SAFETY PROFILE: Questionable carcinogen with experimental neoplastigenic data. Mutation data reported. When heated to decomposition it emits acrid smoke and fumes.

ECS000   CAS: 72074-69-2
(±)-3-α,4-α-EPOXY-1,2,3,4-TETRAHYDRO-1-β,2-α-PHENANTHRENEDIOL
mf: $C_{14}H_{12}O_3$ mw: 228.26

SYN: (±)-1-β,2-α-DIHYDROXY-3-α,4-α-EPOXY-1,2,3,4-TETRAHYDROPHENANTHRENE

TOXICITY DATA with REFERENCE

ETA: ipr-mus TDLo:59 mg/kg/15D-I   CNREA8
39,5063,79

SAFETY PROFILE: Questionable carcinogen with experimental tumorigenic data. When heated to decomposition it emits acrid smoke and fumes.

ECT600   CAS: 16967-79-6
EPOXY-1,1,2-TRICHLOROETHANE
mf: C_2HCl_3O mw: 147.38

SYNS: TCEO ◇ 1,1,2-TRICHLOROEPOXYETHANE ◇ TRICHLOROETHYLENE EPOXIDE ◇ TRICHLOROETHYLENE OXIDE ◇ TRICHLORO-OXIRANE

TOXICITY DATA with REFERENCE

CAR: scu-mus TDLo:20 mg/kg/78W-I   CNREA8
43,159,83

MUT: mmo-ssp 500 μmol/L   45OHAA -,333,80

MUT: msc-ham:lng 50 μmol/L   45OHAA -,333,80

MUT: otr-ham:emb 1100 μmol/L   JJIND8
69,531,82

SAFETY PROFILE: Questionable carcinogen with experimental carcinogenic data. Mutation data reported. When heated to decomposition it emits toxic fumes of Cl^-.

ECV000   CAS: 517-09-9
EQUILENIN
mf: $C_{18}H_{18}O_2$ mw: 266.36

PROP: Leaflets from acetone and ethanol; very sltly sol in water.

SYNS: EQUILENINA (SPANISH) ◇ EQUILENINE ◇ 3-HYDROXYESTRA-1,3,5(10),6,8-PENATEN-17-ONE

TOXICITY DATA with REFERENCE

ETA: imp-gpg TD:17 mg/kg:TER   RBBIAL
5,1,45

ETA: imp-gpg TDLo:1600 μg/kg:TER
BSBSAS 8,142,51

ETA: imp-ham TDLo:640 mg/kg/38W-I
CNREA8 43,5200,83

SAFETY PROFILE: Questionable carcinogen with experimental tumorigenic and teratogenic data. When heated to decomposition it emits acrid smoke and irritating fumes.

ECV500   CAS: 604-58-0
EQUILENIN BENZOATE
mf: $C_{25}H_{22}O_3$ mw: 370.47

PROP: Crystalline. Mp: 223° (in vacuo).

SYN: 3-HYDROXYESTRA-1,3,5,7,9-PENTAEN-17-ONE BENZOATE

TOXICITY DATA with REFERENCE

NEO: scu-mus TDLo:162 mg/kg/81W-I
ZEKBAI 56,482,49

ETA: par-mus TDLo: 86 mg/kg/43W-I CRSBAW
122,183,36

ETA: scu-mus TD: 120 mg/kg/30W-I: TER
YJBMAU 12,213,39

SAFETY PROFILE: Questionable carcinogen with experimental neoplastigenic, tumorigenic, and teratogenic data. When heated to decomposition it emits acrid smoke and irritating fumes.

ECW000   CAS: 474-86-2
EQUILIN
mf: $C_{18}H_{20}O_2$ mw: 268.38

SYNS: 1,3,5,7-ESTRATETRAEN-3-OL-17-ONE ◇ 3-HY-DROXYESTRA-1,3,5(10),7-TETRAEN-17-ONE

TOXICITY DATA with REFERENCE
NEO: scu-mus TDLo: 112 mg/kg/56W-I
ZEKBAI 56,482,49

ETA: imp-ham TDLo: 640 mg/kg/38W-I
CNREA8 43,5200,83

ETA: scu-mus TDLo: 168 mg/kg/42W-I
YJBMAU 12,213,39

SAFETY PROFILE: Questionable carcinogen with experimental neoplastigenic and tumorigenic data. When heated to decomposition it emits acrid smoke and irritating fumes.

ECW500   CAS: 6030-80-4
EQUILIN BENZOATE
mf: $C_{25}H_{24}O_3$ mw: 372.49

SYN: 3-HYDROXYESTRA-1,3,5(10),7-TETRAEN-17-ONE BENZOATE

TOXICITY DATA with REFERENCE
NEO: scu-mus TDLo: 96 mg/kg/48W-I ZEKBAI
56,482,49

ETA: par-mus TDLo: 42 mg/kg/21W-I CRSBAW
122,183,36

ETA: scu-mus TD: 148 mg/kg/37W-I: TER
YJBMAU 12,213,39

SAFETY PROFILE: Questionable carcinogen with experimental neoplastigenic, tumorigenic, and teratogenic data. When heated to decomposition it emits acrid smoke and irritating fumes.

EDB500   CAS: 129-51-1
ERGOT
mf: $C_{19}H_{23}N_3O_2 \cdot C_4H_4O_4$ mw: 441.53

PROP: Composition: ergot amine, ergosine, ergocristine, ergocryptine, ergocornine, ergosinine, ergocristinine, ergocryptinine, ergotaminine, etc.

SYNS: CORNOCENTIN ◇ CRUDE ERGOT ◇ ERGOMET-RINE ACID MALEATE ◇ ERGOMETRINE MALEATE ◇ ERGONOVINE, MALEATE (1:1) (SALT) ◇ ERGOTRATE ◇ ERGOTRATE MALEATE ◇ OXYTOCIC

TOXICITY DATA with REFERENCE
ETA: orl-rat TD: 773 g/kg/44W-C CNREA8
2,11,42

ETA: orl-rat TDLo: 669 g/kg/96W-C CNREA8
2,11,42

SAFETY PROFILE: Questionable carcinogen with experimental tumorigenic data. Human poison by unspecified route. Experimental poison by intravenous route. Experimental reproductive effects. Can cause vomiting, diarrhea, thirst, tachycardia, confusion, coma, central nervous system symptoms, gastrointestinal disturbances, gangrene; circulatory changes can follow ingestion. When heated to decomposition it emits toxic fumes of NO_x.

EDO500   CAS: 57-91-0
17-α-ESTRADIOL
mf: $C_{18}H_{24}O_2$ mw: 272.42

SYNS: 3,17-DIHYDROXYESTRATRIENE ◇ 3,17-α-DIHY-DROXYOESTRA-1,3,5(10)-TRIENE ◇ ESTRA-1,3,5(10)-TRIENE-3,17-α-DIOL ◇ 1,3,5-ESTRATRIENE-3,17-α-DIOL ◇ OESTRADIOL-17-α

TOXICITY DATA with REFERENCE
ETA: imp-gpg TD: 3 mg/kg: TER RBBIAL 5,1,45
MUT: dni-hmn: oth 100 mg//L JTEHD6
10,143,82

SAFETY PROFILE: Questionable carcinogen with experimental tumorigenic and teratogenic data. Human mutation data reported. When heated to decomposition it emits acrid smoke and irritating fumes. A steroid.

EDP500   CAS: 63042-19-3
ESTRADIOL-17-BENZOATE-3,n-BUTYRATE
mf: $C_{29}H_{34}O_4$ mw: 446.63

SYNS: 17-BENZOATE-3-n-BUTYRATE d'OESTRADIOL (FRENCH) ◇ ESTRA-1,3,5(10)-TRIENE-3,17-β-DIOL-17-BENZOATE-3-n-BUTYRATE

TOXICITY DATA with REFERENCE
ETA: scu-gpg TDLo: 7 mg/kg/12W-I CRSBAW
130,1466,39

SAFETY PROFILE: Questionable carcinogen with experimental tumorigenic data. When

heated to decomposition it emits acrid smoke and irritating fumes.

EDQ000   CAS: 8000-03-1
ESTRADIOL-3-BENZOATE mixed with PROGESTERONE (1:14 moles)

SYNS: ESTRADIOL BENZOATE mixed with PROGESTER-
ONE (1:14 moles) ◇ ESTRA-1,3,5(10)-TRIETNE-3,17-β-DIOL-
3-BENZOATE mixed with PROGESTERONE (1:14 moles)
◇ PROGESTERONE mixed with ESTRADIOL BENZOATE (14:
1 moles) ◇ PROGESTERONE mixed with ESTRA-1,3,5(10)-
TRIENE-3,17-β-DIOL-3-BENZOATE (14:1 moles)

TOXICITY DATA with REFERENCE
ETA: scu-mus TDLo:338 mg/kg/39W-I:TER
   YJBMAU 12,213,39

SAFETY PROFILE: Questionable carcinogen with experimental tumorigenic and teratogenic data. When heated to decomposition it emits acrid smoke and irritating fumes.

EDQ500   CAS: 63042-22-8
ESTRADIOL-17-CAPRYLATE
mf: $C_{26}H_{38}O_3$ mw: 398.64

SYNS: CAPRYLATE d'OESTRADIOL (FRENCH)
◇ ESTRA-1,3,5(10)-TRIENE-3,17,β-DIOL-17-OCTANOATE

TOXICITY DATA with REFERENCE
ETA: imp-gpg TDLo:2800 μg/kg   RCBIAS
   3,108,44
ETA: scu-gpg TDLo:800 μg/kg/13W-I:TER
   CRSBAW 130,1466,39

SAFETY PROFILE: Questionable carcinogen with experimental tumorigenic and teratogenic data. When heated to decomposition it emits acrid smoke and irritating fumes.

EDR500   CAS: 22966-79-6
ESTRADIOL MUSTARD
mf: $C_{42}H_{50}Cl_4N_2O_4$ mw: 788.74

PROP: Mp: 40-65° (freeze dried).

SYNS: BIS((4-(BIS(2-CHLOROETHYL)AMINO)BENZENE)
ACETATE)ESTRA-1,3,5(10)-TRIENE-3,17-DIOL(17-β) ◇ BIS
((4-(BIS(2-CHLOROETHYL)AMINO)BENZENE)ACETATE)
OESTRA-1,3,5(10)-TRIENE-3,17-DIOL(17-β) ◇ BIS((p-(BIS
(2-CHLOROETHYL)AMINO)PHENYL)ACETATE)ESTRA-
DIOL ◇ BIS((p-(BIS(2-CHLOROETHYL)AMINO)PHENYL)
ACETATE)ESTRA-1,3,5(10)-TRIENE-3,17-β-DIOL ◇ BIS((p-
(BIS(2-CHLOROETHYL)AMINO)PHENYL)ACETATE)OES-
TRADIOL ◇ BIS((p-BIS(2-CHLOROETHYL)AMINOPHENYL)
ACETATE)OESTRA-1,3,5(10)-TRIENE-3,17-β-DIOL
◇ NCI-C01570 ◇ NSC 112259 ◇ OESTRADIOL MUSTARD

TOXICITY DATA with REFERENCE
CAR: orl-mus TD:4680 mg/kg/1Y-I
   NCITR* NCI-CG-TR-59,78
CAR: orl-mus TDLo:2340 mg/kg/52W-I
   NCITR* NCI-CG-TR-59,78
NEO: ipr-mus TDLo:480 mg/kg/8W-I   CNREA8
   33,3069,73

CONSENSUS REPORTS: IARC Cancer Review: GROUP 3 IMEMDT 7,56,87; Animal Limited Evidence IMEMDT 9,217,75. NCI Carcinogenesis Bioassay (gavage); Clear Evidence: mouse NCITR* NCI-CG-TR-59,78; No Evidence: rat NCITR* NCI-CG-TR-59,78.

SAFETY PROFILE: Questionable carcinogen with experimental carcinogenic and neoplastigenic data. When heated to decomposition it emits very toxic fumes of Cl⁻ and NO_x.

EDT500   CAS: 6639-99-2
α-ESTRA-1,3,5,7,9-PENTANE-3,17-DIOL
mf: $C_{18}H_{19}O_2$ mw: 267.37

SYNS: α-DIHYDROEQUILENIN ◇ α-DIHYDROEQUILE-
NINA (SPANISH)

TOXICITY DATA with REFERENCE
ETA: imp-gpg TDLo:20 mg/kg:TER   RBBIAL
   5,1,45

SAFETY PROFILE: Questionable carcinogen with experimental tumorigenic and teratogenic data. When heated to decomposition it emits acrid smoke and irritating fumes.

EDU000   CAS: 1423-97-8
β-ESTRA-1,3,5,7,9-PENTANE-3,17-DIOL
mf: $C_{18}H_{19}O_2$ mw: 267.37

SYNS: β-DIHYDROEQUILENIN ◇ β-DIHYDROEQUILE-
NINA (SPANISH)

TOXICITY DATA with REFERENCE
ETA: imp-gpg TDLo:24 mg/kg:TER   RBBIAL
   5,1,45

SAFETY PROFILE: Questionable carcinogen with experimental tumorigenic and teratogenic data. When heated to decomposition it emits acrid smoke and irritating fumes.

EEF000   CAS: 17088-21-0
1-ETHENYL PYRENE
mf: $C_{18}H_{12}$ mw: 228.2

SYNS: 1-VINYLPYRENE ◇ 3-VINYLPYRENE

TOXICITY DATA with REFERENCE
ETA: skn-mus TDLo: 3651 μg/kg   CNREA8
40,642,80

MUT: mma-sat 10 nmol/plate   CNREA8 40,642,80

SAFETY PROFILE: Questionable carcinogen with experimental tumorigenic data. Mutation data reported. When heated to decomposition it emits acrid smoke and irritating fumes.

EEF500   CAS: 73529-25-6
4-ETHENYL PYRENE
mf: $C_{18}H_{12}$ mw: 228.2

SYN: 4-VINYLPYRENE

TOXICITY DATA with REFERENCE
ETA: skn-mus TDLo: 3651 μg/kg   CNREA8
40,642,80

SAFETY PROFILE: Questionable carcinogen with experimental tumorigenic data. When heated to decomposition it emits acrid smoke and irritating fumes.

EEG000   CAS: 88-12-0
1-ETHENYL-2-PYRROLIDINONE
mf: C_6H_9NO mw: 111.16

PROP: Colorless liquid, water-sol. Bp: 148° @ 100 mm, fp: 13.5°, flash p: 209°F (OC), d: 1.04 @ 25°, autoign temp: 687°F, vap d: 3.8, fire p: 213°F.

SYNS: VINYLBUTYROLACTAM ◇ N-VINYLPYRROLIDI-
NONE ◇ N-VINYL-2-PYRROLIDINONE ◇ 1-VINYL-2-PYRRO-
LIDINONE ◇ VINYLPYRROLIDONE ◇ N-VINYLPYRROLI-
DONE ◇ N-VINYL-2-PYRROLIDONE ◇ 1-VINYL-2-
PYRROLIDONE ◇ V-PYROL

CONSENSUS REPORTS: IARC Cancer Review: GROUP 3 IMEMDT 7,56,87. Reported in EPA TSCA Inventory.

SAFETY PROFILE: Questionable carcinogen. Moderately toxic by ingestion, inhalation and skin contact. A severe eye irritant. Probably irritating and narcotic in high concentrations. Combustible when exposed to heat or flame; can react vigorously with oxidizing materials. To fight fire, use alcohol foam, CO_2, dry chemical. When heated to decomposition it emits highly toxic fumes of NO_x.

EEH575   CAS: 8064-76-4
ETHINYLOESTRADIOL mixed with LYNOESTRENOL
mf: $C_{20}H_{28}O$ • C20-H24-O2   mw: 580.92

SYNS: Ba 49249 ◇ C 49249Ba ◇ ETHYNYLESTRADIOL-
LYNESTRENOL mixture ◇ FISIOQUENS ◇ FYSIOQUENS
◇ LYNOESTRENOL mixed with ETHINYLOESTRADIOL
◇ MINILYN ◇ OVOSTAT ◇ OVOSTAT 1375 ◇ OVOSTAT E
◇ YERMONIL

TOXICITY DATA with REFERENCE
CAR: orl-wmn TDLo: 77112 μg/kg/6Y-I
LANCAO 1,273,80

SAFETY PROFILE: Questionable human carcinogen producing liver tumors. Human reproductive effects. When heated to decomposition it emits acrid smoke and irritating fumes.

EEH900
ETHISTERONE and DIETHYLSTILBESTROL
mf: $C_{21}H_{28}O_2 \cdot C_{18}H_{20}O_2$ mw: 580.87

SYNS: DIETHYLSTILBESTROL and ETHISTERONE
◇ DIETHYLSTILBESTROL and PRANONE ◇ PRANONE and
DIETHYLSTILBESTROL ◇ PRANONE and STILBESTROL
◇ 17-α-PREGN-4-EN-20-YN-3-ONE, 17-HYDROXY-, and trans-
α-α'-DIETHYL-4,4'-STILBENEDIOL ◇ STILBESTROL and
PRANONE

TOXICITY DATA with REFERENCE
CAR: unr-wmn TDLo: 164 mg/kg/9Y-I   BJOGAS
82,421,75

SAFETY PROFILE: Questionable human carcinogen producing uterine tumors. Human reproductive effects. When heated to decomposition it emits acrid smoke and irritating fumes.

EEM000   CAS: 938-73-8
2-ETHOXYBENZAMIDE
mf: $C_9H_{11}NO_2$ mw: 165.21

SYNS: ANOVIGAM ◇ ETAMIDE ◇ ETHBENZAMIDE
◇ ETHENZAMID ◇ ETHENZAMIDE ◇ ETHOSALICYL
◇ o-ETHOXYBENZAMIDE ◇ ETOCIL ◇ ETOSALICIL
◇ ETOSALICYL ◇ EUSAL ◇ H.P. 209 ◇ KATAGRIPPE
◇ LINDATOX ◇ LUCAMIDE ◇ PIROSOLVINA ◇ PROTOPY-
RIN ◇ TRANCALGYL

TOXICITY DATA with REFERENCE
CAR: orl-mus TDLo: 544 g/kg/54W-C   JJIND8
76,115,86

MUT: cyt-ham: fbr 500 mg/L   ESKHA5 96,55,78
MUT: cyt-ham: lng 500 mg/L/48H   GMCRDC
27,95,81

CONSENSUS REPORTS: Reported in EPA TSCA Inventory.

SAFETY PROFILE: Questionable carcinogen with experimental carcinogenic data. Poison by intraperitoneal route. Moderately toxic by ingestion. Mutation data reported. When heated to decomposition it emits toxic fumes of NO_x.

EER400   CAS: 83053-57-0
11-ETHOXY-15,16-DIHYDRO-17-CYCLOPENTA(a)PHENANTHREN-17-ONE
mf: $C_{19}H_{16}O_2$ mw: 276.35

TOXICITY DATA with REFERENCE
ETA: skn-mus TDLo: 1600 µg/kg   CRNGDP
3,677,82
MUT: mma-sat 20 µg/plate   CRNGDP 3,677,82

SAFETY PROFILE: Questionable carcinogen with experimental tumorigenic data. Mutation data reported. When heated to decomposition it emits acrid smoke and irritating fumes.

EEV000   CAS: 63019-29-4
10-ETHOXYMETHYL-1:2-BENZANTHRACENE
mf: $C_{21}H_{18}O$ mw: 286.39

SYN: 7-(ETHOXYMETHYL)BENZ(a)ANTHRACENE

TOXICITY DATA with REFERENCE
ETA: skn-mus TDLo: 1200 mg/kg/50W-I
PRLBA4 129,439,40

SAFETY PROFILE: Questionable carcinogen with experimental tumorigenic data. When heated to decomposition it emits acrid smoke and irritating fumes.

EEX000   CAS: 63020-27-9
7-ETHOXY METHYL-12-METHYL BENZ(a)ANTHRACENE
mf: $C_{22}H_{20}O$ mw: 300.42

SYN: 9-METHYL-10-ETHOXYMETHYL-1,2-BENZAN-THRACENE

TOXICITY DATA with REFERENCE
ETA: scu-mus TDLo: 80 mg/kg   CNREA8 6,454,46

SAFETY PROFILE: Questionable carcinogen with experimental tumorigenic data. When heated to decomposition it emits acrid smoke and irritating fumes.

EEX500   CAS: 22960-71-0
N-ETHOXYMORPHOLINO DIAZENIUM FLUOROBORATE
mf: $C_6H_{13}N_2O_2 \cdot BF_4$ mw: 232.02

TOXICITY DATA with REFERENCE
CAR: scu-rat TDLo: 559 mg/kg   ZKKOBW 80,17,73

SAFETY PROFILE: Questionable carcinogen with experimental carcinogenic data. Moderately toxic by subcutaneous route. When heated to decomposition it emits very toxic NO_x and F^-.

EFE000   CAS: 150-69-6
4-ETHOXYPHENYLUREA
mf: $C_9H_{12}N_2O_2$ mw: 180.23

PROP: Needle-like crystals. Mp: 174°.

SYNS: p-AETHOXYPHYLHARNSTOFF (GERMAN)
◇ DULCINE ◇ N-(4-ETHOXYPHENYL)UREA ◇ p-ETHOXY-PHENYLUREA ◇ NCI-C02073 ◇ PHENETHYLCARBAMID (GERMAN) ◇ p-PHENETOLCARBAMID (GERMAN)
◇ p-PHENETOLCARBAMIDE ◇ p-PHENETOLECARBAMIDE ◇ p-PHENETYLUREA ◇ SUCROL ◇ SUESSSTOFF ◇ VALZIN

TOXICITY DATA with REFERENCE
ETA: orl-rat TDLo: 232 g/kg/59W-C   JAPMA8
40,583,51

CONSENSUS REPORTS: IARC Cancer Review: Animal Inadequate Evidence IMEMDT 12,97,76.

SAFETY PROFILE: Questionable carcinogen with experimental tumorigenic data. Human poison by ingestion. Moderately toxic experimentally by ingestion. Human systemic effects by ingestion: somnolence, hallucinations, distorted perceptions and changes in motor activity. In adults 20 to 40 grams produces dizziness, nausea, methemoglobinemia, cyanosis, and hypotension. When heated to decomposition it emits toxic fumes of NO_x.

EGO000   CAS: 56961-62-7
5-ETHYL-1,2-BENZANTHRACENE
mf: $C_{20}H_{16}$ mw: 256.36

SYN: 8-ETHYLBENZ(a)ANTHRACENE

TOXICITY DATA with REFERENCE
ETA: skn-mus TDLo: 650 mg/kg/27W-I
PRLBA4 123,343,37

SAFETY PROFILE: Questionable carcinogen with experimental tumorigenic data. When heated to decomposition it emits acrid smoke and irritating fumes.

EGO500   CAS: 3697-30-1
10-ETHYL-1,2-BENZANTHRACENE
mf: $C_{20}H_{16}$ mw: 256.36

SYN: 7-ETHYLBENZ(a)ANTHRACENE

TOXICITY DATA with REFERENCE
ETA: scu-mus TDLo: 600 mg/kg   JNCIAM 1,303,40
MUT: mma-sat 50 μg/plate   MUREAV 206,55,88

SAFETY PROFILE: Questionable carcinogen with experimental tumorigenic data. Mutation data reported. When heated to decomposition it emits acrid smoke and irritating fumes.

EGP000   CAS: 18868-66-1
12-ETHYLBENZ(a)ANTHRACENE
mf: $C_{20}H_{16}$ mw: 256.36

TOXICITY DATA with REFERENCE
ETA: ims-rat TDLo: 50 mg/kg   CNREA8 29,506,69

SAFETY PROFILE: Questionable carcinogen with experimental tumorigenic data. When heated to decomposition it emits acrid smoke and irritating fumes.

EGS500   CAS: 59965-27-4
2-ETHYL-3:4-BENZPHENANTHRENE
mf: $C_{20}H_{16}$ mw: 256.36

SYN: 5-ETHYLBENZO(c)PHENANTHRENE

TOXICITY DATA with REFERENCE
ETA: skn-mus TDLo: 620 mg/kg/26W-I
    PRLBA4 131,170,42

SAFETY PROFILE: Questionable carcinogen with experimental tumorigenic data. When heated to decomposition it emits acrid smoke and irritating fumes.

EGV000   CAS: 105-36-2
ETHYL BROMACETATE
DOT: 1603
mf: $C_4H_7BrO_2$ mw: 167.02

PROP: Colorless to straw-colored liquid. Bp: 158.8°, fp: <−20°, flash p: 118°F, d: 1.514 @ 13°/4°, vap d: 5.8. Insol in water; misc in alc and ether.

SYNS: BROMOACETIC ACID, ETHYL ESTER ◊ ETHOXY-CARBONYLMETHYL BROMIDE ◊ ETHYL BROMOACETATE ◊ ETHYL-α-BROMOACETATE ◊ ETHYL MONOBROMO-ACETATE

TOXICITY DATA with REFERENCE
NEO: scu-mus TDLo: 252 mg/kg/63W-I
    JNCIAM 53,695,74

CONSENSUS REPORTS: Reported in EPA TSCA Inventory.

DOT Classification: Poison B; Label: Flammable Liquid and Poison.

SAFETY PROFILE: Questionable carcinogen with experimental neoplastigenic data. A poison. An irritant to skin, eyes, and mucous membranes. Flammable when exposed to heat, flame and oxidizers. Will react with water or steam to produce toxic and corrosive fumes. To fight fire, use water as a fire blanket. When heated to decomposition or on contact with acid or acid fumes, it emits highly toxic fumes of Br^-.

EHA100   CAS: 591-62-8
ETHYL BUTYLCARBAMATE
mf: $C_7H_{15}NO_2$ mw: 145.23

SYNS: BUR ◊ 1-BUTYLURETHAN ◊ BUTYLURETHANE ◊ N-BUTYLURETHANE ◊ 1-BUTYLURETHANE ◊ ETHYL-N,N-BUTYLCARBAMATE

TOXICITY DATA with REFERENCE
ETA: scu-rat TDLo: 100 mg/kg (15-21D preg)
    GANNA2 71,811,80
MUT: dnr-bcs 5 g/L   MUREAV 42,19,77
MUT: mmo-bcs 5 g/L   MUREAV 42,19,77

CONSENSUS REPORTS: EPA Genetic Toxicology Program.

SAFETY PROFILE: Questionable carcinogen with experimental tumorigenic data. Poison by intraperitoneal route. Experimental reproductive effects. Mutation data reported. When heated to decomposition it emits toxic fumes of NO_x.

EHC000   CAS: 4549-44-4
ETHYL-N-BUTYLNITROSAMINE
mf: $C_6H_{14}N_2O$ mw: 130.22

SYNS: AETHYL-N-BUTYL-NITROSOAMIN (GERMAN) ◊ N-ETHYL-N-NITROSOBUTYLAMINE ◊ N-NITROSO-N-BUTYLETHYLAMINE ◊ N-NITROSOETHYL-N-BUTYLAMINE

TOXICITY DATA with REFERENCE
CAR: orl-mus TDLo: 2360 mg/kg/34W-C
    NATWAY 50,717,63
ETA: ipr-rat TDLo: 1 g/kg/20W-I   ZEKBAI
    74,110,70
ETA: ivn-rat TDLo: 1000 mg/kg/40W-I
    ARZNAD 19,1077,69
ETA: orl-rat TDLo: 1000 mg/kg/29W-C
    ARZNAD 19,1077,69
MUT: dni-mus-ipr 20 g/kg   ARGEAR 51,605,81
MUT: dns-rat: lvr 1 mmol/L   ENMUDM 3,11,81
MUT: mmo-sat 769 μmol/L   ENMUDM 3,11,81

SAFETY PROFILE: Questionable carcinogen with experimental carcinogenic and tumorigenic data. Poison by ingestion and intravenous routes. Mutation data reported. When heated to decomposition it emits toxic fumes of NO_x.

EHC800
ETHYL N-BUTYL-N-NITROSOSUCCINAMATE
mf: $C_{10}H_{18}N_2O_4$ mw: 230.30

SYNS: N-BUTYL-N-NITROSOSUCCINAMIC ACID ETHYL ESTER ◇ EBNS ◇ N-NITROSO-N-(3-CARBOETHOXYPROPIONYL)BUTYLAMINE

TOXICITY DATA with REFERENCE
CAR: scu-rat TD:87 mg/kg/10W-I   IAPUDO 41,619,82
CAR: scu-rat TDLo:70500 μg/kg/10W-I
   GANNA2 73,687,82

SAFETY PROFILE: Questionable carcinogen with experimental carcinogenic data. When heated to decomposition it emits toxic fumes of NO_x.

EHD000   CAS: 63019-12-5
α-ETHYL-α′,sec-BUTYLSTILBENE
mf: $C_{20}H_{24}$ mw: 264.44

SYN: α-ETHYL-β-sec-BUTYLSTILBENE

TOXICITY DATA with REFERENCE
ETA: skn-mus TDLo:1250 mg/kg/52W-I
   NATUAS 148,142,41

SAFETY PROFILE: Questionable carcinogen with experimental tumorigenic data. When heated to decomposition it emits acrid smoke and irritating fumes.

EHG500   CAS: 105-39-5
ETHYL CHLORACETATE
DOT: 1181
mf: $C_4H_7ClO_2$ mw: 122.56

PROP: Colorless liquid; fruity, pungent odor. Bp: 143.6°, fp: −26.6° flash p: 100°F, d: 1.159 @ 20°/4°, vap press: 10 mm @ 37.5° vap d: 4.3. Insol in water; misc in alcohol and ether.

SYNS: CHLOROACETIC ACID, ETHYL ESTER ◇ ETHYL CHLOROACETATE ◇ ETHYL-α-CHLOROACETATE ◇ ETHYL CHLOROETHANOATE ◇ ETHYL MONOCHLORACETATE ◇ ETHYL MONOCHLOROACETATE

TOXICITY DATA with REFERENCE
NEO: ipr-mus TDLo:2940 mg/kg/8W-I
   CNREA8 39,391,79

CONSENSUS REPORTS: Reported in EPA TSCA Inventory.

DOT Classification: Combustible Liquid; Label: None; Poison B; Label: Flammable Liquid and Poison.

SAFETY PROFILE: Questionable carcinogen with experimental neoplastigenic data. Poison by skin contact and subcutaneous routes. A severe eye irritant. A dangerous fire hazard when exposed to heat or flame; can react vigorously with oxidizing materials. Will react with water or steam to produce toxic and corrosive fumes. To fight fire, use water, foam, CO_2, dry chemical. When heated to decomposition it emits highly toxic fumes of Cl^-.

EHI500   CAS: 4310-69-4
7-(2-(ETHYL-2-CHLOROETHYL)AMINOETHYLAMINO)BENZ(c)ACRIDINE DIHYDROCHLORIDE
mf: $C_{23}H_{24}ClN_3 \cdot 2ClH$ mw: 450.87

SYNS: N′-BENZ(c)ACRIDIN-7-YL-N-(2-CHLOROETHYL)-N-ETHYL-1,2-ETHANEDIAMINE DIHYDROCHLORIDE ◇ 7-(2-(2-CHLOROETHYLEHTYLAMINO)ETHYLAMINO)BENZ(c)ACRIDINE DIHYDROCHLORIDE ◇ ICR 311

TOXICITY DATA with REFERENCE
NEO: ivn-mus TDLo:4500 μg/kg   CNREA8 36,2423,76

SAFETY PROFILE: Questionable carcinogen with experimental neoplastigenic data. Poison by intravenous route. When heated to decomposition it emits very toxic fumes of NO_x and Cl^-.

EHJ000   CAS: 4251-89-2
7-(3-(ETHYL-2-(CHLOROETHYLAMINO)PROPYLAMINO))BENZ(c)ACRIDINE DIHYDROCHLORIDE
mf: $C_{24}H_{26}ClN_3 \cdot 2ClH$ mw: 464.90

SYN: ICR 292

TOXICITY DATA with REFERENCE
NEO: ivn-mus TDLo:4650 μg/kg   CNREA8 36,2423,76
MUT: mmo-sat 500 ng/plate   MUREAV 136,185,84
MUT: msc-ham:ovr 1 g/L   CNREA8 39,4875,79
MUT: pic-esc 60 ng/plate   CNREA8 43,2819,83

CONSENSUS REPORTS: EPA Genetic Toxicology Program.

SAFETY PROFILE: Questionable carcinogen with experimental neoplastigenic data. Poison by intravenous route. Mutation data reported. When heated to decomposition it emits very toxic fumes of NO_x and Cl^-.

EHJ500 CAS: 38915-14-9
9-(3-ETHYL-2-CHLOROETHYL) AMINOPROPYLAMINO)-4-METHOXYACRIDINE DIHYDROCHLORIDE
mf: $C_{21}H_{26}ClN_3O \cdot 2ClH$ mw: 444.87

SYNS: ICR 377 ◇ 4-METHOXY-9-(3-(ETHYL-2-CHLORO-ETHYL)

TOXICITY DATA with REFERENCE
NEO: ivn-mus TDLo: 2200 μg/kg CNREA8 36,2423,76
MUT: mmo-sat 500 ng/plate MUREAV 136,185,84

SAFETY PROFILE: Questionable carcinogen with experimental neoplastigenic data. Poison by intravenous route. Mutation data reported. When heated to decomposition it emits very toxic fumes of Cl^- and NO_x.

EHL000 CAS: 63019-53-4
7-ETHYL-10-CHLORO-11-METHYLBENZ(c)ACRIDINE
mf: $C_{20}H_{16}ClN$ mw: 305.82

SYN: 2-CHLORO-1-METHYL-10-ETHYL-7,8-BENZACRI-DINE (FRENCH)

TOXICITY DATA with REFERENCE
ETA: scu-mus TD: 30 mg/kg/4W-I ACRSAJ 4,315,56
ETA: scu-mus TDLo: 10 mg/kg AICCA6 11,736,55

SAFETY PROFILE: Questionable carcinogen with experimental tumorigenic data. When heated to decomposition it emits very toxic fumes of Cl^- and NO_x.

EHM000 CAS: 7511-54-8
3-ETHYLCHOLANTHRENE
mf: $C_{22}H_{18}$ mw: 282.40

SYNS: 3-ETHYL-CHOLANTHRENE ◇ 20-ETHYLCHOLAN-THRENE

TOXICITY DATA with REFERENCE
ETA: scu-mus TDLo: 400 mg/kg AJCAA7 33,499,38

SAFETY PROFILE: Questionable carcinogen with experimental tumorigenic data. When heated to decomposition it emits acrid smoke and irritating fumes.

EHW000 CAS: 63021-33-0
1-ETHYLDIBENZ(a,h)ACRIDINE
mf: $C_{23}H_{17}N$ mw: 307.41

SYN: 1'-ETHYL-1,2,5,6-DIBENZACRIDINE (FRENCH)

TOXICITY DATA with REFERENCE
ETA: skn-mus TDLo: 780 mg/kg/26W-I BAFEAG 42,186,55

SAFETY PROFILE: Questionable carcinogen with experimental tumorigenic data. When heated to decomposition it emits toxic fumes of NO_x.

EHW500 CAS: 63021-35-2
1-ETHYL-DIBENZ(a,j)ACRIDINE
mf: $C_{23}H_{17}N$ mw: 307.41

SYN: 1'-ETHYL-3,4,5,6-DIBENZACRIDINE (FRENCH)

TOXICITY DATA with REFERENCE
ETA: skn-mus TD: 780 mg/kg/32W-I BAFEAG 42,186,55
ETA: skn-mus TDLo: 384 mg/kg/32W-I ACRSAJ 4,315,56

SAFETY PROFILE: Questionable carcinogen with experimental tumorigenic data. When heated to decomposition it emits toxic fumes of NO_x.

EHX000 CAS: 73927-60-3
8-ETHYL DIBENZ(a,h)ACRIDINE
mf: $C_{23}H_{17}N$ mw: 307.41

SYN: 1''-ETHYLDIBENZ(a,h)ACRIDINE

TOXICITY DATA with REFERENCE
ETA: scu-mus TDLo: 27 mg/kg/26W-I ACRSAJ 4,315,56
ETA: skn-mus TDLo: 312 mg/kg/26W-I ACRSAJ 4,315,56

SAFETY PROFILE: Questionable carcinogen with experimental tumorigenic data. When heated to decomposition it emits toxic fumes of NO_x.

EIB000 CAS: 3553-80-8
ETHYL-N,N-DIETHYL CARBAMATE
mf: $C_7H_{15}NO_2$ mw: 145.23

TOXICITY DATA with REFERENCE
ETA: ipr-mus TDLo: 4875 mg/kg/13W-I JNCIAM 9,35,48

SAFETY PROFILE: Questionable carcinogen with experimental tumorigenic data. Moderately

toxic by subcutaneous route. When heated to decomposition it emits toxic fumes of NO_x.

EIB500   CAS: 4928-41-0
4'-ETHYL-N,N-DIETHYL-p-(PHENYLAZO)ANILINE
mf: $C_{18}H_{23}N_3$ mw: 281.44

SYN: 4'-ETHYL-N,N-DIMETHYL-4-AMINOAZOBENZENE

TOXICITY DATA with REFERENCE
ETA: orl-rat TDLo:7400 mg/kg/26W-C

ARZNAD 12,270,62

MUT: otr-ham:kdy 2500 µg/L   BJCAAI 38,34,78

SAFETY PROFILE: Questionable carcinogen with experimental tumorigenic data. Mutation data reported. When heated to decomposition it emits toxic fumes of NO_x.

EIF450   CAS: 93023-34-8
2'-ETHYL-4-DIMETHYLAMINOAZOBENZENE
mf: $C_{16}H_{19}N_3$ mw: 253.38

SYNS: ANILINE, p-((o-ETHYLPHENYL)AZO)-N,N-DI-METHYL- ◇ BENZENAMINE, N,N-DIMETHYL-2'-ETHYL-4-(PHENYLAZO)- ◇ BENZENAMINE, 4-((2-ETHYLPHE-NYL)AZO)-N,N-DIMETHYL- ◇ N,N-DIMETHYL-p-((o-ETHYLPHENYL)AZO)ANILINE

TOXICITY DATA with REFERENCE
CAR: orl-rat TDLo:13541 mg/kg/52W-C

CBINA8 53,107,85

SAFETY PROFILE: Questionable carcinogen with experimental carcinogenic data. When heated to decomposition it emits toxic fumes of NO_x.

EII500   CAS: 687-48-9
ETHYL-N,N-DIMETHYL CARBAMATE
mf: $C_5H_{11}NO_2$ mw: 117.17

SYNS: DIMETHYLCARBAMIC ACID ETHYL ESTER ◇ DI-N-METHYL ETHYL CARBAMATE

TOXICITY DATA with REFERENCE
ETA: ipr-mus TDLo:6500 mg/kg/13W-I

JNCIAM 9,35,48

SAFETY PROFILE: Questionable carcinogen with experimental tumorigenic and teratogenic data. Moderately toxic by subcutaneous and intraperitoneal routes. Experimental reproductive effects. When heated to decomposition it emits toxic fumes of NO_x.

EIR000   CAS: 12122-67-7
ETHYLENE BIS(DITHIOCARBAMATO) ZINC
mf: $C_4H_6N_2S_4$•Zn   mw: 275.73

PROP: Light-colored powder, insol in water.

SYNS: ASPOR ◇ ASPORUM ◇ BERCEMA ◇ BLIGHTOX ◇ BLITEX ◇ BLIZENE ◇ CARBADINE ◇ CHEM ZINEB ◇ CINEB ◇ CRITTOX ◇ CYNKOTOX ◇ DAISEN ◇ DIPHER ◇ DITHANE Z ◇ DITIAMINA ◇ ENT 14,874 ◇ ((1,2-ETHANEDIYLBIS(CARBAMODITHIOATO))(2-)ZINC ◇ 1,2-ETHANEDIYLBIS(CARBAMODITHIOATO) (2-)-S,S'-ZINC ◇ 1,2-ETHANEDIYLBISCARBAMODITHIOIC ACID, ZINC COMPLEX ◇ 1,2-ETHANEDIYLBISCARBAMOTHIOIC ACID, ZINC SALT ◇ ETHYLENEBIS(DITHIOCARBAMIC ACID), ZINC SALT ◇ ETHYL ZIMATE ◇ HEXATHANE ◇ KUPRATSIN ◇ KYPZIN ◇ LIROTAN ◇ LONACOL ◇ MICIDE ◇ MILTOX ◇ MILTOX SPECIAL ◇ NOVIZIR ◇ NOVOSIR N ◇ PAMOSOL 2 FORTE ◇ PARZATE ◇ PEROSIN ◇ POLYRAM Z ◇ SPERLOX-Z ◇ THIODOW ◇ TIEZENE ◇ TRITOFTOROL ◇ TSINEB (RUSSIAN) ◇ Z-78 ◇ ZEBENIDE ◇ ZEBTOX ◇ ZIDAN ◇ ZIMATE ◇ ZINC ETHYLENEBISDITHIOCARBAMATE ◇ ZINC ETHYLENE-1,2-BIS DITHIOCARBAMATE ◇ ZINEB ◇ ZINK-(N,N'-AETHYLEN-BIS(DITHIOCARBAMAT)) (GERMAN) ◇ ZINOSAN

TOXICITY DATA with REFERENCE
CAR: orl-rat TDLo:53580 mg/kg/94W-I

VPITAR 29,71,70

ETA: imp-rat TDLo:80 mg/kg   VPITAR 29,71,70
ETA: ipr-mus TDLo:2600 mg/kg/13W-I

VRDEA5 (9),100,66

ETA: orl-mus TDLo:7800 mg/kg/5W-I   GISAAA 37(9),25,72

MUT: cyt-mus-orl 10 mg/kg   GISAAA 45(1),80,80
MUT: mmo-bcs 1 nmol/plate   MSERDS 5,93,81
MUT: mmo-omi 1000 ppm   MMAPAP 50,233,73
MUT: sce-hmn:lym 10 mg/L   GESKAC 12,118,79

CONSENSUS REPORTS: IARC Cancer Review: Animal Inadequate Evidence IMEMDT 12,245,76. Community Right-To-Know List. EPA Genetic Toxicology Program.

SAFETY PROFILE: Questionable carcinogen with experimental carcinogenic, tumorigenic, and teratogenic data. Moderately toxic by ingestion and possibly other routes. Experimental reproductive effects. Human mutation data reported. Used as a fungicide. When heated to decomposition it emits very toxic fumes of NO_x, ZnO and SO_x.

EJP000   CAS: 1072-53-3
ETHYLENE SULFATE
mf: $C_2H_4O_4S$ mw: 124.12

SYNS: 2,2-DIOXIDE-1,3,2-DIOXATHIOLANE ◇ ETHYL-ENE GLYCOL, CYCLIC SULFATE ◇ GLYCOL SULFATE ◇ SULFURIC ACID, CYCLIC ETHYLENE ESTER

TOXICITY DATA with REFERENCE
NEO: scu-mus TDLo: 840 mg/kg/42W-I
JNCIAM 53,695,74
ETA: ipr-mus TDLo: 128 mg/kg/64W-I   JNCIAM 53,695,74
MUT: hma-mus/sat 5 mmol/kg   CBINA8 19,241,77
MUT: mmo-sat 1 μmol/plate   CBINA8 19,241,77

CONSENSUS REPORTS: EPA Genetic Toxicology Program.

SAFETY PROFILE: Questionable carcinogen with experimental tumorigenic and neoplastigenic data. Mutation data reported. When heated to decomposition it emits toxic fumes of SO_x.

EJP500   CAS: 420-12-2
ETHYLENE SULFIDE
mf: C_2H_4S mw: 60.12

PROP: Colorless liquid. Bp: 55-56° decomp, d: 1.0368 @ 0°/4°, vap d: 2.07.

SYNS: AETHYLENSULFID (GERMAN) ◇ 2,3-DIHYDRO-THIIRENE ◇ ETHYLENE EPISULFIDE ◇ ETHYLENE EPISUL-PHIDE ◇ ETHYLENE SULPHIDE ◇ THIACYCLOPROPANE ◇ THIIRANE

TOXICITY DATA with REFERENCE
ETA: scu-rat TDLo: 400 mg/kg/50W-I   ZEKBAI 74,241,70

CONSENSUS REPORTS: IARC Cancer Review: GROUP 3 IMEMDT 7,56,87; Animal Limited Evidence IMEMDT 11,257,76. Reported in EPA TSCA Inventory.

SAFETY PROFILE: Questionable carcinogen with experimental tumorigenic data. Poison by ingestion, intraperitoneal, and subcutaneous routes. Mildly toxic by inhalation. A skin, eye, and mucous membrane irritant. When heated to decomposition, or on contact with acid or acid fumes, it emits highly toxic fumes of SO_x.

EJS000   CAS: 19780-35-9
ETHYL-2,3-EPOXYBUTYRATE
mf: $C_6H_{10}O_3$ mw: 130.16

SYN: 2,3-EPOXYBUTYRIC ACID, ETHYL ESTER

TOXICITY DATA with REFERENCE
ETA: scu-mus TDLo: 272 mg/kg/68W-I
JNCIAM 46,143,71
MUT: mmo-sat 5 g/L   MUREAV 89,269,81

SAFETY PROFILE: Questionable carcinogen with experimental tumorigenic data. Moderately toxic by ingestion and skin contact. Mutation data reported. When heated to decomposition it emits acrid smoke and irritating fumes.

EJT000   CAS: 67466-28-8
ETHYL ESTER of 1,2,5,6-DIBENZANTHRACENE-endo-α,β-SUCCINO GLYCINE
mf: $C_{30}H_{21}NO_4$ mw: 459.52

TOXICITY DATA with REFERENCE
ETA: scu-mus TDLo: 200 mg/kg   CNREA81,685,41

SAFETY PROFILE: Questionable carcinogen with experimental tumorigenic data. When heated to decomposition it emits toxic fumes of NO_x.

EJT500
ETHYL ESTER of 3-METHYLCHOLANTHRENE-endo-α,β-SUCCINOGLYCINE
mf: $C_{29}H_{23}NO_4$ mw: 449.53

TOXICITY DATA with REFERENCE
ETA: scu-mus TDLo: 200 mg/kg   CNREA81,685,41

SAFETY PROFILE: Questionable carcinogen with experimental tumorigenic data. When heated to decomposition it emits toxic fumes of NO_x.

EJT575
11-β-ETHYLESTRADIOL
mf: $C_{20}H_{28}O_2$ mw: 300.48

SYNS: ESTRA-1,3,5(10)-TRIENE-3,17-β-DIOL, 11-β-ETHYL- ◇ 11-β-ETHYLESTRA-1,3,5(10)-TRIENE-3,17-β-DIOL

TOXICITY DATA with REFERENCE
NEO: imp-ham TDLo: 400 mg/kg/30W-C
CNREA8 47,2583,87
MUT: otr-mus: fbr 30 μmol/L   CNREA8 47,2583,87

SAFETY PROFILE: Questionable carcinogen with experimental neoplastigenic data. Mutation data reported. When heated to decomposition it emits acrid smoke and irritating fumes.

EJV400
11-β-ETHYL-17-α-ETHINYLESTRADIOL
mf: $C_{22}H_{28}O_2$ mw: 324.50

SYN: 11-β-ETHYL-19-NOR-17-α-PREGNA-1,3,5(10)-TRIEN-20-YNE-3,17-DIOL

TOXICITY DATA with REFERENCE
CAR: imp-ham TDLo: 400 mg/kg/39W-C

 CNREA8 47,2583,87

SAFETY PROFILE: Questionable carcinogen with experimental carcinogenic data. When heated to decomposition it emits acrid smoke and irritating fumes.

EJW500   CAS: 623-78-9
ETHYL-N-ETHYL CARBAMATE
mf: $C_5H_{11}NO_2$ mw: 117.17

SYN: ETHYLCARBAMIC ACID, ETHYL ESTER

TOXICITY DATA with REFERENCE
ETA: ipr-mus TDLo: 6500 mg/kg/13W-I

 JNCIAM 9,35,48

CONSENSUS REPORTS: Reported in EPA TSCA Inventory.

SAFETY PROFILE: Questionable carcinogen with experimental tumorigenic data. Moderately toxic by subcutaneous routes. When heated to decomposition it emits toxic fumes of NO_x.

EKL000   CAS: 109-94-4
ETHYL FORMATE
DOT: 1190
mf: $C_3H_6O_2$ mw: 74.09

PROP: Colorless liquid; sharp, rum-like odor. Mp: $-79°$, bp: $54.3°$, lel: 2.7%, uel: 13.5%, flash p: $-4°F$ (CC), d: 0.9236 @ $20°/20°$, refr index: 1.359, autoign temp: 851°F, vap press: 100 mm @ $5.4°$, vap d: 2.55. Sol in fixed oils, propylene glycol, water (decomp); sltly sol in mineral oil; insol in glycerin @ $54°$.

SYNS: AETHYLFORMIAT (GERMAN) ◊ AREGINAL ◊ ETHYLE (FORMIATE d') (FRENCH) ◊ ETHYLFORMIAAT (DUTCH) ◊ ETHYL FORMIC ESTER ◊ ETHYL METHANOATE ◊ ETILE (FORMIATO di) (ITALIAN) ◊ FEMA No. 2434 ◊ FORMIC ACID, ETHYL ESTER ◊ FORMIC ETHER ◊ MROWCZAN ETYLU (POLISH)

TOXICITY DATA with REFERENCE
ETA: skn-mus TDLo: 110 g/kg/9W-I   BJCAAI
 9,177,55

CONSENSUS REPORTS: Reported in EPA TSCA Inventory.

OSHA PEL: TWA 100 ppm   ACGIH TLV: TWA 100 ppm   DFG MAK: 100 ppm (300 mg/m³)   DOT Classification: Flammable Liquid; Label: Flammable Liquid.

SAFETY PROFILE: Questionable carcinogen with experimental tumorigenic data. Moderately

toxic by ingestion and subcutaneous routes. Mildly toxic by skin contact and inhalation. A powerful inhalation irritant in humans. A skin and eye irritant. Highly flammable liquid. A very dangerous fire and explosion hazard when exposed to heat, flame or oxidizers. To fight fire, use alcohol foam, spray, mist, dry chemical. When heated to decomposition it emits acrid smoke and irritating fumes.

EKL250   CAS: 74920-78-8
1-ETHYL-1-FORMYLHYDRAZINE
mf: $C_3H_8N_2O$ mw: 88.13

SYNS: EFH ◊ N-ETHYL-N-FORMYLHYDRAZINE ◊ FORMIC ACID, 1-ETHYLHYDRAZIDE

TOXICITY DATA with REFERENCE
CAR: orl-mus TDLo: 18345 mg/kg/52W-C

 CRNGDP 1,61,80

SAFETY PROFILE: Questionable carcinogen with experimental carcinogenic data. When heated to decomposition it emits toxic fumes of NO_x.

EKL500   CAS: 2407-43-4
5-ETHYL-2(5H)-FURANONE
mf: $C_6H_8O_2$ mw: 112.14

SYN: 4-HYDROXYHEX-2-ENOIC ACID LACTONE

TOXICITY DATA with REFERENCE
ETA: scu-rat TDLo: 2560 mg/kg/64W-I   BJCAAI
 15,85,61

SAFETY PROFILE: Questionable carcinogen with experimental tumorigenic data. When heated to decomposition it emits acrid smoke and irritating fumes.

ELB400   CAS: 72214-01-8
2-ETHYLHEXYL SULFATE
mf: $C_8H_{18}O_4S$ mw: 210.32

SYN: SULFURIC ACID, MONO(2-ETHYLHEXYL)ESTER

TOXICITY DATA with REFERENCE
ETA: orl-mus TDLo: 1747 g/kg/2Y-C   EVHPAZ
 65,271,86

SAFETY PROFILE: Questionable carcinogen with experimental tumorigenic data. Moderately toxic by ingestion. When heated to decomposition it emits toxic fumes of SO_x.

ELC000   CAS: 18413-14-4
ETHYLHYDRAZINE HYDROCHLORIDE
mf: $C_2H_8N_2 \cdot ClH$ mw: 96.58

TOXICITY DATA with REFERENCE
CAR: orl-mus TDLo: 11 g/kg/64W-C   IJCNAW
13,500,74

SAFETY PROFILE: Questionable carcinogen with experimental carcinogenic data. When heated to decomposition it emits very toxic fumes of HCl and NO_x.

ELD500 CAS: 2497-34-9
4'-ETHYL-4-HYDROXYAZOBENZENE
mf: $C_{14}H_{14}N_2O$ mw: 226.30

TOXICITY DATA with REFERENCE
ETA: orl-rat TDLo: 9780 mg/kg/43W-C
ARZNAD 12,270,62

SAFETY PROFILE: Questionable carcinogen with experimental tumorigenic data. When heated to decomposition it emits toxic fumes of NO_x.

ELE500 CAS: 54897-62-0
N-ETHYL-N-(4-HYDROXYBUTYL) NITROSOAMINE
mf: $C_6H_{14}N_2O_2$ mw: 146.22

SYNS: EHBN ◇ 4-(ETHYLNITROSOAMINO)-1-BUTANOL

TOXICITY DATA with REFERENCE
CAR: orl-mus TD: 7000 mg/kg/20W-C   GANNA2
72,647,81
CAR: orl-mus TD: 9800 mg/kg/14W-C   GANNA2
72,647,81
CAR: orl-mus TDLo: 4900 mg/kg/14W-C
GANNA2 72,647,81
ETA: orl-ham TDLo: 24 g/kg/20W-C   GANNA2
67,175,76
ETA: orl-mus TD: 7 g/kg/120W-C   GANNA2
67,175,76
ETA: orl-rat TD: 59 g/kg/20W-C   GANNA2
67,825,76
ETA: orl-rat TD: 4704 mg/kg/20W-C   GANNA2
72,539,81
ETA: orl-rat TD: 5300 mg/kg/20W-I   GANNA2
65,565,74
ETA: orl-rat TDLo: 4375 mg/kg/20W-C
GANNA2 67,175,76
MUT: mma-sat 35 μmol/plate   CNREA8 37,399,77

CONSENSUS REPORTS: EPA Genetic Toxicology Program.

SAFETY PROFILE: Questionable carcinogen with experimental carcinogenic and tumorigenic data. Mutation data reported. When heated to decomposition it emits toxic fumes of NO_x.

ELO000 CAS: 539-71-9
ETHYLIDENE DIURETHAN
mf: $C_8H_{16}N_2O_4$ mw: 204.26

SYNS: N,N'-ETHYLIDENE-BIS(ETHYL CARBAMATE)
◇ ETHYLIDENEDICARBAMIC ACID, DIETHYL ESTER

TOXICITY DATA with REFERENCE
ETA: ipr-mus TDLo: 6500 mg/kg/13W-I
JNCIAM 9,35,48

SAFETY PROFILE: Questionable carcinogen with experimental tumorigenic data. When heated to decomposition it emits toxic fumes of NO_x.

ELX500 CAS: 16339-04-1
ETHYLISOPROPYLNITROSOAMINE
mf: $C_5H_{12}N_2O$ mw: 116.19

SYNS: AETHYL-ISOPROPYL-NITROSOAMIN (GERMAN)
◇ 1-METHYL-N-NITROSODIETHYLAMINE ◇ N-NITROSO-ETHYLISOPROPYLAMINE

TOXICITY DATA with REFERENCE
CAR: orl-rat TDLo: 3920 mg/kg/56W-C
NATWAY 50,100,63
ETA: orl-rat TD: 3700 mg/kg/53W-C   ARZNAD
19,1077,69

SAFETY PROFILE: Questionable carcinogen with experimental carcinogenic and tumorigenic data. Moderately toxic by ingestion. When heated to decomposition it emits toxic fumes of NO_x.

EMM000 CAS: 63039-89-4
7-ETHYL-9-METHYLBENZ(c)ACRIDINE
mf: $C_{20}H_{17}N$ mw: 271.38

SYNS: 3-METHYL-10-ETHYLBENZ(c)ACRIDINE
◇ 3-METHYL-10-ETHYL-7,8-BENZACRIDINE (FRENCH)

TOXICITY DATA with REFERENCE
NEO: scu-mus TDLo: 72 mg/kg/9W-I   MUREAV
66,307,79
ETA: scu-mus TD: 250 mg/kg/10D-I   BAFEAG
34,22,47
ETA: skn-mus TDLo: 348 mg/kg/29W-I
ACRSAJ 4,315,56

SAFETY PROFILE: Questionable carcinogen with experimental neoplastigenic and tumorigenic data. When heated to decomposition it emits toxic fumes of NO_x.

EMM500 CAS: 16354-50-0
7-ETHYL-12-METHYLBENZ(a) ANTHRACENE
mf: $C_{21}H_{18}$ mw: 270.39

TOXICITY DATA with REFERENCE
NEO: ims-rat TDLo: 50 mg/kg   PNASA6 58,2253,67
ETA: ims-rat TD: 50 mg/kg   BCPCA6 16,607,67
MUT: cyt-rat-ivn 50 mg/kg   GANNA2 64,637,73

SAFETY PROFILE: Questionable carcinogen with experimental neoplastigenic and tumorigenic data. Mutation data reported. When heated to decomposition it emits acrid smoke and irritating fumes.

EMN000   CAS: 16354-55-5
12-ETHYL-7-METHYLBENZ(a) ANTHRACENE
mf: $C_{21}H_{18}$ mw: 270.39

TOXICITY DATA with REFERENCE
NEO: ims-rat TDLo: 50 mg/kg   PNASA6 58,2253,67
MUT: cyt-rat-ivn 50 mg/kg   GANNA2 64,637,73

SAFETY PROFILE: Questionable carcinogen with experimental neoplastigenic data. Mutation data reported. When heated to decomposition it emits acrid smoke and irritating fumes.

EMQ500   CAS: 105-40-8
ETHYL-N-METHYL CARBAMATE
mf: $C_4H_9NO_2$ mw: 103.14

PROP: Needles. Mp: 54°, bp: 177°.

SYNS: METHYLCARBAMIC ACID, ETHYL ESTER
◇ N-METHYL URETHAN

TOXICITY DATA with REFERENCE
ETA: ipr-mus TDLo: 6500 mg/kg/13W-I
   JNCIAM 9,35,48
ETA: skn-mus TDLo: 10 g/kg/1W-I   BJCAAI
   9,177,55

CONSENSUS REPORTS: Reported in EPA TSCA Inventory.

SAFETY PROFILE: Questionable carcinogen with experimental tumorigenic and teratogenic data. Moderately toxic by subcutaneous route. Experimental reproductive effects. When heated to decomposition it emits toxic fumes of NO_x.

EMS000   CAS: 6030-03-1
4'-ETHYL-2-METHYL-4-DIMETHYLAMINOAZOBENZENE
mf: $C_{17}H_{21}N_3$ mw: 267.41

SYN: 4'-ETHYL-N,N-DIMETHYL-4-(PHENYLAZO)-m-TOLUIDINE

TOXICITY DATA with REFERENCE
ETA: orl-rat TDLo: 4040 mg/kg/15W-C
   ARZNAD 12,270,62

SAFETY PROFILE: Questionable carcinogen with experimental tumorigenic data. When heated to decomposition it emits toxic fumes of NO_x.

ENB000   CAS: 2058-66-4
N-ETHYL-N-METHYL-p-(PHENYLAZO) ANILINE
mf: $C_{15}H_{17}N_3$ mw: 239.35

SYNS: p-ETHYLMETHYLAMINOAZOBENZENE
◇ N-ETHYL-N-METHYL-p-AMINOAZOBENZENE
◇ 4-ETHYLMETHYLAMINOAZOBENZENE ◇ 4-(METHYL-ETHYL)AMINOAZOBENZENE ◇ N-METHYL-N-ETHYL-p-AMINOAZOBENZENE

TOXICITY DATA with REFERENCE
CAR: orl-rat TDLo: 4684 mg/kg/17W-C
   JEMEAV 87,139,48
ETA: orl-rat TD: 2100 mg/kg/16W-C   CNREA8
   8,141,48
MUT: dni-mus-orl 20 g/kg   ARGEAR 51,605,81

SAFETY PROFILE: Questionable carcinogen with experimental carcinogenic and tumorigenic data. Mutation data reported. When heated to decomposition it emits toxic fumes of NO_x.

ENR000   CAS: 35363-12-3
3-ETHYL-4-NITROPYRIDINE-1-OXIDE
mf: $C_7H_8N_2O_3$ mw: 168.17

TOXICITY DATA with REFERENCE
ETA: scu-mus TDLo: 1840 mg/kg/15W-I
   GANNA2 70,799,79
MUT: dnd-mus: fbr 500 μmol/L   CNREA8
   35,521,75

SAFETY PROFILE: Questionable carcinogen with experimental tumorigenic data. Mutation data reported. When heated to decomposition it emits toxic fumes of NO_x.

ENR500   CAS: 65986-80-3
(ETHYLNITROSAMINO)METHYL ACETATE
mf: $C_5H_{10}N_2O_3$ mw: 146.17

SYNS: ACETOXYMETHYLETHYLNITROSAMINE
◇ N-(ACETOXY)METHYL-N-ETHYLNITROSAMINE
◇ N-ACETOXYMETHYL-N-NITROSOETHYLAMINE
◇ N-(1-ACETOXYMETHYL)-N-NITROSOETHYL AMINE
◇ AETHYL ACETOXYMETHYLNITROSAMIN (GERMAN)
◇ EAMN ◇ ETHYL ACETOXYMETHYLNITROSAMINE
◇ N-ETHYL-N-(ACETOXYMETHYL)NITROSAMINE

TOXICITY DATA with REFERENCE
CAR: scu-rat TD: 55 mg/kg/10W-I   IAPUDO
   41,619,82

CAR: scu-rat TDLo:50 mg/kg/10W-I   JCROD7
104,13,82

ETA: orl-rat TDLo:380 mg/kg/90D-I   ZKKOBW
91,317,78

MUT: dnd-mus:fbr 70 μmol/L   GANNA273,565,82

MUT: dnr-bcs 5 μmol/plate   GANNA2 70,663,79

MUT: dns-rat:oth 10 μmol/L   CBINA8 53,99,85

MUT: mmo-esc 1 μmol/plate   GANNA2 71,124,80

MUT: msc-ham:lng 100 μmol/L   GANNA2
72,531,81

SAFETY PROFILE: Questionable carcinogen with experimental carcinogenic and tumorigenic data. Moderately toxic by ingestion. Mutation data reported. When heated to decomposition it emits toxic fumes of NO_x.

ENS500   CAS: 20689-96-7
N-ETHYL-N-NITROSOBENZYLAMINE
mf: $C_9H_{12}N_2O$ mw: 164.23

SYNS: N-NITROSO-N-ETHYLBENZYLAMIN (GERMAN)
◇ N-NITROSO-N-ETHYLBENZYLAMINE

TOXICITY DATA with REFERENCE
ETA: orl-rat TDLo:250 mg/kg/36W-C
ZKKOBW 92,235,78

SAFETY PROFILE: Questionable carcinogen with experimental tumorigenic data. Poison by ingestion. Many N-nitroso compounds are carcinogens. When heated to decomposition it emits toxic fumes of NO_x.

ENT000   CAS: 32976-88-8
N-ETHYL-N-NITROSOBIURET
mf: $C_4H_8N_4O_3$ mw: 160.16

SYNS: ENBU ◇ ETHYLNITROSOBIURET ◇ N-NITROSO-
N-ETHYL BIURET

TOXICITY DATA with REFERENCE
ETA: orl-rat TD:100 mg/kg (15D preg):TER
ZKKOBW 76,45,71

ETA: orl-rat TDLo:400 mg/kg ZKKOBW76,45,71

SAFETY PROFILE: Questionable carcinogen with experimental carcinogenic, tumorigenic, and teratogenic data. Moderately toxic by ingestion. Experimental reproductive effects. When heated to decomposition it emits toxic fumes of NO_x.

ENT500   CAS: 38434-77-4
ETHYLNITROSOCYANAMIDE
mf: $C_3H_5N_3O$ mw: 99.11

SYNS: N-CYANO-N-NITROSOETHYLAMINE ◇ ENC
◇ NITROSOETHANECARBAMONITRILE

TOXICITY DATA with REFERENCE
NEO: orl-rat TDLo:1800 mg/kg/52W-I   JJIND8
62,1523,79

CONSENSUS REPORTS: EPA Genetic Toxicology Program. Cyanide and its compounds are on the Community Right-To-Know List.

SAFETY PROFILE: Questionable carcinogen with experimental neoplastigenic data. Poison by intraperitoneal route. Many N-nitroso compounds are carcinogens. When heated to decomposition it emits toxic fumes of NO_x and CN^-.

ENU000   CAS: 4245-77-6
N-ETHYL-N-NITROSO-N'-NITROGUANIDINE
mf: $C_3H_7N_5O_3$ mw: 161.15

SYNS: N-AETHYL-N'-NITRO-N-NITROSOGUANIDIN
(GERMAN) ◇ ENNG ◇ N-ETHYL-N'-NITRO-N-NITROSO-
GUANIDINE

TOXICITY DATA with REFERENCE
CAR: orl-mus TDLo:3 g/kg/43W-C   JNCIAM
52,519,74

NEO: orl-dog TD:560 mg/kg/12W-C   JCREA8
110,87,85

NEO: orl-mus TD:6300 mg/kg/63D-C
GANMAX 25,89,80

NEO: scu-rat TDLo:55 mg/kg/5W-I   GANNA2
69,277,78

NEO: skn-mus TDLo:630 mg/kg/21W-I
JNCIAM 46,973,71

ETA: ipr-mus TDLo:160 mg/kg   BJCAAI
23,757,69

ETA: orl-dog TD:191 g/kg/34W-I   ZEKBAI
90,241,77

ETA: orl-dog TD:1200 mg/kg/34W-C   GANNA2
71,349,80

ETA: orl-dog TD:1500 mg/kg/17W-C   GANNA2
72,880,81

ETA: orl-dog TD:2400 mg/kg/34W-C   NIPAA4
79,765,82

ETA: orl-dog TD:3000 mg/kg/34W-C   GANNA2
65,163,74

ETA: orl-dog TD:5320 mg/kg/73W-I   GANNA2
66,683,75

ETA: orl-dog TDLo:195 mg/kg/37W-C
RKGEDW 1,571,81

ETA: orl-ham TDLo:1900 mg/kg/33W-C
ZEKBAI 81,29,74

ETA: orl-mky TDLo:2600 mg/kg/48W-C
JJIND8 77,179,86

ETA: orl-mus TD:780 mg/kg/26W-I   SACAB7
24,413,80

ETA: orl-rat TDLo: 504 mg/kg/12W-C   JJCREP
78,126,87

ETA: rec-dog TD: 1440 mg/kg/26W-I   IJCNAW
32,255,83

ETA: rec-dog TDLo: 1275 mg/kg/23W-I
IJCNAW 32,255,83

MUT: dnd-ham: ovr 20 μmol/L   MUREAV
132,41,84

MUT: mma-sat 5 μg/plate   TCMUE9 1,13,84

MUT: mmo-esc 2 μg/plate   KSRNAM 19,4465,85

MUT: pic-esc 200 μg/L   TCMUE9 1,91,84

MUT: sce-ham-orl 10 mg/kg   MUREAV 113,33,83

MUT: sce-ham: lng 10 mg/L   CNREA8 44,3270,84

MUT: sce-hmn: lym 1 μmol/L   NGCJAK 15,1085,80

CONSENSUS REPORTS: EPA Genetic Toxicology Program.

SAFETY PROFILE: Questionable carcinogen
with experimental carcinogenic, neoplastigenic,
and tumorigenic data. Human mutation data reported. When heated to decomposition it emits
toxic fumes of NO_x.

EOH500   CAS: 2058-67-5
N-ETHYL-p-(PHENYLAZO)ANILINE
mf: $C_{14}H_{15}N_3$ mw: 225.32

SYNS: EAB ◇ 4-(ETHYLAMINOAZOBENZENE)
◇ N-ETHYL-4-AMINOAZOBENZENE ◇ N-ETHYL-4-(PHE-
NYLAZO)BENZENAMINE

TOXICITY DATA with REFERENCE
ETA: orl-rat TDLo: 376 mg/kg/5W-I   CNREA8
39,3411,79

SAFETY PROFILE: Questionable carcinogen
with experimental tumorigenic and teratogenic
data. Experimental reproductive effects. When
heated to decomposition it emits toxic fumes
of NO_x.

EOI000   CAS: 17010-65-0
p-((m-ETHYLPHENYL)AZO)-N,N-
DIMETHYLANILINE
mf: $C_{16}H_{19}N_3$ mw: 253.38

SYNS: N,N-DIMETHYL-p-(m-ETHYLPHENYL)AZO)ANI-
LINE ◇ N,N-DIMETHYL-p-(3'-ETHYLPHENYLAZO)ANILINE
◇ N,N-DIMETHYL-3'-ETHYL-4-(PHENYLAZO)BENZEN-
AMINE ◇ 3'-ETHYL-DAB ◇ 3'-ETHYL-4-DIMETHYLAMINO-
AZOBENZENE

TOXICITY DATA with REFERENCE
CAR: orl-rat TD: 4858 mg/kg/17W-C   CRNGDP
1,419,80

CAR: orl-rat TDLo: 3175 mg/kg/12W-C
CBINA8 53,107,85

ETA: orl-rat TD: 2261 mg/kg/17W-I   CNREA8
30,1520,70

SAFETY PROFILE: Questionable carcinogen
with experimental carcinogenic and tumorigenic
data. When heated to decomposition it emits
toxic fumes of NO_x.

EOI500   CAS: 5302-41-0
p-((p-ETHYLPHENYL)AZO)-N,N-
DIMETHYLANILINE
mf: $C_{16}H_{19}N_3$ mw: 253.38

SYNS: N,N-DIMETHYL-4'-ETHYL-4-AMINOAZOBEN-
ZENE ◇ N,N-DIMETHYL-p-((4-ETHYLPHENYL)AZO)ANI-
LINE ◇ 4'-ETHYL-DAB ◇ 4'-ETHYL-4-DIMETHYLAMINO-
AZOBENZENE

TOXICITY DATA with REFERENCE
CAR: orl-rat TDLo: 4858 mg/kg/17W-C
CRNGDP 1,419,80

ETA: orl-rat TD: 2142 mg/kg/17W-C   JNCIAM
27,663,61

SAFETY PROFILE: Questionable carcinogen
with experimental carcinogenic and tumorigenic
data. When heated to decomposition it emits
toxic fumes of NO_x.

EOJ000   CAS: 55398-27-1
p-(4-ETHYLPHENYLAZO)-N-
METHYLANILINE
mf: $C_{15}H_{17}N_3$ mw: 239.35

SYNS: 4'-ETHYL-N-METHYL-4-AMINOAZOBENZENE
◇ N-METHYL-4'-ETHYL-p-AMINOAZOBENZENE

TOXICITY DATA with REFERENCE
ETA: orl-rat TDLo: 1890 mg/kg/15W-C
JNCIAM 15,67,54

ETA: scu-rat TDLo: 181 mg/kg/8W-I   CNREA8
35,880,75

SAFETY PROFILE: Questionable carcinogen
with experimental tumorigenic data. When
heated to decomposition it emits toxic fumes
of NO_x.

EOJ500   CAS: 6368-72-5
N-ETHYL-1-((p-(PHENYLAZO)
PHENYL)AZO)-2-NAPHTHYLAMINE
mf: $C_{24}H_{21}N_5$ mw: 379.50

SYNS: CERES RED 7B ◇ C.I. 26050 ◇ C.I. SOLVENT RED
19 ◇ N-ETHYL-1-((p-(PHENYLAZO)PHENYL)AZO)-2-NAPH-
THALENAMINE ◇ N-ETHYL-1-((4-(PHENYLAZO)PHE-
NYL)AZO)-2-NAPHTHALENAMINE ◇ N-ETHYL-1-((4-(PHE-
NYLAZO)PHENYL)AZO)-2-NAPHTHYLAMINE ◇ FAT RED
7B ◇ HEXATYPE CARMINE B ◇ LACQUER RED V3B

◇ OIL VIOLET ◇ ORGANOL BORDEAUX B ◇ (PHENYLAZO-4-PHENYLAZO)-1-ETHYLAMINO-2-NAPHTHALENE ◇ 1-(4-PHENYLAZO-PHENYLAZO)-2-ETHYLAMINONAPH-THALENE ◇ SOLVENT RED 19 ◇ SPECIAL BLUE X 2137 ◇ SUDAN RED 7B ◇ SUDANROT 7B ◇ TYPOGEN CARMINE

TOXICITY DATA with REFERENCE

ETA: orl-rat TDLo: 15 g/kg/50W-C   XPHPAW 149,403,69

MUT: mma-mus: lym 300 mg/L   EPASR* 8EHQ-0982-0455

MUT: mma-sat 500 μg/plate   EPASR* 8EHQ-0982-0455

CONSENSUS REPORTS: IARC Cancer Review: Animal Inadequate Evidence IMEMDT 8,253,75. Reported in EPA TSCA Inventory.

SAFETY PROFILE: Questionable carcinogen with experimental tumorigenic data. Mutation data reported. When heated to decomposition it emits toxic fumes of NO_x.

EPC050   CAS: 623-85-8
ETHYL-N,N-PROPYLCARBAMATE
mf: $C_6H_{13}NO_2$ mw: 131.20

SYN: N,N-PROPYL ETHYL CARBAMATE

TOXICITY DATA with REFERENCE

ETA: ipr-mus TDLo: 6500 mg/kg/13W-I   JNCIAM 9,35,48

SAFETY PROFILE: Questionable carcinogen with experimental tumorigenic data. Moderately toxic by subcutaneous route. When heated to decomposition it emits toxic fumes of NO_x.

EPC950   CAS: 75236-19-0
4'-ETHYL-4-N-PYRROLIDINYLAZOBENZENE
mf: $C_{18}H_{21}N_3$ mw: 279.42

SYN: PYRROLIDINE, 1-(p-((p-ETHYLPHENYL)AZO)PHE-NYL)-

TOXICITY DATA with REFERENCE

CAR: orl-rat TDLo: 11 g/kg/34W-C   CRNGDP 1,419,80

MUT: mma-sat 10 μg/plate   CRNGDP 3,559,82

SAFETY PROFILE: Questionable carcinogen with experimental carcinogenic data. Mutation data reported. When heated to decomposition it emits toxic fumes of NO_x.

EPI300   CAS: 842-00-2
4-(ETHYLSULFONYL)-1-NAPHTHALENE SULFONAMIDE
mf: $C_{12}H_{13}NO_4S_2$ mw: 299.38

SYNS: ENS ◇ 4-ETHYLSULPHONYLNAPHTHALENE-1-SULFONAMIDE ◇ 4-ETHYLSULPHONYLNAPHTHALENE-1-SULPHONAMIDE ◇ HPA

TOXICITY DATA with REFERENCE

CAR: imp-mus TDLo: 77 mg/kg   BJCAAI 19,311,65

CAR: orl-mus TD: 12 g/kg/86W-C   BJCAAI 28,227,73

CAR: orl-mus TDLo: 4200 mg/kg/50W-C   BJCAAI 23,772,69

NEO: orl-mus TD: 440 mg/kg/52W-C   JNCIAM 51,2007,73

ETA: orl-mus TD: 4368 mg/kg/39W-C   BJURAN 39,26,64

ETA: orl-mus TD: 5460 mg/kg/65W-C   BCPCA6 16,619,67

MUT: cyt-mus-orl 40 mg/kg   CTKIAR 2,249,69

MUT: dns-mus-orl 20 mg/kg   BIJOAK 111,12P,69

MUT: oms-mus-orl 20 mg/kg   BIJOAK 111,12P,69

SAFETY PROFILE: Questionable carcinogen with experimental carcinogenic, neoplastigenic, and tumorigenic data. Mutation data reported. When heated to decomposition it emits very toxic fumes of NO_x and SO_x.

EPJ000   CAS: 20941-65-5
ETHYL TELLURAC
mf: $C_{20}H_{40}N_4S_8 \cdot Te$ mw: 720.72

PROP: Orange-yellow powder. D: 1.44, mp: 108-118°.

SYNS: DIETHYLDITHIO CARBAMIC ACID TELLURIUM SALT ◇ NCI-C02857 ◇ TELLURIUM DIETHYLDITHIOCAR-BAMATE ◇ TETRAKIS(DIETHYLCARBAMODITHIOATO-S,S')TELLURIUM ◇ TETRAKIS(DIETHYLDITHIOCAR-BAMATO)TELLURIUM

TOXICITY DATA with REFERENCE

ETA: orl-mus TDLo: 113 g/kg/107W-C   NCITR* NCI-CG-TR-152,79

CONSENSUS REPORTS: IARC Cancer Review: Animal Inadequate Evidence IMEMDT 12,115,76. NCI Carcinogenesis Bioassay (feed); No Evidence: mouse, rat NCITR* NCI-CG-TR-152,79; Results Indefinite: Mouse, Rat (NCITR* NCI-CG-TR-152,79). Reported in EPA TSCA Inventory.

OSHA PEL: TWA 0.1 mg(Te)/m³   ACGIH TLV: TWA 0.1 mg(Te)/m³

SAFETY PROFILE: Questionable carcinogen with experimental tumorigenic data. When heated to decomposition it emits very toxic fumes of NO_x, SO_x and Te.

EPQ000   CAS: 536-33-4
2-ETHYLTHIOISONICOTINAMIDE
mf: $C_8H_{10}N_2S$ mw: 166.26

SYNS: AETINA ◊ AETIVA ◊ AMIDAZIN ◊ BAYER 5312
◊ ETH ◊ ETHIMIDE ◊ ETHINA ◊ ETHINAMIDE
◊ ETHIONIAMIDE ◊ α-ETHYLISONICOTINIC ACID
THIOAMIDE ◊ 2-ETHYLISONICOTINIC ACID THIOAMIDE
◊ 2-ETHYLISONICOTINIC THIOAMIDE ◊ α-ETHYLISONI-
COTINOYLTHIOAMIDE ◊ ETHYLISOTHIAMIDE ◊ α-ETH-
YLISOTHIONICOTINAMIDE ◊ 2-ETHYLISOTHIONICOTIN-
AMIDE ◊ 2-ETHYL-4-PYRIDINECARBOTHIOAMIDE
◊ 2-ETHYL-4-THIOAMIDYLPYRIDINE ◊ 2-ETHYL-4-THIO-
CARBAMOYLPYRIDINE ◊ α-ETHYLTHIOISONICOTINAM-
IDE ◊ ETHYONOMIDE ◊ ETIMID ◊ ETIOCIDAN
◊ ETIONAMID ◊ ETIONIZINA ◊ ETP ◊ FATOLIAMID
◊ F.I. 58-30 ◊ IRIDOCIN ◊ IRIDOZIN ◊ ISOTHIN
◊ ISOTIAMIDA ◊ ITIOCIDE ◊ NCI-C01694 ◊ NICOTION
◊ NISOTIN ◊ NIZOTIN ◊ RIGENICID ◊ SERTINON
◊ TEBERUS ◊ TH 1314 ◊ THIANIDE ◊ THIOAMIDE
◊ THIONIDEN ◊ TRECATOR ◊ TRESCATYL ◊ TRESCAZIDE
◊ TUBERMIN ◊ TUBEROID ◊ TUBEROSON

TOXICITY DATA with REFERENCE
CAR: orl-mus TDLo: 24 g/kg/50W-I   LAPPA5
  24,145,64
MUT: cyt-ham: fbr 400 mg/L   ESKHA5
  96,55,78
MUT: cyt-ham: lng 540 mg/L   GMCRDC
  27,95,81

CONSENSUS REPORTS: IARC Cancer Review: GROUP 3 IMEMDT 7,56,87; Animal
Limited Evidence IMEMDT 13,83,77. NCI
Carcinogenesis Bioassay (feed); No Evidence:
mouse, rat NCITR* NCI-CG-TR-46,78.

SAFETY PROFILE: Questionable carcinogen
with experimental carcinogenic and teratogenic
data. A human systemic poison. Moderately
toxic by ingestion, intraperitoneal, and subcutaneous routes. Human systemic effects by ingestion: jaundice and liver function impairment.
It affects the human peripheral nervous system.
Experimental reproductive effects. Mutation
data reported. Used to treat tuberculosis. When
heated to decomposition it emits very toxic
fumes of SO_x and NO_x.

EPT500   CAS: 17010-63-8
p-((3-ETHYL-p-TOLYL)AZO)-N,N-
DIMETHYLANILINE
mf: $C_{17}H_{21}N_3$ mw: 267.41

SYNS: N,N-DIMETHYL-p-(3'-ETHYL-4'-METHYLPHE-
NYLAZO)ANILINE ◊ N,N-DIMETHYL-p-((3-ETHYL-p-
TOLYL)AZO)ANILINE

TOXICITY DATA with REFERENCE
CAR: orl-rat TDLo: 6497 mg/kg/17W-C
  CBINA8 53,107,85
ETA: orl-rat TDLo: 2005 mg/kg/50D-I   CNREA8
  30,1520.70

SAFETY PROFILE: Questionable carcinogen
with experimental carcinogenic and tumorigenic
data. When heated to decomposition it emits
toxic fumes of NO_x.

EPU000   CAS: 17010-62-7
p-((4-ETHYL-m-TOLYL)AZO)-N,N-
DIMETHYLANILINE
mf: $C_{17}H_{21}N_3$ mw: 266.40

SYNS: N,N-DIMETHYL-p-(4'-ETHYL-3'-METHYLPHE-
NYLAZO)ANILINE ◊ N,N-DIMETHYL-p-((4-ETHYL-m-TOLY-
L)AZO) ANILINE

TOXICITY DATA with REFERENCE
CAR: orl-rat 1109 mg/kg/8W-C   CBINA8 53,107,85
ETA: orl-rat TDLo: 500 mg/kg/50D-I   CNREA8
  30,1520.70

SAFETY PROFILE: Questionable carcinogen
with experimental carcinogenic and tumorigenic
data. When heated to decomposition it emits
toxic fumes of NO_x.

EPW000   CAS: 50707-40-9
1-ETHYL-3-p-TOLYLTRIAZENE
mf: $C_9H_{13}N_3$ mw: 163.25

TOXICITY DATA with REFERENCE
NEO: ipr-mus TDLo: 20 mg/kg/I   JNCIAM
  54,495,75

SAFETY PROFILE: Questionable carcinogen
with experimental neoplastigenic data. Poison
by intraperitoneal route. When heated to decomposition it emits toxic fumes of NO_x.

EPW500   CAS: 80-40-0
ETHYL TOSYLATE
mf: $C_9H_{12}O_3S$ mw: 200.27

PROP: Liquid. Mp: 33°, bp: 221.3°, flash p:
316°F (CC), d: 1.17, vap d: 6.98.

SYNS: ETHYL-p-METHYL BENZENESULFONATE
◊ ETHYL PTS ◊ ETHYL-p-TOLUENESULFONATE
◊ ETHYL-p-TOSYLATE ◊ p-TOLUOLSULFONSAEUREA-
ETHYL ESTER (GERMAN)

TOXICITY DATA with REFERENCE
ETA: scu-rat TD: 3250 mg/kg/65W-I   ZEKBAI
  74,241,70

ETA: scu-rat TDLo:50 mg/kg   FCTXAV 6,576,68
MUT: dnr-esc 50 mg/L   JNCIAM 62,873,79
MUT: mma-sat 4700 μg/plate   PNASA6 72,5135,75
MUT: mmo-sat 2000 μg/plate   JNCIAM 62,893,79
MUT: mrc-smc 1 pph   JNCIAM 62,901,79
MUT: otr-ham:emb 500 μg/L   CRNGDP 1,323,80

CONSENSUS REPORTS: Reported in EPA TSCA Inventory. EPA Genetic Toxicology Program.

SAFETY PROFILE: Questionable carcinogen with experimental tumorigenic data. Moderately toxic by subcutaneous and intraperitoneal routes. Mutation data reported. Combustible when exposed to heat or flame; can react with oxidizing materials. To fight fire, use CO_2, dry chemical. When heated to decomposition it emits highly toxic fumes of SO_x.

EPZ000   CAS: 313-93-9
3-ETHYLTRICYCLOQUINAZOLINE
mf: $C_{23}H_{16}N_4$ mw: 348.43

TOXICITY DATA with REFERENCE
CAR: skn-mus TDLo:1200 mg/kg/50W-I
   BCPCA6 14,323,65

SAFETY PROFILE: Questionable carcinogen with experimental carcinogenic data. When heated to decomposition it emits toxic fumes of NO_x.

EQJ000
ETHYNERONE mixed with MESTRANOL (20:1)
mf: $C_{20}H_{23}ClO_2 \cdot C_{21}H_{26}O_2$ (20:1)   mw: 641.0

SYN: MESTRANOL mixed with ETHYNERONE (1:20)

TOXICITY DATA with REFERENCE
ETA: orl-dog TDLo:243 mg/kg/47W-I   JJIND8 65,137,80

SAFETY PROFILE: Questionable carcinogen with experimental tumorigenic data. When heated to decomposition it emits toxic fumes of Cl^-.

EQK010
ETHYNODIOL DIACETATE mixed with MESTRANOL
SYNS: MESTRANOL mixed with ETHYNODIOL DIACE-TATE ◇ 19-NOR-17-α-PREGN-4-EN-20-YNE-3-β,17-DIOL DI-ACETATE mixed with 3-METHYOXY-19-NOR-17-α-PREGNA-1,3,5(10)-TRIEN-20-YN-17-OL

TOXICITY DATA with REFERENCE
NEO: orl-wmn TDLo:15 mg/kg/78W-I:LIV
   JAMAAP 235,730,76

SAFETY PROFILE: Questionable carcinogen producing liver tumors. Moderately toxic by intraperitoneal route. A steroid.

EQK100   CAS: 8056-92-6
ETHYNODIOL mixed with MESTRANOL
mf: $C_{24}H_{32}O_4 \cdot C_{21}H_{26}O_2$ mw:695.03

SYNS: MESTRANOL mixed with ETHYNODIOL ◇ 10-NOR-17-α-PREGN-4-EN-20-YNE-3-β,17-DIOL mixed with 3-ME-THOXY-17-α-19-NORPREGNA-1-3-5(10)-TRIEN-20-YN-17-OL ◇ OVULEN

TOXICITY DATA with REFERENCE
CAR: orl-wmn TDLo:63504 μg/kg/12Y-I: LIV,MET   LANCAO 1,273,80
NEO: orl-mus TDLo:186 mg/kg/93W-C
   GMCRDC 17,205,75

SAFETY PROFILE: Questionable carcinogen producing liver tumors. Experimental neoplastigenic data. Human systemic effects by ingestion: skin dermatitis, weight loss or decreased weight gain. A steroid. When heated to decomposition it emits acrid smoke and fumes.

EQM500   CAS: 37270-71-6
ETHYNYLESTRADIOL mixed with NORETHINDRONE
mf: $C_{20}H_{26}O_2 \cdot C_{20}H_{24}O_2$ mw:594.90

SYNS: GYNOVLAR ◇ NORETHINDRONE mixed with ETH-YNYLESTRADIOL ◇ NORETHISTERONE mixed with ETHI-NYL OESTRADIOL (60:1) ◇ 19-NOR-17-α-PREGN-4-EN-20-YN-3-ONE, 17-HYDROXY-, mixed with 19-NOR-17-α-PREGNA-1,3,5(10)-TRIEN-2-YNE-3,17-DIOL (60:1)

TOXICITY DATA with REFERENCE
CAR: orl-wmn TD:138 mg/kg/9Y-I:LIV
   BMJOAE 4,496,75
CAR: orl-wmn TDLo:138 mg/kg/9Y-I:LIV
   LANCAO 1,273,80
ETA: orl-mus TDLo:120 mg/kg/84W-I   SCIEAS 154,402,66
MUT: oms-ctl:oth 17410 μg/L   AJOGAH 120,390,74
MUT: oms-dom:oth 17410 μg/L   AJOGAH 120,390,74
MUT: oms-mam:oth 10100 μg/L   AJOGAH 120,390,74

SAFETY PROFILE: Questionable human carcinogen producing liver tumors. Experimental tumorigenic data. Human teratogenic effects by an unspecified route: developmental abnormalities of the urogenital system. Human systemic effects by ingestion: dyspnea, nausea or vomiting, and fever. Experimental reproductive effects. Mutation data reported. A steroid. When heated to decomposition it emits acrid smoke and irritating fumes.

EQN225
α-ETHYNYL-p-METHOXYBENZYL ALCOHOL ACETATE

mf: $C_{12}H_{12}O_3$ mw: 204.24

SYN: 1'-ACETOXY-2',3'-DEHYDROESTRAGOLE

TOXICITY DATA with REFERENCE
NEO: ipr-mus TDLo:10212 µg/kg   CNREA8
47,2275,87

MUT: mmo-sat 150 nmol/plate   CRNGDP 7,2089,86

SAFETY PROFILE: Questionable carcinogen with experimental neoplastigenic data. Mutation data reported. When heated to decomposition it emits acrid smoke and irritating fumes.

EQR500
EUGENOL

CAS: 97-53-0

mf: $C_{10}H_{12}O_2$ mw: 164.22

PROP: Colorless or yellowish liquid; pungent, clove odor. D: 1.064-1.070, refr index: 1.540, bp: 253.5°, flash p: 219°F. Sol in alc, chloroform, ether, volatile oils; very sltly sol in water.

SYNS: 4-ALLYLGUAIACOL ◇ 4-ALLYL-1-HYDROXY-2-METHOXYBENZENE ◇ 4-ALLYL-2-METHOXYPHENOL ◇ CARYOPHYLLIC ACID ◇ EUGENIC ACID ◇ Fa 100 ◇ FEMA No. 2467 ◇ 1-HYDROXY-2-METHOXY-4-ALLYL-BENZENE ◇ 4-HYDROXY-3-METHOXYALLYLBENZENE ◇ 1-HYDROXY-2-METHOXY-4-PROP-2-ENYLBENZENE ◇ 2-METHOXY-4-ALLYLPHENOL ◇ 2-METHOXY-4-PROP-2-ENYLPHENOL ◇ 2-METHOXY-4-(2-PROPENYL)PHENOL ◇ 2-METOKSY-4-ALLILOFENOL (POLISH) ◇ NCI-C50453 ◇ SYNTHETIC EUGENOL

TOXICITY DATA with REFERENCE
ETA: orl-mus TDLo:37080 mg/kg/2Y-I
NTPTR* NTP-TR-223,82

MUT: cyt-ham:fbr 125 mg/L   FCTOD7 22,623,84
MUT: cyt-ham:ovr 400 mg/L   CALEDQ 14,251,81
MUT: mma-sat 50 µg/plate   NTIS** AD-A116-715
MUT: oms-ham:ovr 400 mg/L   CALEDQ 14,251,81

CONSENSUS REPORTS: IARC Cancer Review: GROUP 3 IMEMDT 7,56,87; Animal Limited Evidence IMEMDT 36,75,85. NTP

Carcinogenesis Studies (feed); Equivocal Evidence: mouse NTPTR* NTP-TR-223,83; No Evidence: rat NTPTR* NTP-TR-223,83. Reported in EPA TSCA Inventory. EPA Genetic Toxicology Program.

SAFETY PROFILE: Questionable carcinogen with experimental carcinogenic and tumorigenic data. Moderately toxic by ingestion, intraperitoneal, and subcutaneous routes. Human mutation data reported. A human skin irritant. Combustible liquid. When heated to decomposition it emits acrid smoke and irritating fumes.

EQT500
EUPHORBIA ABYSSINICA LATEX

PROP: Acetone soluble portion of *Euphorbia abyssinica* latex.

TOXICITY DATA with REFERENCE
ETA: skn-mus TDLo:2600 mg/kg/26W-I
CNREA8 21,338,61

SAFETY PROFILE: Questionable carcinogen with experimental tumorigenic data.

EQU000
EUPHORBIA CANARIENSIS LATEX

PROP: Acetone soluble fraction of latex from *Euphorbia canariensis*.

TOXICITY DATA with REFERENCE
ETA: skn-mus TDLo:2600 mg/kg/26W-I
CNREA8 21,338,61

SAFETY PROFILE: Questionable carcinogen with experimental tumorigenic data.

EQU500
EUPHORBIA CANDELABRIUM LATEX

PROP: Acetone soluble portion of latex from *Euphorbia candelabrum*.

TOXICITY DATA with REFERENCE
ETA: skn-mus TDLo:2600 mg/kg/26W-I
CNREA8 21,338,61

SAFETY PROFILE: Questionable carcinogen with experimental tumorigenic data.

EQV000
EUPHORBIA ESULA LATEX

PROP: Acetone soluble portion of latex from *Euphorbia esula*.

TOXICITY DATA with REFERENCE
ETA: skn-mus TDLo:3500 mg/kg/20W-I
TUMOAB 64,99,78

SAFETY PROFILE: Questionable carcinogen with experimental tumorigenic data.

EQV500
EUPHORBIA GRANDIDENS LATEX

PROP: Acetone soluble fraction of latex from *Euphorbia grandides*.

TOXICITY DATA with REFERENCE
ETA: skn-mus TDLo:2600 mg/kg/26W-I
  CNREA8 21,338,61

SAFETY PROFILE: Questionable carcinogen with experimental tumorigenic data.

EQW000
EUPHORBIA LATHYRIS LATEX

PROP: Oil from the seeds of *Euphorbia lathyris*.

SYN: CAPER SPURGE

TOXICITY DATA with REFERENCE
ETA: skn-mus TDLo:5680 mg/kg/W-I   CNREA8
  28,2338,68

SAFETY PROFILE: Questionable carcinogen with experimental tumorigenic data. A skin irritant.

EQW500
EUPHORBIA OBOVALIFOLIA LATEX

PROP: Acetone soluble portion of latex from *Euphorbia obovalifolia*.

TOXICITY DATA with REFERENCE
ETA: skn-mus TDLo:2600 mg/kg/26W-I
  CNREA8 21,338,61

SAFETY PROFILE: Questionable carcinogen with experimental tumorigenic data.

EQX500
EUPHORBIA SERRATA LATEX

PROP: Acetone soluble fraction of latex from *Euphorbia serrata*.

TOXICITY DATA with REFERENCE
ETA: skn-mus TDLo:6400 mg/kg/16W-I
  TUMOAB 64,99,78

SAFETY PROFILE: Questionable carcinogen with experimental tumorigenic data.

EQY000
EUPHORBIA TIRUCALLI LATEX

PROP: Acetone soluble portion of *Euphorbia tirucalli* latex. Contains all biological activity.

SYN: BLEISTIFTBAUMS (GERMAN)

TOXICITY DATA with REFERENCE
ETA: skn-mus TD:2800 mg/kg/28W-I   CNREA8
  21,338,61
ETA: skn-mus TDLo:2400 mg/kg/12W-I
  PLMEAA 22,241,72

SAFETY PROFILE: Questionable carcinogen with experimental tumorigenic data. A skin irritant.

EQY500
EUPHORIA WULFENII LATEX

PROP: Acetone soluble portion of latex from *Euphoria wulfenii*.

TOXICITY DATA with REFERENCE
ETA: skn-mus TDLo:2600 mg/kg/26W-I
  CNREA8 21,338,61

SAFETY PROFILE: Questionable carcinogen with experimental tumorigenic data.

FAC025
FAMFOS
CAS: 13171-21-6

mf: $C_{10}H_{19}ClNO_5P$ mw: 299.72

SYNS: APAMIDON ◇ C 570 ◇ (2-CHLOOR-3-DIETHYL-AMINO-1-METHYL-3-OXO-PROP-1-EN-YL)-DIMETHYL-FOSFAAT ◇ (2-CHLOR-3-DIAETHYLAMINO-1-METHYL-3-OXO-PROP-1-EN-YL)-DIMETHYL-PHOSPHAT ◇ 2-CHLORO-2-DIETHYLCARBAMOYL-1-METHYLVINYL DIMETHYLPHOSPHATE ◇ 1-CHLORO-DIETHYLCARBA-MOYL-1-PROPEN-2-YL DIMETHYL PHOSPHATE ◇ (2-CLORO-3-DIETILAMINO-1-METIL-3-OXO-PROP-1-EN-IL)-DIMETIL-FOSFATO ◇ CIBA 570 ◇ CROTONAMIDE, 2-CHLORO-N,N-DIETHYL-3-HYDROXY-, DIMETHYL PHOS-PHATE ◇ DIMECRON ◇ DIMECRON 100 ◇ DIMETHYL 2-CHLORO-2-DIETHYLCARBAMOYL-1-METHYLVINYL PHOSPHATE ◇ O,O-DIMETHYL O-(2-CHLORO-2-(N,N-DIE-THYLCARBAMOYL)-1-METHYLVINYL) PHOSPHATE ◇ DIMETHYL DIETHYLAMIDO-1-CHLOROCROTONYL (2) PHOSPHATE ◇ O,O-DIMETHYL-O-(1-METHYL-2-CHLOR-2-N,N-DIAETHYL-CARBAMOYL)-VINYL-PHOSPHAT ◇ (O,O-DIMETHYL-O-(1-METHYL-2-CHLORO-2-DIETHYL-CARBAMOYL-VINYL) PHOSPHATE) ◇ DIMETHYL PHOS-PHATE of 2-CHLORO-N,N-DIETHYL-3-HYDROXYCROTO-NAMIDE ◇ DIXON ◇ ENT 25,515 ◇ FOSFAMIDON ◇ FOSFAMIDONE ◇ FOSZFAMIDON ◇ ML 97 ◇ NCI-C00588 ◇ OMS 1325 ◇ OR 1191 ◇ PHOSPHAMIDON ◇ PHOSPHATE de DIMETHYLE et de (2-CHLORO-2-DIETHYLCARBAMOYL-1-METHYL-VINYLE)

TOXICITY DATA with REFERENCE

ETA: orl-rat TDLo: 5400 mg/kg/80W-C NCITR*
NCI-TR-16,79

MUT: bfa-rat: sat 5800 μg/kg IJEBA6 24,305,86
MUT: cyt-hmn: leu 5 μmol/L IJEBA6 18,1145,80
MUT: cyt-hmn: lyms 1900 μg/L MUREAV
31,103,75
MUT: mma-sat 9 mg/plate ENMUDM 5(Suppl 1),3,83
MUT: mmo-sat 5 μg/plate IJEBA6 24,305,86
MUT: mnt-mus-orl 10 mg/kg/24H BECTA6
25,277,80

CONSENSUS REPORTS: NTP Carcinogenesis Bioassay (feed): No Evidence: mouse NCITR* NCI-TR-16,79; Inadequate Studies: rat NCITR* NCI-TR-16,79

SAFETY PROFILE: Questionable carcinogen with experimental tumorigenic data. Poison by ingestion and most other routes. Experimental reproductive data. Mutation data reported. When heated to decomposition it emits toxic fumes of NO_x and PO_x.

FAE000   CAS: 3844-45-9
FD&C BLUE No. 1
mf: $C_{37}H_{36}N_2O_9S_3 \cdot 2Na$ mw: 794.91

PROP: Dark purple to bronze powder. Sol in water, ether, conc sulfuric acid.

SYNS: ACID SKY BLUE A ◇ AIZEN FOOD BLUE No. 2 ◇ 1206 BLUE ◇ BRILLIANT BLUE FCD No. 1 ◇ BRILLIANT BLUE FCF ◇ CANACERT BRILLIANT BLUE FCF ◇ C.I. 42090 ◇ C.I. ACID BLUE 9, DISODIUM SALT ◇ C.I. FOOD BLUE 2 ◇ COGILOR BLUE 512.12 ◇ COSMETIC BLUE LAKE ◇ D&C BLUE No. 4 ◇ DISPERSED BLUE 12195 ◇ DOLKWAL BRILLIANT BLUE ◇ EDICOL BLUE CL 2 ◇ ERIOGLAUCINE G ◇ FENAZO BLUE XI ◇ FOOD BLUE 2 ◇ FOOD BLUE DYE No. 1 ◇ HEXACOL BRILLIANT BLUE A ◇ INTRACID PURE BLUE L ◇ MERANTINE BLUE EG ◇ USACERT BLUE No. 1

TOXICITY DATA with REFERENCE

NEO: scu-rat TDLo: 5500 mg/kg/97W-I
ZEKBAI 64,287,61
ETA: par-rat TDLo: 4580 mg/kg/62W-I
FAONAU 38B,27,66
ETA: scu-rat TD: 2 g/kg/94W-I FAONAU
38B,27,66
MUT: cyt-ham: lng 4400 mg/L GMCRDC
27,95,81

CONSENSUS REPORTS: IARC Cancer Review: GROUP 3 IMEMDT 7,56,87; Animal Sufficient Evidence IMEMDT 16,171,78. Reported in EPA TSCA Inventory.

SAFETY PROFILE: Questionable carcinogen with experimental neoplastigenic and tumorigenic data. Mutation data reported. When heated to decomposition it emits very toxic fumes of NO_x, Na_2O and SO_x.

FAE100   CAS: 860-22-0
FD&C BLUE No. 2
mf: $C_{16}H_{10}N_2O_8S_2 \cdot 2Na$ mw: 468.38

PROP: Blue-brown to red-brown powder. Sol in water, conc sulfuric acid; sltly sol in alc.

SYNS: ACID BLUE W ◇ ACID LEATHER BLUE IC ◇ A.F. BLUE No. 2 ◇ AIRDALE BLUE IN ◇ AMACID BRILLIANT BLUE ◇ ANILINE CARMINE POWDER ◇ ATUL INDIGO CARMINE ◇ 1311 BLUE ◇ 12070 BLUE ◇ BUCACID INDIGOTINE B ◇ CANACERT INDIGO CARMINE ◇ CARMINE BLUE (BIOLOGICAL STAIN) ◇ C.I. 73015 ◇ C.I. 7581 ◇ C.I. ACID BLUE 74 ◇ C.I. FOOD BLUE 1 ◇ DISODIUM INDIGO-5,5-DISULFONATE ◇ DISODIUM SALT of 1-INDIGOTIN-S,S'-DISULPHONIC ACID ◇ DOLKWAL INDIGO CARMINE ◇ E 132 ◇ GRAPE BLUE A GEIGY ◇ INDIGO CARMINE ◇ INDIGO CARMINE (BIOLOGICAL STAIN) ◇ INDIGO CARMINE DISODIUM SALT ◇ INDIGO EXTRACT ◇ INDIGO-KARMIN (GERMAN) ◇ 5,5'-INDIGOTIN DISULFONIC ACID ◇ INDIGOTINE ◇ INDIGOTINE DISODIUM SALT ◇ INTENSE BLUE ◇ L-BLAU 2 (GERMAN) ◇ MAPLE INDIGO CARMINE ◇ SACHSISCHBLAU ◇ SCHULTZ Nr. 1309 (GERMAN) ◇ SODIUM 5,5'-INDIGOTIDISULFONATE ◇ SOLUBLE INDIGO ◇ USACERT BLUE No.2

TOXICITY DATA with REFERENCE

NEO: scu-rat TDLo: 9 g/kg/2Y-I TXAPA9
8,29,66
MUT: cyt-ham: fbr 12 g/L FCTOD7 22,623,84
MUT: cyt-ham: ovr 20 μmol/L/5H-C ENMUDM
1,27,79

CONSENSUS REPORTS: Reported in EPA TSCA Inventory. EPA Genetic Toxicology Program.

SAFETY PROFILE: Questionable carcinogen with experimental neoplastigenic data. Poison by intravenous route. Moderately toxic by ingestion and subcutaneous routes. Mutation data reported. When heated to decomposition it emits very toxic fumes of SO_x, NO_x, and Na_2O.

FAE950   CAS: 4680-78-8
FD&C GREEN 1
mf: $C_{37}H_{36}N_2O_6S_2 \cdot Na$ mw: 691.86

SYNS: ACIDAL GREEN G ◊ ACID GREEN ◊ ACID GREEN 3 ◊ A.F. GREEN No. 1 ◊ BRILLIANT GREEN 3EMBL ◊ BUCACID GUINEA GREEN BA ◊ C.I. ACID GREEN 3, MONOSODIUM SALT ◊ C.I. FOOD GREEN 1 ◊ GUINEA GREEN B ◊ HISPACID GREEN GB ◊ LEATHER GREEN B ◊ NAPHTHALENE GREEN G ◊ PONTACYL GREEN BL ◊ SULFACID BRILLIANT GREEN 1B

TOXICITY DATA with REFERENCE
ETA: orl-rat TDLo: 660 g/kg/43W-C   GASTAB 23,1,53
MUT: mma-sat 320 μg/plate   MUREAV 89,21,81

CONSENSUS REPORTS: IARC Cancer Review: GROUP 3 IMEMDT 7,56,87; Animal Sufficient Evidence IMEMDT 16,199,78. Reported in EPA TSCA Inventory. Community Right-To-Know List.

SAFETY PROFILE: Questionable carcinogen with experimental tumorigenic data. Mutation data reported. When heated to decomposition it emits very toxic fumes of SO_x, Na_2O and NO_x.

FAF000   CAS: 5141-20-8
FD&C GREEN No. 2
mf: $C_{37}H_{36}N_2O_9S_3 \cdot 2Na$ mw: 794.91

SYNS: ACIDAL LIGHT GREEN SF ◊ ACID BRILLIANT GREEN SF ◊ ACID GREEN A ◊ ACILAN GREEN SFG ◊ A.F. GREEN No. 2 ◊ AMACID GREEN G ◊ C.I. 42095 ◊ C.I. ACID GREEN 5 ◊ C.I. ACID GREEN 5, DISODIUM SALT ◊ C.I. FOOD GREEN 2 ◊ D&C GREEN No. 4 ◊ FAST ACID GREEN N ◊ FD&C GREEN No. 2-ALUMINUM LAKE ◊ FENAZO GREEN 7G ◊ FOOD GREEN 2 ◊ GREEN No. 203 ◊ LEATHER GREEN SF ◊ LICHTGRUEN (GERMAN) ◊ LIGHT GREEN FCF YELLOWISH ◊ LIGHT GREEN LAKE ◊ LIGHT SF YELLOWISH (BIOLOGICAL STAIN) ◊ LISSAMINE LAKE GREEN SF ◊ MERANTINE GREEN SF ◊ MY/68 ◊ PENCIL GREEN SF ◊ SULFO GREEN J ◊ SUMITOMO LIGHT GREEN SF YELLOWISH ◊ WOOL BRILLIANT GREEN SF

TOXICITY DATA with REFERENCE
CAR: orl-rat TDLo: 1300 g/kg/86W-C   GASTAB 23,1,53
NEO: scu-rat TDLo: 6825 mg/kg/46W-I   JNCIAM 24,769,60
MUT: mma-sat 320 μg/plate   MUREAV 89,21,81

CONSENSUS REPORTS: IARC Cancer Review: GROUP 3 IMEMDT 7,56,87; Animal Sufficient Evidence IMEMDT 16,209,78. Reported in EPA TSCA Inventory. EPA Genetic Toxicology Program.

SAFETY PROFILE: Questionable carcinogen with experimental carcinogenic and neoplastigenic data. Moderately toxic by intravenous route. Mutation data reported. When heated to decomposition it emits very toxic fumes of NO_x, Na_2O, and SO_x.

FAG000   CAS: 2353-45-9
FD&C GREEN No. 3
mf: $C_{37}H_{36}N_2O_{10}S_3 \cdot 2Na$ mw: 810.91

PROP: Red to brown-violet powder. Sol in water, conc sulfuric acid.

SYNS: AIZEN FOOD GREEN No. 3 ◊ C.I. 42053 ◊ C.I. FOOD GREEN 3 ◊ FAST GREEN FCF ◊ 1724 GREEN ◊ SOLID GREEN FCF

TOXICITY DATA with REFERENCE
NEO: scu-rat TDLo: 5925 mg/kg/48W-I   JNCIAM 24,769,60
MUT: cyt-ham: fbr 4 g/L   FCTOD7 22,623,84
MUT: cyt-ham: lng 2 g/L   GMCRDC 27,95,81
MUT: cyt-ham: ovr 20 μmol/L/5H-C   ENMUDM 1,27,79
MUT: mma-sat 10 mg/plate   FCTOD7 22,623,84

CONSENSUS REPORTS: IARC Cancer Review: GROUP 3 IMEMDT 7,56,87; Animal Sufficient Evidence IMEMDT 16,187,78. Reported in EPA TSCA Inventory. EPA Genetic Toxicology Program.

SAFETY PROFILE: Questionable carcinogen with experimental neoplastigenic data. Mutation data reported. When heated to decomposition it emits very toxic fumes of NO_x and SO_x.

FAG010   CAS: 523-44-4
FD&C ORANGE No. 1
mf: $C_{16}H_{11}N_2O_4S \cdot Na$ mw: 350.34

SYNS: ACID LEATHER ORANGE I ◊ ACID PHOSPHINE CL ◊ A.F. ORANGE No. 1 ◊ AIZEN FOOD ORANGE No. 1 ◊ AIZEN NAPHTHOL ORANGE I ◊ AIZEN ORANGE I ◊ CERTIQUAL ORANGE I ◊ C.I. 14600 ◊ C.I. ACID ORANGE 20 ◊ C.I. ACID ORANGE 20, MONOSODIUM SALT ◊ D&C ORANGE No. 3 ◊ DYE ORANGE No. 1 ◊ EGACID ORANGE GG ◊ ELGACID ORANGE 2G ◊ ENIACID ORANGE I ◊ EXT. D&C ORANGE No.3 ◊ FDC ORANGE I ◊ HISPACID ORANGE 1 ◊ 4-((4-HYDROXY-1-NAPHTHALENYL)AZO)BENZENESULPHONIC ACID, MONOSODIUM SALT ◊ p-((4-HYDROXY-1-NAPHTHYL)AZO)BENZENESULFONIC ACID, MONOSODIUM SALT ◊ p-((4-HYDROXY-1-NAPHTHYL)AZO)BENZENESULPHONIC ACID, MONOSODIUM SALT ◊ p-((4-HYDROXY-1-NAPHTHYL)AZO)BENZENESULPHONIC ACID, SODIUM SALT ◊ JAVA ORANGE I ◊ NANKAI ACID ORANGE I ◊ NAPHTHA-

LENE ORANGE I ◇ NAPHTHOL ORANGE ◇ α-NAPHTHOL ORANGE ◇ NEKLACID ORANGE 1 ◇ 1333 ORANGE ◇ ORANGE I ◇ SODIUM AZO-α-NAPHTHOLSUL-FANILATE ◇ SODIUM AZO-α-NAPHTHOLSULPHANILATE ◇ 4-p-SULFOPHENYLAZO-1-NAPHTHOL MONOSODIUM SALT ◇ TERTRACID ORANGE I ◇ TROPAEOLIN 1

TOXICITY DATA with REFERENCE

ETA: scu-rat TDLo:9360 mg/kg/2Y-I   FEPRA7 16,367,57

MUT: mma-sat 100 μg/plate   MUREAV 56,249,78

CONSENSUS REPORTS: IARC Cancer Review: GROUP 3 IMEMDT 7,56,87; Animal Limited Evidence IMEMDT 8,173,75. Reported in EPA TSCA Inventory. EPA Genetic Toxicology Program.

SAFETY PROFILE: Questionable carcinogen with experimental tumorigenic data. Mutation data reported. When heated to decomposition it emits very toxic fumes of NO_x, SO_x, and Na_2O.

FAG020   CAS: 915-67-3
FD&C RED No. 2
mf: $C_{20}H_{11}N_2O_{10}S_3 \cdot 3Na$ mw: 604.48

SYNS: ACETACID RED 2BR ◇ ACID AMARANTH ◇ ACILAN RED SE ◇ AIZEN AMARANTH ◇ AMACID AMARANTH ◇ AMARANT ◇ AMARANTH ◇ AMARANTHE USP (biological stain) ◇ AZO RED R ◇ BORDEAUX ◇ CALCOCID AMARANTH ◇ CANACERT AMARANTH ◇ CERVEN KYSELA 27 ◇ CERVEN POTRAVINARSKA 9 ◇ C.I. 184 ◇ C.I. 16185 ◇ C.I. ACID RED 27 ◇ C.I. FOOD RED 9 ◇ CILEFA RUBINE 2B ◇ DAISHIKI AMARANTH ◇ D&C RED 2 ◇ DOLKWAL AMARANTH ◇ DYE FDC RED 2 ◇ DYE RED RASPBERRY ◇ EDICOL AMARANTH ◇ EUROCERT AMARANTH ◇ FD&C RED No. 2-ALUMINIUM LAKE ◇ FOOD RED 2 ◇ FOOD RED 9 ◇ FRUIT RED A GEIGY ◇ HD AMARANTH B ◇ HEXACERT RED No. 2 ◇ HIDACID AMARANTH ◇ 2-HYDROXY-1,1'-AZONAPH-THALENE-3,6,4'-TRISULFONIC ACID TRISODIUM SALT ◇ 3-HYDROXY-4-((4-SULFO-1-NAPHTHALENYL)AZO)-2,7-NAPHTHLENEDISULFONIC ACID, TRISODIUM SALT ◇ 3-HYDROXY-4-((4-SULFO-1-NAPHTHYL)AZO)-2,7-NAPHTHALENEDISULFONIC ACID, TRISODIUM SALT ◇ 3-HYDROXY-4-((4-SULPHO-1-NAPHTHALENYL)AZO)-2,7-NAPHTHALENEDISULPHONIC ACID, TRISODIUM SALT ◇ 3-HYDROXY-4-((4-SULPHO-1-NAPHTHYL)AZO)-2,7-NAPHTHALENEDISULPHONIC ACID, TRISODIUM SALT ◇ JAVA AMARANTH ◇ KAYAKU AMARANTH ◇ KCA FOODCOL AMARANTH A ◇ KITON RUBINE S ◇ LISSAMINE AMARANTH AC ◇ MAPLE AMARANTH ◇ NAPHTHOL RED B ◇ NAPTHOLROT S ◇ NEKLACID RED A

◇ RAKUTO AMARANTH ◇ RASPBERRY RED for JELLIES ◇ RED DYE No. 2 ◇ RED No. 2 ◇ SHIKISO AMARANTH ◇ 1-(4-SULPHO-1-NAPHTHYLAZO)-2-NAPHTHOL-3,6-DI-SULPHONIC ACID, TRISODIUM SALT ◇ TAKAOKA AMARANTH ◇ TERTRACID RED A ◇ TOYO AMARANTH ◇ TRISODIUM SALT of 1-(4-SULFO-1-NAPHTHYLAZO)-2-NAPHTHOL-3,6-DISULFONIC ACID ◇ VICTORIA RUBINE O ◇ WHORTLEBERRY RED ◇ WOOL BORDEAUX 6RK ◇ WOOL RED

TOXICITY DATA with REFERENCE

CAR: orl-rat TD:1200 g/kg/78W-C   GASTAB 23,1,53

ETA: orl-rat TD:1643 g/kg/78W-C   NEZAAQ 37,714,82

ETA: orl-rat TDLo:680 g/kg/14W-I   VPITAR 29,61,70

MUT: cyt-ham:fbr 1 g/L/48H   MUREAV 48,337,77

MUT: mmo-esc 20 μg/L   ENVIDV 9,145,83

MUT: mrc-smc 20 mg/L   ENVIDV 9,145,83

CONSENSUS REPORTS: IARC Cancer Review: GROUP 3 IMEMDT 7,56,87, Animal Inadequate Evidence IMEMDT 8,41,75. Reported in EPA TSCA Inventory.

SAFETY PROFILE: Questionable carcinogen with experimental carcinogenic and tumorigenic data. Moderately toxic by intraperitoneal route. Mutation data reported. When heated to decomposition it emits toxic fumes of NO_x and SO_x.

FAG040   CAS: 16423-68-0
FD&C RED No. 3
mf: $C_{20}H_6I_4O_5 \cdot 2Na$ mw: 879.84

PROP: Brown powder. Sol in water, conc sulfuric acid.

SYNS: AIZEN ERYTHROSINE ◇ CALCOCID ERYTHROSINE N ◇ CANACERT ERYTHROSINE BS ◇ 9-(o-CARBOXY-PHENYL)-6-HYDROXY-2,4,5,7-TETRAIODO-3-ISOXAN-THONE ◇ C.I. 45430 ◇ C.I. ACID RED 51 ◇ CILEFA PINK B ◇ D&C RED No. 3 ◇ DOLKWAL ERYTHROSINE ◇ DYE FD&C RED No. 3 ◇ E 127 ◇ EBS ◇ EDICOL SUPRA ERYTHROSINE A ◇ ERYTHROSIN ◇ ERYTHROSINE B-FO (BIOLOGICAL STAIN) ◇ FOOD RED 14 ◇ HEXACERT RED No. 3 ◇ HEXACOL ERYTHROSINE BS ◇ LB-ROT 1 ◇ MAPLE ERYTHROSINE ◇ NEW PINK BLUISH GEIGY ◇ 1427 RED ◇ 1671 RED ◇ 2',4',5',7'-TETRAIODOFLUORES-CEIN, DISODIUM SALT ◇ TETRAIODOFLUORESCEIN SODIUM SALT ◇ USACERT RED No. 3

TOXICITY DATA with REFERENCE

NEO: orl-rat TDLo:1798 g/kg/2Y-C   FCTOD7 25,723,87

MUT: cyt-ham:fbr 600 mg/L   FCTOD7 22,623,84

MUT: cyt-ham:lng 1100 mg/L   GMCRDC 27,95,81

MUT: dni-hmn:leu 500 mg/L   NEZAAQ 30,574,75

MUT: dnr-bcs 2 mg/disc   TRENAF 27,153,76

MUT: mrc-smc 100 mg/L   MUREAV 138,153,84

CONSENSUS REPORTS: Reported in EPA TSCA Inventory. EPA Genetic Toxicology Program.

SAFETY PROFILE: Questionable carcinogen with experimental tumorigenic data. Poison by intravenous route. Moderately toxic by ingestion and possibly other routes. Human mutation data reported. When heated to decomposition it emits very toxic fumes of Na_2O and I^-.

FAG050   CAS: 4548-53-2
FD&C RED No. 4
mf: $C_{18}H_{14}N_2O_7S_2 \cdot 2Na$ mw: 480.44

SYNS: CERTICOL PONCEAU SXS ◇ CERVEN POTRAVI-NARSKA 1 ◇ C.I. 14700 ◇ C.I. FOOD RED 1 ◇ C.I. FOOD RED 1, DISODIUM SALT ◇ 3-((2,4-DIMETHYL-5-SULFOPHE-NYL)AZO)-4-HYDROXY-1-NAPHTHALENESULFONIC ACID, DISODIUM SALT ◇ 3-((2,4-DIMETHYL-5-SULPHOPHE-NYL)AZO)-4-HYDROXY-1-NAPHTHALENESULPHONIC ACID, DISODIUM SALT ◇ DYE FD & C RED No. 4 ◇ DYE FD AND C RED No. 4 ◇ EDICOL SUPRA PONCEAU SX ◇ FD & C RED No. 4-ALUMINIUM LAKE ◇ FOOD RED 4 ◇ HEXACOL PONCEAU SX ◇ 4-HYDROXY-3-((5-SULPHO-2,4-XYLYL)AZO)-1-NAPHTHALENESULPHONIC ACID, DI-SODIUM SALT ◇ 4-HYDROXY-3-((5-SULFO-2,4-XYLYL) AZO)-1-NAPHTHALENESULFONIC ACID, DISODIUM SALT ◇ PONCEAU SX ◇ PURPLE 4R ◇ 1306 RED ◇ 12101 RED ◇ RED No. 1 ◇ RED No. 4 ◇ 2-(6-SULFO-2,4-XYLYLAZO)-1-NAPHTHOL-4-SULFONIC ACID, DISODIUM SALT ◇ USACERT FD & C RED No. 4

TOXICITY DATA with REFERENCE
CAR: orl-rat TDLo: 1200 g/kg/78W-C   GASTAB 23,1,53

ETA: orl-rat TD: 524 g/kg/73W-C   VPITAR 29,61,70

CONSENSUS REPORTS: IARC Cancer Review: GROUP 3 IMEMDT 7,56,87; Animal Sufficient Evidence IMEMDT 8,207,75. Reported in EPA TSCA Inventory.

SAFETY PROFILE: Questionable carcinogen with experimental carcinogenic and tumorigenic data. When heated to decomposition it emits toxic fumes of NO_x and SO_x.

FAG070   CAS: 81-88-9
FD&C RED No. 19
mf: $C_{28}H_{31}N_2O_3 \cdot Cl$ mw: 479.06

SYNS: ACID BRILLIANT PINK B ◇ ADC RHODAMINE B ◇ AIZEN RHODAMINE BH ◇ AKIRIKU RHODAMINE B ◇ BASIC VIOLET 10 ◇ BRILLIANT PINK B ◇ CALCOZINE RED BX ◇ CALCOZINE RHODAMINE BX ◇ 9-o-CARBOXY-PHENYL-6-DIETHYLAMINO-3-ETHYLIMINO-3-ISOXAN-THENE, 3-ETHOCHLORIDE ◇ (9-(o-CARBOXYPHENYL)-6-(DIETHYLAMINO)-3H-XANTHEN-3-YLIDENE) DIETHY-LAMMONIUM CHLORIDE ◇ CERISE TONER X1127 ◇ CERTIQUAL RHODAMIEN ◇ C.I. 749 ◇ C.I. BASIC VIOLET 10 ◇ C.I. FOOD RED 15 ◇ COGILOR RED 321.10 ◇ COSMETIC BRILLIANT PINK BLUISH D CONC ◇ DIABASIC RHODA-MINE B ◇ DIETHYL-m-AMINO-PHENOLPHTHALEIN HY-DROCHLORIDE ◇ EDICOL SUPRA ROSE B ◇ ELCOZINE RHODAMINE B ◇ ERIOSIN RHODAMINE B ◇ FOOD RED 15 ◇ GERANIUM LAKE N ◇ HEXACOL RHODAMINE B EX-TRA ◇ IKADA RHODAMINE B ◇ IRAGEN RED L-U ◇ MITSUI RHODAMINE BX ◇ 11411 RED ◇ RED NO 213 ◇ RHEONINE B ◇ RHODAMINE ◇ RHODAMINE S (RUSSIAN) ◇ SICILIAN CERISE TONER A-7127 ◇ SYMULEX MAGENTA F ◇ SYMULEX PINK F ◇ TAKAOKA RHODAMINE B ◇ TETRAETHYLDIAMINO-o-CARBOXY-PHENYL-XANTHE-NYL CHLORIDE ◇ TETRAETHYLRHODAMINE

TOXICITY DATA with REFERENCE
ETA: scu-rat TD: 3870 mg/kg/68W-I   GANNA2 46,369,55

ETA: scu-rat TDLo: 3600 mg/kg/68W-I   GANNA2 47,51,56

MUT: cyt-ham: ovr 20 μmol/L/5H-C   ENMUDM 1,27,79

MUT: cyt-mam: fbr 2 mg/L   MUREAV 88,211,81

MUT: dnd-ham: ovr 900 μmol/plate   AMNTA4 87,295,53

MUT: mma-sat 50 μg/plate   MUREAV 66,181,79

MUT: sln-dmg-orl 1000 ppm   AMNTA4 87,295,53

CONSENSUS REPORTS: IARC Cancer Review: GROUP 3 IMEMDT 7,80,87; Animal Sufficient Evidence IMEMDT 16,221,78. Reported in EPA TSCA Inventory. EPA Genetic Toxicology Program.

SAFETY PROFILE: Questionable carcinogen with experimental tumorigenic data. Poison by intraperitoneal and intravenous routes. Moderately toxic by ingestion. Mutation data reported. When heated to decomposition it emits very toxic fumes of NO_x, NH_3 and Cl^-.

FAG080   CAS: 85-82-5
FD&C RED No. 32
mf: $C_{18}H_{16}N_2O$ mw: 276.36

SYNS: FD&C ACID RED 32 ◇ OIL RED XO ◇ 1-XYLYLAZO-2-NAPHTHOL ◇ 1-(2,5-XYLYLAZO)-2-NAPHTHOL

TOXICITY DATA with REFERENCE
ETA: orl-mus TDLo: 29 g/kg/52W   BJCAAI
10,653,56

SAFETY PROFILE: Questionable carcinogen with experimental tumorigenic data. When heated to decomposition it emits toxic fumes of NO_x.

FAG130   CAS: 85-84-7
FD&C YELLOW No. 3
mf: $C_{16}H_{13}N_3$ mw: 247.32

SYNS: A.F YELLOW No. 2 ◊ 1-BENZENE-AZO-β-NAPH-THYLAMINE ◊ 1-BENZENEAZO-2-NAPHTHYLAMINE ◊ CERISOL YELLOW AB ◊ C.I. 11380 ◊ C.I. FOOD YELLOW 10 ◊ C.I. SOLVENT YELLOW 5 ◊ DOLKWAL YELLOW AB ◊ EXT. D&C YELLOW No. 9 ◊ GRASAL YELLOW ◊ JAUNE AB ◊ OIL YELLOW A ◊ 1-(PHENYLAZO)-2-NAPH-THALENAMINE ◊ 1-(PHENYLAZO)-2-NAPHTHYLAMINE ◊ YELLOW AB ◊ YELLOW No. 2

TOXICITY DATA with REFERENCE
ETA: orl-rat TDLo: 8190 mg/kg/65W-C
JPPMAB 7,591,55
MUT: dns-rat-orl 500 mg/kg   ENMUDM 7,101,85

CONSENSUS REPORTS: IARC Cancer Review: Animal No Evidence IMEMDT 8,279,75. Reported in EPA TSCA Inventory. EPA Genetic Toxicology Program.

SAFETY PROFILE: Questionable carcinogen with experimental tumorigenic data. Moderately toxic by ingestion and subcutaneous routes. Mutation data reported. When heated to decomposition it emits toxic fumes of NO_x.

FAG135   CAS: 131-79-3
FD&C YELLOW No. 4
mf: $C_{17}H_{15}N_3$ mw: 261.35

SYNS: A.F. YELLOW No. 3 ◊ CERISOL YELLOW TB ◊ C.I. 11390 ◊ C.I. FOOD YELLOW 11 ◊ DOLKWAL YELLOW OB ◊ EXT. D&C YELLOW No. 10 ◊ JAUNE OB ◊ 1-(2-METHYLPHENYL)AZO-2-NAPHTHALENAMINE ◊ 1-((2-METHYLPHENYL)AZO)-2-NAPHTHALENAMINE ◊ 1-(2-METHYLPHENYL)AZO-2-NAPHTHYLAMINE ◊ OIL YELLOW OB ◊ o-TOLUENE-1-AZO-2-NAPHTHYLAMINE ◊ 1-(o-TOLYLAZO)-2-NAPHTHYLAMINE ◊ YELLOW OB

TOXICITY DATA with REFERENCE
ETA: scu-rat TDLo: 700 mg/kg/2Y-I   FEPRA7
16,367,57
MUT: mma-sat 50 μg/plate   CANCAR 49,1970,82

CONSENSUS REPORTS: IARC Cancer Review: GROUP 3 IMEMDT 7,56,87; Animal

Sufficient Evidence IMEMDT 8,287,75. EPA Genetic Toxicology Program.

SAFETY PROFILE: Questionable carcinogen with experimental tumorigenic data. Moderately toxic by ingestion, intraperitoneal, and subcutaneous routes. Mutation data reported. When heated to decomposition it emits toxic fumes of NO_x.

FAG150   CAS: 2783-94-0
FD&C YELLOW No. 6
mf: $C_{16}H_{10}N_2O_7S_2Na_2$ mw: 452.36

PROP: Orange powder. Sol in water, conc sulfuric acid; sltly sol in abs alc.

SYNS: ACID YELLOW TRA ◊ AIZEN FOOD YELLOW No. 5 ◊ CANACERT SUNSET YELLOW FCF ◊ C.I. 15985 ◊ GELBORANGE-S (GERMAN) ◊ SUNSET YELLOW FCF

TOXICITY DATA with REFERENCE
MUT: cyt-ham: lng 2 g/l   GMCRDC 27,95,81

CONSENSUS REPORTS: IARC Cancer Review: GROUP 3 IMEMDT 7,56,87; Animal Inadequate Evidence IMEMDT 8,257,75. Reported in EPA TSCA Inventory.

SAFETY PROFILE: Questionable carcinogen. Moderately toxic by intraperitoneal route. When heated to decomposition it emits very toxic fumes of NO_x and SO_x.

FAO200   CAS: 7698-97-7
FENESTREL
mf: $C_{16}H_{20}O_2$ mw: 244.36

SYNS: 2-METHYL-3-ETHYL-4-PHENYL-4-CYCLOHEXENE CARBOXYLIC ACID ◊ 2-METHYL-3-ETHYL-4-PHENYL-Δ⁴-CYCLOHEXENECARBOXYLIC ACID ◊ ORF 3858

TOXICITY DATA with REFERENCE
ETA: orl-rat TDLo: 27 mg/kg/52W-C   TXAPA9
19,412,71

SAFETY PROFILE: Questionable carcinogen with experimental tumorigenic data. Poison by intravenous and intraperitoneal routes. Moderately toxic by ingestion. Experimental reproductive effects. When heated to decomposition it emits acrid smoke and irritating fumes.

FAQ999   CAS: 55-38-9
FENTHION
mf: $C_{10}H_{15}O_3PS_2$ mw: 278.34

SYNS: BAY 29493 ◊ BAYCID ◊ BAYER 9007 ◊ BAY-TEX ◊ O,O-DIMETHYL-O-4-(METHYLMERCAPTO)-3-

METHYLPHENYL PHOSPHOROTHIOATE ◇ O,O-DI-
METHYL-p-4-(METHYLMERCAPTO)-3-METHYLPHENYL
THIOPHOSPHATE ◇ O,O-DIMETHYL-O-(3-METHYL-4-
METHYLMERCAPTOPHENYL)PHOSPHOROTHIOATE
◇ O,O-DIMETHYL-O-(3-METHYL-4-METHYLTHIO-FENYL)-
MONOTHIOFOSFAAT (DUTCH) ◇ O,O-DIMETHYL-O-(3-
METHYL-4-METHYLTHIOPHENYL)-MONOTHIOPHOSPHAT
(GERMAN) ◇ O,O-DIMETHYL-O-3-METHYL-4-METHYL-
THIOPHENYL PHOSPHOROTHIOATE ◇ O,O-DIMETHYL-
O-(3-METHYL-4-METHYLTHIO-PHENYL)-THIONOPHOS-
PHAT (GERMAN) ◇ O,O-DIMETHYL-O-(4-METHYLTHIO-
3-METHYLPHENYL) PHOSPHOROTHIOATE ◇ O,O-DI-
METHYL-O-(4-(METHYLTHIO)-m-TOLYL) PHOSPHORO-
THIOATE ◇ O,O-DIMETIL-O-(3-METIL-4-METILTIO-
FENIL)-MONOTIOFOSFATO (ITALIAN) ◇ DMTP ◇ ENT
25,540 ◇ ENTEX ◇ LEBAYCID ◇ MERCAPTOPHOS
◇ 4-METHYLMERCAPTO-3-METHYLPHENYL DIMETHYL
THIOPHOSPHATE ◇ MPP ◇ NCI-C08651 ◇ OMS 2
◇ PHOSPHOROTHIOIC ACID-O,O-DIMETHYL-O-(3-METH-
YL-4-METHYLTHIOPHENYLE) (FRENCH) ◇ QUELETOX
◇ S 1752 ◇ SPOTTON ◇ TALODEX ◇ THIOPHOSPHATE
de O,O-DIMETHYLE et de O-(3-METHYL-4-METHYLTHIO-
PHENYLE) (FRENCH) ◇ TIGUVON

TOXICITY DATA with REFERENCE
ETA: orl-mus TDLo:1730 mg/kg/103W-C
NCITR* NCI-CG-TR-103,79
MUT: mma-sat 333 μg/plate   ENMUDM 8(Suppl 7),1,86
MUT: sce-ham:lng 40 mg/L   ENMUDM 4,621,82

CONSENSUS REPORTS: NCI Carcinogenesis Bioassay Completed; Results Negative: rat (NCITR* NCI-CG-TR-103,79); Indefinite: mouse (NCITR* NCI-CG-TR-103,79). EPA Genetic Toxicology Program.

OSHA PEL: TWA 0.2 mg/m³ (skin) ACGIH TLV: TWA 0.2 mg/m³ (skin) DFG MAK: 0.2 mg/m³

SAFETY PROFILE: Questionable carcinogen with experimental tumorigenic and teratogenic data. A human poison by an unspecified route. Poison experimentally by ingestion, skin contact, intraperitoneal, intravenous, and intramuscular routes. Moderately toxic by inhalation. Experimental reproductive effects. Mutation data reported. When heated to decomposition it emits very toxic fumes of PO_x and SO_x.

FAS000   CAS: 14484-64-1
FERBAM
mf: $C_9H_{18}N_3S_6 \cdot Fe$ mw: 416.51
PROP: Black solid, sltly sol in water. Mp: decomp 180°.

SYNS: AAFERTIS ◇ BERCEMA FERTAM 50 ◇ CARBA-
MATE ◇ DIMETHYLCARBAMODITHIOIC ACID, IRON COM-
PLEX ◇ DIMETHYLCARBAMODITHIOIC ACID, IRON(3+)
SALT ◇ DIMETHYLDITHIOCARBAMIC ACID, IRON SALT
◇ DIMETHYLDITHIOCARBAMIC ACID, IRON(3+) SALT
◇ EISENDIMETHYLDITHIOCARBAMAT (GERMAN)
◇ EISEN(III)-TRIS(N,N-DIMETHYLDITHIOCARBAMAT)
(GERMAN) ◇ ENT 14,689 ◇ FERBAM 50 ◇ FERBAM, IRON
SALT ◇ FERBECK ◇ FERMATE FERBAM FUNGICIDE
◇ FERMOCIDE ◇ FERRADOW ◇ FERRIC DIMETHYLDI-
THIOCARBAMATE ◇ FUKLASIN ULTRA ◇ HEXAFERB
◇ HOKMATE ◇ IRON DIMETHYLDITHIOCARBAMATE
◇ KARBAM BLACK ◇ KNOCKMATE ◇ NIACIDE
◇ SUP'R FLO FERBAM FLOWABLE ◇ TRIFUNGOL
◇ TRIS(DIMETHYLCARBAMODITHIOATO-S,S')IRON
◇ TRIS)DIMETHYLDITHIOCARBAMATO)IRON ◇ TRIS(N,N-
DIMETHYLDITHIOCARBAMATO) IRON(111) ◇ VANCIDE
FE95

TOXICITY DATA with REFERENCE
CAR: scu-mus TDLo:100 mg/kg   NTIS** PB223-159
ETA: orl-mus TDLo:3500 mg/kg/78W-I
NTIS** PB223-159
MUT: mmo-omi 1000 ppm   MMAPAP 50,233,73
MUT: mmo-sat 50 μg/plate   CSHCAL 4,267,77
MUT: mrc-bcs 2 μg/disc/24H   MUREAV 40,19,76

CONSENSUS REPORTS: IARC Cancer Review: Animal Inadequate Evidence IMEMDT 12,121,76. Reported in EPA TSCA Inventory. EPA Genetic Toxicology Program.

OSHA PEL: (Transitional: TWA Total Dust: 15 mg/m³; Respirable Fraction: 5 mg/m³) TWA Total Dust: 10 mg/m³; Respirable Fraction: 5 mg/m³ ACGIH TLV: TWA 10 mg/m³ DFG MAK: 15 mg/m³

SAFETY PROFILE: Questionable carcinogen with experimental carcinogenic, tumorigenic, and teratogenic data. Poison by intraperitoneal route. Moderately toxic by ingestion. Experimental reproductive effects. Mutation data reported. A fungicide. When heated to decomposition it emits very toxic fumes of NO_x and SO_x.

FAY000
FERRIC HYDROXIDE
NITRILOTRIPROPIONIC ACID COMPLEX
PROP: Complex with 20.0% Fe (ONCOBS 19,239,65).
SYN: IRON(+3) HYDROXIDE COMPLEX with NITRILO-TRI-PROPIONIC ACID

TOXICITY DATA with REFERENCE
ETA: ims-mus TDLo:45 mg(Fe)/kg/3W-I
ONCOAR 19,239,65

SAFETY PROFILE: Questionable carcinogen
with experimental tumorigenic data. When
heated to decomposition it emits toxic fumes
of NO_x.

FAZ000
FERRIC NITROSODIMETHYL
DITHIOCARBAMATE and
TETRAMETHYL THIURAM DISULFIDE

PROP: 58.5% main component, 6.5% secondary component (NTIS** PB223-159).

SYNS: BIS(DIMETHYLTHIOCARBAMOYL)DISULFIDE and
NITROSOTRIS(DIMETHYLDITHIOCARBAMATO)IRON
◇ TETRAMETHYLTHIURAM DISULFIDE mixed with FERRIC
NITROSODIMETHYLDITHIOCARBAMATE ◇ VANGUARD
GF

TOXICITY DATA with REFERENCE
CAR: orl-mus TDLo:27 g/kg/78W-I   NTIS**
PB223-159
ETA: scu-mus TDLo:46 mg/kg   NTIS** PB223-
159

SAFETY PROFILE: Questionable carcinogen
with experimental carcinogenic and tumorigenic
data. When heated to decomposition it emits
very toxic fumes of NO_x and SO_x.

FBB000   CAS: 9007-73-2
FERRITIN

PROP: Prepared from rat liver protein by precip-
itation with a cadmium salt (BECCAN 39,
74,61).

TOXICITY DATA with REFERENCE
NEO: scu-rat TDLo:224 mg/kg/15W-I   BJCAAI
18,667,64
MUT: cyt-ham:ovr 27 mg/L   CNREA8 41,1628,81

CONSENSUS REPORTS: Reported in EPA
TSCA Inventory.

SAFETY PROFILE: Questionable carcinogen
with experimental neoplastigenic data. Mutation
data reported. When heated to decomposition
it emits very toxic fumes of Cd.

FBB100
FERRLECIT

TOXICITY DATA with REFERENCE
CAR: ipl-rat TD:80 mg/kg   CNREA8 2,157,86

SAFETY PROFILE: Questionable carcinogen
with experimental carcinogenic data. Poison by
intraperterional route. When heated to decomposition it emits acrid smoke and irritating fumes.

FBC000   CAS: 102-54-5
FERROCENE
mf: $C_{10}H_{10}Fe$ mw: 186.05

PROP: Orange crystals, camphor odor, insol
in water, sol in alcohol and ether. Mp: 174°,
sublimes @ >100°, volatile in steam.

SYNS: BISCYCLOPENTADIENYLIRON ◇ DI-2,4-CYCLO-
PENTADIEN-1-YL IRON ◇ DICYCLOPENTADIENYL IRON
(OSHA, ACGIH) ◇ IRON BIS(CYCLOPENTADIENE)
◇ IRON DICYCLOPENTADIENYL

TOXICITY DATA with REFERENCE
ETA: ims-rat TDLo:5175 mg/kg/2Y-I   NCIUS*
PH 43-64-886,AUG,69
MUT: sce-ham:ovr 130 μg/L   ENMUDM 7,1,85
MUT: sln-dmg-par 100 ppm   ENMUDM 7,87,85
MUT: trn-dmg-par 100 ppm   ENMUDM 7,87,85

CONSENSUS REPORTS: Reported in EPA
TSCA Inventory.

OSHA PEL: (Transitional: TWA Total Dust:
15 mg/m^3; Respirable Fraction: 5 mg/m^3) TWA
Total Dust: 10 mg/m^3; Respirable Fraction: 5
mg/m^3 ACGIH TLV: TWA 10 mg/m^3

SAFETY PROFILE: Questionable carcinogen
with experimental tumorigenic data. Poison by
intraperitoneal and intravenous routes. Moderately toxic by ingestion. Mutation data reported.
Flammable. When heated to decomposition it
emits acrid smoke and irritating fumes.

FBD000   CAS: 11114-46-8
FERROCHROME (exothermic)

SYNS: CARBON FERROCHROMIUM ◇ CHROME FER-
ROALLOY ◇ CHROMIUM ALLOY, Cr,C,Fe,N,Si ◇ CHRO-
MIUM ALLOY, BASE, Cr,C,Fe,N,Si (FERROCHROMIUM)
◇ exothermic FERROCHROME (DOT) ◇ FERROCHROME
◇ FERROCHROME, exothermic (DOT) ◇ FERROCHROMIUM

CONSENSUS REPORTS: IARC Cancer Review: Animal Inadequate Evidence IMEMDT
23,205,80. Reported in EPA TSCA Inventory.
Chromium and its compounds are on the Community Right-To-Know List.

OSHA PEL: TWA 1 mg(Cr)/m^3 ACGIH TLV:
TWA 0.5 mg(Cr)/m^3 DOT Classification:
ORM-C; Label: None.

SAFETY PROFILE: Questionable carcinogen. Poison by inhalation.

FBG200 CAS: 15669-07-5
FERROTREMOLITE
mf: $Ca_2Fe_5H_2O_{24}Si_8$ mw: 970.15

SYN: FERROACTINOLITE

TOXICITY DATA with REFERENCE
CAR: ipl-rat TDLo: 80 mg/kg   TOLED5 13,143,82
CAR: itr-rat TDLo: 24 mg/kg/12W-I   TOLED5
13,143,82

SAFETY PROFILE: Questionable carcinogen with experimental carcinogenic data.

FBK000 CAS: 299-29-6
FERROUS GLUCONATE
mf: $C_{12}H_{22}O_{14} \cdot Fe \cdot H_2O$ mw: 482.17

PROP: Yellowish-gray or pale greenish-yellow, fine powder or granules with slt odor of burned sugar. Sol in water and glycerin; insol in alc.

SYNS: FERGON ◇ FERGON PREPARATIONS ◇ FERLU-CON ◇ FERRONICUM ◇ GLUCO-FERRUM ◇ IROMIN ◇ IRON GLUCONATE ◇ IROX (GADOR) ◇ NIONATE ◇ RAY-GLUCIRON

TOXICITY DATA with REFERENCE
ETA: scu-mus TDLo: 2600 mg/kg/13W-I: TER
JNCIAM 24,109,60

CONSENSUS REPORTS: Reported in EPA TSCA Inventory.

OSHA PEL: TWA 1 mg(Fe)/m^3 ACGIH TLV: TWA 1 mg(Fe)/m^3

SAFETY PROFILE: Questionable carcinogen with experimental tumorigenic and teratogenic data. Poison by intraperitoneal and intravenous routes. Moderately toxic by ingestion. Human systemic effects by ingestion: hypermotility, diarrhea, nausea, and vomiting. When heated to decomposition it emits acrid smoke and irritating fumes.

FBM000 CAS: 2896-87-9
FERROUS GLUTAMATE
mf: $C_5H_9FeNO_4$ mw: 203.00

SYN: GLUTAMIC ACID, IRON (2+) SALT (1:1)

TOXICITY DATA with REFERENCE
ETA: scu-mus TDLo: 2600 mg/kg/I   BECCAN
40,30,62

SAFETY PROFILE: Questionable carcinogen with experimental tumorigenic data. When heated to decomposition it emits toxic fumes of NO_x.

FBN100 CAS: 7720-78-7
FERROUS SULFATE
DOT: 9125
mf: $O_4S \cdot Fe$ mw: 151.91

PROP: Grayish white to buff powder. Slowly sol in water; insol in alc.

SYNS: COPPERAS ◇ DURETTER ◇ DUROFERON ◇ EXSICCATED FERROUS SULFATE ◇ EXSICCATED FER-ROUS SULPHATE ◇ FEOSOL ◇ FEOSPAN ◇ FER-IN-SOL ◇ FERO-GRADUMET ◇ FERRALYN ◇ FERRO-GRADUMET ◇ FERROSULFAT (GERMAN) ◇ FERROSULFATE ◇ FERRO-THERON ◇ FERSOLATE ◇ GREEN VITRIOL ◇ IRON MONOSULFATE ◇ IRON PROTOSULFATE ◇ IRON(II) SULFATE (1:1) ◇ IRON VITRIOL ◇ IROSPAN ◇ IROSUL ◇ SLOW-FE ◇ SULFERROUS ◇ SULFURIC ACID, IRON(2$^+$) SALT (1:1)

TOXICITY DATA with REFERENCE
ETA: scu-mus TDLo: 1600 mg/kg/16W-I
JNCIAM 24,109,60
MUT: cyt-ham: fbr 1250 mg/L   FCTOD7 22,623,84
MUT: cyt-ham: ovr 5 mmol/L   CNREA8
41,1628,81
MUT: dnd-omi 2 μmol/L   BBRCA9 77,1150,77
MUT: mmo-smc 100 mmol/L   MUREAV
117,149,83
MUT: mrc-smc 100 mmol/L   MUREAV 117,149,83
MUT: otr-ham: emb 900 μmol/L   CNREA8
39,193,79

CONSENSUS REPORTS: Reported in EPA TSCA Inventory. EPA Genetic Toxicology Program.

OSHA PEL: TWA 1 mg/(Fe)/m^3 ACGIH TLV: TWA 1 mg/(Fe)/m^3 DOT Classification: ORM-E; Label: None.

SAFETY PROFILE: Questionable carcinogen with experimental tumorigenic data. A human poison by ingestion. Moderately toxic to humans by an unspecified route. An experimental poison by ingestion, intraduodenal, intraperitoneal, intravenous, and subcutaneous routes. Human systemic effects by ingestion: aggression, somnolence, brain recording changes, diarrhea, nausea or vomiting, bleeding from the stomach, coma. Experimental reproductive effects. Mutation data reported. When heated to decomposition it emits toxic fumes of SO_x.

FBQ000
FIBROUS GLASS

PROP: Is of a borosilicate variety, of low alkalinity and consists of calcia-alumina-silicate (85INA8 5,270,86).

SYNS: FIBERGLASS ◇ FIBROUS GLASS DUST (ACGIH) ◇ GLASS ◇ GLASS FIBERS

TOXICITY DATA with REFERENCE
CAR: ihl-rat TCLo: 5 mg/m³/7H/90W-I   NTIS** PB83-258111
NEO: imp-rat TDLo: 200 mg/kg   JJIND8 67,965,81
ETA: imp-mus TD: 1600 mg/kg   BJURAN 36,225,64
ETA: imp-rat TD: 200 mg/kg   IARCCD 8,289,73
ETA: ipl-rat TD: 100 mg/kg   IAPUDO 30,311,80
ETA: ipr-ham TDLo: 400 mg/kg   IAPUDO 30,337,80
ETA: ipr-rat TDLo: 50 mg/kg   IAPUDO 30,337,80
ETA: ipr-rbt TDLo: 25 mg/kg   IAPUDO 30,337,80
MUT: oms-ham: ovr 10 mg/L   MUREAV 116,369,83
MUT: oms-hmn: fbr 10 mg/L   MUREAV 116,369,83

OSHA PEL: TWA 15 mg/m³ (total dust); 5 mg/m³ (nuisance dust)   ACGIH TLV: TWA 10 mg/m³ (dust)   NIOSH REL: TWA 5 mg/m³ (total fibrous glass)

SAFETY PROFILE: Questionable carcinogen with experimental carcinogenic, neoplastigenic, and tumorigenic data by inhalation and other routes. Human mutation data reported. Used as thermal and acoustistical insulation.

FBU000   CAS: 59536-65-1
FIREMASTER BP-6

PROP: Consists mainly of penta-, hexa-, and heptabromobiphenyl, with lesser ammounts of tetra- and other brominated biphenyls. (ENVRAL 10,390,75)

SYNS: HEXABROMOBIPHENYL (TECHNICAL GRADE) ◇ PBB ◇ POLYBROMINATED BIPHENYLS

TOXICITY DATA with REFERENCE
CAR: orl-rat TD: 1200 mg/kg/18W-I   JJIND8 66,535,81
ETA: orl-rat TD: 1000 mg/kg   EVHPAZ 23,265,78
MUT: dnd-sal: oth 8 μmol/L   EVHPAZ 23,51,78

CONSENSUS REPORTS: IARC Cancer Review: Animal Inadequate Evidence IMEMDT

18,107,78.   Polybrominated biphenyl compounds are on the Community Right-To-Know List.

SAFETY PROFILE: Questionable carcinogen with experimental carcinogenic, tumorigenic, and teratogenic data. Poison by ingestion. Experimental reproductive effects. Mutation data reported. When heated to decomposition it emits very toxic Br⁻.

FDF000   CAS: 206-44-0
FLUORANTHENE
mf: $C_{16}H_{10}$ mw: 202.26

PROP: A polycyclic hydrocarbon. Colorless solid. Mp: 120°, bp: 367°, vap press: 0.01 mm @ 20°.

SYNS: 1,2-BENZACENAPHTHENE ◇ BENZO(jk)FLUORENE ◇ IDRYL ◇ 1,2-(1,8-NAPHTHALENEDIYL)BENZENE ◇ 1,2-(1,8-NAPHTHYLENE)BENZENE ◇ RCRA WASTE NUMBER U120

TOXICITY DATA with REFERENCE
ETA: skn-mus TDLo: 280 mg/kg/58W-I   JNCIAM 56,1237,76
MUT: mma-sat 5 μg/plate   MUREAV 156,61,85
MUT: msc-ham: ovr 20 mg/L   ENMUDM 6,539,84
MUT: msc-hmn: lym 2 μmol/L   DTESD7 10,277,82

CONSENSUS REPORTS: IARC Cancer Review: GROUP 3 IMEMDT 7,56,87; Animal No Evidence IMEMDT 32,355,83. Reported in EPA TSCA Inventory. EPA Genetic Toxicology Program.

SAFETY PROFILE: Questionable carcinogen with experimental tumorigenic data. Poison by intravenous route. Moderately toxic by ingestion and skin contact. Human mutation data reported. Combustible when exposed to heat or flame. When heated to decomposition it emits acrid smoke and irritating fumes.

FDM000   CAS: 525-64-4
FLUORENE-2,7-DIAMINE
mf: $C_{13}H_{11}N_2$ mw: 195.26

SYNS: 2,7-DIAMINOFLUORENE ◇ 2,7-FLUORENEDIAMINE ◇ 2,7-FLUOROENEDIAMINE

TOXICITY DATA with REFERENCE
CAR: orl-rat TD: 3600 mg/kg/27D-I   CNREA8 28,924,68
CAR: orl-rat TDLo: 1000 mg/kg   CNREA8 26,619,66

MUT: dnd-mus:ast 5 μmol/L   MUREAV 89,95,81
MUT: dns-hmn:lym 10 μmol/L   SHYCD4
(40),47,83
MUT: dns-rat:lvr 500 nmol/L   ENMUDM 3,11,81
MUT: mma-sat 5 μg/plate   MUREAV 143,213,85
MUT: mmo-sat 10 μg/plate   MUREAV 143,213,85

CONSENSUS REPORTS: EPA Genetic Toxicology Program.

SAFETY PROFILE: Questionable carcinogen with experimental carcinogenic data. Moderately toxic by ingestion. Human mutation data reported. When heated to decomposition it emits toxic fumes of NO_x.

FDO000   CAS: 486-25-9
9H-FLUOREN-9-ONE
mf: $C_{13}H_8O$ mw: 180.21

PROP: Yellow, rhombic crystals. Mp: 83-4°, bp: 341.5°. Insol in water; very sol in alc and ether.

SYNS: FLUOREN-9-ONE ◇ 9-FLUORENONE

TOXICITY DATA with REFERENCE
ETA: scu-rat TDLo: 300 mg/kg/26W-I   CNREA8
7,453,47

CONSENSUS REPORTS: Reported in EPA TSCA Inventory. EPA Genetic Toxicology Program.

SAFETY PROFILE: Questionable carcinogen with experimental tumorigenic data. When heated to decomposition it emits acrid smoke and irritating fumes.

FDP000   CAS: 206-00-8
FLUORENO(9,1-gh)QUINOLINE
mf: $C_{19}H_{11}N$ mw: 253.31

SYN: PYRIDO(3',2':3,4)FLUORANTHENE

TOXICITY DATA with REFERENCE
ETA: scu-mus TDLo: 72 mg/kg/9W-I   COREAF
259,3387,64

SAFETY PROFILE: Questionable carcinogen with experimental tumorigenic data. When heated to decomposition it emits toxic fumes of NO_x.

FDQ000   CAS: 28314-03-6
N-FLUOREN-1-YL ACETAMIDE
mf: $C_{15}H_{13}NO$ mw: 223.29

SYNS: 1-FLUORENYLACETAMIDE ◇ N-1-FLUORENYL-ACETAMIDE

TOXICITY DATA with REFERENCE
ETA: ipr-rat TDLo: 627 mg/kg/4W-I   CNREA8
30,1485,70
ETA: orl-rat TDLo: 4400 mg/kg/44W-C:TER
JNCIAM 24,149,60

SAFETY PROFILE: Questionable carcinogen with experimental tumorigenic and teratogenic data. When heated to decomposition it emits toxic fumes of NO_x.

FDS000   CAS: 6292-55-3
3-FLUORENYL ACETAMIDE
mf: $C_{15}H_{13}NO$ mw: 223.29

SYNS: N-3-FLUORENYL ACETAMIDE ◇ N-FLUOREN-3-YL ACETAMIDE ◇ N-9H-FLUOREN-3-YL ACETAMIDE

TOXICITY DATA with REFERENCE
ETA: imp-rat TDLo: 22 mg/kg   CNREA8 37,111,77
ETA: ipr-rat TDLo: 654 mg/kg/4W-I   CNREA8
30,1485,70
ETA: orl-rat TDLo: 6100 mg/kg/66W-C
JNCIAM 24,149,60

SAFETY PROFILE: Questionable carcinogen with experimental tumorigenic data. When heated to decomposition it emits toxic fumes of NO_x.

FDT000   CAS: 22251-01-0
1-FLUORENYL ACETHYDROXAMIC ACID
mf: $C_{15}H_{13}NO_2$ mw: 239.29

SYNS: N-FLUOREN-1-YL ACETOHYDROXAMIC ACID ◇ N-HYDROXY-1-FLUORENYL ACETAMIDE

TOXICITY DATA with REFERENCE
NEO: ipr-rat TDLo: 603 mg/kg/4W-I   CNREA8
30,1485,70

SAFETY PROFILE: Questionable carcinogen with experimental neoplastigenic data. When heated to decomposition it emits toxic fumes of NO_x.

FDU000   CAS: 22225-32-7
3-FLUORENYL ACETHYDROXAMIC ACID
mf: $C_{15}H_{13}NO_2$ mw: 239.29

SYNS: N-FLUOREN-3-YL ACETOHYDROXAMIC ACID ◇ N-HYDROXY-3-FAA ◇ N-HYDROXY-3-FLUORENYL ACETAMIDE

TOXICITY DATA with REFERENCE
CAR: ipr-rat TDLo: 280 mg/kg/4W-I   JNCIAM
60,433,78

CAR: orl-rat TDLo: 3000 mg/kg/21W-C
CNREA8 35,447,75

NEO: imp-rat TDLo: 24 mg/kg   CNREA8
37,111,77

NEO: ipr-rat TD: 270 mg/kg/4W-I   CNREA8
30,1485,70

ETA: imp-rat TD: 24 mg/kg   CNREA8 33,2489,73

ETA: imp-rat TD: 40 mg/kg   JNCIAM 60,433,78

SAFETY PROFILE: Questionable carcinogen with experimental carcinogenic, neoplastigenic, and tumorigenic data. When heated to decomposition it emits toxic fumes of NO_x.

FDU875   CAS: 14751-87-2
N-FLUOREN-2-YLACETOHYDROXAMIC ACID, COBALT(2+) COMPLEX
mf: $C_{30}H_{24}N_2O_4 \cdot Co$ mw: 535.49

SYNS: COBALT, BIS(N-9H-FLUOREN-2-YL-N-HY-DROXYACETAMIDATO-O,O')-(9CI) ◇ COBALT N-FLUO-REN-2-YLACETOHYDROXAMATE ◇ COBALT SALTS ◇ N-HYDROXY-2-ACETYLAMINOFLUORENE, COBAL-TOUS CHELATE

TOXICITY DATA with REFERENCE
NEO: scu-rat TDLo: 160 mg/kg/4W-I   CNREA8
25,527,65

SAFETY PROFILE: Questionable carcinogen with experimental neoplastigenic data. When heated to decomposition it emits toxic fumes of NO_x and Co.

FDV000   CAS: 16808-85-8
N-FLUOREN-2-YL ACETOHYDROXAMIC ACID SULFATE
mf: $C_{15}H_{13}NO_5S$ mw: 319.35

SYNS: SULFATE ESTER of N-HYDROXY-N-2-FLUORENYL ACETAMIDE ◇ N-SULFONOXY-AAF ◇ N-SULFONOXY-N-ACETYL-2-AMINOFLUORENE

TOXICITY DATA with REFERENCE
ETA: scu-rat TDLo: 255 mg/kg/15W-I   CNREA8
37,1461,77

CONSENSUS REPORTS: EPA Genetic Toxicology Program.

SAFETY PROFILE: Questionable carcinogen with experimental tumorigenic data. When heated to decomposition it emits very toxic fumes of NO_x and SO_x.

FDX000   CAS: 3671-78-1
N-(2-FLUORENYL)BENZAMIDE
mf: $C_{20}H_{15}NO$ mw: 285.36

SYNS: 2-BENZOYLAMINOFLUORENE ◇ N-FLUOREN-2-YL BENZAMIDE ◇ N-9H-FLUOREN-2-YL-BENZAMIDE (9CI)

TOXICITY DATA with REFERENCE
ETA: ipr-rat TD: 540 mg/kg/4W-I   NATUAS
209,202,66

ETA: ipr-rat TDLo: 540 mg/kg/4W-I   CNREA8
27,1443,67

MUT: mma-sat 100 ng/plate   BBRCA9 71,1201,76

SAFETY PROFILE: Questionable carcinogen with experimental tumorigenic data. Mutation data reported. When heated to decomposition it emits toxic fumes of NO_x.

FDY000   CAS: 29968-64-7
N-FLUOREN-1-YL BENZOHYDROXAMIC ACID
mf: $C_{20}H_{15}NO_2$ mw: 301.36

SYN: N-HYDROXY-1-FLUORENYL BENZAMIDE

TOXICITY DATA with REFERENCE
NEO: ipr-rat TDLo: 823 mg/kg/4W-I   CNREA8
30,1485,70

SAFETY PROFILE: Questionable carcinogen with experimental neoplastigenic data. When heated to decomposition it emits toxic fumes of NO_x.

FDZ000   CAS: 3671-71-4
N-FLUOREN-2-YL BENZOHYDROXAMIC ACID
mf: $C_{20}H_{15}NO_2$ mw: 301.36

SYNS: N-BENZOYLOXY-ACETYLAMINOFLUORENE ◇ N-(2-FLUORENYL)BENZOHYDROXAMIC ACID ◇ N-9H-FLUOREN-2-YL-N-HYDROXYBENZAMIDE ◇ N-HYDROXY-2-BENZOYLAMINOFLUORENE ◇ N-HY-DROXY-N-2-FLUORENYLBENZAMIDE

TOXICITY DATA with REFERENCE
CAR: ipr-rat TD: 540 mg/kg/4W-I   NATUAS
209,202,66

CAR: ipr-rat TDLo: 540 mg/kg/4W-I   CNREA8
27,1443,67

CAR: orl-rat TDLo: 5200 mg/kg/23W-I   CNREA8
30,1485,70

MUT: mma-sat 1500 ng/plate   CBINA8 54,71,85

MUT: mmo-bcs 10 mol   MOPMA3 4,411,68

MUT: oms-bcs 10 mol   MOPMA3 4,411,68

SAFETY PROFILE: Questionable carcinogen with experimental carcinogenic data. Mutation data reported. When heated to decomposition it emits toxic fumes of NO_x.

FEE000 CAS: 391-57-1
**N,N'-FLUOREN-2,7-YLENE
BIS(TRIFLUOROACETAMIDE)**
mf: $C_{17}H_{10}F_6N_2O_2$ mw: 388.29

TOXICITY DATA with REFERENCE
CAR: orl-rat TDLo:4850 mg/kg/37W-C

JNCIAM 30,143,63
ETA: orl-rat TD:5 g/kg/48W-C JJIND8 71,211,83

SAFETY PROFILE: Questionable carcinogen
with experimental carcinogenic and tumorigenic
data. When heated to decomposition it emits
toxic fumes of F^- and NO_x.

FEF000 CAS: 6957-71-7
N-FLUOREN-2-YL FORMAMIDE
mf: $C_{14}H_{11}NO$ mw: 209.26

SYNS: N,2-FLUORENYL FORMAMIDE ◇ 2-FORMYLAMI-
NOFLUORENE

TOXICITY DATA with REFERENCE
CAR: orl-rat TDLo:4400 mg/kg/35W-C

CNREA8 22,1002,62
MUT: mma-sat 100 ng/plate BBRCA9 71,1201,76

SAFETY PROFILE: Questionable carcinogen
with experimental carcinogenic data. Mutation
data reported. When heated to decomposition
it emits toxic fumes of NO_x.

FEG000 CAS: 67176-33-4
**N-(2-FLUORENYL)
FORMOHYDROXAMIC ACID**
mf: $C_{14}H_{11}NO_2$ mw: 225.26

SYNS: N-FORMYL-N-2-FLUORENYLHYDROXYLAMINE
◇ N-HYDROXY-N-2-FORMYLAMINOFLUORENE

TOXICITY DATA with REFERENCE
CAR: par-rat TDLo:2253 µg/kg NTIS** PB86-
115920
CAR: par-rat TDLo:2815 µg/kg CRNGDP
3,233,82
MUT: mma-sat 5 µg/plate CNREA8 40,1204,80
MUT: mmo-sat 10 µg/plate CRNGDP 3,233,82

SAFETY PROFILE: Questionable carcinogen
with experimental carcinogenic data. Mutation
data reported. When heated to decomposition
it emits toxic fumes of NO_x.

FEH000 CAS: 51029-30-2
3-FLUORENYLHYDROXYLAMINE
mf: $C_{13}H_{11}NO$ mw: 197.25

SYNS: N-FLUOREN-3-YL HYDROXYLAMINE ◇ N-HY-
DROXY-3-AMINOFLUORENE

TOXICITY DATA with REFERENCE
ETA: imp-rat TDLo:20 mg/kg CNREA8
33,2489,73

SAFETY PROFILE: Questionable carcinogen
with experimental tumorigenic data. When
heated to decomposition it emits toxic fumes
of NO_x.

FEI000 CAS: 34461-49-9
**N-FLUOREN-2-YLHYDROXYLAMINE-o-
GLUCURONIDE**
mf: $C_{19}H_{19}NO_8$ mw: 389.39

SYN: N-2-FLUORENYLHYDROXYLAMINE-o-GLUCURO-
NIDE

TOXICITY DATA with REFERENCE
ETA: scu-rat TDLo:750 mg/kg/9W-I CNREA8
31,1645,71

SAFETY PROFILE: Questionable carcinogen
with experimental tumorigenic data. When
heated to decomposition it emits toxic fumes
of NO_x.

FEI500 CAS: 63019-68-1
2-FLUORENYLMONOMETHYLAMINE
mf: $C_{14}H_{13}N$ mw: 195.28

SYNS: 2-METHYLAMINOFLUORENE ◇ N-MONO-
METHYL-2-AMINOFLUORENE ◇ 2-MONOMETHYL-
AMINOFLUORENE

TOXICITY DATA with REFERENCE
ETA: orl-rat TD:4300 mg/kg/47W-C JBCHA3
221,845,56
ETA: orl-rat TDLo:1260 mg/kg/24W-I BJCAAI
6,89,52

SAFETY PROFILE: Questionable carcinogen
with experimental tumorigenic data. When
heated to decomposition it emits toxic fumes
of NO_x.

FEM000 · CAS: 63224-45-3
**N-(2-FLUORENYL)
MYRISTOHYDROXAMIC ACID ACETATE**
mf: $C_{29}H_{39}NO_3$ mw: 449.69

SYNS: N-ACETOXY-2-MYRISTOYL-AMINOFLUORENE
◇ N-(ACETYLOXY)-N-9H-FLUOREN-2-YL-TETRADECAN-
AMIDE

TOXICITY DATA with REFERENCE
CAR: scu-rat TDLo:114 mg/kg/6W-I CNREA8
37,1461,77
MUT: dns-hmn:fbr 100 mmol/L/5H IJCNAW
16,284,75

MUT: mma-sat 20 nmol/plate   CNREA8
37,1461,77

CONSENSUS REPORTS: EPA Genetic Toxicology Program.

SAFETY PROFILE: Questionable carcinogen with experimental carcinogenic data. Human mutation data reported. When heated to decomposition it emits toxic fumes of NO_x.

FEN000   CAS: 2485-10-1
N-FLUORENYL-2-PHTHALIMIC ACID
mf: $C_{21}H_{15}NO_3$ mw: 329.37

SYNS: 2-BENZOYLAMIDOFLUORENE-2'-CARBOXYLATE ◇ 2-BENZOYLAMINOFLUORENE-2'-CARBOXYLATE ◇ N-(2-FLUORENYL)PHTHALAMIC ACID

TOXICITY DATA with REFERENCE
ETA: orl-rat TD:6000 mg/kg/42W-C   CNREA8
20,1252,60
ETA: orl-rat TDLo:5000mg/kg/42W-C   AICCA6
20,1364,64

SAFETY PROFILE: Questionable carcinogen with experimental tumorigenic data. When heated to decomposition it emits toxic fumes of NO_x.

FEO000   CAS: 52663-84-0
N-(2-FLUORENYL) PROPIONOHYDROXAMIC ACID
mf: $C_{16}H_{15}NO_2$ mw: 253.32

SYNS: N-HYDROXY-N-2-PROPIONYLAMINO FLUORENE ◇ N-PROPIONYL-N-2-FLUORENYLHYDROXYLAMINE

TOXICITY DATA with REFERENCE
CAR: par-rat TDLo:2533 μg/kg   NTIS** PB86-
115920
ETA: par-rat TDLo:3166 μg/kg   CRNGDP
3,233,82
MUT: mma-sat 5 μg/plate   CNREA8 40,1204,80
MUT: mmo-sat 10 μg/plate   CRNGDP 3,233,82

SAFETY PROFILE: Questionable carcinogen with experimental carcinogenic and tumorigenic data. Mutation data reported. When heated to decomposition it emits toxic fumes of NO_x.

FEP000   CAS: 59935-47-6
N-2-FLUORENYL SUCCINAMIC ACID
mf: $C_{17}H_{15}NO_3$ mw: 281.33

TOXICITY DATA with REFERENCE
NEO: orl-rat TDLo:6200 mg/kg/72W-C
JNCIAM 24,149,60

SAFETY PROFILE: Questionable carcinogen with experimental neoplastigenic data. When heated to decomposition it emits toxic fumes of NO_x.

FER000   CAS: 363-17-7
N-FLUOREN-2-YL-2,2,2-TRIFLUOROACETAMIDE
mf: $C_{15}H_{10}F_3NO$ mw: 277.26

SYNS: N-(2-FLUORENYL)-2,2,2-TRIFLUOROACETAMIDE ◇ 2-TRIFLUOROACETYLAMINOFLUORENE ◇ 2,2,2-TRI-FLUORO-N-(FLUOREN-2-YL)ACETAMIDE

TOXICITY DATA with REFERENCE
CAR: orl-rat TD:4500 mg/kg/26W-C   CNREA8
22,1002,62
CAR: orl-rat TDLo:3750 mg/kg/44W-C
JNCIAM 24,149,60

SAFETY PROFILE: Questionable carcinogen with experimental carcinogenic data. When heated to decomposition it emits very toxic F^- and NO_x.

FEW000   CAS: 518-47-8
FLUORESCEIN SODIUM
mf: $C_{20}H_{10}O_5 \cdot 2Na$ mw: 376.28

PROP: Orange-red powder; sol in water; sltly sol in alcohol.

SYNS: AIZEN URANINE ◇ CALCOCID URANINE B4315 ◇ 9-o-CARBOXYPHENYL-6-HYDROXY-3-ISOXANTHONE, DISODIUM SALT ◇ CERTIQUAL FLUORESCEINE ◇ C.I. 766 ◇ C.I. ACID YELLOW 73 ◇ C.I. 45350 DISODIUM SALT ◇ D&C YELLOW No. 8 ◇ DISODIUM-6-HYDROXY-3-OXO-9-XANTHENE-o-BENZOATE ◇ FLUORESCEIN SODIUM B.P ◇ FLUORESCEIN, SOLUBLE ◇ FLUOR-I-STRIP A.T. ◇ FUL-GLO ◇ FUNDUSCEIN ◇ FURANIUM ◇ HIDACID URA-NINE ◇ NCI-C54706 ◇ RESORCINOL PHTHALEIN SODIUM ◇ SODIUM FLUORESCEIN ◇ SODIUM FLUORESCEINATE ◇ SODIUM SALT of HYDROXY-o-CARBOXY-PHENYL-FLUO-RONE ◇ SOLUBLE FLUORESCEIN ◇ SPIRO(ISOBENZOFU-RAN-1(3H),9'-(9H)XANTHENE-3-ONE, 3',6'-DIHYDROXY-DISODIUM SALT ◇ URANIN ◇ URANINE A EXTRA ◇ URANINE USP XII ◇ URANINE YELLOW ◇ 11824 YELLOW ◇ 12417 YELLOW

TOXICITY DATA with REFERENCE
ETA: scu-rat TD:16 g/kg/1Y-I   GANNA2
47,51,56
ETA: scu-rat TDLo:19 g/kg/79W-I   GANNA2
45,446,54
MUT: dnd-esc 15 μmol/L   MUREAV 89,95,81

CONSENSUS REPORTS: Reported in EPA TSCA Inventory.

SAFETY PROFILE: Questionable carcinogen with experimental tumorigenic data. Moderately toxic by intraperitoneal route. Mildly toxic by ingestion. Experimental reproductive effects. Mutation data reported. When heated to decomposition it emits toxic fumes of Na_2O.

FFG000   CAS: 343-89-5
7-FLUORO-2-ACETAMIDO-FLUORENE
mf: $C_{15}H_{12}FNO$ mw: 241.28

SYNS: 7-FLUORO-2-ACETYLAMINOFLUORENE ◇ N-(7-FLUOROFLUORENE-2-YL)ACETAMIDE

TOXICITY DATA with REFERENCE
CAR: orl-rat TD: 1200 mg/kg/14W-C   CNREA8 15,188,55
CAR: orl-rat TDLo: 450 mg/kg/11W-C   CNREA8 26,2239,66
ETA: orl-rat TD: 1200 mg/kg/15W-C   CNREA8 18,469,58
MUT: dnd-rat-par 27 μmol/kg   CBINA8 40,27,82

SAFETY PROFILE: Questionable carcinogen with experimental carcinogenic and tumorigenic data. Mutation data reported. When heated to decomposition it emits toxic fumes of F^- and NO_x.

FFL000   CAS: 2824-10-4
1-FLUORO-2-ACETYLAMINOFLUORENE
mf: $C_{15}H_{12}FNO$ mw: 241.28

SYNS: 1-FLUORO-2-FAA ◇ N-(1-FLUOROFLUOREN-2-YL)ACETAMIDE

TOXICITY DATA with REFERENCE
CAR: orl-rat TDLo: 1400 mg/kg/19W-C
CNREA8 22,1002,62

SAFETY PROFILE: Questionable carcinogen with experimental carcinogenic data. When heated to decomposition it emits very toxic fumes of F^- and NO_x.

FFM000   CAS: 2823-93-0
3-FLUORO-2-ACETYLAMINOFLUORENE
mf: $C_{15}H_{12}FNO$ mw: 241.28

SYNS: 3-FLUORO-2-FAA ◇ N-(3-FLUOROFLUOREN-2-YL)ACETAMIDE

TOXICITY DATA with REFERENCE
CAR: orl-rat TDLo: 3900 mg/kg/26W-C
CNREA8 22,1002,62

SAFETY PROFILE: Questionable carcinogen with experimental carcinogenic data. When heated to decomposition it emits very toxic fumes of F^- and NO_x.

FFN000   CAS: 2823-91-8
4-FLUORO-2-ACETYLAMINOFLUORENE
mf: $C_{15}H_{12}FNO$ mw: 241.28

SYNS: 4-FLUORO-2-FAA ◇ N-(4-FLUOROFLUOREN-2-YL)ACETAMIDE

TOXICITY DATA with REFERENCE
CAR: orl-rat TDLo: 2560 mg/kg/17W-C
CNREA8 22,1002,62

SAFETY PROFILE: Questionable carcinogen with experimental carcinogenic data. When heated to decomposition it emits very toxic fumes of F^- and NO_x.

FFO000   CAS: 2823-90-7
5-FLUORO-2-ACETYLAMINOFLUORENE
mf: $C_{15}H_{12}FNO$ mw: 241.28

SYNS: 5-FLUORO-2-FAA ◇ N-(5-FLUOROFLUOREN-2-YL)ACETAMIDE

TOXICITY DATA with REFERENCE
CAR: orl-rat TDLo: 3900 mg/kg/26W-C
CNREA8 22,1002,62

SAFETY PROFILE: Questionable carcinogen with experimental carcinogenic data. When heated to decomposition it emits very toxic fumes of F^- and NO_x.

FFP000   CAS: 2823-94-1
6-FLUORO-2-ACETYLAMINOFLUORENE
mf: $C_{15}H_{12}FNO$ mw: 241.28

SYNS: 6-FLUORO-2-FAA ◇ N-(6-FLUOROFLUOREN-2-YL)ACETAMIDE

TOXICITY DATA with REFERENCE
CAR: orl-rat TDLo: 3900 mg/kg/26W-C
CNREA8 22,1002,62

SAFETY PROFILE: Questionable carcinogen with experimental carcinogenic data. When heated to decomposition it emits very toxic fumes of F^- and NO_x.

FFQ000   CAS: 2823-95-2
8-FLUORO-2-ACETYLAMINOFLUORENE
mf: $C_{15}H_{12}FNO$ mw: 241.28

SYNS: 8-FLUORO-2-FAA ◇ N-(8-FLUOROFLUOREN-2-YL)ACETAMIDE

TOXICITY DATA with REFERENCE
CAR: orl-rat TDLo: 3900 mg/kg/26W-C
CNREA8 22,1002,62

SAFETY PROFILE: Questionable carcinogen with experimental carcinogenic data. When heated to decomposition it emits very toxic fumes of F^- and NO_x.

FFZ000   CAS: 388-72-7
4-FLUOROBENZANTHRACENE
mf: $C_{18}H_{11}F$ mw: 246.29

SYNS: 4-FLUOROBENZ(a)ANTHRACENE ◇ 4'-FLUORO-1,2-BENZANTHRACENE

TOXICITY DATA with REFERENCE
NEO: scu-rat TDLo: 8 mg/kg   CNREA8 23,229,63
ETA: scu-mus TDLo: 41 mg/kg   CNREA8 23,229,63

SAFETY PROFILE: Questionable carcinogen with experimental neoplastigenic and tumorigenic data. When heated to decomposition it emits toxic fumes of F^-.

FGB000   CAS: 52831-45-5
2-FLUORO-BENZO(e)(1) BENZOTHIOPYRANO(4,3-b)INDOLE
mf: $C_{19}H_{10}FNS$ mw: 303.36

TOXICITY DATA with REFERENCE
NEO: scu-mus TDLo: 72 mg/kg/9W-I   MUREAV 66,307,79
MUT: mma-sat 30 µg/plate   MUREAV 66,307,79

SAFETY PROFILE: Questionable carcinogen with experimental neoplastigenic data. Mutation data reported. When heated to decomposition it emits very toxic fumes of SO_x, NO_x, and F^-.

FGC000   CAS: 52831-56-8
3-FLUORO-BENZO(e)(1) BENZOTHIOPYRANO(4,3-b)INDOLE
mf: $C_{19}H_{10}FNS$ mw: 303.36

TOXICITY DATA with REFERENCE
NEO: scu-mus TDLo: 72 mg/kg/9W-I   MUREAV 66,307,79
MUT: mma-sat 30 µg/plate   MUREAV 66,307,79

SAFETY PROFILE: Questionable carcinogen with experimental neoplastigenic data. Mutation data reported. When heated to decomposition it emits very toxic fumes of NO_x, SO_x, and F^-.

FGD000   CAS: 52831-68-2
4-FLUORO-BENZO(e)(1) BENZOTHIOPYRANO(4,3-b)INDOLE
mf: $C_{19}H_{10}FNS$ mw: 303.36

TOXICITY DATA with REFERENCE
NEO: scu-mus TDLo: 72 mg/kg/9W-I   MUREAV 66,307,79
MUT: mma-sat 30 µg/plate   MUREAV 66,307,79

SAFETY PROFILE: Questionable carcinogen with experimental neoplastigenic data. Mutation data reported. When heated to decomposition it emits very toxic fumes of F^-, NO_x, and SO_x.

FGF000   CAS: 52831-53-5
3-FLUORO-BENZO(g)(1) BENZOTHIOPYRANO(4,3-b)INDOLE
mf: $C_{19}H_{10}FNS$ mw: 303.36

TOXICITY DATA with REFERENCE
NEO: scu-mus TDLo: 92 mg/kg/9W-I   MUREAV 66,307,79
MUT: mma-sat 30 µg/plate   MUREAV 66,307,79

SAFETY PROFILE: Questionable carcinogen with experimental neoplastigenic data. Mutation data reported. When heated to decomposition it emits very toxic fumes of NO_x, SO_x, and F^-.

FGG000   CAS: 52831-65-9
4-FLUORO-BENZO(g)(1) BENZOTHIOPYRANO(4,3-b)INDOLE
mf: $C_{19}H_{10}FNS$ mw: 303.36

TOXICITY DATA with REFERENCE
NEO: scu-mus TDLo: 72 mg/kg/9W-I   MUREAV 66,307,79
MUT: mma-sat 30 µg/plate   MUREAV 66,307,79

SAFETY PROFILE: Questionable carcinogen with experimental neoplastigenic data. Mutation data reported. When heated to decomposition it emits very toxic fumes of F^-, NO_x, and SO_x.

FGI000   CAS: 61735-77-1
3-FLUOROBENZO(rst)PENTAPHENE
mf: $C_{24}H_{13}F$ mw: 320.37

TOXICITY DATA with REFERENCE
NEO: scu-mus TDLo: 20 mg/kg   JFLCAR 8,513,76

SAFETY PROFILE: Questionable carcinogen with experimental neoplastigenic data. When heated to decomposition it emits toxic fumes of F^-.

FGJ000   CAS: 52831-39-7
2-FLUORO-(1)BENZOTHIOPYRANO(4,3-b)INDOLE
mf: $C_{15}H_8FNS$ mw: 253.30

SYN: 2-FLUOROTHIOPYRANO(4,3-b)BENZ(e)INDOLE

TOXICITY DATA with REFERENCE
NEO: scu-mus TDLo:72 mg/kg/9W-I   MUREAV
66,307,79
MUT: mma-sat 30 μg/plate   MUREAV 66,307,79

SAFETY PROFILE: Questionable carcinogen with experimental neoplastigenic data. Mutation data reported. When heated to decomposition it emits very toxic fumes such as F^-, SO_x, and NO_x.

FGL000   CAS: 52831-62-6
4-FLUORO-(1)BENZOTHIOPYRANO(4,3-b)INDOLE
mf: $C_{15}H_8FNS$ mw: 253.30

SYN: 4-FLUOROTHIOPYRANO(4,3-b)BENZ(e)INDOLE

TOXICITY DATA with REFERENCE
NEO: scu-mus TDLo:72 mg/kg/9W-I   MUREAV
66,307,79
MUT: mma-sat 30 μg/plate   MUREAV 66,307,79

SAFETY PROFILE: Questionable carcinogen with experimental neoplastigenic data. Mutation data reported. When heated to decomposition it emits very toxic fumes such as F^-, SO_x, and NO_x.

FGO000   CAS: 52831-58-0
4-FLUORO-6H-(1)BENZOTHIOPYRANO (4,3-b)QUINOLINE
mf: $C_{16}H_{10}FNS$ mw: 267.33

TOXICITY DATA with REFERENCE
NEO: scu-mus TDLo:72 mg/kg/9W-I   MUREAV
66,307,79
MUT: mma-sat 90 μg/plate   MUREAV 66,307,79

SAFETY PROFILE: Questionable carcinogen with experimental neoplastigenic data. Mutation data reported. When heated to decomposition it emits very toxic fumes such as F^-, NO_x, and SO_x.

FHH025   CAS: 67639-45-6
5-FLUORO-7-CHLOROMETHYL-12-METHYLBENZ(a)ANTHRACENE
mf: $C_{20}H_{14}ClF$ mw: 308.79

SYN: 7-(CHLOROMETHYL)-5-FLUORO-12-METHYL-BENZ(a)ANTHRACENE

TOXICITY DATA with REFERENCE
NEO: ivn-mus TDLo:1239 μg/kg   CNREA8
40,782,80

SAFETY PROFILE: Questionable carcinogen with experimental neoplastigenic data. When heated to decomposition it emits toxic fumes of Cl^- and F^-.

FHP000   CAS: 1764-39-2
6-FLUORODIBENZ(a,h)ANTHRACENE
mf: $C_{22}H_{13}F$ mw: 296.35

SYN: 4-FLUORO-1,2:5,6-DIBENZANTHRACENE

TOXICITY DATA with REFERENCE
ETA: scu-mus TDLo:200 mg/kg/I   BECCAN
40,30,62

SAFETY PROFILE: Questionable carcinogen with experimental tumorigenic data. When heated to decomposition it emits toxic fumes of F^-.

FHQ000   CAS: 321-25-5
2-FLUORO-4-DIMETHYLAMINOAZOBENZENE
mf: $C_{14}H_{14}FN_3$ mw: 243.31

SYN: N,N-DIMETHYL-2-FLUORO-4-PHENYLAZOANILINE

TOXICITY DATA with REFERENCE
ETA: orl-rat TDLo:3200 mg/kg/12W-C
CNREA8 13,93,53

SAFETY PROFILE: Questionable carcinogen with experimental tumorigenic data. When heated to decomposition it emits toxic fumes of NO_x and F^-.

FHQ010   CAS: 331-91-9
2'-FLUORO-4-DIMETHYLAMINOAZOBENZENE
mf: $C_{14}H_{14}FN_3$ mw: 243.31

SYN: N,N-DIMETHYL-p-(2-FLUOROPHENYLAZO)ANI-LINE

TOXICITY DATA with REFERENCE
ETA: orl-rat TD:3200 mg/kg/12W-C   CNREA8
13,93,53
ETA: orl-rat TDLo:3150 mg/kg/13W-C
CNREA8 9,652,49

SAFETY PROFILE: Questionable carcinogen with experimental tumorigenic data. When heated to decomposition it emits very toxic fumes of F^- and NO_x.

FHQ100   CAS: 332-54-7
3'-FLUORO-4-DIMETHYLAMINOAZOBENZENE
mf: $C_{14}H_{14}FN_3$ mw: 243.31

SYN: m-FLUORODIMETHYLAMINOAZOBENZENE

TOXICITY DATA with REFERENCE
NEO: orl-rat TDLo:5300 mg/kg/21W-C
  CNREA8 17,387,57
ETA: orl-rat TD:3150 mg/kg/13W-C   CNREA8
  9,652,49
ETA: orl-rat TD:3200 mg/kg/12W-C   CNREA8
  13,93,53

SAFETY PROFILE: Questionable carcinogen
with experimental neoplastigenic and tumorigenic data. Moderately toxic by subcutaneous
route. Experimental reproductive effects. When
heated to decomposition it emits toxic fumes
of F$^-$ and NO$_x$.

FHR000   CAS: 64038-39-7
10-FLUORO-9,12-DIMETHYLBENZ(a)
ACRIDINE
mf: $C_{19}H_{14}FN$ mw: 275.34
SYNS: 2,10-DIMETHYL-3-FLUORO-5,6-BENZACRIDINE
◇ 9,12-DIMETHYL-10-FLUOROBENZ(a)ACRIDINE
◇ 3-FLUORO-2,10-DIMETHYL-5,6-BENZACRIDINE

TOXICITY DATA with REFERENCE
ETA: skn-mus TD:370 mg/kg/31W-I   ACRSAJ
  4,315,56
ETA: skn-mus TDLo:324 mg/kg/27W-I
  AICCA6 11,736,55

SAFETY PROFILE: Questionable carcinogen
with experimental tumorigenic data. When
heated to decomposition it emits toxic F$^-$ and
NO$_x$.

FHS000   CAS: 68141-57-1
1-FLUORO-7,12-DIMETHYLBENZ(a)
ANTHRACENE
mf: $C_{20}H_{15}F$ mw: 274.35
SYN: 7,12-DIMETHYL-1-FLUOROBENZ(a)ANTHRACENE

TOXICITY DATA with REFERENCE
ETA: skn-mus TDLo:110 µg/kg   CNREA8
  39,411,79
MUT: msc-ham:lng 1 mg/L   MUREAV 136,65,84

CONSENSUS REPORTS: EPA Genetic Toxicology Program.

SAFETY PROFILE: Questionable carcinogen
with experimental tumorigenic data. Mutation
data reported. When heated to decomposition
it emits toxic fumes of F$^-$.

FHU000   CAS: 959-73-9
2'-FLUORO-N,N-DIMETHYL-4-
STILBENAMINE
mf: $C_{16}H_{16}FN$ mw: 241.33

SYNS: 2'-FLUORO-4-DIMETHYLAMINOSTILBENE
◇ 2-FLUORO-4-STILBENYL-N,N-DIMETHYLAMINE

TOXICITY DATA with REFERENCE
ETA: orl-rat TDLo:490 mg/kg/46W-C   ABMGAJ
  9,87,62

SAFETY PROFILE: Questionable carcinogen
with experimental tumorigenic data. When
heated to decomposition it emits very toxic
fumes of F$^-$ and NO$_x$.

FHV000   CAS: 405-86-7
4'-FLUORO-N,N-DIMETHYL-4-
STILBENAMINE
mf: $C_{16}H_{16}FN$ mw: 241.33
SYNS: 4'-FLUORO-4-DIMETHYLAMINOSTILBENE
◇ 4'-FLUORO-4-STILBENYL-N,N-DIMETHYLAMINE

TOXICITY DATA with REFERENCE
ETA: orl-rat TDLo:440 mg/kg/42W-C   ABMGAJ
  9,87,62

SAFETY PROFILE: Questionable carcinogen
with experimental tumorigenic data. When
heated to decomposition it emits very toxic
fumes of F$^-$ and NO$_x$.

FIA500   CAS: 1881-37-4
4-FLUOROESTRADIOL
mf: $C_{18}H_{23}FO_2$ mw: 290.41
SYNS: ESTRA-1,3,5(10)-TRIENE-3,17-DIOL, 4-FLUORO-,
(17-β)-(9CI) ◇ 4-FLUOROESTRA-1,3,5-(10)-TRIENE-3,17-β-
DIOL

TOXICITY DATA with REFERENCE
CAR: imp-ham TDLo:360 mg/kg/15W-I
  MOPMA3 23,278,83

SAFETY PROFILE: Questionable carcinogen
with experimental carcinogenic data. When
heated to decomposition it emits toxic fumes
of F$^-$.

FIT200   CAS: 2508-18-1
7-FLUORO-2-N-(FLUORENYL)
ACETHYDROXAMIC ACID
mf: $C_{15}H_{12}FNO_2$ mw: 257.28
SYNS: 7-FLUORO-2-FAA ◇ 7-FLUORO-N-(FLUOREN-2-
YL)ACETOHYDROXAMIC ACID ◇ N-(7-FLUORO-2-FLUO-
RENYL)ACETOHYDROXAMIC ACID ◇ 7-FLUORO-N-HY-
DROXY-N-2-ACETYLAMINOFLUORENE ◇ N-HYDROXY-7-
FLUORO-2-ACETYLAMINOFLUORENE

TOXICITY DATA with REFERENCE
CAR: orl-rat TDLo:675 mg/kg/10W-C   CNREA8
  26,2239,66

MUT: mma-sat 20 nmol/plate   MUREAV 67,85,79
MUT: mmo-sat 15 nmol/plate   MUREAV 67,85,79

SAFETY PROFILE: Questionable carcinogen with experimental carcinogenic data. Mutation data reported. When heated to decomposition it emits toxic fumes of NO_x and F^-.

FJN000   CAS: 1994-57-6
2-FLUORO-7-METHYLBENZ(a) ANTHRACENE
mf: $C_{19}H_{13}F$ mw: 260.32

SYN: 7-METHYL-2-FLUOROBENZ(a)ANTHRACENE

TOXICITY DATA with REFERENCE
NEO: ims-rat TDLo: 10 mg/kg   NATUAS
   273,566,78

SAFETY PROFILE: Questionable carcinogen with experimental neoplastigenic data. When heated to decomposition it emits toxic fumes of F^-.

FJO000   CAS: 2606-87-3
3-FLUORO-7-METHYLBENZ(a) ANTHRACENE
mf: $C_{19}H_{13}F$ mw: 260.32

SYN: 3'-FLUORO-10-METHYL-1,2-BENZANTHRACENE

TOXICITY DATA with REFERENCE
NEO: scu-mus TDLo: 43 mg/kg   CNREA8
   23,229,63
NEO: scu-rat TDLo: 9 mg/kg   CNREA8 23,229,63
ETA: skn-mus TDLo: 120 mg/kg/20W-I
   CNREA8 23,229,63

SAFETY PROFILE: Questionable carcinogen with experimental neoplastigenic and tumorigenic data. When heated to decomposition it emits toxic fumes of F^-.

FJP000   CAS: 2541-68-6
6-FLUORO-7-METHYLBENZ(a) ANTHRACENE
mf: $C_{19}H_{13}F$ mw: 260.32

TOXICITY DATA with REFERENCE
NEO: ims-rat TDLo: 10 mg/kg   NATUAS
   273,566,78
NEO: scu-mus TDLo: 43 mg/kg   CNREA8
   23,229,63
NEO: scu-rat TDLo: 9 mg/kg   CNREA8 23,229,63
NEO: skn-mus TDLo: 120 mg/kg/20W-I
   CNREA8 23,229,63

SAFETY PROFILE: Questionable carcinogen

with experimental neoplastigenic data. When heated to decomposition it emits toxic fumes of F^-.

FJQ000   CAS: 1881-75-0
9-FLUORO-7-METHYLBENZ(a) ANTHRACENE
mf: $C_{19}H_{13}F$ mw: 260.32

SYN: 6-FLUORO-10-METHYL-1,2-BENZANTHRACENE

TOXICITY DATA with REFERENCE
NEO: ims-rat TDLo: 10 mg/kg   NATUAS
   273,566,78
NEO: skn-mus TDLo: 120 mg/kg/20W-I
   CNREA8 23,229,63

SAFETY PROFILE: Questionable carcinogen with experimental neoplastigenic data. When heated to decomposition it emits toxic fumes of F^-.

FJR000   CAS: 1881-76-1
7-FLUORO-10-METHYL-1,2- BENZANTHRACENE
mf: $C_{19}H_{13}F$ mw: 260.32

SYN: 10-FLUORO-7-METHYLBENZ(a)ANTHRACENE

TOXICITY DATA with REFERENCE
NEO: scu-mus TDLo: 43 mg/kg   CNREA8
   23,229,63
NEO: scu-rat TDLo: 9 mg/kg   CNREA8 23,229,63
NEO: skn-mus TDLo: 120 mg/kg/20W-I
   CNREA8 23,229,63

SAFETY PROFILE: Questionable carcinogen with experimental neoplastigenic data. When heated to decomposition it emits toxic fumes of F^-.

FJT000   CAS: 52831-60-4
4-FLUORO-7-METHYL-6H-(1) BENZOTHIOPYRANO(4,3-b)QUINOLINE
mf: $C_{17}H_{12}FNS$ mw: 281.36

TOXICITY DATA with REFERENCE
NEO: scu-mus TDLo: 72 mg/kg/9W-I   MUREAV
   66,307,79
MUT: mma-sat 100 µg/plate   MUREAV 66,307,79

SAFETY PROFILE: Questionable carcinogen with experimental neoplastigenic data. Mutation data reported. When heated to decomposition it emits very toxic fumes of F^-, SO_x, and NO_x.

FJU000   CAS: 73771-72-9
2-FLUORO-3-METHYLCHOLANTHRENE
mf: $C_{21}H_{15}F$ mw: 286.36

TOXICITY DATA with REFERENCE
NEO: ims-rat TDLo:50 mg/kg   NATUAS
273,566,78

SAFETY PROFILE: Questionable carcinogen
with experimental neoplastigenic data. When
heated to decomposition it emits toxic fumes
of F⁻.

FJV000   CAS: 73771-73-0
6-FLUORO-3-METHYLCHOLANTHRENE
mf: $C_{21}H_{15}F$ mw: 286.36

TOXICITY DATA with REFERENCE
NEO: ims-rat TDLo:50 mg/kg   NATUAS
273,566,78

SAFETY PROFILE: Questionable carcinogen
with experimental neoplastigenic data. When
heated to decomposition it emits toxic fumes
of F⁻.

FJW000   CAS: 73771-74-1
9-FLUORO-3-METHYLCHOLANTHRENE
mf: $C_{21}H_{15}F$ mw: 286.36

TOXICITY DATA with REFERENCE
NEO: ims-rat TDLo:50 mg/kg   NATUAS
273,566,78

SAFETY PROFILE: Questionable carcinogen
with experimental neoplastigenic data. When
heated to decomposition it emits toxic fumes
of F⁻.

FJY000   CAS: 64977-44-2
1-FLUORO-5-METHYLCHRYSENE
mf: $C_{19}H_{13}F$ mw: 260.32

TOXICITY DATA with REFERENCE
ETA: skn-mus TD:40 mg/kg/I   CALEDQ 1,147,76
ETA: skn-mus TDLo:1200 µg/kg/20D-I
CNREA8 38,1694,78
MUT: mma-sat 20 µg/plate   JMCMAR 21,38,78

CONSENSUS REPORTS: EPA Genetic Toxicology Program.

SAFETY PROFILE: Questionable carcinogen
with experimental tumorigenic data. Mutation
data reported. When heated to decomposition
it emits toxic fumes of F⁻.

FKA000   CAS: 64977-46-4
6-FLUORO-5-METHYLCHRYSENE
mf: $C_{19}H_{13}F$ mw: 260.32

TOXICITY DATA with REFERENCE
ETA: skn-mus TD:1200 µg/kg/20W-I   JJIND8
63,855,79

ETA: skn-mus TDLo:1200 µg/kg/20D-I
CNREA8 38,1694,78
MUT: mma-sat 20 µg/plate   JMCMAR 21,38,78

CONSENSUS REPORTS: EPA Genetic Toxicology Program.

SAFETY PROFILE: Questionable carcinogen
with experimental tumorigenic data. Mutation
data reported. When heated to decomposition
it emits toxic fumes of F⁻.

FKB000   CAS: 64977-47-5
7-FLUORO-5-METHYLCHRYSENE
mf: $C_{19}H_{13}F$ mw: 260.32

TOXICITY DATA with REFERENCE
ETA: skn-mus TDLo:1200 µg/kg/20W-I
JJIND8 63,855,79
ETA: skn-mus TDLo:4000 µg/kg/20D-I
CNREA8 38,1694,78
MUT: mma-sat 20 µg/plate   JJIND8 63,855,79

SAFETY PROFILE: Questionable carcinogen
with experimental tumorigenic data. Mutation
data reported. When heated to decomposition
it emits toxic fumes of F⁻.

FKC000   CAS: 64977-48-6
9-FLUORO-5-METHYLCHRYSENE
mf: $C_{19}H_{13}F$ mw: 260.32

TOXICITY DATA with REFERENCE
ETA: skn-mus TD:1200 µg/kg/20W-I
JJIND8 63,855,79
ETA: skn-mus TDLo:1200 µg/kg/20D-I
CNREA8 38,1694,78
MUT: mma-sat 20 µg/plate   JMCMAR 21,38,78

CONSENSUS REPORTS: EPA Genetic Toxicology Program.

SAFETY PROFILE: Questionable carcinogen
with experimental tumorigenic data. Mutation
data reported. When heated to decomposition
it emits toxic fumes of F⁻.

FKD000   CAS: 64977-49-7
11-FLUORO-5-METHYLCHRYSENE
mf: $C_{19}H_{13}F$ mw: 260.32

TOXICITY DATA with REFERENCE
ETA: skn-mus TD:1200 µg/kg/20W-I   JJIND8
63,855,79
ETA: skn-mus TDLo:1200 µg/kg/20D-I
CNREA8 38,1694,78
MUT: mma-sat 20 µg/plate   JMCMAR 21,38,78

CONSENSUS REPORTS: EPA Genetic Toxicology Program.

SAFETY PROFILE: Questionable carcinogen with experimental tumorigenic data. Mutation data reported. When heated to decomposition it emits toxic fumes of F⁻.

FKE000 CAS: 61413-38-5
12-FLUORO-5-METHYLCHRYSENE
mf: $C_{19}H_{13}F$ mw: 260.32

TOXICITY DATA with REFERENCE
NEO: skn-mus TDLo:4 mg/kg/I CALEDQ
1,147,76
ETA: skn-mus TD:40 mg/kg/3W-I CCSUDL
1,325,76
MUT: mma-sat 20 μg/plate JMCMAR 21,38,78

CONSENSUS REPORTS: EPA Genetic Toxicology Program.

SAFETY PROFILE: Questionable carcinogen with experimental neoplastigenic and tumorigenic data. Mutation data reported. When heated to decomposition it emits toxic fumes of F⁻.

FKF800 CAS: 937-25-7
p-FLUORO-N-METHYL-N-NITROSOANILINE
mf: $C_7H_7FN_2O$ mw: 154.16

SYN: N-NITROSO-N-METHYL-4-FLUOROANILINE

TOXICITY DATA with REFERENCE
ETA: orl-ratTDLo:1140mg/kg/50W-I CRNGDP
4,157,83
MUT: mma-sat 500 μg/plate MUREAV 89,255,81

SAFETY PROFILE: Questionable carcinogen with experimental tumorigenic data. Mutation data reported. When heated to decomposition it emits toxic fumes of NO_x and F⁻.

FKO000 CAS: 17576-63-5
3-FLUORO-4-NITROQUINOLINE-1-OXIDE
mf: $C_9H_5FN_2O_3$ mw: 208.16

TOXICITY DATA with REFERENCE
ETA: scu-mus TDLo:347 mg/kg/I CPBTAL
17,544,69
MUT: cyt-omi 10 μmol/L GANNA2 60,155,69
MUT: cyt-rat:ast 100 nmol/L GMCRDC 17,31,75
MUT: dns-ham:oth 2 μmol/L NATUAS
229,416,71

CONSENSUS REPORTS: EPA Genetic Toxicology Program.

SAFETY PROFILE: Questionable carcinogen with experimental tumorigenic data. Mutation

data reported. When heated to decomposition it emits very toxic fumes of F⁻ and NO_x.

FKP000 CAS: 19789-69-6
8-FLUORO-4-NITROQUINOLINE-1-OXIDE
mf: $C_9H_5FN_2O_3$ mw: 208.16

TOXICITY DATA with REFERENCE
ETA: scu-mus TDLo:60 mg/kg/I CPBTAL
17,544,69

SAFETY PROFILE: Questionable carcinogen with experimental tumorigenic data. When heated to decomposition it emits very toxic fumes of F⁻ and NO_x.

FKV000 CAS: 371-41-5
4-FLUOROPHENOL
mf: C_6H_5FO mw: 112.11

TOXICITY DATA with REFERENCE
CAR: skn-mus TDLo:10 g/kg/25W-I CNREA8
19,413,59

CONSENSUS REPORTS: Reported in EPA TSCA Inventory.

SAFETY PROFILE: Questionable carcinogen with experimental carcinogenic data. When heated to decomposition it emits toxic fumes of F⁻.

FKX000 CAS: 725-04-2
2'-FLUORO-4'-PHENYLACETANILIDE
mf: $C_{14}H_{12}FNO$ mw: 229.27

SYN: 3-FLUORO-4-ACETYLAMINOBIPHENYL

TOXICITY DATA with REFERENCE
CAR: orl-rat TDLo:3700 mg/kg/26W-C
CNREA8 22,1002,62

SAFETY PROFILE: Questionable carcinogen with experimental carcinogenic data. When heated to decomposition it emits very toxic fumes of NO_x and F⁻.

FKY000 CAS: 725-06-4
4'-(m-FLUOROPHENYL)ACETANILIDE
mf: $C_{14}H_{12}FNO$ mw: 229.27

SYN: 3'-FLUORO-4-ACETYLAMINOBIPHENYL

TOXICITY DATA with REFERENCE
CAR: orl-rat TDLo:2580 mg/kg/21W-C
CNREA8 22,1002,62

SAFETY PROFILE: Questionable carcinogen with experimental carcinogenic data. When

heated to decomposition it emits very toxic fumes of F^- and NO_x.

FKZ000   CAS: 398-32-3
4'-(p-FLUOROPHENYL)ACETANILIDE
mf: $C_{14}H_{12}FNO$ mw: 229.27

SYNS: 4'-FLUORO-4-ACETYLAMINOBIPHENYL
◊ N-4-(4'-FLUORO)BIPHENYLACETAMIDE ◊ N-(4'-FLUORO-4-BIPHENYLYL)ACETAMIDE

TOXICITY DATA with REFERENCE
ETA: orl-rat TD:5040 mg/kg/36W-C   JNCIAM 54,1223,75
ETA: orl-rat TD:5 g/kg/36W-I   JNCIAM 54,427,75
ETA: orl-rat TD:6048 mg/kg/36W-C   BECTA6 23,464,79
ETA: orl-rat TD:6048 mg/kg/36W-C   EXPEAM 32,217,76
ETA: orl-rat TD:8064 mg/kg/48W-C   JJIND8 64,1537,80
ETA: orl-rat TDLo:4032 mg/kg/24W-C   AJPAA4 100,317,80

SAFETY PROFILE: Questionable carcinogen with experimental tumorigenic data. When heated to decomposition it emits very toxic fumes of NO_x and F^-.

FLY000   CAS: 10010-36-3
4'-FLUORO-4-STILBENAMINE
mf: $C_{14}H_{12}FN$ mw: 213.27

TOXICITY DATA with REFERENCE
ETA: scu-rat TDLo:200 mg/kg/W-I   BMBUAQ 14,141,58

SAFETY PROFILE: Questionable carcinogen with experimental tumorigenic data. When heated to decomposition it emits very toxic fumes of F^- and NO_x.

FMB000   CAS: 17902-23-7
5-FLUORO-1-(TETRAHYDROFURAN-2-YL)URACIL
mf: $C_8H_9FN_2O_3$ mw: 200.19

SYNS: CARZONAL ◊ CITOFUR ◊ COPAROGIN
◊ EXONAL ◊ FENTAL ◊ F-5-FU ◊ FLUOROFUR
◊ 5-FLUORO-1-(TETRAHYDRO-2-FURANYL)-2,4-PYRIMI-DINEDIONE ◊ 5-FLUORO-1-(TETRAHYDRO-2-FURANYL)-2,4(1H,3H)-PYRIMIDINEDIONE ◊ 5-FLUORO-1-(TETRA-HYDRO-3-FURYL)URACIL ◊ FRANROZE ◊ FTORAFUR
◊ FULAID ◊ FULFEEL ◊ FURAFLUOR ◊ FUROFUTRAN
◊ FUTRAFUL ◊ LAMAR ◊ LIFRIL ◊ MJF-12264 ◊ NEBERK
◊ NITOBANIL ◊ NSC-148958 ◊ PYRIMIDINE-DEOXYRIBOSE
N1-2'-FURANIDYL-5-FLUOROURACIL ◊ RIOL ◊ SINOFLU-ROL ◊ SUNFRAL ◊ TEFSIEL C ◊ TEGAFUR ◊ 1-(TETRAHY-DROFURAN-2-YL)-5-FLUOROURACIL ◊ N(^{1})-(2-TETRAHY-DROFURYL)-5-FLUOROURACIL ◊ THFU

TOXICITY DATA with REFERENCE
CAR: orl-man TDLo:11046 mg/kg/4.7Y-C: GIT   ARSUAX 118,1454,83
MUT: cyt-ham:fbr 100 nmol/L   MUREAV 88,241,81
MUT: cyt-mus-ipr 40 mg/kg   MUREAV 88,301,81
MUT: dns-hmn:fbr 1 g/L   STBIBN 78,165,80
MUT: oms-hmn:hla 200 mg/L   JMCMAR 22,1096,79
MUT: slt-dmg-mul 10 mg/L   TAKHAA 44,96,85

CONSENSUS REPORTS: Reported in EPA TSCA Inventory.

SAFETY PROFILE: Questionable human carcinogen producing gastrointestinal tumors. Experimental carcinogenic and teratogenic data. Poison by ingestion and possibly other routes. Moderately toxic to humans by intravenous route. Moderately toxic experimentally by intraperitoneal, intravenous and subcutaneous routes. Human systemic effects by ingestion and intravenous route: hallucinations and distorted perceptions. Experimental reproductive effects. Human mutation data reported. Used as an anticancer agent. When heated to decomposition it emits very toxic fumes of F^- and NO_x.

FMF000   CAS: 313-95-1
2-FLUOROTRICYCLOQUINAZOLINE
mf: $C_{21}H_{11}FN_4$ mw: 338.36

TOXICITY DATA with REFERENCE
ETA: skn-mus TDLo:48 mg/kg   BECCAN 41,420,63

SAFETY PROFILE: Questionable carcinogen with experimental tumorigenic data. When heated to decomposition it emits very toxic fumes of NO_x and F^-.

FMG000   CAS: 803-57-6
3-FLUORO-TRICYCLOQUINAZOLINE
mf: $C_{21}H_{11}FN_4$ mw: 338.36

TOXICITY DATA with REFERENCE
NEO: skn-mus TDLo:920 mg/kg/1Y-I   BJCAAI 16,275,62

SAFETY PROFILE: Questionable carcinogen with experimental neoplastigenic data. When heated to decomposition it emits very toxic fumes of F^- and NO_x.

FMM000 CAS: 51-21-8
FLUOROURACIL
mf: $C_4H_3FN_2O_2$ mw: 130.09

SYNS: ADRUCIL ◇ ARUMEL ◇ CARZONAL ◇ EFFLU-
DERM (FREE BASE) ◇ EFUDEX ◇ EFUDIX ◇ 5-FLUORACIL
(GERMAN) ◇ FLUOROBLASTIN ◇ FLUOROPLEX
◇ 5-FLUORPROPYRIMIDINE-2,4-DIONE ◇ 5-FLUORO-2,4-
PYRIMIDINEDIONE ◇ 5-FLUORO-2,4(1H,3H)-PYRIMIDINE-
DIONE ◇ 5-FLUOROURACIL ◇ 5-FLUURURACIL (GERMAN)
◇ FLURACIL ◇ FLURI ◇ FLURIL ◇ 5-FU ◇ NSC-19893
◇ RO 2-9757 ◇ TIMAZIN ◇ U-8953 ◇ ULUP

TOXICITY DATA with REFERENCE
MUT: dnd-hmn:leu 2600 nmol/L CNREA8
43,5145,83
MUT: dnr-bcs 300 µg/plate TAKHAA 44,96,85
MUT: dnr-esc 100 µg/L PCJOAU 16,721,82
MUT: dns-hmn:oth 1 mmol/L CNREA8
44,3414,84
MUT: mnt-ham-ipr 41 mg/kg PHARAT
38,353,83
MUT: par-ham LD10:140 mg/kg JSONAU
15,355,80

CONSENSUS REPORTS: IARC Cancer Review: GROUP 3 IMEMDT 7,210,87; Human
Inadequate Evidence IMEMDT 26,217,81; Animal Inadequate Evidence IMEMDT 26,217,81.
Reported in EPA TSCA Inventory. EPA Genetic
Toxicology Program. EPA Extremely Hazardous Substances List.

SAFETY PROFILE: Questionable carcinogen.
Poison by ingestion, intraperitoneal, subcutaneous, intravenous and possibly other routes.
Moderately toxic by parenteral and rectal routes.
An experimental teratogen. Human systemic effects by ingestion, intravenous and possibly
other routes: EKG changes, bone marrow
changes, cardiac, pulmonary and gastrointestinal effects. Experimental reproductive effects.
Human mutation data reported. A human skin
irritant. When heated to decomposition it emits
very toxic fumes of F^- and NO_x.

FMR700 CAS: 76050-49-2
FOGARD

SYN: FOGARD S

TOXICITY DATA with REFERENCE
ETA: ipr-mus TDLo:2600 µg/kg/39D-I
PATHAB 73,707,81
ETA: scu-mus TDLo:2600 µg/kg/39D-I
PATHAB 73,707,81

SAFETY PROFILE: Questionable carcinogen
with experimental tumorigenic data. When
heated to decomposition it emits acrid smoke
and irritating fumes.

FMU059 CAS: 2650-18-2
FOOD BLUE 1
mf: $C_{37}H_{36}N_2O_9S_3 \cdot 2H_3N$ mw: 783.01

SYNS: ACID BLUE 9 ◇ ACILAN TURQUOISE BLUE AE
◇ A.F. BLUE No. 1 ◇ AIZEN BRILLIANT BLUE FCF
◇ ALPHAZURINE ◇ AMACID BLUE FG CONC ◇ BLEU BRIL-
LIANT FCF ◇ 11388 BLUE ◇ BRILLIANT BLUE ◇ BUCACID
AZURE BLUE ◇ CALCOCID BLUE EG ◇ C.I. 671
◇ C.I. 42090 ◇ C.I. ACID BLUE 9, DIAMMONIUM SALT
◇ C.I. DIRECT BROWN 78, DIAMMONIUM SALT
◇ C.I. FOOD BLUE 2 ◇ D&C BLUE No. 4 ◇ DISULPHINE
LAKE BLUE EG ◇ EDICOL SUPRA BLUE E6 ◇ ERIOGLAU-
CINE ◇ ERIOSKY BLUE ◇ FENAZO BLUE XR ◇ HIDACID
AZURE BLUE ◇ H.K. FORMULA No. K. 7117 ◇ KITON PURE
BLUE L ◇ MAPLE BRILLIANT BLUE FCF ◇ NEPTUNE BLUE
BRA CONCENTRATION ◇ PATENT BLUE AE ◇ PEACOCK
BLUE X-1756 ◇ SCHULTZ No. 770 ◇ TRIANTINE LIGHT
BROWN 3RN ◇ XYLENE BLUE VSG

TOXICITY DATA with REFERENCE
NEO: scu-rat TDLo:10 g/kg/77W-I TXAPA9
8,29,66
ETA: par-rat TDLo:4580 mg/kg/62W-I
FAONAU 38B,22,66
ETA: scu-rat TD:2 g/kg/94W-I FAONAU
38B,29,66
MUT: cyt-ham:fbr 5 g/L FCTOD7 22,623,84
MUT: dns-rat-orl 500 mg/kg ENMUDM 7,101,85
MUT: dns-rat:lvr 200 µmol/L ENMUDM
7,101,85

CONSENSUS REPORTS: Community Right-
To-Know List. Reported in EPA TSCA Inventory. EPA Genetic Toxicology Program.

SAFETY PROFILE: Questionable carcinogen
with experimental neoplastigenic and tumorigenic data. Human poison by intravenous route.
Human systemic effects by intravenous route:
muscle contractions or spasticity and dyspnea.
Mutation data reported. When heated to decomposition it emits very toxic fumes of NH_3, NO_x
and SO_x.

FMU070 CAS: 3761-53-3
FOOD RED No. 101
mf: $C_{18}H_{14}N_2O_7S_2 \cdot 2Na$ mw: 480.44

SYNS: ACETACID RED J ◇ ACIDAL PONCEAU G
◇ ACID LEATHER RED KPR ◇ ACID PONCEAU R

◇ ACID RED 26 ◇ ACID SCARLET ◇ ACILAN PONCEAU RRL ◇ AHCOCID FAST SCARLET R ◇ AIZEN PONCEAU RH ◇ AMACID LAKE SCARLET 2R ◇ BRILLIANT PONCEAU G ◇ CALCOCID 2RIL ◇ CALCOLAKE SCARLET 2R ◇ CERTICOL PONCEAU MXS ◇ CERVEN KYSELA 26 ◇ C.I. 79 ◇ C.I. 16150 ◇ C.I. ACID RED 26 ◇ C.I. ACID RED 26, DISODIUM SALT ◇ C.I. FOOD RED 5 ◇ COLACID PONCEAU SPECIAL ◇ D&C RED No. 5 ◇ 4-((2,4-DIMETHYL-PHENYL)AZO)-3-HYDROXY-2,7-NAPHTHALENEDISUL-FONIC ACID, DISODIUM SALT ◇ 4-((2,4-DIMETHYLPHE-NYL)AZO)-3-HYDROXY-2,7-NAPHTHALENEDISULPHONIC ACID, DISODIUM SALT ◇ DISODIUM (2,4-DIMETHYLPHE-NYLAZO)-2-HYDROXYNAPHTHALENE-3,6-DISULFONATE ◇ DISODIUM (2,4-DIMETHYLPHENYLAZO)-2-HYDROXY-NAPHTHALENE-3,6-DISULPHONATE ◇ DISODIUM SALT of 1-(2,4-XYLYLAZO)-2-NAPHTHOL-3,6-DISULFONIC ACID ◇ DISODIUM SALT of 1-(2,4-XYLYLAZO)-2-NAPHTHOL-3,6-DISULPHONIC ACID ◇ EDICOL PONCEAU RS ◇ FENAZO SCARLET 2R ◇ HEXACOL PONCEAU MX ◇ HIDACID SCAR-LET 2R ◇ 3-HYDROXY-4-(2,4-XYLYLAZO)-3,7-NAPHTHAL-ENEDISULFONIC ACID, DISODIUM SALT ◇ 3-HYDROXY-4-(2,4-XYLYLAZO)-3,7-NAPHTHALENEDISULPHONIC ACID, DISODIUM SALT ◇ JAVA PONCEAU 2R ◇ KITON PONCEAU R ◇ LAKE PONCEAU ◇ NAPHTHALENE LAKE SCARLET R ◇ NEKLACID RED RR ◇ NEW PONCEAU 4R ◇ PAPER RED HRR ◇ PIGMENT PONCEAU R ◇ PONCEAU BNA ◇ PONCEAU R (BIOLOGICAL STAIN) ◇ PONCEAU XY-LIDINE (BIOLOGICAL STAIN) ◇ 1695 RED ◇ RED R ◇ SCARLET R ◇ SCHULTZ No. 95 ◇ TERTRACID PONCEAU 2R ◇ XYLIDINE PONCEAU ◇ 1-XYLYLAZO-2-NAPHTHOL-3,6-DISULFONIC ACID, DISODIUM SALT ◇ 1-(2,4-XYLY-LAZO)-2-NAPHTHOL-3,6-DISULPHONIC ACID, DISODIUM SALT ◇ 1-(2,4-XYLYLAZO)-2-NAPHTHOL-3,6-DISUL-PHONIC ACID, DISODIUM SALT ◇ 1-XYLYLAZO-2-NAPHTHOL-3,6-DISULPHONIC ACID, DISODIUM SALT

TOXICITY DATA with REFERENCE
CAR: orl-mus TDLo: 136 g/kg/81W-C   FCTXAV
   6,591,68
ETA: orl-mus TD: 35 g/kg/52W   BJCAAI
   10,653,56
MUT: mma-sat 100 μg/plate   CANCAR
   49,1970,82
MUT: oth-esc 300 μmol/L   SKEZAP 12,298,71

CONSENSUS REPORTS: IARC Cancer Review: GROUP 3 IMEMDT 7,56,87; Animal Sufficient Evidence IMEMDT 8,189,75. Reported in EPA TSCA Inventory.

SAFETY PROFILE: Questionable carcinogen with experimental carcinogenic and tumorigenic data. Moderately toxic by intraperitoneal route. Mutation data reported. When heated to decomposition it emits toxic fumes of NO_x and SO_x.

FMU080   CAS: 2611-82-7
FOOD RED No. 102
mf: $C_{20}H_{14}N_2O_{10}S_3$•3Na   mw: 607.51

SYNS: ACIDAL BRIGHT PONCEAU 3R ◇ ACID BRILLIANT SCARLET 3R ◇ ACID PONCEAU 4R ◇ ACID RED 18 ◇ ACID SCARLET 3R ◇ ACILAN SCARLET V3R ◇ AIZEN BRILLIANT SCARLET 3RH ◇ ATUL ACID SCARLET 3R ◇ BRILLIANT PONCEAU 3R ◇ BRILLIANT SCARLET ◇ BUCACID BRILLIANT SCARLET 3R ◇ CALCOCID BRIL-LIANT SCARLET 3RN ◇ CERTICOL PONCEAU 4RS ◇ CERVEN KOSENILOVA A ◇ CILEFA PONCEAU 4R ◇ COCCINE ◇ COCHENILLEROT A ◇ COCHINEAL RED A ◇ COLACID PONCEAU 4R ◇ C.I. 185 ◇ C.I. 16255 ◇ C.I. ACID RED 18 ◇ C.I. FOOD RED 7 ◇ CRIMSON SX ◇ CUROL BRIGHT RED 4R ◇ DAISHIKI BRILLIANT SCAR-LET 3R ◇ EDICOL SUPRA PONCEAU 4R ◇ EUROCERT COCHINEAL RED A ◇ FENAZO SCARLET 3R ◇ FOOD RED 6 ◇ FOOD RED 7 ◇ HD PONCEAU 4R ◇ HEXACOL PONCEAU 4R ◇ HIDACID FAST SCARLET 3R ◇ HISPACID BRILLIANT SCARLET 3RF ◇ JAVA SCARLET 3R ◇ KAYAKU ACID BRIL-LIANT SCARLET 3R ◇ KITON SCARLET 4R ◇ KOCHINEAL RED A FOR FOOD ◇ NAPHTHALENE INK SCARLET 4R ◇ 1,3-NAPHTHALENEDISULFONIC ACID, 7-HYDROXY-8-((4-SULFO-1-NAPHTHYL)AZO)-, TRISODIUM SALT ◇ NEKLACID RED 3R ◇ NEUCOCCIN ◇ NEW COCCIN ◇ PONCEAU 4R ◇ PONCEAU 4R ALUMINUM LAKE ◇ PONTACYL SCARLET RR ◇ PURPLE RED ◇ ROUGE de COCHENILLE A ◇ SAN-EI BRILLIANT SCARLET 3R ◇ STRAWBERRY RED A GEIGY ◇ SYMULON ACID BRIL-LIANT SCARLET 3R ◇ TAKAOKA BRILLIANT SCARLET 3R ◇ VICTORIA SCARLET 3R

TOXICITY DATA with REFERENCE
ETA: orl-rat TDLo: 428 g/kg/64W-I   VPITAR
   29,61,70
MUT: cyt-ham:fbr 1 g/L   FCTOD7 22,623,84

CONSENSUS REPORTS: Reported in EPA TSCA Inventory.

SAFETY PROFILE: Questionable carcinogen with experimental tumorigenic data. Moderately toxic by intraperitoneal route. Mutation data reported. When heated to decomposition it emits toxic fumes of NO_x and SO_x.

FNB000   CAS: 32852-21-4
FORMIC ACID (2-(4-METHYL-2-THIAZOLYL)HYDRAZIDE
mf: $C_5H_7N_3OS$ mw: 157.21

TOXICITY DATA with REFERENCE
NEO: orl-rat TDLo: 11 g/kg/46W-C   JNCIAM
   47,437,71
MUT: pic-esc 10 mg/L   MUREAV 26,3,74

CONSENSUS REPORTS: EPA Genetic Toxicology Program.

SAFETY PROFILE: Questionable carcinogen with experimental neoplastigenic data. Mutation data reported. When heated to decomposition it emits very toxic fumes of SO_x and NO_x.

FNK000   CAS: 63040-55-1
6-FORMYLANTHANTHRENE
mf: $C_{25}H_{14}O$ mw: 330.39

SYN: DIBENZO(def,mno)CHRYSENE-12-CARBOXALDE-HYDE

TOXICITY DATA with REFERENCE
ETA: scu-mus TDLo: 72 mg/kg 9W-I   COREAF
252,1711,61

SAFETY PROFILE: Questionable carcinogen with experimental tumorigenic data. When heated to decomposition it emits acrid smoke and irritating fumes.

FNN000   CAS: 624-84-0
FORMYLHYDRAZINE
mf: CH_4N_2O mw: 60.07

PROP: Mp: 54°. Very sol in alc and ether; sol in benzene.

SYNS: CARBAZALDEHYDE ◇ FORMAL HYDRAZINE ◇ FORMHYDRAZID (GERMAN) ◇ FORMHYDRAZIDE ◇ FORMIC ACID, HYDRAZIDE ◇ FORMIC HYDRAZIDE ◇ FORMOHYDRAZIDE ◇ FORMYLHYDRAZIDE ◇ N-FORMYLHYDRAZINE ◇ HYDRAZINECARBOXALDEHYDE

TOXICITY DATA with REFERENCE
NEO: orl-mus TDLo: 73 g/kg/43W-C   BJCAAI
37,960,78

CONSENSUS REPORTS: Reported in EPA TSCA Inventory.

SAFETY PROFILE: Questionable carcinogen with experimental neoplastigenic data. Poison by intraperitoneal and subcutaneous routes. When heated to decomposition it emits toxic fumes of NO_x.

FNQ000   CAS: 63040-58-4
6-FORMYL-12-METHYLANTHANTHRENE
mf: $C_{26}H_{16}O$ mw: 344.42

SYN: 6-METHYLDIBENZO(def,mno)CHRYSENE-12-CARBOXALDEHYDE

TOXICITY DATA with REFERENCE
ETA: scu-mus TDLo: 72 mg/kg/9W-I   COREAF
252,1711,61

SAFETY PROFILE: Questionable carcinogen with experimental tumorigenic data. When heated to decomposition it emits acrid smoke and irritating fumes.

FNR000   CAS: 2732-09-4
7-FORMYL-9-METHYLBENZ(c)ACRIDINE
mf: $C_{19}H_{13}NO$ mw: 271.33

SYN: 9-METHYLBENZ(c)ACRIDINE-7-CARBOXALDE-HYDE

TOXICITY DATA with REFERENCE
ETA: scu-mus TDLo: 120 mg/kg/9W-I   CHDDAT
267,981,68

SAFETY PROFILE: Questionable carcinogen with experimental tumorigenic data. When heated to decomposition it emits toxic fumes of NO_x.

FNS000   CAS: 18936-78-2
7-FORMYL-11-METHYLBENZ(c)ACRIDINE
mf: $C_{19}H_{13}NO$ mw: 271.33

SYN: 11-METHYLBENZ(c)ACRIDINE-7-CARBOXALDE-HYDE

TOXICITY DATA with REFERENCE
ETA: scu-mus TDLo: 120 mg/kg/9W-I   CHDDAT
267,981,68

SAFETY PROFILE: Questionable carcinogen with experimental tumorigenic data. When heated to decomposition it emits toxic fumes of NO_x.

FNT000   CAS: 13345-61-4
7-FORMYL-12-METHYLBENZ(a)ANTHRACENE
mf: $C_{20}H_{14}O$ mw: 270.34

SYN: 12-METHYLBENZ(a)ANTHRACENE-7-CARBOXALDEHYDE

TOXICITY DATA with REFERENCE
CAR: scu-mus TDLo: 120 mg/kg/6W-I   IJCNAW
2,500,67
NEO: scu-rat TDLo: 20 mg/kg/39D-I   CNREA8
31,1951,71
NEO: skn-mus TDLo: 8000 μg/kg   JJIND8
61,135,78
MUT: dni-omi 200 μg/L   PNASA6 74,1378,77

SAFETY PROFILE: Questionable carcinogen with experimental carcinogenic and neoplasti-

genic data. Mutation data reported. When heated to decomposition it emits acrid smoke and irritating fumes.

FNU000   CAS: 63040-56-2
5-FORMYL-8-METHYL-3,4:9,10-DIBENZOPYRENE
mf: $C_{26}H_{16}O$ mw: 344.42

SYN: 8-METHYLBENZO(rst)PENTAPHENE-5-CARBOXAL-DEHYDE

TOXICITY DATA with REFERENCE
ETA: scu-mus TDLo: 72 mg/kg/9W-I   COREAF
   252,1236,61

SAFETY PROFILE: Questionable carcinogen with experimental tumorigenic data. When heated to decomposition it emits acrid smoke and irritating fumes.

FNV000   CAS: 63040-57-3
5-FORMYL-10-METHYL-3,4,:8,9-DIBENZOPYRENE
mf: $C_{26}H_{16}O$ mw: 344.42

SYN: 14-METHYLDIBENZO(b,def)CHRYSENE-7-CARBOX-ALDEHYDE

TOXICITY DATA with REFERENCE
ETA: scu-mus TDLo: 72 mg/kg/9W-I   COREAF
   252,1711,61

SAFETY PROFILE: Questionable carcinogen with experimental tumorigenic data. When heated to decomposition it emits acrid smoke and irritating fumes.

FNX000   CAS: 4845-14-1
N-FORMYL-N-METHYL-p-(PHENYLAZO)ANILINE
mf: $C_{14}H_{13}N_3O$ mw: 239.30

SYN: 4-FORMYLMONOMETHYLAMINOAZOBENZENE

TOXICITY DATA with REFERENCE
ETA: orl-rat TDLo: 9100 mg/kg/34W-C
   CNREA8 9,652,49

SAFETY PROFILE: Questionable carcinogen with experimental tumorigenic data. When heated to decomposition it emits toxic fumes of NO_x.

FOJ000   CAS: 2302-84-3
1-FORMYL-3-THIOSEMICARBAZIDE
mf: $C_2H_5N_3OS$ mw: 119.16

TOXICITY DATA with REFERENCE
ETA: orl-rat TDLo: 43 g/kg/46W-C   JNCIAM
   47,437,71

CONSENSUS REPORTS: Reported in EPA TSCA Inventory.

SAFETY PROFILE: Questionable carcinogen with experimental tumorigenic data. When heated to decomposition it emits very toxic fumes of NO_x and SO_x.

FOP100
FUEL OIL, pyrolyzate

SYN: WATER QUENCH PYROLYSIS FUEL OIL

TOXICITY DATA with REFERENCE
CAR: skn-mus TDLo: 977 g/kg/8W-I   AIHAAP
   38,730,77

SAFETY PROFILE: Questionable carcinogen with experimental carcinogenic data. When heated to decomposition it emits acrid smoke and irritating fumes.

FQC000   CAS: 523-50-2
2H-FURO(2,3-h)(1)BENZOPYRAN-2-ONE
mf: $C_{11}H_6O_3$ mw: 186.17

SYNS: ANGECIN ◇ ANGELICIN (COUMARIN DERIV) ◇ FURO(5',4',7,8)COUMARIN ◇ ISOPSORALIN

TOXICITY DATA with REFERENCE
MUT: dnd-mam: lym 20 μmol/L   CBINA8
   21,103,78
MUT: dnd-omi 20 μmol/L   CBINA8 21,103,78
MUT: dnd-sal: spr 20 μmol/L   CBINA8 21,103,78
MUT: mmo-esc 40 mg/L   MUREAV 58,23,78
MUT: mmo-smc 50 μmol/L   BUCABS 67,245,80
MUT: mrc-smc 100 μmol/L   BUCABS 67,245,80

CONSENSUS REPORTS: IARC Cancer Review: GROUP 3 IMEMDT 7,56,87; Animal Inadequate Evidence IMEMDT 40,291,86. EPA Genetic Toxicology Program.

SAFETY PROFILE: Questionable carcinogen. Poison by ingestion and intraperitoneal routes. Mutation data reported. A tranquilizer, sedative and anticonvulsant. When heated to decomposition it emits acrid smoke and irritating fumes.

FQJ000   CAS: 2578-75-8
FUROTHIAZOLE
mf: $C_8H_6N_4O_4S$ mw: 254.24

SYN: N-(5-(5-NITRO-2-FURYL)-1,3,4-THIADIAZOL-2-YL)ACETAMIDE

TOXICITY DATA with REFERENCE
CAR: orl-rat TDLo: 33 g/kg/40W-C   JNCIAM
   54,841,75

NEO: orl-mus TDLo:80 g/kg/46W-C CNREA8
33,1593,73
MUT: dnr-sat 500 nmol/L CNREA8 34,2266,74
MUT: mma-sat 100 ng/plate MUREAV 48,295,77
MUT: mmo-esc 300 nmol/L CNREA8 34,2266,74
MUT: mrc-esc 500 nmol/L CNREA8 34,2266,74

SAFETY PROFILE: Questionable carcinogen with experimental carcinogenic and neoplastigenic data. Mutation data reported. When heated to decomposition it emits very toxic fumes of SO_x and NO_x.

FQQ100   CAS: 75884-37-6
**N-(4-(2-FURYL)-2-THIAZOLYL)
ACETAMIDE**
mf: $C_9H_8N_2O_2S$ mw: 208.25
SYN: FTA

TOXICITY DATA with REFERENCE
ETA: orl-mus TDLo:1008 mg/kg/12W-C
CNREA8 41,1397,81

SAFETY PROFILE: Questionable carcinogen with experimental tumorigenic data. When heated to decomposition it emits toxic fumes of NO_x and SO_x.

FQQ400   CAS: 77503-17-4
**N-(4-(2-FURYL)-2-THIAZOLYL)
FORMAMIDE**
mf: $C_8H_6N_2O_2S$ mw: 194.22
SYN: FAFT

TOXICITY DATA with REFERENCE
ETA: orl-mus TDLo:1008 mg/kg/12W-C
CNREA8 41,1397,81

SAFETY PROFILE: Questionable carcinogen with experimental tumorigenic data. When heated to decomposition it emits toxic fumes of NO_x and SO_x.

FQR000   CAS: 23255-69-8
FUSARENONE X
mf: $C_{17}H_{22}O_8$ mw: 354.39
PROP: Isolated from the culture filtrate of *Fusarium nivale* (34ZHAD -,163,71).

SYNS: 4-ACETYLOXY-12,13-EPOXY-3,7,15-TRIHY-
DROXY-(3-α,4-β,7-β)-TRICHOTHEC-9-EN-8-ONE ◇ NIVALE-
NOL-4-O-ACETATE ◇ 3,7,15-TRIHYDROXY-4-ACETOXY-8-
OXO-12,13-EPOXY-Δ⁹-TRICHOTHECENE ◇ 3,7,15-TRIHY-
DROXYSCIRP-4-ACETOXY-9-EN-8-ONE

TOXICITY DATA with REFERENCE
ETA: orl-rat TD:153 mg/kg 1Y-C JJEMAG
50,293,80

ETA: orl-rat TDLo:146 mg/kg/2Y-C JJEMAG
50,293,80
MUT: dnd-hmn:hla 32 mg/L/1H JJEMAG
42,527,72

SAFETY PROFILE: Questionable carcinogen with experimental tumorigenic data. Poison by ingestion, subcutaneous, intravenous, intraperitoneal, and possibly other routes. Experimental reproductive effects. Human mutation data reported. When heated to decomposition it emits acrid smoke and irritating fumes.

FQS000   CAS: 21259-20-1
FUSARIOTOXIN T 2
mf: $C_{24}H_{34}O_9$ mw: 466.58

PROP: A strain of *F. tricinctum* isolated from infected corn (AJVRAH 32,1843,71).

SYNS: 4,15-DIACETOXY-8-(3-METHYLBUTYRYLOXY)-
12,13-EPOXY-Δ-9-TRICHOTHECEN-3-OL ◇ 4-β,15-DIACE-
TOXY-8-α-(3-METHYLBUTYRYLOXY)-3-α-HYDROXY-
12,13-EPOXYTRICHOTHEC-9-ENE ◇ 3-HYDROXY-4,15-DIA-
CETOXY-8-(3-METHYLBUTYRYLOXY)-12,13-EPOXY-Δ⁹-
TRICHOTHECENE ◇ INSARIOTOXIN ◇ 8-ISOVALERATE
◇ 8-(3-METHYLBUTYRYLOXY)-DIACETOXYSCIRPENOL
◇ NSC 138780 ◇ T-2 MYCOTOXIN ◇ TOXIN T2 ◇ T (²)-
TRICHOTHECENE

TOXICITY DATA with REFERENCE
NEO: orl-mus TDLo:179 mg/kg/71W-C
FCTOD7 25,593,87
MUT: cyt-ham-ipr 1700 μg/kg HEREAY
93,329,80
MUT: dnd-mus-ipr 3 mg/kg MUREAV 88,115,81
MUT: dnd-mus:lym 5 μg/L MUREAV 88,115,81
MUT: dnd-mus:oth 5 μg/L MUREAV 88,115,81
MUT: ims-mky LD20: 650 μg/kg TXAPA9
82,532,86
MUT: sln-dmg-orl 31 mg/L HEREAY 92,163,80

CONSENSUS REPORTS: IARC Cancer Review: GROUP 3 IMEMDT 7,56,87; Animal Inadequate Evidence IMEMDT 31,265,83. EPA Genetic Toxicology Program.

SAFETY PROFILE: Questionable carcinogen with experimental neoplastigenic data. Poison by ingestion, intramuscular, subcutaneous, intraperitoneal, intracerebral, and intravenous routes. Moderately toxic by inhalation. An experimental teratogen. Experimental reproductive effects. Mutation data reported. A skin irritant. When heated to decomposition it emits acrid smoke and irritating fumes.

FQU875   CAS: 13674-87-8
FYROL FR 2
mf: $C_9H_{15}Cl_6O_4P$ mw: 430.91

PROP: Viscous liquid. Bp: (5) 236-237°, n (20/D) 1.5022. Solubility in water: 100 ppm.

SYNS: 1,3-DICHLORO-2-PROPANOL PHOSPHATE (3:1) ◊ EMULSION 212 ◊ FOSFORAN TROJ-(1,3-DWUCHLOROI-ZOPROPYLOWY) (POLISH) ◊ PF 38 ◊ PHOSPHORIC ACID TRIS(1,3-DICHLORO-2-PROPYL)ESTER ◊ TCPP ◊ TDCPP ◊ TRIS(1-CHLOROMETHYL-2-CHLOROETHYL)PHOSPHATE ◊ TRIS(1,3-DICHLOROISOPROPYL)PHOSPHATE ◊ TRIS--(1,3-DICHLORO-2-PROPYL)-PHOSPHATE

TOXICITY DATA with REFERENCE
CAR: orl-rat TDLo: 58400 mg/kg/2Y-C   EPASR*
8EHQ-1280-0401S
MUT: mma-sat 100 μg/plate   SCIEAS 200,785,78
MUT: mmo-sat 100 μmol/plate   MUREAV
66,373,79
MUT: otr-ham: emb 20 μmol/L   APTOA6 56,20,85

CONSENSUS REPORTS: EPA Genetic Toxicology Program. Reported in EPA TSCA Inventory.

SAFETY PROFILE: Questionable carcinogen with experimental carcinogenic data. Moderately toxic by ingestion. Experimental reproductive effects. Mutation data reported. When heated to decomposition it emits toxic fumes of Cl^- and PO_x.

GAF000   CAS: 7440-54-2
GADOLINIUM
af: Gd   aw: 157.25

PROP: A yellow-white, malleable, and ductile metallic element. A rare earth, stable in dry air; reacts slowly with H_2O. Mp: 1312°, bp: 3233°, d: 7.898 @ 25°.

TOXICITY DATA with REFERENCE
ETA: imp-mus TDLo: 25 g/kg   PSEBAA 135,426,70

CONSENSUS REPORTS: Reported in EPA TSCA Inventory.

SAFETY PROFILE: Questionable carcinogen with experimental tumorigenic data. It may act as an anticoagulant. It can react violently with air and halogens.

GAT000   CAS: 1772-03-8
d-GALACTOSAMINE HYDROCHLORIDE
mf: $C_6H_{13}NO_5 \cdot ClH$ mw: 215.66

SYN: 2-AMINO-2-DEOXY-d-GALACTOSE HYDROCHLORIDE

TOXICITY DATA with REFERENCE
ETA: ipr-rat TDLo: 135 g/kg/77W-I   VAAZA2
12,285,73

CONSENSUS REPORTS: Reported in EPA TSCA Inventory.

SAFETY PROFILE: Questionable carcinogen with experimental tumorigenic data. Moderately toxic by intraperitoneal route. When heated to decomposition it emits very toxic fumes of NO_x and Cl^-.

GBW000   CAS: 64741-44-2
GAS OIL

PROP: Yellow liquid. Flash p: 150°F, d: 1, lel: 6.0%, uel: 13.5%, autoign temp: 640°F, boiling range: 230-250°.

TOXICITY DATA with REFERENCE
CAR: skn-mus TDLo: 114 g/kg/38W-I   FAATDF3
7,228,86

CONSENSUS REPORTS: Reported in EPA TSCA Inventory.

SAFETY PROFILE: Questionable carcinogen with experimental carcinogenic data. Pulmonary aspiration can cause severe pneumonitis. Combustible when exposed to heat or flame; can react vigorously with oxidizing materials. A moderate explosion hazard when exposed to heat or flame. To fight fire use foam, CO_2, dry chemical.

GBW010   CAS: 64742-86-5
**GAS OILS (petroleum),
hydrodesulfurized heavy vacuum**

SYN: HYDRODESULFURIZED HEAVY VACUUM GAS OIL

TOXICITY DATA with REFERENCE
NEO: skn-mus TDLo: 104 g/kg/26W I   EPASR*
8EHQ-0887-0687

SAFETY PROFILE: Questionable carcinogen with experimental neoplastigenic data data. When heated to decomposition it emits acrid smoke and irritating fumes.

GBW025   CAS: 64741-58-8
GAS OILS (petroleum), light vacuum

SYN: LIGHT GAS OIL

TOXICITY DATA with REFERENCE
CAR: skn-mus TDLo: 306 g/kg/2Y-I   FAATDF
7,228,86

CONSENSUS REPORTS: Reported in EPA TSCA Inventory.

SAFETY PROFILE: Questionable carcinogen with experimental carcinogenic data. Pulmonary aspiration can cause severe pneumonitis. Flammable liquid. When heated to decomposition it emits acrid smoke and irritating fumes.

GBY000
GASOLINE
CAS: 8006-61-9

DOT: 1203/1257

PROP: Clear, aromatic, volatile liquid; a mixture of aliphatic HC. Flash p: −50°F, d: <1.0, vap d: 3.0-4.0, ulc: 95-100, lel: 1.3%, uel: 6.0%, autoign temp: 536-853°F, bp: Initially 39°, after 10% distilled = 60°, after 50% = 110°, after 90% = 170°, final bp: 204°. Insol in water, freely sol in absolute alc, ether, chloroform, benzene.

SYNS: CASING HEAD GASOLINE (DOT) ◇ MOTOR FUEL (DOT) ◇ MOTOR SPIRIT (DOT) ◇ NATURAL GASOLINE (DOT) ◇ PETROL (DOT)

CONSENSUS REPORTS: Reported in EPA TSCA Inventory.

OSHA PEL: TWA 300 ppm; STEL 500 ppm ACGIH TLV: TWA 300 ppm; STEL 500 ppm DOT Classification: Flammable Liquid; Label: Flammable Liquid.

SAFETY PROFILE: Questionable carcinogen. Mildly toxic by inhalation. Human systemic effects by inhalation: cough, conjunctiva irritation, hallucinations or distorted perceptions. Repeated or prolonged dermal exposure causes dermatitis. Can cause blistering of skin. Inhalation or ingestion can cause central nervous system depression. A human eye irritant. A very dangerous fire and explosion hazard when exposed to heat or flame; can react vigorously with oxidizing materials. To fight fire use foam, CO_2, dry chemical.

GCE000
GASOLINE ENGINE EXHAUST "TAR"

SYNS: AUTOMOBILE EXHAUST CONDENSATE ◇ GASOLINE ENGINE EXHAUST CONDENSATE

TOXICITY DATA with REFERENCE
CAR: skn-mus TDLo: 110 g/kg/69W-I CANCAR 15,103,62
NEO: itr-ham TD: 860 mg/kg/60W-I CANCAR 40,203,77

NEO: itr-ham TDLo: 469 mg/kg/60W-I CANCAR 40,203,77
ETA: itr-ham TD: 420 mg/kg/78W-I JCROD7 105,24,83
ETA: itr-ham TD: 643 mg/kg/78W-I JCROD7 105,24,83

SAFETY PROFILE: Questionable carcinogen with experimental carcinogenic, neoplastigenic, and tumorigenic data.

GCK300
GEMFIBROZIL
CAS: 25812-30-0

mf: $C_{15}H_{22}O_3$ mw: 250.37

PROP: Crystals from hexane. Mp: 61-63°, bp: 158-159°.

SYNS: CI-719 ◇ 5-(2,5-DIMETHYLPHENOXY)-2,2-DIMETHYLPENTANOIC ACID (9CI) ◇ 2,2-DIMETHYL-5-(2,5-XYLYLOXY)VALERIC ACID ◇ GEVILON ◇ LIPUR ◇ LOPID

TOXICITY DATA with REFERENCE
CAR: orl-rat TDLo: 218 g/kg/2Y-C JJIND8 67,1105,81
NEO: orl-rat TD: 22 g/kg/2Y-C JJIND8 67,1105,81
ETA: orl-mus TDLo: 16 g/kg/78W-C JJIND8 67,1105,81

SAFETY PROFILE: Questionable carcinogen with experimental carcinogenic, neoplastigenic, and tumorigenic data. Moderately toxic by ingestion.

GEM000
GIBBERELLIC ACID
CAS: 77-06-5

mf: $C_{19}H_{22}O_6$ mw: 346.41

PROP: A plant growth-promoting hormone. White crystals or crystalline powder. Mp: 233-235°. Sltly sol in water, ether; sol in methanol, ethanol, acetone, aqueous solns of sodium bicarbonate and sodium acetate; modderately sol in ethyl acetate.

SYNS: BERELEX ◇ BRELLIN ◇ CEKUGIB ◇ FLORALTONE ◇ GA ◇ GIBBERELLIN ◇ GIBBREL ◇ GIB-SOL ◇ GIB-TABS ◇ GROCEL ◇ NCI-C55823 ◇ PRO-GIBB ◇ 2,4a,7-TRIHYDROXY-1-METHYL-8-METHYLENEGIBB-3-ENE-1,10-CARBOXYLIC ACID 1-4-LACTONE

TOXICITY DATA with REFERENCE
ETA: orl-mus TDLo: 142 g/kg/78W-I NTIS** PB223-159
MUT: dnd-mam: lym 1 mmol/L PYTCAS 11,3135,72

MUT: dnd-sal: spr 1 mmol/L   PYTCAS 11,3135,72

CONSENSUS REPORTS: EPA Genetic Toxicology Program. Reported in EPA TSCA Inventory.

SAFETY PROFILE: Questionable carcinogen with experimental tumorigenic data. Mildly toxic by ingestion. Mutation data reported. When heated to decomposition it emits acrid smoke and irritating fumes.

GFA000   CAS: 15879-93-3
α-d-GLUCOCHLORALOSE
mf: $C_8H_{11}Cl_3O_6$ mw: 309.54

SYNS: AGC ◇ ALFAMAT ◇ ANHYDROGLUCOCHLORAL ◇ APHOSAL ◇ CHLORALOSANE ◇ α-CHLORALOSE ◇ CHLOROALOSANE ◇ DULCIDOR ◇ GLUCOCHLORAL ◇ GLUCOCHLORALOSE ◇ KALMETTUMSOMNIFERUM ◇ MONOTRICHLOR-AETHYLIDEN-α-GLUCOSE (GERMAN) ◇ MUREX ◇ SOMIO ◇ 1,2-o-(2,2,2-TRICHLOROETHYLIDENE)-α-d-GLUCOFURANOSE

TOXICITY DATA with REFERENCE
ETA: scu-mus TDLo: 215 mg/kg   NTIS** PB223-159

CONSENSUS REPORTS: Reported in EPA TSCA Inventory.

SAFETY PROFILE: Questionable carcinogen with experimental tumorigenic data. Poison by ingestion, subcutaneous and intraperitoneal routes. When heated to decomposition it emits toxic fumes of Cl^-.

GFG000   CAS: 50-99-7
d-GLUCOSE
mf: $C_6H_{12}O_6$ mw: 180.18

PROP: Colorless crystals or white crystalline or granular powder; odorless with sweet taste. D: 1.544, mp: 146°. Sol in water; sltly sol in alc. α Form: (monohydrate) crystals from water. Mp: 83°. α Form: (anhydrous) crystals from hot ethanol or water. Mp: 146°. Very sparingly sol in abs alc, ether, acetone; sol in hot glacial acetic acid, pyridine, aniline. β Form: crystals from hot H_2O + ethanol, from dil acetic acid or from pyridine; mp: 148-155°.

SYNS: ANHYDROUS DEXTROSE ◇ CARTOSE ◇ CERELOSE ◇ CORN SUGAR ◇ DEXTROPUR ◇ DEXTROSE (FCC) ◇ DEXTROSE, ANHYDROUS ◇ DEXTROSOL ◇ GLUCOLIN ◇ GLUCOSE ◇ d-GLUCOSE, ANHYDROUS ◇ GLUCOSE LIQUID ◇ GRAPE SUGAR ◇ SIRUP

TOXICITY DATA with REFERENCE
ETA: scu-rat TDLo: 15400 g/kg/22W-C
GANNA2 30,419,36

MUT: mmo-sat 25 mg/plate   NARHAD 12,2127,84
MUT: oms-omi 1 mol/L   ARMKA7 91,305,73

CONSENSUS REPORTS: Reported in EPA TSCA Inventory. EPA Genetic Toxicology Program.

SAFETY PROFILE: Questionable carcinogen with experimental tumorigenic data. Mildly toxic by ingestion. Experimental reproductive effects. Mutation data reported. When heated to decomposition it emits acrid smoke and irritating fumes.

GFO100
N²-(γ-l-(+)-GLUTAMYL)-4-CARBOXYPHENYLHYDRAZINE
mf: $C_{12}H_{15}N_3O_5$ mw: 281.30

SYNS: ANTHGLUTIN ◇ l-GLUTAMIC ACID, 5-(2-(4-CARBOXYPHENYL)HYDRAZIDE)

TOXICITY DATA with REFERENCE
CAR: orl-mus TDLo: 72800 mg/kg/52W-I
ANTRD4 6,917,86

SAFETY PROFILE: Questionable carcinogen with experimental carcinogenic data. When heated to decomposition it emits toxic fumes of NO_x.

GGY000   CAS: 17526-74-8
GLYCIDYL ESTER of HEXANOIC ACID
mf: $C_9H_{16}O_3$ mw: 172.25

TOXICITY DATA with REFERENCE
ETA: scu-rat TDLo: 2000 mg/kg/7W-I   ANYAA9 68,750,58

SAFETY PROFILE: Questionable carcinogen with experimental tumorigenic data. When heated to decomposition it emits acrid smoke and irritating fumes.

GIS000   CAS: 7440-57-5
GOLD
af: Au   aw: 196.97

PROP: Cubic, yellow, ductile, metallic crystals. Mp: 1064.76°, bp: 2700°, d: 19.3 (liquid) 17.0 @ 1063°, vap press: 1 mm @ 1869°, Hardness (Mohs') 2.5-3.0; (Brinell's) 18.5.

SYNS: BURNISH GOLD ◇ COLLOIDAL GOLD ◇ GOLD FLAKE ◇ GOLD LEAF ◇ GOLD POWDER ◇ MAGNESIUM GOLD PURPLE ◇ SHELL GOLD

TOXICITY DATA with REFERENCE
ETA: imp-mus TDLo: 21 g/kg   NATWAY 42,75,55

ETA: imp-rat TD: 4730 mg/kg   NATWAY
42,75,55

ETA: imp-rat TDLo: 200 mg/kg   NATWAY
42,75,55

CONSENSUS REPORTS: Reported in EPA
TSCA Inventory.

SAFETY PROFILE: Questionable carcinogen
with experimental tumorigenic data by implantation. Poison by intravenous route. Experimental
reproductive effects.

GJU000   CAS: 8016-20-4
GRAPEFRUIT OIL

PROP: From the fresh peel of *Citrus paradisi*
Macfayden (*Citrus decumana* L.). Yellow liquid. Sol in fixed oils, mineral oil; sltly sol in
propylene glycol; insol in glycerin.

SYNS: GRAPEFRUIT OIL, COLDPRESSED ◇ GRAPEFRUIT
OIL, EXPRESSED ◇ OIL of GRAPEFRUIT ◇ OIL of SHAD-
DOCK

TOXICITY DATA with REFERENCE
ETA: skn-mus TDLo: 280 g/kg/33W-I   JNCIAM
24,1389,60

MUT: dnr-bcs 20 mg/disc   TOFOD5 8,91,85

CONSENSUS REPORTS: Reported in EPA
TSCA Inventory.

SAFETY PROFILE: Questionable carcinogen
with experimental tumorigenic data. Mutation
data reported. A skin irritant. When heated to
decomposition it emits acrid smoke and irritating
fumes.

GKE900   CAS: 14567-61-4
GRUNERITE

TOXICITY DATA with REFERENCE
ETA: ipl-rat TDLo: 80 mg/kg   CNREA8 2,157,86

SAFETY PROFILE: Questionable carcinogen
with experimental tumorigenic data.

GLI000   CAS: 73-40-5
GUANINE
mf: $C_5H_5N_5O$ mw: 151.15

PROP: Usually amorphous. Decomp: >360°
with partial sublimation; very sol in ammonia
water, aq KOH solns, dil acids; very sltly sol
in alc, ether. Insol in water.

SYNS: 2-AMINOHYPOXANTHINE ◇ MEARLMAID

TOXICITY DATA with REFERENCE
ETA: scu-rat TDLo: 1300 mg/kg/26W-I: TER

CNREA8 27,925,67

MUT: cyt-mus-ipr 15 ng/kg   NULSAK 19,40,76
MUT: sln-hmn: lym 30 μmol/L   MUTAEX 1,99,86

CONSENSUS REPORTS: Reported in EPA
TSCA Inventory. EPA Genetic Toxicology Program.

SAFETY PROFILE: Questionable carcinogen
with experimental tumorigenic and teratogenic
data. Human mutation data reported. When
heated to decomposition it emits toxic fumes
of NO_x.

GLM000   CAS: 5227-68-9
GUANINE-7-N-OXIDE
mf: $C_5H_5N_5O_2$ mw: 167.15

SYN: 7-HYDROXYGUANINE

TOXICITY DATA with REFERENCE
NEO: scu-rat TDLo: 390 mg/kg/26W-I   CNREA8
27,925,67

SAFETY PROFILE: Questionable carcinogen
with experimental neoplastigenic data. Poison
by intraperitoneal route. When heated to decomposition it emits very toxic fumes of NO_x.

GLO000   CAS: 19039-44-2
GUANINE-3-N-OXIDE
HEMIHYDROCHLORIDE
mf: $C_5H_5O_2 \cdot 1/2ClH$ mw: 115.33

TOXICITY DATA with REFERENCE
NEO: scu-rat TDLo: 1040 mg/kg/24W-I
CNREA8 30,184,70

SAFETY PROFILE: Questionable carcinogen
with experimental neoplastigenic data. When
heated to decomposition it emits toxic fumes
of Cl^-.

GLW000
GUAVA

PROP: Material extracted with hot water from
the unripe fruits of *P. guajava* (JNCIAM
60,683,78).

SYN: PSIDIUM GUAJAVA

TOXICITY DATA with REFERENCE
ETA: scu-rat TDLo: 10 g/kg/72W-I   JNCIAM
60,683,78

SAFETY PROFILE: Questionable carcinogen
with experimental tumorigenic data. When
heated to decomposition it emits acrid smoke
and irritating fumes.

HAD000   CAS: 14456-34-9
HAFNIUM CHLORIDE OXIDE
OCTAHYDRATE
mf: $Cl_2HfO \cdot 8H_2O$ mw: 409.55

PROP: Colorless crystals.

SYN: HAFNIUM OXYCHLORIDE OCTAHYDRATE

TOXICITY DATA with REFERENCE
ETA: idr-mus TDLo:800 µg/kg   CNREA8
  33,287,73

SAFETY PROFILE: Questionable carcinogen with experimental tumorigenic data. When heated to decomposition it emits very toxic fumes of Cl^-.

HAF375   CAS: 12068-50-7
HALLOYSITE

TOXICITY DATA with REFERENCE
ETA: imp-rat TDLo:200 mg/kg   JJIND8 67,965,81

SAFETY PROFILE: Questionable carcinogen with experimental tumorigenic data.

HAL000   CAS: 20004-62-0
HELIOMYCIN
mf: $C_{22}H_{16}O_6$ mw: 376.38

PROP: Yellow needles from dioxane. Decomp 315°, sublimes at 200-205° (0.001 mm). Stable to hot conc H_2SO_4 or hot KOH. Weakly acid. Slt soly in water; fair in ether, benzene, alc, acetone, acetic acid.

SYNS: A 3733A ◊ ANTIBIOTIC A 3733A ◊ CROCEOMYCIN ◊ GELIOMYCIN ◊ ITAMYCIN ◊ RESISTOMYCIN ◊ X-340

TOXICITY DATA with REFERENCE
CAR: imp-rat TDLo:20750 µg/kg   JJIND8
  71,539,83

SAFETY PROFILE: Questionable carcinogen with experimental carcinogenic data. Poison by intraperitoneal route. Moderately toxic by ingestion. When heated to decomposition it emits toxic fumes of NO_x.

HAL500   CAS: 303-33-3
HELIOTRINE
mf: $C_{16}H_{27}NO_5$ mw: 313.44

SYN: HELIOTRON

TOXICITY DATA with REFERENCE
ETA: orl-rat TDLo:460 mg/kg/6D-I   CNREA8
  35,2020,75

MUT: cyt-mam:leu 50 µmol/L   AJBSAM
  21,469,68
MUT: dni-hmn:lvr 25 mg/L   IJEVAW 1,107,71
MUT: mma-sat 1 mg/plate   MUREAV 68,211,79
MUT: oms-hmn:lvr 10 mg/L   IJEVAW 1,107,71
MUT: sce-ham:lng 1200 µg/L   MUREAV
  142,209,85

CONSENSUS REPORTS: EPA Genetic Toxicology Program.

SAFETY PROFILE: Questionable carcinogen with experimental tumorigenic and teratogenic data. A poison by ingestion, intravenous, intraperitoneal, and possibly other routes. Other experimental reproductive effects. Human mutation data reported. When heated to decomposition it emits toxic fumes of NO_x.

HAM000
HELIOTROPIUM SUPINUM L.

PROP: Crude alkaloidal fraction (CNREA8 30,2127,70).

TOXICITY DATA with REFERENCE
ETA: orl-rat TD:400 mg/kg   JNCIAM 47,1037,71
ETA: orl-rat TDLo:300 mg/kg   CNREA8
  30,2127,70

SAFETY PROFILE: Questionable carcinogen with experimental tumorigenic data. When heated to decomposition it emits toxic fumes.

HAP500   CAS: 517-28-2
HEMATOXYLIN
mf: $C_{16}H_{14}O_6$ mw: 302.30

SYN: NCI-C55889

TOXICITY DATA with REFERENCE
ETA: orl-rat TDLo:400 mg/kg/26W-C   GASTAB
  23,1,53

CONSENSUS REPORTS: Reported in EPA TSCA Inventory.

SAFETY PROFILE: Questionable carcinogen with experimental tumorigenic data. When heated to decomposition it emits acrid smoke and fumes.

HAR500
HEPTACHLOR (TECHNICAL GRADE)

PROP: Mixture of 73% heptachlor, 22% trans-chlordane, and 5% nonachlor (NCITR* NCI-CG-TR-9).

SYN: 1,4,5,6,7,8,8-HEPTACHLORO-3a,4,7,7a-TETRAHY-DRO 4,7-METHANOINDENE (technical grade)

TOXICITY DATA with REFERENCE
CAR: orl-mus TDLo: 410 mg/kg/80W-C
NCITR* NCI-CG-TR-9,77

SAFETY PROFILE: Questionable carcinogen with experimental carcinogenic data. Poison by ingestion. Moderately toxic by skin contact. When heated to decomposition it emits toxic fumes of Cl⁻.

HBN000 CAS: 63019-32-9
8-HEPTYLBENZ(a)ANTHRACENE
mf: $C_{25}H_{26}$ mw: 326.51

SYN: 5-n-HEPTYLBENZ(1:2)BENZANTHRACENE

TOXICITY DATA with REFERENCE
ETA: skn-mus TDLo: 1970 mg/kg/82W-I
PRLBA4 131,170,42

SAFETY PROFILE: Questionable carcinogen with experimental tumorigenic data. When heated to decomposition it emits acrid smoke and fumes.

HBP000 CAS: 16338-99-1
HEPTYLMETHYLINITROSAMINE
mf: $C_8H_{18}N_2O$ mw: 158.28

SYNS: METHYLHEPTYLNITROSAMIN (GERMAN) ◊ N-METHYL-N-NITROSOHEPTYLAMINE ◊ N-NITROSO-N-METHYLHEPTYLAMINE

TOXICITY DATA with REFERENCE
ETA: orl-rat TDLo: 1960 mg/kg/30W-I JCROD7
106,171,83
ETA: scu-rat TDLo: 4600 mg/kg/58W-I ZEKBAI
69,103,67
MUT: mma-sat 50 μg/plate TCMUD8 1,295,80

SAFETY PROFILE: Questionable carcinogen with experimental tumorigenic data. Moderately toxic by subcutaneous route. Mutation data reported. Many N-nitroso compounds are carcinogens. When heated to decomposition it emits toxic fumes of NO_x.

HBP250 CAS: 24346-78-9
1-HEPTYL-1-NITROSOUREA
mf: $C_8H_{17}N_3O_2$ mw: 187.28

SYN: n-HEPTYL NITROSUREA

TOXICITY DATA with REFERENCE
ETA: orl-rat TDLo: 600 mg/kg ANYAA9
381,250,82
ETA: scu-rat TDLo: 650 mg/kg ANYAA9
381,250,82

SAFETY PROFILE: Questionable carcinogen with experimental tumorigenic data. When heated to decomposition it emits toxic fumes of NO_x.

HCD000 CAS: 35065-27-1
2,2′,4,4′,5′5′-HEXACHLORO-1,1′-BIPHENYL
mf: $C_{12}H_4Cl_6$ mw: 360.86

SYNS: 2,2′,4,4′5,5′-HEXACHLOROBIPHENYL ◊ 2,4,5, 2′,4′,5′-HEXACHLOROBIPHENYL

TOXICITY DATA with REFERENCE
ETA: orl-rat TDLo: 3650 mg/kg/104W-C
TXAPA9 48,A181,79
MUT: dnd-mus-orl 36400 μg/kg/5D CBINA8
27,99,79
MUT: oms-mus-orl 36400 μg/kg/5D CBINA8
27,99,79

SAFETY PROFILE: Questionable carcinogen with experimental tumorigenic data. Experimental reproductive effects. Mutation data reported. When heated to decomposition it emits toxic fumes of Cl⁻.

HCE400
HEXACHLOROCYCLOHEXANE, delta and epsilon mixture
mf: $C_6H_6Cl_6$ mw: 290.82

SYN: Δ-HEXACHLOROCYCLOHEXANE mixed with epsilon-HEXACHLOROCYCLOHEXANE

TOXICITY DATA with REFERENCE
CAR: orl-mus TDLo: 12960 mg/kg/26W-C
CMSHAF 1,279,72

SAFETY PROFILE: Questionable carcinogen with experimental carcinogenic data. When heated to decomposition it emits toxic fumes of Cl⁻.

HCF000 CAS: 57653-85-7
1,2,3,4,7,8-HEXACHLORODIBENZO-p-DIOXIN
mf: $C_{12}H_2Cl_6O_2$ mw: 390.84

CONSENSUS REPORTS: IARC Cancer Review: Animal Inadequate Evidence IMEMDT 15,41,77.

SAFETY PROFILE: Questionable carcinogen. A deadly poison by ingestion. When heated to decomposition it emits toxic fumes of Cl⁻.

HCI000 CAS: 67-72-1
HEXACHLOROETHANE
DOT: 9037
mf: C_2Cl_6 mw: 236.72

PROP: Rhombic, triclinic or cubic crystals, colorless, camphor-like odor. Mp: 186.6° (sublimes), d: 2.091, vap press: 1 mm @ 32.7°, bp: 186.8° (triple point). Sol in alc, benzene, chloroform, ether, oils; insol in water.

SYNS: AVLOTANE ◇ CARBON HEXACHLORIDE ◇ DISTOKAL ◇ DISTOPAN ◇ DISTOPIN ◇ EGITOL ◇ ETHANE HEXACHLORIDE ◇ ETHYLENE HEXACHLORIDE ◇ FALKITOL ◇ FASCIOLIN ◇ HEXACHLOR-AETHAN (GERMAN) ◇ 1,1,1,2,2,2-HEXACHLOROETHANE ◇ HEXACHLOROETHYLENE ◇ MOTTENHEXE ◇ NCI-C04604 ◇ PERCHLOROETHANE ◇ PHENOHEP ◇ RCRA WASTE NUMBER U131

TOXICITY DATA with REFERENCE
CAR: orl-mus TD:460 g/kg/78W-I   NCITR*
    NCI-CG-TR-68,78
CAR: orl-mus TDLo:230 g/kg/78W-I   NCITR*
    NCI-CG-TR-68,78

CONSENSUS REPORTS: IARC Cancer Review: GROUP 3 IMEMDT 7,56,87; Animal Limited Evidence IMEMDT 20,467,79. NCI Carcinogenesis Bioassay (gavage); Clear Evidence: mouse NCITR* NCI-CG-TR-68,78. NCI Carcinogenesis Bioassay (gavage); No Evidence: rat NCITR* NCI-CG-TR-68,78. Community Right-To-Know List. Reported in EPA TSCA Inventory. EPA Genetic Toxicology Program.

OSHA PEL: TWA 1 ppm (skin)   ACGIH TLV: TWA 1 ppm   DFG MAK: 1 ppm (10 mg/m^3)   NIOSH REL: (Hexachloroethane) Reduce to lowest level   DOT Classification: ORM-A; Label: None.

SAFETY PROFILE: Questionable carcinogen with experimental carcinogenic data. A poison by intravenous route. Moderately toxic by intraperitoneal route. Mildly toxic by ingestion. Experimental reproductive effects. An insecticide. When heated to decomposition it emits highly toxic fumes of Cl$^-$ and phosgene.

HCL000   CAS: 70-30-4
HEXACHLOROPHENE
DOT: 2875
mf: $C_{13}H_6Cl_6O_2$ mw: 406.89

PROP: Crystals, water insol. Mp: 165°. Sol in alc, acetone, ether, chloroform, propylene glycol, polyethylene glycols, olive oil, cottonseed oil, dil solns of alkalies.

SYNS: ACIGENA ◇ ALMEDERM ◇ AT 7 ◇ B32 ◇ BILEVON ◇ BIS(2-HYDROXY-3,5,6-TRICHLOROPHENYL)

METHANE ◇ BIS-2,3,5-TRICHLOR-6-HYDROXYFENYL-METHAN (CZECH) ◇ BIS(3,5,6-TRICHLORO-2-HYDROXYPHENYL)METHANE ◇ COMPOUND G-11 ◇ COTOFILM ◇ DERMADEX ◇ 2,2'-DIHYDROXY-3,3',5,5',6,6'-HEXACHLORODIPHENYLMETHANE ◇ 2,2'-DIHYDROXY-3,5,6,-3',5',6'-HEXACHLORODIPHENYLMETHANE ◇ EXOFENE ◇ FOMAC ◇ FOSTRIL ◇ G-11 ◇ GAMOPHENE ◇ G-ELEVEN ◇ GERMA-MEDICA ◇ HCP ◇ HEXABALM ◇ 2,2',3,3',5,5'-HEXACHLORO-6,6'-DIHYDROXYDIPHENYLMETHANE ◇ HEXACHLOROFEN (CZECH) ◇ HEXACHLOROPHANE ◇ HEXACHLOROPHEN ◇ HEXACHLOROPHENE (DOT) ◇ HEXAFEN ◇ HEXIDE ◇ HEXOPHENE ◇ HEXOSAN ◇ ISOBAC 20 ◇ 2,2'-METHYLENEBIS(3,4,6-TRICHLOROPHENOL) ◇ NABAC ◇ NCI-C02653 ◇ NEOSEPT ◇ PHISO-DANV ◇ PHISOHEX ◇ RCRA WASTE NUMBER U132 ◇ RITOSEPT ◇ SEPTISOL ◇ SEPTOFEN ◇ STERAL ◇ STERASKIN ◇ SURGI-CEN ◇ SUROFENE ◇ TERSASEPTIC ◇ TRICHLOROPHENE ◇ TURGEX

TOXICITY DATA with REFERENCE
NEO: ihl-rat TCLo:33500 µg/m^3/52W
    VOONAW 33(1),62,87
ETA: skn-mus TDLo:8400 mg/kg/21W-I
    CNREA8 19,413,59

CONSENSUS REPORTS: IARC Cancer Review: Human Inadequate Evidence IMEMDT 20,241,79. NCI Carcinogenesis Bioassay (feed); No Evidence: rat NCITR* NCI-CG-TR-40,78. Reported in EPA TSCA Inventory. Chlorophenols are on the Community Right-To-Know List.

DOT Classification: IMO: Poison B; Label: St. Andrews Cross.

SAFETY PROFILE: Questionable carcinogen with experimental neoplastigenic, tumorigenic, and teratogenic data. A human poison by ingestion. An experimental poison by ingestion, intraperitoneal, and intravenous routes. Moderately toxic by skin contact. Human systemic effects by ingestion: cardiomyopathy (damage to the heart muscle), nausea or vomiting, diarrhea, shock. Unspecified human reproductive effects. Experimental reproductive effects. An eye and hunan skin irritant. Used as a germicidal agent. When heated to decomposition it emits toxic fumes of Cl$^-$.

HCX000   CAS: 604-88-6
HEXAETHYLBENZENE
mf: $C_{18}H_{30}$ mw: 246.48

PROP: Colorless crystals. Mp: 130°, bp: 298°, d: 0.831 @ 130°, vap press: 10 mm @ 150.3°. Insol in water; very sol in benzene.

TOXICITY DATA with REFERENCE
ETA: imp-mus TDLo:1000 mg/kg   CNREA 8
   26,105,66

CONSENSUS REPORTS: Reported in EPA
TSCA Inventory.

SAFETY PROFILE: Questionable carcinogen
with experimental tumorigenic data. Flammable
when exposed to heat or flame; can react with
oxidizing materials. When heated to decomposition it emits acrid smoke and fumes.

HDH000   CAS: 63041-92-9
1,2,4,5,6,7-
HEXAHYDROBENZ(e)ACEANTHRYLENE
mf: $C_{20}H_{18}$ mw: 258.38

SYN: 1′,2′,3′,4′ -TETRAHYDRO-4,10-ACE-1,2-BENZAN-
THRACENE

TOXICITY DATA with REFERENCE
ETA: scu-mus TDLo:200 mg/kg   AJCAA7
   33,499,38

SAFETY PROFILE: Questionable carcinogen
with experimental tumorigenic data. When
heated to decomposition it emits acrid smoke
and fumes.

HDK000   CAS: 153-32-2
1,2,3,4,12,13-
HEXAHYDRODIBENZ(a,h)ANTHRACENE
mf: $C_{22}H_{20}$ mw: 284.42

TOXICITY DATA with REFERENCE
NEO: skn-mus TDLo:152 mg/kg/50W-I
   JNCIAM 34,1,65
MUT: mma-sat 1 μg/plate   MUREAV 51,311,78

SAFETY PROFILE: Questionable carcinogen
with experimental neoplastigenic data. Mutation
data reported. When heated to decomposition
it emits acrid smoke and fumes.

HDR500   CAS: 35281-27-7
6,7,8,9,10,12b-HEXAHYDRO-3-METHYL
CHOLANTHRENE
mf: $C_{21}H_{22}$ mw: 274.43

SYN: 1,2,6,7,8,9,10,12b-OCTAHYDRO-3-METHYL-
BENZ(j)ACEANTHRYLENE

TOXICITY DATA with REFERENCE
CAR: skn-mus TDLo:140 mg/kg/50W-I
   ZKKOBW 77,226,72
MUT: mma-sat 1 μg/plate   MUREAV 51,311,78

SAFETY PROFILE: Questionable carcinogen

with experimental carcinogenic data. Mutation
data reported. When heated to decomposition
it emits acrid smoke and fumes.

HDV500   CAS: 13980-04-6
HEXAHYDRO-1,3,5-s-TRIAZINE
mf: $C_3H_6N_6O_3$ mw: 174.15

SYNS: HEXAHYDRO-1,3,5-TRINITROSO-s-TRIAZINE
◇ HEXAHYDRO-1,3,5-TRINITROSO-1,3,5-TRIAZINE
◇ 1,3,5-TRINITROSO-1,3,5-TRIAZACYCLOHEXANE
◇ TRINITROSOTRIMETHYLENETRIAMINE ◇ TRINITROSO-
TRIMETHYLENTRIAMIN (GERMAN) ◇ TTT

TOXICITY DATA with REFERENCE
ETA: orl-rat TDLo:765 mg/kg/52W-I   ARGEAR
   46,657,76

SAFETY PROFILE: Questionable carcinogen
with experimental tumorigenic data. A poison
by ingestion. Explodes on contact with sulfuric
acid. When heated to decomposition it emits
toxic fumes of NO_x.

HEC000   CAS: 87-85-4
HEXAMETHYLBENZENE
mf: $C_{12}H_{18}$ mw: 162.30

PROP: Plates from ethanol. Mp: 165.5°, bp:
265°. Insol in water; very sol in ether.

TOXICITY DATA with REFERENCE
NEO: imp-mus TDLo:1000 mg/kg   CNREA8
   26,105,66

CONSENSUS REPORTS: Reported in EPA
TSCA Inventory.

SAFETY PROFILE: Questionable carcinogen
with experimental neoplastigenic data. Mildly
toxic by ingestion. When heated to decomposition it emits acrid smoke and fumes.

HEC500   CAS: 7641-77-2
HEXAMETHYLBICYCLO(2.2.0)HEXA-2,5-
DIENE
mf: $C_{12}H_{18}$ mw: 162.30

SYNS: 2-BUTIN HEXAMETHYL-DEWAR-BENZOL (GER-
MAN) ◇ HEXAMETHYL-BICYCLO(2.2.0)HEXA-2,5-DIEN
(GERMAN)

TOXICITY DATA with REFERENCE
ETA: scu-mus TDLo:800 mg/kg/15W-I
   ZEKBAI 74,100,70

SAFETY PROFILE: Questionable carcinogen
with experimental tumorigenic data. When

heated to decomposition it emits acrid smoke and fumes.

HED500   CAS: 999-97-3
HEXAMETHYLDISILAZANE
mf: $C_6H_{19}NSi_2$ mw: 161.44

PROP: Flash p: 57.2°F.

SYNS: BIS(TRIMETHYLSILYL)AMINE ◇ HEXAMETHYL-SILAZANE ◇ HMDS ◇ OAP ◇ 1,1,1-TRIMETHYL-N-(TRI-METHYLSILYL)SILANAMINE

TOXICITY DATA with REFERENCE
ETA: ipr-mus TDLo: 1 g/kg/I   JNCIAM 54,495,75

CONSENSUS REPORTS: Reported in EPA TSCA Inventory.

SAFETY PROFILE: Questionable carcinogen with experimental tumorigenic data. Moderately toxic by intraperitoneal route. A dangerous fire hazard when exposed to heat or flame; can react vigorously with oxidizing materials. When heated to decomposition it emits toxic fumes of NO_x.

HEI500   CAS: 100-97-0
HEXAMETHYLENETETRAMINE
DOT: 1328
mf: $C_6H_{12}N_4$ mw: 140.22

PROP: Odorless, rhombic crystals from alcohol. Mp: 280° (sublimes), flash p: 482°F, d: 1.33 @ −5°. Very sltly sol in hot ether.

SYNS: ACETO HMT ◇ AMINOFORM ◇ AMMOFORM ◇ AMMONIOFORMALDEHYDE ◇ CYSTAMIN ◇ CYSTOGEN ◇ ESAMETILENTETRAMINA (ITALIAN) ◇ FORMAMINE ◇ FORMIN ◇ HEXAFORM ◇ HEXAMETHYLENAMINE ◇ HEXAMETHYLENEAMINE ◇ HEXAMETHYLENE-TETRAAMINE ◇ HEXAMETHYLENTETRAMIN (GERMAN) ◇ HEXAMINE (DOT) ◇ HEXILMETHYLENAMINE ◇ HMT ◇ METHAMIN ◇ METHENAMINE ◇ PREPARATION AF ◇ RESOTROPIN ◇ 1,3,5,7-TETRAAZAADAMANTANE ◇ URITONE ◇ UROTROPIN ◇ UROTROPINE

TOXICITY DATA with REFERENCE
ETA: scu-rat TDLo: 140 g/kg/78W-I   FAONAU 50A,77,72
MUT: cyt-hmn: hla 1 mmol/L   HUMAA7 4,112,67
MUT: dlt-mus-ipr 25 g/kg   DMWOAX 92,2315,67
MUT: dlt-mus-orl 25 g/kg   HUMAA7 4,112,67
MUT: dnr-bcs 1 mg/disc   SAIGBL 26,147,84
MUT: dnr-esc 6 mg/well/16H   CBINA8 15,219,76
MUT: otr-ham: kdy 10 mg/L   CRNGDP 4,457,83

CONSENSUS REPORTS: EPA Genetic Toxicology Program. Reported in EPA TSCA Inventory.

DOT Classification: IMO: Flammable Solid; Label: Flammable Solid.

SAFETY PROFILE: Questionable carcinogen with experimental tumorigenic data. A poison by subcutaneous route. Moderately toxic by ingestion and intraperitoneal routes. Human mutation data reported. An irritant to skin, eyes, and mucous membranes. Some persons suffer a skin rash if they come in contact with this material or the fumes evolved when it is heated. Its major industrial use is in the manufacture of phenolic resins. Combustible. When heated to decomposition it emits toxic fumes of formaldehyde and NO_x.

HEJ500   CAS: 645-05-6
HEXAMETHYLMELAMINE
mf: $C_9H_{18}N_6$ mw: 210.33

PROP: A solid material, insol in water, sol in acetone.

SYNS: ALTRETAMINE ◇ ENT 50,852 ◇ HEMEL ◇ N,N,N′,N′,N′,N′′-HEXAMETHYL-1,3,5-TRIAZINE-2,4,6-TRIAMINE ◇ HEXASTAT ◇ HMM ◇ NCI-C50259 ◇ NSC 13875 ◇ 2,4,6-TRIS(DIMETHYLAMINO)-s-TRIAZINE ◇ 2,4,6-TRIS(DIMETHYLAMINO)-1,3,5-TRIAZINE

TOXICITY DATA with REFERENCE
NEO: orl-rat TDLo: 7 g/kg/46W-C   JNCIAM 51,403,73
MUT: cyt-hmn: leu 250 μmol/L   CHROAU 24,314,68
MUT: dlt-oin-par 5 mmol/L   MUREAV 4,255,67
MUT: dnd-mam: lym 250 μmol/L   CNREA8 43,500,83
MUT: ipr-mus LD10: 200 mg/kg   CNREA8 40,2762,80
MUT: mma-sat 200 μg/plate   MUREAV 142,121,85
MUT: sln-dmg-par 150 ppm   IMSUAI 38,442,69

CONSENSUS REPORTS: EPA Genetic Toxicology Program.

SAFETY PROFILE: Questionable carcinogen with experimental neoplastigenic data. A poison by ingestion, intraperitoneal, and intravenous routes. An experimental teratogen. Other experimental reproductive effects. Human mutation data reported. Human systemic effects by ingestion: nausea or vomiting and leukopenia (reduced white blood cell count). When heated to decomposition it emits toxic fumes of NO_x.

HEM500   CAS: 628-02-4
HEXANAMIDE
mf: $C_6H_{13}NO$ mw: 115.20

SYNS: CAPROAMIDE ◇ CAPRONAMIDE ◇ NCI-C02142

TOXICITY DATA with REFERENCE
CAR: orl-mus TDLo:438 g/kg/1Y-C JEPTDQ 3(5-6),149,80

CONSENSUS REPORTS: Reported in EPA TSCA Inventory.

SAFETY PROFILE: Questionable carcinogen with experimental carcinogenic data. Moderately toxic by ingestion. When heated to decomposition it emits toxic fumes such as NO_x.

HET500 CAS: 131-73-7
2,4,6,2',4',6'-
HEXANITRODIPHENYLAMINE
mf: $C_{12}H_5N_7O_{12}$ mw: 439.24

SYNS: BIS(2,4,6-TRINITRO-PHENYL)-AMIN (GERMAN) ◇ DPA ◇ ESANITRODIFENILAMINA (ITALIAN) ◇ HEXANI-TRODIFENYLAMINE (DUTCH) ◇ HEXANITRODIPHENYL-AMINE ◇ HEXANITRODIPHENYLAMINE (FRENCH) ◇ 2,2',4,4',6,6'-HEXANITRODIPHENYLAMINE ◇ HEXYL (GERMAN, DUTCH)

TOXICITY DATA with REFERENCE
NEO: orl-rat TDLo:14 g/kg/76W-C NATUAS 180,509,57
MUT: mma-sat 456 nmol/plate MUREAV 136,209,84
MUT: mmo-sat 228 nmol/plate MUREAV 136,209,84

CONSENSUS REPORTS: Reported in EPA TSCA Inventory.

SAFETY PROFILE: Questionable carcinogen with experimental neoplastigenic data. Mutation data reported. A powerful and violent explosive used as a booster explosive; its use is superior to TNT. It is not as good for this purpose as tetryl, but is extremely stable and much safer to handle.

HEW000 CAS: 45776-10-1
1-HEXANOYLAZIRIDINE
mf: $C_8H_{15}NO$ mw: 141.24

SYNS: 1-CAPROYLAZIRIDINE ◇ CAPROYLETHYLENEI-MINE ◇ HEXANOYLETHYLENEIMINE

TOXICITY DATA with REFERENCE
NEO: scu-rat TD:525 mg/kg/17W-I BJPCAL 9,306,54
NEO: scu-rat TDLo:495 mg/kg/19W-I BJPCAL 9,306,54
ETA: scu-mus TDLo:360 mg/kg/41W-I BJPCAL 9,306,54

MUT: cyt-rat-ipr 50 mg/kg BJPCAL 9,306,54

SAFETY PROFILE: Questionable carcinogen with experimental neoplastigenic and tumorigenic data. Mutation data reported. When heated to decomposition it emits toxic fumes of NO_x.

HFL000 CAS: 63019-34-1
5-n-HEXYL-1,2-BENZANTHRACENE
mf: $C_{24}H_{24}$ mw: 312.48

SYN: 8-HEXYL-BENZ(a)ANTHRACENE

TOXICITY DATA with REFERENCE
ETA: skn-mus TDLo:1050 mg/kg/44W-I PRLBA4 129,439,40

SAFETY PROFILE: Questionable carcinogen with experimental tumorigenic data. When heated to decomposition it emits acrid smoke and fumes.

HFS500 CAS: 18774-85-1
1-HEXYL-1-NITROSOUREA
mf: $C_7H_{15}N_3O_2$ mw: 173.25

SYN: NITROSO-N-HEXYLUREA

TOXICITY DATA with REFERENCE
CAR: skn-mus TDLo:693 mg/kg/50W-I JCROD7 102,13,81
ETA: orl-rat TDLo:550 mg/kg ANYAA9 381,250,82
ETA: scu-rat TDLo:410 mg/kg ANYAA9 381,250,82
MUT: mma-sat 10 μg/plate TCMUE9 1,13,84
MUT: mmo-sat 1 μg/plate MUREAV 68,1,79

CONSENSUS REPORTS: EPA Genetic Toxicology Program.

SAFETY PROFILE: Questionable carcinogen with carcinogenic and tumorigenic data. Mutation data reported. When heated to decomposition it emits toxic fumes of NO_x.

HFV500 CAS: 136-77-6
HEXYLRESORCINOL
mf: $C_{12}H_{18}O_2$ mw: 194.30

PROP: Colorless liquid to pale yellow, heavy liquid becoming solid on standing at room temp; needles from benzene or petr ether. Pungent odor, sharp astringent taste. Bp: 179°, mp: 67.5-69°. Very sol in water; sol in benzene, ether, acetone, chloroform, alc, vegetable oils; sltly sol in petr ether.

SYNS: ASCARYL ◇ CAPROKOL ◇ CRYSTOIDS ◇ CYSTOIDS ANTHELMINTIC ◇ 4-HEXYL-1,3-BENZENE

DIOL ◇ 4-HEXYL-1,3-DIHYDROXYBENZENE ◇ HEXYLRE-
SORCIN (GERMAN) ◇ 4-HEXYLRESORCINE ◇ p-HEXYLRE-
SORCINOL ◇ 4-HEXYLRESORCINOL ◇ 4-n-HEXYLRESOR-
CINOL ◇ NCI-C55787 ◇ S.T. 37 ◇ SUCRETS ◇ WORM-AGEN

TOXICITY DATA with REFERENCE

ETA: orl-mus TDLo: 64 g/kg/2Y-C   NTPTR*
  NTP-TR-330,88
MUT: dnr-esc 3 mg/disc   MUREAV 188,111,87
MUT: mma-mus: lyms 5 μg/L   NTPTR*
  NTP-TR-330,88
MUT: sce-ham: ovr 18 μg/L   NTPTR*
  NTP-TR-330,88

CONSENSUS REPORTS: Reported in EPA
TSCA Inventory.

SAFETY PROFILE: Questionable carcinogen
with experimental tumorigenic data. A poison
by ingestion, intraperitoneal, and possibly other
routes. Moderately toxic by subcutaneous route.
Experimental reproductive effects. Mutation
data reported. An eye irritant. Concentrated solutions can cause burns on the skin and mucous
membranes in humans. An anthelmintic and topical antiseptic. When heated to decomposition
it emits acrid smoke and fumes.

HGC000   CAS: 1936-15-8
HISPACID FAST ORANGE 2G
mf: $C_{16}H_{10}N_2O_7S_2 \cdot 2Na$ mw: 452.38

SYNS: ACIDAL FAST ORANGE ◇ ACID FAST ORANGE
EGG ◇ ACID LEATHER ORANGE PGW ◇ ACID LIGHT OR-
ANGE G ◇ ACID ORANGE 10 ◇ ACILAN ORANGE GX
◇ APOCID ORANGE 2G ◇ ATUL ACID CRYSTAL ORANGE
G ◇ BRASILAN ORANGE 2G ◇ BUCACID FAST ORANGE
G ◇ CALCOCID FAST LIGHT ORANGE 2G ◇ CERTICOL
ORANGE GS ◇ CETIL LIGHT ORANGE GG ◇ C.I. 27
◇ C.I. ACID ORANGE 10 ◇ C.I. FOOD ORANGE 4
◇ CRYSTAL ORANGE 2G ◇ D&C ORANGE No. 3
◇ ENIACID LIGHT ORANGE G ◇ ERIO FAST ORANGE AS
◇ FAST LIGHT ORANGE GA ◇ HEXACOL ORANGE GG
CRYSTALS ◇ HIDACID FAST ORANGE G ◇ 7-HYDROXY-
8-(PHENYLAZO)-1,3-NAPHTHALENEDISULFONIC ACID, DI-
SODIUM SALT ◇ 7-HYDROXY-8-(PHENYLAZO)-1,3-
NAPHTHALENEDISULPHONIC ACID, DISODIUM SALT
◇ INK ORANGE JSN ◇ INTRACID FAST ORANGE G
◇ JAVA ORANGE 2G ◇ KITON FAST ORANGE G
◇ NAPHTHALENE FAST ORANGE 2GS ◇ NCI-C53838
◇ NEKLACID FAST ORANGE 2G ◇ ORANGE #10
◇ ORANGE G (BIOLOGICAL STAIN) ◇ ORANGE G DYE
◇ ORANGE G (INDICATOR) ◇ ORANZ G (POLISH)
◇ 1-PHENYLAZO-2-NAPHTHOL-6,8-DISULFONIC ACID, DI-
SODIUM SALT ◇ 1-PHENYLAZO-2-NAPHTHOL-6,8-DISUL-

PHONIC ACID, DISODIUM SALT ◇ SCHULTZ NO. 39
◇ SOLAR LIGHT ORANGE GX ◇ STANDACOL ORANGE G
◇ SULFACID LIGHT ORANGE J ◇ TERTRACID LIGHT OR-
ANGE G ◇ UNITERTRACID LIGHT ORANGE G ◇ VENDACID
LIGHT ORANGE 2G ◇ WOOL ORANGE 2G ◇ XYLENE FAST
ORANGE G

TOXICITY DATA with REFERENCE

MUT: cyt-ham: ovr 20 μmol/L/5H-C   ENMUDM
  1,27,79
MUT: pic-esc 100 mmol/L   MDMIAZ 31,11,79

CONSENSUS REPORTS: IARC Cancer Review: GROUP 3 IMEMDT 7,56,87; Animal
Inadequate Evidence IMEMDT 8,181,75. Reported in EPA TSCA Inventory. EPA Genetic
Toxicology Program.

SAFETY PROFILE: Questionable carcinogen.
Experimental reproductive effects. Mutation
data reported. Used as a drug and cosmetic colorant. When heated to decomposition it emits
very toxic SO_x, Na_2O and NO_x.

HGE500
HISTAMINE HYDROCHLORIDE
mf: $C_5H_9N_3 \cdot xClH$ mw: 366.39

SYNS: 4-AMINOETHYLIMIDAZOLE HYDROCHLORIDE
◇ CHLORHYDRATE D'HISTAMINE (FRENCH)

TOXICITY DATA with REFERENCE

ETA: scu-mus TDLo: 1140 mg/kg/28W-I
  BAFEAG 36,305,49

SAFETY PROFILE: Questionable carcinogen
with experimental tumorigenic data. When
heated to decomposition it emits very toxic
fumes of NO_x and HCl.

HGM000
HUMAN SPERM

TOXICITY DATA with REFERENCE

CAR: ipr-mus TDLo: 56 g/kg/15D-I   13BYAH
  279,62

SAFETY PROFILE: Questionable carcinogen
with experimental carcinogenic data. Slightly
toxic by intraperitoneal route.

HGO500   CAS: 23255-93-8
HYCANTHONE METHANESULFONATE
mf: $C_{20}H_{24}N_2O_2S \cdot CH_4O_3S$; mw: 452.63

SYNS: 1-((2-(DIETHYLAMINO)ETHYL)AMINO)-4-(HY-
DROXYMETHYL)-9H-THIOXANTHEN-9-ONE MONOMETH-
ANE-SULFONATE (SALT) ◇ ETRENOL ◇ HCT ◇ HYCAN-

THONE MESYLATE ◇ HYCANTHONE METHANESULPHO-
NATE ◇ HYCANTHONE MONOMETHANESULPHONATE

TOXICITY DATA with REFERENCE
CAR: ipr-mus TDLo:815 mg/kg/33W-I
IJCNAW 23,97,79
ETA: ims-mus TDLo:350 mg/kg/30W-I
IJCNAW 23,97,79
MUT: cyt-hmn:leu 1 μmol/L   MUREAV 21,287,73
MUT: cyt-hmn:lym 2400 μg/L   JTEHD6 1,211,76
MUT: dni-hmn:lym 50 mg/L   BCPCA6 22,1253,73
MUT: dnr-esc 16 μg/well   ENMUDM 3,429,81
MUT: otr-rat-ipr 30 mg/kg   CNREA8 40,1157,80
MUT: sln-dmg-orl 4400 μmol/L   MUREAV
82,111,81
MUT: sln-dmg-par 4400 μmol/L   MUREAV
82,111,81

CONSENSUS REPORTS: IARC Cancer Review: Animal Inadequate Evidence IMEMDT
13,91,77. EPA Genetic Toxicology Program.

SAFETY PROFILE: Questionable carcinogen
with experimental carcinogenic, tumorigenic,
and teratogenic data. A poison by intraperitoneal, subcutaneous, intravenous, and intramuscular routes. Moderately toxic by ingestion. Human systemic effects by intramuscular route:
hallucinations, muscle weakness, nausea or
vomiting. Human mutation data reported. When
heated to decomposition it emits very toxic
fumes of SO_x.

HGU000   CAS: 57-56-7
HYDRAZINECARBOXAMIDE
mf: CH_5N_3O mw: 75.09

SYNS: AMINOUREA ◇ CARBAMIC ACID HYDRAZIDE
◇ CARBAMOYLHYDRAZINE ◇ CARBAMYLHYDRAZINE
◇ CARBAZAMIDE ◇ SEMICARBAZIDE

TOXICITY DATA with REFERENCE
ETA: orl-mus TDLo:25 g/kg/30W-C   GANNA2
51,83,60
MUT: cyt-grh-par 100 mmol/L   MUREAV
40,237,76
MUT: dnd-mam:lym 2 mmol/L/25H   BBACAQ
123,458,66
MUT: mma-sat 67 μmol/plate   CNREA8 41,1469,81
MUT: mmo-sat 67 μmol/plate   CNREA8 41,1469,81
MUT: sln-grh-par 100 mmol/L   MUREAV
40,237,76
MUT: spm-grh-par 100 mmol/L   MUREAV
40,237,76

CONSENSUS REPORTS: Reported in EPA
TSCA Inventory.

SAFETY PROFILE: Questionable carcinogen
with experimental tumorigenic data. A poison
by ingestion, intraperitoneal, subcutaneous, and
intravenous routes. Human systemic effects by
intravenous route: convulsions. Mutation data
reported. When heated to decomposition it emits
toxic fumes of NO_x.

HGU500   CAS: 7803-57-8
HYDRAZINE HYDRATE
mf: $H_4N_2 \bullet H_2O$ mw: 50.08

PROP: Colorless fuming, refractive liquid. Mp:
−51.7°, bp: 118.5° @ 740 mm. D: 1.03 @
21°. Faint characteristic odor. A strong base,
very corrosive; attacks glass, rubber, and cork.
Very powerful reducing agent. Misc with water
and alc; insol in chloroform and ether.

SYNS: HYDRAZINE MONOHYDRATE ◇ IDRAZINA
IDRATA (ITALIAN)

TOXICITY DATA with REFERENCE
CAR: skn-mus TDLo:80 g/kg/43W-I   LAPPA5
25,149,65
MUT: cyt-rat-ihl 850 μg/m^3/5H/16W-I   GISAAA
49(9),25,84
MUT: dnd-mus-ipr 1560 nmol/kg   CNREA8
41,1469,81
MUT: mma-sat 800 μg/plate   NEZAAQ 33,474,78
MUT: mmo-esc 20 μmol/L   ARTODN 46,277,80
MUT: mmo-sat 10 μmol/plate   CNREA8
41,1469,81

CONSENSUS REPORTS: EPA Genetic Toxicology Program.

NIOSH REL: (Hydrazines) CL 0.04 mg/m^3/2H

SAFETY PROFILE: Questionable carcinogen
with experimental carcinogenic data. A poison
by ingestion and intravenous routes. Experimental reproductive effects. Mutation data reported.
A corrosive irritant to the eyes, skin, and mucous
membranes. When heated to decomposition it
emits toxic fumes of NO_x.

HHB000   CAS: 26049-71-8
**2-HYDRAZINO-4-(p-AMINOPHENYL)
THIAZOLE**
mf: $C_9H_{10}N_4S$ mw: 206.29

SYN: 2-HYDRAZINO-4-(4-AMINOPHENYL)THIAZOLE

TOXICITY DATA with REFERENCE
CAR: orl-rat TDLo:12 g/kg/24W-C   CNREA8
30,897,70

ETA: orl-mus TDLo: 8000 mg/kg/46W-C
CNREA8 33,1593,73

SAFETY PROFILE: Questionable carcinogen with experimental carcinogenic and tumorigenic data. When heated to decomposition it emits very toxic fumes of NO_x and SO_x.

HHC000   CAS: 109-84-2
2-HYDRAZINOETHANOL
mf: $C_2H_8N_2O$ mw: 76.12

PROP: Colorless, sltly viscous liquid. Mp: −70°, bp: 145-153° @ 25 mm, flash p: 224°F, vap d: 2.63, d: 1.11. Misc with water. Sol in lower alcs; sltly sol in ether.

SYNS: BOH ◇ HYDROXYETHYL HYDRAZINE ◇ β-HYDROXYETHYLHYDRAZINE ◇ N-(2-HYDROXY-ETHYL)HYDRAZINE

TOXICITY DATA with REFERENCE
CAR: orl-mus TDLo: 572 mg/kg/78W-I-C
JNCIAM 42,1101,69
MUT: cyt-ham: lng 100 μmol/L   MUREAV 78,177,80
MUT: dni-mus-orl 200 mg/kg   MUREAV 46,305,77
MUT: mma-esc 500 μg/plate   MUREAV 116,185,83
MUT: mma-sat 1100 μg/plate   PNASA6 72,5135,75
MUT: mmo-esc 1 pph   MUREAV 40,19,76
MUT: mrc-bcs 5 pph/24H   MUREAV 40,19,76
MUT: sce-ham: lng 100 μmol/L   MUREAV 78,177,80

CONSENSUS REPORTS: Reported in EPA TSCA Inventory. EPA Genetic Toxicology Program.

SAFETY PROFILE: Questionable carcinogen with experimental carcinogenic data. Poison by ingestion. Mutation data reported. Combustible when exposed to heat or flame; can react with oxidizing materials. To fight fire, use foam, CO_2, dry chemical. When heated to decomposition it emits toxic fumes such as NO_x.

HHD500   CAS: 26049-68-3
2-HYDRAZINO-4-(5-NITRO-2-FURYL) THIAZOLE
mf: $C_7H_6N_4O_3S$ mw: 226.23

SYNS: HNT ◇ 2-HYDRAZINO-4-(5-NITRO-2-FURANYL) THIAZOLE

TOXICITY DATA with REFERENCE
CAR: orl-rat TD: 21 g/kg/46W-C   CNREA8 30,897,70

CAR: orl-rat TDLo: 14 g/kg/44W-C   PAACA3 10,15,69
NEO: orl-mus TDLo: 38 g/kg/46W-C   CNREA8 33,1593,73
NEO: orl-rat TD: 21 g/kg/46W-C   JNCIAM 47,437,71
MUT: mmo-esc 10 μg/plate   MUREAV 26,3,74
MUT: pic-esc 100 μg/L   MUREAV 26,3,74

CONSENSUS REPORTS: EPA Genetic Toxicology Program.

SAFETY PROFILE: Questionable carcinogen with experimental carcinogenic and neoplastigenic data. Mutation data reported. When heated to decomposition it emits very toxic fumes of NO_x and SO_x.

HHE000   CAS: 26049-70-7
2-HYDRAZINO-4-(4-NITROPHENYL) THIAZOLE
mf: $C_9H_8N_4O_2S$ mw: 236.27

TOXICITY DATA with REFERENCE
CAR: orl-rat TD: 29 g/kg/44W-C   PAACA3 10,15,69
CAR: orl-rat TD: 37 g/kg/46W-C   CNREA8 30,897,70
CAR: orl-rat TDLo: 2700 mg/kg/46W-C   JNCIAM 51,403,73
ETA: orl-mus TDLo: 8000 mg/kg/46W-C   CNREA8 33,1593,73

SAFETY PROFILE: Questionable carcinogen with experimental carcinogenic and tumorigenic data. When heated to decomposition it emits very toxic fumes of NO_x and SO_x.

HHH000   CAS: 13529-51-6
2,2′-HYDRAZONODIETHANOL
mf: $C_4H_{12}N_2O_2$ mw: 120.18

SYNS: 1,1-BIS(2-HYDROXYETHYL)HYDRAZINE ◇ DEH ◇ 1,1-DIETHANOLHYDRAZINE

TOXICITY DATA with REFERENCE
ETA: scu-ham TDLo: 742 mg/kg   CALEDQ 4,55,77

SAFETY PROFILE: Questionable carcinogen with experimental tumorigenic data. A poison by subcutaneous route. When heated to decomposition it emits toxic fumes such as NO_x.

HHK000   CAS: 9034-34-8
HYDROCELLULOSE

SYN: REGENERATED CELLULOSE

TOXICITY DATA with REFERENCE
NEO: imp-rat TDLo:2 film disc/rat ZENBAX
7,353,52

SAFETY PROFILE: Questionable carcinogen with experimental neoplastigenic data. When heated to decomposition it emits acrid smoke and fumes.

HHW509
HYDROGENATED COAL OIL FRACTION 1

PROP: Centrifugation residue obtained through the direct hydrogenation of coal by Bergius process; liquid phase, highly viscous, black material (IMSUAI 25,51,56).

SYN: BERGIUS COAL HYDROGENATION PRODUCTS FRACTION 1

TOXICITY DATA with REFERENCE
ETA: ims-rat TDLo:600 mg/kg/32W-I IMSUAI 25,51,56
ETA: skn-mus TDLo:443 mg/kg/60W-I IMSUAI 25,51,56
ETA: skn-rbt TDLo:8703 mg/kg/94W-I IMSUAI 25,51,56

SAFETY PROFILE: Questionable carcinogen with experimental tumorigenic data by skin contact and intramuscular routes. A fire hazard. When heated to decomposition it emits acrid smoke and fumes.

HHW519
HYDROGENATED COAL OIL FRACTION 3

PROP: Light oil bottoms obtained through the direct hydrogenation of coal by the Bergius process, liquid phase; a viscous, brown oil containing a scaly admixture (IMSUAI 25,51,56).

SYN: BERGIUS COAL HYDROGENATION PRODUCTS FRACTION 3

TOXICITY DATA with REFERENCE
ETA: ims-rat TDLo:600 mg/kg/32W-I IMSUAI 25,51,56
ETA: skn-mus TDLo:480 mg/kg/60W-I IMSUAI 25,51,56
ETA: skn-rbt TDLo:9429 mg/kg/94W-I IMSUAI 25,51,56

SAFETY PROFILE: Questionable carcinogen with experimental tumorigenic data by skin contact and intramuscular routes. A fire hazard.

When heated to decomposition it emits acrid smoke and fumes.

HHW529
HYDROGENATED COAL OIL FRACTION 4

PROP: Middle oil obtained through the direct hydrogenation of coal by the Bergius process; liquid phase, a thin, reddish-brown oil having an aromatic odor (IMSUAI 25,51,56).

SYN: BERGIUS COAL HYDROGENATION PRODUCTS FRACTION 4

TOXICITY DATA with REFERENCE
ETA: ims-rat TDLo:600 mg/kg/32W-I:TER IMSUAI 25,51,56
ETA: skn-mus TDLo:343 mg/kg/43W-I IMSUAI 25,51,56
ETA: skn-rbt TDLo:9429 mg/kg/94W-I IMSUAI 25,51,56

SAFETY PROFILE: Questionable carcinogen with experimental tumorigenic data by skin contact and intramuscular routes data. An experimental teratogen. A fire hazard. When heated to decomposition it emits acrid smoke and fumes.

HHW539
HYDROGENATED COAL OIL FRACTION 7

PROP: Raw gasoline obtained through the direct hydrogenation of coal by the Bergius process; a thin dark brown liquid which quickly evaporates leaving a brownish-red, oily residue (IMSUAI 25,51,56).

SYN: BERGIUS COAL HYDROGENATION PRODUCTS FRACTION 7

TOXICITY DATA with REFERENCE
ETA: ims-rat TDLo:600 mg/kg/32W-I IMSUAI 25,51,56
ETA: skn-mus TDLo:480 mg/kg/60W-I IMSUAI 25,51,56
ETA: skn-rbt TDLo:9429 mg/kg/94W-I IMSUAI 25,51,56

SAFETY PROFILE: Questionable carcinogen with experimental tumorigenic data by skin contact and intramuscular routes data. A dangerous fire hazard. When heated to decomposition it emits acrid smoke and fumes.

HHW549
HYDROGENATED COAL OIL FRACTION 9

PROP: Pitch flash distillation residue obtained through the direct hydrogenation of coal by the Bergius process; a solid, black, coke-like material (IMSUAI 25,51,56).

SYN: BERGIUS COAL HYDROGENATION PRODUCTS FRACTION 4

TOXICITY DATA with REFERENCE
ETA: ims-rat TDLo: 600 mg/kg/32W-I   IMSUAI 25,51,56
ETA: skn-mus TDLo: 206 mg/kg/26W-I   IMSUAI 25,51,56
ETA: skn-rbt TDLo: 2571 mg/kg/26W-I   IMSUAI 25,51,56

SAFETY PROFILE: Questionable carcinogen with experimental tumorigenic data by skin contact and intramuscular routes data. Flammable. When heated to decomposition it emits acrid smoke and fumes.

HIB000   CAS: 7722-84-1
HYDROGEN PEROXIDE
DOT: 2015
mf: H_2O_2 mw: 34.02

PROP: Colorless, heavy liquid, or, at low temp, a crystalline solid; bitter taste. D: 1.71 @ $-20°$, 1.46 @ 0°, vap press: 1 mm @ 15.3°, unstable. Mp: $-0.43°$, bp: 152°. Misc with water, sol in ether; insol in petr ether. Decomposed by many organic solvents.

SYNS: ALBONE ◇ DIHYDROGEN DIOXIDE ◇ HIOXYL ◇ HYDROGEN DIOXIDE ◇ HYDROGEN PEROXIDE, SOLUTION (over·52% peroxide) (DOT) ◇ HYDROGEN PEROXIDE, STABILIZED (over 60% peroxide) (DOT) ◇ HYDROPEROXIDE ◇ INHIBINE ◇ OXYDOL ◇ PERHYDROL ◇ PERONE ◇ PEROSSIDO di IDROGENO (ITALIAN) ◇ PEROXAN ◇ PEROXIDE ◇ PEROXYDE d'HYDROGENE (FRENCH) ◇ SUPEROXOL ◇ T-STUFF ◇ WASSERSTOFFPEROXID (GERMAN) ◇ WATERSTOFPEROXYDE (DUTCH)

TOXICITY DATA with REFERENCE
ETA: orl-mus TD: 168 g/kg/30W-C   GANNA2 75,17,84
ETA: orl-mus TDLo: 144 g/kg/26W-C   GANNA2 75,17,84
MUT: dnd-hmn: fbr 28 μmol/L   BBACAQ 781,56,84
MUT: dnd-hmn: oth 100 μmol/L   CNREA8 45,2522,85

MUT: dni-hmn: fbr 1 mg/L   CRNGDP 4,1317,83
MUT: dni-hmn: oth 1200 μmol/L   CNREA8 45,2522,85
MUT: dns-hmn: lng 600 μg/L   ENMUDM 5,177,83
MUT: oms-hmn: oth 1200 μmol/L   CNREA8 45,2522,85

CONSENSUS REPORTS: IARC Cancer Review: GROUP 3 IMEMDT 7,56,87; Animal Limited Evidence IMEMDT 28,151,82. EPA Extremely Hazardous Substances List. Reported in EPA TSCA Inventory. EPA Genetic Toxicology Program.

OSHA PEL: TWA 1 ppm   ACGIH TLV: TWA 1 ppm   DFG MAK: 1 ppm ($1.4 mg/m^3$)   DOT Classification: Oxidizer; Label: Oxidizer and Corrosive.

SAFETY PROFILE: Questionable carcinogen with experimental tumorigenic data. Moderately toxic by inhalation, ingestion, and skin contact. A corrosive irritant to skin, eyes, and mucous membranes. Human mutation data reported. A very powerful oxidizer. A dangerous fire hazard by chemical reaction with flammable materials.

HIB010   CAS: 7722-84-1
HYDROGEN PEROXIDE, 30%
DOT: 2014
mf: H_2O_2 mw: 34.02

SYNS: ALBONE 35 ◇ ALBONE 50 ◇ ALBONE 70 ◇ ALBONE 35CG ◇ ALBONE 50CG ◇ ALBONE 70CG ◇ HYDROGEN PEROXIDE SOLUTION 30% ◇ HYDROGEN PEROXIDE SOLUTION (8% to 40% PEROXIDE) (DOT) ◇ INTEROX ◇ KASTONE ◇ PERONE 30 ◇ PERONE 35 ◇ PERONE 50

TOXICITY DATA with REFERENCE
CAR: orl-mus TDLo: 622 g/kg/2Y-C   HIUN** 17(1),53,74
MUT: cyt-hmn: emb 20 μmol/L   MUREAV 172,245,86
MUT: msc-ham: lng 1 mmol/L   MUREAV 192,65,87
MUT: oth-hmn: emb 50 μmol/L   MUREAV 172,245,86

CONSENSUS REPORTS: IARC Cancer Review: GROUP 3 IMEMDT 7,56,87, Animal Limited Evidence IMEMDT 36,285,85. Reported in EPA TSCA Inventory.

DOT Classification: Oxidizer; LABEL: Oxidizer

SAFETY PROFILE: Questionable carcinogen with experimental carcinogenic data. Mutation data reported.

HID500 CAS: 2207-76-3
6-HYDROPEROXY-4-CHOLESTEN-3-ONE
mf: $C_{27}H_{44}O_3$ mw: 416.71

SYNS: 6-β-HYDROPEROXYCHOLEST-4-EN-3-ONE ◇ 6-β-HYDROPEROXY-Δ⁴CHOLESTEN-3-ONE

TOXICITY DATA with REFERENCE
CAR: scu-mus TDLo: 600 mg/kg/72W-I
JNCIAM 19,977,57
ETA: scu-mus TD: 600 mg/kg/W-I JCSOA9
77,3928,55

SAFETY PROFILE: Questionable carcinogen with experimental carcinogenic and tumorigenic data. When heated to decomposition it emits acrid smoke and fumes.

HIE000 CAS: 4096-33-7
1-HYDROPEROXYCYCLOHEX-3-ENE
mf: $C_6H_{10}O_2$ mw: 114.16

SYN: 1-HYDROPEROXY-3-CYCLOHEXENE

TOXICITY DATA with REFERENCE
NEO: skn-mus TDLo: 6960 mg/kg/58W-I
JNCIAM 35,707,65
ETA: skn-mus TD: 8880 mg/kg/74W-I 14JTAF
275,64

SAFETY PROFILE: Questionable carcinogen with experimental neoplastigenic and tumorigenic data. When heated to decomposition it emits acrid smoke and fumes.

HIE570 CAS: 74955-23-0
N-(HYDROPEROXYMETHYL)-N-NITROSOPROPYLAMINE
mf: $C_4H_{10}N_2O_3$ mw: 134.16

SYN: N-PROPYL-N-(HYDROPEROXYMETHYL)NITROSAMINE

TOXICITY DATA with REFERENCE
CAR: ivn-rat TDLo: 50 mg/kg/10W-I CRNGDP
7,1313,86
MUT: msc-ham: lng 100 μmol/L GANNA2
73,522,82

SAFETY PROFILE: Questionable carcinogen with experimental carcinogenic data. Mutation data reported. When heated to decomposition it emits toxic fumes of NO_x.

HIE600 CAS: 74940-23-1
HYDROPEROXY-N-NITROSODIBUTYLAMINE
mf: $C_8H_{18}N_2O_3$ mw: 190.28

SYNS: BHPBN ◇ N-BUTYL-N-(1-HYDROPEROXYBUTYL) NITROSAMINE

TOXICITY DATA with REFERENCE
CAR: scu-rat TD: 72 mg/kg/10W-I IAPUDO
41,619,82
CAR: scu-rat TDLo: 70500 μg/kg/10W-I
GANNA2 73,687,82
MUT: msc-ham: lng 50 μmol/L GANNA2
73,522,82

SAFETY PROFILE: Questionable carcinogen with experimental carcinogenic data. Mutation data reported. When heated to decomposition it emits toxic fumes of NO_x.

HIE700 CAS: 74940-26-4
1-(HYDROPEROXY)-N-NITROSODIMETHYLAMINE
mf: $C_2H_6N_2O_3$ mw: 106.10

SYN: N-METHYL-N-(HYDROPEROXYMETHYL)NITROSAMINE

TOXICITY DATA with REFERENCE
CAR: ivn-rat TDLo: 50 mg/kg/10W-I CRNGDP
7,1313,86
MUT: msc-ham: lng 50 μmol/L GANNA2
73,522,82

SAFETY PROFILE: Questionable carcinogen with experimental carcinogenic data. Mutation data reported. When heated to decomposition it emits toxic fumes of NO_x.

HIF575 CAS: 3736-26-3
1-HYDROPEROXY-1-VINYLCYCLOHEX-3-ENE
mf: $C_8H_{12}O_2$ mw: 140.20

SYN: 4-HYDROPEROXY-4-VINYL-1-CYCLOHEXENE

TOXICITY DATA with REFERENCE
NEO: skn-mus TDLo: 1440 mg/kg/24W-I
14JTAF -,275,64
ETA: skn-mus TD: 1440 mg/kg/24W-I JNCIAM
31,41,63

SAFETY PROFILE: Questionable carcinogen with experimental neoplastigenic and tumorigenic data. When heated to decomposition it emits acrid smoke and fumes.

HIH000 CAS: 123-31-9
HYDROQUINONE
DOT: 2662
mf: $C_6H_6O_2$ mw: 110.12

PROP: Colorless, hexagonal prisms. Mp: 170.5°, bp: 286.2°, flash p: 329°F (CC), d: 1.358 @ 20°/4°, autoign temp: 960°F (CC), vap press: 1 mm @ 132.4°, vap d: 3.81. Very sol in alc, ether. Sltly sol in benzene. Keep well closed and protected from light.

SYNS: ARCTUVIN ◇ p-BENZENEDIOL ◇ 1,4-BENZENE-DIOL ◇ BENZOHYDROQUINONE ◇ BENZOQUINOL ◇ BLACK AND WHITE BLEACHING CREAM ◇ 1,4-DIHYDROXY-BENZEEN (DUTCH) ◇ 1,4-DIHYDROXYBENZEN (CZECH) ◇ DIHYDROXYBENZENE ◇ p DIHYDROXYBENZENE ◇ 1,4-DIHYDROXYBENZENE ◇ 1,4-DIHYDROXY-BENZOL (GERMAN) ◇ 1,4-DIIDROBENZENE (ITALIAN) ◇ p-DIOXOBENZENE ◇ ELDOPAQUE ◇ ELDOQUIN ◇ HYDROCHINON (CZECH, POLISH) ◇ HYDROQUINOL ◇ α-HYDROQUINONE ◇ p-HYDROQUINONE ◇ p-HYDROXYPHENOL ◇ IDROCHINONE (ITALIAN) ◇ NCI-C55834 ◇ β-QUINOL ◇ TECQUINOL ◇ TENOX HQ ◇ USAF EK-356

TOXICITY DATA with REFERENCE
MUT: dns-rat-orl 8 g/kg   JJIND8 74,1283,85
MUT: mnt-mus-orl 200 mg/kg   AJIMD8 7,475,85
MUT: oms-hmn:lym 5 μmol/L   CNREA8 45,2471,85
MUT: oms-mus:lym 10 μmol/L   TOLED5 29,161,85
MUT: sce-hmn:lym 5 μmol/L   CNREA8 45,2471,85

CONSENSUS REPORTS: IARC Cancer Review: GROUP 3 IMEMDT 7,56,87; Animal Inadequate Evidence IMEMDT 15,155,77. Community Right-To-Know List. EPA Extremely Hazardous Substances List. EPA Genetic Toxicology Program. Reported in EPA TSCA Inventory.

OSHA PEL: TWA 2 mg/m³ ACGIH TLV: TWA 2 mg/m³ DFG MAK: 2 mg/m³ NIOSH REL: (Hydroquinone) CL 2.0 mg/m³/15M DOT Classification: IMO: Poison B; Label: St. Andrews Cross.

SAFETY PROFILE: Questionable carcinogen. A human poison by ingestion. An experimental poison by ingestion, intraperitoneal, intravenous, parenteral, subcutaneous and possibly other routes. Human systemic effects by ingestion: pulse rate increase without fall in blood pressure, cyanosis, coma. An active allergen and a strong skin irritant. Human mutation data reported. A severe human skin irritant. Experimental reproductive data. Combustible. To fight fire, use water, CO_2, dry chemical.

HIJ400   CAS: 2784-86-3
1-HYDROXY-2-ACETAMIDOFLUORENE
mf: $C_{15}H_{13}NO_2$ mw: 239.29

SYN: N-(1-HYDROXY-2-FLUORENYL)ACETAMIDE

TOXICITY DATA with REFERENCE
CAR: imp-mus TDLo:96 mg/kg   GANMAX 17,383,75
ETA: imp-mus TD:75 mg/kg   CALEDQ 6,21,79

SAFETY PROFILE: Questionable carcinogen with experimental carcinogenic and tumorigenic data. When heated to decomposition it emits toxic fumes of NO_x.

HIK000   CAS: 843-34-5
trans-4′-HYDROXY-4-ACETAMIDOSTILBENE
mf: $C_{16}H_{15}NO_2$ mw: 253.32

SYNS: trans-4′-HYDROXY-AAS ◇ (E)-4′-(p-HYDROXYSTY-RYL) ACETANILIDE

TOXICITY DATA with REFERENCE
ETA: orl-rat TDLo:713 mg/kg/36W-C   BJCAAI 22,133,68

SAFETY PROFILE: Questionable carcinogen with experimental tumorigenic data. When heated to decomposition it emits toxic fumes of NO_x.

HIK500   CAS: 363-49-5
7-HYDROXY-2-ACETAMINOFLUORENE
mf: $C_{15}H_{13}NO_2$ mw: 239.290

SYNS: 7OH-2AAF ◇ 7-HYDROXY-N-2-FLUORENYLACE-TAMIDE

TOXICITY DATA with REFERENCE
NEO: orl-rat TDLo:14 g/kg/2Y-C   BJCAAI 1,391,47
MUT: dnr-esc 10 mg/L   JJIND8 62,873,79
MUT: mma-sat 250 μg/plate   JJIND8 62,893,79

CONSENSUS REPORTS: EPA Genetic Toxicology Program.

SAFETY PROFILE: Questionable carcinogen with experimental neoplastigenic data. Mutation data reported. When heated to decomposition it emits toxic fumes of NO_x.

HIN000   CAS: 19315-64-1
N-HYDROXY-p-ACETOPHENETIDIDE
mf: $C_{10}H_{13}NO_3$ mw: 195.24

SYNS: N-(4-ETHOXYPHENYL)ACETOHYDROXAMIC ACID ◇ N-(4-ETHOXYPHENYL)-N-HYDROXYACETAMIDE ◇ N-HYDROXYPHENACETIN

TOXICITY DATA with REFERENCE
NEO: orl-rat TDLo: 15 g/kg/73W-C   PTLGAX
8,1,76
MUT: mma-sat 500 μg/plate   MUREAV 58,387,78
MUT: otr-mus:emb 100 μg/L   NCIMAV 58,21,81

CONSENSUS REPORTS: IARC Cancer Review: Animal Limited Evidence IMEMDT 13,141,77; IMEMDT 24,135,80.

SAFETY PROFILE: Questionable carcinogen with experimental neoplastigenic data. Moderately toxic by intraperitoneal route. Mutation data reported. When heated to decomposition it emits toxic fumes of NO_x.

HIO875   CAS: 1838-56-8
3-HYDROXY-N-ACETYL-2-AMINOFLUORENE
mf: $C_{15}H_{13}NO_2$ mw: 239.29

SYNS: 3-HO-AAF ◇ N-(3-HYDROXY-2-FLUORENYL) ACETAMIDE

TOXICITY DATA with REFERENCE
CAR: imp-mus TDLo: 96 mg/kg   GMCRDC
17,383,75
ETA: imp-mus TD: 75 mg/kg   CALEDQ 6,21,79
MUT: slt-dmg-par 10 mmol/L   IJCNAW 9,284,72

CONSENSUS REPORTS: EPA Genetic Toxicology Program.

SAFETY PROFILE: Questionable carcinogen with experimental carcinogenic and tumorigenic data by implantation. Mutation data reported. When heated to decomposition it emits toxic fumes of NO_x.

HIP500   CAS: 14751-90-7
N-HYDROXY-2-ACETYLAMINOFLUORENE, CUPRIC CHELATE
mf: $C_{30}H_{24}N_2O_4 \cdot Cu$ mw: 540.10

SYNS: COPPER CHELATE of N-HYDROXY-2-ACETYLAMI-NOFLUORENE ◇ CUPRIC CHELATE of 2-N-HYDROXY-FLUORENYL ACETAMIDE ◇ N-FLUOREN-2-YL ACETOHY-DROXAMIC ACID, COPPER(2+) COMPLEX ◇ N-HYDROXY-N-2-FLUORENYL ACETAMIDE, CUPRIC CHELATE ◇ 2-N-HYDROXYFLUORENYL ACETAMIDE, CUPRIC CHELATE

TOXICITY DATA with REFERENCE
NEO: scu-rat TDLo: 160 mg/kg/4W-I   CNREA8
25,527,65
ETA: orl-rat TDLo: 12 g/kg/17W-C   CNREA8
25,527,65

ETA: scu-rbt TDLo: 120 mg/kg/6W-I   CNREA8
27,838,67

CONSENSUS REPORTS: Copper and its compounds are on the Community Right-To-Know List.

SAFETY PROFILE: Questionable carcinogen with experimental tumorigenic and neoplastigenic data. When heated to decomposition it emits toxic fumes of NO_x.

HIQ000   CAS: 63904-81-4
N-HYDROXY-2-ACETYLAMINOFLUORENE, FERRIC CHELATE
mf: $C_{45}H_{36}N_3O_6 \cdot Fe$ mw: 770.69

SYNS: N-FLUOREN-2-YL ACETOHYDROXAMIC ACID, IRON(3+) COMPLEX ◇ IRON complex with N-FLUOREN-2-YL ACETOHYDROXAMIC ACID

TOXICITY DATA with REFERENCE
NEO: scu-rat TDLo: 160 mg/kg/4W-I   CNREA8
25,527,65

SAFETY PROFILE: Questionable carcinogen with experimental neoplastigenic data. When heated to decomposition it emits toxic fumes of NO_x.

HIQ500   CAS: 2495-54-7
N-HYDROXY-2-ACETYLAMINOFLUORENE-o-GLUCURONIDE
mf: $C_{21}H_{21}NO_9$ mw: 431.43

SYN: ACETOHYDROXAMIC ACID, FLUOREN-2-YL-o-GLUCURONIDE

TOXICITY DATA with REFERENCE
CAR: scu-rat TDLo: 850 mg/kg/9W-I   CNREA8
31,1645,71

SAFETY PROFILE: Questionable carcinogen with experimental carcinogenic data. When heated to decomposition it emits toxic fumes of NO_x.

HIR000   CAS: 14751-74-7
N-HYDROXY-2-ACETYLAMINOFLUORENE, MANGANOUS CHELATE
mf: $C_{30}H_{24}N_2O_4 \cdot Mn$ mw: 531.50

SYNS: N-FLUOREN-2-YL ACETOHYDROXAMIC ACID, MANGANESE(2+) COMPLEX ◇ MANGANESE complex with N-FLUOREN-2-YL ACETOHYDROXAMIC ACID

TOXICITY DATA with REFERENCE
NEO: scu-rat TDLo:160 mg/kg/4W-I   CNREA8
25,527,65

CONSENSUS REPORTS: Manganese and its compounds are on the Community Right-To-Know List.

OSHA PEL: CL 5 mg(Mn)/m^3 ACGIH TLV: TWA 5 mg(Mn)/m^3

SAFETY PROFILE: Questionable carcinogen with experimental neoplastigenic data. When heated to decomposition it emits toxic fumes of NO_x.

HIR500   CAS: 14751-76-9
N-HYDROXY-2-ACETYLAMINOFLUORENE, NICKELOUS CHELATE
mf: $C_{30}H_{24}N_2O_4 \cdot Ni$ mw: 535.27

SYNS: N-FLUOREN-2-YL ACETOHYDROXAMIC ACID, NICKEL(2+) COMPLEX ◇ NICKEL COMPLEX with N-FLUOREN-2-YL ACETOHYDROXAMIC ACID

TOXICITY DATA with REFERENCE
NEO: scu-rat TDLo:160 mg/kg/4W-I   CNREA8
25,527,65

CONSENSUS REPORTS: Nickel and its compounds are on the Community Right-To-Know List.

NIOSH REL: (Inorganic Nickel) TWA 0.015 mg(Ni)/m^3

SAFETY PROFILE: Questionable carcinogen with experimental neoplastigenic data. When heated to decomposition it emits toxic fumes of NO_x.

HIS000   CAS: 6023-26-3
N-HYDROXY-2-ACETYLAMINOFLUORENE, POTASSIUM SALT
mf: $C_{15}H_{13}NO_2 \cdot K$ mw: 278.39

SYNS: N-FLUOREN-2-YL ACETOHYDROXAMIC ACID, POTASSIUM SALT ◇ POTASSIUM N-FLUOREN-2-YL ACETOHYDROXAMATE

TOXICITY DATA with REFERENCE
ETA: scu-rat TDLo:160 mg/kg/4W-I   CNREA8
25,527,65

SAFETY PROFILE: Questionable carcinogen with experimental tumorigenic data. When heated to decomposition it emits toxic fumes of NO_x.

HIU500   CAS: 53-94-1
N-HYDROXY-2-AMINOFLUORENE
mf: $C_{13}H_{11}NO$ mw: 197.25

SYNS: 2-FLUORENYL HYDROXYLAMINE ◇ N-FLUOREN-2-YLHYDROXYLAMINE

TOXICITY DATA with REFERENCE
CAR: ipr-gpg TDLo:1600 mg/kg/17W-I
CNREA8 24,2018,64
NEO: scu-rat TDLo:420 mg/kg/9W-I   CNREA8
31,1645,71
MUT: dnd-mus:lvr 5 μmol/L   CRNGDP
5,797,84
MUT: dnd-rat:lvr 40 μmol/L   CNREA8
44,1098,84
MUT: dns-hmn:oth 100 nmol/L   JJIND8
72,847,84
MUT: dns-rbt:oth nmol/L   CNREA8 45,221,85
MUT: mmo-sat 50 ng/plate   CBINA8 54,71,85
MUT: msc-ham:ovr 500 μmol/L   CNREA8
45,5461,85
MUT: sce-ham:ovr 275 μmol/L   CNREA8
45,5461,85

CONSENSUS REPORTS: EPA Genetic Toxicology Program.

SAFETY PROFILE: Questionable carcinogen with experimental carcinogenic and neoplastigenic data. Human mutation data reported. When heated to decomposition it emits toxic fumes of NO_x.

HIV000   CAS: 13442-07-4
4-(HYDROXYAMINO)-5-METHYLQUINOLINE-1-OXIDE
mf: $C_{10}H_{10}N_2O_2$ mw: 190.22

SYN: 5-METHYL-4-HYDROXYLAMINOQUINOLINE-1-OXIDE

TOXICITY DATA with REFERENCE
ETA: scu-mus TDLo:120 mg/kg/50D-I   BCPCA6
16,631,67

SAFETY PROFILE: Questionable carcinogen with experimental tumorigenic data. When heated to decomposition it emits toxic fumes of NO_x.

HIV500   CAS: 13442-08-5
4-(HYDROXYAMINO)-6-METHYLQUINOLINE-1-OXIDE
mf: $C_{10}H_{10}N_2O_2$ mw: 190.22

SYN: 6-METHYL-4-HYDROXYLAMINOQUINOLINE-1-OXIDE

TOXICITY DATA with REFERENCE
ETA: scu-mus TDLo: 120 mg/kg/50D-I   BCPCA6
16,631,67
MUT: pic-esc 5100 µg/L   EXPEAM 24,1245,68

SAFETY PROFILE: Questionable carcinogen with experimental tumorigenic data. Mutation data reported. When heated to decomposition it emits toxic fumes of NO_x.

HIW000   CAS: 13442-09-6
4-(HYDROXYAMINO)-7-METHYLQUINOLINE-1-OXIDE
mf: $C_{10}H_{10}N_2O_2$ mw: 190.22

SYN: 7-METHYL-4-HYDROXYLAMINOQUINOLINE-1-OXIDE

TOXICITY DATA with REFERENCE
ETA: scu-mus TDLo: 120 mg/kg/50D-I   BCPCA6
16,631,67

SAFETY PROFILE: Questionable carcinogen with experimental tumorigenic data. When heated to decomposition it emits toxic fumes of NO_x.

HIW500   CAS: 13442-10-9
4-(HYDROXYAMINO)-8-METHYLQUINOLINE-1-OXIDE
mf: $C_{10}H_{10}N_2O_2$ mw: 190.22

SYN: 8-METHYL-4-HYDROXYLAMINOQUINOLINE-1-OXIDE

TOXICITY DATA with REFERENCE
ETA: scu-mus TDLo: 120 mg/kg/50D-I   BCPCA6
16,631,67

SAFETY PROFILE: Questionable carcinogen with experimental tumorigenic data. When heated to decomposition it emits toxic fumes of NO_x.

HIX000   CAS: 607-30-7
N-HYDROXY-1-AMINONAPHTHALENE
mf: $C_{10}H_9NO$ mw: 159.20

SYNS: N-HYDROXY-1-NAPHTHYLAMINE
◇ 1-NAPHTHYLHYDROXYLAMINE ◇ N-1-NAPHTHYLHYDROXYLAMINE

TOXICITY DATA with REFERENCE
NEO: ipr-rat TDLo: 1300 mg/kg/13W-I   CNREA8
28,535,68
NEO: skn-mus TDLo: 40 mg/kg   ANYAA9
163,828,69
ETA: ipr-rat TD: 1200 mg/kg/12W-I   CNREA8
31,1461,71

MUT: dnd-rat-scu 106 µmol/kg   CNREA8
44,1172,84
MUT: mma-sat 1 µg/plate   PNASA6 72,5135,75
MUT: mmo-sat 1 µg/plate   MUREAV 122,243,83
MUT: oms-rat-scu 106 µmol/kg   CNREA8
44,1172,84
MUT: otr-hmn: oth 2 mg/L   ITCSAF 17,719,81

CONSENSUS REPORTS: EPA Genetic Toxicology Program.

SAFETY PROFILE: Questionable carcinogen with experimental neoplastigenic and tumorigenic data. Human mutation data reported. When heated to decomposition it emits toxic fumes of NO_x.

HIX500   CAS: 13442-15-4
4-(HYDROXYAMINO)-6-NITROQUINOLINE-1-OXIDE
mf: $C_9H_7N_3O_4$ mw: 221.19

SYN: 6-NITRO-4-HYDROXYLAMINOQUINOLINE-1-OXIDE

TOXICITY DATA with REFERENCE
ETA: scu-mus TD: 120 mg/kg/50D-I   BCPCA6
16,631,67
ETA: scu-mus TDLo: 60 mg/kg/I   CPBTAL
17,544,69

SAFETY PROFILE: Questionable carcinogen with experimental tumorigenic data. When heated to decomposition it emits toxic fumes of NO_x.

HIY000   CAS: 13442-16-5
4-(HYDROXYAMINO)-7-NITROQUINOLINE-1-OXIDE
mf: $C_9H_7N_3O_4$ mw: 221.19

SYN: 7-NITRO-4-HYDROXYLAMINOQUINOLINE-1-OXIDE

TOXICITY DATA with REFERENCE
ETA: scu-mus TDLo: 120 mg/kg/50D-I   BCPCA6
16,631,67

SAFETY PROFILE: Questionable carcinogen with experimental tumorigenic data. When heated to decomposition it emits toxic fumes of NO_x.

HIY500   CAS: 4637-56-3
4-(HYDROXYAMINO)QUINOLINE-1-OXIDE
mf: $C_9H_8N_2O_2$ mw: 176.19

SYNS: 4HAQO ◇ N-(4-QUINOLYL)HYDROXYLAMINE-1'-OXIDE

TOXICITY DATA with REFERENCE

CAR: imp-rat TD:20 mg/kg   CANCAR 50,2057,82
CAR: imp-rat TD:40 mg/kg   CANCAR 50,2057,82
CAR: imp-rat TDLo:10 mg/kg   CANCAR 50,2057,82
CAR: ivn-rat TD:7 mg/kg   NAIZAM 33,549,83
CAR: par-rat TD:20 mg/kg   CANCAR 50,2057,82
CAR: par-rat TDLo:10 mg/kg   CANCAR 50,2057,82
CAR: scu-rat TDLo:16 mg/kg/4W-I   IGAYAY 120,1218,82
NEO: imp-rat TD:32 mg/kg   JJIND8 68,859,82
NEO: scu-rat TD:16 mg/kg/4W-I   JJIND8 68,859,82
NEO: scu-rat TDLo:4 mg/kg   PSEBAA 136,1206,71
NEO: skn-mus TDLo:1350 mg/kg/18W-C   GANNA2 60,161,69
ETA: ipr-rat TDLo:5 mg/kg   JNCIAM 53,159,74
ETA: ivn-rat TD:7 mg/kg   CRNGDP 4,17,83
ETA: ivn-rat TDLo:7 mg/kg   INSSDM 15,317,80
ETA: orl-mus TD:200 mg/kg/9W-I   GANNA2 58,551,67
ETA: orl-mus TD:200 mg/kg/9W-I   GANNA2 58,551,67
ETA: orl-mus TDLo:100 mg/kg/9W-I   GANNA2 58,551,67
ETA: scu-mus TDLo:7 mg/kg/60D-I   GANNA2 56,85,65
MUT: dnd-ckn:emb 200 μmol/L   CBINA8 47,123,83
MUT: dnd-hmn:fbr 10 μmol/L   BBACAQ 781,273,84
MUT: dns-hmn:oth 100 nmol/L   JJIND8 69,557,82
MUT: dns-rat-ivn 7 mg/kg   CBINA8 56,125,85
MUT: mma-esc 10 μg/plate   ENMUDM 6(Suppl 2),1,84
MUT: mmo-sat 300 ng/plate   ENMUDM 6(Suppl 2),1,84

CONSENSUS REPORTS: EPA Genetic Toxicology Program.

SAFETY PROFILE: Questionable carcinogen with experimental carcinogenic, neoplastigenic, and tumorigenic data. A poison by intravenous route. Human mutation data reported. When heated to decomposition it emits toxic fumes of NO_x.

HIZ000   CAS: 1010-61-3
4-(HYDROXYAMINO)QUINOLINE-1-OXIDE, HYDROCHLORIDE
mf: $C_9H_8N_2O_2 \cdot ClH$ mw: 212.65

SYNS: 4-HYDROXYAMINOQUINOLINE-1-OXIDE HYDRO-CHLORIDE ◇ 4-HYDROXYAMINOQUINOLINE-1-OXIDE MONOHYDROCHLORIDE ◇ 4-(HYDROXYAMINO)QUINO-LINE-1-OXIDE MONOHYDROCHLORIDE ◇ 4-HYDROXY-QUINOLINAMINE-1-OXIDE MONOHYDROCHLORIDE ◇ N-HYDROXY-4-QUINOLINAMINE-1-OXIDE MONOHY-DROCHLORIDE ◇ NSC 78572

TOXICITY DATA with REFERENCE

CAR: scu-mus TDLo:451 μg/kg   JJEMAG 40,475,70
NEO: ivn-rat TDLo:6 mg/kg   GANNA2 62,329,71
NEO: scu-rat TDLo:16 mg/kg/2W-I   PSEBAA 136,1206,71
ETA: ivn-rat TD:7 mg/kg   GANNA2 67,91,76
ETA: orl-mus TDLo:240 mg/kg/50D-I   GANNA2 60,151,69
ETA: orl-rat TDLo:150 mg/kg/45W-I   GANNA2 60,627,69
MUT: cyt-omi 495 μmol/L   GANNA2 60,155,69
MUT: mmo-esc 25 mg/L   CPBTAL 13,610,65
MUT: mmo-smc 26 mg/L   TXAPA9 15,451,69

SAFETY PROFILE: Questionable carcinogen with experimental carcinogenic, neoplastigenic, and tumorigenic data. Poison by intraperitoneal route. Mutation data reported. When heated to decomposition it emits very toxic fumes of NO_x and HCl.

HJA000   CAS: 60462-51-3
trans-N-HYDROXY-4-AMINOSTILBENE
mf: $C_{14}H_{13}NO$ mw: 211.28

SYNS: (E)-N-(p-STYRYLPHENYL)HYDROXYLAMINE ◇ trans-N-(p-STYRYLPHENYL)HYDROXYLAMINE ◇ trans-N-(4-STYRYLPHENYL)HYDROXYLAMINE

TOXICITY DATA with REFERENCE

NEO: scu-rat TDLo:18 mg/kg/1W-I   CNREA8 24,128,64

SAFETY PROFILE: Questionable carcinogen with experimental neoplastigenic data. When heated to decomposition it emits toxic fumes of NO_x.

HJB100   CAS: 571-22-2
17-β-HYDROXY-5-β-ANDROSTAN-3-ONE
mf: $C_{19}H_{30}O_2$ mw: 290.49

SYNS: 5-β-DHT ◇ 5-β-DIHYDROTESTOSTERONE ◇ ETIOCHOLANE-17-β-OL-3-ONE ◇ ETIOCHOLAN-17-β-OL-3-ONE

TOXICITY DATA with REFERENCE
NEO: scu-mus TDLo: 240 mg/kg/5D-I CNREA8
37,4456,77
MUT: dni-hmn:lym 50 μmol/L PSEBAA
146,401,74

SAFETY PROFILE: Questionable carcinogen with experimental neoplastigenic and teratogenic data. Human mutation data reported. A steroid. When heated to decomposition it emits acrid smoke and irritating fumes.

HJC500   CAS: 17672-21-8
3-HYDROXYANTHRANILIC ACID METHYL ESTER
mf: $C_8H_9NO_3$ mw: 167.18

SYNS: 2-AMINO-3-HYDROXYBENZOIC ACID, METHYL ESTER ◇ METHYL-3-HYDROXYANTHRANILATE

TOXICITY DATA with REFERENCE
ETA: imp-mus TDLo: 80 mg/kg BJCAAI
11,212,57

SAFETY PROFILE: Questionable carcinogen with experimental tumorigenic data. When heated to decomposition it emits toxic fumes of NO_x.

HJD000   CAS: 484-78-6
3-(3-HYDROXYANTHRANILOYL) ALANINE
mf: $C_{10}H_{12}N_2O_4$ mw: 224.24

SYNS: α,2-DIAMINO-3-HYDROXY-γ-OXOBENZENEBUTANOIC ACID ◇ HYDROXYKYNURENINE ◇ 3-HYDROXYKYNURENINE

TOXICITY DATA with REFERENCE
NEO: imp-mus TDLo: 80 mg/kg BJCAAI
11,212,57
MUT: cyt-hmn:emb 50 mg/L BEXBAN 67,200,69
MUT: cyt-mus-scu 10 mg/L NATUAS 222,484,69

SAFETY PROFILE: Questionable carcinogen with experimental neoplastigenic data. Human mutation data reported. When heated to decomposition it emits toxic fumes of NO_x.

HJD500   CAS: 606-14-4
3-(3-HYDROXYANTHRANILOYL)-l-ALANINE
mf: $C_{10}H_{12}N_2O_4$ mw: 224.24

SYNS: l-3-HYDROXYKYNURENINE ◇ 3-HYDROXY-l-KYNURENINE

TOXICITY DATA with REFERENCE
CAR: imp-mus TDLo: 160 mg/kg ANYAA9
108,924,63

ETA: scu-mus TDLo: 4408 mg/kg/21D-I
JCROD7 96,163,80

SAFETY PROFILE: Questionable carcinogen with experimental carcinogenic and tumorigenic data. When heated to decomposition it emits toxic fumes of NO_x.

HJE575   CAS: 42028-33-1
3-HYDROXY-8-AZAXANTHINE
mf: $C_4H_3N_5O_3$ mw: 169.12

SYN: 4-HYDROXY-3H-o-TRIAZOLO(4,5-d)PYRIMIDINE-5,7(4H-6H)-DIONE

TOXICITY DATA with REFERENCE
ETA: scu-rat TDLo: 237 mg/kg/22W-I CNREA8
33,1113,73

SAFETY PROFILE: Questionable carcinogen with experimental tumorigenic data. When heated to decomposition it emits toxic fumes of NO_x.

HJF000   CAS: 1689-82-3
4-HYDROXYAZOBENZENE
mf: $C_{12}H_{10}N_2O$ mw: 198.24

PROP: Orange, rhombic crystals from ethanol. Mp: 155-156°, bp: 220-230°, very sol in ether.

SYNS: p-BENZENEAZOPHENOL ◇ C.I. SOLVENT YELLOW 7 ◇ p-HYDROXYAZOBENZENE ◇ p-PHENYLAZOPHENOL ◇ 4-PHENYLAZOPHENOL

CONSENSUS REPORTS: IARC Cancer Review: GROUP 3 IMEMDT 7,56,87; Animal Inadequate Evidence IMEMDT 8,157,75. Reported in EPA TSCA Inventory.

SAFETY PROFILE: Questionable carcinogen. A poison by intraperitoneal route. When heated to decomposition it emits toxic fumes of NO_x.

HJF500   CAS: 3567-69-9
4-HYDROXY-3,4'-AZODI-1-NAPHTHALENESULFONIC ACID, DISODIUM SALT
mf: $C_{20}H_{12}N_2O_7S_2 \cdot 2Na$ mw: 502.44

SYNS: ACETACID RED B ◇ ACID BRILLIANT RUBINE 2G ◇ ACID CHROME BLUE BA ◇ ACID FAST RED FB ◇ ACID RUBINE ◇ AIREDALE CARMOISINE ◇ AMACID CHROME BLUE R ◇ ATUL CRYSTAL RED F ◇ AZORUBIN ◇ BRASILAN AZO RUBINE 2NS ◇ BRILLIANT CRIMSON RED ◇ CARMOISIN (GERMAN) ◇ CARMOISINE ALUMINUM LAKE ◇ CARMOISINE SUPRA ◇ CERTICOL CARMOISINE S ◇ CHROME FAST BLUE 2R ◇ C.I. 14720 ◇ C.I. ACID

RED 14, DISODIUM SALT ◊ C.I. FOOD RED 3 ◊ CRIMSON EMBL ◊ DIADEM CHROME BLUE R ◊ DISODIUM SALT of 2-(4-SULPHO-1-NAPHTHYLAZO)-1-NAPHTHOL-4-SUL-PHONIC ACID ◊ DISODIUM 2-(4-SULFO-1-NAPHTHYLAZO) 1-NAPHTHOL-4-SULFONATE ◊ DISODIUM 2-(4-SULPHO-1-NAPHTHYLAZO)-1-NAPHTHOL-4-SULPHONATE ◊ EDICOL SUPRA CARMOISINE WS ◊ ENIACID BRILLIANT RUBINE 3B ◊ EUROCERT AZORUBINE ◊ EXTRACT D&C RED NO. 10 ◊ FENAZO RED C ◊ FOOD RED 5 ◊ FRUIT RED A EXTRA YELLOWISH GEIGY ◊ HEXACOL CARMOISINE ◊ HIDACID AZO RUBINE ◊ 4-HYDROXY-3,4′-AZODI-1-NAPHTHALENE-SULPHONIC ACID, DISODIUM SALT ◊ 4-HYDROXY-3-((4-SULFO-1-NAPHTHALENYL)AZO)-1-NAPHTHALENESUL-FONIC ACID, DISODIUM SALT ◊ JAVA RUBINE N ◊ KARMESIN ◊ KENACHROME BLUE 2R ◊ KITON CRIM-SON 2R ◊ LIGHTHOUSE CHROME BLUE 2R ◊ NACARAT A EXPORT ◊ NCI-C53849 ◊ NEKLACID RUBINE W ◊ NYLOMINE ACID RED P4B ◊ OMEGA CHROME BLUE FB ◊ POLOXAL RED 2B ◊ PONTACYL RUBINE R ◊ RED #14 ◊ 11959 RED ◊ SCHULTZ Nr. 208 (GERMAN) ◊ SOLAR RUBINE ◊ SOLOCHROME BLUE FB ◊ STANDA-COL CARMOISINE ◊ 2-(4-SULFO-1-NAPHTHYLAZO)-1-NAPHTHOL-4-SULFONIC ACID, DISODIUM SALT ◊ TERTRACID RED CA ◊ TERTROCHROME BLUE FB

TOXICITY DATA with REFERENCE
MUT: mmo-esc 100 mg/L   MUREAV 53,289,78
MUT: mmo-sat 1 g/L   MUREAV 53,289,78

CONSENSUS REPORTS: IARC Cancer Review: GROUP 3 IMEMDT 7,56,87; Animal Inadequate Evidence IMEMDT 8,83,75. NTP Carcinogenesis Bioassay (feed); No Evidence: mouse, rat NTPTR* NTP-TR-220,82. Reported in EPA TSCA Inventory. EPA Genetic Toxicology Program.

SAFETY PROFILE: Questionable carcinogen. Moderately toxic by intraperitoneal and intravenous routes. Mutation data reported. When heated to decomposition it emits very toxic fumes of SO_x, Na_2O and NO_x.

HJG000   CAS: 57598-00-2
4′-HYDROXY-2,3′-AZOTOLUENE
mf: $C_{14}H_{14}N_2O$ mw: 226.30

SYN: p-(o-TOLYLAZO)-o-CRESOL

TOXICITY DATA with REFERENCE
ETA: mul-mus TDLo:400 mg/kg/I   CNREA8
  1,397,41

SAFETY PROFILE: Questionable carcinogen with experimental tumorigenic data. When heated to decomposition it emits toxic fumes of NO_x.

HJH500   CAS: 7340-50-3
N-HYDROXYBENZENESULFONANILIDE
mf: $C_{12}H_{11}NO_3S$ mw: 249.30

SYN: N-HYDROXYPHENYLBENZENESULFONAMIDE

TOXICITY DATA with REFERENCE
ETA: ipr-rat TDLo:623 mg/kg/4W-I   CNREA8
  30,1485,70

SAFETY PROFILE: Questionable carcinogen with experimental tumorigenic data. When heated to decomposition it emits very toxic fumes of NO_x and SO_x.

HJP500   CAS: 26690-77-7
N-HYDROXY-4-BIPHENYLYLBENZAMIDE
mf: $C_{19}H_{15}NO_2$ mw: 289.35

SYNS: N-4-BIPHENYLYLBENZOHYDROXAMIC ACID ◊ N-HYDROXY-4-BIPHENYLBENZAMIDE

TOXICITY DATA with REFERENCE
CAR: ipr-rat TDLo:561 mg/kg/4W-I   CNREA8
  30,1485,70

SAFETY PROFILE: Questionable carcinogen with experimental carcinogenic data. When heated to decomposition it emits toxic fumes of NO_x.

HJS400   CAS: 61424-17-7
4-HYDROXYBUTYL(2-PROPENYL)NITROSAMINE
mf: $C_7H_{14}N_2O_2$ mw: 158.23

SYNS: 4-(ALLYLNITROSAMINO)-1-BUTANOL ◊ 1-BUTA-NOL, 4-(NITROSO-2-PROPENYLAMINO)-

TOXICITY DATA with REFERENCE
CAR: scu-ham TDLo:22500 mg/kg/75W-I
  CDPRD4 4,79,81

SAFETY PROFILE: Questionable carcinogen with experimental carcinogenic data. When heated to decomposition it emits toxic fumes of NO_x.

HJS850   CAS: 1083-57-4
3-HYDROXY-p-BUTYROPHENETIDIDE
mf: $C_{12}H_{17}NO_3$ mw: 223.30

SYNS: BETADID ◊ BUCETIN ◊ BUTANAMIDE, N-(4-ETHOXYPHENYL)-3-HYDROXY- ◊ BUTYRANILIDE, 4′-ETHOXY-3-HYDROXY- ◊ 4′-ETHOXY-3-HYDROXYBUTYR-ANILIDE ◊ β-HYDROXYBUTYRIC ACID-p-PHENETIDIDE ◊ β-OXYBUTTERSAEURE-p-PHENETIDID

TOXICITY DATA with REFERENCE
CAR: orl-mus TDLo:958 g/kg/76W-C   JJIND8 79,1151,87

NEO: orl-mus TD:479 g/kg/76W-C   JJIND8 79,1151,87

MUT: mma-sat 2 µmol/plate   CPBTAL 33,2877,85

CONSENSUS REPORTS: Reported in EPA TSCA Inventory.

SAFETY PROFILE: Questionable carcinogen with experimental carcinogenic and neoplastigenic data. Moderately toxic by ingestion and intraperitoneal routes. Mutation data reported. When heated to decomposition it emits toxic fumes of NO_x.

HJV500   CAS: 69853-71-0
6-HYDROXYCHOLEST-4-EN-3-ONE
mf: $C_{27}H_{44}O_2$ mw: 400.71

TOXICITY DATA with REFERENCE
ETA: scu-mus TDLo:600 mg/kg/72W-I

JNCIAM 19,977,57

SAFETY PROFILE: Questionable carcinogen with experimental tumorigenic data. When heated to decomposition it emits acrid smoke and fumes.

HKA300   CAS: 25316-40-9
HYDROXYDAUNORUBICIN HYDROCHLORIDE
mf: $C_{27}H_{29}NO_{11}$•ClH   mw: 580.03

SYNS: ADM HYDROCHLORIDE ◇ ADR ◇ ADRIACIN ◇ ADRIAMYCIN ◇ ADRIAMYCIN, HYDROCHLORIDE ◇ ADRIBLASTIN ◇ ADRIBLASTINE ◇ DOX HYDROCHLORIDE ◇ DOXORUBICIN ◇ DOXORUBICIN HYDROCHLORIDE ◇ FI 106 ◇ FI 6804

TOXICITY DATA with REFERENCE
ETA: ivn-mky TDLo:27 mg/kg/2Y-I   PHMGBN 20,9,80

MUT: dni-ckn:emb 900 nmol/L   JMCMAR 26,638,83

MUT: dni-mus:leu 1500 nmol/L   JMCMAR 22,912,79

MUT: oms-mus:leu 580 nmol/L   JMCMAR 22,912,79

CONSENSUS REPORTS: EPA Genetic Toxicology Program.

SAFETY PROFILE: Questionable carcinogen with experimental tumorigenic data. Poison by subcutaneous, intramuscular, intravenous, and intraperitoneal routes. Moderately toxic by ingestion. Mutation data reported. An antineoplastic and immunosuppressive agent. When heated to decomposition it emits toxic fumes of NO_x and HCl.

HKA700   CAS: 19115-30-1
1'-HYDROXY-2',3'-DEHYDROESTRAGOLE
mf: $C_{10}H_{10}O_2$ mw: 162.20

SYNS: BENZENEMETHANOL, α-ETHYNYL-4-METHOXY- ◇ α-ETHYNYL-p-METHOXYBENZYL ALCOHOL

TOXICITY DATA with REFERENCE
CAR: ipr-mus TDLo:1632 µg/kg   CNREA8 47,2275,87

MUT: dnd-mus-ipr 100 µmol/kg   PAACA3 25,88,84

MUT: oth-mus-ipr 100 µmol/kg   PAACA3 25,88,84

SAFETY PROFILE: Questionable carcinogen with experimental carcinogenic data. Mutation data reported. When heated to decomposition it emits acrid smoke and irritating fumes.

HKB000   CAS: 71609-22-8
N-HYDROXY-N,N'-DIACETYLBENZIDINE
mf: $C_{16}H_{16}N_2O_3$ mw: 284.34

SYNS: N-(4'-ACETAMIDOBIPHENYLYL)ACETOHYDROXAMIC ACID ◇ NOHDABZ

TOXICITY DATA with REFERENCE
CAR: ipr-rat TDLo:68 mg/kg/4W-I   CRNGDP 2,747,81

MUT: mma-sat 250 nmol/plate   CNREA8 39,3107,79

MUT: mmo-sat 250 nmol/plate   CNREA8 39,3107,79

SAFETY PROFILE: Questionable carcinogen with experimental carcinogenic data. Mutation data reported. When heated to decomposition it emits toxic fumes of NO_x.

HKC000   CAS: 75-60-5
HYDROXYDIMETHYLARSINE OXIDE
DOT: 1572
mf: $C_2H_7AsO_2$ mw: 138.01

PROP: Colorless crystals, odorless and sol in water. Mp: 192°.

SYNS: ACIDE CACODYLIQUE (FRENCH) ◇ ACIDE DIMETHYLARSINIQUE (FRENCH) ◇ AGENT BLUE ◇ ANSAR

◇ ARSAN ◇ BOLLS-EYE ◇ CACODYLIC ACID (DOT)
◇ CHEXMATE ◇ DILIC ◇ DIMETHYLARSENIC ACID
◇ DIMETHYLARSINIC ACID ◇ DMAA ◇ ERASE ◇ PHYTAR
◇ RAD-E-CATE 25 ◇ RCRA WASTE NUMBER U136
◇ SALVO ◇ SILVISAR 510

TOXICITY DATA with REFERENCE
ETA: scu-mus TDLo:464 mg/kg   NTIS** PB223-159

MUT: mma-smc 2 pph   NTIS** PB84-138973
MUT: mmo-smc 2 pph   NTIS** PB84-138973
MUT: mnt-mus-ipr 7900 mg/kg/24H   NTIS** PB84-138973
MUT: mrc-smc 5 pph   NTIS** PB268-647
MUT: msc-mus:lym 1080 mg/L   NTIS** PB84-138973

CONSENSUS REPORTS: IARC Cancer Review: Animal Inadequate Evidence IMEMDT 23,39,80. Arsenic and its compounds are on the Community Right-To-Know List. Reported in EPA TSCA Inventory. EPA Genetic Toxicology Program.

OSHA PEL: TWA 0.5 mg(As)/m^3 ACGIH TLV: TWA 0.2 mg(As)/m^3 DOT Classification: IMO: Poison B; Label: Poison.

SAFETY PROFILE: Questionable carcinogen with experimental tumorigenic and teratogenic data. A suspected carcinogenic. Poison by an unspecified route. Moderately toxic by ingestion and intraperitoneal routes. Experimental reproductive effects. A skin and eye irritant. Mutation data reported. Used as an herbicide, defoliant, and silvicide. Hazardous when water solution is in contact with active metals, i.e., Fe; Al; Zn. When heated to decomposition it emits toxic fumes of As.

HKF000   CAS: 101-73-5
p-HYDROXYDIPHENYLAMINE ISOPROPYL ETHER
mf: $C_{15}H_{17}NO$ mw: 227.33

SYNS: AGERITE 150 ◇ AGERITE ISO ◇ p-ISOPROPOXYDI-PHENYLAMINE ◇ 4-ISOPROPOXYDIPHENYLAMINE ◇ N-(4-ISOPROPOXYPHENYL)ANILINE

TOXICITY DATA with REFERENCE
NEO: orl-mus TDLo:332 g/kg/78W-I   NTIS** PB223-159

CONSENSUS REPORTS: Reported in EPA TSCA Inventory.

SAFETY PROFILE: Questionable carcinogen with experimental neoplastigenic data. When

heated to decomposition it emits toxic fumes of NO$_x$.

HKG000   CAS: 28094-15-7
6-HYDROXYDOPAMINE HYDROCHLORIDE
mf: $C_8H_{11}NO_3$•ClH   mw: 205.66

SYNS: 4-(2-AMINOETHYL)-1,2,3-BENZENETRIOL HYDROCHLORIDE ◇ 3,4,5-TRIHYDROXYPHENETHYLAMINE HYDROCHLORIDE

TOXICITY DATA with REFERENCE
NEO: scu-mus TDLo:100 mg/kg/52W-I   RCOCB8 17,411,77

SAFETY PROFILE: Questionable carcinogen with experimental neoplastigenic data. When heated to decomposition it emits very toxic fumes of NO$_x$ and HCl.

HKH850   CAS: 5976-61-4
4-HYDROXYESTRADIOL
mf: $C_{18}H_{24}O_3$ mw: 288.42

SYNS: 4-HYDROXY-17-β-ESTRADIOL ◇ 4-OH-E2 ◇ 4-OH-ESTRADIOL

TOXICITY DATA with REFERENCE
ETA: imp-ham TDLo:900 mg/kg/90D-I   JSTBBK 24,353,86

SAFETY PROFILE: Questionable carcinogen with experimental tumorigenic data. Experimental reproductive data. When heated to decomposition it emits acrid smoke and irritating fumes.

HKI000   CAS: 51410-44-7
1'-HYDROXYESTRAGOLE
mf: $C_{10}H_{12}O_2$ mw: 164.22

SYN: p-METHOXY-α-VINYLBENZYL ALCOHOL

TOXICITY DATA with REFERENCE
CAR: ipr-mus TDLo:16422 µg/kg   CNREA8 47,2275,87
CAR: orl-mus TDLo:106 g/kg/1Y-C   CNREA8 43,1124,83
CAR: scu-mus TDLo:131 mg/kg/22D-I   JNCIAM 57,1323,76
MUT: mma-sat 1 µmol/plate   MUREAV 60,143,79
MUT: mmo-sat 1 µmol/plate   MUREAV 60,143,79

CONSENSUS REPORTS: EPA Genetic Toxicology Program.

SAFETY PROFILE: Questionable carcinogen with experimental carcinogenic data. Mutation

data reported. When heated to decomposition it emits acrid smoke and fumes.

HKI075 CAS: 730771-71-0
1'-HYDROXY-ESTRAGOLE-2',3'-OXIDE
mf: $C_{10}H_{12}O_3$ mw: 180.22

SYN: α-(EPOXYETHYL)-p-METHOXYBENZYL ALCOHOL

TOXICITY DATA with REFERENCE
NEO: ipr-mus TDLo: 43 mg/kg/12W-I CNREA8
43,1124,83
MUT: mmo-sat 200 nmol/plate MUREAV
60,143,79

SAFETY PROFILE: Questionable carcinogen with experimental neoplastigenic data. Mutation data reported. When heated to decomposition it emits acrid smoke and irritating fumes.

HKO000 CAS: 33389-36-5
4-(2-HYDROXYETHYLAMINO)-2-(5-NITRO-2-THIENYL)QUINAZOLINE
mf: $C_{14}H_{12}N_4O_3S$ mw: 316.36

TOXICITY DATA with REFERENCE
CAR: orl-rat TDLo: 13 g/kg/58W-C JNCIAM
57,277,76
MUT: mma-sat 1250 µg/plate CNREA8
35,3611,75

SAFETY PROFILE: Questionable carcinogen with experimental carcinogenic data. Mutation data reported. When heated to decomposition it emits very toxic fumes of NO_x and SO_x.

HKQ025 CAS: 589-41-3
N-HYDROXY ETHYL CARBAMATE
mf: $C_3H_7NO_3$ mw: 105.11

SYNS: ETHYL-N-HYDROXYCARBAMATE ◇ HYDROXY-CARBAMIC ACID ETHYL ESTER ◇ N-HYDROXYURETHAN ◇ N-HYDROXYURETHANE ◇ NHU ◇ NSC-83629 ◇ NSC-71045 ◇ SQ 16819

TOXICITY DATA with REFERENCE
NEO: ipr-mus TD: 2400 mg/kg/4W-I CNREA8
29,2184,69
NEO: ipr-mus TD: 5800 mg/kg/10W-I IJCNAW
4,318,69
NEO: ipr-mus TDLo: 2400 mg/kg/2W-I
CNREA8 29,2184,69
NEO: ipr-rat TDLo: 500 mg/kg RRCRBU
52,29,75
NEO: unr-mus TDLo: 1 mg/kg (21D preg):
REP 40YJAX -,141,76
ETA: ipr-mus TD: 1 g/kg VOONAW 15(2),66,69

ETA: ipr-mus TD: 2900 mg/kg/5W-I IJCNAW
4,318,69
ETA: scu-rat TDLo: 8 g/kg/8W-I JNCIAM
43,749,75
MUT: cyt-hmn: leu 333 µmol/L/48H CNREA8
25,980,65
MUT: dni-hmn: hla 1320 µmol/L BCPCA6
14,205,65
MUT: dns-rat: lvr 10 mmol/L MUREAV
145,201,85
MUT: mma-ham: lng 20 mmol/L MUREAV
152,225,85
MUT: mmo-esc 10 mmol/L MUREAV 151,201,85
MUT: sce-ham-ipr 400 mg/kg MUREAV
126,159,84
MUT: sce-rat-ipr 400 mg/kg MUREAV 126,159,84

CONSENSUS REPORTS: EPA Genetic Toxicology Program.

SAFETY PROFILE: Questionable carcinogen with experimental neoplastigenic and tumorigenic data. Moderately toxic by intraperitoneal route. Experimental teratogenic and reproductive effects. Human mutation data reported. When heated to decomposition it emits toxic fumes of NO_x.

HKQ300
HYDROXYETHYL CNU METHANESULFONATE
mf: $C_5H_{10}ClN_3O_3 \cdot CH_4O_3S$ mw: 291.74

SYNS: HECNU-MS ◇ HYDROXY CNU METHANESULPHONATE

TOXICITY DATA with REFERENCE
ETA: ivn-rat TD: 32 mg/kg/60W-I DTESD7
8,273,80
ETA: ivn-rat TD: 51 mg/kg/24W-I DTESD7
8,273,80
ETA: ivn-rat TD: 64 mg/kg/60W-I DTESD7
8,273,80
ETA: ivn-rat TDLo: 16 mg/kg/60W-I DTESD7
8,273,80

SAFETY PROFILE: Questionable carcinogen with experimental tumorigenic data. When heated to decomposition it emits toxic fumes of Cl^-, SO_x, and NO_x.

HKU000 CAS: 13345-58-9
7-(2-HYDROXYETHYL)-12-METHYLBENZ(a)ANTHRACENE
mf: $C_{21}H_{18}O$ mw: 286.39

SYN: 12-METHYL BENZ(A)ANTHRACENE-7-ETHANOL

TOXICITY DATA with REFERENCE
ETA: ims-rat TDLo: 50 mg/kg   BCPCA6 16,607,67

SAFETY PROFILE: Questionable carcinogen with experimental tumorigenic data. When heated to decomposition it emits acrid smoke and fumes.

HKV000   CAS: 21600-45-3
3-(2-HYDROXYETHYL)-3-METHYL-1-PHENYLTRIAZENE
mf: $C_9H_{13}N_3O$ mw: 179.25

SYNS: 1-PHENYL-3-METHYL-3-(2-HYDROXYAETHYL) TRIAZEN (GERMAN) ◇ 1-PHENYL-3-METHYL-3-(2-HY-DROXYETHYL)TRIAZENE

TOXICITY DATA with REFERENCE
CAR: scu-rat TDLo: 1200 mg/kg/54W-I
   ZKKOBW 81,285,74

SAFETY PROFILE: Questionable carcinogen with experimental carcinogenic data. A poison by subcutaneous route. When heated to decomposition it emits toxic fumes of NO_x.

HKW345   CAS: 40343-32-6
N-(2-HYDROXYETHYL)-3-NITROBENZYLIDENIMINE N-OXIDE
mf: $C_9H_{10}N_2O_4$ mw: 210.21

SYN: 2-((m-NITROBENZYLIDENE)AMINO)ETHANOL N-OXIDE

TOXICITY DATA with REFERENCE
ETA: orl-rat TDLo: 551 g/kg/46W-C   FEPRA7
   38,1403,79

SAFETY PROFILE: Questionable carcinogen with experimental tumorigenic data. When heated to decomposition it emits toxic fumes of NO_x.

HKW350   CAS: 40343-30-4
N-(2-HYDROXYETHYL)-4-NITROBENZYLIDENIMINE N-OXIDE
mf: $C_9H_{10}N_2O_4$ mw: 210.21

SYN: 2-((p-NITROBENZYLIDENE)AMINO)ETHANOL N-OXIDE

TOXICITY DATA with REFERENCE
ETA: orl-rat TDLo: 551 g/kg/46W-C   FEPRA7
   38,1403,79

SAFETY PROFILE: Questionable carcinogen with experimental tumorigenic data. When heated to decomposition it emits toxic fumes of NO_x.

HKW450   CAS: 19561-70-7
N-(2-HYDROXYETHYL)-α-(5-NITRO-2-FURYL)NITRONE
mf: $C_7H_8N_2O_5$ mw: 200.17

SYNS: ETHANOL, 2-(((5-NITRO-2-FURANYL)METHY-LENE)AMINO)-, N-OXIDE (9CI) ◇ ETHANOL, 2-((5-NITRO-FURFURYLIDENE)AMINO)-, N-OXIDE ◇ NIFURATRONE ◇ 2-(5-NITRO-2-FURFURYLIDENE)AMINOETHANOL N-OXIDE

TOXICITY DATA with REFERENCE
ETA: orl-rat TDLo: 522 g/kg/46W-C   FEPRA7
   38,1403,79
MUT: dnr-esc 500 nmol/well   CNREA8
   34,2266,74
MUT: dnr-sat 500 nmol/well   CNREA8
   34,2266,74
MUT: mmo-esc 10 μg/plate   MUREAV 26,3,74
MUT: mmo-sat 100 ng/plate   MUREAV 40,9,76

SAFETY PROFILE: Questionable carcinogen with experimental tumorigenic data. Mutation data reported. When heated to decomposition it emits toxic fumes of NO_x.

HKW475
1-((2-HYDROXYETHYL)NITROSAMINO)2-PROPANOL
mf: $C_5H_{12}N_2O_4$ mw: 164.19

SYNS: NIEA ◇ N-NITROSOETHANOLISOPROPANOLAMINE ◇ N-NITROSO-(2-HYDROXYPROPYL)-(2-HYDROXYETHYL)AMINE ◇ NITROSOISOPROPANOL-ETHANOLAMINE

TOXICITY DATA with REFERENCE
CAR: orl-rat TDLo: 5 g/kg/50W-C   CRNGDP
   5,167,84
MUT: mma-sat 500 μg/plate   MUREAV 111,135,83

SAFETY PROFILE: Questionable carcinogen with experimental carcinogenic data. Mutation data reported. When heated to decomposition it emits toxic fumes of NO_x.

HKY000   CAS: 58989-02-9
N-HYDROXY-N-ETHYL-p-(PHENYLAZO) ANILINE
mf: $C_{14}H_{15}N_3O$ mw: 241.32

SYNS: N-ETHYL-N-(p-(PHENYLAZO)PHENYL)HYDROXYLAMINE ◇ N-HY-DROXY-EAB ◇ N-HYDROXY-N-ETHYL-4-AMINOAZOBEN-ZENE

TOXICITY DATA with REFERENCE
ETA: orl-rat TDLo: 424 mg/kg/5W-I   CNREA8
   39,3411,79

SAFETY PROFILE: Questionable carcinogen with experimental tumorigenic data. When heated to decomposition it emits toxic fumes of NO_x.

HLE450 CAS: 14461-87-1
N-(7-HYDROXYFLUOREN-2-YL)ACETOHYDROXAMIC ACID
mf: $C_{15}H_{13}NO_3$ mw: 255.29

SYN: N-HYDROXY-N-(7-HYDROXY-2-FLUORENYL) ACETAMIDE

TOXICITY DATA with REFERENCE
CAR: ipr-rat TDLo:540 mg/kg/4W-I CNREA8 27,1443,67

SAFETY PROFILE: Questionable carcinogen with experimental carcinogenic data. When heated to decomposition it emits toxic fumes of NO_x.

HLE500 CAS: 26630-60-4
N-HYDROXY-2-FLUORENYLBENZENESULFONAMIDE
mf: $C_{19}H_{15}NO_3S$ mw: 337.41

SYN: N-HYDROXY-N-FLUORENYLBENZENESULFON-AMIDE

TOXICITY DATA with REFERENCE
CAR: ipr-rat TDLo:192 mg/kg/4W-I CNREA8 30,1485,70
CAR: orl-rat TDLo:3660 mg/kg/29W CNREA8 31,778,71

SAFETY PROFILE: Questionable carcinogen with experimental carcinogenic data. When heated to decomposition it emits very toxic fumes of NO_x and SO_x.

HLE650 CAS: 78281-06-8
N-HYDROXY-4-FORMYLAMINOBIPHENYL
mf: $C_{13}H_{11}NO_2$ mw: 213.25

SYNS: N-(4-BIPHENYLYL)FORMOHYDROXAMIC ACID ◇ FORMAMIDE, N-(1,1'-BIPHENYL)-4-YL-N-HYDROXY- ◇ N-HYDROXY-FABP

TOXICITY DATA with REFERENCE
CAR: ipr-rat TDLo:85 mg/kg CNREA8 41,2450,81

SAFETY PROFILE: Questionable carcinogen with experimental carcinogenic data. When heated to decomposition it emits toxic fumes of NO_x.

HLE750 CAS: 89947-76-2
N-HYDROXY-N-GLUCURONOSYL-2-AMINOFLUORENE
mf: $C_{19}H_{19}NO_7$ mw: 373.39

SYNS: β-D-GLUCOPYRANURONIC ACID, 1-DEOXY-1-(9H-FLUOREN-2-YLHYDROXYAMINO)- ◇ GLUCURONIC ACID, 1-DEOXY-1-(2-FLUORENYLHYDROXYAMINO)- ◇ N-GLUCURONIDE of N-HYDROXY-2-AMINOFLUORENE ◇ N-HYDROXY-2-AMINOFLUORENE N-GLUCURONIDE

TOXICITY DATA with REFERENCE
CAR: par-rat TDLo:5600 μg/kg/30W-C CNREA8 47,3406,87
MUT: dns-hmn:oth 100 nmol/L JJIND8 72,847,84

SAFETY PROFILE: Questionable carcinogen with experimental carcinogenic data. Mutation data reported. When heated to decomposition it emits toxic fumes of NO_x.

HLF000 CAS: 3393-34-8
4-HYDROXYHEX-4-ENOIC ACID LACTONE
mf: $C_6H_8O_2$ mw: 112.14

SYN: 5-ETHYLIDENEDIHYDRO-2(3H)-FURANONE

TOXICITY DATA with REFERENCE
ETA: scu-rat TDLo:1160 mg/kg/58W-I BJCAAI 15,85,61

SAFETY PROFILE: Questionable carcinogen with experimental tumorigenic data. When heated to decomposition it emits acrid smoke and fumes.

HLJ000 CAS: 54-16-0
5-HYDROXYINDOLYLACETIC ACID
mf: $C_{10}H_9NO_3$ mw: 191.20

SYN: 5-HYDROXYINDOLEACETIC ACID

TOXICITY DATA with REFERENCE
ETA: scu-mus TDLo:2000 mg/kg/20W-I AICCA6 19,660,63

SAFETY PROFILE: Questionable carcinogen with experimental tumorigenic data. Moderately toxic by intraperitoneal route. When heated to decomposition it emits toxic fumes of NO_x.

HLR000 CAS: 78265-95-9
N-HYDROXY-3-METHOXY-4-AMINOAZOBENZENE
mf: $C_{13}H_{13}N_3O_2$ mw: 243.29

SYNS: 4-HYDROXY-3-METHOXY-4-AMINOAZOBEN-ZENE ◇ N-HYDROXY-2-METHOXY-4-(PHENYLAZO)BENZE

NAMINE ◇ N-(2-METHOXY-4-(PHENYLAZO)PHENYL)HY-DROXYLAMINE

TOXICITY DATA with REFERENCE
CAR: scu-mus TDLo: 623 mg/kg/8W-I   GANNA2 73,136,82

ETA: scu-mus TD: 1246 mg/kg/8W-I   GANNA2 73,136,82

MUT: mma-sat 50 nmol/plate   GANNA2 72,921,81

MUT: mmo-sat 100 nmol/plate   GANNA2 68,373,77

SAFETY PROFILE: Questionable carcinogen with experimental carcinogenic and tumorigenic data. Mutation data reported. When heated to decomposition it emits toxic fumes of NO_x.

HLR500   CAS: 63040-24-4
3-HYDROXY-4'-METHOXY-4-AMINODIPHENYL
mf: $C_{13}H_{13}NO_2$ mw: 215.27

SYN: 4-AMINO-4'-METHOXY-3-BIPHENYLOL

TOXICITY DATA with REFERENCE
CAR: imp-mus TDLo: 67 mg/kg   AICCA6 18,538,62

SAFETY PROFILE: Questionable carcinogen with experimental carcinogenic data. When heated to decomposition it emits toxic fumes of NO_x.

HLT500   CAS: 2929-14-8
4-HYDROXY-8-METHOXYQUINALDIC ACID
mf: $C_{11}H_9NO_4$ mw: 219.21

SYNS: 8-METHOXY-4-HYDROXYQUINOLINE-2-CAR-BOXYLIC ACID ◇ 8-METHYL ETHER of XANTHURENIC ACID ◇ XANTHURENIC ACID-8-METHYL ETHER

TOXICITY DATA with REFERENCE
CAR: scu-mus TDLo: 5280 mg/kg/44W-I   CNREA8 28,183,68

NEO: imp-mus TDLo: 89 mg/kg   BJCAAI 11,212,57

ETA: imp-mus TD: 80 mg/kg   BJCAAI 11,212,57

SAFETY PROFILE: Questionable carcinogen with experimental carcinogenic, neoplastigenic, and tumorigenic data. When heated to decomposition it emits toxic fumes of NO_x.

HLV000   CAS: 1910-36-7
N-HYDROXY-N-METHYL-4-AMINOAZOBENZENE
mf: $C_{13}H_{13}N_3O$ mw: 227.29

SYNS: N-HYDROXY-MAB ◇ N-METHYL-N-(p-(PHENYLAZO)PHENYL)HYDROXYLAMINE

TOXICITY DATA with REFERENCE
CAR: orl-rat TDLo: 466 mg/kg/5W-I   CNREA8 39,3411,79

ETA: ipr-rat TDLo: 28 mg/kg   CNREA8 39,3411,79

ETA: scu-rat TDLo: 149 mg/kg/12W-I   CNREA8 39,3411,79

MUT: mma-sat 100 nmol/plate   CALEDQ 1,91,75

MUT: mmo-sat 100 nmol/plate   CALEDQ 1,91,75

SAFETY PROFILE: Questionable carcinogen with experimental carcinogenic and tumorigenic data. Mutation data reported. When heated to decomposition it emits toxic fumes of NO_x.

HLX550   CAS: 69321-16-0
4-(N-HYDROXY-N-METHYLAMINO)QUINOLINE 1-OXIDE
mf: $C_{10}H_{10}N_2O_2$ mw: 190.22

SYNS: HYDROXYLAMINE, N-METHYL-N-(4-QUINOLI-NYL)-, 1-OXIDE ◇ 4-(N-METHYLHYDROXYAMINO)-QUINO-LINE-1-OXIDE ◇ 4-QUINOLINAMINE, N-HYDROXY-N-METHYL-, 1-OXIDE

TOXICITY DATA with REFERENCE
ETA: scu-mus TDLo: 60 mg/kg/10W-I   GANNA2 69,835,78

MUT: mma-esc 200 μmol/L   CPBTAL 34,1755,86

SAFETY PROFILE: Questionable carcinogen with experimental tumorigenic data. Mutation data reported. When heated to decomposition it emits toxic fumes of NO_x.

HLX900
4-(HYDROXYMETHYL) BENZENEDIAZONIUM SULFATE
mf: $C_7H_7N_2O \cdot 1/2H_2O_4S$ mw: 184.15

SYNS: HMBD ◇ BENZENEDIAZONIUM, 4-(HYDROXY-METHYL)-, SULFATE (2:1)

TOXICITY DATA with REFERENCE
CAR: scu-mus TDLo: 1300 mg/kg/26W-I   PAACA3 25,115,84

SAFETY PROFILE: Questionable carcinogen with experimental carcinogenic data. When heated to decomposition it emits toxic fumes of NO_x and SO_x.

HLY000   CAS: 68041-18-9
6-HYDROXYMETHYLBENZO(a)-PYRENESULFATE ESTER (SODIUM SALT)
mf: $C_{21}H_{13}O_4S \cdot Na$ mw: 384.39

TOXICITY DATA with REFERENCE
NEO: skn-mus TDLo: 56 mg/kg/40W-I   CBINA8
22(1),53,78

MUT: mmo-sat 1 nmol/plate   CBINA8 58,253,86

SAFETY PROFILE: Questionable carcinogen with experimental neoplastigenic data. Mutagenic data reported. When heated to decomposition it emits toxic fumes of SO_x and Na_2O.

HMA000   CAS: 3342-98-1
1-HYDROXY-3-METHYLCHOLANTHRENE
mf: $C_{21}H_{16}O$ mw: 284.37

SYNS: 15-HYDROXY-20-METHYLCHOLANTHRENE ◇ 3-METHYLCHOLANTHREN-1-OL ◇ 3-METHYL-1-CHO-LANTHRENOL

TOXICITY DATA with REFERENCE
CAR: skn-mus TDLo: 91 mg/kg/20W-I   CBINA8
22(1),69,78
NEO: scu-mus TDLo: 120 mg/kg/6W-I   IJCNAW
2,505,67
MUT: mma-sat 20 nmol/plate   CNREA8 38,3398,78

CONSENSUS REPORTS: EPA Genetic Toxicology Program.

SAFETY PROFILE: Questionable carcinogen with experimental carcinogenic and neoplastigenic data. Mutation data reported. When heated to decomposition it emits acrid smoke and fumes.

HMA500   CAS: 3308-64-3
2-HYDROXY-3-METHYLCHOLANTHRENE
mf: $C_{21}H_{16}O$ mw: 284.37

SYN: 3-METHYLCHOLANTHREN-2-OL

TOXICITY DATA with REFERENCE
CAR: skn-mus TDLo: 91 mg/kg/20W-I   CBINA8
22,69,78
NEO: scu-mus TDLo: 120 mg/kg/6W-I   IJCNAW
2,505,67
MUT: mma-ham: lng 15 nmol/plate   CNREA8
38,3398,78
MUT: mma-sat 20 nmol/plate   CNREA8
38,3398,78

CONSENSUS REPORTS: EPA Genetic Toxicology Program.

SAFETY PROFILE: Questionable carcinogen with experimental carcinogenic and neoplastigenic data. Mutation data reported. When heated

to decomposition it emits acrid smoke and fumes.

HMB595   CAS: 35282-68-9
2'-HYDROXYMETHYL-N,N-DIMETHYL-4-AMINOAZOBENZENE
mf: $C_{15}H_{17}N_3O$ mw: 255.35

SYNS: BENZENEMETHANOL, 2-((4-(DIMETHYLAMINO) PHENYL)AZO)-(9CI) ◇ o-((p-DIMETHYLAMINOPHENYL) AZO)BENZYL ALCOHOL

TOXICITY DATA with REFERENCE
NEO: orl-rat TDLo: 3600 mg/kg/17W-C   JJIND8
79,1159,87
MUT: dns-rat: lvr 1 μmol/L   CNREA8 46,1654,86
MUT: mma-sat 500 nmol/plate   MUREAV
121,95,83

SAFETY PROFILE: Questionable carcinogen with experimental neoplastigenic data. Mutation data reported. When heated to decomposition it emits toxic fumes of NO_x.

HMB600   CAS: 35282-69-0
3'-HYDROXYMETHYL-N,N-DIMETHYL-4-AMINOAZOBENZENE
mf: $C_{15}H_{17}N_3O$ mw: 255.35

SYNS: m-((p-DIMETHYLAMINOPHENYL)AZO)BENZYL ALCOHOL ◇ 3-((p-DIMETHYLAMINO)PHENYLAZO)BEN-ZYL ALCOHOL ◇ 3'-HYDROXYMETHYL-4-(DIMETHYL-AMINO)AZOBENZENE

TOXICITY DATA with REFERENCE
CAR: orl-rat TD: 3600 mg/kg/17W-C   JJIND8
79,1159,87
CAR: orl-rat TD: 5240 mg/kg/90D-C   CRNGDP
1,533,80
NEO: orl-rat TD: 2563 mg/kg/30D-C   CRNGDP
1,533,80
NEO: orl-rat TD: 4880 mg/kg/13W-C   GANNA2
72,160,81
NEO: orl-rat TDLo: 2280 mg/kg/13W-C
GANNA2 72,160,81
MUT: dns-rat: lvr 1 μmol/L   CNREA8 46,1654,86
MUT: mma-sat 1 μmol/L   CPBTAL 32,3641,84
MUT: mmo-sat 1 μmol/plate   CRNGDP 4,1487,83

SAFETY PROFILE: Questionable carcinogen with experimental carcinogenic and neoplastigenic data. Mutation data reported. When heated to decomposition it emits toxic fumes of NO_x.

HMC500   CAS: 63885-07-4
3-HYDROXY-1-METHYLGUANINE
mf: $C_6H_7N_5O_2$ mw: 181.18

TOXICITY DATA with REFERENCE
NEO: scu-rat TDLo: 96 mg/kg/8W-I   CNREA8 33,1113,73

SAFETY PROFILE: Questionable carcinogen with experimental neoplastigenic data. When heated to decomposition it emits toxic fumes of NO_x.

HMD000   CAS: 30345-27-8
3-HYDROXY-7-METHYLGUANINE
mf: $C_6H_7N_5O_2$ mw: 181.18

SYN: 2-AMINO-3-HYDROXY-1,7-DIHYDRO-7-METHYL-6H-PURIN-6-ONE

TOXICITY DATA with REFERENCE
ETA: scu-rat TDLo: 96 mg/kg/8W-I   CNREA8 33,1113,73

SAFETY PROFILE: Questionable carcinogen with experimental tumorigenic data. When heated to decomposition it emits toxic fumes of NO_x.

HMD500   CAS: 30345-28-9
3-HYDROXY-9-METHYLGUANINE
mf: $C_6H_7N_5O_2$ mw: 181.18

SYN: 2-AMINO-3-HYDROXY-1,7-DIHYDRO-8-METHYL-6H-PURIN-6-ONE

TOXICITY DATA with REFERENCE
ETA: scu-rat TDLo: 96 mg/kg/8W-I   CNREA8 33,1113,73

SAFETY PROFILE: Questionable carcinogen with experimental tumorigenic data. When heated to decomposition it emits toxic fumes of NO_x.

HMF000   CAS: 568-75-2
7-HYDROXYMETHYL-12-METHYLBENZ(a)ANTHRACENE
mf: $C_{20}H_{16}O$ mw: 272.36

SYNS: 7-HM-12-MBA ◇ 12-METHYBENZ(a)ANTHRA-CENE-7-METHANOL ◇ 7-OHM-MBA ◇ 7-OHM-12-MBA

TOXICITY DATA with REFERENCE
CAR: scu-mus TDLo: 400 mg/kg/10W-I
   IJCNAW 2,500,67
NEO: scu-rat TDLo: 150 mg/kg/39D-I   CNREA8 31,1951,71
ETA: ivn-mus TDLo: 100 mg/kg   KIDZAK 23(Suppl 1),35,71
ETA: ivn-rat TDLo: 25 mg/kg   KIDZAK 23(Suppl 1),35,71

ETA: orl-rat TDLo: 50 mg/kg   BJCAAI 22,122,68
ETA: skn-mus TDLo: 16 mg/kg/17W-I
   VOONAW 21(10),50,75
MUT: dnd-mus-skn 16 μmol/kg   CNREA8 43,4221,83
MUT: dnd-mus: emb 50 mg/L   CNREA8 39,1154,79
MUT: dnd-rat-ipr 100 μmol/kg   CRNGDP 3,297,82
MUT: dnr-esc 250 mg/L   JJIND8 62,873,79
MUT: mma-ham: lng 400 nmol/L   PNASA6 76,862,79
MUT: msc-ham: lng 100 nmol/L   PNASA6 76,862,79

CONSENSUS REPORTS: EPA Genetic Toxicology Program.

SAFETY PROFILE: Questionable carcinogen with experimental carcinogenic, neoplastigenic, tumorigenic, and teratogenic data. Poison by intravenous route. Other experimental reproductive effects. Mutation data reported. When heated to decomposition it emits acrid smoke and fumes.

HMF500   CAS: 568-70-7
12-HYDROXYMETHYL-7-METHYLBENZ(a)ANTHRACENE
mf: $C_{20}H_{16}O$ mw: 272.36

SYNS: 12-HM-7-MBA ◇ 7-METHYLBENZ(a)ANTHRA-CENE-12-METHANOL ◇ 7-METHYL-12-HYDROXYMETHYL-BENZ(a)ANTHRACENE

TOXICITY DATA with REFERENCE
CAR: scu-mus TDLo: 400 mg/kg/10W-I
   IJCNAW 2,500,67
ETA: orl-rat TDLo: 150 mg/kg   BJCAAI 22,122,68
ETA: par-mus TDLo: 400 mg/kg/10W-I
   NATUAS 207,816,65
ETA: skn-mus TDLo: 32683 ng/kg   CNREA8 40,3661,80
MUT: mma-ham: lng 400 nmol/L   PNASA6 76,862,79
MUT: mma-sat 10 nmol/plate   46OJAN -,675,81

CONSENSUS REPORTS: EPA Genetic Toxicology Program.

SAFETY PROFILE: Questionable carcinogen with experimental carcinogenic and tumorigenic data. Mutation data reported. When heated to decomposition it emits acrid smoke and fumes.

HMI500 CAS: 18857-59-5
**3-HYDROXYMETHYL-1-((3-(5-NITRO-2-FURYL)ALLYLIDENE)AMINO)
HYDANTOIN**
mf: $C_{11}H_{10}N_4O_6$ mw: 294.25

TOXICITY DATA with REFERENCE
CAR: orl-rat TDLo:51 g/kg/49W-C CNREA8 33,2894,73

SAFETY PROFILE: Questionable carcinogen with experimental carcinogenic data. When heated to decomposition it emits toxic fumes of NO_x.

HMP000 CAS: 5756-69-4
3-HYDROXY-3-METHYL-1-PHENYLTRIAZENE
mf: $C_7H_9N_3O$ mw: 151.19

SYNS: 1-PHENYL-3-METHYL-3-HYDROXY-TRIAZEN (GERMAN) ◇ 1-PHENYL-3-METHYL-3-HYDROXY-TRIAZENE

TOXICITY DATA with REFERENCE
CAR: scu-rat TD:3300 mg/kg/I ZKKOBW 81,285,74
CAR: scu-rat TDLo:420 mg/kg ZKKOBW 81,285,74

SAFETY PROFILE: Questionable carcinogen with experimental carcinogenic data. Moderately toxic by subcutaneous route. When heated to decomposition it emits toxic fumes of NO_x.

HMQ500 CAS: 65229-18-7
**d-N,N'-(1-HYDROXYMETHYLPROPYL)
ETHYLENEDINITROSAMINE**
mf: $C_{10}H_{22}N_4O_4$ mw: 262.36

SYNS: DDETA ◇ 2,2'-(ETHYLENEBIS(NITROSOIMINO))BISBUTANOL ◇ d-N,N'-(1-IDROSSIMETIL PROPIL)-ETILENDINITROSAMINA (ITALIAN)

TOXICITY DATA with REFERENCE
CAR: scu-mus TDLo:4320 mg/kg/36W-C LAPPA5 35,45,75

SAFETY PROFILE: Questionable carcinogen with experimental carcinogenic data. When heated to decomposition it emits toxic fumes of NO_x.

HMU000 CAS: 32766-75-9
N-HYDROXY-N-MYRISTOYL-2-AMINOFLUORENE
mf: $C_{27}H_{37}NO_2$ mw: 407.65

SYNS: N-FLUOREN-2-YL-N-TETRADECANOYLHYDROXAMIC ACID ◇ N-HYDROXY-N-TETRADECANOYL-2-AMINOFLUORENE

TOXICITY DATA with REFERENCE
NEO: scu-rat TDLo:104 mg/kg/5W-I CNREA8 37,1461,77
MUT: mma-sat 20 nmol/plate CNREA8 37,1461,77

CONSENSUS REPORTS: EPA Genetic Toxicology Program.

SAFETY PROFILE: Questionable carcinogen with experimental neoplastigenic data. Mutation data reported. When heated to decomposition it emits toxic fumes of NO_x.

HNB500 CAS: 30310-80-6
trans-4-HYDROXY-1-NITROSO-l-PROLINE
mf: $C_5H_8N_2O_4$ mw: 160.15

SYN: N-NITROSOHYDROXYPROLINE

CONSENSUS REPORTS: IARC Cancer Review: GROUP 3 IMEMDT 7,56,87; Animal Inadequate Evidence IMEMDT 17,303,78.

SAFETY PROFILE: Questionable carcinogen. When heated to decomposition it emits toxic fumes of NO_x.

HNI500 CAS: 129-20-4
p-HYDROXYPHENYLBUTAZONE
mf: $C_{19}H_{20}N_2O_3$ mw: 324.41

SYNS: ARTROFLOG ◇ BM 1 ◇ BUTAFLOGIN ◇ BUTANOVA ◇ BUTAPIRONE ◇ BUTILENE ◇ 4-BUTYL-2-(4-HYDROXYPHENYL)-1-PHENYL-3,5-DIOXOPYRAZOLIDINE ◇ 4-BUTYL-1-(p-HYDROXYPHENYL)-2-PHENYL-3,5-PYRAZOLIDINEDIONE ◇ 4-BUTYL-1-(4-HYDROXYPHENYL)-2-PHENYL-3,5-PYRAZOLIDINEDIONE ◇ 4-BUTYL-2-(p-HYDROXYPHENYL)-1-PHENYL-3,5-PYRAZOLIDINEDIONE ◇ CROVARIL ◇ DEFLOGIN ◇ 3,5-DIOXO-1-PHENYL-2-(p-HYDROXYPHENYL)-4-N-BUTYLPYRAZOLIDENE ◇ ETROZOLIDINA ◇ FLAMARIL ◇ FLANARIL ◇ GLOGAL ◇ FLOGHENE ◇ FLOGISTIN ◇ FLOGITOLO ◇ FLOGODIN ◇ FLOGORIL ◇ FLOGOSTOP ◇ FLOPIRINA ◇ FRABEL ◇ G 27202 ◇ 1-(p-HYDROXYPHENYL)-2-PHENYL-4-BUTYL-3,5-PYRAZOLIDINEDIONE ◇ 1-p-HYDROXYPHENYL-2-PHENYL-3,5-DIOXO-4-N-BUTYLPYRAZOLIDINE ◇ IDROBUTAZINA ◇ INFAMIL ◇ IPABUTONA ◇ IRIDIL ◇ ISOBUTAZINA ◇ ISOBUTIL ◇ METABOLITE I ◇ NEO-FARMADOL ◇ NEOFEN ◇ OFFITRIL ◇ OXALID ◇ OXAZOLIDIN ◇ OXAZOLIDIN-GEIGY ◇ OXIBUTOL ◇ OXI-FENIBUTOL ◇ OXIFENYLBUTAZON ◇ OXYPHENBUTAZONE ◇ OXYPHENYLBUTAZONE ◇ 1-PHENYL-2-(p-HYDROXY

PHENYL)-3,5-DIOXO-4-BUTYLPYRAZOLIDINE ◇ PIRABU-TINA ◇ PIRAFLOGIN ◇ POLIFLOGIL ◇ REMAZIN ◇ REUMOX ◇ RUMAPAX ◇ TANDACOTE ◇ TANDALGESIC ◇ TANDEARIL ◇ TANDERAL ◇ TELIDAL ◇ TENDEARIL ◇ VALIOIL ◇ VISUBUTINA ◇ USAF GE-14

TOXICITY DATA with REFERENCE
MUT: sln-asn 1 g/L   MUREAV 26,159,74

CONSENSUS REPORTS: IARC Cancer Review: GROUP 3 IMEMDT 7,56,87; Human Inadequate Evidence IMEMDT 13,183,77.

SAFETY PROFILE: Questionable carcinogen. A poison by ingestion, intraperitoneal and intravenous routes. Moderately toxic to humans by ingestion. Human systemic effects by ingestion: salivary gland changes, diarrhea, nausea or vomiting, hepatitis, hemorrhage, agranulocytosis, thrombocytopenia, dermatitis, fever, and unspecified endocrine system effects. Experimental reproductive effects. Mutation data reported. Used as an anti-inflammatory agent. When heated to decomposition it emits toxic fumes of NO_x.

HNL000   CAS: 306-23-0
p-HYDROXYPHENYLLACTIC ACID
mf: $C_9H_{10}O_4$ mw: 182.19

TOXICITY DATA with REFERENCE
CAR: scu-mus TD: 2800 mg/kg/10W-I   GETRE8 28(2),50,83
CAR: scu-mus TDLo: 800 mg/kg (15-21D post): TER   BEXBAN 87,46,79
CAR: scu-mus TDLo: 1600 mg/kg/8W-I   VOONAW 22(6),47,76

SAFETY PROFILE: Questionable carcinogen with experimental carcinogenic and teratogenic data. When heated to decomposition it emits acrid smoke and fumes.

HNL500   CAS: 156-39-8
p-HYDROXYPHENYLPYRUVIC ACID
mf: $C_9H_8O_4$ mw: 180.17

TOXICITY DATA with REFERENCE
ETA: scu-mus TDLo: 1600 mg/kg/8W-I   VOONAW 22(6),47,76

SAFETY PROFILE: Questionable carcinogen with experimental tumorigenic data. When heated to decomposition it emits acrid smoke and fumes.

HNT500   CAS: 630-56-8
HYDROXYPROGESTERONE CAPROATE
mf: $C_{27}H_{40}O_4$ mw: 428.67

PROP: Dense needles. Mp: 119-121°.

SYNS: CAPRON ◇ CORLUTIN L.A. ◇ DELALUTIN ◇ DEPO-PROLUTON ◇ DURALUTON ◇ ESTRALUTIN ◇ GESTEROL L.A. ◇ 17-α-HEXANOYLOXYPREGN-4-ENE-3,20-DIONE ◇ HORMOFORT ◇ HPC ◇ 17-HYDROXYPREGN-4-ENE-3,20-DIONE HEXANOATE ◇ 17-α-HYDROXYPROGESTERONE CAPROATE ◇ 17-α-HYDROXY PROGESTERONE-N-CAPROATE ◇ 17-α-HYDROXYPROGESTERONE HEXANOATE ◇ HYDROXON ◇ HYLUTIN ◇ HYPROVAL-PA ◇ IDROGESTENE ◇ LUETOCRIN DEPOT ◇ LUTATE ◇ LUTEOCRIN ◇ LUTOPRON ◇ NEOLUTIN ◇ NSC-17592 ◇ 17-((1-OXOHEXYL)OXY)PREGN-4-ENE-3,20-DIONE ◇ PRIMOLUT DEPOT ◇ PROGESTERONE CAPROATE ◇ PROGESTERONE RETARD PHARLON ◇ PROLUTON DEPOT ◇ RELUTIN ◇ SQUIBB ◇ SYNGYNON ◇ TERALUTIL

CONSENSUS REPORTS: IARC Cancer Review: Animal Inadequate Evidence IMEMDT 21,399,79.

SAFETY PROFILE: Questionable carcinogen. Human reproductive effects by an unknown route: behavioral effects on newborn. Experimental teratogenic and reproductive effects. A steroid. Used to treat menstrual disorders, threatened abortion and sterility. When heated to decomposition it emits acrid smoke and fumes.

HOB000   CAS: 54643-52-6
3-HYDROXYPURIN-2(3H)-ONE
mf: $C_5H_4O_2$ mw: 96.09

SYN: 3-HYDROXY-2-OXOPURINE

TOXICITY DATA with REFERENCE
ETA: scu-rat TDLo: 96 mg/kg/8W-I   CBINA8 25,369,79

SAFETY PROFILE: Questionable carcinogen with experimental tumorigenic data. When heated to decomposition it emits acrid smoke and fumes.

HOE000   CAS: 1571-30-8
8-HYDROXYQUINALDIC ACID
mf: $C_{10}H_7NO_3$ mw: 189.18

TOXICITY DATA with REFERENCE
NEO: imp-mus TDLo: 160 mg/kg   ANYAA9 108,924,63

SAFETY PROFILE: Questionable carcinogen with experimental neoplastigenic data. When heated to decomposition it emits toxic fumes of NO_x.

HOE500 CAS: 59901-91-6
1'-HYDROXYSAFROLE-2',3'-OXIDE
mf: $C_{10}H_{10}O_4$ mw: 194.20

SYN: α-EPOXYETHYL-1,3-BENZODIOXOLE-5-METHA-NOL

TOXICITY DATA with REFERENCE
CAR: scu-rat TDLo: 1554 mg/kg/10W-I
  CNREA8 43,1124,83
NEO: ipr-mus TDLo: 47 mg/kg/12W-I CNREA8 43,1124,83
NEO: skn-mus TDLo: 700 mg/kg/6W-I CNREA8 37,1883,77
MUT: mma-sat 20 nmol/plate CRSBAW 171,1041,77
MUT: mmo-sat 200 nmol/plate MUREAV 60,143,79

CONSENSUS REPORTS: EPA Genetic Toxicology Program.

SAFETY PROFILE: Questionable carcinogen with experimental carcinogenic and neoplastigenic data. Mutation data reported. When heated to decomposition it emits acrid smoke and fumes.

HOF000 CAS: 26782-43-4
HYDROXYSENKIRKINE
mf: $C_{19}H_{27}NO_7$ mw: 381.47

PROP: Isolated from the plant *Crotalaria laburnifolia*.

SYN: 8,12,18-TRIHYDROXY-4-METHYL-11,16-DIOXOSE-NECIONANIUM

TOXICITY DATA with REFERENCE
ETA: ipr-rat TDLo: 300 mg/kg JNCIAM 49,665,72

CONSENSUS REPORTS: IARC Cancer Review: Animal Inadequate Evidence IMEMDT 10,265,76.

SAFETY PROFILE: Questionable carcinogen with experimental tumorigenic data. Poison by ingestion. When heated to decomposition it emits toxic fumes of NO_x.

HOG000 CAS: 106-14-9
12-HYDROXYSTEARIC ACID
mf: $C_{18}H_{36}O_3$ mw: 300.54

TOXICITY DATA with REFERENCE
NEO: scu-mus TDLo: 160 mg/kg/40W-I
  CNREA8 30,1037,70

CONSENSUS REPORTS: Reported in EPA TSCA Inventory.

SAFETY PROFILE: Questionable carcinogen with experimental neoplastigenic data. When heated to decomposition it emits acrid smoke and fumes.

HOG500 CAS: 141-23-1
12-HYDROXYSTEARIC ACID, METHYL ESTER
mf: $C_{19}H_{38}O_3$ mw: 314.57

SYN: METHYL-12-HYDROXYSTEARATE

TOXICITY DATA with REFERENCE
ETA: scu-mus TDLo: 1600 mg/kg/40W-I
  CNREA8 30,1037,70

CONSENSUS REPORTS: Reported in EPA TSCA Inventory.

SAFETY PROFILE: Questionable carcinogen with experimental tumorigenic data. When heated to decomposition it emits acrid smoke and fumes.

HOI000 CAS: 2058-46-0
5-HYDROXYTETRACYCLINE HYDROCHLORIDE
mf: $C_{22}H_{24}N_2O_9 \cdot ClH$ mw: 496.94

SYNS: BISOLVOMYCIN ◇ HYDROCYCLIN ◇ LIQUAMYCIN INJECTABLE ◇ NSC 9169 ◇ OTETRYN ◇ OXLOPAR ◇ OXYJECT 100 ◇ OXYTETRACYCLINE HYDROCHLORIDE ◇ TERAMYCIN HYDROCHLORIDE ◇ TETRAMINE ◇ TETRAN HYDROCHLORIDE

TOXICITY DATA with REFERENCE
ETA: orl-rat TDLo: 1802 g/kg/2Y NTPTR* NTP-TR-315,87
MUT: dnd-bcs 10 μmol/L BIORAK 39,587,74
MUT: dnd-mam: lym 20 mg/L BIORAK 39,587,74
MUT: dnd-omi 10 μmol/L BIORAK 39,587,74
MUT: dns-mam: lym 20 mg/L BIORAK 39,587,74
MUT: mnt-mus-orl 100 mg/kg/24H-I MUREAV 117,193,83

CONSENSUS REPORTS: NTP Carcinogenesis Studies (feed); Equivocal Evidence: rat NTPTR* NTP-TR-315,87. NTP Carcinogenesis Studies (feed); No Evidence: mouse NTPTR* NTP-TR-315,87. Reported in EPA TSCA Inventory.

SAFETY PROFILE: Questionable carcinogen with experimental tumorigenic data. Poison by intravenous route. Moderately toxic by subcutaneous route. Mildly toxic by ingestion. Experimental teratogenic and reproductive effects. Mutation data reported. When heated to decomposition it emits very toxic fumes of HCl and NO_x.

HOJ000   CAS: 1012-82-4
7-HYDROXYTHEOPHYLLINE
mf: $C_7H_8N_4O_3$ mw: 196.19

SYNS: 3,7-DIHYDRO-7-HYDROXY-1,3-DIMETHYL-1H-PURINE-2,6-DIONE (9CI) ◇ 7-HYDROXYTHEOPHYLLIN (GERMAN)

TOXICITY DATA with REFERENCE
ETA: scu-mus TDLo:700 mg/kg/24W-I
ARZFAN 21,356,71

SAFETY PROFILE: Questionable carcinogen with experimental tumorigenic data. When heated to decomposition it emits toxic fumes of NO_x.

HOO500   CAS: 127-07-1
HYDROXYUREA
mf: $CH_4N_2O_2$ mw: 76.07

PROP: Needles from ethanol. Mp: 133-136°, bp: decomp. Very sol in water; sol in hot alc.

SYNS: N-(AMINOCARBONYL)HYDROXYLAMINE ◇ BIOSUPRESSIN ◇ CARBAMOHYDROXAMIC ACID ◇ CARBAMOHYDROXIMIC ACID ◇ CARBAMOHY-DROXYAMIC ACID ◇ CARBAMOYL OXIME ◇ N-CARBAM-OYLHYDROXYLAMINE ◇ CARBAMYL HYDROXAMATE ◇ HIDRIX ◇ HYDREA ◇ HYDROXYCARBAMINE ◇ HYDROXYLUREA ◇ N-HYDROXYUREA ◇ HYDURA ◇ LITALER ◇ NCI-C04831 ◇ NSC 32065 ◇ ONCO-CARBIDE ◇ OXYUREA ◇ SK 22591 ◇ SQ 1089

TOXICITY DATA with REFERENCE
ETA: ipr-mus TDLo:9750 mg/kg/26W-I
CANCAR 40(Suppl 4),1935,77
ETA: ipr-rat TDLo:2500 mg/kg/7W-I CANCAR 40(Suppl 4),1935,77
ETA: scu-mus TDLo:500 mg/kg IJCAAR 10,26,73
MUT: dni-hmn-orl 50 mg/kg/10H-C PAACA3 24,262,83
MUT: dni-hmn:fbr 1300 μmol/L TXCYAC 21,151,81
MUT: dni-hmn:hla 1 μmol/L/4H BECTA6 32,220,84
MUT: mmo-smc 7600 mg/L MUREAV 160,19,86
MUT: mrc-smc 7600 mg/L MGGEAE 140,339,75
MUT: scu-mus LD10:2400 mg/kg EJCAAH 10,667,74

CONSENSUS REPORTS: NCI Carcinogenesis Studies (ipr); No Evidence: mouse CANCAR 40,1935,77. NCI Carcinogenesis Studies (ipr); Equivocal Evidence: rat CANCAR 40,1935,77. EPA Genetic Toxicology Program.

SAFETY PROFILE: Questionable carcinogen with experimental tumorigenic data. Human systemic effects by ingestion, intravenous, and possibly other routes: nausea or vomiting, microcytosis (smaller than normal red blood cells), normocytic anemia (reduced red blood cell count), leukopenia (reduced white blood cell count), thrombocytopenia (decrease in the number of blood platelets), and other blood effects. Experimental teratogenic and reproductive effects. Mildly toxic by several routes. Human mutation data reported. When heated to decomposition it emits toxic fumes of NO_x.

HOO875   CAS: 22151-75-3
3-HYDROXYURIC ACID
mf: $C_5H_4N_4O_4$ mw: 184.13

TOXICITY DATA with REFERENCE
ETA: scu-rat TDLo:440 mg/kg/22W-I BICHAW 10,4463,71

SAFETY PROFILE: Questionable carcinogen with experimental tumorigenic data. When heated to decomposition it emits toxic fumes of NO_x.

HOP000   CAS: 13479-29-3
3-HYDROXYXANTHINE
mf: $C_5H_4N_4O_3$ mw: 168.13

SYNS: 3,7-DIHYDRO-3-HYDROXY-1H-PURINE-2,6-DIONE ◇ XANTHINE-x-N-OXIDE ◇ XANTHINE-3-N-OXIDE

TOXICITY DATA with REFERENCE
CAR: ipr-rat TDLo:96 mg/kg/8W-I CNREA8 38,2038,78
CAR: ipr-rat TDLo:500 mg/kg (19-22D preg): TER JJIND8 61,1405,78
NEO: scu-rat TD:96 mg/kg/8W-I CNREA8 38,2038,78
NEO: scu-rat TDLo:500 mg/kg (19-22D preg): TER JJIND8 61,1411,78
NEO: scu-rat TDLo:9600 μg/kg/8W-I CNREA8 38,2038,78
MUT: dnd-rat-ipr 50 mg/kg CBINA8 10,19,75

SAFETY PROFILE: Questionable carcinogen with experimental carcinogenic and neoplastigenic data. A poison by intraperitoneal route. Moderately toxic by subcutaneous route. Experimental teratogenic effects. Mutation data reported. When heated to decomposition it emits toxic fumes of NO_x.

HOP259   CAS: 16870-90-9
7-HYDROXYXANTHINE
mf: $C_5H_4N_4O_3$ mw: 168.13

SYN: XANTHINE-7-N-OXIDE

TOXICITY DATA with REFERENCE
CAR: ipr-rat TDLo: 96 mg/kg/8W-I   CNREA8
38,2038,78
NEO: scu-rat TD: 390 mg/kg/26W-I   CNREA8
27,925,67
NEO: scu-rat TDLo: 96 mg/kg/8W-I   CNREA8
38,2038,78

SAFETY PROFILE: Questionable carcinogen with experimental carcinogenic and neoplastigenic data. Poison by intraperitoneal route. When heated to decomposition it emits toxic fumes of NO_x.

HOQ000   CAS: 64038-48-8
1-HYDROXYXANTHINE DIHYDRATE
mf: $C_5H_4N_4O_3 \cdot 2H_2O$ mw: 204.17

TOXICITY DATA with REFERENCE
NEO: scu-rat TDLo: 1040 mg/kg/26W-I
CNREA8 30,184,70

SAFETY PROFILE: Questionable carcinogen with experimental neoplastigenic data. When heated to decomposition it emits toxic fumes of NO_x.

HOQ500   CAS: 64038-49-9
3-HYDROXYXANTHINE HYDRATE
mf: $C_5H_4N_4O_3 \cdot H_2O$ mw: 186.15

SYN: 3-HYDROXYXANTHINE

TOXICITY DATA with REFERENCE
NEO: scu-rat TDLo: 60 mg/kg/24W-I   CNREA8
30,184,70

SAFETY PROFILE: Questionable carcinogen with experimental neoplastigenic data. When heated to decomposition it emits toxic fumes of NO_x.

IAE000   CAS: 38915-28-5
ICR 340
mf: $C_{20}H_{24}Cl_2N_4O \cdot 2ClH$ mw: 480.30

SYN: 7-CHLORO-10-(3-(N-(2-CHLOROETHYL)-N-ETHYL)
AMINOPROPYLAMINO)-2-METHOXY-
BENZO(B)(1,5)NAPHTHYRIDINE DIHYDROCHLORIDE

TOXICITY DATA with REFERENCE
NEO: ivn-mus TDLo: 4800 μg/kg   CNREA8
36,2423,76
MUT: mmo-sat 500 ng/plate   MUREAV
136,185,84
MUT: msc-ham: ovr 1 μmol/L   CNREA8
39,4875,79

SAFETY PROFILE: Questionable carcinogen with experimental neoplastigenic data. Poison by intravenous route. Mutation data reported. When heated to decomposition it emits very toxic fumes of HCl and NO_x.

IAS000   CAS: 120-93-4
2-IMIDAZOLIDINONE
mf: $C_3H_6N_2O$ mw: 86.11

PROP: Needles. Mp: 131°; sol in water, hot alc; very sltly sol in ether.

SYNS: 1,3-ETHYLENE UREA ◇ ETHYLENE UREA
◇ 2-IMIDAZOLIDONE

TOXICITY DATA with REFERENCE
CAR: scu-mus TDLo: 1000 mg/kg   NTIS**PB223-
159

CONSENSUS REPORTS: Reported in EPA TSCA Inventory.

SAFETY PROFILE: Questionable carcinogen with experimental carcinogenic data. Moderately toxic by intraperitoneal route. Experimental reproductive effects. When heated to decomposition it emits toxic fumes of NO_x.

IBZ100   CAS: 99520-58-8
INDENO(1,2,3-cd)PYREN-8-OL
mf: $C_{22}H_{12}O$ mw: 292.34

SYN: 8-HYDROXYINDENO(1,2,3-cd)PYRENE

TOXICITY DATA with REFERENCE
ETA: skn-mus TDLo: 40 mg/kg/20D-I   CRNGDP
7,1761,86
MUT: mma-sat 10 μg/plate   CNREA8 45,5421,85

SAFETY PROFILE: Questionable carcinogen with experimental tumorigenic data. Mutation data reported. When heated to decomposition it emits acrid smoke and irritating fumes.

ICD000   CAS: 2642-37-7
INDICAN (POTASSIUM SALT)
mf: $C_8H_6NO_4S \cdot K$ mw: 251.31

PROP: Light brown plates from aq alc. Decomp @ 179-180° (subl), very sol in H_2O, insol in cold alc.

SYNS: INDOL-3-OL, HYDROGEN SULFATE (ESTER), PO-
TASSIUM SALT ◇ INDOL-3-OL, POTASSIUM SULFATE
◇ INDOL-3-YL POTASSIUM SULFATE ◇ INDOL-3-YL SUL-
FATE, POTASSIUM SALT ◇ POTASSIUM INDOL-3-YL SUL-
FATE ◇ URINARY INDICAN

TOXICITY DATA with REFERENCE
ETA: scu-mus TDLo:3500 mg/kg/26W-I
   KLWOAZ 36,1056,58

SAFETY PROFILE: Questionable carcinogen
with experimental tumorigenic data. When
heated to decomposition it emits very toxic
fumes of NO_x, K_2O and SO_x.

ICE000   CAS: 520-18-3
INDIGO YELLOW
mf: $C_{15}H_{10}O_6$ mw: 286.25

SYNS: PELARGIDENOLON ◇ RHAMNOLUTEIN
◇ RHAMNOLUTIN ◇ 3,4′,5,7-TETRAHYDROXYFLAVONE
◇ 5,7,4′-TRIHYDROXYFLAVONOL

TOXICITY DATA with REFERENCE
MUT: mma-sat 166 nmol/plate   MUREAV
   54,297,78
MUT: mnt-mus-ipr 200 mg/kg   MUREAV 89,69,81

CONSENSUS REPORTS: IARC Cancer Review: GROUP 3 IMEMDT 7,56,87; Animal
Inadequate Evidence IMEMDT 31,171,83.

SAFETY PROFILE: Questionable carcinogen.
Mutation data reported. When heated to decomposition it emits acrid smoke and fumes.

ICM000   CAS: 120-72-9
INDOLE
mf: C_8H_7N mw: 117.16

PROP: Colorless to yellowish scales; intense
fecal odor. Mp: 52°, bp: 253°; volatile with
steam. Sol in hot water, alc, ether, petroleum
ether; insol in mineral oil, glycerin.

SYNS: 1-AZAINDENE ◇ 1-BENZAZOLE ◇ BENZOPYR-
ROLE ◇ 2,3-BENZOPYRROLE ◇ FEMA No. 2593 ◇ INDOL
(GERMAN) ◇ KETOLE

TOXICITY DATA with REFERENCE
CAR: scu-mus TDLo:1000 mg/kg/25W-I
   KLWOAZ 35,504,57
ETA: scu-mus TD:120 mg/kg/12W-I   VOONAW
   10(9),70,64
ETA: scu-mus TD:1200 mg/kg/93W-C
   VOONAW 10(9),70,64
ETA: scu-mus TD:2000 mg/kg/20W-I   AICCA6
   19,660,63

CONSENSUS REPORTS: Reported in EPA
TSCA Inventory.

SAFETY PROFILE: Questionable carcinogen
with experimental carcinogenic and tumorigenic
data. A poison by intraperitoneal and subcutaneous routes. Moderately toxic by ingestion and
skin contact. When heated to decomposition it
emits toxic fumes of NO_x.

ICN000   CAS: 87-51-4
1H-INDOLE-3-ACETIC ACID
mf: $C_{10}H_9NO_2$ mw: 175.20

PROP: Colorless leaves from benzene. Mp:
165-168°. Very sltly sol in cold water; sol in
alc, ether and acetic acid; insol in chloroform.

SYNS: HETEROAUXIN ◇ IAA ◇ β-INDOLEACETIC ACID
◇ β-INDOLE-3-ACETIC ACID ◇ 3-INDOLEACETIC ACID
◇ α-INDOL-3-YL-ACETIC ACID ◇ INDOLYACETIC ACID
◇ β-INDOLYLACETIC ACID ◇ INDOLYL-3-ACETIC ACID
◇ 3-INDOLYLACETIC ACID ◇ RHIZOPIN ◇ φ-SKATOLE
CARBOXYLIC ACID

TOXICITY DATA with REFERENCE
ETA: scu-mus TDLo:2000 mg/kg/20W-I
   AICCA6 19,660,63
MUT: dnd-mam:lym 250 µmol/L   PYTCAS
   11,3135,72
MUT: dnd-sal:spr 250 µmol/L   PYTCAS
   11,3135,72
MUT: mrc-asn 1150 µmol/L   CRNGDP 4,1409,83
MUT: sln-asn 1150 µmol/L   CRNGDP 4,1409,83

CONSENSUS REPORTS: Reported in EPA
TSCA Inventory.

SAFETY PROFILE: Questionable carcinogen
with experimental tumorigenic and teratogenic
data. A poison by intraperitoneal route. Mutation data reported. When heated to decomposition it emits toxic fumes of NO_x.

ICO000   CAS: 1204-06-4
INDOLE-3-ACRYLIC ACID
mf: $C_{11}H_9NO_2$ mw: 187.21

SYNS: 3-INDOLYLACRYLIC ACID ◇ 3-(1-H-INDOL-3-YL)
2-PROPENOIC ACID

TOXICITY DATA with REFERENCE
CAR: scu-mus TDLo:1600 mg/kg/8W-I
   VOONAW 22(6),47,76
NEO: scu-ham TDLo:1600 mg/kg/10W-I
   VOONAW 22(6),52,76
ETA: scu-gpg TDLo:1100 mg/kg/13W-I
   BEXBAN 84,1156,77

MUT: cyt-hmn:leu 100 mg/L   TSITAQ 15,1505,73
MUT: cyt-mky-scu 15 mg/kg/2D-I   TSITAQ 15,1505,73

SAFETY PROFILE: Questionable carcinogen with experimental carcinogenic, neoplastigenic, and tumorigenic data. Human mutation data reported. When heated to decomposition it emits toxic fumes of NO_x.

IDW000   CAS: 144-48-9
IODOACETAMIDE
mf: C_2H_4INO mw: 184.97

SYNS: α-IODOACETAMIDE ◇ 2-IODOACETAMIDE ◇ MONOIODOACETAMIDE ◇ SURAUTO ◇ USAF D-1

TOXICITY DATA with REFERENCE
ETA: skn-mus TDLo:1480 mg/kg/20W-I
    BJCAAI 7,482,53
MUT: dnd-esc 20 ppm   MUREAV 24,365,74
MUT: dni-hmn:lym 10 μmol/L   STBIBN 50,97,75

CONSENSUS REPORTS: EPA Genetic Toxicology Program. Reported in EPA TSCA Inventory.

SAFETY PROFILE: Questionable carcinogen with experimental tumorigenic data. A poison by ingestion, intraperitoneal, and intravenous routes. Human mutation data reported. When heated to decomposition it emits very toxic fumes of I^- and NO_x.

IDZ000   CAS: 64-69-7
IODOACETIC ACID
mf: $C_2H_3IO_2$ mw: 185.95

PROP: Colorless or white crystals. Mp: 82-83°. Sol in water and alc. Very sltly sol in ether.

SYNS: IA ◇ IODOACETATE ◇ MIA ◇ MONOIODOACETATE ◇ MONOIODOACETIC ACID

TOXICITY DATA with REFERENCE
NEO: skn-mus TDLo:5800 mg/kg/27W-I
    BJCAAI 7,482,53
ETA: scu-mus TDLo:480 mg/kg/14W-I
    GANNA2 45,601,54
ETA: skn-mus TD:480 mg/kg/8W-I   AICCA6 11,699,55
MUT: cyt-ham:fbr 100 μg/L   CRNGDP 3,499,82
MUT: cyt-smc 5 mg/L   NATUAS 294,263,81
MUT: dni-hmn:hla 500 μmol/L   RAREAE 37,334,69
MUT: dni-mus:ast 2143 μmol/L   JPMSAE 67,1235,78

CONSENSUS REPORTS: Reported in EPA TSCA Inventory.

SAFETY PROFILE: Questionable carcinogen with experimental neoplastigenic and tumorigenic data. A poison by ingestion, subcutaneous, and intravenous routes. Experimental teratogenic effects. Human mutation data reported. When heated to decomposition it emits toxic fumes of I^-.

IEH000   CAS: 513-48-4
2-IODOBUTANE
DOT: 2390
mf: C_4H_9I mw: 184.03
PROP: Flash p: 14°F.
SYN: sec-BUTYL IODIDE

TOXICITY DATA with REFERENCE
NEO: ipr-mus TDLo:6000 mg/kg/8W-I
    CNREA8 35,1411,75
MUT: dnr-esc 25 μL/well/16H   CBINA8 15,219,76

CONSENSUS REPORTS: Reported in EPA TSCA Inventory. EPA Genetic Toxicology Program.

DOT Classification: Flammable Liquid; Label: Flammable Liquid.

SAFETY PROFILE: Questionable carcinogen with experimental neoplastigenic data. Mutation data reported. A very dangerous fire hazard when exposed to heat or flame; can react vigorously with oxidizing materials. When heated to decomposition it emits toxic fumes of I^-.

IEO000   CAS: 14722-22-6
N-(3-IODO-2-FLUORENYL)ACETAMIDE
mf: $C_{15}H_{12}INO$ mw: 349.18
SYN: 3-IODO-2-FAA

TOXICITY DATA with REFERENCE
CAR: orl-rat TDLo:3400 mg/kg/44W-C
    JNCIAM 24,149,60

SAFETY PROFILE: Questionable carcinogen with experimental carcinogenic data. When heated to decomposition it emits very toxic fumes of I^- and NO_x.

IER000   CAS: 27018-50-4
7-IODOMETHYL-12-METHYLBENZ(a) ANTHRACENE
mf: $C_{20}H_{15}I$ mw: 382.25

TOXICITY DATA with REFERENCE
NEO: scu-rat TDLo:150 mg/kg/39D-I   CNREA8 31,1951,71

SAFETY PROFILE: Questionable carcinogen with experimental neoplastigenic data. When heated to decomposition it emits toxic fumes of I⁻.

IEW000   CAS: 540-38-5
4-IODOPHENOL
mf: C_6H_5IO mw: 220.01

PROP: Needles or water. Mp: 93-94°, d: 1.857, bp: decomp. Sltly sol in water; very sol in alc and ether.

SYN: p-IODOPHENOL

TOXICITY DATA with REFERENCE
NEO: skn-mus TDLo: 7200 mg/kg/18W-I
CNREA8 19,413,59

CONSENSUS REPORTS: Reported in EPA TSCA Inventory.

SAFETY PROFILE: Questionable carcinogen with experimental neoplastigenic data. Moderately toxic by intraperitoneal route. When heated to decomposition it emits toxic fumes of I⁻.

IEY000   CAS: 141-76-4
3-IODOPROPIONIC ACID
mf: $C_3H_5IO_2$ mw: 199.98

PROP: (a) Needles from water. D: 1.857, mp: 93-94°, bp: decomp. Sltly sol in water; very sol in alc and ether. (b) Needles. Mp: 44.5-45.5°, bp: 105°. Very sltly sol in water; sol in alc, ether.

TOXICITY DATA with REFERENCE
ETA: skn-mus TDLo: 5700 mg/kg/3W-I
CNREA8 28,653,68
MUT: mmo-sat 50 μg/plate   DHEFDK FDA-78-
1046,78

CONSENSUS REPORTS: Reported in EPA TSCA Inventory.

SAFETY PROFILE: Questionable carcinogen with experimental tumorigenic data. Moderately toxic by skin contact. Mutation data reported. When heated to decomposition it emits toxic fumes of I⁻.

IGK800   CAS: 7439-89-6
IRON
af: Fe   aw: 55.85

PROP: From decomposition of iron pentacarbonyl: dark grey powder. From electrodeposition: lusterless, gray black powder. From chemical reduction: gray-black powder.

SYNS: ANCOR EN 80/150 ◇ ARMCO IRON ◇ CARBONYL IRON ◇ IRON, CARBONYL (FCC) ◇ IRON, ELECTROLYTIC ◇ IRON, ELEMENTAL ◇ IRON, REDUCED (FCC)

TOXICITY DATA with REFERENCE
ETA: itr-rat TDLo: 450 mg/kg/15W-I   SAIGBL
16,380,74

CONSENSUS REPORTS: Reported in EPA TSCA Inventory.

SAFETY PROFILE: Questionable carcinogen with experimental tumorigenic data. Poison by intraperitoneal route. Iron is potentially toxic in all forms and by all routes of exposure. The inhalation of large amounts of iron dust results in iron pneumoconiosis (arc welder's lung). Chronic exposure to excess levels of iron (> 50-100 mg Fe/day) can result in pathological deposition of iron in the body tissues, the symptoms of which are fibrosis of the pancreas, diabetes mellitus, and liver cirrhosis.

IGT000
IRON DEXTRAN GLYCEROL GLYCOSIDE

TOXICITY DATA with REFERENCE
NEO: scu-rat TDLo: 2500 mg(Fe)/kg/24W-I
BJCAAI 22,521,68

SAFETY PROFILE: Questionable carcinogen with experimental neoplastigenic data. Moderately toxic by intraperitoneal route.

IGU000   CAS: 9004-51-7
IRON-DEXTRIN COMPLEX

PROP: For human use, it is a clear, brown, colloidal solvent. Approximate molecular weight is 230,000 (IARC** 2,161,72).

SYNS: ASTRAFER ◇ DEXTRIFERRON ◇ DEXTRIFERRON INJECTION ◇ FERRIGEN ◇ IRON CARBOHYDRATE COMPLEX ◇ IRON DEXTRIN INJECTION

TOXICITY DATA with REFERENCE
NEO: ims-rat TDLo: 1150 mg/kg/17W-I
BJCAAI 15,838,61
ETA: scu-mus TDLo: 1200 mg(Fe)/kg/27W-I
BMJOAE 1,1800,62

CONSENSUS REPORTS: IARC Cancer Review: GROUP 3 IMEMDT 7,56,87; Animal Sufficient Evidence IMEMDT 2,161,73.

SAFETY PROFILE: Questionable carcinogen with experimental neoplastigenic and tumorigenic data. A poison by intravenous route. Moderately toxic by intraperitoneal route.

IGW500   CAS: 79-69-6
α-IRONE
mf: $C_{14}H_{22}O$ mw: 206.36

SYNS: 3-BUTEN-2-ONE, 4-(2,5,6,6-TETRAMETHYL-2-CY-
CLOHEXEN-1-YL)-(9CI) ◇ 4-(2,5,6,6-TETRAMETHYL-2-CY-
CLO-HEXEN-1-YL)-3-BUTEN-2-ONE

TOXICITY DATA with REFERENCE
ETA: ipr-mus TDLo: 1950 mg/kg/8W-I   CNREA8
33,3069,73

CONSENSUS REPORTS: Reported in EPA
TSCA Inventory.

SAFETY PROFILE: Questionable carcinogen
with experimental tumorigenic data. When
heated to decomposition it emits acrid smoke
and irritating fumes.

IHA000
IRON(III)HYDROXIDE-POLYMALTOSE

SYN: EISEN-III-HYDROXID-POLYMALTOSE (GERMAN)

TOXICITY DATA with REFERENCE
ETA: imp-rat TDLo: 1000 mg(Fe)/kg/10W-I
SMWOAS 92,130,62

SAFETY PROFILE: Questionable carcinogen
with experimental tumorigenic data by implant.

IHC100   CAS: 16448-54-7
IRON NITRILOTRIACETATE
mf: $C_6H_6FeNO_6$ mw: 243.98

SYNS: ACETIC ACID, NITRILOTRI-, IRON(III) chelate
◇ FERRIC NITRILOTRIACETATE ◇ IRON, (N,N-
BIS(CARBOXYMETHYL)GLYCINATO(3-)-N,O,O',O'')-,
(T-4)-(9CI) ◇ IRON-NITRILOTRIACETATE CHELATE
◇ IRON(3+) NTA

TOXICITY DATA with REFERENCE
CAR: ipr-mus TDLo: 566 mg/kg/12W-I
CNREA8 47,1867,87
CAR: ipr-rat TDLo: 1988 mg/kg/65D-C   JJIND8
,5,107,86
MUT: cyt-ham: ovr 2 mmol/L   CNREA8
41,1628,81

SAFETY PROFILE: Questionable carcinogen
with experimental carcinogenic data. Mutation
data reported. When heated to decomposition
it emits toxic fumes of NO_x.

IHD000   CAS: 1309-37-1
IRON OXIDE
mf: Fe_2O_3 mw: 159.70

SYNS: ANCHRED STANDARD ◇ ANHYDROUS IRON OX-
IDE ◇ ANHYDROUS OXIDE of IRON ◇ ARMENIAN BOLE

◇ BAUXITE RESIDUE ◇ BLACK OXIDE of IRON ◇ BLENDED
RED OXIDES of IRON ◇ BURNTISLAND RED ◇ BURNT
SIENNA ◇ BURNT UMBER ◇ CALCOTONE RED ◇ CAPUT
MORTUUM ◇ C.I. 77491 ◇ C.I. PIGMENT RED 101
◇ COLCOTHAR ◇ COLLOIDAL FERRIC OXIDE ◇ CROCUS
MARTIS ADSTRINGENS ◇ DEANOX ◇ EISENOXYD
◇ ENGLISH RED ◇ FERRIC OXIDE ◇ FERRUGO ◇ INDIAN
RED ◇ IRON(III) OXIDE ◇ IRON OXIDE RED ◇ IRON SESQUI-
OXIDE ◇ JEWELER'S ROUGE ◇ LEVANOX RED 130A
◇ LIGHT RED ◇ MANUFACTURED IRON OXIDES
◇ MARS BROWN ◇ MARS RED ◇ NATURAL IRON OXIDES
◇ NATURAL RED OXIDE ◇ OCHRE ◇ PRUSSIAN BROWN
◇ RADDLE ◇ 11554 RED ◇ RED IRON OXIDE ◇ RED OCHRE
◇ ROUGE ◇ RUBIGO ◇ SIENNA ◇ SPECULAR IRON
◇ STONE RED ◇ SUPRA ◇ SYNTHETIC IRON OXIDE
◇ VENETIAN RED ◇ VITRIOL RED ◇ VOGEL'S IRON RED
◇ YELLOW FERRIC OXIDE ◇ YELLOW OXIDE of IRON

TOXICITY DATA with REFERENCE
ETA: scu-rat TDLo: 135 mg/kg   PBPHAW
14,47,78

CONSENSUS REPORTS: IARC Cancer Re-
view: GROUP 3 IMEMDT 7,216,87; Human
Limited Evidence IMEMDT 1,29,72; Animal
No Evidence IMEMDT 1,29,72. Reported in
EPA TSCA Inventory.

OSHA PEL: Dust and Fume: TWA 10 mg(Fe)/
m^3; Rouge (Transitional: Total Dust: 15 mg/
m^3; Respirable Fraction: 5 mg/m^3) TWA Total
Dust: 10 mg/m^3; Respirable Fraction: 5 mg/m^3
ACGIH TLV: TWA 5 mg(Fe)/m^3 (vapor, dust);
Rouge: 10 mg/m^3 DFG MAK: 6 mg/m^3

SAFETY PROFILE: Questionable carcinogen
with experimental tumorigenic data. A poison
by subcutaneous route.

IHH000
IRON-POLYSACCHARIDE COMPLEX

PROP: Solution of iron and synthetically prepared polysaccharide with a mean molecular
weight of about 20,000 (BJCAAI 21,448,67).

SYN: MUSCULARON

TOXICITY DATA with REFERENCE
ETA: ims-mus TD: 2000 mg(Fe)/kg/9W-I
BJCAAI 21,448,67
ETA: ims-mus TDLo: 1000 mg(Fe)/kg/9W-I
BJCAAI 21,448,67
ETA: scu-mus TDLo: 1000 mg(Fe)/kg/9W-I
BJCAAI 21,448,67

SAFETY PROFILE: Questionable carcinogen
with experimental tumorigenic data. A poison
by intravenous and intraperitoneal routes. When

heated to decomposition it emits acrid smoke and fumes.

IHK000
IRON SODIUM GLUCONATE

SYNS: FERRIC SODIUM GLUCONATE COMPLEX ◊ OSMOFERRIN

TOXICITY DATA with REFERENCE
NEO: scu-mus TDLo: 3000 mg(Fe)/kg/16W-I
BJCAAI 22,521,68
ETA: scu-mus TD: 40 g/kg/I   BECCAN 40,30,62

SAFETY PROFILE: Questionable carcinogen with experimental neoplastigenic and tumorigenic data. When heated to decomposition it emits toxic fumes of Na_2O.

IHL000   CAS: 1338-16-5
IRON SORBITOL CITRATE
mf: $C_6H_{14}O_6 \cdot C_6H_8O_7 \cdot xFe$ mw: 765.29

SYNS: ESZ ◊ IRON SORBITEX ◊ IRON-SORBITOL-CITRIC ACID

CONSENSUS REPORTS: IARC Cancer Review: GROUP 3 IMEMDT 7,56,87; Animal No Evidence IMEMDT 2,161,73.

OSHA PEL: TWA 1 mg/(Fe)/m^3 ACGIH TLV: TWA 1 mg/(Fe)/m^3

SAFETY PROFILE: Questionable carcinogen. A poison by subcutaneous and intravenous routes. Moderately toxic by ingestion and intramuscular routes. When heated to decomposition it emits acrid smoke and fumes.

IHP000   CAS: 123-51-3
ISOAMYL ALCOHOL
DOT: 1105
mf: $C_5H_{12}O$ mw: 88.17

PROP: Clear liquid; pungent, repulsive taste. Bp: 132°, ULC: 35-40, lel: 1.2%, uel: 9.0% @ 212°F, flash p: 109°F (CC), d: 0.813, autoign temp: 662°F, vap d: 3.04, mp: −117.2°. Sol in water @ 14°; misc in alc and ether.

SYNS: ALCOOL AMILICO (ITALIAN) ◊ ALCOOL ISOAMYLIQUE (FRENCH) ◊ AMYLOWY ALKOHOL (POLISH) ◊ FERMENTATION AMYL ALCOHOL ◊ ISOAMYL ALKOHOL (CZECH) ◊ ISO-AMYLALKOHOL (GERMAN) ◊ ISOAMYLOL ◊ ISOBUTYLCARBINOL ◊ ISOPENTANOL ◊ ISOPENTYL ALCOHOL ◊ 2-METHYL-4-BUTANOL ◊ 3-METHYL BUTANOL ◊ 3-METHYLBUTAN-1-OL ◊ 3-METHYL-1-BUTANOL (CZECH) ◊ 3-METIL-BUTANOLO (ITALIAN)

TOXICITY DATA with REFERENCE
CAR: orl-rat TDLo: 27 g/kg/75W-I   ARGEAR 45,19,75
CAR: scu-rat TDLo: 3800 mg/kg/85W-I
ARGEAR 45,19,75
MUT: cyt-smc 10 mmol/tube   HEREAY 33,457,47

CONSENSUS REPORTS: Reported in EPA TSCA Inventory.

OSHA PEL: TWA 100 ppm; STEL 125 ppm ACGIH TLV: TWA 100 ppm; STEL 125 ppm DFG MAK: 100 ppm (360 mg/m^3) DOT Classification: Flammable or Combustible Liquid; Label: Flammable Liquid.

SAFETY PROFILE: Questionable carcinogen with experimental carcinogenic data. A poison by intraperitoneal and intravenous routes. Moderately toxic by ingestion and skin contact. A skin and human eye irritant. Human systemic effects by inhalation: olfactory effects, conjunctiva irritation, respiratory changes. Mutation data reported. Flammable when exposed to heat or flame; can react vigorously with reducing materials. To fight fire, use alcohol foam, CO_2, dry chemical. When heated to decomposition it emits acrid smoke and fumes. Used as a flotation agent, a solvent, and in organic synthesis.

IHX400   CAS: 2883-98-9
trans-ISOASARONE
mf: $C_{12}H_{16}O_3$ mw: 208.28

SYNS: ASARON ◊ ASARONE ◊ ASARONE, trans- ◊ α-ASARONE ◊ trans-ASARONE ◊ ASARUM CAMPHOR ◊ BENZENE, 1,2,4-TRIMETHOXY-5-PROPENYL-, (E)- ◊ BENZENE, 1,2,4-TRIMETHOXY-5-PROPENYL-, trans- ◊ ETHEROPHENOL

TOXICITY DATA with REFERENCE
CAR: ipr-mus TDLo: 156 mg/kg   CNREA8 47,2275,87

SAFETY PROFILE: Questionable carcinogen with experimental carcinogenic data. Moderately toxic by ingestion, intravenous, and intraperitoneal routes. When heated to decomposition it emits acrid smoke and irritating fumes.

IIL000   CAS: 78-83-1
ISOBUTYL ALCOHOL
DOT: 1212
mf: $C_4H_{10}O$ mw: 74.14

PROP: Clear mobile liquid; sweet odor. Bp: 107.90°, flash p: 82°F, ULC: 40-45, lel: 1.2%, uel: 10.9% @ 212°F, fp: −108°, d: 0.800, autoign temp: 800°F, vap press: 10 mm @ 21.7°, vap d: 2.55. Sltly sol in water; misc with alc and ether.

SYNS: ALCOOL ISOBUTYLIQUE (FRENCH) ◇ FEMA No. 2179 ◇ FERMENTATION BUTYL ALCOHOL ◇ 1-HYDROXY-METHYLPROPANE ◇ ISOBUTANOL (DOT) ◇ ISOBUTYLAL-KOHOL (CZECH) ◇ ISOPROPYLCARBINOL ◇ 2-METHYL PROPANOL ◇ 2-METHYL-1-PROPANOL ◇ 2-METHYLPRO-PAN-1-OL ◇ 2-METHYLPROPYL ALCOHOL ◇ RCRA WASTE NUMBER U140

TOXICITY DATA with REFERENCE
CAR: scu-rat TDLo: 9 g/kg/I   ARGEAR 45,19,75
ETA: orl-rat TDLo: 29 g/kg/I   ARGEAR 45,19,75
MUT: cyt-smc 20 mmol/tube   HEREAY 33,457,47
MUT: mmo-esc 25000 ppm   ABMGAJ 23,843,69

CONSENSUS REPORTS: Reported in EPA TSCA Inventory.

OSHA PEL: (Transitional: TWA 100 mg/m^3) TWA 50 ppm ACGIH TLV: TWA 50 ppm DFG MAK: 100 ppm (300 mg/m^3)   DOT Classification: Flammable or Combustible Liquid; Label: Flammable Liquid.

SAFETY PROFILE: Questionable carcinogen with experimental carcinogenic and tumorigenic data. Poison by intravenous and intraperitoneal routes. Moderately toxic by ingestion and skin contact. Mildly toxic by inhalation. A severe skin and eye irritant. Mutation data reported. Flammable liquid. Dangerous fire hazard when exposed to heat or flame. To fight fire, use alcohol foam, CO_2, dry chemical. When heated to decomposition it emits acrid smoke and fumes.

IIV000   CAS: 6104-30-9
ISOBUTYLIDENEDIUREA
mf: $C_6H_{14}N_4O_2$ mw: 174.24

SYNS: 1,1-DIUREIDISOBUTANE ◇ DIUREIDOISOBUTANE ◇ IBDU ◇ ISOBUTYLDIUREA ◇ ISOBUTYLENEDIUREA ◇ 1,1'-ISOBUTYLIDENEBISUREA ◇ ISODUR ◇ N,N''-(2-METHYLPROPYLIDENE)BISUREA (9CI)

TOXICITY DATA with REFERENCE
ETA: orl-mus TDLo: 32 g/kg/20W-I   VPITAR 37(2),72,79
ETA: orl-rat TDLo: 64 g/kg/20W-I   VPITAR 37(2),72,79

CONSENSUS REPORTS: Reported in EPA TSCA Inventory.

SAFETY PROFILE: Questionable carcinogen with experimental tumorigenic data. When heated to decomposition it emits toxic fumes of NO_x.

IJF000   CAS: 760-60-1
N-ISOBUTYL-N-NITROSOUREA
mf: $C_5H_{11}N_3O_2$ mw: 145.19

SYNS: ISO-BNU ◇ 1-ISO-BUTYL-1-NITROSOUREA ◇ N-(2-METHYLPROPYL)-N-NITROSOUREA ◇ N-NITROSO-ISO-BUTYLUREA

TOXICITY DATA with REFERENCE
CAR: orl-rat TD: 675 mg/kg/49W-C   GANNA2 74,342,83
CAR: orl-rat TDLo: 447 mg/kg/64W-C   GANNA2 74,342,83
MUT: cyt-ham: fbr 25 mg/L/48H   MUREAV 48,337,77
MUT: mma-sat 10 μg/plate   TCMUE9 1,13,84
MUT: mmo-sat 1 μg/plate   MUREAV 68,1,79

CONSENSUS REPORTS: EPA Genetic Toxicology Program.

SAFETY PROFILE: Questionable carcinogen with experimental carcinogenic data. Mutation data reported. When heated to decomposition it emits toxic fumes of NO_x.

IKE000   CAS: 513-37-1
ISOCROTYL CHLORIDE
mf: C_4H_7Cl mw: 90.56

PROP: Liquid. D: 0.919 @ 20°/4°, bp: 68°.

SYNS: α-CHLOROISOBUTYLENE ◇ 1-CHLORO-2-METHYLPROPENE ◇ 1-CHLORO-2-METHYL-1-PROPENE ◇ β,β-DIMETHYLVINYL CHLORIDE ◇ NCI-C54819

TOXICITY DATA with REFERENCE
CAR: orl-mus TDLo: 51 g/kg/2Y-I   NTPTR* NTP-TR-316,86
CAR: orl-rat TDLo: 51500 mg/kg/2Y-I   NTPTR* NTP-TR-316,86
NEO: orl-mus TD: 102 g/kg/2Y-I   NTPTR* NTP-TR-316,86
MUT: msc-mus: lyms 400 μg/L   NTPTR* NTP-TR-316,86
MUT: sce-ham: ovr 500 mg/L   NTPTR* NTP-TR-316,86
MUT: trn-oin-dmg 12750 ppm/3D-C   NTPTR* NTP-TR-316,86

CONSENSUS REPORTS: NTP Carcinogenesis Studies (gavage); Clear Evidence: mouse, rat NTPTR* NTP-TR-316,86.

SAFETY PROFILE: Questionable carcinogen with experimental carcinogenic and neoplastigenic data. Mildly toxic by inhalation. A local irritant and narcotic in high concentration. When heated to decomposition it emits toxic fumes of Cl^-.

ILD000   CAS: 54-85-3
ISONICOTINIC ACID HYDRAZIDE
mf: $C_6H_7N_3O$ mw: 137.16

PROP: Consists of 12% w/v each of dodecylamine hydrochloride, trimethyl alkyl ammonium chloride, and methyl alkyl dipolyoxypropylene ammonium methyl sulfate (TXAPA9 4,44,62).

SYNS: AMIDON ◇ ANDRAZIDE ◇ ANTIMICINA ◇ ANTITUBERKULOSUM ◇ ARMACIDE ◇ ATCOTIBINE ◇ AZUREN ◇ BACILLIN ◇ CEDIN ◇ CEMIDON ◇ CHEMIAZID ◇ CHEMIDON ◇ CORTINAZINE ◇ COTINAZIN ◇ COTINIZIN ◇ DEFONIN ◇ DIBUTIN ◇ DIFORIN ◇ DINACRIN ◇ DITUBIN ◇ EBIDENE ◇ ERALON ◇ ERTUBAN ◇ EUTIZON ◇ EVALON ◇ FIMALENE ◇ HIDRANIZIL ◇ HIDRASONIL ◇ HIDRULTA ◇ HIDRUN ◇ HYCOZID ◇ HYDRAZID ◇ HYDRAZIDE ◇ HYOZID ◇ HYZYD ◇ IDRAZIDE DELL'ACIDO ISONICOTINICO ◇ IDRAZIL ◇ ISCOTIN ◇ ISIDRINA ◇ ISMAZIDE ◇ ISOBICINA ◇ ISOCID ◇ ISOCIDENE ◇ ISOCOTIN ◇ ISOLYN ◇ ISONERIT ◇ ISONEX ◇ ISONIACID ◇ ISONIAZID ◇ ISONIAZIDE ◇ ISONICAZIDE ◇ ISONICID ◇ ISONICO ◇ ISONICOTAN ◇ ISONICOTIL ◇ ISONICOTINHYDRAZID ◇ ISONICOTINOYL HYDRAZIDE ◇ ISONICOTINOYLHYDRAZINE ◇ ISONICOTINSAEUREHYDRAZID ◇ ISONICOTINYL HYDRAZIDE ◇ ISONIDE ◇ ISONIDRIN ◇ ISONIKAZID ◇ ISONILEX ◇ ISONIN ◇ ISONINDON ◇ ISONIRIT ◇ ISONITON ◇ ISONIZIDE ◇ ISOTEBE ◇ ISOTEBEZID ◇ ISOTINYL ◇ ISOZIDE ◇ ISOZYD ◇ LANIAZID ◇ LANIOZID ◇ MYBASAN ◇ NEOTEBEN ◇ NEOXIN ◇ NEUMANDIN ◇ NEVIN ◇ NIADRIN ◇ NICAZIDE ◇ NICETAL ◇ NICIZINA ◇ NICONYL ◇ NICOTIBINA ◇ NICOTIBINE ◇ NICOZIDE ◇ NIDATON ◇ NIDRAZID ◇ NIKOZID ◇ NIPLEN ◇ NITADON ◇ NITEBAN ◇ NSC 9659 ◇ NYDRAZID ◇ NYSCOZID ◇ PELAZID ◇ PERCIN ◇ PHTHISEN ◇ PYCAZIDE ◇ PYREAZID ◇ PYRICIDIN ◇ PYRIDICIN ◇ 4-PYRIDINECARBOXYLIC ACID, HYDRAZIDE ◇ PYRIZIDIN ◇ RAUMANON ◇ RAZIDE ◇ RETOZIDE ◇ RIFAMATE ◇ RIMICID ◇ RIMIFON ◇ RIMITSID ◇ ROBISELIN ◇ ROBISELLIN ◇ ROXIFEN ◇ SANOHIDRAZINA ◇ SAUTERAZID ◇ SAUTERZID ◇ STANOZIDE ◇ TEBECID ◇ TEBENIC ◇ TEBEXIN ◇ TEBOS ◇ TEEBACONIN ◇ TEKAZIN ◇ TIBAZIDE ◇ TIBEMID ◇ TIBINIDE ◇ TIBISON ◇ TIBIVIS ◇ TIBIZIDE ◇ TIBUSAN ◇ TISIN ◇ TISIODRAZIDA ◇ TIZIDE ◇ TUBAZID ◇ TUBAZIDE ◇ TUBECO ◇ TUBERCID ◇ TUBERIAN ◇ TUBICON ◇ TUBOMEL ◇ TYVID ◇ UNICOCYDE ◇ USAF CB-2 ◇ VAZADRINE ◇ VEDERON ◇ ZINADON ◇ ZONAZIDE

TOXICITY DATA with REFERENCE
CAR: ipr-mus TDLo: 2200 mg/kg/8W-I   UICMAI 7,180,67
CAR: orl-mus TD: 93 g/kg/70W-C   CNREA8 26,1473,66
CAR: orl-mus TD: 79576 mg/kg/98W-C   TUMOAB 56,315,70
CAR: orl-mus TDLo: 1892 mg/kg (multi)   JCREA8 105,258,83
CAR: orl-mus TDLo: 18524 mg/kg/84W-I   JCREA8 105,258,83
NEO: ipr-mus TD: 2240 mg/kg/32W-C   JLCMAK 60,1025,62
NEO: orl-mus TD: 9 g/kg/17W-I   IJCNAW 21,381,78
NEO: orl-mus TD: 15 g/kg/30W-C   GANNA2 51,83,60
NEO: orl-mus TD: 27 g/kg/49W-C   JNCIAM 41,331,68
NEO: orl-mus TD: 2240 mg/kg/4W-I   BJCAAI 18,543,64
NEO: orl-mus TD: 6720 mg/kg/32W-C   JLCMAK 60,1025,62
NEO: orl-rat TDLo: 55 g/kg/45W-C   JNCIAM 41,331,68
NEO: scu-mus TDLo: 5040 mg/kg/18W-C   GANNA2 51,83,60
NEO: unr-mus TDLo: 27400 mg/kg/39W-C   PAPOAC 12,53,61
ETA: orl-mus TD: 8880 mg/kg/19W-C   GANNA2 50,107,59
ETA: scu-mus TD: 269 mg/kg/21D-I   JCREA8 96,163,80
MUT: dni-hmn: fbr 10 mmol/L   MUREAV 89,9,81
MUT: dns-hmn: fbr 500 μmol/L   MUREAV 89,9,81
MUT: dns-hmn: lvr 100 μmol/L   CALEDQ 30,103,86
MUT: mma-omi 1500 mg/L   MUREAV 173,233,86
MUT: mma-sat 2 mg/plate   CRNGDP 5,391,84
MUT: mmo-omi 156 mg/L   MUREAV 173,233,86
MUT: mmo-sat 1 mg/plate   CRNGDP 5,391,84

CONSENSUS REPORTS: IARC Cancer Review: GROUP 3 IMEMDT 7,227,87, Animal Sufficient Evidence IMEMDT 4,159,74. EPA Genetic Toxicology Program.

SAFETY PROFILE: Questionable carcinogen with experimental carcinogenic, neoplastigenic, and tumorigenic data. A human poison by ingestion. An experimental poison by ingestion, intravenous, subcutaneous, intraperitoneal, and intramuscular routes. Experimental teratogenic and reproductive effects. Human systemic effects by ingestion: peripheral nerve sensory changes, somnolence, respiratory depression, anorexia, sweating, urine changes, toxic psychosis, hepatitis, dermatitis. Human mutation data reported. A skin irritant. Used as an antitubercular, antibacterial and anti-actinomycotic agent. When heated to decomposition it emits toxic fumes of NO_x and NH_3.

ILE000   CAS: 54-92-2
ISONICOTINIC ACID-2-ISOPROPYLHYDRAZIDE
mf: $C_9H_{13}N_3O$ mw: 179.25

SYNS: EUPHOZID ◇ FOSFAZIDE ◇ IIH ◇ IPN ◇ IPRAZID ◇ IPRONIAZID ◇ IPRONID ◇ IPRONIN ◇ 1-ISONICOTINOYL-2-ISOPROPYLHYDRAZINE ◇ 1-ISONICOTINYL-2-ISOPRO-PYLHYDRAZINE ◇ N-ISOPROPYL ISONICOTINHYDRAZIDE ◇ LH ◇ MARSALID ◇ MARSILID ◇ P 887 ◇ RIVIVOL ◇ RO 2-4572 ◇ YATROZIDE

TOXICITY DATA with REFERENCE
ETA: orl-mus TDLo: 10 g/kg/36W-I   34ZRA9 -,869,66
MUT: oms-bcs 10 mmol/L   MUREAV 5,343,68

SAFETY PROFILE: Questionable carcinogen with experimental tumorigenic and teratogenic data. A human poison by ingestion. An experimental poison by ingestion, intraperitoneal, intravenous, and possibly other routes. Moderately toxic by skin contact, intramuscular, and subcutaneous routes. Human systemic effects by ingestion: constipation, anuria, metabolic changes, change in liver function. Human reproductive effects by ingestion: impotence. Experimental reproductive effects. Mutation data reported. Used as an antidepressant. When heated to decomposition it emits toxic fumes of NO_x.

ILF000   CAS: 16887-79-9
ISONICOTINIC ACID, SODIUM SALT
mf: $C_6H_4NO_2 \cdot Na$ mw: 145.10

SYN: SODIUM SALT of ISONICOTINIC ACID

TOXICITY DATA with REFERENCE
ETA: orl-mus TDLo: 13 g/kg/46W-I   NATUAS 194,488,62

SAFETY PROFILE: Questionable carcinogen with experimental tumorigenic data. When heated to decomposition it emits toxic fumes of NO_x and Na_2O.

ILG000   CAS: 63041-19-0
4-(ISONICOTINOYLHYDRAZONE) PIMELIC ACID
mf: $C_{13}H_{15}N_3O_5$ mw: 293.31

SYNS: ACIDO-4-(ISONICOTINIL-IDRAZONE)PIMELICO (ITALIAN) ◇ 4-OXOHEPTANEDIOIC ACID, ISONICOTINOYL HYDRAZONE

TOXICITY DATA with REFERENCE
ETA: orl-mus TDLo: 12 g/kg/30W-I   LAPPA5 24,39,64

SAFETY PROFILE: Questionable carcinogen with experimental tumorigenic data. When heated to decomposition it emits toxic fumes of NO_x.

ILO000   CAS: 25168-26-7
ISOOCTYL-2,4-DICHLOROPHENOXYACETATE
mf: $C_{16}H_{22}Cl_2O_3$ mw: 333.28

SYNS: 2,4-DICHLOROPHENOXYACETIC ACID ISOOCTYL ESTER ◇ 2,4-D ISOOCTYL ESTER ◇ ISOOCTYL ALCOHOL (2,4-DICHLOROPHENOXY)ACETATE ◇ REED LV 2,4-D ◇ REED LV 400 2,4-D ◇ REED LV 600 2,4-D ◇ WEEDTRINE-II

TOXICITY DATA with REFERENCE
CAR: scu-mus TDLo: 21 mg/kg   NTIS** PB223-159
ETA: orl-mus TDLo: 14 g/kg/78W-I   NTIS** PB223-159
MUT: sce-hmn: lym 50 nL/L   DBABEF 8,105,84

CONSENSUS REPORTS: IARC Cancer Review: Animal Inadequate Evidence IMEMDT 15,111,77.

SAFETY PROFILE: Questionable carcinogen with experimental carcinogenic, tumorigenic, and teratogenic data. A poison by ingestion. Other experimental reproductive effects. Human mutation data reported. An herbicide. When heated to decomposition it emits toxic fumes of Cl^-.

IMF400   CAS: 78-59-1
ISOPHORONE
mf: $C_9H_{14}O$ mw: 138.23

PROP: Practically water-white liquid. Bp: 215.2°, flash p: 184°F (OC), d: 0.9229, autoign temp: 864°F, vap press: 1 mm @ 38.0°, vap d: 4.77, lel: 0.8%, uel: 3.8%.

SYNS: ISOACETOPHORONE ◇ ISOFORON ◇ ISOFORONE (ITALIAN) ◇ IZOFORON (POLISH) ◇ NCI-C55618

◊ 1,1,3-TRIMETHYL-3-CYCLOHEXENE-5-ONE ◊ 3,5,5-TRI-
METHYL-2-CYCLOHEXENE-1-ONE ◊ 3,5,5-TRIMETHYL-2-
CYCLOHEXEN-1-ON (GERMAN, DUTCH) ◊ 3,5,5-TRIMETIL-
2-CICLOESEN-1-ONE (ITALIAN)

TOXICITY DATA with REFERENCE
CAR: orl-mus TDLo:258 g/kg/2Y-I   TXCYAC
  39,207,86

MUT: msc-mus:lym 1 g/L   NTPTR* NTP-TR-291,86
MUT: sce-ham:ovr 1 g/L   NTPTR* NTP-TR-291,86

CONSENSUS REPORTS: NTP Carcinogen-
esis Studies (gavage); Some Evidence: rat
NTPTR* NTP-TR-291,86; (gavage); Equivocal
Evidence: mouse NTPTR* NTP-TR-291,86.
Reported in EPA TSCA Inventory.

OSHA PEL: (Transitional: TWA 25 ppm) TWA
4 ppm   ACGIH TLV: CL 5 ppm   DFG MAK:
5 ppm (28 mg/m^3)   NIOSH REL: TWA (Ketones) 23 mg/m^3

SAFETY PROFILE: Questionable carcinogen
with experimental carcinogenic data. Moderately toxic by ingestion and skin contact. Mildly
toxic by inhalation. Human systemic effects by
inhalation: olfactory changes, conjunctiva irritation, and respiratory changes. Human systemic
irritant by inhalation. A skin and severe eye
irritant. Mutation data reported. It can cause
irritation, lachrimation, possible opacity of the
cornea and necrosis of the cornea (experimental). Flammable and explosive when exposed
to heat or flame. To fight fire, use foam, CO_2,
dry chemical.

INA400   CAS: 83053-59-2
**11-ISOPROPOXY-15,16-DIHYDRO-17-
CYCLOPENTA(a)PHENANTHREN-17-
ONE**
mf: $C_{20}H_{18}O_2$ mw: 290.38

TOXICITY DATA with REFERENCE
ETA: skn-mus TDLo:1600 μg/kg   CRNGDP
  3,677,82
MUT: mma-sat 20 μg/plate   CRNGDP 3,677,82

SAFETY PROFILE: Questionable carcinogen
with experimental tumorigenic data. Mutation
data reported. When heated to decomposition
it emits acrid smoke and irritating fumes.

INJ000   CAS: 67-63-0
ISOPROPYL ALCOHOL
DOT: 1219
mf: C_3H_8O mw: 60.11

PROP: Clear, colorless liquid; slt odor, sltly
bitter taste. Mp: −88.5 to −89.5°, bp: 82.5°,

lel: 2.5%, uel: 12%, flash p: 53°F (CC), d:
0.7854 @ 20°/4°, refr index: 1.377 @ 20°,
vap d: 2.07, ULC: 70. fp: −89.5°; autoign temp:
852°F. Misc with water, alc, ether, chloroform;
insol in salt solns.

SYNS: ALCOOL ISOPROPILICO (ITALIAN) ◊ ALCOOL
ISOPROPYLIQUE (FRENCH) ◊ DIMETHYLCARBINOL
◊ ISOHOL ◊ ISOPROPANOL (DOT) ◊ ISO-PROPYLALKO-
HOL (GERMAN) ◊ LUTOSOL ◊ PETROHOL ◊ PROPAN-2-
OL ◊ 2-PROPANOL ◊ i-PROPANOL (GERMAN) ◊ sec-PRO-
PYL ALCOHOL (DOT) ◊ i-PROPYLALKOHOL (GERMAN)
◊ SPECTRAR

TOXICITY DATA with REFERENCE
MUT: cyt-rat-ihl 1030 μg/m^3/16W-I   GTPZAB
  25(7),33,81
MUT: cyt-smc 200 mmol/tube   HEREAY 33,457,47

CONSENSUS REPORTS: IARC Cancer Review: GROUP 3 IMEMDT 7,229,87. The isopropyl alcohol strong acid manufacturing process is on the Community Right-To-Know List.
EPA Genetic Toxicology Program. Reported
in EPA TSCA Inventory.

OSHA PEL: (Transitional: TWA 400 ppm)
TWA 400 ppm; STEL 500 ppm   ACGIH TLV:
TWA 400 ppm; STEL 500 ppm   DFG MAK:
400 ppm (980 mg/m^3)   NIOSH REL: (Isopropyl Alcohol) TWA 400 ppm; CL 800 ppm/
15M   DOT Classification: Flammable Liquid;
Label: Flammable Liquid.

SAFETY PROFILE: Questionable carcinogen.
Poison by ingestion and subcutaneous routes.
Moderately toxic to humans by an unspecified
route. Moderately toxic experimentally by intravenous and intraperitoneal routes. Mildly
toxic by skin contact. Human systemic effects
by ingestion or inhalation: flushing, pulse rate
decrease, blood pressure lowering, anesthesia,
narcosis, headache, dizziness, mental depression, hallucinations, distorted perceptions,
dyspnea, respiratory depression, nausea or vomiting, coma. Experimental teratogenic and reproductive effects. Mutation data reported. An
eye and skin irritant. Flammable liquid. To fight
fire, use CO_2, dry chemical, alcohol foam.
When heated to decomposition it emits acrid
smoke and fumes.

INS000   CAS: 54-80-8
**α-((ISOPROPYLAMINO)METHYL)-2-
NAPHTHALENEMETHANOL**
mf: $C_{15}H_{19}NO$ mw: 229.35

SYNS: ALDERLIN ◇ COMPOUND 38,174 ◇ INETOL
◇ 2-ISOPROPYLAMINO-1-(NAPHTH-2-YL)ETHANOL
◇ 2-ISOPROPYLAMINO-1-(2-NAPHTHYL)ETHANOL
◇ (2-NAPHTHYL)-1-ISOPROPYLAMINOETHANOL
◇ NAPHTHYLISOPROTERENOL ◇ NEATHALIDE
◇ NETALID ◇ NETH ◇ NETHALIDE ◇ PRONETALOL
◇ PRONETHALOL

TOXICITY DATA with REFERENCE
CAR: orl-rat TDLo:15 g/kg/30W-C   PSDTAP
10,175,69
ETA: orl-mus TD:72 g/kg/43W-C   PSDTAP
4,30,64
ETA: orl-mus TDLo:28080 mg/kg/33W-C
PSDTAP 10,175,69
ETA: unr-mus TDLo:200 mg/kg   BMJOAE
2,1266,63
MUT: dns-hmn:hla 100 μmol/L   CNREA8
38,2621,78

CONSENSUS REPORTS: EPA Genetic Toxicology Program.

SAFETY PROFILE: Questionable carcinogen
with experimental carcinogenic and tumorigenic
data. Poison by ingestion, intravenous, and intraperitoneal routes. Human mutation data reported. When heated to decomposition it emits
toxic fumes of NO_x.

INT000   CAS: 51-02-5
α-((ISOPROPYLAMINO)METHYL) NAPHTHALENEMETHANOL, HYDROCHLORIDE
mf: $C_{15}H_{19}NO_2 \cdot ClH$ mw: 265.81

SYNS: ALDERLIN HYDROCHLORIDE ◇ ICI 38174
◇ I.C.I. HYDROCHLORIDE ◇ INETOL ◇ 2-ISOPROPYL-
AMINO-1-(2-NAPHTHYL)ETHANOL HYDROCHLORIDE
◇ α-(((1-METHYLETHYL)AMINO)METHYL)-2-NAPHTHA-
LENEMETHANOL, HYDROCHLORIDE ◇ NAPHTHYLISO-
PROTERENOL HYDROCHLORIDE ◇ NETHALIDE HYDRO-
CHLORIDE ◇ PRONETHALOL ◇ PRONETHALOL HYDRO-
CHLORIDE

TOXICITY DATA with REFERENCE
ETA: orl-mus TDLo:10 g/kg/25W-C   NATUAS
207,594,65

CONSENSUS REPORTS: IARC Cancer Review: GROUP 3 IMEMDT 7,56,87; Animal
Limited Evidence IMEMDT 13,227,77.

SAFETY PROFILE: Questionable carcinogen
with experimental tumorigenic data. A poison
by intravenous and intraperitoneal routes. Moderately toxic by ingestion. When heated to de-

composition it emits very toxic fumes of NO_x
and HCl.

INZ000   CAS: 63020-47-3
5-ISOPROPYL-1:2-BENZANTHRACENE
mf: $C_{21}H_{18}$ mw: 270.39

SYN: 8-ISOPROPYLBENZ(a)ANTHRACENE

TOXICITY DATA with REFERENCE
ETA: scu-mus TDLo:3000 mg/kg/45W-I
PRLBA4 129,439,40
ETA: skn-mus TDLo:840 mg/kg/35W-I
PRLBA4 129,439,40

SAFETY PROFILE: Questionable carcinogen
with experimental tumorigenic data. When
heated to decomposition it emits acrid smoke
and fumes.

IOA000   CAS: 63020-48-4
6-ISOPROPYL-1:2-BENZANTHRACENE
mf: $C_{21}H_{18}$ mw: 270.39

SYN: 9-ISOPROPYLBENZ(a)ANTHRACENE

TOXICITY DATA with REFERENCE
ETA: skn-mus TDLo:700 mg/kg/29W-I
PRLBA4 111,485,32

SAFETY PROFILE: Questionable carcinogen
with experimental tumorigenic data. When
heated to decomposition it emits acrid smoke
and fumes.

IOB000   CAS: 80-15-9
ISOPROPYLBENZENE HYDROPEROXIDE
DOT: 2116
mf: $C_9H_{12}O_2$ mw: 152.21

PROP: Bp: 153°, flash p: 175°F, d: 1.05. The
hydroperoxide of cumene.

SYNS: CUMEENHYDROPEROXYDE (DUTCH) ◇ CUMENE
HYDROPEROXIDE (DOT) ◇ CUMENE HYDROPEROXIDE,
TECHNICALLY PURE (DOT) ◇ CUMENT HYDROPEROXIDE
◇ CUMENYL HYDROPEROXIDE ◇ CUMOLHYDROPEROXID
(GERMAN) ◇ CUMYL HYDROPEROXIDE ◇ α-CUMYL HY-
DROPEROXIDE ◇ CUMYL HYDROPEROXIDE, TECHNICAL
PURE (DOT) ◇ α,α-DIMETHYLBENZYL HYDROPEROXIDE
(MAK) ◇ HYDROPEROXYDE de CUMENE (FRENCH)
◇ HYDROPEROXYDE de CUMYLE (FRENCH) ◇ IDROPEROS-
SIDO di CUMENE (ITALIAN) ◇ IDROPEROSSIDO di CUMOLO
(ITALIAN) ◇ RCRA WASTE NUMBER U096

TOXICITY DATA with REFERENCE
ETA: scu-mus TDLo:8844 mg/kg/67W-I
JNCIAM 37,825,66
ETA: unr-mus TDLo:304 mg/kg   RARSAM
3,193,63
MUT: mma-sat 100 μg/plate   ABCHA6 44,1989,00
MUT: mmo-sat 100 μg/plate   PNASA6 79,7445,82

CONSENSUS REPORTS: Community Right-To-Know List. Reported in EPA TSCA Inventory. EPA Genetic Toxicology Program.

DFG MAK: Moderate Skin Effects. DOT Classification: Organic Peroxide; Label: Organic Peroxide.

SAFETY PROFILE: Questionable carcinogen with experimental tumorigenic data. A poison by ingestion and intraperitoneal routes. Moderately toxic by skin contact, inhalation and subcutaneous routes. Mutation data reported. A skin and eye irritant. A strong oxidizing agent. Flammable when exposed to heat or flame; can react with reducing materials. When heated to decomposition it emits acrid smoke and fumes. To fight fire, use foam, CO_2, dry chemical.

IOF000   CAS: 63020-53-1
2-ISOPROPYL-3:4-BENZPHENANTHRENE
mf: $C_{21}H_{18}$ mw: 270.39

TOXICITY DATA with REFERENCE
ETA: scu-mus TDLo:4600 mg/kg/69W-I
PRLBA4 129,439,40
ETA: skn-mus TDLo:720 mg/kg/30W-I
PRLBA4 129,439,40

SAFETY PROFILE: Questionable carcinogen with experimental tumorigenic data. When heated to decomposition it emits acrid smoke and fumes.

IOJ000   CAS: 1746-77-6
ISOPROPYL CARBAMATE
mf: $C_4H_9NO_2$ mw: 103.14

PROP: Prisms. Mp: 60-61°, bp: 200°C. Very sol in water, alc, and ether.

SYNS: CARBAMIC ACID, ISOPROPYL ESTER ◇ CARBAMIC ACID-1-METHYLETHYL ESTER

TOXICITY DATA with REFERENCE
NEO: ipr-mus TD:6500 mg/kg/13W-I   JNCIAM
8,99,47
NEO: ipr-mus TDLo:2400 mg/kg/4W-I
CNREA8 29,2184,69

MUT: dni-mus-ipr 1 g/kg   CNREA8 29,994,69
MUT: mmo-esc 25000 ppm   CRSBAW 143,776,49
MUT: sce-mus-ipr 4400 μmol/kg   CNREA8
41,4489,81

CONSENSUS REPORTS: Reported in EPA TSCA Inventory.

SAFETY PROFILE: Questionable carcinogen with experimental neoplastigenic data. Moderately toxic by subcutaneous route. Mutation data reported. When heated to decomposition it emits toxic fumes of NO_x.

ION000   CAS: 63041-70-3
20-ISOPROPYLCHOLANTHRENE
mf: $C_{23}H_{20}$ mw: 296.43

SYN: 3-ISOPROPYLCHOLANTHRENE

TOXICITY DATA with REFERENCE
ETA: scu-mus TDLo:80 mg/kg   JNCIAM 2,99,41

SAFETY PROFILE: Questionable carcinogen with experimental tumorigenic data. When heated to decomposition it emits acrid smoke and fumes.

IOR000   CAS: 10457-59-7
14-ISOPROPYLDIBENZ(a,j)ACRIDINE
mf: $C_{24}H_{19}N$ mw: 321.44

SYN: 10-ISOPROPYL-3,4,5,6-DIBENZACRIDINE (FRENCH)

TOXICITY DATA with REFERENCE
ETA: skn-mus TD:1280 mg/kg/53W-I
BAFEAG 42,186,55
ETA: skn-mus TDLo:636 mg/kg/53W-I
ACRSAJ 4,315,56

SAFETY PROFILE: Questionable carcinogen with experimental tumorigenic data. When heated to decomposition it emits toxic fumes of NO_x.

IOT875   CAS: 24596-38-1
4'-ISOPROPYL-4-DIMETHYLAMINOAZOBENZENE
mf: $C_{17}H_{21}N_3$ mw: 267.41

SYN: p-(p-CUMENYLAZO)-N,N-DIMETHYLANILINE

TOXICITY DATA with REFERENCE
ETA: orl-rat TDLo:2142 mg/kg/17W-C
JNCIAM 27,663,61

SAFETY PROFILE: Questionable carcinogen with experimental tumorigenic data. When

heated to decomposition it emits toxic fumes of NO_x.

IOY000   CAS: 94-11-1
ISOPROPYL-2,4-D ESTER
mf: $C_{11}H_{12}Cl_2O_3$ mw: 263.13

SYNS: (2,4-DICHLOROPHENOXY)ACETIC ACID, ISOPRO-PYL ESTER ◇ (2-4-DICHLOROPHENOXY)ACETIC ACID-1-METHYLETHYL ESTER (9CI) ◇ 2,4-D ISOPROPYL ESTER ◇ ESTERON 44 ◇ WEEDONE 128

TOXICITY DATA with REFERENCE
ETA: orl-mus TDLo:12 g/kg/78W-I   NTIS**
   PB223-159

CONSENSUS REPORTS: IARC Cancer Review: Animal Inadequate Evidence IMEMDT 15,111,77.

SAFETY PROFILE: Questionable carcinogen with experimental tumorigenic data. Moderately toxic by ingestion. Experimental teratogenic and reproductive effects. Used as a pesticide. When heated to decomposition it emits toxic fumes of Cl^-.

IPA000   CAS: 2594-20-9
ISOPROPYL ETHYL URETHAN
mf: $C_6H_{13}NO_2$ mw: 131.20

PROP: Liquid. Bp: 192-193°.

SYN: ISOPROPYLCARBAMIC ACID, ETHYL ESTER

TOXICITY DATA with REFERENCE
ETA: ipr-mus TDLo:6500 mg/kg/13W-I
   JNCIAM 9,35,48

SAFETY PROFILE: Questionable carcinogen with experimental tumorigenic data. When heated to decomposition it emits toxic fumes of NO_x.

IPL000   CAS: 3173-79-3
4-ISOPROPYLIDENE-3,3-DIMETHYL-2-OXETANONE
mf: $C_8H_{12}O_2$ mw: 140.20

SYN: 3-HYDROXY-2,2,4-TRIMETHYL-3-PENTENOIC ACID, β-LACTONE

TOXICITY DATA with REFERENCE
ETA: scu-rat TDLo:39 g/kg/78W-I   JNCIAM
   39,1213,67

SAFETY PROFILE: Questionable carcinogen with experimental tumorigenic data. When heated to decomposition it emits acrid smoke and fumes.

IPS000   CAS: 75-30-9
ISOPROPYL IODIDE
mf: C_3H_7I mw: 170.00

PROP: Colorless liquid. Readily discolors in air and light. D: 1.703 @ 20°/4°, mp: −90°, bp: 89-90°. Sltly sol in water; misc with alc, benzene, chloroform, and ether.

SYNS: 2-IODOPROPANE ◇ i-PROPYL IODIDE

TOXICITY DATA with REFERENCE
NEO: ipr-mus TDLo:1190 mg/kg/8W-I
   CNREA8 35,1411,75

CONSENSUS REPORTS: Reported in EPA TSCA Inventory.

SAFETY PROFILE: Questionable carcinogen with experimental neoplastigenic data. Moderately toxic by intraperitoneal route. Mildly toxic by inhalation. When heated to decomposition it emits toxic fumes of I^-.

IQB000   CAS: 2235-59-8
N-ISOPROPYL-α-(2-METHYLAZO)-p-TOLUAMIDE
mf: $C_{12}H_{17}N_3O$ mw: 219.32

TOXICITY DATA with REFERENCE
NEO: orl-mus TDLo:2800mg/kg/8W-I   JNCIAM
   42,337,69

SAFETY PROFILE: Questionable carcinogen with experimental neoplastigenic data. When heated to decomposition it emits toxic fumes of NO_x.

IQJ000   CAS: 4427-56-9
2-ISOPROPYL-4-METHYLPHENOL
mf: $C_{10}H_{14}O$ mw: 150.24

TOXICITY DATA with REFERENCE
ETA: skn-mus TDLo:3840 mg/kg/12W-I
   CNREA8 19,413,59

CONSENSUS REPORTS: Reported in EPA TSCA Inventory.

SAFETY PROFILE: Questionable carcinogen with experimental tumorigenic data. When heated to decomposition it emits acrid smoke and fumes.

IRN000   CAS: 779-47-5
N-ISOPROPYL TEREPHTHALAMIC ACID
mf: $C_{11}H_{13}NO_3$ mw: 207.25

SYNS: 4-(((1-METHYLETHYL)AMINO)CARBONYL)-BEN-ZOIC ACID (9CI) ◇ TEREPHTHALIC ACID ISOPROPYLAMIDE

TOXICITY DATA with REFERENCE
ETA: orl-mus TDLo: 1936 mg/kg/8W-I   JNCIAM
   42,337,69

SAFETY PROFILE: Questionable carcinogen
with experimental tumorigenic data. When
heated to decomposition it emits toxic fumes
of NO_x.

IRZ000   CAS: 120-58-1
ISOSAFROLE

mf: $C_{10}H_{10}O_2$ mw: 162.20

PROP: Liquid, odor of anise. Bp: 253°, mp:
8.2°.

SYNS: 1,2-METHYLENEDIOXY-4-PROPENYLBENZENE
◇ 3,4-METHYLENEDIOXY-1-PROPENYL BENZENE
◇ 5-(1-PROPENYL)-1,3-BENZODIOXOLE ◇ 4-PROPENYLCA-
TECHOL METHYLENE ETHER ◇ 4-PROPENYL-1,2-METHY-
LENEDIOXYBENZENE ◇ RCRA WASTE NUMBER U141

TOXICITY DATA with REFERENCE
CAR: orl-mus TDLo: 61 g/kg/81W-C   JNCIAM
   42,1101,69
ETA: orl-mus TD: 101 g/kg/81W-C   FCTXAV
   19,130,81

CONSENSUS REPORTS: IARC Cancer Review: GROUP 3 IMEMDT 7,56,87; Animal
Sufficient Evidence IMEMDT 1,169,72. Reported in EPA TSCA Inventory. EPA Genetic
Toxicology Program.

SAFETY PROFILE: Questionable carcinogen
with experimental carcinogenic and tumorigenic
data. Poison by intraperitoneal and intravenous
routes. Moderately toxic by ingestion and subcutaneous routes. A skin irritant. Used as a pesticide. When heated to decomposition it emits
acrid smoke and fumes.

ISA000   CAS: 120-62-7
ISOSAFROLE-n-OCTYLSULFOXIDE

mf: $C_{18}H_{28}O_3S$ mw: 324.52

PROP: Water-insol, sltly sol in petroleum oils,
sol in most organic solvents.

SYNS: ENT 16,634 ◇ ISOSAFROLE, OCTYL SULFOXIDE
◇ 1,2-(METHYLENEDIOXY)-4-(2-(OCTYLSULFINYL)PRO-
PYL)BENZENE ◇ 1-METHYL-2-(3,4-METHYLENEDIOXY-
PHENYL)ETHYL OCTYL SULFOXIDE ◇ NCI-C02824
◇ n-OCTYLISOSAFROLE SULFOXIDE ◇ PIPERONYL SULF-
OXIDE ◇ SULFOX-CIDE ◇ SULFOXIDE ◇ SULFOXYL
◇ SULPHOXIDE

TOXICITY DATA with REFERENCE
CAR: orl-mus TDLo: 31 g/kg/2Y-C   NCITR*
   NCI-CG-TR-124,79

ETA: orl-mus TD: 62 g/kg/2Y-C   NCITR* NCI-
   CG-TR-124,79

CONSENSUS REPORTS: NCI Carcinogen-
esis Bioassay (feed); No Evidence: rat NCITR*
NCI-CG-TR-124,79. NCI Carcinogenesis
Bioassay (feed); Clear Evidence: mouse
NCITR* NCI-CG-TR-124,79.

SAFETY PROFILE: Questionable carcinogen
with experimental carcinogenic, tumorigenic,
and teratogenic data. Moderately toxic by ingestion. Slightly toxic by skin contact. An insecticide. When heated to decomposition it emits
highly toxic fumes of SO_x.

ITE000
IVORY

TOXICITY DATA with REFERENCE
ETA: imp-mus TDLo: 10 g/kg   NATWAY 42,75,55
ETA: imp-rat TDLo: 2330 mg/kg   NATWAY
   42,75,55

SAFETY PROFILE: Questionable carcinogen
with experimental tumorigenic data by implant.

JAK000   CAS: 6870-67-3
JACOBINE

mf: $C_{18}H_{25}NO_6$ mw: 351.44

PROP: An alkaloid isolated from *S. Jacobaea*
(RETOAE 5,55,49).

SYNS: 15,20-EPOXY-15,30-DIHYDRO-12-HYDROXYSENE-
CIONAN-11,16-DIONE ◇ NSC 89936

TOXICITY DATA with REFERENCE
MUT: dns-rat: lvr 1 μmol/L   CNREA8 45,3125,85
MUT: sln-dmg-par 20 μmol/L   ZEVBA5 91,74,60

CONSENSUS REPORTS: IARC Cancer Re-
view: GROUP 3 IMEMDT 7,56,87; Animal
Inadequate Evidence IMEMDT 10,275,76.
EPA Genetic Toxicology Program.

SAFETY PROFILE: Questionable carcinogen.
Poison by intravenous and possibly other routes.
Mutation data reported. When heated to decom-
position it emits toxic fumes of NO_x.

JDA135
JET FUEL JP-4

PROP: A mixture of aliphatic and aromatic hydrocarbon compounds which meet the requirement of military specification MIL-J-5624E
(AMRL** TR-74-78,74)   AMRL** TR-74-78,74

TOXICITY DATA with REFERENCE
CAR: ihl-rat TCLo:500 mg/m³/2Y JETPEZ
108,387,86

SAFETY PROFILE: Questionable carcinogen with experimental carcinogenic data. Moderately toxic by ingestion. When heated to decomposition it emits acrid smoke and irritating fumes.

KDK000 CAS: 9002-83-9
KEL-F
mf: (C₂ClF₃)ₙ

SYN: VOLTALEF 10

TOXICITY DATA with REFERENCE
ETA: imp-rat TDLo:36 mg/kg CNREA8 15,333,55

SAFETY PROFILE: Questionable carcinogen with experimental tumorigenic data. A relatively inert chloro-fluorocarbon polymer. When heated to decomposition it emits very toxic fumes of Cl⁻ and F⁻.

KGK150 CAS: 16694-30-7
4-KETOSTEARIC ACID
mf: C₁₈H₃₄O₃ mw: 298.52

TOXICITY DATA with REFERENCE
ETA: scu-mus TDLo:2000 mg/kg/25W-I
CNREA8 30,1037,70

SAFETY PROFILE: Questionable carcinogen with experimental tumorigenic data. When heated to decomposition it emits acrid smoke and irritating fumes.

LAL000 CAS: 5905-52-2
LACTIC ACID, IRON(2+) SALT (2:1)
mf: C₆H₁₀O₆•Fe mw: 234.01

PROP: Greenish-white crystals; slight peculiar odor. Moderately sol in water; sltly sol in alc.

SYNS: FERROUS LACTATE ◇ IRON(2+) LACTATE

TOXICITY DATA with REFERENCE
ETA: scu-mus TDLo:4200 mg/kg/21W-I
JNCIAM 24,109,60

OSHA PEL: TWA 1 mg(Fe)/m³ ACGIH TLV: TWA 1 mg(Fe)/m³

SAFETY PROFILE: Questionable carcinogen with experimental tumorigenic data. Poison by ingestion. When heated to decomposition it emits acrid smoke and irritating fumes.

LAR000 CAS: 63-42-3
LACTOSE
mf: C₁₂H₂₂O₁₁ mw: 342.34

PROP: Colorless, rhombic crystals; faintly sweet taste. D: 1.525 @ 20°, mp: 202° (anhydrous), bp: decomp. Sol in water; insol in alc and ether.

SYNS: 4-(β-d-GALACTOSIDO)-d-GLUCOSE ◇ LACTIN ◇ d-LACTOSE ◇ LACTOBIOSE ◇ MILK SUGAR ◇ SACCHARUM LACTIN

TOXICITY DATA with REFERENCE
ETA: scu-mus TDLo:1 kg/kg/29W-C GANNA2
46,363,55

CONSENSUS REPORTS: Reported in EPA TSCA Inventory.

SAFETY PROFILE: Questionable carcinogen with experimental tumorigenic and teratogenic data. Moderately toxic by intravenous route. Experimental reproductive effects. Mixtures with oxidants (e.g., potassium chlorate; potassium nitrate; or potassium perchlorate) may be explosion hazards. When heated to decomposition it emits acrid smoke and irritating fumes.

LBE000
LARAHA

PROP: Aqueous extract from the dried leaves of the plant.

SYN: CITRUS AURANTIUM

TOXICITY DATA with REFERENCE
ETA: ims-rat TDLo:45 g/kg/1Y-I JNCIAM
46,1131,71

SAFETY PROFILE: Questionable carcinogen with expermental tumorigenic data. When heated to decomposition it emits acrid smoke and irritating fumes.

LBL000 CAS: 143-07-7
LAURIC ACID
mf: C₁₂H₂₄O₂ mw: 200.36

PROP: Colorless, needle-like crystals; slt odor of bay oil. Mp: 48°, bp: 225° @ 100 mm, d: 0.883, vap press: 1 mm @ 121.0°. Insol in water; sol in chloroform, benzene, alc, ether, and petroleum ether.

SYNS: DODECANOIC ACID ◇ DODECOIC ACID ◇ DUODECYLIC ACID ◇ HYDROFOL ACID 1255 ◇ HYSTRENE 9512 ◇ LAUROSTEARIC ACID ◇ NEO-FAT

12 ◇ NINOL AA62 EXTRA ◇ 1-UNDECANECARBOXYLIC ACID ◇ WECOLINE 1295

TOXICITY DATA with REFERENCE
NEO: skn-mus TDLo: 108 g/kg/15W-I   APMIAL 46,51,59

MUT: cyt-smc 10 mg/L   NATUAS 294,263,81

CONSENSUS REPORTS: Reported in EPA TSCA Inventory.

SAFETY PROFILE: Questionable carcinogen with experimental neoplastigenic data. Poison by intravenous route. Mildly toxic by ingestion. Mutation data reported. Combustible when exposed to heat or flame; can react with oxidizing materials. When heated to decomposition it emits acrid smoke and irritating fumes.

LBM000   CAS: 1984-77-6
LAURIC ACID-2,3-EPOXYPROPYL ESTER
mf: $C_{15}H_{28}O_3$ mw: 256.43

SYN: GLYCIDYL LAURATE

TOXICITY DATA with REFERENCE
NEO: scu-mus TDLo: 16 mg/kg/40W-I: TER
CNREA8 30,1037,70

SAFETY PROFILE: Questionable carcinogen with experimental neoplastigenic and teratogenic data. When heated to decomposition it emits acrid smoke and irritating fumes.

LBQ000   CAS: 48163-10-6
LAUROYLETHYLENEIMINE
mf: $C_{14}H_{27}NO$ mw: 225.42

SYN: 1-LAUROYLAZIRIDINE

TOXICITY DATA with REFERENCE
ETA: scu-rat TDLo: 1000 mg/kg/32D-I   BJPCAL 9,306,54

MUT: cyt-rat-ipr 100 mg/kg   BJPCAL 9,306,54

SAFETY PROFILE: Questionable carcinogen with experimental tumorigenic data. Mutation data reported. When heated to decomposition it emits toxic fumes of NO_x.

LBR000   CAS: 105-74-8
LAUROYL PEROXIDE
DOT: 2124
mf: $C_{24}H_{46}O_4$ mw: 398.70

PROP: White, tasteless, coarse powder; faint odor. Mp: 53-55°.

SYNS: ALPEROX C ◇ BIS(1-OXODODECYL)PEROXIDE ◇ DILAUROYL PEROXIDE ◇ DILAUROYL PEROXIDE,

TECHNICAL PURE (DOT) ◇ DODECANOYL PEROXIDE ◇ DYP-97 F ◇ LAUROX ◇ LAUROYL PEROXIDE, TECHNICALLY PURE (DOT) ◇ LAURYDOL ◇ LYP 97 ◇ PEROXYDE de LAUROYLE (FRENCH)

TOXICITY DATA with REFERENCE
ETA: scu-mus TDLo: 184 mg/kg/46W-I
JNCIAM 37,825,66

ETA: unr-mus TDLo: 638 mg/kg   RARSAM 3,193,63

CONSENSUS REPORTS: IARC Cancer Review: Animal Inadequate Evidence IMEMDT 36,315,85. Reported in EPA TSCA Inventory.

DFG MAK: Mild skin effects. DOT Classification: Organic Peroxide; Label: Organic Peroxide.

SAFETY PROFILE: Questionable carcinogen with experimental tumorigenic data. A powerful oxidizing agent. It is a corrosive irritant to the eyes and mucous membranes and can cause burns. A dangerous fire hazard. When heated to decomposition it emits acrid smoke and fumes.

LCE000   CAS: 64083-05-2
LD-813

PROP: Commercial mixture of aromatic amines containing approx 40% MOCA.

TOXICITY DATA with REFERENCE
CAR: orl-rat TDLo: 37 g/kg/2Y-C   TXAPA9 31,159,75

SAFETY PROFILE: Questionable carcinogen with experimental carcinogenic data. When heated to decomposition it emits toxic fumes of NO_x.

LCH000   CAS: 1335-32-6
LEAD ACETATE, BASIC
mf: $C_4H_{10}O_8Pb_3$ mw: 807.71

PROP: White powder.

SYNS: BASIC LEAD ACETATE ◇ BIS(ACETO)DIHYDROXYTRILEAD ◇ BIS(ACETATO)TETRAHYDROXYTRILEAD ◇ BLA ◇ LEAD MONOSUBACETATE ◇ LEAD SUBACETATE ◇ MONOBASIC LEAD ACETATE ◇ RCRA WASTE NUMBER U146 ◇ SUBACETATE LEAD

TOXICITY DATA with REFERENCE
CAR: orl-rat TDLo: 350 g/kg/90W-C   BJCAAI 16,289,62

NEO: ipr-mus TD: 150 mg/kg/5W-I   CNREA8 36,1744,76

NEO: ipr-mus TDLo:38 mg/kg/6W-I   TXAPA9 82,19,86

NEO: orl-rat TD:30 g/kg/77W-C   BJCAAI 16,289,62

ETA: orl-mus TDLo:90 g/kg/2Y-C   BJCAAI 23,765,69

ETA: orl-rat TD:300 g/kg/48W-C   APJAAG 23,87,73

MUT: mmo-sat 250 mg/L   ENMUDM 2,234,80

CONSENSUS REPORTS: IARC Cancer Review: GROUP 3 IMEMDT 7,230,87; Animal Sufficient Evidence IMEMDT 23,325,80; IMEMDT 1,40,72; Human Limited Evidence IMEMDT 23,325,80. Lead and its compounds are on the Community Right-To-Know List. Reported in EPA TSCA Inventory. EPA Genetic Toxicology Program.

SAFETY PROFILE: Questionable carcinogen with experimental experimental carcinogenic, neoplastigenic, and tumorigenic data. Experimental reproductive effects. Mutation data reported. When heated to decomposition it emits toxic fumes of Pb.

LCP000   CAS: 598-63-0
LEAD CARBONATE
mf: $CO_3 \cdot Pb$ mw: 267.20

PROP: White, heavy powder. D: 6.61, decomp @ 400° leaving residue of PbO. Insol in water, alc, sol in acetic acid, dil HNO_3 (effervescence).

SYNS: CARBONIC ACID, LEAD(2+) SALT (1:1) ◇ CERUSSETE ◇ DIBASIC LEAD CARBONATE ◇ LEAD(2+) CARBONATE ◇ WHITE LEAD

CONSENSUS REPORTS: IARC Cancer Review: Animal Inadequate Evidence IMEMDT 23,325,80; IMEMDT 1,40,72. Lead and its compounds are on the Community Right-To-Know List. Reported in EPA TSCA Inventory.

OSHA PEL: TWA 0.05 mg(Pb)/m^3 ACGIH TLV: TWA 0.15 mg(Pb)/m^3 NIOSH REL: (Inorganic Lead) TWA 0.10 mg(Pb)/m^3

SAFETY PROFILE: Questionable carcinogen. Moderately toxic by ingestion. Human systemic effects by ingestion: gastrointestinal contractions and jaundice. Experimental reproductive effects. Ignites spontaneously and burns fiercely in fluorine. When heated to decomposition it emits toxic fumes of Pb.

LCQ000   CAS: 7758-95-4
LEAD CHLORIDE
DOT: 2291
mf: Cl_2Pb mw: 278.09

PROP: White crystals. Mp: 501°, bp: 950°, d: 5.85, vap press: 1 mm @ 547°. Somewhat sol in cold water, more sol in hot water. Very sol in ammonium chloride, NH_4NO_3, alkali hydroxides.

SYNS: LEAD (2+) CHLORIDE ◇ LEAD (II) CHLORIDE ◇ LEAD DICHLORIDE ◇ PLUMBOUS CHLORIDE

TOXICITY DATA with REFERENCE
MUT: dnd-mam:lym 100 μmol/L   SCIEAS 198,513,77

MUT: dnd-omi 100 μmol/L   SCIEAS 198,513,77
MUT: dni-hmn:hla 250 μmol/L   TXCYAC 5,167,75
MUT: dni-mus:fbr 20 μmol/L   ZHPMAT 161,26,75
MUT: mmo-smc 1 mmol/L   CPBTAL 33,1571,85
MUT: oms-hmn:hla 250 μmol/L   TXCYAC 5,167,75

CONSENSUS REPORTS: IARC Cancer Review: Animal Inadequate Evidence IMEMDT 23,325,80. Lead and its compounds are on the Community Right-To-Know List. Reported in EPA TSCA Inventory. EPA Genetic Toxicology Program.

OSHA PEL: TWA 0.05 mg(Pb)/m^3 ACGIH TLV: TWA 0.15 mg(Pb)/m^3 NIOSH REL: (Inorganic Lead) TWA 0.10 mg(Pb)/m^3 DOT Classification: ORM-B; Label: None.

SAFETY PROFILE: Questionable carcinogen. Moderately toxic by ingestion. An experimental teratogen. Experimental reproductive effects. Human mutation data reported. When heated to decomposition it emits very toxic fumes of Pb and Cl^-.

LCW000   CAS: 19010-66-3
LEAD DIMETHYLDITHOCARBAMATE
mf: $C_6H_{12}N_2S_4 \cdot Pb$ mw: 447.63

PROP: Solid. Mp: 258°, d: 2.5.

SYNS: BIS(DIMETHYLCARBAMODITHIOATO-S,S')LEAD ◇ BIS(DIMETHYLDITHIOCARBAMIATO)LEAD ◇ DIMETHYLDITHIOCARBAMIC ACID, LEAD SALT ◇ METHYL LEDATE ◇ NCI-C02891

TOXICITY DATA with REFERENCE
ETA: scu-mus TDLo:1000 mg/kg   NTIS** PB223-159
MUT: mma-sat 33 μg/plate   NTPTB* JAN 82
MUT: mmo-sat 100 μg/plate   ENMUDM 5(Suppl 1),3,83

CONSENSUS REPORTS: IARC Cancer Review: Animal Inadequate Evidence IMEMDT

12,131,76. NCI Carcinogenesis Bioassay (feed); No Evidence: mouse, rat NCITR* NCI-CG-TR-151,79. Lead and its compounds are on the Community Right-To-Know List. Reported in EPA TSCA Inventory.

NIOSH REL: (Inorganic Lead) TWA 0.10 mg(Pb)/m^3

SAFETY PROFILE: Questionable carcinogen with experimental tumorigenic data. Mutation data reported. Combustible when exposed to heat or flame. When heated to decomposition it emits very toxic fumes of Pb, NO$_x$, and SO$_x$.

LDM000   CAS: 12709-98-7
LEAD-MOLYBDENUM CHROMATE

SYNS: CHROMIC ACID, LEAD and MOLYBDENUM SALT ◇ CHROMIC ACID LEAD SALT with LEAD MOLYBDATE ◇ C.I. PIGMENT RED 104 ◇ LEAD CHROMATE, SULPHATE and MOLYBDATE ◇ MOLYBDENUM-LEAD CHROMATE ◇ MOLYBDENUM ORANGE

TOXICITY DATA with REFERENCE
NEO: scu-rat TDLo:135 mg/kg   ANYAA9 271,431,81

ETA: scu-rat TD:135 mg/kg   PBPHAW 14,47,78
MUT: cyt-ham:ovr 5 mg/L   BJCAAI 44,219,81
MUT: cyt-hmn:oth 500 mg/L   BJCAAI 44,219,81
MUT: dni-ham:kdy 150 mg/L   BJCAAI 44,219,81
MUT: mmo-sat 2 mg/plate   CRNGDP 2,283,81
MUT: oms-ham:kdy 150 mg/L   BJCAAI 44,219,81
MUT: oms-hmn:oth 500 mg/L   BJCAAI 44,219,81
MUT: sce-ham:ovr 100 μg/L   MUREAV 156,219,85

CONSENSUS REPORTS: Lead and its compounds, as well as chromium and its compounds, are on the Community Right-To-Know List.

OSHA PEL: TWA CL 0.1 mg(CrO$_3$)/m^3; TWA 0.05 mg(Pb)/m^3; TWA 5 mg(Mo)/m^3 ACGIH TLV: TWA 0.05 mg(Cr)/m^3; TWA 5 mg(Mo)/m^3; TWA 0.15 mg(Pb)/m^3 NIOSH REL: (Chromium(VI)) TWA 0.001 mg(Cr(VI))/m^3; (Inorganic Lead) TWA 0.10 mg(BrPb)/m^3

SAFETY PROFILE: Questionable carcinogen with experimental neoplastigenic and tumorigenic data. Human mutation data reported. A powerful oxidizer. Probably a severe eye, skin, and mucous membrane irritant. When heated to decomposition it emits toxic fumes of Pb, chromium trioxide, and Mo.

LDN000   CAS: 1317-36-8
LEAD MONOXIDE
mf: OPb   mw: 223.19

PROP: Exists in 2 forms: (1) red to reddish-yellow, tetragonal crystals; stable at ordinary temps. (2) Yellow, orthorhombic crystals; stable > 489°. D: 9.53, mp: 888°. Insol in H$_2$O, alc, sol in acetic acid, dil HNO$_3$, warm solns of fixed alkali hydroxides.

SYNS: C.I. 77577 ◇ C.I. PIGMENT YELLOW 46 ◇ LEAD OXIDE ◇ LEAD(II) OXIDE ◇ LEAD OXIDE YELLOW ◇ LEAD PROTOXIDE ◇ LITHARGE ◇ LITHARGE YELLOW L-28 ◇ MASSICOT ◇ MASSICOTITE ◇ PLUMBOUS OXIDE ◇ YELLOW LEAD OCHER

TOXICITY DATA with REFERENCE
MUT: dnd-ham:emb 50 μmol/L   CNREA8 39,193,79
MUT: otr-ham:emb 50 μmol/L   CNREA8 39,193,79

CONSENSUS REPORTS: IARC Cancer Review: Animal Inadequate Evidence IMEMDT 23,325,80. Reported in EPA TSCA Inventory. EPA Genetic Toxicology Program. Lead and its compounds are on the Community Right-To-Know List.

OSHA PEL: TWA 0.05 mg(Pb)/m^3 ACGIH TLV: TWA 0.15 mg(Pb)/m^3 NIOSH REL: (Inorganic Lead) TWA 0.10 mg(Pb)/m^3

SAFETY PROFILE: Questionable carcinogen. Moderately toxic by ingestion and intraperitoneal routes. Mutation data reported. A skin irritant. Avoid breathing dust. When heated to decomposition it emits toxic fumes of Pb. Used in manufacturing of storage batteries, ceramic products, paints and rubber.

LDO000   CAS: 10099-74-8
LEAD(II) NITRATE (1:2)
DOT: 1469
mf: N$_2$O$_6$•Pb   mw: 331.21

PROP: White crystals. Mp: decomp @ 470°, d: 4.53 @ 20°.

SYNS: LEAD DINITRATE ◇ LEAD NITRATE ◇ LEAD (2+) NITRATE ◇ LEAD(II) NITRATE ◇ NITRATE de PLOMB (FRENCH) ◇ NITRIC ACID, LEAD (2+) SALT

TOXICITY DATA with REFERENCE
MUT: cyt-mus-par 200 μg/kg   MILEDM 17,29,81
MUT: cyt-rat:oth 300 μmol/L   CBINA8 30,237,80
MUT: dni-rat:lvr 100 μmol/L   JTEHD6 4,503,78
MUT: msc-mus:lym 450 mg/L   JTEHD6 9,367,82
MUT: pic-esc 320 μmol/L   ENMUDM 6,59,84

CONSENSUS REPORTS: IARC Cancer Review: Animal Inadequate Evidence IMEMDT

23,325,80. Reported in EPA TSCA Inventory. Lead and its compounds are on the Community Right-To-Know List.

OSHA PEL: TWA 0.05 mg(Pb)/m^3 ACGIH TLV: TWA 0.15 mg(Pb)/m^3 NIOSH REL: (Inorganic Lead) TWA 0.10 mg(Pb)/m^3 DOT Classification: Oxidizer; Label: Oxidizer, Poison.

SAFETY PROFILE: Questionable carcinogen. Poison by intraperitoneal route. Moderately toxic by ingestion and possibly other routes. Probably a severe eye, skin and mucous membrane irritant. An experimental teratogen. Experimental reproductive effects. Mutation data reported. A powerful oxidizer. Used as a mordant, a chemical reagent, and in production of matches and pyrotechnics.

LEI000 CAS: 8008-56-8
LEMON OIL

PROP: Expressed from the peel of the fruit of *Citrus limon* L. Burmann filius (Fam. *Rutaceae*). Pale yellow liquid; taste and odor of lemon peel. D: 0.849, refr index: 1.473 @ 20°. Misc with dehydrated alc, glacial acetic acid.

SYNS: CEDRO OIL ◇ LEMON OIL, COLDPRESSED (FCC) ◇ LEMON OIL, EXPRESSED ◇ OIL of LEMON ◇ ZITRONEN OEL (GERMAN)

TOXICITY DATA with REFERENCE
ETA: skn-mus TDLo: 280 g/kg/33W-I JNCIAM 24,1389,60

CONSENSUS REPORTS: Reported in EPA TSCA Inventory.

SAFETY PROFILE: Questionable carcinogen with experimental tumorigenic data. Moderately toxic by ingestion. A skin irritant. When heated to decomposition it emits acrid smoke and irritating fumes.

LEY000 CAS: 57-22-7
LEUROCRISTINE
mf: C$_{46}$H$_{56}$N$_4$O$_{10}$ mw: 825.06

SYNS: LCR ◇ NCI-C04864 ◇ NSC-67574 ◇ ONCOVIN ◇ 22-OXOVINCALEUKOBLASTINE ◇ VCR ◇ VINCRISTINE ◇ VINCRYSTINE ◇ VINKRISTIN

TOXICITY DATA with REFERENCE
ETA: ipr-mus TDLo: 5850 μg/kg/26W-I CANCAR 40(Suppl 4),1935,77
ETA: ipr-rat TDLo: 1200 μg/kg/7W-I CANCAR 40(Suppl 4),1935,77

MUT: dnd-hmn: fbr 1 mg/L BBACAQ 824,117,85
MUT: dns-mus: oth 500 nmol/L CNREA8 43,3591,83
MUT: mnt-mus-ipr 125 μg/kg MUREAV 120,127,83
MUT: par-ham LD10: 350 μg/kg JSONAU 15,355,80
MUT: sce-hmn: leu 20 μg/L MUREAV 138,55,84
MUT: spm-mus-ipr 160 μg/kg MUREAV 138,55,84

CONSENSUS REPORTS: NCI Carcinogenesis Studies (ipr); No Evidence: mouse, rat CANCAR 40,1935,77. EPA Genetic Toxicology Program.

SAFETY PROFILE: Questionable carcinogen with experimental tumorigenic and teratogenic data. Poison by parenteral, intraperitoneal, and intravenous routes. Human systemic effects by parenteral, intravenous, and possibly other routes: sensory change involving peripheral nerves, flaccid paralysis without anesthesia, somnolence, anorexia, convulsions or effect on seizure threshold, nausea or vomiting, changes in blood cell count and bone marrow, pulmonary and gastrointestinal changes. Experimental reproductive effects. Human mutation data reported. A skin irritant. When heated to decomposition it emits toxic fumes of NO$_x$.

LEZ000 CAS: 2068-78-2
LEUROCRISTINE SULFATE (1:1)
mf: C$_{46}$H$_{56}$N$_4$O$_{10}$•H$_2$O$_4$S mw: 923.14

SYNS: KYOCRISTINE ◇ LILLY 37231 ◇ NSC 67574 ◇ ONCOVIN ◇ VCR SULFATE ◇ VINCRISTINE SULFATE ONCORIN ◇ VINCRISTINSULFAT (GERMAN) ◇ VINCRISUL

TOXICITY DATA with REFERENCE
MUT: dni-hmn: otr 69120 pmol/L CNREA8 38,560,78
MUT: mnt-ham-ipr 200 μg/kg HEREAY 93,329,80
MUT: otr-ham: emb 1 μg/L CRNGDP 7,131,86
MUT: sce-ham: ovr 50 μg/L ENMUDM 4,65,82
MUT: sln-ham: emb 3 μg/L CRNGDP 7,131,86

CONSENSUS REPORTS: IARC Cancer Review: GROUP 3 IMEMDT 7,372,87; Human Inadequate Evidence IMEMDT 26,365,81; Animal Inadequate Evidence IMEMDT 26,365,81.

SAFETY PROFILE: Questionable carcinogen. Poison by intraperitoneal and intravenous routes. An experimental teratogen. Experimental reproductive effects. Human mutation data reported. When heated to decomposition it emits very toxic fumes of NO_x and SO_x.

LFI000   CAS: 7660-25-5
LEVULOSE
mf: $C_6H_{12}O_6$ mw: 180.18

PROP: White, hygroscopic crystals or crystalline powder; odorless with sweet taste. D: 1.6. Sol in methanol, ethanol, water.

SYNS: FRUCTOSE (FCC) ◇ FRUIT SUGAR ◇ FRUTABS ◇ LAEVORAL ◇ LAEVOSAN ◇ LEVUGEN

TOXICITY DATA with REFERENCE
ETA: scu-mus TDLo:5000 mg/kg   GANNA2 46,371,55

SAFETY PROFILE: Questionable carcinogen with experimental tumorigenic data. When heated to decomposition it emits acrid smoke and fumes.

LFU000   CAS: 5989-27-5
d-LIMONENE
mf: $C_{10}H_{16}$ mw: 136.26

PROP: Colorless liquid; citrus odor. Bp: 175.5-176°, d: 0.8402 @ 25°/4°, refr index: 1.471. Misc with alc, fixed oils; sltly sol in glycerin; insol in propylene glycol, water.

SYNS: FEMA No. 2633 ◇ (+)-4-ISOPROPENYL-1-METHYL-CYCLOHEXENE ◇ d-(+)-LIMONENE ◇ (+)-R-LIMONENE ◇ d-p-MENTHA-1,8-DIENE ◇ p-MENTHA-1,8-DIENE ◇ (R)-1-METHYL-4-(1-METHYLETHENYL)-CYCLOHEXENE ◇ NCI-C55572

TOXICITY DATA with REFERENCE
ETA: orl-mus TDLo:67 g/kg/39W-I   JNCIAM 35,771,65

CONSENSUS REPORTS: Reported in EPA TSCA Inventory.

SAFETY PROFILE: Questionable carcinogen with experimental tumorigenic and teratogenic data. Poison by intravenous route. Moderately toxic by intraperitoneal and intraduodenal routes. Mildly toxic by ingestion. Experimental reproductive effects. When heated to decomposition it emits acrid smoke and irritating fumes. Used as a food additive, flavor agent, packaging material, as an inhibitor of tetrafluoroethylene polymerization, and as a gallstone solubilizer.

LFV000   CAS: 96-08-2
LIMONENE DIOXIDE
mf: $C_{10}H_{16}O_2$ mw: 168.26

SYNS: 1,2,8,9-DIEPOXYLIMONENE ◇ 1,2:8,9-DIEPOXYMENTHANE ◇ 1,2:8,9-DIEPOXY-p-MENTHANE ◇ DIPENTENE DIOXIDE ◇ EPOXIDE 269 ◇ 4-(1,2-EPOXY-1-METHYLETHYL)-1-METHYL-7-OXABICYCLO(4.1.0) HEPTANE ◇ UNOXAT EPOXIDE 269

TOXICITY DATA with REFERENCE
ETA: unr-mus TDLo:6700 mg/kg   RARSAM 3,193,63

CONSENSUS REPORTS: Reported in EPA TSCA Inventory.

SAFETY PROFILE: Questionable carcinogen with experimental tumorigenic data. Moderately toxic by skin contact and intramuscular routes. Mildly toxic by ingestion. A skin irritant. When heated to decomposition it emits acrid smoke and irritating fumes.

LGI000
LINOLEIC ACID mixed with OLEIC ACID

SYNS: (Z)-9-OCTADECENOIC ACID mixed with (Z,Z)-9,12-OCTADECADIENOIC ACID ◇ OLEIC ACID mixed with LINOLEIC ACID

TOXICITY DATA with REFERENCE
ETA: orl-mus TDLo:33 g/kg/52W-C   PAACA3 14,35,73

SAFETY PROFILE: Questionable carcinogen with experimental tumorigenic data. When heated to decomposition it emits acrid smoke and irritating fumes.

LGM200
LIQUIPRON

PROP: A yeast (CANDIDA MALTOSA) protein concentrate   TOERD9 3,305,81

TOXICITY DATA with REFERENCE
CAR: orl-rat TDLo:15525 g/kg/3Y-C   TOERD9 3,305,81
ETA: orl-rat TD:2628 g/kg/2Y-C   TOERD9 3,305,81

SAFETY PROFILE: Questionable carcinogen with experimental carcinogenic and tumorigenic data. When heated to decomposition it emits acrid smoke and irritating fumes.

LGZ000   CAS: 554-13-2
LITHIUM CARBONATE (2:1)
mf: $CO_3 \cdot 2Li$ mw: 73.89

PROP: White, light alkaline, crystalline powder. D: 2.11 @ 17.5°; mp: 618°. Insol in alc. @ 17.5°.

SYNS: CAMCOLIT ◇ CANDAMIDE ◇ CARBOLITH ◇ CARBONIC ACID, DILITHIUM SALT ◇ CARBONIC ACID LITHIUM SALT ◇ CEGLUTION ◇ CP-15467-61 ◇ DILITHIUM CARBONATE ◇ ESKALITH ◇ HYPNOREX ◇ LIMAS ◇ LISKONUM ◇ LITHANE ◇ LITHICARB ◇ LITHINATE ◇ LITHIUM CARBONATE ◇ LITHOBID ◇ LITHONATE ◇ LITHOTABS ◇ NSC-16895 ◇ PLENUR ◇ PRIADEL ◇ QUILONUM RETARD

TOXICITY DATA with REFERENCE
CAR: orl-man TD: 6132 mg/kg/2Y-C: BLD
  HAEMAX 67,944,82
CAR: orl-wmn TD: 21 g/kg/3.5Y-C: END
  ANZJB8 10,62,80
CAR: orl-wmn TD: 5940 mg/kg/47W-C: BLD
  AIMEAS 92,262,80
CAR: orl-wmn TDLo: 3600 mg/kg/21W-C:
  BLD   NEJMAG 302,808,80
MUT: cyt-hmn-unr 12800 μg/kg/12W-I
  TJADAB 13,131,76
MUT: dnd-hmn: fbr 500 mg/L   MUREAV 169,171,86
MUT: dni-hmn: fbr 2 g/L   MUREAV 169,171,86
MUT: msc-ham: lng 2 g/L   MUREAV 169,171,86

CONSENSUS REPORTS: Reported in EPA TSCA Inventory.

SAFETY PROFILE: Questionable carcinogen producing leukemia and thyroid tumors. Human carcinogenic and teratogenic data. Poison by intraperitoneal and intravenous routes. Moderately toxic by ingestion, subcutaneous and possibly other routes. Human systemic effects by ingestion and possibly other routes: toxic psychosis, tremors, changes in fluid intake, muscle weakness, increased urine volume, and gastrointestinal changes. Human reproductive effects by ingestion and possibly other routes: effects on newborn including apgar score changes and other neonatal measures or effects. Human teratogenic effects by ingestion and possibly other routes: developmental abnormalities of the cardiovascular system, central nervous system, musculoskeletal and gastrointestinal systems. Experimental reproductive effects. Human mutation data reported. Used in the treatment of manic-depressive psychoses.

LHB000   CAS: 7447-41-8
LITHIUM CHLORIDE
mf: ClLi   mw: 42.39

PROP: Cubic, white, deliquescent crystals. Mp: 605°, bp: 1350°, d: 2.068 @ 25°, vap press: 1 mm @ 547°.

SYNS: CHLORKU LITU (POLISH) ◇ CHLORURE de LITHIUM (FRENCH)

TOXICITY DATA with REFERENCE
NEO: ipr-mus TDLo: 882 mg/kg/7D-I   PWPSA8
  22,343,79
MUT: cyt-hmn: lym 50 mg/L   TJADAB 13,131,76
MUT: dni-hmn: hla 70 mmol/L   MUREAV
  92,427,82
MUT: dni-hmn: lym 50 mg/L   TJADAB 13,131,76
MUT: mrc-smc 9 mmol/L   MUTAEX 1,21,86
MUT: orl-rbt LD90: 850 mg/kg   BEXBAN
  74,914,73
MUT: sln-smc 3 mmol/L   MUTAEX 1,21,86

CONSENSUS REPORTS: Reported in EPA TSCA Inventory. EPA Genetic Toxicology Program.

SAFETY PROFILE: Questionable carcinogen with experimental neoplastigenic and teratogenic data. Human poison by ingestion. Experimental poison by intravenous and intracerebral routes. Moderately toxic by subcutaneous and intraperitoneal routes. Human systemic effects by ingestion: somnolence, tremors, nausea or vomiting. Experimental reproductive effects. Human mutation data reported. An eye and severe skin irritant. When heated to decomposition it emits toxic fumes of Cl⁻. Used for dehumidification in the air conditioning industry. Also used to obtain lithium metal.

LIJ000   CAS: 39456-76-3
LSP 1

SYNS: LAC LSP-1 ◇ OIL-SHALE PYROLYSE LAC LSP-1

TOXICITY DATA with REFERENCE
ETA: skn-mus TDLo: 80 g/kg/25W-I   GTPPAF
  8,175,72

SAFETY PROFILE: Questionable carcinogen with experimental tumorigenic data.

LIM000   CAS: 3105-97-3
LUCANTHONE METABOLITE
mf: $C_{20}H_{24}N_2O_2S$ mw: 356.52

SYNS: 1-((2-(DIETHYLAMINO)ETHYL)AMINO)-4-(HYDROXYMETHYL)THIOXANTHEN-9-ONE ◇ 1-((2-(DIETHYLAMINO)ETHYL)AMINO)-4-(HYDROXYMETHYL)9H-THIOXANTHEN-9-ONE ◇ HYCANTHON ◇ HYCANTHONE ◇ NSC-134434 ◇ WIN 24933

TOXICITY DATA with REFERENCE
CAR: ims-mus TDLo: 180 mg/kg/60D-I   JPETAB
  197,703,76

MUT: dni-hmn:hla 1 mmol/L   MUREAV 93,447,82

MUT: dnr-bcs 200 µg/disc   AEMIDF 43,177,82

MUT: dns-rbt-ivn 12500 µg/kg   ARTODN 46,139,80

MUT: oms-hmn:lym 5 mg/L   BCPCA6 22,1253,73

MUT: sln-smc 20 µmol/L   ENMUDM 7,121,85

MUT: slt-ham:ovr 1 mg/L   MUREAV 136,137,84

CONSENSUS REPORTS: EPA Genetic Toxicology Program.

SAFETY PROFILE: Questionable carcinogen with experimental carcinogenic and teratogenic data. Poison by subcutaneous, intravenous and intramuscular routes. Moderately toxic by ingestion. Experimental reproductive effects. Human mutation data reported. When heated to decomposition it emits very toxic fumes of NO_x and SO_x.

LIV000   CAS: 21884-44-6
LUTEOSKYRIN
mf: $C_{30}H_{22}O_{12}$ mw: 574.52

PROP: Yellow rectangular crystals. Mp: 278° (decomp). Anthraquinoid hepatotoxin of *Penicillium islandicum sopp* (JJEMAG 41,177,71).

SYNS: 5H,6H-6,5A,13A,14-(1,2,3,4)BUTANETETRAY-CYCLOOCTA(1,2-B:5,6-B′)DINAPHTHALENE ◇ 8,8′-DIHYDROXY-RUGULOSIN ◇ FLAVOMYCELIN ◇ (−)-LUTEOSKYRIN

TOXICITY DATA with REFERENCE

NEO: orl-mus TDLo:1356 mg/kg/32W-C FCTXAV 10,193,72

ETA: orl-mus TD:1200 mg/kg/27W-I   NGGKED 32,187,73

MUT: cyt-hmn:leu 1 mg/L   HUMAA7 7,344,69

MUT: cyt-mus:ast 1 mg/L   ECREAL 57,19,69

MUT: dni-mus:ast 1 mg/L   ECREAL 57,19,69

MUT: dns-mus:lvr 10 µmol/L   CNREA8 44,2918,84

MUT: mmo-smc 10 µmol/L   CPBTAL 22,2258,74

MUT: mrc-bcs 100 µg/disc   CNREA8 36,445,76

MUT: pic-esc 500 ng/plate   CNREA8 43,2819,83

CONSENSUS REPORTS: IARC Cancer Review: GROUP 3 IMEMDT 7,56,87; Animal Limited Evidence IMEMDT 10,163,76.

SAFETY PROFILE: Questionable carcinogen with experimental carcinogenic and tumorigenic data. Poison by ingestion, intraperitoneal, subcutaneous, and intravenous routes. Human mu-

tation data reported. When heated to decomposition it emits acrid smoke and irritating fumes.

MAC250   CAS: 632-99-5
MAGENTA
mf: $C_{20}H_{19}N_3 \cdot ClH$ mw: 337.88

PROP: Green powder or greenish crystals with a bronze luster, faint odor. D: 1.22, mp: decomp >200°; sol in water, alc and HCl; insol in ether.

SYNS: FUCHSIN ◇ ORIENT BASIC MAGENTA ◇ ROSANILINE CHLORIDE ◇ ROSANILINE HYDROCHLORIDE ◇ ROSANILINIUM CHLORIDE

TOXICITY DATA with REFERENCE

MUT: mma-sat 32 µg/plate   MUREAV 89,21,81

CONSENSUS REPORTS: IARC Cancer Review: GROUP 3 IMEMDT 7,238,87; Animal Inadequate Evidence IMEMDT 4,57,74; Human Inadequate Evidence IMEMDT 4,57,74. Reported in EPA TSCA Inventory.

SAFETY PROFILE: Questionable carcinogen. Mutation data reported. When heated to decomposition it emits very toxic fumes of HCl and NO_x.

MAH500   CAS: 1309-48-4
MAGNESIUM OXIDE
mf: MgO   mw: 40.31

PROP: White, bulky, very fine powder; odorless. Mp: 2500-2800°, d: 3.65-3.75. Very sltly sol in water; sol in dil acids; insol in alc.

SYNS: CALCINED BRUCITE ◇ CALCINED MAGNESIA ◇ CALCINED MAGNESITE ◇ MAGNESIA ◇ MAGNESIA USTA ◇ MAGNEZU TLENEK (POLISH) ◇ SEAWATER MAGNESIA

TOXICITY DATA and REFERENCE

ETA: itr-ham TDLo:480 mg/kg/30W-I   CNREA8 33,2209,73

CONSENSUS REPORTS: Reported in EPA TSCA Inventory.

OSHA PEL: Fume: (Transitional: TWA Total Dust: 15 mg/m³; Respirable Fraction: 5 mg/m³) Total Dust: 10 mg/m³; Respirable Fraction: 5 mg/m³ ACGIH TLV: TWA 10 mg/m³ (fume) DFG MAK: 6 mg/m³ (fume)

SAFETY PROFILE: Questionable carcinogen with experimental tumorigenic data. Inhalation of the fumes can produce a febrile reaction and leukocytosis in humans.

MAI250   CAS: 1661-03-6
MAGNESIUM PHTHALOCYANINE
mf: $C_{32}H_{16}MgN_8$ mw: 536.87

SYN: (PHTHALOCYANINATO(2−))MAGNESIUM

TOXICITY DATA and REFERENCE
ETA: scu-mus TDLo:1000 mg/kg/I   BECCAN
40,30,62

CONSENSUS REPORTS: Reported in EPA TSCA Inventory.

SAFETY PROFILE: Questionable carcinogen with experimental tumorigenic data. When heated to decomposition it emits toxic fumes of NO_x.

MAK700   CAS: 121-75-5
MALATHION
DOT: 2783
mf: $C_{10}H_{19}O_6PS_2$ mw: 330.38

PROP: Brown to yellow liquid; characteristic odor. D: 1.23 @ 25°/4°, mp: 2.9°, bp: 156° @ 0.7 mm. Miscible in organic solvents, sltly water-sol.

SYNS: AMERICAN CYANAMID 4,049 ◇ S-(1,2-BIS (AETHOXY-CARBONYL)-AETHYL)-O,O-DIMETHYL-DI-THIOPHASPHAT (GERMAN) ◇ S-(1,2-BIS(CARBETHOXY) ETHYL)-O,O-DIMETHYL DITHIOPHOSPHATE ◇ S-(1,2-BIS (ETHOXY-CARBONYL)-ETHYL)-O,O-DIMETHYL-DITHIO-FOSFAAT (DUTCH) ◇ S-(1,2-BIS(ETHOXYCARBONYL)E-THYL)-O,O-DIMETHYL PHOSPHORODITHIOATE ◇ S-1,2-BI-S(ETHOXYCARBONYL)ETHYL-O,O-DIMETHYL THIOPHOSPHATE ◇ S-(1,2-BIS(ETOSSI-CARBONIL)-ETIL)-O,O-DIMETIL-DITIOFOSFATO (ITALIAN) ◇ CALMATHION ◇ CARBETHOXY MALATHION ◇ CARBETOVUR ◇ CARBETOX ◇ CARBOFOS ◇ CARBOPHOS ◇ CELTHIGN ◇ CHEMATHION ◇ CIMEXAN ◇ COMPOUND 4049 ◇ CYTHION ◇ DETMOL MA ◇ DETMOL MA 96% ◇ S-(1,2-DICARBETHOXYETHYL)-O,O-DIMETHYLDITHIO-PHOSPHATE ◇ DICARBOETHOXYETHYL-O,O-DIMETHYL PHOSPHORODITHIOATE ◇ 1,2-DI(ETHOXYCARBONYL) ETHYL-O,O-DIMETHYL PHOSPHORODITHIOATE ◇ S-(1,2-DI(ETHOXYCARBONYL)ETHYL DIMETHYL PHOS-PHOROTHIOLOTHIONATE ◇ DIETHYL (DIMETHOXYPHOS-PHINOTHIOYLTHIO) BUTANEDIOATE ◇ DIETHYL (DIMETHOXYPHOSPHINOTHIOYLTHIO)SUCCINATE ◇ DIETHYL MERCAPTOSUCCINATE-O,O-DIMETHYL DI-THIOPHOSPHATE, S-ESTER ◇ DIETHYL MERCAPTOSUCCI-NATE-O,O-DIMETHYL PHOSPHORODITHIOATE ◇ DIETHYL MERCAPTOSUCCINATE-O,O-DIMETHYL THIOPHOSPHATE ◇ DIETHYL MERCAPTOSUCCINATE-S-ESTER with O,O-DI-METHYLPHOSPHORODITHIOATE ◇ DIETHYL MERCAPTO-SUCCINIC ACID O,O-DIMETHYL PHOSPHORODITHIOATE

◇ (DIMETHOXYPHOSPHINOTHIOYL)THIO)BUTANEDIOIC ACID DIETHYL ESTER ◇ O,O-DIMETHYL-S-(1,2-BIS (ETHOXYCARBONYL)ETHYL)DITHIOPHOSPHATE ◇ O,O-DIMETHYL-S-1,2-(DICARBAETHOXYAETHYL)-DITHIO-PHOSPHAT (GERMAN) ◇ O,O-DIMETHYL-S-(1,2-DICAR-BETHOXYETHYL) DITHIOPHOSPHATE ◇ O,O-DIMETHYL -S-(1,2-DICARBETHOXYETHYL)PHOSPHORODITHIOATE ◇ O,O-DIMETHYL-S-(1,2-DICARBETHOXYETHYL) THIO-THIONOPHOSPHATE ◇ O,O-DIMETHYL-S-1,2-DI(ETHOXY-CARBAMYL)ETHYL PHOSPHORODITHIOATE ◇ O,O-DI-METHYL-S-1,2-DIKARBETOXYLETHYLDITIOFOSFAT (CZECH) ◇ O,O-DIMETHYLDITHIOPHOSPHATE DIETHYL-MERCAPTOSUCCINATE ◇ DITHIOPHOSPHATE de O,O-DI-METHYLE et de S-(1,2-DICARBOETHOXYETHYLE) (FRENCH) ◇ EL 4049 ◇ EMMATOS ◇ EMMATOS EXTRA ◇ ENT 17,034 ◇ S-ESTER with O,O-DIMETHYL PHOSPHO-ROTHIOATE ◇ ETHIOLACAR ◇ ETIOL ◇ EXPERIMENTAL INSECTICIDE 4049 ◇ EXTERMATHION ◇ FORMAL ◇ FORTHION ◇ FOSFOTHION ◇ FOSFOTION ◇ FOUR THOU-SAND FORTY-NINE ◇ FYFANON ◇ HILTHION ◇ HILTHION 25WDP ◇ INSECTICIDE No. 4049 ◇ KARBOFOS ◇ KOP-THION ◇ KYPFOS ◇ MALACIDE ◇ MALAFOR ◇ MALA-GRAN ◇ MALAKILL ◇ MALAMAR ◇ MALAMAR 50 ◇ MALAPHELE ◇ MALAPHOS ◇ MALASOL ◇ MALASPRAY ◇ MALATHION ◇ MALATHION ULV CONCENTRATE ◇ MALATHIOZOO ◇ MALATHON ◇ MALATHYL LV CON-CENTRATE & ULV CONCENTRATE ◇ MALATION (POLISH) ◇ MALATOL ◇ MALATOX ◇ MALDISON ◇ MALMED ◇ MALPHOS ◇ MALTOX ◇ MALTOX MLT ◇ MERCAPTO-SUCCINIC ACID DIETHYL ESTER ◇ MERCAPTOTHION ◇ MERCAPTOTION (SPANISH) ◇ MLT ◇ MOSCARDA ◇ NCI-C00215 ◇ OLEOPHOSPHOTHION ◇ ORTHO MALA-THION ◇ PHOSPHORODITHIOIC ACID-O,O-DIMETHYL ESTER-S-ESTER with DIETHYL MERCAPTOSUCCINATE ◇ PHOSPHOTHION ◇ PRIODERM ◇ SADOFOS ◇ SADOPHOS ◇ SF 60 ◇ SIPTOX I ◇ SUMITOX ◇ TAK ◇ TM-4049 ◇ VEGFRU MALATOX ◇ VETIOL ◇ ZITHIOL

TOXICITY DATA with REFERENCE
MUT: cyt-mus-ipr 230 mg/kg   MUREAV 122,163,83
MUT: cyt-ofs-mul 200 nL/L   JFIBA9 26,13,85
MUT: mmo-bcs 1 nmol/plate   MSERDS 5,93,81
MUT: mmo-sat 10 mg/L   TGANAK 15(3),68,81
MUT: oms-hmn:leu 200 mg/L   PSEBAA 142,36,73
MUT: sce-hmn:lym 40 mg/L   MUREAV 88,307,81

CONSENSUS REPORTS: IARC Cancer Review: GROUP 3 IMEMDT 7,56,87; Animal No Evidence IMEMDT 30,103,83; NCI Carcinogenesis Bioassay (feed); No Evidence: mouse, rat NCITR* NCI-CG-TR-24,78; No Evidence: rat NCITR* NCI-CG-TR-192,79. EPA Genetic Toxicology Program.

OSHA PEL: (Transitional: TWA Total Dust: 15 mg/m³; Respirable Fraction: 5 mg/m³ (skin))

TWA Total Dust:10 mg/m^3' Respirable Fraction: 5 mg/m^3 (skin)   ACGIH TLV: TWA 10 mg/m^3 (skin)   DFG MAK: 15 mg/m^3 NIOSH REL: (Malathion) TWA 15 mg/m^3 DOT Classification: ORM-A; Label: None.

SAFETY PROFILE: Questionable carcinogen. A human poison by ingestion. An experimental poison by ingestion, inhalation, intraperitoneal, intravenous, intraarterial, subcutaneous, and possibly other routes. Human systemic effects by ingestion: coma, blood pressure depression, and difficulty in breathing. Human mutation data reported. Has caused allergic sensitization of the skin. An organic phosphate cholinesterase inhibitor. When heated to decomposition it emits toxic fumes of PO$_x$ and SO$_x$.

MAM000   CAS: 108-31-6
MALEIC ANHYDRIDE
DOT: 2215
mf: C$_4$H$_2$O$_3$ mw: 98.06

PROP: Fused black or white crystals. Mp: 52.8°, bp: 202°, flash p: 215°F (CC), d: 1.48 @ 20°/4°, autoign temp: 890°F, vap press: 1 mm @ 44.0°, vap d: 3.4, lel: 1.4%, uel: 7.1%. Sol in dioxane, water @ 30° forming maleic acid; very sltly sol in alc.

SYNS: cis-BUTENEDIOIC ANHYDRIDE ◇ 2,5-DIHYDRO-FURAN-2,5-DIONE ◇ 2,5-FURANDIONE ◇ MALEIC ACID ANHYDRIDE (MAK) ◇ RCRA WASTE NUMBER U147 ◇ TOXILIC ANHYDRIDE

TOXICITY DATA and REFERENCE
ETA: scu-rat TDLo: 1220 mg/kg/61W-I   BJCAAI 17,100,63

CONSENSUS REPORTS: Community Right-To-Know List. Reported in EPA TSCA Inventory.

OSHA PEL: TWA 0.25 ppm   ACGIH TLV: TWA 0.25 ppm DFG MAK: 0.2 ppm (0.8 mg/m^3)   DOT Classification: ORM-A; Label: None; IMO: Corrosive Material; Label: None.

SAFETY PROFILE: Questionable carcinogen with experimental tumorigenic data. Poison by ingestion and intraperitoneal routes. Moderately toxic by skin contact. A corrosive irritant to eyes, skin, and mucous membranes. Can cause pulmonary edema. A pesticide. Combustible when exposed to heat or flame; can react vigorously on contact with oxidizing materials. To

fight fire, use alcohol foam. When heated to decomposition (above 150°C) it emits acrid smoke and irritating fumes.

MAN700   CAS: 24382-04-5
MALONALDEHYDE SODIUM SALT
mf: C$_3$H$_3$O$_2$•Na   mw: 94.05

SYNS: 3-HYDROXY-2-PROPENAL SODIUM SALT ◇ MALONALDEHYDE, ION(1-), SODIUM ◇ PROPANE-DIAL, ION(1-), SODIUM (9CI) ◇ SODIUM MALONDIAL-DEHYDE

TOXICITY DATA and REFERENCE
CAR: orl-rat TDLo: 51500 mg/kg/2Y-I   NTPTR* NTP-TR-331,88
MUT: cyt-rat: fbr 100 umol/L   MUREAV 101,237,82
MUT: mnt-rat: fbr 100 umol/L   MUREAV 101,237,82

CONSENSUS REPORTS: NTP Carcinogenesis Studies (gavage): Clear Evidence: rat NTPTR* NTP-TR-331,88; No Evidence: mouse NTPTR* NTP-TR-331,88

SAFETY PROFILE: Questionable carcinogen with experimental carcinogenic data. Mutation data reported. When heated to decomposition it emits acrid smoke and irritating fumes.

MAO500   CAS: 69-79-4
MALTOSE
mf: C$_{12}$H$_{22}$O$_{11}$ mw: 342.31

PROP: Colorless needles. D: 1.540 @ 17°, mp: decomp. Very sol in water; very sltly sol in cold alc; insol in ether.

SYNS: 4-(α-d-GLUCOPYRANOSIDO)-α-GLUCOPYRA-NOSE ◇ 4-(α-d-GLUCOSIDO)-d-GLUCOSE ◇ MALTOBIOSE ◇ d-MALTOSE ◇ MALT SUGAR ◇ α-MALT SUGAR

TOXICITY DATA and REFERENCE
ETA: scu-mus TDLo: 1750 mg/kg/50W-C   GANNA2 48,556,57

CONSENSUS REPORTS: Reported in EPA TSCA Inventory.

SAFETY PROFILE: Questionable carcinogen with experimental tumorigenic and teratogenic data. Experimental reproductive effects. When heated to decomposition it emits acrid smoke and irritating fumes.

MAP750   CAS: 7439-96-5
MANGANESE
af: Mn   aw: 54.94

PROP: Reddish-grey or silvery, brittle, metallic element. Mp: 1260°, bp: 1900°, d: 7.20, vap press: 1 mm @ 1292°.

SYNS: COLLOIDAL MANGANESE ◇ MAGNACAT ◇ MANGAN (POLISH) ◇ MANGAN NITRIDOVANY (CZECH) ◇ TRONAMANG

TOXICITY DATA and REFERENCE
ETA: ims-rat TDLo:400 mg/kg/1Y-I NCIUS*
PH 43-64-886,SEPT,71
MUT: mrc-smc 8 mmol/L/18H MUREAV 42,343,77

CONSENSUS REPORTS: Manganese and its compounds are on the Community Right-To-Know List. Reported in EPA TSCA Inventory.

OSHA PEL: Fume: (Transitional: CL 5 mg/m^3) TWA 1 mg/m^3; STEL 3 mg/m^3; Compounds: CL 5 mg/m^3 ACGIH TLV: Fume: 1 mg/m^3; STEL 3 mg/m^3; Dust and Compounds: TWA 5 mg/m^3 DFG MAK: 5 mg/m^3

SAFETY PROFILE: Questionable carcinogen with experimental tumorigenic data. Human systemic effects by inhalation: degenerative brain changes, change in motor activity, muscle weakness. A skin and eye irritant. Mutation data reported. Flammable and moderately explosive in the form of dust or powder when exposed to flame. The dust may be pyrophoric in air. To fight fire, use special dry chemical.

MAQ500 CAS: 14024-58-9
MANGANESE ACETYLACETONATE
mf: C$_{10}$H$_{14}$O$_4$Mn mw: 253.18

SYN: MANGANOUS ACETYLACETONATE

TOXICITY DATA and REFERENCE
NEO: ims-rat TDLo:1200 mg/kg/26W-I
JNCIAM 60,1171,78
ETA: ims-rat TD:1350 mg/kg/21W-I NCIUS*
PH 43-64-886,SEPT,71

CONSENSUS REPORTS: Manganese and its compounds are on the Community Right-To-Know List. Reported in EPA TSCA Inventory.

OSHA PEL: CL 5 mg(Mn)/m^3 ACGIH TLV: TWA 5 mg(Mn)/m^3

SAFETY PROFILE: Questionable carcinogen with experimental neoplastigenic and tumorigenic data. When heated to decomposition it emits acrid smoke and irritating fumes.

MAR000 CAS: 7773-01-5
MANGANESE(II) CHLORIDE (1:2)
mf: Cl$_2$Mn mw: 125.84

PROP: Cubic, deliquescent, pink crystals. Mp: 650°, bp: 1190°, d: 2.977 @ 25°. Sol in water.

SYNS: MANGANESE DICHLORIDE ◇ MANGANOUS CHLORIDE

TOXICITY DATA and REFERENCE
CAR: ipr-mus TDLo:2080 mg/kg/26W-I
FEPRA7 23,393,64
CAR: scu-mus TDLo:2080 mg/kg/26W-I
FEPRA7 23,393,64
MUT: dlt-rat-orl 106 mg/kg/30W-C GISAAA
49(11),80,84
MUT: mmo-esc 5 μmol/L MUREAV 126,9,84
MUT: msc-mus:lym 40 mg/L JTEHD6 9,367,82
MUT: pic-esc 1600 μmol/L ENMUDM 6,59,84
MUT: sln-rat-orl 10640 μg/kg/30W-C GISAAA
49(11),80,84

CONSENSUS REPORTS: Manganese and its compounds are on the Community Right-To-Know List. Reported in EPA TSCA Inventory. EPA Genetic Toxicology Program.

OSHA PEL: CL 5 mg(Mn)/m^3 ACGIH TLV: TWA 5 mg(Mn)/m^3

SAFETY PROFILE: Questionable carcinogen with experimental carcinogenic and teratogenic data. Poison by intraperitoneal, subcutaneous, intramuscular, intravenous, parenteral, and possibly other routes. Moderately toxic by ingestion. Mutation data reported. Experimental reproductive effects. When heated to decomposition it emits toxic fumes of Cl$^-$.

MAS500 CAS: 12427-38-2
MANGANESE(II) ETHYLENEBIS (DITHIOCARBAMATE)
DOT: 2210/2968
mf: C$_4$H$_7$N$_2$S$_4$•Mn mw: 266.31

PROP: Yellow powder or crystals; water-sol.

SYNS: AAMANGAN ◇ AKZO CHEMIE MANEB ◇ BASF-MANEB SPRITZPULVER ◇ CHEM NEB ◇ CHLORO-BLE M ◇ CR 3029 ◇ DITHANE M 22 SPECIAL ◇ ENT 14,875 ◇ 1,2-ETHANEDIYLBIS(CARBAMODITHIOATO)(2−)-MAN-GANESE ◇ 1,2-ETHANEDIYLBISCARBAMODITHIOIC ACID MANGANESE COMPLEX ◇ 1,2-ETHANEDIYLBISCARBAMO-DITHIOIC ACID, MANGANESE(2+) SALT (1:1) ◇ 1,2-ETH-ANEDIYLBISMANEB, MANGANESE (2+) SALT (1:1) ◇ ETHYLENEBISDITHIOCARBAMATE MANGANESE ◇ N,N′-ETHYLENE BIS(DITHIOCARBAMATE MANGA-NEUX) (FRENCH) ◇ ETHYLENEBIS(DITHIOCARBAMATO) MANGANESE ◇ ETHYLENEBIS(DITHIOCARBAMIC ACID) MANGANESE SALT ◇ ETHYLENEBIS(DITHIOCARBAMIC

ACID) MANGANOUS SALT ◇ 1,2-ETHYLENEDIYLBIS
(CARBAMODITHIOATO)MANGANESE ◇ N,N′-ETILEN-BIS
(DITIOCARBAMMATO) di MANGANESE (ITALIAN)
◇ F 10 (PESTICIDE) ◇ GRIFFIN MANEX ◇ KYPMAN 80
◇ LONOCOL M ◇ MANAM ◇ MANEB ◇ MANEB, STABI-
LIZED AGAINST SELF-HEATING (DOT) ◇ MANEB, WITH
NOT LESS THAN 60% MANEB (DOT) ◇ MANEBE
(FRENCH) ◇ MANGAAN(II)-(N,N′-ETHYLEEN-BIS(DITHIO-
CARBAMAAT)) (DUTCH) ◇ MANGAN(II)-(N,N′-AETHYLEN-
BIS(DITHIOCARBAMATE)) (GERMAN) ◇ MANGANESE
ETHYLENE-1,2-BISDITHIOCARBAMATE ◇ MANGANESE(II)
ETHYLENE DI(DITHIOCARBAMATE) ◇ MANZATE
◇ MANZATE MANEB FUNGICIDE ◇ MEB ◇ NESPOR
◇ PLANTIFOG 160M ◇ POLYRAM M ◇ REMASAN CHLORO-
BLE M ◇ TRIMANGOL ◇ UNICROP MANEB ◇ VANCIDE

TOXICITY DATA and REFERENCE
CAR: orl-rat TDLo:62980 mg/kg/94W-I
  VPITAR 29,71,70
ETA: imp-rat TDLo:50 mg/kg   VPITAR
  29,71,70
ETA: orl-mus TDLo:3600 mg/kg/5W-L
  GISAAA 37(9),25,72
MUT: cyt-ham:lng 31 mg/L   GMCRDC
  27,95,81
MUT: mmo-omi 1000 ppm   MMAPAP
  50,233,73
MUT: mmo-smc 5 ppm   RSTUDV 6,161,76

CONSENSUS REPORTS: IARC Cancer Review: Animal Inadequate Evidence IMEMDT
12,137,76. Community Right-To-Know List.
EPA Genetic Toxicology Program.

OSHA PEL: CL 5 mg(Mn)/m^3 ACGIH TLV:
TWA 5 mg(Mn)/m^3 DOT Classification:
Flammable Solid; Label: Spontaneously Com-
bustible, Danger When Wet.

SAFETY PROFILE: Questionable carcinogen
with experimental carcinogenic, tumorigenic,
and teratogenic data. Moderately toxic by ingestion and possibly other routes. Experimental
reproductive effects. Mutation data reported. A
fungicide. May ignite spontaneously in air. Dangerous; when heated to decomposition it emits
highly toxic fumes of NO$_x$ and SO$_x$.

MAU250   CAS: 7785-87-7
MANGANESE(II) SULFATE (1:1)
mf: O$_4$S•Mn   mw: 151.00

PROP: Pink granular powder; odorless. Mp:
700°, bp: decomp @ 850°. d: 3.25. Very sol
in water, more so in boiling water; insol in
alc.

SYNS: MANGANOUS SULFATE ◇ MAN-GRO ◇ NCI-
C61143 ◇ SORBA-SPRAY Mn ◇ SULFURIC ACID,
MANGANESE(2+) SALT

TOXICITY DATA and REFERENCE
MUT: dni-smc 10 mmol/L   MGGEAE 151,69,77
MUT: dnr-bcs 50 mmol/L   MUREAV 31,185,75
MUT: mmo-omi 10 mmol/L   JMOBAK 14,453,65
MUT: mmo-smc 40 µmol/L   MUREAV 137,47,84
MUT: mrc-smc 40 µmol/L   MUREAV 137,47,84

CONSENSUS REPORTS: Manganese and its
compounds are on the Community Right-To-
Know List. Reported in EPA TSCA Inventory.
EPA Genetic Toxicology Program.

OSHA PEL: CL 5 mg(Mn)/m^3 ACGIH TLV:
TWA 5 mg(Mn)/m^3

SAFETY PROFILE: Questionable carcinogen
with experimental neoplastigenic data. Poison
by intraperitoneal route. Mutation data reported.
When heated to decomposition it emits toxic
fumes of SO$_x$ and manganese.

MAW750   CAS: 551-74-6
MANNOMUSTINE DIHYDROCHLORIDE
mf: C$_{10}$H$_{23}$Cl$_2$N$_2$O$_4$•2ClH   mw: 378.13

PROP: Crystals from 80% ethanol. Decomp
@ 239-241°. Sol in H$_2$O; sltly sol in ethanol.

SYNS: 1,6-BIS-(CHLOROETHYLAMINO)-1,6-DESOXY-d-
MANNITOLDIHYDROCHLORIDE ◇ 1,6-BIS-(CHLORO-
ETHYLAMINO)-1,6-DIDEOXY-d-MANNITEDIHYDROCHLO-
RIDE ◇ 1,6-DIDEOXY-1,6-DI(2-CHLOROETHYLAMINO)-d-
MANNITOLDIHYDROCHLORIDE ◇ MANNITOL MUSTARD
DIHYDROCHLORIDE ◇ NSC-9698

TOXICITY DATA and REFERENCE
CAR: ipr-mus TDLo:23 mg/kg/4W   JNCIAM
  36,915,66
NEO: ipr-mus TDLo:7265 µg/kg/4W-I   JNCIAM
  36,915,66
MUT: cyt-hmn:lym 10 µmol/L   IPPABX 17,131,81
MUT: dnd-mus-ipr 200 mg/kg   FOBLAN 25,380,79
MUT: hma-mus:esc 1 mg/kg   MUREAV 21,190,73
MUT: sce-hmn:lym 3 µmol/L   IPPABX 17,131,81

CONSENSUS REPORTS: IARC Cancer Review: GROUP 3 IMEMDT 7,56,87; Animal
Sufficient Evidence IMEMDT 9,157,75.

SAFETY PROFILE: Questionable carcinogen
with experimental carcinogenic, and neoplastigenic data. Poison by intravenous, subcutaneous, and parenteral routes. Experimental reproductive effects. Human mutation data reported.

A drug used for the treatment of malignant neoplasms. When heated to decomposition it emits very toxic fumes of HCl^- and NO_x.

MAX000   CAS: 63710-10-1
MARCELLOMYCIN
mf: $C_{42}H_{55}NO_{17}$ mw: 845.98

TOXICITY DATA and REFERENCE
CAR: ivn-rat TDLo:15 mg/kg   CNREA8
43,5248,83
MUT: dnd-rat:lvr 11300 nmol/L   MOPMA3
14,290,78
MUT: dni-mus:leu 950 nmol/L   JANTAJ
34,1596,81
MUT: oms-mus:leu 50 nmol/L   JANTAJ
34,1596,81

SAFETY PROFILE: Questionable carcinogen with experimental carcinogenic data. Poison by intraperitoneal and intravenous routes. Mutation data reported. When heated to decomposition it emits toxic fumes of NO_x.

MBU750
MARSH ROSEMARY EXTRACT

PROP: Tannin containing extract of root (JNCIAM 57,207,76).

SYNS: LIMONIUM NASHII ◇ TANNIN from LIMONIUM NASHII ◇ TANNIN from MARSH ROSEMARY

TOXICITY DATA and REFERENCE
NEO: scu-rat TDLo:530 mg/kg/66W-I   JNCIAM
57,207,76

SAFETY PROFILE: Questionable carcinogen with experimental neoplastigenic data. When heated to decomposition it emits acrid smoke and irritating fumes.

MBV500   CAS: 64521-14-8
7-MBA-3,4-DIHYDRODIOL
mf: $C_{18}H_{16}O_2$ mw: 264.34

SYN: trans-3,4-DIHYDRO-3,4-DIHYDROXY-7-METHYL-BENZ(a)ANTHRACENE

TOXICITY DATA and REFERENCE
NEO: skn-mus TD:4230 μg/kg   CNREA8
40,1981,80
NEO: skn-mus TDLo:1000 μg/kg   CALEDQ
3,247,77
MUT: mma-sat 10 μmol/L   BBRCA9 75,427,77
MUT: msc-ham:lng 1 mg/L   IJCNAW 19,828,77
MUT: msc-ham:ovr 10 mg/L   IJCNAW 19,828,77

MUT: otr-mus:fbr 1 mg/L   IJCNAW 19,828,77
MUT: sce-ham:ovr 4 mg/L   MUREAV 129,365,84

CONSENSUS REPORTS: EPA Genetic Toxicology Program.

SAFETY PROFILE: Questionable carcinogen with experimental neoplastigenic data by skin contact. Mutation data reported. When heated to decomposition it emits acrid smoke and irritating fumes.

MCA500   CAS: 8064-66-2
MEGESTROL ACETATE +
ETHINYLOESTRADIOL

SYNS: 17-HYDROXY-6-METHYLPREGNA-4,6-DIENE-3,20-DIONE ACETATE mixed with 19-NOR-17-α-PREGNA-1,3,5(10)-TRIEN-2-YNE-3,17-DIOL ◇ MEGESTROL ACETATE 4 MG., ETHINYLOESTRADIOL 50 μg ◇ MENOQUENS ◇ NEODELPREGNIN ◇ ORACONAL ◇ SERIAL ◇ TRI-ERVONUM ◇ VOLDYS ◇ VOLIDAN

TOXICITY DATA and REFERENCE
CAR: orl-wmn TD:41 mg/kg/2Y-I:LIV
BMJOAE 4,496,75
CAR: orl-wmn TDLo:10584 μg/kg/2Y-I:
LIV,BLD   LANCAO 1,273,80

SAFETY PROFILE: Questionable human carcinogen producing normocytic anemia and liver tumors. Human reproductive effects by ingestion: female fertility effects. An oral contraceptive. When heated to decomposition it emits acrid smoke and irritating fumes.

MCB000   CAS: 108-78-1
MELAMINE
mf: $C_3H_6N_6$ mw: 126.15

PROP: Monoclinic, colorless prisms. Mp: <250°, bp: sublimes, d: 1.573 @ 250°, vap press: 50 mm @ 315°, vap d: 4.34. Sltly sol in water; very sltly sol in hot alc; insol in ether.

SYNS: AERO ◇ CYANURAMIDE ◇ CYANUROTRIAMIDE ◇ CYANUROTRIAMINE ◇ CYMEL ◇ NCI-C50715 ◇ 2,4,6-TRIAMINO-s-TRIAZINE

TOXICITY DATA and REFERENCE
CAR: orl-rat TD:197 g/kg/2Y-C   NTPTR* NTP-TR-245,83
CAR: orl-rat TDLo:195 g/kg/2Y-C   TXAPA9
72,292,84
ETA: orl-rat TD:162 g/kg/2Y-C   TXAPA9
72,292,84
MUT: mnt-mus-orl 1 g/kg   ENMUDM 4,342,82

CONSENSUS REPORTS: IARC Cancer Review: Animal Inadequate Evidence IMEMDT 39,333,86. NTP Carcinogenesis Bioassay (feed); No Evidence: mouse NTPTR* NTP-TR-245,83; (feed); Clear Evidence: rat NTPTR* NTP-TR-245,83. Community Right-To-Know List. Reported in EPA TSCA Inventory.

SAFETY PROFILE: Questionable carcinogen with experimental carcinogenic and tumorigenic data. Moderately toxic by ingestion and intraperitoneal routes. An eye, skin, and mucous membrane irritant. Causes dermatitis in humans. Mutation data reported. When heated to decomposition it emits toxic fumes of NO_x and CN^-.

MCB350   CAS: 73-31-4
MELATONIN
mf: $C_{13}H_{16}N_2O_2$ mw: 232.31

PROP: A hormone of the pineal gland, also produced by extra-pineal tissues, that lightens skin color in amphibians by reversing the darkening effect of MSH (melanotropin). Pale yellow leaflets from benzene. Mp: 116-118°.

SYNS: N-ACETYL-5-METHOXYTRYPTAMINE ◇ MELA-TONINE ◇ 5-METHOXY-N-ACETYLTRYPTAMINE

TOXICITY DATA and REFERENCE
CAR: scu-mus TDLo:4200 mg/kg/20W-I
    GETRE8 28(2),47,83

SAFETY PROFILE: Questionable carcinogen with experimental carcinogenic data by skin contact. Poison by intravenous route. Experimental reproductive effects. When heated to decomposition it emits toxic fumes of NO_x.

MCE000   CAS: 80-47-7
p-MENTHANE-8-HYDROPEROXIDE
mf: $C_{10}H_{20}O_2$ mw: 172.30

PROP: Clear, pale yellow liquid. D: 0.910-0.925 @ 15.5°/4°.

SYN: p-MENTHANE HYDROPEROXIDE

TOXICITY DATA and REFERENCE
ETA: unr-mus TDLo:620 mg/kg   RARSAM
    3,193,63

SAFETY PROFILE: Questionable carcinogen with experimental tumorigenic data. When heated to decomposition it emits acrid smoke and irritating fumes. An irritant and powerful oxidizer.

MCO500   CAS: 60-56-0
2-MERCAPTO-1-METHYLIMIDAZOLE
mf: $C_4H_6N_2S$ mw: 114.18

SYNS: BASOLAN ◇ DANANTIZOL ◇ FAVISTAN ◇ FRENTIROX ◇ MERCAPTAZOLE ◇ MERCAZOLYL ◇ METAZOLO ◇ METHIAMAZOLE ◇ 1-METHYLIMIDA-ZOLE-2-THIOL ◇ 1-METHYL-2-MERCAPTOIMIDAZOLE ◇ METIZOL ◇ METOTHYRINE ◇ 1-METYLO-2-MERKAP-TOIMIDAZOLEM (POLISH) ◇ STRUMAZOLE ◇ TAPAZOLE ◇ THACAPZOL ◇ THIAMAZOLE ◇ THYCAPSOL ◇ USAF EL-30

TOXICITY DATA and REFERENCE
NEO: orl-mus TDLo:33 g/kg/1Y-C   CANCAR
    40,2188,77
NEO: orl-rat TD:2700 mg/kg/26W-C   CRSBAW
    174,268,80
NEO: orl-rat TDLo:1100 mg/kg/2Y-C   FCTXAV
    11,649,73
MUT: cyt-mus:mmr 3200 μmol/L/24H-C
    JTSCDR 5,141,80

CONSENSUS REPORTS: Reported in EPA TSCA Inventory.

SAFETY PROFILE: Questionable carcinogen with experimental neoplastigenic data. Poison by subcutaneous route. Moderately toxic by ingestion and intraperitoneal routes. Human teratogenic effects. An experimental teratogen. Experimental reproductive effects. Mutation data reported. An antithyroid drug. When heated to decomposition it emits very toxic fumes of NO_x and SO_x.

MCR750   CAS: 52-67-5
d,3-MERCAPTOVALINE
mf: $C_5H_{11}NO_2S$ mw: 149.23

SYNS: CUPRENIL ◇ CUPRIMINE ◇ DEPEN ◇ DIMETHYL-CYSTEINE ◇ β,β-DIMETHYLCYSTEINE ◇ d-MERCAPTO-VALINE ◇ METALCAPTASE ◇ PCA ◇ d-PENAMINE ◇ PENICILLAMIN ◇ (S)-PENICILLAMIN ◇ PENICILLAMINE ◇ d-PENICILLAMINE ◇ REDUCED-d-PENICILLAMINE ◇ TROLOVOL

TOXICITY DATA and REFERENCE
CAR: orl-chd TDLo:122 g/kg/3Y-C:BLD
    JAMAAP 248,467,82
ETA: ipr-mus TDLo:2 g/kg/4W-I   LANCAO
    2,1356,76
MUT: mma-sat 1 mg/plate   ABCHA6 45,2157,81
MUT: mmo-sat 60 μmol/plate   BCPCA6 34,3725,85

SAFETY PROFILE: Questionable human carcinogen producing leukemia. Poison by intraperitoneal route. Moderately toxic by subcutaneous and intravenous routes. Mildly toxic by ingestion. An experimental teratogen. Human systemic effects by ingestion: leukopenia, thrombocytopenia, proteinuria, dermatitis, and fever. Human teratogenic effects by an unspecified route: developmental abnormalities of the craniofacial areas, skin and skin appendages, and body wall. Experimental reproductive effects. Mutation data reported. Used in the treatment of rheumatoid arthritis, metal poisonings, and cystinuria. When heated to decomposition it emits very toxic fumes of NO_x and SO_x.

MCW250   CAS: 7439-97-6
MERCURY
DOT: 2809
af: Hg   aw: 200.59

PROP: Silvery, heavy, mobile liquid. A liquid metallic element. Mp: −38.89°, bp: 356.9°, d: 13.534 @ 25°, vap press: 2×10^{-3} mm @ 25°. Solid: tin-white, ductile, malleable mass which can be cut with a knife.

SYNS: COLLOIDAL MERCURY ◇ KWIK (DUTCH) ◇ MERCURE (FRENCH) ◇ MERCURIO (ITALIAN) ◇ MERCURY, METALLIC (DOT) ◇ NCI-C60399 ◇ QUECKSILBER (GERMAN) ◇ QUICK SILVER ◇ RCRA WASTE NUMBER U151 ◇ RTEC (POLISH)

TOXICITY DATA and REFERENCE
ETA: ipr-rat TDLo:400 mg/kg/14D-I   ZEKBAI 61,511,57
MUT: cyt-man-unr 150 µg/m³   AEHLAU 34,461,79

CONSENSUS REPORTS: Mercury and its compounds are on the Community Right-To-Know List.

OSHA PEL: Vapor: (Transitional: CL 1 mg/10m³) 0.05 mg/m³ (skin)   ACGIH TLV: TWA 0.05 mg(Hg)/m³ (vapor, skin)   DFG MAK: 0.1 mg/m³; BAT: 5 µg/dL in blood.   NIOSH REL: (Inorganic Mercury) TWA 0.05 mg(Hg)/m³   DOT Classification: Corrosive Material; Label: Corrosive.

SAFETY PROFILE: Questionable carcinogen with experimental tumorigenic data. Poison by inhalation. Corrosive to skin, eyes, and mucous membranes. Human systemic effects by inhalation: wakefulness, muscle weakness, anorexia, headache, tinnitus, hypermotility, diarrhea, liver changes, dermatitis, fever. An experimental teratogen. Experimental reproductive effects. Human mutation data reported. Used in dental

applications, electronics, and chemical synthesis. When heated to decomposition it emits toxic fumes of Hg.

MDD750   CAS: 115-09-3
MERCURY METHYLCHLORIDE
mf: CH_3ClHg mw: 251.08

PROP: White crystals, characteristic odor. D: 4.063, mp: 170°.

SYNS: CASPAN ◇ CHLOROMETHYLMERCURY ◇ METHYLMERCURIC CHLORIDE ◇ METHYLMERCURY CHLORIDE ◇ MMC ◇ MONOMETHYL MERCURY CHLORIDE

TOXICITY DATA and REFERENCE
CAR: orl-mus TD:660 mg/kg/2Y-C   NJUZA9 48,127,86
CAR: orl-mus TD:668 mg/kg/53W-C   CALEDQ 12,305,81
CAR: orl-mus TD:731 mg/kg/58W-C   TOLED5 18(Suppl 1),114,83
CAR: orl-mus TD:5359 mg/kg/58W-C   TOLED5 18(Suppl 1),114,83
CAR: orl-mus TDLo:402 mg/kg/58W-C   JTSCDR 8,329,83
MUT: cyt-hmn:lym 1 µmol/L   ESKGA2 26,99,80
MUT: dni-mus:lym 10 nmol/L   TXCYAC 36,297,85
MUT: dni-mus:oth 50 µmol/L   TXAPA9 53,24,80
MUT: oms-hmn:leu 1 ppm   JIDZA9 20,256,76

CONSENSUS REPORTS: Mercury and its compounds are on the Community Right-To-Know List. EPA Genetic Toxicology Program.

OSHA PEL: (Transitional: CL 1 mg/10m³) TWA 0.01 mg(Hg)/m³; STEL 0.03 mg/m³ (skin)   ACGIH TLV: TWA 0.01 mg(Hg)/m³; STEL 0.03 mg(Hg)/m³   NIOSH REL: TWA 0.05 mg(Hg)/m³

SAFETY PROFILE: Questionable carcinogen with experimental carcinogenic and teratogenic data. Poison by ingestion, intramuscular, intravenous, and intraperitoneal routes. Human mutation data reported. Experimental reproductive effects. When heated to decomposition it emits very toxic fumes of Cl^- and Hg.

MDI000   CAS: 54-64-8
MERTHIOLATE SODIUM
mf: $C_9H_9HgO_2S \cdot Na$ mw: 404.82

SYNS: ((o-CARBOXYPHENYL)THIO)ETHYLMERCURY SODIUM SALT ◇ ELCIDE 75 ◇ ELICIDE ◇ o-(ETHYLMERCURITHIO)BENZOIC ACID SODIUM SALT ◇ ETHYLMERCURI-

THIOSALICYLIC ACID SODIUM SALT ◇ MERCUROTHIO-
LATE ◇ MERFAMIN ◇ MERTHIOLATE ◇ MERTHIOLATE
SALT ◇ MERTORGAN ◇ MERZONIN SODIUM ◇ SET
◇ SODIUM ETHYLMERCURIC THIOSALICYLATE
◇ SODIUM-o-(ETHYLMERCURITHIO)BENZOATE ◇ SO-
DIUM ETHYLMERCURITHIOSALICYLATE ◇ SODIUM MER-
THIOLATE ◇ THIMEROSALATE ◇ THIMEROSOL
◇ THIOMERSALATE

TOXICITY DATA and REFERENCE
NEO: scu-rat TDLo: 104 mg/kg/1Y-I   CTOXAO
4,185,71

CONSENSUS REPORTS: Mercury and its
compounds are on the Community Right-To-
Know List. EPA Genetic Toxicology Program.

OSHA PEL: (Transitional: CL 1 mg/10m^3) CL
0.1 mg(Hg)/m^3 (skin)   ACGIH TLV: TWA 0.1
mg(Hg)/m^3 (skin)   NIOSH REL: TWA 0.05
mg(Hg)/m^3

SAFETY PROFILE: Questionable carcinogen
with experimental neoplastigenic and teratogenic data. Poison by ingestion, subcutaneous,
intravenous, and possibly other routes. Experimental reproductive effects. An eye irritant. An
ophthalmic preservative, a topical anti-infec-
tive, topical veterinary antibacterial and antifun-
gal agent. An FDA over-the-counter drug. When
heated to decomposition it emits very toxic
fumes of Hg, Na$_2$O and SO$_x$.

MDJ250   CAS: 34807-41-5
MESEREIN
mf: C$_{38}$H$_{38}$O$_{10}$ mw: 654.76

SYNS: MEZEREIN ◇ (12-β(E,E))-12-((1-OXO-5-PHENYL-
2,4-PENTADIENYL)OXY)-DAPHNETOXIN

TOXICITY DATA and REFERENCE
NEO: skn-mus TD: 18 mg/kg/20W-I   CNREA8
39,4791,79
NEO: skn-mus TDLo: 3560 μg/kg/20W-I
CNREA8 39,4791,79
MUT: dns-mus-skn 340 nmol/kg   CNREA8
43,4126,83
MUT: mrc-smc 20 mg/L   NATUAS 294,263,81
MUT: otr-mus: fbr 100 μg/L   FACOEB 1,179,84
MUT: otr-mus: oth 16 nmol/L   CRNGDP 4,1507,83

SAFETY PROFILE: Questionable carcinogen
with experimental neoplastigenic data. Mutation
data reported. When heated to decomposition
it emits acrid smoke and irritating fumes.

MDL750   CAS: 8015-29-0
MESTRANOL mixed with
NORETHINDRONE

SYNS: ETHYNYLESTRADIOL-3-METHYL ETHER and 17-
α-ETHYNYL-17-HYDROXYESTREN-3-ONE ◇ ETHYNYLES-
TRADIOL-3-METHYL ETHER and 17-α-ETHYNYL-19-NOR-
TESTOSTERONE ◇ 17-α-ETHYNYL-17-HYDROXYESTREN-3-
ONE and ETHYNYLESTRADIOL 3-METHYL ETHER
◇ 17-α-ETHYNYL-19-NORTESTOSTERONE and ETHYNYLES-
TRADIOL 3-METHYL ETHER ◇ MESTRANOL mixed with
NORETHISTERONE ◇ NORETHINDRONE mixed with MES-
TRANOL ◇ NORETHISTERONE mixed with MESTRANOL
◇ NORINYL-1 ◇ ORTHO-NOVUM ◇ SOPHIA

TOXICITY DATA and REFERENCE
CAR: orl-wmn TD: 53 mg/kg/7Y-I: LIV,BLD
LANCAO 1,365,80
CAR: orl-wmn TDLo: 26460 μg/kg/5Y-I: LIV
LANCAO 1,310,80
NEO: orl-rat TDLo: 5639 mg/kg/2Y-C   NAIZAM
25,684,74
NEO: orl-wmn TD: 71 mg/kg/7Y-I: LIV
ANSUA5 183,239,76
NEO: orl-wmn TDLo: 40 mg/kg/4Y-I: LIV
JAMAAP 235,730,76

SAFETY PROFILE: Questionable human carcinogen producing liver tumors. An experimental
neoplastigenic. Human systemic effects by ingestion: thrombocytopenia (decrease in the number of blood platelets), dyspnea, nausea or
vomiting, fever. Human teratogenic and
reproductive effects by ingestion: developmental
abnormalities of the urogenital system; spermatogenesis; impotence; breast development in
males; changes in the uterus, cervix, or vagina;
female fertility effects. Experimental reproductive effects.

MDM000   CAS: 7660-71-1
MESUPRINE HYDROCHLORIDE
mf: C$_{19}$H$_{26}$N$_2$O$_5$S•ClH   mw: 430.99

SYN: 2'-HYDROXY-5'-(1-HYDROXY-2-(p-
METHOXYPHENETHYL)AMINO)PROPYL)METHANESULFO-
NANILIDE HCl

TOXICITY DATA and REFERENCE
ETA: orl-rat TDLo: 22 g/kg/78W-C   TXAPA9
22,276,72

SAFETY PROFILE: Questionable carcinogen
with experimental tumorigenic data. When
heated to decomposition it emits very toxic
fumes of NO$_x$, SO$_x$ and HCl.

MDM750
METANICOTINE
CAS: 538-79-4

mf: $C_{10}H_{14}N_2$ mw: 162.26

TOXICITY DATA and REFERENCE
ETA: itr-rat TDLo:75 mg/kg   BJCAAI 16,453,62

SAFETY PROFILE: Questionable carcinogen with experimental tumorigenic data. When heated to decomposition it emits toxic fumes of NO_x.

MDT000
METHAPYRILENE mixed with SODIUM NITRITE (1:2)

SYN: SODIUM NITRITE mixed with METHAPYRILENE (2:1)

TOXICITY DATA and REFERENCE
CAR: orl-rat TDLo:121 g/kg/90W-I   FCTXAV 15,269,77

SAFETY PROFILE: Questionable carcinogen with experimental carcinogenic data. When heated to decomposition it emits toxic fumes of Na_2O and NO_x.

MDT600
METHEDRINE
CAS: 51-57-0

mf: $C_{10}H_{15}N \cdot ClH$ mw: 185.72

SYNS: ADIPEX ◇ DEOFED ◇ d-DEOXYEPHEDRINE HYDROCHLORIDE ◇ DESOXO-5 ◇ d-DESOXYEPHEDRINE HYDROCHLORIDE ◇ DESOXYFED ◇ DESOXYN ◇ DESOXYNE ◇ DESTIM ◇ DESYPHED ◇ DEXOVAL ◇ DEXTIM ◇ DOXYFED ◇ DRINALFA ◇ EFROXINE ◇ EUFODRIANL ◇ GERVOT ◇ ISOPHEN ◇ METAMPHETAMINE HYDROCHLORIDE ◇ (+)-METHAMPHETAMINE CHLORIDE ◇ (+)-METHAMPHETAMINE HYDROCHLORIDE ◇ METHAMPHETAMINE HYDROCHLORIDE ◇ d-METHAMPHETAMINE HYDROCHLORIDE ◇ METHAMPHETAMINIUM CHLORIDE ◇ METHEDRINE HYDROCHLORIDE ◇ METHYLAMPHETAMINE HYDROCHLORIDE ◇ d-METHYLAMPHETAMINE HYDROCHLORIDE ◇ N-METHYLAMPHETAMINE HYDROCHLORIDE ◇ METHYLISOMYN ◇ NORODIN HYDROCHLORIDE ◇ PERVITIN ◇ PHILOPON ◇ SOXYSYMPAMINE ◇ SYNDROX ◇ TONEDRON

TOXICITY DATA and REFERENCE
NEO: scu-rat TDLo:400 mg/kg (1-21D preg/19D post)   EAGRDS 5,509,79

CONSENSUS REPORTS: EPA Genetic Toxicology Program. Reported in EPA TSCA Inventory.

SAFETY PROFILE: Questionable carcinogen with experimental neoplastigenic data. Poison by ingestion, subcutaneous, intravenous, and intraperitoneal routes. Experimental reproductive effects. When heated to decomposition it emits toxic fumes of NO_x and HCl.

MDV500
METHOTREXATE
CAS: 59-05-2

mf: $C_{20}H_{22}N_8O_5$ mw: 454.50

SYNS: AMETHOPTERIN ◇ 4-AMINO-4-DEOXY-N[10]-METHYLPTEROYLGLUTAMATE ◇ 4-AMINO-4-DEOXY-N[10]-METHYLPTEROYLGLUTAMIC ACID ◇ 4-AMINO-10-METHYLFOLIC ACID ◇ 4-AMINO-N[10]-METHYLPTEROYLGLUTAMIC ACID ◇ ANTIFOLAN ◇ N-BISMETHYLPTEROYLGLUTAMIC ACID ◇ CL-14377 ◇ l-(+)-N-(p-(((2,4-DIAMINO-6-PTERIDINYL)METHYL)METHYLAMINO)BENZOYL)GLUTAMIC ACID ◇ EMT 25,299 ◇ EMTEXATE ◇ HDMTX ◇ METHOPTERIN ◇ METHOTEXTRATE ◇ METHYLAMINOPTERIN ◇ MTX ◇ NCI-C04671 ◇ NSC-740 ◇ R 9985

TOXICITY DATA and REFERENCE
CAR: orl-cld TDLo:125 mg/kg/6Y-I   JAMAAP 238,2631,77
CAR: orl-man TD:74 mg/kg/48W-I: BLD,SKN   ARDEAC 103,501,71
CAR: orl-man TD:8260 µg/kg/44W-I:BLD   SJHAAQ 24,234,80
CAR: orl-man TDLo:7 mg/kg/12W-C:BLD   ONCOBS 40,268,83
CAR: orl-mus TDLo:51 mg/kg/4Y-C   ARDEAC 103,505,71
ETA: orl-ham TDLo:210 mg/kg/50W-C   TXAPA9 26,392,73
ETA: orl-mus TD:55 mg/kg/78W-C   DEGEA3 26,219,71
ETA: orl-mus TD:139 mg/kg/55W-C   TXAPA9 26,392,73
MUT: cyt-ham:ovr 5 mg/L   ENMUDM 2,455,80
MUT: cyt-hmn:lym 100 nmol/L   MUREAV 139,67,84
MUT: dni-mus-ipr 2000 mg/kg   CNREA8 44,2278,84
MUT: dnr-bcs 400 µg/plate   TAKHAA 44,96,85

CONSENSUS REPORTS: IARC Cancer Review: Animal Inadequate Evidence IMEMDT 26,267,81; Human Inadequate Evidence IMEMDT 26,267,81. NCI Carcinogenesis Studies (ipr); No Evidence: mouse, rat CANCAR 40,1935,77. Reported in EPA TSCA Inventory.

SAFETY PROFILE: Questionable human carcinogen producing leukemia, Hodgkin's disease, and skin tumors. Experimental tumorigenic and teratogenic data. A human poison by intraspinal route. Poison experimentally by ingestion, intravenous, subcutaneous, and intraperitoneal routes. Human teratogenic effects by ingestion: developmental abnormalities of the craniofacial area and the musculoskeletal system. Human systemic effects by multiple routes: thrombocytopenia (decrease in the number of blood platelets), bone marrow changes, other blood changes, cerebral spinal fluid effects, eye effects, blood pressure lowering, cough, dyspnea, fibrosis (pneumoconiosis), cyanosis, gastrointestinal effects, fatty liver degeneration, hepatitis, liver function tests impaired, other liver changes, fever, effects on inflammation or mediation of inflammation. Human mutation data reported. Experimental reproductive effects. A human eye irritant. An FDA proprietary drug. A chemotherapeutic agent. When heated to decomposition it emits toxic fumes including NO_x.

MDZ000   CAS: 5834-17-3
2-METHOXY-3-AMINODIBENZOFURAN
mf: $C_{13}H_{11}NO_2$ mw: 213.25

SYN: 2-AMINO-3-METHOXYDIPHENYLENOXYD (GERMAN)

TOXICITY DATA and REFERENCE
CAR: orl-rat TDLo: 13 g/kg/56W-C   ZEKBAI 61,45,56

SAFETY PROFILE: Questionable carcinogen with experimental carcinogenic data. When heated to decomposition it emits toxic fumes of NO_x.

MEA000   CAS: 56970-24-2
3-METHOXY-4-AMINODIPHENYL
mf: $C_{13}H_{13}NO$ mw: 199.27

SYN: 3-METHOXYBIPHENYLAMINE

TOXICITY DATA and REFERENCE
ETA: scu-rat TDLo: 4400 mg/kg/W-I   BMBUAQ 14,141,58

SAFETY PROFILE: Questionable carcinogen with experimental tumorigenic data. When heated to decomposition it emits toxic fumes of NO_x.

MEA750   CAS: 67293-86-1
METHOXYAZOXYMETHANOLACETATE
mf: $C_4H_8N_2O_4$ mw: 148.14

TOXICITY DATA and REFERENCE
ETA: par-rat TDLo: 1800 μg/kg/9W-I   PAACA3 14,55,73
MUT: sln-dmg-orl 47 ng   PSEBAA 125,988,67

SAFETY PROFILE: Questionable carcinogen with experimental tumorigenic data. Mutation data reported. When heated to decomposition it emits toxic fumes of NO_x.

MEB000   CAS: 56183-20-1
3-METHOXY-1,2-BENZANTHRACENE
mf: $C_{19}H_{14}O$ mw: 258.33

SYN: 5-METHOXY-BENZ(a)ANTHRACENE

TOXICITY DATA and REFERENCE
ETA: scu-mus TDLo: 400 mg/kg   JNCIAM 1,303,40

SAFETY PROFILE: Questionable carcinogen with experimental tumorigenic data. When heated to decomposition it emits acrid smoke and irritating fumes.

MEB250   CAS: 63019-69-2
5-METHOXY-1,2-BENZANTHRACENE
mf: $C_{19}H_{14}O$ mw: 258.33

SYNS: 5-METHOXY-1,2-BENZ(a)ANTHRACENE ◇ 8-METHOXY-BENZ(a)ANTHRACENE

TOXICITY DATA and REFERENCE
ETA: scu-mus TDLo: 60 mg/kg   BJCAAI 9,457,55

SAFETY PROFILE: Questionable carcinogen with experimental tumorigenic data. When heated to decomposition it emits acrid smoke and irritating fumes.

MEB500   CAS: 6366-20-7
10-METHOXY-1,2-BENZANTHRACENE
mf: $C_{19}H_{14}O$ mw: 258.33

SYN: 7-METHOXY-BENZ(a)ANTHRACENE

TOXICITY DATA and REFERENCE
ETA: scu-mus TDLo: 600 mg/kg   JNCIAM 1,303,40

SAFETY PROFILE: Questionable carcinogen with experimental tumorigenic data. When heated to decomposition it emits acrid smoke and irritating fumes.

MEC500   CAS: 52351-96-9
6-METHOXYBENZO(a)PYRENE
mf: $C_{21}H_{14}O$ mw: 282.35

TOXICITY DATA and REFERENCE
ETA: skn-mus TDLo: 180 mg/kg/40W-I   CBINA8 22(1),53,78
ETA: unr-mus TDLo: 80 mg/kg/8D-I   BEBMAE 88(11),592,79
MUT: mma-sat 18 nmol/plate   BBRCA9 85,351,78

SAFETY PROFILE: Questionable carcinogen with experimental tumorigenic data. Mutation data reported. When heated to decomposition it emits acrid smoke and irritating fumes.

MED000 CAS: 38860-48-9
**N-(4-METHOXY)
BENZOYLOXYPIPERIDINE**
mf: $C_{13}H_{17}NO_3$ mw: 235.31

TOXICITY DATA and REFERENCE
NEO: skn-mus TDLo: 19 mg/kg JNCIAM 54,491,75

SAFETY PROFILE: Questionable carcinogen with experimental neoplastigenic data. When heated to decomposition it emits toxic fumes of NO_x.

MED250 CAS: 63059-68-7
8-METHOXY-3,4-BENZPYRENE
mf: $C_{21}H_{14}O$ mw: 282.35

TOXICITY DATA and REFERENCE
ETA: scu-mus TDLo: 20 mg/kg BJCAAI 6,400,52
ETA: scu-rat TDLo: 16 mg/kg/13W-I BJCAAI 6,400,52

SAFETY PROFILE: Questionable carcinogen with experimental tumorigenic data. When heated to decomposition it emits acrid smoke and irritating fumes.

MEI000 CAS: 100700-29-6
**N-(3-METHOXYCARBONYLPROPYL)-
N-(1-ACETOXYBUTYL)NITROSAMINE**
mf: $C_{11}H_{20}N_2O_5$ mw: 260.2

SYNS: N-(3-CARBOMETHOXYPROPYL)-N-(1-ACETOXY-BUTYL)NITROSAMINE ◇ CMPABN ◇ 4-((4-HYDROXY-BUTYL)NITROSAMINO)BUTYRIC ACID METHYL ESTER ACETATE (ESTER)

TOXICITY DATA and REFERENCE
CAR: scu-rat TDLo: 99 mg/kg 10W-I IAPUDO 41,619,82
ETA: scu-rat TD: 70500 μg/kg/10W-I GANNA2 73,687,82
MUT: mmo-esc 1 μmol/plate GANNA2 71,124,80
MUT: mmo-sat 1 μmol/plate GANNA2 71,124,80
MUT: mrc-bcs 1 μmol/plate GANNA2 71,124,80

SAFETY PROFILE: Questionable carcinogen with experimental carcinogenic and tumorigenic data. Mutation data reported. When heated to decomposition it emits toxic fumes of NO_x.

MEJ500 CAS: 61413-39-6
5-METHOXYCHRYSENE
mf: $C_{19}H_{14}O$ mw: 258.33

TOXICITY DATA and REFERENCE
NEO: skn-mus TD: 40 mg/kg/I CALEDQ 1,147,76
NEO: skn-mus TDLo: 1200 μg/kg/I CALEDQ 1,147,76
ETA: skn-mus TD: 40 mg/kg/3W-I CCSUDL 1,325,76

SAFETY PROFILE: Questionable carcinogen with experimental neoplastigenic and tumorigenic data by skin contact. When heated to decomposition it emits acrid smoke and irritating fumes.

MEK700 CAS: 865-04-3
**10-METHOXY-11-
DESMETHOXYRESERPINE**
mf: $C_{33}H_{40}N_2O_9$ mw: 608.75

SYNS: CANESCINE 10-METHOXYDERIVATIVE ◇ DEASERPYL ◇ DECASERPIL ◇ DECASERPINE ◇ DECASERPYL ◇ DECASERPYL PLUS ◇ DECOSERPYL ◇ DESERPIDINE, 10-METHOXY- ◇ 10-MD ◇ METHOSER-PEDINE ◇ METHOSERPIDINE ◇ 10-METHOXYDESERPIDINE ◇ MINORAN ◇ R 694 ◇ 3-β,20-α-YOHIMBAN-16-β-CARBOX-YLIC ACID, 18-β-HYDROXY-10,17-α-DIMETHOXY-, METHYL ESTER, 3,4,5-TRIMETHOXYBENZOATE (ester)

TOXICITY DATA and REFERENCE
NEO: orl-wmn TD: 1168 mg/kg/8Y-C LANCAO 2,672,74
NEO: orl-wmn TD: 1752 mg/kg/8Y-C LANCAO 2,672,74
NEO: orl-wmn TDLo: 438 mg/kg/3Y-C LANCAO 2,672,74

SAFETY PROFILE: Questionable human carcinogen producing colon, nose, and skin tumors. Poison by intraperitoneal and intravenous routes. When heated to decomposition it emits toxic fumes of NO_x.

MEK750 CAS: 63019-72-7
5-METHOXYDIBENZ(a,h)ANTHRACENE
mf: $C_{23}H_{16}O$ mw: 308.39

SYNS: 3-METHOXY-DBA ◇ 3-METHOXY-1,2:5,6-DIBEN-ZANTHRACENE

TOXICITY DATA and REFERENCE
ETA: scu-mus TDLo: 80 mg/kg CNREA8 22,78,62
ETA: skn-mus TDLo: 300 mg/kg/30W-I CNREA8 22,78,62

SAFETY PROFILE: Questionable carcinogen with experimental tumorigenic data. When

heated to decomposition it emits acrid smoke and irritating fumes.

MEL000   CAS: 63041-72-5
7-METHOXYDIBENZ(a,h)ANTHRACENE
mf: $C_{23}H_{16}O$ mw: 308.39

SYNS: 9-METHOXY-DBA ◊ 9-METHOXY-1,2,5,6-DIBEN-ZANTHRACENE

TOXICITY DATA and REFERENCE
NEO: skn-mus TDLo:400 mg/kg/40W-I
  CNREA8 22,78,62
ETA: scu-mus TDLo:80 mg/kg   CNREA8 22,78,62
ETA: skn-mus TD:620 mg/kg/26W-I   PRLBA4
  111,485,32
ETA: skn-mus TD:1030 mg/kg/43W-I   PRLBA4
  117,318,35

SAFETY PROFILE: Questionable carcinogen with experimental neoplastigenic and tumorigenic data. When heated to decomposition it emits acrid smoke and irritating fumes.

MEL570
2-METHOXY-7,12-DIMETHYLBENZ(a)ANTHRACENE
mf: $C_{21}H_{18}O$ mw: 286.39

SYN: 2-METHOXY-DMBA

TOXICITY DATA and REFERENCE
CAR: skn-mus TDLo:440 mg/kg/50W-I
  CRNGDP 4,1221,83
MUT: mma-sat 5 μg/plate   CRNGDP 4,1221,83

SAFETY PROFILE: Questionable carcinogen with experimental carcinogenic data. Mutation data reported. When heated to decomposition it emits acrid smoke and irritating fumes.

MEL580
3-METHOXY-7,12-DIMETHYLBENZ(a)ANTHRACENE
mf: $C_{21}H_{18}O$ mw: 286.39

SYN: 3-METHOXY-DMBA

TOXICITY DATA and REFERENCE
ETA: skn-mus TDLo:440 mg/kg/50W-I
  CRNGDP 4,1221,83
MUT: mma-sat 2500 ng/plate   CRNGDP
  4,1221,83

SAFETY PROFILE: Questionable carcinogen with experimental tumorigenic data. Mutation data reported. When heated to decomposition it emits acrid smoke and irritating fumes.

MEL600
4-METHOXY-7,12-DIMETHYLBENZ(a)ANTHRACENE
mf: $C_{21}H_{18}O$ mw: 286.39

SYN: 4-METHOXY-DMBA

TOXICITY DATA and REFERENCE
CAR: skn-mus TDLo:440 mg/kg/50W-I
  CRNGDP 4,1221,83
MUT: mma-sat 5 μg/plate   CRNGDP 4,1221,83

SAFETY PROFILE: Questionable carcinogen with experimental carcinogenic data. Mutation data reported. When heated to decomposition it emits acrid smoke and irritating fumes.

MEN750   CAS: 63020-60-0
3-METHOXY-10-ETHYL-1,2-BENZANTHRACENE
mf: $C_{21}H_8O$ mw: 276.29

SYN: 7-ETHYL-5-METHOXY-BENZ(a)ANTHRACENE

TOXICITY DATA and REFERENCE
NEO: scu-mus TDLo:900 mg/kg   JNCIAM1,303,40

SAFETY PROFILE: Questionable carcinogen with experimental neoplastigenic data. When heated to decomposition it emits acrid smoke and irritating fumes.

MEO000   CAS: 1616-88-2
METHOXYETHYL CARBAMATE
mf: $C_4H_9NO_3$ mw: 119.24

SYNS: 2-METHOXYETHYL ESTER CARBAMIC ACID
◊ N-METHOXYURETHANE

TOXICITY DATA and REFERENCE
ETA: ipr-mus TD:3300 mg/kg/5W-I   IJCNAW
  4,318,69
ETA: ipr-mus TDLo:6600 mg/kg/10W-I
  IJCNAW 4,318,69

CONSENSUS REPORTS: Reported in EPA TSCA Inventory.

SAFETY PROFILE: Questionable carcinogen with experimental tumorigenic data. Mildly toxic by ingestion. A skin irritant. When heated to decomposition it emits toxic fumes of NO_x.

MEO500   CAS: 61738-03-2
1-METHOXY ETHYL ETHYLNITROSAMINE
mf: $C_5H_{12}N_2O_2$ mw: 132.19

SYN: 1-METHOXY-AETHYL-AETHYLNITROSAMIN (GERMAN)

TOXICITY DATA and REFERENCE
CAR: orl-rat TD:800 mg/kg/23W-I ZKKOBW
88,25,76
CAR: orl-rat TDLo:400 mg/kg/23W-I ZKKOBW
88,25,76

SAFETY PROFILE: Questionable carcinogen with experimental carcinogenic data. Moderately toxic by ingestion. When heated to decomposition it emits toxic fumes of NO_x.

MEP500   CAS: 61738-05-4
1-METHOXY ETHYL METHYLNITROSAMINE
mf: $C_4H_{10}N_2O_2$ mw: 118.16

SYN: 1-METHOXY-AETHYL-METHYLNITROSAMIN (GERMAN)

TOXICITY DATA and REFERENCE
CAR: orl-rat TDLo:920 mg/kg/60W-I ZKKOBW
88,25,76

SAFETY PROFILE: Questionable carcinogen with experimental carcinogenic data. Poison by ingestion. When heated to decomposition it emits toxic fumes of NO_x.

MEQ750   CAS: 6893-24-9
1-METHOXY-2-FLUORENAMINE HYDROCHLORIDE
mf: $C_{14}H_{13}NO \cdot ClH$ mw: 247.74

SYN: 1-METHOXYFLUOREN-2-AMINE HYDROCHLORIDE

TOXICITY DATA and REFERENCE
CAR: orl-rat TDLo:3370 mg/kg/23W-C
CNREA8 28,234,68
ETA: ipr-rat TDLo:450 mg/kg/4W-I CNREA8
28,234,68

SAFETY PROFILE: Questionable carcinogen with experimental carcinogenic and tumorigenic data. When heated to decomposition it emits very toxic fumes of Cl^- and NO_x.

MER000   CAS: 6893-20-5
N-(1-METHOXYFLUOREN-2-YL)ACETAMIDE
mf: $C_{16}H_{15}NO_2$ mw: 253.32

SYNS: 1-METHOXY-2-ACETAMIDOFLUORENE ◇ 1-METHOXY-2-FAA ◇ N-(1-METHOXY-2-FLUORENYL)ACETAMIDE

TOXICITY DATA and REFERENCE
CAR: orl-rat TDLo:3300 mg/kg/23W-C
CNREA8 28,234,68

SAFETY PROFILE: Questionable carcinogen with experimental carcinogenic data. When heated to decomposition it emits toxic fumes of NO_x.

MER250   CAS: 16690-44-1
N-(7-METHOXY-2-FLUORENYL)ACETAMIDE
mf: $C_{16}H_{15}NO_2$ mw: 253.32

SYNS: 7-METHOXY-2-FAA ◇ N-(7-METHOXYFLUOREN-2-YL)ACETAMIDE ◇ 7-METHOXY-N-2-FLUORENYL-ACETAMIDE

TOXICITY DATA and REFERENCE
CAR: orl-rat TD:3940 mg/kg/43W-C JNCIAM
24,149,60
CAR: orl-rat TDLo:2740 mg/kg/22W-C
CNREA8 28,234,68

SAFETY PROFILE: Questionable carcinogen with experimental carcinogenic data. When heated to decomposition it emits toxic fumes of NO_x.

MES850   CAS: 3471-31-6
5-METHOXYINDOLEACETIC ACID
mf: $C_{11}H_{11}NO_3$ mw: 205.23

SYNS: METHOXYINDOLEACETIC ACID ◇ 5-METHOXY-INDOLE-3-ACETIC ACID

TOXICITY DATA and REFERENCE
NEO: scu-mus TDLo:4 g/kg/13W-I BEBMAE
101,605,86
ETA: scu-mus TDLo:2 g/kg (10-21D post)
BEBMAE 101,605,86

SAFETY PROFILE: Questionable carcinogen with experimental neoplastigenic and tumorigenic data. Poison by intraperitoneal route. When heated to decomposition it emits toxic fumes of NO_x.

MET875   CAS: 83876-56-6
3-METHOXY-7-METHYLBENZ(c)ACRIDINE
mf: $C_{19}H_{15}NO$ mw: 273.35

SYN: BENZ(c)ACRIDINE, 3-METHOXY-7-METHYL-

TOXICITY DATA and REFERENCE
ETA: scu-mus TDLo:72 mg/kg/12W-I JMCMAR
26,303,83

SAFETY PROFILE: Questionable carcinogen with experimental tumorigenic data. When heated to decomposition it emits toxic fumes of NO_x.

MEU000   CAS: 966-48-3
3-METHOXY-10-METHYL-1,2-BENZANTHRACENE
mf: $C_{20}H_{16}O$ mw: 272.36

SYN: 5-METHOXY-7-METHYL-BENZ(a)ANTHRACENE

TOXICITY DATA and REFERENCE
ETA: scu-mus TDLo:140 mg/kg   JNCIAM
   1,303,40

SAFETY PROFILE: Questionable carcinogen with experimental tumorigenic data. When heated to decomposition it emits acrid smoke and irritating fumes.

MEU250   CAS: 63020-61-1
5-METHOXY-10-METHYL-1,2-BENZANTHRACENE
mf: $C_{20}H_{16}O$ mw: 272.36

SYN: 8-METHOXY-7-METHYL-BENZ(a)ANTHRACENE

TOXICITY DATA and REFERENCE
ETA: scu-mus TDLo:80 mg/kg   CNREA8
   6,454,46

SAFETY PROFILE: Questionable carcinogen with experimental tumorigenic data. When heated to decomposition it emits acrid smoke and irritating fumes.

MEU500   CAS: 16354-47-5
7-METHOXY-12-METHYLBENZ(a)ANTHRACENE
mf: $C_{20}H_{16}O$ mw: 272.36

TOXICITY DATA and REFERENCE
NEO: ims-rat TD:50 mg/kg   PNASA6 58,2253,67
NEO: ims-rat TDLo:50 mg/kg   CNREA8 29,506,69

SAFETY PROFILE: Questionable carcinogen with experimental neoplastigenic data. When heated to decomposition it emits acrid smoke and irritating fumes.

MEU750   CAS: 5831-08-3
3-METHOXY-17-METHYL-15H-CYCLOPENTAPHENANTHRENE
mf: $C_{19}H_{16}O$ mw: 260.35

SYN: 3-METHOXY-17-METHYL 15H-CYCLOPENTA(a)PHE-NANTHRENE

TOXICITY DATA and REFERENCE
ETA: skn-mus TDLo:108 mg/kg/1Y-I   PEXTAR
   11,69,69
MUT: mma-sat 50 µg/plate   CNREA8 36,4525,76

CONSENSUS REPORTS: EPA Genetic Toxicology Program.

SAFETY PROFILE: Questionable carcinogen with experimental tumorigenic data. Mutation data reported. When heated to decomposition it emits acrid smoke and irritating fumes.

MEV000   CAS: 5831-12-9
11-METHOXY-17-METHYL-15H-CYCLOPENTA(a)PHENANTHRENE
mf: $C_{19}H_{16}O$ mw: 260.35

TOXICITY DATA and REFERENCE
CAR: skn-mus TDLo:108 mg/kg/1Y-I   PEXTAR
   11,69,69
MUT: mma-sat 50 µg/plate   CNREA8 36,4525,76

CONSENSUS REPORTS: EPA Genetic Toxicology Program.

SAFETY PROFILE: Questionable carcinogen with experimental carcinogenic data. Mutation data reported. When heated to decomposition it emits acrid smoke and irritating fumes.

MEV250   CAS: 24684-49-9
6-METHOXY-11-METHYL-15,16-DIHYDRO-17H-CYCLOPENTA(a)PHENANTHREN-17-ONE
mf: $C_{19}H_{16}O_2$ mw: 276.35

SYN: 15,16-DIHYDRO-11-METHYL-6-METHOXY-17H-CYCLOPENTA(a)PHENANTHREN-17-ONE

TOXICITY DATA and REFERENCE
NEO: skn-mus TDLo:120 mg/kg/50W-I
   CNREA8 33,832,73
MUT: mma-sat 50 µg/plate   CNREA8
   36,4525,76

CONSENSUS REPORTS: EPA Genetic Toxicology Program.

SAFETY PROFILE: Questionable carcinogen with experimental neoplastigenic data. Mutation data reported. When heated to decomposition it emits acrid smoke and irritating fumes.

MEV750   CAS: 61738-04-3
METHOXYMETHYL ETHYL NITROSAMINE
mf: $C_4H_{10}N_2O_2$ mw: 118.16

SYN: METHOXYMETHYL-AETHYLNITROSAMINE (GERMAN)

TOXICITY DATA and REFERENCE
CAR: orl-rat TD:1890 mg/kg/17W-I   ZKKOBW
   88,25,76

CAR: orl-rat TDLo: 1240 mg/kg/23W-I
ZKKOBW 88,25,76

SAFETY PROFILE: Questionable carcinogen with experimental carcinogenic data. Moderately toxic by ingestion. When heated to decomposition it emits toxic fumes of NO_x.

MEW000   CAS: 13345-60-3
7-METHOXYMETHYL-12-METHYLBENZ(a)ANTHRACENE
mf: $C_{21}H_{18}O$ mw: 286.39

SYN: 9-METHYL-10-METHOXYMETHYL-1,2-BENZANTHRACENE

TOXICITY DATA and REFERENCE
ETA: orl-rat TDLo: 100 mg/kg   JMCMAR 10,932,67
ETA: scu-mus TDLo: 80 mg/kg   CNREA8 6,454,46
ETA: scu-rat TDLo: 150 mg/kg/39D-I   CNREA8 31,1951,71

SAFETY PROFILE: Questionable carcinogen with experimental tumorigenic data. When heated to decomposition it emits acrid smoke and irritating fumes.

MEW250   CAS: 39885-14-8
METHOXYMETHYL METHYLNITROSAMINE
mf: $C_3H_8N_2O_2$ mw: 104.13

SYNS: METHOXYMETHYL-METHYLNITROSAMIN (GERMAN) ◇ METHYL(METHOXYMETHYL)NITROSAMINE ◇ N-NITROSO-N-METHOXYMETHYLMETHYLAMINE

TOXICITY DATA and REFERENCE
CAR: orl-rat TDLo: 1470 mg/kg/50W-I
ZKKOBW 88,25,76
ETA: ipr-rat TDLo: 417 mg/kg   MCEBD4 6,2716,86
ETA: ipr-rat TDLo: 448 mg/kg   PAACA3 16,32,75

SAFETY PROFILE: Questionable carcinogen with experimental carcinogenic and tumorigenic data. Moderately toxic by ingestion and intraperitoneal routes. When heated to decomposition it emits toxic fumes of NO_x.

MEW975   CAS: 86539-71-1
7-METHOXY-1-METHYL-2-NITRONAPHTHO(2,1-b)FURAN
mf: $C_{14}H_{11}NO_4$ mw: 257.26

SYN: R 7372

TOXICITY DATA and REFERENCE
CAR: scu-rat TDLo: 168 mg/kg/42W-I   CALEDQ 35,59,87

MUT: mmo-sat 1 nmol/plate   MUTAEX 1,217,86
MUT: msc-ham: ovr 1 μmol/L   MUTAEX 1,217,86
MUT: oth-esc 1 nmol/tube   MUTAEX 1,217,86

SAFETY PROFILE: Questionable carcinogen with experimental carcinogenic data. Mutation data reported. When heated to decomposition it emits toxic fumes of NO_x.

MFA000   CAS: 3178-03-8
1-METHOXY-2-NAPHTHYLAMINE
mf: $C_{11}H_{11}NO$ mw: 173.23

SYN: 2-AMINO-1-METHOXYNAPHTHALENE

TOXICITY DATA and REFERENCE
CAR: imp-mus TDLo: 100 mg/kg   BMBUAQ 14,147,58

SAFETY PROFILE: Questionable carcinogen with experimental carcinogenic data. When heated to decomposition it emits toxic fumes of NO_x.

MFA250   CAS: 63020-03-1
1-METHOXY-2-NAPHTHYLAMINE HYDROCHLORIDE
mf: $C_{11}H_{11}NO \cdot ClH$ mw: 209.69

SYNS: 1-METHOXY-2-AMINONAPHTHALENE ◇ o-METHYL-2-AMINO-1-NAPHTHOL HYDROCHLORIDE ◇ NEOSONE D ◇ PHENYL-β-NAPHTHALAMINE

TOXICITY DATA and REFERENCE
CAR: imp-mus TDLo: 50 mg/kg   BJCAAI 12,222,58
NEO: scu-mus TDLo: 12500 mg/kg/52W   BJCAAI 10,653,56

SAFETY PROFILE: Questionable carcinogen with experimental neoplastigenic and carcinogenic data. When heated to decomposition it emits very toxic fumes of HCl and NO_x.

MFE250   CAS: 104-01-8
p-METHOXYPHENYLACETIC ACID
mf: $C_9H_{10}O_3$ mw: 166.19

SYNS: ANISYL FORMATE ◇ 2-(p-ANISYL)ACETIC ACID ◇ HOMOANISIC ACID ◇ 4-METHOXYBENZENEACETIC ACID ◇ p-METHOXYBENZYL FORMATE ◇ 4-METHOXY-PHENYLACETIC ACID ◇ MOPA

TOXICITY DATA and REFERENCE
NEO: orl-mus TDLo: 63 g/kg/78W-I   NTIS** PB223-159

CONSENSUS REPORTS: Reported in EPA TSCA Inventory.

SAFETY PROFILE: Questionable carcinogen with experimental neoplastigenic data. Moderately toxic by ingestion and intraperitoneal routes. When heated to decomposition it emits acrid smoke and irritating fumes.

MFF250   CAS: 3647-17-4
N-(p-METHOXYPHENYL)-1-AZIRIDINECARBOXAMIDE
mf: $C_{10}H_{12}N_2O_2$ mw: 192.24

SYNS: 1-(1-AZIRIDINYL)-N-(p-METHOXYPHENYL)FOR-MAMIDE ◇ p-METHOXYPHENYL-N-CARBAMOYLAZIRI-DINE

TOXICITY DATA and REFERENCE
NEO: ipr-mus TDLo: 240 mg/kg/4W-I   CNREA8 29,2184,69

SAFETY PROFILE: Questionable carcinogen with experimental neoplastigenic data. Poison by intravenous route. When heated to decomposition it emits toxic fumes of NO_x.

MFF500   CAS: 3544-23-8
2-METHOXY-4-PHENYLAZOANILINE
mf: $C_{13}H_{13}N_3O$ mw: 227.29

SYNS: 4-AMINO-3-METHOXYAZOBENZENE ◇ 4-(PHENY-LAZO)-o-ANISIDINE

TOXICITY DATA and REFERENCE
CAR: orl-rat TD: 19 g/kg/49W-C   GANNA2 59,131,68
CAR: orl-rat TDLo: 7950 mg/kg/34W-C   CNREA8 21,1068,61
NEO: orl-mus TD: 40320 mg/kg/56W-I   GANNA2 73,136,82
NEO: orl-mus TDLo: 40 g/kg/56W-C   GANNA2 73,136,82
NEO: skn-rat TDLo: 1490 mg/kg/93W-I   CNREA8 26,2406,66
ETA: orl-mus TD: 30 g/kg/56W-C   GANNA2 73,136,82
ETA: orl-mus TD: 30400 mg/kg/56W-I   GANNA2 73,136,82
ETA: orl-rat TD: 8 g/kg/22W-C   GANNA2 59,131,68
ETA: orl-rat TD: 18 g/kg/66W-I   CNREA8 24,1279,64
MUT: dns-mus: lvr 1 μmol/L   GANNA2 72,930,81
MUT: hma-mus/sat 50 mg/kg   JNCIAM 62,911,79
MUT: mma-sat 50 nmol/plate   CALEDQ 8,71,79

CONSENSUS REPORTS: EPA Genetic Toxicology Program.

SAFETY PROFILE: Questionable carcinogen with experimental carcinogenic, neoplastigenic, and tumorigenic data. Mutation data reported. When heated to decomposition it emits toxic fumes of NO_x.

MFF750   CAS: 16143-89-8
2-(p-METHOXYPHENYL)-3,3-DIPHENYLACRYLONITRILE
mf: $C_{22}H_{17}NO$ mw: 311.40

SYN: α-(p-METHOXYPHENYL)-β,β-DIPHENYLACRYLO-NITRILE

TOXICITY DATA and REFERENCE
CAR: scu-mus TDLo: 94 mg/kg/26W-I   MMJJAI 11,95,61
ETA: par-mus TDLo: 320 mg/kg/1Y-I   NNGZAZ 33,53,57

CONSENSUS REPORTS: Cyanide and its compounds are on the Community Right-To-Know List.

SAFETY PROFILE: Questionable carcinogen with experimental carcinogenic and tumorigenic data. When heated to decomposition it emits toxic fumes of NO_x and CN^-

MFG400   CAS: 25355-59-3
1-(p-METHOXYPHENYL)-3-METHYL-3-NITROSOUREA
mf: $C_9H_{11}N_3O_3$ mw: 209.23

SYN: N-METHYL-N′-(p-METHOXYPHENYL)-N-NITRO-SOUREA

TOXICITY DATA and REFERENCE
CAR: skn-mus TDLo: 621 mg/kg/7W-I   CNREA8 44,1027,84
MUT: mmo-sat 33500 pmol/plate   CNREA8 39,5147,79

SAFETY PROFILE: Questionable carcinogen with experimental carcinogenic data. Mutation data reported. When heated to decomposition it emits toxic fumes of NO_x.

MFP500   CAS: 73928-02-6
3-METHOXY-4-STILBENAMINE
mf: $C_{15}H_{15}NO$ mw: 225.31

SYN: 3-METHOXY-4-AMINOSTILBENE

TOXICITY DATA and REFERENCE
ETA: scu-rat TDLo: 250 mg/kg/W-I   BMBUAQ 14,141,58

SAFETY PROFILE: Questionable carcinogen with experimental tumorigenic data. When

heated to decomposition it emits toxic fumes of NO_x.

MFQ750   CAS: 313-96-2
2-METHOXYTRICYCLOQUINAZOLINE
mf: $C_{22}H_{14}N_4O$ mw: 350.40

TOXICITY DATA and REFERENCE
ETA: skn-mus TDLo: 1240 mg/kg/1Y-I   BJCAAI
16,275,62

SAFETY PROFILE: Questionable carcinogen with experimental tumorigenic data. When heated to decomposition it emits toxic fumes of NO_x.

MFR000   CAS: 2642-50-4
3-METHOXYTRICYCLOQUINAZOLINE
mf: $C_{22}H_{14}N_4O$ mw: 350.40

TOXICITY DATA and REFERENCE
NEO: skn-mus TDLo: 1200 mg/kg/50W-I
BCPCA6 14,323,65

SAFETY PROFILE: Questionable carcinogen with experimental neoplastigenic data. When heated to decomposition it emits toxic fumes of NO_x.

MFW500   CAS: 520-45-6
METHYLACETOPYRONONE
mf: $C_8H_8O_4$ mw: 168.16

PROP: White crystals or crystalline powder. Mp: 109°, bp: 269.0°, vap press: 1 mm @ 91.7°, vap d: 5.8. Moderately sol in water and organic solvents.

SYNS: 2-ACETYL-5-HYDROXY-3-OXO-4-HEXENOIC ACID Δ-LACTONE ◇ 3-ACETYL-6-METHYL-2,4-PYRAN-DIONE ◇ 3-ACETYL-6-METHYLPYRANDIONE-2,4 ◇ 3-ACETYL-6-METHYL-2H-PYRAN-2,4(3H)-DIONE ◇ DEHYDRACETIC ACID ◇ DEHYDROACETIC ACID (FCC) ◇ DHA ◇ DHS

TOXICITY DATA and REFERENCE
ETA: scu-rat TDLo: 592 mg/kg/37W-I   BJCAAI
20,134,66

CONSENSUS REPORTS: Reported in EPA TSCA Inventory.

SAFETY PROFILE: Questionable carcinogen with experimental tumorigenic data. Poison by ingestion and intravenous routes. Moderately toxic by intraperitoneal route. Combustible when exposed to heat or flame. When heated to decomposition it emits acrid smoke and irritating fumes.

MFX725   CAS: 72586-67-5
N-METHYL-N'-(p-ACETYLPHENYL)-N-NITROSOUREA
mf: $C_{10}H_{11}N_3O_3$ mw: 221.24

SYN: 1-(p-ACETYLPHENYL)-3-METHYL-3-NITROSOUREA

TOXICITY DATA and REFERENCE
CAR: skn-mus TDLo: 657 mg/kg/7W-I   CNREA8
44,1027,84
MUT: mmo-sat 33500 pmol/plate   CNREA8
39,5147,79

SAFETY PROFILE: Questionable carcinogen with experimental carcinogenic data. Mutation data reported. When heated to decomposition it emits toxic fumes of NO_x.

MGA500   CAS: 96-33-3
METHYL ACRYLATE
DOT: 1919
mf: $C_4H_6O_2$ mw: 86.10

PROP: Colorless liquid; acrid odor. D: 0.9561 @ 20°/4°, mp: −76.5°, bp: 70° @ 608 mm, lel: 2.8%, uel: 25%, fp: −75°, flash p: 27°F (OC), vap press: 100 mm @ 28°, vap d: 2.97, sol in alc and ether.

SYNS: ACRYLATE de METHYLE (FRENCH) ◇ ACRYLIC ACID METHYL ESTER (MAK) ◇ ACRYLSAEUREMETHYLES-TER (GERMAN) ◇ CURITHANE 103 ◇ METHOXYCARBON-YLETHYLENE ◇ METHYLACRYLAAT (DUTCH) ◇ METHYL-ACRYLAT (GERMAN) ◇ METHYL ACRYLATE, INHIBITED (DOT) ◇ METHYL PROPENATE ◇ METHYL PROPENOATE ◇ METHYL-2-PROPENOATE ◇ METILACRILATO (ITALIAN) ◇ PROPENOIC ACID METHYL ESTER ◇ 2-PROPENOIC ACID METHYL ESTER

TOXICITY DATA with REFERENCE
MUT: cyt-ham: lng 6500 μg/L   GMCRDC 27,95,81
MUT: cyt-mus: lym 22 mg/L   ENMUDM 8(Suppl 6),4,86
MUT: mma-mus: lym 22 mg/L   ENMUDM 8(Suppl 6),4,86
MUT: mnt-mus-ipr 37500 μg/kg   MUREAV 135,189,84
MUT: msc-mus: lym 22 mg/L   ENMUDM 8(Suppl 6),4,86

CONSENSUS REPORTS: IARC Cancer Review: GROUP 3 IMEMDT 7,56,87; Animal Inadequate Evidence IMEMDT 39,99,86; Human Inadequate Evidence IMEMDT 19,47,79.

Community Right-To-Know List. Reported in EPA TSCA Inventory.

OSHA PEL: TWA 10 ppm (skin) ACGIH TLV: TWA 10 ppm (skin)   DFG MAK: 5 ppm (18 mg/m³)   DOT Classification: Flammable Liquid; Label: Flammable Liquid.

SAFETY PROFILE: Questionable carcinogen. Poison by ingestion and intraperitoneal routes. Moderately toxic by skin contact. Mildly toxic by inhalation. Human systemic effects by inhalation: olfaction effects, eye effects and respiratory effects. A skin and eye irritant. Mutation data reported. Chronic exposure has produced injury to lungs, liver, and kidneys in experimental animals. Dangerously flammable when exposed to heat, flame or oxidizers. Dangerous explosion hazard in the form of vapor when exposed to heat, sparks, or flame. To fight fire, use foam, CO_2, dry chemical. When heated to decomposition it emits acrid smoke and irritating fumes.

MGE000   CAS: 63019-98-7
3-METHYL-4-AMINOBIPHENYL
mf: $C_{13}H_{13}N$ mw: 183.27

SYN: 3-METHYL-4-AMINODIPHENYL

TOXICITY DATA and REFERENCE
ETA: scu-rat TD: 1600 mg/kg   AICCA6 10,174,54
ETA: scu-rat TDLo: 1200 mg/kg/W-I   BMBUAQ 14,141,58

SAFETY PROFILE: Questionable carcinogen with experimental tumorigenic data. When heated to decomposition it emits toxic fumes of NO_x.

MGF500   CAS: 63019-97-6
2-METHYL-4-AMINODIPHENYL
mf: $C_{13}H_{13}N$ mw: 183.27

SYN: 2-METHYL-4-PHENYLANILINE

TOXICITY DATA and REFERENCE
ETA: scu-rat TDLo: 2400 mg/kg/W-I   BMBUAQ 14,141,58

SAFETY PROFILE: Questionable carcinogen with experimental tumorigenic data. When heated to decomposition it emits toxic fumes of NO_x.

MGF750   CAS: 1204-78-0
4′-METHYL-4-AMINODIPHENYL
mf: $C_{13}H_{13}N$ mw: 183.27

SYN: 4′-METHYLBIPHENYLAMINE

TOXICITY DATA and REFERENCE
ETA: scu-rat TDLo: 10 g/kg/W-I   BMBUAQ 14,141,58

SAFETY PROFILE: Questionable carcinogen with experimental tumorigenic data. When heated to decomposition it emits toxic fumes of NO_x.

MGO000
METHYLANILINE and SODIUM NITRITE (1.2:1)

SYN: SODIUM NITRITE and METHYLANILINE (1:1.2)

TOXICITY DATA and REFERENCE
CAR: orl-mus TDLo: 81 g/kg/28W-C   JNCIAM 46,1029,71

SAFETY PROFILE: Questionable carcinogen with experimental carcinogenic data. When heated to decomposition it emits toxic fumes of NO_x.

MGO250
N-METHYLANILINE mixed with SODIUM NITRITE (1:35)

SYNS: N-METHYLANILIN UND NATRIUMNITRIT (GERMAN) ◊ NATRIUMNITRAT UND N-METHYLANILIN (GERMAN) ◊ SODIUM NITRITE mixed with N-METHYLANILINE (35:1)

TOXICITY DATA and REFERENCE
CAR: orl-rat TDLo: 124 g/kg/16W-C   ARZNAD 21,1572,71

SAFETY PROFILE: Questionable carcinogen with experimental carcinogenic data. When heated to decomposition it emits toxic fumes of NO_x.

MGP250   CAS: 31927-64-7
6-METHYLANTHANTHRENE
mf: $C_{23}H_{14}$ mw: 290.37

SYN: 12-METHYL DIBENZO(def,mno)CHRYSENE

TOXICITY DATA and REFERENCE
ETA: scu-mus TDLo: 72 mg/kg/9W-I   COREAF 246,1477,58

SAFETY PROFILE: Questionable carcinogen with experimental tumorigenic data. When heated to decomposition it emits acrid smoke and irritating fumes.

MGP750   CAS: 779-02-2
9-METHYLANTHRACENE
mf: $C_{15}H_{12}$ mw: 192.27

TOXICITY DATA and REFERENCE
ETA: ipr-mus TDLo: 11 mg/kg   CANCAR 14,308,61
MUT: dnd-esc 10 μmol/L   PNCCA2 5,39,65
MUT: dnd-mam: lym 100 μmol   BIPMAA 9,689,70
MUT: mma-sat 5 μg/plate   MUREAV 156,61,85
MUT: msc-hmn: lym 9 μmol/L   DTESD7 10,277,82

CONSENSUS REPORTS: Reported in EPA TSCA Inventory.

SAFETY PROFILE: Questionable carcinogen with experimental tumorigenic data. Human mutation data reported. When heated to decomposition it emits acrid smoke and irritating fumes.

MGS500   CAS: 11069-34-4
METHYL-AZOXY-BUTANE
mf: $C_5H_{12}N_2O$ mw: 116.19

TOXICITY DATA and REFERENCE
ETA: scu-rat TDLo: 2130 mg/kg/71W-I
PPTCBY 2,73,72

SAFETY PROFILE: Questionable carcinogen with experimental tumorigenic data. Poison by an unspecified route. When heated to decomposition it emits toxic fumes of NO_x.

MGS700   CAS: 71856-48-9
METHYLAZOXYMETHANOL-β-D-GLUCOSIDURONIC ACID
mf: $C_8H_{14}N_2O_8$ mw: 266.24

SYNS: β-D-GLUCOPYRANOSIDURONIC ACID, (METHYL-ONN-AZOXY)METHYL- ◇ (METHYL-ONN-AZOXY)ME-THYL-β-D-GLUCOPYRANOSIDURONIC ACID

TOXICITY DATA and REFERENCE
CAR: orl-rat TD: 282 mg/kg/4W-I   JJIND8 67,1053,81
CAR: orl-rat TDLo: 71 mg/kg   JJIND8 67,1053,81
MUT: mma-sat 20 nmol/plate   CNREA8 39,3780,79

SAFETY PROFILE: Questionable carcinogen with experimental carcinogenic data. Mutation data reported. When heated to decomposition it emits toxic fumes of NO_x.

MGS925   CAS: 3527-05-7
METHYLAZOXYMETHYL BENZOATE
mf: $C_9H_{10}N_2O_3$ mw: 194.21

SYN: METHANOL, (METHYL-ONN-AZOXY)-, BENZOATE (ester) (9CI)

TOXICITY DATA and REFERENCE
ETA: orl-rat TDLo: 250 mg/kg/4W-I   IGKEAO
44,211,74

ETA: scu-rat TDLo: 125 mg/kg/2W-I   IGKEAO
44,211,74

SAFETY PROFILE: Questionable carcinogen with experimental tumorigenic data. When heated to decomposition it emits toxic fumes of NO_x.

MGT000   CAS: 54405-61-7
METHYLAZOXYOCTANE
mf: $C_9H_{20}N_2O$ mw: 172.31

SYNS: METHYLOCTYLDIAZENE 1-OXIDE ◇ OCTANE-1-NNO-AZOXYMETHANE

TOXICITY DATA and REFERENCE
CAR: ipr-mus TDLo: 2450 mg/kg/14W-I
JNCIAM 53,1181,74

SAFETY PROFILE: Questionable carcinogen with experimental carcinogenic data. When heated to decomposition it emits toxic fumes of NO_x.

MGT250   CAS: 28390-42-3
METHYL-AZULENO(5,6,7-c,d) PHENALENE
mf: $C_{21}H_{14}$ mw: 266.35

TOXICITY DATA and REFERENCE
ETA: scu-mus TDLo: 80 mg/kg/4W-I   NATWAY
57,499,70

SAFETY PROFILE: Questionable carcinogen with experimental tumorigenic data. When heated to decomposition it emits acrid smoke and irritating fumes.

MGT400
3-METHYLBENZ(e) ACEPHENANTHRYLENE
mf: $C_{21}H_{14}$ mw: 266.35

SYN: 3-METHYLBENZO(b)FLUORANTHENE

TOXICITY DATA and REFERENCE
ETA: skn-mus TDLo: 4262 μg/kg/20D-I
CRNGDP 6,1023,85
MUT: mma-sat 125 nmol/plate   CRNGDP
6,1023,85

SAFETY PROFILE: Questionable carcinogen with experimental tumorigenic data. Mutation data reported. When heated to decomposition it emits acrid smoke and irritating fumes.

MGT410
7-METHYLBENZ(e) ACEPHENANTHRYLENE
mf: $C_{21}H_{14}$ mw: 266.35

SYN: 7-METHYLBENZO(b)FLUORANTHENE

TOXICITY DATA and REFERENCE
ETA: skn-mus TDLo:426 μg/kg/20D-I
  CRNGDP 6,1023,85

SAFETY PROFILE: Questionable carcinogen
with experimental tumorigenic data. When
heated to decomposition it emits acrid smoke
and irritating fumes.

MGT415
8-METHYLBENZ(e)
ACEPHENANTHRYLENE
mf: $C_{21}H_{14}$ mw: 266.35

SYN: 8-METHYLBENZO(b)FLUORANTHENE

TOXICITY DATA and REFERENCE
ETA: skn-mus TDLo:426 μg/kg/20D-I
  CRNGDP 6,1023,85

SAFETY PROFILE: Questionable carcinogen
with experimental tumorigenic data. When
heated to decomposition it emits acrid smoke
and irritating fumes.

MGT420
12-METHYLBENZ(e)
ACEPHENANTHRYLENE
mf: $C_{21}H_{14}$ mw: 266.35

SYN: 12-METHYLBENZO(b)FLUORANTHENE

TOXICITY DATA and REFERENCE
ETA: skn-mus TDLo:1065 μg/kg/20D-I
  CRNGDP 6,1023,85

SAFETY PROFILE: Questionable carcinogen
with experimental tumorigenic data. When
heated to decomposition it emits acrid smoke
and irritating fumes.

MGT500   CAS: 3340-94-1
7-METHYLBENZ(c)ACRIDINE
mf: $C_{18}H_{13}N$ mw: 243.32

SYNS: 9-METHYL-3,4-BENZACRIDINE ◇ 10-METHYL-7,8-
BENZACRIDINE (FRENCH) ◇ 7-METHYLBENZO(c)ACRI-
DINE

TOXICITY DATA and REFERENCE
ETA: scu-mus TDLo:200 mg/kg   VOONAW
  1,52,55
ETA: skn-mus TDLo:240 mg/kg/20W-I
  ACRSAJ 4,315,56
MUT: mma-ham:lng 1 μmol/L   CRNGDP 7,23,86
MUT: mma-sat 100 μg/plate   MUREAV 66,307,79

MUT: sce-ham:lng 5 μmol/L   CRNGDP 7,23,86

SAFETY PROFILE: Questionable carcinogen
with experimental tumorigenic data. Mutation
data reported. When heated to decomposition
it emits toxic fumes of NO_x.

MGU500   CAS: 3340-93-0
12-METHYLBENZ(a)ACRIDINE
mf: $C_{18}H_{13}N$ mw: 243.32

SYNS: 9-METHYL-1,2-BENZACRIDINE ◇ 10-METHYL-5,6-
BENZACRIDINE

TOXICITY DATA and REFERENCE
ETA: scu-mus TDLo:200 mg/kg   VOONAW
  1,52,55

SAFETY PROFILE: Questionable carcinogen
with experimental tumorigenic data. When
heated to decomposition it emits toxic fumes
of NO_x.

MGU550   CAS: 92145-26-1
7-METHYLBENZ(c)ACRIDINE 3,4-
DIHYDRODIOL
mf: $C_{18}H_{15}NO_2$ mw: 277.34

SYNS: trans-3,4-DIHYDRO-3,4-DIHYDROXY-7-METHYL-
BENZ(c)ACRIDINE ◇ trans-3,4-DIHYDROXY-3,4-DIHYDRO-
7-METHYLBENZ(c)ACRIDINE

TOXICITY DATA and REFERENCE
NEO: ipr-mus TDLo:3883 μg/kg   CNREA8
  46,4552,86
MUT: mma-sat nmol/plate   CRNGDP 7,23,86
MUT: sce-ham:lng 5 μmol/L   CRNGDP 7,23,86

SAFETY PROFILE: Questionable carcinogen
with experimental neoplastigenic data. Mutation
data reported. When heated to decomposition
it emits acrid smoke and irritating fumes.

MGU750   CAS: 2498-77-3
1-METHYLBENZ(a)ANTHRACENE
mf: $C_{19}H_{14}$ mw: 242.33

SYN: 1'-METHYL-1,2-BENZANTHRACENE

TOXICITY DATA and REFERENCE
ETA: scu-mus TDLo:200 mg/kg   AIHAAP
  26,475,65
ETA: scu-rat TDLo:18 mg/kg   JNCIAM 25,387,60
MUT: mma-sat 20 μg/plate   CNREA8 36,4525,76

CONSENSUS REPORTS: EPA Genetic Toxicology Program.

SAFETY PROFILE: Questionable carcinogen
with experimental tumorigenic data. Mutation

data reported. When heated to decomposition it emits acrid smoke and irritating fumes.

MGV000   CAS: 2498-76-2
2-METHYLBENZ(a)ANTHRACENE
mf: $C_{19}H_{14}$ mw: 242.33

SYN: 2'-METHYL-1,2-BENZANTHRACENE

TOXICITY DATA and REFERENCE
ETA: scu-mus TDLo:200 mg/kg   AIHAAP 26,475,65
ETA: skn-mus TDLo:210 mg/kg/33W-I
CNREA8 11,892,51
MUT: dnd-omi 1800 μmol/L   ZKKOBW 90,37,77
MUT: mma-sat 10 μg/plate   CNREA8 36,4525,76

SAFETY PROFILE: Questionable carcinogen with experimental tumorigenic data. Mutation data reported. When heated to decomposition it emits acrid smoke and irritating fumes.

MGV250   CAS: 2498-75-1
3-METHYLBENZ(a)ANTHRACENE
mf: $C_{19}H_{14}$ mw: 242.33

TOXICITY DATA and REFERENCE
ETA: scu-mus TDLo:200 mg/kg   AIHAAP 26,475,65
MUT: mma-sat 5 μg/plate   CNREA8 36,4525,76

CONSENSUS REPORTS: EPA Genetic Toxicology Program.

SAFETY PROFILE: Questionable carcinogen with experimental tumorigenic data. Mutation data reported. When heated to decomposition it emits acrid smoke and irritating fumes.

MGV500   CAS: 316-49-4
4-METHYLBENZ(a)ANTHRACENE
mf: $C_{19}H_{14}$ mw: 242.33

SYN: 4'-METHYL-1:2-BENZANTHRACENE

TOXICITY DATA and REFERENCE
ETA: imp-mus TDLo:80 mg/kg   JNCIAM 2,241,41
ETA: scu-rat TDLo:18 mg/kg   JNCIAM 25,387,60
ETA: skn-mus TDLo:2100 mg/kg/89W-I
PRLBA4 129,439,40
MUT: mma-sat 20 μg/plate   CNREA8 36,4525,76

CONSENSUS REPORTS: EPA Genetic Toxicology Program.

SAFETY PROFILE: Questionable carcinogen with experimental tumorigenic data. Mutation data reported. When heated to decomposition it emits acrid smoke and irritating fumes.

MGV750   CAS: 2319-96-2
5-METHYLBENZ(a)ANTHRACENE
mf: $C_{19}H_{14}$ mw: 242.33

SYN: 3-METHYL-1,2-BENZANTHRACENE

TOXICITY DATA and REFERENCE
ETA: scu-mus TD:200 mg/kg   AIHAAP 26,475,65
ETA: scu-mus TD:1360 mg/kg/20W-I   PRLBA4 129,439,40
ETA: scu-mus TDLo:72 mg/kg/9W-I   BAFEAG 49,312,62
ETA: scu-rat TDLo:18 mg/kg   JNCIAM 25,387,60
ETA: skn-mus TDLo:1750 mg/kg/73W-I
PRLBA4 129,439,40
MUT: mma-sat 10 μg/plate   CNREA8 36,4525,76

CONSENSUS REPORTS: EPA Genetic Toxicology Program.

SAFETY PROFILE: Questionable carcinogen with experimental tumorigenic data. Mutation data reported. When heated to decomposition it emits acrid smoke and irritating fumes.

MGW000   CAS: 316-14-3
6-METHYLBENZ(a)ANTHRACENE
mf: $C_{19}H_{14}$ mw: 242.33

SYN: 4-METHYL-1,2-BENZANTHRACENE

TOXICITY DATA and REFERENCE
CAR: scu-mus TDLo:200 mg/kg   AIHAAP 26,475,65
ETA: scu-mus TD:72 mg/kg/9W-I   BAFEAG 49,312,62
ETA: scu-rat TDLo:18 mg/kg   JNCIAM 25,387,60
ETA: skn-mus TDLo:1080 mg/kg/45W-I
PRLBA4 117,318,35
MUT: mma-sat 10 μg/plate   CNREA8 36,4525,76

CONSENSUS REPORTS: EPA Genetic Toxicology Program.

SAFETY PROFILE: Questionable carcinogen with experimental carcinogenic and tumorigenic data. Mutation data reported. When heated to decomposition it emits acrid smoke and irritating fumes.

MGW250   CAS: 2381-31-9
8-METHYLBENZ(a)ANTHRACENE
mf: $C_{19}H_{14}$ mw: 242.33

SYN: 5-METHYL-1,2-BENZANTHRACENE

TOXICITY DATA and REFERENCE
CAR: scu-mus TDLo:200 mg/kg   AIHAAP 26,475,65

ETA: scu-mus TD: 200 mg/kg AJCAA7 33,499,38
ETA: scu-rat TDLo: 18 mg/kg JNCIAM 25,387,60
ETA: skn-mus TDLo: 1250 mg/kg/52W-I
 PRLBA4 117,318,35
MUT: mma-sat 20 µg/plate CNREA8 36,4525,76

CONSENSUS REPORTS: EPA Genetic Toxicology Program.

SAFETY PROFILE: Questionable carcinogen with experimental carcinogenic and tumorigenic data. Mutation data reported. When heated to decomposition it emits acrid smoke and irritating fumes.

MGW500   CAS: 2381-16-0
9-METHYLBENZ(a)ANTHRACENE
mf: $C_{19}H_{14}$ mw: 242.33

SYN: 6-METHYL-1,2-BENZANTHRACENE

TOXICITY DATA and REFERENCE
ETA: scu-mus TDLo: 200 mg/kg AIHAAP
 26,475,65
ETA: scu-rat TDLo: 18 mg/kg JNCIAM 25,387,60
ETA: skn-mus TD: 1250 mg/kg/52W-I PRLBA4
 117,318,35
ETA: skn-mus TDLo: 860 mg/kg/43W-I
 JPBAA7 57,467,45
MUT: mma-sat 20 µg/plate CNREA8 36,4525,76

CONSENSUS REPORTS: EPA Genetic Toxicology Program.

SAFETY PROFILE: Questionable carcinogen with experimental tumorigenic data. Mutation data reported. When heated to decomposition it emits acrid smoke and irritating fumes.

MGW750   CAS: 2541-69-7
10-METHYL-1,2-BENZANTHRACENE
mf: $C_{19}H_{14}$ mw: 242.33

SYNS: 7-MBA ◇ 10-METHYL-1,2-BENZANTHRACEN (GERMAN) ◇ 7-METHYLBENZ(a)ANTHRACENE

TOXICITY DATA and REFERENCE
CAR: scu-mus TDLo: 200 mg/kg AIHAAP
 26,475,65
NEO: scu-mus TD: 10 mg/kg CNREA8 23,229,63
NEO: scu-mus TD: 40 mg/kg CNREA8 23,229,63
NEO: scu-mus TD: 40 mg/kg PSEBAA 124,915,67
NEO: scu-mus TD: 400 mg/kg/10W-I IJCNAW
 2,500,67
NEO: scu-rat TD: 8 mg/kg CNREA8 23,229,63
NEO: scu-rat TDLo: 8 mg/kg PSEBAA 124,915,67
NEO: skn-mus TD: 112 mg/kg/20W-I CNREA8
 23,229,63

NEO: skn-mus TD: 1000 µg/kg CALEDQ 3,247,77
NEO: skn-mus TDLo: 112 mg/kg/20W-I
 PSEBAA 124,915,67
ETA: orl-rat TDLo: 1000 mg/kg SCIEAS
 137,257,62
ETA: scu-mus TD: 2 mg/kg JNCIAM 1,45,40
ETA: scu-rat TD: 18 mg/kg JNCIAM 25,387,60
ETA: skn-mus TD: 360 mg/kg/15W-I PRLBA4
 129,439,40
MUT: dnd-mus-skn 40 µmol/kg IJCNAW
 23,201,69
MUT: msc-ham: fbr 1 mg/L DTESD7 8,121,80
MUT: sce-ham: ovr 8 mg/L MUREAV 50,367,78

CONSENSUS REPORTS: EPA Genetic Toxicology Program.

SAFETY PROFILE: Questionable carcinogen with experimental carcinogenic, neoplastigenic, and tumorigenic data. Mutation data reported. When heated to decomposition it emits acrid smoke and irritating fumes.

MGX000   CAS: 2381-15-9
10-METHYLBENZ(a)ANTHRACENE
mf: $C_{19}H_{14}$ mw: 242.33

SYN: 7-METHYL-1,2-BENZANTHRACENE

TOXICITY DATA and REFERENCE
ETA: scu-mus TD: 2900 mg/kg/44W-I PRLBA4
 129,439,40
ETA: scu-mus TDLo: 880 mg/kg/35W-I
 AJCAA7 33,499,38
ETA: scu-rat TD: 19 mg/kg SCPHA4 22,224,54
ETA: scu-rat TDLo: 18 mg/kg JNCIAM 25,387,60
ETA: skn-mus TDLo: 1920 mg/kg/80W-I
 PRLBA4 129,439,40
MUT: mma-sat 10 µg/plate CNREA8 36,4525,76
MUT: otr-ham: emb 10 mg/L JNCIAM 35,641,65

CONSENSUS REPORTS: EPA Genetic Toxicology Program.

SAFETY PROFILE: Questionable carcinogen with experimental tumorigenic data. Mutation data reported. When heated to decomposition it emits acrid smoke and irritating fumes.

MGX250   CAS: 6111-78-0
11-METHYLBENZ(a)ANTHRACENE
mf: $C_{19}H_{14}$ mw: 242.33

SYN: 8-METHYL-1:2-BENZANTHRACENE

TOXICITY DATA and REFERENCE
CAR: scu-mus TDLo: 200 mg/kg AIHAAP
 26,475,65

ETA: skn-mus TDLo:1180 mg/kg/49W-I
PRLBA4 129,439,40

MUT: mma-sat 50 µg/plate   CNREA8 36,4525,76

CONSENSUS REPORTS: EPA Genetic Toxicology Program.

SAFETY PROFILE: Questionable carcinogen with carcinogenic and tumorigenic data. Mutation data reported. When heated to decomposition it emits acrid smoke and irritating fumes.

MGX500   CAS: 2422-79-9
12-METHYLBENZ(a)ANTHRACENE
mf: $C_{19}H_{14}$ mw: 242.33

SYN: 9-METHYL-1,2-BENZANTHRACENE

TOXICITY DATA and REFERENCE
CAR: scu-mus TDLo:200 mg/kg   AIHAAP
26,475,65

ETA: orl-rat TDLo:1000 mg/kg   SCIEAS
137,257,62

ETA: scu-mus TD:140 mg/kg/70D-I   AJCAA7
33,499,38

ETA: scu-rat TDLo:18 mg/kg   JNCIAM 25,387,60

ETA: skn-mus TDLo:900 mg/kg/38W-I
PRLBA4 129,439,40

MUT: mma-sat 20 µg/plate   CNREA8 36,4525,76

CONSENSUS REPORTS: EPA Genetic Toxicology Program.

SAFETY PROFILE: Questionable carcinogen with experimental carcinogenic and tumorigenic data. Mutation data reported. When heated to decomposition it emits acrid smoke and irritating fumes.

MGX750   CAS: 64082-43-5
10-METHYL-1,2-BENZANTHRACENE-5-CARBONAMIDE
mf: $C_{20}H_{15}NO$ mw: 285.36

SYN: 7-METHYLBENZ(a)ANTHRACEN-8-YL CARBAMIDE

TOXICITY DATA and REFERENCE
ETA: scu-mus TDLo:4 mg/kg   JNCIAM 1,45,40

SAFETY PROFILE: Questionable carcinogen with experimental tumorigenic data. When heated to decomposition it emits toxic fumes of NO_x.

MGY000   CAS: 63018-70-2
7-METHYLBENZ(a)ANTHRACENE-8-CARBONITRILE
mf: $NC_{20}H_{13}$ mw: 267.34

SYNS: 5-CYANO-10-METHYL-1,2-BENZANTHRACENE
◇ 8-CYANO-7-METHYLBENZ(a)ANTHRACINE

TOXICITY DATA and REFERENCE
ETA: scu-mus TDLo:200 mg/kg   JNCIAM
1,303,40

CONSENSUS REPORTS: Cyanide and its compounds are on the Community Right-To-Know List.

SAFETY PROFILE: Questionable carcinogen with experimental tumorigenic data. When heated to decomposition it emits toxic fumes of NO_x and CN^-.

MGY250   CAS: 6366-23-0
7-METHYLBENZ(a)ANTHRACENE-10-CARBONITRILE
mf: $C_{20}H_{13}N$ mw: 267.34

SYN: 7-CYANO-10-METHYL-1,2-BENZANTHRACENE

TOXICITY DATA and REFERENCE
ETA: scu-mus TDLo:400 mg/kg   JNCIAM
1,303,40

CONSENSUS REPORTS: Cyanide and its compounds are on the Community Right-To-Know List.

SAFETY PROFILE: Questionable carcinogen with experimental tumorigenic data. When heated to decomposition it emits toxic fumes of NO_x and CN^-.

MGY500   CAS: 17513-40-5
7-METHYLBENZ(a)ANTHRACENE-12-CARBOXALDEHYDE
mf: $C_{20}H_{14}O$ mw: 270.34

SYN: 12-FORMYL-7-METHYLBENZ(a)ANTHRACENE

TOXICITY DATA and REFERENCE
NEO: skn-mus TDLo:8000 mg/kg   JJIND8
61,135,78

MUT: dni-omi 200 µg/L   PNASA6 74,1378,77

SAFETY PROFILE: Questionable carcinogen with experimental neoplastigenic data. Mutation data reported. When heated to decomposition it emits acrid smoke and irritating fumes.

MGZ000   CAS: 1155-38-0
7-METHYLBENZ(a)ANTHRACENE-5,6-OXIDE
mf: $C_{19}H_{14}O$ mw: 258.33

SYN: 5,6-EPOXY-5,6-DIHYDRO-7-METHYLBENZ(A) ANTHRACENE

TOXICITY DATA and REFERENCE
NEO: scu-mus TDLo:400 mg/kg/10W-I
  IJCNAW 2,500,67
ETA: scu-mus TD:43 mg/kg   PSEBAA 124,915,67
ETA: skn-mus TDLo:120 mg/kg/20W-I
  PSEBAA 124,915,67
MUT: dnd-mam:lym 2 mg   CBINA8 14,13,76
MUT: dnr-esc 100 μmol/L   ZKKOBW 92,157,78
MUT: dns-esc 1 mmol/L   ZKKOBW 92,157,78
MUT: mma-sat 500 ng/plate   CNREA8 45,2600,85

CONSENSUS REPORTS: EPA Genetic Toxicology Program.

SAFETY PROFILE: Questionable carcinogen with experimental neoplastigenic and tumorigenic data. Mutation data reported. When heated to decomposition it emits acrid smoke and irritating fumes.

MHA000   CAS: 66964-37-2
S-(12-METHYL-7-BENZ(a) ANTHRYLMETHYL)HOMOCYSTEINE
mf: $C_{24}H_{23}NO_2S$ mw: 389.54

TOXICITY DATA and REFERENCE
ETA: ivn-mus TDLo:5800 mg/kg   JMCMAR
  19,1422,76

SAFETY PROFILE: Questionable carcinogen with experimental tumorigenic data. When heated to decomposition it emits very toxic fumes of NO_x and SO_x.

MHD000   CAS: 21064-50-6
6-METHYL-3,4-BENZOCARBAZOLE
mf: $C_{17}H_{13}N$ mw: 231.31

SYN: 10-METHYL-7H-BENZO(c)CARBAZOLE

TOXICITY DATA and REFERENCE
ETA: scu-mus TDLo:120 mg/kg/9W-I   BAFEAG
  42,3,55

SAFETY PROFILE: Questionable carcinogen with experimental tumorigenic data. When heated to decomposition it emits toxic fumes of NO_x.

MHD250   CAS: 13127-50-9
9-METHYL-1:2-BENZOCARBAZOLE
mf: $C_{17}H_{13}N$ mw: 231.31

SYN: 11-METHYL-11H-BENZO(a)CARBAZOLE

TOXICITY DATA and REFERENCE
ETA: skn-mus TDLo:400 mg/kg/17W-I
  CRSBAW 141,635,47

SAFETY PROFILE: Questionable carcinogen with experimental tumorigenic data. When heated to decomposition it emits toxic fumes of NO_x.

MHE250   CAS: 33942-88-0
5-METHYLBENZO(rat)PENTAPHENE
mf: $C_{25}H_{16}$ mw: 316.41

SYN: 5-METHYL-3,4,9,10-DIBENZPYRENE (FRENCH)

TOXICITY DATA and REFERENCE
ETA: scu-mus TDLo:72 mg/kg/9W-I   COREAF
  244,273,57

SAFETY PROFILE: Questionable carcinogen with experimental tumorigenic data. When heated to decomposition it emits acrid smoke and irritating fumes.

MHE500   CAS: 41699-09-6
METHYL-1,12-BENZOPERYLENE
mf: $C_{23}H_{14}$ mw: 290.37

TOXICITY DATA and REFERENCE
ETA: scu-mus TDLo:24 mg/kg   COREAF
  245,991,57

SAFETY PROFILE: Questionable carcinogen with experimental tumorigenic data. When heated to decomposition it emits acrid smoke and irritating fumes.

MHE750   CAS: 1492-55-3
7-METHYLBENZO(a)PHENALENO (1,9-hi)ACRIDINE
mf: $C_{28}H_{17}N$ mw: 367.46

SYN: 7-METHYL-BENZO(a)PHENALENO(1,9-hi)ACRIDINE

TOXICITY DATA and REFERENCE
ETA: scu-mus TDLo:72 mg/kg/9W-I   BAFEAG
  52,49,65

SAFETY PROFILE: Questionable carcinogen with experimental tumorigenic data. When heated to decomposition it emits toxic fumes of NO_x.

MHF000   CAS: 1492-54-2
7-METHYLBENZO(h)PHENALENO (1,9-bc)ACRIDINE
mf: $C_{28}H_{17}N$ mw: 367.46

TOXICITY DATA and REFERENCE
ETA: scu-mus TDLo:72 mg/kg/9W-I   BAFEAG
  52,49,65

SAFETY PROFILE: Questionable carcinogen with experimental tumorigenic data. When

heated to decomposition it emits toxic fumes of NO_x.

MHF250   CAS: 652-04-0
5-METHYLBENZO(c)PHENANTHRENE
mf: $C_{19}H_{14}$ mw: 242.33

SYN: 2-METHYL-3,4-BENZPHENANTHRENE

TOXICITY DATA and REFERENCE
NEO: ivn-mus TDLo: 10 mg/kg   JNCIAM 1,225,40
ETA: orl-mus TDLo: 10 g/kg/51W-I   PRLBA4
   129,439,40
ETA: scu-mus TDLo: 1800 mg/kg/27W-I
   PRLBA4 129,439,40
ETA: skn-mus TDLo: 480 mg/kg/17W-I
   PRLBA4 123,343,37

SAFETY PROFILE: Questionable carcinogen with experimental neoplastigenic and tumorigenic data. When heated to decomposition it emits acrid smoke and irritating fumes.

MHF500   CAS: 2381-34-2
6-METHYLBENZO(c)PHENANTHRENE
mf: $C_{19}H_{14}$ mw: 242.33

SYN: 1-METHYL-3,4-BENZPHENANTHRENE

TOXICITY DATA and REFERENCE
ETA: skn-mus TDLo: 720 mg/kg/30W-I
   PRLBA4 129,439,40

SAFETY PROFILE: Questionable carcinogen with experimental tumorigenic data. When heated to decomposition it emits acrid smoke and irritating fumes.   ☼

MHG250   CAS: 40568-90-9
1-METHYLBENZO(a)PYRENE
mf: $C_{21}H_{14}$ mw: 266.35

SYN: 1-METHYL-BP

TOXICITY DATA and REFERENCE
NEO: skn-mus TDLo: 2130 µg/kg   CNREA8
   40,1073,80

SAFETY PROFILE: Questionable carcinogen with experimental neoplastigenic data. When heated to decomposition it emits acrid smoke and irritating fumes.

MHG500   CAS: 16757-82-7
2-METHYLBENZO(a)PYRENE
mf: $C_{21}H_{14}$ mw: 266.35

SYN: 9-METHYL-3,4-BENZPYRENE

TOXICITY DATA and REFERENCE
ETA: scu-mus TDLo: 72 mg/kg/13W-I   IJCNAW
   3,238,68

SAFETY PROFILE: Questionable carcinogen with experimental tumorigenic data. When heated to decomposition it emits acrid smoke and irritating fumes.

MHG750   CAS: 16757-83-8
4-METHYLBENZO(a)PYRENE
mf: $C_{21}H_{14}$ mw: 266.35

TOXICITY DATA and REFERENCE
ETA: scu-mus TDLo: 72 mg/kg/13W-I   IJCNAW
   3,238,68

SAFETY PROFILE: Questionable carcinogen with experimental tumorigenic data. When heated to decomposition it emits acrid smoke and irritating fumes.

MHH000   CAS: 63041-77-0
4'-METHYLBENZO(a)PYRENE
mf: $C_{21}H_{14}$ mw: 266.35

SYNS: 7-METHYLBENZO(a)PYRENE ◇ 4'-METHYL-3:4-BENZPYRENE

TOXICITY DATA and REFERENCE
NEO: ims-rat TDLo: 4 mg/kg   NATUAS 273,566,78
NEO: ivn-mus TDLo: 10 mg/kg   JNCIAM 1,225,40
ETA: imp-mus TDLo: 400 mg/kg   AJCAA7
   36,211,39
MUT: msc-ham: lng 500 nmol/L   CRNGDP4,321,83

SAFETY PROFILE: Questionable carcinogen with experimental neoplastigenic and tumorigenic data. Mutation data reported. When heated to decomposition it emits acrid smoke and irritating fumes.

MHH200   CAS: 31647-36-6
5-METHYLBENZO(a)PYRENE
mf: $C_{21}H_{14}$ mw: 266.35
SYN: 5-METHYL-BP

TOXICITY DATA and REFERENCE
NEO: skn-mus TDLo: 2130 µg/kg   CNREA8
   40,1073,80
MUT: mma-sat 25 µg/plate   CNREA8 47,1509,87

SAFETY PROFILE: Questionable carcinogen with experimental neoplastigenic data. Mutation data reported. When heated to decomposition it emits acrid smoke and irritating fumes.

MHH500   CAS: 63104-32-5
10-METHYLBENZO(a)PYRENE
mf: $C_{21}H_{14}$ mw: 266.35

SYN: 10-MONOMETHYLBENZO(a)PYRENE

TOXICITY DATA and REFERENCE
NEO: ims-rat TDLo: 10 mg/kg   NATUAS 273,566,78
ETA: skn-mus TDLo: 2000 μg/kg/20D-I
  CALEDQ 5,179,78
MUT: mma-sat 2900 pmol/plate   BBRCA9
  85,351,78

SAFETY PROFILE: Questionable carcinogen with experimental neoplastigenic and tumorigenic data. Mutation data reported. When heated to decomposition it emits acrid smoke and irritating fumes.

MHH750   CAS: 16757-80-5
11-METHYLBENZO(a)PYRENE
mf: $C_{21}H_{14}$ mw: 266.35

SYN: 6-METHYL-3,4-BENZPYRENE

TOXICITY DATA and REFERENCE
ETA: scu-mus TDLo: 72 mg/kg/13W-I   IJCNAW
  3,238,68
MUT: msc-ham: lng 500 nmol/L   CRNGDP 4,321,83

SAFETY PROFILE: Questionable carcinogen with experimental tumorigenic data. Mutation data reported. When heated to decomposition it emits acrid smoke and irritating fumes.

MHI000   CAS: 4514-19-6
12-METHYLBENZO(a)PYRENE
mf: $C_{21}H_{14}$ mw: 266.35

TOXICITY DATA and REFERENCE
ETA: scu-mus TDLo: 72 mg/kg/13W-I   IJCNAW
  3,238,68

SAFETY PROFILE: Questionable carcinogen with experimental tumorigenic data. When heated to decomposition it emits acrid smoke and irritating fumes.

MHJ750   CAS: 1541-60-2
7-METHYL-6H-(1)
BENZOTHIOPYRANO(4,3-b)
QUINOLINE
mf: $C_{17}H_{13}NS$ mw: 263.37

TOXICITY DATA and REFERENCE
NEO: scu-mus TDLo: 72 mg/kg/9W-I   MUREAV
  66,307,79
MUT: mma-sat 30 μg/plate   MUREAV
  66,307,79

SAFETY PROFILE: Questionable carcinogen with experimental neoplastigenic data. Mutation

data reported. When heated to decomposition it emits very toxic fumes of NO_x and SO_x.

MHL250   CAS: 2606-85-1
6-METHYL-3:4-BENZPHENANTHRENE
mf: $C_{19}H_{14}$ mw: 242.33

TOXICITY DATA and REFERENCE
ETA: orl-mus TDLo: 11 g/kg/56W-I   PRLBA4
  129,439,40
ETA: scu-mus TDLo: 4400 mg/kg/67W-I
  PRLBA4 129,439,40
ETA: skn-mus TDLo: 2100 mg/kg/88W-I
  PRLBA4 129,439,40

SAFETY PROFILE: Questionable carcinogen with experimental tumorigenic data. When heated to decomposition it emits acrid smoke and irritating fumes.

MHL500   CAS: 2381-19-3
7-METHYL-3,4-BENZPHENANTHRENE
mf: $C_{19}H_{14}$ mw: 242.33

TOXICITY DATA and REFERENCE
ETA: skn-mus TDLo: 1850 mg/kg/77W-I
  PRLBA4 129,439,40

SAFETY PROFILE: Questionable carcinogen with experimental tumorigenic data. When heated to decomposition it emits acrid smoke and irritating fumes.

MHL750   CAS: 4076-40-8
8-METHYL-3:4-BENZPHENANTHRENE
mf: $C_{19}H_{14}$ mw: 242.33

SYN: 4-METHYLBENZO(c)PHENANTHRENE

TOXICITY DATA and REFERENCE
ETA: orl-mus TDLo: 14 g/kg/71W-I   PRLBA4
  129,439,40
ETA: scu-mus TDLo: 4600 mg/kg/68W-I
  PRLBA4 129,439,40
ETA: skn-mus TDLo: 1460 mg/kg/61W-I
  PRLBA4 129,439,40

SAFETY PROFILE: Questionable carcinogen with experimental tumorigenic data. When heated to decomposition it emits acrid smoke and irritating fumes.

MHM000   CAS: 2381-39-7
5-METHYL-3,4-BENZPYRENE
mf: $C_{21}H_{14}$ mw: 266.35

SYNS: 6-METHYLBENZO(a)PYRENE ◇ 5-METHYL-3,4-BENZOPYRENE

TOXICITY DATA and REFERENCE
CAR: skn-mus TDLo: 43 mg/kg/20W-I CBINA8 22,53,78
NEO: scu-mus TDLo: 40 mg/kg BJCAAI 26,506,72
NEO: scu-rat TDLo: 479 μg/kg/60D-I CBINA8 29,159,80
NEO: skn-mus TD: 4260 μg/kg CRNGDP 3,371,78
ETA: scu-mus TD: 80 mg/kg JNCIAM 1,303,40
ETA: skn-mus TD: 32 mg/kg/20W-I BEXBAN 87,474,79
ETA: skn-mus TD: 32 mg/kg/20W-I BEXBAN 87,474,79
ETA: skn-mus TD: 170 mg/kg/20W-I PAACA3 18,59,77
ETA: unr-mus TDLo: 80 mg/kg/8D-I BEBMAE 88(11),592,79
MUT: dnd-mus-skn 8 μmol/kg CBINA8 47,111,83
MUT: dnd-uns: lyms 30 μmol/L CBINA8 47,87,83
MUT: mma-ham: lng 3800 nmol/L PNASA6 73,607,76
MUT: mma-sat 6250 ng/plate CNREA8 47,1509,87

CONSENSUS REPORTS: EPA Genetic Toxicology Program.

SAFETY PROFILE: Questionable carcinogen with experimental carcinogenic, neoplastigenic, and tumorigenic data by skin contact. Mutation data reported. When heated to decomposition it emits toxic fumes of NO_x.

MHM250 CAS: 16757-81-6
8-METHYL-3,4-BENZPYRENE
mf: $C_{21}H_{14}$ mw: 266.35

SYN: 3-METHYLBENZO(a)PYRENE

TOXICITY DATA and REFERENCE
ETA: scu-mus TDLo: 40 mg/kg BJCAAI 6,400,52
MUT: sln-dmg-par 5 mmol/L CNREA8 33,302,73

CONSENSUS REPORTS: EPA Genetic Toxicology Program.

SAFETY PROFILE: Questionable carcinogen with experimental tumorigenic data. Mutation data reported. When heated to decomposition it emits acrid smoke and irritating fumes.

MHN000
N-METHYLBENZYLAMINE mixed with SODIUM NITRITE (1:1)

SYN: SODIUM NITRITE mixed with N-METHYLBENZYL-AMINE (1:1)

TOXICITY DATA and REFERENCE
ETA: orl-rat TD: 44 g/kg/16W-I IAPUDO41,679,82
ETA: orl-rat TD: 139 g/kg/37W-I IAPUDO 41,679,82
ETA: orl-rat TDLo: 28 g/kg/8W-C ZEKBAI 73,54,69

SAFETY PROFILE: Questionable carcinogen with experimental tumorigenic data. When heated to decomposition it emits very toxic fumes of NO_x and Na_2O.

MHN250
METHYLBENZYLAMINE mixed with SODIUM NITRITE (2:3)

SYNS: N-METHYLBENZYLAMINE mixed with SODIUM NITRITE (2:3) ◇ SODIUM NITRITE mixed with METHYLBENZ-YLAMINE (3:2)

TOXICITY DATA and REFERENCE
ETA: orl-mus TDLo: 4800 mg/kg/16D-I IARCCD 4,159,73
ETA: orl-rat TDLo: 25 g/kg/22W-I IARCCD 4,159,73

SAFETY PROFILE: Questionable carcinogen with experimental tumorigenic data. When heated to decomposition it emits very toxic fumes of NO_x and Na_2O.

MHN750 CAS: 10309-79-2
1-METHYL-2-BENZYLHYDRAZINE
mf: $C_8H_{12}N_2$ mw: 136.22

SYN: 1-BENZYL-2-METHYLHYDRAZINE

TOXICITY DATA and REFERENCE
CAR: scu-rat TDLo: 15 mg/kg (15D preg): TER IARCCD 4,45,73
ETA: scu-rat TDLo: 520 mg/kg/27W-I 23HZAR -,267,70
MUT: cyt-mus/ast 320 μg/kg CNREA8 32,1133,72
MUT: cyt-mus/leu 6400 μg/kg CNREA8 32,1133,72

SAFETY PROFILE: Questionable carcinogen with experimental carcinogenic, tumorigenic, and teratogenic data. Poison by subcutaneous route. Mutation data reported. When heated to decomposition it emits toxic fumes of NO_x.

MHP250 CAS: 937-40-6
N-METHYL-N-BENZYLNITROSAMINE
mf: $C_8H_{10}N_2O$ mw: 150.20

SYNS: METHYL-BENZYL-NITROSOAMIN (GERMAN) ◇ N-METHYL-N-NITROSOBENZYLAMINE ◇ N-NITROSO-

BENZYLMETHYLAMINE ◇ N-NITROSOMETHYLBENZYL-
AMINE

TOXICITY DATA and REFERENCE
ETA: ipr-rat TDLo: 16 mg/kg/4W-I · CRNGDP
8,1129,87
ETA: orl-rat TD: 40 mg/kg/8W   CALEDQ 33,107,86
ETA: orl-rat TD: 100 mg/kg/81W-I   XENOBH
3,271,73
ETA: orl-rat TD: 108 mg/kg/86W-I   PPTCBY
2,73,72
ETA: orl-rat TD: 116 mg/kg/22W-I   JJIND8
68,681,82
ETA: orl-rat TD: 120 mg/kg/69W-C   ARZNAD
19,1077,69
ETA: orl-rat TD: 200 mg/kg/29W-C   IARCCD
14,453,76
ETA: orl-rat TD: 250 mg/kg/36W-C   ZEKBAI
88,231,77
ETA: orl-rat TDLo: 16 mg/kg/4W-I   JJIND8
61,145,78
ETA: par-mus TDLo: 10 mg/kg   IARCCD 4,159,73
ETA: scu-rat TD: 50 mg/kg/20W-I   JJIND8
61,1471,78
ETA: scu-rat TDLo: 37500 μg/kg/15W-I
ARZNAD 31,677,81
MUT: mma-esc 5 μmol/plate   GANNA2 75,8,84
MUT: mma-ham: lng 200 μmol/L   CRNGDP
6,1731,85
MUT: mma-sat 50 μg/plate   JMCMAR 29,40,86
MUT: sce-ham: lng 1 mmol/L   CRNGDP 6,1731,85

CONSENSUS REPORTS: EPA Genetic Toxicology Program.

SAFETY PROFILE: Questionable carcinogen
with experimental tumorigenic data. Poison by
ingestion. Mutation data reported. When heated
to decomposition it emits toxic fumes of NO_x.

MHS375   CAS: 20680-07-3
1-METHYL-3-(p-BROMOPHENYL)UREA
mf: $C_8H_9BrN_2O$ mw: 229.10

SYNS: BROMDEFENURON ◇ 1-(p-BROMOPHENYL)-3-
METHYLUREA ◇ 1-METHYL-3-(p-BROMPHENYL)HARNS-
TOFF ◇ UREA, N-(4-BROMOPHENYL)-N'-METHYL-(9CI)

TOXICITY DATA and REFERENCE
ETA: orl-rat TDLo: 722 mg/kg/87W-   ARGEAR
53,329,83

SAFETY PROFILE: Questionable carcinogen
with experimental tumorigenic data. When
heated to decomposition it emits toxic fumes
of NO_x and Br^-

MHW000   CAS: 20240-62-4
METHYLBUTYL HYDRAZINE
mf: $C_5H_{14}N_2$ mw: 102.21

TOXICITY DATA and REFERENCE
ETA: orl-rat TDLo: 1425 mg/kg/57W-I   PPTCBY
2,73,72
ETA: scu-rat TDLo: 1500 mg/kg/60W-I
PPTCBY 2,73,72

SAFETY PROFILE: Questionable carcinogen
with experimental tumorigenic data. When
heated to decomposition it emits toxic fumes
of NO_x.

MHW250   CAS: 73454-79-2
1-METHYL-2-BUTYL-HYDRAZINE
DIHYDROCHLORIDE
mf: $C_5H_{14}N_2 \cdot 2ClH$ mw: 175.13

SYN: 1-BUTYL-2-METHYL-HYDRAZINE DIHYDROCHLO-
RIDE

TOXICITY DATA and REFERENCE
ETA: orl-rat TDLo: 1425 mg/kg/57W-I   23HZAR
-,267,70
ETA: scu-rat TDLo: 1275 mg/kg/51W-I   23HZAR
-,267,70

SAFETY PROFILE: Questionable carcinogen
with experimental tumorigenic data. Moderately
toxic by an unspecified route. When heated to
decomposition it emits very toxic fumes of Cl^-
and NO_x.

MHW500   CAS: 7068-83-9
METHYLBUTYLNITROSAMINE
mf: $C_5H_{12}N_2O$ mw: 116.19

SYNS: MBNA ◇ METHYL-BUTYL-NITROSAMIN (GER-
MAN) ◇ METHYL-N-BUTYLNITROSAMINE ◇ N-METHYL-
N-NITROSOBUTYLAMINE ◇ N-NITROSO-N-BUTYL-
METHYLAMINE ◇ N-NITROSOMETHYL-N-BUTYLAMINE
◇ NMBA

TOXICITY DATA and REFERENCE
CAR: orl-mus TDLo: 182 mg/kg/1Y-C   85DUA4
-,129,70
ETA: ihl-rat TD: 69 mg/kg/23W   ARZNAD
19,1077,69
ETA: ihl-rat TD: 69 mg/kg/23W-I   ZEKBAI
71,135,68
ETA: ihl-rat TD: 100 mg/kg/24W-I   ZEKBAI
75,221,71
ETA: ihl-rat TDLo: 31 mg/kg/30W-I   ZEKBAI
75,221,71
ETA: orl-rat TD: 128 mg/kg/20W-I   JCROD7
106,171,83

ETA: orl-rat TD: 160 mg/kg/20W-I   JJIND8 70,959,83

ETA: orl-rat TDLo: 128 mg/kg/20W-I   CRNGDP 1,157,80

ETA: scu-mus TDLo: 90 mg/kg/50W-I   85DUA4 -,129,70

ETA: scu-rat TDLo: 150 mg/kg/30W-I   IJPBAR 17,180,74

MUT: mma-esc 100 μmol/L   MUREAV 26,361,74

MUT: mma-sat 10 μmol/plate   TCMUE9 1,13,84

MUT: mmo-sat 1 mg/plate   TCMUD8 1,295,80

MUT: pic-esc 100 mg/L   TCMUE9 1,91,84

CONSENSUS REPORTS: EPA Genetic Toxicology Program.

SAFETY PROFILE: Questionable carcinogen with experimental carcinogenic and tumorigenic data. Poison by ingestion, inhalation, intraperitoneal, and subcutaneous routes. Mutation data reported. When heated to decomposition it emits toxic fumes of NO_x.

MHZ000   CAS: 598-55-0
METHYL CARBAMATE
mf: $C_2H_5NO_2$ mw: 75.07

PROP: Needles. Bp: 177°, mp: 52-54°. Very sol in water, alc.

SYNS: BENDIOCARB ◇ METHYLURETHAN ◇ METHYLURETHANE ◇ NCI-C55594 ◇ URETHYLANE

TOXICITY DATA and REFERENCE
CAR: orl-rat TDLo: 102 g/kg/2Y   NTPTR* NTP-TR-328,87

ETA: skn-mus TDLo: 45 mg/kg/14W-I   BJCAAI 9,177,55

MUT: mmo-esc 50 g/L/3H   CRSUBM 3,69,55

MUT: oms-mus-par 375 mg/kg   ZKKOBW 76,69,71

MUT: otr-rat:emb 120 μg/L   JJIND8 67,1303,81

CONSENSUS REPORTS: IARC Cancer Review: Animal Inadequate Evidence IMEMDT 12,151,76. EPA Genetic Toxicology Program. Reported in EPA TSCA Inventory.

SAFETY PROFILE: Questionable carcinogen with experimental carcinogenic and tumorigenic data. Poison by ingestion and intraperitoneal routes. Mutation data reported. When heated to decomposition it emits toxic fumes of NO_x.

MIF250   CAS: 61445-55-4
N-METHYL-N-(3-CARBOXYPROPYL)NITROSAMINE
mf: $C_5H_{10}N_2O_3$ mw: 146.17

SYNS: 4-(METHYLNITROSOAMINO)BUTYRIC ACID ◇ N-NITROSOMETHYL-3-CARBOXYPROPYLAMINE

TOXICITY DATA and REFERENCE
NEO: par-rat TDLo: 4500 mg/kg/30W-I   JJCREP 79,309,88

ETA: orl-rat TD: 8500 mg/kg/57W-I   JJIND8 70,959,83

ETA: orl-rat TDLo: 6800 mg/kg/57W-I   JJIND8 70,959,83

MUT: mma-sat 48 μmol/plate   CNREA8 37,399,77

MUT: mmo-smc 16260 mg/L   IAPUDO 57,721,84

SAFETY PROFILE: Questionable carcinogen with experimental neoplastigenic and tumorigenic data. Mutation data reported. When heated to decomposition it emits toxic fumes of NO_x.

MIH275   CAS: 71-55-6
METHYL CHLOROFORM
DOT: 2831
mf: $C_2H_3Cl_3$ mw: 133.40

PROP: Colorless liquid. Bp: 74.1°, fp: −32.5°, flash p: none, d: 1.3376 @ 20°/4°, vap press: 100 mm @ 20.0°. Insol in water; sol in acetone, benzene, carbon tetrachloride, methanol, ether.

SYNS: AEROTHENE TT ◇ CHLOROETENE ◇ CHLOROETHENE ◇ CHLOROTHANE NU ◇ CHLOROTHENE ◇ CHLOROTHENE (INHIBITED) ◇ CHLOROTHENE NU ◇ CHLOROTHENE VG ◇ CHLORTEN ◇ INHIBISOL ◇ METHYLCHLOROFORM ◇ METHYLTRICHLOROMETHANE ◇ NCI-C04626 ◇ RCRA WASTE NUMBER U226 ◇ SOLVENT 111 ◇ STROBANE ◇ α-T ◇ 1,1,1-TCE ◇ 1,1,1-TRICHLOORETHAAN (DUTCH) ◇ 1,1,1-TRICHLORAETHAN (GERMAN) ◇ TRICHLORO-1,1,1-ETHANE (FRENCH) ◇ 1,1,1-TRICHLOROETHANE ◇ α-TRICHLOROETHANE ◇ 1,1,1-TRICLOROETANO (ITALIAN) ◇ TRI-ETHANE

TOXICITY DATA with REFERENCE
MUT: dnr-esc 500 mg/L   PMRSDJ 1,195,81

MUT: otr-mus:emb 20 mg/L   CALEDQ 28,85,85

CONSENSUS REPORTS: IARC Cancer Review: GROUP 3 IMEMDT 7,56,87; Animal Inadequate Evidence IMEMDT 20,515,79. NCI Carcinogenesis Bioassay (gavage); Inadequate Studies: mouse, rat NCITR* NCI-CG-TR-3,77. Community Right-To-Know List. Reported in EPA TSCA Inventory. EPA Genetic Toxicology Program.

OSHA PEL: (Transitional: TWA 350 ppm) TWA 350 ppm; STEL 450 ppm   ACGIH TLV: TWA 350 ppm; STEL 450 ppm (Proposed: BEI:

10 mg/L trichloroacetic acid in urine at end of workweek.)   DFG MAK: 200 ppm (1080 mg/m^3); BAT: 55 μg/dL in blood after several shifts.   NIOSH REL: (1,1,1-Trichloroethane) CL 350 ppm/15M DOT Classification: ORM-A; Label: None; Poison B; Label: St. Andrews Cross.

SAFETY PROFILE: Questionable carcinogen. Poison by intravenous route. Moderately toxic by ingestion, inhalation, skin contact, subcutaneous and intraperitoneal routes. An experimental teratogen. Human systemic effects by ingestion and inhalation: conjunctiva irritation, hallucinations or distorted perceptions, motor activity changes, irritability, aggression, hypermotility, diarrhea, nausea or vomiting and other gastrointestinal changes. Experimental reproductive effects. Mutation data reported. A human skin irritant. An experimental skin and severe eye irritant. Narcotic in high concentrations. When heated to decomposition it emits toxic fumes of Cl$^-$. Used as a cleaning solvent, a chemical intermediate to produce vinylidene chloride, and as a propellant in aerosol cans.

MIH500   CAS: 4274-06-0
4-METHYL-6-(((2-CHLORO-4-NITRO)PHENYL)AZO)-m-ANISIDINE
mf: $C_{14}H_{13}ClN_4O_3$ mw: 320.76

SYNS: AZO DYE NO. 6945 ◊ BROWN SALT NV ◊ 2-CHLORO-4-NITROBENZENEAZO-2′-AMINO-4′-METHOXY-5′-METHYLBENZENE ◊ C.I. 37200 ◊ C.I. AZOIC DIAZO COMPONENT 21 ◊ FAST BROWN SALT RR

TOXICITY DATA and REFERENCE
ETA: orl-rat TDLo:49 g/kg/119W-C   ZEKBAI 57,530,51

SAFETY PROFILE: Questionable carcinogen with experimental tumorigenic data. When heated to decomposition it emits very toxic fumes of Cl$^-$ and NO$_x$.

MIK000   CAS: 63041-78-1
5-METHYLCHOLANTHRENE
mf: $C_{21}H_{16}$ mw: 268.37

PROP: Yellow needles from benzene. Mp: 176.5-177.5°.

TOXICITY DATA and REFERENCE
ETA: scu-mus TD:80 mg/kg   CNREA8 1,685,41
ETA: scu-mus TDLo:40 mg/kg   CNREA8 1,695,41
MUT: dnd-mus:oth 400 nmol   CNREA8 42,1239,82

SAFETY PROFILE: Questionable carcinogen with experimental tumorigenic data. Mutation data reported. When heated to decomposition it emits acrid smoke and irritating fumes.

MIK250   CAS: 17012-89-4
22-METHYLCHOLANTHRENE
mf: $C_{21}H_{16}$ mw: 268.37

SYN: 4-METHYLCHOLANTHRENE

TOXICITY DATA and REFERENCE
CAR: scu-mus TD:80 mg/kg   CNREA8 1,685,41
CAR: scu-mus TDLo:40 mg/kg   CNREA8 1,695,41

SAFETY PROFILE: Questionable carcinogen with experimental carcinogenic data. When heated to decomposition it emits acrid smoke and irritating fumes.

MIK500
20-METHYLCHOLANTHRENE CHOLEIC ACID
mf: $C_{96}H_{160}O_{16}•C_{21}H_{16}$ mw: 1838.93

TOXICITY DATA and REFERENCE
ETA: scu-mus TDLo:400 mg/kg   JNCIAM 2,99,41
MUT: cyt-mus:fbr 1 mg/L   AJCAA7 39,149,40

SAFETY PROFILE: Questionable carcinogen with experimental tumorigenic data. Mutation data reported. When heated to decomposition it emits acrid smoke and irritating fumes.

MIK750   CAS: 3342-99-2
cis-3-METHYLCHOLANTHRENE-1,2-DIOL
mf: $C_{21}H_{16}O_2$ mw: 300.37

SYN: cis-1,2-DIHYDROXY-3-METHYLCHOLANTHRENE

TOXICITY DATA and REFERENCE
NEO: scu-mus TDLo:120 mg/kg/6W-I   IJCNAW 2,505,67

SAFETY PROFILE: Questionable carcinogen with experimental neoplastigenic data. When heated to decomposition it emits acrid smoke and irritating fumes.

MIL250   CAS: 3343-08-6
3-METHYLCHOLANTHRENE-2-ONE
mf: $C_{21}H_{14}O$ mw: 282.35

SYN: 3-METHYLCHOLANTHREN-2-ONE

TOXICITY DATA and REFERENCE
CAR: skn-mus TDLo:90 mg/kg/20W-I   CBINA8 22(1),69,78

NEO: scu-mus TDLo: 120 mg/kg/6W-I IJCNAW
2,505,67

MUT: mma-ham: lng 15 nmol/plate CNREA8
38,3398,78

MUT: mma-sat 20 nmol/plate CNREA8
38,3398,78

CONSENSUS REPORTS: EPA Genetic Toxicology Program.

SAFETY PROFILE: Questionable carcinogen with experimental carcinogenic and neoplastigenic data. Mutation data reported. When heated to decomposition it emits acrid smoke and irritating fumes.

MIL500　　　　CAS: 3416-21-5
3-METHYLCHOLANTHRENE-11,12-OXIDE
mf: $C_{21}H_{16}O$　　mw: 284.37

SYNS: 11,12-DIHYDRO-11,12-EPOXY-3-METHYLCHOL-ANTHRENE ◇ 11,12-EPOXY-11,12-DIHYDRO-3-METHYL-CHOLANTHRENE

TOXICITY DATA and REFERENCE
NEO: scu-mus TDLo: 40 mg/kg/6W-I IJCNAW
2,505,67

MUT: dnd-hmn: oth 10 μmol/L CNREA836,272,76
MUT: otr-mus: oth 750 μg/L PNASA6 68,1098,71
MUT: sln-dmg-par 5 mmol/L CNREA8 33,2354,73
MUT: slt-dmg-par 5 mmol/L CNREA8 33,2354,73

CONSENSUS REPORTS: EPA Genetic Toxicology Program.

SAFETY PROFILE: Questionable carcinogen with experimental neoplastigenic data. Human mutation data reported. When heated to decomposition it emits acrid smoke and irritating fumes.

MIL750　　　　CAS: 63041-80-5
20-METHYLCHOLANTHRENE PICRATE
mf: $C_{21}H_{16} \cdot C_6H_3N_3O_7$　　mw: 497.49

SYNS: 1,2-DIHYDRO-3-METHYLBENZ(j)ACEANTHRYL-ENE COMPOUND with 2,4,6-TRINITROPHENOL (1:1) ◇ 3-METHYLCHOLANTHRENE COMPOUND with PICRIC ACID (1:1) ◇ 2,4,6-TRINITROPHENOL COMPOUND with 1,2-DIHYDRO-3-METHYLBENZ(j)ACEANTHRYLENE

TOXICITY DATA and REFERENCE
ETA: scu-mus TDLo: 200 mg/kg XPHPAW
149,319,51

SAFETY PROFILE: Questionable carcinogen with experimental tumorigenic data. When

heated to decomposition it emits toxic fumes of NO_x.

MIM000　　　　CAS: 63040-09-5
20-METHYLCHOLANTHRENE-TRINITROBENZENE
SYN: 3-METHYLCHOLANTHRENE COMPOUND with 1,3,5-TRINITROBENZENE (1:1)

TOXICITY DATA and REFERENCE
NEO: scu-mus TDLo: 60 mg/kg XPHPAW
149,319,51

SAFETY PROFILE: Questionable carcinogen with experimental neoplastigenic data. When heated to decomposition it emits toxic fumes of NO_x.

MIM250　　　　CAS: 3343-07-5
20-METHYLCHOLANTHREN-15-ONE
mf: $C_{21}H_{14}O$　　mw: 282.35

SYNS: 15-KETO-20-METHYLCHOLANTHRENE ◇ 3-ME-THYLCHOLANTHREN-1-ONE

TOXICITY DATA and REFERENCE
NEO: scu-mus TDLo: 120 mg/kg/6W-I IJCNAW
2,505,67

ETA: skn-mus TDLo: 340 mg/kg/42W-I
PRLBA4 129,439,40

MUT: mma-ham: lng 15 nmol/plate CNREA8
38,3398,78

MUT: mma-sat 20 nmol/plate CNREA8 38,3398,78

CONSENSUS REPORTS: EPA Genetic Toxicology Program.

SAFETY PROFILE: Questionable carcinogen with experimental neoplastigenic and tumorigenic data. Mutation data reported. When heated to decomposition it emits acrid smoke and irritating fumes.

MIM500　　　　CAS: 3351-28-8
1-METHYLCHRYSENE
mf: $C_{19}H_{14}$　　mw: 242.33

TOXICITY DATA and REFERENCE
ETA: skn-mus TDLo: 40 mg/kg/3W-I CCSUDL
1,325,76

MUT: mma-sat 10 μg/plate CNREA8 36,4525,76

CONSENSUS REPORTS: IARC Cancer Review: Animal Inadequate Evidence IMEMDT 32,379,83. EPA Genetic Toxicology Program.

SAFETY PROFILE: Questionable carcinogen with experimental tumorigenic data. Mutation

data reported. When heated to decomposition it emits acrid smoke and irritating fumes.

MIM750   CAS: 3351-32-4
2-METHYLCHRYSENE
mf: $C_{19}H_{14}$ mw: 242.33

TOXICITY DATA and REFERENCE
ETA: skn-mus TD:480 mg/kg/40W-I   JNCIAM 53,1121,74
ETA: skn-mus TDLo:40 mg/kg/3W-I   CCSUDL 1,325,76
MUT: mma-sat 10 μg/plate   CNREA8 36,4525,76

CONSENSUS REPORTS: IARC Cancer Review: Animal Limited Evidence IMEMDT 32,379,83. EPA Genetic Toxicology Program.

SAFETY PROFILE: Questionable carcinogen with experimental tumorigenic and possible carcinogenic data. Mutation data reported. When heated to decomposition it emits acrid smoke and irritating fumes.

MIN000   CAS: 3351-31-3
3-METHYLCHRYSENE
mf: $C_{19}H_{14}$ mw: 242.33

TOXICITY DATA with REFERENCE
NEO: skn-mus TDLo:40 mg/kg/3W-I   CCSUDL 1,325,76
ETA: skn-mus TD:180 mg/kg/15W-I   JNCIAM 53,1121,74
MUT: mma-sat 20 μg/plate   CNREA8 36,4525,76

CONSENSUS REPORTS: IARC Cancer Review: GROUP 3 IMEMDT 7,56,87; Animal Limited Evidence IMEMDT 32,379,83. EPA Genetic Toxicology Program.

SAFETY PROFILE: Questionable carcinogen with experimental neoplastigenic and tumorigenic data. Mutation data reported. When heated to decomposition it emits acrid smoke and irritating fumes.

MIN250   CAS: 3351-30-2
4-METHYLCHRYSENE
mf: $C_{19}H_{14}$ mw: 242.33

TOXICITY DATA and REFERENCE
ETA: scu-mus TDLo:80 mg/kg   CNREA8 3,606,43
ETA: skn-mus TD:660 mg/kg/55W-I   JNCIAM 53,1121,74
ETA: skn-mus TDLo:40 mg/kg/3W-I   CCSUDL 1,325,76
MUT: mma-sat 10 μg/plate   CNREA8 36,4525,76

CONSENSUS REPORTS: IARC Cancer Review: Animal Limited Evidence IMEMDT 32,379,83. EPA Genetic Toxicology Program.

SAFETY PROFILE: Questionable carcinogen with experimental tumorigenic data. Mutation data reported. When heated to decomposition it emits acrid smoke and irritating fumes.

MIN500   CAS: 3697-24-3
5-METHYLCHRYSENE
mf: $C_{19}H_{14}$ mw: 242.33

TOXICITY DATA and REFERENCE
CAR: scu-mus TDLo:20 mg/kg/20W-I   CCSUDL 1,325,76
CAR: skn-mus TD:40 mg/kg/62W-I   CCSUDL 1,147,76
CAR: skn-mus TD:40 mg/kg/62W-I   CCSUDL 1,147,76
CAR: skn-mus TDLo:32 μg/kg   CNREA8 45,6406,85
NEO: skn-mus TD:40 mg/kg/30W-I   CCSUDL 1,325,76
NEO: skn-mus TD:40 mg/kg/30W-I   CCSUDL 1,325,76
ETA: scu-mus TD:80 mg/kg   CNREA8 3,606,43
ETA: skn-mus TD:132 mg/kg/11W-I   JNCIAM 53,1121,74
MUT: dnd-mus-skn 467 μmol/L   CRNGDP 4,843,83
MUT: mma-sat 3 μg/plate   CRNGDP 7,673,86

CONSENSUS REPORTS: IARC Cancer Review: GROUP 3 IMEMDT 7,56,87; Animal Sufficient Evidence IMEMDT 32,379,83. EPA Genetic Toxicology Program.

SAFETY PROFILE: Questionable carcinogen with experimental carcinogenic, neoplastigenic, and tumorigenic data. Mutation data reported. When heated to decomposition it emits acrid smoke and irritating fumes.

MIN750   CAS: 1705-85-7
6-METHYLCHRYSENE
mf: $C_{19}H_{14}$ mw: 242.33

TOXICITY DATA with REFERENCE
ETA: imp-mus TDLo:160 mg/kg/40W   JNCIAM 2,241,41
ETA: skn-mus TD:240 mg/kg/20W-I   JNCIAM 53,1121,74
ETA: skn-mus TDLo:40 mg/kg/3W-I   CCSUDL 1,325,76
MUT: mma-sat 10 μg/plate   CNREA8 36,4525,76

CONSENSUS REPORTS: IARC Cancer Review: Animal Limited Evidence IMEMDT 32,379,83. EPA Genetic Toxicology Program.

SAFETY PROFILE: Questionable carcinogen with experimental tumorigenic data. Mutation data reported. When heated to decomposition it emits acrid smoke and irritating fumes.

MIO975   CAS: 21340-68-1
METHYL CLOFENAPATE
mf: $C_{17}H_{17}ClO_3$ mw: 304.79

SYNS: ICI 54856 METHYL ESTER ◇ METHYL-2-(4-(p-CHLOROPHENYL)PHENOXY)-2-METHYLPROPIONATE ◇ PROPANOIC ACID, 2-((4'-CHLORO(1,1'-BIPHENYL)-4-YL)OXY)-2-METHYL-, METHYL ESTER (9CI)

TOXICITY DATA and REFERENCE
CAR: orl-rat TDLo: 31500 mg/kg/75W-C
CNREA8 42,259,82

SAFETY PROFILE: Questionable carcinogen with experimental carcinogenic data. When heated to decomposition it emits toxic fumes of Cl⁻.

MIQ250   CAS: 63020-25-7
9-METHYL-10-CYANO-1,2-BENZANTHRACENE
mf: $C_{20}H_{14}N$ mw: 268.35

SYN: 7-CYANO-12-METHYL-BENZ(a)ANTHRACENE

TOXICITY DATA and REFERENCE
ETA: scu-mus TDLo: 1600 mg/kg/24W-I
PRLBA4 129,439,40
ETA: skn-mus TDLo: 620 mg/kg/26W-I
PRLBA4 129,439,40

CONSENSUS REPORTS: Cyanide and its compounds are on the Community Right-To-Know List.

SAFETY PROFILE: Questionable carcinogen with experimental tumorigenic data. When heated to decomposition it emits toxic fumes of NO_x and CN⁻.

MIU750   CAS: 3353-08-0
17-METHYL-15H-CYCLOPENTA(a) PHENANTHRENE
mf: $C_{18}H_{14}$ mw: 230.32

TOXICITY DATA and REFERENCE
ETA: skn-mus TDLo: 125 mg/kg/52W-I
NATUAS 210,1281,66
MUT: mma-sat 50 μg/plate   CNREA8 36,4525,76

CONSENSUS REPORTS: EPA Genetic Toxicology Program.

SAFETY PROFILE: Questionable carcinogen with experimental tumorigenic data. Mutation data reported. When heated to decomposition it emits acrid smoke and irritating fumes.

MIV250   CAS: 63020-76-8
10-METHYL-1,2-CYCLOPENTENOPHENANTHRENE
mf: $C_{18}H_{16}$ mw: 232.34

SYN: 16,17-DIHYDRO-7-METHYL-15H-CYCLOPENTA(a)PHENANTHRENE

TOXICITY DATA and REFERENCE
ETA: skn-mus TDLo: 1200 mg/kg/37W-I
ARGEAR 6,1,53

SAFETY PROFILE: Questionable carcinogen with experimental tumorigenic data. When heated to decomposition it emits acrid smoke and irritating fumes.

MIX000   CAS: 63991-70-8
2-METHYLDIACETYLBENZIDINE
mf: $C_{17}H_{18}N_2O_2$ mw: 282.37

SYN: 2-METHYL-N,N'-DIACETYLBENZIDINE

TOXICITY DATA and REFERENCE
CAR: orl-rat TDLo: 5600 mg/kg/35W-C
CNREA8 16,525,56

SAFETY PROFILE: Questionable carcinogen with experimental carcinogenic data. When heated to decomposition it emits toxic fumes of NO_x.

MIY000   CAS: 59652-21-0
7-METHYLDIBENZ(c,h)ACRIDINE
mf: $C_{22}H_{15}N$ mw: 293.38

SYN: 9-METHYL-3,4,5,6-DIBENZACRIDINE

TOXICITY DATA and REFERENCE
ETA: scu-mus TDLo: 72 mg/kg/9W-I   COREAF 251,1322,60
ETA: scu-mus TDLo: 200 mg/kg   VOONAW 1,52,55

SAFETY PROFILE: Questionable carcinogen with experimental tumorigenic data. When heated to decomposition it emits toxic fumes of NO_x.

MIY200   CAS: 79543-29-6
14-METHYLDIBENZ(a,h)ACRIDINE
mf: $C_{22}H_{15}N$ mw: 293.38

SYN: 10-METHYL-1,2:5,6-DIBENZACRIDINE

TOXICITY DATA and REFERENCE
ETA: scu-mus TDLo:48 mg/kg/4W-I   COREAF
251,1322,60

SAFETY PROFILE: Questionable carcinogen with experimental tumorigenic data. When heated to decomposition it emits toxic fumes of NO_x.

MIY250   CAS: 59652-20-9
14-METHYLDIBENZ(a,j)ACRIDINE
mf: $C_{22}H_{15}N$ mw: 293.38

SYN: 10-METHYL-3,4,5,6-DIBENZACRIDINE

TOXICITY DATA and REFERENCE
ETA: skn-mus TDLo:280 mg/kg/23W-I
ACRSAJ 4,315,56

SAFETY PROFILE: Questionable carcinogen with experimental tumorigenic data. When heated to decomposition it emits toxic fumes of NO_x.

MIY500   CAS: 63041-83-8
2-METHYLDIBENZ(a,h)ANTHRACENE
mf: $C_{23}H_{16}$ mw: 292.39

SYN: 2'-METHYL-1:2:5:6-DIBENZANTHRACENE

TOXICITY DATA and REFERENCE
ETA: skn-mus TDLo:1250 mg/kg/52W-I
PRLBA4 111,485,32

SAFETY PROFILE: Questionable carcinogen with experimental tumorigenic data. When heated to decomposition it emits acrid smoke and irritating fumes.

MIY750   CAS: 63041-84-9
3-METHYLDIBENZ(a,h)ANTHRACENE
mf: $C_{23}H_{16}$ mw: 292.39

SYN: 3'-METHYL-1:2:5:6-DIBENZANTHRACENE

TOXICITY DATA and REFERENCE
ETA: skn-mus TD:1250 mg/kg/52W-I   PRLBA4
111,485,32
ETA: skn-mus TDLo:552 mg/kg/23W-I
PRLBA4 111,455,32

SAFETY PROFILE: Questionable carcinogen with experimental tumorigenic data. When heated to decomposition it emits acrid smoke and irritating fumes.

MIZ000   CAS: 63041-85-0
4-METHYL-1,2,5,6-DIBENZANTHRACENE
mf: $C_{23}H_{16}$ mw: 292.39

SYN: 6-METHYL DIBENZ(a,h)ANTHRACENE

TOXICITY DATA and REFERENCE
ETA: skn-mus TDLo:1010 mg/kg/42W-I
PRLBA4 117,318,35

SAFETY PROFILE: Questionable carcinogen with experimental tumorigenic data. When heated to decomposition it emits acrid smoke and irritating fumes.

MJA000   CAS: 17278-93-2
10-METHYLDIBENZ(a,c)ANTHRACENE
mf: $C_{23}H_{16}$ mw: 292.39

TOXICITY DATA and REFERENCE
ETA: scu-mus TDLo:72 mg/kg/9W-I   EJCAAH
4,123,68

SAFETY PROFILE: Questionable carcinogen with experimental tumorigenic data. When heated to decomposition it emits acrid smoke and irritating fumes.

MJA250   CAS: 27093-62-5
N-METHYL-3:4:5:6-DIBENZCARBAZOLE
mf: $C_{21}H_{15}N$ mw: 281.37

SYN: N-METHYL-7H-DIBENZO(c,g)CARBAZOLE

TOXICITY DATA and REFERENCE
ETA: scu-mus TDLo:24 mg/kg/4W-I   BJEPA5
27,179,46
ETA: skn-mus TDLo:1350 mg/kg/33W-C
BJEPA5 27,179,46

SAFETY PROFILE: Questionable carcinogen with experimental tumorigenic data. When heated to decomposition it emits toxic fumes of NO_x.

MJA500   CAS: 33942-87-9
5-METHYL-DIBENZO(b,def)CHRYSENE
mf: $C_{25}H_{16}$ mw: 316.41

SYN: 5-METHYL-3,4:8,9-DIBENZOPYRENE (FRENCH)

TOXICITY DATA and REFERENCE
ETA: scu-mus TDLo:72 mg/kg/9W-I   COREAF
246,1477,58

SAFETY PROFILE: Questionable carcinogen with experimental tumorigenic data. When heated to decomposition it emits acrid smoke and irritating fumes.

MJA750   CAS: 2869-12-7
7-METHYLDIBENZO(h,rst)PENTAPHENE
mf: $C_{29}H_{18}$ mw: 366.47

SYN: 2'-METHYL-1,2:4,5:8,9-TRIBENZOPYRENE

TOXICITY DATA and REFERENCE
ETA: scu-mus TDLo:72 mg/kg/9W-I   COREAF
259,3899,64

SAFETY PROFILE: Questionable carcinogen with experimental tumorigenic data. When heated to decomposition it emits acrid smoke and irritating fumes.

MJB000   CAS: 2869-60-5
5-METHYL-1,2,3,4-DIBENZOPYRENE
mf: C$_{25}$H$_{16}$ mw: 316.41

SYN: 10-METHYLDIBENZO(def,p)CHRYSENE

TOXICITY DATA and REFERENCE
ETA: scu-mus TDLo:72 mg/kg/9W-I   COREAF
259,3899,64

SAFETY PROFILE: Questionable carcinogen with experimental tumorigenic data. When heated to decomposition it emits acrid smoke and irritating fumes.

MJB250   CAS: 63041-95-2
7-METHYL-1:2:3:4-DIBENZPYRENE
mf: C$_{25}$H$_{16}$ mw: 316.41

TOXICITY DATA and REFERENCE
ETA: skn-mus TDLo:980 mg/kg/41W-I
PRLBA4 123,343,37

SAFETY PROFILE: Questionable carcinogen with experimental tumorigenic data. When heated to decomposition it emits acrid smoke and irritating fumes.

MJD000   CAS: 63041-05-4
METHYL DIEPOXYDIALLYLACETATE
mf: C$_9$H$_{14}$O$_4$ mw: 186.23

SYN: 4,5-EPOXY-2-(2,3-EPOXYPROPYL)VALERIC ACID, METHYL ESTER

TOXICITY DATA and REFERENCE
ETA: unr-mus TDLo:3700 mg/kg   RARSAM
3,193,63

SAFETY PROFILE: Questionable carcinogen with experimental tumorigenic data. When heated to decomposition it emits acrid smoke and irritating fumes.

MJD610   CAS: 68688-87-9
trans-3-METHYL-9,10-DIHYDROCHOLANTHRENE-9,10-DIOL
mf: C$_{21}$H$_{18}$O$_2$ mw: 302.39

SYN: trans-9,10-DIHYDRO-9,10-DIHYDROXY-3-METHYL-CHOLANTHRENE

TOXICITY DATA and REFERENCE
ETA: skn-mus TDLo:378 ng/kg   CALEDQ
28,223,85
MUT: mma-sat 10 μmol/L   BBRCA9 85,1568,78
MUT: msc-ham:lng 2 mg/L   BBRCA9 85,1568,78
MUT: otr-mus:fbr 250 μg/L   BBRCA9 85,1568,78
MUT: sce-ham:ovr 500 μg/L   CALEDQ 7,45,79

SAFETY PROFILE: Questionable carcinogen with experimental tumorigenic data. Mutation data reported. When heated to decomposition it emits acrid smoke and irritating fumes.

MJD750   CAS: 24684-41-1
11-METHYL-15,16-DIHYDRO-17H-CYCLOPENTA(a)PHENANTHRENE
mf: C$_{18}$H$_{16}$ mw: 232.34

PROP: Crystals from acetic acid. Mp: 126-127°.

SYN: 16,17-DIHYDRO-11-METHYL-15H-CYCLOPENTA (a)PHENANTHRENE

TOXICITY DATA and REFERENCE
ETA: skn-mus TDLo:1440 mg/kg/45W-I
ARGEAR 6,1,53
MUT: mma-sat 20 ng/plate   CNREA8 36,4525,76

SAFETY PROFILE: Questionable carcinogen with experimental tumorigenic data. Mutation data reported. When heated to decomposition it emits acrid smoke and irritating fumes.

MJF000   CAS: 3732-90-9
3-METHYL-4-DIMETHYLAMINOAZOBENZENE
mf: C$_{15}$H$_{17}$N$_3$ mw: 239.35

SYNS: N,N-DIMETHYL-4-(PHENYLAZO)-o-TOLUIDINE
◇ 3-METHYL-4-DAB

TOXICITY DATA and REFERENCE
CAR: orl-rat TDLo:749 mg/kg/2Y-C   TOPADD
13,257,85
ETA: orl-rat TD:3900 mg/kg/17W-C   EXPEAM
19,316,63
ETA: orl-rat TDLo:3024 mg/kg/12W-C
VAAZA2 46,21,84
MUT: dni-rat:lvr 10 μmol/L   CNREA8 45,337,85

SAFETY PROFILE: Questionable carcinogen with experimental carcinogenic and tumorigenic data. Mutation data reported. When heated to decomposition it emits toxic fumes of NO$_x$.

MJF500   CAS: 17400-69-0
3'-METHYL-5'-(p-DIMETHYLAMINOPHENYLAZO) QUINOLINE
mf: $C_{18}H_{18}N_4$ mw: 290.40

SYNS: 5-((p-(DIMETHYLAMINO)PHENYL)AZO)-3-METHYLQUINOLINE ◇ N,N-DIMETHYL-4-(5-(3'-METHYLQUINOLYL)AZO)ANILINE

TOXICITY DATA and REFERENCE
CAR: orl-rat TDLo: 3276 mg/kg/26W-C
  JNCIAM 40,891,68

SAFETY PROFILE: Questionable carcinogen with experimental carcinogenic data. When heated to decomposition it emits toxic fumes of NO_x.

MJF750   CAS: 17400-70-3
6'-METHYL-5'-(p-DIMETHYLAMINOPHENYLAZO) QUINOLINE
mf: $C_{18}H_{18}N_4$ mw: 290.40

SYNS: 5-((p-(DIMETHYLAMINO)PHENYL)AZO)-6-METHYLQUINOLINE ◇ N,N-DIMETHYL-4-(5'-(6'-METHYLQUINOLYL)AZO)ANILINE

TOXICITY DATA and REFERENCE
ETA: orl-rat TDLo: 4914 mg/kg/39W-C
  JNCIAM 40,891,68

SAFETY PROFILE: Questionable carcinogen with experimental tumorigenic data. When heated to decomposition it emits toxic fumes of NO_x.

MJG000   CAS: 17416-20-5
8'-METHYL-5'-(p-DIMETHYLAMINOPHENYLAZO) QUINOLINE
mf: $C_{18}H_{18}N_4$ mw: 290.40

SYNS: 5-((p-(DIMETHYLAMINO)PHENYL)AZO)-8-METHYLQUINOLINE ◇ N,N-DIMETHYL-4-(5'-(8'-METHYLQUINOLYL)AZO)ANILINE

TOXICITY DATA and REFERENCE
CAR: orl-rat TDLo: 378 mg/kg/9W-C   JNCIAM
  40,891,68

SAFETY PROFILE: Questionable carcinogen with experimental carcinogenic data. When heated to decomposition it emits toxic fumes of NO_x.

MJG750   CAS: 99-80-9
N-METHYL-N,p-DINITROSOANILINE
mf: $C_7H_7N_3O_2$ mw: 165.17.

PROP: Mp: 101°. Contains 30% Contains 30% N-methyl-N,p-dinitrosoaniline (JNCIAM 41,985,68).

SYNS: N,4-DINITROSO-N-METHYLANILINE ◇ ELASTO-PAR ◇ ELASTOPAX ◇ HEAT PRE ◇ N-METHYL-N,4-DINITROSOANILINE ◇ N-METHYL-N,4-DINITROSOBENZENAMINE ◇ METHYL-(4-NITROSOPHENYL)NITROSAMINE ◇ N-NITROSO-N-METHYL-4-NITROSO-ANILINE ◇ NITROZAN K

TOXICITY DATA and REFERENCE
ETA: ipr-rat TDLo: 520 mg/kg/26W-I   EJCAAH
  4,233,68
ETA: scu-rat TDLo: 29 g/kg/78W-I   VOONAW
  19(8),80,73
MUT: dni-mus-ipr 20 g/kg   ARGEAR 51,605,81
MUT: mma-sat 5 μg/plate   PCBRD2 141,407,84

CONSENSUS REPORTS: IARC Cancer Review: Animal Inadequate Evidence IMEMDT 1,141,72.

SAFETY PROFILE: Questionable carcinogen with experimental tumorigenic data. Mutation data reported. When heated to decomposition it emits toxic fumes of NO_x.

MJH000   CAS: 55556-94-0
2-METHYLDINITROSOPIPERAZINE
mf: $C_5H_{11}N_4O_2$ mw: 159.20

SYN: 2-METHYL-DNPZ

TOXICITY DATA and REFERENCE
ETA: orl-rat TDLo: 1650 mg/kg/33W-I   CNREA8
  35,1270,75
MUT: mma-sat 50 μg/plate   TCMUE9 1,13,84
MUT: mma-smc 50 μmol/plate   MUREAV
  77,143,80

CONSENSUS REPORTS: EPA Genetic Toxicology Program.

SAFETY PROFILE: Questionable carcinogen with experimental tumorigenic data. Mutation data reported. When heated to decomposition it emits toxic fumes of NO_x.

MJM250   CAS: 64049-29-2
4,4'-METHYLENE-BIS(2-CHLOROANILINE) HYDROCHLORIDE
mf: $C_{13}H_{12}Cl_2N_2 \cdot ClH$ mw: 303.63

TOXICITY DATA and REFERENCE
CAR: orl-mus TDLo: 66 g/kg/78W-C   TXAPA9
  31,47,75
ETA: orl-rat TDLo: 14 g/kg/78W-C   TXAPA9
  31,47,75

SAFETY PROFILE: Questionable carcinogen with experimental carcinogenic and tumorigenic data. When heated to decomposition it emits very toxic fumes of Cl^- and NO_x.

MJO000 CAS: 1807-55-2
4,4'-METHYLENEBIS(N-METHYLANILINE)
mf: $C_{15}H_{18}N_2$ mw: 226.35

SYNS: BIS(N-METHYLANILINE)METHANE ◇ BIS(N-METHYLANILINO)METHAN (GERMAN) ◇ DIMETHYLDIAMINODIPHENYLMETHANE

TOXICITY DATA and REFERENCE
ETA: scu-rat TDLo: 850 mg/kg ZEKBAI 71,105,68

CONSENSUS REPORTS: Reported in EPA TSCA Inventory.

SAFETY PROFILE: Questionable carcinogen with experimental tumorigenic data. When heated to decomposition it emits toxic fumes of NO_x.

MJP400 CAS: 101-68-8
METHYLENE BISPHENYL ISOCYANATE
DOT: 2489
mf: $C_{15}H_{10}N_2O_2$ mw: 250.27

PROP: Crystals or yellow fused solid. Mp: 37.2°, bp: 194-199° @ 5 mm, d: 1.19 @ 50°, vap press: 0.001 mm @ 40°.

SYNS: BIS(p-ISOCYANATOPHENYL)METHANE ◇ BIS(1,4-ISOCYANATOPHENYL)METHANE ◇ BIS(4-ISO-CYANATOPHENYL)METHANE ◇ CARADATE 30 ◇ DESMO-DUR 44 ◇ DIFENIL-METAN-DIISOCIANATO (ITALIAN) ◇ DIFENYLMETHAAN-DISSOCYANAAT (DUTCH) ◇ 4-4'-DIISOCYANATE de DIPHENYLMETHANE (FRENCH) ◇ 4,4'-DIISOCYANATODIPHENYLMETHANE ◇ DIPHENYL-METHAN-4,4'-DIISOCYANAT (GERMAN) ◇ DIPHENYL METHANE DIISOCYANATE ◇ p,p'-DIPHENYLMETHANE DI-ISOCYANATE ◇ 4,4'-DIPHENYLMETHANE DIISOCYANATE ◇ DIPHENYLMETHANE 4,4'-DIISOCYANATE (DOT) ◇ HYLENE M50 ◇ ISONATE ◇ MDI ◇ METHYLENEBIS(4-ISOCYANATOBENZENE) ◇ 1,1-METHYLENEBIS(4-ISO-CYANATOBENZENE) ◇ METHYLENEBIS(4-PHENYLENE ISOCYANATE) ◇ METHYLENEBIS(p-PHENYLENE ISO-CYANATE) ◇ p,p'-METHYLENEBIS(PHENYL ISOCYA-NATE) ◇ METHYLENEBIS(p-PHENYL ISOCYANATE) ◇ METHYLENEBIS(4-PHENYL ISOCYANATE) ◇ 4,4'-METHYLENEBIS(PHENYL ISOCYANATE) ◇ 4,4'-METHYL-ENEDIPHENYL DIISOCYANATE ◇ METHYLENEDI-p-PHENYLENE DIISOCYANATE ◇ METHYLENEDI-p-PHENYL-ENE ISOCYANATE ◇ 4,4'-METHYLENEDIPHENYL ISO-CYANATE ◇ 4,4'-METHYLENEDIPHENYLENE ISO-CYANATE ◇ METHYLENE DI(PHENYLENE ISOCYA-NATE) (DOT) ◇ NACCONATE 300 ◇ NCI-C50668 ◇ RUBI-NATE 44

TOXICITY DATA with REFERENCE
MUT: eye-rbt 100 μg MLD AIHAAP 43,89,82
MUT: mma-sat 50 μg/plate SWEHDO 6,221,80
MUT: orl-mus LD16: 10700 mg/kg TPKVAL 15,128,79

CONSENSUS REPORTS: IARC Cancer Review: GROUP 3 IMEMDT 7,56,87. Reported in EPA TSCA Inventory. Community Right-To-Know List.

OSHA PEL: CL 0.02 ppm ACGIH TLV: 0.005 ppm DFG MAK: 0.01 ppm (0.1 mg/m³) NIOSH REL: (Diisocyanates) TWA 0.005 ppm; CL 0.02 ppm/10M DOT Classification: Poison B; Label: St. Andrews Cross.

SAFETY PROFILE: Questionable carcinogen. Poison by inhalation. Mildly toxic by ingestion. Human systemic effects by inhalation: increased immune response and body temperature. Mutation data reported. A skin and eye irritant. An allergic sensitizer. When heated to decomposition it emits toxic fumes of NO_x and SO_x.

MJQ250 CAS: 34481-84-0
METHYLENEDIANTHRANILIC ACID DIMETHYL ESTER
mf: $C_{17}H_{18}N_2O_4$ mw: 314.37

SYNS: MBMA ◇ METHYLENEBIS(2-AMINO-BENZOIC ACID) DIMETHYL ESTER (9CI) ◇ 4,4'-METHYLENEBIS(2-CARBOMETHOXYANILINE) ◇ METHYLENE-BIS(METHYL ANTHRANILATE)

TOXICITY DATA and REFERENCE
CAR: orl-rat TDLo: 490 g/kg/78W-C JEPTDQ 1(3),199,78
ETA: orl-rat TD: 410 g/kg/78W-C JEPTDQ 1(3),199,78

SAFETY PROFILE: Questionable carcinogen with experimental carcinogenic and tumorigenic data. When heated to decomposition it emits toxic fumes of NO_x.

MJQ750 CAS: 5625-90-1
4,4'-METHYLENEDIMORPHOLINE
mf: $C_9H_{18}N_2O_2$ mw: 186.29

SYNS: BIS(MORPHOLINO-)METHAN (GERMAN) ◇ BISMORPHOLINO METHANE

TOXICITY DATA and REFERENCE
ETA: scu-rat TD: 2000 mg/kg/40W-I ZEKBAI 71,105,68

ETA: scu-rat TDLo: 50 mg/kg   FCTXAV 6,576,68

SAFETY PROFILE: Questionable carcinogen with experimental tumorigenic data. Moderately toxic by subcutaneous route. When heated to decomposition it emits toxic fumes of NO_x.

MJT750   CAS: 3693-53-6
METHYLENE DIURETHAN
mf: $C_7H_{14}N_2O_4$ mw: 190.23

SYN: N,N-METHYLENE-BIS(ETHYL CARBAMATE)

TOXICITY DATA and REFERENCE
ETA: ipr-mus TDLo: 6500 mg/kg/13W-I
    JNCIAM 9,35,48

SAFETY PROFILE: Questionable carcinogen with experimental tumorigenic data. When heated to decomposition it emits toxic fumes of NO_x.

MJU000   CAS: 533-31-3
METHYLENE ETHER of OXYHYDROQUINONE
mf: $C_7H_6O_3$ mw: 138.13

SYN: SESAMOL

TOXICITY DATA and REFERENCE
ETA: orl-rat TDLo: 4608 mg/kg/82W-C
    JAFCAU 6,600,58

CONSENSUS REPORTS: Reported in EPA TSCA Inventory.

SAFETY PROFILE: Questionable carcinogen with experimental tumorigenic data. When heated to decomposition it emits acrid smoke and irritating fumes.

MJW000   CAS: 112-61-8
METHYL ESTER STEARIC ACID
mf: $C_{19}H_{38}O_2$ mw: 298.57

PROP: Liquid to semi-solid. Mp: 38°, bp: 215° @ 15 mm, flash p: 307°F (CC), d: 0.860. Sol in water and ether.

SYNS: EMERY 2218 ◇ METHOLENE 2218 ◇ METHYL OC-TADECANOATE ◇ METHYL STEARATE ◇ OCTADECANOIC ACID, METHYL ESTER

TOXICITY DATA and REFERENCE
ETA: scu-mus TD: 5200 mg/kg/26W-I   CNREA8 30,1037,70
ETA: scu-mus TDLo: 5200 mg/kg/26W-I
    CNREA8 32,880,72

CONSENSUS REPORTS: Reported in EPA TSCA Inventory.

SAFETY PROFILE: Questionable carcinogen with experimental tumorigenic data. Combustible when exposed to heat or flame; can react with oxidizing materials. To fight fire, use CO_2, dry chemical. When heated to decomposition it emits acrid smoke and irritating fumes.

MJW875   CAS: 13655-95-3
11-β-METHYL-17-α-ETHINYLESTRADIOL
mf: $C_{21}H_{26}O_2$ mw: 310.47

SYN: 11-β-METHYL-19-NOR-17-α-PREGNA-1,3,5(10)-TRIEN-20-YNE-3,17-DIOL

TOXICITY DATA and REFERENCE
CAR: imp-ham TDLo: 400 mg/kg/39W-C
    CNREA8 47,2583,87

SAFETY PROFILE: Questionable carcinogen with experimental carcinogenic data. When heated to decomposition it emits acrid smoke and irritating fumes.

MJX000   CAS: 16354-48-6
9-METHYL-10-ETHOXYMETHYL-1,2-BENZANTHRACENE
mf: $C_{21}H_{18}O$ mw: 286.39

SYN: 7-ETHOXY-12-METHYLBENZ(a)ANTHRACENE

TOXICITY DATA and REFERENCE
NEO: ims-rat TD: 50 mg/kg   PNASA6 58,2253,67
NEO: ims-rat TDLo: 50 mg/kg   CNREA8 29,506,69

SAFETY PROFILE: Questionable carcinogen with experimental neoplastigenic data. When heated to decomposition it emits acrid smoke and irritating fumes.

MJY250   CAS: 56961-65-0
7-METHYL-9-ETHYLBENZ(c)ACRIDINE
mf: $C_{20}H_{17}N$ mw: 271.38

SYN: 10-METHYL-3-ETHYL-7,8-BENZACRIDINE (FRENCH)

TOXICITY DATA and REFERENCE
ETA: skn-mus TD: 530 mg/kg/22W-I   BAFEAG 42,180,55
ETA: skn-mus TDLo: 275 mg/kg/22W-I
    ACRSAJ 4,315,56

SAFETY PROFILE: Questionable carcinogen with experimental tumorigenic data. When heated to decomposition it emits toxic fumes of NO_x.

MKA500   CAS: 1338-23-4
METHYL ETHYL KETONE PEROXIDE
mf: $C_8H_{16}O_4$ mw: 176.24

SYNS: HI-POINT 90 ◇ LUPERSOL ◇ MEKP ◇ MEK PEROX-IDE ◇ METHYLETHYLKETONHYDROPEROXIDE ◇ NCI-C55447 ◇ QUICKSET EXTRA ◇ RCRA WASTE NUMBER U160 ◇ SPRAYSET MEKP ◇ THERMACURE

TOXICITY DATA and REFERENCE
ETA: unr-mus TDLo:282 mg/kg   RARSAM 3,193,63

CONSENSUS REPORTS: Reported in EPA TSCA Inventory.

OSHA PEL: CL 0.7 ppm   ACGIH TLV: CL 0.2 ppm   DFG MAK: Organic Peroxide, moderate skin irritant.   DOT Classification: Forbidden.

SAFETY PROFILE: Questionable carcinogen with experimental tumorigenic data. Poison by intraperitoneal route. Moderately toxic by ingestion and inhalation. Human systemic effects by ingestion: changes in structure or function of esophagus, nausea or vomiting, other gastrointestinal effects. A moderate skin and eye irritant. A shock-sensitive explosive. When heated to decomposition it emits acrid smoke and irritating fumes.

MKB500   CAS: 14551-09-8
N-METHYL-N-ETHYL-4-(4′-(PYRIDYL-1′OXIDE)AZO)ANILINE
mf: $C_{14}H_{16}N_4O$ mw: 256.34

SYN: 4-((((4-ETHYL-4-METHYL)AMINO)PHENYL)AZO) PYRIDINE 1-OXIDE

TOXICITY DATA and REFERENCE
NEO: orl-rat TDLo:2142 mg/kg/17W-C
JNCIAM 37,365,66

SAFETY PROFILE: Questionable carcinogen with experimental neoplastigenic data. When heated to decomposition it emits toxic fumes of NO_x.

MKC500   CAS: 33543-31-6
2-METHYLFLUORANTHENE
mf: $C_{17}H_{12}$ mw: 216.29

TOXICITY DATA with REFERENCE
ETA: skn-mus TDLo:624 mg/kg/52W-I
JNCIAM 49,1165,72
MUT: mma-sat 50 μg/plate   CRNGDP 3,841,82

CONSENSUS REPORTS: IARC Cancer Review: Animal Limited Evidence IMEMDT 32,399,83.

SAFETY PROFILE: Suspected carcinogen with experimental tumorigenic data. Mutation data

reported. When heated to decomposition it emits acrid smoke and irritating fumes.

MKC750   CAS: 1706-01-0
3-METHYLFLUORANTHENE
mf: $C_{17}H_{12}$ mw: 216.29

TOXICITY DATA and REFERENCE
NEO: skn-mus TDLo:40 mg/kg/20D   JNCIAM 49,1165,72
MUT: mma-sat 10 μg/plate   CRNGDP 3,841,82

CONSENSUS REPORTS: IARC Cancer Review: Animal Inadequate Evidence IMEMDT 32,399,83.

SAFETY PROFILE: Questionable carcinogen with experimental neoplastigenic data. Mutation data reported. When heated to decomposition it emits acrid smoke and irritating fumes.

MKD250   CAS: 482-41-7
7-METHYL-9-FLUOROBENZ(c)ACRIDINE
mf: $C_{18}H_{12}FN$ mw: 261.31

SYN: 3-FLUORO-10-METHYL-7,8-BENZACRIDINE (FRENCH)

TOXICITY DATA and REFERENCE
ETA: scu-mus TD:60 mg/kg/9W-I   ACRSAJ 4,315,56
ETA: scu-mus TDLo:20 mg/kg   AICCA6 11,736,55
ETA: skn-mus TD:216 mg/kg/18W-I   AICCA6 11,736,55
ETA: skn-mus TDLo:132 mg/kg/11W-I
ACRSAJ 4,315,56

SAFETY PROFILE: Questionable carcinogen with experimental tumorigenic data. When heated to decomposition it emits very toxic fumes of F^- and NO_x.

MKD500   CAS: 439-25-8
7-METHYL-11-FLUOROBENZ(c)ACRIDINE
mf: $C_{18}H_{12}FN$ mw: 261.31

SYN: 1-FLUORO-10-METHYL-7,8-BENZACRIDINE

TOXICITY DATA and REFERENCE
ETA: scu-mus TD:60 mg/kg/9W-I   ACRSAJ 4,315,56
ETA: scu-mus TDLo:20 mg/kg   AICCA6 11,736,55

SAFETY PROFILE: Questionable carcinogen with experimental tumorigenic data. When heated to decomposition it emits very toxic fumes of F⁻ and NO_x.

MKD750 CAS: 436-30-6
10-METHYL-3-FLUORO-5,6-BENZACRIDINE
mf: $C_{18}H_{12}FN$ mw: 261.31

SYNS: 3-FLUORO-10-METHYL-5,6-BENZACRIDINE ◇ 10-FLUORO-12-METHYLBENZ(a)ACRIDINE

TOXICITY DATA and REFERENCE
ETA: scu-mus TD:60 mg/kg/9W-I ACRSAJ 4,315,56
ETA: scu-mus TDLo:20 mg/kg AICCA6 11,736,55
ETA: skn-mus TD:552 mg/kg/46W-I AICCA6 11,736,55
ETA: skn-mus TDLo:245 mg/kg/20W-I AICCA6 11,736,55

SAFETY PROFILE: Questionable carcinogen with experimental tumorigenic data. When heated to decomposition it emits very toxic fumes of F⁻ and NO_x.

MKH500 CAS: 591-11-7
5-METHYL-2(5H)-FURANONE
mf: $C_5H_6O_2$ mw: 98.11

SYNS: β-ANGELICA LACTONE ◇ Δ¹-ANGELICA LACTONE ◇ 4-HYDROXY-2-PENTENOIC ACID γ-LACTONE ◇ γ-METHYL-α,β-CROTONOLACTONE

TOXICITY DATA and REFERENCE
ETA: scu-rat TDLo:2600 mg/kg/65W-I BJCAAI 19,392,65

SAFETY PROFILE: Questionable carcinogen with experimental tumorigenic data. Moderately toxic by intraperitoneal route. When heated to decomposition it emits acrid smoke and irritating fumes.

MKI000 CAS: 31959-87-2
METHYL GAG
SYNS:
1,1'-(METHYLETHANEDILIDENEDINITRILO)BIGUANIDINE DIHYDROCHLORIDE DIHYDRATE ◇ NSC 32946

TOXICITY DATA and REFERENCE
NEO: orl-rat TDLo:3900 mg/kg/1Y-I JNCIAM 41,985,68

SAFETY PROFILE: Questionable carcinogen with experimental neoplastigenic by ingestion

data. Human systemic effects by an unspecified route: gastrointestinal changes and dermatitis. A skin irritant. When heated to decomposition it emits very toxic fumes of HCl and NO_x.

MKJ000 CAS: 65272-47-1
METHYLGUANIDINE mixed with SODIUM NITRITE (1:1)

SYN: SODIUM NITRITE mixed with METHYLGUANIDINE (1:1)

TOXICITY DATA and REFERENCE
NEO: orl-rat TDLo:70 g/kg/63W-C ZKKOBW 91,189,78
MUT: mmo-sat 80 mmol/L GANNA2 65,45,74

SAFETY PROFILE: Questionable carcinogen with experimental neoplastigenic data. Mutation data reported. When heated to decomposition it emits very toxic fumes of NO_x and Na_2O.

MKN500 CAS: 302-15-8
METHYL HYDRAZINE SULFATE
mf: $CH_6N_2 \cdot H_2O_4S$ mw: 144.17

PROP: Crystals from methyl alcohol. Mp: 142°. Very sol in water; very sltly sol in alc.

TOXICITY DATA and REFERENCE
NEO: orl-mus TDLo:2092 mg/kg/83W-C IJCNAW 9,109,72

CONSENSUS REPORTS: Reported in EPA TSCA Inventory.

SAFETY PROFILE: Questionable carcinogen with experimental neoplastigenic data. Poison by intraperitoneal route. When heated to decomposition it emits very toxic fumes of SO_x and NO_x.

MKN750 CAS: 366-71-2
(α-(2-METHYLHYDRAZINO)-p-TOLUOYL)UREA, MONOHYDROBROMIDE
mf: $C_{10}H_{14}N_4O_2 \cdot BrH$ mw: 303.20

SYNS: 1-(p-ALLOPHANOYLBENZYL)-2-METHYLHYDRAZINE HYDROBROMIDE ◇ N-AMINOCARBONYL)-4-((2-METHYLHYDRAZINO)METHYL)BENZAMIDE MONOHYDROBROMIDE ◇ 1-METHYL-2-(p-ALLOPHANOYLBENZYL)HYDRAZINE HYDROBROMIDE ◇ NSC 77517

TOXICITY DATA and REFERENCE
CAR: orl-rat TDLo:900 mg/kg/30D-I CNREA8 28,924,68

SAFETY PROFILE: Questionable carcinogen with experimental carcinogenic and teratogenic lata. Moderately toxic by ingestion. Experimenal reproductive effects. When heated to decomposition it emits very toxic fumes of HBr and NO_x.

MKP000   CAS: 51938-16-0
N-METHYL-N-(4-HYDROXYBUTYL)NITROSAMINE
mf: $C_5H_{12}N_2O_2$ mw: 132.19

SYN: N-NITROSO-N-METHYL-(4-HYDROXYBUTYL) AMINE

TOXICITY DATA and REFERENCE
ETA: orl-rat TDLo:53 g/kg/20W-C   GANNA2 67,825,76

MUT: mma-sat 40 μmol/plate   CNREA8 37,399,77

CONSENSUS REPORTS: EPA Genetic Toxicology Program.

SAFETY PROFILE: Questionable carcinogen with experimental tumorigenic data. Mutation data reported. When heated to decomposition it emits toxic fumes of NO_x.

MKR000   CAS: 10482-16-3
2-METHYL-4-HYDROXYLAMINOQUINOLINE 1-OXIDE
mf: $C_{10}H_{10}N_2O_2$ mw: 190.22

SYN: 4-(HYDROXYLAMINO)-2-METHYL-QUINOLINE, 1-OXIDE

TOXICITY DATA and REFERENCE
ETA: scu-mus TDLo:120 mg/kg/50D-I   BCPCA6 16,631,67

SAFETY PROFILE: Questionable carcinogen with experimental tumorigenic data. When heated to decomposition it emits toxic fumes of NO_x.

MKR500   CAS: 23324-72-3
METHYL HYDROXYOCTADECADIENOATE
mf: $C_{19}H_{34}O_3$ mw: 310.53

SYN: 13-HYDROXY-9,11-OCTADECADIENOIC METHYL ESTER

TOXICITY DATA and REFERENCE
ETA: skn-mus TDLo:64 g/kg/53W-I   AMBPBZ 82,127,74

SAFETY PROFILE: Questionable carcinogen with experimental tumorigenic data. When heated to decomposition it emits acrid smoke and irritating fumes.

MLH500   CAS: 66-27-3
METHYL MESYLATE
mf: $C_2H_6O_3S$ mw: 110.14

PROP: Liquid. D: 1.046 @ 16°/4° bp: 126.5° @ 756 mm. Decomp in water; sol in alc and ether.

SYNS: as-DIMETHYL SULPHATE ◇ METHANESULPHONIC ACID METHYL ESTER ◇ METHYL ESTER of METHANESULFONIC ACID ◇ METHYL ESTER of METHANESULPHONIC ACID ◇ METHYLMETHANSULFONAT (GERMAN) ◇ METHYL METHANESULFONATE ◇ METHYL METHANE-SULPHONATE ◇ METHYL METHANSULFONATE ◇ METHYL METHANSULPHONATE ◇ MMS ◇ NSC-50256

TOXICITY DATA and REFERENCE
NEO: orl-mus TD:14 g/kg/78W-C   SCIEAS 161,913,68
NEO: orl-mus TDLo:300 mg/kg/8W-I   TXAPA9 82,19,86
ETA: ipr-rat TDLo:72 mg/kg   NATUAS 223,947,69
ETA: ivn-rat TDLo:20 mg/kg/(15D preg):TER   EJCAAH 8,641,72
ETA: ivn-rat TDLo:20 mg/kg:REP   EJCAAH 8,641,72
ETA: ivn-rat TDLo:30 mg/kg (21D preg):TER   43XWAI -,15,78
ETA: ivn-rat TDLo:30 mg/kg:REP   43XWAI-,15,78
ETA: ivn-rat TDLo:96 mg/kg   ANYAA9 163,717,69
ETA: ivn-rat TDLo:96 mg/kg   ANYAA9 163,717,69
ETA: orl-rat TDLo:420 mg/kg/2W-C   CRNGDP 6,1529,85
ETA: scu-rat TDLo:184 mg/kg/46W-I   ZEKBAI 74,241,70
ETA: unr-rat TD:75 mg/kg/10W-I   BJCAAI 50,63,84
ETA: unr-rat TDLo:20 mg/kg/(15D preg):TER   IARCCD 4,143,73
MUT: dnd-mus:emb 250 nmol/L   AJOGAH 148,929,84
MUT: dnr-smc 900 nmol/L   CNJGA8 24,771,82
MUT: dns-dmg:emb 4500 μmol/L   MUREAV 112,215,83
MUT: dns-hmn:fbr 2400 μmol/L   ENMUDM 7,267,85
MUT: dns-hmn:oth 100 μmol/L   TXAPA979,28,85
MUT: mma-sat 100 μg/plate   ENMUDM 6(Suppl 2),1,84
MUT: mmo-sat 1 μL/plate   MUREAV 130,79,84
MUT: pic-bcs 50 mmol/L   IJEBA6 22,338,84

MUT: sce-nml-skn 500 μmol/L   MUREAV
105,235,82

CONSENSUS REPORTS: IARC Cancer Review: GROUP 3 IMEMDT 7,56,87; Animal Sufficient Evidence IMEMDT 7,253,74. Reported in EPA TSCA Inventory. EPA Genetic Toxicology Program.

SAFETY PROFILE: Questionable carcinogen with experimental carcinogenic, neoplastigenic, tumorigenic, and teratogenic data. Poison by ingestion, intraperitoneal, intravenous, and subcutaneous routes. Human mutation data reported. Experimental reproductive effects. When heated to decomposition it emits toxic fumes of SO_x.

MLH750   CAS: 80-62-6
METHYL METHACRYLATE
DOT: 1247
mf: $C_5H_8O_2$ mw: 100.13

PROP: Colorless liquid, very sltly sol in water. Mp: −50°, bp: 101.0°, flash p: 50°F (OC), d: 0.936 @ 20°/4°, vap press: 40 mm @ 25.5°, vap d: 3.45, lel: 2.1%, uel: 12.5%.

SYNS: DIAKON ◇ METAKRYLAN METYLU (POLISH) ◇ METHACRYLATE de METHYLE (FRENCH) ◇ METHACRYLIC ACID, METHYL ESTER (MAK) ◇ METHACRYLSAEUREMETHYL ESTER (GERMAN) ◇ METHYLMETHACRYLAAT (DUTCH) ◇ METHYL-METHACRYLAT (GERMAN) ◇ METHYL METHACRYLATE MONOMER, INHIBITED (DOT) ◇ METHYL-α-METHYLACRYLATE ◇ METHYL-2-METHYL-2-PROPENOATE ◇ 2-METHYL-2-PROPENOIC ACID METHYL ESTER ◇ METIL METACRILATO (ITALIAN) ◇ MME ◇ "MONOCITE" METHACRYLATE MONOMER ◇ NCI-C50680 ◇ RCRA WASTE NUMBER U162

TOXICITY DATA and REFERENCE
ETA: imp-rat TDLo: 1620 mg/kg   CORTBR
88,223,72
MUT: cyt-rat-ihl 4 mg/m³/16W   BZARAZ27,102,74
MUT: mma-mus: lym 500 mg/L   ENMUDM8(Suppl 6),4,86
MUT: mma-sat 34 mmol/L   JBJSA3 61-A,1203,79

CONSENSUS REPORTS: IARC Cancer Review: Human Inadequate Evidence IMEMDT 19,187,79; Animal Inadequate Evidence IMEMDT 19,187,79. NTP Carcinogenesis Studies (inhalation); No Evidence: mouse, rat NTPTR* NTP-TR-314,86. Reported in EPA TSCA Inventory. Community Right-To-Know List.

OSHA PEL: TWA 100 ppm   ACGIH TLV: TWA 100 ppm   DFG MAK: 50 ppm (210 mg/m³)   DOT Classification: Flammable Liquid; Label: Flammable Liquid.

SAFETY PROFILE: Questionable carcinogen with experimental tumorigenic and teratogenic data. Moderately toxic by inhalation and intraperitoneal routes. Mildly toxic by ingestion. Human systemic effects by inhalation: sleep effects, excitement, anorexia and blood pressure decrease. Experimental reproductive effects. Mutation data reported. A skin and eye irritant. A very dangerous fire hazard when exposed to heat or flame; can react with oxidizing materials. To fight fire, use foam, CO_2, dry chemical. When heated to decomposition it emits acrid smoke and irritating fumes.

MLK750   CAS: 53499-68-6
N-METHYL-4'-(p-METHYLAMINOPHENYLAZO)
ACETANILIDE
mf: $C_{16}H_{18}N_4O$ mw: 282.38

SYNS: 4-(N-ACETYL-N-METHYL)AMINO-4'-N-METHYL-AMINOAZOBENZENE ◇ N'-ACETYL-N'-MONOMETHYL-4'-AMINO-N-MONOMETHYL-4-AMINOAZOBENZENE ◇ N-METHYL-N-(4-((4-(METHYLAMINO)PHENYL)AZO)PHENYLACETAMIDE)

TOXICITY DATA and REFERENCE
ETA: orl-rat TDLo: 2500 mg/kg/17W-C
CNREA8 34,2274,74
MUT: dns-rat: lvr 1 μmol/L   CNREA8 46,1654,86
MUT: mma-sat 250 nmol/plate   CNREA8
46,1654,86

SAFETY PROFILE: Questionable carcinogen with experimental tumorigenic data. Mutation data reported. When heated to decomposition it emits toxic fumes of NO_x.

MLL250   CAS: 80-48-8
METHYL-p-METHYLBENZENESULFONATE
mf: $C_8H_{10}O_3S$ mw: 186.24

PROP: Light brown crystals; crystals of ethyl ligroin. D: 1.230-1.238 @ 25°/25°, vap d: 6.45, mp: 28°. Insol in water; sol in benzene, very sol in alc and ether.

SYNS: METHYLESTER KYSELINY p-TOLUENSULFONOVE (CZECH) ◇ METHYL-4-METHYLBENZENESULFONATE ◇ METHYL-p-TOLUENESULFONATE ◇ METHYL TOLUENE-4-SULFONATE ◇ METHYL TOSYLATE ◇ METHYL-p-TOSYLATE ◇ p-TOLUOLSULFONSAEURE METHYL ESTER (GERMAN)

TOXICITY DATA and REFERENCE
ETA: orl-rat TDLo:1400 mg/kg/2Y ZEKBAI 74,241,70
ETA: scu-rat TD:800 mg/kg/54W-I ZEKBAI 74,241,70
ETA: scu-rat TDLo:50 mg/kg FCTXAV 6,576,68

CONSENSUS REPORTS: Reported in EPA TSCA Inventory.

SAFETY PROFILE: Questionable carcinogen with experimental tumorigenic data. Poison by ingestion and subcutaneous route. An eye and severe skin irritant. A vesicant and skin sensitizer. When heated to decomposition it emits toxic fumes of SO_x.

MLN500 CAS: 63041-88-3
10-METHYL-1′,9-METHYLENE-1,2-BENZANTHRACENE
mf: $C_{20}H_{14}$ mw: 254.34

SYN: 6-METHYL-11H-BENZ(bc)ACEANTHRYLENE

TOXICITY DATA and REFERENCE
ETA: scu-mus TDLo:40 mg/kg CNREA8 6,454,46

SAFETY PROFILE: Questionable carcinogen with experimental tumorigenic data. When heated to decomposition it emits acrid smoke and irritating fumes.

MLY250 CAS: 64-01-7
3-METHYL-4-MONOMETHYLAMINOAZOBENZENE
mf: $C_{14}H_{14}N_3$ mw: 224.31

SYN: N-METHYL-3-METHYL-p-AMINOAZOBENZENE

TOXICITY DATA and REFERENCE
NEO: orl-rat TDLo:9864 mg/kg/39W-C JEMEAV 87,139,48

SAFETY PROFILE: Questionable carcinogen with experimental neoplastigenic data. When heated to decomposition it emits toxic fumes of NO_x.

MMD000 CAS: 2869-09-2
5-METHYLNAPHTHO(1,2,3,4-def)CHRYSENE
mf: $C_{25}H_{16}$ mw: 316.41

SYN: 2′-METHYL-1,2:4,5-DIBENZOPYRENE

TOXICITY DATA and REFERENCE
ETA: scu-mus TDLo:72 mg/kg/9W-I COREAF 259,3899,64

SAFETY PROFILE: Questionable carcinogen with experimental tumorigenic data. When heated to decomposition it emits acrid smoke and irritating fumes.

MMD250 CAS: 2869-10-5
6-METHYLNAPHTHO(1,2,3,4-def)CHRYSENE
mf: $C_{25}H_{16}$ mw: 316.41

SYN: 3′-METHYL-1,2:4,5-DIBENZOPYRENE

TOXICITY DATA and REFERENCE
ETA: scu-mus TDLo:72 mg/kg/9W-I COREAF 259,3899,64

SAFETY PROFILE: Questionable carcinogen with experimental tumorigenic data. When heated to decomposition it emits acrid smoke and irritating fumes.

MMD500 CAS: 58-27-5
2-METHYL-1,4-NAPHTHOQUINONE
mf: $C_{11}H_8O_2$ mw: 172.19

SYNS: AQUAKAY ◇ AQUINONE ◇ HEMODAL ◇ KAERGONA ◇ KANONE ◇ KAPPAXAN ◇ KARCON ◇ KAREON ◇ KATIV-G ◇ KAYKLOT ◇ KAYQUINONE ◇ KIPCA ◇ KLOTTONE ◇ KOAXIN ◇ KOLKLOT ◇ K-THROMBYL ◇ K-VITAN ◇ MENADION ◇ MENADIONE ◇ MENAPHTHON ◇ MENAPHTONE ◇ 2-METHLY-1,4-NAPHTHALENDIONE ◇ 2-METHLY-1,4-NAPHTHALENEDIONE ◇ 2′-METHYL-1,4-NAPHTHOCHINON (GERMAN) ◇ 3-METHYL-1,4-NAPHTHOQUINONE ◇ MITENON ◇ MNQ ◇ NSC 4170 ◇ PANOSINE ◇ PROKAYVIT ◇ SYNKAY ◇ THYLOQUINONE ◇ USAF EK-5185 ◇ VITAMIN K2(O) ◇ VITAMIN K3

TOXICITY DATA and REFERENCE
ETA: skn-mus TD:8400 mg/kg/21W-I CNREA8 19,413,59
ETA: skn-mus TDLo:1860 mg/kg/27W-I BJCAAI 7,482,53
MUT: dnd-hmn:fbr 20 μmol/L TOLED5 28,37,85
MUT: dnd-rat:lvr 10 μmol/L TOLED5 28,37,85
MUT: mma-sat 30 nmol/plate BBRCA9 94,737,80
MUT: mmo-sat 4 μg/plate ABCHA6 45,327,81

CONSENSUS REPORTS: Reported in EPA TSCA Inventory.

SAFETY PROFILE: Questionable carcinogen with experimental tumorigenic and teratogenic data. Poison by ingestion, intraperitoneal, and subcutaneous routes. Moderately toxic by intravenous route. Experimental reproductive effects. Human mutation data reported. When

heated to decomposition it emits acrid smoke and irritating fumes.

MME750   CAS: 5096-18-4
3-METHYL-2-NAPHTHYLAMINE HYDROCHLORIDE
mf: $C_{11}H_{11}N \cdot ClH$ mw: 193.69

TOXICITY DATA and REFERENCE
CAR: orl-rat TD:5250 mg/kg/21W-I   JNCIAM 41,985,68
CAR: orl-rat TDLo:1500 mg/kg   CNREA8 26,619,66

SAFETY PROFILE: Questionable carcinogen with experimental carcinogenic data. Moderately toxic by ingestion. When heated to decomposition it emits very toxic fumes of NO_x and HCl.

MME800   CAS: 27636-33-5
N-METHYL NAPHTHYLCARBAMATE
mf: $C_{12}H_{11}NO_2$ mw: 201.24

SYN: CARBAMIC ACID, METHYL-, NAPHTHALENYL ESTER

TOXICITY DATA and REFERENCE
ETA: ipr-mus TDLo:240 mg/kg/4W-I   CNREA8 29,2184,69

SAFETY PROFILE: Questionable carcinogen with experimental tumorigenic data. When heated to decomposition it emits toxic fumes of NO_x.

MMJ000   CAS: 21638-36-8
4-METHYL-1-((5-NITROFURFURYLIDENE)AMINO-2-IMIDAZOLIDINONE
mf: $C_8H_{10}N_4O_4$ mw: 226.22

TOXICITY DATA and REFERENCE
NEO: orl-rat TDLo:14 g/kg/46W-C   JNCIAM 51,403,73
MUT: dnr-sat 500 nmol/well   CNREA8 34,2266,74
MUT: mma-sat 100 ng/plate   MUREAV 48,295,77
MUT: mmo-esc 500 nmol/well   CNREA8 34,2266,74
MUT: mrc-esc 500 nmol/well   CNREA8 34,2266,74

CONSENSUS REPORTS: EPA Genetic Toxicology Program.

SAFETY PROFILE: Questionable carcinogen with experimental neoplastigenic data. Mutation data reported. When heated to decomposition it emits toxic fumes of NO_x.

MMJ950   CAS: 7194-19-6
5-METHYL-3-(5-NITRO-2-FURYL)ISOXAZOLE
mf: $C_8H_6N_2O_4$ mw: 194.16

TOXICITY DATA and REFERENCE
ETA: orl-rat TDLo:37674 mg/kg/46W-C
    PAACA3 21,75,80

SAFETY PROFILE: Questionable carcinogen with experimental tumorigenic data. When heated to decomposition it emits toxic fumes of NO_x.

MMJ960   CAS: 5052-75-5
5-METHYL-3-(5-NITRO-2-FURYL)PYRAZOLE
mf: $C_8H_7N_3O_3$ mw: 193.18

TOXICITY DATA and REFERENCE
ETA: orl-rat TDLo:37352 mg/kg/46W-C
    PAACA3 21,75,80
MUT: dnd-mus:fbr 300 μmol/L   BJCAAI 3,124,78

SAFETY PROFILE: Questionable carcinogen with experimental tumorigenic data. Mutation data reported. When heated to decomposition it emits toxic fumes of NO_x.

MMJ975   CAS: 53757-29-2
2-METHYL-4-(5-NITRO-2-FURYL)THIAZOLE
mf: $C_8H_6N_2O_3S$ mw: 210.22

TOXICITY DATA and REFERENCE
ETA: orl-rat TDLo:40572 mg/kg/46W-C
    PAACA3 21,75,80
MUT: dnr-esc 500 nmol/well   CNREA8 34,2266,74
MUT: dnr-sat 500 nmol/well   CNREA8 34,2266,74
MUT: mmo-esc 300 nmol/well   CNREA8 34,2266,74
MUT: mmo-sat 100 ng/plate   MUREAV 40,9,76

SAFETY PROFILE: Questionable carcinogen with experimental tumorigenic data. Mutation data reported. When heated to decomposition it emits toxic fumes of SO_x.

MML500
1-METHYL-3-NITROGUANIDINE mixed with SODIUM NITRITE (1:1)

SYN: SODIUM NITRITE mixed with 1-METHYL-3-NITROGUANIDINE (1:1)

TOXICITY DATA and REFERENCE
CAR: orl-rat TDLo:90 g/kg/67W-C   VOONAW 23(8),54,77

MUT: dns-hmn:fbr 100 μmol/L/3H   IJCNAW
16,284,75

SAFETY PROFILE: Questionable carcinogen
with experimental carcinogenic data. Human
mutation data reported. When heated to decomposition it emits very toxic fumes of NO_x and
Na_2O.

MMP500   CAS: 5470-66-6
2-METHYL-4-NITROPYRIDINE-1-OXIDE
mf: $C_6H_6N_2O_3$ mw: 154.14

TOXICITY DATA and REFERENCE
ETA: scu-mus TDLo: 1800 mg/kg/15W-I
GANNA2 70,799,79
MUT: dnd-mus:fbr 50 μmol/L   CNREA8 35,521,75
MUT: mmo-esc 500 μmol/L   GANNA2 70,799,79
MUT: mmo-sat 1 μmol/plate   GANNA2 70,799,79

SAFETY PROFILE: Questionable carcinogen
with experimental tumorigenic data. Mutation
data reported. When heated to decomposition
it emits toxic fumes of NO_x.

MMP750   CAS: 1074-98-2
3-METHYL-4-NITROPYRIDINE-1-OXIDE
mf: $C_6H_6N_2O_3$ mw: 154.14

TOXICITY DATA and REFERENCE
ETA: scu-mus TD: 1680 mg/kg/15W-I   GANNA2
70,799,79
ETA: scu-mus TDLo: 1680 mg/kg/28W-I
GANNA2 62,325,71
MUT: dnd-mus:fbr 50 μmol/L   CNREA8 35,521,75
MUT: dnr-esc 500 μg/well   CNREA8 32,2369,72
MUT: mmo-esc 500 μmol/L   GANNA2 70,799,79
MUT: mmo-sat 100 nmol/plate   GANNA2 70,799,79
MUT: mmo-smc 500 μg/well   CNREA8 32,2369,72
MUT: mrc-esc 500 μg/well   CNREA8 32,2369,72

SAFETY PROFILE: Questionable carcinogen
with experimental tumorigenic data. Mutation
data reported. When heated to decomposition
it emits toxic fumes of NO_x.

MMQ250   CAS: 4831-62-3
2-METHYL-4-NITROQUINOLINE-1-OXIDE
mf: $C_{10}H_8N_2O_3$ mw: 204.20

SYN: 4-NITROQUINALDINE-N-OXIDE

TOXICITY DATA and REFERENCE
ETA: scu-mus TDLo: 120 mg/kg/50D-I   BCPCA6
16,631,67
ETA: skn-mus TDLo: 60 mg/kg/10W-I   GANNA2
49,33,58

MUT: cyt-hmn:lvr 5260 nmol/L   JNCIAM
47,367,71
MUT: cyt-omi 195 μmol/L   GANNA2 60,155,69
MUT: dnd-mam:lym 50 μmol/L   GANNA2
60,97,69
MUT: dnd-mus:fbr 10 μmol/L   CNREA8 35,521,75
MUT: dns-ham:oth 500 μmol/L   NATUAS
229,416,71
MUT: dns-hmn:fbr 1 nmol/L/90M   IJCNAW
16,284,75
MUT: mmo-smc 200 μg/L   IGSBAL 85,127,72

SAFETY PROFILE: Questionable carcinogen
with experimental tumorigenic data. Human
mutation data reported. When heated to decomposition it emits toxic fumes of NO_x.

MMQ500   CAS: 14073-00-8
3-METHYL-4-NITROQUINOLINE-1-OXIDE
mf: $C_{10}H_8N_2O_3$ mw: 204.20

TOXICITY DATA and REFERENCE
ETA: skn-mus TDLo: 600 mg/kg/10W-I
GANNA2 60,523,69
MUT: cyt-rat:lvr 100 μg/L   PMRSDJ 1,570,81
MUT: dnd-hmn:fbr 250 μmol/L   CRNGDP
3,1463,82
MUT: dns-hmn:fbr 1100 μg/L   PMRSDJ 1,517,81
MUT: dns-rat:lvr 50 μmol/L   ENMUDM 3,11,81
MUT: sce-ham:ovr 115 mg/L   PMRSDJ 1,551,81

CONSENSUS REPORTS: EPA Genetic Toxicology Program.

SAFETY PROFILE: Questionable carcinogen
with experimental tumorigenic data. Poison by
intraperitoneal route. Human mutation data reported. When heated to decomposition it emits
toxic fumes of NO_x.

MMQ750   CAS: 14094-43-0
5-METHYL-4-NITROQUINOLINE-1-OXIDE
mf: $C_{10}H_8N_2O_3$ mw: 204.20

TOXICITY DATA and REFERENCE
ETA: scu-mus TDLo: 120 mg/kg/50D-I   BCPCA6
16,631,67
MUT: dns-ham:oth 500 nmol/L   NATUAS
229,416,71
MUT: mmo-sat 800 μmol/L   CPBTAL 31,959,83

CONSENSUS REPORTS: EPA Genetic Toxicology Program.

SAFETY PROFILE: Questionable carcinogen
with experimental tumorigenic data. Mutation

data reported. When heated to decomposition it emits toxic fumes of NO_x.

MMR000   CAS: 715-48-0
6-METHYL-4-NITROQUINOLINE-1-OXIDE
mf: $C_{10}H_8N_2O_3$ mw: 204.20

TOXICITY DATA and REFERENCE
ETA: scu-mus TDLo: 120 mg/kg/50D-I BCPCA6 16,631,67
MUT: cyt-hmn: lvr 5260 nmol/L JNCIAM 47,367,71
MUT: dnd-mus-orl 10 mg/kg IJCNAW 17,765,76
MUT: dnd-mus: fbr 10 µmol/L CNREA8 35,521,75
MUT: dns-ham: oth 500 nmol/L NATUAS 229,416,71
MUT: mmo-sat 8 µmol/L CPBTAL 31,959,83
MUT: mmo-smc 200 mg/L IGSBAL 85,127,72

CONSENSUS REPORTS: EPA Genetic Toxicology Program.

SAFETY PROFILE: Questionable carcinogen with experimental tumorigenic data. Poison by intraperitoneal route. Human mutation data reported. When heated to decomposition it emits toxic fumes of NO_x.

MMR250   CAS: 14753-13-0
7-METHYL-4-NITROQUINOLINE-1-OXIDE
mf: $C_{10}H_8N_2O_3$ mw: 204.20

TOXICITY DATA and REFERENCE
ETA: scu-mus TDLo: 120 mg/kg/50D-I BCPCA6 16,631,67
MUT: cyt-hmn: lvr 5260 nmol/L JNCIAM 47,367,71
MUT: dnd-mus: fbr 10 µmol/L CNREA8 35,521,75
MUT: dns-ham: oth 500 µmol/L NATUAS 229,416,71
MUT: mmo-smc 200 mg/L IGSBAL 85,127,72

SAFETY PROFILE: Questionable carcinogen with experimental tumorigenic data. Human mutation data reported. When heated to decomposition it emits toxic fumes of NO_x.

MMR500   CAS: 14094-45-2
8-METHYL-4-NITROQUINOLINE-1-OXIDE
mf: $C_{10}H_8N_2O_3$ mw: 204.20

TOXICITY DATA and REFERENCE
ETA: scu-mus TDLo: 120 mg/kg/50D-I BCPCA6 16,631,67

MUT: dns-ham: oth 8 µmol/L NATUAS 229,416,71
MUT: mmo-smc 100 µg/L TXAPA9 15,451,69

SAFETY PROFILE: Questionable carcinogen with experimental tumorigenic data. Mutation data reported. When heated to decomposition it emits toxic fumes of NO_x.

MMR750   CAS: 16699-07-3
1-(4-N-METHYL-N-NITROSAMINOBENZYLIDENE)INDENE
mf: $C_{17}H_{14}N_2O$ mw: 262.33

SYNS: 4-(1-H-INDEN-1-YLIDENEMETHYL)-N-METHYL-N-NITROSOBENZENAMINE ◇ NSC-101983

TOXICITY DATA and REFERENCE
CAR: orl-rat TDLo: 238 g/kg/34W-C JNCIAM 51,1313,73

SAFETY PROFILE: Questionable carcinogen with experimental carcinogenic data. When heated to decomposition it emits toxic fumes of NO_x.

MMR800
1-(METHYLNITROSAMINO)-2-BUTANONE
mf: $C_5H_{10}N_2O_2$ mw: 130.17

SYNS: M-2-OB ◇ N-NITROSOMETHYL(2-OXOBUTYL) AMINE

TOXICITY DATA and REFERENCE
CAR: scu-ham TD: 100 mg/kg CNREA8 43,4885,83
CAR: scu-ham TDLo: 67 mg/kg/29W-I CNREA8 43,4885,83
MUT: msc-ham: lng 700 µmol/L 50EYAN-,241,83

SAFETY PROFILE: Questionable carcinogen with experimental carcinogenic data. Poison by subcutaneous route. Mutation data reported. When heated to decomposition it emits toxic fumes of NO_x.

MMR810
4-(METHYLNITROSAMINO)-2-BUTANONE
mf: $C_5H_{10}N_2O_2$ mw: 130.17

SYNS: M-3-OB ◇ N-NITROSOMETHYL(3-OXOBUTYL) AMINE

TOXICITY DATA and REFERENCE
CAR: scu-ham TD: 1377 mg/kg/34W-I CNREA8 43,4885,83
CAR: scu-ham TDLo: 770 mg/kg/38W-I CNREA8 43,4885,83

MUT: mma-ham:lng 600 μmol/L   MUREAV
163,303,86

MUT: msc-ham:lng 700 μmol/L   50EYAN-,241,83

SAFETY PROFILE: Questionable carcinogen with experimental carcinogenic data. Moderately toxic by subcutaneous route. Mutation data reported. When heated to decomposition it emits toxic fumes of NO_x.

MMS000   CAS: 67557-57-7
METHYLNITROSAMINOMETHYL-d3 ESTER ACETIC ACID
mf: $C_4H_5D_3N_2O_3$ mw: 135.14

SYNS:
ACETOXYMETHYLTRIDEUTEROMETHYLNITROSAMINE ◇ 1-ACETOXY-N-NITROSO-N-TRIDEUTEROMETHYL-METHYLAMINE ◇ NITROSO-N-(1-ACETOXYMETHYL)TRIDEUTEROMETHYLAMINE ◇ TRIDEUTEROMETHYL ACETOXYMETHYLNITROS-AMINE

TOXICITY DATA and REFERENCE
ETA: orl-rat TDLo:51 mg/kg/90D-I   ZKKOBW
91,317,78

SAFETY PROFILE: Questionable carcinogen with experimental tumorigenic data. Poison by ingestion. When heated to decomposition it emits toxic fumes of NO_x.

MMS250   CAS: 64091-90-3
4-(N-METHYL-N-NITROSAMINO)-4-(3-PYRIDYL)BUTANAL
mf: $C_{10}H_{13}N_3O_2$ mw: 207.26

SYNS: γ-(METHYLNITROSAMINO)-3-PYRIDINEBUTYR-ALDEHYDE ◇ γ-(METHYLNITROSOAMINO)-3-PYRIDINE-BUTANAL ◇ 4-(N-NITROSO-N-METHYLAMINO)-4-(3-PYRI-DYL)BUTANAL ◇ NNA

TOXICITY DATA and REFERENCE
NEO: ipr-mus TDLo:880 mg/kg/I   IARCCD
19,395,78

ETA: ipr-mus TD:880 mg/kg/7W-I   JNCIAM
60,819,78

CONSENSUS REPORTS: IARC Cancer Review: Animal Inadequate Evidence IMEMDT 37,205,85.

SAFETY PROFILE: Questionable carcinogen with experimental neoplastigenic and tumorigenic data. When heated to decomposition it emits toxic fumes of NO_x.

MMS750   CAS: 16699-10-8
4-(4-N-METHYL-N-NITROSAMINOSTYRYL)QUINOLINE
mf: $C_{18}H_{15}N_3O$ mw: 289.36

SYNS: N-METHYL-N-NITROSO-4-(2-(4-QUINOLINY-L)ETHENYL)BENZENAMINE ◇ NSC-101984

TOXICITY DATA and REFERENCE
CAR: orl-rat TDLo:12 g/kg/34W-C   JNCIAM
51,1313,73

SAFETY PROFILE: Questionable carcinogen with experimental carcinogenic data. When heated to decomposition it emits toxic fumes of NO_x.

MMT000   CAS: 7417-67-6
METHYLNITROSOACETAMIDE
mf: $C_3H_6N_2O_2$ mw: 102.11

SYNS: N-METHYL-N-NITROSOACETAMIDE ◇ METHYL-NITROSOACETAMID (GERMAN) ◇ N-NITROSO-N-METHY-LACETAMIDE

TOXICITY DATA and REFERENCE
ETA: orl-rat TD:506 mg/kg/72W-C   ZEKBAI
69,103,67

ETA: orl-rat TDLo:375 mg/kg/75W-I   PPTCBY
2,73,72

MUT: mma-sat 2 nmol/plate   CNREA8 39,1328,79

MUT: mmo-smc 100 μmol/L   ZEVBA5 95,55,65

MUT: sln-dmg-par 3000 ppm   BPYKAU 4,90,67

CONSENSUS REPORTS: EPA Genetic Toxicology Program.

SAFETY PROFILE: Questionable carcinogen with experimental tumorigenic data. Poison by ingestion. Mutation data reported. When heated to decomposition it emits toxic fumes of NO_x.

MMT250   CAS: 21928-82-5
N-METHYL-N-NITROSOADENINE
mf: $C_6H_6N_6O$ mw: 178.18

SYNS: 6-(METHYLNITROSAMINO)PURINE ◇ N-METHYL-N-NITROSO-1H-PURIN-6-AMINE ◇ 6-MNA ◇ N^6-METHYL-N^6-NITROSO-1H-PURIN-6-AMINE

TOXICITY DATA and REFERENCE
CAR: orl-mus TDLo:10263 mg/kg/72W-I
IJCNAW 24,319,79

NEO: orl-mus TD:15 g/kg/2Y-I   IAPUDO31,787,80

NEO: orl-mus TD:485 g/kg/34W-I   PAACA3
18,79,77

SAFETY PROFILE: Questionable carcinogen with experimental carcinogenic and neoplasti-

genic data. When heated to decomposition it emits toxic fumes of NO$_x$.

MMT300
N^6-(METHYLNITROSO)ADENOSINE
mf: C$_{11}$H$_{14}$N$_6$O$_5$ mw: 310.31

SYN: N^6-METHYL-N^6-NITROSO-9b-d-RIBOFURANOSYL-9H-PURIN-6-AMINE

TOXICITY DATA and REFERENCE
CAR: orl-mus TD: 17856 mg/kg/72W-I IJCNAW 24,319,79
CAR: orl-mus TDLo: 16368 mg/kg/66W-I IJCNAW 24,319,79
NEO: orl-mus TD: 26 g/kg/2Y-I IAPUDO 31,787,80

SAFETY PROFILE: Questionable carcinogen with experimental carcinogenic and neoplastigenic data. When heated to decomposition it emits toxic fumes of NO$_x$.

MMT500   CAS: 4549-43-3
N-METHYL-N-NITROSOALLYLAMINE
mf: C$_4$H$_8$N$_2$O   mw: 100.14

SYNS: METHYLALLYLNITROSAMIN (GERMAN) ◇ METHYLALLYLNITROSAMINE ◇ N-METHYL-N-NITROSO-2-PROPEN-1-AMINE ◇ N-NITROSOALLYLMETHYLAMINE ◇ NITROSOMETHYLALLYLAMINE ◇ N-NITROSOMETHYLALLYLAMINE

TOXICITY DATA and REFERENCE
ETA: ivn-rat TDLo: 380 mg/kg/38W-I ZEKBAI 69,103,67
ETA: orl-rat TDLo: 800 mg/kg/76W-C ARZNAD 19,1077,69
MUT: dns-rat: lvr 500 μmol/L ENMUDM 3,11,81
MUT: mmo-esc 40 μmol/L ENMUDM 3,11,81
MUT: mmo-sat 40 μmol/L ENMUDM 3,11,81

SAFETY PROFILE: Questionable carcinogen with experimental tumorigenic data. Poison by ingestion and intravenous routes. Mutation data reported. When heated to decomposition it emits toxic fumes of NO$_x$.

MMT750   CAS: 3684-97-7
2-(N-METHYL-N-NITROSO)AMINOACETONITRILE
mf: C$_3$H$_5$N$_3$O   mw: 99.11

SYNS: N-NITROSOMETHYLAMINACETONITRIL (GERMAN) ◇ N-NITROSOMETHYLAMINOACETONITRILE

TOXICITY DATA and REFERENCE
ETA: orl-rat TDLo: 620 mg/kg/89W-C ZEKBAI 69,103,67

CONSENSUS REPORTS: Cyanide and its compounds are on the Community Right-To-Know List.

SAFETY PROFILE: Questionable carcinogen with experimental tumorigenic data. Poison by ingestion. When heated to decomposition it emits toxic fumes of NO$_x$ and CN$^-$.

MMU500   CAS: 63412-06-6
N-METHYL-N-NITROSOBENZAMIDE
mf: C$_8$H$_8$N$_2$O$_2$ mw: 164.18

SYN: MNB

TOXICITY DATA and REFERENCE
CAR: orl-rat TDLo: 2800 mg/kg/52W-I JJIND8 62,1523,79
MUT: mmo-sat 340 nmol/L MUREAV 48,131,77

CONSENSUS REPORTS: EPA Genetic Toxicology Program.

SAFETY PROFILE: Questionable carcinogen with experimental carcinogenic data. Poison by intraperitoneal route. Mutation data reported. When heated to decomposition it emits toxic fumes of NO$_x$.

MMV000   CAS: 13860-69-0
N-METHYL-N-NITROSOBIURET
mf: C$_3$H$_6$N$_4$O$_3$ mw: 146.13

SYNS: 1-METHYL-1-NITROSOBIURET ◇ N-METHYL-N-NITROSO-N'-CARBAMOYLUREA ◇ N-NITROSO-N-METHYLBIURET

TOXICITY DATA and REFERENCE
ETA: orl-rat TD: 1200 mg/kg/1Y-I ZEKBAI 75,229,71
ETA: orl-rat TD: 1300 mg/kg/52W-I PPTCBY 2,73,72
ETA: orl-rat TDLo: 25 mg/kg ZEKBAI 75,229,71
MUT: mmo-omi 1 pph ANTBAL 27,738,82
MUT: mmo-omi 500 ppm/2H-C ANTBAL 24,168,79
MUT: mmo-omi 2500 ppm/2H-C ANTBAL 24,168,79
MUT: mmo-omi 5000 ppm/2H ANTBAL 21,795,76
MUT: mmo-omi 5000 ppm/4H-C ANTBAL 24,168,79

CONSENSUS REPORTS: EPA Genetic Toxicology Program.

SAFETY PROFILE: Questionable carcinogen with experimental tumorigenic data. Moderately

toxic by ingestion. Mutation data reported. When heated to decomposition it emits toxic fumes of NO_x.

MMX000 CAS: 33868-17-6
METHYLNITROSOCYANAMIDE
mf: $C_2H_3N_3O$ mw: 85.08

SYN: MNC

TOXICITY DATA and REFERENCE
ETA: orl-rat TD: 11 g/kg/51W-C   PJACAW 50,497,74
ETA: orl-rat TDLo: 490 mg/kg/28W-C   GANNA2 68,813,77
MUT: cyt-ham: emb 2 mmol/L/24H   MUREAV 43,429,77
MUT: mmo-esc 5 µmol/L   CNREA8 38,4630,78
MUT: mmo-sat 2500 µmol/L   GMCRDC 17,17,75

CONSENSUS REPORTS: EPA Extremely Hazardous Substances List.

SAFETY PROFILE: Questionable carcinogen with experimental tumorigenic data. Poison by ingestion. Mutation data reported. When heated to decomposition it emits toxic fumes of NO_x.

MMX200 CAS: 75881-22-0
N-METHYL-N-NITROSODECYLAMINE
mf: $C_{11}H_{24}N_2O$ mw: 200.37

SYN: NITROSOMETHYL-n-DECYLAMINE

TOXICITY DATA and REFERENCE
ETA: orl-rat TDLo: 5200 mg/kg/2Y-C   CNREA8 41,1288,81
MUT: mma-sat 25 µg/plate   TCMUD8 1,295,80

SAFETY PROFILE: Questionable carcinogen with experimental tumorigenic data. Mutation data reported. When heated to decomposition it emits toxic fumes of NO_x.

MMX500 CAS: 31364-55-3
N-METHYL-N-NITROSO-β-d-GLUCOSAMINE
mf: $C_7H_{14}N_2O_6$ mw: 222.23

SYNS: N-METHYL-N-NITROSO-β-d-GLUCOSYLAMIN (GERMAN) ◊ N-METHYL-N-NITROSO-β-d-GLUCOSYL-AMINE

TOXICITY DATA and REFERENCE
ETA: orl-rat TDLo: 2500 mg/kg/25W-I   ZEKBAI 75,296,71

SAFETY PROFILE: Questionable carcinogen with experimental tumorigenic data. When

heated to decomposition it emits toxic fumes of NO_x.

MMX750 CAS: 16339-21-2
4-METHYL-4-N-NITROSOMETHYLAMINO)-2-PENTANONE
mf: $C_7H_{14}N_2O_2$ mw: 158.23

SYNS: METHYL-1,1-DIMETHYLBUTANON(3)-NITRO-SAMIN (GERMAN) ◊ 2-METHYLNITROSAMINO-2-METHYLPENTANON(4) (GERMAN)

TOXICITY DATA and REFERENCE
ETA: orl-rat TDLo: 16 g/kg/89W-C   ZEKBAI 69,103,67

SAFETY PROFILE: Questionable carcinogen with experimental tumorigenic data. Moderately toxic by ingestion. When heated to decomposition it emits toxic fumes of NO_x.

MMY250 CAS: 16339-01-8
N-METHYL-N-NITROSO-4-(PHENYLAZO)ANILINE
mf: $C_{13}H_{12}N_4O$ mw: 240.29

SYNS: 4-METHYLAMINO-N-NITROSOAZOBENZENE ◊ N-NITROSO-4-METHYLAMINOAZOBENZENE ◊ N-NITROSO-4-METHYLAMINOAZOBENZOL (GERMAN)

TOXICITY DATA and REFERENCE
ETA: orl-rat TDLo: 100 mg/kg   ZEKBAI 69,103,67
MUT: dni-mus-orl 20 g/kg   ARGEAR 51,605,81

SAFETY PROFILE: Questionable carcinogen with experimental tumorigenic data. Moderately toxic by ingestion. Mutation data reported. When heated to decomposition it emits toxic fumes of NO_x.

MMY750 CAS: 13603-07-1
3-METHYLNITROSOPIPERIDINE
mf: $C_6H_{12}N_2O$ mw: 128.20

SYN: 1-NITROSO-3-PIPECOLINE

TOXICITY DATA and REFERENCE
ETA: orl-rat TDLo: 2520 mg/kg/50W-I   IJCNAW 16,318,75
MUT: mma-sat 1 µmol/plate   MUREAV 56,131,77
MUT: mma-smc 25 mmol/L/24H   MUREAV 57,155,78
MUT: sce-hmn: lym 10 mmol/L   TCMUE9 1,129,84
MUT: sln-dmg-orl 5 mmol/L/24H   MUREAV 67,27,79

CONSENSUS REPORTS: EPA Genetic Toxicology Program.

SAFETY PROFILE: Questionable carcinogen with experimental tumorigenic data. Human mutation data reported. When heated to decomposition it emits toxic fumes of NO_x.

MMZ000   CAS: 15104-03-7
4-METHYLNITROSOPIPERIDINE
mf: $C_6H_{12}N_2O$ mw: 128.20

SYN: 1-NITROSO-4-PIPECOLINE

TOXICITY DATA and REFERENCE
ETA: orl-rat TDLo: 2016 mg/kg/40W-I   IJCNAW 16,318,75
MUT: mma-sat 200 μg/plate   MUREAV 56,131,77
MUT: mma-smc 25 mmol/L/24H   MUREAV 57,155,78
MUT: sln-dmg-orl 5 mmol/L/24H   MUREAV 67,27,79

CONSENSUS REPORTS: EPA Genetic Toxicology Program.

SAFETY PROFILE: Questionable carcinogen with experimental tumorigenic data. Mutation data reported. When heated to decomposition it emits toxic fumes of NO_x.

MMZ800   CAS: 71677-48-0
3-METHYL-1-NITROSO-4-PIPERIDONE
mf: $C_6H_{10}N_2O_2$ mw: 142.18

SYN: NITROSO-3-METHYL-4-PIPERIDONE

TOXICITY DATA and REFERENCE
ETA: orl-rat TDLo: 1640 mg/kg/26W-I   CRNGDP 5,1351,84
MUT: mma-sat 250 μg/plate   TCMUD8 1,295,80

SAFETY PROFILE: Questionable carcinogen with experimental tumorigenic data. Mutation data reported. When heated to decomposition it emits toxic fumes of NO_x.

MNA250   CAS: 16395-80-5
N-METHYL-N-NITROSOPROPIONAMIDE
mf: $C_4H_8N_2O_2$ mw: 116.14

SYNS: METHYLNITROSO-PROPIONAMIDE ◊ METHYL-NITROSOPROPIONSAEUREAMID (GERMAN) ◊ METHYLNI-TROSOPROPIONYLAMIDE

TOXICITY DATA and REFERENCE
ETA: ivn-rat TDLo: 62 mg/kg/31W-I   EJCAAH 13,1183,77

ETA: orl-rat TDLo: 445 mg/kg/89W-I   PPTCBY 2,73,72

SAFETY PROFILE: Questionable carcinogen with experimental tumorigenic data. When heated to decomposition it emits toxic fumes of NO_x.

MNA650   CAS: 23139-00-6
1-METHYL-1-NITROSO-3-(p-TOLYL)UREA
mf: $C_9H_{11}N_3O_2$ mw: 193.23

SYN: N-METHYL-N'-(p-METHYLPHENYL)-N-NITRO-SOUREA

TOXICITY DATA and REFERENCE
CAR: skn-mus TDLo: 574 mg/kg/7W-I   CNREA8 44,1027,84
MUT: mmo-sat 33500 pmol/plate   CNREA8 39,5147,79

SAFETY PROFILE: Questionable carcinogen with experimental carcinogenic data. Mutation data reported. When heated to decomposition it emits toxic fumes of NO_x.

MNF250   CAS: 21308-79-2
METHYL-12-OXO-trans-10-OCTADECENOATE
mf: $C_{19}H_{34}O_3$ mw: 310.53

SYNS: 12-OXO-trans-10-OCTADECENOIC ACID, METHYL ESTER ◊ (E)-12-OXO-10-OCTADECENOIC ACID, METHYL ESTER

TOXICITY DATA and REFERENCE
ETA: skn-mus TDLo: 55 g/kg/46W-I   AMBPBZ 82,127,74

SAFETY PROFILE: Questionable carcinogen with experimental tumorigenic data. When heated to decomposition it emits acrid smoke and irritating fumes.

MNG250   CAS: 27343-29-9
11-METHYL-1-OXO-1,2,3,4-TETRAHYDROCHRYSENE
mf: $C_{19}H_{16}O$ mw: 260.35

SYN: 1,2,3,4-TETRAHYDRO-11-METHYLCHRYSEN-1-ONE

TOXICITY DATA and REFERENCE
NEO: skn-mus TD: 65 mg/kg/27W-I   CNREA8 34,1315,74
NEO: skn-mus TDLo: 62 mg/kg/26W-I   CNREA8 33,832,73
ETA: skn-mus TD: 16 mg/kg/4D-C   BJCAAI 38,148,78

MUT: mma-sat 50 μg/plate   CNREA8
36,4525,76

CONSENSUS REPORTS: EPA Genetic Toxicology Program.

SAFETY PROFILE: Questionable carcinogen with experimental neoplastigenic and tumorigenic data. Mutation data reported. When heated to decomposition it emits acrid smoke and irritating fumes.

MNH000   CAS: 298-00-0
METHYL PARATHION
DOT: 2783
mf: $C_8H_{10}NO_5PS$ mw: 263.22

PROP: Crystals. Vap d: 9.1, mp: 37-38°, d: 1.358 @ 20°/4°. Sol in most organic solvents.

SYNS: A-GRO ◊ AZOFOS ◊ AZOPHOS ◊ BAY E-601 ◊ BAY 11405 ◊ BLADAN-M ◊ CEKUMETHION ◊ DALF ◊ DEVITHION ◊ O,O-DIMETHYL-O-p-NITROFENYLESTER KYSELINY THIOFOSFORECNE (CZECH) ◊ O,O-DIMETHYL-O-(4-NITROFENYL)-MONOTHIOFOSFAAT (DUTCH) ◊ DIMETHYL p-NITROPHENYL MONOTHIOPHOSPHATE ◊ O,O-DIMETHYL-O-(4-NITRO-PHENYL)-MONOTHIO-PHOSPHAT (GERMAN) ◊ O,O-DIMETHYL-O-(p-NITRO-PHENYL) PHOSPHOROTHIOATE ◊ O,O-DIMETHYL-O-(4-NITROPHENYL) PHOSPHOROTHIOATE ◊ DIMETHYL 4-NITROPHENYL PHOSPHOROTHIONATE ◊ O,O-DIMETHYL-O-(p-NITROPHENYL)-THIONOPHOSPHAT (GERMAN) ◊ O,O-DIMETHYL-O-(4-NITROPHENYL)-THIONOPHOSPHAT (GERMAN) ◊ DIMETHYL-p-NITROPHENYL THIONPHOSPHATE ◊ DIMETHYL p-NITROPHENYL THIOPHOSPHATE ◊ O,O-DIMETHYL-O-p-NITROPHENYL THIOPHOSPHATE ◊ DIMETHYL PARATHION ◊ O,O-DIMETIL-O-(4-NITRO-FENIL)-MONOTIOFOSFATO (ITALIAN) ◊ DREXEL METHYL PARATHION 4E ◊ ENT 17,292 ◊ FOLIDOL M ◊ GEARPHOS ◊ ME-PARATHION ◊ MEPATON ◊ MEPTOX ◊ METACIDE ◊ METAFOS ◊ METAPHOR ◊ METAPHOS ◊ METHYL-E 605 ◊ METHYL FOSFERNO ◊ METHYL NIRAN ◊ METHYLTHIOPHOS ◊ METILPARATION (HUNGARIAN) ◊ METRON ◊ METYLOPARATION (POLISH) ◊ METYLPARATION (CZECH) ◊ NCI-C02971 ◊ p-NITROPHENYLDIMETHYLTHIONOPHOSPHATE ◊ NITROX ◊ OLEOVOFOTOX ◊ PARAPEST M-50 ◊ PARATAF ◊ M-PARATHION ◊ PARATHION METHYL ◊ PARATHION-METILE (ITALIAN) ◊ PARATOX ◊ PENNCAP-M ◊ RCRA WASTE NUMBER P071 ◊ SINAFID M-48 ◊ SIXTY-THREE SPECIAL E.C. INSECTICIDE ◊ TEKWAISA ◊ THIOPHENIT ◊ THIOPHOSPHATE de O,O-DIMETHYLE et de O-(4-NITROPHENYLE) (FRENCH) ◊ THYLFAR M-50 ◊ TOLL ◊ VERTAC METHYL PARATHION TECHNISCH 80% ◊ VOFATOX ◊ WOFATOS ◊ WOFATOX ◊ WOFOTOX

TOXICITY DATA with REFERENCE
MUT: dnr-omi 50 μL/plate   BIZNAT 95,463,76
MUT: mmo-sat 667 μg/plate   ENMUDM 5(Suppl 1),3,83
MUT: mnt-mus-ipr 1 mg/kg   MUREAV 155,131,85
MUT: sce-ham:lng 10 mg/L   MUREAV 88,307,81
MUT: sce-hmn:lym 10 mg/L   MUREAV 88,307,81

CONSENSUS REPORTS: IARC Cancer Review: GROUP 3 IMEMDT 7,56,87; Animal No Evidence IMEMDT 30,131,83. NCI Carcinogenesis Bioassay (feed); No Evidence: mouse, rat NCITR* NCI-CG-TR-157,79. EPA Genetic Toxicology Program. EPA Extremely Hazardous Substances List.

OSHA PEL: TWA 0.2 mg/m³ (skin)   ACGIH TLV: TWA 0.2 mg/m³ (skin)   NIOSH REL: (Methyl Parathion) TWA 0.2 mg/m³   DOT Classification: Poison B; Label: Poison.

SAFETY PROFILE: Questionable carcinogen. Poison by inhalation, ingestion, skin contact, subcutaneous, intravenous, intraperitoneal, and possibly other routes. An experimental teratogen. Experimental reproductive effects. Human mutation data reported. A cholinesterase inhibitor type of insecticide. When heated to decomposition it emits very toxic fumes of NO_x, PO_x, and SO_x.

MNN500   CAS: 832-69-9
1-METHYLPHENANTHRENE
mf: $C_{15}H_{12}$ mw: 192.27

TOXICITY DATA with REFERENCE
MUT: mma-sat 5 μg/plate   MUREAV 156,61,85
MUT: msc-hmn:lym 25 μmol/L   MUREAV 128,221,84

CONSENSUS REPORTS: IARC Cancer Review: GROUP 3 IMEMDT 7,56,87; Animal Inadequate Evidence IMEMDT 32,405,83.

SAFETY PROFILE: Questionable carcinogen. Human mutation data reported. When heated to decomposition it emits acrid smoke and irritating fumes.

MNO250   CAS: 21917-91-9
2-METHYLPHENANTHRO(2,1-d)THIAZOLE
mf: $C_{16}H_{11}NS$ mw: 249.34

TOXICITY DATA and REFERENCE
ETA: skn-mus TDLo:800 mg/kg/31W-I
VOONAW 15(8),54,69

SAFETY PROFILE: Questionable carcinogen with experimental tumorigenic data. When heated to decomposition it emits very toxic fumes of NO_x and SO_x.

MNR500   CAS: 621-90-9
N-METHYL-p-(PHENYLAZO)ANILINE
mf: $C_{13}H_{13}N_3$ mw: 211.29

SYNS: MAB ◇ 4-(METHYLAMINO)AZOBENZENE ◇ N-METHYL-4-AMINOAZOBENZENE ◇ N-METHYL-p-AMINOAZOBENZENE ◇ p-MONOMETHYLAMINOAZOBEN-ZENE ◇ 4-MONOMETHYLAMINOAZOBENZENE

TOXICITY DATA and REFERENCE
CAR: ipr-rat TDLo: 317 mg/kg/3W-I   CNREA8 44,2540,84
CAR: orl-rat TD: 2100 mg/kg/5W-C   CRNGDP 8,577,87
NEO: ipr-mus TD: 11 mg/kg   CNREA8 44,2540,84
NEO: ipr-mus TDLo: 3592 μg/kg   CNREA8 44,2540,84
NEO: orl-rat TDLo: 634 mg/kg/5W-I   CNREA8 39,3411,79
NEO: skn-rat TDLo: 930 mg/kg/58W-I   CNREA8 26,2406,66
ETA: ipr-rat TDLo: 38 mg/kg   CNREA8 39,3411,79
ETA: orl-rat TD: 13 g/kg/34W-C   GANNA2 59,131,68
ETA: orl-rat TD: 2550 mg/kg/19W-C   CNREA8 8,141,48
ETA: orl-rat TD: 2600 mg/kg/15W-C   CNREA8 5,235,45
ETA: orl-rat TD: 3400 mg/kg/27W-C   JNCIAM 15,67,54
ETA: orl-rat TD: 3700 mg/kg/17W-C   CNREA8 5,227,45
ETA: scu-rat TDLo: 480 mg/kg/12W-I   CNREA8 27,1600,67
MUT: dnd-mam: lvr 830 μmol/L   CNREA8 33,529,73
MUT: dnd-mam: lym 250 μmol/L   CNREA8 33,529,73
MUT: dnd-rat-orl 200 μmol/kg   CBINA8 31,1,80
MUT: dnd-rat: lvr 790 μmol/L   CNREA8 33,529,73
MUT: dnd-smc 830 μmol/L   CNREA8 33,529,73
MUT: dns-rat: lvr 1 μmol/L   GANNA2 72,930,81
MUT: mma-sat 200 μg/plate   PNASA6 72,5135,75

CONSENSUS REPORTS: EPA Genetic Toxicology Program.

SAFETY PROFILE: Questionable carcinogen with experimental carcinogenic, neoplastigenic, tumorigenic, and teratogenic data. Moderately toxic by subcutaneous route. Experimental re-productive effects. Mutation data reported. When heated to decomposition it emits toxic fumes of NO_x.

MNS000   CAS: 10121-94-5
N-METHYL-4-(PHENYLAZO)-o-ANISIDINE
mf: $C_{14}H_{15}N_3O$ mw: 241.32

SYNS: 3-METHOXYMETHYLAMINOAZOBENZENE ◇ 3-METHOXY-4-MONOMETHYLAMINOAZOBENZENE

TOXICITY DATA and REFERENCE
NEO: skn-rat TDLo: 660 mg/kg/41W-I   CNREA8 26,2406,66
ETA: orl-rat TD: 13 g/kg/47W-I   CNREA8 24,1279,64
ETA: orl-rat TDLo: 9300 mg/kg/34W-C   CNREA8 21,1068,61

SAFETY PROFILE: Questionable carcinogen with experimental tumorigenic and neoplastigenic data. When heated to decomposition it emits toxic fumes of NO_x.

MNS250   CAS: 21075-41-2
5-METHYL-7-PHENYL-1:2-BENZACRIDINE
mf: $C_{24}H_{17}N$ mw: 319.42

SYNS: 7-METHYL-9-PHENYLBENZ(c)ACRIDINE ◇ 3-PHENYL-10-METHYL-7:8 BENZACRIDINE (FRENCH)

TOXICITY DATA and REFERENCE
ETA: scu-mus TDLo: 20 mg/kg   AICCA6 7,184,50
ETA: skn-mus TD: 410 mg/kg/34W-I   ACRSAJ 4,315,56
ETA: skn-mus TDLo: 390 mg/kg/32W-I   AICCA6 7,184,50

SAFETY PROFILE: Questionable carcinogen with experimental tumorigenic data. When heated to decomposition it emits toxic fumes of NO_x.

MNT500   CAS: 20240-98-6
1-(2-METHYLPHENYL)-3,3-DIMETHYLTRIAZENE
mf: $C_9H_{13}N_3$ mw: 163.25

SYNS: 3,3-DIMETHYL-1-(o-METHYLPHENYL)TRIAZENE ◇ 3,3-DIMETHYL-1-(o-TOLYL)TRIAZENE ◇ 1-(o-METHYL-PHENYL)-3,3-DIMETHYL-TRIAZEN (GERMAN) ◇ 1-(o-METHYLPHENYL)-3,3-DIMETHYL-TRIAZENE

TOXICITY DATA and REFERENCE
CAR: orl-rat TDLo: 300 mg/kg   ZKKOBW 81,285,74

CAR: scu-rat TD:1620 mg/kg/45W-I ZKKOBW 81,285,74

CAR: scu-rat TDLo:500 mg/kg ZKKOBW 81,285,74

SAFETY PROFILE: Questionable carcinogen with experimental carcinogenic data. Poison by ingestion. Moderately toxic by subcutaneous route. When heated to decomposition it emits toxic fumes of NO_x.

MNU250 CAS: 13256-11-6
METHYL-PHENYLETHYL-NITROSAMINE
mf: $C_9H_{12}N_2O$ mw: 164.23

SYNS: N-METHYL-N-NITROSOPHENETHYLAMINE ◇ METHYL(2-PHENYLAETHYL)NITROSAMIN (GERMAN) ◇ N-NITROSO-N-METHYL-2-PHENYLETHYLAMINE

TOXICITY DATA and REFERENCE
CAR: orl-rat TD:78 mg/kg/33W-I FCTOD7 20,393,82

CAR: orl-rat TD:14400 μg/kg/33W-I FCTOD7 20,393,82

CAR: orl-rat TDLo:5200 μg/kg/33W-I FCTOD7 20,393,82

ETA: orl-rat TD:124 mg/kg/33W-I FCTOD7 20,393,82

ETA: orl-rat TD:124 mg/kg/33W-I JJIND8 68,681,82

ETA: orl-rat TD:160 mg/kg/46W-C ARZNAD 19,1077,69

ETA: orl-rat TD:165 mg/kg/33W-I XENOBH 3,271,73

ETA: orl-rat TD:312 mg/kg/28W-I JJIND8 68,681,82

ETA: orl-rat TD:336 mg/kg/33W-I FCTOD7 20,393,82

MUT: mma-sat 10 μg/plate MUREAV 66,1,79

SAFETY PROFILE: Questionable carcinogen with experimental carcinogenic and tumorigenic data. Poison by ingestion. Mutation data reported. When heated to decomposition it emits toxic fumes of NO_x.

MNU500 CAS: 637-60-5
4-METHYLPHENYLHYDRAZINE HYDROCHLORIDE
mf: $C_7H_{10}N_2 \cdot ClH$ mw: 158.65

TOXICITY DATA and REFERENCE
CAR: scu-mus TDLo:3640 mg/kg/26W-I ZKKOBW 89,245,77

NEO: orl-mus TDLo:1750 mg/kg/7W-I ZKKOBW 89,245,77

NEO: scu-mus TD:1400 mg/kg/10W-I ZKKOBW 89,245,77

MUT: mma-sat 800 μg/plate NEZAAQ 33,474,78

MUT: mmo-sat 800 μg/plate NEZAAQ 33,474,78

CONSENSUS REPORTS: Reported in EPA TSCA Inventory.

SAFETY PROFILE: Questionable carcinogen with experimental carcinogenic and neoplastigenic data. Mutation data reported. When heated to decomposition it emits very toxic fumes of Cl^- and NO_x.

MNX850 CAS: 20921-41-9
1-METHYL-1-PHENYL-2-PROPYNYL CYCLOHEXANECARBAMATE
mf: $C_{17}H_{21}NO_2$ mw: 271.39

SYNS: CYCLOHEXANECARBAMIC ACID, 1-METHYL-1-PHENYL-2-PROPYNYL ESTER ◇ 1-METHYL-1-PHENYL-2-PROPYNYL-N-CYCLOHEXYLCARBAMATE

TOXICITY DATA and REFERENCE
ETA: orl-rat TDLo:38 g/kg/96W-C JJIND8 71,211,83

SAFETY PROFILE: Questionable carcinogen with experimental tumorigenic data. When heated to decomposition it emits toxic fumes of NO_x.

MOA725 CAS: 16033-21-9
3-METHYL-1-PHENYLTRIAZENE
mf: $C_7H_9N_3$ mw: 135.19

SYNS: 1-PHENYL-3-METHYLTRIAZINE ◇ 1-PHENYL-3-MONOMETHYLTRIAZENE ◇ PMT

TOXICITY DATA and REFERENCE
NEO: scu-mus TDLo:45 mg/kg/4W-I CNREA8 34,1671,74

NEO: skn-mus TDLo:284 mg/kg/8W-I CNREA8 34,1671,74

MUT: dnd-ofs-sal:spr 250 g/L BCPCA6 19,1505,70

MUT: mma-sat 1 mmol/L CNREA8 42,1446,82

MUT: mmo-nsc 600 μmol/L MUREAV 13,276,71

MUT: mmo-sat 100 μmol/L CNREA8 42,1446,82

SAFETY PROFILE: Questionable carcinogen with experimental neoplastigenic data. Poison by ingestion and subcutaneous routes. Mutation data reported. When heated to decomposition it emits toxic fumes of NO_x.

MOU250 CAS: 16354-54-4
12-METHYL-7-PROPYLBENZ(a)ANTHRACENE
mf: $C_{22}H_{20}$ mw: 284.42

TOXICITY DATA and REFERENCE
NEO: ims-rat TDLo:50 mg/kg   PNASA6
   58,2253,67

SAFETY PROFILE: Questionable carcinogen with experimental neoplastigenic data. When heated to decomposition it emits acrid smoke and irritating fumes.

MOW500   CAS: 3690-50-4
METHYL PROTOANEMONIN
mf: $C_6H_6O_2$ mw: 110.12

SYNS: ETHYLIDENE-2(5H)-FURANONE ◇ 4-HYDROXY-HEXA-2,4-DIENOIC ACID LACTONE

TOXICITY DATA and REFERENCE
ETA: scu-rat TDLo:2440 mg/kg/61W-I   BJCAAI
   15,85,61

SAFETY PROFILE: Questionable carcinogen with experimental tumorigenic data. When heated to decomposition it emits acrid smoke and irritating fumes.

MOX875   CAS: 2381-21-7
3-METHYLPYRENE
mf: $C_{17}H_{12}$ mw: 216.29

SYN: 1-METHYLPYRENE

TOXICITY DATA and REFERENCE
NEO: ipr-mus TDLo:42 mg/kg/3D-I   JTEHD6
   21,525,87
MUT: mma-sat 180 μmol/L/2H   CNREA8
   39,4152,79

SAFETY PROFILE: Questionable carcinogen with experimental neoplastigenic data. Mutation data reported. When heated to decomposition it emits acrid smoke and irritating fumes.

MOY500   CAS: 63019-78-3
2-METHYLPYRIDINE-4-AZO-p-DIMETHYLANILINE
mf: $C_{14}H_{16}N_4$ mw: 240.34

TOXICITY DATA and REFERENCE
ETA: orl-rat TDLo:5550 mg/kg/22W-C
   CNREA8 14,715,54

SAFETY PROFILE: Questionable carcinogen with experimental tumorigenic data. When heated to decomposition it emits toxic fumes of NO_x.

MOY750   CAS: 31932-35-1
3-METHYLPYRIDINE-1-OXIDE-4-AZO-p-DIMETHYL-ANILINE
mf: $C_{14}H_{16}N_4O$ mw: 256.34

SYN: N,N-DIMETHYL-4-(4'-(3'-METHYLPYRIDYL-1'-OXIDE)AZO)ANILINE

TOXICITY DATA and REFERENCE
NEO: orl-rat TDLo:3700 mg/kg/35W-C
   JNCIAM 41,855,68
ETA: orl-rat TD:4284 mg/kg/17W-C   JNCIAM
   41,855,68

SAFETY PROFILE: Questionable carcinogen with experimental neoplastigenic and tumorigenic data. When heated to decomposition it emits toxic fumes of NO_x.

MPB175   CAS: 53365-77-8
1-METHYLPYRROLE-2,3-DIMETHANOL
mf: $C_7H_{11}NO_2$ mw: 141.19

SYNS: 1,2-BISHYDROXYMETHYL-1-METHYLPYRROLE ◇ 2,3-BISHYDROXYMETHYL-1-METHYLPYRROLE

TOXICITY DATA and REFERENCE
CAR: skn-mus TDLo:1325 mg/kg/47W-I
   CALEDQ 17,61,82
MUT: dni-rat:lvr 100 μmol/L   CBINA8 30,325,80
MUT: mmo-sat 500 μg/plate   MUREAV 149,485,85
MUT: oth-hmn:hlas 20 μmol/L   CBINA8
   30,325,80
MUT: oth-rat:lvr 20 μmol/L   CBINA8 30,325,80
MUT: otr-ham:kdy 250 μg/L   CRNGDP 1,161,80
MUT: sce-hmn:lyms 5 μmol/L   MUREAV
   149,485,85

SAFETY PROFILE: Questionable carcinogen with experimental carcinogenic data. Mutation data reported. When heated to decomposition it emits toxic fumes of NO_x.

MPJ250   CAS: 73928-03-7
2-METHYL-4-STILBENAMINE
mf: $C_{15}H_{15}N$ mw: 209.31

SYN: 2-METHYL-4-AMINOSTILBENE

TOXICITY DATA and REFERENCE
ETA: scu-rat TDLo:240 mg/kg/W-I   BMBUAQ
   14,141,58

SAFETY PROFILE: Questionable carcinogen with experimental tumorigenic data. When heated to decomposition it emits toxic fumes of NO_x.

MPJ500   CAS: 73928-04-8
3-METHYL-4-STILBENAMINE
mf: $C_{15}H_{15}N$ mw: 209.31

SYN: 3-METHYL-4-AMINOSTILBENE

TOXICITY DATA and REFERENCE

ETA: orl-rat TDLo: 350 mg/kg/W   BMBUAQ
14,141,58

ETA: scu-rat TDLo: 200 mg/kg/W-I   BMBUAQ
14,141,58

SAFETY PROFILE: Questionable carcinogen with experimental tumorigenic data. When heated to decomposition it emits toxic fumes of NO_x.

MPL500   CAS: 27302-90-5
2-((METHYLSULFINYL)ACETYL) PYRIDINE
mf: $C_8H_9NO_2S$ mw: 183.24

SYN: OXISURAN

TOXICITY DATA and REFERENCE

CAR: orl-mus TDLo: 336 g/kg/80W-C   TXCYAC
28,17,83

NEO: orl-rat TDLo: 437 g/kg/2Y-C   TXCYAC
28,17,83

SAFETY PROFILE: Questionable carcinogen with experimental carcinogenic and neoplastigenic data. Moderately toxic by intravenous route. Mildly toxic by ingestion. When heated to decomposition it emits very toxic fumes of SO_x and NO_x.

MPN500   CAS: 58-18-4
17-METHYLTESTOSTERONE
mf: $C_{20}H_{30}O_2$ mw: 302.50

SYNS: ANDROMETH ◇ ANDROSAN ◇ ANDROSAN (tablets) ◇ ANDROSTEN ◇ 4-ANDROSTENE-17-α-METHYL-17-β-OL-3-ONE ◇ ANERTAN ◇ ANERTAN (tablets) ◇ DELATESTRYL ◇ DIANABOL ◇ DUMOGRAN ◇ GLOSSO STERANDRYL ◇ HOMANDREN ◇ HORMALE ◇ 17-β-HYDROXY-17-METHYLANDROST-4-EN-3-ONE ◇ MALESTRONE ◇ MALOGEN ◇ MASENONE ◇ MASTESTONA ◇ MESTERONE ◇ METANDREN ◇ 17-METHYLTESTOSTERON ◇ METHYLTESTOSTERONE ◇ 17-α-METHYLTESTOSTERONE ◇ METRONE ◇ M.T. MUCORETTES ◇ NABOLIN ◇ NEO-HOMBREOL-M ◇ NSC-9701 ◇ NU MAN ◇ ORAVIRON ◇ ORETON-M ◇ ORETON METHYL ◇ STENOLON ◇ STERONYL ◇ SYNANDRETS ◇ SYNANDROTABS ◇ TESTHORMONE ◇ TESTORA ◇ TESTOVIRON ◇ TESTRED

TOXICITY DATA and REFERENCE

CAR: orl-man TDLo: 420 mg/kg/4Y-C: LIV
LANCAO 2,1273,72

CAR: orl-man TDLo: 5366 mg/kg/7Y-C: LIV
BJSUAM 66,212,79

CONSENSUS REPORTS: Reported in EPA TSCA Inventory. EPA Genetic Toxicology Program.

SAFETY PROFILE: Questionable human carcinogen producing liver tumors. Poison by intraperitoneal route. Moderately toxic by ingestion. Human teratogenic effects by ingestion: developmental abnormalities of the urogenital system. An experimental teratogen. Experimental reproductive effects. A synthetic androgenic steroid. When heated to decomposition it emits acrid smoke and irritating fumes.

MPO250   CAS: 63020-37-1
6-METHYL-1,2,3,4-TETRAHYDROBENZ(a)ANTHRACENE
mf: $C_{19}H_{18}$ mw: 246.37

SYN: 4-METHYL-1',2',3',4'-TETRAHYDRO-1,2-BENZANTHRACENE

TOXICITY DATA and REFERENCE

ETA: imp-mus TDLo: 80 mg/kg   JNCIAM
2,241,41

SAFETY PROFILE: Questionable carcinogen with experimental tumorigenic data. When heated to decomposition it emits acrid smoke and irritating fumes.

MPO390   CAS: 101607-49-2
7-METHYL-1,2,3,4-TETRAHYDRODIBENZ(c,h)ACRIDINE
mf: $C_{22}H_{19}N$ mw: 297.42

SYN: 10-METHYL-1,2-TETRAHYDRO-1,2:7,8-BENZACRIDINE

TOXICITY DATA and REFERENCE

ETA: scu-mus TDLo: 72 mg/kg/9W-I   COREAF
251,1322,60

SAFETY PROFILE: Questionable carcinogen with experimental tumorigenic data. When heated to decomposition it emits toxic fumes of NO_x.

MPO400   CAS: 101607-48-1
14-METHYL-8,9,10,11-TETRAHYDRODIBENZ(a,h)ACRIDINE
mf: $C_{22}H_{19}N$ mw: 297.42

SYN: 10-METHYL-1,2-TETRAHYDRO-1,2:5,6-BENZACRIDINE

TOXICITY DATA and REFERENCE

ETA: scu-mus TDLo: 72 mg/kg/9W-I   COREAF
251,1322,60

SAFETY PROFILE: Questionable carcinogen with experimental tumorigenic data. When

heated to decomposition it emits toxic fumes of NO_x.

MPQ500   CAS: 22885-98-9
α-METHYL TETRONIC ACID
mf: $C_5H_6O_3$ mw: 114.11

SYN: 4-HYDROXY-5-METHYL-2(5H)-FURANONE

TOXICITY DATA and REFERENCE
ETA: scu-rat TDLo: 2600 mg/kg/65W-I   BJCAAI 19,392,65

SAFETY PROFILE: Questionable carcinogen with experimental tumorigenic data. When heated to decomposition it emits acrid smoke and irritating fumes.

MPQ750   CAS: 144-82-1
N^1-(5-METHYL-1,3,4-THIADIAZOL-2-YL)-SULFANILAMIDE
mf: $C_9H_{10}N_4O_2S_2$ mw: 270.35

SYNS: 2-(p-AMINOBENZENESULFONAMIDO)-5-METHYLTHIADIAZOLE ◇ 5-METHYL-2-SULFANIL-AMIDO-1,3,4-THIADIAZOLE ◇ SULFAMETHIZOLE ◇ SULFAMETHYLTHIADIAZOLE ◇ 2-SULFANILAMIDO-5-METHYL-1,3,4-THIADIAZOLE

TOXICITY DATA and REFERENCE
ETA: par-mus TDLo: 6000 mg/kg/4W-I
    ACRAAX 37,258,52

CONSENSUS REPORTS: Reported in EPA TSCA Inventory.

SAFETY PROFILE: Questionable carcinogen with experimental tumorigenic data. Moderately toxic by subcutaneous route. When heated to decomposition it emits very toxic fumes of NO_x and SO_x.

MPU000   CAS: 342-69-8
METHYLTHIOINOSINE
mf: $C_{11}H_{14}N_4O_4S$ mw: 298.35

SYNS: 6-METHYLMERCAPTOPURINE RIBONUCLEOSIDE ◇ 6-METHYLMERCAPTOPURINE RIBOSIDE ◇ 6-METHYL-MP-RIBOSIDE ◇ 6-METHYL-9-RIBOFURANOSYLPURINE-6-THIOL ◇ 6-METHYLTHIOINOSINE ◇ 6-(METHYLTHIO)PU-RINE RIBONUCLEOSIDE ◇ 6-METHYLTHIOPURINE RIBO-SIDE ◇ NCI-C04784 ◇ NSC 40774 ◇ β-d-RIBOSYL-6-METHYL-THIOPURINE ◇ SQ 21977

TOXICITY DATA and REFERENCE
ETA: ipr-mus TDLo: 780 mg/kg/26W-I
    CANCAR 40(Suppl 4),1935,77

ETA: ipr-rat TDLo: 44 mg/kg/7W-I   CANCAR
    40(Suppl 4),1935,77

MUT: dni-mus: lym 2 μmol/L   CNREA8 44,2272,84
MUT: oms-mus: lym 3 μmol/L   CNREA8
    43,1587,83
MUT: unr-mus LD10: 20 mg/kg   PMDCAY 7,69,70

CONSENSUS REPORTS: NCI Carcinogenesis Studies (ipr); Equivocal Evidence: mouse CANCAR 40,1935,77; (ipr); No Evidence: rat CANCAR 40,1935,77.

SAFETY PROFILE: Questionable carcinogen with experimental tumorigenic and teratogenic data. Poison by intraperitoneal and possibly other routes. Experimental reproductive effects. Mutation data reported. When heated to decomposition it emits very toxic fumes of SO_x and NO_x.

MPY000   CAS: 2058-62-0
N-METHYL-p-(m-TOLYLAZO)ANILINE
mf: $C_{14}H_{15}N_3$ mw: 225.32

SYNS: N-METHYL-3′-METHYL-p-AMINOAZOBENZENE ◇ N-METHYL-3′-METHYL-4-AMINOAZOBENZENE ◇ 3′-METHYL-4-MONOMETHYLAMINOAZOBENZENE

TOXICITY DATA and REFERENCE
ETA: orl-rat TD: 2550 mg/kg/20W-C   CNREA8
    8,141,48
ETA: orl-rat TDLo: 2520 mg/kg/20W-C
    JNCIAM 15,67,54
MUT: dns-rat: lvr 1 μmol/L   CNREA8 46,1654,86
MUT: mmo-sat 1 μmol/plate   CRNGDP 1,121,80

SAFETY PROFILE: Questionable carcinogen with experimental tumorigenic data. Mutation data reported. When heated to decomposition it emits toxic fumes of NO_x.

MPY250   CAS: 17018-24-5
N-METHYL-p-(o-TOLYLAZO)ANILINE
mf: $C_{14}H_{15}N_3$ mw: 225.32

SYNS: N-METHYL-2′-METHYL-p-AMINOAZOBENZENE ◇ N-METHYL-2′-METHYL-4-AMINOAZOBENZENE

TOXICITY DATA and REFERENCE
ETA: orl-rat TD: 4540 mg/kg/36W-C   JNCIAM
    15,67,54
ETA: orl-rat TD: 7800 mg/kg/34W-C   CNREA8
    17,387,57
ETA: orl-rat TDLo: 2350 mg/kg/14W-C
    CNREA8 8,141,48

SAFETY PROFILE: Questionable carcinogen with experimental tumorigenic data. When

heated to decomposition it emits toxic fumes of NO_x.

MPY500 CAS: 28149-22-6
N-METHYL-p-(p-TOLYLAZO)ANILINE
mf: $C_{14}H_{15}N_3$ mw: 225.32

SYNS: N-METHYL-4'-METHYL-p-AMINOAZOBENZENE ◇ N-METHYL-4'-METHYL-4-AMINOAZOBENZENE

TOXICITY DATA and REFERENCE
ETA: orl-rat TD:4540 mg/kg/36W-C JNCIAM 15,67,54
ETA: orl-rat TDLo:2400 mg/kg/14W-C CNREA8 8,141,48

SAFETY PROFILE: Questionable carcinogen with experimental tumorigenic data. When heated to decomposition it emits toxic fumes of NO_x.

MQB750 CAS: 3413-72-7
5-(3-METHYL-1-TRIAZENO)IMIDAZOLE-4-CARBOXAMIDE
mf: $C_5H_8N_6O$ mw: 168.19

SYNS: MTIC ◇ NSC-407347

TOXICITY DATA and REFERENCE
CAR: orl-rat TDLo:4450 mg/kg/14W-C:TER JNCIAM 54,951,75
ETA: ipr-rat TDLo:10 mg/kg:TER JNCIAM 54,951,75
MUT: dnd-hmn:oth 100 μmol/L CRNGDP 7,259,86
MUT: dni-mus:fbr 10 μmol/L BCPCA6 24,615,75
MUT: mmo-esc 100 μg/plate CRNGDP 3,467,82
MUT: mmo-sat 100 μg/plate CRNGDP 3,467,82
MUT: oms-hmn:oth 60 μmol/L CNREA8 42,1454,82

SAFETY PROFILE: Questionable carcinogen with experimental carcinogenic, tumorigenic, and teratogenic data. Human mutation data reported. When heated to decomposition it emits toxic fumes of NO_x.

MQD000 CAS: 63041-14-5
1-METHYLTRICYCLOQUINAZOLINE
mf: $C_{22}H_{14}N_4$ mw: 334.40

TOXICITY DATA and REFERENCE
NEO: skn-mus TDLo:1240 mg/kg/1Y-I BJCAAI 16,275,62

SAFETY PROFILE: Questionable carcinogen with experimental neoplastigenic data. When heated to decomposition it emits toxic fumes of NO_x.

MQD250 CAS: 28522-57-8
3-METHYLTRICYCLOQUINAZOLINE
mf: $C_{22}H_{14}N_4$ mw: 334.40

TOXICITY DATA and REFERENCE
NEO: skn-mus TDLo:1240 mg/kg/1Y-I BJCAAI 16,275,62

SAFETY PROFILE: Questionable carcinogen with experimental neoplastigenic data. When heated to decomposition it emits toxic fumes of NO_x.

MQD500 CAS: 63041-15-6
4-METHYLTRICYCLOQUINAZOLINE
mf: $C_{22}H_{14}N_4$ mw: 334.40

TOXICITY DATA and REFERENCE
NEO: skn-mus TDLo:1240 mg/kg/1Y-I BJCAAI 16,275,62

SAFETY PROFILE: Questionable carcinogen with experimental neoplastigenic data. When heated to decomposition it emits toxic fumes of NO_x.

MQI250 CAS: 154-06-3
l-5-METHYLTRYPTOPHAN
mf: $C_{12}H_{14}N_2O_2$ mw: 218.28

TOXICITY DATA and REFERENCE
ETA: scu-mus TDLo:2000 mg/kg/20W-I AICCA6 19,660,63

SAFETY PROFILE: Questionable carcinogen with experimental tumorigenic data. When heated to decomposition it emits toxic fumes of NO_x.

MQI750 CAS: 626-48-2
6-METHYLURACIL
mf: $C_5H_6N_2O_2$ mw: 126.13

PROP: Crystals from glacial acetic acid. Decomp above 300°.

SYNS: 6-METHYL-2,4(1H,3H)-PYRIMIDINEDIONE ◇ 4-METHYLURACIL ◇ PSEUDOTHYMINE

TOXICITY DATA and REFERENCE
NEO: orl-rat TDLo:18 g/kg/52W-C VOONAW 8(10),49,62

CONSENSUS REPORTS: Reported in EPA TSCA Inventory.

SAFETY PROFILE: Questionable carcinogen with experimental neoplastigenic and teratogenic data. Moderately toxic by ingestion. Experimental reproductive effects. When heated to decomposition it emits toxic fumes of NO_x.

MQJ250
METHYL UREA and SODIUM NITRITE

SYNS: METHYLHARNSTOFF and NATRIUMNITRIT (GERMAN) ◇ SODIUM NITRITE and METHYL UREA

TOXICITY DATA and REFERENCE
NEO: orl-rat TDLo: 15 g/kg/50D-C   ZAPPAN 121,61,77
ETA: orl-rat TDLo: 12 g/kg/17D-C   ARZNAD 21,1707,71

SAFETY PROFILE: Questionable carcinogen with experimental neoplastigenic, tumorigenic, and teratogenic data. Experimental reproductive effects. When heated to decomposition it emits toxic fumes of Na_2O.

MQL250   CAS: 598-32-3
METHYL VINYL CARBINOL
mf: C_4H_8O mw: 72.12

PROP: Liquid. D: 0.831 20°/4° mp: $<-80°$, bp: 97°. Misc in water.

SYNS: 3-BUTEN-2-OL ◇ 1-METHYL PROPENOL

TOXICITY DATA and REFERENCE
MUT: mmo-sat 50 mmol/L   MUREAV 93,305,82
MUT: mma-sat 50 mmol/L   MUREAV 93,305,82

CONSENSUS REPORTS: Reported in EPA TSCA Inventory.

SAFETY PROFILE: Questionable carcinogen producing nasal tumors. Human systemic effects by inhalation: eye problems. A human eye irritant. Human mutation data reported. When heated to decomposition it emits acrid smoke and irritating fumes.

MQR250
4-o-METPA
mf: $C_{37}H_{58}O_8$ mw: 630.95

TOXICITY DATA and REFERENCE
ETA: skn-mus TD: 970 mg/kg/48W-I   CCSUDL 2,11,78
ETA: skn-mus TDLo: 966 mg/kg/48W-I   CNREA8 39,4183,79

SAFETY PROFILE: Questionable carcinogen with experimental tumorigenic data by skin con-

tact. A skin irritant. When heated to decomposition it emits acrid smoke and irritating fumes.

MQS225   CAS: 3704-09-4
MIBOLERONE
mf: $C_{20}H_{30}O_2$ mw: 302.50

PROP: Crystalline solid. Solubility in deionized water: 0.0454 mg/mL @ 37°.

SYNS: CHEQUE ◇ (7-α,17-β)-17-HYDROXY-7,17-DIMETHYL-ESTR-4-EN-3-ONE (9CI) ◇ 17-β-HYDROXY-7-α, 17-DIMETHYLESTR-4-EN-3-ONE ◇ MATENON ◇ MIBOLERON ◇ U 10997

TOXICITY DATA and REFERENCE
NEO: orl-dog TDLo: 8985 μg/kg/9.6Y-I   TOPADD 13,177,85

SAFETY PROFILE: Questionable carcinogen with experimental neoplastigenic and teratogenic data. Experimental reproductive effects. When heated to decomposition it emits acrid smoke and irritating fumes.

MQV250   CAS: 1401-55-4
MIMOSA TANNIN

SYNS: ACACIA MOLLISSIMA TANNIN ◇ TANNIN from MIMOSA

TOXICITY DATA and REFERENCE
ETA: scu-mus TDLo: 750 mg/kg/12W-I   BJCAAI 14,147,60
ETA: scu-rat TDLo: 350 mg/kg/12W-I   BJCAAI 14,147,60

SAFETY PROFILE: Questionable carcinogen with experimental tumorigenic data. Poison by intravenous and intraperitoneal routes. When heated to decomposition it emits acrid smoke and irritating fumes.

MQV750   CAS: 8012-95-1
MINERAL OIL

PROP: Colorless, oily liquid; practically tasteless and odorless. D: 0.83-0.86 (light), 0.875-0.905 (heavy), flash p: 444°F (OC), ULC: 10-20. Insol in water and alc; sol in benzene, chloroform, and ether. A mixture of liquid hydrocarbons from petroleum.

SYNS: ADEPSINE OIL ◇ ALBOLINE ◇ BAYOL F ◇ BLANDLUBE ◇ CRYSTOSOL ◇ DRAKEOL ◇ FONOLINE ◇ GLYMOL ◇ KAYDOL ◇ KONDREMUL ◇ MINERAL OIL, WHITE (FCC) ◇ MOLOL ◇ NEO-CULTOL ◇ NUJOL ◇ OIL MIST, MINERAL (OSHA, ACGIH) ◇ PAROL ◇ PAROLEINE ◇ PARRAFIN OIL ◇ PENETECK ◇ PENRECO

◇ PERFECTA ◇ PETROGALAR ◇ PETROLATUM, LIQUID ◇ PRIMOL 335 ◇ PROTOPET ◇ SAXOL ◇ TECH PET F ◇ WHITE MINERAL OIL

TOXICITY DATA and REFERENCE
CAR: ihl-man TCLo: 5 mg/m^3/5Y-I: GIT,TER
JOCMA7 23,333,81
ETA: ipr-mus TD: 50 g/kg/9W-I   IJCNAW 6,422,70
ETA: ipr-mus TD: 60 g/kg/17W-I   CNREA8
38,703,78
ETA: ipr-mus TD: 60 g/kg/17W-I   IMMUAM
17,481,69
ETA: ipr-mus TD: 72 g/kg/26W-I   JOIMA3
92,747,62
ETA: ipr-mus TDLo: 14 g/kg   NATUAS 193,1086,62
ETA: skn-mus TDLo: 332 g/mg/20W-I   ANYAA9
132,439,65

CONSENSUS REPORTS: Reported in EPA TSCA Inventory.

OSHA PEL: Oil Mist: TWA 5 mg/m^3 ACGIH TLV: TWA 5 mg/m^3; STEL 10 mg/m^3

SAFETY PROFILE: Questionable human carcinogen producing gastrointestinal tumors. A human teratogen by inhalation which causes testicular tumors in the fetus. Inhalation of vapor or particulates can cause aspiration pneumonia. An eye irritant. Combustible liquid when exposed to heat or flame. To fight fire, use dry chemical, CO_2, foam. When heated to decomposition it emits acrid smoke and fumes.

MQV820   CAS: 64742-63-8
MINERAL OIL, PETROLEUM DISTILLATES, SOLVENT-DEWAXED HEAVY NAPHTHENIC

SYNS: DISTILLATES (PETROLEUM), SOLVENT-DE-WAXED HEAVY NAPHTHENIC (9CI) ◇ SOLVENT-DEWAXED HEAVY NAPHTHENIC DISTILLATE

CONSENSUS REPORTS: IARC Cancer Review: GROUP 3 IMEMDT 7,252,87; Animal No Evidence IMEMDT 33,87,84. Reported in EPA TSCA Inventory.

SAFETY PROFILE: Questionable carcinogen. When heated to decomposition it emits acrid smoke and irritating fumes.

MQV825   CAS: 64742-65-0
MINERAL OIL, PETROLEUM DISTILLATES, SOLVENT-DEWAXED HEAVY PARAFFINIC

SYNS: DISTILLATES (PETROLEUM), SOLVENT-DE-WAXED HEAVY PARAFFINIC (9CI) ◇ PETROLEUM DISTIL-LATES, SOLVENT-DEWAXED HEAVY PARAFFINIC ◇ SOLVENT-DEWAXED HEAVY PARAFFINIC DISTILLATE

TOXICITY DATA and REFERENCE
ETA: skn-mus TD: 389 g/kg/78W-I   BJCAAI
48,429,83
ETA: skn-mus TDLo: 386 g/kg/22W-I   BJCAAI
48,429,83

CONSENSUS REPORTS: IARC Cancer Review: GROUP 3 IMEMDT 7,252,87; Animal No Evidence IMEMDT 33,87,84. Reported in EPA TSCA Inventory.

SAFETY PROFILE: Questionable carcinogen with experimental tumorigenic data. When heated to decomposition it emits acrid smoke and irritating fumes.

MQV845   CAS: 64741-96-4
MINERAL OIL, PETROLEUM DISTILLATES, SOLVENT-REFINED HEAVY NAPHTHENIC

SYNS: DISTILLATES (PETROLEUM), SOLVENT-REFINED HEAVY NAPHTHENIC (9CI) ◇ SOLVENT-REFINED HEAVY NAPHTHENIC DISTILLATE

CONSENSUS REPORTS: IARC Cancer Review: GROUP 3 IMEMDT 7,252,87; Animal No Evidence IMEMDT 33,87,84. Reported in EPA TSCA Inventory.

SAFETY PROFILE: Questionable carcinogen. When heated to decomposition it emits acrid smoke and irritating fumes.

MQV850   CAS: 64741-88-4
MINERAL OIL, PETROLEUM DISTILLATES, SOLVENT-REFINED HEAVY PARAFFINIC

SYNS: DISTILLATES (PETROLEUM), SOLVENT-REFINED HEAVY PARAFFINIC (9CI) ◇ SOLVENT-REFINED HEAVY PARAFFINIC DISTILLATE

CONSENSUS REPORTS: IARC Cancer Review: GROUP 3 IMEMDT 7,252,87; Animal No Evidence IMEMDT 33,87,84. Reported in EPA TSCA Inventory.

SAFETY PROFILE: Questionable carcinogen. When heated to decomposition it emits acrid smoke and irritating fumes.

MRE000   CAS: 1313-27-5
MOLYBDENUM TRIOXIDE
mf: MoO_3 mw: 143.94

PROP: White or yellow to sltly bluish powder or granules. Mp: 795°; bp: 1155°; d: 4.696 @ 26°/4°. Sol in 1000 parts water, in concentration mineral acids, solutions of alkali hydroxides. Sol in ammonia or potassium bitartrate, solidifying to a yellowish-white mass.

SYNS: MOLYBDENUM(VI) OXIDE ◇ MOLYBDIC ANHYDRIDE ◇ MOLYBDIC TRIOXIDE

TOXICITY DATA and REFERENCE
NEO: ipr-mus TDLo:4750 mg/kg/7W-I
    CNREA8 36,1744,76

CONSENSUS REPORTS: Reported in EPA TSCA Inventory. EPA Extremely Hazardous Substances List.

OSHA PEL: TWA 5 mg(Mo)/m^3 ACGIH TLV: TWA 5 mg(Mo)/m^3

SAFETY PROFILE: Questionable carcinogen with experimental neoplastigenic data. Poison by ingestion, subcutaneous, and intraperitoneal routes. Human systemic effects by inhalation: pulmonary fibrosis and cough. A powerful irritant. When heated to decomposition it emits toxic fumes of Mo.

MRI500   CAS: 63041-07-6
MONOGLYCIDYL ETHER of N-PHENYLDIETHANOLAMINE
mf: C$_{13}$H$_{19}$NO$_3$ mw: 237.33

SYN: 2-(N-(2-(2,3-EPOXYPROPOXY)ETHYL)ANILINO)ETHANOL

TOXICITY DATA and REFERENCE
ETA: scu-mus TDLo:17 g/kg/43W-I   FCTXAV 4,365,66

SAFETY PROFILE: Questionable carcinogen with experimental tumorigenic data. When heated to decomposition it emits toxic fumes of NO$_x$.

MRI750   CAS: 39801-14-4
8-MONOHYDRO MIREX
mf: C$_{10}$HCl$_{11}$ mw: 511.06

SYNS: HYDROMIREX ◇ PHOTOMIREX ◇ 1,2,3,4,5,5,-6,7,9,10,10-UNDECACHLOROPENTACYCLO(5.3.0.O^{2,6}.0^{3,9}.0^{4,8})DECANE

TOXICITY DATA and REFERENCE
ETA: orl-rat TDLo:1276 mg/kg/91W-C
    TXAPA9 59,268,81
MUT: spm-mus-ipr 9 mg/kg/5D-C   ENMUDM 8(Suppl 6),39,86

SAFETY PROFILE: Questionable carcinogen with experimental tumorigenic and teratogenic data. Poison by ingestion. Experimental reproductive effects. Mutation data reported. When heated to decomposition it emits toxic fumes of Cl$^-$.

MRJ750   CAS: 5632-47-3
MONONITROSOPIPERAZINE
mf: C$_4$H$_9$N$_3$O   mw: 115.16

SYNS: N-NITROSOPIPERAZINE ◇ 1-NITROSOPIPERAZINE

TOXICITY DATA and REFERENCE
CAR: orl-rat TDLo:5400 mg/kg/60W-I   ZEKBAI 74,179,70
NEO: orl-rat TD:1400 mg/kg/60W-I   ZEKBAI 74,179,70
ETA: orl-mus TDLo:720 mg/kg/20W-I   JNCIAM 55,633,75
MUT: hma-mus/sat 8 mg/kg   CNREA8 37,4572,77
MUT: mma-sat 5 μmol/plate   MUREAV 57,1,78

SAFETY PROFILE: Questionable carcinogen with experimental carcinogenic, neoplastigenic, and tumorigenic data. Moderately toxic by ingestion. Mutation data reported. When heated to decomposition it emits toxic fumes of NO$_x$.

MRK750   CAS: 4390-16-3
MONOSODIUM BARBITURATE
mf: C$_4$H$_4$N$_2$O$_3$•Na   mw: 151.09

SYNS: 2,4,6(1H,3H,5H)-PYRIMIDINETRIONE, MONOSODIUM SALT (9CI) ◇ SODIUM BARBITURATE

TOXICITY DATA and REFERENCE
NEO: orl-rat TDLo:14 g/kg/20W-C   JJIND8 63,1089,79

CONSENSUS REPORTS: Reported in EPA TSCA Inventory.

SAFETY PROFILE: Questionable carcinogen with experimental neoplastigenic data. When heated to decomposition it emits toxic fumes of NO$_x$ and Na$_2$O.

MRN000   CAS: 4166-00-1
MONOTHIOSUCCINIMIDE
mf: C$_4$H$_5$NOS   mw: 115.16

SYNS: THIOSUCCINIMIDE ◇ USAF WI-1

TOXICITY DATA and REFERENCE
ETA: orl-rat TDLo:29 g/kg/2W-C   GANNA2 68,397,77

SAFETY PROFILE: Questionable carcinogen with experimental tumorigenic data. Poison by intraperitoneal route. When heated to decomposition it emits very toxic fumes of NO_x and SO_x.

MRP750   CAS: 110-91-8
MORPHOLINE
DOT: 2054/1760
mf: C_4H_9NO mw: 87.14

PROP: Colorless, hygroscopic oil; amine odor. Bp: 128.9°, fp: −7.5°, flash p: 100°F (OC), autoign temp: 590°F, vap press: 10 mm @ 23°, vap d: 3.00, mp: −4.9°, d: 1.007 @ 20°/4°. Volatile with steam; misc· with water evolving some heat; misc with acetone, benzene, ether, castor oil, methanol, ethanol, ethylene, glycol, linseed oil, turpentine, pine oil. Immiscible with concentrated NaOH solns.

SYNS: DIETHYLENEIMIDE OXIDE ◊ DIETHYLENE IMIDOXIDE ◊ DIETHYLENE OXIMIDE ◊ DIETHYLENI-MIDE OXIDE ◊ MORPHOLINE, AQUEOUS MIXTURE (DOT) ◊ 1-OXA-4-AZACYCLOHEXANE ◊ TETRAHYDRO-p-ISOXA-ZINE ◊ TETRAHYDRO-1,4-ISOXAZINE ◊ TETRAHYDRO-1,4-OXAZINE ◊ TETRAHYDRO-2H-1,4-OXAZINE

TOXICITY DATA and REFERENCE
NEO: orl-mus TDLo: 2560 mg/kg/Y-C   GISAAA
    44(8),15,79

MUT: otr-mus: lym 1 μL/L   ENMUDM 4,390,82

CONSENSUS REPORTS: Reported in EPA TSCA Inventory. EPA Genetic Toxicology Program.

OSHA PEL: (Transitional: TWA 20 ppm (skin) TWA 20 ppm (skin); STEL 30 ppm (skin) ACGIH TLV: TWA 20 ppm; STEL 30 ppm (skin); (Proposed: TWA 20 ppm (skin)) DFG MAK: 20 ppm (70 mg/m³) DOT Classification: Flammable Liquid; Label: Flammable Liquid; Corrosive Material; Label: Corrosive, aqueous solution.

SAFETY PROFILE: Questionable carcinogen with experimental neoplastigenic data. Moderately toxic by ingestion, inhalation, skin contact, intraperitoneal and possibly other routes. Mutation data reported. A corrosive irritant to skin, eyes, and mucous membranes. Can cause kidney damage. Flammable liquid. A very dangerous fire hazard when exposed to flame, heat, or oxidizers; can react with oxidizing materials. To fight fire, use alcohol foam, CO_2, dry chemical. When heated to decomposition it emits highly toxic fumes of NO_x.

MRR775   CAS: 72122-60-2
MORPHOLINO-CNU
mf: $C_7H_{14}ClN_4O_3$ mw: 237.70

SYN: 1-(2-CHLOROETHYL)-3-MORPHOLINO-1-NITRO-SOUREA

TOXICITY DATA and REFERENCE
ETA: ivn-rat TD: 51 mg/kg/24W-I   DTESD7
    8,273,80
ETA: ivn-rat TD: 64 mg/kg/60W-I   DTESD7
    8,273,80
ETA: ivn-rat TD: 102 mg/kg/24W-I   DTESD7
    8,273,80
ETA: ivn-rat TDLo: 32 mg/kg/60W-I   DTESD7
    8,273,80

SAFETY PROFILE: Questionable carcinogen with experimental tumorigenic data. When heated to decomposition it emits toxic fumes of Cl^- and NO_x.

MRR850   CAS: 79867-78-0
MORPHOLINODAUNOMYCIN
mf: $C_{31}H_{35}NO_{11}$ mw: 597.67

SYN: 5,12-NAPHTHACENEDIONE, 7,8,9,10-TETRAHY-DRO-8-ACETYL-1-METHOXY-10-((2,3,6-TRIDEOXY-3-(4-MORPHOLINYL)-α-L-lyxo-HEXOPYRANOSYL)OXY)-6,8,11-TRIHYDROXY-, (8S-cis)-

TOXICITY DATA and REFERENCE
CAR: ivn-rat TDLo: 250 μg/kg   CBTOE2 3,17,87
MUT: dns-rat: lvr 2 mg/L   CNREA8 44,5599,84
MUT: msc-ham: lng 10 μg/L   CNREA8 44,5599,84
MUT: otr-mus: fbr 5 μg/L   CBTOE2 3,17,87

SAFETY PROFILE: Questionable carcinogen with experimental carcinogenic data. Mutation data reported. When heated to decomposition it emits toxic fumes of NO_x.

MRT100   CAS: 80790-68-7
3'-MORPHOLINO-3'-DEAMINODAUNORUBICIN
mf: $C_{31}H_{38}NO_{12}$ mw: 616.70

SYNS: 3'-DEAMINO-3'-MORPHOLINO-ADRIAMYCIN ◊ 3'-DEAMINO-3'-(4-MORPHOLINYL)DAUNORUBICIN ◊ 5,12-NAPHTHACENEDIONE, 7,8,9,10-TETRAHYDRO-8-(HYDROXYACETYL)-1-METHOXY-10-((2,3,6-TRIDEOXY-MORPHOLINO-α-L-lyxo-HEXOPYRANOSYL)OXY)-6,8,11-TRIHYDROXY-

TOXICITY DATA and REFERENCE
ETA: ivn-rat TDLo: 250 μg/kg   PAACA3 27,238,86
MUT: dnd-uns: lyms 2500 nmol/L   CNREA8
    43,1044,83

MUT: dni-hmn:oth 50 nmol/L   CNREA8
43,1044,83

MUT: oth-hmn:oth 50 nmol/L   CNREA8
43,1044,83

SAFETY PROFILE: Questionable carcinogen with experimental tumorigenic data. Poison by ingestion and intraperitoneal routes. Human mutation data reported. When heated to decomposition it emits toxic fumes of NO_x.

MRU000   CAS: 58139-48-3
4-MORPHOLINO-2-(5-NITRO-2-THIENYL)QUINAZOLINE
mf: $C_{16}H_{14}N_4O_3S$ mw: 342.40

TOXICITY DATA and REFERENCE
NEO: orl-rat TDLo:14 g/kg/60W-C   JNCIAM
57,277,76

MUT: mmo-sat 1250 µg/plate   CNREA8 35,3611,75

SAFETY PROFILE: Questionable carcinogen with experimental neoplastigenic data. Mutation data reported. When heated to decomposition it emits very toxic fumes of SO_x and NO_x.

MRU600   CAS: 34816-55-2
MOXESTROL
mf: $C_{21}H_{26}O_3$ mw: 326.47

PROP: Crystals. Mp: 280°.

SYNS: 11-β-METHOXY-19-NOR-17-α-PREGNA-1,3,5(10)-TRIEN-20-YNE-3,17-DIOL ◇ R 2858 ◇ RU 2858 ◇ SURESTRYL

TOXICITY DATA and REFERENCE
CAR: imp-ham TDLo:400 mg/kg/39W-C
CNREA8 47,2583,87

SAFETY PROFILE: Questionable carcinogen with experimental carcinogenic data. Experimental reproductive effects. A steroid. When heated to decomposition it emits acrid smoke and irritating fumes.

MRU900   CAS: 87-56-9
MUCOCHLORIC ACID
mf: $C_4H_2Cl_2O_3$ mw: 168.96

SYNS: ALDEHYDODICHLOROMALEIC ACID ◇ 2-BUTENOIC ACID, 2,3-DICHLOR-4-OXO-, (Z)-(9CI) ◇ α-β-DICHLORO-β-FORMYL ACRYLIC ACID ◇ 3,4-DICHLORO-2-HYDROXYCROTONOLACTONE ◇ 3,4-DICHLORO-2-HYDROXYCROTONOLACTONIC ACID ◇ DICHLOROMALEALDEHYDIC ACID ◇ 2,3-DICHLOROMALEIC ALDEHYDE ACID ◇ 2,3-DICHLORO-4-OXO-2-BUTENOIC ACID ◇ KYSELINA MUKOCHLOROVA ◇ MALEALDEHYDIC ACID, DICHLORO-4-OXO-, (Z)-(9CI)

TOXICITY DATA and REFERENCE
ETA: orl-mus TDLo:6100 mg/kg/78W-I
NTIS** PB223-159

MUT: mmo-sat 100 ng/plate   BECTA6 24,590,80

CONSENSUS REPORTS: Reported in EPA TSCA Inventory.

SAFETY PROFILE: Questionable carcinogen with experimental tumorigenic data. Poison by ingestion. Moderate skin and severe eye irritant. Mutation data reported. When heated to decomposition it emits toxic fumes of Cl^-.

MSA750   CAS: 64817-78-3
9-MYRISTOYL-1,7,8-ANTHRACENETRIOL
mf: $C_{28}H_{36}O_4$ mw: 436.64

SYNS: 1,8-DIHYDROXY-10-MYRISTOYL-9-ANTHRONE ◇ 1,8-DIHYDROXY-10-(1-OXOTETRADECYL)-9(10H)-ANTHRACENONE ◇ 10-MYRISTOYL-1,8,9-ANTHRACENETRIOL

TOXICITY DATA and REFERENCE
NEO: skn-mus TDLo:2621 mg/kg/73W-I
JMCMAR 21,26,78

SAFETY PROFILE: Questionable carcinogen with experimental neoplastigenic data. When heated to decomposition it emits acrid smoke and irritating fumes.

MSB000   CAS: 63021-43-2
1-MYRISTOYLAZIRIDINE
mf: $C_{16}H_{31}NO$ mw: 253.48

SYNS: MYRISTOYLETHYLENEIMINE ◇ TETRADECANOYLETHYLENEIMINE

TOXICITY DATA and REFERENCE
NEO: scu-mus TDLo:4 g/kg/32W-I   BJPCAL
9,306,54

SAFETY PROFILE: Questionable carcinogen with experimental neoplastigenic data. When heated to decomposition it emits toxic fumes of NO_x.

MSB100   CAS: 79127-47-2
N-MYRISTOYLOXY-N-ACETYL-2-AMINO-7-IODOFLUORENE
mf: $C_{29}H_{38}INO_3$ mw: 575.58

SYNS: ACETOHYDROXAMIC ACID, N-(7-IODOFLUOREN-2-YL)-O-MYRISTOYL- ◇ HYDROXYLAMINE, N-ACETYL-N-(7-IODO-2-FLUORENYL)-O-MYRISTOYL- ◇ N-MYRISTOYLOXY-AAIF

TOXICITY DATA and REFERENCE
CAR: scu-rat TDLo: 147 mg/kg/6W-I   CRNGDP
  2,655,81

SAFETY PROFILE: Questionable carcinogen
with experimental carcinogenic data. When
heated to decomposition it emits toxic fumes
of NO_x.

MSB250　　　　CAS: 63224-46-4
N-MYRISTOYLOXY-N-MYRISTOYL-2-AMINOFLUORENE
mf: $C_{41}H_{63}NO_3$　　mw: 618.05

SYN: N-TETRADECANOYL-N-TETRADECANOYLOXY-2-
AMINOFLUORENE

TOXICITY DATA and REFERENCE
NEO: scu-rat TDLo: 157 mg/kg/5W-I   CNREA8
  37,1461,77
MUT: dnr-hmn: fbr 100 μmol/L   CNREA8
  37,1461,77
MUT: dns-hmn: fbr 100 μmol/L/5H   IJCNAW
  16,284,75

SAFETY PROFILE: Questionable carcinogen
with experimental neoplastigenic data. Human
mutation data reported. When heated to decomposition it emits toxic fumes of NO_x.

MSB750
MYROBALANS TANNIN

SYNS: TANNIN from MYROBALANS ◇ TERMINALIA CHE-
BULA RETZ TANNING

TOXICITY DATA and REFERENCE
ETA: scu-mus TDLo: 750 mg/kg/12W-I   BJCAAI
  14,147,60

SAFETY PROFILE: Questionable carcinogen
with experimental tumorigenic data.

MSC000
MYRTAN TANNIN

SYNS: EUCALYPTUS REDUNCA TANNIN ◇ TANNIN from
MYRTAN

TOXICITY DATA and REFERENCE
ETA: scu-mus TDLo: 750 mg/kg/12W-I   BJCAAI
  14,147,60

SAFETY PROFILE: Questionable carcinogen
with experimental tumorigenic data.

NAD500　　　　CAS: 1845-11-0
NAFOXIDINE
mf: $C_{29}H_{31}NO_2$　　mw: 425.61

SYNS: 1-(2-(4-(3,4-DIHYDRO-6-METHOXY-2-PHENYL-1-
NAPHTHALENYL)PHENOXY)ETHYL)PYRROLIDENE
◇ 1-(2-(p-(3,4-DIHYDRO-6-METHOXY-2-PHENYL-1-
NAPHTHYL)PHENOXY)ETHYL)PYRROLIDINE

TOXICITY DATA with REFERENCE
ETA: par-rat TDLo: 200 μg/kg   SCIEAS 197,164,77
ETA: scu-rat TDLo: 500 μg/kg   JSTBBK 12,47,80
MUT: dni-hmn: mmr 1 μmol/L   CNREA8
  45,1611,85

SAFETY PROFILE: Questionable carcinogen
with experimental tumorigenic data. Experimental reproductive effects. Human mutation
data reported. When heated to decomposition
it emits toxic fumes of NO_x.

NAJ500　　　　CAS: 91-20-3
NAPHTHALENE
DOT: 1334/2304
mf: $C_{10}H_8$　　mw: 128.18

PROP: Aromatic odor; white, crystalline, volatile flakes. Mp: 80.1°, bp: 217.9°, flash p: 174°F
(OC), d: 1.162, lel: 0.9%, uel: 5.9%, vap press:
1 mm @ 52.6°, vap d: 4.42, autoign temp:
1053°F (567°C). Sol in alc, benzene; insol in
water; very sol in ether, CCl_4, CS_2, hydro-
naphthalenes, in fixed and volatile oils.

SYNS: CAMPHOR TAR ◇ MIGHTY 150 ◇ MOTH BALLS
◇ MOTH FLAKES ◇ NAFTALEN (POLISH) ◇ NAPHTHA-
LENE, CRUDE or REFINED (DOT) ◇ NAPHTHALENE, MOL-
TEN (DOT) ◇ NAPHTHALIN (DOT) ◇ NAPHTHALINE
◇ NAPHTHENE ◇ NCI-C52904 ◇ RCRA WASTE NUMBER
U165 ◇ TAR CAMPHOR ◇ WHITE TAR

TOXICITY DATA with REFERENCE
ETA: scu-rat TDLo: 3500 mg/kg/12W-I
  APAVAY 329,141,56
MUT: dnd-mus-ipr 200 mg/kg   CBINA8 40,287,82
MUT: dnd-rat-orl 26 μmol/kg   CBINA8 33,301,81

CONSENSUS REPORTS: Reported in EPA
TSCA Inventory. EPA Genetic Toxicology Program. Community Right-To-Know List.

OSHA PEL: (Transitional: TWA 10 ppm) TWA
10 ppm; STEL 15 ppm   ACGIH TLV: TWA
10 ppm; STEL 15 ppm   DFG MAK: 10 ppm
(50 mg/m^3)   DOT Classification: ORM-A; Label: None; Flammable Solid; Label: Flammable
Solid.

SAFETY PROFILE: Questionable carcinogen
with experimental tumorigenic data. Human
poison by ingestion and possibly other routes.
Experimental poison by ingestion, intravenous,

and intraperitoneal routes. Moderately toxic by subcutaneous route. Experimental reproductive effects. Mutation data reported. An eye and skin irritant. Can cause nausea, headache, diaphoresis, hematuria, fever, anemia, liver damage, vomiting, convulsions, and coma. Poisoning may occur by ingestion of large doses, inhalation, or skin absorption. Flammable when exposed to heat or flame; reacts with oxidizing materials. Explosive in the form of vapor or dust when exposed to heat or flame. To fight fire, use water, CO_2, dry chemical. When heated to decomposition it emits acrid smoke and irritating fumes.

NAM500   CAS: 3173-72-6
1,5-NAPHTHALENE DIISOCYANATE
mf: $C_{12}H_6N_2O_2$ mw: 210.20

PROP: White to light yellow crystals.

SYNS: 1,5-DIISOCYANATONAPHTHALENE ◇ ISO-CYANIC ACID-1,5-NAPHTHYLENE ESTER

CONSENSUS REPORTS: IARC Cancer Review: GROUP 3 IMEMDT 7,56,87. Reported in EPA TSCA Inventory.

DFG MAK: 0.01 ppm (0.09 mg/m^3)

SAFETY PROFILE: Questionable carcinogen. A powerful allergen. An irritant. When heated to decomposition it emits toxic fumes of NO_x.

NAS500   CAS: 61790-14-5
NAPHTHENIC ACID, LEAD SALT
mf: $C_7H_{12}O_2$•xPb   mw: 1578.52

PROP: Contains 24% lead (AMIHAB 12,-477,55).

SYNS: CYCLOHEXANECARBOXYLIC ACID, LEAD SALT ◇ LEAD NAPHTHENATE

TOXICITY DATA with REFERENCE
ETA: skn-mus TDLo:50 g/kg/29W-I   BECCAN 39,420,61

CONSENSUS REPORTS: IARC Cancer Review: Animal Inadequate Evidence IMEMDT 23,325,80. Lead and its compounds are on the Community Right-To-Know List. Reported in EPA TSCA Inventory.

NIOSH REL: (Inorganic Lead) TWA 0.10 mg(Pb)/m^3

SAFETY PROFILE: Questionable carcinogen with experimental tumorigenic data. A poison.

Moderately toxic by intraperitoneal route. Mildly toxic by ingestion. When heated to decomposition it emits toxic fumes of lead.

NAU000   CAS: 16566-64-6
NAPHTHO(1,8-gh:4,5-g′h′) DIQUINOLINE
mf: $C_{22}H_{12}N_2$ mw: 304.36

SYNS: 1,12-DIAZADIBENZO(a,i)PYRENE ◇ DIPYRIDO(2,3-d,2,3-1)PYRENE

TOXICITY DATA with REFERENCE
ETA: scu-mus TDLo:72 mg/kg/9W-I   BJCAAI 26,262,72

SAFETY PROFILE: Questionable carcinogen with experimental tumorigenic data. When heated to decomposition it emits toxic fumes of NO_x.

NAU500   CAS: 16566-62-4
NAPHTHO(1,8-gh:5,4-g′h′) DIQUINOLINE
mf: $C_{22}H_{12}N_2$ mw: 304.36

SYNS: 4,11-DIAZADIBENZO(a,h)PYRENE ◇ DIPYRIDO(2,3-D,2,3-K)PYRENE

TOXICITY DATA with REFERENCE
ETA: ipr-rat TDLo:100 mg/kg   NEOLA4 26,23,79
ETA: scu-mus TDLo:72 mg/kg/9W-I   BJCAAI 26,262,72

SAFETY PROFILE: Questionable carcinogen with experimental tumorigenic data. When heated to decomposition it emits toxic fumes of NO_x.

NAZ000   CAS: 224-98-6
NAPHTHO(2,3-f)QUINOLINE
mf: $C_{17}H_{11}N$ mw: 229.29

PROP: Colorless leaflets. Mp: 170°, bp: 446°. Insol in water, sol in alc and ether.

SYN: β-ANTHRAQUINOLINE

TOXICITY DATA with REFERENCE
ETA: scu-rat LDLo:40 mg/kg/4W-I   AJCAA7 35,534,39
MUT: mma-sat 500 μg/plate   CRNGDP 3,947,82

SAFETY PROFILE: Questionable carcinogen with experimental tumorigenic data. Mutation data reported. When heated to decomposition it emits toxic fumes of NO_x.

NBA500   CAS: 130-15-4
1,4-NAPHTHOQUINONE
mf: $C_{10}H_6O_2$ mw: 158.16

PROP: Yellow triclinic; odor of benzoquinone. Mp: 125-126°, D: 1.422. Very sltly sol in cold water; very sol in hot alc; sol in ether, benzene, chloroform, carbon bisulfide, acetic acid, alkali hydroxide solns. Volatile with steam.

SYNS: 1,4-DIHYDRO-1,4-DIKETONAPHTHALENE ◇ 1,4-NAPHTHALENEDIONE ◇ α-NAPHTHOQUINONE ◇ RCRA WASTE NUMBER U166 ◇ USAF CY-10

TOXICITY DATA with REFERENCE
ETA: skn-mus TDLo:800 mg/kg/29W-C
PIATA8 16,309,40

CONSENSUS REPORTS: Reported in EPA TSCA Inventory.

SAFETY PROFILE: Questionable carcinogen with experimental tumorigenic data. Poison by ingestion, intravenous, subcutaneous and intra-peritoneal routes. Experimental reproductive effects. When heated to decomposition it emits acrid smoke and irritating fumes.

NBC000 CAS: 63021-45-4
1-(2-NAPHTHOYL)-AZIRIDINE
mf: $C_{13}H_{11}NO$ mw: 197.25

SYN: β-NAPHTHOYLETHYLENEIMINE

TOXICITY DATA with REFERENCE
NEO: scu-rat TDLo:975 mg/kg/20W-I BJPCAL
9,306,54

SAFETY PROFILE: Questionable carcinogen with experimental neoplastigenic data. Poison by intraperitoneal route. When heated to decomposition it emits toxic fumes of NO_x.

NBD000 CAS: 2508-23-8
N-2-NAPHTHYLACETOHYDROXAMIC ACID
mf: $C_{12}H_{11}NO_2$ mw: 201.24

SYNS: N-ACETYL-2-NAPHTHYLHYDROXYLAMINE ◇ 2-(N-HYDROXYACETAMIDO)NAPHTHALENE ◇ N-HY-DROXY-2-ACETYLAMINONAPHTHALENE ◇ N-HYDROXY-N-2-NAPHTHALENYLACETAMIDE

TOXICITY DATA with REFERENCE
NEO: imp-mus TDLo:160 mg/kg ANYAA9
108,924,63
MUT: dns-hmn:oth 10 μmol/L JJIND8 72,847,84

SAFETY PROFILE: Questionable carcinogen with experimental neoplastigenic data. Human mutation data reported. When heated to decomposition it emits toxic fumes of NO_x.

NBE850 CAS: 86-65-7
2-NAPHTHYLAMINE-6,8-DISULFONIC ACID
mf: $C_{10}H_9NO_6S_2$ mw: 303.32

SYNS: AMIDO-G-ACID ◇ 7-AMINO-1,3-NAPHTHALENE-DISULFONIC ACID

TOXICITY DATA with REFERENCE
NEO: ipr-mus TDLo:7500 mg/kg/8W-I JJIND8
67,1299,81

CONSENSUS REPORTS: Reported in EPA TSCA Inventory.

SAFETY PROFILE: Questionable carcinogen with experimental neoplastigenic data. When heated to decomposition it emits toxic fumes of NO_x and SO_x.

NBG000 CAS: 63978-93-8
4-(1-NAPHTHYLAZO)-2-NAPHTHYLAMINE
mf: $C_{20}H_{15}N_3$ mw: 297.38

TOXICITY DATA with REFERENCE
ETA: orl-rat TDLo:23 g/kg/64W-C ZEKBAI
57,530,51

SAFETY PROFILE: Questionable carcinogen with experimental tumorigenic data. When heated to decomposition it emits toxic fumes of NO_x.

NBG500 CAS: 6416-57-5
4-(1-NAPHTHYLAZO)-m-PHENYLENEDIAMINE
mf: $C_{16}H_{14}N_4$ mw: 262.34

SYNS: C.I. 11285 ◇ FAT BROWN ◇ 1-NAPHTHALENAZO-2',4'-DIAMINOBENZENE ◇ 4-(1-NAPHTHALENYLAZO)-1,3-PHENYLENEDIAMINE ◇ ORGANOL BROWN 2R ◇ RESINOL BROWN RRN ◇ SUDAN BROWN RR

TOXICITY DATA with REFERENCE
ETA: orl-rat TDLo:34 g/kg/89W-C ZEKBAI
57,530,51

CONSENSUS REPORTS: IARC Cancer Review: Animal Inadequate Evidence IMEMDT 8,249,75. Reported in EPA TSCA Inventory.

SAFETY PROFILE: Questionable carcinogen with experimental tumorigenic data. When heated to decomposition it emits toxic fumes of NO_x.

NBI500 CAS: 613-47-8
2-NAPHTHYLHYDROXYLAMINE
mf: $C_{10}H_9NO$ mw: 159.20

SYNS: N-HYDROXY-2-AMINONAPHTHALENE ◇ N-HY-
DROXY-2-NAPHTHYLAMINE ◇ NHA

TOXICITY DATA with REFERENCE
CAR: imp-mus TDLo:80 mg/kg   BJCAAI
17,127,63
NEO: imp-mus TD:160 mg/kg   ANYAA9
108,924,63
NEO: ipr-rat TDLo:1300 mg/kg/13W-I   CNREA8
28,535,68
ETA: par-dog TDLo:30 mg/kg/2Y-I   CNREA8
31,1461,71
ETA: skn-mus TDLo:40 mg/kg   ANYAA9
163,828,69
ETA: skn-rat TDLo:624 mg/kg 52W-I   RCOCB8
18,353,77
MUT: dnd-hmn:fbr 10 μmol/L   GANNA2 75,349,84
MUT: dnd-rat-scu 106 μmol/kg   CNREA8
44,1172,84
MUT: dns-hmn:oth 10 μmol/L   JJIND8 72,847,84
MUT: mmo-sat 1 μg/plate   MUREAV 122,243,83
MUT: msc-ham:ovr 2 mg/L   MUREAV 112,329,83
MUT: oms-rat-scu 106 μmol/kg   CNREA8
44,1172,84

CONSENSUS REPORTS: EPA Genetic Toxicology Program.

SAFETY PROFILE: Questionable carcinogen
with experimental carcinogenic, neoplastigenic,
and tumorigenic data. Human mutation data reported. When heated to decomposition it emits
toxic fumes of NO_x.

NBL000   CAS: 93-46-9
2-NAPHTHYL-p-PHENYLENEDIAMINE
mf: $C_{26}H_{20}N_2$ mw: 360.48

SYNS: ACETO DIPP ◇ AGERITE WHITE ◇ DI-β-
NAPHTHYL-p-PHENYLDIAMINE ◇ DI-β-NAPHTHYL-p-
PHENYLENEDIAMINE ◇ N,N′-DI-β-NAPHTHYL-p-PHENYL-
ENEDIAMINE ◇ sym-DI-β-NAPHTHYL-p-PHENYLENEDI-
AMINE ◇ DNPD ◇ DWU-β-NAFTYLO-p-FENYLODWU-
AMINA (POLISH) ◇ NONOX CL ◇ TISPERSE MB-2X

TOXICITY DATA with REFERENCE
ETA: orl-mus TDLo:31 g/kg/78W-I   NTIS**
PB223-159
MUT: pic-esc 100 mmol/L   MDMIAZ 31,11,79

CONSENSUS REPORTS: Reported in EPA
TSCA Inventory.

SAFETY PROFILE: Questionable carcinogen
with experimental tumorigenic data. Mutation
data reported. A human skin irritant. An experimental skin and eye irritant. When heated to
decomposition it emits toxic fumes of NO_x.

NBO500   CAS: 32524-44-0
5-β-NAPHTHYL-2:4:6-
TRIAMINOAZOPYRIMIDINE
mf: $C_{14}H_{13}N_7$ mw: 279.34

SYN: 5-(β-NAPHTHYLAZO)-2,4,6-TRIAMINOPYRIMIDINE

TOXICITY DATA with REFERENCE
ETA: ipr-rat TDLo:270 mg/kg/14D-I   JRMSAS
74,59,54

SAFETY PROFILE: Questionable carcinogen
with experimental tumorigenic data. When
heated to decomposition it emits toxic fumes
of NO_x.

NBR100
NDPEA
mf: $C_5H_{12}N_2O_4$ mw: 164.19

SYNS: 3-((2-HYDROXYETHYL)NITROSAMINO)-1.2-PRO-
PANEDIOL ◇ N-NITRISO-N-(2,3-DIHYDROXYPROPYL)-N-(2-
HYDROXYETHYL)AMINE ◇ N-NITROSODIHYDROXY-
PROPYLETHANOLAMINE ◇ N-NITROSO-2,3-DIHYDROXY-
PROPYL-2-HYDROXYETHYLAMINE

TOXICITY DATA with REFERENCE
ETA: orl-rat TD:5500 mg/kg/1Y-C   CRNGDP
5,167,84
ETA: orl-rat TDLo:2750 mg/kg/2Y-C   CRNGDP
5,167,84
MUT: mma-sat 50 μg/plate   MUREAV
111,135,83
MUT: mmo-sat 1 mg/plate   MUREAV 111,135,83

SAFETY PROFILE: Questionable carcinogen
with experimental tumorigenic data. Mutation
data reported. Many N-nitroso compounds are
carcinogens. When heated to decomposition it
emits toxic fumes of NO_x.

NBT000   CAS: 1317-43-7
NEMALITE
mf: H_2MgO_2 mw: 58.33

PROP: Dust used was fibrous (NATWAY
59,318,72).

SYNS: BRUCITE ◇ NEMALITH (GERMAN)

TOXICITY DATA with REFERENCE
CAR: ipr-rat TDLo:450 mg/kg/3W-I   ZHPMAT
162,467,76
NEO: ipl-rat TDLo:200 mg/kg   BJCAAI
28,173,73
NEO: ipr-rat TD:450 mg/kg/4W-I   NATWAY
59,318,72

SAFETY PROFILE: Questionable carcinogen with experimental carcinogenic and neoplastigenic data.

NBW000   CAS: 64093-79-4
NEOCHROMIUM
mf: $CrHO_5S$ mw: 165.07

SYNS: BASIC CHROMIC SULFATE ◇ BASIC CHROMIC SULPHATE ◇ BASIC CHROMIUM SULFATE ◇ BASIC CHROMIUM SULPHATE ◇ CHROMIUM HYDROXIDE SULFATE ◇ CHROMIUM SULFATE ◇ CHROMIUM SULFATE, BASIC ◇ CHROMIUM SULPHATE ◇ KOREON ◇ MONOBASIC CHROMIUM SULFATE ◇ MONOBASIC CHROMIUM SULPHATE ◇ SULFURIC ACID, CHROMIUM SALT, BASIC

TOXICITY DATA with REFERENCE
NEO: scu-rat TDLo: 135 mg/kg   ANYAA9 271,431,76
ETA: scu-rat TD: 135 mg/kg   PBPHAW 14,47,78
MUT: cyt-ham: ovr 5 mg/L   BJCAAI 44,219,81
MUT: cyt-hmn: oth 500 mg/L   BJCAAI 44,219,81
MUT: dni-ham: kdy 500 mg/L   BJCAAI 44,219,81
MUT: oms-ham: kdy 500 mg/L   BJCAAI 44,219,81
MUT: oms-hmn: oth 500 mg/L   BJCAAI 44,219,81

CONSENSUS REPORTS: Chromium and its compounds are on the Community Right-To-Know List.

OSHA PEL: TWA 0.5 mg(Cr)/m^3 ACGIH TLV: TWA 0.5 mg(Cr)/m^3

SAFETY PROFILE: Questionable carcinogen with experimental neoplastigenic and tumorigenic data. Human mutation data reported. When heated to decomposition it emits toxic fumes of SO_x.

NCI300   CAS: 17557-23-2
NEOPENTYL GLYCOL DIGLYCIDYL ETHER
mf: $C_{11}H_{20}O_4$ mw: 216.31

SYNS: 1,3-BIS(2,3-EPOXYPROPOXY)-2,2-DIMETHYLPROPANE ◇ DIGLYCIDYL ETHER of NEOPENTYL GLYCOL ◇ 2,2'-((2,2-DIMETHYL-1,3-PROPANEDIYL)BIS(OXYMETHYLENE))BISOXIRANE ◇ HELOXY WC68

TOXICITY DATA with REFERENCE
ETA: skn-mus TD: 11 g/kg/3Y-I   NTIS** ORNL-5762
ETA: skn-mus TD: 17 g/kg/2Y-I   NTIS** ORNL-5762
ETA: skn-mus TD: 25 g/kg/3Y-I   NTIS** ORNL-5762
ETA: skn-mus TDLo: 9393 mg/kg/2Y-I   NTIS** ORNL-5762

CONSENSUS REPORTS: Glycol ether compounds are on the Community Right-To-Know List. Reported in EPA TSCA Inventory.

SAFETY PROFILE: Questionable carcinogen with experimental tumorigenic data. When heated to decomposition it emits acrid smoke and irritating fumes.

NCI500   CAS: 126-99-8
NEOPRENE
DOT: 1991
mf: C_4H_5Cl mw: 88.54

PROP: Colorless liquid. D: 0.958 @ 20°/20°, bp: 59.4°, flash p: −4°F, lel: 4.0%, uel: 20%, vap d: 3.0, brittle point: −35°, softens @ approx 80°. Sltly sol in water; misc in alc and ether. An oil-resistant synthetic rubber made by the polymerization of chloroprene.

SYNS: 2-CHLOOR-1,3-BUTADIEEN (DUTCH) ◇ 2-CHLOR-1,3-BUTADIEN (GERMAN) ◇ CHLOROBUTADIENE ◇ 2-CHLOROBUTA-1,3-DIENE ◇ 2-CHLORO-1,3-BUTADIENE ◇ CHLOROPREEN (DUTCH) ◇ CHLOROPREN (GERMAN, POLISH) ◇ CHLOROPRENE ◇ β-CHLOROPRENE (OSHA, MAK) ◇ CHLOROPRENE, INHIBITED (DOT) ◇ CHLOROPRENE, UNINHIBITED (DOT) ◇ 2-CLORO-1,3-BUTADIENE (ITALIAN) ◇ CLOROPRENE (ITALIAN)

TOXICITY DATA with REFERENCE
MUT: cyt-hmn-unr 1 mg/m^3 MUREAV 147,301,85
MUT: cyt-rat-ihl 1960 μg/m^3/16W   BZARAZ 27,102,74
MUT: dlt-rat-ihl 4 μg/L/48D-I   TNICS* 13,56,73
MUT: mma-sat 2 pph/4H   ARTODN 41,249,79
MUT: mmo-sat 70 μmol/L   NATUAS 255,641,75
MUT: sln-dmg-orl 5700 μmol/L/3D-I   35WYAM -,63,76

CONSENSUS REPORTS: IARC Cancer Review: GROUP 3 IMEMDT 7,160,87; Animal Inadequate Evidence IMEMDT 19,131,79; Human Inadequate Evidence IMEMDT 19,131,79. Reported in EPA TSCA Inventory. Community Right-To-Know List.

OSHA PEL: (Transitional: TWA 25 ppm (skin)) TWA 10 ppm (skin)   ACGIH TLV: TWA 10 ppm (skin)   DFG MAK: 10 ppm (36 mg/m^3)   NIOSH REL: CL (Chloroprene) 1 ppm/15M   DOT Classification: Flammable Liquid; Label: Flammable Liquid, inhibited; Forbidden, uninhibited ; Flammable Liquid; Label: Flammable Liquid, Poison, inhibited.

SAFETY PROFILE: Questionable carcinogen. Poison by ingestion, intravenous, and subcutaneous routes. Moderately toxic by inhalation. An experimental teratogen. Experimental reproductive effects. Human mutation data reported. Human exposure has caused dermatitis, conjunctivitis, corneal necrosis, anemia, temporary loss of hair, nervousness, and irritability. Exposure to the vapor can cause respiratory tract irritation leading to asphyxia. Other effects are central nervous system depression, drop in blood pressure, severe degenerative changes in the liver, kidneys, lungs, and other vital organs. A very dangerous fire hazard when exposed to heat or flame. Explosive in the form of vapor when exposed to heat or flame. To fight fire, use alcohol foam. When heated to decomposition it emits toxic fumes of Cl^-.

NCQ900   CAS: 59-67-6
NIACIN
mf: $C_6H_5NO_2$ mw: 123.12

PROP: The anti-pellagra vitamin. Colorless needles or white crystalline powder; slt odor. Mp: 236°, subl above mp, d: 1.473. Sol in water and boiling alc; insol in most lipid solvents. Nonhygroscopic and stable in air.

SYNS: ACIDE NICOTINIQUE (FRENCH) ◇ ACIDUM NICOTINICUM ◇ AKOTIN ◇ ANTI-PELLAGRA VITAMIN ◇ APELAGRIN ◇ BIONIC ◇ 3-CARBOXYPYRIDINE ◇ DASKIL ◇ DAVITAMON PP ◇ DIREKTAN ◇ EFACIN ◇ NAH ◇ NAOTIN ◇ NICACID ◇ NICAMIN ◇ NICANGIN ◇ NICO ◇ NICO-400 ◇ NICOBID ◇ NICOCAP ◇ NICOCIDIN ◇ NICOCRISINA ◇ NICODAN ◇ NICODELMINE ◇ NICOLAR ◇ NICONACID ◇ NICONAT ◇ NICONAZID ◇ NICOROL ◇ NICOSIDE ◇ NICO-SPAN ◇ NICOSYL ◇ NICOTAMIN ◇ NICOTENE ◇ NICOTIL ◇ NICOTINE ACID ◇ NICOTINIC ACID ◇ NICOTINIPCA ◇ NICOTINOYL HYDRAZINE ◇ NICOTINSAURE (GERMAN) ◇ NICOVASAN ◇ NICOVASEN ◇ NICOVEL ◇ NICYL ◇ NIPELLEN ◇ PELLAGRAMIN ◇ PELLAGRA PREVENTIVE FACTOR ◇ PELLAGRIN ◇ PELONIN ◇ PEVITON ◇ PP FACTOR ◇ P.P. FACTOR-PELLAGRA PREVENTIVE FACTOR ◇ PYRIDINE-3-CARBONIC ACID ◇ PYRIDINE-β-CARBOXYLIC ACID ◇ PYRIDINE-3-CARBOXYLIC ACID ◇ 3-PYRIDINECARBOXYLIC ACID ◇ PYRIDINE-CARBOXYLIQUE-3 (FRENCH) ◇ S115 ◇ SK-NIACIN ◇ TINIC ◇ VITAPLEX N ◇ WAMPOCAP

TOXICITY DATA with REFERENCE
CAR: orl-mus TDLo: 174 g/kg/94W-C   ONCOBS 38,106,81

CONSENSUS REPORTS: Reported in EPA TSCA Inventory.

SAFETY PROFILE: Questionable carcinogen with experimental carcinogenic data. Poison by

intraperitoneal route. Moderately toxic by ingestion, intravenous and subcutaneous routes. When heated to decomposition it emits toxic fumes of NO_x.

NCY100   CAS: 12035-52-8
NICKEL ANTIMONIDE
mf: NiSb   mw: 180.46

SYNS: ANTIMONY, compounded with NICKEL (1:1) ◇ NICKEL MONOANTIMONIDE

TOXICITY DATA with REFERENCE
CAR: ims-rat TDLo: 172 mg/kg   IAPUDO 53,127,84

CONSENSUS REPORTS: Reported in EPA TSCA Inventory.

SAFETY PROFILE: Questionable carcinogen with experimental carcinogenic data. When heated to decomposition it emits toxic fumes of Ni and Sb.

NDB875   CAS: 12035-51-7
NICKEL DISULFIDE
mf: NiS_2 mw: 122.83

SYN: NICKEL SULFIDE

TOXICITY DATA with REFERENCE
CAR: ims-rat TDLo: 117 mg/kg   IAPUDO 53,127,84
NEO: irn-rat TDLo: 58580 μg/kg   CRNGDP 5,1511,84

SAFETY PROFILE: Questionable carcinogen with experimental carcinogenic and neoplastigenic data. When heated to decomposition it emits toxic fumes of SO_x.

NDF000   CAS: 74203-45-5
NICKEL(II) ISODECYL ORTHOPHOSPHATE (3:2)

SYN: PHOSPHORIC ACID, ISODECYL NICKEL(2+) SALT (2:3)

TOXICITY DATA with REFERENCE
NEO: ims-rat TDLo: 320 mg/kg/35W-I   NCIUS* PH 43-64-886,DEC,68
ETA: ims-rat TD: 1260 mg/kg/30W-I   NCIUS* PH 43-64-886,AUG,69

CONSENSUS REPORTS: Nickel and its compounds are on the Community Right-To-Know List.

NIOSH REL: (Inorganic Nickel) TWA 0.015 mg(Ni)/m³

SAFETY PROFILE: Questionable carcinogen with experimental neoplastigenic and tumorigenic data. Poison by intraperitoneal route. When heated to decomposition it emits very toxic fumes of PO_x.

NDF400   CAS: 1314-05-2
NICKEL MONOSELENIDE
mf: NiSe   mw: 137.67

SYN: NICKEL SELENIDE

TOXICITY DATA with REFERENCE
CAR: ims-rat TDLo: 131 mg/kg   IAPUDO 53,127,84

SAFETY PROFILE: Questionable carcinogen with experimental carcinogenic data.

NDL425   CAS: 12142-88-0
NICKEL TELLURIDE
mf: NiTe   mw: 186.31

TOXICITY DATA with REFERENCE
CAR: ims-rat TDLo: 178 mg/kg   IAPUDO 53,127,84
ETA: ims-rat TD: 56 mg/kg   NTIS** DOE/
EV/03140-5

CONSENSUS REPORTS: Reported in EPA TSCA Inventory.

OSHA PEL: TWA 1 mg(Ni)/m^3 ACGIH TLV: TWA 1 mg(Ni)/m^3; 0.1 mg(Te)/m^3 NIOSH REL: TWA 0.015 mg(Ni)/m^3

SAFETY PROFILE: Questionable carcinogen with experimental carcinogenic and tumorigenic data.

NDU500   CAS: 553-53-7
NICOTINIC ACID, HYDRAZIDE
mf: $C_6H_7N_3O$ mw: 137.16

PROP: Needles from dil alc or benzene. Mp: 158-159°. Very sol in water and alc; sltly sol in benzene.

SYNS: NICOTINOYL HYDRAZINE ◇ NICOTINYLHYDRA-ZIDE ◇ 3-PYRIDOYL HYDRAZINE ◇ WS 102

TOXICITY DATA with REFERENCE
CAR: orl-mus TDLo: 124 g/kg/71W-C   ONCOBS 38,106,81

SAFETY PROFILE: Questionable carcinogen with experimental carcinogenic data. Poison by intravenous and parenteral routes. When heated to decomposition it emits toxic fumes of NO_x.

NEL000   CAS: 1777-84-0
3-NITRO-p-ACETOPHENETIDIDE
mf: $C_{10}H_{12}N_2O_4$ mw: 224.24

PROP: Yellow needles in water. M: 103-104°. Sol in abs alc, ether and chloroform.

SYNS: 4-ACETAMINO-2-NITROPHENETOLE ◇ N-(4-ETHOXY-3-NITRO)PHENYLACETAMIDE ◇ N-(4-ETHOXY-PHENYL)-3'-NITROACETAMIDE ◇ NCI C01978 ◇ 2-NITRO-4-ACETAMINOFENETOL (CZECH) ◇ 3-NITRO-p-ACETO-PHENETIDE ◇ 5-NITRO-p-ACETOPHENETIDIDE ◇ 3'-NITRO-p-ACETOPHENETIDIN

TOXICITY DATA with REFERENCE
NEO: orl-mus TDLo: 957 g/kg/78W-C   NCITR*
NCI-CG-TR-133,79
ETA: orl-mus TD: 478 g/kg/78W-C   NCITR*
NCI-CG-TR-133,79
MUT: mma-sat 33 µg/plate   ENMUDM 5(Suppl 1),3,83
MUT: mmo-sat 1 mg/plate   ENMUDM 5(Suppl 1),3,83

CONSENSUS REPORTS: NCI Carcinogenesis Bioassay (feed); Clear Evidence: mouse NCITR* NCI-CG-TR-133,79; (feed); No Evidence: rat NCITR* NCI-CG-TR-133,79. Reported in EPA TSCA Inventory.

SAFETY PROFILE: Questionable carcinogen with experimental carcinogenic, neoplastigenic, and tumorigenic data. Moderately toxic by ingestion. Mutation data reported. An eye irritant. When heated to decomposition it emits toxic fumes of NO_x.

NEM500   CAS: 99-57-0
p-NITRO-o-AMINOPHENOL
mf: $C_6H_6N_2O_3$ mw: 154.14

SYNS: 3-AMINO-4-HYDROXYNITROBENZENE ◇ 2-AMINO-4-NITROPHENOL ◇ 2-HYDROXY-5-NITROANI-LINE ◇ NCI-C55958 ◇ 4-NITRO-2-AMINOFENOL (CZECH) ◇ p-NITROAMINOFENOL (POLISH)

TOXICITY DATA with REFERENCE
NEO: orl-rat TDLo: 64375 mg/kg/2Y-C   NTPTR*
NTP-TR-339,88
MUT: mma-sat 100 µg/plate   PNASA6 72,2423,75
MUT: mmo-sat 20 µg/plate   CMMUAO 8,151,83
MUT: pic-esc 100 mmol/L   MDMIAZ 31,11,79

CONSENSUS REPORTS: Reported in EPA TSCA Inventory. EPA Genetic Toxicology Program.

SAFETY PROFILE: Questionable carcinogen with experimental tumorigenic data. Poison by intraperitoneal route. Moderately toxic by ingestion. Mutation data reported. An eye irritant. When heated to decomposition it emits toxic fumes of NO_x.

NFD500   CAS: 94-52-0
6-NITRO-BENZIMIDAZOLE
mf: $C_7H_5N_3O_2$ mw: 163.15

PROP: Needles from water. Mp: 204°. Sltly sol in water, chloroform, ether, benzene; sol in acid, alkali carbonate.

SYNS: NCI-C01912 ◇ 5-NITRO-1H-BENZIMIDAZOLE

TOXICITY DATA with REFERENCE
CAR: orl-mus TDLo: 160 g/kg/78W-C   NCITR*
NCI-CG-TR-117,79
ETA: orl-mus TD: 79 g/kg/78W-C   NCITR* NCI-
CG-TR-117,79
MUT: mma-sat 33 μg/plate   ENMUDM 8(Suppl
7),1,86
MUT: mmo-sat 33 μg/plate   ENMUDM 8(Suppl
7),1,86

CONSENSUS REPORTS: NCI Carcinogenesis Bioassay (feed); Clear Evidence: mouse NCITR* NCI-CG-TR-117,78; (feed); Negative: rat NCITR* NCI-CG-TR-117,78. Reported in EPA TSCA Inventory.

SAFETY PROFILE: Questionable carcinogen with experimental carcinogenic and tumorigenic data. Moderately toxic by ingestion. Mutation data reported. When heated to decomposition it emits toxic fumes of NO_x.

NFL500   CAS: 38860-52-5
N-(4-NITRO)BENZOYLOXYPIPERIDINE
mf: $C_{12}H_{14}N_2O_4$ mw: 250.28

SYN: p-NITROBENZOIC ACID, PIPERIDINO ESTER

TOXICITY DATA with REFERENCE
NEO: skn-mus TDLo: 50 mg/kg   JNCIAM54,491,75

SAFETY PROFILE: Questionable carcinogen with experimental neoplastigenic data. When heated to decomposition it emits toxic fumes of NO_x.

NFM500   CAS: 63041-90-7
6-NITROBENZ(a)PYRENE
mf: $C_{20}H_{11}NO_2$ mw: 297.32

TOXICITY DATA with REFERENCE
MUT: dnd-mam:lym 35 nmol   GANNA2 74,5,83
MUT: mma-ham:ovr 5 mg/L   CRNGDP 7,681,85
MUT: mma-sat 3 μg/plate   ENMUDM 6,417,84
MUT: otr-ham:emb 6600 nmol/L   CRNGDP
4,357,83
MUT: otr-hmn:fbr 4 μmol/L   CRNGDP 4,353,83

CONSENSUS REPORTS: IARC Cancer Review: GROUP 3 IMEMDT 7,56,87; Animal

Inadequate Evidence IMEMDT 33,187,84. EPA Genetic Toxicology Program.

SAFETY PROFILE: Questionable carcinogen. Human mutation data reported. When heated to decomposition it emits toxic fumes of NO_x.

NFS525   CAS: 100-00-5
p-NITROCHLOROBENZENE
DOT: 1578
mf: $C_6H_4ClNO_2$ mw: 157.56

PROP: D: 1.520, mp: 83°, bp: 242°, flash p: 110°. Insol in water; sltly sol in alc; very sol in CS_2 and ether.

SYNS: 1-CHLOOR-4-NITROBENZEEN (DUTCH)
◇ 1-CHLOR-4-NITROBENZOL (GERMAN) ◇ p-CHLORONI-
TROBENZENE ◇ 4-CHLORONITROBENZENE ◇ 1-CHLORO-
4-NITROBENZENE ◇ 4-CHLORO-1-NITROBENZENE
◇ 1-CLORO-4-NITROBENZENE (ITALIAN) ◇ p-NITRO-
CHLOORBENZEEN (DUTCH) ◇ p-NITROCHLORBENZOL
(GERMAN) ◇ p-NITROCHLOROBENZENE SOLID (DOT)
◇ p-NITROCLOROBENZENE (ITALIAN) ◇ PNCB

TOXICITY DATA with REFERENCE
CAR: orl-mus TD: 390 g/kg/78W-C   JEPTDQ
2(2),325,78
CAR: orl-mus TDLo: 194 g/kg/78W-C   JEPTDQ
2(2),325,78
MUT: dnd-mus-ipr 60 mg/kg   BSIBAC 56,1680,80
MUT: mma-sat 100 μg/plate   ENMUDM 5(Suppl
1),3,83
MUT: mmo-sat 819 μg/plate   MUREAV 116,217,83

CONSENSUS REPORTS: Reported in EPA TSCA Inventory.

OSHA PEL: TWA 1 mg/m^3 (skin) ACGIH TLV: TWA 0.1 ppm (skin) DFG MAK: 1 mg/m^3 DOT Classification: Poison B; Label: Poison.

SAFETY PROFILE: Questionable carcinogen with experimental carcinogenic data. A poison by ingestion. Mutation data reported. May explode on heating. When heated to decomposition it emits very toxic fumes of NO_x and Cl^-.

NFT400   CAS: 7496-02-8
6-NITROCHRYSENE
mf: $C_{18}H_{11}NO_2$ mw: 273.30

TOXICITY DATA with REFERENCE
CAR: ipr-mus TDLo: 9163 μg/kg/2W-I
CRNGDP 6,801,85
MUT: mma-sat 2500 ng/plate   CNREA8 44,3408,84
MUT: mmo-sat 5 μg/plate   CNREA8 44,3408,84

MUT: otr-ham:emb 3700 nmol/L   CRNGDP
4,357,83

CONSENSUS REPORTS: IARC Cancer Review: GROUP 3 IMEMDT 7,56,87; Animal Limited Evidence IMEMDT 33,195,84.

SAFETY PROFILE: Questionable carcinogen with experimental carcinogenic data. Mutation data reported. When heated to decomposition it emits toxic fumes of NO_x.

NGA500   CAS: 3741-14-8
4-NITRO-2-ETHYLQUINOLINE-N-OXIDE
mf: $C_{11}H_{10}N_2O_3$ mw: 218.23

TOXICITY DATA with REFERENCE
ETA: skn-mus TDLo: 69 mg/kg/11W-I   GANNA2
49,33,58

SAFETY PROFILE: Questionable carcinogen with experimental tumorigenic data. When heated to decomposition it emits toxic fumes of NO_x.

NGA700   CAS: 892-21-7
3-NITROFLUORANTHENE

SYN: 4-NITROFLUORANTHENE

TOXICITY DATA with REFERENCE
CAR: scu-rat TDLo: 120 mg/kg/8W-I   CALEDQ
15,1,82
MUT: mma-ham:lng 100 μmol/L   CRNGDP
6,1403,85
MUT: mma-sat 500 ng/plate   MUREAV 91,321,81
MUT: mmo-sat 130 ng/plate   MUREAV 91,321,81
MUT: otr-ham:emb 4100 nmol/L   CRNGDP
4,357,83

CONSENSUS REPORTS: IARC Cancer Review: Animal Inadequate Evidence IMEMDT 33,201,84

SAFETY PROFILE: Questionable carcinogen with experimental carcinogenic data. Mutation data reported. When heated to decomposition it emits toxic fumes of NO_x.

NGB000   CAS: 607-57-8
2-NITROFLUORENE
mf: $C_{13}H_9NO_2$ mw: 211.23

PROP: Needles from 50% acetic acid. Mp: 157-158°.

TOXICITY DATA with REFERENCE
NEO: skn-rat TDLo: 310 mg/kg/79W-I   JNCIAM
10,1201,50

ETA: orl-rat TD: 4000 mg/kg   CNREA8 7,730,47
ETA: orl-rat TDLo: 3400 mg/kg/23W-C
JNCIAM 10,1201,50
MUT: dni-hmn:hla 3 mmol/L   MUREAV 92,427,82
MUT: mma-sat 300 ng/plate   ENMUDM 6(Suppl 2),1,84
MUT: mmo-sat 250 ng/plate   MUREAV 143,213,85
MUT: msc-mus:lym 250 mg/L   MUREAV
125,291,84
MUT: otr-ham:emb 20 mg/L   NCIMAV 58,243,81
MUT: otr-hmn:lvr 80 μg/L   BJCAAI 37,873,78

CONSENSUS REPORTS: Reported in EPA TSCA Inventory. EPA Genetic Toxicology Program.

SAFETY PROFILE: Questionable carcinogen with experimental neoplastigenic and tumorigenic data. Moderately toxic by intraperitoneal route. Human mutation data reported. When heated to decomposition it emits toxic fumes of NO_x.

NGE000   CAS: 67-20-9
NITROFURANTOIN
mf: $C_8H_6N_4O_5$ mw: 238.18

SYNS: BENKFURAN ◇ BERKFURIN ◇ CHEMIOFURAN ◇ CYANTIN ◇ DANTAFUR ◇ FURADANTIN ◇ FURADONIN ◇ FURANTOIN ◇ FUROBACTINA ◇ ITURAN ◇ MACRODANTIN ◇ NCI-C55196 ◇ N-(5-NITROFURFURYLIDENE)-1-AMINOHYDANTOIN ◇ N-(5-NITRO-2-FURFURYLIDENE)-1-AMINOHYDANTOIN ◇ 1-((5-NITROFURFURYLIDENE)AMINO)HYDANTOIN ◇ NSC 2107 ◇ N-TOIN ◇ ORAFURAN ◇ PARFURAN ◇ URIZEPT ◇ USAF EA-2 ◇ WELFURIN ◇ ZOOFURIN

TOXICITY DATA with REFERENCE
NEO: orl-rat TDLo: 135 g/kg/2Y-C   CALEDQ
21,303,84
MUT: dnd-hmn:oth 112 g/L   CBINA8 45,77,83
MUT: dnd-rat:lvr 112 g/L   CBINA8 45,77,83
MUT: dnr-bcs 20 μL/disc   MUREAV 97,1,82
MUT: mma-sat 300 ng/plate   ENMUDM 5(Suppl 1),3,83
MUT: mmo-sat 500 ng/plate   AEMIDF 46,596,83

CONSENSUS REPORTS: Reported in EPA TSCA Inventory. EPA Genetic Toxicology Program.

SAFETY PROFILE: Questionable carcinogen with experimental neoplastigenic and teratogen data. Poison by ingestion and intraperitoneal routes. Human systemic effects by ingestion and possibly other routes: peripheral motor nerve recording changes, ataxia, changes in urine composition and hemolysis with or without anemia. Human reproductive effects by ingestion: spermatogenesis. Experimental reproductive effects. Human mutation data reported. When heated to decomposition it emits toxic fumes of NO_x.

NGG000   CAS: 23256-30-6
4-((5-NITROFURFURYLIDENE)AMINO)-3-METHYLTHIOMORPHOLINE-1,1-DIOXIDE
mf: $C_{10}H_{13}N_3O_5S$ mw: 287.32

SYNS: BAYER 2502 ◇ LAMPIT ◇ 3-METHYL-4-(5'-NITRO-FURYLIDENE-AMINO)-TETRAHYDRO-4H-1,4-THIAZINE-1,1-DIOXIDE ◇ NIFURTIMOX ◇ 1-((5-NITROFURFURYLIDE-NE)AMINO)-2-METHYLTETRAHYDRO-1,4-THIAZINE-4,4-DIOXIDE ◇ TETRAHYDRO-3-METHYL-4-((5-NITROFUR-FURYLIDENE)AMINO)-2H-1,4-THIAZINE-1,1-DIOXIDE

TOXICITY DATA with REFERENCE
ETA: orl-rat TDLo: 11700 mg/kg/47W-I
   ARZNAD 22,1607,72
ETA: scu-rat TDLo: 11700 mg/kg/47W-I
   ARZNAD 22,1607,72
MUT: dnd-omi 100 μmol/L   BCPCA6 34,1457,84
MUT: dnr-esc 500 mg/L   FOMIAZ 25,388,80
MUT: mmo-esc 50 mg/L   MUREAV 77,241,80
MUT: mnt-mus-orl 600 mg/kg   TOLED5 25,259,85

SAFETY PROFILE: Questionable carcinogen with experimental tumorigenic and teratogenic data. Moderately toxic by ingestion. Experimental reproductive effects. Mutation data reported. When heated to decomposition it emits very toxic fumes of NO_x and SO_x.

NGG500   CAS: 67-45-8
3-((5-NITROFURFURYLIDENE)AMINO)-2-OXAZOLIDONE
mf: $C_8H_7N_3O_5$ mw: 225.18

SYNS: BIFURON ◇ CORIZIUM ◇ DIAFURON ◇ ENTERO-TOXON ◇ FURAXONE ◇ FURAZOL ◇ FURAZOLIDON ◇ FURAZOLIDONE (USDA) ◇ FURAZON ◇ FURIDON ◇ FUROVAG ◇ FUROX ◇ FUROXAL ◇ FUROXANE ◇ FUROXONE SWINE MIX ◇ FUROZOLIDINE ◇ GIARDIL ◇ GIARLAM ◇ MEDARON ◇ NEFTIN ◇ NG-180 ◇ NICOLEN ◇ NIFULIDONE ◇ NIFURAN ◇ 3-(((5-NITRO-2-FURANYL) METHYLENE)AMINO)-2-OXAZOLIDINONE ◇ NITROFURA-ZOLIDONE ◇ NITROFURAZOLIDONUM ◇ 3-(5'-NITROFUR-FURALAMINO)-2-OXAZOLIDONE ◇ NITROFUROXON ◇ N-(5-NITRO-2-FURFURYLIDENE)-3-AMINOOXAZOLI-DINE-2-ONE ◇ N-(5-NITRO-2-FURFURYLIDENE)-3-AMINO-2-OXAZOLIDONE ◇ 3-((5-NITROFURYLIDENE)AMINO)-2-OXAZOLIDONE ◇ 5-NITRO-N-(2-OXO-3-OXAZOLIDINYL)-2-

FURANMETHANIMINE ◇ PURADIN ◇ ROPTAZOL ◇ SCLAVENTEROL ◇ TIKOFURAN ◇ TOPAZONE ◇ TRICHOFURON ◇ TRICOFURON ◇ USAF EA-1 ◇ VIOFURAGYN

TOXICITY DATA with REFERENCE
MUT: bfa-rat/sat 62500 μg/kg   CRNGDP 6,967,85
MUT: cyt-hmn: lym 2 mg/L/72H   MUREAV
   59,139,79
MUT: dnd-omi 500 μg/L   CBINA8 45,315,83
MUT: mmo-asn 200 μg/plate   MUREAV 97,293,82
MUT: mmo-omi 7 mg/L   CBINA8 45,315,83
MUT: pic-esc 2 mg/L   MUREAV 156,69,85
MUT: sce-hmn: lym 200 μg/L/72H   MUREAV
   59,139,79

CONSENSUS REPORTS: IARC Cancer Review: GROUP 3 IMEMDT 7,56,87; Animal Inadequate Evidence IMEMDT 31,141,83. Reported in EPA TSCA Inventory. EPA Genetic Toxicology Program.

SAFETY PROFILE: Questionable carcinogen. Poison by ingestion and intraperitoneal routes. Human systemic effects by ingestion: dyspnea, respiratory depression and rosinophillis. Experimental reproductive effects. Human mutation data reported. When heated to decomposition it emits toxic fumes of NO_x.

NGK000   CAS: 2122-86-3
5-(5-NITRO-2-FURYL)-1,3,4-OXADIAZOLE-2-OL
mf: $C_6H_3N_3O_5$ mw: 197.12

TOXICITY DATA with REFERENCE
NEO: orl-rat TDLo: 12 g/kg/46W-C   JNCIAM
   54,841,75

SAFETY PROFILE: Questionable carcinogen with experimental neoplastigenic data. When heated to decomposition it emits toxic fumes of NO_x.

NGK500   CAS: 36133-88-7
N-((3-(5-NITRO-2-FURYL)-1,2,4-OXADIAZOLE-5-YL)METHYL)ACETAMIDE
mf: $C_9H_8N_4O_5$ mw: 252.21

TOXICITY DATA with REFERENCE
CAR: orl-rat TDLo: 11 g/kg/46W-C   JNCIAM
   54,841,75
MUT: dnr-sat 500 nmol/well   CNREA8 34,2266,74
MUT: mma-sat 1 μg/plate   MUREAV 40,9,76
MUT: mmo-esc 300 nmol/well   CNREA8
   34,2266,74

MUT: mrc-esc 500 nmol/well   CNREA8 34,2266,74

CONSENSUS REPORTS: EPA Genetic Toxicology Program.

SAFETY PROFILE: Questionable carcinogen with experimental carcinogenic data. Mutation data reported. When heated to decomposition it emits toxic fumes of NO_x.

NGL000   CAS: 53757-31-6
3-(5-NITRO-2-FURYL)-2-PHENYLACRYLAMIDE
mf: $C_{13}H_{10}N_2O_4$ mw: 258.25

SYN: 3-(5-NITRO-2-FURYL)-2-PHENYL-2-PROPENAMIDE

TOXICITY DATA with REFERENCE
ETA: orl-rat TDLo:474 g/kg/46W-C   FEPRA7
    38,1403,79
MUT: dnr-sat 500 nmol/well   CNREA8 34,2266,74
MUT: mma-sat 1 μg/plate   MUREAV 40,9,76
MUT: mmo-esc 300 nmol/well   CNREA8
    34,2266,74
MUT: mrc-esc 500 nmol/well   CNREA8 34,2266,74

SAFETY PROFILE: Questionable carcinogen with experimental tumorigenic data. Mutation data reported. When heated to decomposition it emits toxic fumes of NO_x.

NGL500   CAS: 710-25-8
3-(5-NITRO-2-FURYL)-2-PROPENAMIDE
mf: $C_7H_6N_2O_4$ mw: 182.15

SYNS: 5-NITRO-2-FURANACRYLAMIDE ◇ 3-(5-NITRO-2-FURYL)ACRYLAMIDE ◇ 5-NITRO-2-FURYLACRYLAMIDE

TOXICITY DATA with REFERENCE
ETA: orl-rat TDLo:475 g/kg/46 W-C   FEPRA7
    38,1403,79
MUT: dnr-sat 500 mmol/well   CNREA8 34,2266,74
MUT: mma-sat 100 ng/plate   MUREAV 40,9,76
MUT: mmo-esc 300 nmol/well   CNREA8
    34,2266,74
MUT: mmo-sat 10 μg/plate   JOPHDQ 1,15,78
MUT: mrc-esc 500 nmol/well   CNREA8 34,2266,74

CONSENSUS REPORTS: EPA Genetic Toxicology Program.

SAFETY PROFILE: Questionable carcinogen with experimental tumorigenic data. Mutation data reported. When heated to decomposition it emits toxic fumes of NO_x.

NGM400   CAS: 53757-28-1
4-(5-NITRO-2-FURYL)THIAZOLE
mf: $C_7H_4N_2O_3S$ mw: 196.19

TOXICITY DATA with REFERENCE
ETA: orl-rat TDLo:37996 mg/kg/46W-C
    PAACA3 21,75,80
MUT: dnr-esc 500 nmol/well   CNREA8 34,2266,74
MUT: dnr-sat 500 nmol/well   CNREA8 34,2266,74
MUT: mmo-sat 10 ng/plate   CNREA8 41,2648,81

SAFETY PROFILE: Questionable carcinogen with experimental tumorigenic data. Mutation data reported. When heated to decomposition it emits toxic fumes of NO_x and SO_x.

NGN000   CAS: 18523-69-8
(4-(5-NITRO-2-FURYL)THIAZOL-2-YL)HYDRAZONOACETONE
mf: $C_{10}H_{10}N_4O_3S$ mw: 266.30

SYN: 2-(2-ISOPROPYLIDENEHYDRAZONO)-4-(5-NITRO-2-FURYL)-THIAZOLE

TOXICITY DATA with REFERENCE
NEO: orl-rat TDLo:16 g/kg/45W-C   FEPRA7
    25,419,66

SAFETY PROFILE: Questionable carcinogen with experimental neoplastigenic data. When heated to decomposition it emits very toxic fumes of NO_x and SO_x.

NGY000   CAS: 55-63-0
NITROGLYCERIN
DOT: 0143
mf: $C_3H_5N_3O_9$ mw: 227.11

PROP: Colorless to yellow liquid; sweet taste. Mp: 13°, bp: explodes @ 218°, d: 1.599 @ 15°/15°, vap press: 1 mm @ 127°, vap d: 7.84, autoign temp:518°F, decomp @ 50-60°, volatile @ 100°. Misc with ether, acetone, glacial acetic acid, ethyl acetate, benzene, nitrobenzene, pyridine, chloroform, ethylene bromide, dichloroethylene; sltly sol in petr ether, glycerol.

SYNS: ANGININE ◇ BLASTING GELATIN (DOT) ◇ BLASTING OIL ◇ GLONOIN ◇ GLYCERINTRINITRATE (CZECH) ◇ GLYCEROL, NITRIC ACID TRIESTER ◇ GLYCEROL TRINITRATE ◇ GLYCEROL(TRINITRATE de) (FRENCH) ◇ GLYCEROLTRINTRAAT (DUTCH) ◇ GLYCERYL NITRATE ◇ GLYCERYL TRINITRATE ◇ GLYCERYL TRINITRATE, solution up to 1% in alcohol (DOT) ◇ GTN ◇ KLAVI KORDAL ◇ MYOCON ◇ NG ◇ NIGLYCON ◇ NIONG ◇ NITRIC ACID TRIESTER of GLYCEROL ◇ NITRINE-TDC ◇ NITROGLICERINA (ITALIAN) ◇ NITROGLICERYNA (POLISH) ◇ NITROGLYCERIN, LIQUID, DESENSITIZED (DOT) ◇ NITROGLYCERIN, LIQUID, NOT DESENSITIZED (DOT) ◇ NITROGLYCERINE ◇ NITROGLYCEROL ◇ NITROGLYN ◇ NITROL ◇ NITRO

LINGUAL ◇ NITROLOWE ◇ NITRONET ◇ NITRONG ◇ NITRO-SPAN ◇ NITROSTAT ◇ NK-843 ◇ NTG ◇ PERGLOTTAL ◇ 1,2,3-PROPANETRIOL, TRINITRATE ◇ 1,2,3-PROPANETRIYL NITRATE ◇ RCRA WASTE NUMBER P081 ◇ SK-106N ◇ SOUP ◇ TNG ◇ TRINITRIN ◇ TRINITROGLYCERIN ◇ TRINITROGLYCEROL

TOXICITY DATA with REFERENCE
ETA: orl-rat TD:438 g/kg/2Y-C   ATSUDG 4,88,80
ETA: orl-rat TDLo:36500 mg/kg/2Y-C
   ATSUDG 4,88,80
MUT: mma-sat 50 μg/well   CBINA8 19,77,77

CONSENSUS REPORTS: Reported in EPA TSCA Inventory. Community Right-To-Know List.

OSHA PEL: (Transitional: TWA CL 0.2 ppm (skin)) STEL: 0.1 mg/m^3 (skin)   ACGIH TLV: TWA 0.05 ppm (skin)   DFG MAK: 0.05 ppm (0.5 mg/m^3) (skin)   NIOSH REL: CL (Nitroglycerin or EGDN) 0.1 mg/m^3/20M   DOT Classification: Flammable Liquid; Label: Explosive A, desensitized; Forbidden, not desensitized; Flammable Liquid; Label: Flammable Liquid.

SAFETY PROFILE: Questionable carcinogen with experimental tumorigenic and teratogenic data. Human poison by an unspecified route. Poison experimentally by ingestion, intraperitoneal, subcutaneous and intravenous routes. Experimental reproductive effects. A skin irritant. Mutation data reported. Used as a vasodilator and as an explosive. A very dangerous fire hazard when exposed to heat or flame or by spontaneous chemical reaction. When heated to decomposition it emits toxic fumes of NO$_x$.

NHE000   CAS: 4812-22-0
3-NITRO-3-HEXENE
mf: C$_6$H$_{11}$NO$_2$ mw: 129.18

TOXICITY DATA with REFERENCE
NEO: ihl-mus TCLo:200 ppb/63W-I   TXAPA9 5,445,63

SAFETY PROFILE: Questionable carcinogen with experimental neoplastigenic data. Poison by intraperitoneal route. Moderately toxic by ingestion and skin contact. A severe eye and skin irritant. When heated to decomposition it emits toxic fumes of NO$_x$.

NHF500   CAS: 4008-48-4
5-NITRO-8-HYDROXYQUINOLINE
mf: C$_9$H$_6$N$_2$O$_3$ mw: 190.17

SYN: 5-NITRO-8-QUINOLINOL

TOXICITY DATA with REFERENCE
ETA: orl-rat TD:26 g/kg/52W-I   TXAPA9 8,343,66
ETA: orl-rat TD:52 g/kg/52W-I   TXAPA9 8,343,66
ETA: orl-rat TDLo:13 g/kg/52W-C   TXAPA9 8,343,66

SAFETY PROFILE: Questionable carcinogen with experimental tumorigenic data. Poison by ingestion. When heated to decomposition it emits its toxic fumes of NO$_x$.

NHK800   CAS: 24458-48-8
NITROL
mf: C$_{10}$H$_{13}$N$_3$O$_3$ mw: 223.26

SYNS: BENZENAMINE, N-(2-METHYL-2-NITROPROPYL)-p-NITROSO-(9CI) ◇ CP 25017 ◇ N-(2-METHYL-2-NITROPROPYL)-p-NITROSOANILINE ◇ N-(2-METHYL-2-NITROPROPYL)-4-NITROSOBENZAMINE ◇ NITROL (PROMOTER) ◇ N-(p-NITROSOANILINOMETHYL)-2-NITROPROPANE

TOXICITY DATA with REFERENCE
CAR: unr-rat TDLo:81800 mg/kg/2Y   EPASR* 8EHQ-0183-0165

CONSENSUS REPORTS: Reported in EPA TSCA Inventory.

SAFETY PROFILE: Questionable carcinogen with experimental carcinogenic data. Moderately toxic by ingestion. When heated to decomposition it emits toxic fumes of NO$_x$.

NHQ950   CAS: 69267-51-2
2-NITRONAPHTHO(2,1-b)FURAN
mf: C$_{12}$H$_7$NO$_3$ mw: 213.20

SYN: R6597

TOXICITY DATA with REFERENCE
ETA: skn-mus TDLo:10489 μg/kg   JJCREP 78,565,87
MUT: mma-sat 1 nmol/plate   MUREAV 88,355,81
MUT: mmo-sat 1 nmol/plate   MUREAV 88,355,81
MUT: msc-ham:lng 500 μg/L   CNREA8 44,1969,84
MUT: pic-sat 100 pmol/plate   MUREAV 104,1,82
   CNREA8 44,1969,84

SAFETY PROFILE: Questionable carcinogen with experimental tumorigenic data. Mutation data reported. When heated to decomposition it emits toxic fumes of NO$_x$.

NHR500   CAS: 13115-28-1
3-NITRO-2-NAPHTHYLAMINE
mf: C$_{10}$H$_8$N$_2$O$_2$ mw: 188.20

TOXICITY DATA with REFERENCE
CAR: orl-rat TDLo:38 g/kg/51W-I   JNCIAM
41,985,68
NEO: orl-rat TD:130 mg/kg/1Y-I   JNCIAM
41,985,68

SAFETY PROFILE: Questionable carcinogen with experimental carcinogenic and neoplastigenic data. When heated to decomposition it emits toxic fumes of NO$_x$.

NIB000   CAS: 943-39-5
p-NITROPEROXYBENZOIC ACID
mf: $C_7H_5NO_5$ mw: 183.13

TOXICITY DATA with REFERENCE
ETA: scu-mus TD:52 mg/kg/26W-I   CNREA8
32,880,72
ETA: scu-mus TDLo:228 mg/kg/57W-I
CNREA8 30,1037,70

SAFETY PROFILE: Questionable carcinogen with experimental tumorigenic data. When heated to decomposition it emits toxic fumes of NO$_x$.

NIK000   CAS: 2581-69-3
4-((p-NITROPHENYL)AZO) DIPHENYLAMINE
mf: $C_{18}H_{14}N_4O_2$ mw: 318.36

TOXICITY DATA with REFERENCE
ETA: orl-rat TDLo:31 g/kg/88W-C   ZEKBAI
57,530,51

CONSENSUS REPORTS: Reported in EPA TSCA Inventory.

SAFETY PROFILE: Questionable carcinogen with experimental tumorigenic data. When heated to decomposition it emits toxic fumes of NO$_x$.

NIK500   CAS: 63019-77-2
7-((p-NITROPHENYLAZO) METHYLBENZ(c)ACRIDINE
mf: $C_{24}H_{16}N_4O_2$ mw: 392.44

SYN: 9-METHYL-φ-(p-NITROBENZENEAZO)-3,4-BENZ-ACRIDINE

TOXICITY DATA with REFERENCE
ETA: scu-mus TDLo:200 mg/kg   VOONAW
1,52,55

SAFETY PROFILE: Questionable carcinogen with experimental tumorigenic data. When

heated to decomposition it emits toxic fumes of NO$_x$.

NIW400   CAS: 3704-42-5
4-(4-NITROPHENYL)THIAZOLE
mf: $C_9H_6N_2O_2S$ mw: 206.23

TOXICITY DATA with REFERENCE
ETA: orl-rat TDLo:39928 mg/kg/46W-C
PAACA3 21,75,80

SAFETY PROFILE: Questionable carcinogen with experimental tumorigenic data. When heated to decomposition it emits toxic fumes of NO$_x$ and SO$_x$.

NIY500   CAS: 504-88-1
3-NITROPROPIONIC ACID
mf: $C_3H_5NO_4$ mw: 119.09

SYNS: BNP ◇ BOVINOCIDIN ◇ HIPTAGENIC ACID ◇ NCI-C03076 ◇ β-NITROPROPIONIC ACID

TOXICITY DATA with REFERENCE
NEO: orl-rat TDLo:1870 mg/kg/2Y-I   NCITR*
NCI-CG-TR-52,78
MUT: dns-rat:lvr 100 mg/L   MUREAV 97,359,82
MUT: mma-sat 100 µg/plate   ENMUDM 7(Suppl 5),1,85
MUT: mmo-sat 100 µg/plate   IAPUDO 27,283,80
MUT: otr-rat:emb 970 ng/plate   JJATDK 1,190,81

CONSENSUS REPORTS: NCI Carcinogenesis Bioassay (gavage); Some Evidence: rat NCITR* NCI-CG-TR-52,78; (gavage); No Evidence: mouse NCITR* NCI-CG-TR-52,78. EPA Genetic Toxicology Program.

SAFETY PROFILE: Questionable carcinogen with experimental neoplastigenic data. Poison by intravenous and intraperitoneal routes. Mutation data reported. When heated to decomposition it emits toxic fumes of NO$_x$.

NJA100   CAS: 57835-92-4
4-NITROPYRENE
mf: $C_{16}H_9NO_2$ mw: 247.26

TOXICITY DATA with REFERENCE
CAR: ipr-mus TDLo:27700 µg/kg/15D-I
CRNGDP 7,1317,86
MUT: dnr-bcs 100 ng/disc   MUREAV 174,89,86
MUT: mmo-sat 1 nmol/plate   MUREAV 143,173,85

SAFETY PROFILE: Questionable carcinogen with experimental carcinogenic data. Mutation data reported. When heated to decomposition it emits toxic fumes of NO$_x$.

NJA500   CAS: 1124-33-0
4-NITROPYRIDINE-N-OXIDE
mf: $C_5H_4N_2O_3$ mw: 140.11

SYN: 4-NITROPYRIDINE-1-OXIDE

TOXICITY DATA with REFERENCE
ETA: scu-mus TDLo:960 mg/kg/15W-I
   GANNA2 70,799,79
MUT: dnd-mus:fbr 50 μmol/L   CNREA8
   35,521,75
MUT: dnr-esc 500 μg/plate   CNREA8 32,2369,72
MUT: mmo-esc 500 μmol/L   GANNA2 70,799,79
MUT: mmo-sat 25 μg/plate   MUREAV 58,371,78
MUT: mrc-esc 500 μg/plate   CNREA8 32,2369,72

CONSENSUS REPORTS: EPA Extremely
Hazardous Substances List. EPA Genetic Toxicology Program. Reported in EPA TSCA Inventory.

SAFETY PROFILE: Questionable carcinogen
with experimental tumorigenic data. Poison by
ingestion and skin contact. Mutation data reported. Mixtures with diethyl-1,4-dihydro-2,
6-dimethylpyridine-3,5-dicarboxylate explode
when heated above 130°C. When heated to decomposition it emits toxic fumes of NO_x.

NJB500   CAS: 18714-34-6
2-NITROQUINOLINE
mf: $C_9H_6N_2O_2$ mw: 174.17

TOXICITY DATA with REFERENCE
ETA: scu-mus TDLo:680 mg/kg/31W-I
   GANNA2 60,609,69

SAFETY PROFILE: Questionable carcinogen
with experimental tumorigenic data. When
heated to decomposition it emits toxic fumes
of NO_x.

NJD500   CAS: 607-35-2
8-NITROQUINOLINE
mf: $C_9H_6N_2O_2$ mw: 174.17

PROP: Monoclinic crystals from alcohol. Mp:
88-89°. Sol in hot water, alc, ether, and benzene.

TOXICITY DATA with REFERENCE
CAR: orl-rat TD:42 g/kg/48W-C   CALEDQ
   4,265,78
CAR: orl-rat TD:36400 mg/kg/2Y-C   CALEDQ
   14,115,81
CAR: orl-rat TD:43680 mg/kg/2Y-C   CALEDQ
   14,115,81
CAR: orl-rat TDLo:17 g/kg/48W-C   CALEDQ
   4,265,78

MUT: dnr-sat 350 μg/disc   MUREAV 39,285,77
MUT: mma-sat 100 nmol/plate   MUREAV 58,11,78
MUT: mmo-sat 50 μg/plate   MUREAV 39,285,77

CONSENSUS REPORTS: EPA Genetic Toxicology Program. Reported in EPA TSCA Inventory.

SAFETY PROFILE: Questionable carcinogen
with experimental carcinogenic data. Poison by
intraperitoneal route. Mutation data reported.
When heated to decomposition it emits toxic
fumes of NO_x.

NJI850   CAS: 75881-17-3
1-NITROSO-4-ACETYL-3,5-
DIMETHYLPIPERAZINE
mf: $C_8H_{15}N_3O_2$ mw: 185.26

SYN: 1-ACETYL-4-NITROSO-2,6-DIMETHYLPIPERAZINE

TOXICITY DATA with REFERENCE
CAR: orl-rat TDLo:1950 mg/kg/30W-I   CNREA8
   41,1034,81

SAFETY PROFILE: Questionable carcinogen
with experimental carcinogenic data. When
heated to decomposition it emits toxic fumes
of NO_x.

NJJ500   CAS: 57644-85-6
NITROSOALDICARB
mf: $C_7H_{13}N_3O_3S$ mw: 219.29

SYNS: 2-METHYL-2-(METHYLTHIO)PROPANAL-
o-((METHYLNITROSOAMINO)CARBONYL)OXIME
◇ 2-METHYL-2-(METHYLTHIO)PROPIONALDEHYDE-o-
((METHYLNITROSO)CARBAMOYL) OXIME

TOXICITY DATA with REFERENCE
ETA: orl-rat TDLo:40 mg/kg/2W-I   EESADV
   2,413,78
MUT: dnd-hmn:fbr 10 μmol/L   MUREAV 44,1,77
MUT: mma-sat 1 μg/plate   TCMUE9 1,13,84
MUT: mmo-esc 100 μmol/L   IARCCD 14,425,76
MUT: mmo-sat 1 μg/plate   TCMUE9 1,13,84
MUT: pic-esc 100 μg/L   TCMUE9 1,91,84

SAFETY PROFILE: Questionable carcinogen
with experimental tumorigenic data. Human
mutation data reported. Many N-nitroso compounds are carcinogens. When heated to decomposition it emits very toxic fumes of SO_x and
NO_x.

NJJ875
N-NITROSOALLYLETHANOLAMINE
mf: $C_5H_{10}N_2O_2$ mw: 130.17

TOXICITY DATA with REFERENCE
ETA: orl-rat TDLo: 4375 mg/kg/50W-I CALEDQ
22,281,84
MUT: mma-sat 10 μg/plate TCMUE9 1,13,84
MUT: mmo-sat 10 μg/plate TCMUE9 1,13,84

SAFETY PROFILE: Questionable carcinogen with experimental tumorigenic data. Mutation data reported. Many N-nitroso compounds are carcinogens. When heated to decomposition it emits toxic fumes of NO_x.

NJJ950
N-NITROSOALLYL-2-HYDROXYPROPYLAMINE
mf: $C_6H_{12}N_2O_2$ mw: 144.20

SYNS: NAHP ◊ NITROSO-ALLYL-2-HYDROXYPROPYL-AMINE ◊ N-NITROSO-N-ALLYL-N-(2-HYDROXYPROPYL)-AMINE

TOXICITY DATA with REFERENCE
ETA: orl-rat TDLo: 4950 mg/kg/50W-I CALEDQ
22,281,84

SAFETY PROFILE: Questionable carcinogen with experimental tumorigenic data. When heated to decomposition it emits toxic fumes of NO_x.

NJK150
1-NITROSOANABASINE
CAS: 1133-64-8
mf: $C_{10}H_{13}N_3O$ mw: 191.26

SYNS: NAB ◊ N-NITROSOANABASINE ◊ N'-NITRO-SOANABASINE ◊ N-NITROSO-2-(3'-PYRIDYL)PIPERIDINE ◊ PYRIDINE, 3-(1-NITROSO-2-PIPERIDINYL)-, (S)-(9CI)

TOXICITY DATA with REFERENCE
CAR: orl-rat TDLo: 6000 mg/kg/50W-I BJCAAI
18,265,64

SAFETY PROFILE: Questionable carcinogen with experimental carcinogenic data. When heated to decomposition it emits toxic fumes of NO_x.

NJK500
1-NITROSOAZACYCLOTRIDECANE
CAS: 40580-89-0
mf: $C_{12}H_{24}N_2O$ mw: 212.38

SYNS: NDMI ◊ N-NITROSODODECAMETHYLENEIMINE ◊ NITROSODODECAMETHYLENIMINE ◊ N-NITROSODO-DECAMETHYLENIMINE

TOXICITY DATA with REFERENCE
CAR: orl-rat TD: 1300 mg/kg/1Y-I CRNGDP
5,537,84
CAR: orl-rat TD: 3440 mg/kg/64W-I CRNGDP
5,537,84

CAR: orl-rat TDLo: 1040 mg/kg/1Y-I CRNGDP
5,537,84
ETA: orl-mus TDLo: 2500 mg/kg/52W-I
IJCNAW 11,369,73
ETA: orl-rat TD: 12 g/kg/50W-I EESADV 2,407,78
MUT: mma-esc 7500 μmol/L IAPUDO 41,543,82
MUT: mma-sat 10 μg/plate TCMUE9 1,13,84

SAFETY PROFILE: Questionable carcinogen with experimental carcinogenic and tumorigenic data. Mutation data reported. When heated to decomposition it emits toxic fumes of NO_x.

NJL000
1-NITROSOAZETIDINE
CAS: 15216-10-1
mf: $C_3H_6N_2O$ mw: 86.11

SYNS: N-NITROSAZETIDINE ◊ NITROSO-AZETIDIN (GERMAN) ◊ NITROSOAZETIDINE ◊ N-NITROSOAZETI-DINE ◊ NITROSOTRIMETHYLENEIMINE ◊ N-NITROSOTRI-METHYLENEIMINE

TOXICITY DATA with REFERENCE
ETA: orl-ham TD: 4306 mg/kg/64W-I IAPUDO
57,617,84
ETA: orl-ham TDLo: 4 g/kg/50W-I CRNGDP
5,875,84
ETA: orl-mus TDLo: 960 mg/kg/48D-C
NATWAY 54,518,67
ETA: orl-rat TD: 920 mg/kg/46D-C NATWAY
54,518,67
ETA: orl-rat TD: 3444 mg/kg/53W-I IAPUDO
57,617,84
ETA: orl-rat TDLo: 198 mg/kg/17W-I ZKKOBW
89,215,77
MUT: mma-sat 250 μg/plate MUREAV 67,21,79
MUT: mmo-sat 1 μg/plate MUREAV 51,319,78

SAFETY PROFILE: Questionable carcinogen with experimental tumorigenic data. Moderately toxic by ingestion. Mutation data reported. Many N-nitroso compounds are carcinogens. When heated to decomposition it emits toxic fumes of NO_x.

NJL850
1-NITROSO-4-BENZOYL-3,5-DIMETHYLPIPERAZINE
CAS: 61034-40-0
mf: $C_{13}H_{18}N_3O_2$ mw: 248.34

SYNS: 4-BENZOYL-3,5-DIMETHYL-N-NITROSOPIPERA-ZINE ◊ N-NITROSO-4-BENZOYL-3,5-DIMETHYLPIPERA-ZINE ◊ PIPERAZINE, 1-BENZOYL-2,6-DIMETHYL-4-NITRO-SO-(9CI)

TOXICITY DATA with REFERENCE
NEO: orl-rat TDLo: 4300 mg/kg/50W-I CNREA8
41,1034,81

MUT: mma-sat 250 μg/plate   MUREAV
111,135,83

SAFETY PROFILE: Questionable carcinogen with experimental neoplastigenic data. Mutation data reported. When heated to decomposition it emits toxic fumes of NO_x.

NJM000   CAS: 775-11-1
NITROSOBENZYLUREA
mf: $C_8H_9N_3O_2$ mw: 179.20

SYNS: 1-BENZYL-1-NITROSOUREA ◇ N-NITROSO-N-(PHENYLMETHYL)UREA

TOXICITY DATA with REFERENCE
ETA: orl-rat TDLo:1600 mg/kg/92W-I
ZKKOBW 91,63,78
ETA: par-rat TDLo:1200 mg/kg/66W-I
ZKKOBW 91,63,78
MUT: mma-sat 250 μg/plate   TCMUE9 1,13,84
MUT: mmo-sat 1 μg/plate   MUREAV 68,1,79

SAFETY PROFILE: Questionable carcinogen with experimental tumorigenic data. Mutation data reported. Many N-nitroso compounds are carcinogens. When heated to decomposition it emits toxic fumes of NO_x.

NJM500   CAS: 60414-81-5
N-NITROSOBIS(2-ACETOXYPROPYL)AMINE
mf: $C_{10}H_{18}N_2O_5$ mw: 246.30

SYNS: BAP ◇ 1,1-(N-NITROSOIMINO)DI-2-PROPANOL, DIACETATE

TOXICITY DATA with REFERENCE
CAR: scu-mus TD:17 g/kg/17W-I   CALEDQ
9,257,80
CAR: scu-mus TD:7350 mg/kg/15W-I   CALEDQ
9,257,80
CAR: scu-mus TDLo:6370 mg/kg/26W-I
CALEDQ 9,257,80
NEO: scu-ham TDLo:3500 mg/kg/20W-I
CNREA8 36,2877,76
ETA: scu-ham TD:4200 mg/kg/6W-I   CALEDQ
1,197,76
ETA: skn-ham TDLo:14 g/kg/41W-I   CALEDQ
3,109,77
MUT: dns-rat:lvr 1 mmol/L   MUREAV 144,197,85
MUT: mma-sat 1 mg/palte   CRNGDP 6,415,85

SAFETY PROFILE: Questionable carcinogen with experimental carcinogenic, neoplastigenic, and tumorigenic data. Mutation data reported. When heated to decomposition it emits toxic fumes of NO_x.

NJN300   CAS: 83335-32-4
N-NITROSO-BIS-(4,4,4-TRIFLUORO-n-BUTYL)AMINE
mf: $C_8H_{12}F_6N_2O$ mw: 266.22

SYNS: F-6-NDBA ◇ 4,4,4,4',4',4'-HEXAFLUORO-N-NITROSODIBUTYLAMINE ◇ N-NITROSO-4,4,4,4',4',4'-HEXAFLUORODIBUTYLAMINE

TOXICITY DATA with REFERENCE
CAR: orl-rat TD:3150 mg/kg/32W-I   CRNGDP
3,1219,82
CAR: orl-rat TDLo:960 g/kg/32W-I   CRNGDP
3,1219,82
MUT: dnd-esc 100 nmol/tube   CRNGDP 3,781,82
MUT: mma-sat 1 μmol/plate   CRNGDP 3,781,82

SAFETY PROFILE: Questionable carcinogen with experimental carcinogenic data. Moderately toxic by ingestion. Mutation data reported. When heated to decomposition it emits toxic fumes of F^- and NO_x.

NJO150
N-NITROSO-N-BUTYLBUTYRAMIDE
mf: $C_8H_{16}N_2O_2$ mw: 172.26

SYNS: N-BUTYL-N-NITROSOBUTYRAMIDE ◇ N-BUTYL-N-(1-OXOBUTYL)NITROSAMINE ◇ NBBA ◇ N-NITROSO-N-BUTYROXY-BUTYLAMINE

TOXICITY DATA with REFERENCE
CAR: scu-rat TDLo:65 mg/kg/10W-I   IAPUDO
41,619,82
ETA: scu-rat TD:70500 μg/kg/10W-I   GANNA2
73,687,82

SAFETY PROFILE: Questionable carcinogen with experimental carcinogenic and tumorigenic data. When heated to decomposition it emits toxic fumes of NO_x.

NJO200   CAS: 73487-24-8
N-NITROSO-N-(BUTYL-N-BUTYROLACTONE)AMINE
mf: $C_8H_{14}N_2O_3$ mw: 186.24

SYNS: BBAL ◇ N-n-BUTYL-N-4-(1,4-BUTYROLACTONE) NITROSAMINE ◇ 4-(N-BUTYLNITROSAMINO)-4-HYDROXYBUTYRIC ACID LACTONE

TOXICITY DATA with REFERENCE
CAR: scu-rat TD:70 mg/kg/10W-I   IAPUDO
41,619,82
CAR: scu-rat TDLo:70500 μg/kg/10W-I
GANNA2 73,687,82
MUT: dnr-bcs 100 nmol/plate   CNREA8 40,162,80
MUT: dns-rat:oth 1 mmol/L   CBINA8 53,99,85
MUT: mmo-esc 500 nmol/plate   CNREA8
40,162,80

MUT: mmo-sat 50 nmol/plate   CNREA8 40,162,80

SAFETY PROFILE: Questionable carcinogen with experimental carcinogenic data. Mutation data reported. When heated to decomposition it emits toxic fumes of NO_x.

NJO300   CAS: 46061-25-0
N-NITROSO-4-tert-BUTYLPIPERIDINE
mf: $C_9H_{18}N_2O$ mw: 170.29

SYNS: 4-tert-BUTYL-1-NITROSOPIPERIDINE ◇ PIPERI-DINE, 4-tert-BUTYL-1-NITROSO   —

TOXICITY DATA with REFERENCE
CAR: orl-rat TDLo:4500 mg/kg/2Y-I   CRNGDP 2,1045,81

MUT: mma-sat 250 µg/plate   MUREAV 111,135,83

SAFETY PROFILE: Questionable carcinogen with experimental carcinogenic data. Mutation data reported. When heated to decomposition it emits toxic fumes of NO_x.

NJO500   CAS: 71752-66-4
NITROSO-sec-BUTYLUREA
mf: $C_5H_{11}N_3O_2$ mw: 145.19

SYN: 1-sec-BUTYL-1-NITROSOUREA

TOXICITY DATA with REFERENCE
ETA: skn-mus TDLo:585 mg/kg/50W-I
   JCROD7 102,13,81
MUT: mma-sat 500 µg/plate   TCMUE9 1,13,84
MUT: mmo-sat 100 µg/plate   MUREAV 68,1,79

SAFETY PROFILE: Questionable carcinogen with experimental tumorigenic data. Mutation data reported. Many N-nitroso compounds are carcinogens. When heated to decomposition it emits toxic fumes of NO_x.

NJP000   CAS: 62573-59-5
NITROSO-BUX-TEN

SYN: 3-(1-ETHYLPROPYL)PHENOL METHYLNITROSO-CARBAMATE mixed with 3-(1-METHYLBUTYL)PHENYL METHYLNITROSOCARBAMATE

TOXICITY DATA with REFERENCE
ETA: orl-rat TDLo:660 mg/kg/10W-I   IARCCD 19,495,78

CONSENSUS REPORTS: EPA Genetic Toxicology Program. EPA Genetic Toxicology Program.

SAFETY PROFILE: Questionable carcinogen with experimental tumorigenic data. Many N-

nitroso compounds are carcinogens. When heated to decomposition it emits toxic fumes of NO_x.

NJQ000   CAS: 13256-15-0
N-NITROSO-N'-CARBETHOXYPIPERAZINE
mf: $C_7H_{13}N_3O_3$ mw: 187.23

SYNS: ETHYL 4-NITROSO-1-PIPERAZINECARBOXYLATE ◇ N-NITROSO-N'-CARBAETHOXYPIPERAZIN (GERMAN)

TOXICITY DATA with REFERENCE
ETA: scu-rat TDLo:2300 mg/kg/66W-I   ZEKBAI 69,103,67

SAFETY PROFILE: Questionable carcinogen with experimental tumorigenic data. Poison by subcutaneous route. Many N-nitroso compounds are carcinogens. When heated to decomposition it emits toxic fumes of NO_x.

NJQ500   CAS: 62593-23-1
NITROSOCARBOFURAN
mf: $C_{12}H_{14}N_2O_4$ mw: 250.28

SYNS: 2,3-DIHYDRO-2,2-DIMETHYL-7-BENZOFURANYL NITROSO-METHYL CARBAMATE ◇ METHYLNITROSOCAR-BAMIC ACID-2,3-DIHYDRO-2,3-DIMETHYL-7-BENZOFURA-NYL ESTER

TOXICITY DATA with REFERENCE
CAR: orl-rat TDLo:380 mg/kg/23W-I   EESADV 2,413,78
MUT: cyt-ham:ovr 50 nmol/L   JTEHD6 7,519,81
MUT: dnd-hmn:fbr 10 µmol/L   MUREAV 44,1,77
MUT: mma-sat 10 µg/plate   TCMUE9 1,13,84
MUT: mmo-esc 100 µmol/L   IARCCD 14,425,76
MUT: mmo-sat 2500 ng/plate   TCMUE9 1,13,84
MUT: sce-ham:500 nmol/L   JTEHD6 7,519,81

SAFETY PROFILE: Questionable carcinogen with experimental carcinogenic data. Human mutation data reported. When heated to decomposition it emits toxic fumes of NO_x.

NJR000   CAS: 69113-00-4
NITROSOCHLOROETHYLDIETHYLUREA
mf: $C_7H_{14}ClN_3O_2$ mw: 207.69

TOXICITY DATA with REFERENCE
ETA: orl-rat TDLo:176 mg/kg/46W-I   JCROD7 94,131,79

SAFETY PROFILE: Questionable carcinogen with experimental tumorigenic data. Many N-nitroso compounds are carcinogens. When heated to decomposition it emits very toxic fumes of Cl^- and NO_x.

NJR500   CAS: 59960-30-4
NITROSOCHLOROETHYL-DIMETHYLUREA
mf: $C_5H_{10}ClN_3O_2$ mw: 179.63

SYN: 1-NITROSO-1-(2-CHLOROETHYL)-3,3-DIMETHYL-UREA

TOXICITY DATA with REFERENCE
ETA: orl-rat TDLo: 168 mg/kg/50W-I   JCROD7 94,131,79

SAFETY PROFILE: Questionable carcinogen with experimental tumorigenic data. Many N-nitroso compounds are carcinogens. When heated to decomposition it emits very toxic fumes of Cl^- and NO_x.

NJS300   CAS: 73785-40-7
NITROSOCIMETIDINE
mf: $C_{10}H_{15}N_7OS$ mw: 281.38

SYN: N-NITROSOCIMETIDINE

TOXICITY DATA with REFERENCE
CAR: orl-mus TDLo: 1316 mg/(pre-post): TER   CNREA8 45,3561,85
MUT: cyt-ham: ovr 1200 nmol/L   CALEDQ 14,71,81
MUT: dnd-hmn: lym 350 μmol/L   CBINA8 38,87,81
MUT: dnd-mus: oth 1 mmol/L   CALEDQ 10,223,80
MUT: dni-hmn: lym 170 μmol/L   CBINA8 38,87,81
MUT: dns-hmn: lym 180 μmol/L   CBINA8 38,87,81
MUT: mma-sat 1 mg/plate   TOLED5 12,281,82
MUT: pic-esc 10 mg/L   TCMUE9 1,91,84
MUT: sce-ham: ovr 1200 nmol/L   CALEDQ 14,71,81
MUT: sce-hmn: lym 260 μmol/L   MUREAV 156,117,85

SAFETY PROFILE: Questionable carcinogen with experimental carcinogenic and teratogenic data. Human mutation data reported. Many N-nitroso compounds are carcinogens. When heated to decomposition it emits toxic fumes of SO_x and NO_x.

NJV000   CAS: 877-31-6
NITROSOCYCLOHEXYLUREA
mf: $C_7H_{13}N_3O_2$ mw: 171.23

SYN: 1-CYCLOHEXYL-1-NITROSOUREA

TOXICITY DATA with REFERENCE
ETA: skn-mus TDLo: 685 mg/kg/50W-I   JCROD7 102,13,81
MUT: mma-sat 250 μg/plate   TCMUE9 1,13,84
MUT: mmo-sat 100 μg/plate   MUREAV 68,1,79
MUT: pic-esc 10 mg/L   TCMUE9 1,91,84

SAFETY PROFILE: Questionable carcinogen with experimental tumorigenic data. Mutation data reported. Many N-nitroso compounds are carcinogens. When heated to decomposition it emits toxic fumes of NO_x.

NJV500   CAS: 16338-97-9
N-NITROSODIALLYL AMINE
mf: $C_6H_{10}N_2O$ mw: 126.18

SYNS: DIALLYINITROSAMIN (GERMAN) ◇ DIALLYLNI-TROSAMINE

TOXICITY DATA with REFERENCE
CAR: orl-ham TDLo: 805 g/kg/37W-I   JJIND8 74,1043,85
NEO: scu-ham TDLo: 500 mg/kg   JNCIAM 59,1569,77
ETA: orl-rat TDLo: 11760 mg/kg/42W-C   JCROD7 109,5,85
MUT: dni-mus-ipr 20 g/kg   ARGEAR 51,605,81
MUT: mma-esc 5 mmol/L   MUREAV 89,209,81
MUT: mma-sat 10 μg/plate   MUREAV 66,1,79
MUT: mmo-omi 1 pph/48H-C   SOGEBZ 10,522,74

CONSENSUS REPORTS: EPA Genetic Toxicology Program.

SAFETY PROFILE: Questionable carcinogen with experimental carcinogenic, neoplastigenic, and tumorigenic data. Moderately toxic by ingestion and subcutaneous routes. Mutation data reported. When heated to decomposition it emits toxic fumes of NO_x.

NJW000   CAS: 5350-17-4
NITROSODI-sec-BUTYLAMINE
mf: $C_8H_{18}N_2O$ mw: 158.28

SYN: N-NITROSO-DI-sec-BUTYLAMINE

TOXICITY DATA with REFERENCE
ETA: orl-rat TDLo: 2750 mg/kg/50W-I   JJIND8 62,407,79

SAFETY PROFILE: Questionable carcinogen with experimental tumorigenic data. Many N-nitroso compounds are carcinogens. When

heated to decomposition it emits toxic fumes of NO_x.

NJX000 CAS: 3276-41-3
N-NITROSO-3,6-DIHYDRO-1,2-OXAZINE
mf: $C_4H_6N_2O_2$ mw: 114.12

SYNS: 3,6-DIHYDRO-2-NITROSO-2H-1,2-OXAZINE ◇ N-NITROSO-3,6-DIHYDROOXAZIN-1,2 (GERMAN)

TOXICITY DATA with REFERENCE
NEO: orl-rat TDLo: 22 g/kg/94W-I   ZKKOBW 79,114,73

SAFETY PROFILE: Questionable carcinogen with experimental neoplastigenic data. Moderately toxic by ingestion. Many N-nitroso compounds are carcinogens. When heated to decomposition it emits toxic fumes of NO_x.

NJY000 CAS: 16813-36-8
1-NITROSO-5,6-DIHYDROURACIL
mf: $C_4H_5N_3O_3$ mw: 143.12

SYNS: DIHYDRO-1-NITROSO-2,4(1H,3H)-PYRIMIDINE-DIONE ◇ 5,6-DIHYDRO-1-NITROSOURACIL ◇ NDHU ◇ NO-DHU

TOXICITY DATA with REFERENCE
CAR: orl-rat TD: 3000 mg/kg/32W-I   ZKKOBW 79,304,73
CAR: orl-rat TDLo: 440 mg/kg/41W-I   JJIND8 62,1523,79
ETA: ipr-rat TD: 1200 mg/kg/1W-I   JJIND8 62,1523,79
ETA: ipr-rat TDLo: 1200 mg/kg/8D-I   TUMOAB 61,509,75
MUT: dnd-rat-ipr 1 mg/kg   BBRCA9 53,773,73
MUT: dns-rat: lvr 7 mmol/L   JJIND8 73,515,84
MUT: mmo-sat 2900 nmol/L   MUREAV 48,131,77

CONSENSUS REPORTS: EPA Genetic Toxicology Program.

SAFETY PROFILE: Questionable carcinogen with experimental carcinogenic and tumorigenic data. Moderately toxic by intraperitoneal route. Mutation data reported. When heated to decomposition it emits toxic fumes of NO_x.

NJY500 CAS: 88208-16-6
N-NITROSO-2,3-DIHYDROXYPROPYLALLYLAMINE
mf: $C_6H_{12}N_2O_3$ mw: 160.20

SYNS: 3-(ALLYLNITROSAMINO)-1,2-PROPANEDIOL ◇ N-NITROSOALLYL-2,3-DIHYDROXYPROPYLAMINE ◇ 1,2-PROPANEDIOL, 3-(NITROSO-2-PROPENYLAMINO)-

TOXICITY DATA with REFERENCE
ETA: orl-rat TDLo: 5500 mg/kg/50W-I   CALEDQ 22,281,84
MUT: mma-sat 250 μg/plate   MUREAV 111,135,83

SAFETY PROFILE: Questionable carcinogen with experimental tumorigenic data. Mutation data reported. When heated to decomposition it emits toxic fumes of NO_x.

NJY550
NITROSO-DIHYDROXYPROPYL-OXOPROPYLAMINE
mf: $C_6H_{12}N_2O_4$ mw: 176.20

SYNS: 1-((2,3-DIHYDROXYPROPYL)NITROSAMINO)-2-PROPANONE ◇ N-NITROSODIHYDROXYPROPYL-2-OXO-PROPYLAMINE ◇ N-NITROSO-2-OXOPROPYL-2,3-DIHY-DROXYPROPYLAMINE

TOXICITY DATA with REFERENCE
ETA: orl-ham TDLo: 2290 mg/kg/38W-I   IAPUDO 57,617,84
ETA: orl-rat TDLo: 528 mg/kg/26W-I   IAPUDO 57,617,84
MUT: mma-sat 50 μg/plate   TCMUE9 1,13,84

SAFETY PROFILE: Questionable carcinogen with experimental tumorigenic data. Mutation data reported. Many N-nitroso compounds are carcinogens. When heated to decomposition it emits toxic fumes of NO_x.

NKA695 CAS: 69091-16-3
cis-NITROSO-2,6-DIMETHYLMORPHOLINE
mf: $C_6H_{12}N_2O_2$ mw: 144.20

SYNS: MORPHOLINE, 2,6-DIMETHYL-N-NITROSO-, (cis)- ◇ MORPHOLINE, 2,6-DIMETHYL-4-NITROSO-, (Z)- ◇ cis-N-NITROSO-2,6-DIMETHYLMORPHOLINE

TOXICITY DATA with REFERENCE
ETA: orl-gpg TDLo: 252 mg/kg/30W-I   CALEDQ 14,7,81
ETA: orl-rat TDLo: 190 mg/kg/30W-I   CRNGDP 1,501,80
MUT: mma-sat 100 nmol/plate   MUREAV 77,215,80

SAFETY PROFILE: Questionable carcinogen with experimental tumorigenic data. Mutation data reported. When heated to decomposition it emits toxic fumes of NO_x.

NKA700 CAS: 69091-15-2
trans-NITROSO-2,6-DIMETHYLMORPHOLINE
mf: $C_6H_{12}N_2O_2$ mw: 144.20

SYN: trans-N-NITROSO-2,6-DIMETHYLMORPHOLINE

TOXICITY DATA with REFERENCE
ETA: orl-gpg TDLo: 127 mg/kg/W-I   CALEDQ
14,7,81
ETA: orl-rat TDLo: 100 mg/kg/30W-I   CRNGDP
1,501,80
MUT: mma-sat 1 mg/plate   TCMUD8 1,295,80
MUT: pic-esc 100 mg/L   TCMUE9 1,91,84

SAFETY PROFILE: Questionable carcinogen
with experimental tumorigenic data. Mutation
data reported. Many N-nitroso compounds are
carcinogens. When heated to decomposition it
emits toxic fumes of NO_x.

NKA850   CAS: 67774-31-6
1-NITROSO-3,5-DIMETHYLPIPERAZINE
mf: $C_6H_{13}N_3O$ mw: 143.22

SYNS: 3,5-DIMETHYL-1-NITROSOPIPERAZINE
◇ NITROSO-3,5-DIMETHYLPIPERAZINE ◇ N-NITROSO-3,5-
DIMETHYLPIPERAZINE

TOXICITY DATA with REFERENCE
CAR: orl-rat TDLo: 1450 mg/kg/29W-I   CNREA8
41,1034,81
MUT: mma-sat 10 μg/plate   TCMUE9 1,13,84

SAFETY PROFILE: Questionable carcinogen
with experimental carcinogenic data. Mutation
data reported. When heated to decomposition
it emits toxic fumes of NO_x.

NKC300   CAS: 71785-87-0
N-NITROSO-3,4-EPOXYPIPERIDINE
mf: $C_5H_8N_2O_2$ mw: 128.15

SYN: 3-NITROSO-7-OXA-3-AZABICYCLO(4.1.0)HEPTANE

TOXICITY DATA with REFERENCE
ETA: orl-rat TDLo: 700 mg/kg/30W-I   CRNGDP
1,753,80
MUT: mma-sat 50 μg/plate   TCMUE9 1,13,84
MUT: mmo-sat 100 μg/plate   TCMUE9 1,13,84

SAFETY PROFILE: Questionable carcinogen
with experimental tumorigenic data. An experimental carcinogenic. Mutation data reported.
Many N-nitroso compounds are carcinogens.
When heated to decomposition it emits toxic
fumes of NO_x.

NKC500   CAS: 56235-95-1
NITROSOETHOXYETHYLAMINE
mf: $C_4H_{10}N_2O_2$ mw: 118.16

SYNS: o,N-DIETHYL-N-NITROSOHYDROXYLAMINE
◇ N-NITROSO-o,N-DIAETHYLHYDROXYLAMIN (GERMAN)
◇ N-NITROSO-o,N-DIETHYLHYDROXYLAMINE

TOXICITY DATA with REFERENCE
CAR: orl-rat TDLo: 7800 mg/kg/39W-I
ZKKOBW 83,205,75

Moderately toxic by ingestion. When heated
to decomposition it emits toxic fumes of
NO_x.

NKD500   CAS: 3398-69-4
N-NITROSOETHYL-tert-BUTYLAMINE
mf: $C_6H_{14}N_2O$ mw: 130.22

SYNS: AETHYL-tert-BUTYL-NITROSOAMIN (GERMAN)
◇ EBNA ◇ ETHYL-tert-BUTYLNITROSAMINE ◇ N-ETHYL-
N-NITROSO-tert-BUTANAMINE ◇ N-NITROSO-tert-BUTYL-
ETHYLAMINE

TOXICITY DATA with REFERENCE
ETA: orl-rat TDLo: 370 mg/kg   NATWAY 50,735,63

CONSENSUS REPORTS: EPA Genetic Toxicology Program.

SAFETY PROFILE: Questionable carcinogen
with experimental tumorigenic data. Moderately
toxic by ingestion. Many N-nitroso compounds
are carcinogens. When heated to decomposition
it emits toxic fumes of NO_x.

NKE000   CAS: 54897-63-1
N-NITROSO-ETHYL(3-CARBOXYPROPYL)AMINE
mf: $C_6H_{12}N_2O_3$ mw: 160.20

SYNS: ECPN ◇ N-ETHYL-N-(3-CARBOXYPROPYL)NITRO-
SOAMINE ◇ 4-(ETHYLNITROSOAMINO)BUTYRIC ACID
◇ N-NITROSO-N-(3-CARBOXYPROPYL)ETHYLAMINE

TOXICITY DATA with REFERENCE
ETA: orl-rat TD: 64 g/kg/20W-C   GANNA2
67,825,76
ETA: orl-rat TDLo: 5800 mg/kg/20W-I
GANNA2 65,565,74
MUT: mma-sat 10 μmol/plate   CNREA8 37,399,77

CONSENSUS REPORTS: EPA Genetic Toxicology Program.

SAFETY PROFILE: Questionable carcinogen
with experimental tumorigenic data. Mutation
data reported. Many N-nitroso compounds are
carcinogens. When heated to decomposition it
emits toxic fumes of NO_x.

NKE500   CAS: 614-95-9
N-NITROSO-N-ETHYLURETHAN
mf: $C_5H_{10}N_2O_3$ mw: 146.17

SYNS: AETHYLNITROSOURETHAN (GERMAN)
◇ ENU ◇ ETHYLNITROSOCARBAMIC ACID, ETHYL ESTER

◇ N-ETHYL-N-NITROSOCARBAMIC ACID ETHYL ESTER
◇ N-ETHYL-N-NITROSOURETHANE ◇ NEU ◇ NITROSO-
ETHYLURETHAN

TOXICITY DATA with REFERENCE
CAR: orl-rat TD: 1024 mg/kg/39W-C GANNA2 73,48,82

CAR: orl-rat TD: 1680 mg/kg/32W-C GANNA2 73,48,82

CAR: orl-rat TDLo: 630 mg/kg/48W-C GANNA2 73,48,82

ETA: ipr-rat TDLo: 66 mg/kg/41W-I BJCAAI 22,316,68

ETA: orl-mus TDLo: 240 mg/kg/39W-I NATUAS 199,190,63

ETA: orl-rat TD: 744 mg/kg/10W-I GANNA2 70,653,79

ETA: orl-rat TD: 1600 mg/kg/10W-I CALEDQ 1,275,76

ETA: skn-rat TDLo: 8100 mg/kg/27W-I GANNA2 70,653,79

MUT: cyt-ham: fbr 15 mg/L/24H MUREAV 48,337,77

MUT: cyt-ham: lng 11 mg/L GMCRDC 27,95,81

MUT: mma-sat 5 μg/plate TCMUE9 1,13,84

MUT: pic-esc 1 mg/L TCMUE9 1,91,84

MUT: slt-mus-ipr 150 mg/kg MUREAV 92,193,82

CONSENSUS REPORTS: EPA Genetic Toxicology Program.

SAFETY PROFILE: Questionable carcinogen with experimental carcinogenic, tumorigenic, and teratogenic data. Poison by intravenous route. Experimental reproductive effects. Mutation data reported. When heated to decomposition it emits toxic fumes of NO$_x$.

NKF000   CAS: 13256-13-8
N-NITROSO-N-ETHYLVINYLAMINE
mf: C$_4$H$_8$N$_2$O   mw: 100.14

SYNS: AETHYL-VINYL-NITROSOAMIN (GERMAN)
◇ N-ETHYL-N-NITROSOETHENAMINE ◇ N-ETHYL-N-NI-
TROSOETHENYLAMINE ◇ N-ETHYL-N-NITROSOVINYL-
AMINE ◇ ETHYLVINYLNITROSAMINE ◇ N-NITROSO-
ETHYLVINYLAMINE ◇ VINYLETHYLNITROSAMIN (GER-
MAN) ◇ VINYLETHYLNITROSAMINE

TOXICITY DATA with REFERENCE
CAR: scu-ham TD: 55 mg/kg/44W-I JCROD7 102,227,82

CAR: scu-ham TD: 82 mg/kg/33W-I JCROD7 102,227,82

CAR: scu-ham TD: 135 mg/kg/27W-I JCROD7 102,227,82

CAR: scu-ham TDLo: 31 mg/kg/50W-I JCROD7 102,227,82

CAR: scu-ham TDLo: 120 mg/kg/12W-I JNCIAM 58,439,77

ETA: ivn-rat TDLo: 250 mg/kg/25W-I ZEKBAI 69,103,67

ETA: orl-gpg TDLo: 335 mg/kg/37W-C ZEKBAI 69,103,67

ETA: orl-rat TDLo: 230 mg/kg/25W-C ARZNAD 19,1077,69

CONSENSUS REPORTS: EPA Genetic Toxicology Program.

SAFETY PROFILE: Questionable carcinogen with experimental carcinogenic, tumorigenic, and teratogenic data. Poison by ingestion, intravenous, and subcutaneous routes. Experimental reproductive effects. When heated to decomposition it emits toxic fumes of NO$_x$.

NKF500   CAS: 2508-20-5
2-NITROSOFLUORENE
mf: C$_{13}$H$_9$NO   mw: 195.23

TOXICITY DATA with REFERENCE
CAR: scu-rat TDLo: 200 mg/kg/8W-I PSEBAA 120,538,65

NEO: ipr-rat TDLo: 160 mg/kg/4W-I CNREA8 30,1485,70

MUT: dnd-esc 10 μmol/L MUREAV 89,95,81

MUT: mma-sat 150 ng/plate CBINA8 54,71,85

MUT: mmo-bcs 500 μg/L CMMUAO 9,165,84

MUT: mmo-sat 50 ng/plate CBINA8 54,71,85

MUT: pic-esc 1950 ng/plate MGBUA3 41,3,76

MUT: pic-sat 500 μmol/L MOPMA3 8,645,72

CONSENSUS REPORTS: EPA Genetic Toxicology Program.

SAFETY PROFILE: Questionable carcinogen with experimental carcinogenic and neoplastigenic data. Mutation data reported. When heated to decomposition it emits toxic fumes of NO$_x$.

NKG000   CAS: 69112-98-7
NITROSOFLUOROETHYLUREA
mf: C$_3$H$_6$FN$_3$O$_2$ mw: 135.12

SYN: 1-(2-FLUOROETHYL)-1-NITROSO-UREA

TOXICITY DATA with REFERENCE
CAR: skn-mus TDLo: 108 mg/kg/50W-I JCROD7 102,13,81

ETA: skn-mus TD: 216 mg/kg/50W-I JCROD7 102,13,81

MUT: mma-sat 2500 ng/plate TCMUE9 1,13,84

MUT: mmo-sat 1 μg/plate   MUREAV 68,1,79
MUT: pic-esc 2 mg/L   TCMUE9 1,91,84

SAFETY PROFILE: Questionable carcinogen with experimental carcinogenic and tumorigenic data. Mutation data reported. When heated to decomposition it emits very toxic fumes of F⁻ and NO$_x$.

NKG450   CAS: 29291-35-8
NITROSOFOLIC ACID
mf: $C_{19}H_{18}N_8O_7$ mw: 470.45

SYN: GLUTAMIC ACID, N-NITROSO-N-PTEROYL-, l-

TOXICITY DATA with REFERENCE
NEO: ipr-mus TDLo: 375 mg/kg/7D-I   CNREA8 35,1981,75
MUT: mma-sat 100 μg/plate   BJCAAI 37,873,78
MUT: otr-ham: kdy 10 mg/L   BJCAAI 37,873,78

CONSENSUS REPORTS: IARC Cancer Review: GROUP 3 IMEMDT 7,56,87; Animal Inadequate Evidence IMEMDT 7,217,78.

SAFETY PROFILE: Questionable carcinogen with experimental neoplastigenic data. Mutation data reported. When heated to decomposition it emits toxic fumes of NO$_x$.

NKH500   CAS: 55557-02-3
NITROSOGUVACOLINE
mf: $C_7H_{10}N_2O_3$ mw: 170.19

SYNS: N-NITROSOGUVACINE ◇ N-NITROSOGUVACO-
LINE ◇ 1-NITROSO-1,2,5,6-TETRAHYDRONICOTINIC ACID
METHYL ESTER ◇ 1,2,5,6-TETRAHYDRO-1-NITROSO-3-
PYRIDINECARBOXYLIC ACID METHYL ESTER

TOXICITY DATA with REFERENCE
MUT: mma-sat 10 μg/plate   MUREAV 111,135,83
MUT: sce-hmn: lym 1 mmol/L   TCMUE9 1,129,84

CONSENSUS REPORTS: IARC Cancer Review: GROUP 3 IMEMDT 7,56,87; Animal Inadequate Evidence IMEMDT 37,263,85. EPA Genetic Toxicology Program.

SAFETY PROFILE: Questionable carcinogen. Human mutation data reported. When heated to decomposition it emits toxic fumes of NO$_x$.

NKI500   CAS: 60391-92-6
NITROSO HYDANTOIC ACID
mf: $C_3H_5N_3O_4$ mw: 147.11

SYNS: N-(AMINOCARBONYL)-N-NITROGLYCINE
◇ N-CARBAMOYL-N-NITROSOGLYCINE ◇ CARBOXY-
METHYLNITROSOUREA ◇ 1-(CARBOXYMETHYL)-1-NI-
TROSOUREA

TOXICITY DATA with REFERENCE
CAR: orl-rat TD: 12390 mg/kg/59W-C   JCROD7 106,12,83
CAR: orl-rat TDLo: 6720 mg/kg/64W-C   JCROD7 106,12,83
NEO: orl-rat TD: 4 g/kg/74W-I   JJIND8 62,1523,79
MUT: cyt-ham: fbr 125 mg/L/48H   MUREAV 48,337,77
MUT: cyt-ham: lng 50 mg/L   GMCRDC 27,95,81
MUT: mmo-esc 5 mmol/L   GANNA2 70,705,79

CONSENSUS REPORTS: EPA Genetic Toxicology Program.

SAFETY PROFILE: Questionable carcinogen with experimental carcinogenic and neoplastigenic data. Poison by intraperitoneal route. Mutation data reported. When heated to decomposition it emits toxic fumes of NO$_x$.

NKJ000   CAS: 42579-28-2
1-NITROSOHYDANTOIN
mf: $C_3H_3N_3O_3$ mw: 129.09

SYN: NHYD

TOXICITY DATA with REFERENCE
NEO: orl-rat TDLo: 5900 mg/kg/52W-I   JJIND8 62,1523,79
MUT: mmo-sat 12 μmol/L/48H   MUREAV 48,131,77

CONSENSUS REPORTS: EPA Genetic Toxicology Program.

SAFETY PROFILE: Questionable carcinogen with experimental neoplastigenic data. Moderately toxic by intraperitoneal route. Mutation data reported. Many nitroso compounds are carcinogens. When heated to decomposition it emits toxic fumes of NO$_x$.

NKJ050   CAS: 96806-34-7
1-NITROSO-1-HYDROXYETHYL-3-
CHLOROETHYLUREA
mf: $C_5H_{10}ClN_3O_3$ mw: 195.63

SYNS: CHNU-I ◇ 1-NITROSO-1-(2-HYDROXYETHYL)-3-(2-
CHLOROETHYL)UREA

TOXICITY DATA with REFERENCE
MUT: mmo-sat 50 μg/plate   MUREAV 178,157,87
CAR: orl-rat TDLo: 656 mg/kg/40W-I   JCREA8 112,221,86
MUT: mmo-sat 50 μg/plate   MUREAV 178,157,87

SAFETY PROFILE: Questionable carcinogen with experimental carcinogenic data. Mutation

data reported. When heated to decomposition it emits toxic fumes of NO_x and Cl^-.

NKJ100 CAS: 96806-35-8
1-NITROSO-1-HYDROXYPROPYL-3-CHLOROETHYLUREA
mf: $C_6H_{12}ClN_3O_3$ mw: 209.66

SYNS: CPNU-I ◇ 1-NITROSO-1-(2-HYDROXYPROPYL)-3-(2-CHLOROETHYL)UREA

TOXICITY DATA with REFERENCE
CAR: orl-rat TDLo: 1104 mg/kg/30W-I JCREA8 112,221,86
MUT: mmo-sat 50 μg/plate MUREAV 178,157,87

SAFETY PROFILE: Questionable carcinogen with experimental carcinogenic data. Mutation data reported. When heated to decomposition it emits toxic fumes of NO_x and Cl^-.

NKK000 CAS: 71752-70-0
NITROSO-3-HYDROXYPROPYLUREA
mf: $C_4H_9N_3O_3$ mw: 147.16

SYNS: 1-(3-HYDROXYPROPYL)-1-NITROSOUREA ◇ NITROSO-3-HYDROXY-N-PROPYLUREA

TOXICITY DATA with REFERENCE
CAR: skn-mus TDLo: 530 mg/kg/45W-I CNREA8 43,214,83
ETA: orl-ham TDLo: 589 mg/kg/37W-I PAACA3 24,92,83
MUT: mmo-sat 25 μg/plate MUREAV 68,1,79

SAFETY PROFILE: Questionable carcinogen with experimental carcinogenic and tumorigenic data. Mutation data reported. When heated to decomposition it emits toxic fumes of NO_x.

NKK500 CAS: 3715-92-2
N-NITROSOIMIDAZOLIDINETHIONE
mf: $C_3H_5ON_3S$ mw: 131.17

SYNS: N-NITROSOETHYLENETHIOUREA ◇ NO-ETU

TOXICITY DATA with REFERENCE
NEO: orl-mus TDLo: 530 mg/kg/9W-I CALEDQ 7,339,79
MUT: dlt-mus-orl 500 mg/kg/5D-I MUREAV 54,258,78
MUT: mnt-mus-ipr 120 mg/kg MUREAV 48,225,77
MUT: sce-ham: lng 50 μmol/L MUREAV 78,177,80

CONSENSUS REPORTS: EPA Genetic Toxicology Program.

SAFETY PROFILE: Questionable carcinogen with experimental neoplastigenic and terato-genic data. Poison by ingestion. Experimental reproductive effects. Mutation data reported. Many N-nitroso compounds are carcinogens. When heated to decomposition it emits very toxic fumes of NO_x and SO_x.

NKL000 CAS: 3844-63-1
1-NITROSOIMIDAZOLIDINONE
mf: $C_3H_5N_3O_2$ mw: 115.11

SYNS: ETHYLENENITROSOUREA ◇ 1-NITROSO-2-IMIDA-ZOLIDINONE ◇ N-NITROSO-IMIDAZOLIDON (GERMAN) ◇ N-NITROSOIMIDAZOLIDONE ◇ N-NITRO-2-IMIDAZOLI-DONE ◇ 1-NITRO-2-IMIDAZOLIDONE ◇ NSC 73438 ◇ SRI 1869

TOXICITY DATA with REFERENCE
ETA: scu-rat TDLo: 600 mg/kg/20W-I ZEKBAI 69,103,67
MUT: mmo-sat 16 μmol/L/48H MUREAV 48,131,77
MUT: mmo-smc 400 mg/L/30M GENTAE 78,1101,74
MUT: mrc-smc 5 mmol/L ZEVBA5 98,230,66

CONSENSUS REPORTS: EPA Genetic Toxicology Program.

SAFETY PROFILE: Questionable carcinogen with experimental tumorigenic data. Poison by intraperitoneal and subcutaneous routes. Mutation data reported. Many N-nitroso compounds are carcinogens. When heated to decomposition it emits toxic fumes of NO_x.

NKL300 CAS: 77698-19-2
1,1'-(NITROSOIMINO)BIS-2-BUTANONE
mf: $C_8H_{14}N_2O_3$ mw: 186.24

SYNS: BOB ◇ N-NITROSOBIS(2-OXOBUTYL)AMINE

TOXICITY DATA with REFERENCE
ETA: scu-ham TDLo: 200 mg/kg CALEDQ 12,223,81
MUT: mma-sat 5 mg/plate JJCREP 77,107,86

SAFETY PROFILE: Questionable carcinogen with experimental tumorigenic data. Poison by subcutaneous route. Mutation data reported. Many N-nitroso compounds are carcinogens. When heated to decomposition it emits toxic fumes of NO_x.

NKL500 CAS: 16339-18-7
2,2'-(N-NITROSOIMINO)DIACETONITRILE
mf: $C_4H_4N_4O$ mw: 124.12

SYNS: N-NITROSAMINO DIACETONITRIL (GERMAN) ◇ NITROSIMINODIACETONITRILE ◇ N-NITROSODIACE-TONITRILE ◇ N-NITROSODI(CYANOMETHYL)AMINE ◇ 2,2'-(NITROSOIMINO)BISACETONITRILE

TOXICITY DATA with REFERENCE
ETA: orl-rat TDLo: 1584 mg/kg/2Y-C: TER
ZEKBAI 69,103,67

CONSENSUS REPORTS: Cyanide and its compounds are on The Community Right-To-Know List.

SAFETY PROFILE: Questionable carcinogen with experimental tumorigenic and teratogenic data. Poison by ingestion. Many N-nitroso compounds are carcinogens. When heated to decomposition it emits toxic fumes of NO_x and CN^-.

NKM500   CAS: 13256-19-4
N-NITROSO-2,2'-IMINODIETHANOLDIACETATE
mf: $C_8H_{14}N_2O_5$ mw: 218.24

SYNS: ACETIC ACID, ESTER with N-NITROSO-2,2'-IMINO-DIETHANOL ◇ BIS-(ACETOXYAETHYL)NITROSAMIN (GERMAN) ◇ N-NITROSOBIS(ACETOXYETHYL)AMINE

TOXICITY DATA with REFERENCE
ETA: orl-rat TDLo: 40 g/kg/58W-C   ZEKBAI 69,103,67
MUT: mmo-sat 100 μg/plate   MUREAV 89,217,81

SAFETY PROFILE: Questionable carcinogen with experimental tumorigenic data. Mildly toxic by ingestion. Mutation data reported. Many N-nitroso compounds are carcinogens. When heated to decomposition it emits toxic fumes of NO_x.

NKN000   CAS: 7633-57-0
N-NITROSOINDOLINE
mf: $C_8H_8N_2O$ mw: 148.18

SYNS: N-NITROSOINDOLIN (GERMAN) ◇ 1-NITROSOIN-DOLINE

TOXICITY DATA with REFERENCE
ETA: orl-rat TDLo: 20 g/kg/2Y-C   ZEKBAI 69,103,67

SAFETY PROFILE: Questionable carcinogen with experimental tumorigenic data. Poison by ingestion. Many N-nitroso compounds are carcinogens. When heated to decomposition it emits toxic fumes of NO_x.

NKO425   CAS: 16830-14-1
NITROSOISOPROPYLUREA
mf: $C_4H_9N_3O_2$ mw: 131.16

SYNS: 1-ISOPROPYL-1-NITROSOUREA ◇ N-(1-METHYL-ETHYL)-N-NITROSO-UREA (9CI)

TOXICITY DATA with REFERENCE
CAR: skn-mus TDLo: 525 mg/kg/50W-I
JCROD7 102,13,81
MUT: mma-sat 100 μg/plate   TCMUE9 1,13,84
MUT: mmo-sat 100 μg/plate   TCMUE9 1,13,84
MUT: pic-esc 4 mg/L   TCMUE9 1,91,84

SAFETY PROFILE: Questionable carcinogen with experimental carcinogenic data. Mutation data reported. When heated to decomposition it emits toxic fumes of NO_x.

NKO600   CAS: 73239-98-2
N-NITROSO-2-METHOXY-2,6-DIMETHYLMORPHOLINE
mf: $C_7H_{14}N_2O_3$ mw: 174.23

SYN: 2,6-DIMETHYL-2-METHOXY-4-NITROSO-MORPHO-LINE

TOXICITY DATA with REFERENCE
ETA: par-ham TD: 250 mg/kg   CALEDQ 13,233,81
ETA: par-ham TDLo: 50 mg/kg   CALEDQ 13,233,81
MUT: bfa-ham/sat 100 mg/kg   JJIND8 64,157,80
MUT: mma-sat 200 nmol/plate   JJIND8 64,157,80

SAFETY PROFILE: Questionable carcinogen with experimental tumorigenic data. Moderately toxic by parenteral route. Mutation data reported. Many N-nitroso compounds are carcinogens. When heated to decomposition it emits toxic fumes of NO_x.

NKO900   CAS: 108278-70-2
1-NITROSOMETHOXYETHYLUREA
mf: $C_4H_9N_3O_3$ mw: 147.16

SYNS: N-(2-METHOXYETHYL)-N-NITROSOUREA ◇ 1-(2-METHOXYETHYL)-1-NITROSOUREA ◇ NITROSO-2-METHOXYETHYLUREA ◇ UREA, N-(2-METHOXYETHYL)-N-NITROSO-

TOXICITY DATA with REFERENCE
CAR: orl-rat TDLo: 480 mg/kg/30W-I   JJCREP 79,181,88
MUT: mmo-sat 10 μg/plate   MUREAV 178,157,87
MUT: pic-esc 250 mg/L   MUREAV 178,157,87

SAFETY PROFILE: Questionable carcinogen with experimental carcinogenic data. Mutation data reported. When heated to decomposition it emits toxic fumes of NO_x.

NKQ000   CAS: 16219-98-0
2-NITROSOMETHYLAMINOPYRIDINE
mf: $C_6H_7N_3O$ mw: 137.16

SYNS: 2-(METHYLNITROSAMINO)PYRIDINE ◇ N-
METHYL-N-NITROSO-2-AMINOPYRIDINE ◇ N-NITROSO-N-
METHYL-2-AMINOPYRIDINE

TOXICITY DATA with REFERENCE
CAR: orl-rat TDLo: 250 mg/kg/50W-I   JJIND8
62,153,79
MUT: hma-mus/esc 60 mg/kg   CRNGDP 3,415,82
MUT: mma-sat 20 mmol/L   CRNGDP 3,415,82

SAFETY PROFILE: Questionable carcinogen
with experimental carcinogenic data. Poison by
ingestion. Mutation data reported. When heated
to decomposition it emits toxic fumes of NO_x.

NKQ500   CAS: 13256-21-8
N-NITROSOMETHYLAMINOSULFOLANE
mf: $C_5H_{10}N_2O_3S$ mw: 178.23

SYNS: 3-(N-NITROSOMETHYLAMINO)SULFOLAN (GER-
MAN) ◇ TETRAHYDRO-N-METHYL-N-NITROSO-3-
THIOPHENAMINE 1,1-DIOXIDE

TOXICITY DATA with REFERENCE
ETA: orl-rat TDLo: 2700 mg/kg/48W-C
ARZNAD 19,1077,69

SAFETY PROFILE: Questionable carcinogen
with experimental tumorigenic data. Moderately
toxic by ingestion. Many N-nitroso compounds
are carcinogens. When heated to decomposition
it emits very toxic fumes of NO_x and SO_x.

NKR000   CAS: 51542-33-7
**N-NITROSO-N-METHYL-N'-(2-
BENZOTHIAZOLYL)UREA**
mf: $C_9H_8N_4OS$ mw: 220.27

SYNS: N-(2-BENZOTHIAZOLYL)-N'-METHYL-
N'NITROSOUREA ◇ N-METHYL-N-NITROSO-N'-(2-BENZO-
THIAZOLYL)-HARNSTOFF (GERMAN) ◇ N-METHYL-N-NI-
TROSO-N'-(2-BENZOTHIAZOLYL)-UREA ◇ N-NITROSO-
BENZTHIAZURON

TOXICITY DATA with REFERENCE
CAR: orl-rat TDLo: 1156 mg/kg/64W-I   IARCCD
14,429,76
ETA: orl-rat TD: 429 mg/kg/86W-I   IARCCD
14,429,76
ETA: orl-rat TDLo: 400 mg/kg   ZKKOBW
81,217,74
MUT: slt-smc 4 mmol/L/16H   MUREAV 22,121,74

SAFETY PROFILE: Questionable carcinogen
with experimental carcinogenic and tumorigenic
data. Moderately toxic by ingestion. Mutation
data reported. Many N-nitroso compounds are

carcinogens. When heated to decomposition it
emits very toxic fumes of SO_x and NO_x.

NKR500   CAS: 62783-48-6
**N-NITROSO-N-(2-METHYLBENZYL)
METHYLAMINE**
mf: $C_9H_{12}N_2O$ mw: 164.23

SYNS: N,o-DIMETHYL-N-NITROSOBENZYLAMINE
◇ N-NITROSO-N-(2-METHYLBENZYL)-METHYLAMIN (GER-
MAN)

TOXICITY DATA with REFERENCE
ETA: orl-rat TD: 31640 mg/kg/2Y-C   JCROD7
95,123,79
ETA: orl-rat TDLo: 300 mg/kg/29W-C
ZKKOBW 88,231,77

SAFETY PROFILE: Questionable carcinogen
with experimental tumorigenic data. Poison by
ingestion. Many N-nitroso compounds are carcinogens. When heated to decomposition it emits
toxic fumes of NO_x.

NKS000   CAS: 62783-49-7
**N-NITROSO-N-(3-METHYLBENZYL)
METHYLAMINE**
mf: $C_9H_{12}N_2O$ mw: 164.23

SYNS: N,m-DIMETHYL-N-NITROSOBENZYLAMINE
◇ N-NITROSO-N-(3-METHYLBENZYL)-METHYLAMIN (GER-
MAN)

TOXICITY DATA with REFERENCE
ETA: orl-rat TD: 158 g/kg/2Y-C   JCROD795,123,79
ETA: orl-rat TD: 405 mg/kg/39W-C   ZKKOBW
88,231,77
ETA: orl-rat TDLo: 170 mg/kg/49W-C
ZKKOBW 88,231,77
MUT: mma-sat 100 µg/plate   JMCMAR 29,40,86

SAFETY PROFILE: Questionable carcinogen
with experimental tumorigenic data. Moderately
toxic by ingestion. Mutation data reported.
Many N-nitroso compounds are carcinogens.
When heated to decomposition it emits very
toxic fumes of NO_x.

NKS500   CAS: 62783-50-0
**N-NITROSO-N-(4-METHYLBENZYL)
METHYLAMINE**
mf: $C_9H_{12}N_2O$ mw: 164.23

SYNS: N,p-DIMETHYL-N-NITROSOBENZYLAMINE
◇ N-NITROSO-N-(4-METHYLBENZYL)-METHYLAMIN (GER-
MAN)

TOXICITY DATA with REFERENCE
ETA: orl-rat TD: 330 mg/kg/31W-C   ZKKOBW
88,231,77

ETA: orl-rat TD:31640 mg/kg/2Y-C   JCROD7
95,123,79

ETA: orl-rat TDLo:155 mg/kg/44W-C
ZKKOBW 88,231,77

MUT: mma-sat 500 µg/plate   JMCMAR 26,309,83

SAFETY PROFILE: Questionable carcinogen with experimental tumorigenic data. Poison by ingestion. Mutation data reported. Many N-nitroso compounds are carcinogens. When heated to decomposition it emits toxic fumes of NO_x.

NKT000   CAS: 69112-99-8
NITROSOMETHYLBIS(CHLOROETHYL) UREA
mf: $C_6H_{11}Cl_2N_3O_2$ mw: 228.10

SYN: 1-NITROSO-1-METHYL-3,3-BIS-(2-CHLORO-ETHYL)UREA

TOXICITY DATA with REFERENCE
ETA: orl-rat TDLo:76 mg/kg/6W-I   JCROD7
94,131,79

SAFETY PROFILE: Questionable carcinogen with experimental tumorigenic data. Many N-nitroso compounds are carcinogens. When heated to decomposition it emits very toxic fumes of Cl^- and NO_x.

NKT100   CAS: 75016-34-1
N-NITROSO-N-METHYL-N-n-BUTYL-1-d^2-AMINE
SYN: NMBA-d2

TOXICITY DATA with REFERENCE
ETA: orl-rat TDLo:132 mg/kg/20W-I   CRNGDP
1,157,80

SAFETY PROFILE: Questionable carcinogen with experimental tumorigenic data. When heated to decomposition it emits toxic fumes of NO_x.

NKT105   CAS: 75016-36-3
NITROSOMETHYL-d^3-n-BUTYLAMINE
mf: $C_5H_9D_3N_2O$ mw: 119.19

SYN: NMBA-d3

TOXICITY DATA with REFERENCE
ETA: orl-rat TDLo:152 mg/kg/23W-I   CRNGDP
1,157,80

SAFETY PROFILE: Questionable carcinogen with experimental tumorigenic data. When heated to decomposition it emits toxic fumes of NO_x. ?

NKT500   CAS: 5432-28-0
N-NITROSO-N-METHYLCYCLOHEXYLAMINE
mf: $C_7H_{14}N_2O$ mw: 142.23

SYNS: METHYLCYCLOHEXYLNITROSAMIN (GERMAN) ◇ METHYLCYCLOHEXYLNITROSAMINE ◇ N-METHYL-N-NITROSOCYCLOHEXYLAMINE ◇ N-NITROSOMETHYLCYCLOHEXYLAMINE

TOXICITY DATA with REFERENCE
ETA: orl-rat TD:190 mg/kg/45W-C   JJIND8
64,1535,80

ETA: orl-rat TD:750 mg/kg/45W-C   JJIND8
64,1535,80

ETA: orl-rat TDLo:150 mg/kg/54W-C   ARZNAD
19,1077,69

MUT: mma-sat 1 µg/plate   MUREAV 51,319,78

MUT: pic-esc 100 mg/L   TCMUE9 1,91,84

SAFETY PROFILE: Questionable carcinogen with experimental tumorigenic data. Poison by ingestion, intravenous, and intraperitoneal routes. Mutation data reported. Many N-nitroso compounds are carcinogens. When heated to decomposition it emits toxic fumes of NO_x.

NKU000   CAS: 55090-44-3
NITROSOMETHYL-n-DODECYLAMINE
mf: $C_{13}H_{28}N_2O$ mw: 228.43

SYNS: N-METHYL-N-NITROSOLAURYLAMINE ◇ N-NITROSO-N-METHYL-N-DODECYLAMIN (GERMAN) ◇ N-NITROSO-N-METHYL-N-DODECYLAMINE ◇ NMDDA

TOXICITY DATA with REFERENCE
CAR: orl-gpg TDLo:8000 mg/kg/40W-I
CNREA8 40,1879,80

CAR: orl-ham TD:3500 mg/kg/58W-I   ZKKOBW
90,227,77

CAR: orl-ham TDLo:2000 mg/kg/67W-I
ZKKOBW 90,227,77

CAR: orl-rat TD:2688 mg/kg/28W-I   ANTRD4
1,389,81

CAR: scu-ham TD:3828 mg/kg/29W-I   CALEDQ
13,165,81

CAR: scu-ham TDLo:3384 mg/kg/24W-I
CALEDQ 13,165,81

ETA: orl-rat TD:4800 mg/kg/50W-I   CNREA8
35,958,75

ETA: orl-rat TD:6000 mg/kg/50W-I   CNREA8
35,958,75

ETA: orl-rat TD:6720 mg/kg/2Y-C   CNREA8
41,1288,81

ETA: orl-rat TDLo: 3600 mg/kg/30W-I   FCTOD7
21,601,83

MUT: mma-sat 1 μg/plate   MUREAV 51,319,78

CONSENSUS REPORTS: EPA Genetic Toxicology Program.

SAFETY PROFILE: Questionable carcinogen with experimental carcinogenic and tumorigenic data. Moderately toxic by ingestion. Mutation data reported. When heated to decomposition it emits toxic fumes of NO$_x$.

NKU350   CAS: 26921-68-6
N-NITROSOMETHYLETHANOLAMINE
mf: C$_3$H$_8$N$_2$O$_2$ mw: 104.13

SYNS: METHYL-2-HYDROXYETHYLNITROSAMINE ◇ METHYL-2-HYDROXYETHYLNITROSOAMINE ◇ 2-(METHYLNITROSOAMINO)ETHANOL ◇ N-NITROSO-METHYL-(2-HYDROXYETHYL)AMINE

TOXICITY DATA with REFERENCE
CAR: orl-rat TDLo: 1602 mg/kg/60W-I   CNREA8
48,1533,88

MUT: dnd-rat-orl 30 μmol/kg   PAACA3 27,105,86

SAFETY PROFILE: Questionable carcinogen with experimental carcinogenic data. Mutation data reported. When heated to decomposition it emits toxic fumes of NO$_x$.

NKU400   CAS: 28538-70-7
NITROSOMETHYL-n-HEXYLAMINE
mf: C$_7$H$_{16}$N$_2$O   mw: 144.25

SYNS: N-METHYL-N-NITROSO-1-HEXANAMINE ◇ N-METHYL-N-NITROSOHEXYLAMINE ◇ NITROSO-n-HEXYLMETHYLAMINE

TOXICITY DATA with REFERENCE
ETA: orl-ham TDLo: 3462 mg/kg/56W-I
IAPUDO 57,617,84

ETA: orl-rat TD: 866 mg/kg/31W-I   IAPUDO
57,617,84

ETA: orl-rat TDLo: 420 mg/kg/21W-I   JCROD7
106,171,83

MUT: mma-sat 10 μg/plate   TCMUE9 1,13,84
MUT: pic-esc 50 mg/L   TCMUE9 1,91,84

SAFETY PROFILE: Questionable carcinogen with experimental tumorigenic data. Mutation data reported. Many N-nitroso compounds are carcinogens. When heated to decomposition it emits toxic fumes of NO$_x$.

NKU500   CAS: 75411-83-5
N-NITROSOMETHYL-2-HYDROXYPROPYLAMINE
mf: C$_4$H$_{10}$N$_2$O$_2$ mw: 118.16

SYNS: 2-HYDROXYPROPYLMETHYLNITROSAMINE ◇ 1-(METHYLNITROSOAMINO)-2-PROPANOL ◇ MHP ◇ NMHP

TOXICITY DATA with REFERENCE
NEO: par-rat TDLo: 600 mg/kg/30W-I   JJCREP
79,309,88

ETA: orl-ham TDLo: 354 mg/kg/25W-I   IAPUDO
57,617,84

ETA: orl-rat TD: 375 mg/kg/30W-I   CALEDQ
22,83,84

ETA: orl-rat TD: 532 mg/kg/29W-I   IAPUDO
57,617,84

ETA: orl-rat TD: 1100 mg/kg/22W-I   JJIND8
70,959,83

ETA: orl-rat TDLo: 300 mg/kg/30W-I   CALEDQ
22,83,84

MUT: dns-rat: lvr 1 mmol/L   MUREAV 144,197,85
MUT: mma-sat 10 μg/plate   TCMUE9 1,13,84
MUT: mmo-sat 500 μg/plate   TCMUE9 1,13,84
MUT: msc-ham: lng 200 μmol/L   CNREA8
40,3463,80

SAFETY PROFILE: Questionable carcinogen with experimental neoplastigenic and tumorigenic data. Mutation data reported. Many N-nitroso compounds are carcinogens. When heated to decomposition it emits toxic fumes of NO$_x$.

NKU550   CAS: 75881-16-2
NITROSO-2-METHYLMORPHOLINE
mf: C$_5$H$_{10}$N$_2$O$_2$ mw: 130.17

SYNS: 2-METHYL-4-NITROSOMORPHOLINE ◇ N-NITROSO-2-METHYLMORPHOLINE

TOXICITY DATA with REFERENCE
CAR: orl-rat TDLo: 146 g/kg/50W-I   CRNGDP
3,911,82

ETA: orl-ham TD: 1302 mg/kg/34W-I   IAPUDO
57,617,84

ETA: orl-ham TDLo: 1296 mg/kg/30W-I
CRNGDP 5,875,84

ETA: orl-rat TD: 456 mg/kg/27W-I   IAPUDO
57,617,84

MUT: mma-sat 250 μg/plate   TCMUD8 1,295,80
MUT: mmo-sat 1 mg/plate   TCMUD8 1,295,80

SAFETY PROFILE: Questionable carcinogen with experimental carcinogenic and tumorigenic data. Mutation data reported. When heated to decomposition it emits toxic fumes of NO$_x$.

NKU570   CAS: 31820-22-1
NITROSOMETHYLNEOPENTYLAMINE
mf: C$_6$H$_{14}$N$_2$O   mw: 130.22

SYNS: NMNA ◇ N,2,2-TRIMETHYL-N-NITROSO-1-PRO-
PYLAMINE

TOXICITY DATA with REFERENCE
ETA: orl-rat TDLo: 200 mg/kg/22W-I   JJIND8
68,681,82

SAFETY PROFILE: Questionable carcinogen
with experimental tumorigenic data. When
heated to decomposition it emits toxic fumes
of NO_x.

NKU580   CAS: 75881-19-5
NITROSO-N-METHYL-n-NONYLAMINE
mf: $C_{10}H_{22}N_2O$ mw: 186.34

SYNS: NITROSOMETHYL-n-NONYLAMINE ◇ N-NITRO-
SOMETHYL-n-NONYLAMINE ◇ 1-NONYLAMINE, N-
METHYL-N-NITROSO-

TOXICITY DATA with REFERENCE
ETA: orl-rat TDLo: 4800 mg/kg/51W-C
CNREA8 41,1288,81
MUT: mma-sat 25 μg/plate   TCMUD8 1,295,80

SAFETY PROFILE: Questionable carcinogen
with experimental tumorigenic data. When
heated to decomposition it emits toxic fumes
of NO_x.

NKU590   CAS: 34423-54-6
NITROSO-N-METHYL-n-OCTYLAMINE
mf: $C_9H_{20}N_2O$ mw: 172.31

SYNS: N-METHYL-N-NITROSOOCTYLAMINE ◇ NITRO-
SOMETHYL-n-OCTYLAMINE ◇ N-NITROSOMETHYL-n-OC-
TYLAMINE ◇ 1-OCTYLAMINE, N-METHYL-N-NITROSO-

TOXICITY DATA with REFERENCE
ETA: orl-rat TDLo: 4480 mg/kg/43W-C
CNREA8 41,1288,81
MUT: mma-sat 50 μg/plate   TCMUD8 1,295,80

SAFETY PROFILE: Questionable carcinogen
with experimental tumorigenic data. Mutation
data reported. When heated to decomposition
it emits toxic fumes of NO_x.

NKU600   CAS: 39884-53-2
NITROSO-2-METHYL-1,3-OXAZOLIDINE
mf: $C_4H_8N_2O_2$ mw: 116.14

SYNS: 2-METHYL-3-NITROSO-1,3-OXAZOLIDINE
◇ N-NITROSO-2-METHYL-1,3-OXAZOLIDINE

TOXICITY DATA with REFERENCE
CAR: orl-rat TDLo: 250 mg/kg/50W-I   CRNGDP
3,911,82

MUT: mma-sat 250 μg/plate   TCMUD8 1,295,80
MUT: mmo-sat 500 μg/plate   TCMUD8 1,295,80

SAFETY PROFILE: Questionable carcinogen
with experimental carcinogenic data. Mutation
data reported. When heated to decomposition
it emits toxic fumes of NO_x.

NKV100
N-NITROSOMETHYL-
PENTYLNITROSAMINE
mf: $C_6H_{13}N_3O_2$ mw: 159.22

SYNS: MPN ◇ N-NITROSO-N-(NITROSOMETHYL)
PENTYLAMINE

TOXICITY DATA with REFERENCE
ETA: scu-rat TDLo: 200 mg/kg/20W-I   SACAB7
25,66,81

SAFETY PROFILE: Questionable carcinogen
with experimental tumorigenic data. Poison by
ingestion. Many N-nitroso compounds are carcinogens. When heated to decomposition it emits toxic fumes of NO_x.

NKV500   CAS: 68426-46-0
NITROSOMETHYLPHENYLCARBAMATE
mf: $C_8H_8N_2O_3$ mw: 180.18

SYNS: N-METHYL-N-NITROSOCARBAMIC ACID, PHE-
NYL ESTER ◇ N-NITROSO-N-METHYLPHENYLCARBA-
MATE ◇ PHENYL METHYLNITROSOCARBAMATE

TOXICITY DATA with REFERENCE
CAR: orl-rat TDLo: 470 mg/kg/10W-I   EESADV
2,413,78
MUT: mma-sat 5 μg/plate   TCMUE9 1,13,84
MUT: mmo-sat 1 μg/plate   MUREAV 68,1,79
MUT: pic-esc 100 μg/L   TCMUE9 1,91,84

SAFETY PROFILE: Questionable carcinogen
with experimental carcinogenic data. Mutation
data reported. When heated to decomposition
it emits toxic fumes of NO_x.

NKW000   CAS: 68690-89-1
N-NITROSO-N-METHYL-1-(1-
PHENYL)ETHYLAMINE
mf: $C_9H_{12}N_2O$ mw: 164.23

SYNS: α,N-DIMETHYL-N-NITROSOBENZYLAMINE
◇ N-METHYL-N-NITROSO-1-PHENYLETHYLAMINE
◇ N-NITROSO-N-METHYL-(1-PHENYL)-ETHYLAMIN (GER-
MAN)

TOXICITY DATA with REFERENCE
ETA: orl-rat TDLo: 610 mg/kg/59W-C
ZKKOBW 92,235,78

SAFETY PROFILE: Questionable carcinogen with experimental tumorigenic data. Moderately toxic by ingestion. Many N-nitroso compounds are carcinogens. When heated to decomposition it emits toxic fumes of NO_x.

NKW500 CAS: 16339-07-4
1-NITROSO-4-METHYLPIPERAZINE
mf: $C_5H_{11}N_3O$ mw: 129.19

SYNS: N'-METHYL-N-NITROSOPIPERAZINE ◇ 1-METHYL-4-NITROSOPIPERAZINE ◇ N-NITROSO-N'-METHYLPIPERAZIN (GERMAN) ◇ N-NITROSO-N'-METHYL-PIPERAZINE

TOXICITY DATA with REFERENCE
ETA: orl-rat TD:11440 mg/kg/22W-I JJIND8 71,165,83
ETA: orl-rat TD:20800 mg/kg/40W-I PAACA3 24,53,83
ETA: orl-rat TDLo:10 g/kg/59W-C ZEKBAI 69,103,67
MUT: hma-mus/sat 1 mmol/kg CNREA8 32,1598,72
MUT: mma-ham:lng 10 mmol/L CNREA8 37,1004,77
MUT: mma-sat 50 nmol/plate MUREAV 57,1,78
MUT: mma-smc 50 μmol/plate MUREAV 77,143,80
MUT: sln-dmg-orl 5 mmol/L/24H FOBLAN 16,225,70
MUT: sln-dmg-par 5 mmol/L FOBLAN 16,225,70

SAFETY PROFILE: Questionable carcinogen with experimental tumorigenic data. Poison by ingestion. Mutation data reported. Many N-nitroso compounds are carcinogens. When heated to decomposition it emits toxic fumes of NO_x.

NKW800 CAS: 75881-20-8
N-NITROSO-N-METHYL-n-TETRADECYLAMINE
mf: $C_{15}H_{32}N_2O$ mw: 256.49

TOXICITY DATA with REFERENCE
ETA: orl-rat TDLo:6720 mg/kg/2Y-C CNREA8 41,1288,81
MUT: mma-sat 50 μg/plate MUREAV 111,135,83

SAFETY PROFILE: Questionable carcinogen with experimental tumorigenic data. When heated to decomposition it emits toxic fumes of NO_x.

NKX000 CAS: 57117-24-5
NITROSO-2-METHYLTHIOPROPIONALDEHYDE-o-METHYL CARBAMOYL-OXIME
mf: $C_5H_9N_3O_3S$ mw: 191.23

SYNS: N-((METHYLNITROSOCARBAMOYL)OXY)-2-METHYLTHIOACETIMIDIC ACID ◇ NITROSO-METHOMYL

TOXICITY DATA with REFERENCE
CAR: orl-rat TDLo:500 mg/kg/10W-I EESADV 2,413,78
ETA: orl-rat TD:500 mg/kg/10W-I IARCCD 19,495,78
MUT: dnd-hmn:fbr 10 μmol/L MUREAV 44,1,77
MUT: mma-sat 1 μg/plate TCMUE9 1,13,84
MUT: mmo-esc 100 μmol/L IARCCD 14,425,76
MUT: mmo-sat 1 μg/plate TCMUE9 1,13,84
MUT: pic-esc 100 μg/L TCMUE9 1,91,84

CONSENSUS REPORTS: EPA Genetic Toxicology Program.

SAFETY PROFILE: Questionable carcinogen with experimental carcinogenic and tumorigenic data. Human mutation data reported. When heated to decomposition it emits very toxic fumes of NO_x and SO_x.

NKX300 CAS: 819-35-2
NITROSOMETHYL-2-TRIFLUOROETHYLAMINE
mf: $C_3H_5F_3N_2O$ mw: 142.10

TOXICITY DATA with REFERENCE
ETA: orl-rat TD:700 mg/kg/28W-I JJIND8 68,681,82
ETA: orl-rat TDLo:300 mg/kg/30W-I JJIND8 68,681,82
MUT: mma-sat 1 mg/plate TCMUD8 1,295,80
MUT: mmo-sat 250 μg/plate TCMUD8 1,295,80

SAFETY PROFILE: Questionable carcinogen with experimental tumorigenic data. Mutation data reported. Many nitroso compounds are carcinogens. When heated to decomposition it emits toxic fumes of F^- and NO_x.

NKX500 CAS: 68107-26-6
NITROSOMETHYLUNDECYLAMINE
mf: $C_{12}H_{26}N_2O$ mw: 214.40

SYN: N-METHYL-N-NITROSOUNDECYLAMINE

TOXICITY DATA with REFERENCE
CAR: orl-rat TDLo:5600 mg/kg/30W-I
CALEDQ 5,209,78

MUT: mma-sat 1 μg/plate   MUREAV 51,319,78

SAFETY PROFILE: Questionable carcinogen with experimental carcinogenic data. Mutation data reported. When heated to decomposition it emits toxic fumes of NO_x.

NLA000   CAS: 21711-65-9
1-NITROSONAPHTHALENE
mf: $C_{10}H_7NO$ mw: 157.18

TOXICITY DATA with REFERENCE
ETA: ipr-rat TDLo: 350 mg/kg/5W-I   CNREA8 31,1461,71
ETA: skn-rat TDLo: 624 mg/kg/52W-I   RCOCB8 18,353,77
MUT: mma-sat 1 μg/plate   MUREAV 94,315,82

SAFETY PROFILE: Questionable carcinogen with experimental tumorigenic data. Mutation data reported. When heated to decomposition it emits toxic fumes of NO_x.

NLA500   CAS: 6610-08-8
2-NITROSONAPHTHALENE
mf: $C_{10}H_7NO$ mw: 157.18

TOXICITY DATA with REFERENCE
NEO: scu-mus TDLo: 250 mg/kg   CNREA8 31,1461,71
ETA: skn-rat TDLo: 624 mg/kg/52W-I   RCOCB8 18,353,77
MUT: dni-sat 100 μmol/L   CNREA8 34,3102,74
MUT: mma-sat 100 μg/plate   PNASA6 72,5135,75
MUT: mmo-sat 50 μg/plate   PNASA6 69,3128,72
MUT: pic-sat 100 μmol/L/2M   CNREA8 34,3102,74

CONSENSUS REPORTS: EPA Genetic Toxicology Program.

SAFETY PROFILE: Questionable carcinogen with experimental neoplastigenic and tumorigenic data. Mutation data reported. Many nitroso compounds are carcinogens. When heated to decomposition it emits toxic fumes of NO_x.

NLB500   CAS: 132-53-6
2-NITROSO-1-NAPHTHOL
mf: $C_{10}H_7NO_2$ mw: 173.18

TOXICITY DATA with REFERENCE
ETA: orl-rat TDLo: 31 g/kg/1Y-I: TER   JNCIAM 41,985,68

CONSENSUS REPORTS: Reported in EPA TSCA Inventory.

SAFETY PROFILE: Questionable carcinogen with experimental tumorigenic and teratogenic

data. Many nitroso compounds are carcinogens. When heated to decomposition it emits toxic fumes of NO_x.

NLC000   CAS: 13010-08-7
1-NITROSO-3-NITRO-1-BUTYLGUANIDINE
mf: $C_5H_{11}N_5O_3$ mw: 189.21

SYNS: N-BUTYL-N'-NITRO-N-NITROSOGUANIDINE
◇ N-NITROSO-N'-NITRO-N-BUTYLGUANIDINE

TOXICITY DATA with REFERENCE
ETA: scu-rat TDLo: 69 mg/kg/5W-I   GANNA2 69,277,78
MUT: cyt-ham: fbr 15 mg/L/24H   MUREAV 48,337,77
MUT: cyt-ham: lng 17 mg/L   GMCRDC 27,95,81
MUT: dnr-smc 2 μmol/well   IDZAAW 50,403,75
MUT: mmo-esc 5 mg/L   ESKHA5 88,118,70
MUT: mmo-omi 500 ppm   SOGEBZ 11,183,75
MUT: mmo-sat 100 nmol/plate   IDZAAW 50,403,75
MUT: pic-esc 10 mg/L   ESKHA5 88,118,70

CONSENSUS REPORTS: EPA Genetic Toxicology Program.

SAFETY PROFILE: Questionable carcinogen with experimental tumorigenic data. Mutation data reported. Many N-nitroso compounds are carcinogens. When heated to decomposition it emits toxic fumes of NO_x.

NLC500   CAS: 13010-10-1
1-NITROSO-3-NITRO-1-PENTYLGUANIDINE
mf: $C_6H_{13}N_5O_3$ mw: 203.24

SYNS: 3-NITRO-1-NITROSO-1-PENTYLGUANIDINE
◇ 1-PENTYL-3-NITRO-1-NITROSOGUANIDINE

TOXICITY DATA with REFERENCE
ETA: scu-rat TDLo: 69 mg/kg/5W-I   GANNA2 69,277,78
MUT: cyt-ham: fbr 30 mg/L/24H   MUREAV 48,337,77
MUT: cyt-ham: lng 16 mg/L   GMCRDC 27,95,81
MUT: dnr-smc 2 μmol/well   IDZAAW 50,403,75
MUT: mmo-esc 5 mg/L   ESKHA5 88,118,70
MUT: mmo-sat 100 nmol/plate   IDZAAW 50,403,75
MUT: pic-esc 10 mg/L   ESKHA5 88,118,70

CONSENSUS REPORTS: EPA Genetic Toxicology Program.

SAFETY PROFILE: Questionable carcinogen with experimental tumorigenic data. Mutation

data reported. Many nitroso compounds are carcinogens. When heated to decomposition it emits very toxic fumes of NO_x.

NLD000 CAS: 71598-10-2
3-NITROSO-1-NITRO-1-PROPYLGUANIDINE

mf: $C_4H_9N_5O_3$ mw: 175.18

SYNS: PNNG ◇ N-PROPYL-N'-NITRO-N-NITROSOGUANI-DINE

TOXICITY DATA with REFERENCE
NEO: orl-rat TD: 2172 mg/kg/52W-C JCROD7
94,201,79
NEO: orl-rat TDLo: 2172 mg/kg/52W-C
GANNA2 70,181,79
ETA: orl-rat TD: 3080 mg/kg/44W-C JCROD7
98,153,80
ETA: orl-rat TD: 3665 mg/kg/44W-C NIPAA4
76,1253,79
ETA: scu-rat TDLo: 60 mg/kg/5W-I GANNA2
69,277,78
MUT: cty-ham: fbr 30 mg/L/24H MUREAV
48,337,77
MUT: cyt-ham: lng 10 mg/L GMCRDC 27,95,81
MUT: dns-rat-orl 1 g/kg BANRDU 13,123,82
MUT: dns-rat: lvr 10 μmol/L ENMUDM 3,11,81
MUT: mmo-esc 300 nmol/L ENMUDM 3,11,81
MUT: mmo-sat 300 nmol/L ENMUDM 3,11,81

SAFETY PROFILE: Questionable carcinogen with experimental neoplastigenic and tumorigenic data. Mutation data reported. Many N-nitroso compounds are carcinogens. When heated to decomposition it emits toxic fumes of NO_x.

NLD525
N'-NITROSONORNICOTINE-1-N-OXIDE

mf: $C_9H_{11}N_3O_2$ mw: 193.23

SYNS: NICOTINE, 1'-DEMETHYL-1'-NITROSO-, 1-OXIDE ◇ NNN-1-N-OXIDE

TOXICITY DATA with REFERENCE
ETA: orl-ham TDLo: 3242 mg/kg/31W-C
CALEDQ 20,333,83
ETA: orl-rat TDLo: 2799 mg/kg/36W-C
CALEDQ 20,333,83

SAFETY PROFILE: Questionable carcinogen with experimental tumorigenic data. When heated to decomposition it emits toxic fumes of NO_x.

NLD800 CAS: 18207-29-9
1-NITROSO-1-OCTYLUREA

mf: $C_9H_{19}N_3O_2$ mw: 201.31

SYN: n-OCTYL NITROSUREA

TOXICITY DATA with REFERENCE
ETA: orl-rat TDLo: 800 mg/kg ANYAA9
381,250,82
ETA: scu-rat TDLo: 600 mg/kg ANYAA9
381,250,82

SAFETY PROFILE: Questionable carcinogen with experimental tumorigenic data. Moderately toxic by subcutaneous route. When heated to decomposition it emits toxic fumes of NO_x.

NLE400 CAS: 77698-20-5
N-NITROSO(2-OXOBUTYL)(2-OXOPROPYL)AMINE

mf: $C_7H_{12}N_2O_3$ mw: 172.21

SYN: OBOB

TOXICITY DATA with REFERENCE
ETA: scu-ham TDLo: 100 mg/kg CALEDQ
12,223,81

SAFETY PROFILE: Questionable carcinogen with experimental tumorigenic data. Poison by subcutaneous route. When heated to decomposition it emits toxic fumes of NO_x.

NLE500 CAS: 61734-86-9
N-NITROSO-N-PENTYL-(4-HYDROXYBUTYL)AMINE

mf: $C_9H_{20}N_2O_2$ mw: 188.31

SYNS: N-PENTYL-N-(4-HYDROXYBUTYL)NITROSAMINE ◇ 4-(PENTYLNITROSAMINO)-1-BUTANOL

TOXICITY DATA with REFERENCE
ETA: orl-rat TDLo: 76 g/kg/20W-C GANNA2
67,825,76
MUT: mma-sat 10 μmol/plate CNREA8 37,399,77

CONSENSUS REPORTS: EPA Genetic Toxicology Program.

SAFETY PROFILE: Questionable carcinogen with experimental tumorigenic data. Mutation data reported. Many N-nitroso compounds are carcinogens. When heated to decomposition it emits toxic fumes of NO_x.

NLG500 CAS: 6268-32-2
NITROSOPHENYLUREA

mf: $C_7H_7N_3O_2$ mw: 165.17

SYNS: N-NITROSO-N-PHENYLUREA ◇ PHENYL-NI-TROSO-HANRSTOFF (GERMAN) ◇ N-PHENYL-N-NITRO-SOUREA

TOXICITY DATA with REFERENCE
ETA: scu-rat TDLo: 150 mg/kg   ZEKBAI 71,63,68
ETA: skn-mus TDLo: 661 mg/kg/50W-I
  JCROD7 102,13,81
MUT: mma-sat 10 μg/plate   TCMUE9 1,13,84
MUT: mmo-sat 10 μg/plate   TCMUE9 1,13,84

SAFETY PROFILE: Questionable carcinogen with experimental tumorigenic data. Poison by subcutaneous route. Mutation data reported. Many N-nitroso compounds are carcinogens. When heated to decomposition it emits toxic fumes of NO_x.

NLH000   CAS: 13256-23-0
N-NITROSO-4-PICOLYLETHYLAMINE
mf: $C_8H_{11}N_3O$ mw: 165.22

SYNS: AETHYL-4-PICOLYLNITROSAMIN (GERMAN) ◇ 4-((ETHYLNITROSAMINO)METHYL)PYRIDINE

TOXICITY DATA with REFERENCE
ETA: ivn-rat TDLo: 160 mg/kg/27W-I   ARZNAD
  19,1077,69
ETA: orl-rat TDLo: 1200 mg/kg/43W-C
  ARZNAD 19,1077,69

SAFETY PROFILE: Questionable carcinogen with experimental tumorigenic data. Poison by ingestion and intravenous routes. Many N-nitroso compounds are carcinogens. When heated to decomposition it emits toxic fumes of NO_x.

NLI000   CAS: 7247-89-4
1-NITROSO-2-PIPECOLINE
mf: $C_6H_{12}N_2O$ mw: 128.20

SYN: 2-METHYLNITROSOPIPERIDINE

TOXICITY DATA with REFERENCE
ETA: orl-rat TDLo: 2520 mg/kg/50W-I   IJCNAW
  16,318,75
MUT: mma-smc 50 mmol/L/24H   MUREAV
  57,155,78
MUT: sln-dmg-orl 5 mmol/L/24H   MUREAV
  67,27,79

SAFETY PROFILE: Questionable carcinogen with experimental tumorigenic data. Mutation data reported. Many nitroso compounds are carcinogens. When heated to decomposition it emits toxic fumes of NO_x.

NLI500   CAS: 14026-03-0
R(−)-N-NITROSO-α-PIPECOLINE
mf: $C_6H_{12}N_2O$ mw: 128.20

SYNS: R(−)-N-NITROSO-2-METHYL-PIPERIDIN (GERMAN) ◇ R(−)-N-NITROSO-2-METHYLPIPERIDINE

TOXICITY DATA with REFERENCE
CAR: orl-rat TDLo: 6300 mg/kg/40W-I
  ZKKOBW 79,118,73

SAFETY PROFILE: Questionable carcinogen with experimental carcinogenic data. Moderately toxic by ingestion. When heated to decomposition it emits toxic fumes of NO_x.

NLJ000   CAS: 36702-44-0
s(+)-N-NITROSO-α-PIPECOLINE
mf: $C_6H_{12}N_2O$ mw: 128.20

SYNS: s(+)-N-NITROSO-2-METHYL-PIPERIDIN (GERMAN) ◇ s(+)-N-NITROSO-2-METHYLPIPERIDINE

TOXICITY DATA with REFERENCE
CAR: orl-rat TDLo: 5700 mg/kg/37W-I
  ZKKOBW 79,118,73

SAFETY PROFILE: Questionable carcinogen with experimental carcinogenic data. Moderately toxic by ingestion. When heated to decomposition it emits toxic fumes of NO_x.

NLK000   CAS: 55556-85-9
NITROSO-3-PIPERIDINOL
mf: $C_5H_{10}N_2O_2$ mw: 130.17

SYNS: N-NITROSO-3-HYDROXYPIPERIDINE ◇ N-NITROSO-3-PIPERIDINOL

TOXICITY DATA with REFERENCE
ETA: orl-rat TDLo: 1666 mg/kg/36W-I   JNCIAM
  55,705,75
MUT: mma-sat 1 μmol/plate   MUREAV 56,131,77
MUT: sce-hmn: lym 10 mmol/L   TCMUE9 1,129,84

CONSENSUS REPORTS: EPA Genetic Toxicology Program.

SAFETY PROFILE: Questionable carcinogen with experimental tumorigenic data. Human mutation data reported. Many N-nitroso compounds are carcinogens. When heated to decomposition it emits toxic fumes of NO_x.

NLK500   CAS: 55556-93-9
NITROSO-4-PIPERIDINOL
mf: $C_5H_{10}N_2O_2$ mw: 130.17

TOXICITY DATA with REFERENCE
ETA: orl-rat TDLo: 1666 mg/kg/36W-I   JNCIAM
  55,705,75
MUT: mma-sat 1 μmol/plate   MUREAV 56,131,77

SAFETY PROFILE: Questionable carcinogen with experimental tumorigenic data. Mutation

data reported. Many nitroso compounds are carcinogens. When heated to decomposition it emits toxic fumes of NO_x.

NLL000 CAS: 55556-91-7
NITROSO-4-PIPERIDONE
mf: $C_5H_8N_2O_2$ mw: 128.15

SYNS: N-NITROSO-4-PIPERIDINONE ◇ NITROSO-4-PIPERIDINONE ◇ 1-NITROSO-4-PIPERIDONE

TOXICITY DATA with REFERENCE
ETA: orl-rat TD:1725 mg/kg/30W-I CRNGDP 5,1351,84
ETA: orl-rat TDLo:1640 mg/kg/36W-I JNCIAM 55,705,75
MUT: mma-sat 250 µg/plate TCMUE9 1,13,84

SAFETY PROFILE: Questionable carcinogen with experimental tumorigenic data. Mutation data reported. Many N-nitroso compounds are carcinogens. When heated to decomposition it emits toxic fumes of NO_x.

NLL500 CAS: 7519-36-0
1-NITROSO-I-PROLINE
mf: $C_5H_8N_2O_3$ mw: 144.15

SYNS: N-NITROSO-l-PROLINE ◇ NO-Pro ◇ NPRO

TOXICITY DATA with REFERENCE
ETA: orl-rat TDLo:770 mg/kg/8W-I JMCMAR 16,583,73

CONSENSUS REPORTS: IARC Cancer Review: Animal Inadequate Evidence IMEMDT 17,303,78.

SAFETY PROFILE: Questionable carcinogen with experimental tumorigenic data. Poison by intraperitoneal route. Many nitroso compounds are carcinogens. When heated to decomposition it emits toxic fumes of NO_x.

NLN000 CAS: 51938-12-6
N-NITROSO-N-PROPYL-(4-HYDROXYBUTYL)AMINE
mf: $C_7H_{16}N_2O_2$ mw: 160.25

SYNS: PHBN ◇ PROPYL(4-HYDROXYBUTYL)NITROSAMINE ◇ 4-(PROPYLNITROSAMINO)-1-BUTANOL

TOXICITY DATA with REFERENCE
ETA: orl-rat TDLo:5200 mg/kg/20W-C GANNA2 65,13,74
MUT: mma-sat 20 µmol/plate CNREA8 37,399,77

CONSENSUS REPORTS: EPA Genetic Toxicology Program.

SAFETY PROFILE: Questionable carcinogen with experimental tumorigenic data. Mutation data reported. Many N-nitroso compounds are carcinogens. When heated to decomposition it emits toxic fumes of NO_x.

NLN500 CAS: 65792-56-5
N-NITROSO-N-PROPYLPROPIONAMIDE
mf: $C_6H_{12}N_2O_2$ mw: 144.20

SYNS: N-NITROSO-N-PROPYL-PROPRIONAMID (GERMAN) ◇ 1-OXOPROPYLPROPYLNITROSAMINE ◇ 1-OXOPROPYLPROPYLNITROSAMIN (GERMAN)

TOXICITY DATA with REFERENCE
ETA: scu-ham TDLo:125 mg/kg ZKKOBW 90,221,77

SAFETY PROFILE: Questionable carcinogen with experimental tumorigenic data. Poison by subcutaneous route. Many N-nitroso compounds are carcinogens. When heated to decomposition it emits toxic fumes of NO_x.

NLP000 CAS: 29291-35-0
N-NITROSO-N-PTEROYL-I-GLUTAMIC ACID
mf: $C_{19}H_{18}N_8O_7$ mw: 470.45

SYNS: N-(p-(((2-AMINO-4-OXO-6-PTERIDINYL)METHYL)-N-NITROSOAMINO)BENZOYL)-l-GLUTAMIC ACID ◇ NITROSOFOLIC ACID

TOXICITY DATA with REFERENCE
NEO: ipr-mus TDLo:375 mg/kg/7D-I CNREA8 35,1981,75
MUT: mma-sat 100 µg/plate BJCAAI 37,873,78
MUT: otr-ham:kdy 80 µg/L BJCAAI 37,873,78

CONSENSUS REPORTS: IARC Cancer Review: Animal Inadequate Evidence IMEMDT 17,217,78.

SAFETY PROFILE: Questionable carcinogen with experimental neoplastigenic data. Poison by intraperitoneal route. Mutation data reported. Many N-nitroso compounds are carcinogens. When heated to decomposition it emits toxic fumes of NO_x.

NLP375 CAS: 86674-51-3
1-NITROSOPYRENE
mf: $C_{16}H_{19}NO$ mw: 241.36

TOXICITY DATA with REFERENCE
CAR: orl-rat TDLo:386 mg/kg/16W-I CNREA8 48,4256,88

MUT: dnd-hmn:fbr 900 nmol/L   CRNGDP
7,1279,86

MUT: mma-sat 2500 ng/plate   CNREA8 43,3132,83
MUT: mmo-sat 500 ng/plate   CNREA8 43,3132,83
MUT: msc-hmn:fbr 42 μmol/L   CRNGDP 7,89,86
MUT: oth-ham:lng 1250 μg/L   MUTAEX 2,23,87

SAFETY PROFILE: Questionable carcinogen
with experimental carcinogenic data. Human
mutation data reported. When heated to decomposition it emits toxic fumes of NO_x.

NLP480   CAS: 35884-45-8
NITROSOPYRROLIDINE
mf: $C_4H_8N_2O$ mw: 100.14

SYN: PYRROLIDINE, NITROSO-

TOXICITY DATA with REFERENCE
CAR: orl-rat TDLo:2804 mg/kg/84W-C
CNREA8 46,1285,86

MUT: mma-esc 2500 mg/L   MUREAV 89,35,81
MUT: mma-sat 10 μg/plate   TCMUE9 1,13,84
MUT: msc-ham:ovr 5 mmol/L   TCMUE9 1,129,84
MUT: msc-mus:lyms 1 g/L   MUREAV 125,291,84
MUT: pic-esc 20 mg/L   TCMUE9 1,91,84

SAFETY PROFILE: Questionable carcinogen
with experimental carcinogenic data. Mutation
data reported. When heated to decomposition
it emits toxic fumes of NO_x.

NLP600   CAS: 54634-49-0
N-NITROSO-2-PYRROLIDINE
mf: $C_4H_6N_2O_2$ mw: 114.12

SYN: 1-NITROSO-2-PYRROLIDINONE

TOXICITY DATA with REFERENCE
ETA: orl-rat TDLo:1460 mg/kg/52W-C
YKKZAJ 97,320,77

MUT: dnr-bcs 1500 μg/disc   YKKZAJ 97,320,77

CONSENSUS REPORTS: EPA Genetic Toxicology Program.

SAFETY PROFILE: Questionable carcinogen
with experimental tumorigenic data. Poison by
ingestion. Mutation data reported. Many N-nitroso compounds are carcinogens. When heated
to decomposition it emits toxic fumes of NO_x.

NLP700   CAS: 56222-35-6
1-NITROSO-3-PYRROLIDINOL
mf: $C_4H_8N_2O_2$ mw: 116.14

SYNS: 3-HYDROXYNITROSOPYRROLIDINE ◇ N-NI-
TROSO-3-HYDROXYPYRROLIDINE

TOXICITY DATA with REFERENCE
CAR: orl-rat TDLo:1778 mg/kg/2Y-I   IAPUDO
31,657,80

MUT: mma-sat 500 μg/plate   MUREAV 89,35,81

SAFETY PROFILE: Questionable carcinogen
with experimental carcinogenic data. Mutation
data reported. When heated to decomposition
it emits toxic fumes of NO_x.

NLQ000   CAS: 10552-94-0
N-NITROSO-3-PYRROLINE
mf: $C_4H_6N_2O$ mw: 98.12

SYNS: 2,5-DIHYDRO-1-NITROSO-1H-PYRROLE
◇ NITROSO-3-PYRROLIN (GERMAN)

TOXICITY DATA with REFERENCE
ETA: orl-rat TDLo:2700 mg/kg/60W-I
ZKKOBW 77,257,72

MUT: mma-esc 2500 mg/L   MUREAV 89,35,81
MUT: mma-sat 1 μg/plate   MUREAV 51,319,78

SAFETY PROFILE: Questionable carcinogen
with experimental tumorigenic data. Mutation
data reported. Many N-nitroso compounds are
carcinogens. When heated to decomposition it
emits toxic fumes of NO_x.

NLQ500   CAS: 1130-69-4
4-NITROSOQUINOLINE-1-OXIDE
mf: $C_9H_6N_2O_2$ mw: 174.17

TOXICITY DATA with REFERENCE
ETA: scu-mus TDLo:60 mg/kg/9W-I   GANNA2
69(4),499,78

SAFETY PROFILE: Questionable carcinogen
with experimental tumorigenic data. Many nitroso compounds are carcinogens. When heated
to decomposition it emits toxic fumes of NO_x.

NLS000   CAS: 13344-50-8
N-NITROSOSARCOSINE, ETHYL ESTER
mf: $C_5H_{10}N_2O_3$ mw: 146.17

SYN: NITROSO-SARKOSIN-AETHYLESTER

TOXICITY DATA with REFERENCE
CAR: orl-rat TD:160 g/kg/8W-I   JJIND8 71,75,83
ETA: ivn-rat TDLo:3900 mg/kg/39W-I   ZEKBAI
69,103,67

ETA: orl-rat TD:21 g/kg/8W-I   PUMTAG 16,355,82
ETA: orl-rat TD:9700 mg/kg/28W-C   ARZNAD
19,1077,69

ETA: orl-rat TD:9700 mg/kg/28W-C   ARZNAD
19,1077,69

ETA: orl-rat TDLo: 7900 mg/kg/23W-C
NATWAY 50,99,63

SAFETY PROFILE: Questionable carcinogen with experimental carcinogenic and tumorigenic data. Moderately toxic by ingestion and intravenous routes. Many N-nitroso compounds are carcinogens. When heated to decomposition it emits toxic fumes of NO_x.

NLT500 CAS: 40548-68-3
N-NITROSO-TETRAHYDRO-1,2-OXAZINE
mf: $C_4H_8N_2O_2$ mw: 116.14

SYNS: N-NITROSO-TETRAHYDROOXAZIN-1,2 (GERMAN) ◇ N-NITROSOTETRAHYDRO-1,2-OXAZIN ◇ 2-NITROSOTETRAHYDRO-2H-1,2-OXAZINE ◇ TETRAHYDRO-2-NITROSO-2H-1,2-OXAZINE

TOXICITY DATA with REFERENCE
CAR: orl-rat TDLo: 18 g/kg/63W-I ZKKOBW
79,114,73

SAFETY PROFILE: Questionable carcinogen with experimental carcinogenic data. Moderately toxic by ingestion. When heated to decomposition it emits toxic fumes of NO_x.

NLU000 CAS: 35627-29-3
N-NITROSO-TETRAHYDRO-1,3-OXAZINE
mf: $C_4H_8N_2O_2$ mw: 116.14

SYNS: N-NITROSOTETRAHYDROOXAZIN-1,3 (GERMAN) ◇ 3-NITROSO-TETRAHYDRO-1,3-OXAZINE

TOXICITY DATA with REFERENCE
CAR: orl-rat TDLo: 250 g/kg/50W-I CRNGDP
3,911,82
ETA: orl-rat TD: 2900 mg/kg/24W-I ZKKOBW
82,257,74
MUT: mma-sat 250 µg/plate TCMUE9 1,13,84

SAFETY PROFILE: Questionable carcinogen with experimental carcinogenic and tumorigenic data. Moderately toxic by ingestion. Mutation data reported. When heated to decomposition it emits toxic fumes of NO_x.

NLU480 CAS: 70501-82-5
N-NITROSO-1,2,3,4-TETRAHYDROPYRIDINE
mf: $C_5H_8N_2O$ mw: 112.15

SYNS: N-NITROSO-Δ²-PIPERIDINE ◇ N-NITROSO-Δ²-TETRAHYDROPYRIDINE ◇ 1-NITROSO-1,2,3,4-TETRAHYDROPYRIDINE

TOXICITY DATA with REFERENCE
ETA: orl-rat TDLo: 1250 mg/kg/25W-I CRNGDP
1,753,80
MUT: mma-sat 25 µg/plate TCMUD8 1,295,80
MUT: mmo-sat 25 µg/plate TCMUE9 1,13,84

SAFETY PROFILE: Questionable carcinogen with experimental tumorigenic data. Mutation data reported. When heated to decomposition it emits toxic fumes of NO_x.

NLU500 CAS: 55556-92-8
N-NITROSO-1,2,3,6-TETRAHYDROPYRIDINE
mf: $C_5H_8N_2O$ mw: 112.15

SYNS: N-NITROSO-Δ³-PIPERIDINE ◇ N-NITROSO-Δ³-TETRAHYDROPYRIDINE

TOXICITY DATA with REFERENCE
CAR: orl-rat TD: 50 mg/kg/2Y-I EESADV6,513,82
CAR: orl-rat TD: 1040 mg/kg/26W-I JNCIAM
57,1315,76
CAR: orl-rat TDLo: 33 mg/kg/25W-I EESADV
6,513,82
MUT: mma-sat 1 µg/plate MUREAV 51,319,78
MUT: mmo-sat 50 µg/plate TCMUE9 1,13,84

CONSENSUS REPORTS: EPA Genetic Toxicology Program.

SAFETY PROFILE: Questionable carcinogen with experimental carcinogenic data. Mutation data reported. When heated to decomposition it emits toxic fumes of NO_x.

NLW000 CAS: 26541-51-5
N-NITROSOTHIOMORPHOLINE
mf: $C_4H_8N_2OS$ mw: 132.20

SYN: 4-NITROSOTHIOMORPHOLINE

TOXICITY DATA with REFERENCE
CAR: orl-rat TDLo: 860 mg/kg/38W-I ZEKBAI
74,179,70
MUT: mma-sat 1 µmol/plate MUREAV 57,1,78

SAFETY PROFILE: Questionable carcinogen with experimental carcinogenic data. Mutation data reported. When heated to decomposition it emits very toxic fumes of NO_x and SO_x.

NLW500 CAS: 611-23-4
2-NITROSOTOLUENE
mf: C_7H_7NO mw: 121.15

PROP: Needles or prisms. Mp: 72.5°. Very sol in chloroform, alc, and ether.

SYNS: 1-METHYL-2-NITROSO-BENZENE (9CI)

◇ o-METHYLNITROSOBENZENE ◇ o-NITROSOTOLUENE

TOXICITY DATA with REFERENCE
CAR: orl-rat TDLo: 103 g/kg/73W-C   CALEDQ
16,103,82

MUT: mma-sat 5 μmol/plate   JMCMAR 22,981,79

SAFETY PROFILE: Questionable carcinogen with experimental carcinogenic data. Mutation data reported. Many nitroso compounds are carcinogens. When heated to decomposition it emits toxic fumes of NO_x.

NLX000   CAS: 71752-68-6
NITROSOTRIDECYLUREA
mf: $C_{14}H_{29}N_3O_2$ mw: 271.46

SYN: 1-NITROSO-1-TRIDECYLUREA

TOXICITY DATA with REFERENCE
ETA: skn-mus TDLo: 1085 mg/kg/50W-I
JCROD7 102,13,81

MUT: mma-sat 100 μg/plate   TCMUE9 1,13,84
MUT: mmo-sat 1 μg/plate   MUREAV 68,1,79

SAFETY PROFILE: Questionable carcinogen with experimental tumorigenic data. Mutation data reported. Many nitroso compounds are carcinogens. When heated to decomposition it emits toxic fumes of NO_x.

NLX500   CAS: 50285-70-6
NITROSOTRIETHYLUREA
mf: $C_7H_{15}N_3O_2$ mw: 173.25

SYNS: NITROSOTRIAETHYLHARNSTOFF (GERMAN)
◇ 1,1,3-TRIETHYL-3-NITROSOUREA

TOXICITY DATA with REFERENCE
CAR: orl-rat TDLo: 150 mg/kg   CRNGDP 9,573,88
NEO: ivn-rat TDLo: 150 mg/kg   CRNGDP
9,573,88
ETA: orl-ham TD: 1733 mg/kg/30W-I   IAPUDO
57,617,84
ETA: orl-ham TDLo: 1733 mg/kg/W-I   PAACA3
24,92,83
ETA: orl-rat TD: 1440 mg/kg/50W-I   ZEKBAI
83,315,75
ETA: orl-rat TD: 2079 mg/kg/33W-I   IAPUDO
57,617,84
ETA: orl-rat TD: 2550 mg/kg/31W-C   JJIND8
65,451,80
MUT: mma-sat 1 μg/plate   MUREAV 51,319,78

SAFETY PROFILE: Questionable carcinogen with experimental carcinogenic, neoplastigenic, and tumorigenic data. Mutation data reported. Many nitroso compounds are carcinogens. When heated to decomposition it emits toxic fumes of NO_x.

NLX700   CAS: 82018-90-4
N-NITROSO-2,2,2-
TRIFLUORODIETHYLAMINE
mf: $C_4H_7F_3N_2O$ mw: 156.13

SYN: N-NITROSO-2,2,2-TRIFLUOROETHYL-ETHYLAMINE

TOXICITY DATA with REFERENCE
CAR: orl-rat TD: 1305 mg/kg/44W-I   CRNGDP
4,755,83
CAR: orl-rat TDLo: 945 mg/kg/63W-I   CRNGDP
4,755,83
MUT: mma-sat 20 μmol/plate   CRNGDP 3,155,82

SAFETY PROFILE: Questionable carcinogen with experimental carcinogenic data. Moderately toxic by ingestion. Mutation data reported. When heated to decomposition it emits toxic fumes of F^- and NO_x.

NLY000   CAS: 16339-14-3
1-NITROSO-1,2,2-
TRIMETHYLHYDRAZINE
mf: $C_3H_9N_3O$ mw: 103.15

SYNS: N-NITROSOTRIMETHYLHYDRAZIN (GERMAN)
◇ N-NITROSO-N,N′,N′-TRIMETHYLHYDRAZINE

TOXICITY DATA with REFERENCE
ETA: orl-rat TDLo: 200 mg/kg/75W-C   ZEKBAI
69,103,67

SAFETY PROFILE: Questionable carcinogen with experimental tumorigenic data. Poison by ingestion. Many N-nitroso compounds are carcinogens. When heated to decomposition it emits very toxic fumes of NO_x.

NLY500   CAS: 62178-60-3
NITROSOTRIMETHYLPHENYL-N-
METHYLCARBAMATE
mf: $C_{11}H_{14}N_2O_3$ mw: 222.27

SYNS: LANDRIN, NITROSO DERIVATIVE ◇ N-METHYL-N-NITROSOCARBAMIC ACID, TRIMETHYLPHENYL ESTER
◇ NITROSO-LANDRIN

TOXICITY DATA with REFERENCE
CAR: orl-rat TDLo: 580 mg/kg/10W-I   EESADV
2,413,78
MUT: dnd-hmn: fbr 10 μmol/L   MUREAV 44,1,77
MUT: mma-sat 111 ng/plate   MUREAV 56,1,77

MUT: mmo-sat 1 μg/plate   MUREAV 68,1,79

SAFETY PROFILE: Questionable carcinogen with experimental carcinogenic data. Human mutation data reported. When heated to decomposition it emits toxic fumes of NO_x.

NLZ000   CAS: 69113-01-5
NITROSOTRIS(CHLOROETHYL)UREA
mf: $C_7H_{12}Cl_3N_3O_2$ mw: 276.57

SYN: 1-NITROSO-1,3,3-TRIS-(2-CHLOROETHYL)UREA

TOXICITY DATA with REFERENCE
ETA: orl-rat TDLo:95 mg/kg/17W-I   JCROD7 94,131,79

SAFETY PROFILE: Questionable carcinogen with experimental tumorigenic data. Many nitroso compounds are carcinogens. When heated to decomposition it emits very toxic fumes of Cl^- and NO_x.

NMA000   CAS: 71752-67-5
NITROSOUNDECYLUREA
mf: $C_{12}H_{25}N_3O_2$ mw: 243.40

SYN: N-NITROSO-N-UNDECYLUREA

TOXICITY DATA with REFERENCE
CAR: skn-mus TDLo:974 mg/kg/50W-I
  JCROD7 102,13,81
MUT: mma-sat 100 μg/plate   TCMUE9 1,13,84
MUT: mmo-sat 1 μg/plate   MUREAV 68,1,79

SAFETY PROFILE: Questionable carcinogen with experimental carcinogenic data. Mutation data reported. When heated to decomposition it emits toxic fumes of NO_x.

NMC000   CAS: 4003-94-5
4-NITROSTILBENE
mf: $C_{14}H_{11}NO_2$ mw: 225.26

SYN: 4-NITROSTILBEN (GERMAN)

TOXICITY DATA with REFERENCE
ETA: orl-rat TDLo:2700 mg/kg/57W-C
  NATWAY 42,128,55
MUT: mma-sat 5 μg/plate   CBINA8 26,11,79
MUT: mmo-sat 5 μg/plate   CBINA8 26,11,79

SAFETY PROFILE: Questionable carcinogen with experimental tumorigenic data. Mutation data reported. When heated to decomposition it emits toxic fumes of NO_x.

NMD500   CAS: 63021-48-7
7-(m-NITROSTYRYL)BENZ(c)ACRIDINE
mf: $C_{25}H_{16}N_2O_2$ mw: 376.43

SYN: m-NITROBENZYLIDENE-3,4-BENZ-9-METHYLACRIDINE

TOXICITY DATA with REFERENCE
ETA: scu-mus TDLo:200 mg/kg   VOONAW 1,52,55

SAFETY PROFILE: Questionable carcinogen with experimental tumorigenic data. When heated to decomposition it emits toxic fumes of NO_x.

NME000   CAS: 63021-49-8
7-(o-NITROSTYRYL)BENZ(c)ACRIDINE
mf: $C_{25}H_{16}N_2O_2$ mw: 376.43

SYN: o-NITROBENZYLIDENE-3,4-BENZ-9-METHYLACRIDINE

TOXICITY DATA with REFERENCE
ETA: scu-mus TDLo:200 mg/kg   VOONAW 1,52,55

SAFETY PROFILE: Questionable carcinogen with experimental tumorigenic data. When heated to decomposition it emits toxic fumes of NO_x.

NME500   CAS: 63021-50-1
7-(p-NITROSTYRYL)BENZ(c)ACRIDINE
mf: $C_{25}H_{16}N_2O_2$ mw: 376.43

SYN: p-NITROBENZYLIDENE-3,4-BENZ-9-METHYLACRIDINE

TOXICITY DATA with REFERENCE
ETA: scu-mus TDLo:200 mg/kg   VOONAW 1,52,55

SAFETY PROFILE: Questionable carcinogen with experimental tumorigenic data. When heated to decomposition it emits toxic fumes of NO_x.

NMF000   CAS: 63021-46-5
12-(m-NITROSTYRYL)BENZ(a)ACRIDINE
mf: $C_{25}H_{16}N_2O_2$ mw: 376.43

SYN: m-NITROBENZYLIDENE-1,2-BENZ-9-METHYLACRIDINE

TOXICITY DATA with REFERENCE
ETA: scu-mus TDLo:200 mg/kg   VOONAW 1,52,55

SAFETY PROFILE: Questionable carcinogen with experimental tumorigenic data. When heated to decomposition it emits toxic fumes of NO_x.

NMF500   CAS: 63021-47-6
12-(o-NITROSTYRYL)BENZ(a)ACRIDINE
mf: $C_{25}H_{16}N_2O_2$ mw: 376.43

SYN: o-NITROBENZYLIDENE-1,2-BENZ-9-METHYLACRI-
DINE

TOXICITY DATA with REFERENCE
ETA: scu-mus TDLo: 200 mg/kg   VOONAW
    1,52,55

SAFETY PROFILE: Questionable carcinogen
with experimental tumorigenic data. When
heated to decomposition it emits toxic fumes
of NO_x.

NMG000   CAS: 22188-15-4
12-(p-NITROSTYRYL)BENZ(a)ACRIDINE
mf: $C_{25}H_{16}N_2O_2$ mw: 376.43

SYN: p-NITROBENZYLIDENE-1,2-BENZ-9-METHYLACRI-
DINE

TOXICITY DATA with REFERENCE
ETA: scu-mus TDLo: 200 mg/kg   VOONAW
    1,52,55

SAFETY PROFILE: Questionable carcinogen
with experimental tumorigenic data. When
heated to decomposition it emits toxic fumes
of NO_x.

NMV450   CAS: 86451-37-8
NMDHP

SYNS: 3-(METHYLNITROSAMINO)-1,2-PROPANEDIOL
◇ N-NITROSOMETHYL(2,3-DIHYDROXYPROPYL)AMINE

TOXICITY DATA with REFERENCE
ETA: orl-rat TDLo: 580 mg/kg/40W-I   CALEDQ
    22,83,84
ETA: orl-rat TDLo: 2300 mg/kg/40W-I   JJIND8
    70,959,83
MUT: dns-rat: lvr 5 mmol/L   MUREAV 144,197,85
MUT: mma-sat 100 µg/plate   TCMUE9 1,13,84
MUT: mmo-sat 500 µg/plate   TCMUE9 1,13,84

SAFETY PROFILE: Questionable carcinogen
with experimental tumorigenic data. Mutation
data reported. Many N-nitroso compounds are
carcinogens. When heated to decomposition it
emits toxic fumes of NO_x.

NMV735   CAS: 27753-52-2
NONABROMOBIPHENYL
mf: $C_{12}HBr_9$ mw: 864.32

SYNS: 1,1-BIPHENYL, NONABROMO- ◇ BROMKAL 80-
9D

CAR: orl-mus TDLo: 4469 mg/kg/78W-C
    YACHDS 14,5541,86

CONSENSUS REPORTS: Reported in EPA
TSCA Inventory.

SAFETY PROFILE: Questionable carcinogen
with experimental carcinogenic data. When
heated to decomposition it emits toxic fumes
of Br^-.

NNA000   CAS: 63021-51-2
1-NONANOYLAZIRIDINE
mf: $C_{11}H_{21}NO$ mw: 183.33

SYN: NONANOYLETHYLENEIMINE

TOXICITY DATA with REFERENCE
NEO: scu-rat TD: 860 mg/kg/27W-I   BJPCAL
    9,306,54
NEO: scu-rat TDLo: 720 mg/kg/20W-I   BJPCAL
    9,306,54
ETA: scu-mus TDLo: 500 mg/kg/20W-I   BJPCAL
    9,306,54

SAFETY PROFILE: Questionable carcinogen
with experimental neoplastigenic and tumorigenic data. When heated to decomposition it
emits toxic fumes of NO_x.

NNL500   CAS: 8056-51-7
NORDIOL-28
mf: $C_{21}H_{28}O_2.C_{20}H_{24}O_2$ mw: 608.93

SYNS: DUOLUTON ◇ EDIWAL ◇ ETHINYL ESTRADIOL
mixed with NORGESTREL ◇ ETHINYLESTRADIOL mixed with
dl-NORGESTREL ◇ ETHINYLOESTRADIOL mixed with NOR-
GESTREL ◇ EUGYON ◇ FOLLINYL ◇ GRAVISTAT
◇ LO/OVRAL ◇ MICROGYNON ◇ MINIDRIL ◇ NEOGYNON
◇ NEOVLETTA ◇ NORDETTE ◇ NORDIOL ◇ NORGESTREL
mixed with ETHINYL ESTRADIOL ◇ dl-NORGESTREL mixed
with ETHINYLESTRADIOL ◇ ORASECRON ◇ OVIDON
◇ OVRAL ◇ OVRAL 21 ◇ OVRAL 28 ◇ OVRAN ◇ OVRANETT
◇ PRIMOVLAR ◇ PRO-DUOSTERONE ◇ RIGEVIDON
◇ SEQUILAR ◇ SEQUOSTAT ◇ SH 71121 ◇ SHB 261AB
◇ SHB 264AB ◇ STEDIRIL ◇ STEDIRIL D ◇ TRIQUILAR
◇ WL 20 ◇ WL 33 ◇ WY-E 104

TOXICITY DATA with REFERENCE
CAR: orl-wmn TD: 50 mg/kg/5Y-I: LIV
    JAMAAP 235,730,76
CAR: orl-wmn TDLo: 18144 µg/kg/12Y-I:
    LIV   LANCAO 1,273,80
NEO: orl-wmn TD: 5 mg/kg/26W-I: LIV
    LANCAO 2,926,73
NEO: orl-wmn TD: 756 µg/kg/26W-I: LIV
    MJAUAJ 2,223,78

SAFETY PROFILE: Questionable human carcinogen producing liver tumors. Human reproductive effects by ingestion: menstrual cycle changes or disorders, postpartum changes, mating performance, female fertility index and other fertility changes. Experimental reproductive effects. A steroid used as a pharmaceutical and veterinary drug. When heated to decomposition it emits acrid smoke and irritating fumes.

NNQ000   CAS: 3836-23-5
NORETHISTERONE ENANTHATE
mf: $C_{27}H_{38}O_3$ mw: 410.65

SYNS: 17-α-ETHINYL-19-NORTESTOSTERONE ENANTHATE ◇ 17-α-ETHYNYL-17-β-HEPTANOYLOXY-4-ESTREN-3-ONE ◇ 17-β-HEPTANOYLOXY-19-NOR-17-α-PREGNEN-20-YNONE ◇ NORETHISTERONE OENANTHATE ◇ NORIGEST ◇ NORLUTIN ENANTHATE ◇ SH 393

TOXICITY DATA with REFERENCE
NEO: ims-rat TDLo:7000 mg/kg/70W
  36PYAS-,163,77

SAFETY PROFILE: Questionable carcinogen with experimental tumorigenic data. An experimental teratogen. Human systemic effects by intravenous route: increased intraocular pressure. Human reproductive effects by intramuscular route: menstrual cycle changes or disorders, changes in female fertility. Experimental reproductive effects. When heated to decomposition it emits acrid smoke and irritating fumes.

NNQ500   CAS: 6533-00-2
NORGESTREL
mf: $C_{21}H_{28}O_2$ mw: 312.49

PROP: Crystals from diethyl ether-hexane. Mp: 142-143°.

SYNS: 13-ETHYL-17-α-ETHYNYLGON-4-EN-17-β-OL-3-ONE ◇ 13-ETHYL-17-α-ETHYNYL-17-β-HYDROXY-4-GONEN-3-ONE ◇ dl-13-β-ETHYL-17-α-ETHYNYL-17-β-HYDROXYGON-4-EN-3-ONE ◇ (±)-13-ETHYL-17-α-ETHYNYL-17-HYDROXYGON-4-EN-3-ONE ◇ dl-13-β-ETHYL-17-α-ETHYNYL-19-NORTESTOSTERONE ◇ (±)-13-ETHYL-17-HYDROXY-18,19-DINOR-17-α-PREGN-4-EN-20-YN-3-ONE ◇ 17-ETHYNYL-18-METHYL-19-NORTESTOSTERONE ◇ FH 122-A ◇ 17-β-HYDROXY-18-METHYL-19-NOR-17-α-PREGN-4-EN-20-YN-3-ONE ◇ LD NORGESTREL (FRENCH) ◇ 18-METHYL-17-α-ETHYNYL-19-NORTESTOSTERONE ◇ MONOVAR ◇ d(−)-NORGESTREL ◇ (±)-NORGESTREL ◇ α-NORGESTREL ◇ d-NORGESTREL ◇ dl-NORGESTREL ◇ POSTINOR ◇ SH 850 ◇ SH 70850 ◇ WY 3707

TOXICITY DATA with REFERENCE
NEO: orl-mus TDLo:29 mg/kg/69W-C
  CRSBAW 168,1190,74

CONSENSUS REPORTS: IARC Cancer Review: Animal Inadequate Evidence IMEMDT 6,201,74, IMEMDT 21,479,79; Human Inadequate Evidence IMEMDT 21,479,79.

SAFETY PROFILE: Questionable carcinogen with experimental neoplastigenic data. Human reproductive effects by ingestion and implant: menstrual cycle changes or disorders and female fertility index changes. Experimental reproductive effects. An oral contraceptive. When heated to decomposition it emits acrid smoke and irritating fumes.

NNQ520   CAS: 797-63-7
d(−)-NORGESTREL
mf: $C_{21}H_{28}O_2$ mw: 312.49

SYNS: 17-α-ETHINYL-13-β-ETHYL-17-β-HYDROXY-4-ESTREN-3-ONE ◇ 13-ETHYL-17-α-ETHYNYLGON-4-EN-17-β-OL-3-ONE ◇ 13-ETHYL-17-α-ETHYNYL-17-β-HYDROXY-4-GONEN-3-ONE ◇ 17-ETHYNYL-18-METHYL-19-NORTESTOSTERONE ◇ 17-β-HYDROXY-18-METHYL-19-NOR-17-α-PREGN-4-EN-20-YN-3-ONE ◇ 18-METHYL-17-α-ETHYNYL-19-NORTESTOSTERONE ◇ d-NORGESTREL ◇ D-NORGESTREL ◇ POSTINOR

TOXICITY DATA with REFERENCE
NEO: orl-mus TDLo:29 mg/kg/69W-C
  CRSBAW 168,1190,74

CONSENSUS REPORTS: IARC Cancer Review: Animal Inadequate Evidence IMEMDT 6,201,74; IMEMDT 21,479,79; Human Inadequate Evidence IMEMDT 21,479,79

SAFETY PROFILE: Questionable carcinogen with experimental neoplastigenic data. Human reproductive effects by ingestion: menstrual cycle changes, fertility index. When heated to decomposition it emits acrid smoke and irritating fumes.

NNR000
NORGESTREL mixed with MESTRANOL
SYN: MESTRANOL mixed with NORGESTREL

TOXICITY DATA with REFERENCE
CAR: orl-wmn TDLo:11 mg/kg/Y-I   JAMAAP
  235,730,76

SAFETY PROFILE: Questionable human carcinogen producing liver tumors.

NNT500   CAS: 472-54-8
19-NORPREGN-4-ENE-3,20-DIONE
mf: $C_{20}H_{28}O_2$ mw: 300.48

SYNS: 19-NOR-P ◊ 19-NORPROGESTERONE

TOXICITY DATA with REFERENCE
ETA: imp-mus TD:400 mg/kg/56W-C:TER
   JRPFA4 6,99,63
ETA: imp-mus TDLo:234 mg/kg/56W-C
   NATUAS 212,686,66

SAFETY PROFILE: Questionable carcinogen
with experimental tumorigenic and teratogenic
data. Experimental reproductive effects. When
heated to decomposition it emits acrid smoke
and irritating fumes.

NNV000   CAS: 52-76-6
19-NOR-17-α-PREGN-4-EN-20-YN-17-OL
mf: $C_{20}H_{28}O$ mw: 284.48

SYNS: 3-DESOXYNORLUTIN ◊ ETHINYLESTRENOL
◊ Δ⁴-17-α-ETHINYLESTREN-17-β-OL ◊ 17-α-ETHINYL-17-β-
HYDROXYESTR-4-ENE ◊ 17-α-ETHINYL-17-β-HYDROX-
YOESTR-4-ENE ◊ ETHINYLOESTRANOL ◊ ETHINYL
OESTRENOL ◊ Δ⁴-17-α-ETHINYLOESTREN-17-β-OL ◊ 17-α-
ETHYNIL-Δ⁴-ESTRENE-17-β-OL ◊ ETHYNYLESTRENOL ◊
17-α-ETHYNYLESTRENOL ◊ 17-α-ETHYNYLESTR-4-EN-17-
β-OL ◊ ETHYNLOESTRENOL ◊ 17-α-ETHYNYLOESTRENOL
◊ 17-α-ETHYNYLOESTR-4-EN-17-β-OL ◊ EXLUTEN ◊ EX-
LUTION ◊ EXLUTON ◊ EXLUTONA ◊ LINESTRENOL ◊
LYNENOL ◊ LYNESTRENOL ◊ LYNOESTRENOL ◊ (17-α)-
19-NORPREGN-4-EN-20-YN-17-OL ◊ NSC-37725 ◊ ORG 485-
50 ◊ ORGAMETIL ◊ ORGAMETRIL ◊ ORGAMETROL

CONSENSUS REPORTS: IARC Cancer Review: Animal Inadequate Evidence IMEMDT
21,407,79.

SAFETY PROFILE: Questionable carcinogen.
An experimental teratogen. Human reproductive
effects by ingestion and implant routes: menstrual cycle changes or disorders, female fertility
index and other fertility changes and effects on
females. Experimental reproductive effects.
Used in oral contraceptives and in the treatment
of dysfunctional uterine bleeding. When heated
to decomposition it emits acrid smoke and irritating fumes.

NOC400   CAS: 89911-79-5
NTPA
mf: $C_6H_{14}N_2O_4$ mw: 178.22

SYNS: 3-((2-HYDROXYPROPYL)NITROSAMINO)-1,2-PRO-
PANEDIOL ◊ N-NITROSO-2,3-DIHYDROXYPROPYL-2-HY-

DROXYPROPYLAMINE ◊ NITROSOTRIHYDROXY-DIPRO-
PYLAMINE

TOXICITY DATA with REFERENCE
CAR: orl-rat TD:720 mg/kg/24W-C   CRNGDP
   5,167,84
CAR: orl-rat TDLo:280 mg/kg/37W-C   CRNGDP
   5,167,84
ETA: orl-rat TD:3150 mg/kg/26W-C   CRNGDP
   5,167,84
MUT: mma-sat 25 μg/plate   TCMUE9 1,13,84

SAFETY PROFILE: Questionable carcinogen
with experimental carcinogenic and tumorigenic
data. Mutation data reported. When heated to
decomposition it emits toxic fumes of NO_x.

NOH000   CAS: 63428-83-1
NYLON
mf: $(C_6H_{11}NO)_n$

PROP: Crystalline solid. Sol in phenol, cresols,
xylene, and formic acid. Insol in alc, esters,
ketones, hydrocarbons. Film used for implant
study. (CNREA8 15,333,55).

SYNS: AMILAN ◊ ASHLENE ◊ CAPROLON ◊ ENKALON
◊ GRILON ◊ KAPRON ◊ MIRLON ◊ PERLON ◊ PHRILON
◊ POLYAMID (GERMAN) ◊ SILON ◊ TROGAMID T
◊ VYDYNE

TOXICITY DATA with REFERENCE
ETA: imp-rat TDLo:123 mg/kg   CNREA815,333,55

SAFETY PROFILE: Questionable carcinogen
with experimental tumorigenic data by implant.
When heated to decomposition it emits toxic
fumes of NO_x.

OAJ000   CAS: 3268-87-9
OCTACHLORODIBENZODIOXIN
mf: $C_{12}Cl_8O_2$ mw: 459.72

PROP: Colorless crystals. Mp: 239°.

SYNS: NCI-C03678 ◊ OCDD ◊ OCTACHLORODIBEN-
ZO(b,e)(1,4)DIOXIN ◊ OCTACHLORODIBENZO-p-DIOXIN
◊ 1,2,3,4,6,7,8,9-OCTACHLORODIBENZODIOXIN

TOXICITY DATA with REFERENCE
ETA: skn-mus TDLo:290 mg/kg/60W-I
   EVHPAZ 5,163,73

CONSENSUS REPORTS: IARC Cancer Review: Animal Inadequate Evidence IMEMDT
15,41,77.

SAFETY PROFILE: Questionable carcinogen
with experimental tumorigenic data. Poison by
ingestion. Experimental reproductive effects.

An eye irritant. When heated to decomposition it emits toxic fumes of Cl^-.

OAN000   CAS: 297-78-9
1,3,4,5,6,8,8-OCTACHLORO-1,3,3a,4,7,7a-HEXAHYDRO-4,7-METHANO ISOBENZOFURAN
mf: $C_9H_4Cl_8O$ mw: 411.73

SYNS: CP 14,957 ◇ ENT 25,545 ◇ ENT 25,545-X ◇ ISOBENZAN ◇ OCTACHLORO-HEXAHYDRO-METHANOISOBENZOFURAN ◇ 1,3,4,5,6,7,10,10-OCTACHLORO-4,7-endo-METHYLENE-4,7,8,9-TETRAHYDROPHTHALAN ◇ 1,3,4,5,6,7,8,8-OCTACHLORO-2-OXA-3a,4,7,7a-TETRAHYDRO-4,7-METHANOINDENE ◇ OMTAN ◇ R 6700 ◇ SD 4402 ◇ SHELL 4402 ◇ SHELL WL 1650 ◇ TELODRIN ◇ WL 1650

TOXICITY DATA with REFERENCE
ETA: orl-mus TDLo: 71 g/kg/78W-I   NTIS** PB223-159

SAFETY PROFILE: Questionable carcinogen with experimental tumorigenic data. Poison by ingestion, skin contact, intraperitoneal, intravenous, and possibly other routes. Used as an insecticide. When heated to decomposition it emits toxic fumes of Cl^-.

OAR000   CAS: 124-26-5
OCTADECANNAMIDE
mf: $C_{18}H_{37}NO$ mw: 283.56

SYNS: KEMAMIDE S ◇ STEARAMIDE

TOXICITY DATA with REFERENCE
ETA: imp-mus TDLo: 1000 mg/kg   CNREA8 26,105,66

CONSENSUS REPORTS: Reported in EPA TSCA Inventory.

SAFETY PROFILE: Questionable carcinogen with experimental tumorigenic data. When heated to decomposition it emits toxic fumes of NO_x.

OAX000   CAS: 112-92-5
1-OCTADECANOL
mf: $C_{18}H_{38}O$ mw: 270.56

PROP: Colorless solid or flakes. Mp: 58°, bp: 202° @ 10 mm, d: 0.8124 @ 59°/4°.

SYNS: ADOL ◇ ADOL 68 ◇ ATALCO S ◇ CO-1895 ◇ CO-1897 ◇ CRODACOL-S ◇ DECYL OCTYL ALCOHOL ◇ DYTOL E-46 ◇ LOROL 28 ◇ OCTADECANOL ◇ n-OCTADE-CANOL ◇ OCTA DECYL ALCOHOL ◇ n-OCTADECYL ALCOHOL ◇ POLAAX ◇ SIPOL S ◇ SIPONOL S ◇ STEAROL ◇ STEARYL ALCOHOL ◇ STERAFFINE ◇ USP XIII STEARYL ALCOHOL

TOXICITY DATA with REFERENCE
NEO: imp-mus TDLo: 1000 mg/kg   CNREA8 26,105,66

CONSENSUS REPORTS: Reported in EPA TSCA Inventory.

SAFETY PROFILE: Questionable carcinogen with experimental neoplastigenic data. Mildly toxic by ingestion. Flammable when exposed to heat or flame; can react with oxidizing materials. To fight fire, use foam, CO_2, dry chemical. When heated to decomposition it emits acrid smoke and irritating fumes.

OBW000   CAS: 63021-67-0
OCTAHYDRO-1:2:5:6-DIBENZANTHRACENE
mf: $C_{22}H_{22}$ mw: 286.44

SYN: OCTAHYDRODIBENZ(a,h)ANTHRACENE

TOXICITY DATA with REFERENCE
ETA: skn-mus TDLo: 1250 mg/kg/52W-I
PRLBA4 111,485,32

SAFETY PROFILE: Questionable carcinogen with experimental tumorigenic data. When heated to decomposition it emits acrid smoke and irritating fumes.

OBW509   CAS: 37394-33-5
2,5,5a,6,9,10,10a,1a-OCTAHYDRO-4-HYDROXYMETHYL-1,1,7,9-TETRAMETHYL-5,5a-6-TRIHYDROXY-1H-2,8a-METHANOCYCLOPENTA(a)CYCLOPROPA(e)CYCLODECEN-11-ONE-5-HEXADECANOATE
mf: $C_{36}H_{58}O_6$ mw: 586.94

SYN: INGENANE HEXADECANOATE

TOXICITY DATA with REFERENCE
ETA: skin-mus TDLo: 56 mg/kg/12W-I   85CVA2 5,213,70
MUT: skin-mus 82 ng MLD   85CVA2 5,213,70

SAFETY PROFILE: Questionable carcinogen with experimental tumorigenic data. A skin irritant. When heated to decomposition it emits acrid smoke and irritating fumes.

OBY000   CAS: 20917-49-1
OCTAHYDRO-1-NITROSOAZOCINE
mf: $C_7H_{14}N_2O$ mw: 142.23

SYNS: NHMI ◇ N-NITROSOAZACYCLOOCTANE
◇ NITROSOHEPTAMETHYLENEIMINE ◇ N-NITROSOHEP-
TAMETHYLENEIMINE ◇ NITROSO-HEPTAMETHYLENIMIN
(GERMAN)

TOXICITY DATA with REFERENCE
CAR: scu-ham TD:760 mg/kg/46W-I   JJIND8
  61,239,78
CAR: scu-ham TDLo:650 mg/kg/59W-I   JJIND8
  61,239,78
ETA: orl-ham TDLo:2000 mg/kg/50W-I
  ZEKBAI 74,185,70
ETA: orl-rat TD:495 mg/kg/22W-I   PSEBAA
  130,945,69
ETA: orl-rat TD:1350 mg/kg/30W-I   ZKKOBW
  77,257,72
ETA: orl-rat TDLo:150 mg/kg/20W-I   IJCNAW
  15,301,75
ETA: scu-rat TDLo:133 mg/kg/4W-I   IJCNAW
  15,301,75
MUT: mma-esc 16700 μmol/L   CNREA836,4099,76
MUT: mma-sat 10 μg/plate   TCMUE9 1,13,84
MUT: orl-rat TD:1200 mg/kg/20W-I   ANTRD4
  2,381,82
MUT: otr-rat-orl 150 mg/kg   JJIND8 67,1057,81
MUT: pic-esc 50 mg/L   TCMUE9 1,91,84
MUT: scu-ham TD:66 mg/kg/W-I   AJPAA4
  93,45,78

SAFETY PROFILE: Questionable carcinogen
with experimental carcinogenic and tumorigenic
data. Poison by ingestion and subcutaneous
routes. Mutation data reported. When heated
to decomposition it emits toxic fumes of NO_x.

OCA000   CAS: 20917-50-4
OCTAHYDRO-1-NITROSO-1H-AZONINE
mf: $C_8H_{16}N_2O$ mw: 156.26

SYNS: N-NITROSOAZACYCLONONANE ◇ N-NITRO-
SOOCTAMETHYLENEIMINE

TOXICITY DATA with REFERENCE
ETA: orl-rat TDLo:742 mg/kg/33W-I   PSEBAA
  130,945,69
MUT: mma-sat 10 μg/plate   TCMUE9 1,13,84
MUT: pic-esc 10 mg/L   TCMUE9 1,91,84

SAFETY PROFILE: Questionable carcinogen
with experimental tumorigenic data. Moderately
toxic by ingestion. Mutation data reported.
Many N-nitroso compounds are carcinogens.
When heated to decomposition it emits toxic
fumes of NO_x.

OGK000   CAS: 8015-79-0
OIL of CALAMUS, GERMAN

PROP: Extract of *Acorus calamus L., araceae.*
Containing: asarone, eugenol; esters of acetic
and heptylic acids. Volatile oil. Yellow to yel-
lowish-brown liquid (viscid); aromatic odor, bitter taste. D: 0.960-0.9707 @ 20°/20°. Very sltly
sol in water, misc with alc. Keep well closed,
cool, and protected from light.

SYNS: CALAMUS OIL ◇ KALMUS OEL (GERMAN)
◇ OIL of SWEET FLAG

TOXICITY DATA with REFERENCE
ETA: orl-rat TD:11 g/kg/59W-C   TXAPA9
  10,405,67
ETA: orl-rat TD:21 g/kg/59W-C   PAACA38,24,67
ETA: orl-rat TD:52 g/kg/59W-C   PAACA38,24,67
ETA: orl-rat TD:103 g/kg/59W-C   PAACA3
  8,24,67
ETA: orl-rat TDLo:10 g/kg/59W-C   PAACA3
  8,24,67

CONSENSUS REPORTS: Reported in EPA
TSCA Inventory.

SAFETY PROFILE: Questionable carcinogen
with experimental tumorigenic data. Poison by
intraperitoneal route. Moderately toxic by ingestion. When heated to decomposition it emits
acrid smoke and irritating fumes.

OGO000   CAS: 8008-26-2
OIL of LIME, DISTILLED

PROP: From distillation of juice or crushed
fruit of *Citrus aurantofolia* Swingle. Colorless
to green-yellow liquid. Sol in fixed oils, mineral
oil; insol glycerin, propylene glycol.

SYNS: DISTILLED LIME OIL ◇ LIME OIL ◇ LIME OIL,
DISTILLED (FCC) ◇ OILS, LIME

TOXICITY DATA with REFERENCE
ETA: orl-mus TDLo:67 g/kg/39W-I   JNCIAM
  35,771,65
MUT: dnr-bcs 20 mg/disc   TOFOD5 8,91,85

CONSENSUS REPORTS: Reported in EPA
TSCA Inventory.

SAFETY PROFILE: Questionable carcinogen
with experimental tumorigenic data. Mutation
data reported. A skin irritant. When heated to
decomposition it emits acrid smoke and irritating
fumes.

OGS000
OIL of MUSTARD, EXPRESSED mixed with OIL of ARGEMONE

PROP: Mustard oil mixed with 0.5% argemone oil (IJMRAQ 61,428,73).

SYNS: ARGEMONE OIL mixed with MUSTARD OIL ◇ OIL of ARGEMONE mixed with OIL of MUSTARD

TOXICITY DATA with REFERENCE
ETA: scu-mus TDLo:300 g/kg/32W-I   IJMRAQ 61,428,73
ETA: skn-mus TDLo:2564 g/kg/92W-C
IJCNAW 10,652,72

SAFETY PROFILE: Questionable carcinogen with experimental tumorigenic data. When heated to decomposition it emits acrid smoke and irritating fumes.

OGY000   CAS: 8008-57-9
OIL of ORANGE

PROP: Yellow to deep-orange liquid; characteristic orange taste and odor. D: 0.842-0.846 @ 25°/25°, refr index: 1.472 @ 20°. Sol in 2 vols 90% alc, in 1 vol glacial acetic acid; sltly sol in water; misc with abs alc, carbon disulfide. Keep well closed, cool, and protected from light. Oil expressed from the peel of *Citrus sinensis* L. Osbeck (Fam. *Rutaceae*) (BJCAAI 13,92,59).

SYNS: NEAT OIL of SWEET ORANGE ◇ OIL of SWEET ORANGE ◇ ORANGE OIL ◇ ORANGE OIL, COLDPRESSED (FCC) ◇ SWEET ORANGE OIL

TOXICITY DATA with REFERENCE
NEO: orl-mus TDLo:67 g/kg/40W-I   JNCIAM 35,771,65

CONSENSUS REPORTS: Reported in EPA TSCA Inventory.

SAFETY PROFILE: Questionable carcinogen with experimental neoplastigenic data. A skin irritant. When heated to decomposition it emits acrid smoke and irritating fumes.

OHA000   CAS: 85-86-9
OIL RED
mf: $C_{22}H_{16}N_4O$ mw: 352.42

SYNS: BENZENEAZOBENZENEAZO-β-NAPHTHOL ◇ CERASINROT ◇ C.I. SOLVENT RED 23 ◇ D&C RED NO. 17 ◇ FETTSCHARLACH ◇ OIL SCARLET ◇ ORGANOL SCARLET ◇ 1-((4-(PHENYLAZO)PHENYL)AZO)-2-NAPHTHALENOL ◇ 1-(p-PHENYLAZOPHENYLAZO)-2-NAPHTHOL

◇ ROUGE CERASINE ◇ SOMALIA RED III ◇ SUDAN III ◇ TETRAZOBENZENE-β-NAPHTHOL ◇ TONY RED

TOXICITY DATA with REFERENCE
MUT: cyt-ham:ovr 20 μmol/L/5H-C   ENMUDM 1,27,79

CONSENSUS REPORTS: IARC Cancer Review: GROUP 3 IMEMDT 7,56,87; Animal Inadequate Evidence IMEMDT 8,241,75. Reported in EPA TSCA Inventory.

SAFETY PROFILE: Questionable carcinogen. Poison by intraperitoneal route. Moderately toxic by subcutaneous and intrapleural routes. Mutation data reported. When heated to decomposition it emits toxic fumes of NO_x.

OHK000   CAS: 6370-43-0
OIL YELLOW HA
mf: $C_{14}H_{14}N_2O$ mw: 226.30

SYNS: C.I. 11860 ◇ C.I. SOLVENT YELLOW 12 ◇ OIL YELLOW OPS ◇ OLEAL YELLOW RE

TOXICITY DATA with REFERENCE
ETA: scu-mus TDLo:6000 mg/kg/57W-I
GMJOAZ 30,364,49

SAFETY PROFILE: Questionable carcinogen with experimental tumorigenic data. When heated to decomposition it emits toxic fumes of NO_x.

OHU000   CAS: 112-80-1
OLEIC ACID
mf: $C_{18}H_{34}O_2$ mw: 282.52

PROP: Colorless liquid; odorless when pure. Mp: 6°, bp: 360.0°, flash p: 372°F (CC), d: 0.895 @ 25°/25°, autoign temp: 685°F, vap press: 1 mm @ 176.5°, bp: 286° @ 100 mm. Insol in water; misc in alc and ether.

SYNS: CENTURY CD FATTY ACID ◇ EMERSOL 210 ◇ EMERSOL 213 ◇ EMERSOL 6321 ◇ EMERSOL 233LL ◇ EMERSOL 221 LOW TITER WHITE OLEIC ACID ◇ EMERSOL 220 WHITE OLEIC ACID ◇ GLYCON RO ◇ GLYCON WO ◇ GROCO 2 ◇ GROCO 4 ◇ GROCO 5L ◇ HY-PHI 1055 ◇ HY-PHI 1088 ◇ HY-PHI 2066 ◇ HY-PHI 2088 ◇ HY-PHI 2102 ◇ INDUSTRENE 105 ◇ INDUSTRENE 205 ◇ INDUSTRENE 206 ◇ K 52 ◇ l'ACIDE OLEIQUE (FRENCH) ◇ METAUPON ◇ NEO-FAT 90-04 ◇ NEO-FAT 92-04 ◇ cis-Δ⁹-OCTADECENOIC ACID ◇ cis-OCTADEC-9-ENOIC ACID ◇ cis-9-OCTADECENOIC ACID ◇ 9,10-OCTADECENOIC ACID ◇ PAMOLYN ◇ RED OIL ◇ TEGO-OLEIC 130 ◇ VOPCOLENE 27 ◇ WECOLINE OO ◇ WOCHEM NO. 320

TOXICITY DATA with REFERENCE
ETA: scu-rbt TDLo:390 mg/kg/17W-I

CRSBAW 137,760,43

MUT: cyt-ham:fbr 2500 μg/L   CRNGDP 3,499,82
MUT: cyt-smc 100 mg/L   NATUAS 294,263,81
MUT: dns-mus-rec 35 mg/kg   CALEDQ 23,253,84

CONSENSUS REPORTS: Reported in EPA
TSCA Inventory.

SAFETY PROFILE: Questionable carcinogen
with experimental tumorigenic data. Poison by
intravenous route. Mildly toxic by ingestion.
Mutation data reported. A human and experimental skin irritant. Combustible when exposed
to heat or flame. To fight fire, use CO_2, dry
chemical. When heated to decomposition it
emits acrid smoke and irritating fumes.

OHW000   CAS: 112-62-9
cis-OLEIC ACID, METHYL ESTER
mf: $C_{19}H_{36}O_2$ mw: 296.55

PROP: Oil. D: 0.874 @ 20°/4°, bp: 168-170°.
Insol in water; misc in alc and ether.

SYNS: EMEREST 2301 ◇ EMEREST 2801 ◇ EMERY 2219
◇ EMERY 2310 ◇ EMERY OLEIC ACID ESTER 2301
◇ KEMESTER 105 ◇ KEMESTER 115 ◇ KEMESTER 205
◇ KEMESTER 213 ◇ METHYL-9-OCTADECENOATE
◇ METHYL cis-9-OCTADECENOATE ◇ METHYL (Z)-9-OCTA-
DECENOATE ◇ METHYL OLEATE ◇ (Z)-9-OCTADECENOIC
ACID METHYL ESTER

TOXICITY DATA with REFERENCE
ETA: skn-mus TDLo:54 g/kg/45W-I   AMBPBZ
82,127,74

CONSENSUS REPORTS: Reported in EPA
TSCA Inventory.

SAFETY PROFILE: Questionable carcinogen
with experimental tumorigenic data by skin contact. When heated to decomposition it emits
acrid smoke and irritating fumes.

OIC000   CAS: 63021-11-4
1-OLEOYLAZIRIDINE
mf: $C_{20}H_{37}NO$ mw: 307.58

SYN: OLEOYLETHYLENEIMINE

TOXICITY DATA with REFERENCE
NEO: scu-rat TDLo:1700 mg/kg/49D-I   BJPCAL
9,306,54

SAFETY PROFILE: Questionable carcinogen
with experimental neoplastigenic data. When

heated to decomposition it emits toxic fumes
of NO_x.

OJV525
OROTIC ACID mixed with
CHOLESTEROL and CHOLIC ACID
(2:2:1)
SYNS: CHOLESTEROL mixed with OROTIC ACID mixed
with CHOLIC ACID (2:2:1) ◇ CHOLIC ACID mixed with CHO-
LESTEROL mixed with OROTIC ACID (1:2:2)

TOXICITY DATA with REFERENCE
ETA: orl-rat TDLo:585 g/kg/56W-C   DABBBA
41,515,80

SAFETY PROFILE: Questionable carcinogen
with experimental tumorigenic data. When
heated to decomposition it emits acrid smoke
and irritating fumes.

OLG000   CAS: 63042-11-5
OXALYL-o-AMINOAZOTOLUENE
mf: $C_{16}H_{15}N_3O_3$ mw: 297.34

SYNS: 2'-METHYL-4'-(o-TOLYLAZO)OXANILIC ACID
◇ 4'-OXALYLAMINO-2,3'-DIMETHYLAZOBENZENE

TOXICITY DATA with REFERENCE
ETA: orl-rat TDLo:20 g/kg/17W-C   GANNA2
32,232,38

SAFETY PROFILE: Questionable carcinogen
with experimental tumorigenic data. When
heated to decomposition it emits toxic fumes
of NO_x.

OMM000   CAS: 497-25-6
2-OXAZOLIDINONE
mf: $C_3H_5NO_2$ mw: 87.09

SYNS: (2-HYDROXYETHYL)CARBAMIC ACID,γ-LAC-
TONE ◇ OXAZOLIDONE

TOXICITY DATA with REFERENCE
ETA: ipr-mus TDLo:400 mg/kg   BCPCA62,168,59
ETA: orl-mus TDLo:1000 mg/kg   BCPCA6
2,168,59

SAFETY PROFILE: Questionable carcinogen
with experimental tumorigenic data. When
heated to decomposition it emits toxic fumes
of NO_x.

OMW000   CAS: 503-30-0
OXETANE
mf: C_3H_6O mw: 58.09

PROP: Oil; agreeable odor. D: 0.8930 @ 25°/
4°, bp: 480 @ 750 mm.

SYNS: 1,3-PROPYLENE OXIDE ◇ TRIMETHYLENE OXIDE ◇ TRIMETHYLENOXID (GERMAN)

TOXICITY DATA with REFERENCE
ETA: scu-rat TDLo: 2240 mg/kg/56W-I ZEKBAI 74,241,70

CONSENSUS REPORTS: Reported in EPA TSCA Inventory.

SAFETY PROFILE: Questionable carcinogen with experimental tumorigenic data. Moderately toxic by subcutaneous route. May be narcotic in high concentrations. When heated to decomposition it emits acrid smoke and irritating fumes.

OMY800
3-N-OXIDE PURIN-6-THIOL MONOHYDRATE
mf: $C_5H_4N_4OS \cdot H_2O$ mw: 186.21

SYN: 6-MERCAPTOPURINE 3-N-OXIDE MONOHYDRATE

TOXICITY DATA with REFERENCE
NEO: scu-rat TDLo: 6500 mg/kg/26W-I
CNREA8 27,925,67

SAFETY PROFILE: Questionable carcinogen with experimental neoplastigenic data. When heated to decomposition it emits toxic fumes of NO_x and SO_x.

ONC000   CAS: 61695-72-5
7-OXIRANYLBENZ(a)ANTHRACENE
mf: $C_{20}H_{14}O$ mw: 270.34

SYNS: BENZ(a)ANTHRACEN-7-YL-OXIRANE ◇ 7-BEN-ZANTHRYLOXIRANE ◇ 7-(EPOXYEHTYL)-BENZ(a)AN-THRACENE

TOXICITY DATA with REFERENCE
ETA: scu-rat TDLo: 11 mg/kg/40D-I CALEDQ 1,339,76
MUT: dnd-omi 1100 μmol/L CNREA8 38,3247,78
MUT: mmo-sat 1 nmol/plate CNREA8 38,3247,78

CONSENSUS REPORTS: EPA Genetic Toxicology Program.

SAFETY PROFILE: Questionable carcinogen with experimental tumorigenic data. Mutation data reported. When heated to decomposition it emits acrid smoke and irritating fumes.

ONE000   CAS: 61695-69-0
6-OXIRANYLBENZO(a)PYRENE
mf: $C_{22}H_{14}O$ mw: 294.36

TOXICITY DATA with REFERENCE
ETA: scu-rat TDLo: 12 mg/kg/40D-I CALEDQ 1,339,76

SAFETY PROFILE: Questionable carcinogen with experimental tumorigenic data. When heated to decomposition it emits acrid smoke and irritating fumes.

ONG000   CAS: 61695-74-7
1-OXIRANYLPYRENE
mf: $C_{18}H_{12}O$ mw: 244.30

SYNS: 1-EPOXYETHYLPYRENE ◇ 1-PYRENYLOXIRANE

TOXICITY DATA with REFERENCE
ETA: skn-mus TDLo: 977 μg/kg CNREA8 40,642,80
MUT: dnd-mam: lym 1790 μmol/L BBRCA9 82,929,78
MUT: dnd-omi 27 μmol/L CNREA8 38,3247,78
MUT: mmo-sat 100 pmol/plate CNREA8 40,642,80
MUT: msc-ham: lng 100 μg/L IJCNAW 24,203,79

CONSENSUS REPORTS: EPA Genetic Toxicology Program.

SAFETY PROFILE: Questionable carcinogen with experimental tumorigenic data. Mutation data reported. When heated to decomposition it emits acrid smoke and irritating fumes.

ONO000   CAS: 566-28-9
7-OXOCHOLESTEROL
mf: $C_{27}H_{44}O_2$ mw: 400.71

SYNS: 3-β-HYDROXYCHOLEST-5-EN-7-ONE (8CI) ◇ (3-β)3-HYDROXYCHOLEST-5-EN-7-ONE (9CI) ◇ 7-KETO-CHOLESTEROL ◇ SC 4722

TOXICITY DATA with REFERENCE
ETA: scu-mus TDLo: 600 mg/kg/72W-I
JNCIAM 19,977,57

SAFETY PROFILE: Questionable carcinogen with experimental tumorigenic data. When heated to decomposition it emits acrid smoke and irritating fumes.

OOA000   CAS: 5100-91-4
8-OXO-8H-ISOCHROMENO(4',3': 4,5)PYRROLO(2,3-f)QUINOLINE
mf: $C_{18}H_{10}N_2O_2$ mw: 286.30

TOXICITY DATA with REFERENCE
ETA: scu-mus TDLo: 72 mg/kg/9W-I SCIEAS 158,387,67

SAFETY PROFILE: Questionable carcinogen with experimental tumorigenic data. When

heated to decomposition it emits toxic fumes of NO$_x$.

OOE000   CAS: 1949-20-8
OXOLAMINE CITRATE
mf: $C_{14}H_{19}N_3O \cdot C_6H_8O_7$ mw:437.50

PROP: Crystals. Sltly sol in water and alc.

SYNS: 5-β-DIETHYLAMINOETHYL-3-PHENYL-1,2,4-OX-
ADIAZOLE CITRATE ◊ 3-PHENYL-5-(β-(DIETHYLAMINO)
ETHYL)-1,2,4-OXADIAZOLE CITRATE

TOXICITY DATA with REFERENCE
CAR: orl-rat TDLo: 15 g/kg/1Y-I   EMPSAL 2,1,63

SAFETY PROFILE: Questionable carcinogen with experimental carcinogenic and teratogenic data. Poison by intraperitoneal route. Moderately toxic by ingestion. Experimental reproductive effects. When heated to decomposition it emits toxic fumes of NO$_x$.

OPI200
2,2′-OXYBIS(6-OXABICYCLO(3.1.0) HEXANE) mixed with 2,2-BIS(p-(2,3-EPOXYPROPOXY)PHENYL)PROPANE

SYNS: ARALDITE 6010 mixed with ERR 4205 (1:1)
◊ BIS(2,3-EPOXYCYCLOPENTYL) ETHER mixed with DIGLY-
CIDYL ETHER of BISPHENOL A (1:1) ◊ 2,2-BIS(p-(2,3-EPOXY-
PROPOXY)PHENYL)PROPANE mixed with 2,2′-OXYBIS(6-
OXABICYCLO(3.1.0)HEXANE) ◊ DIGLYCIDYL ETHER of
BISPHENOL A mixed with BIS(2,3-EPOXYCYCLOPENTYL)
ETHER (1:1) ◊ EPI-REZ 508 mixed with ERR 4205 (1:1)
◊ EPON 828 mixed with ERR 4205 (1:1) ◊ ERR 4205 mixed
with ARALDITE 6010 (1:1) ◊ ERR 4205 mixed with EPI-REZ
508 (1:1) ◊ ERR 4205 mixed with EPON 828 (1:1)

TOXICITY DATA with REFERENCE
ETA: skn-mus TD: 142 g/kg/2Y-I   NTIS** ORNL-
5762
ETA: skn-mus TDLo: 72 g/kg/2Y-I   NTIS**
ORNL-5762

SAFETY PROFILE: Questionable carcinogen with experimental tumorigenic data. When heated to decomposition it emits acrid smoke and irritating fumes.

ORG000   CAS: 67-47-0
5-OXYMETHYLFURFUROLE
mf: $C_6H_6O_3$ mw: 126.12

SYNS: HMF ◊ 5-HYDROXYMETHYLFURALDEHYDE
◊ 5-(HYDROXYMETHYL)-2-FURANCARBOXALDEHYDE
◊ 5-(HYDROXYMETHYL)FURFURAL ◊ HYDROXY-
METHYLFURFUROLE

TOXICITY DATA with REFERENCE
ETA: scu-rat TDLo: 200 mg/kg   JNCIAM 47,1037,71

CONSENSUS REPORTS: Reported in EPA TSCA Inventory.

SAFETY PROFILE: Questionable carcinogen with experimental tumorigenic data. When heated to decomposition it emits acrid smoke and irritating fumes.

ORW000   CAS: 10028-15-6
OZONE
af: O_3 aw: 48.00

PROP: Unstable colorless gas or dark blue liquid; characteristic odor. Mp: $-193°$, bp: $-111.9°$, d (gas): 2.144 g/L, 1.71 @ $-183°$. D: (liquid) 1.614 g/mL @ $-195.4°$.

SYNS: OZON (POLISH) ◊ TRIATOMIC OXYGEN

TOXICITY DATA with REFERENCE
NEO: ihl-mus TCLo: 5 ppm/2H/75D-I   AEHLAU
20,16,70
ETA: ihl-mus TC: 608 μg/m^3/24W-I   JJIND8
75,771,85
MUT: cyt-ham-ihl 200 ppb/5H   ENVRAL 4,262,71
MUT: cyt-hmn: leu 7230 ppb/36H   ENVRAL
12,188,76
MUT: cyt-rat-ihl 28 mg/m^3/5D-C   GISAAA
44(9),12,79
MUT: dlt-oin-ihl 30 ppm/3H-C   ENMUDM 4,657,82
MUT: dnd-omi 3300 nmol/L   BBACAQ 655,323,81
MUT: dni-ham: lng 2 ppm/1H   JTEHD6 17,119,86
MUT: dnr-esc 50 ppm/30M   BBRCA9 77,220,77
MUT: mmo-esc 100 ppb/20M   MEHYDY 4,165,78
MUT: sce-hmn: lng 250 ppb/1H-C   ENVRAL
18,336,79

CONSENSUS REPORTS: Reported in EPA TSCA Inventory. EPA Genetic Toxicology Program.

OSHA PEL: (Transitional: TWA 0.1 ppm) TWA 0.1 ppm; STEL 0.3 ppm   ACGIH TLV: TWA CL 0.1 ppm   DFG MAK: 0.1 ppm (0.2 mg/m^3)

SAFETY PROFILE: Questionable carcinogen with experimental neoplastigenic, tumorigenic, and teratogenic data. A human poison by inhalation. Human systemic effects by inhalation: visual field changes, lacrimation, headache, decreased pulse rate with fall in blood pressure, blood pressure decrease, dermatitis, cough, dyspnea, respiratory stimulation and other pulmonary changes. Experimental reproductive effects. Human mutation data reported. A skin, eye, upper respiratory system and mucous membrane irritant. A powerful oxidizing agent. A severe explosion hazard in liquid form when shocked, exposed to heat or flame, or in concentrated form by chemical reaction with powerful reducing agents.

PAD500 CAS: 7647-10-1
PALLADIUM(2$^+$) CHLORIDE
mf: Cl_2Pd mw: 177.30

PROP: Dark brown, deliquescent crystals. D: 4.0 @ 18°, mp: 678-680° (decomp). Sol in water, alc, acetone, and hydrochloric acid.

SYNS: NCI-C60184 ◇ PALLADIUM CHLORIDE ◇ PALLADOUS CHLORIDE

TOXICITY DATA with REFERENCE
CAR: orl-mus TDLo:880 mg/kg/75W-C
JONUAI 101,1431,71
MUT: dni-hmn:lym 600 μmol/L IAAAAM
79,83,86

CONSENSUS REPORTS: Reported in EPA TSCA Inventory. EPA Genetic Toxicology Program.

SAFETY PROFILE: Questionable carcinogen with experimental carcinogenic data. Poison by ingestion, intraperitoneal, intravenous, and intratracheal routes. Experimental reproductive effects. Human mutation data reported. A skin irritant. When heated to decomposition it emits highly toxic fumes of Cl$^-$.

PAE250 CAS: 57-10-3
PALMITIC ACID
mf: $C_{17}H_{32}O_2$ mw: 256.48

PROP: Colorless plates or white crystalline powder; slt characteristic odor and taste. D: 0.849 @ 70°/4°, mp: 63-64°, bp: 271.5° @ 100 mm. Insol in water; very sltly sol in petr ether; sol in absolute ether, chloroform.

SYNS: CETYLIC ACID ◇ EMERSOL 140 ◇ EMERSOL 143 ◇ HEXADECANOIC ACID ◇ n-HEXADECOIC ACID ◇ HEXADECYLIC ACID ◇ HYDROFOL ◇ HYSTRENE 8016 ◇ INDUSTRENE 4516 ◇ 1-PENTADECANECARBOXYLIC ACID

TOXICITY DATA with REFERENCE
NEO: imp-mus TDLo:1000 mg/kg CNREA8
26,105,66

CONSENSUS REPORTS: Reported in EPA TSCA Inventory.

SAFETY PROFILE: Questionable carcinogen with experimental neoplastigenic data. A poison by intravenous route. A human skin irritant. When heated to decomposition it emits acrid smoke and irritating fumes.

PAE750 CAS: 12174-11-7
PALYGORSCITE
SYNS: ATTAPULGITE ◇ PALYGORSKIT (GERMAN)

TOXICITY DATA with REFERENCE
NEO: ipr-rat TDLo:338 mg/kg/2W-I ZHPMAT
162,467,76
ETA: imp-rat TDLo:200 mg/kg JJIND8 67,965,81

SAFETY PROFILE: Questionable carcinogen with experimental neoplastigenic and tumorigenic data by implant route. When heated to decomposition it emits acrid smoke and irritating fumes.

PAF500 CAS: 804-36-4
PANAZONE
mf: $C_{14}H_{12}N_6O_6$ mw: 360.32

SYNS: 1,5-BIS(5-NITRO-2-FURANYL)-1,4-PENTADIEN-3-ONE, (AMINOIMINOMETHYL)HYDRAZONE ◇ BIS(5-NITRO-FURFURYLIDENE)ACETONE GUANYLHYDRAZONE ◇ sym-BIS(5-NITRO-2-FURFURYLIDENE) ACETONE GUA-NYLHYDRAZONE ◇ 1,5-BIS(5-NITRO-2-FURYL)-3-PENTA-DIENONE AMIDINONHYDRAZONE ◇ 1,5-BIS(5-NITRO-2-FURYL)-3-PENTADIENONE GUANYLHYDRAZONE ◇ DIFURAN ◇ DIFURAZONE ◇ ((3-(5-NITRO-2-FURYL)-1--(2-(5-NITRO-2-FURYL)VINYL)ALLYIDENE)AMINO) GUANIDINE ◇ PAYZONE

CONSENSUS REPORTS: IARC Cancer Review: GROUP 3 IMEMDT 7,117,87; Animal Inadequate Evidence IMEMDT 31,185,83.

SAFETY PROFILE: Questionable carcinogen. Poison by intraperitoneal route. Moderately toxic by subcutaneous route. Mildly toxic by ingestion. A growth promoter in chickens. When heated to decomposition it emits very toxic fumes of NO$_x$.

PAH750 CAS: 8002-74-2
PARAFFIN
PROP: Colorless or white, translucent wax; odorless. D: approx 0.90, mp: 50-57°. Insol in water, alc; sol in benzene, chloroform, ether, carbon disulfide, oils; misc with fats.

SYNS: PARAFFIN WAX ◇ PARAFFIN WAX FUME (ACGIH)

TOXICITY DATA with REFERENCE
ETA: imp-mus TD: 560 mg/kg   BJURAN 36,225,64
ETA: imp-mus TD: 640 mg/kg   BJCAAI 17,127,63
ETA: imp-mus TD: 660 mg/kg   CALEDQ 6,21,79
ETA: imp-mus TDLo: 480 mg/kg   85DAAC 5,170,66
ETA: imp-rat TDLo: 120 mg/kg   CNREA8 33,1225,73

CONSENSUS REPORTS: Reported in EPA TSCA Inventory.

OSHA PEL: Fume: TWA 2 mg/m^3 (fume)
  ACGIH TLV: Fume: TWA 2 mg/m^3 (fume)

SAFETY PROFILE: Questionable carcinogen with experimental tumorigenic data by implant route.

PAH810   CAS: 63449-39-8
PARAFFIN WAXES and HYDROCARBON WAXES, CHLORINATED (C23, 43% CHLORINE)

SYN: CHLORINATED PARAFFINS (C23, 43% CHLORINE)

TOXICITY DATA with REFERENCE
CAR: orl-mus TD: 3750 g/kg/2Y-I   FAATDF 9,454,87
CAR: orl-mus TDLo: 2575 g/kg/2Y-I   NTPTR* NTP-TR-305,86
NEO: orl-rat TDLo: 657 g/kg/2Y-I   FAATDF 9,454,87

CONSENSUS REPORTS: NTP Carcinogenesis Studies (gavage): Clear Evidence: mouse NTPTR* NTP-TR-305,86; Equivocal Evidence: rat NTPTR* NTP-TR-305,86. Reported in EPA TSCA Inventory.

SAFETY PROFILE: Questionable carcinogen with experimental carcinogenic and neoplastigenic data. When heated to decomposition it emits acrid smoke and irritating fumes.

PAJ500   CAS: 10048-32-5
PARASCORBIC ACID
mf: C$_6$H$_8$O$_2$ mw: 112.14

PROP: Oily liquid; sweet, aromatic odor. Bp: 104-105° @ 14 mm, 119-123° @ 22 mm; d: 1.079 @ 18°/4°. Sol in water; very sol in alc, ether.

SYNS: (S)-(+)-5,6-DIHYDRO-6-METHYL-2H-PYRAN-2-ONE ◇ γ-HEXENOLACTONE ◇ 2-HEXEN-5,1-OLIDE ◇ D''-HEXENOLLACTONE ◇ 5-HYDROXY-2-HEXENOIC ACID LACTONE ◇ PARASORBIC ACID ◇ (+)-PARASORBIN-SAEURE (GERMAN) ◇ SORBIC OIL

TOXICITY DATA with REFERENCE
NEO: scu-rat TDLo: 1280 mg/kg/32W-I   BJCAAI 17,100,63

CONSENSUS REPORTS: IARC Cancer Review: Animal Limited Evidence IMEMDT 10,199,76.

SAFETY PROFILE: Questionable carcinogen with experimental neoplastigenic data. Poison by intraperitoneal and intravenous routes. Mildly toxic by skin contact. When heated to decomposition it emits acrid smoke and irritating fumes.

PAK000   CAS: 56-38-2
PARATHION
DOT: 2783
mf: C$_{10}$H$_{14}$NO$_5$PS   mw: 291.28

PROP: Pale-yellow liquid. Bp: 375°, mp: 6°. Very sol in alcs, esters, ethers, ketones, aromatic hydrocarbons; insol in water, petr ether, kerosene.

SYNS: AAT ◇ AATP ◇ AC 3422 ◇ ACC 3422 ◇ ALLERON ◇ APHAMITE ◇ ARALO ◇ B 404 ◇ BAY E-605 ◇ BAYER E-605 ◇ BLADAN ◇ BLADAN F ◇ COMPOUND 3422 ◇ COROTHION ◇ CORTHION ◇ CORTHIONE ◇ DANTHION ◇ O,O-DIAETHYL-O-(4-NITROPHENYL)-MONOTHIOPHOSPHAT (GERMAN) ◇ O,O-DIETHYL-O-(4-NITRO-FENIL)-MONOTHIOFOSFAAT (DUTCH) ◇ O,O-DIETHYL-O-p-NITRO-FENYLESTER KYSELINYTHIOFOSFORECNE (CZECH) ◇ O,O-DIETHYL-O-p-NITROFENYLTIOFOSFAT (CZECH) ◇ O,O-DIETHYL-O-4-NITROPHENYLPHOSPHOROTHIOATE ◇ O,O-DIETHYL-O-(p-NITROPHENYL) PHOSPHOROTHIOATE ◇ O,O-DIETHYL-O-(4-NITROPHENYL) PHOSPHOROTHIOATE ◇ DIETHYL-4-NITROPHENYL PHOSPHOROTHIONATE ◇ DIETHYL-p-NITROPHENYLTHIONOPHOSPHATE ◇ DIETHYL-p-NITROPHENYLTHIOPHOSPHATE ◇ O,O-DIETHYL-O-(p-NITROPHENYL)THIONOPHOSPHATE ◇ O,O-DIETHYL-O-p-NITROPHENYL THIOPHOSPHATE ◇ O,O-DIETHYL-O-4-NITROPHENYL THIOPHOSPHATE ◇ DIETHYLPARATHION ◇ O,O-DIETIL-O-(4-NITRO-FENIL)-MONOTIOFOSFATO (ITALIAN) ◇ DNTP ◇ DPP ◇ DREXEL PARATHION 8E ◇ E 605 ◇ ECATOX ◇ EKATIN WF & WF ULV ◇ EKATOX ◇ ENT 15,108 ◇ ETHLON ◇ ETHYL PARATHION ◇ FOLIDOL ◇ FOLIDOL E605 ◇ FOLIDOL E & E 605 ◇ FOSFERMO ◇ FOSFERNO ◇ FOSFEX ◇ FOSFIVE ◇ FOSOVA ◇ FOSTERN ◇ FOSTOX ◇ GEARPHOS ◇ GENITHION ◇ KOLPHOS ◇ KYPHION ◇ LETHALAIRE G-54 ◇ LIROTHION ◇ MURFOS ◇ NCI-C00226 ◇ NIRAN ◇ NIRAN E-4 ◇ p-NITROPHENOL, O-ESTER with O,O-DI-

ETHYLPHOSPHOROTHIOATE ◇ NITROSTIGMIN (GERMAN) ◇ NITROSTIGMINE ◇ NIUIF-100 ◇ NOURITHION ◇ OLEOFOS 20 ◇ OLEOPARAPHENE ◇ OLEOPARATHION ◇ ORTHOPHOS ◇ PAC ◇ PANTHION ◇ PARADUST ◇ PARAMAR ◇ PARAMAR 50 ◇ PARAPHOS ◇ PARATHENE ◇ PARATHION-ETHYL ◇ PARATHION, LIQUID (DOT) ◇ PARAWET ◇ PESTOX PLUS ◇ PETHION ◇ PHOSKIL ◇ PHOSPHEMOL ◇ PHOSPHENOL ◇ PHOSPHOROTHIOIC ACID, O,O-DIETHYL-O-(4-NITROPHENYL) ESTER ◇ PHOSPHOSTIGMINE ◇ RB ◇ RCRA WASTE NUMBER P089 ◇ RHODIASOL ◇ RHODIATOX ◇ RHODIATROX ◇ SELEPHOS ◇ SIXTY-THREE SPECIAL E.C. INSECTICIDE ◇ SNP ◇ SOPRATHION ◇ STABILIZED ETHYL PARATHION ◇ STATHION ◇ STRATHION ◇ SULPHOS ◇ SUPER RODIA-TOX ◇ T-47 ◇ THIOPHOS ◇ THIOPHOS 3422 ◇ THIOPHOS-PHATE de O,O-DIETHYLE et de O-(4-NITROPHENYLE) (FRENCH) ◇ TIOFOS ◇ TOX 47 ◇ VAPOPHOS ◇ VITREX

TOXICITY DATA with REFERENCE
ETA: orl-rat TDLo: 1260 mg/kg/80W-C NCITR* NCI-CG-TR-70,79

MUT: dnd-mus-ipr 3 µg/kg   MUREAV 53,175,78
MUT: dnd-rat-ipr 3 µg/kg   MUREAV 53,175,78
MUT: dnd-rat-orl 10 mg/kg/28D-I   MUREAV 53,175,78
MUT: dnd-rat-orl 20 mg/kg/28D-I   MUREAV 53,175,78
MUT: dns-hmn: fbr 10 µmol/L   NTIS** PB268-647
MUT: mma-sat 500 µg/plate   JTEHD6 16,403,85

CONSENSUS REPORTS: IARC Cancer Review: Human Inadequate Evidence IMEMDT 30,153,83; Animal Inadequate Evidence IMEMDT 30,153,83. NCI Carcinogenesis Bioassay (feed); Clear Evidence: rat NCITR* NCI-CG-TR-70,79; (feed); No Evidence: mouse NCITR* NCI-CG-TR-70,79. EPA Farm Worker Field Reentry FEREAC 39,16888,74. EPA Extremely Hazardous Substances List. Community Right-To-Know List. EPA Genetic Toxicology Program.

OSHA PEL: TWA 0.1 mg/m³ (skin) ACGIH TLV: TWA 0.1 mg/m³ (skin) (Proposed: BEI: 0.5 mg/L total p-nitrophenol in urine at end of shift.) DFG MAK: 0.1 mg/m³; BAT: 500 µg/L p-nitrophenol in urine after several shifts. NIOSH REL: TWA 0.05 mg/m³ DOT Classification: Poison B; Label: Poison.

SAFETY PROFILE: Questionable carcinogen with experimental carcinogenic, tumorigenic, and teratogenic data. A deadly poison by all routes. Human systemic effects by ingestion: general anesthetic; pulmonary effects; and kid-

ney, ureter, bladder effects. Experimental reproductive effects. Human mutation data reported. A cholinesterase inhibitor. Combustible when exposed to heat or flame. Highly dangerous; shock can shatter the container releasing the contents. A broad spectrum insecticide in agricultural applications. When heated to decomposition it emits highly toxic fumes of NO_x, PO_x, SO_x.

PAO000   CAS: 8002-03-7
PEANUT OIL

PROP: Straw-yellow to greenish-yellow or nearly colorless oil; nutty odor and bland taste. Mp: 2.7°, flash p: 540°F, d: 0.92, autoign temp: 833°F. Misc with ether, petr ether, chloroform, carbon disulfide; sol in benzene, carbon tetrachloride, oils; very sltly sol in alc. From seed of Arachis hypogaea (85DIA2 2,201,77).

SYNS: ARACHIS OIL ◇ EARTHNUT OIL ◇ GROUNDNUT OIL ◇ INDIGENOUS PEANUT OIL ◇ KATCHUNG OIL ◇ PECAN SHELL POWDER

TOXICITY DATA with REFERENCE
ETA: orl-mus TD: 1040 g/kg/1Y-I   IJCNAW 10,652,72
ETA: orl-mus TDLo: 952 g/kg/1Y-I   IJMRAQ 61,422,73
ETA: scu-mus TD: 329 g/kg/39W-I   IJMRAQ 61,422,73
ETA: scu-mus TD: 360 g/kg/39W-I   IJCNAW 10,652,72
ETA: scu-mus TDLo: 160 g/kg/17W-I   IJCNAW 10,652,72
ETA: skn-mus TD: 2276 g/kg/81W-C   IJCNAW 10,652,72
ETA: skn-mus TDLo: 1757 g/kg/88W-I   IJMRAQ 61,422,73
MUT: mma-sat 10 µL/plate   FCTXAV 18,467,80

CONSENSUS REPORTS: Reported in EPA TSCA Inventory.

SAFETY PROFILE: Questionable carcinogen with experimental tumorigenic data. A human skin irritant and mild allergen. Mutation data reported. Combustible when exposed to heat or flame; can react with oxidizing materials. To fight fire, use CO_2, dry chemical. When heated to decomposition it emits acrid smoke and irritating fumes.

PAP750   CAS: 90-65-3
PENICILLIC ACID
mf: $C_8H_{10}O_4$ mw: 170.18

PROP: Needles from petr ether. Mp: 83-84°. Sltly sol in cold water, hot petr ether; very sol in hot water, alc, ether, benzene chloroform; insol in pentane-hexane.

SYNS: γ-KETO-β-METHOXY-Δ-METHYLENE-Δα-HEXE-NOIC ACID ◇ 3-METHOXY-5-METHYL-4-OXO-2,5-HEXA-DIENOIC ACID ◇ PA ◇ PENCILLIC ACID

TOXICITY DATA with REFERENCE
NEO: scu-mus TDLo:608 mg/kg/38W-I

BJCAAI 19,342,65

NEO: scu-rat TDLo:960 mg/kg/48W-I   BJCAAI 15,85,61

MUT: cyt-mus:oth 3200 μg/L   GANNA2 68,619,77

MUT: dnd-hmn:hla 320 mg/L/1H   JJEMAG 42,527,72

MUT: dnd-mus:oth 100 mg/L   GANNA2 68,619,77

MUT: mrc-bcs 100 μg/disc   CNREA8 36,445,76

MUT: msc-mus:oth 3200 μg/L   GANNA2 68,619,77

CONSENSUS REPORTS: IARC Cancer Review: GROUP 3 IMEMDT 7,56,87; Animal Sufficient Evidence IMEMDT 10,211,76. EPA Genetic Toxicology Program.

SAFETY PROFILE: Questionable carcinogen with experimental neoplastigenic data. Poison by intravenous, subcutaneous, intraperitoneal, and possibly other routes. Moderately toxic by ingestion. Experimental reproductive effects. Human mutation data reported. When heated to decomposition it emits acrid smoke and irritating fumes.

PAQ875
PENICILLIUM ROQUEFORTI TOXIN

SYNS: P. ROQUEFORTI TOXIN ◇ PR TOXIN ◇ TOXIN, PENICILLIUM ROQUEFORTI

TOXICITY DATA with REFERENCE
ETA: orl-rat TD:139 mg/kg/52D-C   MYCPAH 78,125,82

ETA: orl-rat TDLo:100 mg/kg/52D-C   MYCPAH 78,125,82

MUT: dnd-rat:lvr 25 μmol/L   TOERD9 2,273,79

MUT: mmo-sat 625 ng/plate   MUREAV 130,79,84

MUT: oms-rat-ipr 10 mg/kg   CBINA8 14,207,76

MUT: oms-rat:lvr 35 mg/L   CBINA8 18,153,77

SAFETY PROFILE: Questionable carcinogen with experimental tumorigenic data. Poison by ingestion and intraperitoneal routes. Mutation data reported. When heated to decomposition it emits acrid smoke and irritating fumes.

PAU500   CAS: 1163-19-5
PENTABROMOPHENYL ETHER
mf: $C_{12}Br_{10}O$ mw: 959.22

SYNS: BERKFLAM B 10E ◇ BR 55N ◇ BROMKAL 83-10DE ◇ BROMKAL 82-ODE ◇ DBDPO ◇ DECABROMOBI-PHENYL ETHER ◇ DECABROMOBIPHENYL OXIDE ◇ DECABROMODIPHENYL OXIDE ◇ DECABROMOPHENYL ETHER ◇ DE 83R ◇ FR 300 ◇ FRP 53 ◇ NCI-C55287 ◇ 1,1'-OXYBIS(2,3,4,5,6-PENTABROMOBENZENE (9CI) ◇ SAYTEX 102 ◇ SAYTEX 102E ◇ TARDEX 100

TOXICITY DATA with REFERENCE
NEO: orl-rat TDLo:1092 g/kg/2Y-C   NTPTR* NTP-TR-309,86

CONSENSUS REPORTS: NTP Carcinogenesis Studies (feed); Some Evidence: rat NTPTR* NTP-TR-309,86; (feed); Equivocal Evidence: mouse NTPTR* NTP-TR-309,86. EPA Extremely Hazardous Substances List. Polybrominated biphenyl compounds are on the Community Right-To-Know List. Reported in EPA TSCA Inventory.

SAFETY PROFILE: Questionable carcinogen with experimental neoplastigenic data. Experimental teratogenic and reproductive effects. Used as a flame retardant for thermoplastics. When heated to decomposition it emits toxic fumes of Br^-.

PAW000   CAS: 40321-76-4
1,2,3,7,8-PENTACHLORODIBENZO-p-DIOXIN
mf: $C_{12}H_3Cl_5O_2$ mw: 356.40

CONSENSUS REPORTS: IARC Cancer Review: Animal Inadequate Evidence IMEMDT 15,41,77.

SAFETY PROFILE: Questionable carcinogen. Poison by ingestion. When heated to decomposition it emits toxic fumes of Cl^-.

PAW500   CAS: 76-01-7
PENTACHLOROETHANE
DOT: 1669
mf: C_2HCl_5 mw: 202.28

PROP: Colorless liquid; chloroform-like odor. Mp: −29°, bp: 161-162°, d: 1.6728 @ 25°/4°. Insol in water; misc in alc and ether.

SYNS: ETHANE PENTACHLORIDE ◇ NCI-C53894 ◇ PENTACHLOORETHAAN (DUTCH) ◇ PENTACHLORAE-THAN (GERMAN) ◇ PENTACHLORETHANE (FRENCH) ◇ PENTACLOROETANO (ITALIAN) ◇ PENTALIN ◇ RCRA WASTE NUMBER U184

TOXICITY DATA with REFERENCE
CAR: orl-mus TD:258 g/kg/2Y-I NTPTR* NTP-
TR-232,82
CAR: orl-mus TDLo:129 g/kg/2Y-I NTPTR*
NTP-TR-232,82
MUT: msc-mus:lyms 70 mg/L EMMUEG 12,85,88
MUT: sce-ham:ovr 100 mg/L SCIEAS 236,933,87

CONSENSUS REPORTS: IARC Cancer Review: GROUP 3 IMEMDT 7,56,87; Animal Limited Evidence IMEMDT 41,99,86. NTP Carcinogenesis Bioassay (gavage); Clear Evidence: mouse NTPTR* NTP-TR-232,82; (gavage); No Evidence: rat NTPTR* NTP-TR-232,82. Reported in EPA TSCA Inventory.

DFG MAK: 5 ppm (40 mg/m^3)   DOT Classification: Poison B; Label: Poison.

SAFETY PROFILE: Questionable carcinogen with experimental carcinogenic data. Poison by inhalation and intravenous routes. Moderately toxic by ingestion and subcutaneous routes. An irritant. Flammable when exposed to heat or flame. Moderately explosive by spontaneous chemical reaction. To fight fire, use water, CO_2, dry chemical. When heated to decomposition it emits highly toxic fumes of Cl$^-$.

PAX000   CAS: 82-68-8
PENTACHLORONITROBENZENE
mf: $C_6Cl_5NO_2$ mw: 295.32

PROP: Colorless crystals. Mp: 146°, bp: 328°, vap press: 0.013 mm @ 25°.

SYNS: AVICOL ◇ BATRILEX ◇ BRASSICOL ◇ EARTH-CIDE ◇ FARTOX ◇ FOLOSAN ◇ FOMAC 2 ◇ FUNGICLOR ◇ GC 3944-3-4 ◇ KOBU ◇ KOBUTOL ◇ KP 2 ◇ NCI-C00419 ◇ OLPISAN ◇ PCNB ◇ PENTACHLORNITROBENZOL (GERMAN) ◇ PENTAGEN ◇ PKhNB ◇ QUINTOCENE ◇ QUINTO-ZEN ◇ QUINTOZENE ◇ RCRA WASTE NUMBER U185 ◇ SANICLOR 30 ◇ TERRACHLOR ◇ TERRAFUN ◇ TILCA-REX ◇ TRI-PCNB ◇ TRITISAN

TOXICITY DATA with REFERENCE
CAR: orl-mus TDLo:135 g/kg/77W-C JNCIAM
42,1101,69
MUT: dnd-esc 20 μmol/L MUREAV 89,95,81
MUT: mmo-asn 5 μmol/L PHYTAJ 66,217,76
MUT: mmo-esc 10 mg/plate MUREAV 11,247,71
MUT: mrc-asn 40 μmol/L MUREAV 147,288,85
MUT: sln-asn 17 μmol/L EVHPAZ 31,81,79

CONSENSUS REPORTS: IARC Cancer Review: GROUP 3 IMEMDT 7,56,87; Animal Sufficient Evidence IMEMDT 5,211,74. NCI Carcinogenesis Bioassay (feed); No Evidence: mouse, rat NCITR* NCI-CG-TR-61,78. EPA Extremely Hazardous Substances List. Reported in EPA TSCA Inventory. EPA Genetic Toxicology Program.

ACGIG TLV: (Proposed: 0.5 mg/m^3)

SAFETY PROFILE: Questionable carcinogen with experimental carcinogenic data. Moderately toxic by ingestion and possibly other routes. Experimental reproductive effects. Mutation data reported. Used as a fungicide. Dangerous; when heated to decomposition it emits highly toxic fumes of NO_x and Cl$^-$.

PBC750   CAS: 3524-68-3
PENTAERYTHRITOL TRIACRYLATE
mf: $C_{14}H_{18}O_7$ mw: 298.32

SYNS: ACRYLIC ACID, PENTAERITHRITOL TRIESTER ◇ PETA ◇ 2-PROPENOIC ACID-2-(HYDROXYMETHYL)-2-(((1-OXO-2-PROPENYL)OXY)METHYL)-1,3-PROPANEDIYL ESTER

TOXICITY DATA with REFERENCE
ETA: skn-mus TDLo:16 g/kg/80W-I JTEHD6
19,149,86

CONSENSUS REPORTS: Reported in EPA TSCA Inventory.

SAFETY PROFILE: Questionable carcinogen with experimental tumorigenic data. Moderately toxic by ingestion and skin contact. Skin and severe eye irritant. Used for radiation-cured adhesives, coatings, inks, textiles, photo resists and coatings. When heated to decomposition it emits acrid smoke and irritating fumes.

PBJ875   CAS: 57590-20-2
PENTANAL
METHYLFORMYLHYDRAZONE
mf: $C_7H_{14}N_2O$ mw: 142.23

SYNS: FORMIC ACID, METHYLPENTYLIDENEHYDRA-ZIDE ◇ PENTANAL, N-FORMYL-N-METHYLHYDRAZONE ◇ PENTYLIDENE GYROMITRIN

TOXICITY DATA with REFERENCE
CAR: orl-mus TDLo:2600 mg/kg/52W-I
MYCPAH 98,83,87
NEO: orl-mus TD:2600 mg/kg/52W-I MYCPAH
98,83,87

SAFETY PROFILE: Questionable carcinogen with experimental carcinogenic and neoplastigenic data. Poison by ingestion. When heated to decomposition it emits toxic fumes of NO_x.

PBX250   CAS: 1119-68-2
n-PENTYLHYDRAZINE HYDROCHLORIDE
mf: $C_5H_{14}N_2 \cdot ClH$ mw: 138.67

SYN: n-AMYLHYDRAZINE HYDROCHLORIDE

TOXICITY DATA with REFERENCE
NEO: orl-mus TDLo:11 g/kg/80W-C   BJCAAI 31,492,75

ETA: orl-mus TD:12 mg/kg/W-C   PAACA3 16,61,75

SAFETY PROFILE: Questionable carcinogen with experimental neoplastigenic and tumorigenic data. When heated to decomposition it emits very toxic fumes of NO_x and HCl.

PBX500   CAS: 10589-74-9
n-PENTYLNITROSOUREA
mf: $C_6H_{13}N_3O_2$ mw: 159.22

SYNS: 1-AMYL-1-NITROSOUREA ◇ n-AMYLNITRO-SOUREA ◇ ANU ◇ 1-NITROSO-1-PENTYLUREA ◇ N-PEN-TYLNITROSOUREA

TOXICITY DATA with REFERENCE
CAR: orl-rat TD:570 mg/kg   ANYAA9 381,250,82
CAR: orl-rat TDLo:184 g/kg/49W-I   GANNA2 71,464,80
CAR: skn-mus TDLo:629 mg/kg/50W-I   JCROD7 102,13,81
ETA: orl-rat TD:5200 mg/kg/52W-I   PPTCBY 2,73,72
ETA: scu-rat TDLo:510 mg/kg   ANYAA9 381,250,82
MUT: cyt-ham:fbr 250 mg/L/48H   MUREAV 48,337,77
MUT: mma-sat 25 µg/plate   TCMUE9 1,13,84
MUT: mmo-sat 1 µg/plate   MUREAV 68,1,79
MUT: pic-esc 2 mg/L   TCMUE9 1,91,84

SAFETY PROFILE: Questionable carcinogen with experimental carcinogenic and tumorigenic data. Moderately toxic by ingestion. Mutation data reported. When heated to decomposition it emits toxic fumes of NO_x.

PBX750   CAS: 62573-57-3
m-(3-PENTYL)PHENYL-N-METHYL-N-NITROSOCARBAMATE
mf: $C_{13}H_{18}N_2O_3$ mw: 250.33

SYNS: N-METHYL-N-NITROSOCARBAMIC ACID-m-3-PENTYLPHENYL ESTER ◇ NITROSO-BUX-TEN

TOXICITY DATA with REFERENCE
CAR: orl-rat TDLO:660 mg/kg/10W-I   EESADV 2,413,78

MUT: dnd-hmn:fbr 10 µmol/L   MUREAV 44,1,77
MUT: mma-sat 125 ng/plate   MUREAV 56,1,77
MUT: mmo-esc 100 µmol/L   IARCCD 14,425,75

SAFETY PROFILE: Questionable carcinogen with experimental carcinogenic data. Human mutation data reported. When heated to decomposition it emits toxic fumes of NO_x.

PCB000   CAS: 70384-29-1
PEPLEOMYCIN SULFATE

SYN: NK 631

TOXICITY DATA with REFERENCE
CAR: par-rat TD:33 mg/kg/52W-I   PAACA3 24,96,83
CAR: par-rat TDLo:17 mg/kg/52W-I   PAACA3 24,96,83
CAR: scu-rat TDLo:23 mg/kg/61W-I   ONCOBS 41,114,84

SAFETY PROFILE: Questionable carcinogen with experimental carcinogenic data. Poison by intraperitoneal, subcutaneous, and intravenous routes. When heated to decomposition it emits very toxic fumes of NO_x and SO_x.

PCF250   CAS: 3200-96-2
PERCHLORO-2-CYCLOBUTENE-1-ONE
mf: C_4Cl_4O mw: 205.84

SYN: 2,3,4,5-TETRACHLORO-2-CYCLOBUTEN-1-ONE

TOXICITY DATA with REFERENCE
ETA: scu-mus TDLo:280 mg/kg/70W-I   JNCIAM 46,143,71

SAFETY PROFILE: Questionable carcinogen with experimental tumorigenic data. When heated to decomposition it emits toxic fumes of Cl^-.

PCL500   CAS: 79-21-0
PEROXYACETIC ACID
DOT: 2131
mf: $C_2H_4O_3$ mw: 76.06

PROP: Not over 40% peracetic acid and not over 6% hydrogen peroxide (FEREAC 41,-15972,76). Colorless liquid; strong odor. Bp: 105°, explodes @ 110°, flash p: 105°F (OC), d: 1.15 @ 20°. Water-sol. Powerful oxidizer.

SYNS: ACETYL HYDROPEROXIDE ◇ ACIDE PERACE-TIQUE (FRENCH) ◇ ETHANEPEROXOIC ACID ◇ HYDRO-

PEROXIDE, ACETYL ◇ PERACETIC ACID (MAK) ◇ PERACETIC ACID SOLUTION (DOT) ◇ PEROXYACETIC ACID, maximum concentration 43% in acetic acid (DOT)

TOXICITY DATA with REFERENCE
ETA: skn-mus TDLo: 21 g/kg/26W-I   JNCIAM
55,1359,75

CONSENSUS REPORTS: EPA Extremely Hazardous Substances List. Community Right-To-Know List. Reported in EPA TSCA Inventory.

DFG MAK: Very strong skin effects. DOT Classification: Organic Peroxide; Label: Organic Peroxide, Corrosive.

SAFETY PROFILE: Questionable carcinogen with experimental tumorigenic data by skin contact. Poison by ingestion. Moderately toxic by inhalation and skin contact. A corrosive eye, skin, and mucous membrane irritant. Flammable when exposed to heat or flames. Severe explosion hazard when exposed to heat or by spontaneous chemical reaction. Dangerous; keep away from combustible materials. When heated to decomposition it emits acrid smoke and irritating fumes. To fight fire, use water, foam, CO_2. Used as a polymerization initiator, curing agent, and cross-linking agent.

PCM000   CAS: 93-59-4
PEROXYBENZOIC ACID
mf: $C_7H_6O_3$ mw: 138.13

PROP: Leaflets. Mp: 42°, bp: explodes @ 80-100°. Insol in water; sol in alc and ether.

SYNS: BENZENECARBOPEROXOIC ACID (9CI) ◇ BENZOYLHYDROGEN PEROXIDE ◇ BENZOYL HYDROPEROXIDE ◇ PERBENZOIC ACID

TOXICITY DATA with REFERENCE
ETA: skn-mus TDLo: 1040 mg/kg/26W-I
JNCIAM 55,1359,75

SAFETY PROFILE: Questionable carcinogen with experimental tumorigenic data by skin contact. Moderately irritating to skin, eyes, and mucous membranes by ingestion and inhalation. A dangerous fire hazard when exposed to heat, flame, or reducing materials. A powerful oxidizing agent. Severe explosion hazard when exposed to heat or flame. When heated to decomposition it emits acrid smoke and irritating fumes.

PCN000   CAS: 19356-22-0
PEROXYLINOLENIC ACID
mf: $C_{18}H_{30}O_3$ mw: 294.48

SYNS: LINOLENIC HYDROPEROXIDE ◇ LINOLENATE HYDROPEROXIDE ◇ 9,12,15-OCTADECATRIENEPEROXOIC ACID (Z,Z,Z) (9CI)

TOXICITY DATA with REFERENCE
CAR: scu-rat TDLo: 1 g/kg/45W   FCTXAV
12,451,74
NEO: scu-rat TD: 1765 mg/kg/95W   FCTXAV
12,451,74
MUT: mma-sat 100 μg/plate   ABCHA6 44,1989,80

SAFETY PROFILE: Questionable carcinogen with experimental carcinogenic and neoplastigenic data. Mutation data reported. When heated to decomposition it emits acrid smoke and irritating fumes.

PCP500
PERSIMMON

PROP: Tannin containing fraction of unripe fruit of *Diospyros virginiana* (JNCIAM 57, 207,76).

SYNS: DIOSPYROS VIRGINIANA ◇ TANNIN from PERSIMMON

TOXICITY DATA with REFERENCE
NEO: scu-rat TDLo: 1800 mg/kg/57W-I
JNCIAM 57,207,76

SAFETY PROFILE: Questionable carcinogen with experimental neoplastigenic data. When heated to decomposition it emits acrid smoke and irritating fumes.

PCQ250   CAS: 198-55-0
PERYLENE
mf: $C_{20}H_{12}$ mw: 252.32

SYNS: DIBENZ9(de,kl)ANTHRACENE ◇ PERI-DINAPHTHALENE ◇ PERILENE

TOXICITY DATA with REFERENCE
MUT: cyt-ham: lng 10 mg/L   JNCIAM 59,289,77
MUT: mma-sat 2 μg/plate   CRNGDP 5,925,84
MUT: mmo-sat 25 nmol/plate   TXCYAC 18,219,80

CONSENSUS REPORTS: IARC Cancer Review: GROUP 3 IMEMDT 7,56,87; Animal Inadequate Evidence IMEMDT 32,411,83. Reported in EPA TSCA Inventory. EPA Genetic Toxicology Program.

SAFETY PROFILE: Questionable carcinogen. Mutation data reported. When heated to decomposition it emits acrid smoke and irritating fumes.

PCQ750   CAS: 60102-37-6
PETASITENINE
mf: $C_{19}H_{27}NO_7$ mw: 381.47

PROP: Pyrrolizidine alkaloid isolated from *Petasites japonicus Maxim* (JNCIAM 58, 1155,77).

SYN: FUKINOTOXIN

TOXICITY DATA with REFERENCE
CAR: orl-rat TDLo: 921 mg/kg/13W-C   JNCIAM 58,1155,77
MUT: dns-rat: lvr 2 μmol/L   CNREA8 45,3125,85
MUT: mma-sat 1 mg/plate   MUREAV 68,211,79

CONSENSUS REPORTS: IARC Cancer Review: GROUP 3 IMEMDT 7,56,87; Animal Limited Evidence IMEMDT 31,207,83.

SAFETY PROFILE: Questionable carcinogen with experimental carcinogenic data. Mutation data reported. Used as a food and herbal remedy. When heated to decomposition it emits toxic fumes of NO_x.

PCR250   CAS: 8002-05-9
PETROLEUM
DOT: 1267

PROP: A thick flammable, dark yellow to brown or green-black liquid. D: 0.780-0.970, flash p: 20-90°F. Insol in water; sol in benzene, chloroform, ether. Consists of a mixture of hydrocarbons from C_2H_6 and up, chiefly of the paraffins, cycloparaffins, or of cyclic aromatic hydrocarbons, with small amounts of benzene hydrocarbons, sulfur, and oxygenated compounds (12VXA5 7,788,60)

SYNS: BASE OIL ◇ COAL LIQUID ◇ COAL OIL ◇ CRUDE OIL ◇ PETROLEUM CRUDE ◇ ROCK OIL ◇ SENECA OIL

TOXICITY DATA with REFERENCE
CAR: skn-mus TD: 210 mg/kg/2Y-I   NTIS** CONF-801143
CAR: skn-mus TD: 12480 mg/kg/2Y-I   NTIS** CONF-790334-3
CAR: skn-mus TD: 21216 mg/kg/2Y-I   NTIS** CONF-801143
CAR: skn-mus TDLo: 3744 mg/kg/2Y-I   NTIS** CONF-790334
NEO: skn-mus TD: 3744 mg/kg/2Y-I   JOCMA7 21,614,79
ETA: skn-mus TD: 40 g/kg/10W-I   BECCAN 39,420,61

CONSENSUS REPORTS: Reported in EPA TSCA Inventory.

DOT Classification: Combustible Liquid; Label: None: Flammable Liquid; Label: Flammable Liquid.

SAFETY PROFILE: Questionable carcinogen with experimental carcinogenic, neoplastigenic, and tumorigenic data by skin contact. A dangerous fire hazard when exposed to heat, flame, or powerful oxidizers. To fight fire, use foam, CO_2, dry chemical. When heated to decomposition it emits acrid smoke and irritating fumes.

PCR500   CAS: 8052-42-4
PETROLEUM ASPHALT

PROP: Steam refined asphalt (IMSUAI 34, 255,65).

SYNS: ASPHALT, PETROLEUM ◇ PETROLEUM ROOFING TAR ◇ ROAD ASPHALT

TOXICITY DATA with REFERENCE
NEO: ims-mus TDLo: 12 g/kg/12W-I   ARPAAQ 70,372,60
NEO: ims-rat TDLo: 5400 mg/kg/24W-I   ARPAAQ 70,372,60
NEO: skn-mus TDLo: 905 g/kg/2Y-I   JMSUAT 34,255,65

CONSENSUS REPORTS: Reported in EPA TSCA Inventory.

SAFETY PROFILE: Questionable carcinogen with experimental neoplastigenic data skin contact. When heated to decomposition it emits acrid smoke and irritating fumes.

PCS260   CAS: 64742-44-5
PETROLEUM DISTILLATES, CLAY-TREATED HEAVY NAPHTHENIC

TOXICITY DATA with REFERENCE
ETA: skn-mus TD: 410 g/kg/78W-I   BJCAAI 48,429,83
ETA: skn-mus TDLo: 406 g/kg/22W-I   BJCAAI 48,429,83

CONSENSUS REPORTS: Reported in EPA TSCA Inventory.

SAFETY PROFILE: Questionable carcinogen with experimental tumorigenic data. When heated to decomposition it emits acrid smoke and irritating fumes.

PCS270 CAS: 64742-45-6
PETROLEUM DISTILLATES, CLAY-TREATED LIGHT NAPHTHENIC

TOXICITY DATA with REFERENCE
ETA: skn-mus TDLo:577 g/kg/78W-I BJCAAI
48,429,83

CONSENSUS REPORTS: Reported in EPA TSCA Inventory.

SAFETY PROFILE: Questionable carcinogen with experimental tumorigenic data. When heated to decomposition it emits acrid smoke and irritating fumes.

PCU500 CAS: 551-16-6
PHENACYL-6-AMINOPENICILLINATE
mf: $C_8H_{12}N_2O_3S$ mw: 216.28

PROP: Obtained from *Penicillum chrysogenum* and *Pleurotus ostroeatus* (12VXA5 8,59,68).

SYNS: 6-AMINOPENICILLANIC ACID ◇ PENICIN

TOXICITY DATA with REFERENCE
ETA: scu-rat TDLo:2600 mg/kg/65W-I BJCAAI
19,392,65

CONSENSUS REPORTS: Reported in EPA TSCA Inventory.

SAFETY PROFILE: Questionable carcinogen with experimental tumorigenic data. When heated to decomposition it emits very toxic fumes of NO_x and SO_x.

PCV500 CAS: 189-92-4
PHENALENO(1,9-gh)QUINOLINE
mf: $C_{19}H_{11}N$ mw: 253.31

SYNS: PYRENOLINE ◇ PYRIDO(2',3':4)PYRENE

TOXICITY DATA with REFERENCE
ETA: scu-mus TDLo:72 mg/kg/9W-I COREAF
258,3387,64

SAFETY PROFILE: Questionable carcinogen with experimental tumorigenic data. When heated to decomposition it emits toxic fumes of NO_x.

PCW000 CAS: 7258-91-5
PHENANTHRA-ACENAPHTHENE
mf: $C_{24}H_{16}$ mw: 304.40

SYN: 4,5-DIHYDRONAPHTH(1,2-k)ACEPHENANTHRYLENE

TOXICITY DATA with REFERENCE
ETA: skn-mus TDLo:1250 mg/kg/52W-I
PRLBA4 117,318,35

SAFETY PROFILE: Questionable carcinogen with experimental tumorigenic data by skin contact. When heated to decomposition it emits acrid smoke and irritating fumes.

PCW250 CAS: 85-01-8
PHENANTHRENE
mf: $C_{14}H_{10}$ mw: 178.24

PROP: Solid or monoclinic crystals. Mp: 100°, bp: 339°, d: 1.179 @ 25°, vap press: 1 mm @ 118.3°, vap d: 6.14. Insol in water; sol in CS_2 benzene, hot alc; very sol in ether.

SYNS: PHENANTHREN (GERMAN) ◇ PHENANTRIN

TOXICITY DATA with REFERENCE
NEO: skn-mus TDLo:71 mg/kg JNCIAM
50,1717,73
ETA: skn-mus TD:22 g/kg/10W-I BJCAAI
10,363,56
MUT: cyt-ham:lng 40 mg/L/27H MUREAV
66,277,79
MUT: dnd-ham:fbr 5 mg/L/24H BCPCA6
20,1297,71
MUT: dnd-ham:kdy 5 mg/L BCPCA6 20,1297,71
MUT: mma-sat 100 μg/plate APSXAS 17,189,80
MUT: sce-ham-ipr 900 mg/kg/24H MUREAV
66,65,79
MUT: sce-ham:fbr 10 μmol/L JNCIAM 58,1635,77

CONSENSUS REPORTS: IARC Cancer Review: Animal Inadequate Evidence IMEMDT 32,419,83. Reported in EPA TSCA Inventory. EPA Genetic Toxicology Program.

OSHA PEL: TWA 0.2 mg/m³

SAFETY PROFILE: Questionable carcinogen with experimental neoplastigenic and tumorigenic data by skin contact. Poison by intravenous route. Moderately toxic by ingestion. Mutation data reported. A human skin photosensitizer. Combustible when exposed to heat or flame; can react vigorously with oxidizing materials. To fight fire, use water, foam, CO_2, dry chemical. When heated to decomposition it emits acrid smoke and irritating fumes.

PCW500 CAS: 20057-09-4
PHENANTHRENE-3,4-DIHYDRODIOL
mf: $C_{14}H_{12}O_2$ mw: 212.26

SYNS: 3,4-DIHYDROMORPHOL ◇ 3,4-DIHYDRO-3,4-PHENANTHRENEDIOL

TOXICITY DATA with REFERENCE
ETA: skn-mus TDLo:85 mg/kg CNREA8
39,4069,79

SAFETY PROFILE: Questionable carcinogen with experimental tumorigenic data by skin contact. When heated to decomposition it emits acrid smoke and irritating fumes.

PCX000   CAS: 585-08-0
9,10-PHENANTHRENE OXIDE
mf: $C_{14}H_{10}O$ mw: 194.24

PROP: Colorless needles. Mp: 152-153°. Very sltly sol in water; very sol in alc, ether.

SYNS: 1a,9b-DIHYDROPHENANTHRO(9,10-B)OXIRENE (9CI) ◇ 9,10-EPOXY-9,10-DIHYDROPHENANTHRENE ◇ PHENANTHRENE-9,10-EPOXIDE

TOXICITY DATA with REFERENCE
ETA: skn-mus TDLo:40 mg/kg   JNCIAM 39,1217,67

MUT: dni-omi 100 µg/L   PNASA6 74,1378,77
MUT: mma-sat 100 µg/plate   MUREAV 66,337,79
MUT: mmo-sat 50 µg/plate   MUTAEX 1,35,86

CONSENSUS REPORTS: EPA Genetic Toxicology Program.

SAFETY PROFILE: Questionable carcinogen with experimental tumorigenic data by skin contact. Mutation data reported. When heated to decomposition it emits acrid smoke and irritating fumes.

PCX250   CAS: 84-11-7
PHENANTHRENEQUINONE
mf: $C_{14}H_8O_2$ mw: 208.22

PROP: Orange needles. D: 1.405 @ 4°, mp: 206.5-207.5°, bp: >300° subl. Very sltly sol in water; sol in hot alc, benzene; sltly sol in ether.

SYNS: 9,10-PHENANTHRAQUINONE ◇ 9,10-PHENAN-THRENEDIONE ◇ 9,10-PHENANTHRENEQUINONE

TOXICITY DATA with REFERENCE
ETA: skn-mus TDLo:800 mg/kg/29W-C
   PIATA8 16,309,40
MUT: mma-sat 30 µmol/L   PNASA6 81,1696,84

CONSENSUS REPORTS: Reported in EPA TSCA Inventory. EPA Genetic Toxicology Program.

SAFETY PROFILE: Questionable carcinogen with experimental tumorigenic data by skin contact. Poison by acute intraperitoneal route. Mutation data reported. When heated to decomposition it emits acrid smoke and irritating fumes.

PCY400   CAS: 14635-33-7
PHENANTHRO(2,1-d)THIAZOLE
mf: $C_{15}H_9NS$ mw: 235.31

TOXICITY DATA with REFERENCE
NEO: skn-mus TDLo:400 mg/kg/13W-I
   VOONAW 15(8),54,69

SAFETY PROFILE: Questionable carcinogen with experimental neoplastigenic data. When heated to decomposition it emits toxic fumes of NO_x and SO_x.

PCY500   CAS: 4120-78-9
N-3-PHENANTHRYLACETAMIDE
mf: $C_{16}H_{13}NO$ mw: 235.30

SYNS: 3-ACETAMIDOPHENANTHRENE ◇ 3-ACETAMI-NOPHENANTHRENE ◇ 3-ACETYLAMINOPHENANTHRENE

TOXICITY DATA with REFERENCE
CAR: orl-rat TDLo:4572 mg/kg/32W-C
   CNREA8 15,188,55
ETA: ims-mus TDLo:80 mg/kg   ZEKBAI72,321,69

SAFETY PROFILE: Questionable carcinogen with experimental carcinogenic and tumorigenic data. When heated to decomposition it emits toxic fumes of NO_x.

PCY750   CAS: 4235-09-0
N-9-PHENANTHRYLACETAMIDE
mf: $C_{16}H_{13}NO$ mw: 235.30

SYNS: 9-ACETAMIDOPHENANTHRENE ◇ 9-ACETAMI-NOPHENANTHRENE ◇ 9-ACETYLAMINOPHENANTHRENE ◇ 9-PHENANTHRYLACETAMIDE

TOXICITY DATA with REFERENCE
ETA: ims-mus TDLo:80 mg/kg   ZEKBAI72,321,69

SAFETY PROFILE: Questionable carcinogen with experimental tumorigenic data. When heated to decomposition it emits toxic fumes of NO_x.

PCZ000   CAS: 2438-51-9
N-2-PHENANTHRYLACETO-HYDROXAMIC ACID
mf: $C_{16}H_{13}NO_2$ mw: 251.30

SYNS: 2-(N-HYDROXYACETAMIDO)PHENANTHRENE ◇ N-HYDROXY-2-ACETYLAMINOPHENANTHRENE ◇ N-HYDROXY-N-2-PHENANTHRENYL-ACETAMIDE (9CI) ◇ 2-PHENANTHRYLACETHYDROXAMIC ACID

TOXICITY DATA with REFERENCE
CAR: scu-rat TDLo:30 mg/kg/4W-I   CNREA8 26,2239,66

MUT: dnd-rat-ipr 40 mg/kg CRNGDP 5,231,84
MUT: dns-hmn:fbr 10 μmol/L/5H IJCNAW 16,284,75
MUT: oms-bcs 10 g/L CNREA8 30,1473,70

SAFETY PROFILE: Questionable carcinogen with experimental carcinogenic data. Human mutation data reported. When heated to decomposition it emits toxic fumes of NO_x.

PDA250   CAS: 3366-65-2
2-PHENANTHRYLAMINE
mf: $C_{14}H_{11}N$ mw: 193.26

SYN: 2-AMINOPHENANTHRENE

TOXICITY DATA with REFERENCE
ETA: orl-rat TD:700 mg/kg SCIEAS 137,257,62
ETA: orl-rat TDLo:450 mg/kg/6D-I ZEKBAI 72,321,69
MUT: mma-sat 200 ng/plate CBINA8 26,11,79

SAFETY PROFILE: Questionable carcinogen with experimental tumorigenic data. Mutation data reported. When heated to decomposition it emits toxic fumes of NO_x.

PDA500   CAS: 1892-54-2
3-PHENANTHRYLAMINE
mf: $C_{14}H_{11}N$ mw: 193.26

SYN: 3-AMINOPHENANTHRENE

TOXICITY DATA with REFERENCE
ETA: orl-rat TDLo:450 mg/kg/6D-I ZEKBAI 72,321,69
MUT: mma-sat 200 ng/plate ENMUDM 6,497,84

SAFETY PROFILE: Questionable carcinogen with experimental tumorigenic data. Mutation data reported. When heated to decomposition it emits toxic fumes of NO_x.

PDA750   CAS: 947-73-9
9-PHENANTHRYLAMINE
mf: $C_{14}H_{11}N$ mw: 193.26

SYN: 9-AMINOPHENANTHRENE

TOXICITY DATA with REFERENCE
ETA: orl-rat TDLo:450 mg/kg/6D-I ZEKBAI 72,321,69
MUT: mma-sat 250 ng/plate JJIND8 71,293,83

SAFETY PROFILE: Questionable carcinogen with experimental tumorigenic data. Mutation data reported. When heated to decomposition it emits toxic fumes of NO_x.

PDB500   CAS: 92-82-0
PHENAZINE
mf: $C_{12}H_8N_2$ mw: 180.22

PROP: Pale yellow crystals. Mp: 171°, bp: > 360° (subl). Very sltly sol in water; sol in cold and hot alc, ether.

SYNS: AZOPHENYLENE ◇ DIBENZOPARADIAZINE ◇ DIBENZOPYRAZINE

TOXICITY DATA with REFERENCE
ETA: imp-rat TDLo:7 mg/kg COREAF 240,1738,55

CONSENSUS REPORTS: Reported in EPA TSCA Inventory.

SAFETY PROFILE: Questionable carcinogen with experimental tumorigenic data. Poison by intraperitoneal and intravenous routes. When heated to decomposition it emits toxic fumes of NO_x.

PDI250   CAS: 33384-03-1
N-(p-PHENETHYL) PHENYLACETOHYDROXAMIC ACID
mf: $C_{16}H_{17}NO_2$ mw: 255.34

SYNS: N-HYDROXY-4-ACETYLAMINOBIBENZYL ◇ N-HYDROXY-4'-PHENETHYLACETANILIDE

TOXICITY DATA with REFERENCE
NEO: ipr-rat TDLo:380 mg/kg/3W-I CNREA8 24,128,64
MUT: dns-hmn:fbr 100 μmol/L/5H IJCNAW 16,284,75

SAFETY PROFILE: Questionable carcinogen with experimental neoplastigenic data. Human mutation data reported. When heated to decomposition it emits toxic fumes of NO_x.

PDN750   CAS: 108-95-2
PHENOL
DOT: 1671/2312/2821
mf: C_6H_6O mw: 94.12

PROP: White, crystalline mass which turns pink or red if not perfectly pure; burning taste, distinctive odor. Mp: 40.6°, bp: 181.9°, flash p: 175°F (CC), d: 1.072, autoign temp: 1319°F, vap press: 1 mm @ 40.1°, vap d: 3.24. Sol in water; misc in alc, ether.

SYNS: ACIDE CARBOLIQUE (FRENCH) ◇ BAKER'S P AND S LIQUID and OINTMENT ◇ BENZENOL ◇ CARBOLIC ACID ◇ CARBOLSAURE (GERMAN) ◇ FENOL (DUTCH, POLISH) ◇ FENOLO (ITALIAN) ◇ HYDROXYBENZENE ◇ MONOHY-DROXYBENZENE ◇ MONOPHENOL ◇ NCI-C50124

◇ OXYBENZENE ◇ PHENIC ACID ◇ PHENOL ALCOHOL ◇ PHENOL, MOLTEN (DOT) ◇ PHENOLE (GERMAN) ◇ PHENYL HYDRATE ◇ PHENYL HYDROXIDE ◇ PHENYLIC ACID ◇ PHENYLIC ALCOHOL ◇ RCRA WASTE NUMBER U188

TOXICITY DATA with REFERENCE

CAR: skn-mus TDLo:16 g/kg/40W-I   CNREA8 19,413,59

NEO: skn-mus TD:4000 mg/kg/24W-I   CNREA8 19,413,59

MUT: dnd-mam:lym 250 mmol/L   PNASA6 48,686,62

MUT: dns-rat-orl 4 g/kg   JJIND8 74,1283

MUT: oms-hmn:hla 17 mg/L   WATRAG 19,577,85

MUT: oms-hmn:lym 5 μmol/L   CNREA8 45,2471,85

MUT: oms-rbt:bmr 250 μmol/L   AJIMD8 7,485,85

MUT: sce-hmn:lym 5 μmol/L   CNREA8 45,2471,85

CONSENSUS REPORTS: NCI Carcinogenesis Bioassay (oral); No Evidence: mouse, rat NCITR* NCI-CG-TR-203,80. EPA Extremely Hazardous Substances List. Community Right-To-Know List. Reported in EPA TSCA Inventory. EPA Genetic Toxicology Program.

OSHA PEL: TWA 5 ppm (skin)   ACGIH TLV: TWA 5 ppm (skin); BEI: 250 mg(total phenol)/g creatinine in urine at end of shift.   DFG MAK: 5 ppm (19 mg/m^3); BAT: 300 mg/L at end of shift.   NIOSH REL: TWA 20 mg/m^3; CL 60 mg/m^3/15M   DOT Classification: Poison B; Label: Poison.

SAFETY PROFILE: Questionable carcinogen with experimental carcinogenic and neoplastigenic data. Human poison by ingestion. An experimental poison by ingestion, subcutaneous, intravenous, parenteral, and intraperitoneal routes. Moderately toxic by skin contact. A severe eye and skin irritant. Human mutation data reported. Combustible when exposed to heat, flame, or oxidizers. To fight fire, use alcohol foam, CO_2, dry chemical. When heated to decomposition it emits acrid smoke and irritating fumes.

PDY000   CAS: 2113-47-5
2'-PHENYLACETANILIDE
mf: $C_{14}H_{13}NO$ mw: 211.28

SYNS: ACETAMIDOBIPHENYL ◇ 2-ACETYLAMINOBIPHENYL ◇ N-(2-BIPHENYLYL)ACETAMIDE

TOXICITY DATA with REFERENCE
ETA: orl-rat TDLo:4200 mg/kg/35W-C

CNREA8 16,525,56

MUT: mma-sat 250 μg/plate   MUREAV 118,49,83

SAFETY PROFILE: Questionable carcinogen with experimental tumorigenic data. Mutation data reported. When heated to decomposition it emits toxic fumes of NO_x.

PDY250   CAS: 2113-54-4
3'-PHENYLACETANILIDE
mf: $C_{14}H_{13}NO$ mw: 211.28

SYNS: 3-ACETYLAMINOBIPHENYL ◇ N-(3-BIPHENYLYL)ACETAMIDE

TOXICITY DATA with REFERENCE
ETA: orl-rat TDLo:4200 mg/kg/35W-C

CNREA8 16,525,56

SAFETY PROFILE: Questionable carcinogen with experimental tumorigenic data. When heated to decomposition it emits toxic fumes of NO_x.

PDY500   CAS: 4075-79-0
4'-PHENYLACETANILIDE
mf: $C_{14}H_{13}NO$ mw: 211.28

SYNS: 4-ACETAMIDOBIPHENYL ◇ 4-ACETYLAMINOBIPHENYL ◇ 4-BIPHENYLACETAMIDE ◇ N-4-BIPHENYLACETAMIDE ◇ N-(4-BIPHENYLYL)ACETAMIDE ◇ p-PHENYLACETANILIDE

TOXICITY DATA with REFERENCE
CAR: orl-rat TD:3425 mg/kg/26W-C   CNREA8 22,1002,62

CAR: orl-rat TD:4070 mg/kg/34W-C   CNREA8 16,525,56

CAR: orl-rat TDLo:2770 mg/kg/21W-C

CNREA8 15,188,55

ETA: orl-dog TDLo:13 g/kg/3Y-I   CNREA8 23,921,63

ETA: orl-rat TD:2240 mg/kg/16W-C   CNREA8 21,1465,61

MUT: dnr-ham:fbr 1 μmol/L   JNCIAM 54,1287,75

MUT: mma-sat 100 μg/plate   BBRCA9 73,1025,76

CONSENSUS REPORTS: Reported in EPA TSCA Inventory.

SAFETY PROFILE: Questionable carcinogen with experimental carcinogenic and tumorigenic data. Mutation data reported. When heated to decomposition it emits toxic fumes of NO_x. Used in the manufacture of plastics, resins, rubber, synthetics, dyes, and pigments.

PEB250   CAS: 63040-30-2
4'-PHENYL-o-ACETOTOLUIDE
mf: $C_{15}H_{15}NO$ mw: 225.31

SYN: 3-METHYL-4-ACETYLAMINOBIPHENYL

TOXICITY DATA with REFERENCE
CAR: orl-rat TDLo: 2160 mg/kg/24W-C

CNREA8 22,1002,62

SAFETY PROFILE: Questionable carcinogen with experimental carcinogenic data. When heated to decomposition it emits toxic fumes of NO_x.

PEE600   CAS: 43085-16-1
17-β-PHENYLAMINOCARBONYLOXY-OESTRA-1,3,5(10)-TRIENE-3-METHYL ETHER
mf: $C_{26}H_{31}NO_3$ mw: 405.58
SYN: STS 153

TOXICITY DATA with REFERENCE
ETA: orl-mus TDLo: 100 mg/kg (12-16D post)

AMSHAR 28,209,80

SAFETY PROFILE: Questionable carcinogen with experimental tumorigenic and teratogenic data. Experimental reproductive effects. When heated to decomposition it emits toxic fumes of NO_x.

PEG250   CAS: 613-37-6
p-PHENYLANISOLE
mf: $C_{13}H_{12}O$ mw: 184.25
PROP: Leaves from alc. Mp: 90°. Sol in hot alc.
SYNS: p-METHOXYBIPHENYL ◇ 4-METHOXYBIPHENYL

TOXICITY DATA with REFERENCE
ETA: orl-rat TDLo: 5450 mg/kg/52W-C

ARZNAD 12,270,62

CONSENSUS REPORTS: Reported in EPA TSCA Inventory.

SAFETY PROFILE: Questionable carcinogen with experimental tumorigenic data. When heated to decomposition it emits acrid smoke and irritating fumes.

PEH250   CAS: 13279-22-6
N-PHENYL-1-AZIRIDINECARBOXAMIDE
mf: $C_9H_{10}N_2O$ mw: 162.21
SYNS: 1-AZIRIDINECARBOXANILIDE ◇ N-PHENYLAMI-NOCARBONYL)AZIRIDINE ◇ 1-PHENYLCARBAMOYLAZIR-IDINE ◇ PHENYL-N-CARBAMOYLAZIRIDINE

TOXICITY DATA with REFERENCE
NEO: ipr-mus TDLo: 120 mg/kg/4W-I   CNREA8
29,2184,69

SAFETY PROFILE: Questionable carcinogen with experimental neoplastigenic data. When heated to decomposition it emits toxic fumes of NO_x.

PEH750   CAS: 4128-71-6
4'-PHENYLAZOACETANILIDE
mf: $C_{14}H_{13}N_3O$ mw: 239.30
SYNS: p-ACETAMIDOAZOBENZENE ◇ 4-ACETYLAMI-NOAZOBENZENE ◇ p-PHENYLAZOACETANILIDE

TOXICITY DATA with REFERENCE
ETA: orl-rat TDLo: 4700 mg/kg/52W-C

JNCIAM 24,149,60

SAFETY PROFILE: Questionable carcinogen with experimental tumorigenic data. When heated to decomposition it emits toxic fumes of NO_x.

PEI750   CAS: 36368-30-6
1-PHENYLAZO-2-ANTHROL
mf: $C_{20}H_{14}N_2O$ mw: 298.36
SYN: BENZENEAZO-2-ANTHROL

TOXICITY DATA with REFERENCE
CAR: scu-mus TDLo: 25 g/kg/52W-I   BJCAAI
10,653,56

SAFETY PROFILE: Questionable carcinogen with experimental carcinogenic data. A poison by intramuscular route. When heated to decomposition it emits toxic fumes of NO_x.

PEJ250   CAS: 22670-79-7
N-PHENYLAZO-N-METHYLTAURINE SODIUM SALT
mf: $C_9H_{12}N_3O_3S \cdot Na$ mw: 265.29
SYNS: 3-METHYL-1-PHENYL-3-(2-SULFOETHYL)TRI-AZENE SODIUM SALT ◇ 1-PHENYL-3-METHYL-3-(2-SUL-FOAETHYL) NATRIUM SALZ (GERMAN) ◇ 1-PHENYL-3-METHYL-3-(2-SULFOETHYL)TRIAZENE, SODIUM SALT

TOXICITY DATA with REFERENCE
NEO: scu-rat TDLo: 1170 mg/kg/78W-I

ZKKOBW 81,285,74

SAFETY PROFILE: Questionable carcinogen with experimental neoplastigenic data. Poison by subcutaneous route. When heated to decomposition it emits very toxic fumes of NO_x, Na_2O, and SO_x.

PEJ500   CAS: 842-07-9
1-(PHENYLAZO)-2-NAPHTHOL
mf: $C_{16}H_{12}N_2O$ mw: 248.30

SYNS: ATUL ORANGE R ◇ BENZENEAZO-β-NAPHTHOL ◇ BENZENE-1-AZO-2-NAPHTHOL ◇ 1-BENZENEAZO-2-NAPHTHOL ◇ BENZENE-1-AZO-2-NAPHTHOL ◇ 1-BENZOAZO-2-NAPHTHOL ◇ BRILLIANT OIL ORANGE R ◇ CALCOGAS ORANGE NC ◇ CALCO OIL ORANGE 7078 ◇ CAMPBELLINE OIL ORANGE ◇ CARMINAPH ◇ CERES ORANGE R ◇ CEROTINORANGE G ◇ C.I. 12055 ◇ C.I. SOLVENT YELLOW 14 ◇ DISPERSOL YELLOW PP ◇ DUNKELGELB ◇ ENIAL ORANGE I ◇ FAST OIL ORANGE ◇ FAST ORANGE ◇ FETTORANGE R ◇ GRASAN ORANGE R ◇ HIDACO OIL ORANGE ◇ LACQUER ORANGE VG ◇ MOTIORANGE R ◇ NCI-C53929 ◇ OIL ORANGE ◇ OLEAL ORANGE R ◇ ORANGE A l'HUILE ◇ ORANGE INSOLUBLE OLG ◇ ORANGE PEL ◇ ORANGE RESENOLE NO. 3 ◇ ORANGE SOLUBLE A l'HUILE ◇ ORGANOL ORANGE ◇ ORIENT OIL ORANGE PS ◇ PETROL ORANGE Y ◇ 1-(PHENYLAZO)-2-NAPHTHALENOL ◇ 1-PHENYLAZO-β-NAPHTHOL ◇ PLASTORESIN ORANGE F4A ◇ PYRONALORANGE ◇ RESINOL ORANGE R ◇ RESOFORM ORANGE G ◇ SANSEL ORANGE G ◇ SCHARLACH B ◇ SILOTRAS ORANGE TR ◇ SOLVENT YELLOW 14 ◇ SOMALIA ORANGE I ◇ SOUDAN I ◇ SPIRIT ORANGE ◇ SPIRIT YELLOW I ◇ STEARIX ORANGE ◇ SUDAN ORANGE R ◇ TERTROGRAS ORANGE SV ◇ TOYO OIL ORANGE ◇ WAXAKOL ORANGE GL ◇ WAXOLINE YELLOW I

TOXICITY DATA with REFERENCE

CAR: imp-mus TD:96 mg/kg   GMCRDC 17,383,75
CAR: imp-mus TDLo:80 mg/kg   BJCAAI22,825,68
NEO: orl-rat TD:21630 mg/kg/2Y-C   NTPTR* NTP-TR-226,82
NEO: orl-rat TDLo:10815 mg/kg/2Y-C   NTPTR* NTP-TR-226,82
ETA: imp-mus TD:75 mg/kg   CALEDQ 6,21,79
ETA: scu-mus TDLo:6000 mg/kg/57W-I
    GMJOAZ 30,364,49

CONSENSUS REPORTS: IARC Cancer Review: GROUP 3 IMEMDT 7,56,87; Animal Sufficient Evidence IMEMDT 8,225,75. NTP Carcinogenesis Bioassay (feed); Clear Evidence: rat NTPTR* NTP-TR-226,82. Community Right-To-Know List. Reported in EPA TSCA Inventory. EPA Genetic Toxicology Program.

SAFETY PROFILE: Questionable carcinogen with experimental carcinogenic, neoplastigenic, and tumorigenic data. When heated to decomposition it emits toxic fumes of NO_x. Used for coloring hydrocarbon solvents, oils, fats, waxes, shoe and floor polishes, and gasoline.

PEK000   CAS: 532-82-1
4-PHENYLAZO-m-PHENYLENEDIAMINE
mf: $C_{12}H_{12}N_4 \cdot ClH$ mw: 248.74

SYNS: ASTRA CHRYSOIDINE R ◇ BRASILAZINA ORANGE Y ◇ BRILLIANT OIL ORANGE Y BASE ◇ CALCOZINE CHRYSOIDINE Y ◇ CALCOZINE ORANGE YS ◇ CHRYSOIDIN ◇ CHRYSOIDINE ◇ CHRYSOIDINE A ◇ CHRYSOIDINE B ◇ CHRYSOIDINE C CRYSTALS ◇ CHRYSOIDINE G ◇ CHRYSOIDINE GN ◇ CHRYSOIDINE HR ◇ CHRYSOIDINE(II) ◇ CHRYSOIDINE J ◇ CHRYSOIDINE M ◇ CHRYSOIDINE ORANGE ◇ CHRYSOIDINE PRL ◇ CHRYSOIDINE PRR ◇ CHRYSOIDINE SL ◇ CHRYSOIDINE SPECIAL (biological stain and indicator) ◇ CHRYSOIDINE SS ◇ CHRYSOIDINE Y ◇ CHRYSOIDINE Y BASE NEW ◇ CHRYSOIDINE Y CRYSTALS ◇ CHRYSOIDINE Y EX ◇ CHRYSOIDINE YGH ◇ CHRYSOIDINE YL ◇ CHRYSOIDINE YN ◇ CHRYSOIDINE Y SPECIAL ◇ CHRYSOIDIN FB ◇ CHRYSOIDIN Y ◇ CHRYSOIDIN YN ◇ CHRYZOIDYNA F.B. (POLISH) ◇ C.I. 11270 ◇ C.I. BASIC ORANGE 2 ◇ C.I. BASIC ORANGE 3 ◇ C.I. BASIC ORANGE 2, MONOHYDROCHLORIDE ◇ C.I. SOLVENT ORANGE 3 ◇ 2,4-DIAMINOAZOBENZENE HYDROCHLORIDE ◇ DIAZOCARD CHRYSOIDINE G ◇ ELCOZINE CHRYSOIDINE Y ◇ LEATHER ORANGE HR ◇ 4-(PHENYLAZO)-1,3-BENZENEDIAMINE MONOHYDROCHLORIDE ◇ 4-(PHENYLAZO)-m-PHENYLENEDIAMINE MONOHYDROCHLORIDE ◇ PURE CHRYSOIDINE YBH ◇ PURE CHRYSOIDINE YD ◇ PYRACRYL ORANGE Y ◇ SUGAI CHRYSOIDINE ◇ TERTROPHENE BROWN CG

TOXICITY DATA with REFERENCE

ETA: orl-mus TDLo:94 g/kg/57W-C   XPHPAW 149,365,69
ETA: orl-mus TDLo:93600 mg/kg/56W-C
    LANCAO 1,564,82
MUT: mma-sat 50 μg/plate   MUREAV 44,9,77

CONSENSUS REPORTS: IARC Cancer Review: GROUP 3 IMEMDT 7,169,87; Animal Sufficient Evidence IMEMDT 8,91,75. Reported in EPA TSCA Inventory. EPA Genetic Toxicology Program.

SAFETY PROFILE: Questionable carcinogen with experimental tumorigenic data. Moderately toxic by ingestion and subcutaneous routes. Mutation data reported. When heated to decomposition it emits very toxic fumes of NO_x and HCl. Used as a colorant in textiles, paper, leather, inks, wood, and biological stains.

PEK250   CAS: 94-78-0
3-(PHENYLAZO)-2,6-PYRIDINEDIAMINE
mf: $C_{11}H_{11}N_5$ mw: 213.27

SYNS: AP ◇ 2,6-DIAMINO-3-PHENYLAZOPYRIDINE ◇ DIRIDONE ◇ DPP ◇ GASTRACID ◇ GASTROTEST ◇ MALLOPHENE ◇ NC 150 ◇ PHENAZODINE ◇ PHENAZOPYRIDINE ◇ PHENYLAZO TABLET ◇ PIRID ◇ PYRAZOFEN

◇ PYRIDACIL ◇ PYRIDIUM ◇ PYRIPYRIDIUM ◇ SEDURAL ◇ URIDINAL ◇ URODINE ◇ W 1655

TOXICITY DATA with REFERENCE
NEO: imp-mus TDLo: 80 mg/kg   BJCAAI 11,212,57

CONSENSUS REPORTS: IARC Cancer Review: Animal Inadequate Evidence IMEMDT 8,117,75.

SAFETY PROFILE: Questionable carcinogen with experimental neoplastigenic data. Moderately toxic by intraperitoneal route. Used as a local anesthetic. When heated to decomposition it emits toxic fumes of NO_x.

PEK750   CAS: 19383-97-2
5-PHENYL-1:2-BENZANTHRACENE
mf: $C_{24}H_{16}$ mw: 304.40

SYN: BENZ(a)ANTHRACENE, 8-PHENYL

TOXICITY DATA with REFERENCE
ETA: skn-mus TDLo: 1650 mg/kg/69W-I
PRLBA4 129,439,40

SAFETY PROFILE: Questionable carcinogen with experimental tumorigenic data. When heated to decomposition it emits acrid smoke and irritating fumes.

PEU500   CAS: 13056-98-9
1-PHENYL-3,3-DIETHYLTRIAZENE
mf: $C_{10}H_{15}N_3$ mw: 177.28

SYNS: 3,3-DIETHYL-1-PHENYLTRIAZENE ◇ 1-FENYL-3,3-DIETHYLTRIAZEN (CZECH) ◇ 1-PHENYL-3,3-DIAETHYLTRIAZEN (GERMAN)

TOXICITY DATA with REFERENCE
CAR: scu-rat TD: 1100 mg/kg/70W-I   ZKKOBW 81,285,74
CAR: scu-rat TDLo: 110 mg/kg/(15D preg): TER   IARCCD 4,45,73
CAR: scu-rat TDLo: 300 mg/kg: TER   ZKKOBW 81,285,74
MUT: cyt-ham: lng 10 mg/L   MUREAV 88,197,81
MUT: mnt-mus-ipr 71 mg/kg/24H   MUREAV 56,319,78

CONSENSUS REPORTS: EPA Genetic Toxicology Program.

SAFETY PROFILE: Questionable carcinogen with experimental carcinogenic data. Moderately toxic by ingestion and subcutaneous routes. Experimental teratogenic and reproductive effects. Mutation data reported. When

heated to decomposition it emits toxic fumes of NO_x.

PEY000   CAS: 108-45-2
m-PHENYLENEDIAMINE
DOT: 1673
mf: $C_6H_8N_2$ mw: 108.16

PROP: White crystals. Mp: 63°, bp: 286°, d: 1.139, vap press: 1 mm @ 99.8°. Sol in water, methanol, ethanol, chloroform, acetone; sltly sol in ether, carbon tetrachloride; very sltly sol in benzene, toluene.

SYNS: 3-AMINOANILINE ◇ m-AMINOANILINE ◇ APCO 2330 ◇ m-BENZENEDIAMINE ◇ 1,3-BENZENEDIAMINE ◇ C.I. 76025 ◇ DEVELOPER 11 ◇ m-DIAMINOBENZENE ◇ 1,3-DIAMINOBENZENE ◇ DIRECT BROWN BR ◇ m-FENYLENDIAMIN (CZECH) ◇ METAPHENYLENEDIAMINE ◇ 1,3-PHENYLENEDIAMINE ◇ m-PHENYLENEDIAMINE (DOT) ◇ PHENYLENEDIAMINE, META, SOLID (DOT)

TOXICITY DATA with REFERENCE
ETA: scu-rat TDLo: 1485 mg/kg/47W-I
KJMSAH 13,175,62
MUT: bfa-rat/sat 240 mg/kg   MUREAV 138,137,84
MUT: cyt-ham: lng 12 mg/L   GMCRDC 27,95,81
MUT: dlt-rat-ipr 375 mg/kg/10W-I   MUREAV 68,85,79
MUT: otr-ham: emb 50 μg/L   NCIMAV 58,243,81

CONSENSUS REPORTS: IARC Cancer Review: Animal Inadequate Evidence IMEMDT 16,111,78. EPA Genetic Toxicology Program. Reported in EPA TSCA Inventory.

ACGIH TLV: (Proposed: 0.1 mg/m³)   DOT Classification: Poison B; Label: St. Andrews Cross.

SAFETY PROFILE: Questionable carcinogen with experimental tumorigenic and teratogenic data. Poison by ingestion, intravenous, subcutaneous, intraperitoneal, and possibly other routes. Mildly toxic by skin contact. Mutation data reported. Combustible when exposed to heat or flame. A hair dye ingredient. When heated to decomposition it emits toxic fumes of NO_x.

PEY500   CAS: 106-50-3
p-PHENYLENEDIAMINE
DOT: 1673
mf: $C_6H_8N_2$ mw: 108.16

PROP: White-sltly red crystals. Mp: 146°, flash p: 312°F, vap d: 3.72, bp: 267°. Sol in alc, chloroform, ether.

SYNS: p-AMINOANILINE ◇ 4-AMINOANILINE ◇ BASF URSOL D ◇ p-BENZENEDIAMINE ◇ 1,4-BENZENE-DIAMINE ◇ BENZOFUR D ◇ C.I. 76060 ◇ C.I. DEVELOPER 13 ◇ C.I. OXIDATION BASE 10 ◇ DEVELOPER 13 ◇ DEVELOPER PF ◇ p-DIAMINOBENZENE ◇ 1,4-DIAMINO-BENZENE ◇ DURAFUR BLACK R ◇ FENYLENODWUAMINA (POLISH) ◇ FOURAMINE D ◇ FOURRINE D ◇ FOURRINE 1 ◇ FUR BLACK 41867 ◇ FUR BROWN 41866 ◇ FURRO D ◇ FUR YELLOW ◇ FUTRAMINE D ◇ NAKO H ◇ ORSIN ◇ PARA ◇ PARAPHENYLEN-DIAMINE ◇ PELAGOL D ◇ PELAGOL DR ◇ PELAGOL GREY D ◇ PELTOL D ◇ 1,4-PHENYLENEDIAMINE ◇ PHENYLENEDIAMINE, PARA, SOLID (DOT) ◇ PPD ◇ RENAL PF ◇ SANTOFLEX IC ◇ TERTRAL D ◇ URSOL D ◇ USAF EK-394 ◇ VULKANOX 4020 ◇ ZOBA BLACK D

TOXICITY DATA with REFERENCE
ETA: scu-rat TDLo:2625 mg/kg/30W-C
    KJMSAH 9,94,58
MUT: mma-sat 10 μg/plate   BCPCA6 26,729,77
MUT: otr-rat:emb 1850 ng/plate   JJATDK 1,190,81
MUT: sln-dmg-orl 15500 μmol/L/3D   MUREAV 48,181,77

CONSENSUS REPORTS: IARC Cancer Review: Animal Inadequate Evidence IMEMDT 16,125,78. Community Right-To-Know List. Reported in EPA TSCA Inventory. EPA Genetic Toxicology Program.

OSHA PEL: TWA 0.1 mg/m³ (skin)   ACGIH TLV: TWA 0.1 mg/m³ (skin); (Proposed TWA 0.1 mg/m³)   DFG MAK: 0.1 mg/m³   DOT Classification: ORM-A; Label: None: Poison B; Label: St. Andrews Cross.

SAFETY PROFILE: Questionable carcinogen with experimental tumorigenic data. Poison by ingestion, subcutaneous, intravenous, intraperitoneal, and possibly other routes. Mildly toxic by skin contact. A human skin irritant. Mutation data reported. Combustible when exposed to heat or flame; can react vigorously with oxidizing materials. To fight fire, use water, CO_2, dry chemical. When heated to decomposition it emits acrid smoke and irritating fumes.

PEY600   CAS: 615-28-1
o-PHENYLENEDIAMINE, DIHYDROCHLORIDE
mf: $C_6H_8N_2 \cdot 2ClH$ mw: 181.08
PROP: Needles. Very sol in water.
SYN: USAF EK-678

TOXICITY DATA with REFERENCE
CAR: orl-mus TD:518 g/kg/78W-C   JEPTDQ 2,325,78

CAR: orl-mus TDLo:260 g/kg/78W-C   JEPTDQ 2,325,78
ETA: orl-rat TDLo:130 g/kg/78W-C   JEPTDQ 2,325,78

CONSENSUS REPORTS: Reported in EPA TSCA Inventory.

SAFETY PROFILE: Questionable carcinogen with experimental carcinogenic and tumorigenic data. Poison by intraperitoneal route. When heated to decomposition it emits very toxic fumes of HCl and NO_x.

PEY650   CAS: 624-18-0
p-PHENYLENEDIAMINE DIHYDROCHLORIDE
mf: $C_6H_8N_2 \cdot 2ClH$ mw: 181.08
PROP: Colorless triclinic. Very sol in water; sltly sol in alc; insol in HCl.

SYNS: p-AMINOANILINE DIHYDROCHLORIDE ◇ 4-AMINOANILINE DIHYDROCHLORIDE ◇ p-BENZENEDIAMINE DIHYDROCHLORIDE ◇ 1,4-BENZENEDIAMINE DIHYDROCHLORIDE ◇ C.I. 76061 ◇ C.I. OXIDATION BASE 10A ◇ p-DIAMINOBENZENE DIHYDROCHLORIDE ◇ 1,4-DIAMINOBENZENE DIHYDROCHLORIDE ◇ DURAFUR BLACK RC ◇ FOURINE DS ◇ FOURRINE 64 ◇ NCI-C03930 ◇ OXIDATION BASE 10A ◇ p-PD HCl ◇ p-PDA HCl ◇ PELAGOL CD ◇ PELAGOL GREY CD ◇ 1,4-PHENYLENEDIAMINE DIHYDROCHLORIDE ◇ p-PHENYLENEDIAMINE HYDROCHLORIDE

TOXICITY DATA with REFERENCE
MUT: mma-esc 333 μg/plate   ENMUDM 7(Suppl 5),1,85
MUT: mma-sat 33300 ng/plate   ENMUDM 7(Suppl 5),1,85

CONSENSUS REPORTS: IARC Cancer Review: Animal Inadequate Evidence IMEMDT 16,125,78. NCI Carcinogenesis Bioassay (feed); No Evidence: mouse, rat NCITR* NCI-CG-TR-174,79. Reported in EPA TSCA Inventory.

SAFETY PROFILE: Questionable carcinogen. Poison by ingestion and subcutaneous routes. Mutation data reported. When heated to decomposition it emits very toxic fumes of NO_x and HCl. Used as an analytical reagent.

PEY750   CAS: 541-69-5
m-PHENYLENEDIAMINE HYDROCHLORIDE
mf: $C_6H_8N_2 \cdot 2ClH$ mw: 181.08

PROP: Colorless needles. Very sol in water; sltly sol in alc, ether.

SYNS: m-AMINOANILINE DIHYDROCHLORIDE ◇ 3-AMINOANILINE DIHYDROCHLORIDE ◇ m-BENZENEDI-AMINE DIHYDROCHLORIDE ◇ 1,3-BENZENEDIAMINE HY-DROCHLORIDE ◇ m-DIAMINOBENZENE DIHYDROCHLO-RIDE ◇ 1,3-DIAMINOBENZENE DIHYDROCHLORIDE ◇ 1,3-PHENYLENEDIAMINE DIHYDROCHLORIDE ◇ USAF EK-206

TOXICITY DATA with REFERENCE
ETA: scu-rat TDLo:1800 mg/kg/21W-I
    KJMSAH 13,175,62

CONSENSUS REPORTS: IARC Cancer Review: Animal Inadequate Evidence IMEMDT 16,111,78. Reported in EPA TSCA Inventory.

SAFETY PROFILE: Questionable carcinogen with experimental tumorigenic data. Poison by intraperitoneal and possibly other routes. When heated to decomposition it emits very toxic fumes of HCl and NO_x.

PFC750   CAS: 156-51-4
β-PHENYLETHYLHYDRAZINE SULFATE
mf: $C_8H_{12}N_2 \cdot H_2O_4S$ mw: 234.30

SYNS: ALACINE ◇ ALAZIN ◇ ALAZINE ◇ EP-411 ◇ ESTINERVAL ◇ FELAZINE ◇ FENELZIN ◇ 1-HYDRAZINO-2-PHENYLETHANE HYDROGEN SULPHATE ◇ KALGAN ◇ MAO-REM ◇ MONOPHEN ◇ MONOTEN ◇ N-1544A ◇ NARDELZINE ◇ NARDIL ◇ P 1531 ◇ PHENALZINE ◇ PHENALZINE DIHYDROGEN SULFATE ◇ PHENALZINE HYDROGEN SULPHATE ◇ PHENELZIN ◇ PHENELZINE ACID SULFATE ◇ PHENELZINE BISULPHATE ◇ PHENEL-ZINE SULFATE ◇ PHENETHYLHYDRAZINE SULFATE (1:1) ◇ PHENLINE ◇ PHENODYNE ◇ PHENYLAETHYL-HY-DRAZIN ◇ β-PHENYLETHYLHYDRAZINE DIHYDROGEN SULFATE ◇ 2-PHENYLETHYLHYDRAZINE DIHYDROGEN SULPHATE ◇ β-PHENYLETHYLHYDRAZINE HYDROGEN SULPHATE ◇ PHENYLETHYLHYDRAZINE SULPHATE ◇ S 1544 ◇ STINERVAL

TOXICITY DATA with REFERENCE
NEO: orl-mus TDLo:28 g/kg/77W-C   CNREA8
    36,917,76

CONSENSUS REPORTS: IARC Cancer Review: GROUP 3 IMEMDT 7,312,87; Human Inadequate Evidence IMEMDT 24,175,80; Animal Limited Evidence IMEMDT 24,175,80. EPA Genetic Toxicology Program.

SAFETY PROFILE: Questionable carcinogen with experimental neoplastigenic data. Poison

by ingestion, intraperitoneal, intravenous, and subcutaneous routes. Human systemic effects by ingestion: wakefulness, blood pressure lowering, constipation. Used as a drug for the treatment of depression. When heated to decomposition it emits very toxic fumes of SO_x and NO_x.

PFE900   CAS: 32228-97-0
N-PHENYL-2-FLUORENAMINE
mf: $C_{19}H_{15}N$ mw: 257.35

SYN: N-PHENYL-9H-FLUORENAMINE

TOXICITY DATA with REFERENCE
ETA: ipr-rat TDLo:310 mg/kg/4W-I   CNREA8
    31,778,71

SAFETY PROFILE: Questionable carcinogen with experimental tumorigenic data. When heated to decomposition it emits toxic fumes of NO_x.

PFF000   CAS: 31874-15-4
N-PHENYL-2-FLUORENYLHYDROXYLAMINE
mf: $C_{19}H_{15}NO$ mw: 273.35

SYN: N-PHENYL-N-9H-FLUOREN-2-YLHYDROXYLAMINE

TOXICITY DATA with REFERENCE
ETA: ipr-rat TDLo:450 mg/kg/4W-I   CNREA8
    31,778,71

SAFETY PROFILE: Questionable carcinogen with experimental tumorigenic data. When heated to decomposition it emits toxic fumes of NO_x.

PFI250   CAS: 59-88-1
PHENYLHYDRAZINE HYDROCHLORIDE
mf: $C_6H_8N_2 \cdot ClH$ mw: 144.62

PROP: Leaflet crystals from alc. Mp: 245°. Very sol in water; sol in alc; insol in ether.

SYNS: PHENYLHYDRAZINE MONOHYDROCHLORIDE ◇ PHENYLHYDRAZIN HYDROCHLORID (GERMAN) ◇ PHENYLHYDRAZINIUM CHLORIDE

TOXICITY DATA with REFERENCE
NEO: orl-mus TD:10 g/kg/58W-C   ZKKOBW
    87,267,76
NEO: orl-mus TDLo:8000 mg/kg/42W-I
    34ZRA9 -,869,65
ETA: ipr-mus TDLo:464 mg/kg/8W-I   JNCIAM
    42,337,69
ETA: orl-mus TD:928 mg/kg/8W-I   JNCIAM
    42,337,69

MUT: mma-sat 800 µg/plate   NEZAAQ 33,474,78
MUT: mmo-sat 800 µg/plate   NEZAAQ 33,474,78

CONSENSUS REPORTS: Reported in EPA TSCA Inventory. EPA Extremely Hazardous Substances List.

NIOSH REL: CL 0.6 mg/m^3/2H

SAFETY PROFILE: Questionable carcinogen with experimental neoplastigenic and tumorigenic data. Poison by ingestion and subcutaneous routes. Experimental reproductive effects. Mutation data reported. When heated to decomposition it emits very toxic fumes of NO_x and HCl.

PFS500   CAS: 16033-21-9
1-PHENYL-3-MONOMETHYLTRIAZENE
mf: $C_7H_9N_3$ mw: 135.19

SYN: PMT

TOXICITY DATA with REFERENCE
NEO: scu-mus TDLo: 45 mg/kg/4W-I   CNREA8 34,1671,74
NEO: skn-mus TDLo: 284 mg/kg/8W-I   CNREA8 34,1671,74
MUT: mmo-nsc 600 µmol/L   MUREAV 13,276,71

SAFETY PROFILE: Questionable carcinogen with experimental neoplastigenic data. Poison by subcutaneous route. Mutation data reported. When heated to decomposition it emits toxic fumes of NO_x.

PFT250   CAS: 90-30-2
N-PHENYL-1-NAPHTHYLAMINE
mf: $C_{16}H_{13}N$ mw: 219.30

PROP: Prisms from alc. Mp: 62°, bp: 335° @ 528 mm. Sol in water, benzene, alc, acetic acid, ether, chloroform.

SYNS: ACETO PAN ◇ ADDITIN 30 ◇ 1-ANILINO-NAPHTHALENE ◇ C.I. 44050 ◇ N-(1-NAPHTHYL)ANILINE ◇ NEOZONE A ◇ PANA ◇ PHENYLNAPHTHYLAMINE ◇ PHENYL-α-NAPHTHYLAMINE ◇ N-PHENYL-α-NAPHTHYLAMINE ◇ α-PHENYLNAPHTHYLAMINE ◇ VULKANOX PAN

TOXICITY DATA with REFERENCE
CAR: orl-mus TD: 17280 mg/kg/9W-I   CNREA8 44,3098,84
CAR: orl-mus TDLo: 5400 mg/kg/9W-I   CNREA8 44,3098,84
MUT: dlt-mus-ipr 830 mg/kg/5D-I   NTIS** AD-A041-973

MUT: dns-hmn: lng 50 mg/L   NTIS** AD-A041-973
MUT: mma-sat 500 nL/plate   NTIS** AD-A041-973
MUT: mmo-sat 10 µg/plate   SYSWAE 12,41,79
MUT: otr-hmn: oth 27500 µg/L   ITCSAF 17,719,81

CONSENSUS REPORTS: Reported in EPA TSCA Inventory. EPA Genetic Toxicology Program.

SAFETY PROFILE: Questionable carcinogen with experimental carcinogenic data. Moderately toxic by ingestion. Human mutation data reported. When heated to decomposition it emits toxic fumes of NO_x. Used as a rubber antioxidant.

PFT600   CAS: 6652-04-6
4-PHENYLNITROSOPIPERIDINE
mf: $C_{11}H_{14}N_2O$ mw: 190.27

SYNS: NITROSO-4-PHENYLPIPERIDINE ◇ N-NITROSO-4-PHENYLPIPERIDINE ◇ 1-NITROSO-4-PHENYLPIPERIDINE

TOXICITY DATA with REFERENCE
CAR: orl-rat TDLo: 4175 mg/kg/2Y-I   CRNGDP 2,1045,81
MUT: mma-sat 25 µg/plate   TCMUE9 1,13,84
MUT: pic-esc 2 mg/L   TCMUE9 1,13,84

CONSENSUS REPORTS: EPA Genetic Toxicology Program.

SAFETY PROFILE: Questionable carcinogen with experimental carcinogenic data. Mutation data reported. When heated to decomposition it emits toxic fumes of NO_x.

PGQ000   CAS: 20921-50-0
1-PHENYL-1-(3,4-XYLYL)-2-PROPYNYL
N-CYCLOHEXYLCARBAMATE
mf: $C_{24}H_{27}NO_2$ mw: 361.52

SYN: N-CYCLOHEXYLCARBAMIC ACID 1-PHENYL-1-(3,4-XYLYL)-2-PROPYNYL ESTER

TOXICITY DATA with REFERENCE
ETA: orl-rat TDLo: 20400 mg/kg/45W-C   JJIND8 71,211,83
MUT: dns-hmn: fbr 10 mmol/L/90M   IJCNAW 16,284,75
MUT: mmo-sat 100 µg/plate   PNASA6 72,979,75

CONSENSUS REPORTS: EPA Genetic Toxicology Program.

SAFETY PROFILE: Questionable carcinogen with experimental tumorigenic data. Human mutation data reported. When heated to decomposition it emits toxic fumes of NO_x.

PGR250   CAS: 90-00-6
PHLOROL
mf: $C_8H_{10}O$ mw: 122.18

PROP: Colorless liquid; phenol odor. Mp: $-28°$ d: 1.037 @ 12°, bp: 204.52°, turns solid <18°. Insol in water; misc in alc, benzene, glacial acetic acid, ether.

SYNS: o-ETHYLPHENOL ◇ 2-ETHYLPHENOL

TOXICITY DATA with REFERENCE
NEO: skn-mus TDLo: 3100 mg/kg/12W-I
  CNREA8 19,413,59

CONSENSUS REPORTS: Reported in EPA TSCA Inventory.

SAFETY PROFILE: Questionable carcinogen with experimental neoplastigenic data. Poison by intraperitoneal route. Moderately toxic by ingestion. Human toxic action similar to, but less severe than, that of phenol. When heated to decomposition it emits acrid smoke and irritating fumes.

PGS250   CAS: 17673-25-5
PHORBOL
mf: $C_{20}H_{27}O_6$ mw: 363.47

PROP: Anhydrous crystals. Two forms: mp: 162-163° and 233-234°. decomp @ 250-251°.

TOXICITY DATA with REFERENCE
CAR: ipr-mus TDLo: 400 mg/kg/25W   CNREA8 30,2744,70
ETA: ipr-mus TD: 284 mg/kg/39W-I   JCROD7 95,19,79

CONSENSUS REPORTS: EPA Genetic Toxicology Program.

SAFETY PROFILE: Questionable carcinogen with experimental carcinogenic and tumorigenic data. Experimental reproductive effects. A skin irritant. When heated to decomposition it emits acrid smoke and irritating fumes.

PGS500   CAS: 20839-16-1
PHORBOL ACETATE, LAURATE
mf: $C_{34}H_{52}O_8$ mw: 588.86

SYNS: 5H-CYCLOPROPA(3,4)BENZ(1,2-e)AZULEN-5-ONE, 1,1a,1b,4,4a,7a,7b,8,9,9a-DECAHYDRO-4a,7-β, 9,9a-TETRAHYDROXY-3-(HYDROXYMETHYL)-1,1,6,8-TETRAMETHYL-, 9-ACETATE 9a-LAURATE ◇ PHORBOL MONOACETATE MONOLAURATE

TOXICITY DATA with REFERENCE
NEO: skn-mus TDLo: 20 mg/kg/25W-I
  NATWAY 54,282,67

SAFETY PROFILE: Questionable carcinogen with experimental neoplastigenic data. When heated to decomposition it emits acrid smoke and irritating fumes.

PGS750   CAS: 24928-15-2
PHORBOL-12,13-DIACETATE
mf: $C_{24}H_{32}O_8$ mw: 448.56

TOXICITY DATA with REFERENCE
ETA: skn-mus TDLo: 19 mg/kg/32W-I   CNREA8 31,1074,71
MUT: dnd-esc 200 μg/tube   CNREA8 33,3103,73

SAFETY PROFILE: Questionable carcinogen with experimental tumorigenic data. Mutation data reported. When heated to decomposition it emits acrid smoke and irritating fumes.

PGT000   CAS: 25405-85-0
PHORBOL-12,13-DIBENZOATE
mf: $C_{34}H_{36}O_8$ mw: 572.70

TOXICITY DATA with REFERENCE
ETA: skn-mus TD: 1100 mg/kg/48W-I   CNREA8 39,4183,79
ETA: skn-mus TDLo: 7760 μg/kg/10W-I
  CNREA8 31,1074,71

SAFETY PROFILE: Questionable carcinogen with experimental tumorigenic data. When heated to decomposition it emits acrid smoke and irritating fumes.

PGT250   CAS: 24928-17-4
PHORBOL-12,13-DIDECANOATE
mf: $C_{40}H_{55}O_8$ mw: 663.95

SYN: PDD

TOXICITY DATA with REFERENCE
ETA: skn-mus TD: 17 mg/kg/16W-I   CRNGDP 2,11,78
ETA: skn-mus TD: 318 mg/kg/12W-I   PLMEAA 22,241,72
ETA: skn-mus TDLo: 5472 μg/kg/6W-I
  CNREA8 31,1074,71
MUT: cyt-smc 1 mg/L   NATUAS 294,263,81
MUT: dnd-esc 200 μg/tube   CNREA8 33,3103,73
MUT: dns-rat: lvr 1 μg/L   CNREA8 40,4541,80
MUT: otr-ham: emb 100 μg/L   CALEDQ 17,1,82

SAFETY PROFILE: Questionable carcinogen with experimental tumorigenic data. A skin irritant. Mutation data reported. When heated to decomposition it emits acrid smoke and irritating fumes.

PGT500
PHORBOL-12,13-DIHEXA(Δ-2,4)-DIENOATE
mf: $C_{32}H_{57}O_8$ mw: 569.89

TOXICITY DATA with REFERENCE
ETA: skn-mus TDLo: 55 g/kg/12W-I   PLMEAA
22,241,72

SAFETY PROFILE: Questionable carcinogen with experimental tumorigenic data. A skin irritant. When heated to decomposition it emits acrid smoke and irritating fumes.

PGT750   CAS: 37558-17-1
PHORBOL-12,13-DIHEXANOATE
mf: $C_{32}H_{45}O_8$ mw: 557.77

TOXICITY DATA with REFERENCE
ETA: skn-mus TDLo: 16 g/kg/12W-I   PLMEAA
22,241,72

SAFETY PROFILE: Questionable carcinogen with experimental tumorigenic data. A skin irritant. When heated to decomposition it emits acrid smoke and irritating fumes.

PGU000   CAS: 63040-44-8
PHORBOL LAURATE, (+)-S-2-METHYLBUTYRATE
mf: $C_{37}H_{58}O_8$ mw: 630.95

SYN: PHORBOL MONOLAURATE MONO(S)-(+)-2-METHYLBUTYRATE

TOXICITY DATA with REFERENCE
NEO: skn-mus TDLo: 24 mg/kg/30W-I
NATWAY 54,282,67

SAFETY PROFILE: Questionable carcinogen with experimental neoplastigenic data. When heated to decomposition it emits acrid smoke and irritating fumes.

PGU250   CAS: 16675-05-1
PHORBOL MONOACETATE MONOLAURATE
mf: $C_{34}H_{52}O_8$ mw: 588.86

SYN: PHORBOL ACETATE LAURATE

TOXICITY DATA with REFERENCE
NEO: skn-mus TDLo: 20 mg/kg/25W-I
NATWAY 54,282,67

SAFETY PROFILE: Questionable carcinogen with experimental neoplastigenic data. When heated to decomposition it emits acrid smoke and irritating fumes.

PGU500   CAS: 63040-43-7
PHORBOL MONODECANOATE (S)-(+)-MONO(2-METHYLBUTYRATE)
mf: $C_{35}H_{54}O_8$ mw: 602.89

SYN: PHORBOL CAPRATE, (+)-(S)-2-METHYLBUTYRATE

TOXICITY DATA with REFERENCE
NEO: skn-mus TDLo: 24 mg/kg/30W-I
NATWAY 54,282,67

SAFETY PROFILE: Questionable carcinogen with experimental neoplastigenic data. When heated to decomposition it emits acrid smoke and irritating fumes.

PGU750   CAS: 59086-92-9
(E)-PHORBOL MONODECANOATE MONO(2-METHYLCROTONATE)
mf: $C_{35}H_{52}O_8$ mw: 600.87

SYN: PHORBOL CAPRATE, TIGLATE

TOXICITY DATA with REFERENCE
NEO: skn-mus TDLo: 23 mg/kg/29W-I
NATWAY 54,282,67

SAFETY PROFILE: Questionable carcinogen with experimental neoplastigenic data. When heated to decomposition it emits acrid smoke and irritating fumes.

PGV000   CAS: 16561-29-8
PHORBOL MYRISTATE ACETATE
mf: $C_{36}H_{56}O_8$ mw: 616.92

SYNS: PENTAHYDROXY-TIGLIADIENONE-MONOACE-TATE(C)MONOMYRISTATE(B) ◇ PHORBOL ACETATE, MYRISTATE ◇ PHORBOL MONOACETATE MONOMYRIS-TATE ◇ PMA ◇ 12-TETRADECANOYLPHORBOL-13-ACE-TATE ◇ 12-o-TETRADEKANOYLPHORBOL-13-ACETAT (GERMAN) ◇ TPA

TOXICITY DATA with REFERENCE
CAR: skn-mus TDLo: 30204 μg/kg/72W-I
ACPADQ 91,103,83
NEO: skn-ham TD: 14 mg/kg/22W-I   PEXTAR
26,128,83
NEO: skn-mus TD: 20 mg/kg/25W-I   NATWAY
54,282,67
NEO: skn-mus TD: 1234 μg/kg/25W-I VAAZA2
30,33,79

ETA: imp-dog TDLo: 798 ng/kg/21W-C JJIND8
6,921,80

ETA: ivg-mus TDLo: 51 mg/kg/52W-I CRNGDP
1,707,80

ETA: orl-mus TDLo: 10 mg/kg CNREA8 39,1293,79

ETA: skn-ham TDLo: 7800 μg/kg/26W-I
CNREA8 40,155,80

ETA: skn-mus TD: 19 mg/kg/47W-I PEXTAR
26,128,83

ETA: skn-mus TD: 21 mg/kg/26W-I CNREA8
40,642,80

ETA: skn-mus TD: 22 mg/kg/52W-I BJCAAI
39,276,79

ETA: skn-mus TD: 1680 μg/kg/16W-I BJCAAI
34,523,76

ETA: skn-mus TD: 2960 mg/kg/24W-I CNREA8
39,4183,79

ETA: skn-mus TD: 4520 μg/kg/67W-I CALEDQ
19,21,83

ETA: skn-mus TD: 7200 μg/kg/24W-I CNREA8
38,921,78

MUT: dnd-hmn: fbr 1300 nmol/L CRNGDP
6,1667,85

MUT: dni-hmn: fbr 20 mg/L JNCIAM 55,801,75

MUT: dns-hmn: fbr 100 μg/L CNREA8 39,4477,79

MUT: dns-hmn: oth 10 μg/L CNREA8 44,4078,84

MUT: mmo-esc 1 mg/L JPPMAB 31,69P,79

CONSENSUS REPORTS: EPA Genetic Toxicology Program.

SAFETY PROFILE: Questionable carcinogen with experimental carcinogenic, neoplastigenic, and tumorigenic data. Deadly poison by intravenous route. Experimental reproductive effects. Human mutation data reported. A skin irritant. When heated to decomposition it emits acrid smoke and irritating fumes.

PGV250
PHORBOL-9-MYRISTATE-9a-ACETATE-3-ALDEHYDE
mf: $C_{36}H_{54}O_7$ mw: 598.90

SYN: PAMA

TOXICITY DATA with REFERENCE
ETA: skn-mus TDLo: 32 mg/kg/27W-I CNREA8
39,2644,79

SAFETY PROFILE: Questionable carcinogen with experimental tumorigenic data. When heated to decomposition it emits acrid smoke and irritating fumes.

PGV750   CAS: 37415-55-7
PHORBOL-12-o-TIGLYL-13-BUTYRATE
mf: $C_{28}H_{40}O_8$ mw: 504.68

SYN: 12-o-TIGLYL-PHORBOL-13-BUTYRATE

TOXICITY DATA with REFERENCE
ETA: skn-mus TDLo: 29 mg/kg/12W-I 85CVA2
5,213,70

SAFETY PROFILE: Questionable carcinogen with experimental tumorigenic data. A skin irritant. When heated to decomposition it emits acrid smoke and irritating fumes.

PGW000   CAS: 37394-32-4
PHORBOL-12-o-TIGLYL-13-DODECANOATE
mf: $C_{37}H_{56}O_8$ mw: 628.93

SYN: 12-o-TIGLYL-PHORBOL-13-DODECANOATE

TOXICITY DATA with REFERENCE
ETA: skn-mus TDLo: 12 mg/kg/12W-I 85CVA2
5,213,70

SAFETY PROFILE: Questionable carcinogen with experimental tumorigenic data. A skin irritant. When heated to decomposition it emits acrid smoke and irritating fumes.

PHW000   CAS: 86-54-4
1(2H)-PHTHALAZINONE HYDRAZONE
mf: $C_8H_8N_4$ mw: 160.20

SYNS: APRESOLIN ◇ APPRESSIN ◇ APREZOLIN ◇ BA5968 ◇ C-5068 ◇ C 5968 ◇ CIBA 5968 ◇ HIDRALAZIN ◇ HIPOFTALIN ◇ HYDRALAZINE ◇ HYDRALLAZINE ◇ HYDRAZINOPHTHALAZINE ◇ 1-HYDRAZINOPHTHALAZINE ◇ HYPOPHTHALIN ◇ IDRALAZINA (ITALIAN)

TOXICITY DATA with REFERENCE
MUT: dnr-esc 200 μg/disc MUREAV 68,79,79
MUT: dns-rbt: lvr 5 mmol/L PNASA6 79,1269,82
MUT: mma-sat 500 μg/plate MUREAV 66,247,79
MUT: mmo-sat 500 μg/plate MUREAV 68,79,79
MUT: slt-dmg-unr 200 mmol/L/6H MUREAV
120,233,83

CONSENSUS REPORTS: IARC Cancer Review: GROUP 3 IMEMDT 7,222,87; Human Inadequate Evidence IMEMDT 24,85,80.

SAFETY PROFILE: Questionable carcinogen. Poison by ingestion, intravenous, intraperitoneal, and subcutaneous routes. Human systemic effects by ingestion: allergic dermatitis. Human teratogenic effects by an unspecified route: developmental abnormalities of the blood and lymphatic system. Mutation data reported. When heated to decomposition it emits toxic fumes of NO_x.

PHY000   CAS: 91-15-6
PHTHALONITRILE
mf: $C_8H_4N_2$ mw: 128.14

SYNS: o-DICYANOBENZENE ◇ 1,2-DICYANOBENZENE ◇ PHTHALIC ACID DINITRILE ◇ PHTHALODINITRILE ◇ o-PHTHALODINITRILE ◇ USAF ND-09

TOXICITY DATA with REFERENCE
ETA: orl-mus TDLo:21 g/kg/65W-I   VOONAW 18(1),81,72
ETA: orl-rat TDLo:7425 mg/kg/66W-I
    VOONAW 18(1),81,72
ETA: scu-mus TDLo:7 g/kg/63W-I   VOONAW 18(1),81,72
ETA: scu-rat TDLo:473 mg/kg/21W-I
    VOONAW 18(1),81,72
ETA: skn-mus TDLo:813 mg/kg/46W-I
    VOONAW 18(1),81,72

CONSENSUS REPORTS: Cyanide and its compounds are on the Community Right-To-Know List. Reported in EPA TSCA Inventory.

SAFETY PROFILE: Questionable carcinogen with experimental tumorigenic data. Poison by ingestion, subcutaneous, and intraperitoneal routes. When heated to decomposition it emits toxic fumes of CN^- and NO_x.

PIB750   CAS: 213-46-7
PICENE
mf: $C_{22}H_{14}$ mw: 278.36

PROP: Leaflets. Mp: 364°, bp: 520°. Insol in water; very sltly sol in alc, ether.

SYNS: 3,4-BENZCHRYSENE ◇ BENZO(a)CHRYSENE ◇ β,β-BINAPHTHYLENEETHENE ◇ DIBEN-ZO(a,i)PHENANTHRENE ◇ 1,2:7,8-DIBENZOPHENAN-THRENE

TOXICITY DATA with REFERENCE
NEO: skn-mus TDLo:111 mg/kg   JNCIAM 50,1717,73

SAFETY PROFILE: Questionable carcinogen with experimental neoplastigenic data. When heated to decomposition it emits acrid smoke and irritating fumes.

PIB900   CAS: 1918-02-1
PICLORAM
mf: $C_6H_3Cl_3N_2O_2$ mw: 241.46

PROP: Crystals. Mp: 218°.

SYNS: AMDON GRAZON ◇ 4-AMINO-3,5,6-TRICHLORO-PICOLINIC ACID ◇ 4-AMINO-3,5,6-TRICHLORO-2-PICO-

LINIC ACID ◇ 4-AMINO-3,5,6-TRICHLORPICOLINSAEURE (GERMAN) ◇ ATCP ◇ BOROLIN ◇ CHLORAMP (RUSSIAN) ◇ K-PIN ◇ NCI-C00237 ◇ TORDON ◇ TORDON 10K ◇ TORDON 22K ◇ TORDON 101 MIXTURE ◇ 3,5,6-TRI-CHLORO-4-AMINOPICOLINIC ACID

TOXICITY DATA with REFERENCE
CAR: orl-rat TD:417 g/kg/80W-C   JTEHD6 7,207,81
CAR: orl-rat TDLo:209 mg/kg/80W-C   JTEHD6 7,207,81
NEO: orl-mus TDLo:340 g/kg/80W-C   JTEHD6 7,207,81
NEO: orl-rat TDLo:416 g/kg/80W-C   NCITR* NCI-CG-TR-23,78
ETA: orl-rat TD:208 g/kg/80W-C   NCITR* NCI-CG-TR-23,78
MUT: mmo-smc 100 mg/L   TGANAK 18,455,84

CONSENSUS REPORTS: NCI Carcinogenesis Bioassay (feed); No Evidence: mouse NCITR* NCI-CG-TR-23,78; Clear Evidence: rat NCITR* NCI-CG-TR-23,78

OSHA PEL: (Transitional: Total Dust: 15 mg/m^3; Respirable Fraction: 5 mg/m^3) TWA Total Dust: 10 mg/m^3; Respirable Fraction: 5 mg/m^3 ACGIH TLV: TWA 10 mg/m^3

SAFETY PROFILE: Questionable carcinogen with experimental carcinogenic, neoplastigenic, tumorigenic, and teratogenic data. Moderately toxic by ingestion. Mutation data reported. When heated to decomposition it emits very toxic fumes of Cl^- and NO_x.

PIJ250
PIPERAZINE and SODIUM NITRITE (4:1)
SYN: SODIUM NITRITE and PIPERAZINE (1:4)

TOXICITY DATA with REFERENCE
CAR: orl-mus TDLo:183 g/kg/28W-C   JNCIAM 46,1029,71
ETA: orl-rat TD:130 g/kg/39W-C   IGSBDO 5,321,79
ETA: orl-rat TDLo:90 g/kg/47W-C   IGSBDO 5,321,79

SAFETY PROFILE: Questionable carcinogen with experimental carcinogenic and tumorigenic data. When heated to decomposition it emits toxic fumes of NO_x and Na_2O.

PIX250   CAS: 51-03-6
PIPERONYL BUTOXIDE
mf: $C_{19}H_{30}O_5$ mw: 338.49

PROP: Light brown liquid; mild odor. Bp: 180° @ 1 mm, flash p: 340°F, d: 1.04-1.07 @ 20°/20°. Misc with methanol, ethanol, benzene.

SYNS: BUTACIDE ◇ BUTOCIDE ◇ BUTOXIDE ◇ α-(2-(2-BUTOXYETHOXY)ETHOXY)-4,5-METHYLENEDI-OXY-2-PROPYLTOLUENE ◇ α-(2-(2-n-BUTOXYETHOXY)-ETHOXY)-4,5-METHYLENEDIOXY-2-PROPYLTOLUENE ◇ 5-((2-(2-BUTOXYETHOXY)ETHOXY)METHYL)-6-PROPYL-1,3-BENZODIOXOLE ◇ BUTYL CARBITOL 6-PROPYLPIPER-ONYL ETHER ◇ BUTYL-CARBITYL (6-PROPYLPIPERONYL) ETHER ◇ ENT 14,250 ◇ FAC 5273 ◇ FMC 5273 ◇ 3,4-METHY-LENDIOXY-6-PROPYLBENZYL-n-BUTYL-DIAETHYLEN-GLYKOLAETHER (GERMAN) ◇ (3,4-METHYLENEDIOXY-6-PROPYLBENZYL) (BUTYL) DIETHYLENE GLICOL ETHER ◇ 3,4-METHYLENEDIOXY-6-PROPYLBENZYL n-BUTYL DI-ETHYLENEGLYCOL ETHER ◇ NCI-C02813 ◇ NIA 5273 ◇ NUSYN-NOXFISH ◇ PB ◇ PRENTOX ◇ 6-(PROPYLPIPERO-NYL)-BUTYL CARBITYL ETHER ◇ 6-PROPYLPIPERONYL BUTYL DIETHYLENE GLYCOL ETHER ◇ 5-PROPYL-4-(2,5,8-TRIOXA-DODECYL)-1,3-BENZODIOXOL (GERMAN) ◇ PYBUTHRIN ◇ PYRENONE 606 ◇ SYNPREN-FISH

TOXICITY DATA with REFERENCE
ETA: scu-mus TDLo: 1000 mg/kg   NTIS** PB223-159
MUT: otr-ham:emb 500 µg/L   CRNGDP 4,291,83

CONSENSUS REPORTS: IARC Cancer Review: Animal No Evidence IMEMDT 30, 183,83. NCI Carcinogenesis Bioassay (feed); No Evidence: mouse, rat NCITR* NCI-CG-TR-120,79. Glycol ether compounds are on the Community Right-To-Know List. Reported in EPA TSCA Inventory.

SAFETY PROFILE: Questionable carcinogen with experimental tumorigenic data. Poison by skin contact. Moderately toxic by ingestion and intraperitoneal routes. Experimental reproductive effects. Many glycol ether compounds have dangerous human reproductive effects. Mutation data reported. Combustible when exposed to heat or flame; can react with oxidizing materials. To fight fire, use foam, CO_2, dry chemical. When heated to decomposition it emits acrid smoke and irritating fumes.

PJA250   CAS: 9002-72-6
PITUITARY GROWTH HORMONE

SYNS: ADENOHYPOPHYSEAL GROWTH HORMONE ◇ ANTERIOR PITUITARY GROWTH HORMONE ◇ GROWTH HORMONE ◇ HORMONE SOMATOTROPE (FRENCH) ◇ HYPOPHYSEAL GROWTH HORMONE ◇ PHYOL ◇ PHYONE ◇ SOMACTON ◇ SOMATOTROPIC HORMONE ◇ SOMATOTROPIN

TOXICITY DATA with REFERENCE
CAR: ipr-rat TDLo: 3600 mg/kg/69W-I   CNREA8 10,297,50
MUT: cyt-mus-ipr 31 mg/kg/5D   RRENAR 10,311,73

SAFETY PROFILE: Questionable carcinogen with experimental carcinogenic data. Experimental teratogenic and reproductive effects. Mutation data reported.

PJA500   CAS: 75-98-9
PIVALIC ACID
mf: $C_5H_{10}O_2$ mw: 102.15

PROP: Crystals. Mp: 35.5°, bp: 164°, d: 0.91. Very sol in alc, ether; somewhat sol in water.

SYNS: 2,2-DIMETHYLPROPANOIC ACID ◇ α,α-DI-METHYLPROPIONIC ACID ◇ 2,2-DIMETHYLPROPIONIC ACID ◇ NEOPENTANOIC ACID ◇ tert-PENTANOIC ACID ◇ PROPANOIC ACID ◇ TRIMETHYLACETIC ACID

TOXICITY DATA with REFERENCE
ETA: skn-mus TDLo: 188 mg/kg/47W-I   CALEDQ 17,61,82

CONSENSUS REPORTS: Reported in EPA TSCA Inventory.

SAFETY PROFILE: Questionable carcinogen with experimental tumorigenic data. Moderately toxic by ingestion and skin contact. When heated to decomposition it emits acrid smoke and irritating fumes.

PJD500   CAS: 7440-06-4
PLATINUM
af: Pt   aw: 195.09

PROP: Silvery-white, malleable, ductile metal; stable in air. Mp: 1772°, bp: 3827°, d: 21.45 @ 20°.

SYNS: PLATINUM BLACK ◇ PLATINUM SPONGE ◇ C.I. 77795 ◇ LIQUID BRIGHT PLATINUM ◇ PLATIN (GERMAN)

TOXICITY DATA with REFERENCE
ETA: imp-mus TDLo: 23 g/kg   NATWAY 42,75,55
ETA: imp-rat TDLo: 5250 mg/kg   NATWAY 42,75,55

CONSENSUS REPORTS: Reported in EPA TSCA Inventory.

OSHA PEL: TWA (metal) 1 mg/m³; (soluble salts as Pt) 0.002 mg/m³   ACGIH TLV: TWA (metal) 1 mg/m³; (soluble salts as Pt) 0.002 mg/m³   DFG MAK: 0.002 mg/m³

SAFETY PROFILE: Questionable carcinogen with experimental tumorigenic data by implant route. Finely divided platinum is a powerful catalyst and can be dangerous to handle. Used catalysts are especially dangerous and may be explosive.

PJH500   CAS: 9006-00-2
PLIOFILM
mf: $(C_3H_5Cl)_n$

SYNS: PERMASEAL ◊ RUBBER HYDROCHLORIDE ◊ RUBBER HYDROCHLORIDE POLYMER

TOXICITY DATA with REFERENCE
ETA: imp-rat TDLo: 18 mg/kg   CNREA8 15,333,55

SAFETY PROFILE: Questionable carcinogen with experimental tumorigenic data. When heated to decomposition it emits toxic fumes of Cl^-.

PJJ000   CAS: 9000-55-9
PODOPHYLLIN

PROP: Light yellow powder or small yellow fragile lumps; bitter, acrid taste.

SYNS: PODOPHYLLUM ◊ PODOPHYLLUM RESIN

TOXICITY DATA with REFERENCE
NEO: orl-mus TDLo: 92 g/kg/60W-C   CNREA8 28,2272,68

SAFETY PROFILE: Questionable carcinogen with experimental neoplastigenic data. Poison by ingestion, subcutaneous, intraperitoneal, and possibly other routes. An irritant to skin, eyes, and mucous membranes. Combustible when exposed to heat or flames. When heated to decomposition it emits acrid smoke and irritating fumes.

PJP250   CAS: 61788-33-8
POLYCHLORINATED TERPHENYL

PROP: Kanechlor carbon consists of 95% polychlorinated terphenyl and 5% PCB (CALEDQ 4,271,78).

SYN: KANECHLOR 500

TOXICITY DATA with REFERENCE
CAR: orl-mus TDLo: 11 g/kg/24W-C   CALEDQ 4,271,78
ETA: orl-mus TD: 10 g/kg/24W-C   JTSCDR 3,259,78

CONSENSUS REPORTS: Reported in EPA TSCA Inventory.

SAFETY PROFILE: Questionable carcinogen with experimental carcinogenic and tumorigenic data. When heated to decomposition it emits toxic fumes of Cl^-.

PJQ750   CAS: 26780-96-1
POLY(1,2-DIHYDRO-2,2,4-TRIMETHYLQUINOLINE)
mf: $(C_{11}H_{16}N)_n$

SYNS: TRIMETHYLDIHYDROQUINOLINE POLYMER ◊ 2,2,4-TRIMETHYL-1,2-DIHYDROQUINOLINE POLYMER

TOXICITY DATA with REFERENCE
NEO: orl-rat TDLo: 548 g/kg/2Y-C   TXAPA9 9,583,66

CONSENSUS REPORTS: Reported in EPA TSCA Inventory.

SAFETY PROFILE: Questionable carcinogen with experimental neoplastigenic data. When heated to decomposition it emits toxic fumes of NO_x.

PJR000   CAS: 9016-00-6
POLYDIMETHYL SILOXANE

PROP: A water-insoluble polymer of high viscosity (AMPLAO 67,589,59).

SYNS: DIMETHICONE 350 ◊ DOW CORNING 346 ◊ GEON ◊ GOOD-RITE ◊ GUM ◊ HYCAR ◊ LATEX ◊ METHYL SILICONE ◊ POLY(OXY(DIMETHYLSILYLENE))

TOXICITY DATA with REFERENCE
NEO: imp-rat TDLo: 1500 mg/kg   AMPLAO 67,589,59

SAFETY PROFILE: Questionable carcinogen with experimental neoplastigenic data. Experimental reproductive effects. When heated to decomposition it emits acrid smoke and irritating fumes. Used as a release material, foam preventative, and surface active agent.

PJR250   CAS: 63394-02-5
POLYDIMETHYLSILOXANE RUBBER

PROP: Vulcanized with 2,4-dichlorbenzoyl peroxide, pure silicon dioxide used as filler and plasticizer (ARPAAQ 67,589,59).

SYNS: POLYSILICONE ◊ SILASTIC ◊ SILICONE RUBBER

TOXICITY DATA with REFERENCE
CAR: imp-rat TDLo: 1500 mg/kg   AMPLAO 67,589,59
ETA: imp-rat TD: 900 mg/kg   JNCIAM 33,1005,64

SAFETY PROFILE: Questionable carcinogen with experimental carcinogenic and tumorigenic data. When heated to decomposition it emits acrid smoke and irritating fumes.

PJR750 CAS: 34828-67-6
POLYESTRADIOL PHOSPHATE

SYNS: ESTRADURIN ◇ PEP

TOXICITY DATA with REFERENCE
ETA: scu-mus TDLo: 70 mg/kg/60D-I ATHBA3 12,209,73

SAFETY PROFILE: Questionable carcinogen with experimental tumorigenic data. Human reproductive effects by intramuscular route: testes, epididymis, sperm duct effects. When heated to decomposition it emits very toxic fumes of PO_x.

PJS750 CAS: 9002-88-4
POLYETHYLENE
mf: $(C_2H_4)_n$

PROP: Odorless. The high molecular weight compounds are tough, white leathery, resinous. D: 0.92 @ 20°/4°, mp: 85-110°. Sol in hot benzene; insol in water.

SYNS: AGILENE ◇ ALKATHENE ◇ BAKELITE DYNH ◇ DIOTHENE ◇ ETHENE POLYMER ◇ ETHYLENE HOMO-POLYMER ◇ ETHYLENE POLYMERS ◇ HOECHST PA 190 ◇ MICROTHENE ◇ POLYETHYLENE AS ◇ POLYWAX 1000 ◇ TENITE 800

TOXICITY DATA with REFERENCE
ETA: imp-mus TDLo: 331 mg/kg CNREA8 15,333,55
ETA: imp-rat TD: 1000 mg/kg AJOGAH 96,134,66
ETA: imp-rat TD: 1476 mg/kg CORTBR 88,223,72
ETA: imp-rat TD: 2120 mg/kg BJCAAI 23,401,69
ETA: imp-rat TDLo: 33 mg/kg CNREA8 15,333,55

CONSENSUS REPORTS: IARC Cancer Review: GROUP 3 IMEMDT 7,56,87; Animal Sufficient Evidence IMEMDT 19,157,79; Human Inadequate Evidence IMEMDT 19,157,79. Reported in EPA TSCA Inventory.

SAFETY PROFILE: Questionable carcinogen with experimental tumorigenic data by implant. When heated to decomposition it emits acrid smoke and irritating fumes.

PJT000 CAS: 25322-68-3
POLYETHYLENE GLYCOL
mf: $H(OC_2H_4)_nOH$

PROP: Clear liquid or white solid. D: 1.110-1.140 @ 20°, mp: 4-10°, flash p: 471°F. Sol in organic solvents, aromatic hydrocarbons.

SYNS: ALKAPOL PEG-200 ◇ CARBOWAX ◇ α-HYDROXY-omega-HYDROXY-POLY(OXY-1,2-ETHANEDIYL) ◇ JEFFOX ◇ JORCHEM 400 ML ◇ LUTROL ◇ PEG ◇ PLURACOL P-410 ◇ POLY(ETHYLENE OXIDE) ◇ POLY-G SERIES ◇ POLYOX

TOXICITY DATA with REFERENCE
ETA: ivg-mus TDLo: 416 mg/kg/Y-I BJCAAI 15,252,61
MUT: eye-rbt 500 mg/24H MLD 85JCAE-,1413,86

CONSENSUS REPORTS: Reported in EPA TSCA Inventory. EPA Genetic Toxicology Program.

SAFETY PROFILE: Questionable carcinogen with experimental tumorigenic data. Moderately toxic by intraperitoneal and intravenous routes. Slightly toxic by ingestion. An eye irritant. Combustible liquid when exposed to heat or flame. To fight fire, use water, foam, dry chemical. When heated to decomposition it emits acrid smoke and irritating fumes. See also other polyethylene glycol entries.

PJT250 CAS: 25322-68-3
POLYETHYLENE GLYCOL 1000
mf: $H(OC_2H_4)_nOH$

SYNS: CARBOWAX 1000 ◇ MACROGOL 1000 ◇ PEG 1000 ◇ POLYAETHYLENGLYKOLE 1000 (GERMAN) ◇ POLYGLY-COL 1000 ◇ POLYGLYCOL E1000

TOXICITY DATA with REFERENCE
ETA: ivg-mus TDLo: 416 mg/kg/Y-I BJCAAI 15,252,61

CONSENSUS REPORTS: Reported in EPA TSCA Inventory. EPA Genetic Toxicology Program.

SAFETY PROFILE: Questionable carcinogen with experimental tumorigenic data. Moderately toxic by intraperitoneal and intravenous routes. Mildly toxic by ingestion. When heated to decomposition it emits acrid smoke and irritating fumes.

PJV250 CAS: 9004-99-3
POLYETHYLENE GLYCOL MONOSTEARATE

SYNS: POLYOXYETHYLENE-8-MONOSTEARATE ◇ POLYOXYETHYLENE(8)STEARATE

TOXICITY DATA with REFERENCE

ETA: imp-rat TDLo: 100 mg/kg   AEHLAU 6,484,63

ETA: ipl-rat TDLo: 4000 mg/kg/69W-I   AEHLAU 6,484,63

ETA: orl-mus TDLo: 18250 g/kg/1Y-C   AEHLAU 6,484,63

ETA: orl-rat TDLo: 4015 g/kg/2Y-C   AEHLAU 6,484,63

CONSENSUS REPORTS: Reported in EPA TSCA Inventory.

SAFETY PROFILE: Questionable carcinogen with experimental tumorigenic data. Very slightly toxic by ingestion. When heated to decomposition it emits acrid smoke and irritating fumes.

PJX750
POLYETHYLENE Y-141-A

TOXICITY DATA with REFERENCE

ETA: imp-rat TDLo: 6750 mg/kg   CNREA8 35,1591,75

SAFETY PROFILE: Questionable carcinogen with experimental tumorigenic data by implant route. When heated to decomposition it emits acrid smoke and irritating fumes.

PJY500   CAS: 25038-54-4
POLY(IMINOCARBONYLPENTA-METHYLENE)

mf: $(C_6H_{11}NO)_n$

SYNS: AKULON ◇ ALKAMID ◇ AMILAN CM 1001 ◇ 6-AMINOHEXANOIC ACID HOMOPOLYMER ◇ BONAMID ◇ CAPRAN 80 ◇ CAPROAMIDE POLYMER ◇ CAPROLAC-TAM OLIGOMER ◇ epsilon-CAPROLACTAM POLYMERE (GERMAN) ◇ CAPRON ◇ CHEMLON ◇ DANAMID ◇ DULL 704 ◇ DURETHAN BK ◇ ERTALON 6SA ◇ GRILON ◇ HEXAHYDRO-2H-AZEPIN-2-ONE HOMO-POLYMER ◇ ITAMID ◇ KAPROLIT ◇ KAPROLON ◇ KAPROMIN ◇ KAPRON ◇ MARANYL F 114 ◇ METAMID ◇ MIRAMID WM 55 ◇ NYLON-6 ◇ ORGAMIDE ◇ PA 6 (POLYMER) ◇ PLASKON 201 ◇ POLICAPRAN ◇ POLYAM-IDE 6 ◇ POLY(epsilon-AMINOCAPROIC ACID) ◇ POLYCA-PROAMIDE ◇ POLY(epsilon-CAPROAMIDE) ◇ POLYCAPRO-LACTAM ◇ POLY(epsilon-CAPROLACTAM) ◇ POLY(IMINO(1-OXO-1,6-HEXANEDIYL)) ◇ RELON P ◇ SPENCER 401 ◇ STILON ◇ TARLON XB ◇ TARNAMID T ◇ ULTRAMID BMK ◇ VIDLON ◇ WIDLON ◇ ZYTEL 211

TOXICITY DATA with REFERENCE

NEO: imp-rat TDLo: 5 film disc/rat   ZENBAX 7B,353,52

CONSENSUS REPORTS: IARC Cancer Review: Animal Inadequate Evidence IMEMDT 19,115,75. Reported in EPA TSCA Inventory.

SAFETY PROFILE: Questionable carcinogen with experimental neoplastigenic data by implant route. Moderately toxic by ingestion. Mildly toxic by inhalation. When heated to decomposition it emits toxic fumes of NO_x.

PKA000
POLYMERIC DIALDEHYDE

mf: $(C_6H_8O_5)_n$

TOXICITY DATA with REFERENCE

ETA: scu-mus TDLo: 268 mg/kg/67W-I JNCIAM 46,143,71

SAFETY PROFILE: Questionable carcinogen with experimental tumorigenic data. When heated to decomposition it emits acrid smoke and irritating fumes.

PKA850
POLYMERS, WATER INSOLUBLE

SAFETY PROFILE: Many produce local tumors of the soft tissues surrounding the site of implantation.

PKA860
POLYMERS, WATER SOLUBLE

SAFETY PROFILE: Many produce local tumors of the soft tissues surrounding the site of implantation, in the lungs, mucosal contact areas, organs, and tissues of retention and deposition.

PKB500   CAS: 9011-14-7
POLYMETHYLMETHACRYLATE

mf: $(C_5H_8O_2)_n$

SYNS: ACRYLITE ◇ ACRYPET ◇ ALUTOR M 70 ◇ CMW BONE CEMENT ◇ CRINOTHENE ◇ DEGALAN S 85 ◇ DELPET 50M ◇ DIAKON ◇ DISPASOL M ◇ DV 400 ◇ ELVACITE ◇ KALLOCRYL K ◇ KALLODENT CLEAR ◇ KORAD ◇ LPT ◇ LUCITE ◇ METAPLEX NO ◇ METH-ACRYLIC ACID METHYL ESTER POLYMERS ◇ METHYL METHACRYLATE HOMOPOLYMER ◇ METHYL METHAC-RYLATE POLYMER ◇ METHYL METHACRYLATE RESIN ◇ 2-METHYL-2-PROPENOIC ACID METHYL ESTER HOMO-POLYMER ◇ ORGANIC GLASS E 2 ◇ OSTEOBOND SURGI-CAL BONE CEMENT ◇ PALACOS ◇ PARAGLAS ◇ PARA-PLEX P 543 ◇ PERSPEX ◇ PLEXIGLAS ◇ PLEXIGUM M 920 ◇ PMMA ◇ PONTALITE ◇ REPAIRSIN ◇ RESARIT 4000 ◇ RHOPLEX B 85 ◇ ROMACRYL ◇ SHINKOLITE ◇ SOL ◇ STELLON PINK ◇ SUMIPLEX LG ◇ SUPERACRYL AE ◇ SURGICAL SIMPLEX ◇ TENSOL 7 ◇ VEDRIL

TOXICITY DATA with REFERENCE
ETA: imp-mus TD: 13 g/kg   CNREA8 37,4367,77
ETA: imp-mus TD: 1280 mg/kg   TUMOAB
52,165,66
ETA: imp-mus TDLo: 800 mg/kg   PSEBAA
87,329,54
ETA: imp-rat TD: 1882 mg/kg   BJEPA5 45,21,64
ETA: imp-rat TDLo: 127 mg/kg   CNREA8 15,333,55

CONSENSUS REPORTS: IARC Cancer Review: GROUP 3 IMEMDT 7,56,87; Human Inadequate Evidence IMEMDT 19,187,79; Animal Sufficient Evidence IMEMDT 19,187,79. Reported in EPA TSCA Inventory.

SAFETY PROFILE: Questionable carcinogen with experimental tumorigenic data by implant route. When heated to decomposition it emits acrid smoke and irritating fumes. Used as the main constituent of acrylic sheet, molding, and extrusion powers.

PKF750   CAS: 25038-59-9
POLY(OXYETHYLENEOXY-TEREPHTHALOYL)
mf: $(C_{10}H_8O_4)_n$

SYNS: ALATHON ◇ AMILAR ◇ ARNITE A ◇ CASSAPPRET SR ◇ CELANAR ◇ CLEARTUF ◇ CRASTIN S 330 ◇ DAIYA FOIL ◇ DOWLEX ◇ ESTAR ◇ ESTROFOL ◇ ETHYLENE TEREPHTHALATE POLYMER ◇ FIBER V ◇ HOSTADUR ◇ HOSTAPHAN ◇ IAMBOLEN ◇ KLT 40 ◇ LAVSAN ◇ LAWSONITE ◇ LUMILAR 100 ◇ LUMIRROR ◇ MELIFORM ◇ MELINEX ◇ MYLAR ◇ NITRON LAVSAN ◇ NITRON (POLYESTER) ◇ PEGOTERATE ◇ POLYETHYLENE TEREPHTHALATE ◇ POLYETHYLENE TEREPHTHALATE FILM ◇ POLY(OXY-1,2-ETHANEDIYLOXYCARBONYL-1,4-PHENYLENECARBONYL) ◇ SCOTCH PAR ◇ SUPERFLOC ◇ TEREPHTAHLIC ACID-ETHYLENE GLYCOL POLYESTER ◇ TERFAN ◇ TERGAL ◇ TEROM ◇ TERPHAN ◇ VFR 3801 ◇ VITUF

TOXICITY DATA with REFERENCE
ETA: imp-rat TDLo: 116 mg/kg   CNREA8 15,333,55
MUT: mma-sat 25 µg/plate   TOLED5 3,325,79

CONSENSUS REPORTS: Reported in EPA TSCA Inventory.

SAFETY PROFILE: Questionable carcinogen with experimental tumorigenic data by implant route. Mutation data reported. When heated to decomposition it emits acrid smoke and irritating fumes.

PKH500   CAS: 89957-52-8
POLYPHENOL FRACTION of BETEL NUT

SYN: BETEL NUT, polyphenol fraction

TOXICITY DATA with REFERENCE
CAR: scu-mus TDLo: 988 mg/kg/13W-I   IJEBA6
18,1159,80
ETA: orl-mus TDLo: 380 mg/kg/W-C   BJCAAI
40,922,79

SAFETY PROFILE: Questionable carcinogen with experimental carcinogenic and tumorigenic data. When heated to decomposition it emits acrid smoke and irritating fumes.

PKH850
POLY p-PHENYLENE
TEREPTHALAMIDE ARAMID FIBER

TOXICITY DATA with REFERENCE
ETA: ihl-rat TCLo: 100 fibrils/cc/6H/2Y-I
EPASR* 8EHQ-0485-0550

SAFETY PROFILE: Questionable carcinogen with experimental tumorigenic data. When heated to decomposition it emits acrid smoke and irritating fumes.

PKL030   CAS: 9005-67-8
POLYSORBATE 60
mf: $C_{64}H_{126}O_{26}$ mw: 1311.90

PROP: Lemon to orange colored oily liquid; faint odor and bitter taste. Sol in water, aniline, ethyl acetate, toluene; insol in mineral oil, vegetable oil.

SYNS: CAPMUL ◇ LGYCOSPERSE S-20 ◇ LIPOSORB S-20 ◇ POLYOXYETHYLENE SORBITAN MONOSTEARATE ◇ POLYOXYETHYLENE 20 SORBITAN MONOSTEARATE ◇ SORBITAN, MONOOCTADECANOATE, POLY(OXY-1,2-ETHANEDIYL) DERIVATIVES ◇ TWEEN 60

TOXICITY DATA with REFERENCE
ETA: scu-rat TDLo: 2100 mg/kg/7W-I
13BYAH -,83,62
ETA: skn-mus TDLo: 168 g/kg/35W-I   JNCIAM
25,607,60

CONSENSUS REPORTS: Reported in EPA TSCA Inventory.

SAFETY PROFILE: Questionable carcinogen with experimental tumorigenic data. Moderately toxic by intravenous route. Experimental reproductive effects. When heated to decomposition it emits acrid smoke and irritating fumes.

PKL100   CAS: 9005-65-6
POLYSORBATE 80

PROP: Yellow to orange oily liquid; faint odor, bitter taste. Sol in water, alc, fixed oils, ethyl acetate, toluene; insol in mineral oil.

SYNS: ARMOTAN PMO-20 ◇ ATLOX 1087 ◇ CAPMUL POE-O ◇ CRILL 10 ◇ DREWMULSE POE-SMO ◇ DURFAX 80 ◇ EMSORB 6900 ◇ ETHOXYLATED SORBITAN MONO-OLEATE ◇ GLYCOSPERSE O-20 ◇ HODAG SVO 9 ◇ LIPOSORB O-20 ◇ MONITAN ◇ MONTANOX 80 ◇ NCI-C60286 ◇ NIKKOL TO ◇ OLOTHORB ◇ POLYOXYE-THYLENE SORBITAN MONOOLEATE ◇ POLYOXYETHY-LENE SORBITAN OLEATE ◇ POLYSORBAN 80 ◇ POLYSOR-BATE 80, U.S.P. ◇ PROTASORB O-20 ◇ ROMULGIN O ◇ SORBIMACROGOL OLEATE ◇ SORBITAL O 20 ◇ SORETHYTAN (20) MONOOLEATE ◇ SORLATE ◇ SVO 9 ◇ TWEEN 80

TOXICITY DATA with REFERENCE
ETA: scu-rat TDLo: 10 g/kg/27W-I   FCTXAV 9,463,71
MUT: dni-hmn: lym 20 ppm   BBRCA9 45,630,71
MUT: dni-mus: oth 20 ppm   ENPBBC 5,84,75

CONSENSUS REPORTS: Reported in EPA TSCA Inventory.

SAFETY PROFILE: Questionable carcinogen with experimental tumorigenic data. Moderately toxic by intravenous route. Mildly toxic by ingestion. Experimental reproductive effects. Human mutation data reported. An eye irritant. When heated to decomposition it emits acrid smoke and irritating fumes.

PKL500   CAS: 9009-54-5
POLYURETHANE FOAM

SYNS: ETHERON SPONGE ◇ NCI-C56451 ◇ POLYFOAM PLASTIC SPONGE ◇ POLYFOAM SPONGE ◇ POLYURE-THANE ESTER FOAM ◇ POLYURETHANE ETHER FOAM ◇ POLYURETHANE SPONGE

TOXICITY DATA with REFERENCE
ETA: imp-rat TD: 10 g/kg   BJSUAM 52,49,65
ETA: imp-rat TDLo: 293 mg/kg   JNCIAM 33,1005,64
ETA: itr-rat TDLo: 225 mg/kg   EVHPAZ 11,109,75

CONSENSUS REPORTS: IARC Cancer Review: GROUP 3 IMEMDT 7,56,87; Animal Sufficient Evidence IMEMDT 19,303,79.

SAFETY PROFILE: Questionable carcinogen with experimental tumorigenic data. When heated to decomposition it emits acrid toxic fumes of CN^- and NO_x.

PKO750   CAS: 25748-74-7
POLYURETHANE Y-299

SYNS: 1,4-BUTANEDIOL, POLYMER with 1,6-DIISOCYAN-ATOHEXANE ◇ DURANATE EXP-D 101 ◇ ISOCYANIC ACID,

HEXAMETHYLENE ESTER, POLYMER with 1,4-BUTANE-DIOL ◇ Y 299

TOXICITY DATA with REFERENCE
ETA: imp-rat TDLo: 6000 mg/kg   CNREA8 35,1591,75

SAFETY PROFILE: Questionable carcinogen with experimental tumorigenic data by implant route. When heated to decomposition it emits very toxic fumes of CN^- and NO_x.

PKP500   CAS: 34149-92-3
POLYVINYL ACETATE CHLORIDE

SYNS: ACETIC ACID, VINYL ESTER, CHLOROETHYLENE COPOLYMER ◇ POLYVINYLCHLORIDE ACETATE ◇ VINYL CHLORIDE ACETATE COPOLYMER ◇ VINYL CHLORIDE VINYL ACETATE COPOLYMER

TOXICITY DATA with REFERENCE
CAR: imp-mus TDLo: 240 mg/kg   JNCIAM 58,1443,77
ETA: imp-mus TD: 1656 g/kg   CNREA8 37,4367,77

SAFETY PROFILE: Questionable carcinogen with experimental carcinogenic and tumorigenic data by implant route. When heated to decomposition it emits toxic fumes of Cl^-.

PKP750   CAS: 9002-89-5
POLYVINYL ALCOHOL

PROP: Colorless, amorphous powder. Mp: decomp over 200°, flash p: 175°F (OC), d: 1.329. Polymer of average molecular weight 120,000 (AMPLAO 67,589,59).

SYNS: ELVANOL ◇ ETHENOL HOMOPOLYMER (9CI) ◇ GELVATOLS ◇ GOHSENOLS ◇ POLY(VINYL ALCOHOL) ◇ VINYL ALCOHOL POLYMER

TOXICITY DATA with REFERENCE
CAR: scu-rat TDLo: 2500 mg/kg   AMPLAO 67,589,59
ETA: imp-rat TD: 3768 mg/kg   EXPEAM 19,424,63
ETA: imp-rat TDLo: 10 g/kg   BJSUAM 52,49,65

CONSENSUS REPORTS: IARC Cancer Review: GROUP 3 IMEMDT 7,56,87; Animal Limited Evidence IMEMDT 19,341,79; Human Inadequate Evidence IMEMDT 19,341,79.

SAFETY PROFILE: Questionable carcinogen with experimental carcinogenic and tumorigenic data by implant route. Flammable when exposed to heat or flame; can react with oxidizing materials. To fight fire, use alcohol foam, CO_2, dry chemical. When heated to decomposition it emits acrid smoke and irritating fumes.

PKQ000   CAS: 25951-54-6
POLYVINYLBROMIDE
mf: $(C_2H_3Br)_x$

PROP: Commercial PVBR is a 40% aqueous suspension in which PVBR constitutes about 90% of the solids (CNREA8 38,3236,78).

SYNS: BROMOETHYLENE POLYMER ◇ POLYBROMO-ETHYLENE ◇ PVBR

TOXICITY DATA with REFERENCE
CAR: scu-mus TDLo:44 g/kg/48W-I   CNREA8 38,3236,78

CONSENSUS REPORTS: IARC Cancer Review: Animal Inadequate Evidence IMEMDT 19,367,79.

SAFETY PROFILE: Questionable carcinogen with experimental carcinogenic data. When heated to decomposition it emits toxic fumes of Br⁻.

PKQ059   CAS: 9002-86-2
POLYVINYL CHLORIDE
mf: $(C_2H_3Cl)_n$

PROP: Polymers with molecular weights ranging from 60,000-150,000 (CNREA8 15, 333,55). White powder, d: 1.406.

SYNS: ARMODOUR ◇ ARON COMPOUND HW ◇ ASTRALON ◇ ATACTIC POLY(VINYL CHLORIDE) ◇ BLACAR 1716 ◇ BOLATRON ◇ BONLOID ◇ BREON ◇ CARINA ◇ CHLOROETHENE HOMOPOLYMER ◇ CHLOROETHYLENE POLYMER ◇ CHLOROSTOP ◇ COBEX (POLYMER) ◇ CONTIZELL ◇ CORVIC 55/9 ◇ DACOVIN ◇ DANUVIL 70 ◇ DARVIC 110 ◇ DARVIS CLEAR 025 ◇ DECELITH H ◇ DENKA VINYL SS 80 ◇ DIAMOND SHAMROCK 40 ◇ DORLYL ◇ DUROFOL P ◇ DYNADUR ◇ E 62 ◇ E 66P ◇ EKAVYL SD 2 ◇ E-PVC ◇ ESCAMBIA 2160 ◇ EUROPHAN ◇ EXON 605 ◇ FC 4648 ◇ FLOCOR ◇ GAFCOTE ◇ GENOTHERM ◇ GEON ◇ GEON LATEX 151 ◇ GUTTAGENA ◇ HALVIC 223 ◇ HISHIREX 502 ◇ HISPAVIC 229 ◇ HOSTALIT ◇ IGELITE F ◇ IMPROVED WILT PRUF ◇ KAYLITE ◇ KLEGECELL ◇ KOROSEAL ◇ LONZA G ◇ LUCOFLEX ◇ LUCOVYL PE ◇ LUTOFAN ◇ MARVINAL ◇ MIRREX MCFD 1025 ◇ MOVINYL 100 ◇ MYRAFORM ◇ NCI-C60797 ◇ NIKA-TEMP ◇ NIKAVINYL SG 700 ◇ NIPEON A 21 ◇ NIPOL 576 ◇ NORVINYL ◇ NOVON 712 ◇ ONGROVIL S 165 ◇ OPALON ◇ ORTUDUR ◇ PANTASOTE R 873 ◇ PARCLOID ◇ PATTINA V 82 ◇ PEVIKON D 61 ◇ PLIOVIC ◇ POLIVINIT ◇ POLY(CHLOROETHYLENE) ◇ POLYTHERM ◇ POLYVI-NYLCHLORID (GERMAN) ◇ PROTOTYPE III SOFT ◇ PVC (MAK) ◇ QSAH 7 ◇ QUIRVIL ◇ QYSA ◇ RAVINYL ◇ RUCON B 20 ◇ S 65 (POLYMER) ◇ SCON 5300 ◇ SICRON ◇ S-LON ◇ SOLVIC ◇ SP 60 (CHLOROCARBON) ◇ SUMILIT EXA 13 ◇ SUMITOMO PX 11 ◇ TAKILON ◇ TECHNOPOR ◇ TENNECO 1742 ◇ TK 1000 ◇ TROVIDUR ◇ TROVITHERM HTL ◇ U 1 (POLYMER) ◇ ULTRON ◇ UNICHEM ◇ VERON P 130/1 ◇ VESTOLIT B 7021 ◇ VINIKA KR 600 ◇ VINIKULON ◇ VINIPLAST ◇ VINIPLEN P 73 ◇ VINNOL E 75 ◇ VINOFLEX ◇ VINYLCHLON 4000LL ◇ VINYL CHLORIDE HOMOPOLYMER ◇ VINYL CHLORIDE POLYMER ◇ VYGEN 85 ◇ WELVIC G 2/5 ◇ WILT PRUF ◇ WINIDUR ◇ X-AB ◇ YUGOVINYL

TOXICITY DATA with REFERENCE
ETA: imp-rat TDLo:75 mg/kg   CNREA8 15,333,55
ETA: orl-rat TDLo:210 g/kg/30W-C   PATHAB 73,59,81

CONSENSUS REPORTS: IARC Cancer Review: Human Inadequate Evidence IMEMDT 19,377,79; IARC Cancer Review: Animal Inadequate Evidence IMEMDT 19,377,79. Reported in EPA TSCA Inventory.

DFG MAK: 6 mg/m³ (dust)

SAFETY PROFILE: Questionable carcinogen with experimental tumorigenic data. Chronic inhalation of dusts can cause pulmonary damage, blood effects, abnormal liver function. Can cause allergic dermatitis. When heated to decomposition it emits toxic fumes of Cl⁻ and phosgene.

PKQ250   CAS: 9003-39-8
POLY(1-VINYL-2-PYRROLIDINONE) HOMOPOLYMER
mf: $(C_6H_9ON)_n$

PROP: A free-flowing, white, amorphous powder. D: 1.23-1.29. Sol in water, chlorinated hydrocarbons, alc, amines, nitroparaffins, and lower molecular weight fatty acids.

SYNS: AGENT AT 717 ◇ ALBIGEN A ◇ ALDACOL Q ◇ AT 717 ◇ BOLINAN ◇ 1-ETHENYL-2-PYRROLIDINONE HOMOPOLYMER ◇ 1-ETHENYL-2-PYRROLIDINONE POLYMERS ◇ GANEX P 804 ◇ HEMODESIS ◇ HEMODEZ ◇ K25 (polymer) ◇ KOLLIDON ◇ LUVISKOL ◇ MPK 90 ◇ NCI C60582 ◇ NEOCOMPENSAN ◇ PERAGAL ST ◇ PERISTON ◇ PLASDONE ◇ POLYCLAR L ◇ POLY(1-(2-OXO-1-PYRROLIDINYL)ETHYLENE) ◇ POLYVIDONE ◇ POLY(n-VINYLBUTYROLACTAM) ◇ POLYVINYLPYRRO-LIDONE ◇ POVIDONE (USP XIX) ◇ PROTAGENT ◇ PVP (FCC) ◇ SUBTOSAN ◇ VINISIL ◇ N-VINYLBUTYRO-LACTAM POLYMER ◇ N-VINYLPYRROLIDONE POLYMER

CONSENSUS REPORTS: IARC Cancer Review: GROUP 3 IMEMDT 7,56,87. Reported in EPA TSCA Inventory.

SAFETY PROFILE: Questionable carcinogen. Mildly toxic by intraperitoneal and intravenous routes. When heated to decomposition it emits toxic fumes of NO_x.

PKX250   CAS: 7778-50-9
POTASSIUM BICHROMATE
DOT: 1479
mf: $Cr_2K_2O_7$ mw: 294.20

PROP: Bright, yellowish-red, transparent crystals; bitter, metallic taste. Mp: 398°, bp: decomp @ 500°, d: 2.69.

SYNS: BICHROMATE OF POTASH ◇ CHROMIC ACID, DIPOTASSIUM SALT ◇ DIPOTASSIUM DICHROMATE ◇ IOPEZITE ◇ KALIUMDICHROMAT (GERMAN) ◇ POTASSIUM DICHROMATE(VI)

TOXICITY DATA with REFERENCE
MUT: cyt-ham-ipr 8 mg/kg   BLOAAO 40,651,85
MUT: cyt-hmn:lym 300 μg/L   MUREAV 97,192,82
MUT: dnr-bcs 1050 μg/L   WATRAG 14,1613,80
MUT: dns-hmn:fbr 100 μmol/L   MUREAV 117,279,83
MUT: mnt-mus-ipr 50 mg/kg   CRSBAW 174,889,80
MUT: oms-hmn:lym 3 mg/L   MUREAV 97,192,82
MUT: sce-hmn:lym 300 μg/L   MUREAV 97,192,82
MUT: spm-mus-ipr 4 mg/kg   BLOAAO 40,1151,85

CONSENSUS REPORTS: IARC Cancer Review: Human Inadequate Evidence IMEMDT 23,205,80; Animal Inadequate Evidence IMEMDT 23,205,80. Chromium and its compounds are on the Community Right-To-Know List. Reported in EPA TSCA Inventory. EPA Genetic Toxicology Program.

OSHA PEL: CL 0.1 mg(CrO_3)/m³ ACGIH TLV: TWA 0.05 mg(CrO_3)/m³ NIOSH REL: TWA (Chromium(VI)) 0.025 mg(Cr(VI))/m³; CL 0.05/15M DOT Classification: ORM-A; Label: None.

SAFETY PROFILE: Questionable carcinogen. Human poison by ingestion. An experimental poison by ingestion, intraperitoneal, intravenous, and subcutaneous routes. Human mutation data reported. Flammable by chemical reaction. A powerful oxidizer. Used in photomechanical processing, chrome pigment production and wool preservation methods. When heated to decomposition it emits toxic fumes of K_2O.

PKX500   CAS: 23746-34-1
POTASSIUM BIS(2-HYDROXYETHYL)DITHIOCARBAMATE
mf: $C_5H_{10}NO_2S_2 \cdot K$ mw: 219.38

SYNS: BIS(2-HYDROXYETHYL)CARBAMODITHIOIC ACID, MONOPOTASSIUM SALT ◇ BIS(2-HYDROXYETHYL)DITHIOCARBAMIC ACID, MONOPOTASSIUM SALT ◇ BIS(2-HYDROXYETHYL)DITHOCARBAMIC ACID, POTASSIUM SALT

TOXICITY DATA with REFERENCE
CAR: orl-mus TDLo: 129 g/kg/79W-C   JNCIAM 42,1101,69
ETA: orl-rat TDLo: 82 g/kg/78W-C   JJIND8 67,75,81

CONSENSUS REPORTS: IARC Cancer Review: GROUP 3 IMEMDT 7,56,87; Animal Sufficient Evidence IMEMDT 12,183,76. Reported in EPA TSCA Inventory.

SAFETY PROFILE: Questionable carcinogen with experimental carcinogenic and tumorigenic data. When heated to decomposition it emits very toxic fumes of K_2O, SO_x and NO_x. Used as an analytical reagent for quantitative determination of mercury, gold, and copper.

PLB250   CAS: 7789-00-6
POTASSIUM CHROMATE(VI)
mf: $CrO_4 \cdot 2K$ mw: 194.20

PROP: Rhombic, yellow crystals. Mp: 975°, d: 2.73 @ 18°. Sol in water; insol in alc.

SYNS: BIPOTASSIUM CHROMATE ◇ CHROMATE of POTASSIUM ◇ DIPOTASSIUM CHROMATE ◇ DIPOTASSIUM MONOCHROMATE ◇ NEUTRAL POTASSIUM CHROMATE ◇ TARAPACAITE

TOXICITY DATA with REFERENCE
ETA: orl-mus TDLo: 1600 mg/kg/62W-C   JONUAI 101,1431,71
MUT: cyt-hmn:lym 20 μmol/L   MUREAV 77,157,80
MUT: dnd-hmn:fbr 50 μmol/L/4H   CNREA8 42,145,82
MUT: dnd-hmn:lng 25 μmol/L   CBINA8 36,345,81
MUT: dnr-ssp 60 nmol/L   CNJGA8 24,771,82
MUT: sce-ham:lng 26 μg/L   CRNGDP 4,605,83

CONSENSUS REPORTS: IARC Cancer Review: Human Inadequate Evidence IMEMDT 23,205,80; Animal Inadequate Evidence IMEMDT 23,205,80. Reported in EPA TSCA Inventory. EPA Genetic Toxicology Program.

Chromium and its compounds are on the Community Right-To-Know List.

OSHA PEL: CL 0.1 mg(CrO₃)/m³ ACGIH TLV: TWA 0.05 mg(Cr)/m³ NIOSH REL: TWA 0.025 mg(Cr(VI))/m³; CL 0.05/ 15M DOT Classification: ORM-E; Label: None.

OSHA PEL: CL 0.1 $mg(CrO_3)/m^3$ ACGIH TLV: TWA 0.05 $mg(Cr)/m^3$ NIOSH REL: TWA 0.025 $mg(Cr(VI))/m^3$; CL 0.05/ 15M DOT Classification: ORM-E; Label: None.

SAFETY PROFILE: Questionable carcinogen with experimental tumorigenic data. Poison by intravenous, subcutaneous, and intramuscular routes. Human mutation data reported. A powerful oxidizer. When heated to decomposition it emits toxic fumes of K_2O. Used as a mordant for wool, in the oxidizing and treatment of dyes on materials.

PLR250 CAS: 16731-55-8
POTASSIUM PYROSULFITE
DOT: 2693
mf: $O_5S_2 \cdot K$ mw: 183.22

PROP: Monoclinic plates or white crystalline powder; sulfur dioxide odor. Mp: decomp; d: 2.3. Sol in water; insol in alc.

SYNS: POTASSIUM METABISULFITE (DOT, FCC) ◇ PYROSULFUROUS ACID, DIPOTASSIUM SALT

TOXICITY DATA with REFERENCE
ETA: orl-mus TD:2880 g/kg/2Y-C   EESADV 3,451,79
ETA: orl-mus TDLo:1440 g/kg/2Y-C   EESADV 3,451,79

CONSENSUS REPORTS: Reported in EPA TSCA Inventory. EPA Genetic Toxicology Program.

DOT Classification: ORM-B; Label: None.

SAFETY PROFILE: Questionable carcinogen with experimental tumorigenic data. Experimental reproductive effects. A very irritating material. When heated to decomposition it emits toxic fumes of SO_x and K_2O.

PLW150 CAS: 12056-53-0
POTASSIUM TITANIUM OXIDE
mf: KO_8Ti_4 mw: 358.70

SYN: POTASSIUM OCTATITANATE

TOXICITY DATA with REFERENCE
NEO: imp-rat TDLo:200 mg/kg   JJIND8 67,965,81

SAFETY PROFILE: Questionable carcinogen with experimental neoplastigenic data.

PLW750
POTATO, GREEN PARTS
SYN: SOLANUM TUBEROSUM L

TOXICITY DATA with REFERENCE
CAR: ipr-rat TDLo:136 g/kg/2Y-I   EXPEAM 34,645,78

SAFETY PROFILE: Questionable carcinogen with experimental carcinogenic data. Moderately toxic by ingestion. Experimental teratogenic effects.

PLZ000 CAS: 53-03-2
PREDNISONE
mf: $C_{21}H_{26}O_5$ mw: 358.47

PROP: White, odorless, crystalline powder. Mp: 235° (with some decomp). Very sltly sol in water; sltly sol in alcohol, chloroform, methanol, and dioxane.

SYNS: ANCORTONE ◇ BICORTONE ◇ COLISONE ◇ CORTAN ◇ CORTANCYL ◇ Δ-CORTELAN ◇ CORTIDELT ◇ Δ-CORTISONE ◇ Δ¹-CORTISONE ◇ Δ-CORTONE ◇ COTONE ◇ DACORTIN ◇ DECORTANCYL ◇ DECORTIN ◇ DECORTISYL ◇ Δ-1-DEHYDROCORTISONE ◇ 1-DEHY-DROCORTISONE ◇ DEKORTIN ◇ DELTACORTELAN ◇ DELTACORTISONE ◇ DELTACORTONE ◇ DELTA-DOME ◇ DELTISONE ◇ 17,21-DIHYDROXYPREGNA-1,4-DIENE-3,11,20-TRIONE ◇ ENCORTON ◇ HOSTACORTIN ◇ IN-SONE ◇ JUVASON ◇ LISACORT ◇ METACORTAN-DRACIN ◇ NCI-C04897 ◇ NSC 10023 ◇ ORASONE ◇ PARACORT ◇ PRECORT ◇ PREDNICEN-M ◇ PREDNI-LONGA ◇ PREDNISON ◇ PREDNIZON ◇ 1,4-PREGNADIENE-17-α,21-DIOL-3,11,20-TRIONE ◇ RECTODELT ◇ SERVISONE ◇ SK-PREDNISONE ◇ SUPERCORTIL ◇ U 6020 ◇ ULTRA-CORTEN ◇ WOJTAB ◇ ZENADRID (VETERINARY)

TOXICITY DATA with REFERENCE
ETA: ipr-rat TDLo:860 mg/kg/26W-I   CANCAR 40S,1935,77
MUT: mma-sat 333 μg/plate   ENMUDM 5(Suppl 1),3,83
MUT: mmo-sat 3333 μg/plate   NTPTB*J JAN82

CONSENSUS REPORTS: IARC Cancer Review: Human Inadequate Evidence IMEMDT 26,293,81; Animal Inadequate Evidence IMEMDT 26,293,81. NCI Carcinogenesis Studies (ipr); No Evidence: mouse CANCAR 40, 1935,77; (ipr); Equivocal Evidence: rat CANCAR 40,1935,77. Reported in EPA TSCA Inventory.

SAFETY PROFILE: Questionable carcinogen with experimental tumorigenic data. Poison by intraperitoneal and subcutaneous routes. Moderately toxic by intramuscular route. Human systemic effects by ingestion and possibly other routes: sensory change involving peripheral nerves. Experimental reproductive effects. Mutation data reported. Has been implicated in aplastic anemia.

PMC600   CAS: 40778-40-3
PRIMIDOLOL HYDROCHLORIDE
mf: $C_{17}H_{23}N_3O_4 \cdot ClH$ mw: 369.89

TOXICITY DATA with REFERENCE
CAR: orl-mus TD:6750mg/kg/77W-C   TXCYAC 21,279,81
CAR: orl-mus TDLo:27000 mg/kg/77W-C   TXCYAC 21,279,81
ETA: orl-mus TD:13500 mg/kg/77W-C   TXCYAC 21,279,81

SAFETY PROFILE: Questionable carcinogen with experimental carcinogenic and tumorigenic data. When heated to decomposition it emits toxic fumes of NO_x and HCl.

PMD500   CAS: 1921-70-6
PRISTANE
mf: $C_{19}H_{40}$ mw: 268.59

PROP: Mobile, transparent, stable liquid. D: 0.782 @ 20°/4°; fp: −100°, bp: 296°. Sol in ether, petr ether, benzene, chloroform.

SYN: 2,6,10,14-TETRAMETHYLPENTADECANE

TOXICITY DATA with REFERENCE
NEO: ipr-mus TD:60 mg/kg/26W-I   NATUAS 222,994,69
ETA: ipr-mus TDLo:47 mg/kg   CNREA8 40,579,80

CONSENSUS REPORTS: Reported in EPA TSCA Inventory.

SAFETY PROFILE: Questionable carcinogen with experimental neoplastigenic and tumorigenic data. When heated to decomposition it emits acrid smoke and irritating fumes.

PMH100   CAS: 1811-28-5
PROFLAVINE HEMISULPHATE
mf: $C_{13}H_{11}N_3 \cdot 1/2H_2O_4S$ mw: 258.29

SYNS: 3,6-DIAMINOACRIDINE HEMISULFATE ◊ PROFLAVINE

TOXICITY DATA with REFERENCE
MUT: dnd-mam:lym 15 μmol/L   JMOBAK 13,138,65

MUT: dnd-omi 100 pph   ZNCBDA 29,128,74
MUT: dnd-sal:spr 2 pph   ZNCBDA 29,128,74
MUT: sce-ham:lng 10 mg/L   CNREA8 44,3270,84

CONSENSUS REPORTS: IARC Cancer Review: GROUP 3 IMEMDT 7,56,87; Animal Inadequate Evidence IMEMDT 24,195,80

SAFETY PROFILE: Questionable carcinogen. Poison by subcutaneous route. Mutation data reported. When heated to decomposition it emits toxic fumes of SO_x and NO_x.

PMH250   CAS: 952-23-8
PROFLAVINE MONOHYDROCHLORIDE
mf: $C_{13}H_{11}N_3 \cdot ClH$ mf: 245.73

SYNS: 3,6-ACRIDINEDIAMINE, MONOHYDROCHLORIDE (9CI) ◊ 3,6-DIAMINOACRIDINE MONOHYDROCHLORIDE ◊ 3,6-DIAMINOACRIDINIUM CHLORIDE ◊ 3,6-DIAMINOACRIDINIUM CHLORIDE HYDROCHLORIDE ◊ 2,8-DIAMINOACRIDINIUM CHLORIDE MONOHYDROCHLORIDE ◊ PROFLAVINE HYDROCHLORIDE

TOXICITY DATA with REFERENCE
MUT: mma-esc 10 μg/plate   ENMUDM 7(Suppl 5),1,85
MUT: mma-sat 3 μg/plate   IAPUDO 27,283,80
MUT: mmo-sat 300 ng/plate   IAPUDO 27,283,80

CONSENSUS REPORTS: IARC Cancer Review: Animal Indefinite Evidence IMEMDT 24,195,80.

SAFETY PROFILE: Questionable carcinogen. Poison by subcutaneous route. Mutation data reported. When heated to decomposition it emits very toxic fumes of NO_x and HCl. Used as a drug, as a disinfectant, and as a topical antiseptic.

PMK000   CAS: 542-78-9
PROPANEDIAL
mf: $C_3H_4O_2$ mw: 72.07

SYNS: MALONALDEHYDE ◊ MALONDIALDEHYDE ◊ MALONIC ALDEHYDE ◊ MALONIC DIALDEHYDE ◊ MALONODIALDEHYDE ◊ MALONYLDIALDEHYDE ◊ NCI-C54842 ◊ 1,3-PROPANEDIAL ◊ 1,3-PROPANEDIALDEHYDE ◊ 1,3-PROPANEDIONE

TOXICITY DATA with REFERENCE
CAR: skn-mus TD:30 g/kg/9W-I   JNCIAM 53,1771,74
CAR: skn-mus TDLo:7488 mg/kg/2Y-I   AUODDK 55,3,80
MUT: dnd-hmn:leu 1 mmol/L   CLREAS 23(5),595A,75

MUT: mmo-esc 2 mmol/L   MUREAV 88,23,81
MUT: mmo-sat 13850 nmol/plate   BTERDG2,81,80
MUT: mnt-rat:fbr 100 μmol/L   MUREAV
  101,237,82

CONSENSUS REPORTS: IARC Cancer Review: Animal Inadequate Evidence IMEMDT 36,163,85. EPA Genetic Toxicology Program.

SAFETY PROFILE: Questionable carcinogen with experimental carcinogenic data. Moderately toxic by ingestion. Human mutation data reported. When heated to decomposition it emits acrid smoke and irritating fumes.

PMN850   CAS: 139-40-2
PROPAZINE
mf: $C_9H_{16}ClN_7O_2$ mw: 229.75

SYNS: 2,4-BIS(ISOPROPYLAMINO)-6-CHLORO-s-TRIAZINE ◇ 2,4-BIS(PROPYLAMINO)-6-CHLOR-1,3,5-TRIAZIN (GERMAN) ◇ GESAMIL ◇ MILOGARD ◇ PLANTULIN ◇ PRIMATOL P ◇ PROPASIN ◇ PROZINEX

TOXICITY DATA with REFERENCE
ETA: orl-gpg TDLo: 11 g/kg/78W-I   NTIS**
  PB223-159

SAFETY PROFILE: Questionable carcinogen with experimental tumorigenic data. Moderately toxic by ingestion. Moderate eye irritation. When heated to decomposition it emits toxic fumes of NO_x and Cl^-.

PMO500   CAS: 115-07-1
PROPENE
DOT: 1075/1077
mf: C_3H_6 mw: 42.09

PROP: A gas. D: (gas) 1.49 (air = 1.0), d: (liquid) 0.581 @ 0°. Mp: −185°, bp: −47.7°, autoign temp: 860°F, vap press: 10 atm @ 19.8°, lel: 2.4%, uel: 10.1%, vap d: 1.5, flash p: −162°F.

SYNS: METHYLETHENE ◇ METHYLETHYLENE ◇ NCI-C50077 ◇ 1-PROPENE ◇ PROPYLENE (DOT)

CONSENSUS REPORTS: IARC Cancer Review: GROUP 3 IMEMDT 7,56,87. NTP Carcinogenesis Studies (inhalation); No Evidence: mouse, rat NTPTR* NTP-TR-272,85. EPA Extremely Hazardous Substances List. Reported in EPA TSCA Inventory.

DOT Classification: Flammable Gas; Label: Flammable Gas.

SAFETY PROFILE: Questionable carcinogen. A simple asphyxiant. No irritant effects from high concentrations in gaseous form. When compressed to liquid form, can cause skin burns from freezing effects on tissue of rapid evaporation. Very dangerous fire hazard when exposed to heat, flame, or oxidizers. To fight fire, stop flow of gas. Used in production of fabricated polymers, fibers, and solvents, in production of plastic products and resins.

PMP500   CAS: 9003-07-0
PROPENE POLYMERS
mf: $(C_3H_6)_n$

PROP: Solid material. Mp: about 165°, d: 0.90-0.92. Insol in organic materials.

SYNS: ADMER PB 02 ◇ AMCO ◇ AMERFIL ◇ AMOCO 1010 ◇ ATACTIC POLYPROPYLENE ◇ AVISUN ◇ AZDEL ◇ BEAMETTE ◇ BICOLENE P ◇ CARLONA P ◇ CELGARD 2500 ◇ CHISSO 507B ◇ CLYSAR ◇ COATHYLENE PF 0548 ◇ DAPLEN AD ◇ DEXON E 117 ◇ EASTBOND M 5 ◇ ELPON ◇ ENJAY CD 460 ◇ EPOLENE M 5K ◇ GERFIL ◇ HERCOFLAT 135 ◇ HERCULON ◇ HOSTALEN PP ◇ HULS P 6500 ◇ ICI 543 ◇ ISOTACTIC POLYPROPYLENE ◇ J 400 ◇ LAMBETH ◇ LUPAREEN ◇ MARLEX 9400 ◇ MAURYLENE ◇ MERAKLON ◇ MOPLEN ◇ MOSTEN ◇ NOBLEN ◇ NOVAMONT 2030 ◇ NOVOLEN ◇ OLETAC 100 ◇ PAISLEY POLYMER ◇ PELLON 2506 ◇ POLYPRO 1014 ◇ POLYPROPENE ◇ POLYPROPYLENE ◇ POLYTAC ◇ POPROLIN ◇ PROFAX ◇ PROPATHENE ◇ 1-PROPENE HOMOPOLYMER (9CI) ◇ PROPOLIN ◇ PROPOPHANE ◇ PROPYLENE POLYMER ◇ REXALL 413S ◇ REXENE ◇ SHELL 5520 ◇ SHOALLOMER ◇ SYNDIOTACTIC POLYPROPYLENE ◇ TENITE 423 ◇ TRESPAPHAN ◇ TUFF-LITE ◇ ULSTRON ◇ VISCOL 350P ◇ W 101 ◇ WEX 1242

CONSENSUS REPORTS: IARC Cancer Review: GROUP 3 IMEMDT 7,56,87; Animal Limited Evidence IMEMDT 19,213,79; Human Inadequate Evidence IMEMDT 19,213,79. Reported in EPA TSCA Inventory.

SAFETY PROFILE: Questionable carcinogen. Suspected carcinogen. When heated to decomposition it emits acrid smoke and irritating fumes. Used in injection molding for auto parts, in bottle caps, and container closures.

PMQ250   CAS: 768-03-6
2-PROPENOPHENONE
mf: C_9H_8O mw: 132.17

SYNS: ACRYLOPHENONE ◇ PHENYLVINYL KETONE

TOXICITY DATA with REFERENCE
ETA: scu-rat TDLo: 2520 mg/kg/63W-I   BJCAAI
  19,392,65

SAFETY PROFILE: Questionable carcinogen with experimental tumorigenic data. When heated to decomposition it emits acrid smoke and irritating fumes.

PMQ750   CAS: 104-46-1
p-PROPENYLANISOLE
mf: $C_{10}H_{12}O$ mw: 148.22

PROP: Leaves from alc or light yellow liquid above 23°; sweet taste with anise odor. D: 0.991 @ 20°/20°, refr index: 1.557-1.561, mp: 22.5°, bp: 235.3°, flash p: 198°F. Very sltly sol in water; misc in abs alc, ether, chloroform.

SYNS: ACINTENE O ◊ ANETHOLE (FCC) ◊ ANISE CAMPHOR ◊ ARIZOLE ◊ FEMA No. 2086 ◊ ISOESTRAGOLE ◊ p-METHOXY-β-METHYLSTYRENE ◊ 1-(p-METHOXYPHENYL)PROPENE ◊ 1-METHOXY-4-PROPENYLBENZENE ◊ 4-METHOXYPROPENYLBENZENE ◊ MONASIRUP ◊ NAULI "GUM" ◊ OIL of ANISEED ◊ p-1-PROPENYLANISOLE ◊ 4-PROPENYLANISOLE ◊ p-PROPENYLPHENYL METHYL ETHER

TOXICITY DATA with REFERENCE
ETA: ipr-mus TDLo: 2400 mg/kg/8W-I   CNREA8 33,3069,73

CONSENSUS REPORTS: Reported in EPA TSCA Inventory.

SAFETY PROFILE: Questionable carcinogen with experimental tumorigenic data. Poison by ingestion. Combustible liquid. When heated to decomposition it emits acrid smoke and irritating fumes.

PMR750   CAS: 590-21-6
PROPENYL CHLORIDE
mf: C_3H_5Cl mw: 76.53

PROP: Liquid. Mp: −137.4°, bp: 22.65°, flash p: <21°F, d: 0.9189°, lel: 4.5%, uel: 16%, insol in water.

SYNS: 1-CHLOROPROPENE ◊ 1-CHLORO-1-PROPENE

TOXICITY DATA with REFERENCE
NEO: orl-mus TDLo: 3560 mg/kg/89W-I   JJIND8 63,1433,79
MUT: mma-sat 100 μmol/plate   BCPCA629,2611,80
MUT: mmo-sat 250 μL/plate   DTESD7 2,249,77

CONSENSUS REPORTS: Reported in EPA TSCA Inventory.

SAFETY PROFILE: Questionable carcinogen with experimental neoplastigenic data. Moderately toxic by ingestion. Very mildly toxic by skin contact and inhalation. Mutation data reported. An eye irritant. Very dangerous fire hazard when exposed to heat, flames (sparks) or oxidizers. Explosive in the form of vapor when exposed to heat or flame. To fight fire, use alcohol foam, dry chemical, mist spray, fog. When heated to decomposition it emits toxic fumes of Cl⁻.

PMS250   CAS: 6380-21-8
2-PROPENYLPHENOL
mf: $C_9H_{10}O$ mw: 134.19

SYNS: o-PROPENYLPHENOL ◊ 2-(1-PROPENYL)PHENOL

TOXICITY DATA with REFERENCE
NEO: skn-mus TDLo: 3400 mg/kg/12W-I   CNREA8 19,413,59
MUT: sce-hmn: lym 250 μmol/L   MUREAV 169,129,86

SAFETY PROFILE: Questionable carcinogen with experimental neoplastigenic data. Human mutation data reported. When heated to decomposition it emits acrid smoke and irritating fumes.

PMW760   CAS: 75464-10-7
10-PROPIONYL DITHRANOL
mf: $C_{17}H_{14}O_4$ mw: 282.31

SYNS: 9(10H)-ANTHRACENONE, 1,8-DIHYDROXY-10-(1-OXOPROPYL)- ◊ DITHRANOL, 10-PROPIONYL- ◊ 10-PROPIONYLDITHRANOL

TOXICITY DATA with REFERENCE
ETA: skn-mus TDLo: 126 mg/kg/50W-I   JPETAB 229,255,84
MUT: cyt-hmn: lyms 30 μg/L   ARTODN 59,180,86
MUT: mma-sat 25 μg/plate   ARTODN 59,180,86
MUT: mmo-sat 250 μg/plate   ARTODN 59,180,86

SAFETY PROFILE: Questionable carcinogen with experimental tumorigenic data. Poison by ingestion. Human mutation data reported. When heated to decomposition it emits acrid smoke and irritating fumes.

PMY310   CAS: 38777-13-8
PROPOXUR NITROSO
mf: $C_{11}H_{14}N_2O_4$ mw: 238.27

SYNS: BAYGON, NITROSO derivative ◊ CARBAMIC ACID, METHYLNITROSO-, o-ISOPROPOXYPHENYL ESTER ◊ CARBAMIC ACID, METHYLNITROSO-, 2-(1-METHYLETHOXY)PHENYL ESTER (9CI) ◊ 2-ISOPROPOXYPHENYL N-METHYLCARBAMATE, nitrosated ◊ o-ISOPROPOXYPHENYL

N-METHYL-N-NITROSOCARBAMATE ◇ o-ISOPROPOXY-
PHENYL METHYLNITROSOCARBAMATE ◇ METHYLNI-
TROSOCARBAMIC ACID o-ISOPROPOXYPHENYL ESTER
◇ NITROSO-BAYGON ◇ NITROSOPROPOXUR ◇ SUNCIDE,
nitrosated

TOXICITY DATA with REFERENCE
CAR: orl-rat TDLo: 625 mg/kg/31W-I   EESADV
  2,413,78
MUT: dnd-hmn: fbr 10 μmol/L   MUREAV 44,1,77
MUT: mmo-esc 50 μg/plate   BECTA6 14,389,75
MUT: mmo-sat 92 ng/plate   MUREAV 56,1,77
MUT: mmo-smc 420 nmol/L/4H   MUREAV
  22,121,74
MUT: mrc-bcs 50 ng/plate   BECTA6 14,389,75

SAFETY PROFILE: Questionable carcinogen
with experimental carcinogenic data. Many
N-nitroso compounds are carcinogens. Human
mutation data reported. When heated to decomposition it emits toxic fumes of NO_x.

PND000   CAS: 71-23-8
n-PROPYL ALCOHOL
DOT: 1274
mf: C_3H_8O mw: 60.11

PROP: Clear liquid; alc-like odor. Mp: −127°,
bp: 97.19°, flash p: 59°F (CC), ULC: 55-60,
d: 0.8044 @ 20°/4°, lel: 2.1%, uel: 13.5%,
autoign temp: 824°F, vap press: 10 mm @ 14.7°,
vap d: 2.07. Misc in water, alc, and ether.

SYNS: ALCOOL PROPILICO (ITALIAN) ◇ ALCOOL PRO-
PYLIQUE (FRENCH) ◇ ETHYL CARBINOL ◇ 1-HYDROXY-
PROPANE ◇ OPTAL ◇ OSMOSOL EXTRA ◇ n-PROPANOL
◇ PROPANOL-1 ◇ 1-PROPANOL ◇ PROPANOLE (GERMAN)
◇ PROPANOLEN (DUTCH) ◇ PROPANOLI (ITALIAN)
◇ PROPYL ALCOHOL ◇ 1-PROPYL ALCOHOL ◇ n-PROPYL
ALKOHOL (GERMAN) ◇ PROPYLIC ALCOHOL ◇ PROPY-
LOWY ALKOHOL (POLISH)

TOXICITY DATA with REFERENCE
CAR: orl-rat TDLo: 50 g/kg/81W-I   ARGEAR
  45,19,75
CAR: scu-rat TDLo: 6 g/kg/95W-I   ARGEAR
  45,19,75
MUT: cyt-smc 100 mmol/tube   HEREAY 33,457,47
MUT: mmo-esc 4 pph   ABMGAJ 23,843,69

CONSENSUS REPORTS: Reported in EPA
TSCA Inventory. EPA Genetic Toxicology Program.

OSHA PEL: (Transitional: TWA 200 ppm)
TWA 200 ppm; STEL 250 ppm   ACGIH TLV:
TWA 200 ppm; STEL 250 ppm (skin)   DOT

Classification: Flammable Liquid; Label: Flammable Liquid.

SAFETY PROFILE: Questionable carcinogen
with experimental carcinogenic data. Poison by
subcutaneous route. Moderately toxic by inhalation, ingestion, intraperitoneal, and intravenous
routes. Mildly toxic by skin contact. Mutation
data reported. A skin and severe eye irritant.
Dangerous fire hazard when exposed to heat,
flame, or oxidizers. Explosive in the form of
vapor when exposed to heat or flame. Dangerous
upon exposure to heat or flame; can react vigorously with oxidizing materials. To fight fire,
use alcohol foam, CO_2, dry chemical. When
heated to decomposition it emits acrid smoke
and irritating fumes.

PNE750   CAS: 54889-82-6
5-n-PROPYL-1,2-BENZANTHRACENE
mf: $C_{21}H_{18}$ mw: 270.39

SYN: 8-PROPYLBENZ(a)ANTHRACENE

TOXICITY DATA with REFERENCE
ETA: skn-mus TDLo: 240 mg/kg/10W-I
  PRLBA4 123,343,37

SAFETY PROFILE: Questionable carcinogen
with experimental tumorigenic data. When
heated to decomposition it emits acrid smoke
and irritating fumes.

PNF000   CAS: 63020-32-6
5-PROPYLBENZO(c)PHENANTHRENE
mf: $C_{21}H_{18}$ mw: 270.39

SYN: 2-n-PROPYL-3:4-BENZPHENANTHRENE

TOXICITY DATA with REFERENCE
ETA: scu-mus TDLo: 5000 mg/kg/50W-I
  PRLBA4 131,170,42
ETA: skn-mus TDLo: 1100 mg/kg/46W-I
  PRLBA4 131,170,42

SAFETY PROFILE: Questionable carcinogen
with experimental tumorigenic data. When
heated to decomposition it emits acrid smoke
and irritating fumes.

PNF500   CAS: 1114-71-2
**S-PROPYL
BUTYLETHYLTHIOCARBAMATE**
mf: $C_{10}H_{21}NOS$ mw: 203.38

PROP: Liquid. Bp: 142° @ 20 mm.

SYNS: BUTYLETHYLTHIOCARBAMIC ACID S-PROPYL
ESTER ◇ PEBC ◇ PEBULATE ◇ S-PROPYL-N-AETHYL-N-

BUTYL-THIOCARBAMAT (GERMAN) ◇ PROPYL-ETHYLBU-
TYLTHIOCARBAMATE ◇ N-PROPYL-N-ETHYL-N-(N-BU-
TYL)THIOCARBAMATE ◇ PROPYLETHYL-N-BUTYLTHIO-
CARBAMATE ◇ PROPYL N-ETHYL-N-
BUTYLTHIOCARBAMATE ◇ S-(N-PROPYL)-N-ETHYL-N-N-
BUTYLTHIOCARBAMATE ◇ N-PROPYL-N-ETHYL-N-(N-BU-
TYL)THIOLCARBAMATE ◇ PROPYL ETHYLBUTYLTHIOL-
CARBAMATE ◇ R-2061 ◇ STAUFFER R-2061 ◇ TILLAM
(RUSSIAN) ◇ TILLAM-6-E

TOXICITY DATA with REFERENCE
ETA: scu-mus TDLo:10 mg/kg   NTIS** PB223-
159

SAFETY PROFILE: Questionable carcinogen
with experimental tumorigenic data. Moderately
toxic by ingestion. Causes violent vomiting
when accompanied by alcohol ingestion. When
heated to decomposition it emits highly toxic
fumes of SO_x and NO_x.

PNF750   CAS: 25413-64-3
N-PROPYL-N-BUTYLNITROSAMINE
mf: $C_7H_{16}N_2O$ mw: 144.25

SYNS: N-NITROSO-N-PROPYL-1-BUTANAMINE
◇ N-NITROSO-N-PROPYLBUTYLAMINE

TOXICITY DATA with REFERENCE
ETA: orl-rat TDLo:46 g/kg/16W-C   GANNA2
67,825,76
MUT: mma-sat 5 μmol/plate   MUREAV 48,121,77

CONSENSUS REPORTS: EPA Genetic Toxicology Program.

SAFETY PROFILE: Questionable carcinogen
with experimental tumorigenic data. Mutation
data reported. Many N-nitroso compounds are
carcinogens. When heated to decomposition it
emits toxic fumes of NO_x.

PNG250   CAS: 627-12-3
PROPYL CARBAMATE
mf: $C_4H_9NO_2$ mw: 103.14

PROP: Crystals. Bp: 196°, mp: 60°, vap press:
1 mm @ 52.4°. Very sol in water, alc, ether.

SYNS: CARBAMIC ACID, PROPYL ESTER ◇ N-PROPYL
CARBAMATE ◇ PROPYL URETHANE

TOXICITY DATA with REFERENCE
NEO: ipr-mus TD:2400 mg/kg/4W-I   CNREA8
29,2184,69
NEO: ipr-mus TDLo:650mg/kg/13W-I   JNCIAM
8,99,47
ETA: ipr-mus TD:2850 mg/kg/5W-I   IJCNAW
4,318,69

ETA: ipr-mus TD:5700 mg/kg/10W-I   IJCNAW
4,318,69
MUT: mmo-esc 2 pph/3H   AMNTA4 85,119,51

CONSENSUS REPORTS: IARC Cancer Review: GROUP 3 IMEMDT 7,56,87; Animal
Sufficient Evidence IMEMDT 12,201,76. Reported in EPA TSCA Inventory.

SAFETY PROFILE: Questionable carcinogen
with experimental neoplastigenic and tumorigenic data. Experimental teratogenic and reproductive effects. Moderately toxic by subcutaneous route. Mutation data reported. When heated
to decomposition it emits toxic fumes of NO_x.

PNI500   CAS: 63020-33-7
5-n-PROPYL-9,10-DIMETHYL-1,2-
BENZANTHRACENE
mf: $C_{23}H_{22}$ mw: 298.45

SYN: 7,12-DIMETHYL-8-PROPYL-BENZ(a)ANTHRACENE

TOXICITY DATA with REFERENCE
ETA: scu-mus TDLo:200mg/kg   CNREA81,685,41

SAFETY PROFILE: Questionable carcinogen
with experimental tumorigenic data. When
heated to decomposition it emits acrid smoke
and irritating fumes.

PNJ400   CAS: 78-87-5
PROPYLENE DICHLORIDE
mf: $C_3H_6Cl_2$ mw: 112.99

PROP: Colorless liquid. Bp: 96.8°, flash p:
60°F, d: 1.1593 @ 20°/20°, vap press: 40 mm
@ 19.4°, vap d: 3.9, autoign temp: 1035°F,
lel: 3.4%, uel: 14.5%.

SYNS: BICHLORURE de PROPYLENE (FRENCH)
◇ 1,2-DICHLOROPROPANE ◇ α,β-DICHLOROPROPANE
◇ DWUCHLOROPROPAN (POLISH) ◇ ENT 15,406
◇ NCI-C55141 ◇ PROPYLENE CHLORIDE ◇ α,β-PROPYLENE
DICHLORIDE ◇ RCRA WASTE NUMBER U083

TOXICITY DATA with REFERENCE
CAR: orl-mus TDLo:130 g/kg/2Y-I   NTPTR*
NTP-TR-263,86
MUT: mma-sat 333 μg/plate   ENMUDM 5(Suppl
1),3,83
MUT: mmo-sat 100 μg/plate   ENMUDM 5(Suppl
1),3,83

CONSENSUS REPORTS: IARC Cancer Re-
view: GROUP 3 IMEMDT 7,56,87; Animal
Limited Evidence IMEMDT 41,131,86. NTP
Carcinogenesis Studies (gavage); Equivocal Ev-

idence: rat NTPTR* NTP-TR-263,86; Some Evidence: mouse NTPTR* NTP-TR-263,86. Reported in EPA TSCA Inventory. EPA Genetic Toxicology Program. Community Right-To-Know List.

OSHA PEL: (Transitional: TWA 75 ppm) TWA 75 ppm; STEL 110 ppm   ACGIH TLV: TWA 75 ppm; STEL 110 ppm   DFG MAK: 75 ppm (350 mg/m^3) DOT Classification: Flammable Liquid; Label: Flammable Liquid.

SAFETY PROFILE: Questionable carcinogen with experimental carcinogenic data. Moderately toxic by inhalation and ingestion. Mildly toxic by skin contact. An eye irritant. Mutation data reported. Can cause dermatitis. A very dangerous fire hazard when exposed to heat or flame. To fight fire, use water, foam, CO_2, dry chemical. When heated to decomposition it emits toxic fumes of Cl^-.

PNM650   CAS: 77337-54-3
N-n-PROPYL-N-FORMYLHYDRAZINE
mf: $C_4H_{10}N_2O$ mw: 102.16

SYNS: FORMIC ACID, 1-PROPYLHYDRAZIDE ◇ PFH

TOXICITY DATA with REFERENCE
CAR: orl-mus TD:34944 mg/kg/60W-C
   BJCAAI 42,922,80
CAR: orl-mus TDLo:34944 mg/kg/60W-C
   BJCAAI 42,922,80

SAFETY PROFILE: Questionable carcinogen with experimental carcinogenic data. When heated to decomposition it emits toxic fumes of NO_x.

PNM750   CAS: 121-79-9
n-PROPYL GALLATE
mf: $C_{10}H_{12}O_5$ mw: 212.22

PROP: Odorless, fine, ivory powder or crystals; sltly bitter taste. Mp: 147-149°. Sltly sol in water; sol in alc and ether.

SYNS: GALLIC ACID, PROPYL ESTER ◇ NIPA 49 ◇ NIPAGALLIN P ◇ PROGALLIN P ◇ n-PROPYL ESTER of 3,4,5-TRIHYDROXYBENZOIC ACID ◇ PROPYL GALLATE ◇ n-PROPYL-3,4,5-TRIHYDROXYBENZOATE ◇ TENOX PG ◇ 3,4,5-TRIHYDROXYBENZENE-1-PROPYLCARBOXYLATE ◇ 3,4,5-TRIHYDROXYBENZOIC ACID, n-PROPYL ESTER

TOXICITY DATA with REFERENCE
ETA: orl-mus TDLo:168 g/kg/2Y-C   NKEZA4
   29,25,82

MUT: cyt-ham:fbr 40 mg/L   ESKHA5 96,55,78
MUT: cyt-ham:lng 10 mg/L   ATSUDG (4),41,80
MUT: mma-sat 200 μg/plate   SYSWAE 12,41,79
MUT: mmo-sat 200 μg/plate   SYSWAE 12,41,79

CONSENSUS REPORTS: NTP Carcinogenesis Bioassay (feed); No Evidence: mouse, rat NTPTR* NTP-TR-240,82. Reported in EPA TSCA Inventory.

SAFETY PROFILE: Questionable carcinogen with experimental tumorigenic data. Poison by ingestion and intraperitoneal routes. Experimental teratogenic and reproductive effects. Mutation data reported. Combustible when exposed to heat or flame; can react with oxidizing materials. When heated to decomposition it emits acrid smoke and irritating fumes.

PNO000   CAS: 56795-66-5
N-PROPYLHYDRAZINE
HYDROCHLORIDE
mf: $C_3H_{10}N_2 \cdot ClH$ mw: 110.61

TOXICITY DATA with REFERENCE
NEO: orl-mus TDLo:20 g/kg/58W-C   EJCAAH
   11,473,75
ETA: orl-mus TD:50 mg/kg/W-C   PAACA3
   16,61,75

SAFETY PROFILE: Questionable carcinogen with experimental neoplastigenic and tumorigenic data. When heated to decomposition it emits very toxic fumes of HCl and NO_x.

PNO750   CAS: 107-08-4
n-PROPYL IODIDE
mf: C_3H_7I mw: 170.00

PROP: Colorless liquid. D: 1.743 @ 20°/4°, mp: about -98.7°, bp: 102.5°. Sltly sol in water; misc in alc, ether.

SYN: 1-IODOPROPANE

TOXICITY DATA with REFERENCE
NEO: ipr-mus TDLo:3000 mg/kg/8W-I
   CNREA8 35,1411,75

CONSENSUS REPORTS: Reported in EPA TSCA Inventory.

SAFETY PROFILE: Questionable carcinogen with experimental neoplastigenic data. Poison by intraperitoneal route. Very mildly toxic by inhalation. When heated to decomposition it emits toxic fumes of I^-.

PNP250   CAS: 83-59-0
n-PROPYL ISOMER
mf: $C_{20}H_{26}O_6$ mw: 362.46

SYNS: DI-n-PROPYL MALEATE-ISOSAFROLE CONDEN-
SATE ◇ DI-n-PROPYL 6,7-METHYLENEDIOXY-3-METHYL-
1,2,3,4-TETRAHYDRONAPHTHALENE ◇ DI-n-PROPYL-3-
METHYL-6,7-METHYLENEDIOXY-1,2,3,4-TETRAHYDRO-
NAPHTHALENE-1,2-DICARBOXYLATE ◇ DIPROPYL-5,-
6,7,8-TETRAHYDRO-7-METHYLNAPHTHO(2,3-d)-1,3-
DIOXOLE-5,6-DICARBOXYLATE ◇ ENT 15,266 ◇ PROPYL
ISOMER

TOXICITY DATA with REFERENCE
CAR: scu-mus TDLo: 1000 mg/kg   NTIS**PB223-
159
ETA: orl-mus TDLo: 655 g/kg/78W-I   NTIS**
PB223-159

SAFETY PROFILE: Questionable carcinogen
with experimental carcinogenic and tumorigenic
data. Poison by skin contact. Moderately toxic
by ingestion. When heated to decomposition
it emits acrid smoke and irritating fumes.

PNR250   CAS: 66017-91-2
PROPYLNITROSAMINOMETHYL
ACETATE
mf: $C_6H_{12}N_2O_3$ mw: 160.20

SYNS: ACETOXYMETHYLPROPYLNITROSAMINE
◇ N-(ACETOXY)METHYL-N-n-PROPYLNITROSAMINE
◇ N-NITROSO-N-(1-ACETOXYMETHYL)PROPYL AMINE
◇ PAMN ◇ PROPYL ACETOXYMETHYLNITROSAMINE
◇ N-PROPYL-N-(ACETOXYMETHYL)NITROSAMINE

TOXICITY DATA with REFERENCE
CAR: scu-rat TD: 61 mg/kg/10W-I   IAPUDO
41,619,82
CAR: scu-rat TDLo: 50 mg/kg/10W-I   JCROD7
104,13,82
ETA: orl-rat TDLo: 450 mg/kg/90D-I   ZKKOBW
91,317,78
MUT: dnd-mus: fbr 230 μmol/L   GANNA2
73,565,82
MUT: dnr-bcs 200 nmol/plate   GANNA2 70,663,79
MUT: dns-rat: oth 10 μmol/L   CBINA8 53,99,85
MUT: mmo-esc 1 μmol/plate   GANNA2 71,124,80
MUT: msc-ham: lng 100 μmol/L   GANNA2
72,531,81

SAFETY PROFILE: Questionable carcinogen
with experimental carcinogenic and tumorigenic
data. Moderately toxic by ingestion. Mutation
data reported. When heated to decomposition
it emits toxic fumes of NO_x.

PNR500   CAS: 19935-86-5
N-PROPYL-N-NITROSOURETHANE
mf: $C_6H_{12}N_2O_3$ mw: 160.20

SYN: N-NITROSO-N-PROPYLCARBAMIC ACID ETHYL
ESTER

TOXICITY DATA with REFERENCE
CAR: orl-rat TDLo: 1680 mg/kg/6W-C   BJCAAI
46,423,82
ETA: orl-rat TDLo: 1370 mg/kg/29W-C
GANNA2 67,549,76
MUT: cyt-ham: fbr 30 mg/L/20H   MUREAV
48,337,77
MUT: cyt-ham: lng 19 mg/L   GMCRDC 27,95,81

SAFETY PROFILE: Questionable carcinogen
with experimental carcinogenic and tumorigenic
data. Mutation data reported. When heated to
decomposition it emits toxic fumes of NO_x.

POF800   CAS: 56299-00-4
PR TOXIN
mf: $C_{17}H_{20}O_6$ mw: 320.37

SYNS: PRT ◇ PR TOXINE ◇ SPIRO(NAPHTHALENE-
2(1H),2'-OXIRANE)-3'-CARBOXALDEHYDE, 3,5,6,7,8,8a-
HEXAHYDRO-7-ACETOXY-5,6-EPOXY-3',8,8a-TRIMETHYL-
3-OXO- ◇ TOXIN (PENICILLIUM ROQUEFORTII) ◇ TOXIN
PR

TOXICITY DATA with REFERENCE
ETA: orl-rat TD: 139 mg/kg/52D-C   MYCPAH
78,125,82
ETA: orl-rat TDLo: 100 mg/kg/52D-C   MYCPAH
78,125,82
MUT: dnr-bcs 100 μg/disc   CNREA8 36,445,76
MUT: mmo-nsc 2 mg/L   ENMUDM 1,45,79
MUT: mmo-sat 625 ng/plate   MUREAV 130,79,84

SAFETY PROFILE: Questionable carcinogen
with experimental tumorigenic data. Poison by
ingestion, intravenous, and intraperitoneal
routes. Mutation data reported. When heated
to decomposition it emits acrid smoke and irritating fumes.

POI100   CAS: 87625-62-5
PTAQUILOSIDE
mf: $C_{19}H_{28}O_8$ mw: 384.47

SYN: 1',3'-α,4',7'-α-TETRAHYDRO-7'-α- β-3-GLUCO-
PYRANOSYLOXY)-4'-HYDROXY-2',4',6'-TRIMETHYL-SPI-
RO(CYCLOPROPANE-1,5'-(5H)INDEN)-3',(2'H)-ONE

TOXICITY DATA with REFERENCE
CAR: orl-rat TD: 4680 mg/kg/30W-C   JJIND8
79,1143,87
CAR: orl-rat TD: 1930 mg/kg/10W-I   CALEDQ
21,239,84
CAR: orl-rat TDLo: 1580 mg/kg/9W-I   JJCREP
75,833,84

MUT: dns-rat:lvr 1 μmol/L   MUREAV 143,75,85

CONSENSUS REPORTS: IARC Cancer Review: GROUP 3 IMEMDT 7,56,87; Animal Limited Evidence IMEMDT 40,47,86

SAFETY PROFILE: Questionable carcinogen with experimental carcinogenic data. Mutation data reported. When heated to decomposition it emits acrid smoke and irritating fumes.

POJ250   CAS: 120-73-0
PURINE
mf: $C_5H_4N_4$ mw: 120.13

PROP: Needles. Mp: 216-217°. Very sol in hot alc; sltly sol in hot ethyl acetate, acetone; insol in ether, chloroform.

SYNS: 7H-IMIDAZO(4,5-D)PYRIMIDINE ◇ ISOPURINE ◇ NSC 753 ◇ 7H-PURINE ◇ 9H-PURINE ◇ 3,5,7-TRIAZAINDOLE

TOXICITY DATA with REFERENCE
ETA: scu-rat TDLo:156 mg/kg/8W-I   CNREA8 38,2229,78
MUT: dnd-mam:lym 50 mmol/L   PNASA6 48,686,62
MUT: pic-esc 1 g/L   ZAPOAK 12,583,72

CONSENSUS REPORTS: EPA Genetic Toxicology Program.

SAFETY PROFILE: Questionable carcinogen with experimental tumorigenic data. Poison by intraperitoneal route. Mutation data reported. When heated to decomposition it emits toxic fumes of NO_x.

POJ750   CAS: 28199-55-5
PURINE-3-OXIDE
mf: $C_5H_4N_4O$ mw: 136.13

TOXICITY DATA with REFERENCE
CAR: scu-rat TDLo:1800 mg/kg/8W-I   CNREA8 38,2229,78
ETA: scu-rat TD:18 mg/kg/8W-I   PAACA3 17,147,76
ETA: scu-rat TD:180 mg/kg/8W-I   PAACA3 17,147,76

SAFETY PROFILE: Questionable carcinogen with experimental carcinogenic and tumorigenic data. When heated to decomposition it emits toxic fumes of NO_x.

POK000   CAS: 50-44-2
PURINE-6-THIOL
mf: $C_5H_4N_4S$ mw: 152.19

SYNS: 1,7-DIHYDRO-6H-PURINE-6-THIONE ◇ ISMIPUR ◇ LEUKERAN ◇ LEUPURIN ◇ MERCALEUKIN ◇ MERCAPTOPURIN (GERMAN) ◇ 6-MERCAPTOPURIN ◇ 6-MERCAPTOPURINE ◇ 7-MERCAPTO-1,3,4,6-TETRAZAINDENE ◇ MERCAPURIN ◇ MERN ◇ MP ◇ NCI-C04886 ◇ NSC 755 ◇ PURIMETHOL ◇ 3H-PURINE-6-THIOL ◇ 6-PURINETHIOL ◇ PURINETHOL ◇ THIOHYPOXANTHINE ◇ 6-THIOXOPURINE ◇ U-4748

TOXICITY DATA with REFERENCE
CAR: orl-chd TD:675 mg/kg/39W-C:BLD   JOPDAB 72,409,68
NEO: orl-wmn TDLo:360 mg/kg/34W-C:BLD   AJGAAR 78,316,83
ETA: ipr-mus TDLo:1170 mg/kg/26W-I   CANCAR 40,1935,77
MUT: cyt-hmn:unr 24 mg/kg/8W   HUHEAS 29,100,79
MUT: dni-hmn:hla 10 μmol/L   BBACAQ 366,333,74
MUT: mma-sat 150 μmol/L   EXPEAM 40,370,84
MUT: mms-ham:lng 2 mg/L   MUREAV 157,189,85
MUT: oms-bcs 10 μmol/L   CNREA8 40,4381,80
MUT: oms-hmn:lym 10 nmol/L   CNREA8 43,3655,83
MUT: sce-hmn:lym 10 pmol/L   NGCJAK 15,1085,80

CONSENSUS REPORTS: IARC Cancer Review: Animal Inadequate Evidence IMEMDT 26,249,81; Human Inadequate Evidence IMEMDT 26,249,81. NCI Carcinogenesis Studies (ipr); Equivocal Evidence: rat CANCAR 40,1935,77; (ipr); Clear Evidence: mouse CANCAR 40,1935,77. EPA Genetic Toxicology Program.

SAFETY PROFILE: Questionable human carcinogen producing Hodgkin's disease and leukemia. Poison by ingestion, intraperitoneal, subcutaneous, parenteral and intravenous routes. Human systemic effects by an ingestion: dermatitis. Experimental teratogenic and reproductive effects. Human mutation data reported. When heated to decomposition it emits very toxic fumes of SO_x and NO_x.

POL475   CAS: 26308-28-1
PYRAZAPON
mf: $C_{15}H_{16}N_4O$ mw: 268.35

SYNS: CI-683 ◇ 1-ETHYL-4,6-DIHYDRO-3-METHYL-8-PHENYLPYRAZOLO(4,3-e)(1,4)DIAZEPINE ◇ RIPAZEPAM

TOXICITY DATA with REFERENCE
CAR: orl-mus TDLo:81900 mg/kg/78W-C   FAATDF 4,178,84

SAFETY PROFILE: Questionable carcinogen with experimental carcinogenic data. When heated to decomposition it emits toxic fumes of NO_x.

POL500   CAS: 98-96-4
PYRAZINECARBOXAMIDE
mf: $C_5H_5N_3O$ mw: 123.13

SYNS: ALDINAMID ◇ 2-CARBAMYL PYRAZINE ◇ D-50 ◇ EPRAZIN ◇ MK 56 ◇ NCI-C01785 ◇ PYRAZINA-MIDE ◇ PYRAZINEAMIDE ◇ PYRAZINE CARBOXYLAMIDE ◇ PYRAZINOIC ACID AMIDE ◇ TEBRAZID

TOXICITY DATA with REFERENCE
ETA: orl-mus TD: 756 g/kg/30W-C   GANNA2 51,83,60
ETA: orl-mus TDLo: 328 g/kg/78W-C   NCITR* NCI-CG-TR-48,78
MUT: cyt-hmn: lym 120 mg/L   MUREAV 48,215,77

CONSENSUS REPORTS: NCI Carcinogenesis Bioassay (feed); No Evidence: rat NCITR* NCI-CG-TR-48,78; (feed); Inadequate Studies: mouse NCITR* NCI-CG-TR-48,78. Reported in EPA TSCA Inventory.

SAFETY PROFILE: Questionable carcinogen with experimental tumorigenic data. Moderately toxic by ingestion, subcutaneous, and intraperitoneal routes. Human mutation data reported. When heated to decomposition it emits toxic fumes of NO_x.

PON250   CAS: 129-00-0
PYRENE
mf: $C_{16}H_{10}$ mw: 202.26

PROP: Colorless solid, solutions have a slight blue color. Mp: 156°, d: 1.271 @ 23°, bp: 404°. Insol in water; fairly sol in organic solvents. (A condensed ring hydrocarbon).

SYNS: BENZO(def)PHENANTHRENE ◇ PYREN (GERMAN) ◇ β-PYRINE

TOXICITY DATA with REFERENCE
ETA: skn-mus TDLo: 10 g/kg/3W-I   BJCAAI 10,363,56
MUT: dns-ham: lvr 100 μmol/L   ENMUDM 5,1,83
MUT: dns-hmn: fbr 100 mg/L   TXCYAC 21,151,81
MUT: dns-rat: lvr 250 nmol/L   CNREA8 42,3010,82
MUT: mma-esc 1 μg/plate   PMRSDJ 1,387,81
MUT: mma-sat 300 ng/plate   ENMUDM 6(Suppl 2),1,84
MUT: msc-hmn: oth 12 μmol/L   MUREAV 130,127,84

CONSENSUS REPORTS: IARC Cancer Review: Animal No Evidence IMEMDT 32,-431,83. EPA Extremely Hazardous Substances List. Reported in EPA TSCA Inventory. EPA Genetic Toxicology Program.

OSHA PEL: TWA 0.2 mg/m³

SAFETY PROFILE: Questionable carcinogen with experimental tumorigenic data. Poison by inhalation. Moderately toxic by ingestion and intraperitoneal routes. Human mutation data reported. A skin irritant. When heated to decomposition it emits acrid smoke and irritating fumes.

PON500   CAS: 1732-14-5
N-PYREN-2-YLACETAMIDE
mf: $C_{18}H_{13}NO$ mw: 259.32

SYN: 2-ACETYLAMINOPYRENE

TOXICITY DATA with REFERENCE
NEO: orl-rat TDLo: 5508 mg/kg/32W-C   CNREA8 15,188,55

SAFETY PROFILE: Questionable carcinogen with experimental neoplastigenic data. When heated to decomposition it emits toxic fumes of NO_x.

POP750   CAS: 156-25-2
PYRIDINE-3-AZO-p-DIMETHYLANILINE
mf: $C_{13}H_{14}N_4$ mw: 226.31

SYNS: 3'-(4-DIMETHYLAMINOPHENYL)AZOPYRIDINE ◇ N,N-DIMETHYL-p-(3-PYRIDYLAZO)ANILINE ◇ N,N-DIMETHYL-4-(3'-PYRIDYLAZO)ANILINE

TOXICITY DATA with REFERENCE
ETA: orl-rat TDLo: 3530 mg/kg/28W-C   JNCIAM 15,67,54

SAFETY PROFILE: Questionable carcinogen with experimental tumorigenic data. When heated to decomposition it emits toxic fumes of NO_x.

POQ000   CAS: 63019-82-9
PYRIDINE-4-AZO-p-DIMETHYLANILINE
mf: $C_{13}H_{14}N_4$ mw: 226.31

TOXICITY DATA with REFERENCE
ETA: orl-rat TDLo: 6480 mg/kg/26W-C   CNREA8 14,22,54

SAFETY PROFILE: Questionable carcinogen with experimental tumorigenic data. When

heated to decomposition it emits toxic fumes of NO_x.

POS250   CAS: 59405-47-9
PYRIDINE-1-OXIDE-3-AZO-p-DIMETHYLANILINE
mf: $C_{13}H_{14}N_4O$ mw: 242.31

TOXICITY DATA with REFERENCE
ETA: orl-rat TDLo: 4300 mg/kg/17W-C
CNREA8 14,715,54

SAFETY PROFILE: Questionable carcinogen with experimental tumorigenic data. When heated to decomposition it emits toxic fumes of NO_x.

POS500   CAS: 13520-96-2
PYRIDINE-1-OXIDE-4-AZO-p-DIMETHYLANILINE
mf: $C_{13}H_{14}N_4O$ mw: 242.31

TOXICITY DATA with REFERENCE
NEO: orl-rat TDLo: 1134 mg/kg/9W-C   JNCIAM 37,365,66
ETA: orl-rat TD: 4320 mg/kg/17W-C   CNREA8 14,22,54

SAFETY PROFILE: Questionable carcinogen with experimental neoplastigenic and tumorigenic data. When heated to decomposition it emits toxic fumes of NO_x.

PPI815   CAS: 240-39-1
12H-PYRIDO(2,3-a)THIENO(2,3-i) CARBAZOLE
mf: $N_2SC_{17}H_{10}$ mw: 274.35

TOXICITY DATA with REFERENCE
NEO: scu-mus TDLo: 72 mg/kg/9W-I   CHDDAT 271,1474,70

SAFETY PROFILE: Questionable carcinogen with experimental neoplastigenic data. When heated to decomposition it emits very toxic fumes of NO_x and SO_x.

PPL500   CAS: 19992-69-9
1-(PYRIDYL-3)-3,3-DIMETHYL TRIAZENE
mf: $C_7H_{10}N_4$ mw: 150.21

SYNS: 1-(PYRIDYL-3)-3,3-DIMETHYL-TRIAZEN (GERMAN) ◇ 1-(m-PYRIDYL)-3,3-DIMETHYL-TRIAZENE

TOXICITY DATA with REFERENCE
NEO: orl-rat TDLo: 160 mg/kg   ZKKOBW81,285,74
NEO: scu-rat TD: 500 mg/kg/44W-I   ZKKOBW 81,285,74

NEO: scu-rat TDLo: 150 mg/kg   ZKKOBW 81,285,74
MUT: hma-mus/lng 6250 μg/kg   PSEBAA 158,269,78
MUT: hma-mus/smc 200 μmol/L/Kg   AGACBH 3,99,73
MUT: mnt-mus-ipr 1250 μg/kg/24H   MUREAV 56,319,78
MUT: mrc-smc 33 mmol/L   AGACBH 3,99,73
MUT: sln-dmg-orl 3300 μmol/L   CBINA8 9,365,74

SAFETY PROFILE: Questionable carcinogen with experimental neoplastigenic data. Poison by ingestion and subcutaneous routes. Experimental reproductive effects. Mutation data reported. When heated to decomposition it emits toxic fumes of NO_x.

PPO000   CAS: 144-83-2
N-2-PYRIDYLSULFANILAMIDE
mf: $C_{11}H_{11}N_3O_2S$ mw: 249.31

PROP: Colorless prisms in water. Mp: 191-192°. Sol in water and alc; sltly sol in ether; very sol in alkali and aqueous HCl.

SYNS: ADIPLON ◇ COCCOCLASE ◇ DAGENAN ◇ EUBASIN ◇ EUBASINUM ◇ HAPTOCIL ◇ M+B 695 ◇ N^1-2-PYRIDYLSULFANILAMIDE ◇ RELBAPIRIDINA ◇ RONIN ◇ SEPTIPULMON ◇ 2-SULFANILYL AMINOPYRIDINE ◇ SULFAPYRIDINE ◇ 2-SULFAPYRIDINE ◇ SULFIDINE ◇ THIOSEPTAL ◇ TRIANON

TOXICITY DATA with REFERENCE
ETA: scu-rat TDLo: 135 mg/kg/9W-I   PSEBAA 68,330,48

CONSENSUS REPORTS: Reported in EPA TSCA Inventory.

SAFETY PROFILE: Questionable carcinogen with experimental tumorigenic data. Moderately toxic by intraperitoneal and intravenous routes. Very mildly toxic by ingestion. When heated to decomposition it emits very toxic fumes of NO_x and SO_x.

PPQ500   CAS: 87-66-1
PYROGALLOL
mf: $C_6H_6O_3$ mw: 126.12

PROP: White, lustrous crystals. Bp: 309°, d: 1.453 @ 4°/4°, vap press: 10 mm @ 167.7°, mp: 131-133°. Sltly sol in benzene, chloroform.

SYNS: 1,2,3-BENZENETRIOL ◇ C.I. 76515 ◇ C.I. OXIDATION BASE 32 ◇ FOURAMINE BROWN AP ◇ FOURRINE PG ◇ PYROGALLIC ACID ◇ 1,2,3-TRIHYDROXYBENZEN (CZECH) ◇ 1,2,3-TRIHYDROXYBENZENE

TOXICITY DATA with REFERENCE
ETA: scu-rat TDLo: 3950 mg/kg/58W-I
  PAACA3 20,117,79
MUT: cyt-ham: ovr 100 mg/L   CALEDQ 14,251,81
MUT: mmo-sat 1 μmol/plate   NEZAAQ 35,533,83
MUT: mrc-smc 300 mg/L   MUREAV 135,109,84
MUT: sln-dmg-orl 125 mmol/L   MUREAV 90,91,81

CONSENSUS REPORTS: Reported in EPA
TSCA Inventory.

SAFETY PROFILE: Questionable carcinogen
with experimental tumorigenic data. Human
poison by ingestion and subcutaneous routes.
An experimental poison by ingestion, subcutaneous, intravenous, and intraperitoneal routes.
Experimental teratogenic and reproductive effects. Mutation data reported. Readily absorbed
through the skin. Human systemic effects by
ingestion: convulsions, dyspnea, gastrointestinal effects. A severe skin and eye irritant. When
heated to decomposition it emits acrid smoke
and irritating fumes. Used as a topical antibacterial agent, as an intermediate, hair dye component, and analytical reagent.

PQB500   CAS: 494-98-4
3-PYRROL-2-YLPYRIDINE
mf: $C_9H_8N_2$ mw: 144.19

SYN: NORNICOTYRINE

TOXICITY DATA with REFERENCE
ETA: itr-rat TDLo: 23 mg/kg   BJCAAI 16,453,62

SAFETY PROFILE: Questionable carcinogen
with experimental tumorigenic data. When
heated to decomposition it emits toxic fumes
of NO_x.

QBJ000   CAS: 1401-55-4
QUEBRACHO TANNIN

SYNS: SCHINOPSIS LORENTZII TANNIN ◇ TANNIN from
QUEBRACHO

TOXICITY DATA with REFERENCE
ETA: scu-mus TDLo: 750 mg/kg/12W-I   BJCAAI
  14,147,60
ETA: scu-rat TDLo: 350 mg/kg/12W-I   BJCAAI
  14,147,60

SAFETY PROFILE: Questionable carcinogen
with experimental tumorigenic data. Poison by
intraperitoneal and intravenous routes. When
heated to decomposition it emits acrid smoke
and irritating fumes.

QCA000   CAS: 117-39-5
QUERCETIN
mf: $C_{15}H_{10}O_7$ mw: 302.25

SYNS: C.I. 75670 ◇ C.I. NATURAL RED 1 ◇ C.I. NATURAL
YELLOW 10 ◇ CYANIDELONON 1522 ◇ 2-(3,4-DIHYDROXY-
PHENYL)-3,5,7-TRIHYDROXY-4H-1-BENZOPYRAN-4-ONE
◇ MELETIN ◇ NCI-C60106 ◇ 3,5,7,3′,4′-PENTAHYDROXY-
FLAVONE ◇ QUERCETINE ◇ QUERCETOL ◇ QUERCITIN
◇ QUERTINE ◇ SOPHORETIN ◇ 3′,4′,5,7-TETRAHYDROXY-
FLAVAN-3-OL ◇ T-GELB BZW. GRUN 1 ◇ XANTHAURINE

TOXICITY DATA with REFERENCE
CAR: orl-rat TD: 38235 mg/kg/58W-C   CNREA8
  40,3468,80
CAR: orl-rat TDLo: 33610 mg/kg/58W-C
  CNREA8 40,3468,80
NEO: orl-rat TD: 243 g/kg/3Y-C   PAACA3
  25,95,84
NEO: orl-rat TD: 487 g/kg/3Y-C   PAACA3
  25,95,84
ETA: orl-mus TDLo: 966 g/kg/23W-C   GANNA2
  72,327,81
MUT: cyt-hmn: fbr 5 mg/L   PJABDW 56,443,80
MUT: cyt-hmn: lym 10 mg/L   PJABDW 56,443,80
MUT: dni-hmn: fbr 50 mg/L   BCPCA6 33,3823,84
MUT: msc-hmn: emb 3 mg/L   KIKNAJ (32),51,81
MUT: oms-hmn: fbr 200 mg/L   BCPCA6
  33,3823,84
MUT: sce-ham: ovr 15 mg/L   MUREAV
  113,45,83
MUT: sce-hmn: fbr 1 mg/L   PJABDW 56,443,80
MUT: sce-hmn: lym 8 mg/L   PJABDW 56,443,80

CONSENSUS REPORTS: IARC Cancer Review: GROUP 3 IMEMDT 7,56,87; Animal
Limited Evidence IMEMDT 31,213,83. Reported in EPA TSCA Inventory. EPA Genetic
Toxicology Program.

SAFETY PROFILE: Questionable carcinogen
with experimental carcinogenic, neoplastigenic,
tumorigenic, and teratogenic data. Poison by
ingestion, subcutaneous, and intravenous
routes. Experimental reproductive effects. Human mutation data reported. Used as a pharmaceutical and veterinary drug. When heated to
decomposition it emits acrid smoke and irritating
fumes.

QCA175   CAS: 6151-25-3
QUERCETIN DIHYDRATE
mf: $C_{15}H_{10}O_7 \cdot 2H_2O$ mw: 338.29

TOXICITY DATA with REFERENCE
ETA: orl-rat TD: 4250 g/kg/121W-C   CALEDQ
  13,15,81

ETA: orl-rat TDLo: 1350 g/kg/77W-C CALEDQ 13,15,81

SAFETY PROFILE: Questionable carcinogen with experimental tumorigenic data. Poison by ingestion. When heated to decomposition it emits acrid smoke and irritating fumes.

QCS875 CAS: 10072-24-9
QUINACRINE ETHYL M/2
mf: $C_{18}H_{19}Cl_2N_3O \cdot 2ClH \cdot H_2O$ mw: 455.24

SYNS: ACRIDINE, 9-(2-((2-CHLOROETHYL)AMINO) ETHYLAMINO)-6-CHLORO-2-METHOXY-, DIHYDROCHLORIDE, HYDRATE ◇ 9-(2-((2-CHLOROETHYL)AMINO)ETHYLAMINO)-6-CHLORO-2-METHOXYACRIDINE, DIHYDROCHLORIDE ◇ ICR-125

TOXICITY DATA with REFERENCE
NEO: ipr-mus TDLo: 570 mg/kg/4W-I JNCIAM 36,915,66

SAFETY PROFILE: Questionable carcinogen with experimental neoplastigenic data. When heated to decomposition it emits toxic fumes of NO_x and HCl.

QDS000 CAS: 4213-45-0
QUINACRINE MUSTARD DIHYDROCHLORIDE
mf: $C_{23}H_{28}Cl_3N_3O \cdot 2ClH$ mw: 541.81

SYNS: 9-(4-BIS(2-CHLOROETHYL)AMINO-1-METHYLBUTYLAMINO)-6-CHLORO-2-METHOXYACRIDINE DIHYDROCHLORIDE ◇ ICR 10 ◇ 2-METHOXY-6-CHLORO-9-(4-BIS(2-CHLOROETHYL)AMINO-1-METHYLBUTYLAMINO)ACRIDINE DIHYDROCHLORIDE ◇ 2-METHOXY-6-CHLORO-9-(3-(ETHYL-2-CHLOROETHYL)AMINOPROPYLAMINO) ACRIDINE DIHYDROCHLORIDE ◇ QUINACRINE MUSTARD

TOXICITY DATA with REFERENCE
NEO: ivn-mus TDLo: 2700 µg/kg CNREA8 36,2423,76
MUT: cyt-mam: lng 50 mg/L HEREAY 69,217,71
MUT: dnr-bcs 20 µL/disc MUREAV 97,1,82
MUT: dnr-esc 20 µL/disc MUREAV 97,1,82
MUT: sce-ham: ovr 468 µg/L/2H-C ENMUDM 4,647,82
MUT: sce-hmn-lym 1 mg/L MUREAV 30,273,75
MUT: slt-dmg-par 2 mmol/L MUREAV 1,437,64

CONSENSUS REPORTS: EPA Genetic Toxicology Program. Reported in EPA TSCA Inventory.

SAFETY PROFILE: Questionable carcinogen with experimental neoplastigenic data. Human

mutation data reported. When heated to decomposition it emits very toxic fumes of Cl^- and NO_x.

QMJ000 CAS: 91-22-5
QUINOLINE
DOT: 2656
mf: C_9H_7N mw: 129.17

PROP: Refractive, colorless liquid; peculiar odor. Mp: $-14.5°$, bp: $237.7°$, d: 1.0900 @ 25°/4°, autoign temp: 896°F, vap press: 1 mm @ 59.7°, vap d: 4.45. Sol in water, CS_2; misc in alc, ether.

SYNS: 1-AZANAPHTHALENE ◇ 1-BENZAZINE ◇ 1-BENZINE ◇ BENZO(b)PYRIDINE ◇ CHINOLEINE ◇ CHINOLIN (CZECH) ◇ CHINOLINE ◇ LEUCOL ◇ LEUCOLINE ◇ LEUKOL ◇ USAF EK-218

TOXICITY DATA with REFERENCE
CAR: ipr-mus TDLo: 9042 µg/kg/15D-I JJCREP 78,139,87
NEO: orl-rat TDLo: 7770 mg/kg/37W-C CNREA8 36,329,76
ETA: orl-mus TDLo: 50 g/kg/30W-C GANNA2 68,785,77
ETA: orl-rat TD: 23 g/kg/30W-C GANNA2 68,785,77
MUT: dnd-esc 30 µmol/L MUREAV 89,95,81
MUT: mma-ham: ovr 80 µmol/L ENMUDM 4,395,82
MUT: mma-sat 1 µmol/plate ABCHA6 42,861,78
MUT: sce-ham: ovr 110 µg/L ENMUDM 7,1,85

CONSENSUS REPORTS: Reported in EPA TSCA Inventory. EPA Genetic Toxicology Program. Community Right-To-Know List.

DOT Classification: Poison B; Label: St. Andrews Cross, Flammable Liquid; ORM-E; Label: None.

SAFETY PROFILE: Questionable carcinogen with experimental neoplastigenic and tumorigenic data. Poison by ingestion, subcutaneous, and intraperitoneal routes. Moderately toxic by skin contact. Mutation data reported. A skin and severe eye irritant. Combustible when exposed to heat or flame. Its preparation has caused many industrial explosions. Unpredictably violent. When heated to decomposition it emits toxic fumes of NO_x.

QPA000 CAS: 148-24-3
8-QUINOLINOL
mf: C_9H_7NO mw: 145.17

PROP: White crystals or powder. Mp: 76°, bp: 267°. Very sltly sol in cold water; sltly sol in ether; sol in alc, dilute alkali.

SYNS: BIOQUIN ◇ FENNOSAN ◇ HYDROXYBENZOPYRI-DINE ◇ 8-HYDROXY-CHINOLIN (GERMAN) ◇ 8-HYDROXY-QUINOLINE ◇ NCI-C55298 ◇ 8-OQ ◇ OXINE ◇ OXYBENZO-PYRIDINE ◇ OXYCHINOLIN ◇ o-OXYCHINOLIN (GERMAN) ◇ OXYQUINOLINE ◇ 8-OXYQUINOLINE ◇ PHENOPYRI-DINE ◇ 8-QUINOL ◇ QUINOPHENOL ◇ TUMEX ◇ USAF EK-794

TOXICITY DATA with REFERENCE
CAR: imp-mus TD:100 mg/kg/   BMBUAQ 14,1475,68
CAR: imp-mus TDLo:50 mg/kg   BJCAAI 11,212,57
NEO: imp-mus TD:80 mg/kg   BJCAAI 11,212,57
ETA: ivg-mus TD:17 g/kg/2Y-I:TER   VOONAW 22(3),68,76
ETA: ivg-mus TDLo:5600 mg/kg/35W-I:TER VOONAW 16(8),67,70
ETA: ivg-rat TDLo:33 g/kg/82W-I:TER ARPAAQ 79,245,65
ETA: orl-rat TD:34 g/kg/84W-I:TER   VOONAW 16(8),67,70
ETA: orl-rat TDLo:29 g/kg/48W-I:TER JNCIAM 41,985,68
ETA: scu-mus TDLo:900 mg/kg/21W-I:TER VOONAW 16(8),67,70
ETA: skn-mus TDLo:7200 mg/kg/50W-I:TER VOONAW 16(8),67,70
MUT: bfa-rat/sat 600 mg/kg   TXCYAC 34,231,85
MUT: dnd-esc 10 μmol/L   MUREAV 89,95,81
MUT: dni-hmn:hla 25 μmol/L   MUREAV 92,427,82
MUT: mma-sat 10 μg/plate   MUREAV 39,285,77
MUT: mmo-bcs 10 mmol/L   FAVUAI 6,118,74
MUT: sln-dmg-orl 5 μmol/L/2H   MUREAV 39,285,77

CONSENSUS REPORTS: IARC Cancer Review: Animal Inadequate Evidence IMEMDT 13,101,77. NTP Carcinogenesis Studies (feed); No Evidence: mouse, rat NTPTR* NTP-TR-276,85. Reported in EPA TSCA Inventory. EPA Genetic Toxicology Program.

SAFETY PROFILE: Questionable carcinogen with experimental carcinogenic, neoplastigenic, tumorigenic, and teratogenic data. Poison by intraperitoneal and subcutaneous routes. Moderately toxic by ingestion and possibly other routes. A central nervous system stimulant. Human mutation data reported. Combustible when exposed to heat or flame. When heated to de-

composition it emits highly toxic fumes of NO_x.

QQA000   CAS: 63040-20-0
N-(4-QUINOLYL)ACETOHYDROXAMIC ACID
mf: $C_{11}H_{10}N_2O_2$ mw: 202.23

SYN: MONOACETYL 4-HYDROXYAMINOQUINOLINE

TOXICITY DATA with REFERENCE
NEO: scu-mus TDLo:96 mg/kg/20W-I   JJEMAG 40,475,70

SAFETY PROFILE: Questionable carcinogen with experimental neoplastigenic data. When heated to decomposition it emits toxic fumes of NO_x.

QQS200   CAS: 106-51-4
QUINONE
mf: $C_6H_4O_2$ mw: 108.10

PROP: Yellow crystals; characteristic irritating odor. Mp: 115.7°, bp: sublimes, d: 1.318 @ 20°/4°.

SYNS: BENZO-CHINON (GERMAN) ◇ 1,4-BENZOQUINE ◇ 1,4-BENZOQUINONE ◇ BENZOQUINONE (DOT) ◇ p-BENZOQUINONE ◇ CHINON (DUTCH, GERMAN) ◇ p-CHINON (GERMAN) ◇ CHINONE ◇ CYCLOHEXADEINE-DIONE ◇ 1,4-CYCLOHEXADIENEDIONE ◇ 2,5-CYCLO-HEXADIENE-1,4-DIONE ◇ 1,4-CYCLOHEXADIENE DI-OXIDE ◇ 1,4-DIOSSIBENZENE (ITALIAN) ◇ 1,4-DIOXY-BENZENE ◇ 1,4-DIOXY-BENZOL (GERMAN) ◇ NCI-C55845 ◇ p-QUINONE ◇ RCRA WASTE NUMBER U197 ◇ USAF P-220

TOXICITY DATA with REFERENCE
ETA: skn-mus TDLo:800 mg/kg/29W-C PIATA8 16,309,40
MUT: mmo-sat 8 mg/plate   MUREAV 81,11,81
MUT: oms-hmn:lym 5 μmol/L   CNREA8 45,2471,85
MUT: oms-mus:lym 10 μmol/L   TOLED5 29,161,85
MUT: oms-rbt:bmr 2 μmol/L   AJIMD8 7,485,85
MUT: sce-hmn:lum 5 μmol/L   CNREA8 45,2471,85

CONSENSUS REPORTS: IARC Cancer Review: Animal Inadequate Evidence IMEMDT 15,255,77. Reported in EPA TSCA Inventory. Community Right-To-Know List. EPA Genetic Toxicology Program.

OSHA PEL: TWA 0.01 ppm   ACGIH TLV: TWA 0.1 ppm   DFG MAK: 0.1 ppm (0.4 mg/

m^3)   DOT Classification: Poison B; Label: Poison.

SAFETY PROFILE: Questionable carcinogen with experimental tumorigenic data by skin contact. Poison by ingestion, subcutaneous, intraperitoneal, and intravenous routes. Human mutation data reported. Quinone has a characteristic, irritating odor. Causes severe damage to the skin and mucous membranes by contact with it in the solid state, in solution, or in the form of condensed vapors. Locally, it causes discoloration, severe irritation, erythema, swelling, and the formation of papules and vesicles, whereas prolonged contact may lead to necrosis. When the eyes become involved, it causes dangerous disturbances of vision. The moist material self heats and decomposes exothermically above 60°C. When heated to decomposition it emits acrid smoke and fumes.

QSA000   CAS: 2423-66-7
QUINOXALINE-1,4-DI-N-OXIDE
mf: $C_8H_6N_2O_2$ mw: 162.16

SYNS: GROFAS ◇ QUINDOXIN ◇ QUINOXALINE DIOXIDE ◇ QUINOXALINE DI-N-OXIDE ◇ QUINOXALINE 1,4-DIOXIDE ◇ USAF H-1

TOXICITY DATA with REFERENCE
CAR: orl-rat TDLo:5400 mg/kg/77W-C
   JNCIAM 55,137,75
MUT: dnr-sat 100 μg/plate   AMACCQ 20,151,81
MUT: mma-sat 5 μg/plate   CPBTAL 27,1954,79
MUT: mmo-sat 5 μg/plate   CPBTAL 27,1954,79
MUT: sce-ham:lng 500 mg/L   MUREAV 139,199,84

CONSENSUS REPORTS: EPA Genetic Toxicology Program.

SAFETY PROFILE: Questionable carcinogen with experimental carcinogenic data. Moderately toxic by intraperitoneal route. Mutation data reported. When heated to decomposition it emits toxic fumes of NO_x.

RAF100   CAS: 22248-79-9
RABOND
mf: $C_{10}H_9Cl_4O_4P$ mw: 365.96

PROP: Mp 97-98°. Solubility in water: 11 ppm, in xylene: <15%, 40-50% in chloroform at room temp.

SYNS: APPEX ◇ (Z)-2-CHLORO-1-(2,4,5-TRICHLOROPHENYL)VINYL DIMETHYL PHOSPHATE ◇ CVMP ◇ DEBANTIC

◇ DIETREEN ◇ DUST M ◇ ENT 25,841 ◇ GARDCIDE ◇ GARDONA ◇ GORDONA ◇ (Z)-PHOSPHORIC ACID-2-CHLORO-1-(2,4,5-TRICHLOROPHENYL)ETHENYL DIMETHYL ESTER ◇ RABON ◇ ROL ◇ SD 8447 ◇ STIROFOS ◇ STIROPHOS ◇ 2,4,5-TRICHLORO-α-(CHLOROMETHYLENE)BENZYL PHOSPHATE ESTER

TOXICITY DATA with REFERENCE
MUT: mnt-mus-ipr 200 mg/kg/7D-I   MUREAV
   117,329,83
MUT: mnt-mus-orl 720 mg/kg/24H-C   MUREAV
   117,329,83

CONSENSUS REPORTS: IARC Cancer Review: GROUP 3 IMEMDT 7,56,87; Animal Limited Evidence IMEMDT 30,197,83.

SAFETY PROFILE: Questionable carcinogen. Poison by ingestion. Moderately toxic by an unspecified route. Mutation data reported. Used as an insecticide. A cholinesterase inhibitor. When heated to decomposition it emits toxic fumes of Cl^- and PO_x.

RBZ000
RATON

PROP: Aqueous extract from the dried leaves of the plant (JNCIAM 46,1131,71).

SYN: GLIRICIDIAL SEPIUM

TOXICITY DATA with REFERENCE
ETA: scu-rat TDLo:300 g/kg/1Y-I   JNCIAM
   46,1131,71

SAFETY PROFILE: Questionable carcinogen with experimental tumorigenic data. When heated to decomposition it emits acrid smoke and irritating fumes.

RCA275   CAS: 8059-82-3
RAUTRAX

TOXICITY DATA with REFERENCE
NEO: orl-wmn TD:2190 mg/kg/3Y-C   LANCAO
   2,672,74
NEO: orl-wmn TDLo:1825 mg/kg/5Y-C
   LANCAO 2,672,74

SAFETY PROFILE: Questionable human carcinogen producing lung and skin tumors. When heated to decomposition it emits acrid smoke and irritating fumes.

RCK725
REFRACTORY CERAMIC FIBERS

PROP: A mixture of ALUMINA and SILICA (1:1).

SYN: FIBERS, REFRACTORY CERAMIC

TOXICITY DATA with REFERENCE
ETA: ipr-rat TDLo: 125 mg/kg   EPASR* 8EHQ-0485-0553

SAFETY PROFILE: Questionable carcinogen with experimental tumorigenic data.

RCU000   CAS: 17095-24-8
REMAZOL BLACK B
mf: $C_{26}H_{25}N_5O_{19}S_6 \cdot 4Na$ mw: 995.88

TOXICITY DATA with REFERENCE
ETA: orl-rat TDLo: 72 g/kg/86W-I   TKORAS 3,53,67
ETA: scu-rat TDLo: 20 g/kg/71W-I   TKORAS 3,53,67

CONSENSUS REPORTS: Reported in EPA TSCA Inventory.

SAFETY PROFILE: Questionable carcinogen with experimental tumorigenic data. When heated to decomposition it emits very toxic fumes of Na_2O, NO_x, and SO_x.

RCZ000   CAS: 18976-74-4
REMAZOL YELLOW G
mf: $C_{20}H_{19}ClN_4O_{11}S_3 \cdot 2Na$ mw: 669.04

SYNS: C.I. REACTIVE YELLOW 14 ◇ p-((4-(5-((2-HY-DROXYETHYL)SULFONYL)-2-METHOXYPHENYL)AZO)-5-HYDROXY-3-METHYLPYRAZOL-1-YL)-3-CHLORO-5-METHYL-BENZENESULFONIC ACID, HYDROGEN SUL-FATE (ESTER), DISODIUM SALT ◇ PROCION YELLOW MX 4R

TOXICITY DATA with REFERENCE
ETA: orl-mus TDLo: 38 g/kg/32W-I   TKORAS 3,53,67
ETA: orl-rat TDLo: 52 g/kg/58W-I   TKORAS 3,53,67
ETA: scu-mus TDLo: 20 g/kg/1Y-I   TKORAS 3,53,67
ETA: scu-rat TDLo: 25 g/kg/81W-I   TKORAS 3,53,67

SAFETY PROFILE: Questionable carcinogen with experimental tumorigenic data. When heated to decomposition it emits very toxic fumes of SO_x, Cl^-, Na_2O, and NO_x.

RDF000   CAS: 131-01-1
RESERPIDINE
mf: $C_{32}H_{38}N_2O_8$ mw: 578.72

SYNS: A-11025 ◇ CANESCINE ◇ 11-DEMETHOXYRESER-PINE ◇ DERESPERINE ◇ DESERPINE ◇ DESMETHOXYRES-

ERPINE ◇ 11-DESMETHOXYRESERPINE ◇ ENDURONYL ◇ HARMONYL ◇ LILLY 22641 ◇ RAUNORINE ◇ RECANES-CIN ◇ TRANQUINIL

TOXICITY DATA with REFERENCE
CAR: orl-rat TDLo: 54 mg/kg/77W-C   COREAF 254,1535,62
NEO: orl-wmn TDLo: 16 mg/kg/9Y-C   LANCAO 2,672,74

SAFETY PROFILE: Questionable human carcinogen producing skin tumors. Poison by intravenous and intraperitoneal routes. Moderately toxic by ingestion. Experimental reproductive effects. When heated to decomposition it emits toxic fumes of NO_x.

RDP300   CAS: 99-30-9
RESISAN
mf: $C_6H_4Cl_2N_2O_2$ mw: 207.02

SYNS: AL-50 ◇ ALLISAN ◇ BORTRAN ◇ BOTRAN ◇ CDNA ◇ CNA ◇ DCNA ◇ DCNA (fungicide) ◇ DICHLORAN ◇ DICHLORAN (amine fungicide) ◇ 2,6-DICHLOR-4-NITRO-ANILIN (CZECH) ◇ 2,6-DICHLORO-4-NITROANILINE ◇ 2,6-DICHLORO-4-NITROBENZENAMINE (9CI) ◇ DICLO-RAN ◇ DITRANIL ◇ 4-NITROANILINE, 2,6-DICHLORO- ◇ RD-6584 ◇ U-2069

TOXICITY DATA with REFERENCE
ETA: orl-mus TDLo: 80 g/kg/78W-I   NTIS** PB223-159
MUT: mmo-asn 14 μmol/L   PHYTAJ 66,217,76
MUT: sln-asn 38 μmol/L   EVHPAZ 31,81,79

CONSENSUS REPORTS: EPA Genetic Toxicology Program. Reported in EPA TSCA Inventory.

SAFETY PROFILE: Questionable carcinogen with experimental tumorigenic data. Poison by intravenous route. Moderately toxic by ingestion and possibly other routes. Mutation data reported. Used as a fungicide. When heated to decomposition it emits toxic fumes of Cl^- and NO_x.

REA000   CAS: 108-46-3
RESORCINOL
DOT: 2876
mf: $C_6H_6O_2$ mw: 110.12

PROP: Very white crystals, become pink on exposure to light when not perfectly pure; unpleasant sweet taste. Mp: 110°, bp: 280.5°, flash p: 261°F (CC), d: 1.285 @ 15°, autoign temp: 1126°F, vap press: 1 mm @ 108.4°, vap d:

3.79. Very sol in alc, ether, glycerol; sltly sol in chloroform; sol in water.

SYNS: m-BENZENEDIOL ◇ 1,3-BENZENEDIOL ◇ C.I. 76505 ◇ C.I. DEVELOPER 4 ◇ C.I. OXIDATION BASE 31 ◇ DEVELOPER R ◇ m-DIHYDROXYBENZENE ◇ 1,3-DIHYDROXYBENZENE ◇ m-DIOXYBENZENE ◇ DURAFUR DEVELOPER G ◇ FOURAMINE RS ◇ FOURRINE 79 ◇ m-HYDROQUINONE ◇ 3-HYDROXYCYCLOHEXADIEN-1-ONE ◇ m-HYDROXYPHENOL ◇ 3-HYDROXYPHENOL ◇ NAKO TGG ◇ NCI-C05970 ◇ PELAGOL GREY RS ◇ RCRA WASTE NUMBER U201 ◇ RESORCIN ◇ RESORCINE

TOXICITY DATA with REFERENCE
ETA: skn-mus TDLo:4800 mg/kg/12W-I
CNREA8 19,413,59
MUT: cyt-hmn:lym 80 mg/L ARZNAD 32,533,82
MUT: cyt-hmn:oth 40 mg/L ARZNAD 32,533,82
MUT: mma-sat 20 μmol/plate MUREAV 90,91,81
MUT: mrc-smc 1 g/L MUREAV 135,109,84

CONSENSUS REPORTS: IARC Cancer Review: Animal Inadequate Evidence IMEMDT 15,155,77. Reported in EPA TSCA Inventory. EPA Genetic Toxicology Program.

OSHA PEL: TWA 10 ppm; STEL 20 ppm ACGIH TLV: TWA 10 ppm; STEL 20 ppm DOT Classification: ORM-E; Label: None; Poison B; Label: St. Andrews Cross.

SAFETY PROFILE: Questionable carcinogen with experimental tumorigenic data. Human poison by ingestion. Experimental poison by ingestion, intraperitoneal, parenteral and subcutaneous routes. Moderately toxic experimentally by skin contact and intravenous routes. Human mutation data reported. A skin and severe eye irritant. Used as a topical antiseptic and keratolytic agent. Combustible when exposed to heat or flame; can react with oxidizing materials. To fight fire, use water, CO_2, dry chemical. When heated to decomposition it emits acrid smoke and irritating fumes.

RFK000   CAS: 875-22-9
RETRONECINE HYDROCHLORIDE
mf: $C_8H_{13}NO_2 \cdot ClH$ mw: 191.68

TOXICITY DATA with REFERENCE
ETA: scu-rat TDLo:600 mg/kg JNCIAM 49,665,72

SAFETY PROFILE: Questionable carcinogen with experimental tumorigenic data. Moderately toxic by intraperitoneal and subcutaneous routes. When heated to decomposition it emits very toxic fumes of NO_x and HCl.

RFP000   CAS: 480-54-6
RETRORSINE
mf: $C_{18}H_{25}NO_6$ mw: 351.44

SYNS: 12,18-DIHYDROXY-SENECIONAN-11,16-DIONE ◇ β-LONGILOBINE ◇ cis-RETRONECIC ACID ESTER of RETRONECINE

TOXICITY DATA with REFERENCE
NEO: orl-rat TDLo:560 mg/kg/62W-I BJCAAI 8,458,54
ETA: ipr-rat TDLo:150 mg/kg/22W-I BJCAAI 11,535,57
ETA: orl-rat TD:68 mg/kg/43W-I JNCIAM 47,1037,71
MUT: ctr-ham:kdy 25 μg/L CRNGDP 1,161,80
MUT: sln-dmg-par 10 mmol/L JOGNAU 59,273,66

CONSENSUS REPORTS: IARC Cancer Review: GROUP 3 IMEMDT 7,56,87; Animal Limited Evidence IMEMDT 10,303,76.

SAFETY PROFILE: Questionable carcinogen with experimental neoplastigenic and tumorigenic data. Poison by ingestion, intraperitoneal, intravenous, and possibly other routes. Mutation data reported. When heated to decomposition it emits toxic fumes of NO_x.

RFU000   CAS: 15503-86-3
RETRORSINE-N-OXIDE
mf: $C_{18}H_{25}NO_7$ mw: 367.44

SYNS: ISATIDINE ◇ cis-RETRONECIC ACID ESTER of RETRONECINE-N-OXIDE

TOXICITY DATA with REFERENCE
NEO: orl-rat TDLo:540 mg/kg/60W-I BJCAAI 8,458,54
ETA: mul-rat TDLo:440 mg/kg/64W-I BJCAAI 8,458,54
MUT: sln-dmg-par 10 mmol/L JOGNAU 59,273,66

CONSENSUS REPORTS: IARC Cancer Review: GROUP 3 IMEMDT 7,56,87; Animal Sufficient Evidence IMEMDT 10,269,76.

SAFETY PROFILE: Questionable carcinogen with experimental neoplastigenic and tumorigenic data. Poison by ingestion and intraperitoneal routes. Moderately toxic by intravenous route. Mutation data reported. When heated to decomposition it emits toxic fumes of NO_x.

RGA000   CAS: 84775-95-1
RHATHANI

PROP: Aqueous extract from the root of the plant (JNCIAM 52,1579,74).

SYN: KRAMERIA TRIANDRA

TOXICITY DATA with REFERENCE
NEO: scu-rat TDLo: 1058 mg/kg/49W-I
JNCIAM 52,1579,74

SAFETY PROFILE: Questionable carcinogen
with experimental neoplastigenic data. When
heated to decomposition it emits acrid smoke
and irritating fumes.

RGW000   CAS: 989-38-8
RHODAMINE 6G EXTRA BASE
mf: $C_{28}H_{30}N_2O_3 \cdot ClH$ mw: 479.06

SYNS: C.I. 45160 ◇ C.I. BASIC RED 1, MONOHYDRO-
CHLORIDE ◇ NCI-C56122 ◇ RHODAMINE 6G (biological stain)
◇ RHODAMINE 6GEX ETHYL ESTER

TOXICITY DATA with REFERENCE
ETA: scu-rat TDLo: 100 mg/kg/1Y-I   GANNA2
47,51,56
MUT: dnd-ham: ovr 90 μmol/L   CNREA8
39,4412,79
MUT: mma-sat 20 nmol/plate   CNREA8 39,4412,79

CONSENSUS REPORTS: IARC Cancer Review: GROUP 3 IMEMDT 7,56,87; Animal
Sufficient Evidence IMEMDT 16,233,78. Reported in EPA TSCA Inventory. Community
Right-To-Know List.

SAFETY PROFILE: Questionable carcinogen
with experimental tumorigenic data. Poison by
intraperitoneal route. Mutation data reported.
When heated to decomposition it emits very
toxic fumes of Cl^- and NO_x.

RHK000   CAS: 10049-07-7
RHODIUM(III) CHLORIDE (1:3)
mf: Cl_3Rh mw: 209.26

SYNS: RHODIUM CHLORIDE ◇ RHODIUM TRICHLORIDE

TOXICITY DATA with REFERENCE
CAR: orl-mus TDLo: 940 mg/kg/66W-C
JONUAI 101,1431,71
MUT: mrc-bcs 5 mmol/L   MUREAV 77,109,80

CONSENSUS REPORTS: Reported in EPA
TSCA Inventory. EPA Genetic Toxicology Program.

OSHA PEL: TWA 0.1 mg(Rh)/m^3 ACGIH
TLV: TWA 1 mg(Rh)/m^3

SAFETY PROFILE: Questionable carcinogen
with experimental carcinogenic data. Poison
by ingestion, intraperitoneal, and intravenous

routes. Experimental reproductive effects. Mutation data reported. When heated to decomposition it emits toxic fumes of Cl^-.

RJP000   CAS: 141-22-0
RICINOLEIC ACID
mf: $C_{18}H_{34}O_3$ mw: 298.52

PROP: Liquid. D: 0.940 @ 27.4°/4°, mp: 5.5°
bp: 245° @ 10 mm. Insol in water; misc in
alc, chloroform, ether.

SYNS: l'ACIDE RICINOLEIQUE (FRENCH) ◇ 12-HY-
DROXY-cis-9-OCTADECENOIC ACID ◇ RICINIC ACID
◇ RICINOLIC ACID

TOXICITY DATA with REFERENCE
ETA: scu-rbt TDLo: 390 mg/kg/17W-I   CRSBAW
137,760,43

CONSENSUS REPORTS: Reported in EPA
TSCA Inventory.

SAFETY PROFILE: Questionable carcinogen
with experimental tumorigenic data. When
heated to decomposition it emits acrid smoke
and irritating fumes.

RJZ000   CAS: 23246-96-0
RIDDELLINE
mf: $C_{18}H_{23}NO_6$ mw: 349.42

PROP: An alkaloid isolated from S. riddellii
(RETOAE 5,55,49).

TOXICITY DATA with REFERENCE
ETA: mul-rat TDLo: 210 mg/kg/52W-I   BJCAAI
11,535,57
MUT: dns-rat-orl 125 mg/kg   ENMUDM 7(Suppl
3),73,85
MUT: dns-rat: lvr 3200 μg/L   ENMUDM 5,482,83

CONSENSUS REPORTS: IARC Cancer Review: Animal Inadequate Evidence IMEMDT
10,313,76.

SAFETY PROFILE: Questionable carcinogen
with experimental tumorigenic data. Poison by
ingestion and intravenous routes. Mutation data
reported. When heated to decomposition it emits
toxic fumes of NO_x.

RNZ000   CAS: 83-79-4
ROTENONE
mf: $C_{23}H_{22}O_6$ mw: 394.45

PROP: Orthorhombic plates. Mp: 165-166° (di-
morphic form mp: 185-186°). D: 1.27 @ 20°.
Almost insol in water; sol in alc, acetone, carbon

tetrachloride, chloroform, ether and other organic solvents. Decomp on exposure to light and air.

SYNS: BARBASCO ◇ CENOL GARDEN DUST ◇ CHEM FISH ◇ CHEM-MITE ◇ CUBE ◇ CUBE EXTRACT ◇ CUBE-PULVER ◇ CUBE ROOT ◇ CUBOR ◇ CUREX FLEA DUSTER ◇ DACTINOL ◇ DERIL ◇ DERRIN ◇ DERRIS ◇ DRI-KIL ◇ ENT 133 ◇ EXTRAX ◇ FISH-TOX ◇ GREEN CROSS WARBLE POWDER ◇ HAIARI ◇ LIQUID DERRIS ◇ MEXIDE ◇ NCI-C55210 ◇ NICOULINE ◇ NOXFISH ◇ PARADERIL ◇ POWDER and ROOT ◇ PRENTOX ◇ RO-KO ◇ RONONE ◇ ROTEFIVE ◇ ROTEFOUR ◇ ROTENONA (SPANISH) ◇ ROTESSENOL ◇ ROTOCIDE ◇ TUBATOXIN

TOXICITY DATA with REFERENCE
NEO: ipr-rat TDLo:71 mg/kg/42D-I CNREA8 33,3047,73
ETA: ipr-rat TD:68 mg/kg/40D-I BJCAAI 36,243,77
ETA: orl-rat TDLo:3245 mg/kg/2Y-C NTPTR* NTP-TR-320,88
MUT: mnt-mus:oth 1 mg/L JNCIAM 56,357,76

OSHA PEL: TWA 5 mg/m^3 ACGIH TLV: TWA 5 mg/m^3 DFG MAK: 5 mg/m^3

SAFETY PROFILE: Questionable carcinogen with experimental neoplastigenic, tumorigenic, and teratogenic data. Human poison by ingestion and possibly other routes. Experimental poison by ingestion, intraperitoneal, and possibly other routes. Experimental reproductive effects. Mutation data reported. A skin and eye irritant. Acute poisoning causes numbness, nausea, vomiting, and tremors. Chronic exposure injures liver and kidneys. It is toxic to animals and very toxic to fish, but leaves no harmful residue on vegetable crops. When heated to decomposition it emits acrid smoke and irritating fumes. Used as an insecticide and as a fish poison.

RRA000   CAS: 23537-16-8
RUGULOSIN
mf: $C_{30}H_{20}O_{10}$ mw: 540.50

PROP: Anthraquinoid hepatotoxin of *Penicillium rugulosum Thom* (JJEMAG 41,177,71).

SYNS: RADICALISIN ◇ (+)-RUGULOSIN

TOXICITY DATA with REFERENCE
ETA: orl-mus TDLo:4400 mg/kg/1Y-C ARMIAZ 26,279,72
MUT: mma-sat 18 mg/L/7H JEPTDQ 2(2),313,78
MUT: mmo-sat 10 μg/7H JEPTDQ 2(2),313,78

MUT: mmo-smc 100 μmol/L CPBTAL 22,2258,74
MUT: mrc-bcs 20 μg/disc CNREA8 36,445,76

CONSENSUS REPORTS: IARC Cancer Review: Animal Inadequate Evidence IMEMDT 40,99,86. EPA Genetic Toxicology Program.

SAFETY PROFILE: Questionable carcinogen with experimental tumorigenic data. Poison by intraperitoneal route. Mutation data reported. When heated to decomposition it emits acrid smoke and irritating fumes.

RRK000
RUSSIAN COMFREY LEAVES

PROP: Fresh leaves dried, milled, and mixed with diet (JNCIAM 61,865,78).

SYNS: COMFREY, RUSSIAN ◇ SYMPHYTUM OFFICINALE L

TOXICITY DATA with REFERENCE
CAR: orl-rat TD:9900 g/kg/86W-C JJIND8 61(3),865,78
CAR: orl-rat TDLo:4800 g/kg/86W-C JJIND8 61(3),865,78

CONSENSUS REPORTS: IARC Cancer Review: Animal Limited Evidence IMEMDT 31,239,83

SAFETY PROFILE: Questionable carcinogen with experimental carcinogenic data. When heated to decomposition it emits acrid smoke and irritating fumes.

RSP000
RUTHENIUM SALT of
TETRAMETHYLPHENANTHRENE

TOXICITY DATA with REFERENCE
ETA: scu-mus TDLo:1000 mg/kg/I BECCAN 40,30,62

SAFETY PROFILE: Questionable carcinogen with experimental tumorigenic data. When heated to decomposition it emits very toxic fumes of NO_x and RuO_x.

RSU000   CAS: 153-18-4
RUTIN
mf: $C_{27}H_{30}O_{16}$ mw: 610.57

PROP: Pale yellow needles. Sol in pyridine, formamide and alkaline solutions; sltly sol in alc, acetone, ethyl acetate; insol in chloroform, carbon bisulfide, ether, benzene.

SYNS: BIOFLAVONOID ◊ BIRUTAN ◊ C.I. 75730
◊ ELDRIN ◊ GLOBULARIACITRIN ◊ ILIXATHIN
◊ MELIN ◊ MYRITICALORIN ◊ MYRITICOALORIN
◊ OSYRITRIN ◊ OXYRITIN ◊ PALIUROSIDE ◊ 3,3′,4′,5,7-
PENTAHYDROXYFLAVONE-3-(o-RHAMNOSYLGLUCO-
SIDE) ◊ 3,3′,4′,5,7-PENTAHYDROXYFLAVONE-3-RUTINO-
SIDE ◊ PHYTOMELIN ◊ QUERCETIN-3-(6-o-(6-DEOXY-α-l-
MANNOPYRANOSYL-β-d-GLUCOPYRANOSIDE) ◊ QUER-
CETIN RHAMNOGLUCOSIDE ◊ QUERCETIN-3-
RHAMNOGLUCOSINE ◊ QUERCETIN-3-(6-o-α-l-RHAMNO-
PYRANOSYL-β-d-GLUCOPYRANOSIDE) ◊ QUERCETIN-3-
RUTINOSIDE ◊ RUTINIC ACID ◊ RUTOSIDE ◊ SOPHORIN
◊ TANRUTIN ◊ USAF CF-5 ◊ VIOLAQUERCITRIN
◊ VITAMIN P

TOXICITY DATA with REFERENCE
NEO: orl-rat TDLo: 973 g/kg/3Y-C   PAACA3
25,95,84
MUT: dnr-esc 100 mg/L   FCTXAV 18,223,83
MUT: mma-sat 2 mg/plate   MUREAV 66,223,79
MUT: mma-sat 80 μg/plate   FCTOD7 23,669,85
MUT: slt-dmg-unr 71300 ppm/48H   MUREAV
120,233,83

CONSENSUS REPORTS: Reported in EPA
TSCA Inventory.

SAFETY PROFILE: Questionable carcinogen
with experimental neoplastigenic data. Poison
by intraperitoneal route. Moderately toxic by
intravenous route. Mutation data reported. Used
as a pharmaceutical and veterinary drug. When
heated to decomposition it emits acrid smoke
and irritating fumes.

SAF000   CAS: 89997-47-7
SAGRADO

SYNS: CHENOPODIUM AMBROSIOIDES ◊ JERUSALEM
OAK ◊ WORMWOOD PLANT

TOXICITY DATA with REFERENCE
NEO: scu-rat TDLo: 2320 mg/kg/58W-I
JNCIAM 60,683,78

SAFETY PROFILE: Questionable carcinogen
with experimental neoplastigenic data. When
heated to decomposition it emits acrid smoke
and irritating fumes.

SAF500   CAS: 81295-38-7
SALI

PROP: Aqueous extract from the dried leaves
of the plant *Heliotropium ternatum* (JNCIAM
46,1131,71).

SYNS: HELIOTROPIUM TERNATUM ◊ H. TERNATUM

TOXICITY DATA with REFERENCE
ETA: orl-ham TDLo: 56 g/kg/70W-I   JNCIAM
53,1259,74
ETA: scu-rat TDLo: 300 g/kg/1Y-I   JNCIAM
46,1131,71

SAFETY PROFILE: Questionable carcinogen
with experimental tumorigenic data. When
heated to decomposition it emits acrid smoke
and irritating fumes.

SAX000   CAS: 8013-77-2
SARAN
mf: $(C_4H_5Cl_3)_n$

TOXICITY DATA with REFERENCE
ETA: imp-rat TDLo: 36 mg/kg   CNREA8 15,333,55

SAFETY PROFILE: Questionable carcinogen
with experimental tumorigenic by implant data.
When heated to decomposition it emits toxic
fumes of Cl^-.

SAX200   CAS: 13045-94-8
d-SARCOLYSINE
mf: $C_{13}H_{18}Cl_2N_2O_2$ mw: 305.23

SYNS: 4-(BIS(2-CHLOROETHYL)AMINO)-d-PHENYLALA-
NINE ◊ (+)-3-(p-(BIS(2-CHLOROETHYL)AMINO)PHENYL)
ALANINE ◊ d-3-(p-(BIS(2-CHLOROETHYL)AMINO)PHENY-
L)ALANINE ◊ 3026 C.B. ◊ CB-3026 ◊ p-DI-(2-CHLOROE-
THYL)-AMINO-d-PHENYLALANINE ◊ p-DI(2-CHLOROE-
THYL)AMINO-d-PHENYLALANINE ◊ MEDFALAN
◊ MEDPHALAN ◊ NSC-35051 ◊ d-PHENYLALANINE MUS-
TARD

TOXICITY DATA with REFERENCE
ETA: skn-mus TDLo: 120 mg/kg/9W-I   BJCAAI
10,363,56
MUT: cyt-dmg-par 10 mmol/L   JOGNAU
54,146,56
MUT: sln-dmg-par 8 mmol/L   GENRA8 1,173,60

CONSENSUS REPORTS: EPA Genetic Toxicology Program.

SAFETY PROFILE: Questionable carcinogen
with experimental tumorigenic data. A deadly
poison by intracerebral route. Mutation data reported. When heated to decomposition it emits
toxic fumes of Cl^- and NO_x.

SAX500   CAS: 11031-48-4
SARKOMYCIN
mf: $C_7H_8O_3$ mw: 140.15

PROP: Oily liquid. Sol in water, methanol, ethanol, butanol, ethyl acetate; sltly sol in ether. Isolated from *Streptomyces sp.* (ANTCAO 4,514,54).

SYNS: 2-METHYLENE-3-OXO-CYCLOPENTANECAR-BOXYLIC ACID ◇ SARCOMYCIN

TOXICITY DATA with REFERENCE
ETA: scu-rat TDLo: 8220 μg/kg/21W-I   JAJAAA
8,168,55
MUT: dni-eug 10 μg/L   NEOLA4 19,579,72
MUT: mmo-eug 10 μg/L   NEOLA4 19,579,72

SAFETY PROFILE: Questionable carcinogen with experimental tumorigenic and teratogenic data. Moderately toxic by intravenous, subcutaneous, and intraperitoneal routes. Mildly toxic by ingestion. Experimental reproductive effects. Mutation data reported. Used as an antibiotic. When heated to decomposition it emits acrid smoke and irritating fumes.

SAY900
SASSAFRAS

PROP: A yellowish-reddish, volatile oil; pungent, aromatic odor and taste. D: 1.065-1.077 @ 25°/25°. Sol in alc, ether, chloroform, glacial acetic acid, CS_2. Safrole-free ethanol extract of *Sassafras albidum* root bark (JNCIAM 60,683,78).

SYN: SASSAFRAS ALBIDUM

TOXICITY DATA with REFERENCE
NEO: scu-rat TDLo: 3540 mg/kg/59W-I

JNCIAM 60,683,78

SAFETY PROFILE: Questionable carcinogen with experimental neoplastigenic data. A skin irritant. When heated to decomposition it emits acrid smoke and irritating fumes.

SBC500
SCARLET RED

CAS: 85-83-6

mf: $C_{24}H_{20}N_4O$ mw: 380.48

SYNS: BRASILAZINA OIL RED B ◇ CALCO OIL RED D ◇ C.I. 258 ◇ C.I. SOLVENT RED 24 ◇ 2',3-DIMETHYL-4-(2-HYDROXYNAPHTHYLAZO)AZOBENZENE ◇ FAST OIL RED B ◇ FAT RED B ◇ 1-((2-METHYL-4-((2-METHYLPHENYL)AZO)PHENYL)AZO)-2-NAPHTHALENOL ◇ PHENOPLASTE ORGANOL RED B ◇ RUBRUM SCARLATINUM ◇ 1-((4-(o-TOLYLAZO)-o-TOLYL)AZO)-2-NAPHTHOL) ◇ o-TOLUEN-EAZO-o-TOLUENEAZO-β-NAPHTHOL ◇ o-TOLUENEAZO-o-TOLUENE-β-NAPHTHOL ◇ o-TOLYLAZO-o-TOLYLAZO-β-NAPHTHOL ◇ o-TOLYLAZO-o-TOLYLAZO-2-NAPHTHOL

TOXICITY DATA with REFERENCE
ETA: scu-rat TDLo: 512 mg/kg/58W-C

GANNA2 49,27,58
MUT: mma-sat 100 μg/plate   MUREAV
56,249,78

CONSENSUS REPORTS: IARC Cancer Review: GROUP 3 IMEMDT 7,56,87. Reported in EPA TSCA Inventory.

SAFETY PROFILE: Questionable carcinogen with experimental tumorigenic data. Mutation data reported. When heated to decomposition it emits toxic fumes of NO_x.

SBO500
SELENIUM

CAS: 7782-49-2

DOT: 2658
af: Se   aw: 78.96

PROP: Steel gray, nonmetallic element. Mp: 170-217°, bp: 690°, d: 4.81-4.26, vap press: 1 mm @ 356°. Insol in water and alc; very sltly sol in ether.

SYNS: C.I. 77805 ◇ COLLOIDAL SELENIUM ◇ ELEMENTAL SELENIUM ◇ SELEN (POLISH) ◇ SELENIUM ALLOY ◇ SELENIUM BASE ◇ SELENIUM DUST ◇ SELENIUM ELEMENTAL ◇ SELENIUM HOMOPOLYMER ◇ SELENIUM METAL POWDER, NON-PYROPHORIC (DOT) ◇ VANDEX

TOXICITY DATA with REFERENCE
ETA: orl-mus TDLo: 480 mg/kg/60D-C

YMBUA7 11,368,60

CONSENSUS REPORTS: IARC Cancer Review: GROUP 3 IMEMDT 7,56,87. Selenium and its compounds are on the Community Right-To-Know List. Reported in EPA TSCA Inventory.

OSHA PEL: TWA 0.2 mg(Se)/m^3 ACGIH TLV: TWA 0.2 mg(Se)/m^3 DFG MAK: 0.1 mg/m^3 DOT Classification: Poison B; Label: St. Andrews Cross.

SAFETY PROFILE: Questionable carcinogen with experimental tumorigenic and teratogenic data. Poison by inhalation, intravenous, and possibly other routes. Experimental reproductive effects. Occupational exposure has caused pallor, nervousness, depression, garlic odor of breath and sweat, gastrointestinal disturbances and dermatitis. Selenosis in humans has occurred from ingestion of 3.2 mg selenium per day. Selenium is an essential trace element for many species. When heated to decomposition it emits toxic fumes of Se.

SBP900   CAS: 5456-28-0
SELENIUM DIETHYLDITHIOCARBAMATE
mf: $C_{20}H_{40}N_4S_8 \cdot Se$ mw: 672.08

SYNS: ETHYL SELENAC ◇ ETHYL SELERAM ◇ TETRAKIS(DIETHYLCARBAMODITHIOATO-S,S') SELENIUM ◇ TETRAKIS(DIETHYLDITHIOCARBAMATO) SELENIUM

TOXICITY DATA with REFERENCE
CAR: orl-mus TDLo: 3060 mg/kg/81W-I
   JNCIAM 42,1101,69

CONSENSUS REPORTS: IARC Cancer Review: Animal Inadequate Evidence IMEMDT 9,245,75; IMEMDT 12,107,76; GROUP 3 IMEMDT 7,56,87

OSHA PEL: TWA 0.2 mg(Se)/m^3 ACGIH TLV: TWA 0.2 mg(Se)/m^3

SAFETY PROFILE: Questionable carcinogen with experimental carcinogenic data. When heated to decomposition it emits toxic fumes of NO$_x$ ans Se.

SBW500   CAS: 563-41-7
SEMICARBAZIDE HYDROCHLORIDE
mf: $CH_5N_3O \cdot ClH$ mw: 111.55

PROP: Prisms from dilute alc. Decomp @ 175-185°, mp: 176° (decomp). Very sol in water; very sltly sol in hot alc; insol in anhydrous ether.

SYNS: AMIDOUREA HYDROCHLORIDE ◇ AMINOUREA HYDROCHLORIDE ◇ CARBAMYLHYDRAZINE HYDRO-CHLORIDE ◇ CH ◇ HYDRAZINECARBOXAMIDE MONOHY-DROCHLORIDE

TOXICITY DATA with REFERENCE
NEO: orl-mus TDLo: 67 g/kg/76W-C   EJCAAH
   11,17,75

CONSENSUS REPORTS: IARC Cancer Review: GROUP 3 IMEMDT 7,56,87; Animal Sufficient Evidence IMEMDT 12,209,76. Reported in EPA TSCA Inventory. EPA Extremely Hazardous Substances List.

SAFETY PROFILE: Questionable carcinogen with experimental neoplastigenic and teratogenic data. Poison by ingestion. Experimental

reproductive effects. When heated to decomposition it emits very toxic fumes of NO$_x$ and HCl.

SBW950
SENECIO CANNABIFOLIUS, leaves and stalks

PROP: Herb of the family SENECIONEAE
CALEDQ 20,191,83
CAR: orl-rat TD: 240 g/kg/69W-C   CALEDQ
   20,191,83

SAFETY PROFILE: Questionable carcinogen with experimental carcinogenic data. When heated to decomposition it emits acrid smoke and irritating fumes.

SBX000
SENECIO LONGILOBUS

PROP: Contains pyrrolizidine alkaloids (CNREA8 28,2237,68).

TOXICITY DATA with REFERENCE
ETA: orl-rat TDLo: 33 g/kg/31W-I   CNREA8
   30,2881,70

SAFETY PROFILE: Questionable carcinogen with experimental tumorigenic data. When heated to decomposition it emits toxic fumes of NO$_x$.

SBX200
SENECIO NEMORENSIS FUCHSII, alkaloidal extract

PROP: Alkaloidal extract contains the two pyrrolizidine alkaloids fuchsisenecionine and senecionine (ARZNAD 32,144,82).

TOXICITY DATA with REFERENCE
CAR: orl-rat TD: 20800 mg/kg/2Y-I   ARZNAD
   32,144,82
CAR: orl-rat TDLo: 4160 mg/kg/2Y-I   ARZNAD
   32,144,82
MUT: msc-ham: lng 156 mg/L   ARZNAD 32,144,82

SAFETY PROFILE: Questionable carcinogen with experimental carcinogenic data. Mutation data reported.

SBX500   CAS: 480-81-9
SENECIPHYLLINE
mf: $C_{18}H_{23}NO_5$ mw: 333.42

PROP: Small, rhombic platelets from hot alcohol or acetone. Mp: 217-218°. Easily sol in chloroform, ethylene chloride; less sol in alc, acetone; difficultly sol in ether, ligroin. An alkaloid isolated from *S. stenocephalus* (RETOAE 5,55,49).

SYNS: 13,19-DIDEHYDRO-12-HYDROXY-SENECIONAN-11,16-DIONE ◇ JACOBINE ◇ SENECIPHYLLIN

TOXICITY DATA with REFERENCE
MUT: dns-ham:lvr 1 μmol/L   CNREA8 45,3125,85
MUT: dns-mus:lvr 1 μmol/L   CNREA8 45,3125,85
MUT: dns-rat:lvr 1 μmol/L   CNREA8 45,3125,85
MUT: sce-ham:lng 60 μg/L   MUREAV 142,209,85
MUT: sln-dmg-orl 10 μmol/L/3D-I   FCTOD7 22,223,84

CONSENSUS REPORTS: IARC Cancer Review: GROUP 3 IMEMDT 7,56,87; Animal Inadequate Evidence IMEMDT 10,319,76

SAFETY PROFILE: Questionable carcinogen. Mutation data reported. When heated to decomposition it emits toxic fumes of NO_x.

SCB000   CAS: 8008-74-0
SESAME OIL

PROP: Flash p: 491°F, d: 0.9. From seed of *Sesamum indicum* (85DIA2 2,290,77).

SYNS: GINGILLI OIL ◇ SEXTRA

TOXICITY DATA with REFERENCE
CAR: scu-mus TDLo: 2000 mg/kg/W-I   AVBIB9 22/23,359,79
ETA: scu-mus TD: 2000 mg/kg/W-I   FEPRA7 38,1450,79

CONSENSUS REPORTS: Reported in EPA TSCA Inventory.

SAFETY PROFILE: Questionable carcinogen with experimental carcinogenic and tumorigenic data. Poison by intravenous route. A human skin irritant. Combustible when exposed to heat or flame. To fight fire, use CO_2, dry chemical. Used in cosmetics, lotions, injectables, and flavorants. When heated to decomposition it emits acrid smoke and irritating fumes.

SCE000   CAS: 138-59-0
SHIKIMIC ACID
mf: $C_7H_{10}O_5$ mw: 174.17

PROP: Isolated from Bracken (NATUAS 250,348,74).

SYNS: BRACKEN FERN TOXIC COMPONENT ◇ SHIKIMATE ◇ 3,4,5-TRIHYDROXY-1-CYCLOHEXENE-1-CARBOXYLIC ACID

TOXICITY DATA with REFERENCE
ETA: ipr-mus TDLo: 40 mg/kg   NATUAS 250,348,74
ETA: orl-mus TDLo: 4000 mg/kg   NATUAS 250,348,74
MUT: dlt-mus-ipr 1000 mg/kg   BJLSAF 73,105,76
MUT: dlt-mus-orl 3200 mg/kg   NATUAS250,348,74
MUT: otr-ham:kdy 250 mg/L   TOLED5 19,43,83

CONSENSUS REPORTS: IARC Cancer Review: Animal Inadequate Evidence IMEMDT 40,47,86. EPA Genetic Toxicology Program.

SAFETY PROFILE: Questionable carcinogen with experimental tumorigenic data. Moderately toxic by intraperitoneal route. Mutation data reported. When heated to decomposition it emits acrid smoke and irritating fumes.

SCF000
SHINING SUMAC

PROP: Hot water extract of shining sumac root (JNCIAM 60,683,78).

SYN: RHUS COPALLINA

TOXICITY DATA with REFERENCE
NEO: scu-rat TDLo: 3900 mg/kg/65W-I   JNCIAM 60,683,78

SAFETY PROFILE: Questionable carcinogen with experimental neoplastigenic data. When heated to decomposition it emits acrid smoke and irritating fumes.

SCF025
cis-SHP
mf: $C_6H_{17}N_2O_5Pt$ mw: 392.34

SYN: cis-SULFATO-1,2-DIAMINOCYCLOHEXANEPLATINUM(II)

TOXICITY DATA with REFERENCE
NEO: ipr-mus TD: 11651 μg/kg/10W-I   CNREA8 41,4368,81
NEO: ipr-mus TD: 42368 μg/kg/10W-I   CNREA8 41,4368,81
NEO: ipr-mus TDLo: 10590 μg/kg/10W-I   CNREA8 41,4368,81
MUT: dnd-sat 10 mg/L/20H-C   CNREA841,4368,81
MUT: mmo-sat 20 nmol/plate   CNREA8 41,4368,81
MUT: oms-bcs 1600 nmol/L/3H-C   CNREA8 41,4368,81

SAFETY PROFILE: Questionable carcinogen with experimental neoplastigenic data. Mutation data reported. When heated to decomposition it emits toxic fumes of NO_x.

SCF050
trans(−)-SHP
mf: $C_6H_{17}N_2O_5Pt$ mw: 392.34

SYN: trans(−)-SULFATO-1,2-DIAMINOCYCLOHEXANE-PLATINUM(II)

TOXICITY DATA with REFERENCE
NEO: ipr-mus TD: 11651 μg/kg/10W-I   CNREA8
  41,4368,81
NEO: ipr-mus TDLo: 10590 μg/kg/10W-I
  CNREA8 41,4368,81
ETA: ipr-mus TD: 42368 μg/kg/10W-I   CNREA8
  41,4368,81
MUT: dnd-sat 10 mg/L/20H-C   CNREA8
  41,4368,81
MUT: mmo-sat 20 nmol/plate   CNREA8 41,4368,81
MUT: oms-bcs 1100 nmol/L/3H-C   CNREA8
  41,4368,81

SAFETY PROFILE: Questionable carcinogen with experimental neoplastigenic data. Mutation data reported. When heated to decomposition it emits toxic fumes of NO_x.

SCF075
trans(+)-SHP
mf: $C_6H_{17}N_2O_5Pt$ mw: 392.34

SYN: trans(+)-SULFATO-1,2-DIAMINOCYCLOHEXANE-PLATINUM(II)

TOXICITY DATA with REFERENCE
NEO: ipr-mus TD: 11651 μg/kg/10W-I   CNREA8
  41,4368,81
NEO: ipr-mus TD: 42368 μg/kg/10W-I   CNREA8
  41,4368,81
NEO: ipr-mus TDLo: 10590 μg/kg/10W-I
  CNREA8 41,4368,81
MUT: dnd-sat 10 mg/L/20H-C   CNREA8
  41,4368,81
MUT: mmo-sat 20 nmol/plate   CNREA8 41,4368,81
MUT: oms-bcs 1600 nmol/L/3H-C   CNREA8
  41,4368,81

SAFETY PROFILE: Questionable carcinogen with experimental neoplastigenic data. Mutation data reported. When heated to decomposition it emits toxic fumes of NO_x.

SCH000   CAS: 7631-86-9
SILICA, AMORPHOUS FUMED
mf: O_2Si mw: 60.09

PROP: A finely powdered microcellular silica foam with minimum SiO_2 content of 89.5%. Insol in water; sol in hydrofluoric acid.

SYNS: ACTICEL ◇ AEROSIL ◇ AMORPHOUS SILICA DUST ◇ AQUAFIL ◇ CAB-O-GRIP II ◇ CAB-O-SIL ◇ CAB-O-SPERSE ◇ CATALOID ◇ COLLOIDAL SILICA ◇ COLLOIDAL SILICON DIOXIDE ◇ DAVISON SG-67 ◇ DICALITE ◇ DRI-DIE INSECTICIDE 67 ◇ ENT 25,550 ◇ FLO-GARD ◇ FOSSIL FLOUR ◇ FUMED SILICA ◇ FUMED SILICON DIOXIDE ◇ HI-SEL ◇ LO-VEL ◇ LUDOX ◇ NALCOAG ◇ NYACOL ◇ NYACOL 830 ◇ NYACOL 1430 ◇ SANTOCEL ◇ SG-67 ◇ SILICA AEROGEL ◇ SILICA, AMORPHOUS ◇ SILICIC ANHYDRIDE ◇ SILICON DIOXIDE (FCC) ◇ SILIKILL ◇ SYNTHETIC AMORPHOUS SILICA ◇ VULKASIL

TOXICITY DATA with REFERENCE
CAR: ihl-rat TCLo: 50 mg/m^3/6H/2Y-I   CNREA8
  2,255,86
MUT: bfa-rat: lng 120 mg/kg   ENVRAL
  41,61,86
MUT: dns-rat-itr 120 mg/kg   ENVRAL 41,61,86

CONSENSUS REPORTS: IARC Cancer Review: GROUP 3 IMEMDT 7,341,87; Animal Inadequate Evidence IMEMDT 42,209,88; Human Inadequate Evidence IMEMDT 42,209,88. Reported in EPA TSCA Inventory.

OSHA PEL: (Transitional: TWA 80 mg/m^3/%SiO$_2$) TWA 6 mg/m^3 ACGIH TLV: (Proposed TWA 2 mg/m^3 (Respirable Dust))

SAFETY PROFILE: Questionable carcinogen with experimental carcinogenic data. Poison by intraperitoneal, intravenous, and intratracheal routes. Moderately toxic by ingestion. Much less toxic than crystalline forms. Mutation data reported. Does not cause silicosis. See also other silica entries.

SCL000   CAS: 7699-41-4
SILICA, GEL and AMORPHOUS-PRECIPITATED
mf: H_2O_3Si mw: 78.11

SYNS: KIESELSAURE (GERMAN) ◇ METASILICIC ACID ◇ PRECIPITATED SILICA ◇ SILICA GEL ◇ SILICIC ACID

CONSENSUS REPORTS: IARC Cancer Review: Animal Inadequate Evidence IMEMDT 42,39,87; Human Inadequate Evidence IMEMDT 42,39,87. Reported in EPA TSCA Inventory.

OSHA PEL: (Transitional: TWA 80 mg/m^3/%SiO$_2$) TWA 6 mg/m^3 ACGIH TLV: TWA (nuisance particulate) 10 mg/m^3 of total dust (when toxic impurities are not present, e.g., quartz < 1%).

SAFETY PROFILE: Questionable carcinogen. Poison by intravenous route. An eye irritant and nuisance dust.

SCQ000   CAS: 409-21-2
SILICON CARBIDE
mf: CSi   mw: 40.10

PROP: Bluish-black, iridescent crystals. Mp: 2600°, bp: subl > 2000°, decomp @ 2210°, d: 3.17.

SYNS: CARBOLON ◇ CARBON SILICIDE ◇ CARBORUNDEUM ◇ CARBORUNDUM ◇ KZ 3M ◇ KZ 5M ◇ KZ 7M ◇ SILICON MONOCARBIDE ◇ SILUNDUM

TOXICITY DATA with REFERENCE
NEO: imp-rat TDLo: 200 mg/kg   JJIND8 67,965,81

CONSENSUS REPORTS: Reported in EPA TSCA Inventory.

OSHA PEL: (Transitional: TWA Total Dust: 15 mg/m^3; Respirable Fraction: 5 mg/m^3) TWA Total Dust: 10 mg/m^3; Respirable Fraction: 5 mg/m^3 ACGIH TLV: TWA (nuisance particulate) 10 mg/m^3 of total dust (when toxic impurities are not present, e.g., quartz < 1%).   DFG MAK: 4 mg/m^{3}0

SAFETY PROFILE: Questionable carcinogen with experimental neoplastigenic data.

SDI000
SILK

TOXICITY DATA with REFERENCE
ETA: imp-rat TDLo: 36 mg/kg   CNREA8 15,333,55

SAFETY PROFILE: Questionable carcinogen with experimental tumorigenic data by implant. In the form of dust it is an allergen and a nuisance dust. Flammable when exposed to heat or flame. A moderate explosion hazard. When heated to decomposition it emits acrid smoke and irritating fumes.

SDI500   CAS: 7440-22-4
SILVER
af: Ag   aw: 107.868

PROP: Soft, ductile, malleable, lustrous, white metal. Mp: 961.93°, bp: 2212°, d: 10.50 @ 20°.

SYNS: ARGENTUM ◇ C.I. 77820 ◇ SHELL SILVER ◇ SILBER (GERMAN) ◇ SILVER ATOM

TOXICITY DATA with REFERENCE
ETA: imp-mus TDLo: 11 g/kg   NATWAY 42,75,55
ETA: imp-rat TD: 2570 mg/kg   NATWAY 42,75,55

ETA: imp-rat TDLo: 2400 mg/kg   CNREA8 16,439,56
ETA: mul-rat TDLo: 330 mg/kg/43W-I   ZEKBAI 63,586,60

CONSENSUS REPORTS: Silver and its compounds are on the Community Right-To-Know List. Reported in EPA TSCA Inventory.

OSHA PEL: Metal, Dust, and Fume: TWA 0.01 mg/m^3 ACGIH TLV: TWA (metal) 0.1 mg/m^3, (soluble compounds as Ag) 0.01 mg/m^3 DFG MAK: 0.01 mg/m^3

SAFETY PROFILE: Questionable carcinogen with experimental tumorigenic data. Human systemic effects by inhalation: skin effects. Inhalation of dusts can cause argyrosis. Flammable in the form of dust when exposed to flame or by chemical reaction.

SDS000   CAS: 7761-88-8
SILVER(I) NITRATE (1:1)
DOT: 1493
mf: NO$_3$•Ag   mw: 169.88

PROP: Mp: 212°, bp: 444° (decomp), d: 4.352 @ 19°. Very sol in ammonia, water; sltly sol in ether.

SYNS: LUNAR CAUSTIC ◇ NITRATE d'ARGENT (FRENCH) ◇ NITRIC ACID, SILVER(1+) SALT ◇ SILBERNITRAT ◇ SILVER(1+) NITRATE ◇ SILVER NITRATE (DOT)

TOXICITY DATA with REFERENCE
ETA: skn-mus TDLo: 15 g/kg/19W-I   NCIMAV 10,489,63
MUT: dnd-ham: emb 60 μmol/L   CNREA8 39,193,79
MUT: dni-hmn: lym 76 μmol/L   IAAAAM 79,83,86
MUT: dni-mus-ipr 20 g/kg   ARGEAR 51,605,81
MUT: otr-ham: emb 60 μmol/L   CNREA8 39,193,79
MUT: sln-smc 140 ppb   ANYAA9 407,186,83

CONSENSUS REPORTS: Silver and its compounds are on the Community Right-To-Know List. EPA Genetic Toxicology Program. Reported in EPA TSCA Inventory.

OSHA PEL: TWA 0.01 mg(Ag)/m^3 ACGIH TLV: TWA 0.01 mg(Ag)/m^3 DOT Classification: Oxidizer; Label: Oxidizer.

SAFETY PROFILE: Questionable carcinogen with experimental tumorigenic data. Human poison by an unspecified route. Experiemental poison by ingestion, intravenous, subcutaneous, and intraperitoneal routes. Experimental reproductive effects. Human mutation data reported.

A severe eye irritant. A powerful caustic and irritant to skin, eyes, and mucous membranes. Swallowing can cause severe gastroenteritis that may be fatal. A powerful oxidizer. When heated to decomposition it emits toxic fumes of NO_x.

SFA000   CAS: 26628-22-8
SODIUM AZIDE
DOT: 1687
mf: N_3Na mw: 65.02

PROP: Colorless, hexagonal crystals. Mp: decomp, d: 1.846. Insol in ether; sol in liquid ammonia.

SYNS: AZIDE ◇ AZIUM ◇ AZOTURE de SODIUM (FRENCH) ◇ KAZOE ◇ NATRIUMAZID (GERMAN) ◇ NATRIUMMAZIDE (DUTCH) ◇ NCI-C06462 ◇ NSC 3072 ◇ RCA WASTE NUMBER P105 ◇ SODIUM, AZOTURE de (FRENCH) ◇ SODIUM, AZOTURO di (ITALIAN) ◇ U-3886

TOXICITY DATA with REFERENCE
ETA: orl-rat TD: 5460 mg/kg/78W-C   JJIND8 67,75,81
ETA: orl-rat TDLo: 2730 mg/kg/78W-C   JJIND8 67,75,81
MUT: dni-hmn: fbr 50 mg/L   STBIBN 78,165,80
MUT: dnr-esc 5 g/L   MUREAV 119,135,83
MUT: mma-esc 33300 ng/plate   ENMUDM 6(Suppl 2),1,84
MUT: mmo-esc 150 nmol/L   ENMUDM 3,11,81
MUT: mmo-omi 600 ppm   POASAD 34,114,53
MUT: mmo-sat 10 μg/plate   MUREAV 144,231,85
MUT: msc-rat: lvr 1 mmol/L   MUREAV 77,293,80

CONSENSUS REPORTS: Reported in EPA TSCA Inventory. EPA Genetic Toxicology Program. EPA Extremely Hazardous Substances List.

OSHA PEL: As NH_3: CL 0.1 ppm; As NaN_3: Cl 0.3 mg/m³ (skin)   ACGIH TLV: CL 0.3 mg/m³   DFG MAK: 0.07 ppm (0.2 mg/m³)   DOT Classification: Poison B; Label: Poison

SAFETY PROFILE: Questionable carcinogen with experimental tumorigenic data. Poison by ingestion, skin contact, intraperitoneal, intravenous, subcutaneous and possibly other routes. Human systemic effects by ingestion: general anesthesia, somnolence, and kidney changes. Human mutation data reported. An unstable explosive sensitive to impact. When heated to decomposition it emits very toxic fumes of NO_x and Na_2O.

SFO500   CAS: 9004-32-4
SODIUM CARBOXYMETHYL
CELLULOSE

PROP: A synthetic cellulose gum (the sodium salt of carboxy methyl cellulose not less than 99.5% on a dry weight basis, with maximum substitution of 0.95 carboxymethyl groups per anhydroglucose unit, and with a minimum viscosity of 25 centipoises for 2% weight aqueous solutions at 25°). Colorless, odorless, hygroscopic powder or granules. Insol in most organic solvents.

SYNS: AC-DI-SOL NF ◇ AQUAPLAST ◇ B10 ◇ BLANOSE BWM ◇ B 10 (polysaccharide) ◇ CARBOXYMETHYL CELLULOSE ◇ CARBOXYMETHYL CELLULOSE, SODIUM ◇ CARBOXYMETHYL CELLULOSE, SODIUM SALT ◇ CARMETHOSE ◇ CELLOFAS ◇ CELLOGEL C ◇ CELLPRO ◇ CELLUFIX FF 100 ◇ CELLUGEL ◇ CELLULOSE GLYCOLIC ACID, SODIUM SALT ◇ CELLULOSE GUM ◇ CELLULOSE SODIUM GLYCOLATE ◇ CMC ◇ CM-CELLULOSE Na SALT ◇ CMC 7H ◇ CMC SODIUM SALT ◇ COLLOWELL ◇ COPAGEL PB 25 ◇ COURLOSE A 590 ◇ DAICEL 1150 ◇ FINE GUM HES ◇ GLIKOCEL TA ◇ KMTS 212 ◇ LOVOSA ◇ LUCEL (polysaccharide) ◇ MAJOL PLX ◇ MODOCOLL 1200 ◇ NACM-CELLULOSE SALT ◇ NYMCEL S ◇ POLYFIBRON 120 ◇ SANLOSE SN 20A ◇ SARCELL TEL ◇ S 75M ◇ SODIUM CELLULOSE GLYCOLATE ◇ SODIUM CMC ◇ SODIUM CM-CELLULOSE ◇ SODIUM SALT of CARBOXYMETHYLCELLULOSE ◇ TYLOSE 666 ◇ UNISOL RH

TOXICITY DATA with REFERENCE
NEO: scu-rat TD: 33 g/kg/22W-I   PAACA3 18,225,77
NEO: scu-rat TD: 8600 mg/kg/19W-I   13BYAH -,83,62
NEO: scu-rat TDLo: 1900 mg/kg/19W-I   13BYAH -,83,62

CONSENSUS REPORTS: Reported in EPA TSCA Inventory.

SAFETY PROFILE: Questionable carcinogen with experimental neoplastigenic data. Mildly toxic by ingestion. Experimental reproductive effects. It migrates to food from packaging materials. When heated to decomposition it emits toxic fumes of Na_2O.

SFQ000   CAS: 9005-46-3
SODIUM CASEINATE

PROP: Coarse, white powder; odorless. Insol in water, alc.

SYNS: CASEIN and CASEINATE SALTS (FCC) ◇ CASEIN-SODIUM ◇ CASEIN, SODIUM COMPLEX ◇ CASEINS, SODIUM COMPLEXES ◇ NUTROSE

TOXICITY DATA with REFERENCE
ETA: scu-mus TDLo:45 g/kg/15D-I   JNCIAM 57,1367,76

CONSENSUS REPORTS: Reported in EPA TSCA Inventory.

SAFETY PROFILE: Questionable carcinogen with experimental tumorigenic data. When heated to decomposition it emits toxic fumes of Na_2O.

SFT500   CAS: 7758-19-2
SODIUM CHLORITE
DOT: 1496
mf: $ClNaO_2$ mw: 90.44

PROP: White crystals or crystalline powder. Bp: decomp @ 180-200°.

SYN: TEXTILE

TOXICITY DATA with REFERENCE
CAR: orl-mus TDLo:29750 mg/kg/85W-C
   EVHPAZ 69,221,86
MUT: cyt-ham:fbr 20 mg/L   FCTOD7 22,623,84
MUT: mma-sat 300 μg/plate   FCTOD7 22,623,84

CONSENSUS REPORTS: Reported in EPA TSCA Inventory.

DOT Classification: Oxidizer; Label: Oxidizer

SAFETY PROFILE: Questionable carcinogen with experimental carcinogenic data. Poison by ingestion. An experimental teratogen. Experimental reproductive effects. Mutation data reported. May act as an irritant due to its oxidizing power. A powerful oxidizing agent; ignited by friction, heat or shock. When heated to decomposition it emits highly toxic fumes of Cl^- and Na_2O. Used as a bleaching agent.

SGC000   CAS: 139-05-9
SODIUM CYCLAMATE
mf: $C_6H_{12}NO_3S•Na$ mw: 201.24

PROP: White, crystalline powder; practically odorless. Sol in water. Almost insol in alc, benzene, chloroform, ether.

SYNS: ASSUGRIN ◇ ASSUGRIN FEINUSS ◇ ASSUGRIN VOLLSUSS ◇ ASUGRYN ◇ CYCLAMATE ◇ CYCLAMATE SODIUM ◇ CYCLAMIC ACID SODIUM SALT ◇ CYCLOHEXANESULFAMIC ACID, MONOSODIUM SALT ◇ CYCLO-HEXANESULPHAMIC ACID, MONOSODIUM SALT ◇ CYCLOHEXYL SULPHAMATE SODIUM ◇ DULZOR-ETAS ◇ HACHI-SUGAR ◇ IBIOSUC ◇ NATREEN ◇ NATRIUMZYKLAMATE (GERMAN) ◇ SODIUM CYCLOHEXANESULFAMATE ◇ SODIUM CYCLOHEXANESULPHAMATE ◇ SODIUM CYCLOHEXYL AMIDOSULPHATE ◇ SODIUM CYCLOHEXYL SULFAMATE ◇ SODIUM CYCLOHEXYL SULFAMIDATE ◇ SODIUM CYCLOHEXYL SULPHAMATE ◇ SODIUM SUCARYL ◇ SUCARYL SODIUM ◇ SUCCARIL ◇ SUCROSA ◇ SUESSETTE ◇ SUESTAMIN ◇ SUGARIN ◇ SUGARON

TOXICITY DATA with REFERENCE
NEO: imp-mus TDLo:176 mg/kg   SCIEAS 167,996,70
NEO: orl-rat TD:112 g/kg/8W-C   CNREA8 37,2943,77
NEO: orl-rat TDLo:63 g/kg/9W-C   CNREA8 37,2943,77
ETA: orl-rat TD:610 g/kg/87W-C   CBINA8 11,255,75
MUT: cyt-grb-unr 100 mg/kg   MUREAV 26,199,74
MUT: cyt-ham:fbr 10 mg/L   MUREAV 39,1,76
MUT: cyt-ham:lng 100 mg/L/3D   HEREAY 70,271,72
MUT: cyt-hmn:fbr 500 mg/L   ACYTAN 16,41,72
MUT: cyt-hmn:leu 10 μmol/L/5H   MUREAV 39,1,76
MUT: cyt-rat-orl 250 mg/kg   DBTEAD 19,215,71
MUT: dni-hmn:hla 800 μg/L   INHEAO 9,188,71

CONSENSUS REPORTS: IARC Cancer Review: GROUP 3 IMEMDT 7,178,87; Animal Limited Evidence IMEMDT 22,55,80. Reported in EPA TSCA Inventory. EPA Genetic Toxicology Program.

SAFETY PROFILE: Questionable carcinogen with experimental neoplastigenic, tumorigenic, and teratogenic data. Moderately toxic by intravenous and intraperitoneal routes. Mildly toxic by ingestion. Experimental reproductive effects. Human mutation data reported. When heated to decomposition it emits very toxic fumes of Na_2O, SO_x and NO_x.

SGF000   CAS: 63041-43-0
SODIUM 1,2:5,6-DIBENZANTHRACENE-9, 10-ENDO-α,β-SUCCINATE
mf: $C_{26}H_{16}O_4•2Na$ mw: 438.40

SYN: 1,2,5,6-DIBENZANTHRACENE-9,10-ENDO-α,β-SUCCINIC ACID, SODIUM SALT

TOXICITY DATA with REFERENCE

CAR: scu-mus TDLo:2304 mg/kg/16W-I

JPBAA7 54,321,42

ETA: ipr-mus TDLo:900 mg/kg/8W-I   AJCAA7 27,267,36

ETA: scu-mus TD:1824 mg/kg/13W-I   JPBAA7 47,501,38

MUT: mmo-esc 500 ppm   CRSBAW 142,453,48

SAFETY PROFILE: Questionable carcinogen with experimental carcinogenic and tumorigenic data. Mutation data reported. When heated to decomposition it emits toxic fumes of Na_2O.

SGI500   CAS: 7789-12-0
SODIUM DICHROMATE DIHYDRATE
mf: $Cr_2Na_2O_7 \cdot 2H_2O$ mw: 298.02

PROP: Red crystals. Mp: loses $2H_2O$ @ 100°, mp (anhydrous): 356.7°, bp: decomp @ 400°, d: 2.35 @ 13°.

SYN: CHROMIS ACID ($H_2Cr_2O_7$), DISODIUM SALT, DIHYDRATE (9CI)

TOXICITY DATA with REFERENCE

CAR: itr-rat TDLo:163 mg/kg/130W-I   EXPADD 30,129,86

MUT: slt-dmg-orl 2340 μm/L   MUREAV 157,157,85

CONSENSUS REPORTS: Chromium and its compounds are on the Community Right To Know List.

OSHA PEL: CL 0.1 mg(CrO_3)/m³   ACGIH TLV: TWA 0.05 mg(Cr)/m³   NIOSH REL: TWA 0.025 mg(Cr(VI))/m³; CL 0.05/15M

SAFETY PROFILE: Questionable carcinogen with experimental carcinogenic data. Probably a poison. A caustic irritant. Mutation data reported. When heated to decomposition it emits toxic fumes of Na_2O.

SGJ000   CAS: 148-18-5
SODIUM DIETHYLDITHIOCARBAMATE
mf: $C_5H_{10}NS_2 \cdot Na$ mw: 171.27

PROP: Crystals. Mp: 95°, d: 1.1 @ 20°/20°, vap d: 5.9.

SYNS: CUPRAL ◊ DDC ◊ DEDC ◊ DEDK ◊ DIETHYLCARBAMODITHIOIC ACID, SODIUM SALT ◊ DIETHYLDITHIOCARBAMATE SODIUM ◊ DIETHYLDITHIOCARBAMIC ACID SODIUM ◊ DIETHYLDITHIOCARBAMIC ACID, SODIUM SALT ◊ DIETHYL SODIUM DITHIOCARBAMATE ◊ DITHIOCARB ◊ DITHIOCARBAMATE ◊ NCI-CO2835 ◊ SODIUM DEDT ◊ SODIUM N,N-DIETHYLDITHIOCARBA-

MATE ◊ SODIUM SALT of N,N-DIETHYLDITHIOCARBAMIC ACID ◊ THIOCARB ◊ USAF EK-2596

TOXICITY DATA with REFERENCE

NEO: orl-mus TDLo:76 g/kg/78W-I   NTIS** PB223-159

MUT: cyt-rat-orl 5200 mg/kg   MUREAV 53,212,78

MUT: dnd-hmn:hla 100 μmol/L   BBACAQ 519,65,78

MUT: dni-ckn:emb 4 μmol/L   BBACAQ 519,65,78

MUT: oms-ckn:emb 40 μmol/L   BBACAQ 519,65,78

MUT: oms-omi 100 μmol/L   BBACAQ 519,65,78

CONSENSUS REPORTS: IARC Cancer Review: Animal Inadequate Evidence IMEMDT 12,217,76. NCI Carcinogenesis Bioassay (feed); No Evidence: mouse, rat NCITR* NCI-CG-TR-172,79. Reported in EPA TSCA Inventory.

SAFETY PROFILE: Questionable carcinogen with experimental neoplastigenic and teratogenic data. Moderately toxic by ingestion, intraperitoneal, and subcutaneous routes. Experimental reproductive effects. Human mutation data reported. When heated to decomposition it emits very toxic fumes of NO_x, SO_x, and Na_2O. Used as a pesticide.

SGP500   CAS: 6373-74-6
SODIUM 4-(2,4-DINITROANILINO)DIPHENYLAMINE-2-SULFONATE
mf: $C_{18}H_{14}N_4O_7S \cdot Na$ mw: 453.41

SYNS: ACID FAST YELLOW AG ◊ ACID LEATHER LIGHT BROWN G ◊ ACID ORANGE NO. 3 ◊ ACID YELLOW E ◊ AIREDALE YELLOW E ◊ AMIDO YELLOW EA-CF ◊ ANTHRALAN YELLOW RRT ◊ C.I. 10385 ◊ C.I. ACID ORANGE 3 ◊ DERMA YELLOW P ◊ ERIO FAST YELLOW AEN ◊ FAST LIGHT YELLOW E ◊ FENALAN YELLOW E ◊ KITON FAST YELLOW A ◊ LIGHT FAST YELLOW ES ◊ LISSAMINE FAST YELLOW AE ◊ NCI-C54911 ◊ NYLOMINE ACID YELLOW B-RD ◊ SUPERIAN YELLOW R ◊ TECTILON ORANGE 3GT ◊ TERTRACID LIGHT YELLOW 2R ◊ VONDACID FAST YELLOW AE ◊ XYLENE FAST YELLOW ES

TOXICITY DATA with REFERENCE

CAR: orl-rat TDLo:386 g/kg/2Y-I   NTPTR* NTP-TR-335,88

MUT: mma-sat 667 μg/plate   EMMUEG 11(Suppl 12),1,88

MUT: mmo-sat 100 μg/plate   EMMUEG 11(Suppl 12),1,88

CONSENSUS REPORTS: NTP Carcinogenesis Studies (gavage): Clear Evidence: rat,

NTPTR* NTP-TR-335,88; No Evidence: mouse NTPTR* NTP-TR-335,88. Reported in EPA TSCA Inventory.

SAFETY PROFILE: Questionable carcinogen with experimental carcinogenic data. Mutation data reported. When heated to decomposition it emits very toxic fumes of SO_x, NO_x, and Na_2O.

SHF500
SODIUM FLUORIDE
CAS: 7681-49-4
DOT: 1690
mf: FNa   mw: 41.99

PROP: Clear, lustrous crystals or white powder or balls. Mp: 993°, bp: 1700°, d: 2 @ 41°, vap press: 1 mm @ 1077°.

SYNS: ALCOA SODIUM FLUORIDE ◇ ANTIBULIT ◇ CAVI-TROL ◇ CHEMIFLUOR ◇ CREDO ◇ DISODIUM DI-FLUORIDE ◇ FDA 0101 ◇ F1-TABS ◇ FLORIDINE ◇ FLOROCID ◇ FLOZENGES ◇ FLUORAL ◇ FLUORIDENT ◇ FLUORID SODNY (CZECH) ◇ FLUORIGARD ◇ FLUORI-NEED ◇ FLUORINSE ◇ FLUORITAB ◇ FLUOR-O-KOTE ◇ FLUORURE de SODIUM (FRENCH) ◇ FLURA-GEL ◇ FLURCARE ◇ FUNGOL B ◇ GEL II ◇ GELUTION ◇ GLEEM ◇ IRADICAV ◇ KARIDIUM ◇ KARIGEL ◇ KARI-RINSE ◇ LEA-COV ◇ LEMOFLUR ◇ LURIDE ◇ NAFEEN ◇ NaFPAK ◇ Na FRINSE ◇ NATRIUM FLUORIDE ◇ NCI-C55221 ◇ NUFLUOR ◇ OSSALIN ◇ OSSIN ◇ PEDIAFLOR ◇ PEDIDENT ◇ PENNWHITE ◇ PERGANTENE ◇ PHOS-FLUR ◇ POINT TWO ◇ PREDENT ◇ RAFLUOR ◇ RESCUE SQUAD ◇ ROACH SALT ◇ SODIUM FLUORIDE, solid and solution (DOT) ◇ SODIUM FLUORURE (FRENCH) ◇ SODIUM HYDROFLUORIDE ◇ SODIUM MONOFLUORIDE ◇ SO-FLO ◇ STAY-FLO ◇ STUDAFLUOR ◇ SUPER-DENT ◇ T-FLUORIDE ◇ THERA-FLUR-N ◇ TRISODIUM TRI-FLUORIDE ◇ VILLIAUMITE

TOXICITY DATA with REFERENCE
ETA: orl-mus TD:87 g/kg/97W-C   IARC** 27,237,82

ETA: orl-mus TD:140 mg/kg/43W-C   IARC** 27,237,82

ETA: orl-mus TD:2190 mg/kg/2Y-C   IARC** 27,237,82

ETA: orl-mus TD:4200 mg/kg/30W-C   IARC** 27,237,82

ETA: orl-mus TD:4217 mg/kg/30W-C   IARC** 27,237,82

ETA: orl-mus TD:4242 mg/kg/30W-C   IARC** 27,237,82

ETA: orl-mus TD:4368 mg/kg/30W-C   IARC** 27,237,82

ETA: orl-mus TDLo:14 mg/kg/43W-C   IARC** 27,237,82

MUT: cyt-hmn:fbr 20 mg/L   MUREAV 139,193,84
MUT: cyt-mam:lng 300 μmol/L   HKXUDL 3,94,83
MUT: dnr-bcs 86 mg/L   WATRAG 14,1613,80
MUT: dns-hmn:fbr 100 mg/L   MUREAV 139,193,84
MUT: otr-ham:emb 75 mg/L   CNREA8 44,938,84

CONSENSUS REPORTS: Reported in EPA TSCA Inventory. EPA Genetic Toxicology Program.

OSHA PEL: TWA 2.5 mg(F)/m³ ACGIH TLV: TWA 2.5 mg(F)/m³ NIOSH REL: TWA (Inorganic Fluorides) 2.5 mg(F)/m³ DOT Classification: ORM-B; Label: None; Corrosive Material; Label: Corrosive, solution; Poison B; Label: St. Andrews Cross.

SAFETY PROFILE: Questionable carcinogen with experimental tumorigenic and teratogenic data. Human poison by ingestion and possibly other routes. Experimental poison by ingestion, skin contact, intravenous, intraperitoneal, subcutaneous and intramuscular routes. Human systemic effects by ingestion and intradermal routes: paresthesia, ptosis (drooping of the eyelid from sympathetic innervation), tremors, fluid intake, muscle weakness, headache, EKG changes, cyanosis, respiratory depression, hypermotility, diarrhea, nausea or vomiting, salivary gland changes, changes in teeth and supporting structures and other musculo-skeletal changes, and increased immune response. Human mutation data reported. A corrosive irritant to skin, eyes, and mucous membranes. Experimental reproductive effects. It is very phytotoxic. When heated to decomposition it emits toxic fumes of F^- and Na_2O. Used in chemical cleaning, for fluoridation of drinking water, as a fungicide and insecticide.

SHG000
SODIUM FLUORIDE (solution)
CAS: 7681-49-4
DOT: 1690
mf: FNa   mw: 41.99

CONSENSUS REPORTS: IARC Cancer Review: GROUP 3 IMEMDT 7,208,87; Animal Inadequate Evidence IMEMDT 27,237,82. Reported in EPA TSCA Inventory.

NIOSH REL: TWA 2.5 mg(F)/m³ DOT Classification: Corrosive Material; Label: Corrosive

SAFETY PROFILE: Questionable carcinogen. A corrosive irritant to skin, eyes and mucous membranes. When heated to decomposition it emits very toxic fumes of F^- and Na_2O.

SHX500   CAS: 3565-15-9
SODIUM 5-IODO-2-THIOURACIL
mf: $C_4H_3IN_2OS \cdot Na$ mw: 277.04

SYN: 5-IODO-2-THIOURACIL, SODIUM SALT

TOXICITY DATA with REFERENCE
ETA: orl-rat TDLo:30 g/kg/43W-C   CANCAR
10,690,57

SAFETY PROFILE: Questionable carcinogen
with experimental tumorigenic data. When
heated to decomposition it emits very toxic
fumes of I^-, NO_x, SO_x and Na_2O.

SIC250
**SODIUM LINOLEIC ACID
HYDROPEROXIDE**
mf: $C_{18}H_{32}O_3 \cdot Na$ mw: 319.49

SYNS: PEROXYLINOLEIC ACID, SODIUM SALT
◇ SODIUM LINOLEATE HYDROPEROXIDE

TOXICITY DATA with REFERENCE
CAR: scu-rat TDLo:1 g/kg/45W-I   FCTXAV
12,451,74
NEO: scu-rat TD:1765 mg/kg/95W-I   FCTXAV
12,451,74

SAFETY PROFILE: Questionable carcinogen
with experimental carcinogenic and neoplastigenic data. When heated to decomposition it
emits acrid smoke and irritating fumes.

SIC500   CAS: 13284-86-1
SODIUM LITHOCHOLATE
mf: $C_{24}H_{40}O_3 \cdot Na$ mw: 399.63

SYNS: 3-α-HYDROXY-5-β-CHOLAN-24-OIC ACID, MONO-
SODIUM SALT ◇ (3-α,5-β)-3-HYDROXYCHOLAN-24-OIC
ACID, MONOSODIUM SALT

TOXICITY DATA with REFERENCE
NEO: rec-mus TDLo:115 g/kg/48W-I   CNREA8
39,1521,79

SAFETY PROFILE: Questionable carcinogen
with experimental neoplastigenic data. When
heated to decomposition it emits toxic fumes
of Na_2O.

SIJ000   CAS: 3804-89-5
SODIUM METHANESULFONATE
mf: $C_7H_8N_3O_4S \cdot Na$ mw: 253.23

SYNS: ISONIAZID SODIUM METHANESULFONATE
◇ NEOISCOTIN ◇ NEOTIZIDE ◇ NEO-TIZIDE SODIUM SALT
◇ SODIUM ISONICOTINYL HYDRAZINE METHANSULFO-
NATE

TOXICITY DATA with REFERENCE
CAR: orl-mus TDLo:101 g/kg/30W-C   GANNA2
51,83,60

SAFETY PROFILE: Questionable carcinogen
with experimental carcinogenic data. Poison by
ingestion. Moderately toxic by subcutaneous
route. When heated to decomposition it emits
very toxic fumes of Na_2O, SO_x, and NO_x.

SIN675
**SODIUM MORPHOLINE and
NITRITE (1:1)**

SYN: MORPHOLINE and SODIUM NITRITE (1:1)

TOXICITY DATA with REFERENCE
CAR: orl-mus TDLo:17200 mg/kg/96W-I
EKSODD 8(1),41,86
ETA: orl-mus TDLo:1125 mg/kg   IAPUDO
41,659,82
ETA: orl-rat TDLo:18800 mg/kg/27W-C
FCTXAV 10,887,72
MUT: hma-mus/sat 1450 μmol/kg   CNREA8
37,4572,77
MUT: mse-ham-orl 1 g/kg   BBRCA9 81,310,78
MUT: otr-ham-orl 1 g/kg   BBRCA9 81,310,78

SAFETY PROFILE: Questionable carcinogen
with experimental carcinogenic and tumorigenic
data. Mutation data reported. When heated to
decomposition it emits toxic fumes of NO_x and
Na_2O.

SIO900   CAS: 7631-99-4
SODIUM(I) NITRATE (1:1)
DOT: 1498
mf: $NO_3 \cdot Na$ mw: 85.00

PROP: Colorless, transparent, odorless crystals;
saline, sltly bitter taste. Mp: 306.8°, bp: decomp
@ 380°, d: 2.261. Deliquescent in moist air;
sol in water, sltly sol in alc.

SYNS: CHILE SALTPETER ◇ CUBIC NITER ◇ NITRATE
de SODIUM (FRENCH) ◇ NITRATINE ◇ NITRIC ACID, SO-
DIUM SALT ◇ SODA NITER ◇ SODIUM NITRATE (DOT)

TOXICITY DATA with REFERENCE
ETA: orl-rat TD:913 g/kg/2Y-C   FCTOD7
20,25,82
ETA: orl-rat TD:1825 g/kg/2Y-C   FCTOD7
20,25,82
ETA: orl-rat TDLo:100 g/kg/2Y-C   FCTOD7
22,715,84
MUT: cyt-ham:fbr 7200 mg/L/48H   MUREAV
48,337,77

MUT: cyt-ham:lng 125 mg/L   GMCRDC 27,95,81
MUT: cyt-mus-orl 7067 mg/kg   MUREAV 155,121,85
MUT: cyt-rat-orl 78500 μg/kg   MUREAV 155,121,85
MUT: dns-hmn:hla 6 mmol/L   AEMBAP 177,269,84
MUT: mmo-omi 1000 ppm   POASAD 34,114,53
MUT: mnt-ham-orl 250 mg/kg   MUREAV 66,149,79
MUT: msc-ham-orl 125 mg/kg   MUREAV 66,149,79
MUT: otr-ham-orl 250 mg/kg   MUREAV 66,149,79

CONSENSUS REPORTS: Reported in EPA TSCA Inventory. EPA Genetic Toxicology Program.

DOT Classification: Oxidizer; Label: Oxidizer

SAFETY PROFILE: Questionable carcinogen with experimental tumorigenic data. Poison by intravenous route. Moderately toxic by ingestion. Human mutation data reported. A powerful oxidizer. It will ignite with heat or friction. A dangerous disaster hazard. When heated to decomposition it emits toxic fumes of NO_x and Na_2O.

SIP500   CAS: 5064-31-3
SODIUM NITRILOTRIACETATE
mf: $C_6H_6NO_6 \cdot 3Na$ mw: 257.10

SYNS: HAMPSHIRE NTA ◇ NITRILOTRIACETIC ACID, TRISODIUM SALT ◇ NTA ◇ TRISODIUM NITRILOTRIACE-TATE ◇ TRISODIUM NITRILOTRIACETIC ACID

TOXICITY DATA with REFERENCE
NEO: orl-rat TDLo:70300 mg/kg/2Y-C   JJIND8 66,869,81
MUT: or-rat:emb 495 μg/plate   JJATDK 1,190,81

CONSENSUS REPORTS: Reported in EPA TSCA Inventory.

SAFETY PROFILE: Questionable carcinogen with experimental neoplastigenic data. Poison by intraperitoneal route. Moderately toxic by ingestion. Experimental reproductive effects. Mutation data reported. When heated to decomposition it emits toxic fumes of NO_x and Na_2O.

SIQ500   CAS: 7632-00-0
SODIUM NITRITE
DOT: 1500
mf: $NO_2 \cdot Na$ mw: 69.00

PROP: Sltly yellowish or white crystals, sticks or powder; slt salty taste. Mp: 271°, bp: decomp @ 320°, d: 2.168. Deliquescent in air; sol in water, sltly sol in alc.

SYNS: ANTI-RUST ◇ DIAZOTIZING SALTS ◇ DUSITAN SODNY (CZECH) ◇ ERINITRIT ◇ FILMERINE ◇ NATRIUM NITRIT (GERMAN) ◇ NCI-C02084 ◇ NITRITE de SODIUM (FRENCH) ◇ NITROUS ACID, SODIUM SALT

TOXICITY DATA with REFERENCE
CAR: orl-mus TDLo:2149 mg/(pre-post-birth):TER   CNREA8 45,3561,85
NEO: orl-rat TD:40 g/kg/56W-C   ZKKOBW 91,189,78
NEO: orl-rat TD:100 g/kg/2Y-I   CRNGDP 4,1189,83
NEO: orl-rat TDLo:40 g/kg/56W-C   ZKKOBW 90,87,77
ETA: orl-rat TD:63 g/kg/95W-C   JJIND8 64,1435,80
ETA: orl-rat TD:91 g/kg/2Y-C:TER   FCTOD7 20,25,82
ETA: orl-rat TD:183 g/kg/2Y-C:TER   FCTOD7 20,25,82
MUT: cyt-rat-orl 2730 mg/kg/13D-C   JTEHD6 13,643,84
MUT: dni-ham:lng 100 ppm   NEOLA4 32,341,85
MUT: dni-hmn:fbr 2000 ppm   NEOLA4 32,341,85
MUT: dns-hmn:hla 6 mmol/L   FCTOD7 21,551,83
MUT: mmo-omi 50 mmol/L   JGMIAN 128,1401,82
MUT: msc-ham:lng 1000 ppm   NEOLA4 32,341,85

CONSENSUS REPORTS: Reported in EPA TSCA Inventory. EPA Genetic Toxicology Program.

DOT Classification: Oxidizer; Label: Oxidizer

SAFETY PROFILE: Questionable carcinogen with experimental neoplastigenic, tumorigenic, and teratogenic data. It may react with organic amines in the body to form carcinogenic nitrosamines. Human poison by ingestion. Experimental poison by ingestion, subcutaneous, intravenous, and intraperitoneal routes. Human systemic effects by ingestion: motor activity changes, coma, decreased blood pressure with possible pulse rate increase without fall in blood pressure, arteriolar or venous dilation, nausea or vomiting, and blood methemoglobinemia-carboxhemoglobinemia. Experimental reproductive effects. Human mutation data reported. An eye irritant. Flammable; a strong oxidizing agent. When heated to decomposition it emits toxic fumes of NO_x and Na_2O.

SIQ675
SODIUM NITRITE mixed with 1-(p-BROMOPHENYL)-3-METHYLUREA

SYNS: 1-(p-BROMOPHENYL)-3-METHYLUREA mixed with SODIUM NITRITE ◇ 1-METHYL-3-(p-BROMOPHENYL)UREA mixed with SODIUM NITRITE ◇ SODIUM NITRITE mixed with 1-METHYL-3-(p-BROMOPHENYL)UREA

TOXICITY DATA with REFERENCE
CAR: orl-rat TDLo: 1186 mg/kg/82W-I

ARGEAR 53,329,83

SAFETY PROFILE: Questionable carcinogen with experimental carcinogenic data. When heated to decomposition it emits toxic fumes of NO_x.

SIQ700
SODIUM NITRITE and CARBENDAZIME (1:1)
mf: $C_9H_7N_5O_4$ mw: 249.21

SYNS: CARBENDAZIME and SODIUM NITRITE (1:1) ◇ 2-METHYL-N-NITROSO-BENZIMIDAZOLE CARBAMATE and SODIUM NITRITE (1:1) ◇ SODIUM NITRITE and 2-METHYL-N-NITROSO-BENZIMIDAZOLE CARBA-MATE (1:1)

TOXICITY DATA with REFERENCE
CAR: orl-mus TDLo: 4200 mg/kg (8-14D post)

MGONAD 20,163,76

SAFETY PROFILE: Questionable carcinogen with experimental carcinogenic data. When heated to decomposition it emits toxic fumes of NO_x.

SIS000   CAS: 104639-49-8
SODIUM NITRITE mixed with CHLORDIAZEPOXIDE (1:1)

SYNS: CHLORDIAZEPOXIDE, NITROSATED ◇ CHLOR-DIAZEPOXIDE mixed with SODIUM NITRITE (1:1) ◇ 7-CHLORO-2-METHYLAMINO-5-PHENYL-3H-1,4-BENZO-DIAZEPINE-4-OXIDE, mixed with SODIUM NITRITE (1:1)

TOXICITY DATA with REFERENCE
CAR: orl-rat TDLo: 90 g/kg/50W-I   FCTXAV

15,269,77

MUT: mma-sat 800 nmol/plate   CALEDQ 12,81,81
MUT: mmo-sat 800 nmol/plate   CALEDQ 12,81,81

SAFETY PROFILE: Questionable carcinogen with experimental carcinogenic data. Mutation data reported. When heated to decomposition it emits very toxic fumes of NO_x, Cl^- and Na_2O.

SIS100
SODIUM NITRITE and l-CITRULLINE (1:2)
mf: $C_6H_{13}N_3O_3 \cdot 1/_{2NNaO2}$ mw: 239.68

SYN: l-CITRULLINE and SODIUM NITRITE (2:1)

TOXICITY DATA with REFERENCE
ETA: orl-rat TDLo: 1650 mg/kg (13-23D post)

NCIMAV 51,103,79

SAFETY PROFILE: Questionable carcinogen with experimental tumorigenic data. When heated to decomposition it emits toxic fumes of NO_x.

SIS150
SODIUM NITRITE mixed with DIMETHYLDODECYLAMINE (8:7)

SYN: DIMETHYLDODECYLAMINE HYDROCHLORIDE mixed with SODIUM NITRITE (7:8)

TOXICITY DATA with REFERENCE
CAR: orl-rat TDLo: 135 g/kg/80W-I   FCTXAV

15,269,77

SAFETY PROFILE: Questionable carcinogen with experimental carcinogenic data. When heated to decomposition it emits toxic fumes of NO_x.

SIS200
SODIUM NITRITE mixed with DISULFIRAM
mf: $C_{10}H_{20}N_2S_4 \cdot NNaO_3$ mw: 381.56

SYNS: BIS(DIETHYLTHIOCARBAMOYL)DISULFIDE mixed with SODIUM NITRITE ◇ DISULFIRAM mixed with SO-DIUM NITRITE ◇ SODIUM NITRITE mixed with BIS(DI-ETHYLTHIOCARBAMOYL)DISULFIDE

TOXICITY DATA with REFERENCE
ETA: orl-rat TD: 197 g/kg/78W-C   FCTXAV

18,85,80

ETA: orl-rat TDLo: 164 g/kg/78W-C   FCTXAV

18,85,80

SAFETY PROFILE: Questionable carcinogen with experimental tumorigenic data. When heated to decomposition it emits toxic fumes of NO_x.

SIS500
SODIUM NITRITE mixed with ETHAMBUTOL (1:1)

SYNS: d-N,N'-DI(1-HYDROXYMETHYLPROPYL)ETHYLENEDIAMINE DIHY-DROCHLORIDE mixed with SODIUM NITRITE ◇ ETHAMBU-TOL mixed with SODIUM NITRITE (1:1)

TOXICITY DATA with REFERENCE
CAR: orl-mus TDLo: 8640 mg/kg/36W-C

LAPPA5 35,45,75

SAFETY PROFILE: Questionable carcinogen with experimental carcinogenic data. When heated to decomposition it emits toxic fumes of NO_x, HCl and Na_2O.

SIS650
SODIUM NITRITE mixed with N-METHYLADENOSINE (4:1)
mf: $C_{11}H_{15}N_5O_4 \cdot 4NNaO_2$ mw: 557.31

SYNS: ADENOSINE, N-METHYL-, mixed with SODIUM NITRITE (1:4) ◊ N^6-METHYLADENOSINE mixed with SODIUM NITRITE (1:4) ◊ N-METHYLADENOSINE mixed with SODIUM NITRITE (1:4)

TOXICITY DATA with REFERENCE
CAR: orl-mus TDLo: 33918 mg/kg/34W-I
IJCNAW 24,319,79
NEO: orl-mus TD: 34 g/kg/34W-I   IAPUDO
31,787,80

SAFETY PROFILE: Questionable carcinogen with experimental carcinogenic and neoplastigenic data. When heated to decomposition it emits toxic fumes of NO_x.

SIS675
SODIUM NITRITE and 1-(METHYLETHYL)UREA
mf: $C_8H_{20}N_4O_2 \cdot NNaO_2$ mw: 273.32

SYNS: ISOPROPYLUREA and SODIUM NITRITE ◊ 1-(METHYLETHYL)UREA and SODIUM NITRITE ◊ SODIUM NITRITE and ISOPROPYLUREA

TOXICITY DATA with REFERENCE
NEO: orl-rat TDLo: 180 mg/kg (21D post)
ZAPPAN 121,61,77
NEO: orl-rat TDLo: 25850 mg/kg/47D-C
ZAPPAN 121,61,77

SAFETY PROFILE: Questionable carcinogen with experimental neoplastigenic data. When heated to decomposition it emits toxic fumes of NO_x.

SIS700
SODIUM NITRITE and 1-METHYL-1-NITROSO-3-PHENYLUREA

TOXICITY DATA with REFERENCE
CAR: orl-rat TDLo: 8250 mg/kg/32W-I
CALEDQ 4,299,78
ETA: orl-rat TD: 200 mg/kg   MVMZA8
33,128,78

SAFETY PROFILE: Questionable carcinogen with experimental carcinogenic and tumorigenic data. When heated to decomposition it emits toxic fumes of NO_x and Na_2O.

SIT000
SODIUM NITRITE mixed with OCTAHYDROAZOCINE HYDROCHLORIDE (1:1)

SYNS: HEPTAMETHYLENEIMINE mixed with SODIUM NITRITE ◊ OCTAHYDROAZOCINE HYDROCHLORIDE mixed with SODIUM NITRITE (1:1) ◊ SODIUM NITRITE mixed with HEPTAMETHYLENEIMINE

TOXICITY DATA with REFERENCE
CAR: orl-rat TDLo: 15 g/kg/24W-I   NATUAS
244,176,73

SAFETY PROFILE: Questionable carcinogen with experimental carcinogenic data. When heated to decomposition it emits very toxic fumes of HCl, NO_x, and Na_2O.

SIT750
SODIUM NITRITE and 1-PROPYLUREA
mf: $C_4H_{10}N_2O \cdot 1/_3NNaO2$ mw: 125.13

SYNS: n-PROPYLUREA and SODIUM NITRITE ◊ 1-PROPYLUREA and SODIUM NITRITE ◊ SODIUM NITRITE and n-PROPYLUREA

TOXICITY DATA with REFERENCE
NEO: orl-rat TDLo: 31350 mg/kg/57D-C
ZAPPAN 121,61,77

SAFETY PROFILE: Questionable carcinogen with experimental neoplastigenic data. When heated to decomposition it emits toxic fumes of NO_x.

SIT800
SODIUM NITRITE and TRIFORINE

SYN: TRIFORINE and SODIUM NITRITE

TOXICITY DATA with REFERENCE
CAR: orl-mus TDLo: 19 g/kg/15W-I   IARCCD
19,477,78

SAFETY PROFILE: Questionable carcinogen with experimental carcinogenic data. When heated to decomposition it emits toxic fumes of NO_x and Na_2O.

SJB000   CAS: 64057-57-4
SODIUM PERACETATE
mf: $C_2H_3O_3 \cdot Na$ mw: 98.04

SYNS: SODIUM ETHANEPEROXOATE ◊ SODIUM PEROXYACETATE

TOXICITY DATA with REFERENCE
ETA: unr-mus TDLo: 314 mg/kg   RARSAM
3,193,63

SAFETY PROFILE: Questionable carcinogen with experimental tumorigenic data. An oxidizer. The dry salt explodes spontaneously at room temperature. When heated to decomposition it emits toxic fumes of Na_2O.

SJS500   CAS: 874-21-5
SODIUM SARKOMYCIN
mf: $C_7H_7O_3 \cdot Na$ mw: 162.13

PROP: A metabolite of *Streptomyces erythro-chromogehes* (12VXA5 8,934,68).

SYNS: 2-METHYLENE-3-OXOCYCLOPENTANECAR-BOXYLIC ACID, SODIUM SALT ◇ SARKOMYCIN B*, SODIUM SALT ◇ SARKOMYCIN, SODIUM SALT

TOXICITY DATA with REFERENCE
ETA: scu-rat TDLo: 1680 mg/kg/42W-I   BJCAAI 19,392,65

SAFETY PROFILE: Questionable carcinogen with experimental tumorigenic data. When heated to decomposition it emits toxic fumes of Na_2O.

SJT500   CAS: 10102-18-8
SODIUM SELENITE
DOT: 2630
mf: $O_3Se \cdot 2Na$ mw: 172.94

PROP: White crystals.

SYNS: DISODIUM SELENITE ◇ NATRIUMSELENIT (GERMAN) ◇ SELENIOUS ACID, DISODIUM SALT

TOXICITY DATA with REFERENCE
MUT: cyt-ham-ipr 3 mg/kg   HEREAY 93,101,80
MUT: cyt-hmn:fbr 80 μmol/L   BTERDG 2,81,80
MUT: dni-hmn:hla 25 μmol/L   TOLED5 25,219,85
MUT: dnr-sat 10 μg/plate   CALEDQ 10,75,80
MUT: dns-rat:lvr 100 μmol/L   CALEDQ 10,75,80
MUT: oms-hmn:hla 50 μmol/L   TOLED5 25,219,85
MUT: sce-ham-ipr 3 mg/kg   HEREAY 93,101,80
MUT: sce-hmn:lym 7900 nmol/L   BTERDG 2,81,80

CONSENSUS REPORTS: IARC Cancer Review: GROUP 3 IMEMDT 7,56,87; Animal Inadequate Evidence IMEMDT 9,245,75. Reported in EPA TSCA Inventory. EPA Genetic Toxicology Program. EPA Extremely Hazardous Substances List. Selenium and its compounds are on the Community Right To Know List.

OSHA PEL: TWA 0.2 mg(Se)/m^3 ACGIH TLV: TWA 0.2 mg(Se)/m^3 DFG MAK: 0.1

mg(Se)/m^3 DOT Classification: Poison B; Label: Poison

SAFETY PROFILE: Questionable carcinogen. Poison by ingestion, intraperitoneal, intravenous, subcutaneous, intracervical, parenteral, and intramuscular routes. An experimental teratogen. Experimental reproductive effects. Human mutation data reported. When heated to decomposition it emits toxic fumes of Se and Na_2O.

SKU000   CAS: 110-44-1
SORBIC ACID
mf: $C_6H_8O_2$ mw: 112.14

PROP: Colorless needles or white powder; characteristic odor. Bp: 228° (decomp), mp: 134.5°, flash p: 260°F (COC), vap press: 0.01 mm @ 20°, vap d: 3.87. Sol in hot water; very sol in alc, ether.

SYNS: (2-BUTENYLIDENE)ACETIC ACID ◇ CROTYLI-DENE ACETIC ACID ◇ HEXADIENIC ACID ◇ HEXADIENOIC ACID ◇ 2,4-HEXADIENOIC ACID ◇ trans-trans-2,4-HEXA-DIENOIC ACID ◇ 1,3-PENTADIENE-1-CARBOXYLIC ACID ◇ 2-PROPENYLACRYLIC ACID ◇ SORBISTAT

TOXICITY DATA with REFERENCE
ETA: scu-rat TDLo: 1040 mg/kg/65W-I   BJCAAI 20,134,66
MUT: cyt-ham:lng 1050 mg/L   FCTOD7 22,501,84
MUT: sce-ham:lng 1050 mg/L   FCTOD7 22,501,84

CONSENSUS REPORTS: Reported in EPA TSCA Inventory.

SAFETY PROFILE: Questionable carcinogen with experimental tumorigenic data. Moderately toxic by intraperitoneal and subcutaneous routes. Mildly toxic by ingestion. Experimental reproductive effects. Mutation data reported. A severe human and experimental skin irritant. Combustible when exposed to heat or flame; can react with oxidizing materials. To fight fire, use water. When heated to decomposition it emits acrid smoke and irritating fumes.

SKV000   CAS: 1338-39-2
SORBITAN MONOLAURATE
mf: $C_{18}H_{34}O_6$ mw: 346.52

SYNS: EMSORB 2515 ◇ RADIASURF 7125 ◇ SORBITAN MONODODECANOATE ◇ SPAN 20

TOXICITY DATA with REFERENCE
NEO: skn-mus TD: 2000 mg/kg/25W-I   NCIMAV 10,489,63

NEO: skn-mus TDLo: 1350 mg/kg/24W-I
SCIEAS 120,1075,54

CONSENSUS REPORTS: Reported in EPA TSCA Inventory.

SAFETY PROFILE: Questionable carcinogen with experimental neoplastigenic data. Experimental reproductive effects. When heated to decomposition it emits acrid smoke and irritating fumes.

SKV500
SORSAKA

PROP: Aqueous extract from the dried leaves of the plant *Annona muricata* (JNCIAM 46,-1131,71).

SYNS: ANNONA MURICATA ◇ l-SORSAKA, LEAF and STEM EXTRACT

TOXICITY DATA with REFERENCE
ETA: scu-rat TDLo: 300 g/kg/1Y-I   JNCIAM
46,1131,71

SAFETY PROFILE: Questionable carcinogen with experimental tumorigenic data. When heated to decomposition it emits acrid smoke and irritating fumes.

SKW500
SOTERENOL HYDROCHLORIDE
CAS: 14816-67-2

mf: $C_{12}H_{20}N_2O_4S \cdot ClH$ mw: 324.86

SYNS: 2'-HYDROXY-5'-(1-HYDROXY-2-(ISOPROPYL-AMINO)ETHYL)-METHANESULFONANILIDE MONOHY-DROCHLORIDE ◇ MJ 1992

TOXICITY DATA with REFERENCE
ETA: orl-rat TDLo: 2512 mg/kg/78W-C
TXAPA9 22,279,72

SAFETY PROFILE: Questionable carcinogen with experimental tumorigenic data. Poison by intravenous and intraperitoneal routes. Moderately toxic by ingestion. When heated to decomposition it emits very toxic fumes of NO_x, SO_x, and HCl. A bronchodilator.

SLK000
STEARIC ACID
CAS: 57-11-4

mf: $C_{18}H_{36}O_2$ mw: 284.54

PROP: White, amorphous solid; slt odor and taste of tallow. Mp: 69.3°, bp: 383°, flash p: 385°F (CC), d: 0.847, autoign temp: 743°F, vap press: 1 mm @ 173.7°, vap d: 9.80. Sol in alc, ether, acetone, chloroform; insol in water.

SYNS: CENTURY 1240 ◇ DAR-CHEM 14 ◇ EMERSOL 120 ◇ GLYCON DP ◇ GLYCON S-70 ◇ GLYCON TP ◇ GROCO 54 ◇ 1-HEPTADECANECARBOXYLIC ACID ◇ HYDROFOL ACID 1655 ◇ HY-PHI 1199 ◇ HYSTRENE 80 ◇ INDUSTRENE 5016 ◇ KAM 1000 ◇ KAM 2000 ◇ KAM 3000 ◇ NEO-FAT 18-61 ◇ NEO-FAT 18-S ◇ OCTADECANOIC ACID ◇ PEARL STEARIC ◇ STEAREX BEADS ◇ STEAROPHANIC ACID ◇ TEGOSTEARIC 254

TOXICITY DATA with REFERENCE
ETA: imp-mus TDLo: 400 mg/kg   BJCAAI
17,127,63

CONSENSUS REPORTS: Reported in EPA TSCA Inventory. EPA Genetic Toxicology Program.

SAFETY PROFILE: Questionable carcinogen with experimental tumorigenic data by implantation route. Poison by intravenous route. A human skin irritant. Combustible when exposed to heat or flame. Heats spontaneously. To fight fire, use CO_2, dry chemical. When heated to decomposition it emits acrid smoke and irritating fumes.

SLK500
STEARIC ACID-2,3-EPOXYPROPYL ESTER
CAS: 7460-84-6

mf: $C_{21}H_{40}O_3$ mw: 340.61

SYNS: 2,3-EPOXY-1-PROPANOL STEARATE ◇ 2,3-EPOXYPROPYL ESTER of STEARIC ACID ◇ 2,3-EPOXY-PROPYL STEARATE ◇ GLYCIDOL STEARATE ◇ GLYC-IDYL OCTADECANOATE ◇ GLYCIDYL STEARATE ◇ OXIRANYLMETHYL ESTER of OCTADECANOIC ACID

TOXICITY DATA with REFERENCE
ETA: scu-mus TD: 52 mg/kg/26W-I   CNREA8
32,880,72
ETA: scu-mus TDLo: 52 mg/kg/26W-I   CNREA8
30,1037,70
ETA: scu-rat TDLo: 2500 mg/kg/5W-I   ANYAA9
68,750,58
MUT: cyt-rat-ipr 5 mg/kg   BJPCAL 6,235,51

CONSENSUS REPORTS: IARC Cancer Review: Animal Inadequate Evidence IMEMDT 11,187,76.

SAFETY PROFILE: Questionable carcinogen with experimental tumorigenic data. Mutation data reported. When heated to decomposition it emits acrid smoke and irritating fumes.

SLL400
γ-STEAROLACTONE
CAS: 502-26-1

mf: $C_{18}H_{34}O_2$ mw: 282.52

SYN: DIHYDRO-5-TETRADECYL-2(3H)-FURANONE

TOXICITY DATA with REFERENCE
NEO: scu-mus TDLo:160 mg/kg/40W-I
   CNREA8 30,1037,70
ETA: scu-mus TD:52 mg/kg/26W-I   CNREA8
32,880,72

SAFETY PROFILE: Questionable carcinogen
with experimental neoplastigenic and tumorigenic data. When heated to decomposition it
emits acrid smoke and irritating fumes.

SLM000   CAS: 3891-30-3
1-STEAROYLAZIRIDINE
mf: $C_{20}H_{39}NO$ mw: 309.60

SYN: STEAROYL ETHYLENEIMINE

TOXICITY DATA with REFERENCE
NEO: scu-rat TD:1100 mg/kg/35D-I   BJPCAL
   9,306,54
NEO: scu-rat TDLo:1000 mg/kg/5W-I   BJPCAL
   6,357,51
MUT: cyt-rat-ipr 200 mg/kg   BJPCAL 9,306,54

SAFETY PROFILE: Questionable carcinogen
with experimental neoplastigenic data. Mutation
data reported. When heated to decomposition
it emits toxic fumes of NO_x.

SLP350
STEVIA REBAUDIANA Bertoni, extract

TOXICITY DATA with REFERENCE
ETA: orl-rat TD:99540 mg/kg/79W-C   SKEZAP
   26,169,85
ETA: orl-rat TDLo:41475 mg/kg/79W-C
   SKEZAP 26,169,85

SAFETY PROFILE: Questionable carcinogen
with experimental tumorigenic data. Experimental reproductive effects.

SLQ900   CAS: 834-24-2
4-STILBENAMINE
mf: $C_{14}H_{13}N$ mw: 195.28

SYNS: p-AMINOSTILBENE ◇ 4-AMINOSTILBENE
◇ 4-(2-PHENYLETHENYL)BENZENAMINE ◇ 4-N-STILBEN
AMINE ◇ p-STYRYLANILINE

TOXICITY DATA with REFERENCE
ETA: imp-mus TDLo:80 mg/kg   BJCAAI
   17,127,63
ETA: scu-rat TD:200 mg/kg/W-I   BMBUAQ
   14,141,58

SAFETY PROFILE: Questionable carcinogen
with experimental tumorigenic data. When
heated to decomposition it emits toxic fumes
of NO_x.

SLR500   CAS: 621-96-5
4,4'-STILBENEDIAMINE
mf: $C_{14}H_{14}N_2$ mw: 210.30

SYNS: 4:4'-DIAMINOSTILBENE ◇ 4,4'-VINYLENEDIANI-
LINE

TOXICITY DATA with REFERENCE
ETA: scu-rat TDLo:200 mg/kg/W-I   BMBUAQ
   14,141,58

SAFETY PROFILE: Questionable carcinogen
with experimental tumorigenic data. When
heated to decomposition it emits toxic fumes
of NO_x.

SMQ500   CAS: 9003-53-6
STYRENE POLYMER
mf: $(C_8H_8)_n$
DOT: 2211

SYNS: A 3-80 ◇ AFCOLENE ◇ ATACTIC POLYSTYRENE
◇ BACTOLATEX ◇ BAKELITE SMD 3500 ◇ BASF III
◇ BEXTRENE XL 750 ◇ BICOLASTIC A 75 ◇ BUSTREN
◇ CADCO 0115 ◇ CARINEX GP ◇ COPAL Z ◇ COSDEN
550 ◇ DENKA QP3 ◇ DIAREX 43G ◇ DORVON ◇ DOW
860 ◇ DYLENE ◇ DYLITE F 40 ◇ ESBRITE ◇ ESCOREZ
7404 ◇ ESTYRENE G 20 ◇ ETHENYLBENZENE HOMO-
POLYMER ◇ FOSTER GRANT 834 ◇ GEDEX ◇ HI-STYROL
◇ HOSTYREN S ◇ HT-F 76 ◇ IT 40 ◇ KB (POLYMER)
◇ KRASTEN 1.4 ◇ LACQREN 550 ◇ LUSTREX ◇ MX 5517-
02 ◇ NBS 706 ◇ OWISPOL GF ◇ PICCOLASTIC ◇ POLIGO-
STYRENE ◇ POLYSTROL D ◇ POLYSTYRENE ◇ POLYSTY-
RENE BEADS (DOT) ◇ POLYSTYRENE LATEX ◇ POLY-
STYROL ◇ PRINTEL'S ◇ REXOLITE 1422 ◇ RHODOLNE
◇ SHELL 300 ◇ STYRAFOIL ◇ STYRAGEL ◇ STYRENE
POLYMERS ◇ STYROFOAM ◇ STYROLUX ◇ STYRON
◇ TOPOREX 855-51 ◇ TROLITUL ◇ UBATOL U 2001
◇ VESTYRON ◇ VINYLBENZENE POLYMER ◇ VINYL
PRODUCTS R 3612

TOXICITY DATA with REFERENCE
ETA: imp-rat TDLo:19 mg/kg   CNREA8 15,333,55

CONSENSUS REPORTS: IARC Cancer Review: GROUP 3 IMEMDT 7,56,87; Animal
Limited Evidence IMEMDT 19,231,79. Reported in EPA TSCA Inventory.

DOT Classification: ORM; Label: None.

SAFETY PROFILE: Questionable carcinogen
with experimental tumorigenic data by implant.

When heated to decomposition it emits acrid smoke and irritating fumes.

SMR000 CAS: 9003-55-8
STYRENE POLYMER with 1,3-BUTADIENE

SYNS: AFCOLAC B 101 ◇ ANDREZ ◇ BASE 661 ◇ 1,3-BUTADIENE-STYRENE COPOLYMER ◇ BUTADIENE-STYRENE POLYMER ◇ 1,3-BUTADIENE-STYRENE POLYMER ◇ BUTADIENE-STYRENE RESIN ◇ BUTADIENE-STYRENE RUBBER (FCC) ◇ BUTAKON 85-71 ◇ DIAREX 600 ◇ DIENOL S ◇ DOW 209 ◇ DOW LATEX 612 ◇ DST 50 ◇ DURANIT ◇ EDISTIR RB 268 ◇ ETHENYLBENZENE POLYMER with 1,3-BUTADIENE ◇ GOODRITE 1800X73 ◇ HISTYRENE S 6F ◇ HYCAR LX 407 ◇ K 55E ◇ KOPOLYMER BUTADIEN STYRENOVY (CZECH) ◇ KRO 1 ◇ LITEX CA ◇ LYTRON 5202 ◇ MARBON 9200 ◇ NIPOL 407 ◇ PHAROS 100.1 ◇ PLIOFLEX ◇ PLIOLITE S5 ◇ POLYBUTADIENE-POLYSTYRENE COPOLYMER ◇ POLYCO 2410 ◇ RICON 100 ◇ SBS ◇ SD 354 ◇ S6F HISTYRENE RESIN ◇ SKS 85 ◇ SOIL STABILIZER 661 ◇ SOLPRENE 300 ◇ STYRENE-BUTADIENE COPOLYMER ◇ STY-RENE-1,3-BUTADIENE COPOLYMER ◇ STYRENE-BUTADIENE POLYMER ◇ SYNPOL 1500 ◇ THERMOPLASTIC 125 ◇ TR 201 ◇ UP 1E ◇ VESTYRON HI

CONSENSUS REPORTS: IARC Cancer Review: GROUP 3 IMEMDT 7,56,87; Human Inadequate Evidence IMEMDT 19,231,79. Reported in EPA TSCA Inventory.

SAFETY PROFILE: Questionable carcinogen. An eye irritant. When heated to decomposition it emits acrid smoke and irritating fumes.

SMR500 CAS: 841-18-9
trans-4'-STYRYLACETANILIDE
mf: $C_{16}H_{15}NO$ mw: 237.32

SYNS: 4-ACETAMIDOSTILBENE ◇ trans-4-ACETAMIDOSTILBENE ◇ trans-4-ACETAMINOSTILBENE ◇ 4-ACETYLAMINOSTILBENE ◇ trans-4-ACETYLAMINOSTILBENE ◇ N-(4-(2-PHENYLETHENYL)PHENYL)ACETAMIDE

TOXICITY DATA with REFERENCE
CAR: orl-rat TD:250 mg/kg/13W-I   CNREA8 24,128,64
CAR: orl-rat TD:336 mg/kg/24W-C   BJCAAI 22,133,68
CAR: orl-rat TDLo:48 mg/kg/3W-I   CRNGDP 4,1519,83
CAR: scu-rat TDLo:31 mg/kg/26W-I   CNREA8 24,128,64
ETA: scu-rat TD:27 mg/kg/13W-I   PTRMAD 241,147,48

ETA: scu-rat TD:37 mg/kg/4W-I   BJCAAI 22,133,68
MUT: dnd-rat-orl 25 μmol/kg   CBINA8 24,355,79
MUT: dnr-ham:fbr 1 μmol/L   JNCIAM 54,1287,75
MUT: mma-sat 5 nmol/plate   JMCMAR 25,593,82
MUT: oms-rat-orl 25 μmol/kg   CBINA8 24,355,79

CONSENSUS REPORTS: EPA Genetic Toxicology Program.

SAFETY PROFILE: Questionable carcinogen with experimental carcinogenic and tumorigenic data. Mutation data reported. When heated to decomposition it emits toxic fumes of NO_x.

SMS000 CAS: 63019-73-8
5-STYRYL-3,4-BENZOPYRENE
mf: $C_{28}H_{18}$ mw: 354.46

SYN: 6-STYRYL-BENZO(a)PYRENE

TOXICITY DATA with REFERENCE
ETA: scu-mus TDLo:200 mg/kg   COREAF 245,876,57

SAFETY PROFILE: Questionable carcinogen with experimental tumorigenic data. When heated to decomposition it emits acrid smoke and irritating fumes.

SMT500 CAS: 843-23-2
trans-N-(p-STYRYLPHENYL) ACETOHYDROXAMIC ACID
mf: $C_{16}H_{15}NO_2$ mw: 253.32

SYNS: HAAS ◇ trans-N-HYDROXY-4-ACETAMIDOSTILBENE ◇ trans-N-HYDROXY-4-ACETYLAMINOSTILBENE ◇ trans-N-HYDROXY-ASS

TOXICITY DATA with REFERENCE
CAR: orl-rat TD:273 mg/kg/13W-I   CNREA8 24,128,64
CAR: orl-rat TD:448 mg/kg/32W-C   BJCAAI 22,133,68
CAR: orl-rat TDLo:140 mg/kg/20W-I   ZEKBAI 74,200,70
CAR: scu-rat TD:37 mg/kg/4W-I   BJCAAI 22,133,68
CAR: scu-rat TDLo:34 mg/kg/4W-I   CNREA8 24,128,64
MUT: dnd-rat-ipr 40 mg/kg   CRNGDP 5,231,84
MUT: mma-sat 2500 pmol/plate   JMCMAR 25,593,82
MUT: mrc-smc 10 ppm   ZEKBAI 74,412,70

SAFETY PROFILE: Questionable carcinogen with experimental carcinogenic data. Mutation

data reported. When heated to decomposition it emits toxic fumes of NO_x.

SMU000   CAS: 63021-62-5
trans-N-(p-STYRYLPHENYL) ACETOHYDROXAMIC ACID, COPPER(2+) COMPLEX
mf: $C_{32}H_{28}N_2O_4 \cdot Cu$ mw: 568.16

SYNS: COPPER complex with trans-N-(p-STYRYL-PHENYL)ACETOHYDROXAMIC ACID ◇ trans-N-HY-DROXY-4-ACETYLAMINOSTILBENE CUPRIC CHELATE

TOXICITY DATA with REFERENCE
CAR: scu-rat TD: 75 mg/kg/4W-I   CNREA8 24,128,64
CAR: scu-rat TDLo: 30 mg/kg/1W-I   CNREA8 24,128,64

CONSENSUS REPORTS: Copper and its compounds are on the Community Right To Know List.

SAFETY PROFILE: Questionable carcinogen with experimental carcinogenic data. When heated to decomposition it emits toxic fumes of NO_x.

SNC000   CAS: 108-30-5
SUCCINIC ANHYDRIDE
mf: $C_4H_4O_3$ mw: 100.08

PROP: Colorless needles. Mp: 119.6°, bp: 261°, d: 1.104, vap press: 1 mm @ 92.0°. Very sltly sol in water, petr ether; sltly sol in ether.

SYNS: BERNSTEINSAURE-ANHYDRID (GERMAN) ◇ BUTANEDIOIC ANHYDRIDE ◇ DIHYDRO-2,5-FURAN-DIONE ◇ 2,5-DIKETOTETRAHYDROFURAN ◇ NCI-C55696 ◇ SUCCINIC ACID ANHYDRIDE ◇ SUCCINYL OXIDE ◇ TETRAHYDRO-2,5-DIOXOFURAN

TOXICITY DATA with REFERENCE
NEO: scu-rat TDLo: 2600 mg/kg/65W-I   BJCAAI 19,392,65
MUT: mmo-esc 2 g/L   MUREAV 130,97,84
MUT: otr-ham: emb 100 µg/L   IJCNAW 19,642,77

CONSENSUS REPORTS: IARC Cancer Review: Animal Inadequate Evidence IMEMDT 15,265,77. Reported in EPA TSCA Inventory. EPA Genetic Toxicology Program.

SAFETY PROFILE: Questionable carcinogen with experimental neoplastigenic and teratogenic data. Mutation data reported. A severe eye irritant. When heated to decomposition it emits acrid smoke and irritating fumes.

SND500   CAS: 128-09-6
SUCCINOCHLORIMIDE
mf: $C_4H_4ClNO_2$ mw: 133.54

PROP: Rhombic crystals from benzene; odor of chlorine. D: 1.65, mp: 148°. Acid to litmus (1:50 aq soln). One gram dissolves in about 70 mL water, 150 mL alc, 50 mL benzene. Sparingly sol in ether, chloroform, carbon tetrachloride.

SYNS: 1-CHLORO-2,5-PYRROLIDINEDIONE ◇ N-CHLOR-SUCCINIMIDE ◇ SUCCINCHLORIMIDE

TOXICITY DATA with REFERENCE
ETA: scu-mus TDLo: 840 mg/kg/70W-I   JNCIAM 53,695,74

CONSENSUS REPORTS: EPA Genetic Toxicology Program.

SAFETY PROFILE: Questionable carcinogen with experimental tumorigenic data. Poison by intravenous route. Moderately toxic by ingestion. Stored as a dust it heats spontaneously. When heated to decomposition it emits toxic fumes of Cl^- and NO_x.

SNF500   CAS: 63042-13-7
4'-SUCCINYLAMINO-2,3'-DIMETHYLAZOBENZOL
mf: $C_{18}H_{19}N_3O_3$ mw: 325.40

SYNS: 4'-SUCCINOYLAMINO-2,3'-DIMETHYLAZOBEN-ZENE ◇ N-(4'-o-TOLYL-o-TOLYLAZOSUCCINAMIC ACID

TOXICITY DATA with REFERENCE
ETA: orl-rat TDLo: 94 g/kg/54W-C   GANNA2 33,196,39

SAFETY PROFILE: Questionable carcinogen with experimental tumorigenic data. When heated to decomposition it emits toxic fumes of NO_x.

SNI000   CAS: 58098-08-1
SULFACOMBIN

PROP: Mixture of sulfamerazine (26%), sulfadiazine (37%), and sulfathiazole (37%).

TOXICITY DATA with REFERENCE
ETA: par-rat TDLo: 400 mg/kg   ACRAAX 37,258,52

SAFETY PROFILE: Questionable carcinogen with experimental tumorigenic data. When heated to decomposition it emits very toxic fumes of NO_x and SO_x.

SNJ000   CAS: 57-68-1
SULFADIMETHYLDIAZINE
mf: $C_{12}H_{14}N_4O_2S$ mw: 278.36

PROP: Crystals; odorless. Mp: 176° (also a range reported of from 178-179°, 198-199°, and 205-207°). Sol in acetone, water, ether; sltly sol in alc.

SYNS: A-502 ◇ 2-(p-AMINOBENZENESULFONAMIDO)-4,6-DIMETHYLPYRIMIDINE ◇ 6-(4'-AMINOBENZOL-SUL-FONAMIDO)-2,4-DIMETHYLPYRIMIDIN (GERMAN) ◇ (p-AMINOBENZOLSULFONYL)-2-AMINO-4,6-DIMETHYL-PYRIMIDIN (GERMAN) ◇ AZOLMETAZIN ◇ CREMOME-THAZINE ◇ DIAZYL ◇ N¹-(4,6-DIMETHYL-2-PYRIMIDINYL)SULFANILAMIDE ◇ N-(4,6-DIMETHYL-2-PYRIMIDYL)SULFANILAMIDE ◇ 4,6-DIMETHYL-2-SULFANILAMIDO-PYRIMIDINE ◇ DIMEZATHINE ◇ MERMETH ◇ METAZIN ◇ NCI-C56600 ◇ NEASINA ◇ PIRMAZIN ◇ PRIMAZIN ◇ SA 111 ◇ SEAZINA ◇ SPANBOLET ◇ SULFADIMERAZINE ◇ SULFADIMETHYLDIAZINE ◇ SULFADIMETHYLPYRIMI-DINE ◇ SULFADIMETINE ◇ SULFADIMEZINE ◇ SULFA-DIMIDINE ◇ SULFADINE ◇ SULFADSIMESINE ◇ SULFA-ISODIMERAZINE ◇ SULFAISODIMIDINE ◇ SULFAMETHIA-ZINE ◇ SULFAMETHIN ◇ SULFAMEZATHINE ◇ 2-SULFA-NILAMIDO-4,6-DIMETHYLPYRIMIDINE ◇ SULFISOMIDIN ◇ SULFISOMIDINE ◇ SULFODIMESIN ◇ SULFODIME-ZINE ◇ SULMET ◇ SULPHADIMETHYLPYRIMIDINE ◇ SULPHADIMIDINE ◇ SUPERSEPTIL ◇ VERTOLAN

TOXICITY DATA with REFERENCE
ETA: imp-rat TDLo:5000 mg/kg ACRAAX 37,258,52

CONSENSUS REPORTS: Reported in EPA TSCA Inventory.

SAFETY PROFILE: Questionable carcinogen with experimental tumorigenic and teratogenic data. Moderately toxic by intravenous and intra-peritoneal routes. Mildly toxic by ingestion. Experimental reproductive effects. When heated to decomposition it emits very toxic fumes of SO_x and NO_x.

SNK000   CAS: 723-46-6
SULFAMETHOXAZOL
mf: $C_{10}H_{11}N_3O_3S$ mw: 253.30

SYNS: 4-AMINO-N-(5-METHYL-3-ISOXAZOLYL)BEN-ZENESULFONAMIDE ◇ 3-(p-AMINOPHENYLSULPHONA-MIDO)-5-METHYLISOXAZOLE ◇ AZO-GANTANOL ◇ BAC-TRIM ◇ CO-TRIMOXAZOLE ◇ EUSAPRIM ◇ FECTRIM ◇ GANTANOL ◇ N'-(5-METHYL-3-ISOXAZOLE)SULFA-NILAMIDE ◇ N'-(5-METHYL-3-ISOXAZOLYL)SULFANILA-MIDE ◇ N'-(5-METHYLISOXAZOL-3-YL)SULPHANILA-MIDE ◇ N¹-(5-METHYL-3-ISOXAZOLYL)SULPHANILA-MIDE ◇ 5-METHYL-3-SULFANILAMIDOISOXAZOLE ◇ 5-METHYL-3-SULPHANIL-AMIDOISOXAZOLE

◇ METOXAL ◇ MS 53 ◇ RADONIL ◇ RO 4-2130 ◇ SIM ◇ SINOMIN ◇ SEPTRA ◇ SEPTRAN ◇ SULFAMETHAL-AZOLE ◇ SULFAMETHOXAZOLE ◇ SULFAMETHYL-ISOXAZOLE ◇ 3-SULFANILAMIDO-5-METHYLISOXAZOLE ◇ SULFISOMEZOLE ◇ SULPHAMETHALAZOLE ◇ SULPHA-METHOXAZOL ◇ SULPHAMETHOXAZOLE ◇ SULPHA-METHYLISOXAZOLE ◇ 3-SULPHANILAMIDO-5-METHYL-ISOXAZOLE ◇ SULPHISOMEZOLE ◇ TRIB ◇ TRIMETO-PRIM-SULFA

TOXICITY DATA with REFERENCE
ETA: orl-rat TDLo:21 g/kg/60W-C TXAPA9 24,351,73

CONSENSUS REPORTS: IARC Cancer Review: GROUP 3 IMEMDT 7,348,87; Human Inadequate Evidence IMEMDT 24,285,80; Animal Limited Evidence IMEMDT 24,285,80. Reported in EPA TSCA Inventory.

SAFETY PROFILE: Questionable carcinogen with experimental tumorigenic data. Moderately toxic by ingestion and intraperitoneal routes. When heated to decomposition it emits very toxic fumes of NO_x and SO_x.

SNM500   CAS: 63-74-1
SULFANILAMIDE
mf: $C_6H_8N_2O_2S$ mw: 172.22

PROP: Crystals. Mp: 164.5-166.5°. Sol in glycerol, propylene glycol, HCl; almost insol in chloroform, ether, benzene, petr ether.

SYNS: ALBEXAN ◇ ALBOSAL ◇ AMBESIDE ◇ p-AMINO-BENZENESULFAMIDE ◇ p-AMINOBENZENESULFONAMIDE ◇ 4-AMINOBENZENESULFONAMIDE ◇ p-AMINOPHENYL-SULFONAMIDE ◇ 4-AMINOPHENYLSULFONAMIDE ◇ p-ANILINESULFONAMIDE ◇ ANILINE-p-SULFONIC AMIDE ◇ ANTISTREPT ◇ BACTERAMID ◇ COLLOMIDE ◇ COLSULANYDE ◇ COPTICIDE ◇ DIPRON ◇ ESTREPTO-CIDA ◇ F 1162 ◇ FOURNEAU 1162 ◇ GERISON ◇ GOMBAR-DOL ◇ LUSIL ◇ LYSOCOCCINE ◇ NEOCOCCYL ◇ ORGASEPTINE ◇ PABS ◇ PRONTALBIN ◇ PRONTOSIL I ◇ PROSEPTINE ◇ PROSEPTOL ◇ PYSOCOCCINE ◇ RUBIAZOL A ◇ SEPTAMIDE ALBUM ◇ SEPTINAL ◇ SEPTOPLEX ◇ STOPTON ALBUM ◇ STREPAMIDE ◇ STREPTAGOL ◇ STREPTOCLASE ◇ STREPTOL ◇ STREPTOSIL ◇ STREPTOZONE ◇ STREPTROCIDE ◇ p-SULFAMIDOANILINE ◇ SULFAMIDYL ◇ SULFANA ◇ SULFANALONE ◇ SULFANIL ◇ SULFOCIDINE ◇ SULFONAMIDE ◇ SULFONAMIDE P ◇ SULPHANILAMIDE ◇ THERAPOL ◇ WHITE STREPTOCIDE

TOXICITY DATA with REFERENCE
CAR: scu-rat TDLo:135 mg/kg/9W-I PSEBAA 68,330,48

MUT: dnd-esc 50 μmol/L   MUREAV 89,95,81
MUT: dnd-rat:lvr 30 μmol/L   SinJF# 26OCT82
MUT: mmo-esc 50 μg/disc   APMBAY 6,23,58
MUT: mmo-sat 10 μL/plate   ANYAA9 76,475,58

CONSENSUS REPORTS: Reported in EPA TSCA Inventory. EPA Genetic Toxicology Program.

SAFETY PROFILE: Questionable carcinogen with experimental carcinogenic and teratogenic data. Poison by ingestion and intraperitoneal routes. Moderately toxic by subcutaneous and intravenous routes. Human teratogenic effects by unspecified route: developmental abnormalities of the blood and lymphatic systems (including the spleen and bone marrow). Experimental reproductive effects. Mutation data reported. Implicated in aplastic anemia. When heated to decomposition it emits very toxic fumes of NO_x and SO_x.

SNN500   CAS: 127-69-5
5-SULFANILAMIDO-3,4-DIMETHYL-ISOXAZOLE
mf: $C_{11}H_{13}N_3O_3S$ mw: 267.33

SYNS: ACCUZOLE ◇ AMIDOXAL ◇ 5-(p-AMINOBEN-ZENESULFONAMIDO)-3,4-DIMETHYLISOOXALE ◇ 5-(p-AMINOBENZENESULFONAMIDO)-3,4-DIMETHYLISOXA-ZOLE ◇ 5-(p-AMINOBENZENESULPHONAMIDO)-3,4-DIMETHYLISOXAZOLE ◇ 5-(p-AMINOBENZENESULPHON-AMIDE)-3,4-DIMETHYLISOXAZOLE ◇ 5-(4-AMINOPHENYL-SULFONAMIDO)-3,4-DIMETHYLISOXAZOLE ◇ 5-(4-AMINO-PHENYLSULPHONAMIDO)-3,4-DIMETHYLISOXAZOLE ◇ 4-AMINO-N-(3,4-DIMETHYL-5-ISOXAZOLYL)BENZENE-SULPHONAMIDE ◇ ASTRAZOLO ◇ AZO GANTRISIN ◇ AZOSULFIZIN ◇ BACTESULF ◇ BARAZAE ◇ CHE-MOUAG ◇ 3,4-DIMETHYLISOXALE-5-SULFANILAMIDE ◇ 3,4-DIMETHYLISOXALE-5-SULPHANILAMIDE ◇ N(^{1})-(3,4-DIMETHYL-5-ISOXAZOLYL)SULFANILAMIDE ◇ N′-(3,4)DIMETHYLISOXAZOL-5-YL-SULPHANILAMIDE ◇ N(^{1})(3,4-DIMETHYL-5-ISOXAZOLYL)SULPHANIL-AMIDE ◇ 3,4-DIMETHYL-5-SULFANILAMIDOISOXAZOLE ◇ 3,4-DIMETHYL-5-SULPHANILAMIDOISOXAZOLE ◇ 3,4-DIMETHYL-5-SULPHONAMIDOISOXAZOLE ◇ DORSULFAN ◇ ENTUSIL ◇ GANTRISINE ◇ ISOXAMIN ◇ J-SUL ◇ KORO-SULF ◇ NEOXAZOL ◇ NORIL-GAN-S ◇ NOVOSAXAZOLE ◇ PANCID ◇ RENOSULFAN ◇ RESOXOL ◇ ROXOSUL TABLETS ◇ SAXOSOZINE ◇ SODIZOLE ◇ SOXISOL ◇ STANSIN ◇ SULFADI-METHYLISOXAZOLE ◇ SULFAFURAZOL ◇ SULFAGAN ◇ SULFASOXAZOLE ◇ SULFAZOLE ◇ SULFISIN ◇ SULFISOX-AZOLE ◇ SULFIZOLE ◇ SULPHADIMETHYL-ISOXAZOLE ◇ SULPHAFURAZ ◇ 5-SULPHANILAMIDO-3,4-

DIMETHYL-ISOXAZOLE ◇ SULPHISOXAZOL ◇ SULPHO-FURAZOLE ◇ THIASIN ◇ UNISULF ◇ URISOXIN ◇ URITRI-SIN ◇ UROGAN ◇ VAGILIA

CONSENSUS REPORTS: IARC Cancer Review: GROUP 3 IMEMDT 7,347,87; Human Inadequate Evidence IMEMDT 24,275,80; Animal Inadequate Evidence IMEMDT 24,275,80. NCI Carcinogenesis Bioassay (gavage); No Evidence: mouse, rat NCITR* NCI-CG-TR-138,79. Reported in EPA TSCA Inventory.

SAFETY PROFILE: Questionable carcinogen. Mildly toxic by ingestion. An experimental teratogen. Experimental reproductive effects. When heated to decomposition it emits very toxic fumes of SO_x and NO_x.

SNW800   CAS: 2435-64-5
4-SULFONAMIDE-4′-DIMETHYLAMINOAZOBENZENE
mf: $C_{14}H_{16}N_4O_2S$ mw: 304.40

SYN: BENZENESULFONAMIDE, p-((p-(DIMETHYL-AMINO)PHENYL)AZO)-

TOXICITY DATA with REFERENCE
ETA: orl-rat TDLo: 15 g/kg/55W-C   BJCAAI 10,129,56

SAFETY PROFILE: Questionable carcinogen with experimental tumorigenic data. When heated to decomposition it emits toxic fumes of NO_x and SO_x.

SNX000   CAS: 63019-42-1
4-SULFONAMIDO-3′-METHYL-4′-AMINOAZOBENZENE
mf: $C_{13}H_{14}N_4O_2S$ mw: 290.37

SYN: p-((4-AMINO-m-TOLYL)AZO)BENZENESULFONA-MIDE

TOXICITY DATA with REFERENCE
ETA: orl-rat TDLo: 20 g/kg/87W-C   BJCAAI 10,129,56

SAFETY PROFILE: Questionable carcinogen with experimental tumorigenic data. When heated to decomposition it emits very toxic fumes of SO_x and NO_x.

SNY500   CAS: 77-46-3
4′,4′′′-SULFONYLBIS(ACETANILIDE)
mf: $C_{16}H_{16}N_2O_4S$ mw: 332.40

SYNS: ACEDAPSONE ◇ ACETAMIN ◇ ATILON ◇ BA 2650 ◇ BIS(p-ACETAMIDOPHENYL) SULFONE

◇ BIS(4-ACETAMIDOPHENYL)SULFONE ◇ CAMILAN ◇ C.I. 556 ◇ DADDS ◇ 4,4'-DIACETAMIDODIPHENYL SULFONE ◇ DI-(p-ACETYLAMINOPHENYL)SULFONE ◇ DIACETYLDAPSONE ◇ N,N'-DIACETYLDAPSONE ◇ 4,4'-DIACETYLDIAMINODIPHENYL SULFONE ◇ N,N'-DIACETYL-4,4'-DIAMINODIPHENYL SULFONE ◇ 1399 F ◇ HANSOLAR ◇ RODILONE ◇ SULFADIAMINE ◇ SULFODIAMINE ◇ p,p'-SULFONYLBISACETANILIDE ◇ 4,4'-SULFONYLBISACETANILIDE

TOXICITY DATA with REFERENCE
CAR: orl-rat TDLo:4200 mg/kg/43W-C
    JNCIAM 24,149,60

SAFETY PROFILE: Questionable carcinogen with experimental carcinogenic data. When heated to decomposition it emits very toxic fumes of NO_x and SO_x.

SOA500
4,4'-SULFONYLDIANILINE
CAS: 80-08-0

mf: $C_{12}H_{12}N_2O_2S$ mw: 248.32

PROP: Crystals. Mp: 176°, vap d: 8.3. Nearly insol in water; sol in acetone, alc.

SYNS: AVLOSULPHONE ◇ BIS(p-AMINOPHENYL) SULFONE ◇ BIS(4-AMINOPHENYL) SULFONE ◇ BIS(p-AMINOPHENYL)SULPHONE ◇ BIS(4-AMINOPHENYL)SULPHONE ◇ CROYSULFONE ◇ DADPS ◇ DAPSONE ◇ DDS ◇ DIAMINODIFENILSULFONA (SPANISH) ◇ DIAMINO-4,4'-DIPHENYL SULFONE ◇ p,p'-DIAMINODIPHENYL SULFONE ◇ 4,4'-DIAMINODIPHENYL SULFONE ◇ DIAMINO-4,4'-DIPHENYL SULPHONE ◇ p,p-DIAMINODIPHENYL SULPHONE ◇ DI(p-AMINOPHENYL) SULFONE ◇ DI(4-AMINOPHENYL) SULFONE ◇ DI(p-AMINOPHENYL)SULPHONE ◇ DI(4-AMINOPHENYL)SULPHONE ◇ DIAPHENYLSULFONE ◇ DIAPHENYLSULPHON ◇ DIAPHENYLSULPHONE ◇ DIPHONE ◇ DISULONE ◇ DSS ◇ DUBRONAX ◇ DUMITONE ◇ EPORAL ◇ 1358F ◇ F 1358 ◇ MALOPRIM ◇ METABOLITE C ◇ NCI-C01718 ◇ NOVOPHONE ◇ NSC-6091 ◇ SULFONA ◇ 1,1'-SULFONYLBIS(4-AMINOBENZENE) ◇ 4,4'-SULFONYLBISANILINE ◇ p,p-SULFONYLBISBENZAMINE ◇ 4,4'-SULFONYLBISBENZAMINE ◇ p,p-SULFONYLBISBENZENAMINE ◇ p,p'-SULFONYLDIANILINE ◇ SULPHADIONE ◇ SULPHON-MERE ◇ 1,1'-SULPHONYLBIS(4-AMINOBENZENE) ◇ p,p-SULPHONYLBISBENZAMINE ◇ 4,4'-SULPHONYLBISBENZAMINE ◇ p,p-SULPHONYLBISBENZENAMINE ◇ 4,4'-SULPHONYLBISBENZENAMINE ◇ SULPHONYLDIANILINE ◇ p,p-SULPHONYLDIANILINE ◇ TARIMYL ◇ UDOLAC ◇ WR 448

TOXICITY DATA with REFERENCE
CAR: orl-rat TD:39 g/kg/78W-C NCITR* NCI-CG-TR-20,77
CAR: orl-rat TD:52 g/kg/2Y-I IJCNAW 25,123,80

CAR: orl-rat TD:78450 mg/kg/2Y-C ALEPA8 53,11,73
CAR: orl-rat TDLo:20 g/kg/80W-C NCITR* NCI-CG-TR-20,77
NEO: ipr-mus TDLo:1312 mg/kg/8W-I CNREA8 33,3069,73
NEO: orl-rat TD:21840 mg/kg/2Y-C FCTOD7 25,619,87
MUT: cyt-hmn-leu 4 mg/L IJLEAG 43,41,75

CONSENSUS REPORTS: IARC Cancer Review: GROUP 3 IMEMDT 7,185,87; Animal Limited Evidence IMEMDT 24,59,80; Human Inadequate Evidence IMEMDT 24,59,80. NCI Carcinogenesis Bioassay (feed); No Evidence: mouse NCITR* NCI-CG-TR-20,77; (feed); Clear Evidence: rat NCITR* NCI-CG-TR-20,77. Reported in EPA TSCA Inventory.

SAFETY PROFILE: Questionable carcinogen with experimental carcinogenic and neoplastigenic data. Poison by ingestion, intraperitoneal, and subcutaneous routes. Moderately toxic by unspecified route. Human systemic effects by ingestion: retinal changes, somnolence, cyanosis, jaundice, change in tubules and other kidney changes, hemolysis with or without anemia and effect on joints. Human mutation data reported. Experimental reproductive effects. Can cause hepatitis, dermatitis, and neuritis. Used in leprosy treatment and veterinary medicine. When heated to decomposition it emits very toxic fumes of NO_x and SO_x.

SOD200
SULFOTRINAPHTHYLENOFURAN, SODIUM SALT

mf: $C_{30}H_{14}O_{14}S_3 \cdot 3Na$ mw: 763.59

TOXICITY DATA with REFERENCE
ETA: ipr-mus TDLo:367 mg/kg/43W-I
    VOONAW 29(2),67,83

SAFETY PROFILE: Questionable carcinogen with experimental tumorigenic data. Poison by subcutaneous and intraperitoneal routes. Mildly toxic by ingestion. When heated to decomposition it emits toxic fumes of SO_x and Na_2O.

SOH500
SULFUR DIOXIDE
CAS: 7446-09-5

DOT: 1079
mf: O_2S mw: 64.06

PROP: Colorless gas or liquid under pressure; pungent odor. Mp: −75.5°, bp: −10.0°, d (liquid): 1.434 @ 0°, vap d: 2.264 @ 0°, vap press: 2538 mm @ 21.1°. Sol in water.

SYNS: BISULFITE ◇ FERMENICIDE LIQUID ◇ FERMENICIDE POWDER ◇ SCHWEFELDIOXYD (GERMAN) ◇ SIARKI DWUTLENEK (POLISH) ◇ SULFUROUS ACID ANHYDRIDE ◇ SULFUROUS ANHYDRIDE ◇ SULFUROUS OXIDE ◇ SULFUR OXIDE ◇ SULPHUR DIOXIDE, LIQUEFIED (DOT)

TOXICITY DATA with REFERENCE
ETA: ihl-mus TCLo: 500 ppm/5M/30W-I
    BJCAAI 21,606,67
MUT: dnd-hmn: lym 5700 ppb   MUREAV 39,149,77
MUT: dni-hmn: lym 5700 ppb   MUREAV 39,149,77
MUT: mmo-omi 10 mmol/L   MUREAV 39,149,77
MUT: mmo-smc 5 μmol/L   MUREAV 39,149,77
MUT: oms-esc 2 mmol/L   CBINA8 43,289,83
MUT: oms-hmn: lym 5700 ppb   MUREAV 39,149,77
MUT: sln-dmg-orl 200 μmol/L   MUREAV 39,149,77

CONSENSUS REPORTS: EPA Extremely Hazardous Substances List. Reported in EPA TSCA Inventory. EPA Genetic Toxicology Program.

OSHA PEL: (Transitional: TWA 5 ppm) TWA 2 ppm; STEL 5 ppm   ACGIH TLV: TWA 2 ppm; STEL 5 ppm   DFG MAK: 2 ppm (5 mg/m³)   NIOSH REL: (Sulfur Dioxide) TWA 0.5 ppm   DOT Classification: Nonflammable Gas; Label: Nonflammable Gas; Poison A; Label: Poison Gas

SAFETY PROFILE: Questionable carcinogen with experimental tumorigenic and teratogenic data. A poison gas. Experimental reproductive effects. Human mutation data reported. Human systemic effects by inhalation: pulmonary vascular resistance, respiratory depression and other pulmonary changes. A corrosive irritant to eyes, skin, and mucous membranes. A nonflammable gas. When heated to decomposition it emits toxic fumes of SO_x.

SOT000   CAS: 7791-25-5
SULFURYL CHLORIDE
DOT: 1834
mf: Cl_2O_2S mw: 134.96

PROP: Colorless liquid; pungent odor. Mp: −54.1°, bp: 69.1°, d: 1.6674, vap press: 100 mm @ 17.8°, vap d: 4.65.

SYNS: SULFONYL CHLORIDE ◇ SULFURIC OXYCHLORIDE

TOXICITY DATA with REFERENCE
ETA: skn-mus TDLo: 2850 mg/kg/1Y-I   GISAAA 47(7),9,82

CONSENSUS REPORTS: Reported in EPA TSCA Inventory.

DOT Classification: Corrosive Material; Label: Corrosive

SAFETY PROFILE: Questionable carcinogen with experimental tumorigenic data. A corrosive irritant to skin, eyes, and mucous membranes. Can explode with PbO_2. Will react with water or steam to produce heat and toxic and corrosive fumes. When heated to decomposition it emits highly toxic fumes of Cl^- and SO_x.

SOY500   CAS: 1401-55-4
SWEET GUM

PROP: Tannin containing fraction of leaf used.

SYNS: LIQUIDAMBAR STYRACIFLUA ◇ TANNIN from SWEET GUM

TOXICITY DATA with REFERENCE
NEO: scu-rat TDLo: 1100 mg/kg/56W-I
    JNCIAM 57,207,76

CONSENSUS REPORTS: Reported in EPA TSCA Inventory.

SAFETY PROFILE: Questionable carcinogen with experimental neoplastigenic data.

SPB500   CAS: 22571-95-5
SYMPHYTINE
mf: $C_{20}H_{31}NO_6$ mw: 381.52

SYNS: 2-METHYLBUTENOIC ACID-7-((2,3-DIHYDROXY-2-(1-METHYLETHYL)-1-OXOBUTOXY)METHYL-2,3,5,7a-TETRAHYDRO-1H-PYRROLIZIN-1-YL ESTER ◇ 7-TIGLYL-RETRONECINE VIRIDIFLORATE ◇ 7-TIGLYL-9-VIRIDI-FLORYLRETRONECINE

TOXICITY DATA with REFERENCE
ETA: ipr-rat TDLo: 780 mg/kg/56W-I   JJIND8 63,469,79

CONSENSUS REPORTS: IARC Cancer Review: Animal Inadequate Evidence IMEMDT 31,239,83.

SAFETY PROFILE: Questionable carcinogen with experimental tumorigenic data. Poison by intraperitoneal route. When heated to decomposition it emits toxic fumes of NO_x.

TAB250   CAS: 51481-61-9
TAGAMET
mf: $C_{10}H_{16}N_6S$ mw: 252.38

SYNS: CIMETIDINE ◇ N-CYANO-N'-METHYL-N''-(2-(((5-METHYL-1H-IMIDAZOL-4-YL)METHYL)THIO)ETHYL) GUANIDINE ◇ 1-CYANO-2-METHYL-3-(2-(((5-METHYL-4-IMIDAZOLYL)METHYL)THIO)ETHYL)GUANIDINE ◇ 2-CYANO-1-METHYL-3-(2-(((5-METHYLIMIDAZOL-4-YL)METHYL)THIO)ETHYL)GUANIDINE ◇ EURECEPTOR ◇ FPF 1002 ◇ GASTROMET ◇ SKF 92334 ◇ TAMETIN ◇ TRATUL ◇ ULCEDINE ◇ ULCIMET ◇ ULCOMET

TOXICITY DATA with REFERENCE

ETA: orl-rat TD:39312 mg/kg/2Y-C TXAPA9 61,119,81

ETA: orl-rat TD:98800 mg/kg/2Y-C TXAPA9 61,119,81

ETA: orl-rat TDLo:15600 mg/kg/2Y-C TXAPA9 61,119,81

CONSENSUS REPORTS: Cyanide and its compounds are on the Community Right-To-Know List. EPA Genetic Toxicology Program.

SAFETY PROFILE: Questionable carcinogen with experimental tumorigenic and teratogenic data. Experimental poison by intravenous and intraperitoneal routes. Moderately toxic to humans by ingestion. Moderately toxic experimentally by ingestion and subcutaneous routes. Human systemic effects by ingestion, intravenous, and possibly other routes: anorexia, muscle weakness, blood pressure decrease, gastritis and other gastrointestinal changes, hepatitis, jaundice, tubule changes, endocrine changes, leukopenia, sweating, changes to hair and fever. Human reproductive and teratogenic effects by unspecified route: developmental abnormalities of the hepatobiliary system and effects on newborn including apgar score. Experimental reproductive effects. An antagonist to histamine H2 receptors used in the treatment of peptic ulcers and alergic dermititus. When heated to decomposition it emits very toxic fumes of NO_x, CN^-, and SO_x.

TAB750   CAS: 14807-96-6
TALC (powder)
mf: $H_2O_3Si \cdot 3/4Mg$ mw: 96.33

PROP: White to grayish-white, fine powder; odorless and tasteless. Powdered native hydrous magnesium silicate. Insol in water, cold acids, or alkalies. Containing less than 1% crystalline silica.

SYNS: AGALITE ◇ AGI TALC, BC 1615 ◇ ALPINE TALC USP, BC 127 ◇ ALPINE TALC USP, BC 141 ◇ ALPINE TALC USP, BC 662 ◇ ASBESTINE ◇ C.I. 77718 ◇ DESERTALC 57 ◇ EMTAL 596 ◇ FIBRENE C 400 ◇ LO MICRON TALC 1 ◇ LO MICRON TALC, BC 1621 ◇ LO MICRON TALC USP, BC 2755 ◇ METRO TALC 4604 ◇ METRO TALC 4608 ◇ METRO TALC 4609 ◇ MISTRON FROST P ◇ MISTRON RCS ◇ MISTRON 2SC ◇ MISTRON STAR ◇ MISTRON SUPER FROST ◇ MISTRON VAPOR ◇ MP 12-50 ◇ MP 25-38 ◇ MP 45-26 ◇ NCI-C06008 ◇ NO. 907 METRO TALC ◇ NYTAL ◇ OOS ◇ OXO ◇ PURTALC USP ◇ SIERRA C-400 ◇ SNOWGOOSE ◇ STEAWHITE ◇ SUPREME DENSE ◇ TALCUM

TOXICITY DATA with REFERENCE
ETA: ihl-rat TCLo:11 mg/m³/1Y-I 43GRAK -,389,79

CONSENSUS REPORTS: Reported in EPA TSCA Inventory.

OSHA PEL: (Transitional: TWA 20 mppcf (containing no asbestos fibers)) TWA 2 mg/m³ ACGIH TLV: TWA 2 mg/m³, respirable dust (use asbestos TLV if asbestos fibers are present) DFG MAK: 2 mg/m³

SAFETY PROFILE: Questionable carcinogen with experimental tumorigenic data. The talc with less than 1 percent asbestos is regarded as a nuisance dust. A human skin irritant. Prolonged or repeated exposure can produce a form of pulmonary fibrosis (talc pneumoconiosis) which may be due to asbestos content. A common air contaminant.

TAD750   CAS: 1401-55-4
TANNIC ACID
mf: $C_{76}H_{52}O_{46}$ mw: 1701.28

PROP: From the nutgalls of *Quercus infectoria Oliver* or seed pods of *Caesalpinia spinosa* or the nutgalls of various sumac species. Yellowish-white or brown, bulky powder or flakes; odorless with astringent taste. Mp: 200°, flash p: 390°F (OC), autoign temp: 980°F. Very sol in water, alc, acetone; almost insol in benzene, chloroform, ether, petr ether, carbon disulfide.

SYNS: d'ACIDE TANNIQUE (FRENCH) ◇ GALLOTANNIC ACID ◇ GALLOTANNIN ◇ GLYCERITE ◇ TANNIN

TOXICITY DATA with REFERENCE
CAR: scu-rat TDLo:4450 mg/kg/17W-I AMSHAR 3,353,53
ETA: scu-mus TDLo:750 mg/kg/12W-I BJCAAI 14,147,60
ETA: scu-rat TD:3750 mg/kg/I BAFEAG 37,52,50
ETA: scu-rat TD:4250 mg/kg/17W-I AMSHAR 1,37,51

ETA: scu-rat TD: 4286 mg/kg/20W-I   AMSHAR
1,37,51

MUT: dni-mus-ipr 76 mg/kg   IJEBA6 17,1141,79

MUT: dns-rat-orl 25 g/kg   JJIND8 74,1283,85

CONSENSUS REPORTS: IARC Cancer Review: GROUP 3 IMEMDT 7,56,87; Animal Sufficient Evidence IMEMDT 10,253,76. Reported in EPA TSCA Inventory. EPA Genetic Toxicology Program.

SAFETY PROFILE: Questionable carcinogen with experimental carcinogenic and tumorigenic data. Poison by ingestion, intramuscular, intravenous, and subcutaneous routes. Moderately toxic by parenteral route. Experimental reproductive effects. Mutation data reported. Combustible when exposed to heat or flame. To fight fire, use water. When heated to decomposition it emits acrid smoke and irritating fumes.

TAE250
TANNIN-FREE FRACTION of BRACKEN FERN

SYN: BRACKEN FERN, TANNIN-FREE

TOXICITY DATA with REFERENCE
CAR: orl-rat TDLo: 2000 g/kg/56W-C   JJIND8
65,131,80

SAFETY PROFILE: Questionable carcinogen with experimental carcinogenic data. When heated to decomposition it emits toxic and irritating fumes.

TAE750   CAS: 7440-25-7
TANTALUM
af: Ta   aw: 180.948

PROP: Gray, very hard, malleable, ductile metal. Mp: 2996°; bp: 5429°; d: 16.69. Insol in water.

SYN: TANTALUM-181

TOXICITY DATA with REFERENCE
ETA: imp-rat TDLo: 3760 mg/kg   CNREA8
16,439,56

CONSENSUS REPORTS: Reported in EPA TSCA Inventory.

OSHA PEL: TWA 5 mg/m^3 ACGIH TLV: TWA 5 mg/m^3 DFG MAK: 5 mg/m^3

SAFETY PROFILE: Questionable carcinogen with experimental tumorigenic data. Some industrial skin injuries from tantalum have been reported. Systemic industrial poisoning however, is apparently unknown. The dry powder ignites spontaneously in air.

TAG250
TARWEED

PROP: The seeds containing pyrrolizidine alkaloids are from *Amsinckia intermedia fisch* and *Mey* (JNCIAM 47,1037,71).

SYNS: AMSINCKIA INTERMEDIA ◇ FIDDLE-NECK ◇ SEED of FIDDLENECK

TOXICITY DATA with REFERENCE
ETA: orl-rat TDLo: 275 g/kg (1-22D preg):
REP   JNCIAM 47,1037,71

SAFETY PROFILE: Questionable carcinogen with experimental tumorigenic data. Moderately toxic by ingestion. Experimental reproductive effects. When heated to decomposition it emits acrid smoke and irritating fumes.

TAI250   CAS: 9002-84-0
TEFLON
mf: $(C_2F_4)_n$

PROP: Grayish-white, tough plastic. Chemically very inert.

SYNS: AFLON ◇ ALGLOFLON ◇ ALGOFLON SV ◇ ALKATHENE RXDG33 ◇ AMIP 15m ◇ BALFON 7000 ◇ BDH 29-801 ◇ CHROMOSORB T ◇ DIXON 164 ◇ DLX-6000 ◇ DUROID 5870 ◇ EK 1108GY-A ◇ ETHICON PTFE ◇ FLUO-KEM ◇ FLUON ◇ FLUOROFLEX ◇ FLUOROLON 4 ◇ FLUOROPAK 80 ◇ FLUORPLAST 4 ◇ FTORLON 4 ◇ FTOROPLAST 4 ◇ GORE-TEX ◇ HALON TFEG 180 ◇ HEYDEFLON ◇ HOSTAFLON ◇ MOLYKOTE 522 ◇ POLIFEN ◇ POLITEF ◇ POLY(ETHYLENE TETRAFLUORIDE) ◇ POLYFENE ◇ POLYFLON ◇ POLYTEF ◇ POLYTETRAFLUOROETHENE ◇ POLYTETRAFLUOROETHYLENE ◇ PTFE ◇ SOREFLON 604 ◇ TARFLEN ◇ TEFLON (various) ◇ TETRAFLUOROETHENE HOMOPOLYMER ◇ TETRAFLUOROETHENE POLYMER ◇ TETRAFLUOROETHYLENE HOMOPOLYMER ◇ TETRAFLUOROETHYLENE POLYMERS ◇ TETRAN PTFE ◇ UNON P ◇ VALFLON ◇ VELFLON ◇ ZITEX H 662-124

TOXICITY DATA with REFERENCE
ETA: imp-mus TDLo: 1140 mg/kg   TUMOAB
62,565,76
ETA: imp-rat TDLo: 80 mg/kg   CNREA8 15,333,55

CONSENSUS REPORTS: IARC Cancer Review: GROUP 3 IMEMDT 7,56,87; Animal Sufficient Evidence IMEMDT 19,285,79; Human Inadequate Evidence IMEMDT 19,285,79. Reported in EPA TSCA Inventory.

SAFETY PROFILE: Questionable carcinogen with experimental tumorigenic data by implant. The finished polymerized compound is inert under ordinary conditions. When heated to above 750°F it decomposes to yield highly toxic fumes of F⁻.

TBC500　　CAS: 8001-50-1
TERPENE POLYCHLORINATES

PROP: Chlorinated mixed terpenes (IARC** 4,219,75).

SYNS: DICHLORICIDE MOTHPROOFER ◇ ENT 19,442 ◇ STROBANE

TOXICITY DATA with REFERENCE
CAR: orl-mus TDLo: 1272 mg/kg/79W-I-C
　　JNCIAM 42,1101,69

CONSENSUS REPORTS: IARC Cancer Review: GROUP 3 IMEMDT 7,56,87; Animal Sufficient Evidence IMEMDT 5,219,74.

SAFETY PROFILE: Questionable carcinogen with experimental carcinogenic data. Poison by ingestion and possibly other routes. When heated to decomposition it emits toxic fumes of Cl⁻.

TBD250　　CAS: 64058-92-0
p-TERPHENYL-4-YLACETAMIDE
mf: $C_{20}H_{17}NO$　　mw: 287.38

SYNS: 4-ACETYLAMINO-p-DIPHENYLBENZENE ◇ 4-ACETYLAMINO-p-TERPHENYL

TOXICITY DATA with REFERENCE
ETA: orl-rat TDLo: 7000 mg/kg/43W-C
　　CNREA8 16,525,56

SAFETY PROFILE: Questionable carcinogen with experimental tumorigenic data. When heated to decomposition it emits toxic fumes of NO_x.

TBF750　　CAS: 315-37-7
TESTOSTERONE HEPTANOATE
mf: $C_{26}H_{40}O_3$　　mw: 400.66

SYNS: ANDROTARDYL ◇ ATLATEST ◇ DELATESTRYL ◇ HEPTANOIC ACID, ester with TESTOSTERONE ◇ MALOGEN L.A.200 ◇ NSC-17591 ◇ (17-β)17-((1-OXOHEPTYL)OXY)-ANDROST-4-EN-3-ONE ◇ REPOSO-TMD ◇ TE ◇ TESTATE ◇ TESTOSTERONE ENANTHATE ◇ TESTOSTERONE ETHANATE ◇ TESTOSTERONE HEPTOATE ◇ TESTOSTERONE HEPTYLATE ◇ TESTOSTERONE OENANTHATE ◇ TESTOSTROVAL

TOXICITY DATA with REFERENCE
ETA: ims-rbt TDLo: 409 mg/kg/2Y-I: TER
　　CNREA8 26,474,66

CONSENSUS REPORTS: EPA Genetic Toxicology Program.

SAFETY PROFILE: Questionable carcinogen with experimental tumorigenic and teratogenic data. Poison by intraperitoneal route. Human systemic effects by ingestion: dyspnea. Human reproductive effects by ingestion, intramuscular, parenteral, and possibly other routes: changes in spermatogenesis and paternal effects to testes, epididymis, and sperm duct. Experimental reproductive effects. When heated to decomposition it emits acrid smoke and irritating fumes. A drug used to treat hypoganadism and metastatic breast cancer.

TBG700　　CAS: 2475-45-8
1,4,5,8-TETRAAMINO-9,10-ANTHRACENEDIONE
mf: $C_{14}H_{12}N_4O_2$　　mw: 268.30

SYNS: ACETATE BLUE G ◇ ACETOQUINONE BLUE L ◇ ACETOQUINONE BLUE R ◇ ACETYLON FAST BLUE G ◇ AMACEL BLUE GG ◇ AMACEL PURE BLUE B ◇ ARTISIL BLUE SAP ◇ BRASILAZET BLUE GR ◇ CELANTHRENE PURE BLUE BRS ◇ CELLITON BLUE G ◇ C.I. 64500 ◇ CIBACET SAPPHIRE BLUE G ◇ C.I. DISPERSE BLUE 1 ◇ CILLA BLUE EXTRA ◇ C.I. SOLVENT BLUE 18 ◇ DIACELLITON FAST BLUE R ◇ DISPERSE BLUE NO 1 ◇ DURANOL BRILLIANT BLUE CB ◇ FENACET BLUE G ◇ GRASOL BLUE 2GS ◇ KAYALON FAST BLUE BR ◇ MICROSETILE BLUE EB ◇ MIKETON FAST BLUE ◇ NACELAN BLUE G ◇ NCI-C54900 ◇ NEOSETILE BLUE EB ◇ NYLOQUINONE BLUE 2J ◇ ORACET SAPPHIRE BLUE G ◇ PERLITON BLUE B ◇ SERINYL BLUE 2G ◇ SUPRACET BRILLIANT BLUE 2GN ◇ 1,4,5,8-TETRAAMINOANTHRAQUINONE ◇ 1,4,5,8-TETRAMINOANTHRAQUINONE

TOXICITY DATA with REFERENCE
CAR: orl-rat TD: 180 g/kg/2Y-C　　NTPTR* NTP-TR-299,86
CAR: orl-rat TDLo: 90125 mg/kg/2Y-C　　NTPTR* NTP-TR-299,86
MUT: mmo-sat 33 μg/plate　　NTPTR* NTP-TR-299,86
MUT: mmo-sat 100 μg/plate　　MUREAV 40,203,76

CONSENSUS REPORTS: NTP Carcinogenesis Studies (feed); Equivocal Evidence: mouse NTPTR* NTP-TR-299-86; (feed); Clear Evidence: rat NTPTR* NTP-TR-299,86. Reported in EPA TSCA Inventory.

SAFETY PROFILE: Questionable carcinogen with experimental carcinogenic data. Mutation data reported. When heated to decomposition it emits toxic fumes of NO_x.

TBI750   CAS: 63040-21-1
9,10,14c-15-TETRAAZANAPHTHO(1,2,-3-fg)NAPHTHACENE NITRATE
mf: $C_{21}H_{12}N_4 \cdot xHNO_3$

SYN: ISOTRICYCLOQUINAZOLINE NITRATE

TOXICITY DATA with REFERENCE
ETA: skn-mus TDLo: 1240 mg/kg/Y-I   BJCAAI 17,266,63

SAFETY PROFILE: Questionable carcinogen with experimental tumorigenic data. When heated to decomposition it emits very toxic fumes of NO_x.

TBO500   CAS: 118-75-2
2,3,5,6-TETRACHLORO-1,4-BENZOQUINONE
mf: $C_6Cl_4O_2$ mw: 245.86

PROP: Yellow crystals. Mp: 290°. Insol in water.

SYNS: CHLORANIL ◊ DOW SEED DISINFECTANT NO. 5 ◊ ENT 3,797 ◊ G-25804 ◊ GEIGY-444E ◊ RERANIL ◊ SPERGON I ◊ SPERGON TECHNICAL ◊ TETRACHLORO-BENZOQUINONE ◊ TETRACHLORO-p-BENZOQUINONE ◊ TETRACHLORO-1,4-BENZOQUINONE ◊ 2,3,5,6-TETRA-CHLORO-p-BENZOQUINONE ◊ 2,3,5,6-TETRACHLORO-2,5-CYCLOHEXADIENE-1,4-DIONE ◊ TETRACHLOROQUINONE ◊ TETRACHLORO-p-QUINONE ◊ VULKLOR

TOXICITY DATA with REFERENCE
NEO: orl-mus TDLo: 71 g/kg/78W-I   NTIS** PB223-159

CONSENSUS REPORTS: Reported in EPA TSCA Inventory.

SAFETY PROFILE: Questionable carcinogen with experimental neoplastigenic data. Moderately toxic by ingestion and intraperitoneal routes. Can cause central nervous system depression. May be irritating to skin and mucous membranes. Used as a fungicide. When heated to decomposition it emits highly toxic fumes of Cl^-.

TBQ000   CAS: 630-20-6
1,1,1,2-TETRACHLOROETHANE
mf: $C_2H_2Cl_4$ mw: 167.84

PROP: Liquid. D: 1.588 @ 20/4°, bp: 129-130°. Sol in water; misc in alc, ether.

SYNS: NCI-C52459 ◊ RCRA WASTE NUMBER U208

TOXICITY DATA with REFERENCE
CAR: orl-mus TD: 258 g/kg/2Y-I   NTPTR* NTP-TR-237,82
CAR: orl-mus TDLo: 129 g/kg/2Y-I   NTPTR* NTP-TR-237,82

CONSENSUS REPORTS: IARC Cancer Review: GROUP 3 IMEMDT 7,56,87; Animal Limited Evidence IMEMDT 41,87,86. NTP Carcinogenesis Bioassay (gavage); Clear Evidence: mouse NTPTR* NTP-TR-237,82; (gavage); No Evidence: rat NTPTR* NTP-TR-237,82. Reported in EPA TSCA Inventory.

SAFETY PROFILE: Questionable carcinogen with experimental carcinogenic data. A skin and severe eye irritant. When heated to decomposition it emits very toxic fumes of Cl^-.

TBQ275   CAS: 16650-10-5
TETRACHLOROETHYLENE OXIDE
mf: C_2Cl_4O mw: 181.82

SYNS: EPOXYPERCHLOROVINYL ◊ PCEO ◊ TETRA-CHLOROEPOXYETHANE

TOXICITY DATA with REFERENCE
CAR: skn-mus TDLo: 300 mg/kg/66W-I   CNREA8 43,159,83
ETA: scu-mus TDLo: 20 mg/kg/70W-I   CNREA8 43,159,83
MUT: otr-ham: emb 4300 µmol/L   JJIND8 69,531,82

SAFETY PROFILE: Questionable carcinogen with experimental carcinogenic and tumorigenic data. Mutation data reported. When heated to decomposition it emits toxic fumes of Cl^-.

TBQ750   CAS: 1897-45-6
TETRACHLOROISOPHTHALONITRILE
mf: $C_8Cl_4N_2$ mw: 265.90

SYNS: BRAVO ◊ BRAVO 6F ◊ BRAVO-W-75 ◊ CHLOROALONIL ◊ CHLOROTHALONIL ◊ CHLORTHALONIL (GERMAN) ◊ DAC 2797 ◊ DACONIL ◊ DACONIL 2787 FLOWABLE FUNGICIDE ◊ DACOSOIL ◊ 1,3-DICYANOTETRACHLOROBENZENE ◊ EXOTHERM ◊ EXOTHERM TERMIL ◊ FORTURF ◊ NCI-C00102 ◊ NOPCOCIDE ◊ SWEEP ◊ TCIN ◊ m-TCPN ◊ TERMIL ◊ 2,4,5,6-TETRACHLORO-3-CYANOBENZONITRILE ◊ m-TETRACHLOROPHTHALONITRILE ◊ TPN (pesticide)

TOXICITY DATA with REFERENCE
CAR: orl-rat TDLo: 142 g/kg/80W-C   NCITR*
    NCI-CG-TR-41,78

CONSENSUS REPORTS: IARC Cancer Review: GROUP 3 IMEMDT 7,56,87; Animal Limited Evidence IMEMDT 30,319,83. NCI Carcinogenesis Bioassay (feed); Clear Evidence: rat NCITR* NCI-CG-TR-41,78. Cyanide and its compounds are on the Community Right-To-Know List. Reported in EPA TSCA Inventory. EPA Genetic Toxicology Program.

SAFETY PROFILE: Questionable carcinogen with experimental carcinogenic data. Moderately toxic by intraperitoneal route. Mildly toxic by ingestion. When heated to decomposition it emits very toxic fumes of Cl^-, NO_x, and CN^-.

TBR500   CAS: 3714-62-3
2,3,4,6-TETRACHLORONITROBENZENE
mf: $C_6HCl_4NO_2$ mw: 260.88

SYNS: 4-NITRO-1,2,3,5-TETRACHLORO-BENZENE ◇ 1,2,3,5-TETRACHLORO-4-NITROBENZENE

TOXICITY DATA with REFERENCE
NEO: skn-mus TDLo: 576 mg/kg/12W-I
    CNREA8 26,12,66

SAFETY PROFILE: Questionable carcinogen with experimental neoplastigenic data. When heated to decomposition it emits very toxic fumes of HCl and NO_x.

TBR750   CAS: 117-18-0
2,3,5,6-TETRACHLORONITROBENZENE
mf: $C_6HCl_4NO_2$ mw: 260.88

SYNS: CHIPMAN 3,142 ◇ FOLOSAN ◇ FUSAREX ◇ 3-NITRO-1,2,4,5-TETRACHLOROBENZENE ◇ TCNB ◇ TECNAZEN (GERMAN) ◇ TECNAZENE ◇ 2,3,5,6-TETRACHLOR-3-NITROBENZOL (GERMAN) ◇ 1,2,4,5-TETRACHLORO-3-NITROBENZENE

TOXICITY DATA with REFERENCE
NEO: skn-mus TDLo: 576 mg/kg/12W-I
    CNREA8 26,12,66
MUT: mma-sat 75 μg/plate   ENMUDM 5(Suppl 1),3,83
MUT: mmo-asn 12 μmol/L   PHYTAJ 66,217,76
MUT: mmo-sat 3 μg/plate   ENMUDM 5(Suppl 1),3,83
MUT: sln-asn 24 μmol/L   EVHPAZ 31,81,79

SAFETY PROFILE: Questionable carcinogen with experimental neoplastigenic data. Poison

by unspecified routes. Mildly toxic by ingestion. Mutation data reported. When heated to decomposition it emits very toxic fumes of HCl and NO_x. Used as a pesticide.

TBS000   CAS: 879-39-0
1,2,3,4-TETRACHLORO-5-NITROBENZENE
mf: $C_6HCl_4NO_2$ mw: 260.88

SYNS: DB-905 ◇ FOLOSAN DB-905 FUMITE ◇ FOLSAN ◇ FUSAREX ◇ TCBN ◇ 2,3,4,5-TETRACHLORONITROBENZENE

TOXICITY DATA with REFERENCE
NEO: skn-mus TDLo: 576 mg/kg/12W-I
    CNREA8 26,12,66

SAFETY PROFILE: Questionable carcinogen with experimental neoplastigenic data. When heated to decomposition it emits very toxic fumes of Cl^- and NO_x.

TBX750   CAS: 629-59-4
TETRADECANE
mf: $C_{14}H_{30}$ mw: 198.44

PROP: Colorless liquid. D: 0.765 @ 20/4°, mp: 5.5°, bp: 252-255°, lel: 0.5%, flash p: 212°F, vap press: 1 mm @ 76.4°, vap d: 6.83, autoign temp: 396°F. Insol in water; very sol in alc and ether.

TOXICITY DATA with REFERENCE
ETA: skn-mus TDLo: 9600 mg/kg/20W-I
    TXAPA9 9,70,66

SAFETY PROFILE: Questionable carcinogen with experimental tumorigenic data. Probably irritating and narcotic in high concentrations. Combustible when exposed to heat or flame. Moderate explosion hazard in the form of vapor when exposed to heat or flame. To fight fire, use foam, CO_2, dry chemical. When heated to decomposition it emits acrid smoke and irritating fumes.

TBY500   CAS: 112-72-1
1-TETRADECANOL
mf: $C_{14}H_{30}O$ mw: 214.44

PROP: Opaque leaflets. Mp: 37.62°, bp: 264.1°, flash p: 285°F (OC), d: (solid) 0.8355 @ 20/20°, d: (liquid) 0.8236 @ 38°/4°, vap press: 0.01 mm @ 20°, vap d: 7.39.

SYNS: MYRISIIC ALCOHOL ◇ N-TETRADECANOL-1 ◇ TETRADECYL ALCOHOL ◇ N-TETRADECYL ALCOHOL

TOXICITY DATA with REFERENCE
ETA: skn-mus TDLo: 12 g/kg/24W-I   TXAPA9
9,70,66

CONSENSUS REPORTS: Reported in EPA
TSCA Inventory.

SAFETY PROFILE: Questionable carcinogen
with experimental tumorigenic data. A human
skin irritant. Combustible when exposed to heat
or flame; can react with oxidizing materials.
To fight fire, use CO_2, dry chemical. When
heated to decomposition it emits acrid smoke
and irritating fumes.

TCA250   CAS: 64604-09-7
12-o-TETRADECA-2-cis-4-trans,6,8-
TETRAENOYLPHORBOL-13-ACETATE
mf: $C_{36}H_{48}O_8$ mw: 608.84

SYN: TI-8

TOXICITY DATA with REFERENCE
ETA: skn-mus TDLo: 19 mg/kg/48W-I   CNREA8
39,4183,79

MUT: dns-mus-skn 400 nmol/kg   RCOCB8
24,533,79

SAFETY PROFILE: Questionable carcinogen
with experimental tumorigenic by skin contact.
Mutation data reported. When heated to decomposition it emits acrid smoke and irritating
fumes.

TCF000   CAS: 78-00-2
TETRAETHYL LEAD
DOT: 1649
mf: $C_8H_{20}Pb$ mw: 323.47

PROP: Colorless, oily liquid; pleasant characteristic odor. Mp: 125-150°, bp: 198-202° with
decomp, d: 1.659 @ 18°, vap press: 1 mm @
38.4°, flash p: 200°F.

SYNS: CZTEROETHLEK OLOWIU (POLISH) ◇ NCI-C54988
◇ RCRA WASTE NUMBER P110 ◇ TEL ◇ TETRAETHYL-
PLUMBANE

TOXICITY DATA with REFERENCE
CAR: scu-mus TDLo: 100 mg/kg/21D-I
EXPEAM 24,580,68

CONSENSUS REPORTS: IARC Cancer Review: Animal Inadequate Evidence IMEMDT
23,325,80, IMEMDT 2,150,73. EPA Extremely Hazardous Substances List. Reported
in EPA TSCA Inventory. EPA Genetic Toxicology Program.

OSHA PEL: TWA 0.075 mg(Pb)/m^3 (skin)
ACGIH TLV: TWA 0.1 mg(Pb)/m^3
(skin) DFG MAK: 0.01 ppm (0.075 mg/
m^3) DOT Classification: Poison B; Label: Poison and Poison, Flammable Liquid.

SAFETY PROFILE: Questionable carcinogen
with experimental carcinogenic and teratogenic
data. Human poison by an unspecified route.
Experimental poison by ingestion, intraperitoneal, intravenous, subcutaneous, and parenteral
routes. Moderately toxic by inhalation and skin
contact. Experimental reproductive effects.
Lead compounds are particularly toxic to the
central nervous system. Flammable when exposed to heat, flame, or oxidizers. To fight fire,
use dry chemical, CO_2, mist, foam. When
heated to decomposition it emits toxic fumes
of Pb.

TCH325   CAS: 71292-84-7
3,5,3′,5′-
TETRAFLUORODIETHYLSTILBESTROL
mf: $C_{18}H_{16}F_4O_2$ mw: 340.34

SYNS: trans-α,α′-DIETHYL-3,3′,5,5′-TETRAFLUORO-4,4′-
STILBENEDIOL ◇ α,α′-DIETHYL-3,3′,5,5′-TETRAFLUORO-
4,4′-STILBENEDIOL (E)-

TOXICITY DATA with REFERENCE
CAR: imp-ham TDLo: 360 mg/kg/12W-I
CNREA8 43,2678,83
MUT: dnd-ham: emb 7 mg/L   CRNGDP 7,1329,86
MUT: dns-ham: emb 1 mg/L   CNREA8 44,184,82
MUT: otr-ham: emb 10 μg/L   CNREA8 42,3040,82

SAFETY PROFILE: Questionable carcinogen
with experimental carcinogenic data. Mutation
data reported. When heated to decomposition
it emits toxic fumes of F$^-$.

TCH500   CAS: 116-14-3
TETRAFLUOROETHYLENE
DOT: 1081
mf: C_2F_4 mw: 100.02

PROP: Colorless gas. Mp: −142.5°, bp:
−78.4°. lel: 11%; uel: 60%.

SYNS: FLUOROPLAST 4 ◇ PERFLUOROETHENE
◇ PERFLUOROETHYLENE ◇ TETRAFLUORETHYLENE
◇ TETRAFLUOROETHENE ◇ TETRAFLUOROETHYLENE, in-
hibited (DOT)

CONSENSUS REPORTS: IARC Cancer Review: GROUP 3 IMEMDT 7,56,87. Reported
in EPA TSCA Inventory.

DOT Classification: Flammable Gas; Label: Flammable Gas.

SAFETY PROFILE: Questionable carcinogen. Mildly toxic by inhalation. Can act as an asphyxiant and may have other toxic properties. The gas is flammable when exposed to heat or flame. The inhibited monomer will explode if ignited. Explosive in the form of vapor when exposed to heat or flame. Will explode at pressures above 2. When heated to decomposition it emits highly toxic fumes of F^-.

TCI250   CAS: 63886-77-1
TETRAFLUORO-m-PHENYLENE DIAMINE DIHYDROCHLORIDE
mf: $C_6H_4F_4N_2 \cdot 2ClH$ mw: 253.04

TOXICITY DATA with REFERENCE
CAR: orl-mus TD: 130 g/kg/78W-C   JEPTDQ 2,325,78
CAR: orl-mus TDLo: 65 g/kg/78W-C   JEPTDQ 2,325,78

SAFETY PROFILE: Questionable carcinogen with experimental carcinogenic data. Poison by intraperitoneal route. When heated to decomposition it emits very toxic fumes of F^-, NO_x, and HCl.

TCJ500   CAS: 3570-54-5
1,2,5,6-TETRAHYDROBENZO(j) CYCLOPENT(fg)ACEANTHRYLENE
mf: $C_{22}H_{16}$ mw: 280.38

SYNS: NORSTEARANTHRENE ◇ F-NORSTEARANTHRENE

TOXICITY DATA with REFERENCE
ETA: scu-mus TD: 72 mg/kg/8W-I   NATWAY 53,583,66
ETA: scu-mus TD: 72 mg/kg/9W-I   NATUAS 200,185,63
ETA: scu-mus TDLo: 72 mg/kg/13W-I NATWAY 53,583,66

SAFETY PROFILE: Questionable carcinogen with experimental tumorigenic data. When heated to decomposition it emits acrid smoke and irritating fumes.

TCJ775   CAS: 17750-93-5
7,8,9,10-TETRAHYDROBENZO(a) PYRENE
mf: $C_{20}H_{16}$ mw: 256.36

SYN: 1',2',3',4'-TETRAHYDRO-3,4-BENZOPYRENE

TOXICITY DATA with REFERENCE
ETA: scu-mus TDLo: 72 mg/kg/9W-I   COREAF 251,1322,60

SAFETY PROFILE: Questionable carcinogen with experimental neoplastigenic data. When heated to decomposition it emits acrid smoke and irritating fumes.

TCM250   CAS: 1972-08-3
1-trans-Δ⁹-TETRAHYDROCANNABINOL
mf: $C_{21}H_{30}O_2$ mw: 314.51

SYNS: ABBOTT 40566 ◇ 3-PENTYL-6,6,9-TRIMETHYL-6a,7,8,10a-TETRAHYDRO-6H-DIBENZO(b,d)PYRAN-1-OL ◇ SP 104 ◇ (1)-Δ¹-TETRAHYDROCANNABINOL ◇ Δ¹-TETRAHYDROCANNABINOL ◇ (−)-Δ¹-3,4-trans-TETRAHYDROCANNABINOL ◇ (−)-Δ⁹-trans-TETRAHYDROCANNABINOL ◇ trans-Δ⁹-TETRAHYDROCANNABINOL ◇ Δ⁹-TETRAHYDROCANNABINON ◇ THC ◇ Δ¹-THC ◇ Δ⁹-THC ◇ 6,6,9-TRIMETHYL-3-PENTYL-7,8,9,10-TETRAHYDRO-6H-DIBENZO(B,D)PYRAN-1-OL

TOXICITY DATA with REFERENCE
ETA: scu-mus TD: 800 μg/kg/W-I   AVBIB9 22/23,359,79
ETA: scu-mus TDLo: 800 μg/kg/W-I   FEPRA7 38,1450,79
MUT: cyt-hmn: lym 2500 μmol/L/24H   FEPRA7 36,1748,77
MUT: cyt-mus-ipr 50 mg/kg/5D-I   PHMGBN 21,277,80
MUT: dni-hmn: hla 40 μmol/L   ANTRD4 3,211,83
MUT: mnt-mus-ipr 50 mg/kg/5D-I   PHMGBN 21,277,80
MUT: oms-hmn: fbr 5 μmol/L   ANTRD4 3,211,83
MUT: oms-hmn: hla 40 μmol/L   ANTRD4 3,211,83
MUT: spm-mus-ipr 25 mg/kg/5D-C   PHMGBN 18,143,79

CONSENSUS REPORTS: EPA Genetic Toxicology Program.

SAFETY PROFILE: Questionable carcinogen with experimental tumorigenic and teratogenic data. Poison by intraperitoneal and intravenous routes. Moderately toxic by ingestion. Experimental reproductive effects. Human mutation data reported. An hallucinatory drug. When heated to decomposition it emits acrid smoke and irritating fumes.

TCN750   CAS: 153-39-9
1,2,3,4-TETRAHYDRODIBENZ(a,h) ANTHRACENE
mf: $C_{22}H_{18}$ mw: 282.40

TOXICITY DATA with REFERENCE
NEO: scu-mus TDLo: 16 mg/kg   JNCIAM 44,641,70
NEO: skn-mus TDLo: 74 mg/kg/29W-I   JNCIAM 34,1,65

SAFETY PROFILE: Questionable carcinogen with experimental neoplastigenic data. When heated to decomposition it emits acrid smoke and irritating fumes.

TCO000   CAS: 16310-68-2
1,2,3,4-TETRAHYDRODIBENZ(a,j) ANTHRACENE
mf: $C_{22}H_{18}$ mw: 282.40

TOXICITY DATA with REFERENCE
ETA: scu-mus TDLo: 16 mg/kg   JNCIAM 44,641,70
ETA: skn-mus TDLo: 104 mg/kg/35W-I
JNCIAM 44,641,70

SAFETY PROFILE: Questionable carcinogen with experimental tumorigenic data. When heated to decomposition it emits acrid smoke and irritating fumes.

TCP600   CAS: 67242-54-0
1,2,3,4-TETRAHYDRO-7,12-DIMETHYLBENZ(a)ANTHRACENE
mf: $C_{20}H_{20}$ mw: 260.40

SYNS: 7,12-DIMETHYL-1,2,3,4-TETRAHYDROBENZ(a)-ANTHRACENE ◇ 1,2,3,4-TETRAHYDRO-DMBA ◇ TH-DMBA

TOXICITY DATA with REFERENCE
CAR: skn-mus TDLo: 200 mg/kg/25W-I
CRNGDP 4,1221,83
ETA: skn-mus TD: 104 μg/kg   CRNGDP 3,651,82
MUT: dnd-ham: lng 100 nmol/L   CRNGDP 3,651,82
MUT: mma-sat 2500 ng/plate   CRNGDP 4,1221,83
MUT: mmo-sat 50 μg/plate   JMCMAR 23,278,80
MUT: otr-hmn: fbr 500 μg/L   CALEDQ 13,119,81

SAFETY PROFILE: Questionable carcinogen with experimental carcinogenic and tumorigenic data. Human mutation data reported. When heated to decomposition it emits acrid smoke and irritating fumes.

TCY000   CAS: 1125-78-6
5,6,7,8-TETRAHYDRO-2-NAPHTHOL
mf: $C_{10}H_{12}O$ mw: 148.22

SYNS: 5,6,7,8-TETRAHYDRO-β-NAPHTHOL ◇ TETRALOL ◇ ac-β-TETRALOL

TOXICITY DATA with REFERENCE
CAR: skn-mus TDLo: 9600 mg/kg/30W-I
CNREA8 19,413,59

NEO: skn-mus TD: 4144 mg/kg/14W-I   CNREA8 19,413,59

SAFETY PROFILE: Questionable carcinogen with experimental carcinogenic and neoplastigenic data. When heated to decomposition it emits acrid smoke and irritating fumes.

TDD750   CAS: 61490-68-4
7-β,8-α-9-β,10-β-TETRAHYDROXY-7,8,9,10-TETRAHYDROBENZO(a) PYRENE
mf: $C_{20}H_{16}O_4$ mw: 320.36

SYN: BENZO(a)PYRENE, 7,8,9,10-TETRAHYDRO-7-β,8-α-9-α-10-α-TETRAHYDROXY- ◇ BENZO(a)PYRENE-7-β,8-α-9-α-10-α-TETRAOL

TOXICITY DATA with REFERENCE
NEO: skn-mus TDLo: 5126 μg/kg   CRNGDP 3,371,78

SAFETY PROFILE: Questionable carcinogen with experimental neoplastigenic data. When heated to decomposition it emits acrid smoke and irritating fumes.

TDE000   CAS: 64043-55-6
TETRAIODO-α,α'-DIETHYL-4,4'-STILBENEDIOL
mf: $C_{18}H_{16}I_4O_2$ mw: 771.94

SYN: DIETHYLSTILBESTROL, IODINE DERIVATIVE

TOXICITY DATA with REFERENCE
CAR: scu-mus TDLo: 85 mg/kg/3W-I   AIPUAN 8,207,65

SAFETY PROFILE: Questionable carcinogen with experimental carcinogenic data. When heated to decomposition it emits toxic fumes of I^-.

TDH500   CAS: 55818-96-7
TETRAKIS(HYDROXYMETHYL) PHOSPHONIUM ACETATE mixed with TETRAKIS(HYDROXYMETHYL) PHOSPHONIUM DIHYDROGEN PHOSPHATE (76:24)
mf: $C_4H_{12}O_4P \cdot C_4H_{12}O_4P \cdot C_2H_3O_2 \cdot 1/3O_4P$ mw: 400.97

SYNS: PYROSET FLAME RETARDANT TKP ◇ PYROSET TKP

TOXICITY DATA with REFERENCE
ETA: skn-mus TDLo: 14 g/kg/57W-I   JTEHD6 2,539,77

SAFETY PROFILE: Questionable carcinogen with experimental tumorigenic data. When heated to decomposition it emits toxic fumes of PO_x.

TDJ250 CAS: 73728-78-6
3,2',4',6'-TETRAMETHYLAMINODIPHENYL
mf: $C_{16}H_{19}N$ mw: 225.36

SYN: 3,2',4',6'-TETRAMETHYLBIPHENYLAMINE

TOXICITY DATA with REFERENCE
ETA: scu-rat TDLo: 1400 mg/kg/W-I   BMBUAQ 14,141,58

SAFETY PROFILE: Questionable carcinogen with experimental tumorigenic data. When heated to decomposition it emits toxic fumes of NO_x.

TDK885 CAS: 66552-77-0
2,3,9,10-TETRAMETHYLANTHRACENE
mf: $C_{18}H_{18}$ mw: 234.34

TOXICITY DATA with REFERENCE
CAR: skn-mus TDLo: 40 mg/kg/20D-I   CRNGDP 6,1483,85
MUT: mma-sat 100 µg/plate   CRNGDP 6,1483,85
MUT: mmo-sat 50 µg/plate   CRNGDP 6,1483,85

SAFETY PROFILE: Questionable carcinogen with experimental carcinogenic data. Mutation data reported. When heated to decomposition it emits acrid smoke and irritating fumes.

TDL500 CAS: 51787-44-1
7,8,9,11-TETRAMETHYLBENZ(c) ACRIDINE
mf: $C_{21}H_{19}N$ mw: 285.41

SYN: 1,3,4,10-TETRAMETHYL-7,8-BENZACRIDINE (FRENCH)

TOXICITY DATA with REFERENCE
ETA: scu-mus TD: 250 mg/kg/10D-I   BAFEAG 34,22,47
ETA: scu-mus TDLo: 200 mg/kg/4W-I   ACRSAJ 4,315,56
ETA: skn-mus TDLo: 350 mg/kg/29W-I   ACRSAJ 4,315,56

SAFETY PROFILE: Questionable carcinogen with experimental tumorigenic data. When heated to decomposition it emits toxic fumes of NO_x.

TDL750 CAS: 63020-39-3
5,6,9,10-TETRAMETHYL-1,2-BENZANTHRACENE
mf: $C_{22}H_{20}$ mw: 284.42

SYN: 7,8,9,12-TETRAMETHYLBENZ(a)ANTHRACENE

TOXICITY DATA with REFERENCE
ETA: scu-mus TDLo: 560 mg/kg/22W-I   PRLBA4 129,439,40
ETA: skn-mus TDLo: 340 mg/kg/14W-I   PRLBA4 129,439,40

SAFETY PROFILE: Questionable carcinogen with experimental tumorigenic data. When heated to decomposition it emits acrid smoke and irritating fumes.

TDM000 CAS: 63019-70-5
6,7,9,10-TETRAMETHYL-1,2-BENZANTHRACENE
mf: $C_{22}H_{20}$ mw: 284.42

SYN: 7,9,10,12-TETRAMETHYLBENZ(a)ANTHRACENE

TOXICITY DATA with REFERENCE
ETA: scu-mus TDLo: 120 mg/kg/9W-I   CRSBAW 148,812,54
ETA: skn-mus TDLo: 270 mg/kg/34W-I   CRSBAW 148,812,54

SAFETY PROFILE: Questionable carcinogen with experimental tumorigenic data. When heated to decomposition it emits acrid smoke and irritating fumes.

TDN500 CAS: 140-66-9
p-(1,1,3,3-TETRAMETHYLBUTYL) PHENOL
mf: $C_{14}H_{22}O$ mw: 206.36

SYNS: p-tert-OCTYLPHENOL ◇ p-terc.OKTYLFENOL (CZECH) ◇ p-(1',1',3',3'-TETRAMETHYLBUTYL)FENOL

TOXICITY DATA with REFERENCE
ETA: skn-mus TDLo: 5280 mg/kg/12W-I   CNREA8 19,413,59

CONSENSUS REPORTS: Reported in EPA TSCA Inventory.

SAFETY PROFILE: Questionable carcinogen with experimental tumorigenic data. Moderately toxic by ingestion. A skin and severe eye irritant. When heated to decomposition it emits acrid smoke and irritating fumes.

TDO250 CAS: 933-52-8
TETRAMETHYL-1,3-CYCLOBUTANEDIONE
mf: $C_8H_{12}O_2$ mw: 140.20

PROP: White, crystalline solid. Mp: 116° (sublimes), bp: 159°, vap press: 6 mm @ 52°, d: 1.11. Insol in water; sol in alc, acetic acid.

SYNS: TETRAMETHYLCYCLOBUTA-1,3-DIONE
◊ 2,2,4,4-TETRAMETHYL-1,3-CYCLOBUTANEDIONE

TOXICITY DATA with REFERENCE
NEO: scu-mus TDLo: 308 mg/kg/77W-I

   JNCIAM 46,143,71

CONSENSUS REPORTS: Reported in EPA TSCA Inventory.

SAFETY PROFILE: Questionable carcinogen with experimental neoplastigenic data. When heated to decomposition it emits acrid smoke and irritating fumes.

TDR250   CAS: 61556-82-9
TETRAMETHYLHYDRAZINE HYDROCHLORIDE
mf: $C_4H_{12}N_2 \cdot ClH$ mw: 124.64

TOXICITY DATA with REFERENCE
CAR: orl-mus TDLo: 49 g/kg/34W-C   JNCIAM
57,1179,76

SAFETY PROFILE: Questionable carcinogen with experimental carcinogenic data. When heated to decomposition it emits very toxic fumes of HCl and NO_x.

TDS000   CAS: 6130-93-4
2,2,6,6-TETRAMETHYLNITROSOPIPERIDINE
mf: $C_9H_{18}N_2O$ mw: 170.29

SYN: 1-NITROSO-2,2,6,6-TETRAMETHYLPIPERIDINE

TOXICITY DATA with REFERENCE
ETA: orl-rat TDLo: 3375 mg/kg/50W-I   IJCNAW
16,318,75

SAFETY PROFILE: Questionable carcinogen with experimental tumorigenic data. Poison by ingestion and intravenous routes. When heated to decomposition it emits toxic fumes of NO_x.

TDS750   CAS: 4466-77-7
1:2:3:4-TETRAMETHYLPHENANTHRENE
mf: $C_{18}H_{18}$ mw: 234.36

TOXICITY DATA with REFERENCE
ETA: skn-mus TDLo: 1340 mg/kg/56W-I
PRLBA4 131,170,42

SAFETY PROFILE: Questionable carcinogen with experimental tumorigenic data. When

heated to decomposition it emits acrid smoke and irritating fumes.

TDX000   CAS: 2782-91-4
TETRAMETHYLTHIOUREA
mf: $C_5H_{12}N_2S$ mw: 132.25

SYNS: NA-101 ◊ 1,1,3,3-TETRAMETHYLTHIOUREA
◊ TMTU

TOXICITY DATA with REFERENCE
CAR: orl-rat TDLo: 1848 mg/kg/79W-C
HunNJ# 10May77

CONSENSUS REPORTS: Reported in EPA TSCA Inventory.

SAFETY PROFILE: Questionable carcinogen with experimental carcinogenic and teratogenic data. Moderately toxic by ingestion. Experimental reproductive effects. When heated to decomposition it emits very toxic fumes of NO_x and SO_x.

TEA750   CAS: 630-76-2
TETRAPHENYL METHANE
mf: $C_{25}H_{20}$ mw: 320.45

PROP: Rhombic crystals from cold benzene. Mp: 285°, bp: 431°. Insol in ligroin, alc, ether, acetic acid; sol in hot benzene.

SYN: 1,1',1'',1'''-METHANETHETRAYLTETRAKISBENZENE

TOXICITY DATA with REFERENCE
ETA: skn-mus TDLo: 920 mg/kg/23W-I
AJCAA7 26,754,36

SAFETY PROFILE: Questionable carcinogen with experimental tumorigenic data. When heated to decomposition it emits acrid smoke and irritating fumes.

TEH500   CAS: 50-35-1
THALIDOMIDE
mf: $C_{13}H_{10}N_2O_4$ mw: 258.25

PROP: Needles. Mp: 269-271°. Sltly sol in water, methanol, ethanol, acetone, ethylacrylate; very sol in dioxane; sol in ether.

SYNS: ALGOSEDIV ◊ ASIDON 3 ◊ ASMADION
◊ ASMAVAL ◊ BONBRAIN ◊ CALMORE ◊ CALMOREX
◊ CONTERGAN ◊ CORRONAROBETIN ◊ 2,6-DIOXO-3-PHTHALIMIDOPIPERIDINE ◊ 2-(6-DIOXO-3-PIPERIDINYL)1H-ISOINDOLE-1,3(2H)-DIONE ◊ N-(2,6-DIOXO-3-PIPERIDYL)PHTHALIMIDE ◊ DISTAVAL ◊ DIS-

TAXAL ◇ DISTOVAL ◇ ECTILURAN ◇ ENTEROSEDIV ◇ GASTRINIDE ◇ GLUPAN ◇ GLUTANON ◇ GRIPPEX ◇ HIPPUZON ◇ IMIDA-LAB ◇ IMIDAN (PEYTA) ◇ IMIDENE ◇ ISOMIN ◇ K 17 ◇ KEDAVON ◇ KEVADON ◇ LULAMIN ◇ NEAUFATIN ◇ NEO ◇ NEOSEDYN ◇ NEOSYDYN ◇ NEURODYN ◇ NEUROSEDIN ◇ NEVRODYN ◇ NIBROL ◇ NOCTOSEDIV ◇ NOXODYN ◇ NSC-66847 ◇ PANGUL ◇ PANTOSEDIV ◇ α-PHTHALIMIDOGLUTARIMIDE ◇ 2-PHTHALIMIDOGLUTARIMIDE ◇ α-(N-PHTHALIMIDO) GLUTARIMIDE ◇ 3-PHTHALIMIDOGLUTARIMIDE ◇ N-PHTHALOYLGLUTAMIMIDE ◇ N-PHTHALYLGLU- TAMIC ACID IMIDE ◇ N-PHTHALYL-GLUTAMINSAEURE- IMID (GERMAN) ◇ α-N-PHTHALYLGLUTARAMIDE ◇ POLY-GIRON ◇ POLYGRIPAN ◇ PREDNI-SEDIV ◇ PRO-BAN M ◇ PROFARMIL ◇ PSYCHOLIQUID ◇ PSYCHOTABLETS ◇ QUETIMID ◇ QUIETOPLEX ◇ SANDORMIN ◇ SEDALIS SEDI-LAB ◇ SEDIMIDE ◇ SEDIN ◇ SEDISPERIL ◇ SEDOVAL ◇ SHIN-NAITO S ◇ SHINNIBROL ◇ SLEEPAN ◇ SLIPRO ◇ SOFTENIL ◇ SOFTENON ◇ TALARGAN ◇ TALIMOL ◇ TELAGAN ◇ TELARGAN ◇ TELARGEAN ◇ TENSIVAL ◇ THALIN ◇ THALINETTE ◇ THEOPHILCHOLINE ◇ ULCERFEN ◇ VALGIS ◇ VALGRAINE ◇ YODOMIN

TOXICITY DATA with REFERENCE
ETA: scu-mus TDLo:34 g/kg/57W-I   NATUAS 200,1016,63
MUT: cyt-hmn:lym 1 mg/L   AMSVAZ 177,783,65
MUT: cyt-rat-orl 7600 mg/kg/30D-C   NATUAS 202,1080,64
MUT: dlt-oin-orl 10 pph   EXPEAM 26,796,70
MUT: dns-rat-ipr 80 mg/kg   JPETAB 171,109,70

CONSENSUS REPORTS: EPA Genetic Toxi- cology Program.

SAFETY PROFILE: Questionable carcinogen with experimental tumorigenic and teratogenic data. Poison by ingestion. Moderately toxic by skin contact and intraperitoneal routes. Human teratogenic effects by ingestion: developmental abnormalities of the musculoskeletal, cardiovas- cular and possibly other systems. Experimental reproductive effects. Human mutation data re- ported. When heated to decomposition it emits toxic fumes of NO_x. Used as a sedative and hypnotic.

TEX250   CAS: 72-14-0
N¹-2-THIAZOLYLSULFANILAMIDE
mf: $C_9H_9N_3O_2S_2$ mw: 255.33

SYNS: 2-(p-AMINOBENZENESULFONAMIDO)THIAZOLE ◇ 2-(p-AMINOBENZENESULPHONAMIDO)THIAZOLE ◇ 4-AMINO-N-2-THIAZOLYLBENZENESULFONAMIDE ◇ AZOSEPTALE ◇ CERAZOL (suspension) ◇ CHEMOSEPT

◇ DUATOK ◇ ELEUDRON ◇ FORMOSULFATHIAZOLE ◇ M+B 760 ◇ NEOSTREPSAN ◇ NORSULFASOL ◇ NORSULFAZOLE ◇ PLANOMIDE ◇ POLISEPTIL ◇ RP 2990 ◇ STREPTOSILTHIAZOLE ◇ SULFAMUL ◇ 2-SULFANILAMIDOTHIAZOLE ◇ 2-(SULFANILYLAMI- NO)THIAZOLE ◇ SULFATHIAZOL ◇ SULFATHIAZOLE (USDA) ◇ 2-SULFONAMIDOTHIAZOLE ◇ SULPHATHIA- ZOLE ◇ SULZOL ◇ THIACOCCINE ◇ THIAZAMIDE ◇ THIOZAMIDE ◇ USAF SN-9

TOXICITY DATA with REFERENCE
ETA: orl-mus TDLo:2310 mg/kg/2W-C
ACRAAX 37,258,52
ETA: par-mus TDLo:500 mg/kg   ACRAAX 37,258,52
ETA: par-rat TDLo:500 mg/kg   ACRAAX 37,258,52
MUT: dnd-esc 50 μmol/L   MUREAV 89,95,81
MUT: pic-omi 5 mg/L   JGMIAN 8,116,53

CONSENSUS REPORTS: Reported in EPA TSCA Inventory. EPA Genetic Toxicology Pro- gram.

SAFETY PROFILE: Questionable carcinogen with experimental tumorigenic data. Human poison by unspecified route. Experimental poi- son by intraperitoneal route. Moderately toxic by intravenous, subcutaneous and parenteral routes. Mildly toxic by ingestion. Human sys- temic effects by unspecified route: conjuctiva irritation, tubule changes and allergic skin der- matitis. Mutation data reported. When heated to decomposition it emits very toxic fumes of NO_x and SO_x.

TFD250   CAS: 97-18-7
2,2'-THIOBIS(4,6-DICHLOROPHENOL)
mf: $C_{12}H_6Cl_4O_2S$ mw: 356.04

PROP: White crystalline powder; very faint phenolic odor. Mp: 187-188°, d: 1.61 @ 25°, vap press: 1.1×10^{-9} mm @ 37°.

SYNS: ACTAMER ◇ BIDIPHEN ◇ BIS(2-HYDROXY-3,5- DICHLOROPHENYL) SULFIDE ◇ BITHIONOL ◇ BITHIONOL SULFIDE ◇ BITIN ◇ CP 3438 ◇ 2,2'-DIHYDROXY-3,3',5,5'- TETRACHLORODIPHENYLSULFIDE ◇ 2-HYDROXY-3,5-DI- CHLOROPHENYL SULPHIDE ◇ LOROTHIDOL ◇ NCI-C60628 ◇ NEOPELLIS ◇ TBP ◇ USAF B-22 ◇ VANCIDE BL ◇ XL 7

TOXICITY DATA with REFERENCE
ETA: orl-mus TDLo:12 g/kg/78W-I   NTIS** PB223-159

CONSENSUS REPORTS: EPA Extremely Hazardous Substance List. Chlorophenol compounds are on the Community Right-To-Know List. Reported in EPA TSCA Inventory.

SAFETY PROFILE: Questionable carcinogen with experimental tumorigenic data. Poison by ingestion, intraperitoneal and intravenous routes. A food additive permitted in feed and drinking water of animals and for the treatment of food-producing animals. Also a food additive permitted in food for human consumption. When heated to decomposition it emits very toxic fumes of Cl^- and SO_x.

TFJ250   CAS: 64039-27-6
β-THIOGUANINE DEOXYRIBOSIDE
mf: $C_{10}H_{13}N_5O_3S \cdot H_2O$ mw: 301.36

SYNS: 2-AMINO-9-(2-DEOXY-β-d-RIBOFURANOSYL)-9H-PURINE-6-THIOL HYDRATE ◇ β-DEOXYTHIOGUANOSINE ◇ β-2′-DEOXY-6-THIOGUANOSINE MONOHYDRATE ◇ NSC-71261 ◇ β-TGDR

TOXICITY DATA with REFERENCE
CAR: ipr-rat TDLo:1092 mg/kg/1Y-I   NCITR* NCI-CG-TR-57,78
NEO: ipr-mus TDLo:175 mg/kg/8W-I   CNREA8 33,3069,73

SAFETY PROFILE: Questionable carcinogen with experimental carcinogenic and neoplastigenic data. Poison by intravenous and intraperitoneal routes. Moderately toxic by ingestion. When heated to decomposition it emits very toxic fumes of NO_x and SO_x.

TFQ000   CAS: 79-19-6
THIOSEMICARBAZIDE
mf: CH_5N_3S mw: 91.15

PROP: Needles from water. Mp: 182-184°. Sol in water, alc.

SYNS: N-AMINOTHIOUREA ◇ HYDRAZINECARBOTHIOAMIDE ◇ RCRA WASTE NUMBER P116 ◇ THIOCARBAMYLHYDRAZINE ◇ 3-THIOSEMICARBAZIDE ◇ TSC ◇ USAF EK-1275

TOXICITY DATA with REFERENCE
ETA: orl-rat TD:2048 mg/kg/78W-C   JJIND8 67,75,81
ETA: orl-rat TDLo:1024 mg/kg/78W-C   JJIND8 67,75,81
MUT: dnd-hmn:hla 20 μmol/L   BCPCA6 25,821,76

CONSENSUS REPORTS: EPA Extremely Hazardous Substances List. Reported in EPA TSCA Inventory.

SAFETY PROFILE: Questionable carcinogen with experimental tumorigenic data. Poison by ingestion, intraperitoneal and intravenous routes. Human mutation data reported. When heated to decomposition it emits very toxic fumes of NO_x and SO_x.

TFR250   CAS: 141-90-2
2-THIOURACIL
mf: $C_4H_4N_2OS$ mw: 128.16

PROP: Small crystals; bitter taste. Practically insol in water, alc, ether, acids; sol in alkalies.

SYNS: ANTAGOTHYROID ◇ ANTAGOTHYROIL ◇ DERACIL ◇ 2,3-DIHYDRO-2-THIOXO-4(1H)-PYRIMIDINONE ◇ 6-HYDROXY-2-MERCAPTOPYRIMIDINE ◇ 4-HYDROXY-2(1H)-PYRIMIDINETHIONE ◇ 2-MERCAPTO-4-HYDROXYPYRIMIDINE ◇ 2-MERCAPTO-4-PYRIMIDINOL ◇ 2-MERCAPTO-4-PYRIMIDONE ◇ 2-MERCAPTOPYRIMID-4-ONE ◇ NOBILEN ◇ 2-THIO-6-OXYPYRIMIDINE ◇ 2-THIO-1,3-PYRIMIDIN-4-ONE ◇ THIOURACIL ◇ 6-THIOURACIL ◇ TIOURACYL (POLISH) ◇ TU ◇ 2-TU

TOXICITY DATA with REFERENCE
NEO: orl-mus TDLo:184 g/kg/73W-C   PSEBAA 113,493,63
ETA: orl-rat TDLo:10 g/kg/14W-C   CANCAR 6,111,53
MUT: pic-esc 100 mmol/L   MDMIAZ 31,11,79

CONSENSUS REPORTS: IARC Cancer Review: GROUP 3 IMEMDT 7,56,87; Animal Sufficient Evidence IMEMDT 7,85,74. Reported in EPA TSCA Inventory. EPA Genetic Toxicology Program.

SAFETY PROFILE: Questionable carcinogen with experimental neoplastigenic, tumorigenic, and teratogenic data. Moderately toxic by ingestion. Human teratogenic effects by unspecified routes: developmental abnormalities of the central nervous system, craniofacial area, and endocrine system. Human reproductive effects by unspecified route: effects on newborn including viability index changes. Mutation data reported. When heated to decomposition it emits very toxic fumes of NO_x and SO_x. Used in the treatment of hyperthyroidism, angina pectoris, and congestive heart failure.

TFS350   CAS: 137-26-8
THIRAM
DOT: 2771
mf: $C_6H_{12}N_2S_4$ mw: 240.44

PROP: Crystals. Mp: 156°, d: 1.30, bp: 129° @ 20 mm. Insol in water; sol in alc, ether, acetone, and chloroform.

SYNS: AATACK ◊ ACCELERATOR THIURAM ◊ ACETO TETD ◊ ARASAN ◊ AULES ◊ BIS((DIMETHYLAMINO)CAR-BONOTHIOYL) DISULPHIDE ◊ BIS(DIMETHYL-THIOCAR-BAMOYL)-DISULFID (GERMAN) ◊ BIS(DIMETHYLTHIO-CARBAMOYL) DISULFIDE ◊ CHIPCO THIRAM 75 ◊ CYURAM DS ◊ DISOLFURO DI TETRAMETILTIOURAME (ITALIAN) ◊ DISULFURE de TETRAMETHYLTHIOURAME (FRENCH) ◊ α,α′-DITHIOBIS(DIMETHYLTHIO)FORMAMIDE ◊ 1,1′-DITHIOBIS(N,N-DIMETHYLTHIO)FORMAMIDE ◊ N,N′-(DITHIODICARBONOTHIOYL)BIS(N-METHYLME-THANAMINE) ◊ EKAGOM TB ◊ FALITIRAM ◊ FER-MIDE ◊ FERNACOL ◊ FERNASAN ◊ FERNIDE ◊ FLO PRO T SEED PROTECTANT ◊ HERMAL ◊ HERMAT TMT ◊ HERYL ◊ HEXATHIR ◊ KREGASAN ◊ MERCURAM ◊ METHYL THIRAM ◊ METHYL THIURAMDISULFIDE ◊ METHYL TUADS ◊ NOBECUTAN ◊ NOMERSAN ◊ NORMERSAN ◊ PANORAM 75 ◊ POLYRAM ULTRA ◊ POMARSOL ◊ POMASOL ◊ PURALIN ◊ RCRA WASTE NUMBER U244 ◊ REZIFILM ◊ ROYAL TMTD ◊ SADOPLON ◊ SPOTRETE ◊ SQ 1489 ◊ TERSAN ◊ TERAMETHYL THIURAM DISULFIDE ◊ TETRAMETHYL-DIURANE SULPHITE ◊ TETRAMETHYLENETHIURAM DISULPHIDE ◊ TETRAMETHYLTHIOCARBAMOYLDI-SULPHIDE ◊ TETRAMETHYLTHIORAMDISULFIDE (DUTCH) ◊ TETRAMETHYL-THIRAM DISULFID (GERMAN) ◊ TETRAMETHYLTHIURAM BISULFIDE ◊ TETRAMETHYLTHIURAM DISULFIDE ◊ TETRAMETHYL THIURANE DISULFIDE ◊ TETRA-METHYLTHIURUM DISULFIDE ◊ N,N,N′,N′-TETRA-METHYLTHIURAM DISULFIDE ◊ N,N-TETRAMETHYL-THIURAM DISULPHIDE ◊ TETRAPOM ◊ TETRASIPTON ◊ TETRATHIURAM DISULFIDE ◊ TETRATHIURAM DISUL-PHIDE ◊ THILLATE ◊ THIMER ◊ THIOSAN ◊ THIOTEX ◊ THIOTOX ◊ THIRAM ◊ THIRAMAD ◊ THIRAME (FRENCH) ◊ THIRASAN ◊ THIULIX ◊ THIURAD ◊ THIURAM ◊ THIURAMIN ◊ THIURAMYL ◊ THYLATE ◊ TIRAMPA ◊ TIURAM (POLISH) ◊ TIURAMYL ◊ TMTD ◊ TMTDS ◊ TRAMETAN ◊ TRIDIPAM ◊ TRIPOMOL ◊ TTD ◊ TUADS ◊ TUEX ◊ TULISAN ◊ USAF B-30 ◊ USAF EK-2089 ◊ USAF P-5 ◊ VANCIDA TM-95 ◊ VANCIDE TM ◊ VUAGT-I-4 ◊ VULCAFOR TMTD ◊ VULKACIT MTIC ◊ VULKACIT THIURAM ◊ VULKACIT THIURAM/C

TOXICITY DATA with REFERENCE
ETA: orl-rat TDLo:108 mg/kg/1Y-C   RPZHAW 31,67,80
ETA: scu-mus TDLo:46 mg/kg   NTIS** PB223-159
MUT: cyt-asn 20 ppm   MUREAV 89,297,81

MUT: dnr-sat 50 μg/plate   MUREAV 89,1,81
MUT: mmo-asn 500 ng/plate   MUREAV 89,1,81
MUT: mnt-mus-ipr 100 mg/kg   FCTOD7 23,373,85
MUT: msc-ham:lng 5 mg/L   FCTOD7 23,373,85
MUT: pic-esc 1 ng/tube   MUREAV 89,1,81

CONSENSUS REPORTS: IARC Cancer Review: Human Inadequate Evidence IMEMDT 12,225,76; Animal Inadequate Evidence IMEMDT 12,225,76. EPA Genetic Toxicology Program. Reported in EPA TSCA Inventory.

OSHA PEL: TWA 5 mg/m³   ACGIH TLV: TWA 5 mg/m³ (Proposed: TWA 1 mg/m³) DFG MAK: 5 mg/m³   DOT Classification: ORM-A; Label: None.

SAFETY PROFILE: Questionable carcinogen with experimental tumorigenic and teratogenic data. Poison by ingestion and intraperitoneal routes. Mutation data reported. Affects human pulmonary system. A mild allergen and irritant. Acute poisoning in experimental animals produced liver, kidney, and brain damage.

TFZ000   CAS: 9007-12-9
THYROCALCITONIN
SYN: TCT

TOXICITY DATA with REFERENCE
ETA: ipr-mus TDLo:120 mg/kg/33D-I   ANREAK 175,462,73

SAFETY PROFILE: Questionable carcinogen with experimental tumorigenic data.

TGB250   CAS: 7440-31-5
TIN
af: Sn   aw: 118.71

PROP: Cubic, gray, crystalline metallic element. Mp: 231.9°, stabilizes <18°, d: 7.31, vap press: 1 mm @ 1492°, bp: 2507°.

SYNS: SILVER MATT POWDER ◊ TIN (α) ◊ TIN FLAKE ◊ TIN POWDER ◊ ZINN (GERMAN)

TOXICITY DATA with REFERENCE
ETA: imp-mus TDLo:840 g/kg   RCOCB8 18,201,77
ETA: imp-rat TDLo:395 g/kg   RCOCB8 18,201,77

CONSENSUS REPORTS: Reported in EPA TSCA Inventory.

OSHA PEL: Organic Compounds: TWA 0.1 mg(Sn)/m³ (skin); Inorganic Compounds (except oxides): TWA 2 mg/m³   ACGIH TLV: TWA metal, oxide and inorganic compounds (except SnH_4) as Sn 2 mg/m^3; organic compounds 0.1 mg/m^3 (skin) (Proposed: TWA 0.1 mg(Sn)/m^3; STEL 0.2 mg(Sn)/m^3 (skin))   DFG MAK: Inorganic 2 mg/m^3, organic 0.1 mg/m^3 NIOSH REL: (Organotin Compounds) TWA 0.1 mg(Sn)/m^3

SAFETY PROFILE: Questionable carcinogen with experimental tumorigenic data by implant route. Combustible in the form of dust when exposed to heat or by spontaneous chemical reaction.

TGD000   CAS: 58-14-0
TINDURIN
mf: $C_{12}H_{13}ClN_4$ mw: 248.74

SYNS: CD ◇ CHLORIDIN ◇ CHLORIDINE ◇ 5-(4'-CHLO-ROPHENYL)-2,4-DIAMINO-6-ETHYLPYRIMIDINE ◇ 5-(4-CHLOROPHENYL)-6-ETHYL-2,4-PYRIMIDINEDIAMINE ◇ DARACLOR ◇ DARAPRAM ◇ DARAPRIM ◇ DARAPRIME ◇ 2,4-DIAMINO-5-p-CHLOROPHENYL-6-ETHYLPYRIMI-DINE ◇ 2,4-DIAMINO-5-(4-CHLOROPHENYL)-6-ETHYL-PYRIMIDINE ◇ DIAMINOPYRITAMIN ◇ ERBAPRELINA ◇ KHLORIDIN ◇ MALACID ◇ MALOCID ◇ MALOCIDE ◇ MALOPRIM ◇ NCI-C01683 ◇ NSC 3061 ◇ PIRIMECIDAN ◇ PIRIMETAMINA (SPANISH) ◇ 4753 R.P. ◇ WR 2978

TOXICITY DATA with REFERENCE
MUT: cyt-mus-ipr 100 mg/kg   GNKAA5 9,67,73
MUT: cyt-rat-orl 5 mg/kg   TGANAK 14(6),20,80
MUT: mmo-omi 300 ng/plate   AMACCQ 12,84,77
MUT: mmo-sat 10 μL/plate   ANYAA9 76,475,58
MUT: mnt-rat-orl 2 mg/kg   CYGEDX 14(6),17,80
MUT: oms-hmn:lym 814 nmol/L   BCPCA6 25,1947,76
MUT: oms-rat-orl 2 mg/kg   CYGEDX 14(6),17,80

CONSENSUS REPORTS: IARC Cancer Review: GROUP 3 IMEMDT 7,56,87; Animal Limited Evidence IMEMDT 13,233,77. NCI Carcinogenesis Bioassay (feed); Inadequate Studies: mouse NCITR* NCI-CG-TR-77,78; (feed); No Evidence: rat NCITR* NCI-CG-TR-77,78. EPA Genetic Toxicology Program.

SAFETY PROFILE: Questionable carcinogen. Poison by ingestion, subcutaneous and intraperitoneal routes. An experimental teratogen. Experimental reproductive effects. Human mutation data reported. When heated to decomposition it emits very toxic fumes of Cl^- and NO_x. Used as an antimalarial drug for humans and to treat toxoplasmosis in hogs.

TGD100   CAS: 7783-47-3
TIN FLUORIDE
mf: F_2Sn mw: 156.69

PROP: Monoclinic, lamellar plates. Mp: 213°, d: (25) 4.57. Sol in water (about 30%). Forms an oxyfluoride, $SnOF_2$, on exposure to air.

SYNS: FLUORISTAN ◇ STANNOUS FLUORIDE ◇ TIN BIFLUORIDE ◇ TIN DIFLUORIDE

TOXICITY DATA with REFERENCE
MUT: mma-sat 4 μmol/plate   MUREAV 90,91,81
MUT: sln-dmg-orl 15 pph/24H   FLUOA4 6,113,73

CONSENSUS REPORTS: IARC Cancer Review: GROUP 3 IMEMDT 7,208,87. EPA Genetic Toxicology Program. Reported in EPA TSCA Inventory.

OSHA PEL: TWA 2 mg(Sn)/m^3; 2.5 mg(F)/m^3 ACGIH TLV: TWA 2 mg(Sn)/m^3; 2.5 mg(F)/m^3 NIOSH REL: TWA 2.5 mg(F)/m^3

SAFETY PROFILE: Questionable carcinogen. Poison by ingestion and intraperitoneal routes. Mutation data reported. When heated to decomposition it emits toxic fumes of F^-.

TGF250   CAS: 7440-32-6
TITANIUM
DOT: 2546/2878
af: Ti   aw: 47.90

PROP: Dark gray amorphous powder or lustrous white metal. D: 4.5 @ 20°, autoign temp: 1200° for solid metal in air, 250° for powder, mp: 1677°, bp: 3277°.

SYNS: CONTIMET 30 ◇ C.P. TITANIUM ◇ IMI 115 ◇ NCI-C04251 ◇ OREMET ◇ TITANIUM ALLOY ◇ TITANIUM METAL POWDER, DRY (DOT) ◇ TITANIUM SPONGE GRANULES (DOT) ◇ TITANIUM SPONGE POWDERS (DOT)

TOXICITY DATA with REFERENCE
ETA: ims-rat TD:360 mg/kg/69W-I   NCIUS* PH 43-64-886,AUG,69
ETA: ims-rat TDLo:114 mg/kg/77W-I   NCIUS* PH 43-64-886,JUL,68

CONSENSUS REPORTS: Reported in EPA TSCA Inventory.

DOT Classification: Flammable Solid; Label: Flammable Solid and Spontaneously Combustible.

SAFETY PROFILE: Questionable carcinogen with experimental tumorigenic data. The dust may ignite spontaneously in air. Flammable when exposed to heat or flame or by chemical reaction. Titanium can burn in an atmosphere of carbon dioxide, nitrogen or air. Ordinary extinguishers are often ineffective against titanium fires. Such fires require special extinguishers designed for metal fires. The application of water to burning titanium can cause an explosion. Finely divided titanium dust and powders, like most metal powders, are potential explosion hazards when exposed to sparks, open flame or high heat sources.

TGG760 CAS: 13463-67-7
TITANIUM DIOXIDE
mf: O_2Ti mw: 79.90

PROP: White amorphous powder. Mp: 1860° (decomp), d: 4.26. Insol in water, hydrochloric acid, dil sulfuric acid, alc.

SYNS: 1700 WHITE ◇ A-FIL CREAM ◇ ATLAS WHITE TITANIUM DIOXIDE ◇ AUSTIOX ◇ BAYERITIAN ◇ BAYERTITAN ◇ BAYTITAN ◇ CALCOTONE WHITE T ◇ C.I. 77891 ◇ C.I. PIGMENT WHITE 6 ◇ COSMETIC WHITE C47-5175 ◇ C-WEISS 7 (GERMAN) ◇ FLAMENCO ◇ HOMBITAN ◇ HORSE HEAD A-410 ◇ KH 360 ◇ KRONOS TITANIUM DIOXIDE ◇ LEVANOX WHITE RKB ◇ NCI-C04240 ◇ RAYOX ◇ RUNA RH20 ◇ RUTILE ◇ TIOFINE ◇ TIOXIDE ◇ TITANDIOXID (SWEDEN) ◇ TITANIUM OXIDE ◇ TRIOXIDE(S) ◇ TRONOX ◇ UNITANE O-110 ◇ ZOPAQUE

TOXICITY DATA with REFERENCE
CAR: ihl-rat TCLo: 250 mg/m³/6H/2Y-I TXAPA9 79,179,85
NEO: ims-rat TDLo: 360 mg/kg/2Y-I NCIUS* PH 43-64-886,JUL,68
ETA: ims-rat TD: 260 mg/kg/84W-I NCIUS* PH 43-64-886,AUG,69

CONSENSUS REPORTS: NCI Carcinogenesis Bioassay (feed); No Evidence: mouse, rat NCITR* NCI-CG-TR-97,79. Reported in EPA TSCA Inventory. EPA Genetic Toxicology Program. Community Right-To-Know List.

OSHA PEL: (Transitional: TWA Total Dust: 15 mg/m³; Respirable Fraction: 5 mg/m³) TWA Total Dust: 10 mg/m³; Respirable Fraction: 5 mg/m³ ACGIH TLV: TWA (nuisance particulate) 10 mg/m³ of total dust (when toxic impurities are not present, e.g., quartz < 1%). DFG MAK: 6 mg/m³

SAFETY PROFILE: Questionable carcinogen with experimental carcinogenic, neoplastigenic, and tumorigenic data. A human skin irritant. A common air contaminant and nuisance dust.

TGH500 CAS: 1271-29-0
TITANOCENE
mf: $C_{10}H_{10}Ti$ mw: 178.10

SYN: DI-pi-CYCLOPENTADIENYLTITANIUM

TOXICITY DATA with REFERENCE
ETA: ims-mus TD: 150 mg/kg NCIUS* PH 43-64-886,SEPT,65
ETA: ims-mus TDLo: 75 mg/kg NCIUS* PH 43-64-886, SEPT,65

SAFETY PROFILE: Questionable carcinogen with experimental tumorigenic data. Poison by intramuscular route. When heated to decomposition it emits acrid smoke and irritating fumes.

TGH750 CAS: 8037-19-2
TOBACCO LEAF ABSOLUTE

PROP: An extract of the cured leaves of *Nicotiana affinis* with petroleum or benzene and then with alc (FCTXAV 16,637,78).

SYN: BURLEY TOBACCO

TOXICITY DATA with REFERENCE
ETA: skn-mus TDLo: 31 g/kg/40W-I CNREA8 28,2363,68

CONSENSUS REPORTS: Reported in EPA TSCA Inventory.

SAFETY PROFILE: Questionable carcinogen with experimental tumorigenic data. A skin irritant. When heated to decomposition it emits acrid smoke and irritating fumes.

TGM000 CAS: 95-70-5
TOLUENE-2,5-DIAMINE
mf: $C_7H_{10}N_2$ mw: 122.19

PROP: Colorless, crystalline tablets. Mp: 64°, bp: 274°.

SYNS: 4-AMINO-2-METHYLANILINE ◇ C.I. 76042 ◇ 2,5-DIAMINOTOLUENE ◇ 2-METHYL-1,4-BENZENEDIAMINE ◇ 2-METHYL-p-PHENYLENEDIAMINE ◇ p-TOLUENEDIAMINE ◇ p-TOLUYLENDIAMINE ◇ TOLUYLENE-2,5-DIAMINE ◇ p,m-TOLYLENEDIAMINE

TOXICITY DATA with REFERENCE
MUT: dni-mus-ipr 40 mg/kg MRLEDH 91,75,81
MUT: dns-ham: lvr 10 μmol/L MUREAV 136,255,84
MUT: dns-rat: lvr 10 μmol/L MUREAV 136,255,84
MUT: mma-sat 100 μg/plate PNASA6 72,2423,75

CONSENSUS REPORTS: IARC Cancer Review: GROUP 3 IMEMDT 7,56,87; Animal Inadequate Evidence IMEMDT 16,97,78. Reported in EPA TSCA Inventory. EPA Genetic Toxicology Program.

SAFETY PROFILE: Questionable carcinogen. Poison by ingestion and subcutaneous routes. Mutation data reported. A skin irritant. When heated to decomposition it emits toxic fumes of NO$_x$.

TGM400   CAS: 6369-59-1
p-TOLUENEDIAMINE SULFATE
mf: C$_7$H$_{10}$N$_2$•7H$_2$O$_4$S   mw: 808.75

SYNS: C.I. 76043 ◇ C.I. OXIDATION BASE 4 ◇ FOURA-MINE STD ◇ 2-METHYL-1,4-BENZENEDIAMINE ◇ NCI-C01832 ◇ 2,5-TDS ◇ 2,5-TOULENEDIAMINE SULFATE

TOXICITY DATA with REFERENCE
ETA: orl-mus TDLo:66 g/kg/78W-C   NCITR*
  NCI-CG-TR-126,78
MUT: mma-sat 33300 ng/plate   ENMUDM 7(Suppl 5),1,85

CONSENSUS REPORTS: EPA Genetic Toxicology Program. Reported in EPA TSCA Inventory.

SAFETY PROFILE: Questionable carcinogen with experimental tumorigenic data. Experimental reproductive effects. Mutation data reported. When heated to decomposition it emits toxic fumes of SO$_x$ and NO$_x$.

TGO750   CAS: 100-53-8
α-TOLUENETHIOL
mf: C$_7$H$_8$S   mw: 124.21

PROP: A water-white, mobile liquid; strong odor. Bp: 194.8°, flash p: 158°F (CC), d: 1.058 @ 20°, vap d: 4.28.

SYNS: BENZYL MERCAPTAN ◇ BENZYLTHIOL ◇ (MERCAPTOMETHYL)BENZENE ◇ α-MERCAPTOTOL-UENE ◇ PHENYLMETHANETHIOL ◇ PHENYLMETHYL MERCAPTAN ◇ THIOBENZYL ALCOHOL ◇ α-TOLUOL-THIOL ◇ α-TOLYL MERCAPTAN ◇ USAF EK-1509

TOXICITY DATA with REFERENCE
ETA: skn-mus TDLo:16 g/kg/26W-I   AJCAA7
  15,2149,31

CONSENSUS REPORTS: Reported in EPA TSCA Inventory.

SAFETY PROFILE: Questionable carcinogen with experimental tumorigenic data. Poison by intraperitoneal route. Moderately toxic by ingestion. An eye irritant. Flammable when exposed to heat or flame. Can react vigorously with oxidizing materials. To fight fire, use foam, CO$_2$, dry chemical, water spray, mist, fog. When

heated to decomposition and on contact with acid or acid fumes it emits highly toxic fumes of SO$_x$.

TGS250   CAS: 638-03-9
m-TOLUIDINE HYDROCHLORIDE
mf: C$_7$H$_9$N•ClH   mw: 143.63

PROP: Leaves from water. Mp: 228°, bp: 250°. Sol in water and alc.

TOXICITY DATA with REFERENCE
ETA: orl-mus TD:950 g/kg/78W-C   JEPTDQ
  2,325,78
ETA: orl-mus TDLo:475 g/kg/78W-C   JEPTDQ
  2,325,78

SAFETY PROFILE: Questionable carcinogen with experimental tumorigenic data. Moderately toxic by subcutaneous and intraperitoneal routes. When heated to decomposition it emits very toxic fumes of NO$_x$ and HCl.

TGS750   CAS: 540-23-8
p-TOLUIDINE HYDROCHLORIDE
mf: C$_7$H$_9$N•ClH   mw: 143.63

PROP: Needles from acetic ether. Mp: 243°, bp: 257.5°. Sol in water, alc; insol in ether, benzene.

SYNS: 4-AMINOTOLUENE HYDROCHLORIDE ◇ 4-METHYLANILINE HYDROCHLORIDE ◇ 4-METHYL-BENZENAMINE HYDROCHLORIDE ◇ p-TOLUIDINIUM CHLORIDE

TOXICITY DATA with REFERENCE
CAR: orl-mus TDLo:86 g/kg/78W-C   JEPTDQ
  2(2),325,78
ETA: orl-mus TD:43 g/kg/78W-C   JEPTDQ
  2(2),325,78

CONSENSUS REPORTS: Reported in EPA TSCA Inventory. EPA Genetic Toxicology Program.

SAFETY PROFILE: Questionable carcinogen with experimental carcinogenic and tumorigenic data. Poison by intraperitoneal route. Moderately toxic by ingestion. When heated to decomposition it emits very toxic fumes of NO$_x$ and HCl.

TGU500   CAS: 6424-34-6
TOLUYLENE BLUE MONOHYDRATE
mf: C$_{15}$H$_{19}$N$_4$•Cl•H$_2$O   mw: 308.85

SYNS: AMMONIUM, (4-((4,6-DIAMINO-m-TOLYL)IMINO)-2,5-CYCLOHEXADIEN-1-YLIDENE)DIMETHYL-, CHLO-

RIDE, MONOHYDRATE ◇ (4-((4,6-DIAMINO-m-TOLYL)
IMINO)-2,5-CYCLOHEXADIEN-1-YLIDENE)DIMETHYLAM-
MONIUM CHLORIDE H₂O

TOXICITY DATA with REFERENCE
ETA: scu-rat TDLo: 940 mg/kg/46W-I   GANNA2
  45,447,54

SAFETY PROFILE: Questionable carcinogen
with experimental neoplastigenic data. When
heated to decomposition it emits toxic fumes
of NO_x and Cl^-.

TGV250   CAS: 829-65-2
N-(p-TOLYL)-1-
AZIRIDINECARBOXAMIDE
mf: $C_{10}H_{12}N_2O$ mw: 176.24

SYN: p-TOLYL-N-CARBAMOYLAZIRIDINE

TOXICITY DATA with REFERENCE
NEO: ipr-mus TDLo: 240 mg/kg/4W-I   CNREA8
  29,2184,69

SAFETY PROFILE: Questionable carcinogen
with experimental neoplastigenic data. When
heated to decomposition it emits toxic fumes
of NO_x.

TGV500   CAS: 64046-59-9
m-TOLYLAZOACETANILIDE
mf: $C_{15}H_{16}N_3O$ mw: 254.34

TOXICITY DATA with REFERENCE
ETA: orl-rat TDLo: 4700 mg/kg/52W-C: TER
  JNCIAM 24,149,60

SAFETY PROFILE: Questionable carcinogen
with experimental tumorigenic and teratogenic
data. When heated to decomposition it emits
toxic fumes of NO_x.

TGV750   CAS: 722-25-8
p-(p-TOLYLAZO)-ANILINE
mf: $C_{13}H_{13}N_3$ mw: 211.29

SYNS: 4'-METHYL-4-AMINOAZOBENZENE
◇ 4-((4-METHYLPHENYL)AZO)BENZENAMINE

TOXICITY DATA with REFERENCE
ETA: orl-rat TDLo: 8000 mg/kg   CNREA8
  5,235,45

MUT: dni-mus-ipr 20 g/kg   ARGEAR 51,605,81

SAFETY PROFILE: Questionable carcinogen
with experimental tumorigenic data. Mutation
data reported. When heated to decomposition
it emits toxic fumes of NO_x.

TGW500   CAS: 63980-19-8
2-(o-TOLYLAZO)-p-TOLUIDINE
mf: $C_{14}H_{15}N_3$ mw: 225.32

SYN: 2'-AMINO-2:5'-AZOTOLUENE

TOXICITY DATA with REFERENCE
CAR: orl-mus TDLo: 30 g/kg/57W-C   BJCAAI
  3,387,49
ETA: orl-rat TDLo: 15 g/kg/57W-C   BJCAAI
  3,387,49

SAFETY PROFILE: Questionable carcinogen
with experimental carcinogenic and tumorigenic
data. When heated to decomposition it emits
toxic fumes of NO_x.

TGW750   CAS: 63980-18-7
4-(p-TOLYLAZO)-o-TOLUIDINE
mf: $C_{14}H_{15}N_3$ mw: 225.32

SYN: 4'-AMINO-4-3'-AZOTOLUENE

TOXICITY DATA with REFERENCE
ETA: orl-mus TDLo: 30 g/kg/57W-C   BJCAAI
  3,387,49

SAFETY PROFILE: Questionable carcinogen
with experimental tumorigenic data. When
heated to decomposition it emits toxic fumes
of NO_x.

TGX000   CAS: 63980-27-8
1-((4-TOLYLAZO)TOLYLAZO)-2-
NAPHTHOL
mf: $C_{24}H_{20}N_4O$ mw: 380.48

PROP: Mixture of m-, o-, and p- isomers (ZEK-
BAI 57,530,51).

SYN: D&C RED NO. 14

TOXICITY DATA with REFERENCE
ETA: orl-rat TDLo: 13 g/kg/39W-C   ZEKBAI
  57,530,51

SAFETY PROFILE: Questionable carcinogen
with experimental tumorigenic data. When
heated to decomposition it emits toxic fumes
of NO_x.

THE500   CAS: 80-11-5
p-TOLYLSULFONYLMETHYL-
NITROSAMINE
mf: $C_8H_{10}N_2O_3S$ mw: 214.26

SYNS: DIAZALE ◇ METHYLNITROSO-p-TOLUENESUL-
FONAMIDE ◇ N-NITROSO-N-METHYL-4-TOLYLSULFON-
AMIDE ◇ TOLUENE-p-SULFONYLMETHYLNITROSAMIDE

◇ p-TOLYLSULFONYL-METHYL-NITROSAMID (GERMAN)
◇ p-TOLYLSULFONYLMETHYLNITROSAMIDE

TOXICITY DATA with REFERENCE
ETA: ipr-mus TDLo: 15 mg/kg   CNREA8 30,11,70
MUT: dns-rat: lvr 100 µmol/L   ENMUDM 3,11,81
MUT: mmo-esc 14 µmol/L   ENMUDM 3,11,81
MUT: mmo-sat 14 µmol/L   ENMUDM 3,11,81
MUT: slt-dmg-orl 2330 µmol/kg   MUREAV
144,177,85

CONSENSUS REPORTS: Reported in EPA TSCA Inventory. EPA Genetic Toxicology Program.

SAFETY PROFILE: Questionable carcinogen with experimental tumorigenic data. Poison by intraperitoneal route. Moderately toxic by ingestion. Mutation data reported. Many nitrosamines are carcinogens. When heated to decomposition it emits very toxic fumes of NO_x and SO_x.

THG000   CAS: 622-51-5
p-TOLYLUREA
mf: $C_8H_{10}N_2O$ mw: 150.20

PROP: Plates from alc. Mp: 188°. Very sltly sol in cold water; sol in hot alc.

SYNS: 4-METHYLPHENYLUREA ◇ NCI-C02153
◇ p-TOLYCARBAMIDE ◇ p-TOLYUREA

TOXICITY DATA with REFERENCE
CAR: orl-mus TDLo: 88 g/kg/1Y-C   JEPTDQ
3(5-6),149,80

SAFETY PROFILE: Questionable carcinogen with experimental carcinogenic data. Moderately toxic by ingestion. When heated to decomposition it emits toxic fumes of NO_x.

THP000   CAS: 548-61-8
TRIAMINOTRIPHENYLMETHANE
mf: $C_{19}H_{19}N_3$ mw: 289.41

PROP: Leaves from water. Mp: 148°. Sltly sol in cold water; sol in abs alc, and benzene.

SYNS: LEUCOPARAFUCHSIN ◇ LEUCOPARAFUCHSINE
◇ 4,4′,4′′-METHYLIDYNETRIANILINE ◇ 4,4′,4′′-METHYLI-
DYNETRISBENZENEAMINE ◇ p,p′,p′′-TRIAMINOTRIPHE-
NYLMETHANE ◇ 4,4′,4′′-TRIAMINOTRIPHENYLMETHANE
◇ TRIS-4-AMINOFENYLMETHAN (CZECH)

TOXICITY DATA with REFERENCE
ETA: orl-mus TDLo: 64 g/kg/64W-I   VOONAW
22(9),66,76
ETA: orl-rat TDLo: 26 g/kg/47W-I   VOONAW
22(9),66,76

ETA: scu-mus TDLo: 16 g/kg/39W-I   VOONAW
22(9),66,76
ETA: scu-rat TDLo: 10 g/kg/90W-I   VOONAW
22(9),66,76
ETA: skn-mus TDLo: 6880 mg/kg/43W-I
VOONAW 22(9),66,76

SAFETY PROFILE: Questionable carcinogen with experimental tumorigenic data. Moderately toxic by ingestion. An eye irritant. When heated to decomposition it emits toxic fumes of NO_x.

THQ900   CAS: 5433-44-3
p,p′-TRIAZENYLENEDIBENZENE-SULFONAMIDE
mf: $C_{12}H_{13}N_5O_4S_2$ mw: 355.42

SYNS: 1,3-DI(4-SULFAMOYLPHENYL)TRIAZENE
◇ DSPT

TOXICITY DATA with REFERENCE
ETA: orl-mus TDLo: 9600 mg/kg (13-18D post)   CRNGDP 5,571,84
MUT: cyt-dmg-orl 2800 µmol/L/3D-I   CRNGDP
5,571,84

SAFETY PROFILE: Questionable carcinogen with experimental tumorigenic data. Experimental reproductive effects. Mutation data reported. When heated to decomposition it emits toxic fumes of NO_x and SO_x.

THR750   CAS: 461-89-2
s-TRIAZINE-3,5(2H,4H)-DIONE
mf: $C_3H_3N_3O_2$ mw: 113.09

SYNS: 4(6)-AZAURACIL ◇ 6-AZAURACIL ◇ NSC 3425
◇ USAF CB-30

TOXICITY DATA with REFERENCE
ETA: orl-rat TDLo: 39 g/kg/1Y-I   JNCIAM
41,985,68

SAFETY PROFILE: Questionable carcinogen with experimental tumorigenic data. Poison by intraperitoneal route. When heated to decomposition it emits toxic fumes of NO_x.

THS000   CAS: 108-80-5
s-TRIAZINE-2,4,6-TRIOL
mf: $C_3H_3N_3O_3$ mw: 129.09

PROP: Off-white; odorless crystals. Mp: >360°, d: 2.500 @ 20°/4°.

SYNS: CYANURIC ACID ◇ ISOCYANURIC ACID
◇ KYSELINA KYANUROVA (CZECH) ◇ PSEUDOCYANURIC
ACID ◇ sym-TRIAZINETRIOL ◇ s-2,4,6-TRIAZINETRIOL

◇ s-TRIAZINE-2,4,6(1H,3H,5H)-TRIONE ◇ TRICYANIC ACID
◇ TRIHYDROXYCYANIDINE ◇ 2,4,6-TRIHYDROXY-1,3,5-
TRIAZINE

TOXICITY DATA with REFERENCE
ETA: orl-mus TDLo:130 g/kg/2Y-I   VOONAW
    16(1),82,70
ETA: orl-rat TD:60750 mg/kg/81W-I   AJHEAA
    65,155,74
ETA: orl-rat TDLo:55 g/kg/82W-I   VOONAW
    16(1),82,70
ETA: scu-rat TD:36 g/kg/2Y-I   AJHEAA 65,155,74
ETA: scu-rat TDLo:27 g/kg/2Y-I   VOONAW
    16(1),82,70
ETA: skn-mus TDLo:138 g/kg/2Y-I   VOONAW
    16(1),82,70
ETA: skn-mus TDLo:2400 mg/kg/W-L
    AJHEAA 64,155,74

CONSENSUS REPORTS: Reported in EPA
TSCA Inventory.

SAFETY PROFILE: Questionable carcinogen
with experimental tumorigenic data. Moderately
toxic by ingestion. An eye irritant. Irritating
to abraided skin. When heated to decomposition
it emits very toxic fumes of NO_x and CN^-.
Used to stabilize chlorine solutions used in
swimming pools.

THV250   CAS: 724-31-2
1,3,7-TRIBROMO-2-FLUORENAMINE
mf: $C_{13}H_8Br_3N$ mw: 417.95

SYN: 1,3,7-TRIBROMOFLUOREN-2-AMINE

TOXICITY DATA with REFERENCE
ETA: orl-rat TDLo:360 mg/kg/27D-I   CNREA8
    28,924,68

SAFETY PROFILE: Questionable carcinogen
with experimental tumorigenic data. When
heated to decomposition it emits very toxic
fumes of Br^- and NO_x.

TIG750   CAS: 60-01-5
TRIBUTYRIN
mf: $C_{15}H_{26}O_6$ mw: 302.41

PROP: Colorless, oily liquid; bitter taste. Mp:
−75°, d: 1.0356 @ 20/20°, bp: 305-310°, flash
p: +212°F. Insol in water; very sol in alc, ether,
chloroform.

SYNS: BUTANOIC ACID, 1,2,3-PROPANETRIYL ESTER
◇ BUTYRIC ACID TRIESTER with GLYCERIN ◇ BUTYRYL
TRIGLYCERIDE ◇ FEMA No. 2223 ◇ GLYCEROL TRIBUTY-
RATE ◇ KODAFLEX ◇ TRIBUTYROIN

TOXICITY DATA with REFERENCE
ETA: orl-rat TDLo:177 g/kg/3W-C   JNCIAM
    10,361,49

CONSENSUS REPORTS: Reported in EPA
TSCA Inventory.

SAFETY PROFILE: Questionable carcinogen
with experimental tumorigenic data. Poison by
intravenous route. Moderately toxic by ingestion. Combustible liquid. When heated to decomposition it emits acrid smoke and irritating
fumes.

TII250   CAS: 76-03-9
TRICHLOROACETIC ACID
DOT: 1839/2564
mf: $C_2HCl_3O_2$ mw: 163.38

PROP: Colorless, rhombic, deliquescent crystals. Bp: 197.5°, fp: 57.7°, flash p: none, d:
1.6298 @ 61°/4°, vap press: 1 mm @ 51.0°.

SYNS: ACETO-CAUSTIN ◇ ACIDE TRICHLORACETIQUE
(FRENCH) ◇ ACIDO TRICLOROACETICO (ITALIAN)
◇ AMCHEM GRASS KILLER ◇ DOW SODIUM TCA INHIB-
ITED ◇ KONESTA ◇ SODIUM TCA SOLUTION ◇ TCA
◇ TRICHLOORAZIJNZUUR (DUTCH) ◇ TRICHLORESSIG-
SAEURE (GERMAN) ◇ TRICHLOROACETIC ACID, SOLID
(DOT) ◇ TRICHLOROACETIC ACID SOLUTION (DOT)
◇ TRICHLOROETHANOIC ACID ◇ VARITOX

TOXICITY DATA with REFERENCE
CAR: orl-mus TDLo:427 g/kg/61W-C   TXAPA9
    90,183,87
MUT: mmo-sat 250 μg/plate   CNJGA8 22,35,80

CONSENSUS REPORTS: Reported in EPA
TSCA Inventory. EPA Genetic Toxicology Program.

OSHA PEL: TWA 1 ppm   ACGIH TLV: TWA
1 ppm   DOT Classification: Corrosive Material; Label: Corrosive, solid; Corrosive Material;
Label: Corrosive, solution.

SAFETY PROFILE: Questionable carcinogen
with experimental carcinogenic data. Poison by
ingestion and subcutaneous routes. Moderately
toxic by intraperitoneal route. Mutation data
reported. A corrosive irritant to skin, eyes, and
mucous membranes. When heated to decomposition it emits toxic fumes of Cl^- and Na_2O.
Used as an herbicide.

TIJ000   CAS: 63041-25-8
**10-TRICHLOROACETYL-1,2-
BENZANTHRACENE**
mf: $C_{20}H_{11}Cl_3O$ mw: 373.66

SYNS: 1-(BENZ(a)ANTHRACEN-7-YL)-2,2,2-TRICHLO-
ROETHANONE ◇ BENZ(a)ANTHRACEN-7-YL TRICHLORO-
METHYL KETONE

TOXICITY DATA with REFERENCE
ETA: scu-mus TDLo:80 mg/kg   XPHPAW
149,191,51

ETA: scu-rat TDLo:45 mg/kg   XPHPAW 149,191,51

SAFETY PROFILE: Questionable carcinogen
with experimental tumorigenic data. When
heated to decomposition it emits toxic fumes
of Cl⁻.

TIJ750   CAS: 634-93-5
2,4,6-TRICHLOROANILINE
mf: $C_6H_4Cl_3N$ mw: 196.46

PROP: Needles from liquid. Mp: 77.5-78.5°,
bp: 262° @ 46 mm, Insol in H_3PO_4; sol in
alc, ether.

SYNS: sym-TRICHLOROANILINE ◇ 2,4,6-TRICHLORO-
BENZENAMINE

TOXICITY DATA with REFERENCE
CAR: orl-mus TD:780 g/kg/78W-C   JEPTDQ
2,325,78

CAR: orl-mus TDLo:390 g/kg/78W-C   JEPTDQ
2,325,78

CONSENSUS REPORTS: Reported in EPA
TSCA Inventory.

SAFETY PROFILE: Questionable carcinogen
with experimental carcinogenic data. Moderately toxic by ingestion. When heated to decomposition it emits very toxic fumes of Cl⁻ and
NO_x.

TIO500   CAS: 107-69-7
TRICHLOROETHYL CARBAMATE
mf: $C_3H_4Cl_3NO_2$ mw: 192.43

SYNS: CARBAMIC ACID, 2,2,2-TRICHLOROETHYL ES-
TER ◇ 2,2,2-TRICHLOROETHANOL CARBAMATE
◇ VOLUNTAL

TOXICITY DATA with REFERENCE
NEO: ipr-mus TDLo:3250 mg/kg/13W-I
JNCIAM 8,99,47

SAFETY PROFILE: Questionable carcinogen
with experimental neoplastigenic data. Moderately toxic by ingestion and intraperitoneal
routes. When heated to decomposition it emits
very toxic fumes of Cl⁻ and NO_x.

TIQ250   CAS: 52-68-6
((2,2,2-TRICHLORO-1-HYDROXYETHYL)
DIMETHYLPHOSPHONATE)
mf: $C_4H_8Cl_3O_4P$ mw: 257.44

SYNS: AEROL 1 (PESTICIDE) ◇ AGROFOROTOX
◇ ANTHON ◇ BAY 15922 ◇ BAYER 15922 ◇ BAYER L 13/
59 ◇ BILARCIL ◇ BOVINOX ◇ BRITON ◇ BRITTEN
◇ CEKUFON ◇ CHLORAK ◇ CHLORFOS ◇ CHLOROFOS
◇ CHLOROFTALM ◇ CHLOROPHOS ◇ CHLOROPHTHALM
◇ CHLOROXYPHOS ◇ CICLOSOM ◇ CLOROFOS (RUSSIAN)
◇ COMBOT EQUINE ◇ DANEX ◇ DEP (PESTICIDE)
◇ DEPTHON ◇ DETF ◇ DIMETHOXY-2,2,2-TRICHLORO-1-
HYDROXY-ETHYL-PHOSPHINE OXIDE ◇ O,O-DIMETHYL-
(1-HYDROXY-2,2,2-TRICHLORAETHYL)PHOSPHON-
SAEURE ESTER (GERMAN) ◇ O,O-DIMETHYL-(1-HY-
DROXY-2,2,2-TRICHLORATHYL)-PHOSPHAT (GERMAN)
◇ O,O-DIMETHYL-(1-HYDROXY-2,2,2-TRICHLORO)ETHYL
PHOSPHATE ◇ DIMETHYL-1-HYDROXY-2,2,2-TRICHLORO-
ETHYL PHOSPHONATE ◇ O,O-DIMETHYL-(1-HYDROXY-
2,2,2-TRICHLOROETHYL)PHOSPHONATE ◇ O,O-DI-
METHYL-1-OXY-2,2,2-TRICHLOROETHYL PHOSPHO-
NATE ◇ O,O-DIMETHYL-(2,2,2-TRICHLOOR-1-HYDROXY-
ETHYL)-FOSFONAAT (DUTCH) ◇ O,O-DIMETHYL-(2,2,2-
TRICHLOR-1-HYDROXY-AETHYL)PHOSPHONAT (GER-
MAN) ◇ DIMETHYLTRICHLOROHYDROXYETHYL PHOS-
PHONATE ◇ DIMETHYL-2,2,2-TRICHLORO-1-HYDROXY-
ETHYLPHOSPHONATE ◇ O,O-DIMETHYL-2,2,2-TRICHLO-
RO-1-HYDROXYETHYL PHOSPHONATE ◇ O,O-DIMETIL-
(2,2,2-TRICLORO-1-IDROSSI-ETIL)-FOSFONATO (ITALIAN)
◇ DIMETOX ◇ DIPTERAX ◇ DIPTEREX ◇ DIPTEREX 50
◇ DIPTEVUR ◇ DITRIFON ◇ DYLOX ◇ DYLOX-METASYS-
TOX-R ◇ DYREX ◇ DYVON ◇ ENT 19,763 ◇ EQUINO-ACID
◇ EQUINO-AID ◇ FLIBOL E ◇ FLIEGENTELLER ◇ FOROTOX
◇ FOSCHLOR ◇ FOSCHLOREM (POLISH) ◇ FOSCHLOR R-
50 ◇ 1-HYDROXY-2,2,2-TRICHLOROETHYLPHOSPHONIC
ACID DIMETHYL ESTER ◇ HYPODERMACID ◇ LEIVASOM
◇ LOISOL ◇ MASOTEN ◇ MAZOTEN ◇ METHYL CHLORO-
PHOS ◇ METIFONATE ◇ METRIFONATE ◇ METRIPHO-
NATE ◇ NCI-C54831 ◇ NEGUVON ◇ NEGUVON A
◇ PHOSCHLOR R50 ◇ POLFOSCHLOR ◇ PROXOL
◇ RICIFON ◇ RITSIFON ◇ SATOX 20WSC ◇ SOLDEP
◇ SOTIPOX ◇ TRICHLOORFON (DUTCH) ◇ TRI-
CHLORFON (USDA) ◇ 2,2,2-TRICHLORO-1-HYDROXY-
ETHYL-PHOSPHONATE, DIMETHYL ESTER ◇ (2,2,2-
TRICHLORO-1-HYDROXYETHYL)PHOSPHONIC
ACID DIMETHYL ESTER ◇ TRICHLOROPHON ◇ TRI-
CHLORPHENE ◇ TRICHLORPHON ◇ TRICHLORPHON
FN ◇ TRINEX ◇ TUGON ◇ TUGON FLY BAIT
◇ TUGON STABLE SPRAY ◇ VERMICIDE
BAYER 2349 ◇ VOLFARTOL ◇ VOTEXIT ◇ WEC 50
◇ WOTEXIT

TOXICITY DATA with REFERENCE

CAR: ims-rat TDLo: 183 mg/kg/6W-I ARGEAR 41,311,73

CAR: orl-rat TDLo: 186 mg/kg/6W-I ARGEAR 41,311,73

ETA: skn-rat TDLo: 1950 mg/kg/22W-I ERNFA7 16,515,72

MUT: cyt-mus-ipr 405 mg/kg WMHMAP 31(2),57,82

MUT: dns-hmn: oth 4 mol/L PSSCBG 15,439,84

MUT: mma-ssp 20 mmol/L MUREAV 117,139,83

MUT: mmo-ssp 20 mmol/L MUREAV 117,139,83

MUT: otr-mus: emb 3 mg/L PMRSDJ 5,659,85

MUT: sce-ham: lng 20 mg/L MUREAV 88,307,81

MUT: sce-hmn: lym 20 mg/L MUREAV 88,307,81

CONSENSUS REPORTS: IARC Cancer Review: Animal Inadequate Evidence IMEMDT 30,207,83. Community Right-To-Know List. EPA Genetic Toxicology Program.

DOT Classification: ORM-A; Label: None.

SAFETY PROFILE: Questionable carcinogen with experimental carcinogenic, tumorigenic, and teratogenic data. Poison by ingestion, inhalation, intraperitoneal, subcutaneous, intravenous, and intramuscular routes. Moderately toxic by skin contact and possibly other routes. Experimental reproductive effects. Human mutation data reported. An eye irritant. When heated to decomposition it emits very toxic fumes of Cl^- and PO_x.

TIT250   CAS: 133-07-3
N-(TRICHLOROMETHYLTHIO) PHTHALIMIDE
mf: $C_9H_4Cl_3NO_2S$ mw: 296.55

SYNS: FOLPAN ◇ FOLPET ◇ FTALAN ◇ ORTHOPHALTAN ◇ PHALTAN ◇ PHTHALTAN ◇ THIOPHAL ◇ N-(TRICHLOR-METHYLTHIO)-PHTHALAMID (GERMAN) ◇ N-(TRICHLOROMETHYLMERCPATO)PHTHALIMIDE ◇ 2-((TRICHLOROMETHYL)THIO)-1H-ISOINDOLE-1,3(2H)-DIONE ◇ TROYSAN ANTI-MILDEW O

TOXICITY DATA with REFERENCE

ETA: scu-mus TDLo: 1000 mg/kg NTIS** PB223-159

MUT: cyt-hmn: lym 15 μg/L/15M MUREAV 53,263,78

MUT: dlt-rat-orl 500 mg/kg/5D FCTXAV 10,363,72

MUT: dns-hmn: fbr 100 μmol/L NTIS** PB268-647

MUT: mma-bcs 50 μg/plate JAFCAU 29,268,81

MUT: mmo-bcs 50 μg/plate JAFCAU 29,268,81

MUT: mmo-esc 5 μg/plate NTIS** PB268-647

MUT: mmo-sat 16 nmol/plate CRNGDP 2,283,81

MUT: mrc-bcs 10 μg/disc/24H MUREAV 40,19,76

MUT: msc-ham: ovr 100 mg/L ENMUDM 3,233,81

MUT: sln-dmg-orl 2000 ppm JPFCD2 B15,867,80

CONSENSUS REPORTS: Reported in EPA TSCA Inventory. EPA Genetic Toxicology Program.

SAFETY PROFILE: Questionable carcinogen with experimental tumorigenic and teratogenic data. Poison by intraperitoneal route. Moderately toxic by ingestion. Experimental reproductive effects. Human mutation data reported. When heated to decomposition it emits very toxic fumes of Cl^-, NO_x, and SO_x. Used as a fungicide.

TIX000   CAS: 2122-77-2
2-(2,4,5-TRICHLOROPHENOXY) ETHANOL
mf: $C_8H_7Cl_3O_2$ mw: 241.50

SYNS: KLORINOL ◇ TCPE

TOXICITY DATA with REFERENCE

ETA: orl-mus TDLo: 3480 mg/kg/52W-I IARCCD 25,167,79

MUT: sce-ham: ovr 100 mg/L CRNGDP 5,1725,84

SAFETY PROFILE: Questionable carcinogen with experimental tumorigenic data. Moderately toxic by ingestion. Mutation data reported. When heated to decomposition it emits toxic fumes of Cl^-. Used as an agricultural chemical and pesticide.

TJD750   CAS: 108-77-0
2,4,6-TRICHLOROTRIAZINE
DOT: 2670
mf: $C_3Cl_3N_3$ mw: 184.41

PROP: Monoclinic, colorless crystals; pungent odor. Mp: 145.8°, bp: 190°, d: 1.32 @ 20/4°, vap press: 2 mm @ 70°, vap d: 6.36. Contains 96.9% cyanuric chloride, the remainder is cyanuric acid (VOONAW 12(4),78,66).

SYNS: CHLOROTRIAZINE ◇ CYANURCHLORIDE ◇ CYANURIC ACID CHLORIDE ◇ CYANURIC CHLORIDE (DOT) ◇ CYANURIC TRICHLORIDE (DOT) ◇ CYANURYL CHLORIDE ◇ KYANURCHLORID (CZECH) ◇ s-TRIAZINE TRICHLORIDE ◇ TRICHLOROCYANIDINE ◇ TRICHLORO-

s-TRIAZINE ◊ sym-TRICHLOROTRIAZINE ◊ 1,3,5-TRICHLO-
ROTRIAZINE ◊ 2,4,6-TRICHLORO-s-TRIAZINE ◊ 2,4,6-TRI-
CHLORO-1,3,5-TRIAZINE ◊ sym-TRICHLOTRIAZIN (CZECH)
◊ TRICYANOGEN CHLORIDE

TOXICITY DATA with REFERENCE
ETA: mul-rat TDLo: 16 g/kg/73W-I   VOONAW
   12(4),78,66
ETA: orl-rat TDLo: 20 g/kg/73W-I: TER
   VOONAW 12(4),78,66

CONSENSUS REPORTS: Reported in EPA
TSCA Inventory.

SAFETY PROFILE: Questionable carcinogen
with experimental tumorigenic and teratogenic
data. Poison by ingestion, inhalation, and intravenous routes. A skin and severe eye irritant.
An allergen. Has been reported as causing irritation of mucous membranes and heart rhythm
disturbances in humans. When heated to decomposition it emits toxic fumes of Cl^- and NO_x.

TJH250   CAS: 195-84-6
TRICYCLOQUINAZOLINE
mf: $C_{21}H_{12}N_4$ mw: 320.37

TOXICITY DATA with REFERENCE
CAR: skn-mus TDLo: 380 mg/kg/16W-I
   BJCAAI 13,94,59
NEO: skn-mus TD: 960 mg/kg/40W-I   BJCAAI
   16,275,62
ETA: scu-rat TDLo: 1600 mg/kg/17W-I   BJCAAI
   13,94,59

SAFETY PROFILE: Questionable carcinogen
with experimental carcinogenic, neoplastigenic,
and tumorigenic data. When heated to decomposition it emits toxic fumes of NO_x.

TJI500   CAS: 63978-73-4
**TRIDECANOIC ACID-2,3-EPOXYPROPYL
ESTER**
mf: $C_{16}H_{30}O_3$ mw: 270.46

SYN: GLYCIDYL ESTER of DODECANOIC ACID

TOXICITY DATA with REFERENCE
ETA: scu-rat TDLo: 4400 mg/kg/5W-I   ANYAA9
   68,750,58

SAFETY PROFILE: Questionable carcinogen
with experimental tumorigenic data. When
heated to decomposition it emits acrid smoke
and irritating fumes.

TJK500   CAS: 52338-90-6
1,2,4,5,9,10-TRIEPOXYDECANE
mf: $C_{10}H_{16}O_3$ mw: 184.26

TOXICITY DATA with REFERENCE
NEO: scu-mus TDLo: 1040 mg/kg/26W-I
   JNCIAM 53,695,74
ETA: skn-mus TDLo: 864 mg/kg/72W-I
   JNCIAM 53,695,74

SAFETY PROFILE: Questionable carcinogen
with experimental neoplastigenic and tumorigenic data. When heated to decomposition it
emits acrid smoke and irritating fumes.

TJQ100   CAS: 1680-21-3
TRIETHYLENE GLYCOL DIACRYLATE
mf: $C_{12}H_{18}O_6$ mw: 258.30

SYNS: ACRYLIC ACID, DIESTER with TRIETHYLENE GLY-
COL ◊ 2-PROPENOIC ACID, 1,2-ETHANEDIYLBIS(OXY-2,1-
ETHANEDIYL) ESTER (9CI)

TOXICITY DATA with REFERENCE
ETA: skn-mus TDLo: 16 g/kg/80W-I   JTEHD6
   19,149,86

CONSENSUS REPORTS: Reported in EPA
TSCA Inventory.

SAFETY PROFILE: Questionable carcinogen
with experimental tumorigenic data. Moderately
toxic by ingestion and skin contact. Severe skin
and eye irritant. When heated to decomposition
it emits acrid smoke and irritating fumes.

TJQ333   CAS: 1954-28-5
**TRIETHYLENE GLYCOL DIGLYCIDYL
ETHER**
mf: $C_{12}H_{22}O_6$ mw: 262.34

SYNS: AYERST 62013 ◊ 2,2'-(2,5,8,11-TETRAOXA-1,12-
DODECANE DIYL)BISOXIRANE ◊ 1,2-BIS(2,3-EPOXYPRO-
POXY)ETHOXY)ETHANE ◊ 1,2,15,16-DIEPOXY-4,7,10,13-
TETRAOXAHEXADECANE ◊ DIGLYCIDYLTRIETHYLENE
GLYCOL ◊ EPODYL ◊ ETHOGLUCID ◊ ETHOGLUCIDE
◊ ETOGLUCID ◊ ICI-32865 ◊ OXIRANE, 2,2'-(2,5,8,11-TET-
RAOXADODECANE-1,12-DIYL)BIS- (9CI) ◊ 2,2'-(2,5,8,11-
TETRAOXA-1,2-DODECANEDIYL)BISOXIRANE ◊ TDE

TOXICITY DATA with REFERENCE
NEO: ipr-mus TFLo: 3800 mg/kg/4W   JNCIAM
   36,915,66
MUT: mmo-sat 10 μg/plate   MUREAV 111,99,83

CONSENSUS REPORTS: IARC Cancer Review: GROUP 3 IMEMDT 7,56,87; Animal
Limited Evidence IMEMDT 11,209,76.

SAFETY PROFILE: Questionable carcinogen
with experimental neoplastigenic data. Moderately toxic by intraperitoneal route. A skin irri-

tant. When heated to decomposition it emits acrid smoke and irritating fumes.

TJQ500   CAS: 111-22-8
TRIETHYLENE GLYCOL, DINITRATE
mf: $C_6H_{12}O_4 \cdot N_2O_4$ mw: 240.20

CONSENSUS REPORTS: Reported in EPA TSCA Inventory.

SAFETY PROFILE: Questionable carcinogen with experimental carcinogenic data. Moderately toxic by ingestion, intraperitoneal, and subcutaneous routes. When heated to decomposition it emits toxic fumes of NO_x.

TJY175   CAS: 75-88-7
2,2,2-TRIFLUOROCHLOROETHANE
mf: $C_2H_2ClF_3$ mw: 118.49

SYNS: CFC 133a ◊ 1-CHLORO-2,2,2-TRIFLUOROETHANE ◊ 2-CHLORO-1,1,1-TRIFLUOROETHANE ◊ FC 133a ◊ FREON 133a ◊ GENETRON 133a ◊ R 133a ◊ 1,1,1-TRIFLUORO-2-CHLOROETHANE ◊ 1,1,1-TRIFLUOROETHYL CHLORIDE

TOXICITY DATA with REFERENCE
CAR: orl-rat TDLo: 78 g/kg/1Y-I   TXAPA9 72,15,84

CONSENSUS REPORTS: IARC Cancer Review: GROUP 3 IMEMDT 7,56,87; Animal Limited Evidence IMEMDT 41,253,86. Reported in EPA TSCA Inventory.

SAFETY PROFILE: Questionable carcinogen with experimental carcinogenic data. When heated to decomposition it emits toxic fumes of F^-.

TKC000   CAS: 52833-75-7
4-TRIFLUOROMETHYL-6H-BENZO(e)(1) BENZOTHIOPYRANO(4,3-b)INDOLE
mf: $C_{20}H_{12}F_3NS$ mw: 355.39

TOXICITY DATA with REFERENCE
NEO: scu-mus TDLo: 92 mg/kg/9W-I   MUREAV 66,307,79

SAFETY PROFILE: Questionable carcinogen with experimental neoplastigenic data. When heated to decomposition it emits very toxic fumes of F^-, NO_x, and SO_x.

TKH000   CAS: 318-22-9
2,2,2-TRIFLUORO-N-(9-OXOFLUOREN-2-YL)ACETAMIDE
mf: $C_{15}H_8F_3NO_2$ mw: 291.24

SYN: 2-TRIFLUOROACETYLAMINOFLUOREN-9-ONE

TOXICITY DATA with REFERENCE
CAR: orl-rat TDLo: 6400 mg/kg/35W-C CNREA8 22,1002,62

SAFETY PROFILE: Questionable carcinogen with experimental carcinogenic data. When heated to decomposition it emits very toxic fumes of F^- and NO_x.

TKK000   CAS: 675-14-9
2,4,6-TRIFLUORO-s-TRIAZINE
mf: $C_3F_3N_3$ mw: 135.06

SYN: CYANURIC FLUORIDE

TOXICITY DATA with REFERENCE
CAR: skn-rbt LD50: 160 mg/kg   AIHAAP 33,382,72

CONSENSUS REPORTS: EPA Extremely Hazardous Substances List. Reported in EPA TSCA Inventory.

SAFETY PROFILE: Questionable carcinogen with experimental carcinogenic data. Poison by skin contact and inhalation. When heated to decomposition it emits very toxic fumes of F^- and NO_x.

TKP500   CAS: 102-71-6
TRIHYDROXYTRIETHYLAMINE
mf: $C_6H_{15}NO_3$ mw: 149.22

PROP: Pale yellow viscous liquid. Mp: 21.2°, bp: 360°, flash p: 355°F (CC), d: 1.1258 @ 20/20°, vap press: 10 mm @ 205°, vap d: 5.14.

SYNS: DALTOGEN ◊ NITRILO-2,2',2''-TRIETHANOL ◊ 2,2',2''-NITRILOTRIETHANOL ◊ STEROLAMIDE ◊ THIOFACO T-35 ◊ TRIAETHANOLAMIN-NG ◊ TRIETHANOLAMIN ◊ TRIETHANOLAMINE ◊ TRIETHYLOLAMINE ◊ TRI(HYDROXYETHYL)AMINE ◊ 2,2',2''-TRIHYDROXY-TRIETHYLAMINE ◊ TRIS(2-HYDROXYETHYL)AMINE ◊ TROLAMINE

TOXICITY DATA with REFERENCE
CAR: orl-mus TD: 154 g/kg/61W-C   CNREA8 38,3918,78
CAR: orl-mus TDLo: 16 g/kg/64W-C   CNREA8 38,3918,78

CONSENSUS REPORTS: Cyanide and its compounds are on the Community Right-To-Know List. Reported in EPA TSCA Inventory. EPA Genetic Toxicology Program.

SAFETY PROFILE: Questionable carcinogen with experimental carcinogenic data. Moderately toxic by intraperitoneal route. Mildly toxic by ingestion. Liver and kidney damage has been demonstrated in animals from chronic exposure. A human and experimental skin irritant. An eye irritant. Combustible liquid when exposed to heat or flame; can react vigorously with oxidizing materials. To fight fire, use alcohol foam, CO_2, dry chemical. When heated to decomposition it emits toxic fumes of NO_x and CN^-.

TLA250   CAS: 34346-90-2
3,4,5-TRIMETHOXYCINNAMALDEHYDE
mf: $C_{12}H_{14}O_4$ mw: 222.26

SYNS: TMCA ◇ 3-(3,4,5-TRIMETHOXYPHENYL)-2-PROPENAL

TOXICITY DATA with REFERENCE
ETA: mul-rat TDLo: 250 mg/kg/7D-I   BJCAAI 26,504,72
ETA: scu-rat TDLo: 100 mg/kg   JNCIAM 47,1037,71

SAFETY PROFILE: Questionable carcinogen with experimental tumorigenic data. When heated to decomposition it emits acrid smoke and irritating fumes.

TLC850
3,4,5-TRIMETHOXY-α-VINYLBENZYL ALCOHOL ACETATE
mf: $C_{14}H_{18}O_5$ mw: 266.32

SYN: 1'-ACETOXYELEMICIN

TOXICITY DATA with REFERENCE
CAR: ipr-mus TDLo: 408 mg/kg/4D-I   CNREA8 47,2275,87
MUT: mmo-sat 2 μmol/plate   CRNGDP 7,2089,86

SAFETY PROFILE: Questionable carcinogen with experimental carcinogenic data. Mutation data reported. When heated to decomposition it emits acrid smoke and irritating fumes.

TLD250   CAS: 5096-21-9
2,4,6-TRIMETHYLACETANILIDE
mf: $C_{11}H_{15}NO$ mw: 177.27

SYNS: ACETOMESIDIDE ◇ 2',4',6'-TRIMETHYLACETA-NILIDE ◇ N-(2,4,6-TRIMETHYLPHENYL)ACETAMIDE

TOXICITY DATA with REFERENCE
ETA: orl-rat TDLo: 3500 mg/kg   CNREA8 26,619,66

SAFETY PROFILE: Questionable carcinogen with experimental tumorigenic data. Moderately

toxic by ingestion. When heated to decomposition it emits toxic fumes of NO_x.

TLE750   CAS: 54-88-6
2,N,N-TRIMETHYL-4-AMINOAZOBENZENE
mf: $C_{15}H_{17}N_3$ mw: 239.35

SYNS: N,N-DIMETHYL-4-(PHENYLAZO)-m-TOLUIDINE ◇ 2-MeDAB ◇ 2-METHYL-DAB ◇ 2-METHYL-N,N-DI-METHYL-4-AMINOAZOBENZENE ◇ 2-METHYL-4-DI-METHYLAMINOAZOBENZENE

TOXICITY DATA with REFERENCE
NEO: scu-mus TDLo: 40 mg/kg/5D-I   JNCIAM 47,593,71
MUT: dni-rat-orl 1080 mg/kg/30D-I   CBINA8 48,221,84
MUT: dns-rat: lvr 1 μmol/L   CNREA8 42,3010,82
MUT: mma-sat 120 μg/plate   PNASA6 72,5135,75
MUT: mrc-smc 5 pph   JNCIAM 62,901,79
MUT: oms-rat-orl 1080 mg/kg30D-I   CBINA8 48,221,84
MUT: otr-rat: emb 1200 μg/L   JJIND8 67,1303,81
MUT: sce-rat: lvr 40 μmol/L   MUREAV 93,409,82

CONSENSUS REPORTS: EPA Genetic Toxicology Program.

SAFETY PROFILE: Questionable carcinogen with experimental neoplastigenic data. Poison by intraperitoneal route. Mutation data reported. When heated to decomposition it emits toxic fumes of NO_x.

TLF000   CAS: 73728-79-7
3,2',5'-TRIMETHYL-4-AMINODIPHENYL
mf: $C_{15}H_{17}N$ mw: 211.33

SYN: 3,2',5'-TRIMETHYLBIPHENYLAMINE

TOXICITY DATA with REFERENCE
ETA: scu-rat TDLo: 1400 mg/kg/W-I   BMBUAQ 14,141,58

SAFETY PROFILE: Questionable carcinogen with experimental tumorigenic data. When heated to decomposition it emits toxic fumes of NO_x.

TLG500   CAS: 88-05-1
2,4,6-TRIMETHYLANILINE
mf: $C_9H_{13}N$ mw: 135.23

SYNS: AMINOMESITYLENE ◇ 2-AMINOMESITYLENE ◇ 1-AMINO-2,4,6-TRIMETHYLBENZEN (CZECH) ◇ 2-AMINO-1,3,5-TRIMETHYLBENZENE ◇ MESIDIN (CZECH) ◇ MESIDINE ◇ MESITYLAMINE ◇ MEZIDINE ◇ 2,4,6-TRIMETHYLBENZENAMINE

TOXICITY DATA with REFERENCE
CAR: orl-rat TD:4200 mg/kg/78W-C   AICCA6 20,1364,64

CAR: orl-rat TDLo:4000 mg/kg/78W-C JNCIAM 58,377,77

MUT: dnd-ham:lng 3 mmol/L/2H   MUREAV 77,317,80

CONSENSUS REPORTS: IARC Cancer Review: Animal Inadequate Evidence IMEMDT 27,177,82. EPA Extremely Hazardous Substances List. Reported in EPA TSCA Inventory.

SAFETY PROFILE: Questionable carcinogen with experimental carcinogenic data. Poison by inhalation and possibly other routes. Moderately toxic by ingestion and possibly other routes. Mutation data reported. A skin and severe eye irritant. When heated to decomposition it emits toxic fumes of NO_x.

TLG750   CAS: 21436-97-5
2,4,5-TRIMETHYLANILINE
HYDROCHLORIDE
mf: $C_9H_{13}N \cdot ClH$ mw: 171.69

SYNS: 1-AMINO-2,4,5-TRIMETHYLBENZENE HYDROCHLORIDE ◇ psi-CUMIDINE HYDROCHLORIDE ◇ PSEUDO-CUMIDINE HYDROCHLORIDE ◇ 1,2,4-TRIMETHYL-5-AMINOBENZENE HYDROCHLORIDE ◇ 2,4,5-TRIMETHYL-BENZENAMINE HYDROCHLORIDE

TOXICITY DATA with REFERENCE
CAR: orl-mus TD:130 g/kg/78W-C   JEPTDQ 2,325,78

CAR: orl-mus TD:540 g/kg/77W-C   IARC** 27,177,82

CAR: orl-mus TD:1080 g/kg/77W-C   IARC** 27,177,82

CAR: orl-mus TDLo:65 g/kg/78W-C   JEPTDQ 2,325,78

NEO: orl-rat TDLo:32 g/kg/78W-C   JEPTDQ 2,325,78

ETA: orl-rat TD:65 g/kg/78W-C   JEPTDQ 2,325,78

ETA: orl-rat TD:540 g/kg/77W-C   IARC** 27,177,82

ETA: orl-rat TD:1080 g/kg/77W-C   IARC** 27,177,82

CONSENSUS REPORTS: IARC Cancer Review: Animal Inadequate Evidence IMEMDT 27,177,82.

SAFETY PROFILE: Questionable carcinogen with experimental carcinogenic, neoplastigenic, and tumorigenic data. Poison by intraperitoneal route. Moderately toxic by ingestion. When heated to decomposition it emits very toxic fumes of NO_x and HCl.

TLH100   CAS: 63018-94-0
2,9,10-TRIMETHYLANTHRACENE
mf: $C_{17}H_{16}$ mw: 220.31

TOXICITY DATA with REFERENCE
CAR: skn-mus TDLo:40 mg/kg/20D-I   CRNGDP 6,1483,85

MUT: mma-sat 5 µg/plate   CRNGDP 6,1483,85
MUT: mmo-sat 20 µg/plate   CRNGDP 6,1483,85

SAFETY PROFILE: Questionable carcinogen with experimental carcinogenic data. Mutation data reported. When heated to decomposition it emits acrid smoke and irritating fumes.

TLH350   CAS: 63040-05-1
3,5,9-TRIMETHYL-1:2-BENZACRIDINE
mf: $C_{20}H_{17}N$ mw: 271.38

SYNS: 1,6,10-TRIMETHYL,7:8 BENZACRIDINE (FRENCH) ◇ 5,7,11-TRIMETHYLBENZ(c)ACRIDINE

TOXICITY DATA with REFERENCE
ETA: scu-mus TDLo:20 mg/kg   AICCA6 7,184,50
ETA: skn-mus TD:290 mg/kg/24W-I   ACRSAJ 4,315,56

ETA: skn-mus TDLo:250 mg/kg/21W-I AICCA6 7,184,50

SAFETY PROFILE: Questionable carcinogen with experimental tumorigenic data. When heated to decomposition it emits toxic fumes of NO_x.

TLH500   CAS: 63040-01-7
3,8,12-TRIMETHYLBENZ(a)ACRIDINE
mf: $C_{20}H_{17}N$ mw: 271.38

SYN: 1,10,3'-TRIMETHYL-5,6-BENZACRIDINE (FRENCH)

TOXICITY DATA with REFERENCE
ETA: scu-mus TD:50 mg/kg   BAFEAG 34,22,47
ETA: scu-mus TDLo:40 mg/kg   ACRSAJ 4,315,56

SAFETY PROFILE: Questionable carcinogen with experimental tumorigenic data. When heated to decomposition it emits toxic fumes of NO_x.

TLH750   CAS: 63040-02-8
5,7,8-TRIMETHYL-3:4-BENZACRIDINE
mf: $C_{20}H_{17}N$ mw: 271.38

SYN: 2,3,10 TRIMETHYL,5:6 BENZACRIDINE (FRENCH)

TOXICITY DATA with REFERENCE
ETA: scu-mus TD:20 mg/kg   ACRSAJ 4,315,56
ETA: scu-mus TDLo:20 mg/kg   AICCA6 7,184,50
ETA: skn-mus TDLo:270 mg/kg/22W-I
   AICCA6 7,184,50

SAFETY PROFILE: Questionable carcinogen with experimental tumorigenic data. When heated to decomposition it emits toxic fumes of NO$_x$.

TLI000   CAS: 64038-40-0
7,8,11-TRIMETHYLBENZ(c)ACRIDINE
mf: C$_{20}$H$_{17}$N   mw: 271.38

SYNS: 5,6,9-TRIMETHYL-1:2-BENZACRIDINE ◇ 1,4,10 TRIMETHYL,7:8 BENZACRIDINE (FRENCH)

TOXICITY DATA with REFERENCE
ETA: scu-mus TDLo:20 mg/kg   AICCA6 7,184,50
ETA: skn-mus TD:280 mg/kg/23W-I   AICCA6 7,184,50
ETA: skn-mus TDLo:270 mg/kg/25W-I
   ACRSAJ 4,315,56

SAFETY PROFILE: Questionable carcinogen with experimental tumorigenic data. When heated to decomposition it emits toxic fumes of NO$_x$.

TLI250   CAS: 58430-01-6
7,9,10-TRIMETHYLBENZ(c)ACRIDINE
mf: C$_{20}$H$_{17}$N   mw: 271.38

SYN: 2,3,10-TRIMETHYL-7:8-BENZACRIDINE (FRENCH)

TOXICITY DATA with REFERENCE
ETA: scu-mus TDLo:20 mg/kg   AICCA6 7,184,50
ETA: skn-mus TD:280 mg/kg/23W-I   AICCA6 7,184,50
ETA: skn-mus TDLo:270 mg/kg/25W-I
   ACRSAJ 4,315,56
MUT: mma-sat 1 nmol/plate   GANNA2 70,749,79

SAFETY PROFILE: Questionable carcinogen with experimental tumorigenic data. Mutation data reported. When heated to decomposition it emits toxic fumes of NO$_x$.

TLI500   CAS: 51787-42-9
7,9,11-TRIMETHYLBENZ(c)ACRIDINE
mf: C$_{20}$H$_{17}$N   mw: 271.38

SYN: 1,3,10-TRIMETHYL-7,8-BENZACRIDINE (FRENCH)

TOXICITY DATA with REFERENCE
ETA: scu-mus TD:336 mg/kg/28W-I   BAFEAG 34,22,47

ETA: scu-mus TDLo:200 mg/kg/4W-I   ACRSAJ 4,315,56
ETA: skn-mus TDLo:336 mg/kg/28W-I
   ACRSAJ 4,315,56
MUT: mma-sat 1 nmol/plate   GANNA2 70,749,79

SAFETY PROFILE: Questionable carcinogen with experimental tumorigenic data. Mutation data reported. When heated to decomposition it emits toxic fumes of NO$_x$.

TLI750   CAS: 51787-43-0
8,10,12-TRIMETHYLBENZ(a)ACRIDINE
mf: C$_{20}$H$_{17}$N   mw: 271.38

SYN: 1,3,10-TRIMETHYL-5,6-BENZACRIDINE (FRENCH)

TOXICITY DATA with REFERENCE
ETA: scu-mus TDLo:250 mg/kg/10D-I
   BAFEAG 34,22,47
ETA: skn-mus TDLo:348 mg/kg/29W-I
   ACRSAJ 4,315,56

SAFETY PROFILE: Questionable carcinogen with experimental tumorigenic data. When heated to decomposition it emits toxic fumes of NO$_x$.

TLJ250   CAS: 18429-71-5
4,5,10-TRIMETHYLBENZ(a) ANTHRACENE
mf: C$_{21}$H$_{18}$ mw: 270.39

TOXICITY DATA with REFERENCE
ETA: scu-rat TDLo:18 mg/kg   PSEBAA 128,720,68

SAFETY PROFILE: Questionable carcinogen with experimental tumorigenic data. When heated to decomposition it emits acrid smoke and irritating fumes.

TLJ500   CAS: 35187-24-7
4,7,12-TRIMETHYLBENZ(a) ANTHRACENE
mf: C$_{21}$H$_{18}$ mw: 270.39

TOXICITY DATA with REFERENCE
NEO: ims-rat TDLo:10 mg/kg   NATUAS273,566,78
MUT: mma-sat 20 μg/plate   CNREA8 36,4525,76

SAFETY PROFILE: Questionable carcinogen with experimental neoplastigenic data. Mutation data reported. When heated to decomposition it emits acrid smoke and irritating fumes.

TLJ750   CAS: 20627-33-2
4,9,10-TRIMETHYL-1,2-BENZANTHRACENE
mf: C$_{21}$H$_{18}$ mw: 270.39

SYN: 6,7,12-TRIMETHYLBENZ(a)ANTHRACENE

TOXICITY DATA with REFERENCE
ETA: scu-mus TDLo: 120 mg/kg/9W-I CRSBAW
148,812,54
ETA: skn-mus TDLo: 670 mg/kg/28W-I
CRSBAW 148,812,54
MUT: cyt-rat-ivn 50 mg/kg GANNA2 64,637,73

SAFETY PROFILE: Questionable carcinogen with experimental tumorigenic data. Mutation data reported. When heated to decomposition it emits acrid smoke and irritating fumes.

TLK000   CAS: 20627-32-1
6,7,8-TRIMETHYLBENZ(a) ANTHRACENE
mf: $C_{21}H_{18}$ mw: 270.39

TOXICITY DATA with REFERENCE
NEO: ims-rat TDLo: 50 mg/kg CNREA8 29,506,69

SAFETY PROFILE: Questionable carcinogen with experimental neoplastigenic data. When heated to decomposition it emits acrid smoke and irritating fumes.

TLK500   CAS: 20627-34-3
6,8,12-TRIMETHYLBENZ(a) ANTHRACENE
mf: $C_{21}H_{18}$ mw: 270.39

TOXICITY DATA with REFERENCE
NEO: ims-rat TDLo: 50 mg/kg CNREA8 29,506,69
ETA: ivn-rat TDLo: 175 mg/kg/10W-I JEMEAV
131,321,70
MUT: cyt-rat-ipr 140 mg/kg/10D-I JEMEAV
131,331,70
MUT: cyt-rat-ivn 50 mg/kg GANNA2 64,637,73

SAFETY PROFILE: Questionable carcinogen with experimental neoplastigenic and tumorigenic data. Mutation data reported. When heated to decomposition it emits acrid smoke and irritating fumes.

TLK600   CAS: 24891-41-6
6,9,12-TRIMETHYL-1,2-BENZANTHRACENE
mf: $C_{21}H_{18}$ mw: 270.39
SYN: 7,9,12-TRIMETHYLBENZ(a)ANTHRACENE

TOXICITY DATA with REFERENCE
ETA: ivn-rat TDLo: 175 mg/kg/10W-I JEMEAV
131,321,70
ETA: scu-mus TDLo: 1200 mg/kg/17W-I
PRLBA4 129,439,40

ETA: skn-mus TD: 530 mg/kg/22W-I PRLBA4
131,170,42
ETA: skn-mus TDLo: 310 mg/kg/13W-I
PRLBA4 129,439,40

SAFETY PROFILE: Questionable carcinogen with experimental tumorigenic data. When heated to decomposition it emits acrid smoke and irritating fumes.

TLK750   CAS: 13345-64-7
7,8,12-TRIMETHYLBENZ(a) ANTHRACENE
mf: $C_{21}H_{18}$ mw: 270.39

SYNS: 7,8,12-TMBA ◇ 5:9:10-TRIMETHYL-1:2-BENZAN-THRACENE

TOXICITY DATA with REFERENCE
CAR: ivn-rat TDLo: 175 mg/kg/10W-I JEMEAV
131,321,70
ETA: ivn-mus TDLo: 20 mg/kg: TER MOPMA3
4,427,68
ETA: ivn-rat TD: 35 mg/kg PNASA6 78,1185,81
ETA: ivn-rat TD: 130 mg/kg/30D-I JNCIAM
48,429,72
ETA: ivn-rat TDLo: 39 mg/kg/6D-I CNREA8
29,506,69
ETA: scu-mus TDLo: 1400 mg/kg/22W-I
PRLBA4 129,439,40
ETA: skn-mus TDLo: 48 mg/kg/10W-I PRLBA4
129,439,40
MUT: cyt-rat-ivn 50 mg/kg GANNA2 64,637,73
MUT: cyt-rat-par 140 mg/kg/10D-I JEMEAV
131,331,70
MUT: sce-rat: bmr 270 mg/L JJIND8 67,831,81
MUT: sln-dmg-orl 30 mmol/L/3D MUREAV
125,243,84
MUT: sln-dmg-par 5 mmol/L MUREAV 125,243,84

SAFETY PROFILE: Questionable carcinogen with experimental carcinogenic, tumorigenic, and teratogenic data. Poison by intravenous route. Mutation data reported. When heated to decomposition it emits acrid smoke and irritating fumes.

TLL000   CAS: 35187-27-0
7,10,12-TRIMETHYLBENZ(a) ANTHRACENE
mf: $C_{21}H_{18}$ mw: 270.39

TOXICITY DATA with REFERENCE
ETA: ims-rat TDLo: 50 mg/kg JMCMAR 14,940,71

SAFETY PROFILE: Questionable carcinogen with experimental tumorigenic data. When

heated to decomposition it emits acrid smoke and irritating fumes.

TLM500   CAS: 16757-92-9
1,3,6-TRIMETHYLBENZO(a)PYRENE
mf: $C_{23}H_{18}$ mw: 294.41

TOXICITY DATA with REFERENCE
ETA: scu-mus TDLo: 72 mg/kg/13W-I   IJCNAW
3,238,68

SAFETY PROFILE: Questionable carcinogen with experimental tumorigenic data. When heated to decomposition it emits acrid smoke and irritating fumes.

TLN250   CAS: 75-77-4
TRIMETHYL CHLOROSILANE
DOT: 1298
mf: C_3H_9ClSi mw: 108.66

PROP: Colorless liquid. Bp: 57°, d: 0.854 @ 25/25°, flash p: −18°F. Sol in benzene, ether, perchloroethylene.

SYNS: CHLOROTRIMETHYLSILICANE ◇ TL 1163

TOXICITY DATA with REFERENCE
NEO: ipr-mus TDLo: 1000 mg/kg/I   JNCIAM
54,495,75

MUT: mma-sat 1666 μg/plate   ENMUDM 8(Suppl 7),1,86

MUT: mmo-sat 1 mg/plate   ENMUDM 8(Suppl 7),1,86

CONSENSUS REPORTS: EPA Extremely Hazardous Substances List. Reported in EPA TSCA Inventory.

DOT Classification: Flammable Liquid; Label: Flammable Liquid and Flammable Liquid, Corrosive.

SAFETY PROFILE: Questionable carcinogen with experimental neoplastigenic data. Moderately toxic by inhalation and intraperitoneal routes. Mutation data reported. A corrosive irritant to skin, eyes, and mucous membranes. A very dangerous fire hazard when exposed to heat or flame. Violent reaction with water. To fight fire, use foam, alcohol foam and fog. When heated to decomposition it emits toxic fumes of Cl^-. An intermediate in the production of silicones.

TLP000   CAS: 5831-11-8
11,12-17-TRIMETHYL-15H-CYCLOPENTA(a)PHENANTHRENE
mf: $C_{20}H_{18}$ mw: 258.38

TOXICITY DATA with REFERENCE
CAR: skn-mus TDLo: 108 mg/kg/1Y-I   PEXTAR
11,69,69

MUT: mma-sat 20 μg/plate   CNREA8 36,4525,76

CONSENSUS REPORTS: EPA Genetic Toxicology Program.

SAFETY PROFILE: Questionable carcinogen with experimental carcinogenic data. Mutation data reported. When heated to decomposition it emits acrid smoke and irritating fumes.

TLP250   CAS: 63041-23-6
3,8,13-TRIMETHYLCYCLOQUINAZOLINE
mf: $C_{24}H_{18}N_4$ mw: 362.46

TOXICITY DATA with REFERENCE
ETA: skn-mus TDLo: 440 mg/kg/1Y-I   BJCAAI
16,275,62

SAFETY PROFILE: Questionable carcinogen with experimental tumorigenic data. When heated to decomposition it emits toxic fumes of NO_x.

TLR675   CAS: 2825-82-3
exo-TRIMETHYLENENORBORNANE
mf: $C_{10}H_{16}$ mw: 136.26

SYNS: exo-HEXAHYDRO-4,7-METHANOINDAN ◇ JP-10 ◇ exo-TETRAHYDROBICYCLOPENTADIENE ◇ exo-TETRAHYDRODI(CYCLOPENTADIENE) ◇ exo-TRICYCLO(5.2.1.0^{2,6})DECANE ◇ exo-5,6-TRIMETHYLENE-NORBORNANE

TOXICITY DATA with REFERENCE
CAR: ihl-rat TCLo: 100 ppm/6H/1Y-I   NTIS**
AD-A163-179

ETA: ihl-rat TC: 100 ppm/6H/1Y-I   NTIS** AD-A134-150

ETA: ihl-rat TC: 556 mg/m^3/6H/1Y-I   AETODY
7,133,84

MUT: cyt-ham: ovr 1 mg/L   NTIS** AD-A124-785

CONSENSUS REPORTS: Reported in EPA TSCA Inventory.

SAFETY PROFILE: Questionable carcinogen with experimental carcinogenic and tumorigenic data. Moderately toxic by ingestion. Mildly toxic by inhalation. Experimental reproductive effects. Mutation data reported. Used as a major component of cruise missile fuel. When heated to decomposition it emits acrid smoke and irritating fumes.

TLU750   CAS: 3475-63-6
1,1,3-TRIMETHYL-3-NITROSOUREA
mf: $C_4H_9N_3O_2$ mw: 131.16

SYNS: N-NITROSO-TRIMETHYLHARNSTOFF (GERMAN)
◇ NITROSOTRIMETHYLUREA ◇ N-NITROSOTRIMETHYL-
UREA ◇ TRIMETHYLNITROSOHARNSTOFF (GERMAN)
◇ N-TRIMETHYL-N-NITROSOUREA

TOXICITY DATA with REFERENCE
ETA: ivn-rat TDLo: 1950 mg/kg/48W-I   ZEKBAI
  69,103,67
ETA: orl-rat TD: 1598 mg/kg/I   BTPGAZ 146,33,72
ETA: orl-rat TD: 2950 mg/kg/47W-C   JJIND8
  65,451,80
ETA: orl-rat TDLo: 1070 mg/kg/53W-C
  ZEKBAI 69,103,67
MUT: mma-sat 1 μg/plate   MUREAV 51,319,78
MUT: mmo-sat 7000 μmol/L/48H   MUREAV
  48,131,77

CONSENSUS REPORTS: EPA Genetic Toxicology Program.

SAFETY PROFILE: Questionable carcinogen
with experimental tumorigenic and teratogenic
data. Poison by ingestion and intravenous
routes. Experimental reproductive effects. Mutation data reported. Many N-nitroso compounds are carcinogens. When heated to decomposition it emits toxic fumes of NO_x.

TMF000   CAS: 10416-59-8
N-(TRIMETHYLSILYL)ACETIMIDIC ACID,
TRIMETHYLSILYL ESTER
mf: $C_8H_{21}NOSi_2$ mw: 203.48

SYNS: BIS(TRIMETHYLSILYL)ACETAMIDE ◇ N,o-BIS-
(TRIMETHYLSILYL)ACETAMIDE ◇ BSA ◇ N-(TRIMETHYL-
SILYL)ETHANIMIDIC ACID, TRIMETHYLSILYL ESTER

TOXICITY DATA with REFERENCE
NEO: ipr-mus TDLo: 500 mg/kg/I   JNCIAM
  54,495,75

CONSENSUS REPORTS: Reported in EPA
TSCA Inventory.

SAFETY PROFILE: Questionable carcinogen
with experimental neoplastigenic data. Moderately toxic by intraperitoneal route. When heated
to decomposition it emits toxic fumes of NO_x.

TMF250   CAS: 18156-74-6
N-(TRIMETHYLSILYL)IMIDAZOLE
mf: $C_6H_{12}N_2Si$ mw: 140.29

SYNS: (TRIMETHYLSILYL)IMIDAZOLE ◇ N-(TRI-
METHYLSILYL)-IMIDAZOL ◇ 1-(TRIMETHYLSILYL)

IMIDAZOLE ◇ 1-(TRIMETHYLSILYL)-1H-IMIDAZOLE
◇ TSIM

TOXICITY DATA with REFERENCE
NEO: ipr-mus TDLo: 1000 mg/kg/I   JNCIAM
  54,495,75

CONSENSUS REPORTS: Reported in EPA
TSCA Inventory.

SAFETY PROFILE: Questionable carcinogen
with experimental neoplastigenic data. Moderately toxic by intraperitoneal route. When heated
to decomposition it emits toxic fumes of NO_x.

TMF750   CAS: 63019-09-0
N,N,2'-TRIMETHYL-4-STILBENAMINE
mf: $C_{17}H_{19}N$ mw: 237.37

SYNS: 4-DIMETHYLAMINO-2'-METHYLSTILBENE
◇ N,N-DIMETHYL-2'-METHYLSTILBENAMINE
◇ 2'-METHYL-4-DIMETHYLAMINOSTILBENE

TOXICITY DATA with REFERENCE
NEO: scu-rat TDLo: 80 mg/kg/4W-I   PTRMAD
  241,147,48
ETA: orl-rat TDLo: 750 mg/kg/71W-C   ABMGAJ
  9,87,62
ETA: scu-rat TD: 90 mg/kg/W-I   PTRMAD
  241,147,48

SAFETY PROFILE: Questionable carcinogen
with experimental tumorigenic and neoplastigenic data. When heated to decomposition it
emits toxic fumes of NO_x.

TMG000   CAS: 63040-32-4
N,N,3'-TRIMETHYL-4-STILBENAMINE
mf: $C_{17}H_{19}N$ mw: 237.37

SYN: 3'-METHYL-4-DIMETHYLAMINOSTILBENE

TOXICITY DATA with REFERENCE
ETA: orl-rat TDLo: 560 mg/kg/53W-C   ABMGAJ
  9,87,62

SAFETY PROFILE: Questionable carcinogen
with experimental tumorigenic data. When
heated to decomposition it emits toxic fumes
of NO_x.

TMG250   CAS: 7378-54-3
N,N,4'-TRIMETHYL-4-STILBENAMINE
mf: $C_{17}H_{19}N$ mw: 237.37

SYN: 4'-METHYL-4-DIMETHYLAMINOSTILBENE

TOXICITY DATA with REFERENCE
ETA: orl-rat TDLo: 305 mg/kg/29W-C   ABMGAJ
  9,87,62

SAFETY PROFILE: Questionable carcinogen with experimental tumorigenic data. When heated to decomposition it emits toxic fumes of NO_x.

TMH750   CAS: 2489-77-2
1,1,3-TRIMETHYL-2-THIOUREA
mf: $C_4H_{10}N_2S$ mw: 118.22

PROP: Trimethylthiourea tested in NCITR* NCI-CG-TR-129 contained 15% 1,3-dimethyl-2-thiourea and 5% Zeolex 80 (NCITR* NCI-CG-TR-129,79).

SYNS: NCI-C02186 ◇ TRIMETHYLTHIOUREA ◇ N,N,N'-TRIMETHYLTHIOUREA

TOXICITY DATA with REFERENCE
CAR: orl-rat TDLo: 13 g/kg/77W-C   NCITR* NCI-CG-TR-129,79

CONSENSUS REPORTS: NCI Carcinogenesis Bioassay (feed); No Evidence: mouse NCITR* NCI-CG-TR-129,79. Reported in EPA TSCA Inventory.

SAFETY PROFILE: Questionable carcinogen with experimental carcinogenic data. Poison by ingestion. When heated to decomposition it emits very toxic fumes of NO_x and SO_x.

TMQ250   CAS: 6304-33-2
2,3,3-TRIPHENYLACRYLONITRILE
mf: $C_{21}H_{15}N$ mw: 281.37

SYNS: α,β-DIPHENYLCINNAMONITRILE ◇ α-(DIPHENYLMETHYLENE)BENZENEACETIC ACID ◇ TRIPHENYLACRYLONITRILE ◇ α,β,β-TRIPHENYL-ACRYLONITRILE ◇ TRIPHENYLCYANOETHYLENE

TOXICITY DATA with REFERENCE
CAR: scu-mus TDLo: 94 mg/kg/26W-I   MMJJAI 11,95,61

CONSENSUS REPORTS: Cyanide and its compounds are on the Community Right-To-Know List.

SAFETY PROFILE: Questionable carcinogen with experimental carcinogenic data. Poison by ingestion and intravenous routes. When heated to decomposition it emits toxic fumes of NO_x and CN^-.

TMR000   CAS: 612-71-5
1,3,5-TRIPHENYLBENZENE
mf: $C_{24}H_{18}$ mw: 306.42

PROP: Rhombic crystals. D: 1.205, mp: 170-171°C. Very sol in benzene; sol in absolute alc, ether.

SYNS: 5'-PHENYL-m-TERPHENYL ◇ TRIPHENYLBEN-ZENE ◇ sym-TRIPHENYLBENZENE

TOXICITY DATA with REFERENCE
ETA: scu-mus TDLo: 1400 mg/kg/35W-I   AJCAA7 26,754,36

SAFETY PROFILE: Questionable carcinogen with experimental tumorigenic data. When heated to decomposition it emits acrid smoke and irritating fumes.

TMS000   CAS: 217-59-4
TRIPHENYLENE
mf: $C_{18}H_{12}$ mw: 228.30

SYNS: 9,10-BENZOPHENANTHRENE ◇ BENZO(1) PHENANTHRENE ◇ 9,10-BENZPHENANTHRENE ◇ 1,2,3,4-DIBENZNAPHTHALENE ◇ ISOCHRYSENE

TOXICITY DATA with REFERENCE
MUT: mma-sat 100 mg/L/72H   FCTXAV 17,141,79
MUT: mmo-sat 1 nmol/L   CNREA8 40,1985,80

CONSENSUS REPORTS: IARC Cancer Review: GROUP 3 IMEMDT 7,56,87; Animal Inadequate Evidence IMEMDT 32,447,83.

SAFETY PROFILE: Questionable carcinogen. Mutation data reported. When heated to decomposition it emits acrid smoke and irritating fumes.

TMS250   CAS: 58-72-0
TRIPHENYLETHYLENE
mf: $C_{20}H_{16}$ mw: 256.36

SYN: 1,1,2-TRIPHENYLETHYLENE

TOXICITY DATA with REFERENCE
ETA: scu-mus TD: 3600 mg/kg/18W-I   NATUAS 142,836,38
ETA: scu-mus TD: 4800 mg/kg/40W-I: TER
JPBAA7 56,15,44
ETA: scu-mus TD: 4920 mg/kg/41W-I: TER
JPBAA7 54,149,42
ETA: scu-mus TD: 7200 mg/kg/36W-I: TER
CNREA8 3,92,43
ETA: scu-mus TDLo: 3000 mg/kg/25W-I
JPBAA7 51,9,40
MUT: cyt-hmn: lng 100 μmol/L/8H   MUREAV 4,83,67

CONSENSUS REPORTS: Reported in EPA TSCA Inventory.

SAFETY PROFILE: Questionable carcinogen with experimental tumorigenic and teratogenic data. Experimental reproductive effects. Human mutation data reported. When heated to decomposition it emits acrid smoke and irritating fumes.

TNC725   CAS: 2706-47-0
TRIS(p-AMINOPHENYL)CARBONIUM PAMOATE

mf: $C_{23}H_{14}O_6 \cdot 2C_{19}H_{18}N_3$ mw: 963.17

SYNS: 4,4'-METHYLENEBIS(3-HYDROXY-2-NAPHTHOIC ACID) with TRIS-(p-AMINOPHENYL)CARBONIUM SALT (1:2) ◊ 4,4'-METHYLENEBIS(3-HYDROXY-2-NAPHTHOIC ACID) with TRIS-(p-AMINOPHENYL)METHYLIUM SALT (1:2) ◊ METHYLIUM, TRIS(4-AMINOPHENYL)-, 4,4'-METHYLENEBIS(3-HYDROXY-NAPHTHOATE) (2:1) ◊ TACP ◊ TRIS(p-AMINOPHENYL)CARBONIUM SALT with 4,4-METHYLENEBIS(3-HYDROXY-2-NAPHTHOIC ACID) (2:1) ◊ TRIS(p-AMINOPHENYL)METHYLIUM SALT with 4,4'-METHYLENEBIS(3-HYDROXY-2-NAPHTHOIC ACID) (2:1)

TOXICITY DATA with REFERENCE
NEO: orl-rat TDLo: 100 mg/kg/78W-C   CNREA8 25,1919,65

SAFETY PROFILE: Questionable carcinogen with experimental neoplastigenic data. When heated to decomposition it emits toxic fumes of NO_x.

TNC750   CAS: 2706-47-0
TRIS(p-AMINOPHENYL)METHYLIUM SALT with 4,4'-METHYLENEBIS(3-HYDROXY-2-NAPHTHOIC ACID) (2:1)

mf: $C_{19}H_8N_3 \cdot 1/2C_{24}H_{14}O_6$ mw: 471.48

SYNS: 4,4'-METHYLENEBIS(3-HYDROXY-2-NAPHTHOIC ACID) with TRIS-(p-AMINOPHENYL)CARBONIUM SALT (1:2) ◊ 4,4'-METHYLENEBIS(3-HYDROXY-2-NAPHTHOIC ACID) with TRIS-(p-AMINOPHENYL)METHYLIUM SALT (1:2) ◊ TRIS(p-AMINOPHENYL)CARBONIUM PAMOATE ◊ TRIS-(p-AMINOPHENYL)CARBONIUM SALT with 4,4-METHYLENEBIS(3-HYDRO XY-2-NAPHTHOIC ACID) (2:1)

TOXICITY DATA with REFERENCE
NEO: orl-rat TDLo: 100 mg/kg/78W-C   CNREA8 25,1919,65

SAFETY PROFILE: Questionable carcinogen with experimental neoplastigenic data. When heated to decomposition it emits toxic fumes of NO_x.

TND000   CAS: 68-76-8
TRIS(1-AZIRIDINYL)-p-BENZOQUINONE

mf: $C_{12}H_{13}N_3O_2$ mw: 231.28

SYNS: BAYER 3231 ◊ 1,1',1'' -(3,6-DIOXO-1,4-CYCLO-HEXADIENE-1,2,4-TRIYL)TRISAZIRIDINE ◊ NSC-29215

◊ ONCOVEDEX ◊ PRENIMON ◊ RIKER 601 ◊ 10257 R.P. ◊ TEIB ◊ TRENIMON ◊ TRIAZICHON (GERMAN) ◊ TRIAZIQUINONE ◊ TRIAZIQUONE ◊ 2,3,5-TRI-(1-AZIRIDINYL)-p-BENZOQUINONE ◊ 2,3,5-TRIETHYLENEIMINO-1,4-BENZOQUINONE ◊ TRIETHYLENIMINOBENZOQUINONE ◊ TRISAETHYLENIMINOBENZOCHINON (GERMAN) ◊ 2,3,5-TRIS(AZIRIDINO)-1,4-BENZOQUINONE ◊ 2,3,5-TRIS(1-AZIRIDINO)-p-BENZOQUINONE ◊ TRIS(AZIRIDINYL)-p-BENZOQUINONE ◊ 2,3,5-TRIS(1-AZIRIDINYL)-p-BENZOQUINONE ◊ 2,3,5-TRIS(AZIRIDINYL)-1,4-BENZOQUINONE ◊ 2,3,5-TRIS(1-AZIRIDINYL)-2,5-CYLOHEXADIENE-1,4-DIONE ◊ 2,3,5-TRISETHYLENEIMINOBENZOQUINONE ◊ TRISETHYLENEIMINOQUINONE ◊ 2,3,5-TRIS(ETHYLENIMINO)BENZOQUINONE ◊ 2,3,5-TRIS (ETHYLENIMINO)-p-BENZOQUINONE ◊ 2,3,5-TRIS(ETHYLENIMINO)-1,4-BENZOQUINONE

TOXICITY DATA with REFERENCE
CAR: ivn-rat TDLo: 1560 μg/kg/1Y-I   ARZNAD 20,1461,70
MUT: cyt-hmn: lym 50 nmol/L   MUREAV 149,83,85
MUT: cyt-mus-unr 1840 ng/kg   MUREAV 97,173,82
MUT: dni-hmn: hla 200 nmol/L/30M-C   JEPTDQ 2(1),65,78
MUT: otr-ham: kdy 200 ng/L   TXCYAC 19,55,81
MUT: sln-dmg-orl 50000 ppm   MUREAV 2,29,65
MUT: sln-dmg-par 5 μmol/L   MUREAV 142,29,85
MUT: slt-dmg-unr 300 μmol/L/2H   MUREAV 120,233,83

CONSENSUS REPORTS: IARC Cancer Review: GROUP 3 IMEMDT 7,367,87; Animal Sufficient Evidence IMEMDT 9,67,75; Human Inadequate Evidence IMEMDT 9,67,75. Community Right-To-Know List. EPA Genetic Toxicology Program.

SAFETY PROFILE: Questionable carcinogen with experimental experimental carcinogenic and teratogenic data. Poison by intraperitoneal, intravenous, and parenteral routes. Experimental reproductive effects. Human mutation data reported. When heated to decomposition it emits toxic fumes of NO_x. Used as a drug for the treatment of neoplastic diseases.

TND250   CAS: 545-55-1
TRIS-(1-AZIRIDINYL)PHOSPHINE OXIDE

DOT: 2501
mf: $C_6H_{12}N_3OP$ mw: 173.18

PROP: Colorless crystals. Mp: 41°, bp: 90° @ 23 mm. Sol in water, alc, ether.

SYNS: APHOXIDE ◊ APO ◊ 1-AZIRIDINYL PHOSPHINE OXIDE (TRIS) (DOT) ◊ CBC 906288 ◊ ENT 24,915

◇ IMPERON FIXER T ◇ NSC 9717 ◇ 1,1′,1′′-PHOSPHINYLI-
DYNETRISAZIRIDINE ◇ PHOSPHORIC ACID TRIETHYLENE
IMIDE ◇ PHOSPHORIC ACID TRIETHYLENEIMINE (DOT)
◇ SK-3818 ◇ TEF ◇ TEPA ◇ TRIAETHYLENPHOSPHOR-
SAEUREAMID (GERMAN) ◇ TRIAZIRIDINOPHOSPHINE OX-
IDE ◇ TRI(AZIRIDINYL)PHOSPHINE OXIDE ◇ TRI-1-AZIRI-
DINYL)PHOSPHINE OXIDE ◇ N,N′,N′′-TRI-1,2-
ETHANEDIYL PHOSPHORIC TRIMIDE ◇ TRIETHYLENE-
PHOSPHOROTRIAMIDE ◇ TRIS(1-AZIRIDINE)PHOSPHINE
OXIDE ◇ TRIS(N-ETHYLENE)PHOSPHOROTRIAMIDATE

AMINE ◇ 2,4,6-TRI(ETHYLENEIMINO)-1,3,5-TRIAZINE
◇ 2,4,6-TRIETHYLENEIMINO-s-TRIAZINE ◇ TRIETHYL-
ENEMELAMINE ◇ 2,4,6-TRIETHYLENIMINO-s-TRIAZINE
◇ 2,4,6-TRIETHYLENIMINO-1,3,5-TRIAZINE ◇ 2,4,6-TRIS(1-
AZIRIDINYL)-s-TRIAZINE ◇ 2,4,6-TRIS(1′-AZIRIDINYL)-
1,3,5-TRIAZINE ◇ TRIS(ETHYLENEIMINO)TRIAZINE
◇ 2,4,6-TRIS(ETHYLENEIMINO)-s-TRIAZINE ◇ TRIS-
ETHYLENEIMINO-1,3,5-TRIAZINE ◇ 2,4,6-TRIS(ETHYL-
ENIMINO)-s-TRIAZINE

TOXICITY DATA with REFERENCE

CAR: orl-rat TDLo: 1300 µg/kg/1Y-I   JNCIAM
41,985,68

NEO: orl-rat TD: 3120 µg/kg/1Y-I   JNCIAM
41,985,68

MUT: cyt-ham: lng 33 µmol/L   EVSRBT
25,917,81

MUT: cyt-hmn: leu 100 µmol/L   CHROAU
24,314,68

MUT: cyt-hmn: lym 125 µg/L   BEXBAN
82,1581,76

MUT: sce-hmn: lym 100 ng/L   MUREAV 53,215,78

MUT: sln-dmg-par 500 µg/kg   EVSRBT 25,917,81

MUT: trn-dmg-ipr 500 µg/kg   EVSRBT 25,917,81

CONSENSUS REPORTS: IARC Cancer Review: Animal Inadequate Evidence IMEMDT
9,75,75. EPA Genetic Toxicology Program.

DOT Classification: Label: Corrosive; Poison
B; Label: Poison.

SAFETY PROFILE: Questionable carcinogen
with experimental carcinogenic, neoplastigenic,
and teratogenic data. Poison by ingestion, skin
contact, intravenous, intraperitoneal, and possibly other routes. Experimental reproductive effects. Human mutation data reported. A corrosive irritant to the skin, eyes, and mucous
membranes. When heated to decomposition it
emits very toxic fumes of PO_x and NO_x. Used
as an acaricide and in the permanent press treatment of cotton.

TND500   CAS: 51-18-3
TRISAZIRIDINYLTRIAZINE
mf: $C_9H_{12}N_6$ mw: 204.27

PROP: Small crystals. Water-sol. Decomp @
139°.

SYNS: DRP 859025 ◇ ENT 25,296 ◇ M-9500 ◇ NSC 9706
◇ PERSISTOL ◇ R-246 ◇ SEM (CYTOSTATIC) ◇ SK1133
◇ TRETAMINE ◇ TRIAETHYLENMELAMIN (GERMAN)
◇ TRIAMELIN ◇ 1,1′,1′′-s-TRIAZINE-2,4,6-TRIYLTRISAZIR-
IDINE ◇ TRIAZIRIDINYL TRIAZINE ◇ TRIETHANOMEL-

TOXICITY DATA with REFERENCE

NEO: ipr-mus TD: 3 mg/kg/19D-I   BJPCAL
6,357,51

NEO: ipr-mus TD: 6 mg/kg/42D-I   CNREA8
25,20,65

NEO: ipr-mus TD: 300 µg/kg   PESTD5 16,138,75

NEO: ipr-mus TDLo: 2 mg/kg   CAMEAS 75,26,51

NEO: ivn-mus TDLo: 4 mg/kg/8W-I   CAMEAS
75,26,51

NEO: skn-mus TDLo: 10 mg/kg   BJCAAI
9,177,55

ETA: scu-mus TDLo: 2 mg/kg   CAMEAS 75,26,51

ETA: scu-rat TDLo: 10 mg/kg/I   ANYAA9
68,750,58

MUT: cyt-hmn: leu 5 µmol/L   CHROAU 24,314,68

MUT: dnd-esc 10 µmol/L   MUREAV 89,95,81

MUT: dnd-hmn: hla 100 µmol/L/30M-C
JEPTDQ 2(1),65,78

MUT: mmo-sat 25 µg/plate   TAKHAA 44,96,85

MUT: mnt-rat-ipr 100 µg/kg   EVSRBT 24,943,81

MUT: sln-dmg-orl 5 µmol/L/24H   IDZAAW
56,145,81

MUT: trn-mus-ipr 750 µg/kg/5W-I   CIHPDR
6,425,84

CONSENSUS REPORTS: IARC Cancer Re-
view: GROUP 3 IMEMDT 7,56,87; Animal
Sufficient Evidence IMEMDT 9,95,75. EPA
Genetic Toxicology Program.

SAFETY PROFILE: Questionable carcinogen
with experimental neoplastigenic, tumorigenic,
and teratogenic data. Poison by ingestion, intraperitoneal, intramuscular, intravenous, subcutaneous, and possibly other routes. Experimental
reproductive effects. Human mutation data reported. Can cause gastrointestinal tract disturbances and bone marrow depression. When
heated to decomposition it emits highly toxic
fumes of NO_x. Used as an antineoplastic agent
and as an insect sterilant.

TNF250   CAS: 555-77-1
TRIS(2-CHLOROETHYL)AMINE
mf: $C_6H_{12}Cl_3N$ mw: 204.54

SYNS: TL 145 ◇ TRICHLORMETHINE ◇ TRI-(2-CHLORO-
ETHYL)AMINE ◇ 2,2',2''-TRICHLOROTRIETHYLAMINE
◇ TRIS(β-CHLOROETHYL)AMINE ◇ TS 160

TOXICITY DATA with REFERENCE
CAR: scu-rat TD:45 mg/kg/26W-C   NEOLA4
28,565,81
CAR: scu-rat TD:180 mg/kg/26W-C   NEOLA4
28,565,81
CAR: scu-rat TDLo:18 mg/kg/26W-C NEOLA4
28,565,81
MUT: dni-ham:lng 500 μg/L   MUREAV 116,431,83
MUT: dni-hmn:fbr 10 mg/L   STBIBN 78,165,80
MUT: msc-ham:lng 1 mg/L   MUREAV 116,431,83
MUT: sln-dmg-ihl 100 pph/5M   PREBA3
62B,284,46/47

CONSENSUS REPORTS: EPA Extremely
Hazardous Substances List. EPA Genetic Toxicology Program. Reported in EPA TSCA Inventory.

SAFETY PROFILE: Questionable carcinogen
with experimental carcinogenic data. Experimental poison by ingestion, inhalation, skin contact, subcutaneous, intravenous and possibly
other routes. Moderately toxic to humans by
inhalation. An eye irritant. Human mutation data
reported. When heated to decomposition it emits
very toxic fumes of Cl^- and NO_x.

TNF500   CAS: 817-09-4
**TRIS(2-CHLOROETHYL)AMMONIUM
CHLORIDE**
mf: $C_6H_{12}Cl_3N•ClH$ mw: 241.00

SYNS: LEKAMIN ◇ NSC-30211 ◇ R-47 ◇ SINALOST
◇ SK-100 ◇ TRI(β-CHLOROETHYL)AMINE HYDROCHLO-
RIDE ◇ TRI-(2-CHLOROETHYL)AMINE HYDROCHLORIDE
◇ TRICHLORMETHINE ◇ TRICHLORMETHINIUM CHLO-
RIDE ◇ TRICHLOR-TRIAETHYLAMIN-HYDROCHLORID
(GERMAN) ◇ 2,2',2''-TRICHLOROTRIETHYLAMINE HY-
DROCHLORIDE ◇ TRILLEKAMIN ◇ TRIMITAN ◇ TRIMUS-
TINE ◇ TRIMUSTINE HYDROCHLORIDE ◇ TRIS(β-CHLORO-
ETHYL)AMINE HYDROCHLORIDE ◇ TRIS(2-CHLORO-
ETHYL)AMINE HYDROCHLORIDE ◇ TRIS(2-CHLORO-
ETHYL)AMINE MONOHYDROCHLORIDE ◇ TRIS-N-LOST
◇ TS-160

TOXICITY DATA with REFERENCE
CAR: scu-mus TDLo:10 mg/kg/9W-I   BJCAAI
3,118,49
MUT: dlt-mus-ipr 5 mg/kg   NEOLA4 25,523,78
MUT: dnd-mus-ipr 20 mg/kg   FOBLAN 25,380,79
MUT: pic-esc 200 mg/L   ARMKA7 51,9,65

CONSENSUS REPORTS: IARC Cancer Review: Animal Inadequate Evidence IMEMDT
9,229,75. EPA Genetic Toxicology Program.

SAFETY PROFILE: Questionable carcinogen
with experimental carcinogenic data. Poison by
ingestion, subcutaneous, intravenous, and intraperitoneal routes. Human systemic effects by
ingestion and intravenous routes: somnolence,
anorexia, headache, thrombosis distant from injection site, nausea or vomiting, and leukopenia.
Experimental reproductive effects. Mutation
data reported. When heated to decomposition
it emits very toxic fumes of Cl^-, NH_3 and NO_x.
Used as an antineoplastic agent.

TNI250   CAS: 78-42-2
TRIS(2-ETHYLHEXYL)PHOSPHATE
mf: $C_{24}H_{51}O_4P$ mw: 434.72

PROP: Liquid. Mp: $-74°$, bp: $216°$ @ 5 mm,
flash p: 405°F (OC), d: 0.9262 @ 20/20°, vap
d: 14.95.

SYNS: DISFLAMOLL TOF ◇ 2-ETHYL-1-HEXANOL PHOS-
PHATE ◇ FLEXOL TOF ◇ KRONITEX TOF ◇ NCI-C54751
◇ PHOSPHORIC ACID, TRIS(2-ETHYLHEXYL) ESTER
◇ TOF ◇ TRIETHYLHEXYL PHOSPHATE ◇ TRI(2-ETHYL-
HEXYL)PHOSPHATE ◇ TRIOCTYL PHOSPHATE

TOXICITY DATA with REFERENCE
CAR: orl-mus TDLo:520 g/kg/2Y-I   EVHPAZ
65,271,86

CONSENSUS REPORTS: NTP Carcinogenesis Studies (gavage); Some Evidence: mouse
NTPTR* NTP-TR-274,84; Equivocal Evidence:
rat NTPTR* NTP-TR-274,84. Reported in EPA
TSCA Inventory.

SAFETY PROFILE: Questionable carcinogen
with experimental carcinogenic data. Mildly
toxic by ingestion, skin contact, and possibly
other routes. A skin and eye irritant. Combustible when exposed to heat or flame. Can react
with oxidizing materials. To fight fire, use foam,
CO_2, dry chemical. When heated to decomposition it emits toxic fumes of PO_x.

TNK250   CAS: 57-39-6
**TRIS(1-METHYLETHYLENE)
PHOSPHORIC TRIAMIDE**
mf: $C_9H_{18}N_3OP$ mw: 215.27

PROP: Amber-colored liquid; amine odor. Bp:
118-125° @ 1 mm, d: 1.079 @ 25/25°. Misc
with water and all organic solvents.

SYNS: C 3172 ◇ ENT 50,003 ◇ MAPO ◇ METEPA ◇ METHAPHOXIDE ◇ METHYL APHOXIDE ◇ 1,1′,1″ - PHOSPHINYLIDYNETRIS(2-METHYL)AZRIDINE ◇ TRIS(2-METHYL-1-AZIRIDINYL)PHOSPHINE OXIDE ◇ TRIS(2-ME-THYLAZIRIDIN-1-YL)PHOSPHINE OXIDE ◇ N,N′,N″-TRIS(1-METHYLETHYLENE)PHOSPHORAMIDE

TOXICITY DATA with REFERENCE
CAR: orl-rat TDLo:1000 mg/kg/60W-I
    BWHOA6 34,317,66
MUT: cyt-hmn:lym 20 mg/L   SOGEBZ 8,783,72
MUT: cyt-rat-orl 408 mg/kg/30D   IJEBA6
    16,1000,78
MUT: dlt-dmg-orl 1 mmol/L   RPZHAW 33,215,82
MUT: dni-esc 10 mmol/L   IJEBA6 22,453,84
MUT: spm-mus-ipr 30 mg/kg/5D   PNASA6
    72,4425,75
MUT: spm-oin-unr 50 μg   JMENA6 9,139,72

CONSENSUS REPORTS: IARC Cancer Review: Animal Inadequate Evidence IMEMDT 9,107,75. Reported in EPA TSCA Inventory. EPA Genetic Toxicology Program.

SAFETY PROFILE: Questionable carcinogen with experimental carcinogenic and teratogenic data. Poison by ingestion, skin contact, intraperitoneal, and subcutaneous routes. Human mutation data reported. Experimental reproductive effects. Animal experiments suggest cholinesterase inhibition, possibly due to metabolic products of this material in the body. When heated to decomposition it emits very toxic fumes of NO_x and PO_x.

TNW500   CAS: 54-12-6
dl-TRYPTOPHAN
mf: $C_{11}H_{12}N_2O_2$ mw: 204.25

PROP: White crystals or crystalline powder; odorless. Sol in water, dil acids, alkalies; sltly sol in alc. Optically inactive.

TOXICITY DATA with REFERENCE
CAR: orl-rat TDLo:844 g/kg/92W-C   CNREA8
    39,1207,79

CONSENSUS REPORTS: Reported in EPA TSCA Inventory. EPA Genetic Toxicology Program.

SAFETY PROFILE: Questionable carcinogen with experimental carcinogenic data. When heated to decomposition it emits toxic fumes of NO_x.

TNW950
l-TRYPTOPHAN, pyrolyzate

PROP: Smoke condensate obtained by pyrolysis of l-TRYPTOPHAN (CALEDQ 2,335,77).
MUT: otr-ham:emb 50 mg/L   MUREAV 49,145,78
MUT: cyt-ham:emb 30 mg/L/24H   MUREAV
    49,145,78
NEO: orl-rat TDLo:77600 mg/kg/2Y-C
    CALEDQ 13,181,81
CAR: imp-mus TDLo:80 mg/kg   CALEDQ
    17,101,82

SAFETY PROFILE: Questionable carcinogen with experimental carcinogenic and neoplastigenic data. Mutation data reported. When heated to decomposition it emits acrid smoke and irritating fumes.

TNX000   CAS: 73-22-3
l-TRYPTOPHANE
mf: $C_{11}H_{12}N_2O_2$ mw: 204.25

PROP: An essential amino acid; occurs in isomeric forms. Mp: decomp 289°. The l and dl forms are: White crystals or crystalline powder; slt bitter taste; (dl) sltly sol in water; (l) Sol in water, hot alc, alkali hydroxides; insol in chloroform.

SYNS: 1-α-AMINO-3-INDOLEPROPRIONIC ACID ◇ α′-AMINO-3-INDOLEPROPRIONIC ACID ◇ α-AMINO-IN-DOLE-3-PROPRIONIC ACID ◇ 2-AMINO-3-INDOL-3-YL-PRO-PRIONIC ACID ◇ EH 121 ◇ INDOLE-3-ALANINE ◇ 1-β-3-INDOLYLALANINE ◇ NCI-C01729 ◇ (−)-TRYPTOPHAN ◇ l-TRYPTOPHAN (FCC) ◇ TRYPTOPHANE

TOXICITY DATA with REFERENCE
ETA: imp-mus TDLo:80 mg/kg   CALEDQ
    17,101,82
ETA: scu-rat TDLo:9500 mg/kg/2Y-C:TER
    VOONAW 20(8),75,74
MUT: dni-hmn:lym 1 mmol/L   PNASA6 79,1171,82
MUT: dni-rat:lvr 100 μmol/L   CNREA8 45,337,85
MUT: mmo-omi 5 g/L   MGGEAE 121,117,73

CONSENSUS REPORTS: NCI Carcinogenesis Bioassay (feed); No Evidence: mouse, rat NCITR* NCI-CG-TR-71,78. Reported in EPA TSCA Inventory.

SAFETY PROFILE: Questionable carcinogen with experimental tumorigenic and teratogenic data. Moderately toxic by intraperitoneal route. Experimental reproductive effects. Human mutation data reported. When heated to decomposition it emits toxic fumes of NO_x.

TOD750
TURPENTINE
DOT: 1299

CAS: 8006-64-2

PROP: Colorless liquid, characteristic odor. Bp: 154-170°, lel: 0.8%, flash p: 95°F (CC), d: 0.854-0.868 @ 25/25°, autoign temp: 488°F, vap d: 4.84, ULC: 40-50.

SYNS: OIL of TURPENTINE ◇ OIL of TURPENTINE, RECTIFIED ◇ SPIRIT of TURPENTINE ◇ SPIRITS of TURPENTINE ◇ TEREBENTHINE (FRENCH) ◇ TERPENTIN OEL (GERMAN) ◇ TURPENTINE OIL, RECTIFIER ◇ TURPENTINE STEAM DISTILLED

TOXICITY DATA with REFERENCE
ETA: skn-mus TDLo: 240 g/kg/20W-I   CNREA8 19,413,59

CONSENSUS REPORTS: Reported in EPA TSCA Inventory.

OSHA PEL: TWA 100 ppm   ACGIH TLV: TWA 100 ppm   DFG MAK: 100 ppm (560 mg/m^3)   DOT Classification: Flammable Liquid; Label: Flammable Liquid; Combustible Liquid; Label: None; Flammable or Combustible Liquid; Label: Flammable Liquid.

SAFETY PROFILE: Questionable carcinogen with experimental tumorigenic data. An experimental poison by intravenous route. Moderately toxic to humans by ingestion and possibly other routes. Mildly toxic experimentally by ingestion and inhalation. Human systemic effects by ingestion and inhalation: conjunctiva irritation, other olfactory and eye effects, hallucinations or distorted perceptions, antipsychotic, headache, pulmonary and kidney changes. A human eye irritant. Irritating to skin and mucous membranes. A very dangerous fire hazard when exposed to heat or flame; can react vigorously with oxidizing materials. To fight fire, use foam, CO_2, dry chemical. When heated to decomposition it emits acrid smoke and irritating fumes.

UNJ800
URACIL
mf: $C_4H_4N_2O_2$ mw: 112.10

CAS: 66-22-8

PROP: Needles from water. Mp: 335° with effervescence. Freely sol in hot water; sparingly sol in cold water (100 parts of water at 25° dissolves 0.358 part of uracil); almost insol in alc, ether; sol in ammonia water and in other alkalies.

SYNS: 2,4-DIHYDROXYPYRIMIDINE ◇ 2,4-DIOXOPYRIMIDINE ◇ HYBAR X ◇ PIROD ◇ 2,4-PYRIMIDINEDIOL ◇ 2,4-PYRIMIDINEDIONE ◇ 2,4(1H,3H)-PYRIMIDINEDIONE (9CI) ◇ PYROD

TOXICITY DATA with REFERENCE
ETA: orl-rat TDLo: 235 g/kg/20W-C   CALEDQ 34,249,87
ETA: orl-rat TDLo: 378 g/kg/30W-C   CNREA8 46,2062,86
MUT: cyt-mus-ipr 15 mg/kg   NULSAK 19,40,76
MUT: pic-esc 1 g/L   ZAPOAK 12,583,72

CONSENSUS REPORTS: EPA Genetic Toxicology Program. Reported in EPA TSCA Inventory.

SAFETY PROFILE: Questionable carcinogen with experimental tumorigenic data. Moderately toxic by intraperitoneal route. Experimental reproductive effects. Mutation data reported. When heated to decomposition it emits toxic fumes of NO_x.

USS000
UREA
mf: CH_4N_2O mw: 60.07

CAS: 57-13-6

PROP: White crystals. Mp: 132.7°, bp: decomp, d: (solid) 1.335. Sol in water, alc; sltly sol in ether.

SYNS: CARBAMIDE ◇ CARBAMIDE RESIN ◇ CARBAMIDIC ACID ◇ CARBONYL DIAMIDE ◇ CARBONYLDIAMINE ◇ ISOUREA ◇ NCI-C02119 ◇ PRESPERSION, 75 UREA ◇ PSEUDOUREA ◇ SUPERCEL 3000 ◇ UREAPHIL ◇ UREOPHIL ◇ UREVERT ◇ VARIOFORM II

TOXICITY DATA with REFERENCE
CAR: orl-mus TDLo: 394 g/kg/1Y-C   JEPTDQ 3(5-6),149,80
NEO: orl-rat TDLo: 821 g/kg/1Y-C   JEPTDQ 3(5-6),149,80
MUT: cyt-ham: fbr 16 g/L/24H   MUREAV 48,337,77
MUT: cyt-ham: lng 13 g/L   GMCRDC 27,95,81
MUT: cyt-hmn: leu 50 mmol/L   CNREA8 25,980,65
MUT: dnd-ham: fbr 8 mol/L   SFCRAO 23,346,70
MUT: dni-hmn: lym 600 mmol/L   PNASA6 79,1171,82

CONSENSUS REPORTS: Reported in EPA TSCA Inventory. EPA Genetic Toxicology Program.

SAFETY PROFILE: Questionable carcinogen with experimental carcinogenic and neoplasti-

genic data. Moderately toxic by ingestion, in-travenous, and subcutaneous routes. Human re-productive effects by intraplacental route: fertil-ity effects. Experimental reproductive effects. Human mutation data reported. A human skin irritant. When heated to decomposition it emits toxic fumes of NO_x.

VCK000
VALONEA TANNIN

SYNS: QUERCUS AEGILOPS L. TANNIN ◇ TANNIN from VALONEA

TOXICITY DATA with REFERENCE
CAR: scu-rat TDLo: 750 mg/kg/2W-I   BJCAAI 14,147,60

SAFETY PROFILE: Questionable carcinogen with experimental carcinogenic data. Poison by intraperitoneal, intravenous, subcutaneous, and intramuscular routes.

VCP000   CAS: 7440-62-2
VANADIUM
af: V   aw: 50.94

PROP: A bright, white, soft, ductile metal; sltly radioactive. Bp: 3000°, d: 6.11 @ 18.7°, mp: 1917°. Insol in water.

TOXICITY DATA with REFERENCE
ETA: ims-rat TDLo: 340 mg/kg/43W-I   NCIUS* PH 43-64-886,SEPT,71

CONSENSUS REPORTS: Reported in EPA TSCA Inventory.

OSHA PEL: (Transitional: Respirable Dust: Cl 0.5 mg(V_2O_5)/m^3; Fume: Cl 0.1 mg(V_2O_5)/m^3) Respirable Dust and Fume: TWA 0.05 mg(V_2O_5)/m^3 NIOSH REL: TWA 1.0 mg(V)/m^3

SAFETY PROFILE: Questionable carcinogen with experimental tumorigenic data. Poison by subcutaneous route. Flammable in dust form from heat, flame or sparks. When heated to decomposition it emits toxic fumes of VO_x.

VEZ925   CAS: 149-17-7
VANCIDE
mf: $C_{14}H_{13}N_3O_3$ mw: 271.30

SYNS: FTIVAZID ◇ FTIVAZIDE ◇ ISONICOTINIC ACID, VANILLYLIDENEHYDRAZIDE ◇ PHTIVAZID ◇ PHTIVA-ZIDE ◇ 4-PYRIDINECARBOXYLIC ACID, ((4-HYDROXY-3-

METHOXYPHENYL)METHYLENE)HYDRAZIDE ◇ VANICID ◇ VANILLABERON ◇ VANIZIDE

TOXICITY DATA with REFERENCE
ETA: orl-mus TDLo: 24960 mg/kg/1Y-I VOONAW 18(6),50,72

SAFETY PROFILE: Questionable carcinogen with experimental tumorigenic data. When heated to decomposition it emits toxic fumes of NO_x.

VKA600   CAS: 2185-86-6
VICTORIA LAKE BLUE R
mf: $C_{29}H_{32}ClN_3$ mw: 458.09

SYNS: AIZEN VICTORIA BLUE BOH ◇ BASIC BLUEK ◇ C.I. 44040 ◇ HIDACO VICTORIA BLUE R ◇ N,N'-(N,N'-TETRAMETHYL)-1-DIAMINODIPHENYLNAPHTHYL-AMINOMETHANE HYDROCHLORIDE ◇ VICTORIA BLUE R ◇ VICTORIA BLUE RS

TOXICITY DATA with REFERENCE
CAR: orl-rat TDLo: 4944 mg/kg/73W-I GISAAA 47(4),30,82
CAR: scu-rat TDLo: 2361 mg/kg/66W-I GISAAA 47(4),30,82

SAFETY PROFILE: Questionable carcinogen with experimental carcinogenic data. Moder-ately toxic by ingestion and subcutaneous routes. When heated to decomposition it emits toxic fumes of Cl^- and NO_x.

VKZ000   CAS: 865-21-4
VINCALEUKOBLASTINE
mf: $C_{46}H_{58}N_4O_9$ mw: 811.08

SYNS: NCI-C04842 ◇ NDC 002-1452-01 ◇ NINCALUICOL-FLASTINE ◇ NSC 47842 ◇ VINBLASTIN ◇ VINBLASTINE ◇ VINCALEUCOBLASTIN ◇ VINCOBLASTINE ◇ VLB

TOXICITY DATA with REFERENCE
ETA: ipr-mus TDLo: 7 mg/kg/26W-I CANCAR 40(Suppl 4),1935,77
ETA: ipr-rat TDLo: 2 mg/kg/7W-I CANCAR 40(Suppl 4),1935,77
MUT: cyt-ham: fbr 7800 ng/L   HDSKEK 10,41,85
MUT: cyt-ham: oth 50 μg/L   NATWAY 56,287,69
MUT: cyt-hmn: hla 10 nmol/L   JJEMAG 40,409,70
MUT: cyt-mus-ipr 900 μg/kg   ENMUDM 8,273,86
MUT: cyt-mus-unr 2 mg/kg   MUREAV 85,299,81
MUT: dlt-mus-unr 500 μg/kg   MUREAV 85,299,81
MUT: dni-hmn: oth 200 μg/L   26QZAP 2,377,72
MUT: oms-nml: 500 ppm   COREAF 258,4854,64
MUT: scu-mus LD10: 20 mg/kg   EJCAAH 10,667,74

MUT: slt-dmg-orl 100 μmol/L ENMUDM 6,153,84

CONSENSUS REPORTS: NCI Carcinogenesis Studies (ipr); No Evidence: mouse CANCAR 40,1935,77; (ipr); Clear Evidence: rat CANCAR 40,1935,77. EPA Genetic Toxicology Program.

SAFETY PROFILE: Questionable carcinogen with experimental tumorigenic and teratogenic data. Human poison by intravenous route. Experimental poison by intravenous, subcutaneous, and intraperitoneal routes. Human systemic effects by intravenous, ocular, and possibly other routes: visual field changes, conjunctiva irritation and other eye effects, cardiomyopathy including infarction, and changes in bone marrow. Experimental reproductive effects. Human mutation data reported. When heated to decomposition it emits toxic fumes of NO_x. Used as an antineoplastic agent.

VLA000 CAS: 143-67-9
VINCALEUKOBLASTINE SULFATE (1:1) (SALT)
mf: $C_{46}H_{58}N_4O_9 \cdot H_2O_4S$ mw: 909.16

SYNS: EXAL ◇ 29060 LE ◇ NSC 49842 ◇ VELBAN ◇ VELBE ◇ VINBLASTINE SULFATE ◇ VINCALEUKOBLASTINE SULFATE ◇ VLB MONOSULFATE

TOXICITY DATA with REFERENCE
MUT: cyt-hmn-unr 4 mg/kg/26W STRAAA 148,614,74
MUT: cyt-hmn:hla 10 μg/L PSEBAA 157,206,78
MUT: cyt-hmn:lym 3750 μg/L CUSCAM 54,807,85
MUT: dni-mus:lym 1 mg/L ARZNAD 25,378,75
MUT: pic-esc 500 mg/L APMBAY 12,234,64
MUT: spm-mus-ipr 5 mg/kg/5D PNASA6 72,4425,75

CONSENSUS REPORTS: IARC Cancer Review: GROUP 3 IMEMDT 7,371,87; Animal Inadequate Evidence IMEMDT 26,349,81; Human Inadequate Evidence IMEMDT 26,349,81. EPA Genetic Toxicology Program.

SAFETY PROFILE: Questionable carcinogen. Poison by intraperitoneal and intravenous routes. An experimental teratogen. Human systemic effects by intravenous route: blood luekopenia and hair changes. Experimental reproductive effects. Human mutation data reported. When heated to decomposition it emits very toxic fumes of NO_x and SO_x.

VLU250 CAS: 108-05-4
VINYL ACETATE
DOT: 1301
mf: $C_4H_6O_2$ mw: 86.10

PROP: Colorless, mobile liquid; polymerizes to solid on exposure to light. Mp: -92.8°, bp: 73°, flash p: 18°F, d: 0.9335 @ 20°, autoign temp: 800°F, vap press: 100 mm @ 21.5°, lel: 2.6%, uel: 13.4%, vap d: 3.0. Misc in alc, ether. Somewhat sol in water.

SYNS: ACETIC ACID ETHENYL ESTER ◇ ACETIC ACID VINYL ESTER ◇ 1-ACETOXYETHYLENE ◇ ETHENYL ACETATE ◇ OCTAN WINYLU (POLISH) ◇ VAC ◇ VINILE (ACETATO di) (ITALIAN) ◇ VINYL A MONOMER ◇ VINYLACETAAT (DUTCH) ◇ VINYLACETAT (GERMAN) ◇ VINYLE (ACETATE de) (FRENCH) ◇ VYAC ◇ ZESET T

TOXICITY DATA with REFERENCE
CAR: orl-rat TDLo: 100 g/kg/2Y-C TXAPA9 68,43,83
MUT: cyt-hmn:lym 250 μmol/L MUREAV 159,109,86
MUT: sce-ham:ovr 125 μmol/L CNREA8 45,4816,85
MUT: sce-hmn:lym 100 μmol/L CNREA8 45,4816,85

CONSENSUS REPORTS: IARC Cancer Review: Animal Inadequate Evidence IMEMDT 19,341,79; IMEMDT 39,113,86; Human Inadequate Evidence IMEMDT 39,113,86. Reported in EPA TSCA Inventory. Community Right-To-Know List. EPA Extremely Hazardous Substances List.

OSHA PEL: TWA 10 ppm; STEL 20 ppm ACGIH TLV: TWA 10 ppm; STEL 20 ppm DFG MAK: 10 ppm (35 mg/m^3) NIOSH REL: (Vinyl Acetate) CL 15 mg/m^3/15M DOT Classification: Label: Flammable Liquid.

SAFETY PROFILE: Questionable carcinogen with experimental carcinogenic data. Moderately toxic by ingestion, inhalation, and intraperitoneal routes. A skin and eye irritant. Human mutation data reported. Highly dangerous fire hazard when exposed to heat, flame, or oxidizers. A storage hazard, it may undergo spontaneous exothermic polymerization. Reaction with air or water to form peroxides which catalyze an exothermic polymerization reaction has caused several large industrial explosions.

VMF000   CAS: 61695-70-3
7-VINYLBENZ(a)ANTHRACENE
mf: $C_{20}H_{14}$ mw: 254.34

TOXICITY DATA with REFERENCE
ETA: scu-rat TDLo: 10 mg/kg/40D-I   CALEDQ
1,339,76

SAFETY PROFILE: Questionable carcinogen
with experimental tumorigenic data. When
heated to decomposition it emits acrid smoke
and irritating fumes.

VNK000   CAS: 15805-73-9
VINYL CARBAMATE
mf: $C_3H_5NO_2$ mw: 87.09

SYN: CARBAMIC ACID, VINYL ESTER

TOXICITY DATA with REFERENCE
NEO: ipr-mus TD: 65 mg/kg   CNREA8 38,3793,78
NEO: ipr-mus TDLo: 13 mg/kg   CNREA8
40,1194,80
NEO: skn-mus TD: 400 mg/kg/1W-I   CNREA8
38,3793,78
NEO: skn-mus TDLo: 200 mg/kg/1W-I   CNREA8
38,3793,78
ETA: ipr-mus TD: 3 mg/kg   CNREA8 46,4911,86
MUT: mma-sat 100 μg/plate   CNREA8 38,3793,78
MUT: msc-ham: lng 1 mg/L   CRNGDP 3,1437,82
MUT: sce-ham-ipr 25 mg/kg   MUREAV 126,159,84
MUT: sce-ham: lng 1 mg/L   CRNGDP 3,1437,82
MUT: sce-hmn: lym 10 mmol/L   MUREAV
89,75,81
MUT: sce-rat-ipr 25 mg/kg   MUREAV 126,159,84

SAFETY PROFILE: Questionable carcinogen
with experimental neoplastigenic data. Poison
by intraperitoneal route. Human mutation data
reported. When heated to decomposition it emits
toxic fumes of NO_x.

VOK000   CAS: 872-36-6
VINYLENE CARBONATE
mf: $C_3H_2O_3$ mw: 86.05

SYNS: CARBONIC ACID, cyclic VINYLENE ESTER
◇ 1,3-DIOXOL-4-EN-2-ONE ◇ 1,3-DIOXOL-2-ONE

TOXICITY DATA with REFERENCE
NEO: scu-rat TDLo: 1760 mg/kg/44W-I   BJCAAI
19,392,65

SAFETY PROFILE: Questionable carcinogen
with experimental neoplastigenic data. When
heated to decomposition it emits acrid smoke
and irritating fumes.

VSK000   CAS: 12629-02-6
VITALLIUM

PROP: Alloy of chromium, cobalt, and molybdenum (CNREA8 16,439,56).

SYNS: CHROMIUM-COBALT-MOLYBDENUM ALLOY
◇ COBALT-CHROMIUM-MOLYBDENUM ALLOY ◇ MOLYB-
DENUM-COBALT-CHROMIUM ALLOY ◇ STELLITE

TOXICITY DATA with REFERENCE
ETA: imp-rat TDLo: 2100 mg/kg   CNREA8
16,439,56
ETA: ims-rat TDLo: 140 mg/kg   JBJSB4 55-
B,759,73

CONSENSUS REPORTS: Cobalt and its compounds, as well as chromium and its compounds, are on the Community Right-To-Know
List.

OSHA PEL: (Transitional: TWA Total Dust:
15 mg/m^3; Respirable Fraction: 5 mg/m^3) TWA
Total Dust: 10 mg/m^3; Respirable Fraction: 5
mg/m^3 ACGIH TLV: TWA 10 mg(Mo)/
m^3 NIOSH REL: (Cobalt) TWA 0.1 mg/m^3

SAFETY PROFILE: Questionable carcinogen
with experimental tumorigenic data.

VSK900   CAS: 127-47-9
VITAMIN A ACETATE
mf: $C_{22}H_{32}O_2$ mw: 328.54

SYNS: CRYSTALETS ◇ MYVAK ◇ MYVAX ◇ RETINOL
ACETATE ◇ RETINYL ACETATE ◇ all-trans-RETINYL ACE-
TATE ◇ trans-VITAMIN A ACETATE ◇ VITAMIN A ALCOHOL
ACETATE

TOXICITY DATA with REFERENCE
NEO: orl-rat TD: 95 g/kg/2Y-C   JJIND8 74,715,85
NEO: orl-rat TDLo: 51800 mg/kg/2Y-C   JJIND8
74,715,85
MUT: dni-rat: mmr 3 μmol/L   JJIND8 70,949,83

CONSENSUS REPORTS: Reported in EPA
TSCA Inventory.

SAFETY PROFILE: Questionable carcinogen
with experimental neoplastigenic and teratogenic data. Moderately toxic by ingestion. Experimental reproductive effects. Mutation data reported. When heated to decomposition it emits
acrid smoke and irritating fumes.

VSK950   CAS: 302-79-4
VITAMIN A ACID
mf: $C_{20}H_{28}O_2$ mw: 300.48

PROP: Mp: 180-182°.

SYNS: ABEREL ◇ 3,7-DIMETHYL-9-(2,6,6-TRIMETHYL-1-CYCLOHEXEN-1-YL-2,4,6,8-NONATETRAENOIC ACID ◇ NSC-122758 ◇ β-RA ◇ RETIN-A ◇ RETINOIC ACID ◇ β-RETINOIC ACID ◇ all-trans-RETINOIC ACID ◇ TRETINOIN

TOXICITY DATA with REFERENCE
NEO: skn-mus TDLo:8400 mg/kg/30W-I
   CALEDQ 7,85,79
MUT: dni-hmn:leu 1 μmol/L   CNREA8 46,1388,86
MUT: dni-omi 1 μmol/L   CNREA8 45,2098,85
MUT: dni-rat:mmr 3 μmol/L   JJIND8 70,949,83
MUT: oms-hmn-skn 1000 ppm   26UYA8 -,335,71
MUT: oms-hmn:leu 1 μmol/L   CNREA846,1388,86

CONSENSUS REPORTS: Reported in EPA TSCA Inventory. EPA Genetic Toxicology Program.

SAFETY PROFILE: Questionable carcinogen with experimental neoplastigenic and teratogenic data. Poison by ingestion, intraperitoneal, subcutaneous, and intravenous routes. Experimental reproductive effects. Human mutation data reported. A human skin irritant. When heated to decomposition it emits acrid smoke and irritating fumes. Used to treat acne and other skin problems.

VSZ050   CAS: 13422-55-4
VITAMIN B12, METHYL
mf: $C_{63}H_{91}N_{13}O_{14}P \cdot Co$ mw: 1344.57

SYNS: COBALT-METHYLCOBALAMIN ◇ COBINAMIDE, COBALT-METHYL derivative, HYDROXIDE, DIHYDROGEN PHOSPHATE (ester), inner salt, 3′-ESTER with 5,6-DIMETHYL-1-α-D-RIBOFURANOSYLBENZIMIDAZOLE ◇ MECOBALAMIN ◇ METHYCOBAL ◇ METHYL-B12 ◇ METHYLCOBALAMIN ◇ METHYL COBALAMINE

TOXICITY DATA with REFERENCE
NEO: ims-mus TDLo:10 mg/kg (14-20D post)
   BEBMAE 101,471,86

SAFETY PROFILE: Questionable carcinogen with experimental neoplastigenic data. When heated to decomposition it emits toxic fumes of NO_x and PO_x.

WAT000   CAS: 481-39-0
WALNUT EXTRACT
mf: $C_{10}H_6O_3$ mw: 174.16

SYNS: C.I. 75500 ◇ C.I. NATURAL BROWN 7 ◇ 5-HYDROXY-1,4-NAPHTHALENEDIONE ◇ 5-HYDROXY-1,4-NAPHTHOQUINONE

TOXICITY DATA with REFERENCE
NEO: skn-mus TDLo:394 mg/kg/53W-I
   JMCMAR 21,26,78
MUT: hma-mus/ast 10 mg/kg   PSEBAA 126,583,67

SAFETY PROFILE: Questionable carcinogen with experimental neoplastigenic data. Poison by ingestion. Mutation data reported. When heated to decomposition it emits acrid smoke and irritating fumes.

WBA000   CAS: 84929-34-0
WAX MYRTLE

PROP: Tannin containing fraction of bark used (JNCIAM 57,207,76).

SYNS: MYRICA CERIFERA ◇ SOUTHERN BAYBERRY ◇ SWEET MYRTLE ◇ TANNIN FROM WAX MYRTLE

TOXICITY DATA with REFERENCE
NEO: scu-rat TDLo:560 mg/kg/69W-I   JNCIAM
   57,207,76

SAFETY PROFILE: Questionable carcinogen with experimental neoplastigenic data.

WBS000
WHISKEY

PROP: Light yellow-amber liquid. Pleasant to fruity odor. D: 0.923-0.935 @ 15.56°; 47%-53% of ethanol, by volume, flash p: 80.0°F (CC). Made by distillation of fermented malted grains, i.e., corn, rye, or barley. After distillation, whiskey is aged in wooden containers for up to several years. The aging extracts such components as acids and esters from the wood and promotes oxidation of components of raw whiskey and some reactions between organic components to form new flavors.

SAFETY PROFILE: The carcinogen urethane is sometimes found in whiskey. The whiskey or wine equivalent of 1 ounce of pure ethanol per capita per day is often cited as healthful to adults to relieve stress and promote relaxation. However, it is often abused which can lead to habituation with consequent liver damage, malnutrition, and a wide variety of other physical and mental problems. A fire hazard when exposed to heat or flame. To fight fire, use water, water spray, alcohol foam, CO_2, dry chemical.

WCA000
WINE

PROP: An alcoholic beverage made from the fermented juice of grapes, other fruits or plants.

Contains from 7-20% ethanol by volume. Concentrations of alcohol higher than those produced naturally are obtained by fortifying with pure ethanol. The distinctive colors, tastes, bouquets of wines are usually produced by adding coloring matter, sugar, acetic acid, salts, and higher fatty acids.

SAFETY PROFILE: Some wines contain the carcinogen urethane. Moderately toxic. Some of the additives to wines have been known to cause allergic reactions in humans.

WCB000   CAS: 68916-39-2
WITCH HAZEL

SYNS: HAMAMELIS ◇ NCI-C50544 ◇ SNAPPING HAZEL ◇ SPOTTED ALDER ◇ STRIPED ALDER ◇ TOBACCO WOOD ◇ WINTER BLOOM

TOXICITY DATA with REFERENCE
ETA: scu-rat TDLo: 2920 mg/kg/73W-I   JNCIAM 60,683,78
MUT: mma-sat 100 μg/plate   ENMUDM 8(Suppl 7),1,86
MUT: mmo-sat 5 mg/plate   ENMUDM 8(Suppl7),1,86

CONSENSUS REPORTS: Reported in EPA TSCA Inventory.

SAFETY PROFILE: Questionable carcinogen with experimental tumorigenic data. Mutation data reported. A mild irritant. Combustible when exposed to heat or flame; can react with oxidizing materials. Used as an ingredient in cosmetics. When heated to decomposition it emits acrid smoke and fumes.

WCJ000   CAS: 13983-17-0
WOLLASTONITE
mf: CaH$_2$O$_3$Si   mw: 118.19

PROP: A calcium silicate mineral (12VXA5 9,215,76).

SYNS: CAB-O-LITE 100 ◇ CAB-O-LITE 130 ◇ CAB-O-LITE 160 ◇ CAB-O-LITE F 1 ◇ CAB-O-LITE P 4 ◇ CASIFLUX VP 413-004 ◇ DAB-O-LITE P 4 ◇ F 1 ◇ FW 50 ◇ FW 200 (mineral) ◇ NCI-C55470 ◇ NYAD 10 ◇ NYAD 325 ◇ NYA G ◇ NYCOR 200 ◇ NYCOR 300 ◇ VANSIL W 10 ◇ VANSIL W 20 ◇ VANSIL W 30 ◇ WOLLASTOKUP

TOXICITY DATA with REFERENCE
ETA: imp-rat TDLo: 200 mg/kg   JJIND8 67,965,81

IARC Cancer Review: GROUP 3 IMEMDT 7,377,87; Animal Limited Evidence IMEMDT 42,145,87; Human Inadequate Evidence IMEMDT 42,145,87.

SAFETY PROFILE: Questionable carcinogen with experimental tumorigenic data. When heated to decomposition it emits acrid smoke and irritating fumes.

XCA000   CAS: 69-89-6
XANTHINE
mf: C$_5$H$_4$N$_4$O$_2$ mw: 152.13

PROP: Scales or plates. Decomp on heating without melting, partial sublimation. Sol in water and mineral acids; less sol in alc; very sol in NH$_4$OH and NaOH solns.

SYNS: 3,7-DIHYDRO-1H-PURINE-2,6-DIONE ◇ 2,6-DIOXOPURINE ◇ ISOXANTHINE ◇ PSEUDOXANTHINE ◇ PURINE-2,6-DIOL ◇ 9H-PURINE-2,6-DIOL ◇ 2,6(1,3)-PURINEDION ◇ PURINE-2,6-(1H,3H)-DIONE ◇ USAF CB-17 ◇ XAN ◇ XANTHIC OXIDE

TOXICITY DATA with REFERENCE
NEO: imp-mus TDLo: 80 mg/kg   BJCAAI 11,212,57
NEO: scu-rat TDLo: 3600 mg/kg/18W-I   JNCIAM 24,109,60

CONSENSUS REPORTS: Reported in EPA TSCA Inventory. EPA Genetic Toxicology Program.

SAFETY PROFILE: Questionable carcinogen with experimental neoplastigenic data. Moderately toxic by intraperitoneal route. When heated to decomposition it emits toxic fumes of NO$_x$.

XKJ500   CAS: 105-67-9
2,4-XYLENOL
DOT: 2261
mf: C$_8$H$_{10}$O   mw: 122.18

SYNS: 2,4-DIMETHYLPHENOL ◇ 4,6-DIMETHYLPHENOL ◇ 1-HYDROXY-2,4-DIMETHYLBENZENE ◇ RCRA WASTE NUMBER U101 ◇ m-XYLENOL ◇ m-XYLENOL (DOT)

TOXICITY DATA with REFERENCE
CAR: skn-mus TDLo: 16 g/kg/39W-I   CNREA8 19,413,59

CONSENSUS REPORTS: Reported in EPA TSCA Inventory.

DOT Classification: DOT-IMO: Poison B; Label: Poison.

SAFETY PROFILE: Questionable carcinogen with experimental carcinogenic data. Poison by intravenous and intraperitoneal routes. Moderately toxic by ingestion and skin contact. When heated to decomposition it emits acrid smoke and irritating fumes.

XKS000   CAS: 95-87-4
2,5-XYLENOL
DOT: 2261
mf: $C_8H_{10}O$ mw: 122.18

PROP: Crystals. Mp: 74.5°, bp: 211.5-213.5°.

SYNS: 2,5-DIMETHYLPHENOL ◊ 3,6-DIMETHYLPHENOL
◊ 2,5-DMP ◊ 6-METHYL-m-CRESOL ◊ p-XYLENOL (DOT)
◊ 1,2,5-XYLENOL

TOXICITY DATA with REFERENCE
ETA: skn-mus TDLo:4000 mg/kg/20W-I
    CNREA8 19,413,59

CONSENSUS REPORTS: Reported in EPA
TSCA Inventory.

DOT Classification: Poison B; Label: Poison.

SAFETY PROFILE: Questionable carcinogen
with experimental tumorigenic data. Poison by
ingestion. Moderately toxic by an unspecified
route. When heated to decomposition it emits
acrid smoke and irritating fumes. Used in disinfectants, solvents, pharmaceuticals, plasticizers, and wetting agents.

XLA000   CAS: 576-26-1
2,6-XYLENOL
mf: $C_8H_{10}O$ mw: 122.18

PROP: Needles. Mp: 48-49°, bp: 203°. Sol in
hot water, alc.

SYNS: 2,6-DIMETHYLPHENOL ◊ 2,6-DMP

TOXICITY DATA with REFERENCE
ETA: skn-mus TDLo:4000 mg/kg/20W-I
    CNREA8 19,413,59

CONSENSUS REPORTS: Reported in EPA
TSCA Inventory.

SAFETY PROFILE: Questionable carcinogen
with experimental tumorigenic data. Poison by
ingestion, intravenous, and intraperitoneal
routes. Moderately toxic by skin contact. An
eye irritant. When heated to decomposition it
emits acrid smoke and irritating fumes. Used
in disinfectants, solvents, pharmaceuticals, and
as an antioxidant in gas, oils, and elastomers.

XLJ000   CAS: 95-65-8
3,4-XYLENOL
mf: $C_8H_{10}O$ mw: 122.18

PROP: Prisms from ligroin. D: 1.076 @ 17.5°,
mp: 62.5°, bp: 225°C. Very sltly sol in water;
sol in alc, ether.

SYNS: 3,4-DIMETHYLPHENOL ◊ 4,5-DIMETHYLPHENOL
◊ 3,4-DMP ◊ 1,3,4-XYLENOL

TOXICITY DATA with REFERENCE
ETA: skn-mus TDLo:4000 mg/kg/20W-I
    CNREA8 19,413,59

CONSENSUS REPORTS: Reported in EPA
TSCA Inventory.

SAFETY PROFILE: Questionable carcinogen
with experimental tumorigenic data. Poison by
ingestion. Moderately toxic by unspecified
route. When heated to decomposition it emits
acrid smoke and irritating fumes. Used in production of sulfur dyes, disinfectants, pharmaceuticals, solvents, and as an antioxidant.

XLS000   CAS: 108-68-9
3,5-XYLENOL
mf: $C_8H_{10}O$ mw: 122.18

PROP: White crystals. Mp: 64°, bp: 219.5°,
d: 1.0362, vap press: 1 mm @ 62°. Sltly sol
in water; sol in alc.

SYNS: 3,5-DIMETHYLPHENOL ◊ 3,5-DMP ◊ 1,3,5-XYLE-
NOL

TOXICITY DATA with REFERENCE
ETA: skn-mus TDLo:4000 mg/kg/20W-I
    CNREA8 19,413,59

CONSENSUS REPORTS: Reported in EPA
TSCA Inventory. EPA Genetic Toxicology Program.

SAFETY PROFILE: Questionable carcinogen
with experimental tumorigenic data. Poison by
intraperitoneal route. Moderately toxic by ingestion. A severe eye irritant. When heated to decomposition it emits acrid smoke and irritating
fumes.

XNA000   CAS: 95-78-3
2,5-XYLIDINE
DOT: 1711
mf: $C_8H_{11}N$ mw: 121.20

PROP: Colorless oil. Bp: 214°, d: 0.979 @
21/4°, mp: 155°. Very sltly sol in water.

SYNS: 1-AMINO-2,5-DIMETHYLBENZENE ◊ 3-AMINO-
1,4-DIMETHYLBENZENE ◊ 2-AMINO-1,4-XYLENE
◊ 2,5-DIMETHYLANILINE ◊ 2,5-DIMETHYLBENZENAMINE
◊ 2,5-DIMETHYLPHENYLAMINE ◊ 5-METHYL-o-TOLUI-
DINE ◊ 6-METHYL-m-TOLUIDINE ◊ p-XYLIDINE (DOT)

TOXICITY DATA with REFERENCE
MUT: dni-mus-orl 200 mg/kg   MUREAV 46,305,77
MUT: mma-sat 1 μmol/plate   MUREAV 77,317,80

CONSENSUS REPORTS: IARC Cancer Review: GROUP 3 IMEMDT 7,56,87; Animal Inadequate Evidence IMEMDT 16,377,78. Reported in EPA TSCA Inventory.

DFG MAK: (all isomers except 2,4-xylidene) 5 ppm (25 mg/m^3)   DOT Classification: Poison B; Label: Poison.

SAFETY PROFILE: Questionable carcinogen. A poison. Moderately toxic by ingestion. Mutation data reported. When heated to decomposition it emits toxic fumes of NO$_x$.

XOJ000   CAS: 21436-96-4
2,4-XYLIDINE HYDROCHLORIDE
mf: $C_8H_{11}N \cdot ClH$ mw: 157.66

SYNS: 1-AMINO-2,4-DIMETHYLBENZENE HYDROCHLORIDE ◇ 4-AMINO-1,3-DIMETHYLBENZENE HYDROCHLORIDE ◇ 4-AMINO-3-METHYLTOLUENE HYDROCHLORIDE ◇ 4-AMINO-1,3-XYLENE HYDROCHLORIDE ◇ 2,4-DIMETHYLANILINE HYDROCHLORIDE ◇ 2,4-DIMETHYLBENZENAMINE HYDROCHLORIDE ◇ 4-METHYL-o-TOLUIDINE HYDROCHLORIDE ◇ 2-METHYL-p-TOLUIDINE HYDROCHLORIDE ◇ m-XYLIDINE HYDROCHLORIDE

TOXICITY DATA with REFERENCE
NEO: orl-mus TDLo:12 g/kg/78W-C   JEPTDQ 2,325,78

SAFETY PROFILE: Questionable carcinogen with experimental neoplastigenic data. Moderately toxic by ingestion and intraperitoneal routes. When heated to decomposition it emits very toxic fumes of NO$_x$ and HCl.

XOS000   CAS: 51786-53-9
2,5-XYLIDINE HYDROCHLORIDE
mf: $C_8H_{11}N \cdot ClH$ mw: 157.66

SYNS: 1-AMINO-2,5-DIMETHYLBENZENE HYDROCHLORIDE ◇ 3-AMINO-1,4-DIMETHYLBENZENE HYDROCHLORIDE ◇ 5-AMINO-1,4-DIMETHYLBENZENE HYDROCHLORIDE ◇ 2-AMINO-4-METHYLTOLUENE HYDROCHLORIDE ◇ 2-AMINO-1,4-XYLENE HYDROCHLORIDE ◇ 2,5-DIMETHYLANILINE HYDROCHLORIDE ◇ 2,5-DIMETHYLBENZENAMINE HYDROCHLORIDE ◇ 5-METHYL-o-TOLUIDINE HYDROCHLORIDE ◇ 6-METHYL-m-TOLUIDINE HYDROCHLORIDE ◇ p-XYLIDINE HYDROCHLORIDE

TOXICITY DATA with REFERENCE
CAR: orl-mus TD:780 g/kg/78W-C   JEPTDQ 2,325,78
CAR: orl-mus TDLo:390 g/kg/78W-C   JEPTDQ 2,325,78

ETA: orl-rat TD:248 g/kg/78W-C   JEPTDQ 2,325,78
ETA: orl-rat TDLo:124 g/kg/78W-C   JEPTDQ 2,325,78

SAFETY PROFILE: Questionable carcinogen with experimental carcinogenic and tumorigenic data. Moderately toxic by intraperitoneal route. When heated to decomposition it emits very toxic fumes of NO$_x$ and HCl.

XRA000   CAS: 3118-97-6
1-(2,4-XYLYLAZO)-2-NAPHTHOL
mf: $C_{18}H_{16}N_2O$ mw: 276.36

SYNS: A.F. RED NO. 5 ◇ AIZEN FOOD RED NO. 5 ◇ BRASILAZINA OIL SCARLET 6G ◇ BRILLIANT OIL SCARLET B ◇ CALCO OIL SCARLET BL ◇ CERES ORANGES RR ◇ CERISOL SCARLET G ◇ CEROTINSCHARLACH G ◇ C.I. 12140 ◇ C.I. SOLVENT ORANGE 7 ◇ 1-((2,4-DIMETHYLPHENYL)AZO)-2-NAPHTHALENOL ◇ EXTRACT D&C RED NO. 14 ◇ FAST OIL ORANGE II ◇ FAT RED (YELLOWISH) ◇ FAT SCARLET 2G ◇ FETTORANGE B ◇ GRASAN ORANGE 3R ◇ LACQUER ORANGE VR ◇ MOTIROT G ◇ OIL ORANGE KB ◇ OIL ORANGE N EXTRA ◇ OIL ORANGE R ◇ OIL ORANGE 2R ◇ OIL ORANGE X ◇ OIL ORANGE XO ◇ OIL RED GRO ◇ OIL RED O ◇ OIL RED RO ◇ OIL RED XO ◇ OIL SCARLET ◇ OIL SCARLET 371 ◇ OIL SCARLET APYO ◇ OIL SCARLET BL ◇ OIL SCARLET 6G ◇ OIL SCARLET L ◇ OIL SCARLET YS ◇ ORANGE INSOLUBLE OLG ◇ ORANGE INSOLUBLE RR ◇ ORANGE OIL KB ◇ PONCEAU INSOLUBLE OLG ◇ PYRONALROT R ◇ RED B ◇ RED NO. 5 ◇ RESIN SCARLET 2R ◇ RESOFORM ORANGE R ◇ ROT B ◇ ROT GG FETTLOESLICH ◇ SOMALIA ORANGE A2R ◇ SOMALIA ORANGE 2R ◇ SOUDAN II ◇ SUDAN AX ◇ SUDAN ORANGE ◇ SUDAN ORANGE RPA ◇ SUDAN ORANGE RRA ◇ SUDAN RED ◇ SUDAN SCARLET 6G ◇ SUDAN X ◇ WAXAKOL VERMILION L ◇ 1-XYLYLAZO-2-NAPHTHOL ◇ 1-(o-XYLYLAZO)-2-NAPHTHOL

TOXICITY DATA with REFERENCE
CAR: imp-mus TDLo:80 mg/kg   BJCAAI22,825,68
MUT: mma-sat 50 µg/plate   MUREAV 44,9,77

CONSENSUS REPORTS: IARC Cancer Review: GROUP 3 IMEMDT 7,56,87; Animal Sufficient Evidence IMEMDT 8,233,75. Reported in EPA TSCA Inventory. Community Right-To-Know List. EPA Genetic Toxicology Program.

SAFETY PROFILE: Questionable carcinogen with experimental carcinogenic data. Mutation data reported. When heated to decomposition it emits toxic fumes of NO$_x$.

YCJ000 CAS: 3458-22-8
YOSHI 864
mf: $C_8H_{19}NO_6S_2 \cdot ClH$ mw: 325.86

SYNS: N,N-BIS(METHYLSULFONEPROPOXY)AMINE HYDROCHLORIDE ◇ COMPOUND 864 ◇ 3,3'-IMIDODI-1-PROPANOL, DIMETHANESULFONATE (ester), HYDROCHLORIDE ◇ IPD ◇ NCI-C01547 ◇ NSC 102627 ◇ SAKURAI NO. 864

TOXICITY DATA with REFERENCE
NEO: ipr-mus TD:3840 mg/kg/64W-I NCITR*
NCI-CG-TR-18,78
NEO: ipr-mus TDLo:1100 mg/kg/8W-I
CNREA8 33,3069,73
NEO: ipr-rat TDLo:3744 mg/kg/52W-I NCITR*
NCI-CG-TR-18,78
MUT: ipr-mus LD10:170 mg/kg JMCMAR
20,515,77
MUT: oms-hmn:lym 100 mg/L EJCAAH 14,741,78

CONSENSUS REPORTS: NCI Carcinogenesis Bioassay (ipr); Clear Evidence: mouse, rat NCITR* NCI-CG-TR-18,78

SAFETY PROFILE: Questionable carcinogen with experimental neoplastigenic data. Poison by intraperitoneal and intravenous routes. Human systemic effects by intravenous route: somnolence, hypermotility, diarrhea, nausea or vomiting. Human mutation data reported. When heated to decomposition it emits very toxic fumes of NO_x, SO_x, and HCl.

YDA000 CAS: 7440-64-4
YTTERBIUM
af: Yb aw: 173.04

PROP: A bright, silvery, lustrous soft, malleable, ductile, and fairly stable element. Mp: 824°, bp: 1193°, d: 6.977. A rare earth.

TOXICITY DATA with REFERENCE
ETA: imp-mus TDLo:25 g/kg PSEBAA
135,426,70

CONSENSUS REPORTS: Reported in EPA TSCA Inventory.

SAFETY PROFILE: Questionable carcinogen with experimental tumorigenic data. As a lanthanon it may have an anticoagulant action on blood. Flammable in the form of dust when reacted with air; halogens.

YFA000 CAS: 63938-20-5
YTTRIUM CITRATE
mf: $C_6H_8O_7 \cdot 1/3Y$ mw: 221.75

SYN: CITRIC ACID, YTTRIUM SALT (3:1)

TOXICITY DATA with REFERENCE
ETA: ipr-mus LD50:79 mg/kg AEHLAU
5,437,62

ACGIH TLV: TWA 1 mg(Y)/m^3

SAFETY PROFILE: Questionable carcinogen with experimental tumorigenic data. Poison by intraperitoneal route. When heated to decomposition it emits acrid smoke and irritating fumes.

YFJ000 CAS: 10361-93-0
YTTRIUM(III) NITRATE (1:3)
mf: $N_3O_9 \cdot Y$ mw: 274.94

PROP: Hexahydrate, deliquescent crystals. Sol in water.

SYN: NITRIC ACID, YTTRIUM(3+) SALT

TOXICITY DATA with REFERENCE
ETA: orl-mus TDLo:1300 mg/kg/60W-C
JONUAI 101,1431,71

CONSENSUS REPORTS: Reported in EPA TSCA Inventory.

ACGIH TLV: TWA 1 mg(Y)/m^3

SAFETY PROFILE: Questionable carcinogen with experimental tumorigenic data. Poison by intraperitoneal route. Moderately toxic by intravenous route. Experimental reproductive effects. When heated to decomposition it emits toxic fumes of NO_x.

ZAK000
ZAMIA DEBILIS

PROP: Dried, ground-up zamia tubers were used (85CVA2 5,197,70).

TOXICITY DATA with REFERENCE
ETA: orl-rat TDLo:650 g/kg/77W-C 85CVA2
5,197,70

SAFETY PROFILE: Questionable carcinogen with experimental tumorigenic data.

ZAT000 CAS: 17924-92-4
ZEARALENONE
mf: $C_{18}H_{22}O_5$ mw: 318.40

PROP: l-Form: Crystals. Mp: 164-165°. Sol in aq alkali, ether, benzene, alc; almost insol in water. dl-Form: Crystals. Mp: 187-189°.

SYNS: COMPOUND F-2 ◇ 14,16-DIHYDROXY-3-METHYL-7-OXO-trans-BENZOXACYCLOTETRADEC-11-EN-1-ONE ◇ FES ◇ F-2 TOXIN ◇ FUSARIUM TOXIN ◇ trans-6-(10-HYDROXY-6-OXO-1-UNDECENYL)-mu-LACTONE, RESORCYLIC ACID ◇ 6-(10-HYDROXY-6-OXO-trans-1-UNDECENYL)-β-RESORCYCLIC ACID-N-LACTONE ◇ MYCOTOXIN F2 ◇ NCI-C50226 ◇ (−)-ZEARALENONE ◇ (s)-ZEARALENONE ◇ (10s)-ZEARALENONE ◇ trans-ZEARALENONE

TOXICITY DATA with REFERENCE

NEO: orl-mus TDLo:8652 mg/kg/2Y-C NTPTR* NTP-TR-235,82

ETA: orl-mus TD:4326 mg/kg/2Y-C   NTPTR* NTP-TR-235,82

MUT: dnr-bcs 2500 mg/L   IRLCDZ 7,204,79

MUT: mrc-bcs 100 μg/disc   CNREA8 36,445,76

CONSENSUS REPORTS: IARC Cancer Review: GROUP 3 IMEMDT 7,56,87; Human Inadequate Evidence IMEMDT 31,279,83; Animal Limited Evidence IMEMDT 31,279,83. NTP Carcinogenesis Bioassay (feed); Clear Evidence: mouse NTPTR* NTP-TR-235,82; (feed); No Evidence: rat NTPTR* NTP-TR-235,82. Reported in EPA TSCA Inventory. EPA Genetic Toxicology Program.

SAFETY PROFILE: Questionable carcinogen with experimental carcinogenic, neoplastigenic, tumorigenic, and teratogenic data. Experimental reproductive effects. Mutation data reported. A severe skin irritant. When heated to decomposition it emits acrid smoke and irritating fumes.

ZFA000   CAS: 7646-85-7
ZINC CHLORIDE
DOT: 1840/2331
mf: Cl_2Zn mw: 136.27

PROP: Odorless, cubic, white, deliquescent crystals. Mp: 290°, bp: 732°, d: 2.91 @ 25°, vap press: 1 mm @ 428°.

SYNS: BUTTER of ZINC ◇ CHLORURE de ZINC (FRENCH) ◇ TINNING GLUX (DOT) ◇ ZINC CHLORIDE, ANHYDROUS (DOT) ◇ ZINC CHLORIDE, SOLID (DOT) ◇ ZINC CHLORIDE, SOLUTION (DOT) ◇ ZINC (CHLORURE de) (FRENCH) ◇ ZINC DICHLORIDE ◇ ZINC MURIATE, SOLUTION (DOT) ◇ ZINCO (CLORURO di) (ITALIAN) ◇ ZINKCHLORID (GERMAN) ◇ ZINKCHLORIDE (DUTCH)

TOXICITY DATA with REFERENCE

ETA: par-ckn TDLo:15 mg/kg   CANCAR 6,464,53

ETA: par-ham TDLo:17 mg/kg   CNREA8 34,2612,74

MUT: cyt-hmn:lym 300 μmol/L   TXCYAC 10,67,78

MUT: cyt-mus-orl 18 g/kg/30D-C   CRSBAW 176,563,82

MUT: dni-hmn:lym 360 μmol/L   IAAAAM 77,461,85

MUT: dns-hmn:lym 180 μmol/L   IAAAAM 77,461,85

MUT: hma-mus/sat 6 mg/kg   SOGEBZ 13,1010,77

MUT: mma-sat 90 mmol/L   SOGEBZ 13,1010,77

MUT: otr-ham:emb 180 μmol/L   CNREA8 39,193,79

CONSENSUS REPORTS: Zinc and its compounds are on the Community Right-To-Know List. Reported in EPA TSCA Inventory. EPA Genetic Toxicology Program.

OSHA PEL: Fume: (Transitional: TWA 1 mg/m³) TWA 1 mg/m³; STEL 2 mg/m³   ACGIH TLV: TWA 1 mg/m³; STEL 2 mg/m³ (fume) DOT Classification: Corrosive Material; Label: Corrosive and Corrosive, solution; ORM-E; Label: None, solid.

SAFETY PROFILE: Questionable carcinogen with experimental tumorigenic and teratogenic data. Poison by ingestion, intravenous, subcutaneous and intraperitoneal routes. Human systemic effects by inhalation: pulmonary changes. Experimental reproductive effects. Human mutation data reported. A corrosive irritant to skin, eyes and mucous membranes. Exposure to $ZnCl_2$ fumes or dusts can cause dermatitis, boils, conjunctivitis, gastrointestinal tract upsets. The fumes are highly toxic. When heated to decomposition it emits toxic fumes of Cl^- and ZnO.

ZHJ000   CAS: 14881-92-6
ZINC-N-FLUOREN-2-YLACETOHYDROXAMATE
mf: $C_{30}H_{24}N_2O_4 \cdot Zn$ mw: 541.93

SYNS: N-FLUOREN-2-YLACETOHYDROXAMIC ACID, ZINC COMPLEX ◇ N-HYDROXY-2-ACETYLAMINOFLUORENE, ZINC CHELATE

TOXICITY DATA with REFERENCE

NEO: scu-rat TDLo:160 mg/kg/4W-I   CNREA8 25,527,65

CONSENSUS REPORTS: Zinc and its compounds are on the Community Right-To-Know List.

SAFETY PROFILE: Questionable carcinogen with experimental neoplastigenic data. When heated to decomposition it emits toxic fumes of NO_x and ZnO.

ZJS000   CAS: 557-07-3
ZINC OLEATE (1:2)
mf: $C_{36}H_{68}O_4 \cdot Zn$ mw: 630.41

PROP: White, dry, greasy powder. Insol in water; sol in alc, ether, carbon disulfide, benzene, petr ether.

SYN: OLEIC ACID, ZINC SALT

TOXICITY DATA with REFERENCE
ETA: orl-mus TDLo: 1080 g/kg/1Y-C   FCTXAV 3,271,65

CONSENSUS REPORTS: Zinc and its compounds are on the Community Right-To-Know List. Reported in EPA TSCA Inventory.

SAFETY PROFILE: Questionable carcinogen with experimental tumorigenic data. When heated to decomposition it emits toxic fumes of ZnO.

ZNA000   CAS: 7733-02-0
ZINC SULFATE
DOT: 9161
mf: $O_4S \cdot Zn$ mw: 161.43

PROP: Rhombic, colorless crystals or crystalline powder. Mp: decomp @ 740°, d: 3.74 @ 15°. Sol in water; almost insol in alc.

SYNS: BONAZEN ◇ BUFOPTO ZINC SULFATE
◇ OP-THAL-ZIN ◇ SULFATE de ZINC (FRENCH) ◇ SULFURIC ACID, ZINC SALT (1:1) ◇ VERAZINC ◇ WHITE COPPERAS ◇ WHITE VITRIOL ◇ ZINC SULPHATE ◇ ZINC VITRIOL ◇ ZINKOSITE

TOXICITY DATA with REFERENCE
ETA: scu-rbt TDLo: 3625 μg/kg/5D-C   COREAF 236,1387,53
MUT: dni-hmn: hla 1 μmol/L/4H   BECTA6 32,220,84
MUT: mmo-smc 100 mmol/L   MUREAV 117,149,83
MUT: mrc-smc 100 mmol/L   BECTA6 32,220,84
MUT: otr-ham: emb 200 μmol/L   CNREA8 39,193,79
MUT: sln-dmg-orl 5 mmol/L   MUREAV 90,91,81

CONSENSUS REPORTS: Zinc and its compounds are on the Community Right-To-Know List. Reported in EPA TSCA Inventory. EPA Genetic Toxicology Program.

DOT Classification: ORM-E; Label: None.

SAFETY PROFILE: Questionable carcinogen with experimental tumorigenic and teratogenic data. Poison by intraperitoneal, subcutaneous,

and intravenous routes. Moderately toxic by ingestion. Human systemic effects by ingestion: increased pulse rate without blood pressure decrease, blood pressure decrease, acute pulmonary edema, normocytic anemia, hypermotility, diarrhea and other gastrointestinal changes. Experimental reproductive effects. Human mutation data reported. An eye irritant. When heated to decomposition it emits toxic fumes of SO_x and ZnO.

ZPS000   CAS: 13520-92-8
ZIRCONIUM CHLORIDE OXIDE OCTAHYDRATE
mf: $Cl_2OZr \cdot 8H_2O$ mw: 322.28

SYN: ZIRCONYL CHLORIDE OCTAHYDRATE

TOXICITY DATA with REFERENCE
ETA: idr-mus TDLo: 800 μg/kg   CNREA8 33,287,73

OSHA PEL: (Transitional: TWA 5 mg(Zr)/m³) TWA 5 mg(Zr)/m³; STEL 10 mg(Zr)/m³ ACGIH TLV: TWA 5 mg(Zr)/m³; STEL 10 mg(Zr)/m³ DFG MAK: 5 mg(Zr)/m³

SAFETY PROFILE: Questionable carcinogen with experimental tumorigenic data. When heated to decomposition it emits toxic fumes of Cl^-.

ZSJ000   CAS: 7699-43-6
ZIRCONIUM OXYCHLORIDE
mf: Cl_2OZr mw: 178.12

PROP: Crystals. D: 1.91. Very sol in water, alc.

SYNS: BASIC ZIRCONIUM CHLORIDE ◇ CHLOROZIRCONYL ◇ DICHLOROOXOZIRCONIUM ◇ NCI-C60811 ◇ ZIRCONYL CHLORIDE

TOXICITY DATA with REFERENCE
NEO: idr-mus TDLo: 800 μg/kg   JIDEAE 57,411,71

CONSENSUS REPORTS: Reported in EPA TSCA Inventory.

OSHA PEL: (Transitional: TWA 5 mg(Zr)/m³) TWA 5 mg(Zr)/m³; STEL 10 mg(Zr)/m³ ACGIH TLV: TWA 5 mg(Zr)/m³; STEL 10 mg(Zr)/m³ DFG MAK: 5 mg(Zr)/m³

SAFETY PROFILE: Questionable carcinogen with experimental neoplastigenic data. Poison by intraperitoneal route. Moderately toxic by ingestion and subcutaneous routes. When heated to decomposition it emits toxic fumes of Cl^-. Used as an antiperspirant.

ZTA000   CAS: 63904-82-5
ZIRCONIUM SODIUM LACTATE
mf: $C_9H_{15}NaO_{10}Zr$ mw: 397.45

PROP: Straw colored liquid. D: 1.28.

SYN: SODIUM HYDROGEN TRILACTATOZIRCONYLATE

TOXICITY DATA with REFERENCE
NEO: idr-mus TDLo: 200 mg/kg
   JIDEAE 57,411,71

OSHA PEL: (Transitional: TWA 5 mg(Zr)/m^3)
TWA 5 mg(Zr)/m^3; STEL 10 mg(Zr)/m^3
ACGIH TLV: TWA 5 mg(Zr)/m^3; STEL 10
mg(Zr)/m^3 DFG MAK: 5 mg(Zr)/m^3

SAFETY PROFILE: Questionable carcinogen
with experimental neoplastigenic data. Inhalation produced bronchiolar abcesses, lobar pneumonia and peribronchial granulomas experimentally. When heated to decomposition it emits
acrid smoke and irritating fumes of Na_2O.

Section 3
APPENDIXES

I. Human Carcinogenic Site or Effect Index

angiosarcoma see I:TFT750

aplastic anemia see I:CDP250

appendages see I:DKQ000

application site see I:TFT750

bladder see I:ABG750, I:ARF750, I:ASB250, I:BBX000, I:BIF250, I:EAS500, I:TFT750, I:CPQ625

blood see I:VNP000

brain see I:RDK000

colon see III:CME400, III:MEK700

esophagus see I:ARF750

gastrointestinal see I:EAS500, III:FMB000, III:MQV750

Hodgkin's disease see I:DKQ000, I:EAS500, I:PED750, III:CQH100, III:DAB845, III:MDV500, III:POK000, I:BBL250

kidney see I:ABG750, I:BOT250, I:TFT750

larynx see I:ARF750

leukemia see I:ASB250, I:BRF500, I:CDO500, I:CDP250, I:CHD250, I:EAS500, III:LGZ000, I:PED750, I:RCA375, I:TFQ750, III:MCR750, III:MDV500, III:POK000

lukemia see I:BOT250

lung see I:ARM250, I:ARM268, I:CAE750, I:CMJ500, I:CMK000, I:DKA600, I:EEH520, I:SKS750, I:ZFJ100, I:ZFJ120, III:RCA275

lymphoma see I:BBL250, I:DKQ000, I:TFT750

mouth see I:ARF750

myeloid leukemia see I:BBL250

nasal see I:CMJ500, I:CMK000, III:MQL250

normocytic anemia see III:MCA500

nose see III:MEK700

para nasal sinus see I:ARF750, I:CMJ500

reproductive system see I:DKA600

scrotum see I:SKS750

site of application see I:IGS000

skin see I:BIE250, I:DKA600, I:DKQ000, I:PKV500, I:RCA375, I:RDK000, I:SKS750, III:CMX500, III:DNA200, III:MDV500, III:MEK700, III:RCA275, III:RDF000

spinal cord see III:CMX500

thyroid see III:LGZ000

uterine see I:BOT250, I:DKA600, I:DNX500, III:EEH900

vascular system see I:ECU750

II. CAS Number Cross-Index

1302-76-7 see III:AHF500	1746-77-6 see III:IOJ000	2386-90-5 see III:BJN250
1302-78-9 see III:BAV750	1764-39-2 see III:FHP000	2393-53-5 see II:EDV500
1303-28-2 see I:ARH500	1772-03-8 see III:GAT000	2401-85-6 see III:DUS600
1303-33-9 see III:ARI000	1777-84-0 see III:NEL000	2407-43-4 see III:EKL500
1303-39-5 see I:ZDJ000	1807-55-2 see III:MJ0000	2409-55-4 see III:BQV750
1304-56-9 see I:BFT250	1811-28-5 see III:PMH100	2417-77-8 see III:BN0500
1306-19-0 see I:CAH500	1836-75-5 see I:DFT800	2422-79-9 see III:MGX500
1306-23-6 see I:CAJ750	1838-56-8 see III:HIO875	2423-66-7 see III:QSA000
1307-96-6 see III:CND125	1845-11-0 see III:NAD500	2425-06-1 see III:CBF800
1308-31-2 see I:CMI500	1881-37-4 see III:FIA500	2426-07-5 see III:DHD800
1308-38-9 see II:CMJ900	1881-75-0 see III:FJQ000	2431-50-7 see I:TIL360
1309-37-1 see III:IHD000	1881-76-1 see III:FJR000	2432-99-7 see III:AMW000
1309-48-4 see III:MAH500	1888-89-7 see III:DHC800	2435-64-5 see III:SNW800
1309-64-4 see I:AQF000	1892-54-2 see III:PDA500	2438-49-5 see III:DTK800
1313-27-5 see III:MRE000	1897-45-6 see III:TBQ750	2438-51-9 see III:PCZ000
1313-99-1 see III:NDF500	1910-36-7 see III:HLV000	2439-10-3 see III:DXX400
1314-05-2 see III:NDF400	1912-24-9 see III:ARQ725	2443-39-2 see III:ECD500
1314-06-3 see II:NDH500	1918-02-1 see III:PIB900	2465-27-2 see I:IBA000
1314-20-1 see I:TFT750	1921-70-6 see III:PMD500	2465-29-4 see III:ADK000
1317-36-8 see III:LDN000	1936-15-8 see III:HGC000	2466-76-4 see III:ACO250
1317-42-6 see III:CNE200	1937-37-7 see I:AQP000	2475-45-8 see III:TBG700
1317-43-7 see III:NBT000	1949-20-8 see III:OOE000	2485-10-1 see III:FEN000
1317-60-8 see I:HA0875	1951-12-8 see III:CEW000	2489-77-2 see III:TMH750
1327-53-3 see I:ARI750	1953-56-6 see III:DNX000	2491-76-1 see III:CGD250
1332-10-1 see I:FOM050	1954-28-5 see III:TJQ333	2495-54-7 see III:HIQ500
1332-21-4 see I:ARM250	1955-45-9 see III:DTH000	2497-34-9 see III:ELD500
1333-82-0 see I:CMK000	1972-08-3 see III:TCM250	2498-75-1 see III:MGV250
1333-86-4 see III:CBT750	1984-77-6 see III:LBM000	2498-76-2 see III:MGV000
1335-32-6 see III:LCH000	1994-57-6 see III:FJN000	2498-77-3 see III:MGU750
1336-36-3 see I:PJL750	2023-60-1 see III:DRY800	2508-18-1 see III:FIT200
1338-16-5 see III:IHL000	2023-61-2 see III:DRZ000	2508-20-5 see III:NKF500
1338-23-4 see III:MKA500	2051-89-0 see III:BBY250	2508-23-8 see III:NBD000
1338-39-2 see III:SKV000	2058-46-0 see III:HOI000	2517-98-8 see III:ABR250
1344-28-1 see III:AHE250	2058-62-0 see III:MPY000	2541-68-6 see III:FJP000
1401-55-4 see III:CDM250	2058-66-4 see III:ENB000	2541-69-7 see III:MGW750
1401-55-4 see III:MQV250	2058-67-5 see III:EOH500	2564-65-0 see III:BBF500
1401-55-4 see III:QBJ000	2068-78-2 see III:LEZ000	2578-75-8 see III:FQJ000
1401-55-4 see III:SOY500	2104-09-8 see III:ALP000	2580-78-1 see III:BMM500
1401-55-4 see III:TAD750	2113-47-5 see III:PDY000	2581-69-3 see III:NIK000
1402-68-2 see I:AET750	2113-54-4 see III:PDY250	2586-60-9 see III:CMP000
1421-85-8 see III:EBP500	2114-11-6 see III:AGA750	2594-20-9 see III:IPA000
1423-97-8 see III:EDU000	2122-77-2 see III:TIX000	2597-54-8 see III:ACL000
1425-67-8 see III:CCG000	2122-86-3 see III:NGK000	2602-46-2 see I:CMO000
1455-77-2 see III:DCF200	2130-56-5 see III:BFX250	2606-85-1 see III:MHL250
1456-28-6 see II:DTA000	2164-17-2 see III:DUK800	2606-87-3 see III:FJO000
1464-53-5 see I:BGA750	2185-86-6 see III:VKA600	2611-82-7 see III:FMU080
1491-09-4 see III:BCF750	2185-92-4 see III:BGE325	2642-37-7 see III:ICD000
1491-10-7 see III:BCF500	2191-10-8 see I:CAD750	2642-50-4 see III:MFR000
1492-54-2 see III:MHF000	2198-54-1 see III:ABP500	2642-98-0 see III:CML800
1492-55-3 see III:MHE750	2207-76-3 see III:HID500	2646-17-5 see II:TGW000
1528-74-1 see III:DUS000	2223-82-7 see III:DUL200	2650-18-2 see III:FMU059
1532-19-0 see III:CMV475	2223-93-0 see I:OAT000	2706-47-0 see III:TNC725
1541-60-2 see III:MHJ750	2227-79-4 see III:BBM250	2706-47-0 see III:TNC750
1571-30-8 see III:HOE000	2235-59-8 see III:IQB000	2732-09-4 see III:FNR000
1582-09-8 see III:DUV600	2238-07-5 see II:DKM200	2747-31-1 see III:DTK600
1596-52-7 see III:DVE000	2243-62-1 see II:NAM000	2782-91-4 see III:TDX000
1596-84-5 see II:DQD400	2302-84-3 see III:F0J000	2783-94-0 see III:FAG150
1615-80-1 see II:DJL400	2303-16-4 see III:DBI200	2784-86-3 see III:HIJ400
1616-88-2 see III:ME0000	2303-47-1 see III:DNW800	2784-94-3 see II:BKF250
1628-58-6 see III:DQC400	2307-55-3 see III:DAB020	2823-90-7 see III:FF0000
1633-83-6 see II:BOU250	2318-18-5 see III:DMX200	2823-91-8 see III:FFN000
1638-22-8 see III:BSD750	2319-96-2 see III:MGV750	2823-93-0 see III:FFM000
1661-03-6 see III:MAI250	2353-45-9 see III:FAG000	2823-94-1 see III:FFP000
1675-54-3 see III:BLD750	2373-98-0 see II:DMI400	2823-95-2 see III:FFQ000
1678-25-7 see III:BBR750	2381-15-9 see III:MGX000	2824-10-4 see III:FFL000
1680-21-3 see III:TJQ100	2381-16-0 see III:MGW500	2825-82-3 see III:TLR675
1689-82-3 see III:HJF000	2381-18-2 see III:BBB750	2832-40-8 see II:AAQ250
1694-09-3 see II:FAG120	2381-19-3 see III:MHL500	2835-39-4 see II:ISV000
1705-85-7 see III:MIN750	2381-21-7 see III:M0X875	2855-19-8 see III:DXU000
1706-01-0 see III:MKC750	2381-31-9 see III:MGW250	2869-09-2 see III:MMD000
1715-81-7 see III:APM750	2381-34-2 see III:MHF500	2869-10-5 see III:MMD250
1732-14-5 see III:PON500	2381-39-7 see III:MHM000	2869-12-7 see III:MJA750
1745-81-9 see III:AGQ500	2381-40-0 see III:DQI800	2869-59-2 see III:DCY800
1746-01-6 see I:TAI000	2385-85-5 see I:MQW500	2869-60-5 see III:MJB000

5834-17-3 see III:MDZ000
5834-25-3 see III:DDC000
5836-85-1 see III:DLR200
5837-17-2 see III:DLU600
5905-52-2 see III:LAL000
5929-01-1 see III:BDV750
5959-56-8 see III:ALK500
5976-61-4 see III:HKH850
5989-27-5 see III:LFU000
6018-89-9 see II:NCX500
6023-26-3 see III:HIS000
6030-03-1 see III:EMS000
6030-80-4 see III:ECW500
6052-82-0 see III:DKB100
6055-19-2 see I:CQC675
6080-56-4 see I:LCJ000
6098-44-8 see III:ABL000
6098-46-0 see III:BDP000
6104-30-9 see III:IIV000
6109-97-3 see II:AJV250
6111-78-0 see III:MGX250
6120-10-1 see III:DQF000
6130-93-4 see III:TDS000
6151-25-3 see III:QCA175
6164-98-3 see III:CJJ250
6219-71-2 see III:CEG625
6240-55-7 see III:DFU400
6268-32-2 see III:NLG500
6292-55-3 see III:FDS000
6296-45-3 see III:CHF500
6304-33-2 see III:TMQ250
6325-54-8 see III:CIG250
6334-11-8 see II:TLH000
6341-85-1 see III:DHD200
6358-53-8 see II:DOK200
6366-20-7 see III:MEB500
6366-23-0 see III:MGY250
6366-24-1 see III:CIG500
6368-72-5 see III:EOJ500
6369-59-1 see III:TGM400
6370-43-0 see III:OHK000
6373-74-6 see III:SGP500
6379-46-0 see III:DVI600
6380-21-8 see III:PMS250
6416-57-5 see III:NBG500
6424-34-6 see III:TGU500
6483-64-3 see III:D00400
6509-08-6 see III:EBK500
6533-00-2 see III:NNQ500
6558-78-7 see III:BRZ000
6580-41-2 see III:ASP750
6610-08-8 see III:NLA500
6623-41-2 see III:AMW750
6629-04-5 see III:COJ750
6632-68-4 see III:DPN400
6639-99-2 see III:EDT500
6652-04-6 see III:PFT600
6728-21-8 see III:AGK750
6795-23-9 see I:AEW000
6810-26-0 see III:BGI250
6870-67-3 see III:JAK000
6893-20-5 see III:MER000
6893-24-9 see III:MEQ750
6898-43-7 see III:BCC250
6921-35-3 see III:EBQ500
6957-71-7 see III:FEF000
6959-48-4 see II:CIV000
6965-71-5 see III:DGB200
6972-76-5 see III:DRO200
6976-50-7 see III:DWT400
6986-48-7 see III:BID000
7008-42-6 see III:ADR750
7008-85-7 see III:DCP400
7047-84-9 see III:AHA250

7068-83-9 see III:MHW500
7090-25-7 see I:NBJ500
7093-10-9 see III:BAW000
7099-43-6 see III:CPY750
7119-92-8 see III:DJS500
7129-91-1 see III:CPY500
7194-19-6 see III:MMJ950
7203-90-9 see III:CJI100
7203-92-1 see III:DSN600
7220-81-7 see I:AEU750
7227-91-0 see III:DTP000
7227-92-1 see III:DSX400
7241-98-7 see I:AEV500
7247-89-4 see III:NLI000
7258-91-5 see III:PCW000
7261-97-4 see III:DAB845
7306-46-9 see III:BKM750
7316-37-2 see III:DJH200
7320-37-8 see III:EBX500
7329-29-5 see III:BJN875
7340-50-3 see III:HJH500
7346-14-7 see III:DJB800
7347-46-8 see III:DSS200
7347-47-9 see III:DQD600
7347-48-0 see III:DQD800
7347-49-1 see III:DIP000
7349-99-7 see III:DPP800
7350-86-9 see III:DLA120
7374-66-5 see III:DLY800
7378-50-9 see III:CGL000
7378-54-3 see III:TMG250
7411-49-6 see III:BGK750
7417-67-6 see III:MMT000
7422-80-2 see III:DEC725
7439-89-6 see III:IGK800
7439-92-1 see II:LCF000
7439-96-5 see III:MAP750
7439-97-6 see III:MCW250
7440-02-0 see I:NCW500
7440-06-4 see III:PJD500
7440-22-4 see III:SDI500
7440-25-7 see III:TAE750
7440-29-1 see II:TFS750
7440-31-5 see III:TGB250
7440-32-6 see III:TGF250
7440-36-0 see III:AQB750
7440-38-2 see I:ARA750
7440-41-7 see I:BFO750
7440-43-9 see I:CAD000
7440-47-3 see I:CMI750
7440-48-4 see I:CNA250
7440-50-8 see III:CNI000
7440-54-2 see III:GAF000
7440-57-5 see III:GIS000
7440-62-2 see III:VCP000
7440-64-4 see III:YDA000
7446-09-5 see III:SOH500
7446-27-7 see I:LDU000
7446-34-6 see I:SBT000
7447-41-8 see III:LHB000
7460-84-6 see III:SLK500
7466-54-8 see III:AOV250
7476-08-6 see III:COK500
7495-93-4 see I:CAD500
7496-02-8 see III:NFT400
7499-32-3 see III:DLT000
7505-62-6 see III:BBC750
7511-54-8 see III:EHM000
7519-36-0 see III:NLL500
7568-37-8 see I:MHY550
7572-29-4 see I:DEN600
7631-86-9 see III:SCH000
7631-89-2 see I:ARD750
7631-99-4 see III:SIO900

7632-00-0 see III:SIQ500
7633-57-0 see III:NKN000
7641-77-2 see III:HEC500
7645-25-2 see I:ARC750
7646-79-9 see III:CNB599
7646-85-7 see III:ZFA000
7647-10-1 see III:PAD500
7660-25-5 see III:LFI000
7660-71-1 see III:MDM000
7681-49-4 see III:SHF500
7681-49-4 see III:SHG000
7698-97-7 see III:FA0200
7699-31-2 see III:DJL600
7699-41-4 see III:SCL000
7699-43-6 see III:ZSJ000
7718-54-9 see II:NDH000
7720-78-7 see III:FBN100
7722-84-1 see III:HIB000
7722-84-1 see III:HIB010
7727-43-7 see III:BAP000
7733-02-0 see III:ZNA000
7758-01-2 see II:PKY300
7758-19-2 see III:SFT500
7758-95-4 see III:LCQ000
7758-97-6 see I:LCR000
7758-98-7 see III:CNP250
7761-88-8 see III:SDS000
7763-77-1 see III:CGX000
7773-01-5 see III:MAR000
7773-34-4 see III:DJB200
7774-41-6 see I:ARC500
7778-39-4 see I:ARB250
7778-43-0 see I:ARC000
7778-44-1 see I:ARB750
7778-50-9 see III:PKX250
7782-49-2 see III:SB0500
7783-47-3 see III:TGD100
7784-35-2 see I:ARI250
7784-37-4 see I:MDF350
7784-40-9 see I:LCK000
7784-41-0 see I:ARD250
7784-42-1 see I:ARK250
7784-46-5 see I:SEY500
7784-46-5 see I:SEZ000
7785-87-7 see III:MAU250
7786-81-4 see II:NDK500
7787-47-5 see I:BFQ000
7787-49-7 see I:BFR500
7787-52-2 see I:BFR750
7787-56-6 see I:BFU500
7788-99-0 see III:CMG850
7789-00-6 see III:PLB250
7789-06-2 see I:SMH000
7789-12-0 see III:SGI500
7790-78-5 see I:CAE425
7790-79-6 see I:CAG250
7790-84-3 see I:CAJ250
7791-20-0 see II:NDA000
7791-25-5 see I:SOT000
7803-57-8 see III:HGU500
8000-03-1 see III:EDQ000
8001-28-3 see III:COC250
8001-29-4 see III:CNU000
8001-35-2 see I:CDV100
8001-50-1 see III:TBC500
8001-58-9 see I:CMY825
8002-03-7 see III:PA0000
8002-05-9 see III:PCR250
8002-74-2 see III:PAH750
8003-03-0 see III:ARP250
8006-61-9 see III:GBY000
8006-64-2 see III:TOD750
8007-45-2 see I:CMY800
8007-45-2 see III:CMY805

13410-01-0 see III:DXG000	14504-15-5 see III:BED750	16395-80-5 see III:MNA250
13422-55-4 see III:VSZ050	14551-09-8 see III:MKB500	16423-68-0 see III:FAG040
13442-07-4 see III:HIV000	14567-61-4 see III:GKE900	16448-54-7 see III:IHC100
13442-08-5 see III:HIV500	14579-91-0 see III:BIL250	16543-55-8 see I:NLD500
13442-09-6 see III:HIW000	14635-33-7 see III:PCY400	16561-29-8 see III:PGV000
13442-10-9 see III:HIW500	14708-14-6 see II:NDC000	16566-62-4 see III:NAU500
13442-11-0 see III:CHM500	14722-22-6 see III:IE0000	16566-64-6 see III:NAU000
13442-12-1 see III:CHN000	14751-74-7 see III:HIR000	16568-02-8 see III:AAH000
13442-13-2 see III:DFM200	14751-76-9 see III:HIR500	16650-10-5 see III:TBQ275
13442-14-3 see III:CCF750	14751-87-2 see III:FDU875	16675-05-1 see III:PGU250
13442-15-4 see III:HIX500	14751-90-7 see III:HIP500	16690-44-1 see III:MER250
13442-16-5 see III:HIY000	14753-13-0 see III:MMR250	16694-30-7 see III:KGK150
13442-17-6 see III:DVE200	14753-14-1 see III:CJF250	16699-07-3 see III:MMR750
13446-73-6 see II:RPK000	14807-96-6 see I:TAB775	16699-10-8 see III:MMS750
13463-39-3 see I:NCZ000	14807-96-6 see III:TAB750	16731-55-8 see III:PLR250
13463-67-7 see III:TGG760	14808-60-7 see I:SCJ500	16757-80-5 see III:MHH750
13466-27-8 see I:BFQ250	14816-67-2 see III:SKW500	16757-81-6 see III:MHM250
13477-17-3 see I:CAI000	14881-92-6 see III:ZHJ000	16757-82-7 see III:MHG500
13477-21-9 see I:CAJ500	14901-08-7 see I:COU000	16757-83-8 see III:MHG750
13478-00-7 see II:NDG500	14913-33-8 see III:DEX000	16757-84-9 see III:DQ0200
13479-29-3 see III:H0P000	14938-35-3 see III:A0M250	16757-85-0 see III:DQN000
13483-18-6 see III:BIJ250	15086-94-9 see III:BM0250	16757-86-1 see III:DQN200
13510-49-1 see I:BFU250	15104-03-7 see III:MMZ000	16757-87-2 see III:DQN800
13517-17-4 see I:SFW500	15120-17-9 see I:ARD500	16757-88-3 see III:DQN400
13520-61-1 see II:NDJ000	15131-84-7 see III:CML815	16757-89-4 see III:DQ0400
13520-92-8 see III:ZPS000	15191-85-2 see II:SCN500	16757-90-7 see III:DQN600
13520-96-2 see III:P0S500	15216-10-1 see III:NJL000	16757-91-8 see III:DQ0000
13529-51-6 see III:HHH000	15336-81-9 see III:DKM130	16757-92-9 see III:TLM500
13530-65-9 see I:ZFJ100	15442-77-0 see II:BIX500	16808-85-8 see III:FDV000
13552-44-8 see I:MJQ100	15457-87-1 see II:TFT250	16813-36-8 see III:NJY000
13597-95-0 see I:BFU000	15460-48-7 see III:DGB800	16830-14-1 see III:NK0425
13597-99-4 see I:BFT000	15468-32-3 see I:SCK000	16830-15-2 see III:ARN500
13598-15-7 see I:BFS000	15503-86-3 see III:RFU000	16870-90-9 see III:H0P259
13603-07-1 see III:MMY750	15663-27-1 see II:PJD000	16887-79-9 see III:ILF000
13607-48-2 see III:BGL000	15669-07-5 see III:FBG200	16967-79-6 see III:ECT600
13629-82-8 see III:D0V200	15721-02-5 see II:TB0000	16993-94-5 see III:BBX250
13655-95-3 see III:MJW875	15721-33-2 see I:DN0200	17010-21-8 see I:CAG500
13674-87-8 see III:FQU875	15805-73-9 see III:VNK000	17010-59-2 see III:CIL710
13743-07-2 see II:HKW500	15879-93-3 see III:GFA000	17010-61-6 see III:DFD400
13765-19-0 see I:CAP500	15914-23-5 see III:DRE200	17010-62-7 see III:EPU000
13770-89-3 see II:NDK000	15930-94-6 see I:CMK500	17010-63-8 see III:EPT500
13838-16-9 see III:EAT900	15954-91-3 see I:CAF750	17010-64-9 see III:DJB400
13860-69-0 see III:MMV000	15973-99-6 see III:DVF000	17010-65-0 see III:E0I000
13865-57-1 see III:DRQ000	16033-21-9 see III:M0A725	17012-89-4 see III:MIK250
13909-09-6 see II:CHD250	16033-21-9 see III:PFS500	17012-91-8 see III:BBG750
13927-77-0 see III:BIW750	16039-55-7 see I:CAG750	17018-24-5 see III:MPY250
13980-04-6 see III:HDV500	16071-86-6 see II:CM0750	17025-30-8 see III:DTY200
13983-17-0 see III:WCJ000	16110-13-7 see III:BBH250	17026-81-2 see III:AJT750
13988-26-6 see III:DJD700	16120-70-0 see III:BRK100	17057-98-6 see III:DRY100
14024-58-9 see III:MAQ500	16143-89-8 see III:MFF750	17068-78-9 see I:ARM266
14024-64-7 see III:BGQ750	16219-98-0 see III:NKQ000	17088-21-0 see III:EEF000
14026-03-0 see III:NLI500	16230-71-0 see III:DWI400	17095-24-8 see III:RCU000
14060-38-9 see I:ARJ500	16238-56-5 see III:BNR000	17167-73-6 see III:AAH100
14073-00-8 see III:MMQ500	16301-26-1 see III:ASP000	17168-85-3 see II:THP250
14076-05-2 see III:CHM750	16310-68-2 see III:TC0000	17210-48-9 see III:DNY400
14076-19-8 see III:CJE750	16338-97-9 see III:NJV500	17230-88-5 see III:DAB830
14094-43-0 see III:MMQ700	16338-99-1 see III:HBP000	17247-77-7 see III:DLX800
14094-45-2 see III:MMR500	16339-01-8 see III:MMY250	17278-93-2 see III:MJA000
14094-48-5 see III:DFV200	16339-04-1 see III:ELX500	17309-87-4 see III:DSI800
14100-52-8 see III:CJE500	16339-05-2 see III:BRY250	17372-87-1 see III:BNH500
14173-58-1 see III:BNT500	16339-07-4 see III:NKW500	17400-65-6 see III:DPQ400
14207-78-4 see III:DRF000	16339-12-1 see III:DSZ000	17400-68-9 see III:DQE400
14215-29-3 see I:CAD350	16339-14-3 see III:NLY000	17400-69-0 see III:MJF500
14220-17-8 see II:NDI000	16339-16-5 see III:CIQ500	17400-70-3 see III:MJF750
14239-68-0 see I:BJB500	16339-18-7 see III:NKL500	17401-48-8 see III:DQH800
14264-16-5 see II:BLS250	16339-21-2 see III:MMX750	17416-17-0 see III:DPQ800
14301-11-2 see III:DUC200	16354-47-5 see III:MEU500	17416-18-1 see III:DPQ600
14323-41-2 see II:TBW250	16354-48-6 see III:MJX000	17416-20-5 see III:MJG000
14324-55-1 see III:BJC000	16354-50-0 see III:EMM500	17416-21-6 see III:DQE600
14456-34-9 see III:HAD000	16354-52-2 see III:DIT800	17433-31-7 see III:ADA000
14461-87-1 see III:HLE450	16354-53-3 see III:D0A000	17513-40-5 see III:MGY500
14464-46-1 see I:SCJ000	16354-54-4 see III:M0U250	17526-24-8 see III:BBH500
14484-64-1 see III:FAS000	16354-55-5 see III:EMN000	17526-74-8 see III:GGY000
14486-19-2 see I:CAG000	16361-01-6 see III:DKY200	17557-23-2 see III:NCI300

64977-44-2 see III:FJY000	69321-16-0 see III:HLX550	75884-37-6 see III:FQQ100
64977-46-4 see III:FKA000	69853-71-0 see III:HJV500	75965-74-1 see II:MFB400
64977-47-5 see III:FKB000	70384-29-1 see III:PCB000	76050-49-2 see III:FMR700
64977-48-6 see III:FKC000	70443-38-8 see III:DNC800	76180-96-6 see III:AKT600
64977-49-7 see III:FKD000	70501-82-5 see III:NLU480	77094-11-2 see III:AJQ600
65089-17-0 see II:CLW500	70715-92-3 see III:ABR125	77337-54-3 see III:PNM650
65229-18-7 see III:HMQ500	70786-64-0 see III:DSY800	77500-04-0 see II:AJQ675
65272-47-1 see III:MKJ000	71016-15-4 see III:MHW350	77503-17-4 see III:FQQ400
65445-59-2 see III:DTA600	71292-84-7 see III:TCH325	77536-66-4 see I:ARM260
65445-60-5 see III:CJG375	71435-43-3 see III:DKW400	77536-67-5 see I:ARM264
65445-61-6 see III:CJG500	71598-10-2 see III:NLD000	77536-68-6 see I:ARM280
65700-59-6 see III:DAU200	71609-22-8 see III:HKB000	77698-19-2 see III:NKL300
65734-38-5 see III:ACN500	71677-48-0 see III:MMZ800	77698-20-5 see III:NLE400
65763-32-8 see III:DLD800	71752-66-4 see III:NJ0500	78246-54-5 see II:HLX925
65792-56-5 see III:NLN500	71752-67-5 see III:NMA000	78265-95-9 see III:HLR000
65986-80-3 see III:ENR500	71752-68-6 see III:NLX000	78281-06-8 see III:HLE650
65996-93-2 see I:CMZ100	71752-69-7 see II:NK0400	78338-31-5 see III:DTA690
66017-91-2 see III:PNR250	71752-70-0 see III:NKK000	78338-32-6 see III:DTA700
66104-24-3 see I:BFP500	71785-87-0 see III:NKC300	78776-28-0 see III:DEC775
66267-18-3 see III:DMK200	71856-48-9 see III:MGS700	79127-47-2 see III:MSB100
66267-19-4 see III:DLD400	71964-72-2 see III:DQK900	79543-29-6 see III:MIY200
66289-74-5 see III:DLJ500	72074-66-9 see III:DMS400	79867-78-0 see III:MRR850
66552-77-0 see III:TDK885	72074-67-0 see III:DMS200	80790-68-7 see III:MRT100
66731-42-8 see III:DMB200	72074-69-2 see III:ECS000	81295-38-7 see III:SAF500
66733-21-9 see I:EDC650	72122-60-2 see III:MRR775	82018-90-4 see III:NLX700
66788-01-0 see III:DKU400	72214-01-8 see III:ELB400	83053-57-0 see III:EER400
66788-03-2 see III:DNC400	72254-58-1 see III:ALE750	83053-59-2 see III:INA400
66788-06-5 see III:DMK600	72586-67-5 see III:MFX725	83053-62-7 see III:DLU700
66788-11-2 see III:ECQ150	72586-68-6 see III:DTN875	83053-63-8 see III:DL0950
66826-72-0 see III:DAC975	72589-96-9 see I:CAE375	83335-32-4 see III:NJN300
66826-73-1 see III:DGH500	73239-98-2 see III:NK0600	83463-62-1 see III:BMY800
66964-37-2 see III:MHA000	73419-42-8 see I:CAK250	83768-87-0 see II:VLU200
66997-69-1 see III:ECR500	73454-79-2 see III:MHW250	83876-50-0 see III:DLE500
67176-33-4 see III:FEG000	73487-24-8 see III:NJ0200	83876-56-6 see III:MET875
67195-50-0 see III:BQU750	73529-25-6 see III:EEF500	83876-62-4 see III:ABQ600
67195-51-1 see III:ECA500	73637-16-8 see III:ACA750	84775-95-1 see III:RGA000
67242-54-0 see III:TCP600	73728-78-6 see III:TDJ250	84929-34-0 see III:WBA000
67293-86-1 see III:MEA750	73728-79-7 see III:TLF000	85616-56-4 see III:DLI300
67335-42-6 see III:BBG000	73728-82-2 see III:AKF250	85723-21-3 see III:AAI125
67335-43-7 see III:BBD750	73758-56-2 see III:DEK400	85923-37-1 see III:DRD850
67411-81-8 see III:DLF400	73771-72-9 see III:FJU000	86166-58-7 see III:BQF750
67466-28-8 see III:EJT000	73771-73-0 see III:FJV000	86451-37-8 see III:NMV450
67523-22-2 see III:DLF600	73771-74-1 see III:FJW000	86539-71-1 see III:MEW975
67557-56-6 see III:BSX500	73771-79-6 see III:DNC600	86674-51-3 see III:NLP375
67557-57-7 see III:MMS000	73785-34-9 see III:DBG200	87625-62-5 see III:POI100
67639-45-6 see III:FHH025	73785-40-7 see III:NJS300	88208-15-5 see II:NLY750
67694-88-6 see III:ECQ200	73926-91-7 see III:DGK400	88208-16-6 see III:NJY500
67730-10-3 see II:DWW700	73926-92-8 see III:DGK600	88254-07-3 see III:COP765
67730-11-4 see II:AKS250	73927-60-3 see III:EHX000	89911-79-5 see III:NOC400
67774-31-6 see III:NKA850	73928-01-5 see III:CLE500	89947-76-2 see III:HLE750
67774-32-7 see II:FBU509	73928-02-6 see III:MFP500	89957-52-8 see III:PKH500
67856-65-9 see III:BK0000	73928-03-7 see III:MPJ250	89997-47-7 see III:SAF000
67856-66-0 see III:BJ0250	73928-04-8 see III:MPJ500	91724-16-2 see I:SME500
67856-68-2 see III:BIF500	73941-35-2 see I:THV500	91845-41-9 see III:PCR000
68006-83-7 see II:ALD750	74203-45-5 see III:NDF000	92145-26-1 see III:MGU550
68041-18-9 see III:HLY000	74278-22-1 see I:KHU000	93023-34-8 see III:EIF450
68107-26-6 see III:NKX500	74339-98-3 see III:DKX875	94362-44-4 see III:DCQ650
68141-57-1 see III:FHS000	74340-04-8 see III:DKX900	96806-34-7 see III:NKJ050
68162-13-0 see III:DLD600	74920-78-8 see III:EKL250	96806-35-8 see III:NKJ100
68308-34-9 see I:COD750	74940-23-1 see III:HIE600	99520-58-8 see III:IBZ100
68426-46-0 see III:NKV500	74940-26-4 see III:HIE700	100466-04-4 see III:DKT400
68688-87-9 see III:MJD610	74955-23-0 see III:HIE570	100700-29-6 see III:MEI000
68690-89-1 see III:NKW000	75016-34-1 see III:NKT100	101607-48-1 see III:MP0400
68808-54-8 see II:AJR500	75016-36-3 see III:NKT105	101607-49-2 see III:MP0390
68916-39-2 see III:WCB000	75198-31-1 see II:NGI800	102420-56-4 see III:DLE400
69091-15-2 see III:NKA700	75236-19-0 see III:EPC950	102488-99-3 see I:AEB750
69091-16-3 see III:NKA695	75321-20-9 see II:DVD400	103416-59-7 see III:AAI100
69112-96-5 see III:DFW000	75410-89-8 see III:BMK634	104639-49-8 see III:SIS000
69112-98-7 see III:NKG000	75411-83-5 see III:NKU500	105735-71-5 see III:DUW100
69112-99-8 see III:NKT000	75464-10-7 see III:PMW760	108278-70-2 see III:NK0900
69113-00-4 see III:NJR000	75881-16-2 see III:NKU550	730771-71-0 see III:HKI075
69113-01-5 see III:NLZ000	75881-17-3 see III:NJI850	
69260-83-9 see III:DMX000	75881-19-5 see III:NKU580	
69260-85-1 see III:DML775	75881-20-8 see III:NKW800	
69267-51-2 see III:NHQ950	75881-22-0 see III:MMX200	

III. Synonym Cross-Index

A 100 (pharmaceutical) see I:IGS000
A-139 see III:BDC750
A 361 see III:ARQ725
A 3-80 see III:SMQ500
A-502 see III:SNJ000
688A see II:DDG800
A 688 see I:PDT250
A 2079 see III:BJP000
A 4942 see II:IMH000
A 10846 see III:DUD800
A-11025 see III:RDF000
A 11032 see I:UVA000
A 3733A see III:HAL000
AAB see II:PEI000
AACAPTAN see III:CBG000
AACIFEMINE see II:EDU500
AAF see I:FDR000
2-AAF see I:FDR000
AAFERTIS see III:FAS000
AALINDAN see I:BBQ500
AAMANGAN see III:MAS500
AAPROTECT see III:BJK500
AAT see I:AIC250, III:PAK000
o-AAT see I:AIC250
AATACK see III:TFS350
AATP see III:PAK000
AATREX see III:ARQ725
AATREX 4L see III:ARQ725
AATREX 80W see III:ARQ725
AATREX NINE-O see III:ARQ725
AAVOLEX see III:BJK500
AAZIRA see III:BJK500
ABBOCILLIN see III:BDY669
ABBOTT 40566 see III:TCM250
ABENSANIL see II:HIM000
ABEREL see III:VSK950
ABIROL see III:DAL300
ABRAREX see III:AHE250
ABSOLUTE ETHANOL see I:EFU000
ABSTENSIL see III:DXH250
ABSTINYL see III:DXH250
5-AC see III:ARY000
AC 3422 see III:PAK000
AC 5223 see III:DXX400
AC-12682 see III:DSP400
ACACIA MOLLISSIMA TANNIN see III:MQV250
ACACIA VILLOSA see III:AAD750
ACAMOL see II:HIM000
ACAR see II:DER000
ACARABEN 4E see II:DER000
ACARACIDE see I:SOP500
ACARICYDOL E 20 see III:CJT750
ACARIN see III:BIO750
ACARON see III:CJJ250
ACC 3422 see III:PAK000
ACCELERATOR L see III:BJK500
ACCELERATOR THIURAM see III:TFS350
ACCELERINE see III:DSY600
ACCO FAST RED KB BASE see II:CLK225
ACCUZOLE see III:SNN500
AC-DI-SOL NF see III:SFO500
8:9-ACE-1:2-BENZANTHRACENE see III:BAW000
4,10-ACE-1,2-BENZANTHRACENE see III:AAE000

ACEDAPSONE see III:SNY500
ACENAPHTHANTHRACENE see III:AAF000
5-ACENAPHTHENAMINE see III:AAF250
13H-ACENAPHTHO(1,8-ab)PHENANTHRENE see III:DCR600
ACEPYRENE see III:CPX500
ACEPYRYLENE see III:CPX500
ACETACID RED B see III:HJF500
ACETACID RED J see III:FMU070
ACETACID RED 2BR see III:FAG020
ACETAGESIC see II:HIM000
ACETALDEHYD (GERMAN) see II:AAG250
ACETALDEHYDE see II:AAG250
ACETALDEHYDE-N-FORMYL-N-METHYLHYDRAZONE see III:AAH000
ACETALDEHYDE-N-METHYL-N-FORMYLHYDRAZONE see III:AAH000
ACETALDEHYDE METHYLHYDRAZONE see III:AAH100
ACETALDEHYDE, N-METHYLHYDRAZONE see III:AAH100
ACETALGIN see II:HIM000
ACETAMIDE see II:AAI000
ACETAMIDE, 2-(DIETHYLAMINO)-N-(1,3-DIMETHYL-4-(o-FLUOROBENZOYL)-5-PYRAZOLYL)-, MONOHYDRO-CHLORIDE see III:AAI100
ACETAMIDE, N-(4-(2-FLUOROBENZOYL)-1,3-DIMETHYL-1H-PYRAZOL-5-YL)-2-((3-(2-METHYL-1-PIPERIDI-NYL)PROPYL)AMINO)-, (Z)-2-BUTENEDIOATE (1:2) see III:AAI125
p-ACETAMIDOAZOBENZENE see III:PEH750
ACETAMIDOBIPHENYL see III:PDY000
4-ACETAMIDOBIPHENYL see III:PDY500
N-(4'-ACETAMIDOBIPHENYLYL)ACETOHYDROXAMIC ACID see III:HKB000
3-ACETAMIDODIBENZFURANE see III:DDC000
3-ACETAMIDODIBENZOFURAN see III:DDC000
3-ACETAMIDODIBENZTHIOPHENE see III:DDD600
3-ACETAMIDODIBENZTHIOPHENE OXIDE see III:DDD800
1-ACETAMIDO-4-ETHOXYBENZENE see I:ABG750
3-ACETAMIDOFLUORANTHENE see III:AAK400
2-ACETAMIDOFLUORENE see I:FDR000
(S)-2-(2-ACETAMIDO-4-METHYLVALERAMIDO)-N-(1-FORMYL-4-GUANIDINOBUTYL)-4-M ETHYL-VALER-AMIDE see III:AAL300
5-ACETAMIDO-3-(5-NITRO-2-FURYL)-6H-1,2,4-OXADIA-ZINE see III:AAL500
2-ACETAMIDO-4-(5-NITRO-2-FURYL)THIAZOLE see II:AAL750
3-ACETAMIDOPHENANTHRENE see III:PCY500
9-ACETAMIDOPHENANTHRENE see III:PCY750
2-ACETAMIDOPHENATHRENE see III:AAM250
4-ACETAMIDOPHENOL see II:HIM000
p-ACETAMIDOPHENOL see II:HIM000
4-ACETAMIDOSTILBENE see III:SMR500
trans-4-ACETAMIDOSTILBENE see III:SMR500
ACETAMIN see III:SNY500
ACETAMINE DIAZO BLACK RD see I:DCJ200
ACETAMINE YELLOW CG see II:AAQ250
3-ACETAMINODIBENZOTHIOPHENE see III:DDD600
2-ACETAMINOFLUORENE see I:FDR000
2-ACETAMINO-4-(5-NITRO-2-FURYL)THIAZOLE see II:AAL750
4-ACETAMINO-2-NITROPHENETOLE see III:NEL000

ACETAMINOPHEN see II:HIM000
2-ACETAMINOPHENANTHRENE see III:AAM250
3-ACETAMINOPHENANTHRENE see III:PCY500
9-ACETAMINOPHENANTHRENE see III:PCY750
p-ACETAMINOPHENOL see II:HIM000
trans-4-ACETAMINOSTILBENE see III:SMR500
ACETATE BLUE G see III:TBG700
ACETATE CORTISONE see III:CNS825
ACETATE FAST ORANGE R see I:AKP750
ACETATE de PLOMB (FRENCH) see I:LCG000
ACETATE de TRIPHENYL-ETAIN (FRENCH) see III:ABX250
ACETATO di STAGNO TRIFENILE (ITALIAN) see III:ABX250
ACETATOTRIPHENYLSTANNANE see III:ABX250
ACETIC ACID (N-ACETYL-N-(4-BIPHENYL)AMINO) ESTER
    see III:ABJ750
ACETIC ACID (N-ACETYL-N-(2-FLUORENYL)AMINO) ES-
    TER see III:ABL000
ACETIC ACID(N-ACETYL-N-(4-FLUORENYL)AMINO)ESTER
    see III:ABO500
ACETIC ACID (N-ACETYL-N-(2-PHENANTHRYL)AMINO)ES-
    TER see III:ABK250
ACETIC ACID-(N-ACETYL-N-(p-STYRYLPHENYL)AMINO)
    ESTER see III:ABW500
ACETIC ACID AMIDE see II:AAI000
ACETIC ACID, BENZ(a)ANTHRACENE-7,12-DIMETHANOL
    DIESTER see III:BBF750
ACETIC ACID, BENZ(a)ANTHRACENE-7-METHANOL ESTER
    see III:BBH500
ACETIC ACID BENZYL ESTER see III:BDX000
ACETIC ACID-1-(BUTYLNITROSOAMINO)BUTYL ESTER see
    III:BPV325
ACETIC ACID, CADMIUM SALT see I:CAD250
ACETIC ACID-2,6-DIMETHYL-m-DIOXAN-4-YL ESTER see
    I:ABC250
ACETIC ACID ESTER with N-4-BIPHENYLYLACETOHY-
    DROXAMIC ACID see III:ABJ750
ACETIC ACID ESTER with N-(FLUOREN-3-YL)ACETOHY-
    DROXAMIC ACID see III:ABO250
ACETIC ACID, ESTER with N-(FLUOREN-4-YL)ACETOXYHY-
    DROXAMIC ACID see III:ABO500
ACETIC ACID, ESTER with N-NITROSO-2,2'-IMINODIETHA-
    NOL see III:NKM500
ACETIC ACID ESTER with N-(2-PHENANTHRYL)ACETOHY-
    DROXAMIC ACID see III:ABK250
ACETIC ACID-ESTER with N-(p-STYRYLPHENYL)ACETOHY-
    DROXAMIC ACID see III:ABW500
ACETIC ACID ETHENYL ESTER see III:VLU250
ACETIC ACID ETHENYL ESTER POLYMER with CHLORETH-
    ENE (9CI) see II:AAX175
ACETIC ACID LEAD (2+) SALT see I:LCG000
ACETIC ACID, LEAD(+2) SALT TRIHYDRATE see I:LCJ000
ACETIC ACID METHYLNITROSAMINOMETHYL ESTER see
    II:AAW000
ACETIC ACID, NICKEL(2+) SALT see I:NCX000
ACETIC ACID, NITRILOTRI-, IRON(III) chelate see III:IHC100
ACETIC ACID, (4-OXO-2-THIAZOLIDINYLIDENE)-, BUTYL
    ESTER (9CI) see III:BPI300
ACETIC ACID PHENYLHYDRAZONE see III:ACX750
ACETIC ACID PHENYLMETHYL ESTER see III:BDX000
ACETIC ACID-1-(PROPYLNITROSAMINO)PROPYL ESTER
    see III:ABT750
ACETIC ACID VINYL ESTER see III:VLU250
ACETIC ACID, VINYL ESTER, CHLOROETHYLENE CO-
    POLYMER see III:PKP500
ACETIC ACID, VINYL ESTER, POLYMER with CHLORO-
    ETHYLENE see II:AAX175
ACETIC ALDEHYDE see II:AAG250
ACETIMIDIC ACID see II:AAI000
ACETOAMINOFLUORENE see I:FDR000
ACETO-CAUSTIN see III:TII250
ACETO DIPP see III:NBL000
ACETO DNPT 40 see III:DVF400
ACETO DNPT 80 see III:DVF400
ACETO DNPT 100 see III:DVF400

ACETO HMT see III:HEI500
ACETOHYDROXAMIC ACID, FLUOREN-2-YL-o-GLUCURO-
    NIDE see III:HIQ500
ACETOHYDROXAMIC ACID, N-(7-IODOFLUOREN-2-YL)-O-
    MYRISTOYL- see III:MSB100
ACETOMESIDIDE see III:TLD250
ACETOMETHOXAN see I:ABC250
ACETOMETHOXANE see ABC250
ACETO PAN see III:PFT250
ACETO PBN see II:PFT500
ACETO-p-PHENALIDE see I:ABG750
p-ACETOPHENETIDE see I:ABG750
p-ACETOPHENETIDIDE see I:ABG750
ACETO-p-PHENETIDIDE see I:ABG750
ACETOPHENETIDIN see I:ABG750
ACETOPHENETIDINE see I:ABG750
ACETO-4-PHENETIDINE see I:ABG750
ACETOPHENETIN see I:ABG750
ACETOQUINONE BLUE L see III:TBG700
ACETOQUINONE BLUE R see III:TBG700
ACETOQUINONE LIGHT ORANGE JL see I:AKP750
ACETO TETD see III:TFS350
ACETOTHIOAMIDE see I:TFA000
ACETO TMTM see III:BJL600
N-ACETOXY-4-ACETAMIDOBIPHENYL see III:ABJ750
N-ACETOXY-2-ACETAMIDOFLUORENE see III:ABL000
N-ACETOXY-2-ACETAMIDOPHENANTHRENE see
    III:ABK250
N-ACETOXY-4-ACETAMIDOSTILBENE see III:ABW500
N-ACETOXY-2-ACETYLAMINOFLUORENE see III:ABL000
N-ACETOXY-N-ACETYL-2-AMINOFLUORENE see
    III:ABL000
N-ACETOXY-2-ACETYLAMINOPHENANTHRENE see
    III:ABK250
trans-N-ACETOXY-4-ACETYL-AMINOSTILBENE see
    III:ABL250
N-ACETOXY-4-BIPHENYLACETAMIDE see III:ABJ750
3-β-ACETOXY-BIS NOR-Δ⁵-CHOLENIC ACID see
    III:ABM000
N-(α-ACETOXY)BUTYL-N-BUTYLNITROSAMINE see
    III:BPV325
17-ACETOXY-6-CHLORO-6-DEHYDROPROGESTERONE see
    II:CBF250
17-α-ACETOXY-6-CHLORO-6-DEHYDROPROGESTERONE
    see II:CBF250
17-α-ACETOXY-6-CHLORO-6,7-DEHYDROPROGESTERONE
    see II:CBF250
17-α-ACETOXY-6-CHLORO-1-α,2-α-METHYLENEPREGNA-
    4,6-DIENE-3,20-DIONE see III:CQJ500
17-α-ACETOXY-6-CHLORO-4,6-PREGNADIENE-3,20-DIONE
    see II:CBF250
17-α-ACETOXY-6-CHLOROPREGNA-4,6-DIENE-3,20-DIONE
    see II:CBF250
1'-ACETOXY-2',3'-DEHYDROESTRAGOLE see III:EQN225
17-α-ACETOXY-6-DEHYDRO-6-METHYLPROGESTERONE
    see II:VTF000
11-ACETOXY-15-
    DIHYDROCYCLOPENTA(a)PHENANTHRACEN-17-ONE
    see III:ABN250
1-ACETOXY-1,4-DIHYDRO-4-(HYDROXYAMINO)QUINO-
    LINE ACETATE (ESTER) see III:ABN500
21-ACETOXY-3,20-DIKETOPREGN-4-ENE see III:DAQ800
6-ACETOXY-2,4-DIMETHYL-m-DIOXANE see I:ABC250
α-ACETOXY DIMETHYLNITROSAMINE see II:AAW000
1'-ACETOXYELEMICIN see III:TLC850
1'-ACETOXYESTRAGOLE see III:ABN725
1-ACETOXYETHYLENE see III:VLU250
N-ACETOXYFLUORENYLACETAMIDE see III:ABO250
N-ACETOXY-2-FLUORENYLACETAMIDE see III:ABL000
N-ACETOXY-3-FLUORENYLACETAMIDE see III:ABO250
N-ACETOXY-4-FLUORENYLACETAMIDE see III:ABO500
N-ACETOXY-2-FLUORENYLBENZAMIDE see III:ABO750
21-ACETOXY-17,α-HYDROXYPREGN-4-ENE-3,11,20-
    TRIONE see III:CNS825

21-ACETOXY-17,α-HYDROXY-3,11,20-TRIKETOPREGNENE-4 see III:CNS825
ACETOXYL see III:BDS000
3′,4′-ACETOXYLIDIDE see III:ABP500
4-ACETOXY-7-METHYLBENZ(c)ACRIDINE see III:ABQ600
10-ACETOXYMETHYL-1,2-BENZANTHRACENE see III:BBH500
6-ACETOXY METHYL BENZO(a)PYRENE see III:ACU500
ACETOXYMETHYLBUTYLNITROSAMINE see III:BRX500
N-(ACETOXY)METHYL-N,N-BUTYLNITROSAMINE see III:BRX500
ACETOXYMETHYLETHYLNITROSAMINE see III:ENR500
N-(ACETOXY)METHYL-N-ETHYLNITROSAMINE see III:ENR500
N-(ACETOXYMETHYL)-N-ISOBUTYLNITROSAMINE see III:ABR125
7-ACETOXYMETHYL-12-METHYLBENZ(a)ANTHRACENE see III:ABR250
ACETOXYMETHYL-METHYL-NITROSAMIN (GERMAN) see II:AAW000
ACETOXYMETHYL METHYLNITROSAMINE see II:AAW000
N-α-ACETOXYMETHYL-N-METHYLNITROSAMINE see II:AAW000
N-ACETOXYMETHYL-N-NITROSOETHYLAMINE see III:ENR500
N-(1-ACETOXYMETHYL)-N-NITROSOETHYL AMINE see III:ENR500
ACETOXYMETHYLPHENYLNITROSAMINE see III:ABR625
17-ACETOXY-6-METHYLPREGNA-4,6-DIENE-3,20-DIONE see II:VTF000
17-α-ACETOXY-6-METHYLPREGNA-4,6-DIENE-3,20-DIONE see II:VTF000
17-α-ACETOXY-6-METHYL-4,6-PREGNADIENE-3,20-DIONE see II:VTF000
17-α-ACETOXY-6-α-METHYLPREGN-4-ENE-3,20-DIONE see II:MCA000
17-ACETOXY-6-α-METHYLPROGESTERONE see II:MCA000
ACETOXYMETHYLPROPYLNITROSAMINE see III:PNR250
N-(ACETOXY)METHYL-N-n-PROPYLNITROSAMINE see III:PNR250
ACETOXYMETHYLTRIDEUTEROMETHYLNITROSAMINE see III:MMS000
N-ACETOXY-2-MYRISTOYL-AMINOFLUORENE see III:FEM000
1-ACETOXY-N-NITROSODIBUTYLAMINE see III:BPV325
1-ACETOXY-N-NITROSODIMETHYLAMINE see II:AAW000
1-ACETOXY-N-NITROSODIPROPYLAMINE see III:ABT750
1-ACETOXY-N-NITROSO-N-TRIDEUTEROMETHYLMETH-YLAMINE see III:MMS000
17-ACETOXY-19-NOR-17-α-PREGN-4-EN-20-YN-3-ONE see II:ABU000
17-β-ACETOXY-19-NOR-17-α-PREGN-4-EN-20-YN-3-ONE see II:ABU000
N-ACETOXY-4-PHENANTHRYLACETAMIDE see III:ABK250
3-β-ACETOXYPREGN-6-ENE-20-CARBOXYLIC ACID see III:ABM000
N-(α-ACETOXY)PROPYL-N-N-PROPYLNITROSAMINE see III:ABT750
1′-ACETOXYSAFROLE see III:ACV000
N-ACETOXY-N-(4-STILBENYL) ACETAMIDE see III:ABW500
α-ACETOXYTOLUENE see III:BDX000
ACETOXY-TRIPHENYL-STANNAN (GERMAN) see III:ABX250
ACETOXYTRIPHENYLSTANNANE see III:ABX250
ACETOXY-TRIPHENYLSTANNANE see III:ABX250
ACETOXYTRIPHENYLTIN see III:ABX250
ACETO ZDBD see III:BIX000
ACETO ZDED see III:BJK500
ACETO ZDMD see III:BJK500
ACET-p-PHENALIDE see I:ABG750
ACETPHENETIDIN see I:ABG750

ACET-p-PHENETIDIN see I:ABG750
p-ACETPHENETIDIN see I:ABG750
ACETYLADRIAMYCIN see II:DAC000
4-ACETYLAMINOAZOBENZENE see III:PEH750
2-ACETYLAMINOBIPHENYL see III:PDY000
3-ACETYLAMINOBIPHENYL see III:PDY250
4-ACETYLAMINOBIPHENYL see III:PDY500
3-ACETYLAMINODIBENZOFURAN see III:DDC000
2-ACETYLAMINODIBENZOTHIOPHENE see III:DDD400
3-ACETYLAMINODIBENZOTHIOPHENE see III:DDD600
3-ACETYLAMINODIBENZOTHIOPHENE-5-OXIDE see III:DDD800
2-ACETYLAMINO-9,10-DIHYDROPHENANTHRENE see III:DMA400
4-ACETYLAMINO-p-DIPHENYLBENZENE see III:TBD250
3-ACETYLAMINO-FLUORANTHEN see III:AAK400
3-ACETYLAMINOFLUORANTHENE see III:AAK400
2-ACETYLAMINO-FLUOREN (GERMAN) see I:FDR000
4-ACETYLAMINOFLUOREN (GERMAN) see III:ABY000
4-ACETYLAMINOFLUORENE see III:ABY000
N-ACETYL-2-AMINOFLUORENE see I:FDR000
2-ACETYLAMINOFLUORENE (OSHA) see I:FDR000
2-ACETYLAMINO-9-FLUORENOL see III:ABY150
2-ACETYLAMINOFLUORENONE see III:ABY250
2-ACETYLAMINO-9-FLUORENONE see III:ABY250
2-ACETYLAMINO-4-(5-NITRO-2- FURYL)THIAZOLE see II:AAL750
2-ACETYLAMINOPHENANTHRENE see III:AAM250
3-ACETYLAMINOPHENANTHRENE see III:PCY500
9-ACETYLAMINOPHENANTHRENE see III:PCY750
p-ACETYLAMINOPHENOL see II:HIM000
N-ACETYL-p-AMINOPHENOL see II:HIM000
2-ACETYLAMINOPYRENE see III:PON500
4-ACETYLAMINOSTILBENE see III:SMR500
trans-4-ACETYLAMINOSTILBENE see III:SMR500
4-ACETYLAMINO-p-TERPHENYL see III:TBD250
9-ACETYL-1,7,8-ANTHRACENETRIOL see III:ACA750
10-ACETYL-1,8,9- ANTHRACENETRIOL see III:ACA750
10-ACETYLANTHRALIN see III:ACA750
1-ACETYLAZIRIDINE see III:ACB250
5-ACETYL BENZO(C)PHENANTHRENE see III:ACC750
2-ACETYL-3:4-BENZPHENANTHRENE see III:ACC750
N-ACETYL-4-BIPHENYLHYDROXYLAMINE see III:ACD000
ACETYLENE BLACK see III:CBT750
ACETYLENE TETRABROMIDE see III:ACK250
ACETYLENE TETRACHLORIDE see III:TBQ100
ACETYLENE TRICHLORIDE see II:TIO750
N-ACETYL ETHYL CARBAMATE see III:ACL000
ACETYLETHYLENEIMINE see III:ACB250
N′-ACETYL ETHYLNITROSOUREA see III:ACL500
N-ACETYL-N-9H-FLUOREN-2-YL-ACETAMIDE see II:DBF200
ACETYL HYDROPEROXIDE see III:PCL500
N-ACETYL-N′-(p-HYDROXYMETHYL)PHENYLHYDRAZINE see III:ACN500
2-ACETYL-5-HYDROXY-3-OXO-4-HEXENOIC ACID Δ-LAC-TONE see III:MFW500
1-ACETYLIMIDAZOLE see III:ACO250
N-ACETYLIMIDAZOLE see III:ACO250
ACETYL ISONIAZID see III:ACO750
N-ACETYLISONIAZID see III:ACO750
1-ACETYL-2-ISONICOTINOYLHYDRAZINE see III:ACO750
N-ACETYLISONICOTINYLHYDRAZIDE see III:ACO750
N-ACETYL-N′-ISONICOTINYL HYDRAZIDE see III:ADA000
N-ACETYL-5-METHOXYTRYPTAMINE see III:MCB350
4-(N-ACETYL-N-METHYL)AMINO-4′-(N′,N′-DIMETHYL-AMINO)AZOBENZENE see III:DPQ200
N′-ACETYL-N′-METHYL-4′-AMINO-N,N-DIMETHYL-4-AMINOAZOBENZENE see III:DPQ200
4-(N-ACETYL-N-METHYL)AMINO-4′-N-METHYLAMINO-AZOBENZENE see III:MLK750
ACETYL-METHYL-NITROSO-HARNSTOFF (GERMAN) see III:ACR250

ACETYLMETHYLNITROSOUREA see III:ACR250
N'-ACETYL-METHYLNITROSOUREA see III:ACR250
3-ACETYL-6-METHYL-2,4-PYRANDIONE see III:MFW500
3-ACETYL-6-METHYLPYRANDIONE-2,4 see III:MFW500
3-ACETYL-6-METHYL-2H-PYRAN-2,4(3H)-DIONE see
  III:MFW500
N'-ACETYL-N'-MONOMETHYL-4'-AMINO-N-ACETYL-N-
  MONOMETHYL-4-AMINOAZOBENZENE see III:DQH200
N'-ACETYL-N'-MONOMETHYL-4'-AMINO-N-MONOME-
  THYL-4-AMINOAZOBENZENE see III:MLK750
N-ACETYL-N-MYRISTOYLOXY-2-AMINOFLUORENE see
  III:ACS000
N-ACETYL-2-NAPHTHYLHYDROXYLAMINE see
  III:NBD000
1-ACETYL-4-NITROSO-2,6-DIMETHYLPIPERAZINE see
  III:NJI850
ACETYLON FAST BLUE G see III:TBG700
2-(ACETYLOXY)BENZOIC ACID, mixed with 3,7-DIHYDRO-
  1,3,7-TRIMETHYL-1H-PURINE-2,6-DIONE and N-(4-
  ETHOXYPHENYL)ACETAMIDE see III:ARP250
17-(ACETYLOXY)-6-CHLOROPREGNA-4,6-DIENE-3,20-
  DIONE see II:CBF250
4-ACETYLOXY-12,13-EPOXY-3,7,15-TRIHYDROXY-(3-α,4-
  β,7-β)-TRICHOTHEC-9-EN-8-ONE see III:FQR000
N-(ACETYLOXY)-N-9H-FLUOREN-2-YL-TETRADECANA-
  MIDE see III:FEM000
21-(ACETYLOXY)-17-HYDROXY-PREGN-4-ENE-3,11,20-
  TRIONE (9CI) see III:CNS825
6-ACETYLOXYMETHYLBENZO(a)PYRENE see III:ACU500
(6-α)-17-(ACETYLOXY)-6-METHYLPREG-4-ENE-3,20-DIONE
  see II:MCA000
(17-α)-17-(ACETYLOXY)-19-NORPREGN-4-EN-20-YN-3-ONE
  see II:ABU000
17-ACETYLOXY(17-α)-19-NORPREGN-4-ESTREN-17-β-OL-
  ACETATE-3-ONE see II:ABU000
5-(1-ACETYLOXY-2-PROPENYL)-1,3-BENZODIOXOLE see
  III:ACV000
(ACETYLOXY)TRIPHENYL-STANNANE (9CI) see
  III:ABX250
ACETYL PEROXIDE see III:ACV500
ACETYLPHENETIDIN see I:ABG750
N-ACETYL-p-PHENETIDINE see I:ABG750
ACETYLPHENYLHYDRAZINE see III:ACX750
β-ACETYLPHENYLHYDRAZINE see III:ACX750
1-ACETYL-2-PHENYLHYDRAZINE see III:ACX750
1-(p-ACETYLPHENYL)-3-METHYL-3-NITROSOUREA see
  III:MFX725
12-O-ACETYL-PHORBOL-13-DECA-(Δ-2)-ENOATE see
  III:ACY750
12-O-ACETYL-PHORBOL-13-DECANOATE see III:ACZ000
1-ACETYL-2-PICOLINOLHYDRAZINE see III:ADA000
1-ACETYL-2-PICOLINOYLHYDRAZINE see III:ADA000
o-ACETYLSTERIGMATOCYSTIN see III:ADB250
N-ACETYL-N-TETRADECANOYLOXY-2-AMINOFLUORENE
  see III:ACS000
7-α-ACETYLTHIO-3-OXO-17-α-PREGN-4-ENE-21,17-β-CAR-
  BOLACTONE see III:AFJ500
ACETYLURETHANE see III:ACL000
ACHROCIDIN see I:BG750
ACIDAL BRIGHT PONCEAU 3R see III:FMU080
ACIDAL FAST ORANGE see III:HGC000
ACIDAL GREEN G see III:FAE950
ACIDAL LIGHT GREEN SF see III:FAF000
ACIDAL PONCEAU G see III:FMU070
ACIDAL WOOL GREEN BS see III:ADF000
ACID AMARANTH see III:FAG020
ACID BLUE 1 see III:ADE500
ACID BLUE 9 see III:FMU059
ACID BLUE W see III:FAE100
ACID BRILLIANT GREEN BS see III:ADF000
ACID BRILLIANT GREEN SF see III:FAF000
ACID BRILLIANT PINK B see III:FAG070
ACID BRILLIANT RUBINE 2G see III:HJF500
ACID BRILLIANT SCARLET 3R see III:FMU080

ÁCID CHROME BLUE BA see III:HJF500
ACIDE ARSENIEUX (FRENCH) see I:ARI750
ACIDE ARSENIQUE LIQUIDE (FRENCH) see ARB250
ACIDE CACODYLIQUE (FRENCH) see III:HKC000
ACIDE CARBOLIQUE (FRENCH) see III:PDN750
ACIDE CHLORACETIQUE (FRENCH) see III:CEA000
ACIDE 2-(4-CHLORO-2-METHYL-PHENOXY)PROPIONIQUE
  (FRENCH) see II:CIR500
ACIDE-2,4-DICHLORO PHENOXYACETIQUE (FRENCH) see
  II:DAA800
ACIDE-2-(2,4-DICHLORO-PHENOXY) PROPIONIQUE
  (FRENCH) see II:DGB000
ACIDE DIMETHYLARSINIQUE (FRENCH) see III:HKC000
ACIDE DIMETHYL-ETHYL-ALLENOLIQUE ETHER METH-
  YLIQUE (FRENCH) see III:DRU600
ACIDE MONOCHLORACETIQUE (FRENCH) see III:CEA000
ACIDE NICOTINIQUE (FRENCH) see III:NCQ900
l'ACIDE OLEIQUE (FRENCH) see III:OHU000
ACIDE PERACETIQUE (FRENCH) see III:PCL500
l'ACIDE RICINOLEIQUE (FRENCH) see III:RJP000
d'ACIDE TANNIQUE (FRENCH) see III:TAD750
ACIDE TRICHLORACETIQUE (FRENCH) see III:TII250
ACIDE 2,4,5-TRICHLORO PHENOXYACETIQUE (FRENCH)
  see II:TAA100
ACIDE 2-(2,4,5-TRICHLORO-PHENOXY) PROPIONIQUE
  (FRENCH) see II:TIX500
ACID FAST ORANGE EGG see III:HGC000
ACID FAST RED FB see III:HJF500
ACID FAST YELLOW AG see III:SGP500
ACID GREEN see III:FAE950
ACID GREEN 3 see III:FAE950
ACID GREEN A see III:FAF000
ACID LEAD ARSENATE see I:LCK000
ACID LEAD ORTHOARSENATE see I:LCK000
ACID LEATHER BLUE IC see III:FAE100
ACID LEATHER GREEN S see III:ADF000
ACID LEATHER LIGHT BROWN G see III:SGP500
ACID LEATHER ORANGE I see III:FAG010
ACID LEATHER ORANGE PGW see III:HGC000
ACID LEATHER RED KPR see III:FMU070
ACID LIGHT ORANGE G see III:HGC000
ACIDO 2-(4-CLORO-2-METIL-FENOSSI)-PROPIONICO (ITAL-
  IAN) see II:CIR500
ACIDO (2,4-DICLORO-FENOSSI)-ACETICO (ITALIAN) see
  II:DAA800
ACIDO-2-(2,4-DICLORO-FENOSSI)-PROPIONICO (ITALIAN)
  see II:DGB000
ACIDO DOISYNOLICO (SPANISH) see III:DYB000
ACIDO-5-FENIL-5-ETILBARBITURICO (ITALIAN) see
  II:EOK000
ACIDO-4-(ISONICOTINIL-IDRAZONE)PIMELICO (ITALIAN)
  see III:ILG000
ACIDOMONOCLOROACETICO (ITALIAN) see III:CEA000
ACID ORANGE 10 see III:HGC000
ACID ORANGE No. 3 see III:SGP500
ACIDO TRICLOROACETICO (ITALIAN) see III:TII250
ACIDO (2,4,5-TRICLORO-FENOSSI)-ACETICO (ITALIAN) see
  II:TAA100
ACIDO 2-(2,4,5-TRICLORO-FENOSSI)-PROPIONICO (ITAL-
  IAN) see II:TIX500
ACID PHOSPHINE CL see III:FAG010
ACID PONCEAU 4R see III:FMU080
ACID PONCEAU R see III:FMU070
ACID RED 18 see III:FMU080
ACID RED 26 see III:FMU070
ACID RUBINE see III:HJF500
ACID SCARLET see III:FMU070
ACID SCARLET 3R see III:FMU080
ACID SKY BLUE A see III:FAE000
ACID-TREATED HEAVY NAPHTHENIC DISTILLATE see
  I:MQV760
ACID-TREATED HEAVY PARAFFINIC DISTILLATE see
  I:MQV765
ACID-TREATED LIGHT NAPHTHENIC DISTILLATE see
  I:MQV770

ACID-TREATED LIGHT PARAFFINIC DISTILLATE see
I:MQV775
ACID-TREATED RESIDUAL OIL see I:MQV872
ACIDUM NICOTINICUM see III:NCQ900
ACID VIOLET see II:FAG120
ACID YELLOW E see III:SGP500
ACID YELLOW TRA see III:FAG150
ACIGENA see III:HCL000
ACILAN GREEN SFG see III:FAF000
ACILAN ORANGE GX see III:HGC000
ACILAN PONCEAU RRL see III:FMU070
ACILAN RED SE see III:FAG020
ACILAN SCARLET V3R see III:FMU080
ACILAN TURQUOISE BLUE AE see III:FMU059
ACINTENE O see III:PMQ750
ACNEGEL see III:BDS000
ACNESTROL see I:DKA600
ACONCEN see III:CNV750
ACP-M-728 see III:AJM000
ACQUINITE see III:ADR000, III:CKN500
ACRALDEHYDE see III:ADR000
ACRIDINE, 9-(2-((2-CHLOROETHYL)AMINO)ETHYL-
AMINO)-6-CHLORO-2-METHOXY-, DIHYDROCHLORIDE,
HYDRATE see III:QCS875
3,6-ACRIDINEDIAMINE see III:DBN600
3,6-ACRIDINEDIAMINE, MONOHYDROCHLORIDE (9CI) see
III:PMH250
ACRIDINE MUSTARD see III:ADJ875
ACRIDINE ORANGE see III:BJF000
ACRIDINE ORANGE FREE BASE see III:BJF000
ACRIDINE RED see III:ADK000
ACRIDINE RED 3B see III:ADK000
ACRIDINE RED, HYDROCHLORIDE see III:ADK000
ACRIDINO(2,1,9,8-klmna)ACRIDINE see III:ADK250
ACRIDINO(2,1,9,8-klmna)ACRIDINE SULFATE see
III:DCK200
ACRIFLAVIN see III:DBX400
ACRIFLAVINE mixture with PROFLAVINE see III:DBX400
ACRIFLAVINIUM CHLORIDE see III:DBX400
ACRIFLAVINIUM CHLORIDUM see III:DBX400
ACRIFLAVON see III:DBX400
ACROLEIC ACID see III:ADS750
ACROLEIN see III:ADR000
ACROLEINA (ITALIAN) see III:ADR000
ACROLEINE (DUTCH, FRENCH) see III:ADR000
ACROMONA see I:MMN250
ACROMYCINE see III:ADR750
ACRONINE see III:ADR750
ACRONYCINE see III:ADR750
ACROPOR see III:ADY250
ACRYLALDEHYD (GERMAN) see III:ADR000
ACRYLALDEHYDE see III:ADR000
ACRYLAMIDE see I:ADS250
ACRYLATE d'ETHYLE (FRENCH) see II:EFT000
ACRYLATE de METHYLE (FRENCH) see III:MGA500
ACRYLIC ACID see III:ADS750
ACRYLIC ACID, inhibited (DOT) see III:ADS750
ACRYLIC ACID, DIESTER with TETRAETHYLENE GLYCOL
see III:ADT050
ACRYLIC ACID, DIESTER with TRIETHYLENE GLYCOL see
III:TJQ100
ACRYLIC ACID ETHYL ESTER see II:EFT000
ACRYLIC ACID-2-ETHYLHEXYL ESTER see III:ADU250
ACRYLIC ACID, GLACIAL see III:ADS750
ACRYLIC ACID METHYL ESTER (MAK) see III:MGA500
ACRYLIC ACID, OXYBIS(ETHYLENEOXYETHYLENE) ES-
TER see III:ADT050
ACRYLIC ACID, PENTAERITHRITOL TRIESTER see
III:PBC750
ACRYLIC ACID POLYMER, ZINC SALT see III:ADW250
ACRYLIC ALDEHYDE see III:ADR000
ACRYLIC AMIDE see I:ADS250
ACRYLITE see III:PKB500
ACRYLNITRIL (GERMAN, DUTCH) see I:ADX500

ACRYLONITRILE see I:ADX500
ACRYLONITRILE MONOMER see I:ADX500
ACRYLONITRILE POLYMER with CHLOROETHYLENE see
III:ADY250
ACRYLOPHENONE see III:PMQ250
ACRYLSAEUREAETHYLESTER (GERMAN) see II:EFT000
ACRYLSAEUREMETHYLESTER (GERMAN) see III:MGA500
ACRYPET see III:PKB500
ACT see III:AEB000
ACTAMER see III:TFD250
ACTICEL see III:SCH000
ACTINOLITE ASBESTOS see I:ARM260
ACTINOMYCIN 1048A see I:AEC000
ACTINOMYCIN 2104L see I:AEB750
ACTINOMYCIN D see III:AEB000
ACTINOMYCINDIOIC D ACID, DILACTONE see III:AEB000
ACTINOMYCIN I see III:AEB000
ACTINOMYCIN L see I:AEB750
ACTINOMYCIN S see I:AEC000
ACTIOQUINONE LIGHT YELLOW see II:AAQ250
ACTIVATED ALUMINUM OXIDE see III:AHE250
ACTOR Q see III:DVR200
ACTYBARYTE see III:BAP000
5-ACZ see III:ARY000
AD see III:AEB000
ADAKANE 12 see III:DXT200
ADC AURAMINE O see I:IBA000
ADC RHODAMINE B see III:FAG070
ADDITIN 30 see III:PFT250
A1-DEHYDROMETHYLTESTERONE see III:DAL300
ADENINE-1-N-OXIDE see III:AEH250
ADENOHYPOPHYSEAL GROWTH HORMONE see III:PJA250
ADENOSINE, N-METHYL-, mixed with SODIUM NITRITE (1:4)
see III:SIS650
ADEPSINE OIL see III:MQV750
ADIPAMIDE see III:AEN000
ADIPEX see III:MDT600
ADIPIC ACID BIS(2-ETHYLHEXYL) ESTER see III:AEO000
ADIPIC ACID DIAMIDE see III:AEN000
ADIPIC ACID, POLYMER with 1,4-BUTANEDIOL and METH-
YLENEDI-p-PHENYLENE ISOCYANATE see I:PKM250
ADIPIC ACID, POLYMER with 1,4-BUTANEDIOL, METH-
YLENEDI-p-PHENYLENE ISOCYANATE and 2,2′-(p-PHEN-
YLENEDIOXY)DIETHANOL see I:PKM500
ADIPIC ACID, POLYMER with ETHYLENE GLYCOL and
METHYLENEDI-p-PHENYLENE ISOCYANATE see
I:PKL750
ADIPIC ACID, UREA mixed with CARBOXYMETHYLCELLU-
LOSE ACIDS see III:AER000
ADIPIC DIAMIDE see III:AEN000
ADIPLON see III:PPO000
ADIPOL 2EH see III:AEO000
ADM see I:AES750
ADMER PB 02 see III:PMP500
ADM HYDROCHLORIDE see III:HKA300
2-ADO see III:DDB600
ADOL see III:OAX000
ADOL 68 see III:OAX000
ADONAL see II:EOK000
ADR see III:HKA300
ADRESON see III:CNS825
ADRIACIN see III:HKA300
ADRIAMYCIN see I:AES750, III:HKA300
ADRIAMYCIN-HCl see I:AES750
ADRIAMYCIN, HYDROCHLORIDE see III:HKA300
ADRIAMYCIN SEMIQUINONE see I:AES750
ADRIBLASTIN see III:HKA300
ADRIBLASTINA see I:AES750
ADRIBLASTINE see III:HKA300
ADROIDIN see I:PAN100
ADROYD see I:PAN100
ADRUCIL see III:FMM000
ADUMBRAN see III:CFZ000
ADVASTAB 401 see III:BFW750

AENH (GERMAN) see I:ENV000
AEPHENAL see II:EOK000
AERO see III:MCB000
AERO-CYANAMID see III:CAQ250
AERO CYANAMID GRANULAR see III:CAQ250
AERO CYANAMID SPECIAL GRADE see III:CAQ250
AEROL 1 (pesticide) see III:TIQ250
AEROSIL see III:SCH000
AEROSOL of THERMOVACUUM CADMIUM see I:CAK000
AEROTHENE MM see II:MJP450
AEROTHENE TT see III:MIH275
AETHANOL (GERMAN) see I:EFU000
AETHIONIN see II:EEI000
p-AETHOXYPHYLHARNSTOFF (GERMAN) see III:EFE000
AETHYL ACETOXYMETHYLNITROSAMIN (GERMAN) see
    III:ENR500
AETHYLACRYLAT (GERMAN) see II:EFT000
AETHYL-AETHANOL-NITROSOAMIN (GERMAN) see
    II:ELG500
AETHYLALKOHOL (GERMAN) see I:EFU000
2-AETHYLAMINO-4-CHLOR-6-ISOPROPYLAMINO-1,3,5-
    TRIAZIN (GERMAN) see III:ARQ725
2-AETHYLAMINO-4-ISOPROPYLAMINO-6-CHLOR-1,3,5-
    TRIAZIN (GERMAN) see III:ARQ725
AETHYL-N-BUTYL-NITROSOAMIN (GERMAN) see
    III:EHC000
AETHYL-tert-BUTYL-NITROSOAMIN (GERMAN) see
    III:NKD500
AETHYLCARBAMAT (GERMAN) see I:UVA000
AETHYLENBROMID (GERMAN) see I:EIY500
AETHYLENCHLORID (GERMAN) see I:EIY600
AETHYLENIMIN (GERMAN) see I:EJM900
AETHYLENOXID (GERMAN) see I:EJN500
AETHYLENSULFID (GERMAN) see III:EJP500
AETHYLFORMIAT (GERMAN) see III:EKL000
AETHYLHARNSTOFF und NATRIUMNITRIT (GERMAN) see
    II:EQE000
AETHYLHARNSTOFF und NITRIT (GERMAN) see II:EQE000
AETHYLIDENCHLORID (GERMAN) see III:DFF809
AETHYL-ISOPROPYL-NITROSOAMIN (GERMAN) see
    III:ELX500
N-AETHYL-N'-NITRO-N-NITROSOGUANIDIN (GERMAN) see
    III:ENU000
AETHYLNITROSO-HARNSTOFF (GERMAN) see I:ENV000
AETHYLNITROSOURETHAN (GERMAN) see III:NKE500
AETHYL-4-PICOLYLNITROSAMIN (GERMAN) see
    III:NLH000
AETHYLURETHAN (GERMAN) see I:UVA000
AETHYL-VINYL-NITROSOAMIN (GERMAN) see III:NKF000
AETINA see III:EPQ000
AETIVA see III:EPQ000
AF 101 see III:DXQ500
AF-2 (preservative) see II:FQN000
AFASTOGEN BLUE 5040 see III:DNE400
AFBI see I:AEU250
A.F. BLUE No. 1 see III:FMU059
A.F. BLUE No. 2 see III:FAE100
AFCOLAC B 101 see III:SMR000
AFCOLENE see III:SMQ500
A.F. GREEN No. 1 see III:FAE950
A.F. GREEN No. 2 see III:FAF000
AFICIDE see I:BBQ500
A-FIL CREAM see III:TGG760
AFLATOXICOL see II:AEW500
AFLATOXIN see I:AET750
AFLATOXIN B see I:AEU250
AFLATOXIN B1 see I:AEU250
AFLATOXIN B2 see I:AEU750
AFLATOXIN B1-2,3-DICHLORIDE see III:AEU500
AFLATOXIN G1 see I:AEV000
AFLATOXIN G2 see I:AEV500
AFLATOXIN G1 mixed with AFLATOXIN B1 see I:AEV250
AFLATOXIN M1 see I:AEW000
AFLATOXIN Ro see II:AEW500

AFLON see III:TAI250
A.F. ORANGE No. 1 see III:FAG010
A.F.ORANGE No. 2 see II:TGW000
A.F. RED No. 1 see II:FAG018
A.F. RED No. 5 see III:XRA000
A.F. VIOLET No 1 see II:FAG120
A.F YELLOW No. 2 see III:FAG130
A.F. YELLOW No. 3 see III:FAG135
AGALITE see III:TAB750
AGATE see I:SCJ500
AGC see III:GFA000
AGENT 504 see III:DAI600
AGENT AT 717 see III:PKQ250
AGENT BLUE see III:HKC000
AGERATOCHROMENE see III:AEX850
AGERITE see III:AEY000, III:BLE500
AGERITE 150 see III:HKF000
AGERITE ALBA see III:AEY000
AGERITEDPPD see III:BLE500
AGERITE ISO see III:HKF000
AGERITE POWDER see II:PFT500
AGERITE WHITE see III:NBL000
AGIDOL see III:BFW750
AGILENE see III:PJS750
AGI TALC, BC 1615 see III:TAB750
AGOFOLLIN see I:EDR000
AGOSTILBEN see I:DKA600
AGOVIRIN see I:TBG000
AGREFLAN see III:DUV600
AGRICIDE MAGGOT KILLER (F) see I:CDV100
AGRIFLAN 24 see III:DUV600
AGRISOL G-20 see I:BBQ500
AGRITAN see I:DAD200
AGRITOX see II:CIR250
A-GRO see III:MNH000
AGROCERES see II:HAR000
AGROCIDE see I:BBQ500
AGROFOROTOX see III:TIQ250
AGRONEXIT see I:BBQ500
AGROSOL S see III:CBG000
AGROTECT see II:DAA800
AGROXONE see II:CIR250
AGROX 2-WAY and 3-WAY see III:CBG000
AGRYPNAL see II:EOK000
AH see III:DBM800
AHCOCID FAST SCARLET R see III:FMU070
AHCO DIRECT BLACK GX see I:AQP000
AHCOVAT PRINTING GOLDEN YELLOW see III:DCZ000
AIRDALE BLUE IN see III:FAE100
AIREDALE BLACK ED see I:AQP000
AIREDALE BLUE 2BD see I:CMO000
AIREDALE CARMOISINE see III:HJF500
AIREDALE VIOLET ND see III:CMP000
AIREDALE YELLOW E see III:SGP500
AISELAZINE see II:HGP500
AITC see II:AGJ250
AIZEN AMARANTH see III:FAG020
AIZEN AURAMINE see I:IBA000
AIZEN BRILLIANT BLUE FCF see III:FMU059
AIZEN BRILLIANT SCARLET 3RH see III:FMU080
AIZEN CRYSTAL VIOLET EXTRA PURE see III:AOR500
AIZEN DIRECT BLUE 2BH see I:CMO000
AIZEN DIRECT DEEP BLACK GH see I:AQP000
AIZEN EOSINE GH see III:BNH500, III:BNK700
AIZEN ERYTHROSINE see III:FAG040
AIZEN FOOD BLUE No. 2 see III:FAE000
AIZEN FOOD GREEN No. 3 see III:FAG000
AIZEN FOOD ORANGE No. 1 see III:FAG010
AIZEN FOOD ORANGE No. 2 see II:TGW000
AIZEN FOOD RED No. 5 see III:XRA000
AIZEN FOOD VIOLET No 1 see II:FAG120
AIZEN FOOD YELLOW No. 5 see III:FAG150
AIZEN NAPHTHOL ORANGE I see III:FAG010
AIZEN ORANGE I see III:FAG010

AIZEN PONCEAU RH see III:FMU070
AIZEN PRIMULA BROWN BRLH see II:CMO750
AIZEN RHODAMINE BH see III:FAG070
AIZEN URANINE see III:FEW000
AIZEN VICTORIA BLUE BOH see III:VKA600
AKAR see II:DER000
AKIRIKU RHODAMINE B see III:FAG070
AKOTIN see III:NCQ900
AKROLEIN (CZECH) see III:ADR000
AKROLEINA (POLISH) see III:ADR000
AKRYLAMID (CZECH) see I:ADS250
AKRYLONITRYL (POLISH) see I:ADX500
AKTIKON see III:ARQ725
AKTIKON PK see III:ARQ725
AKTINIT A see III:ARQ725
AKTINIT PK see III:ARQ725
AKTINIT S see III:BJP000
AKULON see III:PJY500
AKZO CHEMIE MANEB see III:MAS500
AL-50 see III:RDP300
ALABASTER see III:CAX750
ALACINE see III:PFC750
ALANINE NITROGEN MUSTARD see I:PED750, III:BHV250
ALAR see II:DQD400
ALAR-85 see II:DQD400
ALATHON see III:PKF750
ALAZIN see III:PFC750
ALAZINE see III:PFC750
ALBA-DOME see III:AEY000
ALBAGEL PREMIUM USP 4444 see III:BAV750
ALBEXAN see III:SNM500
ALBIGEN A see III:PKQ250
ALBOLINE see III:MQV750
ALBONE see III:HIB000
ALBONE 35 see III:HIB010
ALBONE 50 see III:HIB010
ALBONE 70 see III:HIB010
ALBONE 35CG see III:HIB010
ALBONE 50CG see III:HIB010
ALBONE 70CG see III:HIB010
ALBORAL see III:DCK759
ALBOSAL see III:SNM500
ALCOA F 1 see III:AHE250
ALCOA SODIUM FLUORIDE see III:SHF500
ALCOBAM ZM see III:BJK500
ALCOHOL see I:EFU000
ALCOHOL, ANHYDROUS see I:EFU000
ALCOHOL C-10 see III:DAI600
ALCOHOL C-12 see III:DXV600
ALCOHOL, DEHYDRATED see I:EFU000
ALCOOL AMILICO (ITALIAN) see III:IHP000
ALCOOL AMYLIQUE (FRENCH) see III:AOE000
ALCOOL ETHYLIQUE (FRENCH) see I:EFU000
ALCOOL ETILICO (ITALIAN) see I:EFU000
ALCOOL ISOAMYLIQUE (FRENCH) see III:IHP000
ALCOOL ISOBUTYLIQUE (FRENCH) see III:IIL000
ALCOOL ISOPROPILICO (ITALIAN) see III:INJ000
ALCOOL ISOPROPYLIQUE (FRENCH) see III:INJ000
ALCOOL PROPILICO (ITALIAN) see III:PND000
ALCOOL PROPYLIQUE (FRENCH) see III:PND000
ALCOPHOBIN see III:DXH250
ALDACOL Q see III:PKQ250
ALDACTAZIDE see III:AFJ500
ALDACTIDE see III:AFJ500
ALDACTONE see III:AFJ500
ALDACTONE A see III:AFJ500
ALDEHYDE ACETIQUE (FRENCH) see II:AAG250
ALDEHYDE ACRYLIQUE (FRENCH) see III:ADR000
ALDEHYDE FORMIQUE (FRENCH) see I:FMV000
ALDEHYDODICHLOROMALEIC ACID see III:MRU900
ALDEIDE ACETICA (ITALIAN) see II:AAG250
ALDEIDE ACRILICA (ITALIAN) see III:ADR000
ALDEIDE FORMICA (ITALIAN) see I:FMV000
ALDERLIN see III:INS000

ALDERLIN HYDROCHLORIDE see III:INT000
ALDINAMID see III:POL500
ALDO see III:CLY500
ALDOMYCIN see II:NGE500
ALDREX see III:AFK250
ALDREX 30 see III:AFK250
ALDRIN see III:AFK250
ALDRIN, cast solid (DOT) see III:AFK250
ALDRINE (FRENCH) see III:AFK250
ALDRITE see III:AFK250
ALDROSOL see III:AFK250
ALEPSIN see I:DNU000
ALEVIATIN see I:DKQ000
ALFAMAT see III:GFA000
ALFANAFTILAMINA (ITALIAN) see I:NBE000
ALFA-NAFTYLOAMINA (POLISH) see I:NBE000
ALFICETYN see II:CDP250
ALFOL 12 see III:DXV600
ALFUCIN see II:NGE500
ALGISTAT see III:DFT000
ALGLOFLON see III:TAI250
ALGOFLON SV see III:TAI250
ALGOFRENE TYPE 6 see III:CFX500
ALGOSEDIV see III:TEH500
ALGOTROPYL see II:HIM000
ALGRAIN see I:EFU000
ALGYLEN see II:TIO750
ALINDOR see III:BRF500
ALIPHATIC and AROMATIC EPOXIDES see II:AFM250
ALIPHATIC CHLORINATED HYDROCARBONS see
   II:CDV250
ALISEUM see III:DCK759
ALKABUTAZONA see II:BRF500
ALKAMID see III:PJY500
ALKAPOL PEG-200 see III:PJT000
ALKARSODYL see I:HKC500
ALKATHENE see III:PJS750
ALKATHENE RXDG33 see III:TAI250
ALK-AUBS see III:DXH250
ALKERAN see I:PED750
ALKIRON see II:MPW500
ALKOHOL (GERMAN) see I:EFU000
ALKOHOLU ETYLOWEGO (POLISH) see I:EFU000
ALLBRI NATURAL COPPER see III:CNI000
ALLERGAN 211 see III:DAS000
ALLERON see III:PAK000
ALLILE (CLORURO DI) (ITALIAN) see II:AGB250
ALLISAN see III:RDP300
1-(p-ALLOPHANOYLBENZYL)-2-METHYLHYDRAZINE HY-
   DROBROMIDE see III:MKN750
ALLTEX see I:CDV100
ALLTOX see I:CDV100
ALLYL ALDEHYDE see III:ADR000
p-ALLYLANISOLE see III:AFW750
5-ALLYL-1,3-BENZODIOXOLE see I:SAD000
ALLYL CARBAMATE see III:AGA750
ALLYLCATECHOL METHYLENE ETHER see I:SAD000
ALLYLCHLORID (GERMAN) see II:AGB250
ALLYL CHLORIDE see II:AGB250
ALLYLDIOXYBENZENE METHYLENE ETHER see I:SAD000
ALLYLE (CHLORURE D') (FRENCH) see II:AGB250
4-ALLYLGUAIACOL see III:EQR500
ALLYLHYDRAZINE HYDROCHLORIDE see III:AGH500
4-ALLYL-1-HYDROXY-2-METHOXYBENZENE see
   III:EQR500
ALLYL ISORHODANIDE see II:AGJ250
ALLYL ISOSULFOCYANATE see II:AGJ250
ALLYL ISOTHIOCYANATE see II:AGJ250
ALLYL ISOTHIOCYANATE, stabilized (DOT) see II:AGJ250
ALLYL ISOVALERATE see II:ISV000
ALLYL ISOVALERIANATE see II:ISV000
ALLYL MESYLATE see III:AGK750
ALLYL METHANESULFONATE see III:AGK750
4-ALLYL-1-METHOXYBENZENE see III:AFW750

4-ALLYL-2-METHOXYPHENOL see III:EQR500
ALLYL 3-METHYLBUTYRATE see II:ISV000
1-ALLYL-3,4-METHYLENEDIOXYBENZENE see I:SAD000
4-ALLYL-1,2-METHYLENEDIOXYBENZENE see I:SAD000
ALLYL MUSTARD OIL see II:AGJ250
4-(ALLYLNITROSAMINO)-1-BUTANOL see III:HJS400
3-(ALLYLNITROSAMINO)-1,2-PROPANEDIOL see III:NJY500
1-(ALLYLNITROSAMINO)-2-PROPANONE see III:AGM125
4-(ALLYLNITROSOAMINO)BUTRIC ACID see III:CCJ375
N-ALLYL-N-NITROSO-3-BUTENYLAMINE see III:BPD000
2-ALLYL PHENOL see III:AGQ500
o-ALLYL PHENOL see III:AGQ500
m-ALLYLPYROCATECHIN METHYLENE ETHER see I:SAD000
4-ALLYLPYROCATECHOL FORMALDEHYDE ACETAL see I:SAD000
ALLYLPYROCATECHOL METHYLENE ETHER see I:SAD000
ALLYLSENFOEL (GERMAN) see II:AGJ250
ALLYL SEVENOLUM see II:AGJ250
ALLYL THIOCARBONIMIDE see II:AGJ250
ALMEDERM see III:HCL000
ALMITE see III:AHE250
ALON see III:AHE250
ALOPERIDIN see III:CLY500
ALOPERIDOLO see III:CLY500
ALPEROX C see III:LBR000
ALPHANAPHTHYL THIOUREA see III:AQN635
ALPHANAPHTYL THIOUREE (FRENCH) see III:AQN635
ALPHAZURINE see III:FMU059
ALPINE TALC USP, BC 127 see III:TAB750
ALPINE TALC USP, BC 141 see III:TAB750
ALPINE TALC USP, BC 662 see III:TAB750
ALPINYL see II:HIM000
ALQOVERIN see III:BRF500
ALRATO see III:AQN635
ALTADIOL see II:EDS100
ALTAN see III:DMH400
ALTAX see III:BDE750
ALTOX see III:AFK250
ALTRAD see I:EDO000
ALTRETAMINE see III:HEJ500
ALUMINA see III:AHE250
β-ALUMINA see III:AHE250
γ-ALUMINA see III:AHE250
α-ALUMINA (OSHA) see III:AHE250
ALUMINUM ALLOY, Al,Be see I:BFP250
ALUMINUM BERYLLIUM ALLOY see I:BFP250
ALUMINUM DEXTRAN see III:AHA250
ALUMINUM MONOSTEARATE see III:AHA250
ALUMINUM OXIDE see III:AHE250, III:EAL100
α-ALUMINUM OXIDE see III:AHE250
β-ALUMINUM OXIDE see III:AHE250
γ-ALUMINUM OXIDE see III:AHE250
ALUMINUM OXIDE (2:3) see III:AHE250
ALUMINUM OXIDE SILICATE see III:AHF500
ALUMINUM SESQUIOXIDE see III:AHE250
ALUMINUM(III) SILICATE (2:1) see III:AHF500
ALUMITE see III:AHE250
ALUNDUM see III:AHE250
ALUTOR M 70 see III:PKB500
ALVEDON see II:HIM000
ALVIT see III:DHB400
ALZODEF see III:CAQ250
AMABEVAN see III:CBJ000
AMACEL BLUE GG see III:TBG700
AMACEL DEVELOPED NAVY SD see I:DCJ200
AMACEL PURE BLUE B see III:TBG700
AMACEL YELLOW G see II:AAQ250
AMACID AMARANTH see III:FAG020
AMACID BLUE FG CONC see III:FMU059
AMACID BRILLIANT BLUE see III:FAE100
AMACID CHROME BLUE R see III:HJF500

AMACID GREEN G see III:FAF000
AMACID LAKE SCARLET 2R see III:FMU070
AMADIL see II:HIM000
AMANIL BLACK GL see I:AQP000
AMANIL BLUE 2BX see I:CMO000
AMANIL FAST VIOLET N see III:CMP000
AMANIL SKY BLUE see II:CMO250
AMANIL SUPRA BROWN LBL see II:CMO750
AMANTHRENE GOLDEN YELLOW see III:DCZ000
AMARANT see III:FAG020
AMARANTH see III:FAG020
AMARANTHE USP (biological stain) see III:FAG020
AMARTHOL FAST RED TR BASE see II:CLK220, II:CLK235
AMARTHOL FAST RED TR SALT see II:CLK235
AMATIN see I:HCC500
AMAX see III:BDG000
AMBESIDE see III:SNM500
AMBIBEN see III:AJM000
AMBILHAR see II:NML000
AMBOCHLORIN see CDO500
AMBOCLORIN see CDO500
AMBOFEN see II:CDP250
6-AMC see III:CML800
AMCHEM GRASS KILLER see III:TII250
AMCHEM R 14 see I:PKL750
AMCHEM 2,4,5-TP see II:TIX500
AMCO see III:PMP500
AMDON GRAZON see III:PIB900
AMEBAN see III:CBJ000
AMEBARSONE see III:CBJ000
AMEISENATOD see I:BBQ500
AMEISENMITTEL MERCK see I:BBQ500
AMERCIDE see III:CBG000
AMERFIL see III:PMP500
AMERICAN CYANAMID 4,049 see III:MAK700
AMERICAN CYANAMID 5223 see III:DXX400
AMERICAN CYANAMID 12880 see III:DSP400
AMERICAN PENICILLIN see III:BFD250
AMEROL see I:AMY050
AMETHOPTERIN see III:MDV500
AMETHYST see I:SCJ500
AMETYCIN see II:AHK500
AMFH see III:AAH100
AMIANTHUS see I:ARM250
AMIBIARSON see III:CBJ000
AMIDAZIN see III:EPQ000
AMIDAZOPHEN see III:DOT000
AMIDINE BLUE 4B see II:CMO250
AMID KYSELINY OCTOVE see II:AAI000
o-AMIDOAZOTOLUOL (GERMAN) see I:AIC250
o-AMIDOBENZOIC ACID see III:API500
AMIDOFEBRIN see III:DOT000
AMIDO-G-ACID see III:NBE850
AMIDON see III:ILD000
AMIDOPHEN see III:DOT000
AMIDOPHENAZONE see III:DOT000
AMIDOPYRAZOLINE see III:DOT000
AMIDOPYRIN see III:DOT000
AMIDOUREA HYDROCHLORIDE see III:SBW500
AMIDOX see II:DAA800
AMIDOXAL see III:SNN500
AMIDO YELLOW EA-CF see III:SGP500
AMIFUR see II:NGE500
AMILAN see III:NOH000
AMILAN CM 1001 see III:PJY500
AMILAR see III:PKF750
AMINARSON see III:CBJ000
AMINARSONE see III:CBJ000
AMINE 2,4,5-T for rice see II:TAA100
5-AMINOACENAPHTHENE see III:AAF250
2-AMINO-4-ACETAMINIFENETOL (CZECH) see III:AJT750
2-AMINOACETOPHENONE see III:AHR250
φ-AMINOACETOPHENONE see III:AHR250
3-AMINOANILINE see III:PEY000

4-AMINOANILINE see III:PEY500
m-AMINOANILINE see III:PEY000
p-AMINOANILINE see III:PEY500
3-AMINOANILINE DIHYDROCHLORIDE see III:PEY750
4-AMINOANILINE DIHYDROCHLORIDE see III:PEY650
m-AMINOANILINE DIHYDROCHLORIDE see III:PEY750
p-AMINOANILINE DIHYDROCHLORIDE see III:PEY650
2-AMINOANISOLE see II:AOV900
o-AMINOANISOLE see II:AOV900
1-AMINOANTHRACENE see III:APG250
2-AMINOANTHRACENE see II:APG000
α-AMINOANTHRACENE see III:APG250
β-AMINOANTHRACENE see II:APG000
1-AMINO-9,10-ANTHRACENEDIONE see III:AIA750
2-AMINO-9,10-ANTHRACENEDIONE see I:AIB000
1-AMINOANTHRACHINON (CZECH) see III:AIA750
1-AMINOANTHRAQUINONE see III:AIA750
2-AMINOANTHRAQUINONE see I:AIB000
α-AMINOANTHRAQUINONE see III:AIA750
β-AMINOANTHRAQUINONE see I:AIB000
1-AMINO-9,10-ANTHRAQUINONE see III:AIA750
2-AMINO-9,10-ANTRAQUINONE see I:AIB000
4-AMINO-1-ARABINOFURANOSYL-2-OXO-1,2-DIHYDRO-
   PYRIMIDINE see III:AQQ750
4-AMINO-1-β-d-ARABINOFURANOSYL-2(1H)-PYRIMIDI-
   NONE (9CI) see III:AQQ750
AMINOARSON see III:CBJ000
AMINOAZOBENZENE see II:PEI000
4-AMINOAZOBENZENE see II:PEI000
p-AMINOAZOBENZENE see II:PEI000
4-AMINO-1,1'-AZOBENZENE see II:PEI000
4-AMINOAZOBENZOL see II:PEI000
p-AMINOAZOBENZOL see II:PEI000
AMINOAZOTOLUENE (indicator) see I:AIC250
2-AMINO-5-AZOTOLUENE see I:AIC250
p-AMINO-2':3-AZOTOLUENE see III:AIC000
2'-AMINO-2:5'-AZOTOLUENE see III:TGW500
4'-AMINO-2:3'-AZOTOLUENE see I:AIC250
4'-AMINO-3,2'-AZOTOLUENE see III:AIC000
4'-AMINO-4,2'-AZOTOLUENE see III:AIC500
4'-AMINO-4-3'-AZOTOLUENE see III:TGW750
o-AMINOAZOTOLUENE (MAK) see I:AIC250
o-AMINOAZOTOLUENO (SPANISH) see I:AIC250
o-AMINOAZOTOLUOL see I:AIC250
10-AMINOBENZ(a)ACRIDINE see III:AIC750
5-AMINO-1:2-BENZANTHRACENE see III:BBC000
10-AMINO-1,2-BENZANTHRACENE see III:BBB750
AMINOBENZENE see II:AOQ000
p-AMINOBENZENESULFAMIDE see III:SNM500
4-AMINOBENZENESULFONAMIDE see III:SNM500
p-AMINOBENZENESULFONAMIDE see III:SNM500
5-(p-AMINOBENZENESULFONAMIDO)-3,4-DIMETHYL-
   ISOOXALE see III:SNN500
5-(p-AMINOBENZENESULFONAMIDO)-3,4-DIMETHYL-
   ISOXAZOLE see III:SNN500
2-(p-AMINOBENZENESULFONAMIDO)-4,6-DIMETHYLPY-
   RIMIDINE see III:SNJ000
2-(p-AMINOBENZENESULFONAMIDO)-5-METHYLTHIA-
   DIAZOLE see III:MPQ750
2-(p-AMINOBENZENESULFONAMIDO)THIAZOLE see
   III:TEX250
5-(p-AMINOBENZENESULPHONAMIDE)-3,4-DIMETHYL-
   ISOXAZOLE see III:SNN500
5-(p-AMINOBENZENESULPHONAMIDO)-3,4-DIMETHYL-
   ISOXAZOLE see III:SNN500
2-(p-AMINOBENZENESULPHONAMIDO)THIAZOLE see
   III:TEX250
2-AMINOBENZOIC ACID see III:API500
o-AMINOBENZOIC ACID see III:API500
2-AMINOBENZOIC ACID-3-PHENYL-2-PROPENYL ESTER
   see II:API750
6-(4'-AMINOBENZOL-SULFONAMIDO)-2,4-DIMETHYLPY-
   RIMIDIN (GERMAN) see III:SNJ000
(p-AMINOBENZOLSULFONYL)-2-AMINO-4,6-DIMETHYL-
   PYRIMIDIN (GERMAN) see III:SNJ000

4-(4-AMINOBENZYL)ANILINE see I:MJQ000
4-AMINOBIPHENYL see I:AJS100
p-AMINOBIPHENYL see I:AJS100
4-AMINOBIPHENYL DIHYDROCHLORIDE see III:BGE300
4-AMINO-3-BIPHENYLOL see III:AIV750
4'-AMINO-4-BIPHENYLOL see III:AIW000
3-AMINO-4-BIPHENYLOL HYDROCHLORIDE see
   III:AIW250
4-AMINO-3-BIPHENYLOL HYDROGEN SULFATE see
   III:AKF250
1-AMINO-3-BROMOPROPANE HYDROBROMIDE see
   III:AJA000
1-AMINO-BUTAAN (DUTCH) see III:BPX750
1-AMINOBUTAN (GERMAN) see III:BPX750
1-AMINOBUTANE see III:BPX750
AMINOCAPROIC ACID LACTAM see III:CBF700
AMINO-α-CARBOLINE see II:AJD750
2-AMINO-α-CARBOLINE see II:AJD750
(4-((AMINOCARBONYL)AMINO)PHENYL)ARSONIC ACID
   see III:CBJ000
N-(AMINOCARBONYL)HYDROXYLAMINE see III:HOO500
N-AMINOCARBONYL-4-((2-
   METHYLHYDRAZINO)METHYL)BENZAMIDE MONOHY-
   DROBROMIDE see III:MKN750
N-(AMINOCARBONYL)-N-NITROGLYCINE see III:NKI500
1-AMINO-2-CARBOXYBENZENE see III:API500
1-AMINO-4-CHLOROBENZENE see III:CEH680
1-AMINO-3-CHLORO-6-METHYLBENZENE see II:CLK225
2-AMINO-4-CHLOROTOLUENE see II:CLK225
2-AMINO-5-CHLOROTOLUENE see II:CLK220
2-AMINO-5-CHLOROTOLUENE HYDROCHLORIDE see
   II:CLK235
6-AMINOCHRYSENE see III:CML800
3-AMINO-p-CRESOL METHYL ESTER see I:MGO750
m-AMINO-p-CRESOL, METHYL ESTER see I:MGO750
AMINOCYCLOHEXANE see III:CPF500
2-AMINO-2-DEOXY-d-GALACTOSE HYDROCHLORIDE see
   III:GAT000
4-AMINO-4-DEOXY-N10-METHYLPTEROYLGLUTAMATE
   see III:MDV500
4-AMINO-4-DEOXY-N10-METHYLPTEROYLGLUTAMIC
   ACID see III:MDV500
4-AMINO-4-DEOXYPTEROYLGLUTAMATE see III:AMG750
2-AMINO-9-(2-DEOXY-β-d-RIBOFURANOSYL)-9H-PURINE-
   6-THIOL HYDRATE see III:TFJ250
7-AMINODIBENZ(a,h)ANTHRACENE see III:AJL250
9-AMINO-1,2,5,6-DIBENZANTHRACENE see III:AJL250
3-AMINODIBENZOFURAN see III:DDB600
3-AMINO-2,5-DICHLOROBENZOIC ACID see III:AJM000
4-AMINODIFENIL (SPANISH) see I:AJS100
2-AMINO-3-(3,4-DIHYDROXYPHENYL)PROPANOIC ACID
   see III:DNA200
4-AMINO-2',3-DIMETHYLAZOBENZENE see I:AIC250
4'-AMINO-2,3'-DIMETHYLAZOBENZENE see I:AIC250
1-AMINO-2,4-DIMETHYLBENZENE see II:XMS000
1-AMINO-2,5-DIMETHYLBENZENE see III:XNA000
3-AMINO-1,4-DIMETHYLBENZENE see III:XNA000
4-AMINO-1,3-DIMETHYLBENZENE see II:XMS000
1-AMINO-2,4-DIMETHYLBENZENE HYDROCHLORIDE see
   III:XOJ000
1-AMINO-2,5-DIMETHYLBENZENE HYDROCHLORIDE see
   III:XOS000
3-AMINO-1,4-DIMETHYLBENZENE HYDROCHLORIDE see
   III:XOS000
4-AMINO-1,3-DIMETHYLBENZENE HYDROCHLORIDE see
   III:XOJ000
5-AMINO-1,4-DIMETHYLBENZENE HYDROCHLORIDE see
   III:XOS000
3-AMINO-1,4-DIMETHYL-γ-CARBOLINE see II:TNX275
4-AMINO-3',5'-DIMETHYL-4'-HYDROXYAZOBENZENE see
   III:AJQ500
2-AMINO-3,4-DIMETHYLIMIDAZO(4,5-f)QUINOLINE see
   III:AJQ600
2-AMINO-3,8-DIMETHYLIMIDAZO(4,5-f)QUINOXALINE see
   II:AJQ675

2-AMINO-1-NAPHTHYLGLUCOSIDURONIC ACID see III:ALL000

2-AMINO-1-NAPHTHYL HYDROGEN SULFATE see III:ALK750

2-AMINO-1-NAPHTHYL HYDROGEN SULPHATE see III:ALK750

4-AMINO-2-NITROANILINE see II:ALL750

2-AMINO-4-NITROANISOLE see II:NEQ500

4-AMINO-4'-NITROBIPHENYL see III:ALM000

4-AMINO-4'-NITRO-3-BIPHENYLOL HYDROCHLORIDE see III:AKI500

2-AMINO-5-(5-NITRO-2-FURYL)-1,3,4-OXADIAZOLE see III:ALM250

2-AMINO-5-(5-NITRO-2-FURYL)-1,3,4-THIADIAZOLE see II:NGI500

5-AMINO-2-(5-NITRO-2-FURYL)-1,3,4-THIADIAZOLE see II:NGI500

2-AMINO-4-(5-NITRO-2-FURYL)THIAZOLE see III:ALM500

2-AMINO-4-NITROPHENOL see III:NEM500

2-AMINO-5-NITROPHENOL see III:ALO000

4-AMINO-2-NITROPHENOL see II:NEM480

2-((4-AMINO-2-NITROPHENYL)AMINO)ETHANOL see III:ALO750

2-AMINO-4-(p-NITROPHENYL)THIAZOLE see III:ALP000

AMINONITROTHIAZOLE see III:ALQ000

2-AMINO-5-NITROTHIAZOLE see III:ALQ000

AMINONITROTHIAZOLUM see III:ALQ000

2-AMINO-4-NITROTOLUENE see I:NMP500

N-(2-AMINO-2-OXOETHYL)-2-DIAZOACETAMIDE see III:CBK000

N-(p-(((2-AMINO-4-OXO-6-PTERIDINYL)METHYL)-N-NI-TROSOAMINO)BENZOYL)-l-GLUTAMIC ACID see III:NLP000

6-AMINOPENICILLANIC ACID see III:PCU500

4-AMINO-PGA see III:AMG750

AMINOPHEN see II:AOQ000

1-AMINOPHENANTHRENE see III:ALS000

2-AMINOPHENANTHRENE see III:PDA250

3-AMINOPHENANTHRENE see III:PDA500

9-AMINOPHENANTHRENE see III:PDA750

AMINOPHENAZONE see III:DOT000

AMINOPHENAZONE mixed with SODIUM NITRITE (1:1) see III:DOT200

4-AMINOPHENYL ETHER see I:OPM000

p-AMINOPHENYL ETHER see I:OPM000

4-((4-AMINOPHENYL)(4-IMINO-2,5-CYCLOHEXADIEN-1-YLIDENE)METHYL), MONOCHLORIDE see II:RMK020

4-AMINOPHENYLSULFONAMIDE see III:SNM500

p-AMINOPHENYLSULFONAMIDE see III:SNM500

5-(4-AMINOPHENYLSULFONAMIDO)-3,4-DIMETHYLISOX-AZOLE see III:SNN500

5-(4-AMINOPHENYLSULPHONAMIDO)-3,4-DIMETHYL-ISOXAZOLE see III:SNN500

3-(p-AMINOPHENYLSULPHONAMIDO)-5-METHYLISOXA-ZOLE see III:SNK000

3-AMINO-1,3-PROPANEDIOL see III:AMA250

1-AMINOPROPAN-2-OL see III:AMA500

1-AMINO-2-PROPANOL see III:AMA500

AMINOPTERIDINE see III:AMG750

AMINOPTERIN see III:AMG750

4-AMINOPTEROYLGLUTAMIC ACID see III:AMG750

2-AMINO-9H-PYRIDO(2,3-B)INDOLE see II:AJD750

AMINOPYRINE see III:DOT000

AMINOPYRINE mixed with SODIUM NITRITE (1:1) see III:DOT200

AMINOPYRINE SODIUM SULFONATE see III:AMK500

4-AMINO-1-β-d-RIBOFURANOSYL-d-TRIAZIN-2(1H)-ONE see III:ARY000

4-AMINO-1-β-d-RIBOFURANOSYL-1,3,5-TRIAZIN-2(1H)-ONE see III:ARY000

4-AMINOSTILBENE see III:SLQ900

p-AMINOSTILBENE see III:SLQ900

trans-4-AMINOSTILBENE see III:AMO000

4-AMINO-2-STILBENECARBONITRILE see III:COS750

2-(p-AMINOSTYRYL)-6-(p-ACETYLAMINOBENZOYL-AMINO)QUINOLINE METHOACETATE see III:AMO250

4-AMINO-N-2-THIAZOLYLBENZENESULFONAMIDE see III:TEX250

N-AMINOTHIOUREA see III:TFQ000

2-AMINOTOLUENE see I:TGQ750

o-AMINOTOLUENE see I:TGQ750

2-AMINOTOLUENE HYDROCHLORIDE see I:TGS500

4-AMINOTOLUENE HYDROCHLORIDE see III:TGS750

o-AMINOTOLUENE HYDROCHLORIDE see I:TGS500

3-AMINO-p-TOLUIDINE see I:TGL750

5-AMINO-o-TOLUIDINE see I:TGL750

p-((4-AMINO-m-TOLYL)AZO)BENZENESULFONAMIDE see III:SNX000

AMINOTRIACETIC ACID see I:AMT500

AMINOTRIAZOLE see I:AMY050

AMINOTRIAZOLE (plant regulator) see I:AMY050

2-AMINOTRIAZOLE see I:AMY050

3-AMINOTRIAZOLE see I:AMY050

3-AMINO-s-TRIAZOLE see I:AMY050

2-AMINO-1,3,4-TRIAZOLE see I:AMY050

3-AMINO-1,2,4-TRIAZOLE see I:AMY050

3-AMINO-1H-1,2,4-TRIAZOLE see I:AMY050

AMINO TRIAZOLE WEEDKILLER 90 see I:AMY050

AMINOTRIAZOL-SPRITZPULVER see I:AMY050

4-AMINO-3,5,6-TRICHLOROPICOLINIC ACID see III:PIB900

4-AMINO-3,5,6-TRICHLORO-2-PICOLINIC ACID see III:PIB900

4-AMINO-3,5,6-TRICHLORPICOLINSAEURE (GERMAN) see III:PIB900

1-AMINO-2,4,6-TRIMETHYLBENZEN (CZECH) see III:TLG500

1-AMINO-2,4,5-TRIMETHYLBENZENE see I:TLG250

2-AMINO-1,3,5-TRIMETHYLBENZENE see III:TLG500

1-AMINO-2,4,5-TRIMETHYLBENZENE HYDROCHLORIDE see III:TLG750

2-AMINO-1,3-5-TRIMETHYLBENZENE HYDROCHLORIDE see II:TLH000

AMINOUNDECANOIC ACID see III:AMW000

11-AMINOUNDECANOIC ACID see III:AMW000

11-AMINOUNDECYLIC ACID see III:AMW000

AMINOURACIL MUSTARD see II:BIA250

AMINOUREA see III:HGU000

AMINOUREA HYDROCHLORIDE see III:SBW500

2-AMINO-1,4-XYLENE see III:XNA000

4-AMINO-1,3-XYLENE see II:XMS000

2-AMINO-1,4-XYLENE HYDROCHLORIDE see III:XOS000

4-AMINO-1,3-XYLENE HYDROCHLORIDE see III:XOJ000

2-AMINO-4,5-XYLENOL see III:AMW750

AMINOZIDE see II:DQD400

1,2,-AMINOZOPHENYLENE see III:BDH250

AMINZOL SOLUBLE see III:ALQ000

AMIP 15m see III:TAI250

AMIPROL see III:DCK759

AMITOL see I:AMY050

AMITRIL T.L. see I:AMY050

AMITROL see I:AMY050

AMITROL 90 see I:AMY050

AMITROLE see I:AMY050

AMITROLE-T see I:AMY050

AMIZOL see I:AMY050

AMMN see II:AAW000

AMMOFORM see III:HEI500

AMMOIDIN see I:XDJ000

AMMONIOFORMALDEHYDE see III:HEI500

AMMONIUM CADMIUM CHLORIDE see I:AND250

AMMONIUM CARBOXYMETHYL CELLULOSE see III:CCH000

AMMONIUM, (4-((4,6-DIAMINO-m-TOLYL)IMINO)-2,5-CY-CLOHEXADIEN-1-YLIDENE)DIMETHYL-, CHLORIDE, MONOHYDRATE see III:TGU500

AMMONIUM-N-NITROSOPHENYLHYDROXYLAMINE see I:ANO500

AMMONIUM POTASSIUM SELENIDE mixed with AMMONIUM POTASSIUM SULFIDE see III:ANT250
AMMONIUM POTASSIUM SULFIDE mixed with AMMONIUM POTASSIUM SELENIDE see III:ANT250
AMN see II:AOL000
AMNESTROGEN see I:ECU750
AMOBEN see III:AJM000
AMOCO 1010 see III:PMP500
AMOKIN see III:CLD000
AMORPHOUS CROCIDOLITE ASBESTOS see I:ARM275
AMORPHOUS FUSED SILICA see I:SCK600
AMORPHOUS SILICA DUST see III:SCH000
AMOSITE ASBESTOS see I:ARM262
AMOSITE (OBS.) see I:ARM250
AMOTRIL see III:ARQ750
AMOXONE see I:DAA800
AMPHENICOL see II:CDP250
AMPHIBOLE see I:ARM250
AMPHICOL see II:CDP250
AMPROLENE see I:EJN500
AMSECLOR see II:CDP250
AMSINCKIA INTERMEDIA see III:TAG250
AMUDANE see GKE000
AMYL ALCOHOL see III:AOE000
N-AMYL ALCOHOL see III:AOE000
AMYL ALCOHOL, NORMAL see III:AOE000
N-AMYLALKOHOL (CZECH) see III:AOE000
5-n-AMYL-1:2-BENZANTHRACENE see III:AOE750
n-AMYLHYDRAZINE HYDROCHLORIDE see III:PBX250
n-AMYL-N-METHYLNITROSAMINE see II:AOL000
n-AMYLNITROSOUREA see III:PBX500
1-AMYL-1-NITROSOUREA see III:PBX500
n-AMYL-N-NITROSOURETHANE see III:AOL750
AMYLOFENE see II:EOK000
AMYLOPECTINE SULPHATE see III:AOM150
AMYLOPECTIN, HYDROGEN SULFATE see III:AOM150
AMYLOPECTIN SULFATE see III:AOM150
AMYLOPECTIN SULFATE (SN-263) see III:AOM150
AMYLOWY ALKOHOL (POLISH) see III:IHP000
4-n-AMYLPHENOL see III:AOM250
2-sec-AMYLPHENOL see III:AOM500
4-sec-AMYLPHENOL see III:AOM750
AMYL ZIMATE see III:BJK500
ANABOLIN see III:DAL300
ANAC 110 see III:CNI000
ANACETIN see II:CDP250
ANADOMIS GREEN see II:CMJ900
ANADROL see I:PAN100
ANADROYD see I:PAN100
ANAFEBRINA see III:DOT000
ANAFLON see II:HIM000
ANAGESTONE ACETATE mixed with MESTRANOL (10:1) see III:AOO000
ANAGIARDIL see I:MMN250
ANAMENTH see II:TIO750
ANAPAC see I:ABG750
ANAPOLON see I:PAN100
ANASTERON see I:PAN100
ANASTERONAL see I:PAN100
ANASTERONE see I:PAN100
ANATROPIN mixed with MESTRANOL (10:1) see III:AOO000
ANCHRED STANDARD see III:IHD000
ANCOR EN 80/150 see III:IGK800
ANCORTONE see III:PLZ000
ANDRAZIDE see III:ILD000
ANDREZ see III:SMR000
ANDROGEN see I:TBG000
ANDROLIN see I:TBF500
ANDROMETH see III:MPN500
ANDRONAQ see I:TBF500
ANDROSAN see I:TBG000, III:MPN500
ANDROSAN (tablets) see III:MPN500
ANDROSTEN see III:MPN500
Δ-(⁴)-ANDROSTEN-3,17-DIONE see III:AOO425

ANDROSTENEDIONE see III:AOO425
4-ANDROSTENE-3,17-DIONE see III:AOO425
Δ-4-ANDROSTENEDIONE see III:AOO425
Δ(⁴)-ANDROSTENE-3,17-DIONE see III:AOO425
4-ANDROSTENE-17-α-METHYL-17-β-OL-3-ONE see III:MPN500
Δ⁴-ANDROSTENE-17-β-PROPIONATE-3-ONE see I:TBG000
ANDROSTENOLONE see III:AOO450
ANDROST-4-EN-17β-OL-3-ONE see I:TBF500
Δ⁴-ANDROSTEN-17(β)-OL-3-ONE see I:TBF500
ANDROTARDYL see III:TBF750
ANDROTESTON see I:TBG000
ANDROTEST P see I:TBG000
ANDROTEX see III:AOO425
ANDRUSOL see I:TBF500
ANDRUSOL-P see I:TBG000
ANELIX see II:HIM000
ANERTAN see I:TBG000, III:MPN500
ANERTAN (tablets) see III:MPN500
ANERVAL see II:BRF500
ANESTHETIC COMPOUND No. 347 see III:EAT900
ANETHOLE (FCC) see III:PMQ750
ANFRAM 3PB see I:TNC500
ANFT see III:ALM500
ANGECIN see III:FQC000
β-ANGELICA LACTONE see III:MKH500
Δ¹-ANGELICA LACTONE see III:MKH500
ANGELICIN (coumarin deriv) see III:FQC000
ANGIFLAN see III:DBX400
ANGININE see III:NGY000
ANGIOKAPSUL see III:ARQ750
ANG.-STERANTHREN (GERMAN) see III:DCR800
ANG-STERANTHRENE see III:DCR800
ANHIBA see II:HIM000
ANHYDRIDE ARSENIEUX (FRENCH) see I:ARI750
ANHYDRIDE ARSENIQUE (FRENCH) see I:ARH500
ANHYDRIDE CHROMIQUE (FRENCH) see I:CMK000
ANHYDRO-4,4'-BIS(DIETHYLAMINO)TRIPHENYLMETHANOL-2',4''-DI-SULPHONIC ACID,MONOSODIUM SALT see III:ADE500
3,6-ANHYDRO-d-GALACTAN see III:CCL250
ANHYDROGLUCOCHLORAL see III:GFA000
ANHYDROL see I:EFU000
ANHYDRO-o-SULFAMINE BENZOIC ACID see II:BCE500
ANHYDROUS DEXTROSE see III:GFG000
ANHYDROUS HYDRAZINE (DOT) see I:HGS000
ANHYDROUS IRON OXIDE see III:IHD000
ANHYDROUS OXIDE of IRON see III:IHD000
ANICON KOMBI see II:CIR250
ANICON M see II:CIR250
ANIDRIDE CROMICA (ITALIAN) see I:CMK000
ANIDRIDE CROMIQUE (FRENCH) see II:CMJ900
ANILIN (CZECH) see II:AOQ000
ANILINA (ITALIAN, POLISH) see II:AOQ000
ANILINE see II:AOQ000
ANILINE, p-(7-BENZOFURYLAZO)-N,N-DIMETHYL- see III:BCL100
ANILINE, N,N-BIS(2-CHLOROETHYL)-2,3-DIMETHOXY- see III:BIC600
ANILINE, N,N-BIS(2-(2,3-EPOXYPROPOXY)ETHOXY)- see III:BJN850
ANILINE, N,N-BIS(2-(2,3-EPOXYPROPOXY)ETHYL)- see III:BJN875
ANILINE, p-((3-BROMO-4-ETHYLPHENYL)AZO)-N,N-DI-METHYL- see III:BNK275
ANILINE, p-((4-BROMO-3-ETHYLPHENYL)AZO)-N,N-DI-METHYL- see III:BNK100
ANILINE, p-(m-BROMOPHENYLAZO)-N,N-DIMETHYL- see III:BNE600
ANILINE, p-((3-BROMO-p-TOLYL)AZO)-N,N-DIMETHYL- see III:BNQ100
ANILINE, p-((4-BROMO-m-TOLYL)AZO)-N,N-DIMETHYL- see III:BNQ110
ANILINE, p-((p-BUTYLPHENYL)AZO)-N,N-DIMETHYL- see III:BRB450

ANILINE, p-((p-(tert-BUTYL)PHENYL)AZO)-N,N-DIMETHYL- see III:BRB460
ANILINE CARMINE POWDER see III:FAE100
ANILINE CHLORIDE see II:BBL000
ANILINE, N,N-DIMETHYL-p-(4'-CHLORO-3'-METHYLPHE-NYLAZO)- see III:CIL710
ANILINE, N,N-DIMETHYL-p-(3,5-DIFLUOROPHENYLAZO)- see III:DKH100
ANILINE, p-((o-ETHYLPHENYL)AZO)-N,N-DIMETHYL- see III:EIF450
ANILINE HYDROCHLORIDE (DOT) see II:BBL000
ANILINE OIL see II:AOQ000
"ANILINE SALT" see II:BBL000
p-ANILINESULFONAMIDE see III:SNM500
ANILINE-p-SULFONIC AMIDE see III:SNM500
ANILINE VIOLET see III:AOR500
ANILINE YELLOW see II:PEI000
ANILINIUM CHLORIDE see II:BBL000
ANILINONAPHTHALENE see II:PFT500
1-ANILINONAPHTHALENE see III:PFT250
2-ANILINONAPHTHALENE see II:PFT500
ANISE CAMPHOR see III:PMQ750
ANISENE see II:CLO750
ANISIC ACID HYDRAZIDE see III:AOV500
o-ANISIC ACID, HYDRAZIDE see III:AOV250
p-ANISIC ACID, HYDRAZIDE see III:AOV500
ANISIC HYDRAZIDE see III:AOV500
2-ANISIDINE see II:AOV900
o-ANISIDINE see II:AOV900
o-ANISIDINE HYDROCHLORIDE see I:AOX250
p-ANISIDINE HYDROCHLORIDE see III:AOX500
o-ANISIDINE NITRATE see II:NEQ500
ANISOLE, p-(3-BROMOPROPENYL)-, (E)- see III:BMT300
ANISOPYRADAMINE see III:DBM800
ANISOYLHYDRAZINE see III:AOV500
p-ANISOYLHYDRAZINE see III:AOV500
2-(p-ANISYL)ACETIC ACID see III:MFE250
o-ANISYLAMINE see II:AOV900
ANISYL FORMATE see III:MFE250
ANKILOSTIN see II:PCF275
ANN (GERMAN) see II:AAW000
ANNALINE see III:CAX750
ANNONA MURICATA see III:SKV500
(6)ANNULENE see I:BBL250
ANOFEX see I:DAD200
ANOVIGAM see III:EEM000
ANOVLAR 21 see II:EEH520
ANPARTON see III:ARQ750
ANPROLENE see I:EJN500
ANPROLINE see I:EJN500
ANPUZONE see II:BRF500
ANSAR see III:HKC000
ANSAR 160 see I:HKC500
ANSAR 184 see I:DXE600
ANSAR DSMA LIQUID see I:DXE600
ANSIBASE RED KB see II:CLK225
ANSIOLIN see III:DCK759
ANSIOLISINA see III:CFZ000, III:DCK759
ANSIOXACEPAM see III:CFZ000
ANTABUS see III:DXH250
ANTABUSE see III:DXH250
ANTADIX see III:DXH250
ANTADOL see II:BRF500
ANTAENYL see III:DXH250
ANTAETHAN see III:DXH250
ANTAETHYL see III:DXH250
ANTAETIL see III:DXH250
ANTAGOTHYROID see III:TFR250
ANTAGOTHYROIL see III:TFR250
ANTAK see III:DAI600
ANTALCOL see III:DXH250
ANTENE see III:BJK500
ANTERIOR PITUITARY GROWTH HORMONE see III:PJA250
ANTETAN see III:DXH250

ANTETHYL see III:DXH250
ANTETIL see III:DXH250
ANTEYL see III:DXH250
ANTHANTHREN (GERMAN) see III:APE750
ANTHANTHRENE see III:APE750
ANTHGLUTIN see III:GFO100
ANTHISAN MALEATE see III:DBM800
ANTHON see III:TIQ250
ANTHOPHYLITE see I:ARM264
ANTHRA(9,1,2-cde)BENZO(h)CINNOLINE see III:APF750
ANTHRACEN (GERMAN) see III:APG500
1-ANTHRACENAMINE see III:APG250
2-ANTHRACENAMINE see III:APG000
ANTHRACENE see III:APG500
9,10-ANTHRACENEDIONE, 1,4-DIAMINO-5-NITRO-(9CI) see III:DBY700
1,8,9-ANTHRACENETRIOL see III:APH250
9(10H)-ANTHRACENONE, 1,8-DIHYDROXY-10-(1-OXOPRO-PYL)- see III:PMW760
ANTHRACIN see III:APG500
ANTHRACITE PARTICLES see III:CMY635
1-ANTHRACYLAMINE see III:APG250
2-ANTHRACYLAMINE see II:APG000
ANTHRALAN YELLOW RRT see III:SGP500
ANTHRALIN see III:APH250
1-ANTHRAMINE see III:APG250
2-ANTHRAMINE see II:APG000
ANTHRANILIC ACID see III:API500
ANTHRANILIC ACID, CINNAMYL ESTER see II:API750
ANTHRANTHRENE see III:APE750
β-ANTHRAQUINOLINE see III:NAZ000
α-ANTHRAQUINONYLAMINE see III:AIA750
β-ANTHRAQUINONYLAMINE see I:AIB000
1,8,9-ANTHRATRIOL see III:APH250
ANTHRAVAT GOLDEN YELLOW see III:DCZ000
9-ANTHRONOL see III:APM750
ANTHROPODEOXYCHOLIC ACID see III:CDL325
ANTHROPODESOXYCHOLIC ACID see III:CDL325
ANTHROPODODESOXYCHOLIC ACID see III:CDL325
2-ANTHRYLAMINE see II:APG000
ANTIAETHAN see III:DXH250
ANTIBASON see II:MPW500
ANTIBIOTIC A 3733A see III:HAL000
ANTIBIOTIC S 7481F1 see III:CQH100
ANTIBIOTIC U 18496 see III:ARY000
ANTIBULIT see III:SHF500
ANTICARIE see I:HCC500
ANTIETANOL see III:DXH250
ANTIETIL see III:DXH250
ANTIFOLAN see III:MDV500
ANTI-GERM 77 see III:BEN000
ANTIGESTIL see I:DKA600
ANTIHIST see III:DBM800
ANTIKOL see III:DXH250
ANTILEPSIN see I:DNU000
ANTILIPID see III:ARQ750
ANTIMICINA see III:ILD000
ANTIMIT see I:BIE500
ANTIMONIOUS OXIDE see I:AQF000
ANTIMONY see III:AQB750
ANTIMONY BLACK see III:AQB750
ANTIMONY, compounded with NICKEL (1:1) see III:NCY100
ANTIMONY OXIDE see I:AQF000
ANTIMONY PEROXIDE see I:AQF000
ANTIMONY REGULUS see III:AQB750
ANTIMONY SESQUIOXIDE see I:AQF000
ANTIMONY TRIOXIDE (MAK) see I:AQF000
ANTIMONY WHITE see I:AQF000
ANTIMYCIN see III:CMS775
ANTIOXIDANT 29 see III:BFW750
ANTIOXIDANT 116 see II:PFT500
ANTIOXIDANT DBPC see III:BFW750
ANTIOXIDANT PBN see II:PFT500
ANTIPYRINE see III:AQN000

(ANTIPYRINYLMETHYLAMINO)METHANESULFONIC ACID SODIUM SALT see III:AMK500
ANTI-RUST see III:SIQ500
ANTISACER see I:DKQ000, I:DNU000
ANTISEPTOL see III:BEN000
ANTISOL 1 see II:PCF275
ANTISTREPT see III:SNM500
ANTITUBERKULOSUM see III:ILD000
ANTIVITIUM see III:DXH250
ANTRANCINE 12 see II:BQI000
ANTRAPUROL see III:DMH400
ANTU see III:AQN635
ANTURAT see III:AQN635
ANTYMON (POLISH) see III:AQB750
ANTYWYLEGACZ see III:CMF400
ANU see III:PBX500
ANUSPIRAMIN see II:BRF500
ANXIOLIT see III:CFZ000
AO 29 see III:BFW750
AO 4K see III:BFW750
AOM see II:ASP250
AP see III:PEK250
A1-0109 P see III:AHE250
APADODINE see III:DXX400
APADON see II:HIM000
APAMIDE see II:HIM000
APAMIDON see III:FAC025
APAP see II:HIM000
APARSIN see I:BBQ500
APAURIN see III:DCK759
APC see I:ABG750
APC (pharmaceutical) see III:ARP250
APCO 2330 see III:PEY000
APELAGRIN see III:NCQ900
APEX 462-5 see I:TNC500
APGA see III:AMG750
APH see III:ACX750
APHAMITE see III:PAK000
APHENYLBARBIT see II:EOK000
APHENYLETTEN see II:EOK000
APHOSAL see III:GFA000
APHOXIDE see III:TND250
APHTIRIA see I:BBQ500
APLAKIL see III:CFZ000
APLIDAL see I:BBQ500
APO see III:TND250
APOCHOLIC ACID see III:AQO500
APOCID ORANGE 2G see III:HGC000
APOLAN see III:ARQ750
A 15 (POLYMER) see II:AAX175
APOMINE BLACK GX see I:AQP000, I:AQP000
APOZEPAM see III:DCK759
APPEX see III:RAF100
APPRESINUM see II:HGP500
APPRESSIN see III:PHW000
APRELAZINE see II:HGP500
APRESAZIDE see II:HGP500
APRESINE see II:HGP500
APRESOLIN see II:HGP500, III:PHW000
APRESOLINE-ESIDRIX see II:HGP500
APRESOLINE HYDROCHLORIDE see II:HGP500
APREZOLIN see II:HGP500, III:PHW000
APYONINE AURAMINE BASE see I:IBB000
AQUACAT see I:CNA250
AQUACHLORAL see III:CDO000
AQUACRINE see I:EDV000
AQUAFIL see III:SCH000
AQUAKAY see III:MMD500
AQUA-KLEEN see II:DAA800
AQUALINE see III:ADR000
AQUAMYCETIN see II:CDP250
AQUAPLAST see III:SFO500
AQUA-VEX see II:TIX500
AQUAVIRON see I:TBG000

AQUAZINE see III:BJP000
AQUINONE see III:MMD500
ARABINOCYTIDINE see III:AQQ750
1-β-d-ARABINOFURANOSYL-4-AMINO-2(1H)PYRIMIDINONE see III:AQQ750
1-ARABINOFURANOSYLCYTOSINE see III:AQQ750
1-β-ARABINOFURANOSYLCYTOSINE see III:AQQ750
1-(β-d-ARABINOFURANOSYL)CYTOSINE see III:AQQ750
β-d-ARABINOSYLCYTOSINE see III:AQQ750
ARACHIC ACID see III:EAF000
ARACHIDIC ACID see III:EAF000
ARACHIS OIL see III:PAO000
ARACIDE see I:SOP500
ARALDITE ERE 1359 see II:REF000
ARALDITE 6010 mixed with ERR 4205 (1:1) see III:OPI200
ARALEN see III:CLD000
ARALO see III:PAK000
ARAMITE see I:SOP500
ARAMITEARARAMITE-15W see I:SOP500
ARANCIO CROMO (ITALIAN) see I:LCS000
ARASAN see III:TFS350
ARATHANE see III:AQT500
ARATRON see I:SOP500
ARBITEX see I:BBQ500
ARCHIDYN see II:RKP000
ARCTON 4 see III:CFX500
ARCTUVIN see III:HIH000
ARECA CATECHU see II:BFW000
ARECA CATECHU Linn., fruit extract see II:BFW000
ARECA CATECHU Linn., nut extract see II:BFW000
ARECAIDINE METHYL ESTER see III:AQT750
ARECA NUT see III:AQT650
ARECOLINE see III:AQT750
ARECOLINE BASE see III:AQT750
ARECOLINE HYDROCHLORIDE see III:AQU250
AREGINAL see III:EKL000
ARETIT see III:BRE500
ARFICIN see II:RKP000
ARGEMONE OIL mixed with MUSTARD OIL see III:OGS000
ARGENTUM see III:SDI500
ARGEZIN see III:ARQ725
ARISTOLOCHIC ACID see AQY250
ARISTOLOCHIC ACID SODIUM SALT see III:AQY125
ARISTOLOCHINE see AQY250
ARIZOLE see III:PMQ750
ARKOTINE see I:DAD200
ARLANTHRENE GOLDEN YELLOW see III:DCZ000
ARMACIDE see III:ILD000
ARMCO IRON see III:IGK800
ARMENIAN BOLE see III:IHD000
ARMODOUR see III:PKQ059
ARMOTAN PMO-20 see III:PKL100
ARNITE A see III:PKF750
AROCHLOR 1221 see II:PJM000
AROCHLOR 1242 see II:PJM500
AROCHLOR 1254 see II:PJN000
AROCHLOR 1260 see II:PJN250
AROCLOR see I:PJL750
AROCLOR 1232 see II:PJM250
AROCLOR 1242 see II:PJM500
AROCLOR 1248 see II:PJM750
AROCLOR 1254 see II:PJN000
AROCLOR 1260 see II:PJN250
AROCLOR 1262 see II:PJN500
AROCLOR 1268 see II:PJN750
AROCLOR 2565 see II:PJO000
AROCLOR 4465 see II:PJO250
ARON COMPOUND HW see III:PKQ059
ARRHENAL see I:DXE600
ARSAMBIDE see III:CBJ000
ARSAN see III:HKC000
ARSECODILE see I:HKC500
ARSENATE see ARB250
ARSENATE of IRON, FERRIC see I:IGN000

ARSENATE of IRON, FERROUS see I:IGM000
ARSENATE of LEAD see I:LCK000
ARSENENOUS ACID, POTASSIUM SALT see I:PKV500
ARSENENOUS ACID, SODIUM SALT (9CI) see I:SEY500
ARSENIATE de CALCIUM (FRENCH) see I:ARB750
ARSENIATE de MAGNESIUM (FRENCH) see I:ARD000
ARSENIATE de PLOMB (FRENCH) see I:ARC750
ARSENIC see ARA750
ARSENIC-75 see ARA750
ARSENIC ACID see I:ARH500
m-ARSENIC ACID see ARB000
o-ARSENIC ACID see ARB250
ARSENIC ACID ANHYDRIDE see I:ARH500
ARSENIC ACID, CALCIUM SALT (2:3) see I:ARB750
ARSENIC ACID, DISODIUM SALT see I:ARC000
ARSENIC ACID, DISODIUM SALT, HEPTAHYDRATE see
    I:ARC250
o-ARSENIC ACID, HEMIHYDRATE see I:ARC500
ARSENIC ACID, LEAD SALT see I:ARC750
ARSENIC ACID, LIQUID (DOT) see I:ARB250
ARSENIC ACID, MAGNESIUM SALT see I:ARD000
ARSENIC ACID, MONOPOTASSIUM SALT see I:ARD250
ARSENIC ACID, MONOSODIUM SALT see I:ARD500,
    I:ARD600
ARSENIC ACID, SODIUM SALT see I:ARD750
ARSENIC ACID, SODIUM SALT (9CI) see I:ARD500
ARSENIC ACID, SOLID (DOT) see I:ARB250, I:ARC500
ARSENIC(V) ACID, TRISODIUM SALT, HEPTAHYDRATE
    (1:3:7) see I:ARE000
ARSENIC ACID, ZINC SALT see I:ZDJ000
ARSENICAL DUST see III:ARE500
ARSENICAL FLUE DUST see III:ARE500
ARSENICAL FLUE DUST (DOT) see I:ARE750
ARSENICALS see ARA750, I:ARF750
ARSENICAL SOLUTION see I:FOM050
ARSENIC ANHYDRIDE see I:ARH500
ARSENIC BLACK see ARA750
ARSENIC BLANC (FRENCH) see I:ARI750
ARSENIC COMPOUNDS see I:ARF750
ARSENIC FLUORIDE see I:ARI250
ARSENIC HYDRIDE see I:ARK250
ARSENIC OXIDE see I:ARH500, I:ARI750
ARSENIC(III) OXIDE see I:ARI750
ARSENIC(V) OXIDE see I:ARH500
ARSENIC PENTOXIDE see I:ARH500
ARSENIC SESQUIOXIDE see I:ARI750
ARSENIC SESQUISULFIDE see I:ARI000
ARSENIC SULFIDE see I:ARI000
ARSENIC SULFIDE YELLOW see I:ARI000
ARSENIC SULPHIDE see I:ARI000
ARSENIC TRIFLUORIDE see I:ARI250
ARSENIC TRIHYDRIDE see I:ARK250
ARSENIC TRIOXIDE see I:ARI750
ARSENIC TRIOXIDE mixed with SELENIUM DIOXIDE
    (1:1) see I:ARJ000
ARSENIC TRISULFIDE see I:ARI000
ARSENIC YELLOW see I:ARI000
ARSENIGEN SAURE (GERMAN) see I:ARI750
ARSENIOUS ACID (MAK) see I:ARI750
ARSENIOUS ACID SODIUM SALT see I:ARJ500, I:SEY500
ARSENIOUS ACID, SODIUM SALT POLYMERS see I:ARJ500
ARSENIOUS ACID, STRONTIUM SALT see I:SME500
ARSENIOUS ACID, ZINC SALT see I:ZDS000
ARSENIOUS OXIDE see I:ARI750
ARSENIOUS SULPHIDE see I:ARI000
ARSENIOUS TRIOXIDE see I:ARI750
ARSENITE de POTASSIUM (FRENCH) see I:PKV500
ARSENITE de SODIUM (FRENCH) see I:SEY500
ARSENIURETTED HYDROGEN see I:ARK250
ARSENOUS ACID see I:ARI750
ARSENOUS ACID ANHYDRIDE see I:ARI750
ARSENOUS ANHYDRIDE see I:ARI750
ARSENOUS FLUORIDE see I:ARI250
ARSENOUS HYDRIDE see I:ARK250

ARSENOUS OXIDE see I:ARI750
ARSENOUS OXIDE ANHYDRIDE see I:ARI750
ARSENOUS SULFIDE see I:ARI000
ARSENOWODOR (POLISH) see I:ARK250
ARSEN (GERMAN, POLISH) see ARA750
ARSENWASSERSTOFF (GERMAN) see I:ARK250
ARSINE see I:ARK250
ARSINETTE see I:LCK000
ARSINYL see I:DXE600
ARSONIC ACID, POTASSIUM SALT see I:PKV500
ARSONIC ACID, SODIUM SALT (9CI) see I:ARJ500
p-ARSONOPHENYLUREA see III:CBJ000
ARSYCODILE see I:HKC500
ARSYNAL see I:DXE600
ARTERIOFLEXIN see III:ARQ750
ARTEROSOL see III:ARQ750
ARTES see III:ARQ750
ARTEVIL see III:ARQ750
ARTHROCHIN see III:CLD000
ARTIC see II:MIF765
ARTIFICIAL BARITE see III:BAP000
ARTIFICIAL HEAVY SPAR see III:BAP000
ARTIFICIAL MUSTARD OIL see II:AGJ250
ARTIFICIAL SWEETENING SUBSTANZ GENDORF 450 see
    II:SJN700
ARTISIL BLUE SAP see III:TBG700
ARTISIL ORANGE 3RP see I:AKP750
ARTIZIN see II:BRF500
ARTRIONA see III:CNS825
ARTRIZONE see II:BRF500
ARTROFLOG see III:HNI500
ARTROPAN see II:BRF500
ARUMEL see III:FMM000
ARWOOD COPPER see III:CNI000
AS-17665 see II:NDY500
ASA COMPOUND see I:ABG750
ASARON see III:IHX400
ASARONE see III:IHX400
α-ASARONE see III:IHX400
ASARONE, trans- see III:IHX400
trans-ASARONE see III:IHX400
ASARUM CAMPHOR see III:IHX400
ASBEST (GERMAN) see I:ARM250
ASBESTINE see III:TAB750
ASBESTOS see I:ARM250
7-45 ASBESTOS see I:ARM268
ASBESTOS (ACGIH) see I:ARM260, I:ARM262, I:ARM264,
    I:ARM268, I:ARM275, I:ARM280
ASBESTOS, ACTINOLITE see I:ARM260
ASBESTOS, AMOSITE see I:ARM262
ASBESTOS, ANTHOPHYLITE see I:ARM264
ASBESTOS, ANTHOPHYLLITE see I:ARM266
ASBESTOS, CHRYSOTILE see I:ARM268
ASBESTOS, CROCIDOLITE see I:ARM275
ASBESTOS FIBER see I:ARM250
ASBESTOS, TREMOLITE see I:ARM280
ASBESTOS, WHITE (DOT) see I:ARM268
ASCARIDOLE see III:ARM500
ASCARISIN see III:ARM500
ASCARYL see III:HFV500
ASCOPHEN see III:ARP250
ASHLENE see III:NOH000
ASIATICOSIDE see III:ARN500
ASIDON 3 see III:TEH500
ASMADION see III:TEH500
ASMAVAL see III:TEH500
A 1 (SORBENT) see III:AHE250
ASPARAGINASE see III:ARN800
l-ASPARAGINASE see III:ARN800
l-ASPARAGINASE X see III:ARN800
l-ASPARAGINASI (ITALIAN) see III:ARN800
l-ASPARAGINE AMIDOHYDROLASE see III:ARN800
ASPHALT see II:ARO500
ASPHALT, PETROLEUM see III:PCR500

ASPHALTUM see II:ARO500
ASPIRIN, PHENACETIN and CAFFEINE see III:ARP250
ASPON-CHLORDANE see II:CDR750
ASPOR see III:EIR000
ASPORUM see III:EIR000
ASSAM TEA see III:ARP500
ASSIFLAVINE see III:DBX400
ASSIVAL see III:DCK759
ASSUGRIN see III:SGC000
ASSUGRIN FEINUSS see III:SGC000
ASSUGRIN VOLLSUSS see III:SGC000
ASTA see I:EAS500
ASTA B518 see I:EAS500
ASTA Z 4942 see II:IMH000
ASTRA CHRYSOIDINE R see III:PEK000
ASTRAFER see III:IGU000
ASTRALON see III:PKQ059
ASTRAZOLO see III:SNN500
ASTRESS see III:CFZ000
ASUGRYN see III:SGC000
ASURO see III:DBD750
AT see I:AMY050
AT 7 see III:HCL000
o-AT see I:AIC250
AT-290 see I:PED750
AT 717 see III:PKQ250
ATA see I:AMY050
ATACTIC POLYPROPYLENE see III:PMP500
ATACTIC POLYSTYRENE see III:SMQ500
ATACTIC POLY(VINYL CHLORIDE) see III:PKQ059
ATALCO S see III:OAX000
ATAZINAX see III:ARQ725
ATCOTIBINE see III:ILD000
ATCP see III:PIB900
ATECULON see III:ARQ750
ATENSINE see III:DCK759
ATERIOSAN see III:ARQ750
ATHEBRATE see III:ARQ750
ATHEROMIDE see III:ARQ750
ATHEROPRONT see III:ARQ750
ATHRANID-WIRKSTOFF see III:ARQ750
ATILEN see III:DCK759
ATILON see III:SNY500
ATLANTIC BLACK BD see I:AQP000
ATLANTIC BLUE 2B see I:CMO000
ATLANTIC RESIN FAST BROWN BRL see II:CMO750
ATLANTIC VIOLET N see III:CMP000
ATLAS "A" see I:SEY500
ATLAS WHITE TITANIUM DIOXIDE see III:TGG760
ATLATEST see III:TBF750
AT LIQUID see I:AMY050
ATLOX 1087 see III:PKL100
ATRANEX see III:ARQ725
ATRASINE see III:ARQ725
ATRATOL A see III:ARQ725
ATRAZIN see III:ARQ725
ATRAZINE see III:ARQ725
ATRED see III:ARQ725
ATREX see III:ARQ725
ATRIVYL see I:MMN250
ATROLEN see III:ARQ750
ATROMID see III:ARQ750
ATROMIDIN see III:ARQ750
ATROMID S see III:ARQ750
ATROVIS see III:ARQ750
ATTAC 6 see I:CDV100
ATTAC 6-3 see I:CDV100
ATTAPULGITE see III:PAE750
ATUL ACID CRYSTAL ORANGE G see III:HGC000
ATUL ACID SCARLET 3R see III:FMU080
ATUL CRYSTAL RED F see III:HJF500
ATUL DIRECT BLACK E see I:AQP000
ATUL DIRECT BLUE 2B see I:CMO000
ATUL DIRECT VIOLET N see III:CMP000

ATUL FAST YELLOW R see I:DOT300
ATUL INDIGO CARMINE see III:FAE100
ATUL OIL ORANGE T see II:TGW000
ATUL ORANGE R see III:PEJ500
AUBYGEL GS see III:CCL250
AUBYGUM DM see III:CCL250
AULES see III:TFS350
AURAMINE BASE see I:IBB000
AURAMINE HYDROCHLORIDE see I:IBA000
AURAMINE (MAK) see I:IBA000, I:IBB000
AURAMINE O (BIOLOGICAL STAIN) see I:IBA000
AURAMINE YELLOW see I:IBA000
AURANILE see I:DKQ000, I:DNU000
AUREOTAN see I:ART250
AUROMYOSE see I:ART250
AURORA YELLOW see I:CAJ750
AUROTAN see I:ART250
1-AUROTHIO-d-GLUCOPYRANOSE see I:ART250
AUROTHIOGLUCOSE see I:ART250
AURUMINE see I:ART250
AUSTIOX see III:TGG760
AUSTRACIL see II:CDP250
AUSTRACOL see II:CDP250
AUSTRIAN CINNABAR see I:LCS000
AUSTROMINAL see II:EOK000
AUTHRON see I:ART250
AUTOMOBILE EXHAUST CONDENSATE see III:GCE000
AVADEX see III:DBI200
AVERSAN see III:DXH250
AVERZAN see III:DXH250
AVIBEST C see I:ARM268
AVICOL see III:PAX000
AVISUN see III:PMP500
AVLOCLOR see III:CLD000
AVLON see III:DBX400
AVLOSULPHONE see III:SOA500
AVLOTANE see III:HCI000
AWPA #1 see I:CMY825
AY 61123 see III:ARQ750
AYERST 62013 see III:TJQ333
12-AZABENZ(a)ANTHRACENE see III:BAW750
AZACITIDINE see III:ARY000
2-AZACYCLOHEPTANONE see III:CBF700
AZACYCLOPROPANE see I:EJM900
AZACYTIDINE see III:ARY000
5-AZACYTIDINE see III:ARY000
5'-AZACYTIDINE see III:ARY000
7-AZADIBENZ(a,h)ANTHRACENE see I:DCS400
7-AZADIBENZ(a,j)ANTHRACENE see I:DCS600
14-AZADIBENZ(a,j)ANTHRACENE see III:DCS800
7-AZA-7H-DIBENZO(c,g)FLUORENE see I:DCY000
9-AZAFLUORENE see III:CBN000
2-AZAHYPOXANTHINE see III:ARY500
1-AZAINDENE see III:ICM000
1-AZANAPHTHALENE see III:QMJ000
AZANIL RED SALT TRD see II:CLK235
AZANIN see I:ASB250
AZAPICYL see III:ADA000
AZAPLANT see I:AMY050
AZASERIN see II:ASA500
AZASERINE see II:ASA500
l-AZASERINE see II:ASA500
AZATHIOPRINE see I:ASB250
AZATIOPRIN see I:ASB250
6-AZAURACIL see III:THR750
4(6)-AZAURACIL see III:THR750
AZBLLEN ASBESTOS see I:ARM266
AZBOLEN ASBESTOS see I:ARM264
AZDEL see III:PMP500
AZDID see II:BRF500
AZETYLAMINOFLUOREN (GERMAN) see I:FDR000
AZIDE see III:SFA000
AZIDINE BLUE 3B see II:CMO250
AZIMETHYLENE see I:DCP800

AZIMIDOBENZENE see III:BDH250
AZIMINOBENZENE see III:BDH250
AZINE DEEP BLACK EW see I:AQP000
AZINFOS-METHYL (DUTCH) see III:ASH500
AZINPHOS METHYL see III:ASH500
AZINPHOS METHYL, liquid (DOT) see III:ASH500
AZINPHOS-METILE (ITALIAN) see III:ASH500
AZIONYL see III:ARQ750
AZIRANE see I:EJM900
AZIRIDIN (GERMAN) see I:EJM900
AZIRIDINE see I:EJM900
1-AZIRIDINECARBOXANILIDE see III:PEH250
1-AZIRIDINE ETHANOL see III:ASI000
1-(1-AZIRIDINYL)-N-(m-CHLOROPHENYL)FORMAMIDE see
   III:CJR250
6-(1-AZIRIDINYL)-4-CHLORO-2-PHENYLPYRIMIDINE see
   III:CGW750
2-(1-AZIRIDINYL)ETHANOL see III:ASI000
1-(1-AZIRIDINYL)-N-(p-METHOXYPHENYL)FORMAMIDE
   see III:MFF250
1-AZIRIDINYL PHOSPHINE OXIDE (TRIS) (DOT) see
   III:TND250
AZIRIDYL BENZOQUINONE see III:BDC750
AZIUM see III:SFA000
AZOAETHAN (GERMAN) see III:ASN250
AZOAMINE SCARLET see II:NEQ500
AZOBENZEEN (DUTCH) see III:ASL250
AZOBENZEN (CZECH) see III:COX250
AZOBENZENE see III:ASL250
AZOBENZIDE see III:ASL250
AZOBENZOL see III:ASL250
AZOBISBENZENE see III:ASL250
AZOBUTYL see II:BRF500
AZOCARD BLACK EW see I:AQP000
AZOCARD BLUE 2B see I:CMO000
AZOCARD VIOLET N see III:CMP000
AZODIBENZENE see III:ASL250
AZODIBENZENEAZOFUME see III:ASL250
AZODINE see I:PDC250
N,N'-(AZODI-4,1-PHENYLENE)BIS(N-METHYLACET-
   AMIDE) see III:DQH200
AZODIUM see I:PDC250
AZO DYE No. 6945 see III:MIH500
AZODYNE see I:PDC250
AZOENE FAST BLUE BASE see I:DCJ200
AZOENE FAST RED KB BASE see II:CLK225
AZOENE FAST RED TR BASE see II:CLK220
AZOENE FAST RED TR SALT see II:CLK235
AZO ETHANE see III:ASN250
AZOFIX BLUE B SALT see I:DCJ200
AZOFIX SCARLET G SALT see I:NMP500
AZOFOS see III:MNH000
AZO-GANTANOL see III:SNK000
AZO GANTRISIN see I:PDC250, III:SNN500
AZO GASTANOL see I:PDC250
AZOGEN DEVELOPER H see I:TGL750
AZOGENE ECARLATE R see II:NEQ500
AZOGENE FAST RED TR see II:CLK220, II:CLK235
AZOGENE FAST SCARLET G see I:NMP500
AZOGNE FAST BLUE B see I:DCJ200
AZOIC DIAZO COMPONENT 32 see II:CLK225
AZOIC DIAZO COMPONENT 11, BASE see II:CLK220,
   II:CLK235
AZOIC DIAZO COMPONENT 13, BASE see II:NEQ500
AZOIC RED 36 see I:MGO750
AZOLAN see I:AMY050
AZOLE see I:AMY050
AZOLID see II:BRF500
AZOLMETAZIN see III:SNJ000
AZO-MANDELAMINE see I:PDC250
AZOMINE see I:PDC250
AZOMINE BLACK EWO see I:AQP000
AZOMINE BLUE 2B see I:CMO000
1,1'-AZONAPHTHALENE see III:ASN500

2,2'-AZONAPHTHALENE see III:ASN750
AZOPHENYLENE see III:PDB500
AZOPHOS see III:MNH000
AZO RED R see III:FAG020
AZORUBIN see III:HJF500
AZOSEPTALE see III:TEX250
AZO-STANDARD see I:PDC250
AZO-STAT see I:PDC250
AZOSULFIZIN see III:SNN500
AZOTHIOPRINE see I:ASB250
2:3'-AZOTOLUENE see III:DQH000
AZOTOX see I:DAD200
AZOTOYPERITE see I:BIE500
AZOTREX see I:PDC250
AZOTURE de SODIUM (FRENCH) see III:SFA000
AZOXYAETHAN (GERMAN) see III:ASP000
AZOXYETHANE see III:ASP000
AZOXYISOPROPANE see III:ASP510
AZOXYMETHANE see II:ASP250
1-AZOXYPROPANE see III:ASP500
2-AZOXYPROPANE see III:ASP510
1,1'-AZOXYPROPANE see III:ASP500
AZS see II:ASA500
AZTEC BPO see III:BDS000
AZULENO(5,6,7-cd)PHENALENE see III:ASP750
AZUREN see III:ILD000
AZURRO DIRETTO 3B see II:CMO250

B10 see III:SFO500
B 10 (polysaccharide) see III:SFO500
B32 see III:HCL000
B 404 see III:PAK000
B 518 see I:EAS500
B 995 see II:DQD400
BA see I:BBC250
BA 2650 see III:SNY500
BA 5968 see II:HGP500
BA5968 see III:PHW000
BA 32644 see II:NML000
Ba 49249 see III:EEH575
BA 51-090462 see II:DCY400
BABN see III:BPV325
BABROCID see II:NGE500
B(c)AC see III:BAW750
BA 32644 CIBA see II:NML000
BACILLIN see III:ILD000
BACTERAMID see III:SNM500
BACTESULF see III:SNN500
BACTOLATEX see III:SMQ500
BACTRIM see III:SNK000
BACTROL see II:BGJ750
BADEN ACID see III:ALI300
BA-1,2-DIHYDRODIOL see III:BBD250
BA-3,4-DIHYDRODIOL see III:BBD500
BA-5,6-DIHYDRODIOL see III:BBE250
BA-8,9-DIHYDRODIOL see III:BBE750
BA-10,11-DIHYDRODIOL see III:BBF000
BA-5,6-trans-DIHYDRODIOL see III:BBE250
BA 1,2-DIOL-3,4-EPOXIDE-1 see III:DMP000
BA 3,4-DIOL-1,2-EPOXIDE-1 see III:DLE000, III:DLE200
BA 3,4-DIOL-1,2-EPOXIDE-2 see III:DLE000
BA-10,11-DIOL-8,9-EPOXIDE-1 see III:BAD000
BA 8,9-DIOL-10,11-EPOXIDE-1 see III:DMO600
BADISCHE ACID see III:ALI300
BAKELITE DYNH see III:PJS750
BAKELITE LP 70 see II:AAX175
BAKELITE SMD 3500 see III:SMQ500
BAKELITE VLFV see II:AAX175
BAKELITE VMCC see II:AAX175
BAKELITE VYNS see II:AAX175
BAKER'S P AND S LIQUID and OINTMENT see III:PDN750
BAKONTAL see III:BAP000
BALFON 7000 see III:TAI250
BAMN see III:BRX500

BANGTON see III:CBG000
BAN-HOE see III:CBM000
BAP see III:NJM500
BARAZAE see III:SNN500
BARBAPIL see II:EOK000
BARBASCO see III:RNZ000
BARBELLON see II:EOK000
BARBENYL see II:EOK000
BARBILEHAE (BARBILETTAE) see II:EOK000
BARBINAL see II:EOK000
BARBIPHENYL see II:EOK000
BARBITA see II:EOK000
BARBIVIS see II:EOK000
BARBONAL see II:EOK000
BARBOPHEN see II:EOK000
BARDIOL see I:EDO000
BARDORM see II:EOK000
BARHIST see III:DPJ400
BARIDIUM see I:PDC250
BARIDOL see III:BAP000
BARITE see III:BAP000
BARITOP see III:BAP000
BARIUM CHROMATE (1:1) see I:BAK250
BARIUM CHROMATE(VI) see I:BAK250
BARIUM CHROMATE OXIDE see I:BAK250
BARIUM SULFATE see III:BAP000
BAROSPERSE see III:BAP000
BAROTRAST see III:BAP000
BARTOL see II:EOK000
BARYTA WHITE see III:BAP000
BARYTA YELLOW see I:BAK250
BARYTES see III:BAP000
BASANITE see III:BRE500
BASE 661 see III:SMR000
BASECIL see II:MPW500
BASE OIL see III:PCR250
BASETHYRIN see II:MPW500
BASF III see III:SMQ500
BASF-MANEB SPRITZPULVER see III:MAS500
BASF URSOL D see III:PEY500
BASF URSOL SLA see I:DBO400
BASIC BLUEK see III:VKA600
BASIC CHROMIC SULFATE see III:NBW000
BASIC CHROMIC SULPHATE see III:NBW000
BASIC CHROMIUM SULFATE see III:NBW000
BASIC CHROMIUM SULPHATE see III:NBW000
BASIC LEAD ACETATE see III:LCH000
BASIC LEAD CHROMATE see I:LCS000
BASIC NICKEL CARBONATE see I:NCY500
BASIC ORANGE 3RN see III:BJF000
BASIC PARAFUCHSINE see II:RMK020
BASIC VIOLET 10 see III:FAG070
BASIC ZINC CHROMATE see I:ZFJ100
BASIC ZIRCONIUM CHLORIDE see III:ZSJ000
BASOLAN see III:MCO500
BASORA CORRA see III:BAR500
BATASAN see III:ABX250
BATAZINA see III:BJP000
BATRILEX see III:PAX000
BAUXITE RESIDUE see III:IHD000
BAY 9027 see III:ASH500
BAY 11405 see III:MNH000
BAY 15922 see III:TIQ250
BAY 29493 see III:FAQ999
BAYCID see III:FAQ999
BAY E-601 see III:MNH000
BAY E-605 see III:PAK000
BAYER 2502 see III:NGG000
BAYER 3231 see III:TND000
BAYER 5072 see III:DOU600
BAYER 5312 see III:EPQ000
BAYER 5360 see I:MMN250
BAYER 9007 see III:FAQ999
BAYER 15922 see III:TIQ250

BAYER 17147 see III:ASH500
BAYER A 139 see III:BDC750
BAYER E-605 see III:PAK000
BAYERITIAN see III:TGG760
BAYER L 13/59 see III:TIQ250
BAYER R39 SOLUBLE see III:BDC750
BAYERTITAN see III:TGG760
BAYGON, NITROSO derivative see III:PMY310
BAYOL F see III:MQV750
BAYRITES see III:BAP000
BAYTEX see III:FAQ999
BAYTITAN see III:TGG760
BBAL see III:NJO200
BBC 12 see I:DDL800
BBH see I:BBQ500
BBN see I:HJQ350
BBNOH see I:HJQ350
BBP see III:BEC500
BCF-BUSHKILLER see II:TAA100
BCME see I:BIK000
BCNU see I:BIF750
BCPN see I:BQQ250
BCS COPPER FUNGICIDE see III:CNP250
BDCM see II:BND500
BDH 1298 see II:VTF000
BDH 29-801 see III:TAI250
BD(a,h)P see II:DCY200
BE see III:BNI500
BEAMETTE see III:PMP500
BEAN SEED PROTECTANT see III:CBG000
BECOREL see I:PAN100
BEET-KLEEN see III:CBM000, III:CKC000
BEHA see III:AEO000
BEHP see I:DVL700
BELAMINE BLACK GX see I:AQP000
BELAMINE BLUE 2B see I:CMO000
BELT see II:CDR750
BELUSTINE see I:CGV250
BEMACO see III:CLD000
BEMAPHATE see III:CLD000
BEMASULPH see III:CLD000
BENCIDAL BLACK E see I:AQP000
BENCIDAL BLUE 2B see I:CMO000
BENCIDAL BLUE 3B see II:CMO250
BENCIDAL FAST IVOLET N see III:CMP000
BENDIOCARB see III:MHZ000
BENDOPA see III:DNA200
BEN-HEX see I:BBQ500
BENKFURAN see III:NGE000
BENLATE and SODIUM NITRITE see III:BAV500
BENOQUIN see III:AEY000
BENOVOCYLIN see I:EDP000
BENOXYL see III:BDS000
BENSYLYTE see I:PDT250
BENSYLYT NEN see II:DDG800
BENTONITE see III:BAV750
BENTONITE 2073 see III:BAV750
BENTONITE MAGMA see III:BAV750
BENTOX 10 see I:BBQ500
BEN-U-RON see II:HIM000
(5R,6R)-BENXYLPENICILLIN see III:BDY669
BENZAC see III:BDS000
BENZ(l)ACEANTHRENE see III:BAW000
BENZ(j)ACEANTHRYLENE see III:CMC000
BENZ(j)ACEANTHRYLENE, 1,2-DIHYDRO-3,6-DIMETHYL-
   (9CI) see III:DRD850
1,2-BENZACENAPHTHENE see III:FDF000
BENZ(k)ACEPHENANTHRENE see III:AAF000
BENZ(e)ACEPHENANTHRYLENE see I:BAW250
3,4-BENZ(e)ACEPHENANTHRYLENE see I:BAW250
BENZ(a)ACRIDIN-10-AMINE see III:AIC750
BENZ(c)ACRIDINE see III:BAW750
3,4-BENZACRIDINE see III:BAW750
7,8-BENZACRIDINE (FRENCH) see III:BAW750

BENZENECARBOPEROXOIC ACID (9CI) see III:PCM000
BENZENECARBOTHIOAMIDE see III:BBM250
BENZENECARBOXALDEHYDE see III:BBM500
m-BENZENEDIAMINE see III:PEY000
p-BENZENEDIAMINE see III:PEY500
1,3-BENZENEDIAMINE see III:PEY000
1,4-BENZENEDIAMINE see III:PEY500
m-BENZENEDIAMINE DIHYDROCHLORIDE see III:PEY750
p-BENZENEDIAMINE DIHYDROCHLORIDE see III:PEY650
1,4-BENZENEDIAMINE DIHYDROCHLORIDE see
    III:PEY650
1,3-BENZENEDIAMINE HYDROCHLORIDE see III:PEY750
BENZENEDIAZONIUM FLUOBORATE see III:BBO325
BENZENEDIAZONIUM FLUOROBORATE see III:BBO325
BENZENEDIAZONIUM, 4-(HYDROXYMETHYL)-, SULFATE
    (2:1) see III:HLX900
BENZENEDIAZONIUM, 4-(HYDROXYMETHYL)-,
    TETRAFLUOROBORATE(1-) see II:HLX925
BENZENEDIAZONIUM TETRAFLUOROBORATE see
    III:BBO325
1,2-BENZENEDICARBOXYLIC ACID, BUTYL PHENYL-
    METHYL ESTER see III:BEC500
1,4-BENZENE DICARBOXYLIC ACID DIMETHYL ESTER
    (9CI) see III:DUE000
BENZENE-, 1,3-DIISOCYANATOMETHYL- see I:TGM740
m-BENZENEDIOL see III:REA000
o-BENZENEDIOL see III:CCP850
p-BENZENEDIOL see III:HIH000
1,2-BENZENEDIOL see III:CCP850
1,3-BENZENEDIOL see III:REA000
1,4-BENZENEDIOL see III:HIH000
BENZENE HEXACHLORIDE see I:BBP750
BENZENEHEXACHLORIDE (mixed isomers) see I:BBQ750
α-BENZENEHEXACHLORIDE see I:BBQ000
BENZENE HEXACHLORIDE-α-isomer see I:BBQ000
β-BENZENEHEXACHLORIDE see I:BBR000
γ-BENZENE HEXACHLORIDE see I:BBQ500
BENZENE HEXACHLORIDE-γ isomer see I:BBQ500
trans-α-BENZENEHEXACHLORIDE see I:BBR000
BENZENEMETHANOL, 2-((4-(DIMETHYLAMINO)PHE-
    NYL)AZO)-(9CI) see III:HMB595
BENZENEMETHANOL, α-ETHYNYL-4-METHOXY- see
    III:HKA700
BENZENESULFANILIDE see III:BBR750
BENZENESULFONAMIDE, p-((p-(DIMETHYLAMINO)PHE-
    NYL)AZO)- see III:SNW800
BENZENESULFONANILIDE see III:BBR750
BENZENE, 1,2,4-TRIMETHOXY-5-PROPENYL-, (E)- see
    III:IHX400
BENZENE, 1,2,4-TRIMETHOXY-5-PROPENYL-, trans- see
    III:IHX400
1,2,3-BENZENETRIOL see III:PPQ500
BENZENOL see III:PDN750
BENZENYL CHLORIDE see I:BFL250
BENZENYL TRICHLORIDE see I:BFL250
BENZETHONIUM CHLORIDE see III:BEN000
BENZETONIUM CHLORIDE see III:BEN000
BENZEX see I:BBQ750
2,3-BENZFLUORANTHENE see I:BAW250
3,4-BENZFLUORANTHENE see I:BAW250
10,11-BENZFLUORANTHENE see II:BCJ500
BENZ(j)FLUORANTHRENE see III:BCJ500
BENZHORMOVARINE see I:EDP000
BENZHYDRAZIDE see III:BBV250
BENZIDIN (CZECH) see I:BBX000
BENZIDINA (ITALIAN) see I:BBX000
BENZIDINE see I:BBX000
3,3′-BENZIDINEDICARBOXYLIC ACID see III:BFX250
3,3′-BENZIDINE DICARBOXYLIC ACID, DISODIUM SALT
    see III:BBX250
3,3′-BENZIDINE-γ,γ′-DIOXYDIBUTYRIC ACID see
    III:DEK400
γ,γ′-,3,3′-BENZIDINE DIOXYDIBUTYRIC ACID see
    III:DEK400

BENZIDINE HYDROCHLORIDE see II:BBX750
BENZIDINE SULFATE see I:BBY000
BENZIDINE-3-SULFURIC ACID see III:BBY250
BENZIDINE SULPHATE and HYDRAZINE-BENZENE see
    II:BBY300
BENZIDINE-3-SULPHURIC ACID see III:BBY250
BENZIDIN-3-YL ESTER SULFURIC ACID see III:BBY500
BENZIDIN-3-YL HYDROGEN SULFATE see III:BBY500
BENZILAN see II:DER000
BENZILE (CLORURO di) (ITALIAN) see II:BEE375
BENZIMIDAZOLE METHYLENE MUSTARD see III:BCC250
BENZIMIDAZOLE MUSTARD see III:BCC250
BENZIN (OBS.) see I:BBL250
BENZ(e)INDENO(1,2-b)INDOLE see III:BCE000
1-BENZINE see III:QMJ000
BENZINE (OBS.) see I:BBL250
BENZINOFORM see CBY000
BENZINOL see II:TIO750
3-BENZISOTHIAZOLINONE-1,1-DIOXIDE see II:BCE500
1,2-BENZISOTHIAZOL-3(2H)-ONE-1,1-DIOXIDE see
    II:BCE500
BENZISOTRIAZOLE see III:BDH250
3,4-BENZOACRIDINE see III:BAW750
BENZOANTHRACENE see I:BBC250
BENZO(a)ANTHRACENE see I:BBC250
1,2-BENZOANTHRACENE see I:BBC250
BENZO(a)ANTHRACENE-5,6-OXIDE see III:EBP000
17-BENZOATE-3-n-BUTYRATE d′OESTRADIOL (FRENCH)
    see III:EDP500
BENZOATE d′OESTRADIOL (FRENCH) see I:EDP000
BENZOATE d′OESTRONE (FRENCH) see II:EDV500
1-BENZOAZO-2-NAPHTHOL see III:PEJ500
BENZO(f)(1)BENZOTHIENO(3,2-b)QUINOLINE see
    III:BCF500
BENZO(h)(1)BENZOTHIENO(3,2-b)QUINOLINE see
    III:BCF750
BENZO(e)(1)BENZOTHIOPYRANO(4,3-b)INDOLE see
    III:BCG000
BENZO BLUE see II:CMO250
BENZO BLUE GS see I:CMO000
11H-BENZO(a)CARBAZOLE see III:BCG250
8,9-BENZO-γ-CARBOLINE see III:BDB500
BENZO-CHINON (GERMAN) see III:QQS200
BENZO(a)CHRYSENE see III:PIB750
BENZO(b)CHRYSENE see III:BCG500
BENZO(c)CHRYSENE see III:BCG750
BENZO(g)CHRYSENE see III:BCH000
2,3-BENZOCHRYSENE see III:BCG500
BENZO(d,e,f)CHRYSENE see II:BCS750
BENZO(10,11)CHRYSENO(1,2-b)OXIRENE-6-β,7-α-DIHY-
    DRO see III:BCV750
N-6-(3,4-BENZOCOUMARINYL)ACETAMIDE see
    III:BCH250
BENZO(de)CYCLOPENT(a)ANTHRACENE see III:BCI000
1H-BENZO(a)CYCLOPENT(b)ANTHRACENE see III:BCI250
BENZO DEEP BLACK E see I:AQP000
1,3-BENZODIOXOLE-5-(2-PROPEN-1-OL) see II:BCJ000
BENZOEPIN see III:EAQ750
BENZOESTROFOL see I:EDP000
BENZO(1)FLUORANTHENE see II:BCJ500
BENZO(b)FLUORANTHENE see I:BAW250
BENZO(e)FLUORANTHENE see I:BAW250
BENZO(j)FLUORANTHENE see II:BCJ500
BENZO(k)FLUORANTHENE see I:BCJ750
2,3-BENZOFLUORANTHENE see I:BAW250
3,4-BENZOFLUORANTHENE see I:BAW250
7,8-BENZOFLUORANTHENE see I:BCJ500
8,9-BENZOFLUORANTHENE see I:BCJ750
11,12-BENZOFLUORANTHENE see I:BCJ750
11,12-BENZO(k)FLUORANTHENE see I:BCJ750
2,3-BENZOFLUORANTHRENE see I:BAW250
BENZO(jk)FLUORENE see III:FDF000
BENZOFOLINE see I:EDP000
BENZOFORM BLACK BCN-CF see I:AQP000

1,4-BENZOQUINONE see III:QQS200
BENZOQUINONE AZIRIDINE see III:BDC750
1,4-BENZOQUINONE DIOXINE see III:DVR200
o-BENZOSULFIMIDE see II:BCE500
BENZOSULPHIMIDE see II:BCE500
BENZO-2-SULPHIMIDE see II:BCE500
3,4-BENZOTETRACENE see III:BCG500
BENZO(c)TETRAPHENE see III:BCG500
3,4-BENZOTETRAPHENE see III:BCG500
BENZOTHIAMIDE see III:BBM250
BENZOTHIAZOLE DISULFIDE see III:BDE750
2-BENZOTHIAZOLETHIOL see II:BDF000
2-BENZOTHIAZOLETHIOL, ZINC SALT (2:1) see III:BHA750
BENZOTHIAZOLYL DISULFIDE see III:BDE750
2-BENZOTHIAZOLYL DISULFIDE see III:BDE750
N-(2-BENZOTHIAZOLYL)-N'-METHYL-N'NITROSOUREA
    see III:NKR000
2-BENZOTHIAZOLYL-N-MORPHOLINOSULFIDE see
    III:BDG000
2-BENZOTHIAZOLYLSULFENYL MORPHOLINE see
    III:BDG000
4-(2-BENZOTHIAZOLYLTHIO)MORPHOLINE see
    III:BDG000
BENZOTHIOAMIDE see III:BBM250
BENZOTRIAZINEDITHIOPHOSPHORIC ACID DIMETHOXY
    ESTER see III:ASH500
BENZOTRIAZINE derivative of a METHYL DITHIOPHOS-
    PHATE see III:ASH500
1H-BENZOTRIAZOLE see III:BDH250
1,2,3-BENZOTRIAZOLE see III:BDH250
BENZOTRICHLORIDE (DOT, MAK) see I:BFL250
2,5,8-BENZOTRIOXACYCLOUNDECIN-1,9-DIONE, 3,4,6,7-
    TETRAHYDRO-(9CI) see III:DJD700
BENZO(b)TRIPHENYLENE see III:BDH750
BENZO VIOLET N see III:CMP000
BENZOYL see III:BDS000
2-BENZOYLAMIDOFLUORENE-2'-CARBOXYLATE see
    III:FEN000
2-BENZOYLAMINOFLUORENE see III:FDX000
2-BENZOYLAMINOFLUORENE-2'-CARBOXYLATE see
    III:FEN000
BENZOYL CHLORIDE see III:BDM500
BENZOYL CHLORIDE (DOT) see III:BDM500
4-BENZOYL-3,5-DIMETHYL-N-NITROSOPIPERAZINE see
    III:NJL850
BENZOYL HYDRAZIDE see III:BBV250
BENZOYLHYDROGEN PEROXIDE see III:PCM000
BENZOYL HYDROPEROXIDE see III:PCM000
o-BENZOYL-N-METHYL-
    N-(p-(PHENYLAZO)PHENYL)HYDROXYLAMINE see
    III:BDP000
N-BENZOYLOXY-ACETYLAMINOFLUORENE see
    III:FDZ000
3-(BENZOYLOXY)ESTRA-1,3,5(10)-TRIEN-17-ONE see
    II:EDV500
N-BENZOYLOXY-N-ETHYL-4-AMINOAZOBENZENE see
    III:BDO199
N-BENZOYLOXY-4'-ETHYL-N-METHYL-4-AMINOAZOBEN-
    ZENE see III:BDO500
N-BENZOYLOXY-N-METHYL-4-AMINOAZOBENZENE see
    III:BDP000
6-BENZOYLOXYMETHYLBENZO(a)PYRENE see III:BDP500
N-BENZOYLOXY-4'-METHYL-N-METHYL-4-AMINOAZO-
    BENZENE see III:BDQ000
7-BENZOYLOXYMETHYL-12-METHYLBENZ(a)ANTHRA-
    CENE see III:BDQ250
N-(BENZOYLOXY)-N-METHYL-4-(PHENYLAZO)-BENZENA-
    MINE see III:BDP000
BENZOYLPEROXID (GERMAN) see III:BDS000
BENZOYL PEROXIDE see III:BDS000
BENZOYLPEROXYDE (DUTCH) see III:BDS000
o-BENZOYL SULFIMIDE see II:BCE500
o-BENZOYL SULPHIMIDE see II:BCE500
BENZOYL SUPEROXIDE see III:BDS000

1,12-BENZPERYLENE see III:BCR000
BENZ(a)PHENANTHRENE see I:CML810
1,2-BENZPHENANTHRENE see I:CML810
2,3-BENZPHENANTHRENE see I:BBC250
3,4-BENZPHENANTHRENE see III:BCR750
9,10-BENZPHENANTHRENE see III:TMS000
3,4-BENZPYREN (GERMAN) see II:BCS750
BENZ(a)PYRENE see II:BCS750
1,2-BENZPYRENE see III:BCT000
3,4-BENZ(a)PYRENE see II:BCS750
3,4-BENZPYRENE-5-ALDEHYDE see III:BCT250
3,4-BENZPYRENE-5-ALDEHYDE THIOSEMICARBAZONE
    see III:BCT500
BENZ(a)PYRENE 4,5-OXIDE see III:BCV500
12-BENZPYRENE PICRATE see III:BDV750
BENZYDYNA (POLISH) see I:BBX000
BENZYHYDRYLCYANIDE see III:DVX200
BENZYL ACETATE see III:BDX000
BENZYL-6-AMINOPENICILLINIC ACID see III:BDY669
BENZYL BUTYL PHTHALATE see III:BEC500
3-BENZYL-4-CARBAMOYLMETHYLSYDNONE see
    III:BED750
BENZYLCHLORID (GERMAN) see II:BEE375
BENZYL CHLORIDE see II:BEE375
2-(N-BENZYL-2-CHLOROETHYLAMINO)-1-PHENOXYPRO-
    PANE see I:PDT250
2-(N-BENZYL-2-CHLOROETHYLAMINO)-1-PHENOXYPRO-
    PANE HYDROCHLORIDE see I:DDG800
BENZYL(2-CHLOROETHYL)-(1-METHYL-2-PHENOXY-
    ETHYL)AMINE see I:PDT250
BENZYL(2-CHLOROETHYL)(1-METHYL-2-PHENOXYETH-
    YL)AMINE HYDROCHLORIDE see III:DDG800
2-BENZYL-4-CHLOROPHENOL see III:CJU250
o-BENZYL-p-CHLOROPHENOL see III:CJU250
BENZYL DICHLORIDE see II:BAY300
BENZYLDIMETHYL-p-(1,1,3,3-TETRAMETHYLBUTYL)PHE-
    NOXYETHOXY-ETHYLAMMONIUM CHLORIDE see
    III:BEN000
BENZYLDIMETHYL(2-(2-(p-(1,1,3,3-
    TETRAMETHYLBUTYL)PHENOXY)ETHOXY)ETHYL)
    AMMONIUM CHLORIDE see III:BEN000
BENZYLE (CHLORURE de) (FRENCH) see II:BEE375
BENZYLENE CHLORIDE see II:BAY300
BENZYL ETHANOATE see III:BDX000
BENZYLHYDRAZINE DIHYDROCHLORIDE see III:BEQ250
BENZYL HYDROQUINONE see III:AEY000
1,1'-(BENZYLIDENEBIS((2-METHOXY-p-PHENYLENE)
    (AZO))DI-2-NAPHTHOL see III:DOO400
BENZYLIDENE CHLORIDE (DOT) see II:BAY300
BENZYLIDYNE CHLORIDE see I:BFL250
BENZYL MERCAPTAN see III:TGO750
1-BENZYL-2-METHYLHYDRAZINE see III:MHN750
1-BENZYL-1-NITROSOUREA see III:NJM000
p-BENZYLOXYPHENOL see III:AEY000
BENZYLPENICILLIN see III:BDY669
BENZYLPENICILLIN G see III:BDY669
BENZYLPENICILLINIC ACID see III:BDY669
BENZYL PENICILLINIC ACID SODIUM SALT see III:BFD250
BENZYLPENICILLIN SODIUM see III:BFD250
N-BENZYL-N-PHENOXYISOPROPYL-β-CHLORETHYLA-
    MINE HYDROCHLORIDE see II:DDG800
3-BENZYLSYDNONE-4-ACETAMIDE see III:BED750
BENZYLT see I:PDT250
BENZYLTHIOL see III:TGO750
BENZYL TRICHLORIDE see I:BFL250
BENZYL VIOLET see II:FAG120
BENZYL VIOLET 3B see II:FAG120
BENZYLYT see II:DDG800
3,4-BENZYPYRENE see II:BCS750
BEOSIT see III:EAQ750
BEP see III:BJP899
BERCEMA see III:EIR000
BERCEMA FERTAM 50 see III:FAS000
BERELEX see III:GEM000

BERGAPTEN see II:MFN275
BERGIUS COAL HYDROGENATION PRODUCTS FRACTION 1 see III:HHW509
BERGIUS COAL HYDROGENATION PRODUCTS FRACTION 3 see III:HHW519
BERGIUS COAL HYDROGENATION PRODUCTS FRACTION 4 see III:HHW529, III:HHW549
BERGIUS COAL HYDROGENATION PRODUCTS FRACTION 7 see III:HHW539
BERKFLAM B 10E see III:PAU500
BERKFURIN see III:NGE000
BERMAT see III:CJJ250
BERNSTEINSAEURE-2,2-DIMETHYLHYDRAZID (GERMAN) see II:DQD400
BERNSTEINSAURE-ANHYDRID (GERMAN) see III:SNC000
BERTRANDITE see I:BFO250
BERYL see I:BFO500
BERYLLIA see I:BFT250
BERYLLIUM see I:BFO750
BERYLLIUM-9 see I:BFO750
BERYLLIUM, metal powder (DOT) see I:BFO750
BERYLLIUM ACETATE see I:BFP000
BERYLLIUM ACETATE, BASIC see I:BFT500
BERYLLIUM ACETATE, NORMAL see I:BFP000
BERYLLIUM ALUMINOSILICATE see I:BFO500
BERYLLIUM ALUMINUM ALLOY see I:BFP250
BERYLLIUM ALUMINUM SILICATE see I:BFO500
BERYLLIUM CARBONATE see I:BFP500
BERYLLIUM CARBONATE (1:1) see I:BFP750
BERYLLIUM CARBONATE, BASIC see I:BFP500
BERYLLIUM CHLORIDE see I:BFQ000
BERYLLIUM CHLORIDE TETRAHYDRATE see I:BFQ250
BERYLLIUM COMPOUND with NIOBIUM (12:1) see I:BFQ750
BERYLLIUM COMPOUNDS see I:BFQ500
BERYLLIUM COMPOUND with TITANIUM (12:1) see I:BFR000
BERYLLIUM COMPOUND with VANADIUM (12:1) see I:BFR250
BERYLLIUM-COPPER-COBALT ALLOY see I:CNJ000
BERYLLIUM DICHLORIDE see I:BFQ000
BERYLLIUM DIFLUORIDE see I:BFR500
BERYLLIUM DIHYDROXIDE see I:BFS250
BERYLLIUM DINITRATE see I:BFT000
BERYLLIUM FLUORIDE see I:BFR500
BERYLLIUM HYDRATE see I:BFS250
BERYLLIUM HYDRIDE see I:BFR750
BERYLLIUM HYDROGEN PHOSPHATE (1:1) see I:BFS000
BERYLLIUM HYDROXIDE see I:BFS250
BERYLLIUM LACTATE see I:LAH000
BERYLLIUM MANGANESE ZINC SILICATE see I:BFS750
BERYLLIUM MONOXIDE see I:BFT250
BERYLLIUM NITRATE see I:BFT000
BERYLLIUM ORTHOSILICATE see II:SCN500
BERYLLIUM OXIDE see I:BFT250
BERYLLIUM OXIDE ACETATE see I:BFT500
BERYLLIUMOXIDE CARBONATE see I:BFP500
BERYLLIUM OXYACETATE see I:BFT500
BERYLLIUM OXYFLUORIDE see I:BFT750
BERYLLIUM PERCHLORATE see I:BFU000
BERYLLIUM PHOSPHATE see I:BFS000
BERYLLIUM SILICATE see II:SCN500
BERYLLIUM SILICATE HYDRATE see I:BFO250
BERYLLIUM SILICIC ACID see II:SCN500
BERYLLIUM SULFATE (1:1) see I:BFU250
BERYLLIUM SULFATE TETRAHYDRATE (1:1:4) see I:BFU500
BERYLLIUM SULPHATE TETRAHYDRATE see I:BFU500
BERYLLIUM TETRAHYDROBORATE see I:BFU750
BERYLLIUM TETRAHYDROBORATETRIMETHYLAMINE see I:BFV000
BERYLLIUM ZINC SILICATE see I:BFV250
BERYL ORE see I:BFO500

BETADID see III:HJS850
BETA-NAFTYLOAMINA (POLISH) see I:NBE500
BETAPRONE see I:PMT100
BETAZED see II:BRF500
BETEL LEAVES see III:BFV975
BETEL NUT see III:AQT650, II:BFW000
BETEL NUT, polyphenol fraction see I:PKH500
BETEL NUT TANNIN see III:BFW050
BETEL QUID EXTRACT see II:BFW125
BETEL TOBACCO EXTRACT see I:BFW135
BEXOL see I:BBQ500
BEXON see I:MMN250
BEXTRENE XL 750 see III:SMQ500
B(b)F see I:BAW250
B(j)F see II:BCJ500
BFH see III:BRK100
BFV see I:FMV000
3-tert-BHA see III:BQI010
BHA (FCC) see II:BQI000
BHBN see I:HJQ350
BHC see I:BBQ500
BHC (USDA) see I:BBP750
α-BHC see I:BBQ000
β-BHC see I:BBR000
γ-BHC see I:BBQ500
BH 2,4-D see II:DAA800
BHEN see III:BRO000
BH MCPA see II:CIR250
BH MECOPROP see II:CIR500
BHP see II:DNB200
BHPBN see III:HIE600
BHT (food grade) see III:BFW750
BI-58 see III:DSP400
Bi 3411 see III:CDO000
4′,4′′′-BIACETANILIDE see II:BFX000
BIALFLAVINA see III:DBX400
BIALMINAL see II:EOK000
BIALZEPAM see III:DCK759
p,p-BIANILINE see I:BBX000
4,4′-BIANILINE see I:BBX000
N,N′-BIANILINE see I:HHG000
o,p′-BIANILINE see III:BGF109
BIANISIDINE see I:TGJ750
5,5′-BIANTHRANILIC ACID see III:BFX250
BIBENZENE see III:BGE000
BIC see II:IAN000
BICARBURET of HYDROGEN see I:BBL250
BICHLORACETIC ACID see III:DEL000
BICHLORENDO see I:MQW500
BICHLORURE d′ETHYLENE (FRENCH) see I:EIY600
BICHLORURE de PROPYLENE (FRENCH) see III:PNJ400
BICHROMATE OF POTASH see III:PKX250
BICHROMATE OF SODA see I:SGI000
BICHROMATE de SODIUM (FRENCH) see I:SGI000
BICKIE-MOL see II:HIM000
BiCNU see I:BIF750
BICOLASTIC A 75 see III:SMQ500
BICOLENE P see III:PMP500
BICORTONE see III:PLZ000
BICYCLO(4.4.0)DECANE see III:DAE800
BIDIPHEN see III:TFD250
BIETHYLENE see I:BOP500
1,1′-BI(ETHYLENE OXIDE) see I:BGA750
BIFURON see III:NGG500
BIHEXYL see III:DXT200
BILARCIL see III:TIQ250
BILEVON see III:HCL000
(1,1′-BINAPHTHALENE)-2,2′-DIAMINE see III:BGB750
(1,2′-BINAPHTHALENE)-1,2′-DIAMINE see III:BGC000
2,3,1′,8′-BINAPHTHYLENE see I:BCJ750
β,β-BINAPHTHYLENEETHENE see III:PIB750
BINITROBENZENE see II:DUQ200
BIO 5,462 see III:EAQ750
BIOACRIDIN see III:DBX400

BIOCETIN see II:CDP250
BIOCIDE see III:ADR000
BIO-CLAVE see III:CJU250
BIOCORT ACETATE see III:CNS825
BIO-DES see I:DKA600
BIODOPA see III:DNA200
BIOFLAVONOID see III:RSU000
BIOFUREA see II:NGE500
BIOGRISIN-FP see GKE000
BIONIC see III:NCQ900
BIOPHENICOL see II:CDP250
BIOQUIN see III:BLC250, III:QPA000
BIOQUIN 1 see III:BLC250
BIOSCLERAN see III:ARQ750
BIOSUPRESSIN see III:HOO500
BIO-TESTICULINA see I:TBG000
BIOXIRANE see I:BGA750
2,2'-BIOXIRANE see I:BGA750
(R*,S*)-2,2'-BIOXIRANE see II:DHB800
(S-(R*,R*))-2,2'-BIOXIRANE see II:BOP750
BIPHENYL see III:BGE000
1,1'-BIPHENYL see III:BGE000
4-BIPHENYLACETAMIDE see III:PDY500
N-4-BIPHENYLACETAMIDE see III:PDY500
4-BIPHENYLACETHYDROXAMIC ACID see III:ACD000
BIPHENYLAMINE see I:AJS100
4-BIPHENYLAMINE see I:AJS100
p-BIPHENYLAMINE see I:AJS100
(1,1'-BIPHENYL)-4-AMINE see I:AJS100
4-BIPHENYLAMINE, DIHYDROCHLORIDE see III:BGE300
2-BIPHENYLAMINE, HYDROCHLORIDE see III:BGE325
N-4-BIPHENYLBENZAMIDE see III:BGF000
2,4'-BIPHENYLDIAMINE see III:BGF109
4,4'-BIPHENYLDIAMINE see I:BBX000
(1,1'-BIPHENYL)-2,4'-DIAMINE see III:BGF109
(1,1'-BIPHENYL)-4,4'-DIAMINE (9CI) see I:BBX000
(1,1'-BIPHENYL)-4,4'-DIAMINE, DIHYDROCHLORIDE see
    II:BBX750
(1,1'-BIPHENYL)-4,4'-DIAMINE SULFATE (1:1) see
    I:BBY000
4-BIPHENYLDIMETHYLAMINE see III:BGF899
N,N'-(1,1'-BIPHENYL)-4,4'-DIYLBIS-ACETAMIDE 4',4'''-
    BIACETANILIDE see II:BFX000
4,4'-BIPHENYLENEDIAMINE see I:BBX000
4-BIPHENYLHYDROXYLAMINE see III:BGI250
1,1-BIPHENYL, NONABROMO- see III:NMV735
2-BIPHENYLOL see III:BGJ250
4-BIPHENYLOL see III:BGJ500
o-BIPHENYLOL see III:BGJ250
(1,1'-BIPHENYL)-2-OL see III:BGJ250
2-BIPHENYLOL, SODIUM SALT see II:BGJ750
3,3',4,4'-BIPHENYLTETRAMINE see III:BGK500
3,3',4,4'-BIPHENYLTETRAMINE TETRAHYDROCHLORIDE
    see III:BGK750
N-(2-BIPHENYLYL)ACETAMIDE see III:PDY000
N-(3-BIPHENYLYL)ACETAMIDE see III:PDY250
N-(4-BIPHENYLYL)ACETAMIDE see III:PDY500
N-(4-BIPHENYLYL)ACETOHYDROXAMIC ACETATE see
    III:ABJ750
N-4-BIPHENYLYLBENZAMIDE see III:BGF000
N-4-BIPHENYLYLBENZENESULFONAMIDE see III:BGL000
N-4-BIPHENYLYL BENZENESULFONAMIDE see III:BGL000
N-4-BIPHENYLYLBENZOHYDROXAMIC ACID see
    III:HJP500
N,N'-4,4'-BIPHENYLYLENEBISACETAMIDE see II:BFX000
N-(4-BIPHENYLYL)FORMOHYDROXAMIC ACID see
    III:HLE650
N-4-BIPHENYLYL-N-HYDROXYBENZENESULFONAMIDE
    see III:BGN000
N-4-BIPHENYLYLHYDROXYLAMINE see III:BGI250
BIPOTASSIUM CHROMATE see III:PLB250
BIPYRIDINE see III:BGO500
2,2'-BIPYRIDINE see III:BGO500
α,α'-BIPYRIDINE see III:BGO500

2,2'-BIPYRIDYL see III:BGO500
α,α'-BIPYRIDYL see III:BGO500
BIRTHWORT see AQY250
BIRUTAN see III:RSU000
2,7-BIS(ACETAMIDO)FLUORENE see II:BGP250
BIS(4-ACETAMIDOPHENYL)SULFONE see III:SNY500
BIS(p-ACETAMIDOPHENYL) SULFONE see III:SNY500
BIS-4-ACETAMINO PHENYL SELENIUMDIHYDROXIDE see
    III:BGP500
BIS(ACETATO)TETRAHYDROXYTRILEAD see III:LCH000
BIS(ACETATO)TRIHYDROXYTRILEAD see I:LCJ000
BIS(ACETO)DIHYDROXYTRILEAD see III:LCH000
BIS-(ACETOXYAETHYL)NITROSAMIN (GERMAN) see
    III:NKM500
BIS(ACETOXY)CADMIUM see I:CAD250
9,10-BISACETOXYMETHYL-1,2-BENZANTHRACENE see
    III:BBF750
BIS(ACETYLACETONATO) TITANIUM OXIDE see
    III:BGQ750
2,5-BIS(ACETYLAMINO)FLUORENE see III:BGR250
4,4'-BIS(N-ACETYL-N-METHYLAMINO)AZOBENZENE see
    III:DQH200
S-(1,2-BIS(AETHOXY-CARBONYL)-AETHYL)-O,O-DI-
    METHYL-DITHIOPHASPHAT (GERMAN) see III:MAK700
2,4-BIS(AETHYLAMINO)-6-CHLOR-1,3,5-TRIAZIN (GER-
    MAN) see III:BJP000
BIS AMINE see I:MJM200
BIS(4-AMINO-3-CHLOROPHENYL) ETHER see II:BGT000
BIS-p-AMINOFENYLMETHAN (CZECH) see I:MJQ000
4,4'-BIS(1-AMINO-8-HYDROXY-2,4-DISULFO-7-NAPH-
    THYLAZO)-3,3'-BITOLYL, TETRASODIUM SALT see
    III:BGT250
4,4'-BIS(7-(1-AMINO-8-HYDROXY-2,4-DISULFO)NAPH-
    THYLAZO)-3,3' -BITOLYL, TETRASODIUM SALT see
    III:BGT250
4,4'-BIS(1-AMINO-8-HYDROXY-2,4-DISULPHO-7-
    NAPHTHYLAZO)-3,3' -BITOLYL, TETRASODIUM SALT
    see III:BGT250
BIS-4-AMINO-3-METHYLFENYLMETHAN (CZECH) see
    I:MJO250
BIS(2-AMINO-1-NAPHTHYL)SODIUM PHOSPHATE see
    III:BGU000
BIS(4-AMINOPHENYL)ETHER see I:OPM000
BIS(p-AMINOPHENYL)ETHER see I:OPM000
BIS(4-AMINOPHENYL)METHANE see I:MJQ000
BIS(p-AMINOPHENYL)METHANE see I:MJQ000
BIS(4-AMINOPHENYL) SULFIDE see I:TFI000
BIS(p-AMINOPHENYL)SULFIDE see I:TFI000
BIS(4-AMINOPHENYL) SULFONE see III:SOA500
BIS(p-AMINOPHENYL) SULFONE see III:SOA500
BIS(4-AMINOPHENYL) SULPHIDE see I:TFI000
BIS(p-AMINOPHENYL)SULPHIDE see I:TFI000
BIS(4-AMINOPHENYL)SULPHONE see III:SOA500
BIS(p-AMINOPHENYL)SULPHONE see III:SOA500
2,2-BIS(p-ANISYL)-1,1,1-TRICHLOROETHANE see
    II:MEI450
2,5-BIS(1-AZIRIDINYL)-3,6-BIS(2-METHOXYETHOXY)-p-
    BENZOQUINONE see III:BDC750
2,5-BIS(1-AZIRIDINYL)-3,6-BIS(2-METHOXYETHOXY)-2,5-
    CYCLOHEXADIENE-1,4-DIONE see III:BDC750
BIS(BENZOTHIAZOLYL)DISULFIDE see III:BDE750
BIS(2-BENZOTHIAZOLYLTHIO)ZINC see III:BHA750
BIS(2-BENZOTHIAZYL) DISULFIDE see III:BDE750
BIS(2-BENZOYLBENZOATO)BIS(3-(1-METHYL-2-PYRROLI-
    DINYL)PYRIDINE) NICKEL TRIHYDRATE see II:BHB000
BIS((4-(BIS(2-CHLOROETHYL)AMINO)BENZENE)ACE-
    TATE)ESTRA-1,3,5(10)-TRIENE-3,17-DIOL(17-β) see
    III:EDR500
BIS((4-(BIS(2-CHLOROETHYL)AMINO)BENZENE)ACE-
    TATE)OESTRA-1,3,5(10)-TRIENE-3,17-DIOL(17-β)
    see III:EDR500
2,5-BIS(BIS-(2-CHLOROETHYL)AMINOMETHYL)HYDRO-
    QUINONE see III:BHB750
BIS((p-(BIS(2-CHLOROETHYL)AMINO)PHENYL)ACETATE)
    ESTRADIOL see III:EDR500

BIS(CHLOROMETHYL) ETHER see I:BIK000
BIS(2-CHLORO-1-METHYLETHYL) ETHER see III:BII250
BIS(2-CHLORO-1-METHYLETHYL)ETHER mixed with 2-
  CHLORO-1-METHYLETHYL-(2-CHLOROPROPYL) ETHER
  see III:BIK100
1,3-BIS(CHLOROMETHYL)-1,1,3,3-TETRAMETHYLDISILA-
  ZANE see III:BIL250
1,1-BIS(4-CHLOROPHENYL)-2,2-DICHLOROETHANE see
  I:BIM500
1,1-BIS(p-CHLOROPHENYL)-2,2-DICHLOROETHANE see
  I:BIM500
2,2-BIS(4-CHLOROPHENYL)-1,1-DICHLOROETHANE see
  I:BIM500
2,2-BIS(p-CHLOROPHENYL)-1,1-DICHLOROETHANE see
  I:BIM500
2,2-BIS(p-CHLOROPHENYL)-1,1-DICHLOROETHYLENE see
  II:BIM750
BIS(CHLOROPHENYL) ETHER see III:DFQ000
α,α-BIS(p-CHLOROPHENYL)-β,β,β-TRICHLORETHANE see
  I:DAD200
1,1-BIS-(p-CHLOROPHENYL)-2,2,2-TRICHLOROETHANE see
  I:DAD200
2,2-BIS(p-CHLOROPHENYL)-1,1,1-TRICHLOROETHANE see
  I:DAD200
1,1-BIS(CHLOROPHENYL)-2,2,2-TRICHLOROETHANOL see
  III:BIO750
1,1-BIS(4-CHLOROPHENYL)-2,2,2-TRICHLOROETHANOL
  see III:BIO750
1,1-BIS(p-CHLOROPHENYL)-2,2,2-TRICHLOROETHANOL
  see III:BIO750
BIS-CME see I:BIK000
BIS(CYCLOPENTADIENYL)COBALT see III:BIR529
BISCYCLOPENTADIENYLIRON see III:FBC000
cis-BIS(CYCLOPENTYLAMMINE)PLATINUM(II) see
  III:BIS250
BISDEHYDRODOISYNOLIC ACID 7-METHYL ETHER see
  III:BIT030
BISDEHYDROISYNOLIC ACID METHYL ESTER see
  III:BIT000
BIS(DIBUTYLDITHIOCARBAMATO)NICKEL see III:BIW750
BIS(DIBUTYLDITHIOCARBAMATO)ZINC see III:BIX000
BIS(3,4-DICHLOROBENZOATO)NICKEL see II:BIX500
BIS(DIETHYLAMINO)THIOXOMETHYL)DISULPHIDE see
  III:DXH250
BIS(DIETHYLDITHIOCARBAMATO)CADMIUM see
  I:BJB500
BIS(DIETHYLDITHIOCARBAMATO)ZINC see III:BJC000
BIS(DIETHYLTHIOCARBAMOYL) DISULFIDE see
  III:DXH250
BIS(N,N-DIETHYLTHIOCARBAMOYL) DISULFIDE see
  III:DXH250
BIS(DIETHYLTHIOCARBAMOYL)DISULFIDE mixed with SO-
  DIUM NITRITE see III:SIS200
BIS(N,N-DIETHYLTHIOCARBAMOYL)DISULPHIDE see
  III:DXH250
2,8-BISDIMETHYLAMINOACRIDINE see III:BJF000
3,6-BIS(DIMETHYLAMINO)ACRIDINE see III:BJF000
4,4'-BIS(DIMETHYLAMINO)BENZHYDRYLIDENIMINE HY-
  DROCHLORIDE see I:IBA000
4,4'-BIS(DIMETHYLAMINO)BENZOPHENONE see
  I:MQS500
p,p'-BIS(N,N-DIMETHYLAMINO)BENZOPHENONE see
  I:MQS500
4,4'-BIS(DIMETHYLAMINO)BENZOPHENONE-IMINE HY-
  DROCHLORIDE see I:IBA000
BIS((DIMETHYLAMINO)CARBONOTHIOYL) DISULPHIDE
  see III:TFS350
4,4'-BIS(DIMETHYLAMINO)DIPHENYLMETHANE see
  I:MJN000
p,p'-BIS(DIMETHYLAMINO)DIPHENYLMETHANE see
  I:MJN000
BIS(p-(N,N-DIMETHYLAMINO)PHENYL)KETONE see
  I:MQS500
BIS(p-DIMETHYLAMINOPHENYL)METHANE see I:MJN000

BIS(p-(N,N-DIMETHYLAMINO)PHENYL)METHANE see
  I:MJN000
p,p'-BIS(N,N-DIMETHYLAMINOPHENYL)METHANE see
  I:MJN000
BIS(4-(DIMETHYLAMINO)PHENYL)METHANONE see
  I:MQS500
BIS(p-DIMETHYLAMINOPHENYL)METHYLENEIMINE see
  I:IBB000
1,1-BIS(p-DIMETHYLAMINOPHENYL)METHYLENIMINE-
  HYDROCHLORIDE see I:IBA000
BIS(DIMETHYLCARBAMODITHIOATO-S,S')LEAD see
  III:LCW000
BIS(DIMETHYLCARBAMODITHIOATO-S,S')ZINC see
  III:BJK500
BIS(DIMETHYLDITHIOCARBAMATE de ZINC) (FRENCH) see
  III:BJK500
BIS(DIMETHYLDITHIOCARBAMATO)ZINC see III:BJK500
BIS(DIMETHYLDITHIOCARBAMIATO)LEAD see
  III:LCW000
2,6-BIS(1,1-DIMETHYLETHYL)-4-METHYLPHENOL see
  III:BFW750
BIS(DIMETHYL-THIOCARBAMOYL)-DISULFID (GERMAN)
  see III:TFS350
BIS(DIMETHYLTHIOCARBAMOYL) DISULFIDE see
  III:TFS350
BIS(DIMETHYLTHIOCARBAMOYL)DISULFIDE and
  NITROSOTRIS(DIMETHYLDITHIOCARBAMATO)IRON
  see III:FAZ000
BIS(DIMETHYLTHIOCARBAMOYL)SULFIDE see III:BJL600
BIS(DIMETHYLTHIOCARBAMYL) MONOSULFIDE see
  III:BJL600
BIS(N,N-DIMETIL-DITIOCARBAMMATO) DI ZINCO (ITAL-
  IAN) see III:BJK500
($\pm$)-1,2-BIS(3,5-DIOXOPIPERAZINE-1-YL)PROPANE see
  II:PIK250
($\pm$)-1,2-BIS(3,5-DIOXOPIPERAZINYL)PROPANE see
  II:PIK250
BIS(2,3-EPOXYCYCLOPENTYL) ETHER see III:BJN250
BIS(2,3-EPOXYCYCLOPENTYL) ETHER mixed with DIGLYCI-
  DYL ETHER of BISPHENOL A (1:1) see III:OPI200
m-BIS(2,3-EPOXYPROPOXY)BENZENE see II:REF000
1,3-BIS(2,3-EPOXYPROPOXY)BENZENE see II:REF000
2,2'-BIS(2,3-EPOXYPROPOXY)-N-tert-BUTYLDIPROPYLA-
  MINE see III:DKM400
1,3-BIS(2,3-EPOXYPROPOXY)-2,2-DIMETHYLPROPANE see
  III:NCI300
N,N-BIS(2-(2,3-EPOXYPROPOXY)ETHOXY)ANILINE see
  III:BJN850
1,2-BIS(2,3-EPOXYPROPOXY)ETHOXY)ETHANE see
  III:TJQ333
N,N-BIS(2-(2,3-EPOXYPROPOXY)ETHYL)ANILINE see
  III:BJN875
2,2-BIS(p-(2,3-EPOXYPROPOXY)PHENYL)PROPANE mixed
  with 2,2'-OXYBIS(6-OXABICYCLO(3.1.0)HEXANE) see
  III:OPI200
1,3-BIS(2,3-EPOXYPROPYL)-5,5-DIMETHYLHYDANTOIN
  see III:DKM130
BIS(2,3-EPOXYPROPYL)ETHER see II:DKM200
2,2-BIS(4-(2,3-EPOXYPROPYLOXY)PHENYL)PROPANE see
  III:BLD750
N,N-BIS(2,3-EPOXYPROPYL)-p-TOLUENESULFONAMIDE
  see III:DKM800
S-(1,2-BIS(ETHOXY-CARBONYL)-ETHYL)-O,O-DIMETHYL-
  DITHIOFOSFAAT (DUTCH) see III:MAK700
S-(1,2-BIS(ETHOXYCARBONYL)ETHYL)-O,O-DIMETHYL
  PHOSPHORODITHIOATE see III:MAK700
S-1,2-BIS(ETHOXYCARBONYL)ETHYL-O,O-DIMETHYL
  THIOPHOSPHATE see III:MAK700
BIS(2-ETHOXYETHYL)NITROSOAMINE see III:BJO250
2,4-BIS(ETHYLAMINO)-6-CHLORO-s-TRIAZINE see
  III:BJP000
omega,omega'-BIS-(ETHYLENEIMINOSULPHONYL)PRO-
  PANE see III:BJP899
1,3-BIS(ETHYLENIMINOSULFONYL)PROPANE see
  III:BJP899

BIS(2-ETHYLHEXYL) ADIPATE see III:AEO000
BIS(2-ETHYLHEXYL)-1,2-BENZENEDICARBOXYLATE see
  I:DVL700
BIS(2-ETHYLHEXYL) ESTER PHOSPHORUS ACID CADMIUM
  SALT see I:CAD500
BIS(2-ETHYLHEXYL)PHTHALATE see I:DVL700
1,1-BIS(p-ETHYLPHENYL)-2,2-DICHLOROETHANE see
  III:DJC000
2,2-BIS(p-ETHYLPHENYL)-1,1-DICHLOROETHANE see
  III:DJC000
2,2-BIS(ETHYLSULFONYL)BUTANE see III:BJT750
S-(1,2-BIS(ETOSSI-CARBONIL)-ETIL)-O,O-DIMETIL-DITIO-
  FOSFATO (ITALIAN) see III:MAK700
1,1-BIS(4-FLUOROPHENYL)-2-PROPYNYL-N-CYCLOHEP-
  TYLCARBAMATE see III:BJW250
1,1-BIS(4-FLUOROPHENYL)-2-PROPYNYL-N-CYCLOOCTYL
  CARBAMATE see III:BJW500
m-BIS(GLYCIDYLOXY)BENZENE see II:REF000
BIS(4-GLYCIDYLOXYPHENYL)DIMETHYAMETHANE see
  III:BLD750
2,2-BIS(p-GLYCIDYLOXYPHENYL)PROPANE see
  III:BLD750
BIS(β-HYDROXYAETHYL)NITROSAMIN (GERMAN) see
  I:NKM000
BIS(2-HYDROXY-3,5-DICHLOROPHENYL) SULFIDE see
  III:TFD250
4-BIS(2-HYDROXYETHYL)AMINO-2-(5-NITRO-2-FURYL)
  QUINAZOLINE see III:BKB750
4-BIS(2-HYDROXYETHYL)AMINO-2-(5-NITRO-2-THIENYL)
  QUINAZOLINE see III:BKC250
BIS(2-HYDROXYETHYL)CARBAMODITHIOIC ACID, MONO-
  POTASSIUM SALT see III:PKX500
BIS(2-HYDROXYETHYL)DITHIOCARBAMIC ACID, MONO-
  POTASSIUM SALT see III:PKX500
BIS(2-HYDROXYETHYL)DITHOCARBAMIC ACID, POTAS-
  SIUM SALT see III:PKX500
BIS(2-HYDROXYETHYL) ETHER see III:DJD600
1,1-BIS(2-HYDROXYETHYL)HYDRAZINE see III:HHH000
N′,N′-BIS(2-HYDROXYETHYL)-N-METHYL-2-NITRO-p-PHE-
  NYLENEDIAMINE see II:BKF250
BIS(β-HYDROXYETHYL)NITROSAMINE see I:NKM000
3-BIS(HYDROXYMETHYL)AMINO-6-(5-NITRO-2-FURYL-
  ETHENYL)-1,2,4-TRIAZINE see II:BKH500
9:10-BISHYDROXYMETHYL-1:2-BENZANTHRACENE see
  III:BBF500
BIS(HYDROXYMETHYL)FURATRIZINE see II:BKH500
1,2-BISHYDROXYMETHYL-1-METHYLPYRROLE see
  III:MPB175
2,3-BISHYDROXYMETHYL-1-METHYLPYRROLE see
  III:MPB175
BIS(4-HYDROXYPHENYL)DIMETHYLMETHANE DIGLYCI-
  DYL ETHER see III:BLD750
3,4-BIS(4-HYDROXYPHENYL)-2,4-HEXADIENE see
  II:DAL600
3,4-BIS(p-HYDROXYPHENYL)-2,4-HEXADIENE see
  II:DAL600
3,4-BIS(p-HYDROXYPHENYL)HEXANE see III:DLB400
meso-3,4-BIS(p-HYDROXYPHENYL)-n-HEXANE see
  III:DLB400
3,4-BIS(p-HYDROXYPHENYL)-3-HEXENE see I:DKA600
2,2-BIS(4-HYDROXYPHENYL)PROPANE, DIGLYCIDYL
  ETHER see III:BLD750
2,2-BIS(p-HYDROXYPHENYL)PROPANE, DIGLYCIDYL
  ETHER see III:BLD750
N-BIS(2-HYDROXYPROPYL)NITROSAMINE see II:DNB200
2,2′-BISHYDROXYPROPYLNITROSAMINE see II:DNB200
BIS(2-HYDROXY-3,5,6-TRICHLOROPHENYL)METHANE see
  III:HCL000
BIS(4-ISOCYANATOPHENYL)METHANE see III:MJP400
BIS(p-ISOCYANATOPHENYL)METHANE see III:MJP400
BIS(1,4-ISOCYANATOPHENYL)METHANE see III:MJP400
2,4-BIS(ISOPROPYLAMINO)-6-CHLORO-s-TRIAZINE see
  III:PMN850
BISMATE see III:BKW000

BIS(MERCAPTOBENZOTHIAZOLATO)ZINC see III:BHA750
1,4-BIS(METHANESULFONOXY)BUTANE see I:BOT250
BIS(METHANE SULFONYL)-d-MANNITOL see III:BKM500
(1,4-BIS(METHANESULFONYLOXY)BUTANE) see
  I:BOT250
3,4-BIS(METHOXY)BENZYL CHLORIDE see III:BKM750
2,5-BISMETHOXYETHOXY-3,6-BISETHYLENEIMINO-1,4-
  BENZOQUINONE see III:BDC750
3,6-BIS (β-METHOXYETHOXY)-2,5-BIS(ETHYLENEIMINO)-
  p-BENZOQUINONE see III:BDC750
3,6-BIS(β-METHOXYETHOXY)-2,5-BIS(ETHYLENIMINO)-p-
  BENZOQUINONE see III:BDC750
BIS(2-METHOXYETHYL)NITROSOAMINE see III:BKO000
3,4-BIS(p-METHOXYPHENYL)-3-HEXENE see III:DJB200
1,1-BIS(p-METHOXYPHENYL)-2,2,2-TRICHLOROETHANE
  see II:MEI450
2,2-BIS(p-METHOXYPHENYL)-1,1,1-TRICHLOROETHANE
  see II:MEI450
BIS(N-METHYLANILINE)METHANE see III:MJO000
BIS(N-METHYLANILINO)METHAN (GERMAN) see
  III:MJO000
BIS(1-METHYLETHYL)DIAZENE 1-OXIDE see III:ASP510
N-BISMETHYLPTEROYLGLUTAMIC ACID see III:MDV500
N,N-BIS(METHYLSULFONEPROPOXY)AMINE HYDRO-
  CHLORIDE see III:YCJ000
1,6-BIS-o-METHYLSULFONYL-d-MANNITOL see
  III:BKM500
BIS(MORPHOLINO-)METHAN (GERMAN) see III:MJQ750
BISMORPHOLINO METHANE see III:MJQ750
BISMUTH DIMETHYL DITHIOCARBAMATE see
  III:BKW000
1,5-BIS(5-NITRO-2-FURANYL)-1,4-PENTADIEN-3-ONE,
  (AMINOIMINOMETHYL)HYDRAZONE see III:PAF500
BIS(5-NITROFURFURYLIDENE)ACETONE GUANYLHYDRA-
  ZONE see III:PAF500
sym-BIS(5-NITRO-2-FURFURYLIDENE) ACETONE GUANYL-
  HYDRAZONE see III:PAF500
1,5-BIS(5-NITRO-2-FURYL)-3-PENTADIENONE AMIDINON-
  HYDRAZONE see III:PAF500
1,5-BIS(5-NITRO-2-FURYL)-3-PENTADIENONE GUANYLHY-
  DRAZONE see III:PAF500
BISOFLEX 81 see I:DVL700
BISOFLEX DOA see III:AEO000
BISOFLEX DOP see I:DVL700
BISOLVOMYCIN see III:HOI000
BIS(1-OXODODECYL)PEROXIDE see III:LBR000
BIS-(2-OXOPROPYL)-N-NITROSAMINE see II:NJN000
BIS(8-OXYQUINOLINE)COPPER see III:BLC250
BIS(2,4-PENTANEDIONATO)TITANIUM OXIDE see
  III:BGQ750
BISPHENOL A DIGLYCIDYL ETHER see III:BLD750
BISPHENOL DIGLYCIDYL ETHER, MODIFIED see
  III:BLE000
1,4-BIS(PHENYL AMINO)BENZENE see III:BLE500
2,4-BIS(PROPYLAMINO)-6-CHLOR-1,3,5-TRIAZIN (GER-
  MAN) see III:PMN850
BIS(8-QUINOLINATO)COPPER see III:BLC250
BIS(8-QUINOLINOLATO)COPPER see III:BLC250
BIS(8-QUINOLINOLATO-N(¹),O(⁸))-COPPER see III:BLC250
BISTERIL see I:PDC250
BISTHIOCARBAMYL HYDRAZINE see III:BLJ250
BIS(THIOUREA) see III:BLJ250
BIS(TRI-N-BUTYLPHOSPHINE)DICHLORONICKEL see
  II:BLS250
BIS-2,3,5-TRICHLOR-6-HYDROXYFENYLMETHAN (CZECH)
  see III:HCL000
BIS(3,5,6-TRICHLORO-2-HYDROXYPHENYL)METHANE see
  III:HCL000
2,3-BISTRIMETHYLACETOXYMETHYL-1-METHYLPYR-
  ROLE see III:BLQ600
BIS(TRIMETHYLSILYL)ACETAMIDE see III:TMF000
N,o-BIS(TRIMETHYLSILYL)ACETAMIDE see III:TMF000
BIS(TRIMETHYLSILYL)AMINE see III:HED500
BIS(2,4,6-TRINITRO-PHENYL)-AMIN (GERMAN) see
  III:HET500

BIS(TRIPHENYLPHOSPHINE)DICHLORONICKEL see
  II:BLS250
BISULFAN see I:BOT250
BISULFITE see III:SOH500
BISULPHANE see I:BOT250
BITEMOL see III:BJP000
BITEMOL S 50 see III:BJP000
BITHIONOL see III:TFD250
BITHIONOL SULFIDE see III:TFD250
BITIN see III:TFD250
4,4′-BI-o-TOLUIDINE see I:TGJ750
(m,o′-BITOLYL)-4-AMINE see II:BLV250
BITUMEN (MAK) see II:ARO500
BIVINYL see I:BOP500
BIZOLIN 200 see II:BRF500
γ-BL see III:BOV000
BLA see III:LCH000
BLACAR 1716 see III:PKQ059
BLACK AND WHITE BLEACHING CREAM see III:HIH000
BLACK 2EMBL see I:AQP000
BLACK OXIDE of IRON see III:IHD000
BLACOSOLV see II:TIO750
BLADAN see III:PAK000
BLADAN F see III:PAK000
BLADAN-M see III:MNH000
BLANC FIXE see III:BAP000
BLANDLUBE see III:MQV750
BLANOSE BWM see III:SFO500
BLASTING GELATIN (DOT) see III:NGY000
BLASTING OIL see III:NGY000
BLASTOESTIMULINA see III:ARN500
L-BLAU 2 (GERMAN) see III:FAE100
BLEIACETAT (GERMAN) see I:LCG000
BLEIAZETAT (GERMAN) see I:LCJ000
BLEIPHOSPHAT (GERMAN) see I:LDU000
BLEISTIFTBAUMS (GERMAN) see III:EQY000
BLEKIT EVANSA (POLISH) see III:BGT250
BLENDED RED OXIDES of IRON see III:IHD000
BLENOXANE see II:BLY000, III:BLY780
BLEO see II:BLY000
BLEOCIN see II:BLY000
BLEOMYCIN see II:BLY000
BLEOMYCIN SULFATE see III:BLY780
BLEU BRILLIANT FCF see III:FMU059
BLEU DIAMINE see II:CMO250
BLEXANE see III:BLY780
BLIGHTOX see III:EIR000
BLITEX see III:EIR000
BLIZENE see III:EIR000
BLM see II:BLY000
BLO see III:BOV000
BLOCADREN see II:DDG800
BLON see III:BOV000
BLOOD STONE see I:HAO875
BLUE 2B see I:CMO000
BLUE 1084 see III:ADE500
1206 BLUE see III:FAE000
1311 BLUE see III:FAE100
11388 BLUE see III:FMU059
12070 BLUE see III:FAE100
BLUE ASBESTOS (DOT) see I:ARM275
BLUE BN BALSE see I:DCJ200
BLUE COPPER see III:CNP250
BLUE EMB see II:CMO250
BLUE OIL see II:AOQ000, I:COD750
BLUE STONE see III:CNP250
BLUE VITRIOL see III:CNP250
BLU-PHEN see II:EOK000
BM 1 see III:HNI500
7-BMBA see III:BNO750
BN see II:BFW000
B-NINE see II:DQD400
BNP see III:NIY500
BNP 30 see III:BRE500

BNU see II:BSA250
BOB see III:NKL300
BOH see III:HHC000
BOLATRON see III:PKQ059
BOLINAN see III:PKQ250
BOLLS-EYE see I:HKC500, III:HKC000
BONAMID see III:PJY500
BONARE see III:CFZ000
BONAZEN see III:ZNA000
BONBRAIN see III:TEH500
BONIBAL see III:DXH250
BONLOID see III:PKQ059
BONOFORM see III:TBQ100
BOP see II:NJN000
BORDEAUX see III:FAG020
BORDERMASTER see II:CIR250
BORER SOL see I:EIY600
BOROLIN see III:PIB900
BORTRAN see III:RDP300
BOSAN SUPRA see I:DAD200
BOTRAN see III:RDP300
BOVIDERMOL see I:DAD200
BOVINOCIDIN see III:NIY500
BOVINOX see III:TIQ250
BOVOFLAVIN see III:DBX400
BOVOLIDE see III:BMK500
B(e)P see III:BCT000
BPDE-syn see III:DMR000
BP-4,5-DIHYDRODIOL see III:DLB800
BP-7,8-DIHYDRODIOL see III:BCT750, III:DML000,
  III:DML200
BP-9,10-DIHYDRODIOL see III:DLC400
B(e)P-4,5-DIHYDRODIOL see III:DMK400
B(E)P 9,10-DIHYDRODIOL see III:DMK600
trans-BP-7,8-DIHYDRODIOL DIACETATE see III:DBG200
BP-7,8-DIHYDRODIOL-9,10-EPOXIDE (anti) see III:BCU000
anti-BP-7,8-DIHYDRODIOL-9,10-OXIDE see III:BCU000
B(e)P DIOL EPOXIDE-1 see III:DMR150
B(E)P DIOL EPOXIDE-2 see III:DMR200
BP 7,8-DIOL-9,10-EPOXIDE 2 see III:DMP900
B(e)P 9,10-DIOL-11,12-EPOXIDE-1 see III:DMR150
(−)-BP 7-α,8-β-DIOL-9-β,10-β-EPOXIDE 2 see III:DVO175
(−)BP-7,β,8,α-DIOL-9,β,10,β-EPOXIDE 1 see III:DMP800
(+)-BP-7,α,8-β-DIOL-9,α,10,α-EPOXIDE 1 see III:DMP600
(+)-BP-7-β,8-α-DIOL-9-α,10-α-EPOXIDE 2 see III:BMK620
BP-4,5-EPOXIDE see III:BCV500
BP 7,8-EPOXIDE see III:BCV750
B(a)P EPOXIDE I see III:DMR000
B(a)P EPOXIDE II see III:BMK630
B(E)P H4-9,10-DIOL see III:DNC400
B(c)PH DIOL EPOXIDE-1 see III:BMK634
B(c)PH DIOL EPOXIDE-2 see III:BMK635
B(e)P H4-9,10-EPOXIDE see III:ECQ150
BP-3-HYDROXY see III:BCX250
BPL see I:PMT100
BP 4,5-OXIDE see III:BCV500
BP 7,8-OXIDE see III:BCV750
BP-9,10-OXIDE see III:BCW000
BP-11,12-OXIDE see III:BCW250
BP-3,6-QUINONE see III:BCU750
BP-6,12-QUINONE see III:BCV000
BR 55N see III:PAU500
BR-931 see II:CLW500
BRACKEN FERN, CHLOROFORM FRACTION see
  III:BMK750
BRACKEN FERN, DRIED see I:BML000
BRACKEN FERN TANNIN see III:BML250
BRACKEN FERN, TANNIN-FREE see III:TAE250
BRACKEN FERN TOXIC COMPONENT see III:SCE000
BRASILAMINA BLACK GN see I:AQP000
BRASILAMINA BLUE 2B see I:CMO000
BRASILAMINA BLUE 3B see II:CMO250
BRASILAMINA VIOLET 3R see III:CMP000
BRASILAN AZO RUBINE 2NS see III:HJF500

BRASILAN ORANGE 2G see III:HGC000
BRASILAZET BLUE GR see III:TBG700
BRASILAZINA OIL RED B see III:SBC500
BRASILAZINA OIL SCARLET 6G see III:XRA000
BRASILAZINA OIL YELLOW G see II:PEI000
BRASILAZINA OIL YELLOW R see I:AIC250
BRASILAZINA ORANGE Y see III:PEK000
BRASSICOL see III:PAX000
BRAVO see III:TBQ750
BRAVO 6F see III:TBQ750
BRAVO-W-75 see III:TBQ750
BRECOLANE NDG see III:DJD600
BRELLIN see III:GEM000
BRENOL see I:ART250
BRENTAMINE FAST BLUE B BASE see I:DCJ200
BRENTAMINE FAST RED TR BASE see II:CLK220
BRENTAMINE FAST RED TR SALT see II:CLK235
BREON see III:PKQ059
BREON 351 see II:AAX175
BRESIT see III:ARQ750
BRESTAN see III:ABX250
BRICK OIL see I:CMY825
BRIGHT RED see III:CHP500
BRILLIANT ACRIDINE ORANGE E see III:BJF000
BRILLIANT BLUE see III:FMU059
BRILLIANT BLUE FCD No. 1 see III:FAE000
BRILLIANT BLUE FCF see III:FAE000
BRILLIANT BLUE R see III:BMM500
BRILLIANT CRIMSON RED see III:HJF500
BRILLIANT FAST YELLOW see I:DOT300
BRILLIANT GREEN 3EMBL see III:FAE950
BRILLIANT OIL ORANGE R see III:PEJ500
BRILLIANT OIL ORANGE Y BASE see III:PEK000
BRILLIANT OIL SCARLET B see III:XRA000
BRILLIANT OIL YELLOW see I:IBB000
BRILLIANT PINK B see III:FAG070
BRILLIANT PONCEAU 3R see III:FMU080
BRILLIANT PONCEAU G see III:FMU070
BRILLIANT RED see III:CHP500
BRILLIANTSAEURE GRUEN BS (GERMAN) see III:ADF000
BRILLIANT SCARLET see III:CHP500, III:FMU080
BRILLIANT TONER Z see III:CHP500
BRITON see III:TIQ250
BRITTEN see III:TIQ250
BROCADOPA see III:DNA200
BROCIDE see I:EIY600
BROCKMANN, ALUMINUM OXIDE see III:AHE250
10-BROM-1,2-BENZANTHRACEN (GERMAN) see
    III:BMT750
BROMDEFENURON see III:MHS375
BROMEOSIN see III:BMO250
BROMIC ACID, POTASSIUM SALT see II:PKY300
BROMINAL M & PLUS see II:CIR250
BROMKAL 80-9D see III:NMV735
BROMKAL 83-10DE see III:PAU500
BROMKAL 82-ODE see III:PAU500
BROMKAL P 67-6HP see I:TNC500
BROM-METHAN (GERMAN) see III:MHR200
BROMOACETIC ACID, ETHYL ESTER see III:EGV000
BROMO ACID see III:BNH500, III:BNK700
3'-BROMO-trans-ANETHOLE see III:BMT300
BROMO B see III:BNK700
10-BROMO-1,2-BENZANTHRACENE see III:BMT750
6-BROMOBENZO(a)PYRENE see III:BMU500
α-BROMO-β,β-BIS(p-ETHOXYPHENYL)STYRENE see
    III:BMX000
4-BROMO-7-BROMOMETHYLBENZ(a)ANTHRACENE see
    III:BMX250
2-BROMOBUTANE see III:BMX750
BROMOCHLOROACETONITRILE see III:BMY800
BROMOCHLOROMETHYL CYANIDE see III:BMY800
BROMOCRIPTIN see III:BNB250
BROMOCRIPTINE see III:BNB250
BROMODICHLOROMETHANE see II:BND500

3'-BROMO-4-DIMETHYLAMINOAZOBENZENE see
    III:BNE600
3-BROMO-7,12-DIMETHYLBENZ(a)ANTHRACENE see
    III:BNF300
4-BROMO-7,12-DIMETHYLBENZ(a)ANTHRACENE see
    III:BNF310
5-BROMO-9,10-DIMETHYL-1,2-BENZANTHRACENE see
    III:BNF315
3-BROMO-DMBA see III:BNF300
4-BROMO-DMBA see III:BNF310
BROMOEOSIN see III:BMO250
BROMOEOSINE see III:BNH500, III:BNK700
α-BROMOERGOCRIPTINE see III:BNB250
BROMOERGOCRYPTINE see III:BNB250
2-BROMOERGOCRYPTINE see III:BNB250
2-BROMO-α-ERGOKRYPTIN see III:BNB250
BROMOETHANOL see III:BNI500
2-BROMO ETHANOL see III:BNI500
BROMOETHENE see I:VMP000
3'-BROMO-4'-ETHYL-4-DIMETHYLAMINOAZOBENZENE
    see III:BNK275
4'-BROMO-3'-ETHYL-4-DIMETHYLAMINOAZOBENZENE
    see III:BNK100
BROMOETHYLENE see I:VMP000
BROMOETHYLENE POLYMER see III:PKQ000
p-((3-BROMO-4-ETHYLPHENYL)AZO)-N,N-DIMETHYLANI-
    LINE see III:BNK275
p-((4-BROMO-3-ETHYLPHENYL)AZO)-N,N-DIMETHYLANI-
    LINE see III:BNK100
BROMOFLUORESCEIC ACID see III:BMO250, III:BNH500,
    III:BNK700
BROMO FLUORESCEIN see III:BNH500, III:BNK700
BROMOFORM see III:BNL000
BROMOFORME (FRENCH) see III:BNL000
BROMOFORMIO (ITALIAN) see III:BNL000
BROMOFUME see I:EIY500
2-BROMO-12'-HYDROXY-2'-(1-METHYLETHYL)-5'-α-(2-
    METHYLPROPYL)ERGOTAMIN-3',6',18-TRIONE see
    III:BNB250
2-BROMOISOBUTANE see III:BQM250
3'-BROMOISOSAFROLE see III:BOA750
BROMOMETANO (ITALIAN) see III:MHR200
BROMO METHANE see III:MHR200
9-BROMOMETHYLANTHRACENE see III:BNO500
7-BROMO METHYL BENZ(a)ANTHRACENE see III:BNO750
6-BROMOMETHYLBENZO(a)PYRENE see III:BNP000
10-BROMOMETHYL-9-CHLOROANTHRACENE see
    III:BNP850
9-(BROMOMETHYL)-10-CHLOROANTHRACENE see
    III:BNP850
7-BROMOMETHYL-4-CHLOROBENZ(a)ANTHRACENE see
    III:BNQ000
3'-BROMO-4'-METHYL-4-DIMETHYLAMINOAZOBENZENE
    see III:BNQ100
4'-BROMO-3'-METHYL-4-DIMETHYLAMINOAZOBENZENE
    see III:BNQ110
7-BROMOMETHYL-6-FLUOROBENZ(a)ANTHRACENE see
    III:BNQ250
7-BROMOMETHYL-1-METHYLBENZ(a)ANTHRACENE see
    III:BNQ750
12-BROMOMETHYL-7-METHYLBENZ(a)ANTHRACENE see
    III:BNR250
7-BROMO METHYL-12-METHYL BENZ(a)ANTHRACENE see
    III:BNR000
1-BROMO-2-METHYL PROPANE see III:BNR750
2-BROMO-2-METHYLPROPANE (DOT) see III:BQM250
3-BROMO-4-NITROQUINOLINE-1-OXIDE see III:BNT500
BROMO-O-GAS see III:MHR200
4-BROMOPHENOL see III:BNU750
p-BROMOPHENOL see III:BNU750
p-(m-BROMOPHENYLAZO)-N,N-DIMETHYLANILINE see
    III:BNE600
3-(p-BROMOPHENYL)-1-METHYL-1-NITROSOUREA see
    III:BNX125

1-(p-BROMOPHENYL)-3-METHYLUREA see III:MHS375
1-(p-BROMOPHENYL)-3-METHYLUREA mixed with SODIUM
  NITRITE see III:SIQ675
3-BROMO-1-PROPANAMINE HYDROBROMIDE see
  III:AJA000
(E)-p-(3-BROMOPROPENYL)ANISOLE see III:BMT300
5-(3-BROMO-1-PROPENYL)-1,3-BENZODIOXOLE see
  III:BOA750
3-BROMOPROPIONIC ACID see III:BOB250
β-BROMOPROPIONIC ACID see III:BOB250
3-BROMOPROPYLAMINE HYDROBROMIDE see III:AJA000
BROMO SELTZER see I:ABG750
p-((3-BROMO-p-TOLYL)AZO)-N,N-DIMETHYLANILINE see
  III:BNQ100
p-((4-BROMO-m-TOLYL)AZO)-N,N-DIMETHYLANILINE see
  III:BNQ110
3-BROMOTRICYCLOQUINAZOLINE see III:BOI250
BROMURE de METHYLE (FRENCH) see III:MHR200
BROMURE de VINYLE (FRENCH) see I:VMP000
BROMURO di ETILE (ITALIAN) see I:EIY500
BROMURO di METILE (ITALIAN) see III:MHR200
BRONZE BROMO see III:BNH500, III:BNK700
BRONZE POWDER see III:CNI000
BRONZE RED RO see III:CHP500
BRONZE SCARLET see III:CHP500
BROOMMETHAAN (DUTCH) see III:MHR200
BROTOPON see III:CLY500
BROWN SALT NV see III:MIH500
BRUCITE see III:NBT000
BRUFANEUXOL see III:DOT000
BRUSH-OFF 445 MLD VOLATILE BRUSH KILLER see
  II:TAA100
BRUSH RHAP see II:TAA100
BRUSHTOX see II:TAA100
BSA see III:TMF000
B-SELEKTONON M see II:CIR250
B.T.Z. see II:BRF500
BUCACID AZURE BLUE see III:FMU059
BUCACID BRILLIANT SCARLET 3R see III:FMU080
BUCACID FAST ORANGE G see III:HGC000
BUCACID GUINEA GREEN BA see III:FAE950
BUCACID INDIGOTINE B see III:FAE100
BUCETIN see III:HJS850
BUD-NIP see III:CKC000
BUFF-A-COMP see I:ABG750
BUFON see I:DKA600
BUFOPTO ZINC SULFATE see III:ZNA000
BUKS see III:BFW750
BUNSENITE see I:NDF500
BUNT-CURE see I:HCC500
BUNT-NO-MORE see I:HCC500
BUR see III:EHA100
BURLEY TOBACCO see III:TGH750
BURNISH GOLD see III:GIS000
BURNOL see III:DBX400
BURNTISLAND RED see III:IHD000
BURNT SIENNA see III:IHD000
BURNT UMBER see III:IHD000
BUROFLAVIN see III:DBX400
BURTONITE-V-40-E see III:CCL250
BUSONE see II:BRF500
BUSTREN see III:SMQ500
BUTACIDE see III:PIX250
BUTACOMPREN see II:BRF500
BUTACOTE see II:BRF500
BUTADIEEN (DUTCH) see I:BOP500
BUTA-1,3-DIEEN (DUTCH) see I:BOP500
BUTADIEN (POLISH) see I:BOP500
BUTA-1,3-DIEN (GERMAN) see I:BOP500
BUTADIENDIOXYD (GERMAN) see I:BGA750
1,3-BUTADIENE see I:BOP500
BUTA-1,3-DIENE see I:BOP500
α-γ-BUTADIENE see I:BOP500
BUTADIENE DIEPOXIDE see I:BGA750

l-BUTADIENE DIEPOXIDE see II:BOP750
1,3-BUTADIENE DIEPOXIDE see I:BGA750
BUTADIENE DIMER see III:CPD750
BUTADIENE DIOXIDE see I:BGA750
dl-BUTADIENE DIOXIDE see II:DHB600
BUTADIENE MONOXIDE see III:EBJ500
1,3-BUTADIENE-STYRENE COPOLYMER see III:SMR000
BUTADIENE-STYRENE POLYMER see III:SMR000
1,3-BUTADIENE-STYRENE POLYMER see III:SMR000
BUTADIENE-STYRENE RESIN see III:SMR000
BUTADIENE-STYRENE RUBBER (FCC) see III:SMR000
BUTADION see II:BRF500
BUTADIONA see II:BRF500
BUTAFLOGIN see III:HNI500
BUTAGESIC see II:BRF500
BUTAKON 85-71 see III:SMR000
BUTALAN see II:BRF500
BUTALGINA see II:BRF500
BUTALIDON see II:BRF500
BUTALUY see II:BRF500
BUTANAMIDE, N-(4-ETHOXYPHENYL)-3-HYDROXY- see
  III:HJS850
1-BUTANAMINE see III:BPX750
1,4-BUTANEDIAMINE, 2-METHYL-, POLYMER with α-HY-
  DRO-omega-HYDROXYPOLY(OXY-1,4-BUTANEDIYL) and
  1,1'-METHYLENEBIS(4-ISOCYANATOCYCLOHEXANE)
  see I:PKN500
1,4-BUTANEDICARBOXAMIDE see III:AEN000
BUTANE DIEPOXIDE see I:BGA750
BUTANEDIOIC ACID MONO(2,2-DIMETHYLHYDRAZIDE)
  see II:DQD400
BUTANEDIOIC ANHYDRIDE see III:SNC000
1,4-BUTANEDIOL DIMETHANESULPHONATE see I:BOT250
1,4-BUTANEDIOL DIMETHYL SULFONATE see I:BOT250
1,4-BUTANEDIOL, POLYMER with 1,6-DIISOCYANATOHEX-
  ANE see III:PKO750
1,4-BUTANEDIOL POLYMER with 1,1'-METHYLENEBIS(4-
  ISOCYANATOBENZENE) see I:PKP000
BUTANESULFONE see II:BOU250
BUTANE SULTONE see II:BOU250
Δ-BUTANE SULTONE see II:BOU250
1,4-BUTANESULTONE (MAK) see II:BOU250
5H,6H-6,5A,13A,14-(1,2,3,-
  4)BUTANETETRAYCYCLOOCTA(1,2-B:5,6-
  B')DINAPHTHALENE see III:LIV000
BUTANOIC ACID, 1,2,3-PROPANETRIYL ESTER see
  III:TIG750
BUTANOL (4)-BUTYL-NITROSAMINE see I:HJQ350
4-BUTANOLIDE see III:BOV000
1-BUTANOL, 4-(NITROSO-2-PROPENYLAMINO)- see
  III:HJS400
BUTANOVA see III:HNI500
BUTAPHEN see II:BRF500
BUTAPHENE see III:BRE500
BUTAPIRAZOL see II:BRF500
BUTAPIRONE see III:HNI500
BUTAPYRAZOLE see II:BRF500
BUTARECBON see II:BRF500
BUTARTRIL see II:BRF500
BUTARTRINA see II:BRF500
BUTAZATE see III:BIX000
BUTAZATE 50-D see III:BIX000
BUTAZINA see II:BRF500
BUTAZOLIDIN see II:BRF500
BUTAZONA see II:BRF500
BUTAZONE see II:BRF500
BUTE see II:BRF500
2-BUTENAL see II:COB250
cis-BUTENEDIOIC ANHYDRIDE see III:MAM000
2-BUTENE-1,4-DIOL, DIMETHANESULFONATE, (E)- see
  III:DNX000
1-BUTENE OXIDE see III:BOX750
1,2-BUTENE OXIDE see III:BOX750
1-BUTENE, 2,3,4-TRICHLORO- see I:TIL360

2-BUTENOIC ACID, 2,3-DICHLOR-4-OXO-, (Z)-(9CI) see III:MRU900

3-BUTEN-2-OL see III:MQL250

3-BUTEN-2-ONE, 4-(2,5,6,6-TETRAMETHYL-2-CYCLO-HEXEN-1-YL)-(9CI) see III:IGW500

BUTENYL(3-HYDROXYPROPYL)NITROSAMINE see III:BPC600

(2-BUTENYLIDENE)ACETIC ACID see III:SKU000

3-(3-BUTENYLNITROSAMINO)-1-PROPANOL see III:BPC600

3-BUTENYL-(2-PROPENYL)-N-NITROSAMINE see III:BPD000

BUTIDIONA see II:BRF500

n-BUTILAMINA (ITALIAN) see III:BPX750

BUTILENE see III:HNI500

2-BUTIN HEXAMETHYL DEWAR BENZOL (GERMAN) see III:HEC500

BUTIWAS-SIMPLE see II:BRF500

BUTOCIDE see III:PIX250

BUTONE see II:BRF500

BUTOXIDE see III:PIX250

2-BUTOXYCARBONYLMETHYLENE-4-OXOTHIAZOLIDONE see III:BPI300

α-(2-(2-BUTOXYETHOXY)ETHOXY)-4,5-METHYLENEDI-OXY-2-PROPYLTOLUENE see III:PIX250

α-(2-(2-n-BUTOXYETHOXY)-ETHOXY)-4,5-METHYLENEDI-OXY-2-PROPYLTOLUENE see III:PIX250

5-((2-(2-BUTOXYETHOXY)ETHOXY)METHYL)-6-PROPYL-1,3-BENZODIOXOLE see III:PIX250

BUTOZ see II:BRF500

BUTTERCUP YELLOW see I:CMK500, I:PLW500, I:ZFJ100

BUTTER YELLOW see I:AIC250, I:DOT300

BUTTER of ZINC see III:ZFA000

N-BUTYL-N-(1-ACETOXYBUTYL)NITROSAMINE see III:BPV325

BUTYL ACETOXYMETHYLNITROSAMINE see III:BRX500

N-BUTYL-N-(ACETOXYMETHYL)NITROSAMINE see III:BRX500

n-BUTYLAMIN (GERMAN) see III:BPX750

n-BUTYLAMINE see III:BPX750

1-(tert-BUTYLAMINO)3-(3-METHYL-2-NITROPHENOXY)-2-PROPANOL see III:BQF750

BUTYLAMYLNITROSAMIN (GERMAN) see III:BRY250

BUTYLATED HYDROXYANISOLE see II:BQI000

3-tert-BUTYLATED HYDROXYANISOLE see III:BQI010

BUTYLATED HYDROXYTOLUENE see III:BFW750

8-BUTYLBENZ(a)ANTHRACENE see III:BQI500

5-n-BUTYL-1,2-BENZANTHRACENE see III:BQI500

BUTYL BENZYL PHTHALATE see III:BEC500

n-BUTYL BENZYL PHTHALATE see III:BEC500

1-BUTYL BROMIDE see III:BNR750

i-BUTYL BROMIDE see III:BNR750

sec-BUTYL BROMIDE see III:BMX750

tert-BUTYL BROMIDE see III:BQM250

BUTYL-BUTANOL(4)-NITROSAMIN see I:HJQ350

BUTYL-BUTANOL-NITROSAMINE see I:HJQ350

N-n-BUTYL-N-4-(1,4-BUTYROLACTONE)NITROSAMINE see III:NJO200

BUTYL CARBAMATE see III:BQP250

1-(BUTYLCARBAMOYL)-2-BENZIMIDAZOLECARBAMIC ACID METHYL ESTER and SODIUM NITRITE (1:6) see III:BAV500

N-BUTYLCARBINOL see III:AOE000

BUTYL CARBITOL 6-PROPYLPIPERONYL ETHER see III:PIX250

BUTYL-CARBITYL (6-PROPYLPIPERONYL) ETHER see III:PIX250

N-BUTYL-(3-CARBOXY PROPYL)NITROSAMINE see I:BQQ250

sec-BUTYL CHLORIDE see III:CEU250

tert-BUTYL CHLORIDE see III:BQR000

3-tert-BUTYLCHOLANTHRENE see III:BQU750

tert-20-BUTYLCHOLANTHRENE see III:BQU750

2-tert-BUTYL-p-CRESOL see III:BQV750

BUTYL 2,4-D see III:BQZ000

14-n-BUTYL DIBENZ(a,h)ACRIDINE see III:BQY000

10-n-BUTYL-1,2,5,6-DIBENZACRIDINE (FRENCH) see III:BQY000

BUTYL DICHLOROPHENOXYACETATE see III:BQZ000

BUTYL (2,4-DICHLOROPHENOXY)ACETATE see III:BQZ000

4'-n-BUTYL-4-DIMETHYLAMINOAZOBENZENE see III:BRB450

4'-tert-BUTYL-4-DIMETHYLAMINOAZOBENZENE see III:BRB460

1-BUTYL-3,3-DIMETHYL-1-NITROSOUREA see III:BRE000

2-sec-BUTYL-4,6-DINITROPHENOL see III:BRE500

4-BUTYL-1,2-DIPHENYL-3,5-DIOXO PYRAZOLIDINE see II:BRF500

4-BUTYL-1,2-DIPHENYLPYRAZOLIDINE-3,5-DIONE see II:BRF500

4-BUTYL-1,2-DIPHENYL-3,5-PYRAZOLIDINEDIONE see II:BRF500

2-BUTYLENE DICHLORIDE see III:BRG000

1,2-BUTYLENE OXIDE see III:BOX750

1,4-BUTYLENE SULFONE see II:BOU250

BUTYL-9,10-EPOXYSTEARATE see III:BRH250

BUTYL ESTER 2,4-D see III:BQZ000

BUTYLETHYLTHIOCARBAMIC ACID S-PROPYL ESTER see III:PNF500

p-tert-BUTYLFENOL (CZECH) see III:BSE500

N-n-BUTYL-N-FORMYLHYDRAZINE see III:BRK100

n-BUTYLHYDRAZINE HYDROCHLORIDE see III:BRL500

N-BUTYL-N-(1-HYDROPEROXYBUTYL)NITROSAMINE see III:HIE600

6-BUTYL-4-HYDROXYAMINOQUINOLINE-1-OXIDE see III:BRM750

BUTYLHYDROXYANISOLE see II:BQI000

tert-BUTYLHYDROXYANISOLE see II:BQI000

tert-BUTYL-4-HYDROXYANISOLE see II:BQI000

3-tert-BUTYL-4-HYDROXYANISOLE see III:BRN000

2(3)-tert-BUTYL-4-HYDROXYANISOLE see II:BQI000

n-BUTYL-(4-HYDROXYBUTYL)NITROSAMINE see I:HJQ350

N-BUTYL-N-(4-HYDROXYBUTYL)NITROSAMINE see I:HJQ350

BUTYL(2-HYDROXYETHYL)NITROSOAMINE see III:BRO000

4-BUTYL-2-(4-HYDROXYPHENYL)-1-PHENYL-3,5-DIOXO-PYRAZOLIDINE see III:HNI500

4-BUTYL-1-(4-HYDROXYPHENYL)-2-PHENYL-3,5-PYRAZO-LIDINEDIONE see III:HNI500

4-BUTYL-1-(p-HYDROXYPHENYL)-2-PHENYL-3,5-PYRAZO-LIDINEDIONE see III:HNI500

4-BUTYL-2-(p-HYDROXYPHENYL)-1-PHENYL-3,5-PYRAZO-LIDINEDIONE see III:HNI500

BUTYLHYDROXYTOLUENE see III:BFW750

n-BUTYL IODIDE see III:BRQ250

sec-BUTYL IODIDE see III:IEH000

2-tert-BUTYL-p-KRESOL (CZECH) see III:BQV750

2-tert-BUTYL-4-METHOXYPHENOL see III:BRN000

3-tert-BUTYL-4-METHOXYPHENOL see III:BQI010

1-BUTYL-2-METHYL-HYDRAZINE DIHYDROCHLORIDE see III:MHW250

2-tert-BUTYL-4-METHYLPHENOL see III:BQV750

N-BUTYL-N'-NITRO-N-NITROSOGUANIDINE see III:NLC000

6-BUTYL-4-NITROQUINOLINE-1-OXIDE see III:BRW750

4-(BUTYLNITROSAMINO)-1-BUTANOL see I:HJQ350

4-(n-BUTYLNITROSAMINO)-1-BUTANOL see I:HJQ350

2-(BUTYLNITROSAMINO)ETHANOL see III:BRO000

4-(N-BUTYLNITROSAMINO)-4-HYDROXYBUTYRIC ACID LACTONE see III:NJO200

4-(BUTYLNITROSOAMINO)BUTANOIC ACID see I:BQQ250

1-(BUTYLNITROSOAMINO)BUTYL ACETATE see III:BPV325

BUTYLNITROSOAMINOMETHYL ACETATE see III:BRX500

1-(BUTYLNITROSOAMINO)-2-PROPANONE see III:BRY000

N-BUTYL-N-NITROSO AMYL AMINE see III:BRY250
n-BUTYL-N-NITROSO-1-BUTAMINE see I:BRY500
N-BUTYL-N-NITROSOBUTYRAMIDE see III:NJO150
N-BUTYL-N-NITROSO ETHYL CARBAMATE see III:BRZ000
BUTYLNITROSOHARNSTOFF (GERMAN) see II:BSA250
N-BUTYL-N-NITROSOPENTYLAMINE see III:BRY250
4-tert-BUTYL-1-NITROSOPIPERIDINE see III:BRZ200,
    III:NJO300
N-BUTYL-N-NITROSOSUCCINAMIC ACID ETHYL ESTER see
    III:EHC800
n-BUTYLNITROSOUREA see II:BSA250
1-BUTYL-1-NITROSOUREA see II:BSA250
N-n-BUTYL-N-NITROSOUREA see II:BSA250
1-sec-BUTYL-1-NITROSOUREA see III:NJO500
1-BUTYL-1-NITROSOURETHAN see III:BRZ000
N-BUTYL-N-NITROSOURETHAN see III:BRZ000
BUTYLOHYDROKSYANIZOL (POLISH) see II:BQI000
N-BUTYL-N-(1-OXOBUTYL)NITROSAMINE see III:NJO150
N-BUTYL-N-(2-OXOBUTYL)NITROSAMINE see III:BSB500
N-BUTYL-N-(3-OXOBUTYL)NITROSAMINE see III:BSB750
BUTYL(2-OXOPROPYL)NITROSOAMINE see III:BRY000
2-(n-BUTYLOXYCARBONYLMETHYLENE)THIAZOLID-4-
    ONE see III:BPI300
N-BUTYL-N-PENTYLINITROSAMINE see III:BRY250
tert-BUTYLPERBENZOAN (CZECH) see III:BSC500
tert-BUTYL PERBENZOATE see III:BSC500
tert-BUTYL PEROXIDE see III:BSC750
tert-BUTYL PEROXY BENZOATE see III:BSC500
tert-BUTYL PEROXYBENZOATE, technical pure or in concentra-
    tion of more than 75% (DOT) see III:BSC500
BUTYLPHEN see III:BSE500
2-n-BUTYLPHENOL see III:BSD500
4-n-BUTYLPHENOL see III:BSD750
4-tert-BUTYLPHENOL see III:BSE500
o-BUTYLPHENOL, solid (DOT) see III:BSD500
o-BUTYLPHENOL, liquid (DOT) see III:BSD500
p-tert-BUTYLPHENOL (MAK) see III:BSE500
BUTYLPHENOXYISOPROPYL CHLOROETHYL SULFITE see
    I:SOP500
2-(p-BUTYLPHENOXY)ISOPROPYL 2-CHLOROETHYL SUL-
    FITE see I:SOP500
2-(4-tert-BUTYLPHENOXY)ISOPROPYL-2-CHLOROETHYL
    SULFITE see I:SOP500
2-(p-tert-BUTYLPHENOXY)ISOPROPYL 2'-CHLOROETHYL
    SULPHITE see I:SOP500
2-(p-tert-BUTYLPHENOXY)-1-METHYLETHYL 2-CHLORO-
    ETHYL ESTER of SULPHUROUS ACID see I:SOP500
2-(p-BUTYLPHENOXY)-1-METHYLETHYL 2-CHLORO-
    ETHYL SULFITE see I:SOP500
2-(p-tert-BUTYLPHENOXY)-1-METHYLETHYL-2-CHLORO-
    ETHYL SULFITE ESTER see I:SOP500
2-(p-tert-BUTYLPHENOXY)-1-METHYLETHYL 2'-CHLORO-
    ETHYL SULPHITE see I:SOP500
2-(p-tert-BUTYLPHENOXY)-1-METHYLETHYL SULPHITE of
    2-CHLOROETHANOL see I:SOP500
1-(p-tert-BUTYLPHENOXY)-2-PROPANOL-2-CHLOROETHYL
    SULFITE see I:SOP500
p-((p-BUTYLPHENYL)AZO)-N,N-DIMETHYLANILINE see
    III:BRB450
p-((p-tert-BUTYLPHENYL)AZO)-N,N-DIMETHYLANILINE see
    III:BRB460
BUTYLPYRIN see II:BRF500
3-tert-BUTYLTRICYCLOQUINAZOLINE see III:BSR500
1-BUTYLUREA and SODIUM NITRITE (2:1) see II:BSS500
1-BUTYLURETHAN see III:EHA100
BUTYLURETHANE see III:EHA100
1-BUTYLURETHANE see III:EHA100
N-BUTYLURETHANE see III:EHA100
BUTYL ZIMATE see III:BIX000
BUTYL ZIRAM see III:BIX000
BUTYRANILIDE, 4'-ETHOXY-3-HYDROXY- see III:HJS850
BUTYRIC ACID LACTONE see III:BOV000
BUTYRIC ACID TRIESTER with GLYCERIN see III:TIG750

α-BUTYROLACTONE see III:BOV000
β-BUTYROLACTONE see II:BSX000
γ-BUTYROLACTONE (FCC) see III:BOV000
N-(1-BUTYROXYMETHYL)METHYLNITROSAMINE see
    III:BSX500
N-(1-BUTYROXYMETHYL)-N-NITROSOMETHYLAMINE see
    III:BSX500
12-o-BUTYROYL-PHORBOLDODECANOATE see III:BSX750
1-BUTYRYLAZIRIDINE see III:BSY000
1-n-BUTYRYLAZIRIDINE see III:BSY000
BUTYRYLETHYLENEIMINE see III:BSY000
BUTYRYLETHYLENIMINE see III:BSY000
BUTYRYL LACTONE see III:BOV000
BUTYRYL TRIGLYCERIDE see III:TIG750
BUVETZONE see II:BRF500
BUZON see II:BRF500
BUZULFAN see I:BOT250
BW 57-322 see I:ASB250
2,2'-BYPYRIDIN see III:BGO500
BZF-60 see III:BDS000
BZT see III:BEN000

C 570 see III:FAC025
C-854 see III:CJT750
C 1,006 see III:CJT750
C 2059 see III:DUK800
C 3172 see III:TNK250
C-5068 see III:PHW000
C 5968 see III:PHW000
C 6866 see I:BIE500
C 8514 see III:CJJ250
CAB-O-GRIP see III:AHE250
CAB-O-GRIP II see III:SCH000
CAB-O-LITE 100 see III:WCJ000
CAB-O-LITE 130 see III:WCJ000
CAB-O-LITE 160 see III:WCJ000
CAB-O-LITE F 1 see III:WCJ000
CAB-O-LITE P 4 see III:WCJ000
CAB-O-SIL see III:SCH000
CAB-O-SPERSE see III:SCH000
CABRONAL see II:EOK000
CACHALOT L-50 see III:DXV600
CACODYLATE de SODIUM (FRENCH) see I:HKC500
CACODYLIC ACID (DOT) see III:HKC000
CACODYLIC ACID SODIUM SALT see I:HKC500
CACODYL NEW see I:DXE600
CACP see II:PJD000
CADCO 0115 see III:SMQ500
CADDY see I:CAE250
CADET see III:BDS000
CADIA DEL PERRO see III:CAC500
CADMINATE see I:CAI750
CADMIUM see I:CAD000
CADMIUM(II) ACETATE see I:CAD250
CADMIUM ACETATE (DOT) see I:CAD250
CADMIUM AMIDE see I:CAD325
CADMIUM AZIDE see I:CAD350
CADMIUM BIS(2-ETHYLHEXYL) PHOSPHITE see I:CAD500
CADMIUM CAPRYLATE see I:CAD750
CADMIUM CHLORATE see I:CAE000
CADMIUM CHLORIDE see I:CAE250
CADMIUM CHLORIDE, DIHYDRATE see I:CAE375
CADMIUM CHLORIDE, HYDRATE (2:5) see I:CAE425
CADMIUM CHLORIDE, MONOHYDRATE see I:CAE500
CADMIUM COMPOUNDS see I:CAE750
CADMIUM DIACETATE see I:CAD250
CADMIUM DIAMIDE see I:CAD325
CADMIUM DIAZIDE see I:CAD350
CADMIUM DICHLORIDE see I:CAE250
CADMIUM DICYANIDE see I:CAF500
CADMIUM DIETHYL DITHIOCARBAMATE see I:BJB500
CADMIUM DINITRATE see I:CAH000
CADMIUM(II) EDTA COMPLEX see I:CAF750
CADMIUM FLUOBORATE see I:CAG000

CADMIUM FLUORIDE see I:CAG250
CADMIUM FLUOROBORATE see I:CAG000
CADMIUM FLUORURE (FRENCH) see I:CAG250
CADMIUM FLUOSILICATE see I:CAG500
CADMIUM FUME see I:CAH750
CADMIUM GOLDEN 366 see I:CAJ750
CADMIUM LACTATE see I:CAG750
CADMIUM LEMON YELLOW 527 see I:CAJ750
CADMIUM NITRATE see I:CAH000
CADMIUM(II) NITRATE TETRAHYDRATE (1:2:4) see
  I:CAH250
CADMIUM NITRIDE see I:TIH000
CADMIUM ORANGE see I:CAJ750
CADMIUM OXIDE see I:CAH500
CADMIUM OXIDE FUME see I:CAH750
CADMIUM PHOSPHATE see I:CAI000
CADMIUM PHOSPHIDE see I:CAI125
CADMIUM PRIMROSE 819 see I:CAJ750
CADMIUM PROPIONATE see I:CAI250
CADMIUM SELENIDE see I:CAI500
CADMIUM STEARATE see I:OAT000
CADMIUM SUCCINATE see I:CAI750
CADMIUM SULFATE see I:CAJ000
CADMIUM SULFATE (1:1) see I:CAJ000
CADMIUM SULFATE (1:1) HYDRATE (3:8) see I:CAJ250
CADMIUM SULFATE OCTAHYDRATE see I:CAJ250
CADMIUM SULFATE TETRAHYDRATE see I:CAJ500
CADMIUM SULFIDE see I:CAJ750
CADMIUM SULPHATE see I:CAJ000
CADMIUM SULPHIDE see I:CAJ750
CADMIUM THERMOVACUUM AEROSOL see I:CAK000
CADMIUM-THIONEIN see I:CAK250
CADMIUM salt of 2,4-5-TRIBROMOIMIDAZOLE see
  I:THV500
CADMIUM YELLOW see I:CAJ750
CADMOPUR YELLOW see I:CAJ750
CADOX see III:BDS000, III:BSC750
CAF see II:CDP250, III:CEA750
CAFFEIN see III:CAK500
CAFFEINE see III:CAK500
CALAMUS OIL see III:OGK000
CALCINED BRUCITE see III:MAH500
CALCINED DIATOMITE see I:SCJ000
CALCINED MAGNESIA see III:MAH500
CALCINED MAGNESITE see III:MAH500
CALCIUMARSENAT see I:ARB750
CALCIUM ARSENATE (MAK) see I:ARB750
CALCIUM CARBIMIDE see III:CAQ250
CALCIUM CHLORIDE see III:CAO750
CALCIUM CHLORIDE, ANHYDROUS see III:CAO750
CALCIUM CHROMATE see I:CAP500
CALCIUM CHROMATE (VI) see I:CAP500
CALCIUM CHROMATE(VI) DIHYDRATE see I:CAP750
CALCIUM CHROME YELLOW see I:CAP500, I:CAP750
CALCIUM CHROMIUM OXIDE (CaCrO₄) see I:CAP500
CALCIUM CYANAMID see III:CAQ250
CALCIUM CYANAMIDE see III:CAQ250
CALCIUM CYCLAMATE see III:CAR000
CALCIUM CYCLOHEXANESULFAMATE see III:CAR000
CALCIUM CYCLOHEXANE SULPHAMATE see III:CAR000
CALCIUM CYCLOHEXYLSULFAMATE see III:CAR000
CALCIUM CYCLOHEXYLSULPHAMATE see III:CAR000
CALCIUM MONOCHROMATE see I:CAP500
CALCIUM ORTHOARSENATE see I:ARB750
CALCIUM SODIUM METAPHOSPHATE see III:CAX260
CALCIUM(II) SULFATE DIHYDRATE (1:1:2) see III:CAX750
CALCOCID AMARANTH see III:FAG020
CALCOCID BLUE EG see III:FMU059
CALCOCID BRILLIANT SCARLET 3RN see III:FMU080
CALCOCID ERYTHROSINE N see III:FAG040
CALCOCID FAST LIGHT ORANGE 2G see III:HGC000
CALCOCID 2RIL see III:FMU070

CALCOCID URANINE B4315 see III:FEW000
CALCOCID VIOLET 4BNS see II:FAG120
CALCODUR BROWN BRL see II:CMO750
CALCOGAS ORANGE NC see III:PEJ500
C 10 ALCOHOL see III:DAI600
CALCOLAKE SCARLET 2R see III:FMU070
CALCOLOID GOLDEN YELLOW see III:DCZ000
CALCOMINE BLACK see I:AQP000
CALCOMINE BLUE 2B see I:CMO000
CALCOMINE VIOLET N see III:CMP000
CALCO OIL ORANGE 7078 see III:PEJ500
CALCO OIL RED D see III:SBC500
CALCO OIL SCARLET BL see III:XRA000
CALCOSYN YELLOW GC see II:AAQ250
CALCOTONE RED see III:IHD000
CALCOTONE WHITE T see III:TGG760
CALCOZINE CHRYSOIDINE Y see III:PEK000
CALCOZINE MAGENTA N see II:RMK020
CALCOZINE ORANGE YS see III:PEK000
CALCOZINE RED BX see III:FAG070
CALCOZINE RHODAMINE BX see III:FAG070
CALCOZINE YELLOW OX see I:IBA000
CALDON see III:BRE500
CALEDON GOLDEN YELLOW see III:DCZ000
CALEDON PRINTING YELLOW see III:DCZ000
CALIDRIA RG 100 see I:ARM268
CALIDRIA RG 144 see I:ARM268
CALIDRIA RG 600 see I:ARM268
CALMATHION see III:MAK700
CALMETTEN see II:EOK000
CALMINAL see II:EOK000
CALMOCITENE see III:DCK759
CALMORE see III:TEH500
CALMOREX see III:TEH500
CALMPOSE see III:DCK759
CALOMEL and MAGNESIUM SULFATE (5:8) see III:CAZ000
CALPLUS see III:CAO750
CALPOL see II:HIM000
CALTAC see III:CAO750
CAM see II:CDP250
CAMCOLIT see III:LGZ000
CAMELLIA SINENSIS see III:ARP500
CAMILAN see III:SNY500
CAMPAPRIM A 1544 see I:AMY050
CAMPBELLINE OIL ORANGE see III:PEJ500
CAMPHECHLOR see I:CDV100
CAMPHOCHLOR see I:CDV100
CAMPHOCLOR see I:CDV100
CAMPHOFENE HUILEUX see I:CDV100
CAMPHOR TAR see III:NAJ500
CANACERT AMARANTH see III:FAG020
CANACERT BRILLIANT BLUE FCF see III:FAE000
CANACERT ERYTHROSINE BS see III:FAG040
CANACERT INDIGO CARMINE see III:FAE100
CANACERT SUNSET YELLOW FCF see III:FAG150
CANARY CHROME YELLOW 40-2250 see I:LCR000
CANDAMIDE see III:LGZ000
CANDEX see III:ARQ725
CANESCINE see III:RDF000
CANESCINE 10-METHOXYDERIVATIVE see III:MEK700
CANNABIS SMOKE RESIDUE see III:CBD760
CANTHARIDES CAMPHOR see III:CBE750
CANTHARIDIN see III:CBE750
CANTHARIDINE see III:CBE750
CANTHARONE see III:CBE750
CAO 1 see III:BFW750
CAO 3 see III:BFW750
CAP see II:CBF250, II:CDP250, III:CEA750
CAPATHYN see III:DPJ400
CAPER SPURGE see III:EQW000
CAPMUL see III:PKL030
CAPMUL POE-O see III:PKL100
CAPRAN 80 see III:PJY500

CAPRIC ALCOHOL see III:DAI600
CAPRINIC ALCOHOL see III:DAI600
CAPROAMIDE see III:HEM500
CAPROAMIDE POLYMER see III:PJY500
CAPROKOL see III:HFV500
CAPROLACTAM see III:CBF700
6-CAPROLACTAM see III:CBF700
omega-CAPROLACTAM (MAK) see III:CBF700
CAPROLACTAM OLIGOMER see III:PJY500
epsilon-CAPROLACTAM POLYMERE (GERMAN) see
  III:PJY500
CAPROLATTAME (FRENCH) see III:CBF700
CAPROLON see III:NOH000
CAPRON see III:HNT500, III:PJY500
CAPRONAMIDE see III:HEM500
1-CAPROYLAZIRIDINE see III:HEW000
CAPROYLETHYLENEIMINE see III:HEW000
CAPRYLATE d'OESTRADIOL (FRENCH) see III:EDQ500
CAPRYLDINITROPHENYL CROTONATE see III:AQT500
2-CAPRYL-4,6-DINITROPHENYL CROTONATE see
  III:AQT500
CAPSEBON see I:CAJ750
CAPTAF see III:CBG000
CAPTAFOL see III:CBF800
CAPTAN see III:CBG000
CAPTANCAPTENEET 26,538 see III:CBG000
CAPTANE see III:CBG000
CAPTAN-STREPTOMYCIN 7.5-0.1 POTATO SEED PIECE PRO-
  TECTANT see III:CBG000
CAPTAX see II:BDF000
CAPTEX see III:CBG000
CAPTOFOL see III:CBF800
CAPUT MORTUUM see III:IHD000
CARADATE 30 see III:MJP400
CARASTAY see III:CCL250
CARASTAY G see III:CCL250
CARBACRYL see I:ADX500
CARBADINE see III:EIR000
CARBAMATE see III:FAS000
CARBAMIC ACID, ALLYL ESTER see III:AGA750
CARBAMIC ACID, BUTYL ESTER see III:BQP250
CARBAMIC ACID, 1-(4-CHLOROPHENYL)-1-PHENYL-2-PRO-
  PYNYL ESTER see III:CKI500
CARBAMIC ACID, DIMETHYLDITHIO-, ANHYDROSULFIDE
  see III:BJL600
CARBAMIC ACID, DIMETHYLDITHIO-, ZINC SALT (2:) see
  III:BJK500
CARBAMIC ACID, ETHYL ESTER see I:UVA000
CARBAMIC ACID HYDRAZIDE see III:HGU000
CARBAMIC ACID, ISOPROPYL ESTER see III:IOJ000
CARBAMIC ACID-1-METHYLETHYL ESTER see III:IOJ000
CARBAMIC ACID, METHYL-, NAPHTHALENYL ESTER see
  III:MME800
CARBAMIC ACID, METHYLNITROSO-, o-ISOPROPOXYPHE-
  NYL ESTER see III:PMY310
CARBAMIC ACID, METHYLNITROSO-, 2-(1-METHYL-
  ETHOXY)PHENYL ESTER (9CI) see III:PMY310
CARBAMIC ACID, PROPYL ESTER see III:PNG250
CARBAMIC ACID, 2,2,2-TRICHLOROETHYL ESTER see
  III:TIO500
CARBAMIC ACID, VINYL ESTER see III:VNK000
CARBAMIDE see III:USS000
CARBAMIDE RESIN see III:USS000
p-CARBAMIDOBENZENEARSONIC ACID see III:CBJ000
CARBAMIDSAEURE-AETHYLESTER (GERMAN) see
  I:UVA000
CARBAMIMIDIC ACID see III:USS000
p-CARBAMINO PHENYL ARSONIC ACID see III:CBJ000
CARBAMINOPHENYL-p-ARSONIC ACID see III:CBJ000
CARBAMOHYDROXAMIC ACID see III:HOO500
CARBAMOHYDROXIMIC ACID see III:HOO500
CARBAMOHYDROXYAMIC ACID see III:HOO500
N-CARBAMOYLARSANILIC ACID see III:CBJ000
CARBAMOYLHYDRAZINE see III:HGU000

N-CARBAMOYLHYDROXYLAMINE see III:HOO500
N-(CARBAMOYLMETHYL)-2-DIAZOACETAMIDE see
  III:CBK000
N-CARBAMOYL-N-NITROSOGLYCINE see III:NKI500
CARBAMOYL OXIME see III:HOO500
4-CARBAMYLAMINOPHENYLARSONIC ACID see
  III:CBJ000
N-CARBAMYL ARSANILIC ACID see III:CBJ000
CARBAMYLHYDRAZINE see III:HGU000
CARBAMYLHYDRAZINE HYDROCHLORIDE see
  III:SBW500
CARBAMYL HYDROXAMATE see III:HOO500
1-CARBAMYL-2-PHENYLHYDRAZINE see III:CBL000
2-CARBAMYL PYRAZINE see III:POL500
CARBANILIC ACID ETHYL ESTER see III:CBL750
CARBANILIC ACID ISOPROPYL ESTER see III:CBM000
CARBANTHRENE GOLDEN YELLOW see III:DCZ000
CARBARSONE (USDA) see III:CBJ000
CARBARYL see III:CBM750
CARBASONE see III:CBJ000
CARBATOX-60 see III:CBM750
CARBAX see III:BIO750
CARBAZALDEHYDE see III:FNN000
CARBAZAMIDE see III:HGU000
CARBAZINC see III:BJK500
CARBAZOLE see III:CBN000
9H-CARBAZOLE see III:CBN000
CARBENDAZIME and SODIUM NITRITE (1:1) see III:SIQ700
CARBENDAZIM and SODIUM NITRITE (5:1) see II:CBN375
CARBETHOXY MALATHION see III:MAK700
1-(4-CARBETHOXYPHENYL)-3,3-DIMETHYLTRIAZENE see
  III:CBP250
CARBETOVUR see III:MAK700
CARBETOX see III:MAK700
CARBIDE BLACK E see I:AQP000
CARBITOL see III:DJD600
CARBO-CORT see I:CMY800
CARBOFOS see III:MAK700
CARBOLIC ACID see III:PDN750
CARBOLITH see III:LGZ000
CARBOLON see III:SCQ000
CARBOLSAURE (GERMAN) see III:PDN750
4'-CARBOMETHOXY-2,3'-DIMETHYLAZOBENZENE see
  CBS750
4'-CARBOMETHOXY-2,3'-DIMETHYLAZOBENZOL see
  CBS750
N-(3-CARBOMETHOXYPROPYL)-N-(1-ACETOXYBUTYL)NI-
  TROSAMINE see III:MEI000
CARBONA see CBY000
CARBON BICHLORIDE see II:PCF275
CARBON BLACK see III:CBT750
CARBON CHLORIDE see CBY000
CARBON DICHLORIDE see II:PCF275
CARBON FERROCHROMIUM see III:FBD000
CARBON HEXACHLORIDE see III:HCI000
CARBONIC ACID BERYLLIUM SALT (1:1) see I:BFP750
CARBONIC ACID, DILITHIUM SALT see III:LGZ000
CARBONIC ACID, DIPHENYL ESTER see III:DVZ000
CARBONIC ACID, LEAD(2+) SALT (1:1) see III:LCP000
CARBONIC ACID LITHIUM SALT see III:LGZ000
CARBONIC ACID METHYL-4-(o-TOLYLAZO)-o-TOLYL ES-
  TER see CBS750
CARBONIC ACID, NICKEL SALT (1:1) see I:NCY500
CARBONIC ACID, cyclic VINYLENE ESTER see III:VOK000
4,4'-CARBONIMIDOYLBIS(N,N-DIMETHYLBENZENAMINE)
  see III:IBB000
4,4'-CARBONIMIDOYLBIS(N,N-DIMETHYL-
  BENZENAMINE)MONOHYDROCHLORIDE see I:IBA000
CARBON OIL see I:BBL250
CARBON SILICIDE see III:SCQ000
CARBON TET see CBY000
CARBON TETRACHLORIDE see CBY000
CARBONYL DIAMIDE see III:USS000

CARBONYLDIAMINE see III:USS000
CARBONYL IRON see III:IGK800
CARBOPHOS see III:MAK700
CARBORUNDEUM see III:SCQ000
CARBORUNDUM see III:SCQ000
CARBOSPOL see II:AGJ250
CARBOWAX see III:PJT000
CARBOWAX 1000 see III:PJT250
1-(p-CARBOXYAETHYLPHENYL)-3,3-DIMETHYLTRIAZEN
(GERMAN) see III:CBP250
CARBOXYANILINE see III:API500
2-CARBOXYANILINE see III:API500
o-CARBOXYANILINE see III:API500
2-CARBOXY-4'-(DIMETHYLAMINO)AZOBENZENE see
III:CCE500
3'-CARBOXY-4-DIMETHYLAMINOAZOBENZENE see
III:CCE750
S-2-CARBOXYETHYL-1-CYSTEINE see III:CCF250
3-((2-CARBOXYETHYL)THIO)ALANINE see III:CCF250
6-CARBOXYL-4-HYDROXYLAMINOQUINOLINE-1-OXIDE
see III:CCF750
6-CARBOXYL-4-NITROQUINOLINE-1-OXIDE see
III:CCG000
CARBOXYMETHYL CELLULOSE see III:SFO500
CARBOXYMETHYL CELLULOSE, AMMONIUM SALT see
III:CCH000
CARBOXYMETHYLCELLULOSE NORDIC see III:CCH000
CARBOXYMETHYL CELLULOSE, SODIUM see III:SFO500
CARBOXYMETHYL CELLULOSE, SODIUM SALT see
III:SFO500
CARBOXYMETHYLNITROSOUREA see III:CCH500,
III:NKI500
1-(CARBOXYMETHYL)-1-NITROSOUREA see III:NKI500
6-CARBOXY-4-NITROQUINOLINE-1-OXIDE see III:CCG000
9-o-CARBOXYPHENYL-6-DIETHYLAMINO-3-ETHYLIMINO-
3-ISOXANTHENE, 3-ETHOCHLORIDE see III:FAG070
(9-(o-CARBOXYPHENYL)-6-(DIETHYLAMINO)-3H-XAN-
THEN-3-YLIDENE) DIETHYLAMMONIUM CHLORIDE see
III:FAG070
9-o-CARBOXYPHENYL-6-HYDROXY-3-ISOXANTHONE, DI-
SODIUM SALT see III:FEW000
9-(o-CARBOXYPHENYL)-6-HYDROXY-2,4,5,7-TETRAIODO-
3-ISOXANTHONE see III:FAG040
((o-CARBOXYPHENYL)THIO)ETHYLMERCURY SODIUM
SALT see III:MDI000
3-CARBOXYPROPYL(2-PROPENYL)NITROSAMINE see
III:CCJ375
3-CARBOXYPYRIDINE see III:NCQ900
CARCINOLIPIN see III:CCJ500
CARDENAL see II:EOK000
CARFENE see III:ASH500
CARINA see III:PKQ059
CARINEX GP see III:SMQ500
CARLONA P see III:PMP500
CARMETHOSE see III:SFO500
CARMINAPH see III:PEJ500
CARMINE BLUE (BIOLOGICAL STAIN) see III:FAE100
CARMOISIN (GERMAN) see III:HJF500
CARMOISINE ALUMINUM LAKE see III:HJF500
CARMOISINE SUPRA see III:HJF500
CARMUBRIS see I:BIF750
CARMUSTIN see I:BIF750
CARMUSTINE see I:BIF750
CAROLYSINE see I:BIE500
CARPENE see III:DXX400
CARRAGEEN see III:CCL250
kappa-CARRAGEEN see III:CCL350
kappa-CARRAGEENAN see III:CCL350
CARRAGEENAN, DEGRADED see CCL500
CARRAGEENAN (FCC) see III:CCL250
CARRAGEENAN GUM see III:CCL250
kappa-CARRAGEENIN see III:CCL350
CARRAGHEANIN see III:CCL250
CARRAGHEEN see III:CCL250

CARRAGHEENAN see III:CCL250
CARSORON see III:DER800
CARTAGYL see III:ARQ750
CARTOSE see III:GFG000
CARYOLYSIN see I:BIE250
CARYOLYSINE see I:BIE500
CARYOLYSINE HYDROCHLORIDE see I:BIE500
CARYOPHYLLIC ACID see III:EQR500
CARZOL see III:CJJ250
CARZONAL see III:FMB000, III:FMM000
CASALIS GREEN see II:CMJ900
CASEIN and CASEINATE SALTS (FCC) see III:SFQ000
CASEIN-SODIUM see III:SFQ000
CASEIN, SODIUM COMPLEX see III:SFQ000
CASEINS, SODIUM COMPLEXES see III:SFQ000
CASIFLUX VP 413-004 see III:WCJ000
CASING HEAD GASOLINE (DOT) see III:GBY000
CASORON 133 see III:DER800
CASPAN see III:MDD750
CASSAPPRET SR see III:PKF750
CASSIAR AK see I:ARM268
CASTANEA SATIVA MILL TANNIN see III:CDM250
CATALIN CAO-3 see III:BFW750
CATALOID see III:SCH000
CATALYTIC-DEWAXED HEAVY NAPHTHENIC DISTILLATE
see I:MQV865
CATALYTIC-DEWAXED HEAVY PARAFFINIC DISTILLATE
see I:MQV868
CATALYTIC-DEWAXED LIGHT NAPHTHENIC DISTILLATE
see I:MQV867
CATALYTIC-DEWAXED LIGHT PARAFFINIC DISTILLATE
see I:MQV870
CATECHIN see III:CCP850
CATECHOL see III:CCP850
CAT (HERBICIDE) see III:BJP000
CATILAN see II:CDP250
CAUSOIN see I:DKQ000
CAVALITE BRILLIANT BLUE R see III:BMM500
CAVI-TROL see III:SHF500
CB-154 see III:BNB250
CB 1348 see I:CDO500
C.B. 2041 see I:BOT250
CB2058 see III:DNX200
CB 2095 see III:DNX000
CB 2511 see III:BKM500
CB 2562 see I:TFU500
CB 3025 see I:PED750, III:BHV250
3026 C.B. see III:SAX200
CB-3026 see III:SAX200
CB-3307 see II:BHT750
CB-4564 see I:CQC675, I:EAS500
CB-4835 see II:BIA250
C 49249Ba see III:EEH575
CBC 806495 see I:TFQ750
CBC 906288 see III:TND250
CCC see III:CAQ250
CCC PLANT GROWTH REGULANT see III:CMF400
CCHO see III:CPD000
CCNU see I:CGV250
CCS see III:CJT750
CCUCOL see I:ASB250
CD see III:TGD000
CD 68 see II:CDR750
CDA 101 see III:CNI000
CDA 102 see III:CNI000
CDA 110 see III:CNI000
CDA 122 see III:CNI000
CDC see III:CDL325
CDCA see III:CDL325
CDDP see II:PJD000
CDEC see CDO250
CDHA see III:DGT600
CDM see III:CJJ250
CDNA see III:RDP300

CDT see III:BJP000
CE CE CE see III:CMF400
CECENU see I:CGV250
CECOLENE see II:TIO750
CEDIN see III:ILD000
CEDRO OIL see III:LEI000
CEE see I:PMB000
CEENU see I:CGV250
CEGLUTION see III:LGZ000
CEKIURON see III:DXQ500
CEKUDIFOL see III:BIO750
CEKUFON see III:TIQ250
CEKUGIB see III:GEM000
CEKUMETHION see III:MNH000
CEKUSAN see III:BJP000
CEKUTHOATE see III:DSP400
CEKUZINA-S see III:BJP000
CEKUZINA-T see III:ARQ725
CELANAR see III:PKF750
CELANEX see I:BBQ500
CELANTHRENE PURE BLUE BRS see III:TBG700
CELGARD 2500 see III:PMP500
CELLITAZOL B see I:DCJ200
CELLITON BLUE G see III:TBG700
CELLITON FAST YELLOW G see II:AAQ250
CELLITON ORANGE R see I:AKP750
CELLOFAS see III:SFO500
CELLOFOR (CZECH) see III:DWO800
CELLOGEL C see III:SFO500
CELLON see III:TBQ100
CELLOPHANE see III:CCT250
CELLPRO see III:SFO500
CELLUFIX FF 100 see III:SFO500
CELLUGEL see III:SFO500
CELLULOSE GLYCOLIC ACID, SODIUM SALT see
    III:SFO500
CELLULOSE GUM see III:SFO500
CELLULOSE SODIUM GLYCOLATE see III:SFO500
CELLU-QUIN see III:BLC250
CELMIDE see I:EIY500
CELTHIGN see III:MAK700
CEMIDON see III:ILD000
CENOL GARDEN DUST see III:RNZ000
CENTELASE see III:ARN500
CENTRALINE BLUE 3B see II:CMO250
CENTRAX see III:DAP700
CENTURY 1240 see III:SLK000
CENTURY CD FATTY ACID see III:OHU000
CERAMIC FIBRE see III:AHF500
CERASINE YELLOW GG see I:DOT300
CERASINROT see III:OHA000
CERAZOL (suspension) see III:TEX250
CERCINE see III:DCK759
CEREGULART see III:DCK759
CERELOSE see III:GFG000
CEREPAP see III:DNA200
CERES ORANGE R see III:PEJ500
CERES ORANGES RR see III:XRA000
CERES RED 7B see III:EOJ500
CERES YELLOW R see II:PEI000
CERISE TONER X1127 see III:FAG070
CERISOL SCARLET G see III:XRA000
CERISOL YELLOW AB see III:FAG130
CERISOL YELLOW TB see III:FAG135
CERN PRIMA 38 see I:AQP000
CEROTINORANGE G see III:PEJ500
CEROTINSCHARLACH G see III:XRA000
CERTICOL CARMOISINE S see III:HJF500
CERTICOL ORANGE GS see III:HGC000
CERTICOL PONCEAU MXS see III:FMU070
CERTICOL PONCEAU 4RS see III:FMU080
CERTICOL PONCEAU SXS see III:FAG050
CERTIQUAL EOSINE see III:BNH500, III:BNK700
CERTIQUAL FLUORESCEINE see III:FEW000

CERTIQUAL ORANGE I see III:FAG010
CERTIQUAL RHODAMIEN see III:FAG070
CERUBIDIN see II:DAC000
CERUSSETE see III:LCP000
CERVEN KOSENILOVA A see III:FMU080
CERVEN KUMIDINOVA see II:FAG018
CERVEN KYSELA 26 see III:FMU070
CERVEN KYSELA 27 see III:FAG020
CERVEN POTRAVINARSKA 1 see III:FAG050
CERVEN POTRAVINARSKA 9 see III:FAG020
CERVICUNDIN see II:EQJ500
CES see I:ECU750, I:SOP500
CET see III:BJP000
CETADOL see II:HIM000
CETIL LIGHT ORANGE GG see III:HGC000
CETYLIC ACID see III:PAE250
CFC 133a see III:TJY175
CG-1283 see I:MQW500
CH see III:SBW500
CHA see III:CPF500
CHALCEDONY see I:SCJ500
CHANNEL BLACK see III:CBT750
CHA-SULFATE see III:CPF750
CHAVICOL METHYL ETHER see III:AFW750
CHEMAID see I:HKC500
CHEMANOX 11 see III:BFW750
CHEMATHION see III:MAK700
CHEMBUTAZONE see II:BRF500
CHEM FISH see III:RNZ000
CHEM-HOE see III:CBM000
CHEMIAZID see III:ILD000
CHEMICAL 109 see III:AQN635
CHEMICAL MACE see III:CEA750
CHEMICETIN see II:CDP250
CHEMICETINA see II:CDP250
CHEMIDON see III:ILD000
CHEMIFLUOR see III:SHF500
CHEMIOFURAN see III:NGE000
CHEMLON see III:PJY500
CHEM-MITE see III:RNZ000
CHEM NEB see III:MAS500
CHEMOCHIN see III:CLD000
CHEMOFURAN see II:NGE500
CHEMOSEPT see III:TEX250
CHEMOUAG see III:SNN500
CHEMOX GENERAL see III:BRE500
CHEMOX P.E. see III:BRE500
CHEM PELS C see I:SEY500
CHEM-PHENE see I:CDV100
CHEM-SEN 56 see I:SEY500
CHEM-TOL see II:PAX250
CHEM ZINEB see III:EIR000
CHENDAL see III:CDL325
CHENDOL see III:CDL325
CHENIC ACID see III:CDL325
CHENIX see III:CDL325
CHENOCEDON see III:CDL325
CHENODEOXYCHOLIC ACID see III:CDL325
CHENODESOXYCHOLIC ACID see III:CDL325
CHENODESOXYCHOLSAEURE (GERMAN) see III:CDL325
CHENODEX see III:CDL325
CHENODIOL see III:CDL325
CHENOFALK see III:CDL325
CHENOPODIUM AMBROSIOIDES see III:SAF000
CHENOSAURE see III:CDL325
CHENOSSIL see III:CDL325
CHEQUE see III:MQS225
CHERRY BARK OAK see III:CDL750
CHERTS see I:SCJ500
CHESTNUT TANNIN see III:CDM250
17-CHETOVIS see III:AOO450
CHEWING TOBACCO see I:SED400
CHEXMATE see III:HKC000

CHILE SALTPETER see III:SIO900
CHINESE RED see I:LCS000
CHINGAMIN see III:CLD000
CHINOFER see I:IGS000
CHINOLEINE see III:QMJ000
CHINOLIN (CZECH) see III:QMJ000
CHINOLINE see III:QMJ000
p-CHINON (GERMAN) see III:QQS200
CHINON (DUTCH, GERMAN) see III:QQS200
CHINONE see III:QQS200
CHIPCO CRAB KLEEN see I:DXE600
CHIPCO THIRAM 75 see III:TFS350
CHIPCO TURF HERBICIDE "D" see II:DAA800
CHIPCO TURF HERBICIDE MCPP see II:CIR500
CHIPMAN 3,142 see III:TBR750
CHIPTOX see II:CIR250
CHISSO 507B see III:PMP500
CHISSONOX 201 see III:ECB000
CHISSONOX 206 see I:VOA000
CHKHZ 18 see III:DVF400
CHLODITAN see III:CDN000
CHLODITHANE see III:CDN000
CHLOMAPHENE see III:CMX500
CHLOMIN see II:CDP250
CHLOMYCOL see II:CDP250
2-CHLOOR-1,3-BUTADIEEN (DUTCH) see III:NCI500
CHLOORDAAN (DUTCH) see II:CDR750
(2-CHLOOR-3-DIETHYLAMINO-1-METHYL-3-OXO-PROP-1-
    EN-YL)-DIMETHYL-FOSFAAT see III:FAC025
1-CHLOOR-2,3-EPOXY-PROPAAN (DUTCH) see I:EAZ500
CHLOORFENSON (DUTCH) see III:CJT750
(4-CHLOOR-FENYL)-4-CHLOOR-BENZEEN-SULFONAAT
    (DUTCH) see III:CJT750
3-(4-CHLOOR-FENYL)-1,1-DIMETHYLUREUM (DUTCH) see
    III:CJX750
N-(3-CHLOOR-FENYL)-ISOPROPYL CARBAMAAT (DUTCH)
    see III:CKC000
CHLOOR-METHAAN (DUTCH) see II:MIF765
2-(4-CHLOOR-2-METHYL-FENOXY)-PROPIONZUUR
    (DUTCH) see II:CIR500
1-CHLOOR-4-NITROBENZEEN (DUTCH) see III:NFS525
CHLOORPIKRINE (DUTCH) see III:CKN500
CHLOPHEN see I:PJL750
CHLORACETIC ACID see III:CEA000
CHLORACETONITRILE see III:CDN500
N-(2-CHLOROAETHYL)-N'-(2 CHLOROETHYL)-N'-o-PRO-
    PYLEN-PHOSPHORSAUREESTER-DIAMID (GERMAN) see
    II:IMH000
2-CHLORAETHYL-TRIMETHYLAMMONIUMCHLORID see
    III:CMF400
CHLORAK see III:TIQ250
CHLORALDURAT see III:CDO000
CHLORAL HYDRATE see III:CDO000
CHLORALLYL DIETHYLDITHIOCARBAMATE see CDO250
2-CHLORALLYL DIETHYLDITHIOCARBAMATE see
    CDO250
CHLORALLYLENE see II:AGB250
CHLORALOSANE see III:GFA000
α-CHLORALOSE see III:GFA000
CHLORAMBEN see III:AJM000
CHLORAMBUCIL see CDO500
CHLORAMEX see II:CDP250
CHLORAMFICIN see II:CDP250
CHLORAMFILIN see II:CDP250
CHLORAMIFENE see III:CMX500
CHLORAMIN see I:BIE500
CHLORAMINE see I:BIE500
CHLORAMINE BLACK C see I:AQP000
CHLORAMINE BLUE see II:CMO250
CHLORAMINE BLUE 2B see I:CMO000
CHLORAMINE FAST BROWN BRL see II:CMO750
CHLORAMIN HYDROCHLORIDE see I:BIE500
CHLORAMINOPHEN see I:CDO500
CHLORAMINOPHENE see I:CDO500

CHLORAMIPHENE see III:CMX500, III:CMX700
CHLORAMIPHENE CITRATE see III:CMX700
CHLORAMP (RUSSIAN) see III:PIB900
CHLORAMPHENICOL see II:CDP250
d-CHLORAMPHENICOL see II:CDP250
d-threo-CHLORAMPHENICOL see II:CDP250
CHLORAMSAAR see II:CDP250
CHLORANIL see III:TBO500
4-CHLORANILIN (CZECH) see III:CEH680
p-CHLORANILINE see III:CEH680
CHLORAQUINE see III:CLD000
CHLORASOL see II:CDP250
CHLORA-TABS see II:CDP250
CHLORAZOL BLACK E (biological stain) see I:AQP000
CHLORAZOL BLACK EA see I:AQP000
CHLORAZOL BLACK EN see I:AQP000
CHLORAZOL BLUE 3B see II:CMO250
CHLORAZOL BLUE B see I:CMO000
CHLORAZOL SKY BLUE FF see III:BGT250
CHLORAZOL VIOLET N see III:CMP000
CHLORBENZILATE see II:DER000
2-CHLOR-1,3-BUTADIEN (GERMAN) see III:NCI500
4-CHLORBUTAN-1-OL (GERMAN) see III:CEU500
CHLORCHOLINCHLORID see III:CMF400
CHLORCHOLINE CHLORIDE see III:CMF400
CHLORDAN see II:CDR750
γ-CHLORDAN see II:CDR750
CHLORDANE see II:CDR750
CHLORDANE, liquid (DOT) see II:CDR750
CHLORDECONE see I:KEA000
(2-CHLOR-3-DIAETHYLAMINO-1-METHYL-3-OXO-PROP-1-
    EN-YL)-DIMETHYL-PHOSPHAT see III:FAC025
CHLORDIAZEPOXIDE, NITROSATED see III:SIS000
CHLORDIAZEPOXIDE mixed with SODIUM NITRITE (1:1) see
    III:SIS000
CHLORDIMEFORM see III:CJJ250
CHLORDIMETHYLETHER (CZECH) see I:CIO250
CHLOREFENIZON (FRENCH) see III:CJT750
CHLORENDIC ACID see II:CDS000
1-CHLOR-2,3-EPOXY-PROPAN (GERMAN) see I:EAZ500
CHLORESENE see I:BBQ500
CHLORESTROLO see II:CLO750
CHLORETHAMINACIL see II:BIA250
CHLORETHAMINE see I:BIE500
CHLORETHAZINE see I:BIE500
CHLORETHENE see I:VNP000
CHLORETHYLENE see I:VNP000
CHLOREX see III:DFJ050
CHLOREXTOL see I:PJL750
CHLORFENAMIDINE see III:CJJ250
CHLORFENIDIM see III:CJX750
CHLORFENSON see III:CJT750
CHLORFENSONE see III:CJT750
1-p-CHLORFENYL-3,3-DIMETHYLTRIAZEN (CZECH) see
    III:CJI100
CHLORFOS see III:TIQ250
CHLORHYDRATE d'ANILINE (FRENCH) see II:BBL000
CHLORHYDRATE de 4-CHLOROORTHOTOLUIDINE
    (FRENCH) see II:CLK235
CHLORHYDRATE D'HISTAMINE (FRENCH) see III:HGE500
CHLORHYDRIN see III:CDT750
α-CHLORHYDRIN see III:CDT750
CHLORICOL see II:CDP250
CHLORID ANILINU (CZECH) see II:BBL000
CHLORIDIN see III:TGD000
CHLORIDINE see III:TGD000
CHLORIERTE BIPHENYLE, CHLORGEHALT 42% (GERMAN)
    see II:PJM500
CHLORIERTE BIPHENYLE, CHLORGEHALT 54% (GERMAN)
    see II:PJN000
CHLOR-IFC see III:CKC000
CHLORINATED BIPHENYL see I:PJL750
CHLORINATED CAMPHENE see I:CDV100
CHLORINATED DIPHENYL see I:PJL750

CHLORINATED DIPHENYLENE see I:PJL750
CHLORINATED HC, ALIPHATIC see II:CDV250
CHLORINATED HYDROCARBONS, ALIPHATIC see II:CDV250
CHLORINATED HYDROCHLORIC ETHER see III:DFF809
CHLORINATED NAPHTHALENES see III:CDV575
CHLORINATED PARAFFINS (C12, 60% CHLORINE) see II:PAH800
CHLORINATED PARAFFINS (C23, 43% CHLORINE) see III:PAH810
CHLORINATED POLYETHER POLYURETHAN see I:CDV625
CHLORINDAN see II:CDR750
CHLOR-IPC see III:CKC000
CHLOR KIL see II:CDR750
CHLORKU LITU (POLISH) see III:LHB000
CHLORMADINON ACETATE see II:CBF250
CHLORMADINONE ACETATE see II:CBF250
CHLORMADINONE ACETATE mixed with MESTRANOL see III:CNV750
CHLORMADINONU (POLISH) see II:CBF250
CHLORMEQUAT see III:CMF400
CHLORMEQUAT CHLORIDE see III:CMF400
CHLOR-METHAN (GERMAN) see II:MIF765
CHLORMETHINE see I:BIE250
CHLORMETHINE HYDROCHLORIDE see I:BIE500
CHLORMETHINE-N-OXIDE HYDROCHLORIDE see II:CFA750
CHLORMETHINUM see I:BIE500
2-(4-CHLOR-2-METHYL-PHENOXY)-PROPIONSAEURE (GERMAN) see II:CIR500
3-CHLOR-2-METHYL-PROP-1-EN (GERMAN) see II:CIU750
CHLORNAFTINA see I:BIF250
CHLORNAPHAZIN see I:BIF250
CHLORNAPHTHIN see I:BIF250
1-CHLOR-4-NITROBENZOL (GERMAN) see III:NFS525
CHLORNITROMYCIN see II:CDP250
CHLOROACETIC ACID see III:CEA000
α-CHLOROACETIC ACID see III:CEA000
CHLOROACETIC ACID, liquid (DOT) see III:CEA000
CHLOROACETIC ACID, solid (DOT) see III:CEA000
CHLOROACETIC ACID, ETHYL ESTER see III:EHG500
2-CHLOROACETONITRILE see IIi:CDN500
α-CHLOROACETONITRILE see III:CDN500
CHLOROACETONITRILE (DOT) see III:CDN500
1-CHLOROACETOPHENONE see III:CEA750
α-CHLOROACETOPHENONE see III:CEA750
omega-CHLOROACETOPHENONE see III:CEA750
CHLOROACETOPHENONE, gas, liquid or solid (DOT) see III:CEA750
6-CHLORO-17-α-ACETOXY-4,6-PREGNADIENE-3,20-DIONE see II:CBF250
6-CHLORO-Δ⁶-17-ACETOXYPROGESTERONE see II:CBF250
Δ⁶-6-CHLORO-17-α-ACETOXYPROGESTERONE see II:CBF250
6-CHLORO-Δ⁶-(17-α)ACETOXYPROGESTERONE see II:CBF250
α-CHLOROALLYL CHLORIDE see I:DGG950
γ-CHLOROALLYL CHLORIDE see I:DGG950
2-CHLOROALLYL DIETHYLDITHIOCARBAMATE see CDO250
2-CHLOROALLYL-N,N-DIETHYLDITHIOCARBAMATE see CDO250
CHLOROALLYLENE see II:AGB250
CHLOROALONIL see III:TBQ750
CHLOROALOSANE see III:GFA000
CHLOROAMBUCIL see I:CDO500
3-CHLORO-4-AMINOANILINE SULFATE see III:CEG625
4'-CHLORO-4-AMINOBIPHENYL ETHER see III:CEH125
3-CHLORO-4-AMINODIPHENYL see III:CEH000
4-CHLORO-4'-AMINODIPHENYL ETHER see III:CEH125
3-CHLORO-4-AMINOSTILBENE see III:CLE500
4-CHLORO-2-AMINOTOLUENE see II:CLK225
5-CHLORO-2-AMINOTOLUENE see II:CLK220
5-CHLORO-2-AMINOTOLUENE HYDROCHLORIDE see II:CLK235

4-CHLOROANILINE see III:CEH680
p-CHLOROANILINE see III:CEH680
p-CHLOROANILINE, solid (DOT) see III:CEH680
p-CHLOROANILINE, liquid (DOT) see III:CEH680
CHLOROBEN see III:DEP600
α-CHLOROBENZALDEHYDE see III:BDM500
7-CHLOROBENZ(a)ANTHRACENE see III:CEJ000
10-CHLORO-1,2-BENZANTHRACENE see III:CEJ000
4-CHLOROBENZENAMINE see III:CEH680
4-CHLORO BENZENEAMINE see III:CEH680
3-CHLORO-BENZENECARBOPEROXOIC ACID (9CI) see III:CJI750
4-CHLORO-1,3-BENZENEDIAMINE see II:CJS125
2-CHLORO-1,4-BENZENEDIAMINE SULFATE see III:CEG625
4-CHLOROBENZENESULFONATE de 4-CHLOROPHENYLE (FRENCH) see III:CJT750
p-CHLOROBENZENESULFONIC ACID-p-CHLOROPHENYL ESTER see III:CJT750
4-CHLOROBENZENETHIOL see III:CEK425
6-CHLOROBENZENO(a)PYRENE see III:CEK500
2-CHLOROBENZO(e)(1)BENZOTHIOPYRANO(4,3-b)INDOLE see III:CEL000
m-CHLOROBENZOYL HYDROPEROXIDE see III:CJI750
CHLOROBENZYLATE see II:DER000
CHLORO BIPHENYL see I:PJL750
CHLORO-1,1-BIPHENYL see I:PJL750
3-CHLOROBIPHENYLAMINE see III:CEH000
2-CHLORO-4,6-BIS(ETHYLAMINO)-s-TRIAZINE see III:BJP000
1-CHLORO-3,5-BISETHYLAMINO-2,4,6-TRIAZINE see III:BJP000
2-CHLORO-4,6-BIS(ETHYLAMINO)-1,3,5-TRIAZINE see III:BJP000
CHLOROBLE M see III:MAS500
4-CHLORO-7-BROMOMETHYLBENZ(a)ANTHRACENE see III:BNQ000
CHLOROBUTADIENE see III:NCI500
2-CHLOROBUTA-1,3-DIENE see III:NCI500
2-CHLORO-1,3-BUTADIENE see III:NCI500
2-CHLOROBUTANE see III:CEU250
4-CHLORO-1-BUTANE-OL see III:CEU500
3-CHLOROBUTANOIC ACID see III:CEW000
4-CHLOROBUTANOL see III:CEU500
4-CHLORO-1-BUTANOL see III:CEU500
CHLOROBUTIN see I:CDO500
CHLOROBUTINE see I:CDO500
3-CHLOROBUTYRIC ACID see III:CEW000
β-CHLOROBUTYRIC ACID see III:CEW000
CHLOROCAMPHENE see I:CDV100
CHLOROCAPS see II:CDP250
3-CHLOROCARBANILIC ACID, ISOPROPYL ESTER see III:CKC000
m-CHLOROCARBANILIC ACID, ISOPROPYL ESTER see III:CKC000
CHLOROCHIN see III:CLD000
3-CHLOROCHLORDENE see II:HAR000
1-CHLORO-2-(β-CHLOROETHOXY)ETHANE see III:DFJ050
7-CHLORO-10-(3-(N-(2-CHLOROETHYL)-N-ETHYL)AMINO-PROPYLAMINO)-2-METHOXY-BENZO(B)(1,5)NAPH-THYRIDINE DIHYDROCHLORIDE see III:IAE000
6-CHLORO-9-(3-(2-CHLOROETHYL)MERCAPTOPROPYL-AMINO)-2-METHOXYACRIDINE HYDROCHLORIDE see III:CFA250
2-CHLORO-N-(2-CHLOROETHYL)-N-METHYLETHANA-MINE HYDROCHLORIDE see I:BIE500
2-CHLORO-N-(2-CHLOROETHYL)-N-METHYL ETHANA-MINE-N-OXIDE see III:CFA500
2-CHLORO-N-(2-CHLOROETHYL)-N-METHYLETHANA-MINE-N-OXIDE HYDROCHLORIDE see II:CFA750
1-CHLORO-2-(β-CHLOROETHYLTHIO)ETHANE see I:BIH250
CHLORO(CHLOROMETHOXY)METHANE see I:BIK000
9-CHLORO-10-CHLOROMETHYL ANTHRACENE see III:CFB500

cis-2-CHLORO-3-(CHLOROMETHYL)OXIRANE see III:DAC975

trans-2-CHLORO-3-(CHLOROMETHYL)OXIRANE see III:DGH500

4-CHLORO-α-(4-CHLOROPHENYL)-α-(TRICHLORO-METHYL)BENZENEMETHANOL see III:BIO750

CHLOROCHOLINE CHLORIDE see III:CMF400

CHLOROCID see II:CDP250

CHLOROCIDIN C TETRAN see II:CDP250

CHLOROCOL see II:CDP250

4-CHLORO-o-CRESOXYACETIC ACID see II:CIR250

7-CHLORO-1-(CYCLOPROPYLMETHYL)-1,3-DIHYDRO-5-PHENYL-2H-1,4-BENZODIAZEPIN-2-ONE see III:DAP700

7-CHLORO-1-CYCLOPROPYLMETHYL-5-PHENYL-1H-1,4-BENZODIAZEPIN-2(3H)-ONE see III:DAP700

CHLORODANE see II:CDR750

6-CHLORO-6-DEHYDRO-17-α-ACETOXYPROGESTERONE see II:CBF250

6-CHLORO-Δ⁶-DEHYDRO-17-ACETOXYPROGESTERONE see II:CBF250

6-CHLORO-6-DEHYDRO-17-α-ACETOXYPROGESTERONE mixed with MESTRENOL see III:CNV750

6-CHLORO-6-DEHYDRO-17-α-HYDROXYPROGESTERONE ACETATE see II:CBF250

CHLORODEN see III:DEP600

CHLORODEOXYGLYCEROL see III:CDT750

1-CHLORO-2,4-DIAMINOBENZENE see II:CJS125

4-CHLORO-1,2-DIAMINOBENZENE see I:CFK125

1-CHLORO-2,3-DIBROMOPROPANE see I:DDL800

3-CHLORO-1,2-DIBROMOPROPANE see I:DDL800

1-CHLORO-2-(2,2-DICHLORO-1-(4-CHLOROPHENYL)ETHYL)BENZENE see CDN000

1-CHLORO-2,2-DICHLOROETHYLENE see II:TIO750

2-CHLORO-1-(p-(β-DIETHYLAMINOETHOXY)PHENYL)-1,2-DIPHENYLETHYLENE see III:CMX700

7-CHLORO-4-(4-DIETHYLAMINO-1-METHYLBUTYL-AMINO)QUINOLINE see III:CLD000

2-CHLORO-2-DIETHYLCARBAMOYL-1-METHYLVINYL DI-METHYLPHOSPHATE see III:FAC025

1-CHLORO-DIETHYLCARBAMOYL-1-PROPEN-2-YL DI-METHYL PHOSPHATE see III:FAC025

CHLORODIFLUOROMETHANE see III:CFX500

2-CHLORO-1-(DIFLUOROMETHOXY)-1,1,2-TRIFLUORO-ETHANE see III:EAT900

12-CHLORO-7,12-DIHYDRO-8,11-DIMETHYLBENZO(a)PHE-NARSAZINE see III:CGH500

(R)N-((5-CHLORO-3,4-DIHYDRO-8-HYDROXY-3-METHYL-1-OXO-1H-2-BENZOPYRAN-7-YL)PHENYLALANINE see III:CHP750

7-CHLORO-1,3-DIHYDRO-3-HYDROXY-5-PHENYL-2H-1,4-BENZODIAZEPINE-2-ONE see III:CFZ000

7-CHLORO-1,3-DIHYDRO-1-METHYL-5-PHENYL-2H-1,4-BENZODIAZEPIN-2-ONE see III:DCK759

1-CHLORO-2,3-DIHYDROXYPROPANE see III:CDT750

3-CHLORO-1,2-DIHYDROXYPROPANE see III:CDT750

p-CHLORO DIMETHYLAMINOAZOBENZENE see III:CGD250

2'-CHLORO-4-DIMETHYLAMINOAZOBENZENE see III:DRD000

3'-CHLORO-4-DIMETHYLAMINOAZOBENZENE see III:DRC800

4'-CHLORO-4-DIMETHYLAMINOAZOBENZENE see III:CGD250

3'-CHLORO-N,N-DIMETHYLAMINOSTIBEN (GERMAN) see III:CGK750

4'-CHLORO-N,N-DIMETHYLAMINOSTIBEN (GERMAN) see III:CGL000

2'-CHLORO-4-DIMETHYLAMINOSTILBENE see III:CGK500

3'-CHLORO-4-DIMETHYLAMINOSTILBENE see III:CGK750

4'-CHLORO-4-DIMETHYLAMINOSTILBENE see III:CGL000

9-CHLORO-8,12-DIMETHYLBENZ(a)ACRIDINE see III:CGH250

2-CHLORO-1,10-DIMETHYL-5,6-BENZACRIDINE (FRENCH) see III:CGH250

2-CHLORO-1,10-DIMETHYL-7,8-BENZACRIDINE (FRENCH) see III:DRB800

10-CHLORO-6,9-DIMETHYL-5,10-DIHYDRO-3,4-BENZOPHE-NARSAZINE see III:CGH500

2-CHLORO-N,N-DIMETHYLETHYLAMINE HYDROCHLO-RIDE see III:DRC000

((4-CHLORO-6-((2,3-DIMETHYLPHENYL)AMINO)-2-PYRIMI-DINYL)THIO)ACETIC ACID see II:CLW250

2-CHLORO-5-(3,5-DIMETHYLPIPERIDINO SULPHONYL)BENZOIC ACID see III:CGJ250

2'-CHLORO-N,N-DIMETHYL-4-STILBENAMINE see III:CGK500

3'-CHLORO-N,N-DIMETHYL-4-STILBENAMINE see III:CGK750

4'-CHLORO-N,N-DIMETHYL-4-STILBENAMINE see III:CGL000

1-CHLORO-2,4-DINITRONAPHTHALENE see III:DUS600

CHLORODIPHENYL (21% Cl) see II:PJM000

CHLORODIPHENYL (32% Cl) see II:PJM250

CHLORODIPHENYL (48% Cl) see II:PJM750

CHLORODIPHENYL (60% Cl) see II:PJN250

CHLORODIPHENYL (62% Cl) see II:PJN500

CHLORODIPHENYL (68% Cl) see II:PJN750

CHLORODIPHENYL (42% Cl) (OSHA) see II:PJM500

CHLORODIPHENYL (54% Cl) (OSHA) see II:PJN000

2-(4-(2-CHLORO-1,2-DIPHENYLETHENYL)PHENOXY)-N,N-DIETHYLETHANAMINE see III:CMX500

2-(p-(2-CHLORO-1,2-DIPHENYL VINYL)PHENOXY)TRI-ETHYLAMINE CITRATE (1:1) see III:CMX700

CHLOROEPOXYETHANE see III:CGX000

1-CHLORO-2,3-EPOXYPROPANE see I:EAZ500

3-CHLORO-1,2-EPOXYPROPANE see I:EAZ500

cis-1-CHLORO-1,2-EPOXYPROPANE see III:CKS099

trans-1-CHLORO-1,2-EPOXYPROPANE see III:CKS100

CHLOROETENE see III:MIH275

CHLOROETHANOIC ACID see III:CEA000

2-CHLOROETHANOL-2-(p-t-BUTYLPHENOXY)-1-METHYL-ETHYL SULFITE see I:SOP500

2-CHLOROETHANOL ESTER with 2-(p-t-BUTYLPHENOXY)-1-METHYLETHYL SULFITE see I:SOP500

CHLOROETHENE see I:VNP000, III:MIH275

CHLOROETHENE HOMOPOLYMER see III:PKQ059

1,1',1''-(1-CHLORO-1-ETHENYL-2-YLIDENE)-TRIS(4-METHOXYBENZENE) see II:CLO750

17-α-CHLOROETHINYL-17-β-HYDROXYESTRA-4,9-DIEN-3-ONE see III:CHP750

2-CHLORO-4-ETHYLAMINEISOPROPYLAMINE-s-TRIAZINE see III:ARQ725

9-(2-((2-CHLOROETHYL)AMINO)ETHYLAMINO)-6-CHLORO-2-METHOXYACRIDINE, DIHYDROCHLORIDE see III:QCS875

1-CHLORO-3-ETHYLAMINO-5-ISOPROPYLAMINO-s-TRIA-ZINE see III:ARQ725

2-CHLORO-4-ETHYLAMINO-6-ISOPROPYLAMINO-s-TRIA-ZINE see III:ARQ725

1-CHLORO-3-ETHYLAMINO-5-ISOPROPYLAMINO-2,4,6-TRIAZINE see III:ARQ725

2-CHLORO-4-ETHYLAMINO-6-ISOPROPYLAMINO-1,3,5-TRIAZINE see III:ARQ725

β-CHLOROETHYL-β'-(p-tert-BUTYLPHENOXY)-α'-METH-YLETHYL SULFITE see I:SOP500

β-CHLOROETHYL-β-(p-tert-BUTYLPHENOXY)-α-METHYL-ETHYL SULPHITE see I:SOP500

3-(2-CHLOROETHYL)-2-((2-CHLOROETHYL)AMINO)PER-HYDRO-2H-1,3,2-OXAZAPHOSPHORINE OXIDE see II:IMH000

6-CHLORO-9-(3-ETHYL-2-CHLOROETHYL)AMINOPROPYL-AMINO)-2-METHOXYACRIDINE DIHYDROCHLORIDE see III:ADJ875

3-(2-CHLOROETHYL)-2-((2-CHLOROETHYL)AMINO)TET-RAHYDRO-2H-1,3,2-OXAZAPHOSPHORINE-2-OXIDE see II:IMH000

N-(2-CHLOROETHYL)-N'-(2-CHLOROETHYL)-N',O-PROPY-LENEPHOSPHORIC ACID DIAMIDE see II:IMH000

N-(2-CHLOROETHYL)-N'-(2-CHLOROETHYL)-N',O-PROPY-
LENEPHOSPHORIC ACID ESTER DIAMIDE see II:IMH000
CHLOROETHYLCYCLOHEXYLNITROSOUREA see
I:CGV250
((CHLORO-2-ETHYL)-1-CYCLOHEXYL-3-NITROSOUREA see
I:CGV250
1-(2-CHLOROETHYL)-3-CYCLOHEXYL-1-NITROSOUREA
see I:CGV250
N-(2-CHLOROETHYL)-N'-CYCLOHEXYL-N-NITROSOUREA
see I:CGV250
3'-CHLORO-4'-ETHYL-4-DIMETHYLAMINOAZOBENZENE
see III:CGW100
4'-CHLORO-3'-ETHYL-4-DIMETHYLAMINOAZOBENZENE
see III:CGW105
CHLOROETHYLENE see I:VNP000
4-CHLORO-6-ETHYLENEIMINO-2-PHENYLPYRIMIDINE see
III:CGW750
CHLOROETHYLENE OXIDE see III:CGX000
CHLOROETHYLENE POLYMER see III:PKQ059
CHLOROETHYLENEVINYL ACETATE POLYMER see
II:AAX175
CHLOROETHYL ETHER see III:DFJ050
7-(2-(2-CHLOROETHYLETHYLAMINO)ETHYLAMINO)
BENZ(c)ACRIDINE DIHYDROCHLORIDE see III:EHI500
1-(2-CHLOROETHYL)-3-(d-GLUCOPYRANOS-2-YL)-1-NI-
TROSOUREA see III:CLX000
1-(2-CHLOROETHYL)-3-(2-HYDROXYETHYL)-1-NITROSO-
UREA see III:CHB750
2-CHLOROETHYL 1-METHYL-2-(p-tert-BUTYLPHENOXY)
ETHYL SULPHATE see I:SOP500
1-(2-CHLOROETHYL)-3-(4-METHYL-CYCLOHEXYL)-1-NI-
TROSOUREA see II:CHD250
1-(2-CHLOROETHYL)-3-(trans-4-METHYL-CYCLOHEXYL)-1-
NITROSOUREA see II:CHD250
N-(2-CHLOROETHYL)-N'-(trans-4-METHYLCYCLOHEXYL)-
N-NITROSOUREA see II:CHD250
6-CHLORO-N-ETHYL-N'-(1-METHYLETHYL)-1,3,5-TRIA-
ZINE-2,4-DIAMINE (9CI) see III:ARQ725
N-(2-CHLOROETHYL)-N-(1-METHYL-2-
PHENOXYETHYL)BENZENEMETHANAMINE see
I:PDT250
N-(2-CHLOROETHYL)-N-(1-METHYL-2-
PHENOXYETHYL)BENZENEMETHANAMINE HYDRO-
CHLORIDE see II:DDG800
N-(2-CHLOROETHYL)-N-(1-METHYL-2-PHENOXYETHYL)
BENZYLAMINE see I:PDT250
N-(2-CHLOROETHYL)-N-(1-METHYL-2-PHENOXYETHYL)
BENZYLAMINE HYDROCHLORIDE see II:DDG800
1-(2-CHLOROETHYL)-3-MORPHOLINO-1-NITROSOUREA
see III:MRR775
2-((((2-CHLOROETHYL)NITROSOAMINO)CARBONYL)
AMINO)-2-DEOXY-d-GLUCOPYRANOSE see III:CLX000
2-((((2-CHLOROETHYL)NITROSOAMINO)CARBONYL)
AMINO)-2-DEOXY-d-GLUCOSE see III:CLX000
N-(2-CHLOROETHYL)-N-NITROSOETHYLCARBAMATE see
III:CHF500
2-(3-(2-CHLOROETHYL)-3-NITROSOUREIDO)-2-DEOXY-d-
GLUCOSOPYRANOSE see III:CLX000
2-(3-(2-CHLOROETHYL)-3-NITROSOUREIDO)-d-GLUCO-PY-
RANOSE see III:CLX000
N-(β-CHLOROETHYL)-N-NITROSOURETHAN see
III:CHF500
2-CHLOROETHYL-N-NITROSOURETHANE see III:CHF500
p-((3-CHLORO-4-ETHYLPHENYL)AZO)-N,N-DIMETHYLANI-
LINE see III:CGW100
p-((4-CHLORO-3-ETHYLPHENYL)AZO)-N,N-DIMETHYLANI-
LINE see III:CGW105
7-(3-(2-CHLOROETHYL-n-
PROPYLAMINO)PROPYLAMINO)BENZO(b)(1,10)-PHE-
NATHROLINE HYDROCHLORIDE see III:CHH000
2-CHLOROETHYL SULFUROUS ACID-2-(4-(1,1-DIMETHYL-
ETHYL)PHENOXY)-1-METHYLETHYL ESTER see
I:SOP500

2-CHLOROETHYL SULPHITE of 1-(p-tert-BUTYLPHENOXY)-
2-PROPANOL see I:SOP500
(2-CHLOROETHYL)TRIMETHYLAMMONIUM CHLORIDE
see III:CMF400
(β-CHLOROETHYL)TRIMETHYLAMMONIUM CHLORIDE
see III:CMF400
17-α-CHLOROETHYNLY-19-NOR-4,9-ANDROSTADIEN-17-β-
OL-3-ONE see III:CHP750
17-α-CHLOROETHYNYL-17-β-HYDROXY-19-NOR-4,9-AN-
DROSTADIEN-3-ONE see III:CHP750
CHLOROETHYNYL NORGESTREL mixed with MESTRANOL
(20:1) see III:CHP750
4-CHLORO-α-ETHYNYL-α-PHENYLBENZENEMETHANOL
CARBAMATE see III:CKI250, III:CKI500
CHLOROFENIZON see III:CJT750
N-2-(7-CHLORO)FLUORENYLACETAMIDE see III:CHI825
N-(7-CHLORO-2-FLUORENYL)ACETAMIDE see III:CHI825
CHLOROFLUOROMETHANE see I:CHI900
CHLOROFORM see I:CHJ500
CHLOROFORME (FRENCH) see I:CHJ500
CHLOROFORMIC ACID DIMETHYLAMIDE see I:DQY950
CHLOROFOS see III:TIQ250
CHLOROFTALM see III:TIQ250
4-CHLORO-2-HEXYLPHENOL see III:CHL500
α-CHLOROHYDRIN see III:CDT750
epi-CHLOROHYDRIN see I:EAZ500
5-CHLORO-4-(HYDROXYAMINO)QUINOLINE-1-OXIDE see
III:CHM500
6-CHLORO-4-(HYDROXYAMINO)QUINOLINE-1-OXIDE see
III:CHM750
7-CHLORO-4-(HYDROXYAMINO)QUINOLINE-1-OXIDE see
III:CHN000
5-CHLORO-2-HYDROXYDIPHENYLMETHANE see
III:CJU250
(−)-N-((5-CHLORO-8-HYDROXY-3-METHYL-1-OXO-7-ISO-
CHROMANYL)CARBONYL)-3-PHENYLALANINE see
III:CHP250
5-CHLORO-2-((2-HYDROXY-1-NAPHTHALENYL)AZO)-4-
METHYLBENZENE SULFONIC ACID, BARIUM SALT
(2:1) see III:CHP500
5-CHLORO-2-((2-HYDROXY-1-NAPHTHALENYL)AZO)-4-
METHYLBENZENE SULPHONIC ACID, BARIUM SALT see
III:CHP500
5-CHLORO-2-((2-HYDROXY-1-NAPHTHYL)AZO)-p-TO-
LUENE SULFONIC ACID, BARIUM SALT see III:CHP500
21-CHLORO-17-HYDROXY-19-NOR-17-α-PREGNA-4,9-DIEN-
20-YN-3-ONE see III:CHP750
7-CHLORO-3-HYDROXY-5-PHENYL-1,3-DIHYDRO-2H-1,4-
BENZODIAZEPIN-2-ONE see III:CFZ000
6-CHLORO-17-α-HYDROXYPREGNA-4,6-DIENE-3,20-DIONE
ACETATE see III:CBF250
6-CHLORO-17-α-HYDROXY-Δ⁶-PROGESTERONE ACETATE
see II:CBF250
2-CHLOROISOBUTANE see III:BQR000
α-CHLOROISOBUTYLENE see III:IKE000
γ-CHLOROISOBUTYLENF see II:CIU750
2-(α-CHLORO-β-ISOPROPYLAMINE)ETHYLNAPHTHALENE
HYDROCHLORIDE see III:CHT500
β-CHLORO-N-ISOPROPYL-2-NAPHTHALENEETHYLAMINE
HYDROCHLORIDE see III:CHT500
CHLOROJECT L see II:CDP250
CHLOROMADINONE ACETATE see II:CBF250
CHLOROMAX see II:CDP250
CHLOROMETHANE see II:MIF765
7-CHLORO-2-METHYLAMINO-5-PHENYL-3H-1,4-BENZO-
DIAZEPINE-4-OXIDE, mixed with SODIUM NITRITE (1:1)
see III:SIS000
3-CHLORO-6-METHYLANILINE see II:CLK225
4-CHLORO-2-METHYLANILINE see II:CLK220
4-CHLORO-6-METHYLANILINE see II:CLK220
5-CHLORO-2-METHYLANILINE see II:CLK235
4-CHLORO-2-METHYLANILINE HYDROCHLORIDE see
II:CLK235
4-CHLORO-6-METHYLANILINE HYDROCHLORIDE see
II:CLK235

7-CHLOROMETHYL BENZ(a)ANTHRACENE see III:CIG250
8-CHLORO-7-METHYLBENZ(a)ANTHRACENE see III:CIG000
10-CHLORO-7-METHYLBENZ(a)ANTHRACENE see III:CIG500
5-CHLORO-10-METHYL-1,2-BENZANTHRACENE see III:CIG000
7-CHLORO-10-METHYL-1,2-BENZANTHRACENE see III:CIG500
CHLOROMETHYLBENZENE see II:BEE375
4-CHLORO-2-METHYLBENZENEAMINE see II:CLK220
4-CHLORO-2-METHYLBENZENEAMINE HYDROCHLORIDE see II:CLK235
7-CHLORO-1-METHYL-5-3H-1,4-BENZODIAZEPIN-2(1H)-ONE see III:DCK759
6-CHLOROMETHYL BENZO(a)PYRENE see III:CIII000
10-CHLOROMETHYL-9-CHLOROANTHRACENE see III:CFB500
1-(CHLOROMETHYL)-N-((CHLOROMETHYL)DIMETHYL-SILYL)-1,1-DIMETHYL-SILANAMINE see III:BIL250
CHLOROMETHYL CYANIDE see III:CDN500
3'-CHLORO-4'-METHYL-4-DIMETHYLAMINOAZOBENZENE see III:CIL700
4'-CHLORO-3'-METHYL-4-DIMETHYLAMINOAZOBENZENE see III:CIL710
6-CHLORO-1,2-α-METHYLENE-6-DEHYDRO-17-α-HY-DROXYPROGESTERONE ACETATE see III:CQJ500
6-CHLORO-Δ⁶-1,2-α-METHYLENE-17-α-HYDROXYPRO-GESTERONE ACETATE see III:CQJ500
6-CHLORO-1,2-α-METHYLENE-17-α-HYDROXY-Δ⁶-PRO-GESTERONE ACETATE see III:CQJ500
2-CHLORO-1-METHYL-10-ETHYL-7,8-BENZACRIDINE (FRENCH) see III:EHL000
(CHLOROMETHYL)ETHYLENE OXIDE see I:EAZ500
(2-CHLORO-1-METHYLETHYL) ETHER see III:BII250
7-(CHLOROMETHYL)-5-FLUORO-12-METHYLBENZ(a)AN-THRACENE see III:FHH025
CHLOROMETHYLMERCURY see III:MDD750
10-CHLOROMETHYL-9-METHYLANTHRACENE see III:CIN500
7-CHLOROMETHYL-12-METHYL BENZ(a)ANTHRACENE see III:CIN750
CHLOROMETHYL METHYL ETHER see I:CIO250
2-CHLORO-2-METHYL-N-NITROSOETHANAMINE see III:CIQ500
2-CHLORO-N-METHYL-N-NITROSOETHYLAMINE see III:CIQ500
CHLOROMETHYLOXIRANE see I:EAZ500
2-(CHLOROMETHYL)OXIRANE see I:EAZ500
cis-2-CHLORO-3-METHYLOXIRANE see III:CKS099
trans-2-CHLORO-3-METHYLOXIRANE see III:CKS100
7-CHLORO-1-METHYL-2-OXO-5-PHENYL-3H-1,4-BENZO-DIAZEPINE see III:DCK759
(4-CHLORO-2-METHYLPHENOXY)ACETIC ACID see II:CIR250
2-(4-CHLORO-2-METHYLPHENOXY)PROPIONIC ACID see II:CIR500
4-CHLORO-2-METHYLPHENOXY-α-PROPIONIC ACID see II:CIR500
(+)-α-(4-CHLORO-2-METHYLPHENOXY) PROPIONIC ACID see II:CIR500
7-CHLORO-1-METHYL-5-PHENYL-2H-1,4-BENZODIAZEPIN-2-ONE see III:DCK759
7-CHLORO-1-METHYL-5-PHENYL-3H-1,4-BENZODIAZEPIN-2(1H)-ONE see III:DCK759
7-CHLORO-1-METHYL-5-PHENYL-1,3-DIHYDRO-2H-1,4-BENZODIAZEPIN-2-ONE see III:DCK759
N'-(4-CHLORO-2-METHYLPHENYL)-N,N-DIMETHYLMETH-ANIMIDAMIDE see III:CJJ250
CHLOROMETHYL PHENYL KETONE see III:CEA750
2-CHLORO-2-METHYLPROPANE see III:BQR000
1-CHLORO-2-METHYLPROPENE see III:IKE000
3-CHLORO-2-METHYLPROPENE see II:CIU750
1-CHLORO-2-METHYL-1-PROPENE see III:IKE000

3-CHLORO-2-METHYL-1-PROPENE see II:CIU750
3-(CHLOROMETHYL) PYRIDINE HYDROCHLORIDE see II:CIV000
CHLOROMYCETIN see II:CDP250
CHLORONAFTINA see I:BIF250
CHLORONAPHTHINE see I:BIF250
CHLORONITRIN see II:CDP250
2-CHLORONITROBENZENE see III:CJB750
4-CHLORONITROBENZENE see III:NFS525
CHLORO-o-NITROBENZENE see III:CJB750
o-CHLORONITROBENZENE see III:CJB750
p-CHLORONITROBENZENE see III:NFS525
1-CHLORO-2-NITROBENZENE see III:CJB750
1-CHLORO-4-NITROBENZENE see III:NFS525
2-CHLORO-1-NITROBENZENE see III:CJB750
4-CHLORO-1-NITROBENZENE see III:NFS525
o-CHLORONITROBENZENE (DOT) see III:CJB750
2-CHLORO-4-NITROBENZENEAZO-2'-AMINO-4'-ME-THOXY-5'-METHYLBENZENE see III:MIH500
3-CHLORO-4-NITROQUINOLINE-1-OXIDE see III:CJE500
5-CHLORO-4-NITROQUINOLINE-1-OXIDE see III:CJE750
6-CHLORO-4-NITROQUINOLINE-1-OXIDE see III:CJF000
7-CHLORO-4-NITROQUINOLINE-1-OXIDE see III:CJF250
3-CHLORONITROSOPIPERIDINE see III:CJG375
4-CHLORONITROSOPIPERIDINE see III:CJG500
3-CHLORO-1-NITROSOPIPERIDINE see III:CJG375
4-CHLORO-1-NITROSOPIPERIDINE see III:CJG500
CHLOROOXIRANE see III:CGX000
CHLOROPARAFFIN XP-470 see III:CJI000
CHLORO-PDMT see III:CJI100
3-CHLOROPERBENZOIC ACID see III:CJI750
m-CHLOROPERBENZOIC ACID see III:CJI750
3-CHLOROPEROXYBENZOIC ACID see III:CJI750
m-CHLOROPEROXYBENZOIC ACID see III:CJI750
CHLOROPHEN see II:PAX250
CHLOROPHENAMADIN see III:CJJ250
CHLOROPHENAMIDINE see III:CJJ250
CHLOROPHENE see III:CJU250
4-CHLOROPHENE-1,3-DIAMINE see II:CJS125
2-CHLOROPHENOL see III:CJK250
3-CHLOROPHENOL see III:CJK500
m-CHLOROPHENOL see III:CJK500
o-CHLOROPHENOL see III:CJK250
m-CHLOROPHENOL, liquid (DOT) see III:CJK500
m-CHLOROPHENOL, solid (DOT) see III:CJK500
o-CHLOROPHENOL, liquid (DOT) see III:CJK250
o-CHLOROPHENOL, solid (DOT) see III:CJK250
CHLOROPHENOLS see II:CJL000
CHLOROPHENOTHAN see I:DAD200
CHLOROPHENOTHANE see I:DAD200
CHLOROPHENOTOXUM see I:DAD200
4-(4-CHLOROPHENOXY)ANILINE see III:CEH125
p-(p-CHLOROPHENOXY)ANILINE see III:CEH125
4-(4-CHLOROPHENOXY)-BENZENAMINE (9CI) see III:CEH125
α-p-CHLOROPHENOXYISOBUTYRYL ETHYL ESTER see III:ARQ750
2-(4-CHLOROPHENOXY)-2-METHYLPROPANOIC ACID ETHYL ESTER see III:ARQ750
2-(4-CHLOROPHENOXY-2-METHYL)PROPIONIC ACID see II:CIR500
2-(p-CHLOROPHENOXY)-2-METHYLPROPIONIC ACID ETHYL ESTER see III:ARQ750
4-CHLOROPHENYLAMINE see III:CEH680
N-(3-CHLOROPHENYL)-1-AZIRIDINECARBOXAMIDE see III:CJR250
N-(3-CHLORO PHENYL) CARBAMATE D'ISOPROPYLE (FRENCH) see III:CKC000
N-(3-CHLOROPHENYL)CARBAMIC ACID, ISOPROPYL ES-TER see III:CKC000
(3-CHLOROPHENYL)CARBAMIC ACID, 1-METHYLETHYL ESTER see III:CKC000
3-CHLOROPHENYL-N-CARBAMOYLAZIRIDINE see III:CJR250

2-(p-CHLORO-o-TOLYLOXY)PROPIONIC ACID see
  II:CIR500
CHLOROTRIANISENE see II:CLO750
CHLOROTRIANIZEN see II:CLO750
CHLOROTRIAZINE see III:TJD750
2-CHLORO-1-(2,4,5-TRICHLOROPHENYL)VINYL DI-
  METHYL PHOSPHATE see II:TBW100
(Z)-2-CHLORO-1-(2,4,5-TRICHLOROPHENYL)VINYL DI-
  METHYL PHOSPHATE see III:RAF100
2-CHLORO-1-(2,4,5-TRICHLOROPHENYL(VINYL PHOS-
  PHORIC ACID DIMETHYL ESTER see II:TBW100
1-CHLORO-2,2,2-TRIFLUOROETHANE see III:TJY175
2-CHLORO-1,1,1-TRIFLUOROETHANE see III:TJY175
2-CHLORO-1,1,2-TRIFLUOROETHYL DIFLUOROMETHYL
  ETHER see III:EAT900
7-CHLORO-4,6,2′-TRIMETHOXY-6′-METHYLGRIS-2′ EN-
  3,4′-DIONE see GKE000
2-CHLORO-N,N,N-TRIMETHYLETHANAMINIUM CHLO-
  RIDE see III:CMF400
CHLOROTRIMETHYLSILICANE see III:TLN250
CHLOROTRISIN see II:CLO750
CHLOROTRIS(p-METHOXYPHENYL)ETHYLENE see
  II:CLO750
CHLOROVULES see II:CDP250
CHLOROXONE see II:DAA800
(4-CHLORO-6-(2,3-XYLIDINO)-2-PYRIMIDINYLTHIO)
  ACETIC ACID see II:CLW250
2-((4-CHLORO-6-(2,3-XYLIDINO)-2-PYRIMIDINYL)THIO)-
  N-(2-HYDROXYETHYL)ACETAMIDE see II:CLW500
CHLOROXYPHOS see III:TIQ250
CHLOROZIRCONYL see III:ZSJ000
CHLOROZOTOCIN see III:CLX000
CHLORPHENAMIDINE see III:CJJ250
o-CHLORPHENOL (GERMAN) see III:CJK250
4-CHLORPHENYL-4′-CHLORBENZOLSULFONAT (GERMAN)
  see III:CJT750
(4-CHLOR-PHENYL)-4-CHLOR-BENZOL-SULFONATE (GER-
  MAN) see III:CJT750
3-(4-CHLOR-PHENYL)-1,1-DIMETHYL-HARNSTOFF (GER-
  MAN) see III:CJX750
1-(p-CHLOR-PHENYL)-3,3-DIMETHYL-TRIAZEN (GERMAN)
  see III:CJI100
γ-(4-(p-CHLORPHENYL)-4-HYDROXPIPERIDINO)-p-FLUOR-
  BUTYROPHENONE see III:CLY500
N-(3-CHLOR-PHENYL)-ISOPROPYL-CARBAMAT (GERMAN)
  see III:CKC000
CHLOR-O-PIC see III:CKN500
CHLORPIKRIN (GERMAN) see III:CKN500
3-CHLORPROPEN (GERMAN) see II:AGB250
CHLORPROPHAM see III:CKC000
CHLORPROPHAME (FRENCH) see III:CKC000
N-CHLORSUCCINIMIDE see III:SND500
CHLORTEN see III:MIH275
CHLORTHALONIL (GERMAN) see III:TBQ750
CHLORTHIEPIN see III:EAQ750
p-CHLORTHIOFENOL (CZECH) see III:CEK425
α-CHLORTOLUOL (GERMAN) see II:BEE375
N′-(4-CHLOR-o-TOLYL)-N,N-DIMETHYLFORMAMIDIN
  (GERMAN) see III:CJJ250
CHLORTOX see II:CDR750
CHLORTRIANISEN see II:CLO750
CHLORURE de BENZENYLE (FRENCH) see I:BFL250
CHLORURE de BENZYLE (FRENCH) see II:BEE375
CHLORURE de BENZYLIDENE (FRENCH) see II:BAY300
CHLORURE de DICHLORACETYLE (FRENCH) see
  III:DEN400
CHLORURE d'ETHYLENE (FRENCH) see I:EIY600
CHLORURE d'ETHYLIDENE (FRENCH) see III:DFF809
CHLORURE de LITHIUM (FRENCH) see III:LHB000
CHLORURE de METHALLYLE (FRENCH) see II:CIU750
CHLORURE de METHYLE (FRENCH) see II:MIF765
CHLORURE de METHYLENE (FRENCH) see II:MJP450
CHLORURE de VINYLE (FRENCH) see I:VNP000
CHLORURE de VINYLIDENE (FRENCH) see II:VPK000

CHLORURE de ZINC (FRENCH) see III:ZFA000
CHLORYLEA see II:TIO750
CHLZ see III:CLX000
CHNU-I see III:NKJ050
CHOLANORM see III:CDL325
CHOLANTHRENE see III:CMC000
CHOLEIC ACID see III:DAQ400
CHOLEREBIC see III:DAQ400
5,7-CHOLESTADIEN-3-β-OL see III:DAK600
(3-β)CHOLESTA-5,7-DIEN-3-OL see III:DAK600
CHOLESTA-5,7-DIEN-3-β-OL ACETATE see III:DAK800
3-β-CHOLESTANOL see III:DKW000
(3-β,5-β)-CHOLESTAN-3-OL see III:DKW000
CHOLEST-5-EN-3-β-OL see III:CMD750
5-CHOLESTEN-3-β-OL see III:CMD750
7-CHOLESTEN-3-β-OL see III:CMD000
5:6-CHOLESTEN-3-β-OL see III:CMD750
5-α-CHOLEST-7-EN-3-β-OL see III:CMD000
Δ⁷-CHOLESTENOL see III:CMD000
Δ⁵-CHOLESTEN-3-β-OL see III:CMD750
5-CHOLESTEN-3-β-OL 3-(p-(BIS(2-CHLOROETHYL)
  AMINO)PHENYL)ACETATE see II:CME250
CHOLEST-6-EN-3-β-OL-5-α-HYDROPEROXIDE see
  III:CMD250
Δ⁶-CHOLESTEN-3-β-OL-5-α-HYDROPEROXIDE see
  III:CMD250
Δ⁶-CHOLESTEN-3-β-OL-5-α-HYDROPEROXYD (GERMAN)
  see III:CMD250
CHOLESTENONE see III:CMD500
CHOLEST-5-EN-3-ONE see III:CMD500
5-CHOLESTEN-3-ONE see III:CMD500
Δ⁽⁵⁾-CHOLESTENONE see III:CMD500
CHOLESTERIN see III:CMD750
CHOLESTERIN (GERMAN) see III:CMD000
CHOLESTEROL see III:CMD750
Δ⁷-CHOLESTEROL see III:DAK600
Δ⁵,⁷-CHOLESTEROL see III:DAK600
CHOLESTEROL BASE H see III:CMD750
CHOLESTEROL-α-EPOXIDE see III:EBM000
CHOLESTEROL-5-α,6-α-EPOXIDE see III:EBM000
CHOLESTEROL-5-α-HYDROPEROXIDE see III:CMD250
CHOLESTEROL ISOHEPTYLATE see III:CME000
CHOLESTEROL-5-METHYL-1-HEXANOATE see III:CME000
CHOLESTEROL mixed with OROTIC ACID mixed with CHOLIC
  ACID (2:2:1) see III:OJV525
CHOLESTEROL OXIDE see III:EBM000
CHOLESTEROL-α-OXIDE see III:EBM000
CHOLESTERONE see III:CMD500
CHOLESTERYL ALCOHOL see III:CMD750
CHOLESTERYL-p-BIS(2-CHLOROETHYL)AMINO PHENYL-
  ACETATE see II:CME250
CHOLESTERYL-14-METHYLHEXADECANOATE see
  III:CCJ500
CHOLESTRIN see III:CMD750
CHOLESTROL see III:CMD750
CHOLESTYRAMINE see III:CME400
CHOLESTYRAMINE CHLORIDE see III:CME400
CHOLESTYRAMINE RESIN see III:CME400
CHOLIC ACID mixed with CHOLESTEROL mixed with OROTIC
  ACID (1:2:2) see III:OJV525
CHOLIFLAVIN see III:DBX400
CHOLINE DICHLORIDE see III:CMF400
CHOLOREBIC see III:DAQ400
CHONDRUS see III:CCL250
CHONDRUS EXTRACT see III:CCL250
CHORYLEN see II:TIO750
CHROMATE de PLOMB (FRENCH) see I:LCR000
CHROMATE of POTASSIUM see III:PLB250
CHROME see I:CMI750
CHROME ALUM see III:CMG850
CHROME ALUM (DODECAHYDRATE) see III:CMG850
CHROME FAST BLUE 2R see III:HJF500
CHROME FERROALLOY see III:FBD000
CHROME GREEN see I:LCR000, II:CMJ900

CHROME LEATHER BLACK EM see I:AQP000
CHROME LEATHER BLUE 2B see I:CMO000
CHROME LEATHER BLUE 3B see II:CMO250
CHROME LEATHER BROWN BRLL see II:CMO750
CHROME LEMON see I:LCR000
CHROME OCHER see II:CMJ900
CHROME ORANGE see I:LCS000
CHROME ORE see I:CMI500
CHROME OXIDE see II:CMJ900
CHROME OXIDE GREEN see II:CMJ900
CHROME (TRIOXYDE de) (FRENCH) see I:CMK000
CHROME YELLOW see I:LCR000
CHROMIA see II:CMJ900
CHROMIC ACETATE see III:CMH000
CHROMIC ACETATE(III) see III:CMH000
CHROMIC ACID see I:CMK000, II:CMJ900
CHROMIC(VI) ACID see I:CMK000
CHROMIC ACID, solid (DOT) see I:CMK000
CHROMIC ACID, solution (DOT) see I:CMK000
CHROMIC ACID, BARIUM SALT (1:1) see I:BAK250
CHROMIC ACID, CALCIUM SALT (1:1) see I:CAP500
CHROMIC ACID, CALCIUM SALT (1:1), DIHYDRATE see I:CAP750
CHROMIC ACID, CHROMIUM(3+) SALT (3:2) see I:CMI250
CHROMIC ACID, DIPOTASSIUM SALT see III:PKX250
CHROMIC ACID, DISODIUM SALT see I:SGI000
CHROMIC ACID, DISODIUM SALT, DECAHYDRATE see I:SFW500
CHROMIC ACID GREEN see II:CMJ900
CHROMIC ACID, LEAD and MOLYBDENUM SALT see III:LDM000
CHROMIC ACID, LEAD(2+) SALT (1:1) see I:LCR000
CHROMIC ACID LEAD SALT with LEAD MOLYBDATE see III:LDM000
CHROMIC ACID, MERCURY ZINC COMPLEX see I:ZJA000
CHROMIC ACID, POTASSIUM ZINC SALT (2:2:1) see I:PLW500
CHROMIC ACID, STRONTIUM SALT (1:1) see I:SMH000
CHROMIC ACID, ZINC SALT see I:ZFJ100
CHROMIC ACID, ZINC SALT (1:2) see I:CMK500
CHROMIC ANHYDRIDE (DOT) see I:CMK000
CHROMIC CHROMATE see I:CMI250
CHROMIC OXIDE see II:CMJ900
CHROMIC TRIOXIDE (DOT) see I:CMK000
CHROMIS ACID ($H_2Cr_2O_7$), DISODIUM SALT, DIHYDRATE (9CI) see III:SGI500
CHROMITE see I:CMI500
CHROMITE (mineral) see I:CMI500
CHROMITE ORE see I:CMI500
CHROMIUM see I:CMI750
CHROMIUM ACETATE see III:CMH000
CHROMIUM(III) ACETATE see III:CMH000
CHROMIUM ALLOY, BASE, Cr,C,Fe,N,Si (FERROCHROMIUM) see III:FBD000
CHROMIUM ALLOY, Cr,C,Fe,N,Si see III:FBD000
CHROMIUM CARBONYL (MAK) see I:HCB000
CHROMIUM CARBONYL (OC-6-11) (9CI) see I:HCB000
CHROMIUM CHROMATE (MAK) see I:CMI250
CHROMIUM-COBALT ALLOY see I:CNA750
CHROMIUM-COBALT-MOLYBDENUM ALLOY see III:VSK000
CHROMIUM COMPOUNDS see II:CMJ500
CHROMIUM HEXACARBONYL see I:HCB000
CHROMIUM HYDROXIDE SULFATE see III:NBW000
CHROMIUM LEAD OXIDE see I:LCS000
CHROMIUM OXIDE see I:CMK000, II:CMJ900
CHROMIUM(3+) OXIDE see II:CMJ900
CHROMIUM(VI) OXIDE see I:CMK000
CHROMIUM(III) OXIDE see II:CMJ900
CHROMIUM(VI) OXIDE (1:3) see I:CMK000
CHROMIUM(III) OXIDE (2:3) see II:CMJ900
CHROMIUM OXIDE, aerosols see III:CMJ900
CHROMIUM OXIDE, NICKEL OXIDE, and IRON OXIDE FUME see I:IHE000

CHROMIUM POTASSIUM ZINC OXIDE see I:CMK400
CHROMIUM SESQUIOXIDE see II:CMJ900
CHROMIUM SODIUM OXIDE see I:SGI000
CHROMIUM SULFATE see III:NBW000
CHROMIUM SULFATE, BASIC see III:NBW000
CHROMIUM SULPHATE see III:NBW000
CHROMIUM TRIACETATE see III:CMH000
CHROMIUM TRIOXIDE see I:CMK000
CHROMIUM(3+) TRIOXIDE see II:CMJ900
CHROMIUM(6+) TRIOXIDE see I:CMK000
CHROMIUM TRIOXIDE, ANHYDROUS (DOT) see I:CMK000
CHROMIUM YELLOW see I:LCR000
CHROMIUM ZINC OXIDE see I:ZFJ100
CHROMIUM(6+)ZINC OXIDE HYDRATE (1:2:6:1) see I:CMK500
CHROMOFLAVINE see III:DBX400
CHROMOSORB T see III:TAI250
CHROMO (TRIOSSIDO di) (ITALIAN) see I:CMK000
CHROMSAEUREANHYDRID (GERMAN) see I:CMK000
CHROMTRIOXID (GERMAN) see I:CMK000
CHRONOGYN see III:DAB830
CHROOMTRIOXYDE (DUTCH) see I:CMK000
CHROOMZUURANHYDRIDE (DUTCH) see I:CMK000
CHRYSAZIN see III:DMH400
6-CHRYSENAMINE see III:CML800
CHRYSENE see I:CML810
CHRYSENE-5,6-EPOXIDE see III:CML815
CHRYSENE-K-REGION EPOXIDE see III:CML815
CHRYSENE-5,6-OXIDE see III:CML815
CHRYSENEX see III:CML800
α-CHRYSIDINE see III:BAW750
CHRYSOIDIN see III:PEK000
CHRYSOIDINE see III:PEK000
CHRYSOIDINE(II) see III:PEK000
CHRYSOIDINE A see III:PEK000
CHRYSOIDINE B see III:PEK000
CHRYSOIDINE C CRYSTALS see III:PEK000
CHRYSOIDINE G see III:PEK000
CHRYSOIDINE GN see III:PEK000
CHRYSOIDINE HR see III:PEK000
CHRYSOIDINE J see III:PEK000
CHRYSOIDINE M see III:PEK000
CHRYSOIDINE ORANGE see III:PEK000
CHRYSOIDINE PRL see III:PEK000
CHRYSOIDINE PRR see III:PEK000
CHRYSOIDINE SL see III:PEK000
CHRYSOIDINE SPECIAL (biological stain and indicator) see III:PEK000
CHRYSOIDINE SS see III:PEK000
CHRYSOIDINE Y see III:PEK000
CHRYSOIDINE Y BASE NEW see III:PEK000
CHRYSOIDINE Y CRYSTALS see III:PEK000
CHRYSOIDINE Y EX see III:PEK000
CHRYSOIDINE YGH see III:PEK000
CHRYSOIDINE YL see III:PEK000
CHRYSOIDINE YN see III:PEK000
CHRYSOIDINE Y SPECIAL see III:PEK000
CHRYSOIDIN FB see III:PEK000
CHRYSOIDIN Y see III:PEK000
CHRYSOIDIN YN see III:PEK000
CHRYSONEX see III:CML800
CHRYZOIDYNA F.B. (POLISH) see III:PEK000
CHS see III:CPF750
CHWASTOX see II:CIR250
C.I. 27 see III:HGC000
C.I. 79 see III:FMU070
C.I. 184 see III:FAG020
C.I. 185 see III:FMU080
C.I. 258 see III:SBC500
CI-337 see II:ASA500
CI-406 see I:PAN100

C.I. 556 see III:SNY500
CI-588 see III:BGO500
C.I. 671 see III:FMU059
CI-683 see III:POL475
CI-719 see III:GCK300
C.I. 749 see III:FAG070
C.I. 766 see III:FEW000
C.I. 7581 see III:FAE100
C.I. 10385 see III:SGP500
C.I. 11000 see II:PEI000
C.I. 11020 see I:DOT300
C.I. 11050 see III:DHM500
C.I. 11160 see I:AIC250
C.I. 11270 see III:PEK000
C.I. 11285 see III:NBG500
C.I. 11380 see III:FAG130
C.I. 11390 see III:FAG135
C.I. 11855 see II:AAQ250
C.I. 11860 see III:OHK000
C.I. 12055 see III:PEJ500
C.I. 12100 see II:TGW000
C.I. 12140 see III:XRA000
C.I. 12156 see II:DOK200
C.I. 13020 see III:CCE500
C.I. 14600 see III:FAG010
C.I. 14700 see III:FAG050
C.I. 14720 see III:HJF500
C.I. 15985 see III:FAG150
C.I. 16150 see III:FMU070
C.I. 16155 see II:FAG018
C.I. 16185 see III:FAG020
C.I. 16255 see III:FMU080
C.I. 22570 see III:CMP000
C.I. 22610 see I:CMO000
C.I. 23060 see I:DEQ600
C.I. 23850 see II:CMO250
C.I. 23860 see III:BGT250
C.I. 24110 see I:DCJ200
C.I. 26050 see III:EOJ500
C.I. 30145 see II:CMO750
C.I. 30235 see I:AQP000
C.I. 37020 see III:DBR400
C.I. 37077 see I:TGQ750
C.I. 37085 see II:CLK235
C.I. 37105 see I:NMP500
C.I. 37115 see I:AOX250
C.I. 37130 see II:NEQ500
C.I. 37200 see III:MIH500
C.I. 37225 see I:BBX000
C.I. 37230 see I:TGJ750
C.I. 37270 see I:NBE500
C.I. 37275 see III:AIA750
C.I. 41000 see I:IBA000
C.I. 42053 see III:FAG000
C.I. 42090 see III:FAE000, III:FMU059
C.I. 42095 see III:FAF000
C.I. 42500 see II:RMK020
C.I. 42640 see II:FAG120
C.I. 44040 see III:VKA600
C.I. 44050 see III:PFT250
C.I. 44090 see III:ADF000
C.I. 45160 see III:RGW000
C.I. 45380 see III:BNH500, III:BNK700
C.I. 45430 see III:FAG040
C.I. 46005 see III:BJF000
C.I. 59100 see III:DCZ000
C.I. 60700 see I:AKP750
C.I. 61200 see III:BMM500
C.I. 64500 see III:TBG700
C.I. 73015 see III:FAE100
C.I. 75500 see III:WAT000
C.I. 75670 see III:QCA000
C.I. 75730 see III:RSU000
C.I. 76000 see II:AOQ000

C.I. 76025 see III:PEY000
C.I. 76027 see II:CJS125
C.I. 76035 see I:TGL750
C.I. 76042 see I:TGM000
C.I. 76043 see III:DCE600, III:TGM400
C.I. 76050 see I:DBO000
C.I. 76051 see I:DBO400
C.I. 76060 see III:PEY500
C.I. 76061 see III:PEY650
C.I. 76066 see III:CEG625
C.I. 76070 see II:ALL750
C.I. 76500 see III:CCP850
C.I. 76505 see III:REA000
C.I. 76515 see III:PPQ500
C.I. 76535 see III:ALO000
C.I. 76555 see II:NEM480
C.I. 77050 see III:AQB750
C.I. 77086 see I:ARI000
C.I. 77103 see I:BAK250
C.I. 77120 see III:BAP000
C.I. 77180 see I:CAD000
C.I. 77185 see I:CAD250
C.I. 77199 see I:CAJ750
C.I. 77223 see I:CAP500, I:CAP750
C.I. 77231 see III:CAX750
C.I. 77288 see II:CMJ900
C.I. 77320 see I:CNA250
C.I. 77322 see III:CND125
C.I. 77400 see I:CNI000
C.I. 77491 see III:IHD000
C.I. 77575 see II:LCF000
C.I. 77577 see III:LDN000
C.I. 77600 see I:LCR000
C.I. 77601 see I:LCS000
C.I. 77622 see I:LDU000
C.I. 77718 see III:TAB750
C.I. 77775 see I:NCW500
C.I. 77777 see I:NDF500
C.I. 77779 see I:NCY500
C.I. 77795 see III:PJD500
C.I. 77805 see III:SBO500
C.I. 77820 see III:SDI500
C.I. 77891 see III:TGG760
C.I. 77955 see I:ZFJ100
C.I. 11160B see I:AIC250
C.I. 45380:2 see III:BMO250
C.I. ACID BLUE 74 see III:FAE100
C.I. ACID BLUE 9, DIAMMONIUM SALT see III:FMU059
C.I. ACID BLUE 9, DISODIUM SALT see III:FAE000
C.I. ACID BLUE 1, SODIUM SALT see III:ADE500
C.I. ACID GREEN 5 see III:FAF000
C.I. ACID GREEN 5, DISODIUM SALT see III:FAF000
C.I. ACID GREEN 3, MONOSODIUM SALT see III:FAE950
C.I. ACID GREEN 50, MONOSODIUM SALT see III:ADF000
C.I. ACID ORANGE 3 see III:SGP500
C.I. ACID ORANGE 10 see III:HGC000
C.I. ACID ORANGE 20 see III:FAG010
C.I. ACID ORANGE 20, MONOSODIUM SALT see III:FAG010
C.I. ACID RED 2 see III:CCE500
C.I. ACID RED 18 see III:FMU080
C.I. ACID RED 26 see III:FMU070
C.I. ACID RED 27 see III:FAG020
C.I. ACID RED 51 see III:FAG040
C.I. ACID RED 87 see III:BNK700
C.I. ACID RED 14, DISODIUM SALT see III:HJF500
C.I. ACID RED 26, DISODIUM SALT see III:FMU070
C.I. ACID YELLOW 73 see III:FEW000
CIANURO di VINILE (ITALIAN) see I:ADX500
C.I. AZOIC DIAZO COMPONENT 11 see II:CLK235
C.I. AZOIC DIAZO COMPONENT 12 see I:NMP500
C.I. AZOIC DIAZO COMPONENT 13 see II:NEQ500
C.I. AZOIC DIAZO COMPONENT 21 see III:MIH500
C.I. AZOIC DIAZO COMPONENT 48 see I:DCJ200
C.I. AZOIC DIAZO COMPONENT 112 see I:BBX000

C.I. AZOIC DIAZO COMPONENT 113 see I:TGJ750
C.I. AZOIC DIAZO COMPONENT 114 see I:NBE000
C.I. AZOIC RED 83 see I:MGO750
C.I. 41000B see I:IBB000
CIBA 570 see III:FAC025
CIBA 2059 see III:DUK800
CIBA 5968 see II:HGP500, III:PHW000
CIBA 8514 see I:KEA000, III:CJJ250
CIBA 32644 see II:NML000
CIBA 17309 BA see III:DAL300
CIBA 32644-BA see II:NML000
CIBACETE DIAZO NAVY BLUE 2B see I:DCJ200
CIBACET SAPPHIRE BLUE G see III:TBG700
CIBACET YELLOW GBA see II:AAQ250
CIBANONE GOLDEN YELLOW see III:DCZ000
C.I. BASIC ORANGE 2 see III:PEK000
C.I. BASIC ORANGE 3 see III:PEK000
C.I. BASIC ORANGE 14 see III:BJF000
C.I. BASIC ORANGE 2, MONOHYDROCHLORIDE see
   III:PEK000
C.I. BASIC RED 1, MONOHYDROCHLORIDE see
   III:RGW000
C.I. BASIC RED 9, MONOHYDROCHLORIDE see II:RMK020
C.I. BASIC VIOLET 10 see III:FAG070
C.I. BASIC YELLOW 2 see I:IBA000
C.I. BASIC YELLOW 2, FREE BASE see I:IBB000
C.I. BASIC YELLOW 2, MONOHYDROCHLORIDE see
   I:IBA000
CICLOSOM see III:TIQ250
CICLOSPORIN see III:CQH100
CICP see III:CKC000
CIDANCHIN see III:CLD000
CIDANDOPA see III:DNA200
C.I. DEVELOPER 4 see III:REA000
C.I. DEVELOPER 13 see III:PEY500
C.I. DIRECT BLACK 38 see I:AQP000
C.I. DIRECT BLUE 14 see II:CMO250
C.I. DIRECT BLUE 53 see III:BGT250
C.I. DIRECT BLUE 6, TETRASODIUM SALT see I:CMO000
C.I. DIRECT BLUE 14, TETRASODIUM SALT see II:CMO250
C.I. DIRECT BROWN see II:CMO750
C.I. DIRECT BROWN 78, DIAMMONIUM SALT see
   III:FMU059
C.I. DIRECT VIOLET 1, DISODIUM SALT see III:CMP000
C.I. 45350 DISODIUM SALT see III:FEW000
C.I. DISPERSE BLACK 6 see I:DCJ200
C.I. DISPERSE BLACK-6-DIHYDROCHLORIDE see
   II:DOA800
C.I. DISPERSE BLUE 1 see III:TBG700
C.I. DISPERSE ORANGE 11 see I:AKP750
C.I. DISPERSE YELLOW 3 see II:AAQ250
CIDOCETINE see II:CDP250
C.I. FOOD BLUE 1 see III:FAE100
C.I. FOOD BLUE 2 see III:FAE000, III:FMU059
C.I. FOOD GREEN 1 see III:FAE950
C.I. FOOD GREEN 2 see III:FAF000
C.I. FOOD GREEN 3 see III:FAG000
C.I. FOOD GREEN 4 see III:ADF000
C.I. FOOD ORANGE 4 see III:HGC000
C.I. FOOD RED 1 see III:FAG050
C.I. FOOD RED 3 see III:HJF500
C.I. FOOD RED 5 see III:FMU070
C.I. FOOD RED 6 see II:FAG018
C.I. FOOD RED 7 see III:FMU080
C.I. FOOD RED 9 see III:FAG020
C.I. FOOD RED 15 see III:FAG070
C.I. FOOD RED 1, DISODIUM SALT see III:FAG050
C.I. FOOD RED 6, DISODIUM SALT see II:FAG018
C.I. FOOD VIOLET 2 see II:FAG120
C.I. FOOD YELLOW 10 see III:FAG130
C.I. FOOD YELLOW 11 see III:FAG135
CIGARETTE REFINED TAR see II:CMP800
CIGARETTE SMOKE CONDENSATE see I:SEC000
CIGARETTE TAR see II:CMP800

CI-IPC see III:CKC000
CILEFA PINK B see III:FAG040
CILEFA PONCEAU 4R see III:FMU080
CILEFA RUBINE 2B see III:FAG020
CILLA BLUE EXTRA see III:TBG700
CILLA ORANGE R see I:AKP750
CILLORAL see III:BDY669
CILOPEN see III:BDY669
CIMETIDINE see III:TAB250
CIMEXAN see III:MAK700
C.I. NATURAL BROWN 7 see III:WAT000
C.I. NATURAL RED 1 see III:QCA000
C.I. NATURAL YELLOW 10 see III:QCA000
CINEB see III:EIR000
CINNAMENE see II:SMQ000
CINNAMENOL see II:SMQ000
CINNAMYL ALCOHOL ANTHRANILATE see II:API750
CINNAMYL-2-AMINOBENZOATE see II:API750
CINNAMYL-o-AMINOBENZOATE see II:API750
CINNAMYL ANTHRANILATE (FCC) see II:API750
CINNARIZIN see III:ARQ750
C.I. No. 77278 see II:CMJ900
C.I. No. 46005:1 see III:BJF000
CINU see I:CGV250
C.I. OXIDATION BASE see I:TGL750
C.I. OXIDATION BASE 4 see III:TGM400
C.I. OXIDATION BASE 10 see III:PEY500
C.I. OXIDATION BASE 12 see I:DBO000
C.I. OXIDATION BASE 22 see II:ALL750
C.I. OXIDATION BASE 26 see III:CCP850
C.I. OXIDATION BASE 31 see III:REA000
C.I. OXIDATION BASE 32 see III:PPQ500
C.I. OXIDATION BASE 10A see III:PEY650
C.I. OXIDATION BASE 12A see I:DBO400
C.I. OXIDATION BASE 13A see III:CEG625
CIPC see III:CKC000
C.I. PIGMENT BLACK 13 see III:CND125
C.I. PIGMENT GREEN 17 see II:CMJ900
C.I. PIGMENT METAL 2 see III:CNI000
C.I. PIGMENT METAL 4 see II:LCF000
C.I. PIGMENT ORANGE 20 see I:CAJ750
C.I. PIGMENT ORANGE 21 see I:LCS000
C.I. PIGMENT RED see I:LCS000, III:CHP500
C.I. PIGMENT RED 101 see III:IHD000
C.I. PIGMENT RED 104 see III:LDM000
C.I. PIGMENT WHITE 6 see III:TGG760
C.I. PIGMENT WHITE 11 see I:AQF000
C.I. PIGMENT WHITE 21 see III:BAP000
C.I. PIGMENT WHITE 25 see III:CAX750
C.I. PIGMENT YELLOW 31 see I:BAK250
C.I. PIGMENT YELLOW 32 see I:SMH000
C.I. PIGMENT YELLOW 33 see I:CAP500, I:CAP750
C.I. PIGMENT YELLOW 34 see I:LCR000
C.I. PIGMENT YELLOW 36 see I:ZFJ100
C.I. PIGMENT YELLOW 37 see I:CAJ750
C.I. PIGMENT YELLOW 46 see III:LDN000
CIPLAMYCETIN see II:CDP250
CIPROFIBRATE see III:CMS210
CIRAM see III:BJK500
CIRCOSOLV see II:TIO750
C.I. REACTIVE BLUE 19 see III:BMM500
C.I. REACTIVE BLUE 19, DISODIUM SALT see III:BMM500
C.I. REACTIVE YELLOW 14 see III:RCZ000
CISCLOMIPHENE see III:CMX500
C.I. SOLVENT BLUE 7 see II:PEI000
C.I. SOLVENT BLUE 18 see III:TBG700
C.I. SOLVENT ORANGE 2 see II:TGW000
C.I. SOLVENT ORANGE 3 see III:PEK000
C.I. SOLVENT ORANGE 7 see III:XRA000
C.I. SOLVENT ORANGE 15 see III:BJF000
C.I. SOLVENT RED 19 see III:EOJ500
C.I. SOLVENT RED 23 see III:OHA000
C.I. SOLVENT RED 24 see III:SBC500
C.I. SOLVENT RED 43 see III:BMO250

C.I. SOLVENT RED 80 see II:DOK200
C.I. SOLVENT YELLOW 1 see II:PEI000
C.I. SOLVENT YELLOW 2 see I:DOT300
C.I. SOLVENT YELLOW 3 see I:AIC250
C.I. SOLVENT YELLOW 5 see III:FAG130
C.I. SOLVENT YELLOW 7 see III:HJF000
C.I. SOLVENT YELLOW 12 see III:OHK000
C.I. SOLVENT YELLOW 14 see III:PEJ500
C.I. SOLVENT YELLOW 34 see I:IBB000
CISPLATINO (SPANISH) see II:PJD000
CISPLATYL see II:PJD000
CITIFLUS see III:ARQ750
CITOBARYUM see III:BAP000
CITOFUR see III:FMB000
CITOSULFAN see I:BOT250
CITOX see I:DAD200
CITRA-FORT see I:ABG750
CITRAMON see III:ARP250
CITRIC ACID, YTTRIUM SALT (3:1) see III:YFA000
CITRININ see III:CMS775
CITRON YELLOW see I:PLW500, I:ZFJ100
CITRULLAMON see I:DKQ000, I:DNU000
l-CITRULLINE and SODIUM NITRITE (2:1) see III:SIS100
CITRUS AURANTIUM see III:LBE000
CITRUS RED No. 2 see II:DOK200
C.I. VAT YELLOW see III:DCZ000
CL 337 see II:ASA500
CL 12880 see III:DSP400
CL-14377 see III:MDV500
CLAFEN see I:CQC675, I:EAS500
CLAIRFORMIN see III:CMV000
CLAPHENE see I:EAS500
CLARIPEX see III:ARQ750
CLAVACIN see III:CMV000
3′,4′-Cl2-DAB see III:DFD400
CLEARASIL BENZOYL PEROXIDE LOTION see III:BDS000
CLEARASIL BP ACNE TREATMENT see III:BDS000
CLEARTUF see III:PKF750
CLEP see III:CMV475
CLIMATERINE see I:DKA600
CLIMESTRONE see I:ECU750
CLINESTROL see I:DKB000
CLINOPTILOLITE see III:CMV850
CLIVORINE see III:CMV950
CLIXODYNE see II:HIM000
4-Cl-M-PD see II:CJS125
CLOBERAT see III:ARQ750
CLOBRAT see III:ARQ750
CLOBREN-SF see III:ARQ750
CLOFAR see III:ARQ750
CLOFENOTANE see I:DAD200
CLOFIBRAM see III:ARQ750
CLOFIBRAT see III:ARQ750
CLOFIBRATO (SPANISH) see III:ARQ750
CLOFINIT see III:ARQ750
CLOFIPRONT see III:ARQ750
CLOMEPHENE B see III:CMX500
CLOMID see III:CMX700
CLOMIFEN CITRATE see III:CMX700
CLOMIFENE see III:CMX500
CLOMIFENO see III:CMX700
CLOMIPHENE see III:CMX500
CLOMIPHENE CITRATE see III:CMX700
racemic-CLOMIPHENE CITRATE see III:CMX700
CLOMIPHENE DIHYDROGEN CITRATE see III:CMX700
CLOMIPHENE-R see III:CMX700
CLOMIPHINE see III:CMX700
CLOMIVID see III:CMX700
CLOMPHID see III:CMX700
CLONT see I:MMN250
CLOPHEN see I:PJL750
CLOPHEN A-30 see III:CMX845
CLOPHEN A60 see II:PJN250
CLORAMIDINA see II:CDP250

CLORAMIN see I:BIE250
CLOR CHEM T-590 see I:CDV100
CLORDAN (ITALIAN) see II:CDR750
CLORDION see II:CBF250
CLORESTROLO see II:CLO750
CLOREX see III:DFJ050
CLORNAPHAZINE see I:BIF250
CLOROAMFENICOLO (ITALIAN) see II:CDP250
CLOROBEN see III:DEP600
2-CLORO-1,3-BUTADIENE (ITALIAN) see III:NCI500
CLOROCHINA see III:CLD000
(2-CLORO-3-DIETILAMINO-1-METIL-3-OXO-PROP-1-EN-IL)-
    DIMETIL-FOSFATO see III:FAC025
CLORODIFENILI, CLORO 42% (ITALIAN) see II:PJM500
CLORODIFENILI, CLORO 54% (ITALIAN) see II:PJN000
1-CLORO-2,3-EPOSSIPROPANO (ITALIAN) see I:EAZ500
(CLORO-2-ETIL)-1-CICLOESIL-3-NITROSOUREA (ITALIAN)
    see I:CGV250
(4-CLORO-FENIL)-4-CLORO-VENZOL-SOLFONATO (ITAL-
    IAN) see III:CJT750
3-(4-CLORO-FENIL)-1,1-DIMETIL-UREA (ITALIAN) see
    III:CJX750
N-(3-CLORO-FENIL)-ISOPROPIL-CARBAMMATO (ITALIAN)
    see III:CKC000
CLOROFORMIO (ITALIAN) see I:CHJ500
CLOROFOS (RUSSIAN) see III:TIQ250
CLOROMETANO (ITALIAN) see II:MIF765
3-CLORO-2-METIL-PROP-1-ENE (ITALIAN) see II:CIU750
CLOROMISAN see II:CDP250
1-CLORO-4-NITROBENZENE (ITALIAN) see III:NFS525
CLOROPHENE see III:CJU250
CLOROPICRINA (ITALIAN) see III:CKN500
CLOROPRENE (ITALIAN) see III:NCI500
CLOROSINTEX see II:CDP250
CLOROTRISIN see II:CLO750
CLORURO di ETHENE (ITALIAN) see I:EIY600
CLORURO di ETILIDENE (ITALIAN) see III:DFF809
CLORURO di METALLILE (ITALIAN) see II:CIU750
CLORURO di METILE (ITALIAN) see II:MIF765
CLORURO di VINILE (ITALIAN) see I:VNP000
CLOUT see I:DXE600
4-Cl-o-PD see I:CFK125
2-Cl-P-PD see III:CEG625
CLYSAR see III:PMP500
CMA see II:CBF250
CMC see III:SFO500
CMC 7H see III:SFO500
CM-CELLULOSE Na SALT see III:SFO500
CMC SODIUM SALT see III:SFO500
CMME see I:CIO250
CMPABN see III:MEI000
CMPP see II:CIR500
CMU see III:CJX750
CMW BONE CEMENT see III:PKB500
CN see III:CEA750
CN 8676 see II:EEI000
CN-15,757 see II:ASA500
CNA see III:RDP300
CNU-ETHANOL see III:CHB750
CO 12 see III:DXV600
CO-1214 see III:DXV600
CO-1895 see III:OAX000
CO-1897 see III:OAX000
COAL CONVERSION MATERIALS, SRC-II HEAVY DISTIL-
    LATE see II:CMY625
COAL DUST see III:CMY635
COAL FACINGS see III:CMY635
COAL, GROUND BITUMINOUS (DOT) see III:CMY635
COAL LIQUID see III:PCR250
COAL-MILLED see III:CMY635
COAL NAPHTHA see I:BBL250
COAL OIL see III:PCR250
COAL SLAG-MILLED see III:CMY635
COAL TAR see I:CMY800

COAL TAR, AEROSOL see III:CMY805
COAL TAR CREOSOTE see I:CMY825
COAL TAR OIL see I:CMY825
COAL TAR OIL (DOT) see I:CMY825
COAL TAR PITCH VOLATILES see I:CMZ100
COATHYLENE PF 0548 see III:PMP500
COBALT see I:CNA250
COBALT-59 see I:CNA250
COBALT ALLOY, Co, Cr see I:CNA750
COBALT, BIS(N-9H-FLUOREN-2-YL-N-HYDROXYACETAMI-
    DATO-O,O')-(9CI) see III:FDU875
COBALT BLACK see III:CND125
COBALT(II) CHLORIDE see III:CNB599
COBALT-CHROMIUM ALLOY see I:CNA750
COBALT-CHROMIUM-MOLYBDENUM ALLOY see
    III:VSK000
COBALT COMPOUNDS see I:CNB850
COBALT DICHLORIDE see III:CNB599
COBALT DINITRATE see III:CNC500
COBALT N-FLUOREN-2-YLACETOHYDROXAMATE see
    III:FDU875
COBALT-METHYLCOBALAMIN see III:VSZ050
COBALT MONOOXIDE see III:CND125
COBALT MONOSULFIDE see III:CNE200
COBALT MONOXIDE see III:CND125
COBALT MURIATE see III:CNB599
COBALT(II) NITRATE see III:CNC500
COBALTOCENE see III:BIR529
COBALTOUS CHLORIDE see III:CNB599
COBALTOUS DICHLORIDE see III:CNB599
COBALTOUS NITRATE see III:CNC500
COBALTOUS OXIDE see III:CND125
COBALTOUS SULFIDE see III:CNE200
COBALT OXIDE see III:CND125
COBALT(2+) OXIDE see III:CND125
COBALT(II) OXIDE see III:CND125
COBALT SALTS see III:FDU875
COBALT SULFIDE see III:CNE200
COBALT(II) SULFIDE see III:CNE200
COBALT SULFIDE (AMORPHOUS) see III:CNE200
COBEX (POLYMER) see III:PKQ059
COBINAMIDE, COBALT-METHYL derivative, HYDROXIDE,
    DIHYDROGEN PHOSPHATE (ester), inner salt, 3'-ESTER with
    5,6-DIMETHYL-1-α-D-RIBOFURANOSYLBENZIMIDA-
    ZOLE see III:VSZ050
COBRATEC #99 see III:BDH250
COCAFURIN see II:NGE500
COCARTRIT see III:CLD000
COCCINE see III:FMU080
COCCOCLASE see III:PPO000
COCHENILLEROT A see III:FMU080
COCHINEAL RED A see III:FMU080
CODECHINE see I:BBQ500
CODE H 133 see III:DER800
CODEMPIRAL see I:ABG750
CODIBARBITA see II:EOK000
CO-ESTRO see I:ECU750
COFFEIN (GERMAN) see III:CAK500
COFFEINE see III:CAK500
COGILOR BLUE 512.12 see III:FAE000
COGILOR RED 321.10 see III:FAG070
COIR DEEP BLACK C see I:AQP000
COLACID PONCEAU 4R see III:FMU080
COLACID PONCEAU SPECIAL see III:FMU070
COLCOTHAR see III:IHD000
COLESTYRAMIN see III:CME400
COLISONE see III:PLZ000
COLLIRON I.V. see I:IHG000
COLLOID 775 see III:CCL250
COLLOIDAL ARSENIC see ARA750
COLLOIDAL CADMIUM see I:CAD000
COLLOIDAL FERRIC OXIDE see III:IHD000
COLLOIDAL GOLD see III:GIS000
COLLOIDAL MANGANESE see III:MAP750

COLLOIDAL MERCURY see III:MCW250
COLLOIDAL SELENIUM see III:SBO500
COLLOIDAL SILICA see III:SCH000
COLLOIDAL SILICON DIOXIDE see III:SCH000
COLLOMIDE see III:SNM500
COLLOWELL see III:SFO500
COLLUNOSOL see II:TIV750
COLOGNE SPIRIT see I:EFU000
COLOGNE SPIRITS (ALCOHOL) (DOT) see I:EFU000
COLOGNE YELLOW see I:LCR000
COLOMBIAN BLACK TOBACCO CIGARETTE REFINED TAR
    see II:CMP800
COLONATRAST see III:BAP000
COLOR-SET see II:TIX500
COLPOVISTER see II:EDU500
COLSULANYDE see III:SNM500
COLTS FOOT see II:PCR000
COLTSFOOT see III:CNH250
COLUMBIA BLACK EP see I:AQP000
COLYONAL see III:DBD750
COMBOT EQUINE see III:TIQ250
COMESTROL see I:DKA600
COMESTROL ESTROBENE see I:DKA600
COMFREY, RUSSIAN see II:RRP000, III:RRK000
COMITAL see I:DKQ000
COMMOTIONAL see I:ABG750
COMPALOX see III:AHE250
COMPITOX see II:CIR500
COMPOCILLIN G see III:BDY669
COMPOUND 118 see III:AFK250
COMPOUND 269 see III:EAT500
COMPOUND 338 see II:DER000
COMPOUND 347 see III:EAT900
COMPOUND 497 see III:DHB400
COMPOUND 604 see III:DFT000
COMPOUND-666 see I:BBP750
COMPOUND 864 see III:YCJ000
COMPOUND 889 see I:DVL700
COMPOUND 88R see I:SOP500
COMPOUND 923 see III:DFY400
COMPOUND 1189 see I:KEA000
COMPOUND 3422 see III:PAK000
COMPOUND 3956 see I:CDV100
COMPOUND 4049 see III:MAK700
COMPOUND 17309 see III:DAL300
COMPOUND 33355 see I:MKB750
COMPOUND 38,174 see III:INS000
COMPOUND 42339 see III:ADR750
COMPOUND E ACETATE see III:CNS825
COMPOUND F-2 see III:ZAT000
COMPOUND G-11 see III:HCL000
COMYCETIN see II:CDP250
CONDENSATES (PETROLEUM), VACUUM TOWER (9CI) see
    I:MQV755
CONDITION see III:DCK759
CONEST see I:ECU750
CONESTRON see I:ECU750
CONGOBLAU 3B see II:CMO250
CONGO BLUE see II:CMO250
CONJES see I:ECU750
CONJUGATED EQUINE ESTROGEN see I:PMB000
CONJUGATED ESTROGENS see I:ECU750
CONJUTABS see I:ECU750
CONOVID see I:EAP000
CONOVID E see I:EAP000
CONT see I:MMN250
CONTERGAN see III:TEH500
CONTIMET 30 see III:TGF250
CONTIZELL see III:PKQ059
CONTRADOL see I:ABG750
CONTRALIN see III:DXH250
CONTRAPOT see III:DXH250
CONTROVLAR see II:EEH520
CONVUL see I:DKQ000

COOMASSIE VIOLET see II:FAG120
CO-OP HEXA see I:HCC500
COPAGEL PB 25 see III:SFO500
COPAL Z see III:SMQ500
COPAROGIN see III:FMB000
COPPER see III:CNI000
COPPER-8 see III:BLC250
COPPER-AIRBORNE see III:CNI000
COPPER ALLOY, Cu, Be see I:CNI750
COPPER ALLOY, Cu, Be, Co see I:CNJ000
COPPERAS see III:FBN100
COPPER-BERYLLIUM ALLOY see I:CNI750
COPPER BRONZE see III:CNI000
COPPER CHELATE of N-HYDROXY-2-ACETYLAMINO-
    FLUORENE see III:HIP500
COPPER-COBALT-BERYLLIUM see I:CNJ000
COPPER HYDROXYQUINOLATE see III:BLC250
COPPER-8-HYDROXYQUINOLATE see III:BLC250
COPPER-8-HYDROXYQUINOLINATE see III:BLC250
COPPER-8-HYDROXYQUINOLINE see III:BLC250
COPPER-MILLED see III:CNI000
COPPER MONOSULFATE see III:CNP250
COPPER OXINATE see III:BLC250
COPPER (2+) OXINATE see III:BLC250
COPPER OXINE see III:BLC250
COPPER OXYQUINOLATE see III:BLC250
COPPER OXYQUINOLINE see III:BLC250
COPPER QUINOLATE see III:BLC250
COPPER-8-QUINOLATE see III:BLC250
COPPER-8-QUINOLINOL see III:BLC250
COPPER QUINOLINOLATE see III:BLC250
COPPER-8-QUINOLINOLATE see III:BLC250
COPPER SLAG-AIRBORNE see III:CNI000
COPPER SLAG-MILLED see III:CNI000
COPPER complex with trans-N-(p-STYRYLPHENYL)ACETOHY-
    DROXAMIC ACID see III:SMU000
COPPER SULFATE see III:CNP250
COPPER(II) SULFATE (1:1) see III:CNP250
COPROSTANOL see III:DKW000
COPROSTAN-3-β-OL see III:DKW000
COPROSTEROL see III:DKW000
COPTICIDE see III:SNM500
CORDULAN see III:CMD750
COREINE see III:CCL250
CORICIDIN see I:ABG750
CORIFORTE see I:ABG750
CORIZIUM see III:NGG500
CORLUTIN see I:PMH500
CORLUTIN L.A. see III:HNT500
CORLUVITE see I:PMH500
CORNOCENTIN see III:EDB500
CORNOX-M see II:CIR250
CORNOX RD see II:DGB000
CORNOX RK see II:DGB000
CORN SUGAR see III:GFG000
CORODANE see II:CDR750
CORONA COROZATE see III:BJK500
CORONALETTA see II:EOK000
CORONENE see III:CNS250
COROTHION see III:PAK000
COROTRAN see III:CJT750
COROZATE see III:BJK500
CORPORIN see I:PMH500
CORPUS LUTEUM HORMONE see I:PMH500
CORRONAROBETIN see III:TEH500
CORTACET see III:DAQ800
CORTADREN see III:CNS825
CORTAN see III:PLZ000
CORTANCYL see III:PLZ000
CORTATE see III:DAQ800
CORTELAN see III:CNS825
Δ-CORTELAN see III:PLZ000
CORTENIL see III:DAQ800
CORTESAN see III:DAQ800

CORTEXONE ACETATE see III:DAQ800
CORTHION see III:PAK000
CORTHIONE see III:PAK000
CORTIDELT see III:PLZ000
CORTIFAR see III:DAQ800
CORTIGEN see III:DAQ800
CORTILAN-NEU see II:CDR750
CORTINAQ see III:DAQ800
CORTINAZINE see III:ILD000
CORTIRON see III:DAQ800
CORTISAL see III:CNS825
CORTISATE see III:CNS825
Δ-CORTISONE see III:PLZ000
Δ¹-CORTISONE see III:PLZ000
CORTISONE ACETATE see III:CNS825
CORTISONE-21-ACETATE see III:CNS825
CORTISONE MONOACETATE see III:CNS825
CORTISTAB see III:CNS825
CORTISYL see III:CNS825
CORTIVIS see III:DAQ800
CORTIVITE see III:CNS825
CORTIXYL see III:DAQ800
CORTOGEN see III:CNS825
CORTOGEN ACETATE see III:CNS825
CORTONE see III:CNS825
Δ-CORTONE see III:PLZ000
CORTONE ACETATE see III:CNS825
CORUNDUM see III:EAL100
CORVIC 55/9 see III:PKQ059
CORVIC 236581 see II:AAX175
CORYBAN-D see I:ABG750
CORYZOL see III:DPJ400
COSDEN 550 see III:SMQ500
COSMEGEN see III:AEB000
COSMETIC BLUE LAKE see III:FAE000
COSMETIC BRILLIANT PINK BLUISH D CONC see
    III:FAG070
COSMETIC CORAL RED KO BLUISH see III:CHP500
COSMETIC GREEN BLUE R25396 see III:ADE500
COSMETIC WHITE C47-5175 see III:TGG760
COSMOPEN see III:BDY669
COTINAZIN see III:ILD000
COTINIZIN see III:ILD000
COTNION METHYL see III:ASH500
COTOFILM see III:HCL000
COTONE see III:PLZ000
COTORAN see III:DUK800
COTORAN MULTI 50WP see III:DUK800
CO-TRIMOXAZOLE see III:SNK000
COTTONEX see III:DUK800
COTTONSEED OIL (unhydrogenated) see III:CNU000
COTTON VIOLET R see III:CMP000
COUMARIN see III:CNV000
cis-o-COUMARINIC ACID LACTONE see III:CNV000
COUMARINIC ANHYDRIDE see III:CNV000
COURLOSE A 590 see III:SFO500
COXISTAT see II:NGE500
CP see I:EAS500
CP 3438 see III:TFD250
CP 4572 see CDO250
CP 14,957 see III:OAN000
CP 15,336 see III:DBI200
CP 25017 see III:NHK800
CP-15467-61 see III:LGZ000
CPA see I:EAS500, III:CQJ500
CP BASIC SULFATE see III:CNP250
CPCA see III:BIO750
CPCBS see III:CJT750
C.P. CHROME LIGHT 2010 see I:LCS000
C.P. CHROME ORANGE DARK 2030 see I:LCS000
C.P. CHROME ORANGE MEDIUM 2020 see I:LCS000
C.P. CHROME YELLOW LIGHT see I:LCR000
CPDC see II:PJD000
CPDD see II:PJD000

CPH see II:CDP250, III:CBL000
CPIB see III:ARQ750
CPNU-I see III:NKJ100
cis-CPO see III:CKS099
trans-CPO see III:CKS100
C.P. TITANIUM see III:TGF250
C.P. ZINC YELLOW X-883 see I:ZFJ100
C-QUENS see II:CBF250, III:CNV750
CR see III:DDE200
CR 3029 see III:MAS500
CRAB-E-RAD see I:DXE600
CRAG SEVIN see III:CBM750
CRALO-E-RAD see I:DXE600
CRASTIN S 330 see III:PKF750
CRATECIL see II:EOK000
CRAWHASPOL see II:TIO750
CREDO see III:SHF500
CREIN see III:DAL300
CREMOMETHAZINE see III:SNJ000
CREOSOTE see I:CMY825
CREOSOTE, from COAL TAR see I:CMY825
CREOSOTE OIL see I:CMY825
CREOSOTE P1 see I:CMY825
CREOSOTUM see I:CMY825
CRESIDINE see I:MGO750
m-CRESIDINE see II:MGO500
p-CRESIDINE see I:MGO750
2-CRESOL see III:CNX000
3-CRESOL see III:CNW750
4-CRESOL see III:CNX250
m-CRESOL see III:CNW750
o-CRESOL see III:CNX000
p-CRESOL see III:CNX250
CRESORCINOL DIISOCYANATE see I:TGM750
CRESOTINE BLUE 2B see I:CMO000
CRESOTINE BLUE 3B see II:CMO250
CRESTOXO see I:CDV100
m-CRESYLIC ACID see III:CNW750
o-CRESYLIC ACID see III:CNX000
p-CRESYLIC ACID see III:CNX250
CRESYLIC CREOSOTE see I:CMY825
CRILL 10 see III:PKL100
CRIMSON EMBL see III:HJF500
CRIMSON SX see III:FMU080
CRINOTHENE see III:PKB500
CRINOVARYL see I:EDV000
CRISALIN see III:DUV600
CRISATRINA see III:ARQ725
CRISAZINE see III:ARQ725
CRISTALLOSE see II:SJN700
CRISTALLOVAR see I:EDV000
CRISTERONE T see I:TBF500
CRISTOBALITE see I:SCJ000
CRISTOXO 90 see I:CDV100
CRISULFAN see III:EAQ750
CRISURON see III:DXQ500
CRITTOX see III:EIR000
CROCEOMYCIN see III:HAL000
CROCIDOLITE (DOT) see I:ARM275
CROCIDOLITE ASBESTOS see I:ARM275
CROCOITE see I:LCR000
CROCUS MARTIS ADSTRINGENS see III:IHD000
CRODACOL-S see III:OAX000
CROLEAN see III:ADR000
CRONETAL see III:DXH250
CROP RIDER see II:DAA800
CROTALINE see II:MRH000
CROTILIN see II:DAA800
CROTONALDEHYDE see II:COB250
CROTONAMIDE, 2-CHLORO-N,N-DIETHYL-3-HYDROXY-,
 DIMETHYL PHOSPHATE see III:FAC025
CROTONATE de 2,4-DINITRO 6-(1-METHYL-HEPTYL)-PHE-
 NYLE (FRENCH) see III:AQT500
CROTONIC ALDEHYDE see II:COB250

CROTONOEL (GERMAN) see III:COC250
CROTON OIL see III:COC250
CROTON RESIN see III:COC250
CROTON TIGLIUM L. OIL see III:COC250
CROTYLIDENE ACETIC ACID see III:SKU000
CROVARIL see III:HNI500
CROYSULFONE see III:SOA500
CRUDE ARSENIC see I:ARI750
CRUDE COAL TAR see I:CMY800
CRUDE ERGOT see III:EDB500
CRUDE OIL see III:PCR250
CRUDE OIL, synthetic see III:COD725
CRUDE SHALE OILS see I:COD750
CRYOGENINE see III:CBL000
CRYPTOGIL OL see II:PAX250
CRYSTALETS see III:VSK900
CRYSTALLINE DEHYDROXY SODIUM ALUMINUM, CAR-
 BONATE see III:DAC450
CRYSTALLOSE see II:SJN700
CRYSTAL ORANGE 2G see III:HGC000
CRYSTAPEN see III:BFD250
CRYSTHION 2L see III:ASH500
CRYSTHYON see III:ASH500
CRYSTOGEN see I:EDV000
CRYSTOIDS see III:HFV500
CRYSTOSOL see III:MQV750
60-CS-16 see III:CMF400
CSC see I:SEC000
CTA see II:CLO750
CTX see I:EAS500
CUBE see III:RNZ000
CUBE EXTRACT see III:RNZ000
CUBE-PULVER see III:RNZ000
CUBE ROOT see III:RNZ000
CUBIC NITER see III:SIO900
CUBOR see III:RNZ000
CUEMID see III:CME400
CUMAN see III:BJK500
CUMAN L see III:BJK500
CUMEENHYDROPEROXYDE (DUTCH) see III:IOB000
CUMENE HYDROPEROXIDE (DOT) see III:IOB000
CUMENE HYDROPEROXIDE, TECHNICALLY PURE (DOT)
 see III:IOB000
CUMENT HYDROPEROXIDE see III:IOB000
p-(p-CUMENYLAZO)-N,N-DIMETHYLANILINE see
 III:IOT875
CUMENYL HYDROPEROXIDE see III:IOB000
psi-CUMIDINE see I:TLG250
psi-CUMIDINE HYDROCHLORIDE see III:TLG750
CUMOLHYDROPEROXID (GERMAN) see III:IOB000
CUMYL HYDROPEROXIDE see III:IOB000
α-CUMYL HYDROPEROXIDE see III:IOB000
CUMYL HYDROPEROXIDE, TECHNICAL PURE (DOT) see
 III:IOB000
CUNILATE see III:BLC250
CUNILATE 2472 see III:BLC250
CUPFERRON see I:ANO500
CUPRAL see III:SGJ000
CUPRENIL see III:MCR750
CUPRIC CHELATE of 2-N-HYDROXYFLUORENYL ACET-
 AMIDE see III:HIP500
CUPRIC-8-HYDROXYQUINOLATE see III:BLC250
CUPRIC-8-QUINOLINOLATE see III:BLC250
CUPRIC SULFATE see III:CNP250
CUPRIMINE see III:MCR750
CURALIN M see I:MJM200
CURENE 442 see I:MJM200
CURETARD see III:COG250
CURETARD A see III:DWI000
CUREX FLEA DUSTER see III:RNZ000
CURITAN see III:DXX400
CURITHANE see I:MJQ000
CURITHANE 103 see III:MGA500
CURITHANE C126 see I:DEQ600

6,7-CYCLOPENTENO-1,2-BENZANTHRACENE see
   III:BCI250
CYCLOPENTENO(c,d)PYRENE see III:CPX500
CYCLOPHOSPHAMIDE see I:EAS500
CYCLOPHOSPHAMIDE HYDRATE see I:CQC675
CYCLOPHOSPHAMIDE MONOHYDRATE see I:CQC675
CYCLOPHOSPHAMIDUM see I:CQC675, I:EAS500
CYCLOPHOSPHAN see I:CQC675, I:EAS500
CYCLOPHOSPHANE see I:CQC675
CYCLOPHOSPHANUM see I:CQC675
CYCLOPHOSPHORAMIDE see I:EAS500
5H-CYCLOPROPA(3,4)BENZ(1,2-e)AZULEN-5-ONE, 1,-
   1a,1b,4,4a,7a,7b,8,9,9a-DECAHYDRO-4a,7-β, 9,9a-TET-
   RAHYDROXY-3-(HYDROXYMETHYL)-1,1,6,8-TETRA-
   METHYL-, 9-ACETATE 9a-LAURATE see III:PGS500
5H-CYCLOPROPA(3,4)BENZ(1,2-e)AZULEN-5-ONE,1,1a-
   α,1b-β,4,4a,7a-α,7b,8,9,9a-DECAHYDRO-4a-α,7b-α,9a-α-
   TRIHYDROXY-3-HYDROXYMETHYL-1,6,8-α-TRI-
   METHYL-1-ACETOXYMETHYL-,9a-(2-METHYLBUT-2-
   ENOATE) see III:CQD250
CYCLOSPORIN see III:CQH100
CYCLOSPORIN A see III:CQH100
CYCLOSPORINE see III:CQH100
CYCLOSPORINE A see III:CQH100
CYCLOSTIN see I:EAS500
CYCOCEL see III:CMF400
CYCOCEL-EXTRA see III:CMF400
CYCOGAN see III:CMF400
CYCOGAN EXTRA see III:CMF400
CYFOS see II:IMH000
CYGON see III:DSP400
CYGON INSECTICIDE see III:DSP400
CYKAZINE see I:COU000
CY-L 500 see III:CAQ250
CYLAN see III:CAR000
CYLPHENICOL see II:CDP250
CYMATE see III:BJK500
CYMEL see III:MCB000
CYNKOTOX see III:EIR000
CYOCEL see III:CMF400
CYPREX see III:DXX400
CYPREX 65W see III:DXX400
CYPROSTERONE ACETATE see III:CQJ500
CYPROTERONE ACETATE see III:CQJ500
CYPROTERON-R ACETATE see III:CQJ500
CYREN see I:DKA600
CYREN B see I:DKB000
CYSTAMIN see III:HEI500
CYSTAMINE "MCCLUNG" see I:PDC250
CYSTOGEN see III:HEI500
CYSTOIDS ANTHELMINTIC see III:HFV500
CYSTOPYRIN see I:PDC250
CYSTURAL see I:PDC250
CYTHION see III:MAK700
CYTOPHOSPHAN see I:CQC675, I:EAS500
CYTOSINE-β-ARABINOSIDE see III:AQQ750
CYTOSINE β-d-ARABINOSIDE see III:AQQ750
CYTOSTASAN see III:CQM750
CYTOXAL ALCOHOL see II:CQN000
CYTOXAN see I:CQC675, I:EAS500
CYTOXYL ALCOHOL CYCLOHEXYLAMMONIUM SALT see
   II:CQN000
CYTROL see I:AMY050
CYURAM DS see III:TFS350
CZT see III:CLX000
CZTEROCHLOREK WEGLA (POLISH) see CBY000
2,3,7,8-CZTEROCHLORODWUBENZO-p-DWUOKSYNY
   (POLISH) see I:TAI000
1,1,2,2-CZTEROCHLOROETAN (POLISH) see III:TBQ100
CZTEROCHLOROETYLEN (POLISH) see II:PCF275
CZTEROETHLEK OLOWIU (POLISH) see III:TCF000

2,4-D see II:DAA800
D-50 see III:POL500, II:DAA800

D 854 see III:CJT750
DA see III:DNA200
2,4-DAA see I:DBO000
DAAB see III:DWO800
DAAE see III:DCN800
2,4-DAA SULFATE see I:DBO400
DAB see I:DOT300
DABI see III:DOT600
DAB-O-LITE P 4 see III:WCJ000
DAB-N-OXIDE see III:DTK600
DAC 2797 see III:TBQ750
DACAMINE see II:DAA800, II:TAA100
DACARBAZINE see II:DAB600
2,4-D ACID see II:DAA800
DACONIL see III:TBQ750
DACONIL 2787 FLOWABLE FUNGICIDE see III:TBQ750
DACORTIN see III:PLZ000
DACOSOIL see III:TBQ750
DACOVIN see III:PKQ059
DACTINOL see III:RNZ000
DACTINOMYCIN see III:AEB000
DADDS see III:SNY500
DADPE see I:OPM000
DADPS see III:SOA500
DAF 68 see I:DVL700
DAGENAN see III:PPO000
DAGUTAN see II:SJN700
1,1-DAH see III:DBK100
1,2-DAH HYDROCHLORIDE see III:DBK120
DAICEL 1150 see III:SFO500
DAILON see III:DXQ500
DAINICHI CHROME ORANGE R see I:LCS000
DAINICHI CHROME YELLOW G see I:LCR000
DAINICHI FAST SCARLET G BASE see I:NMP500
DAINICHI LAKE RED C see III:CHP500
DAISEN see III:EIR000
DAISHIKI AMARANTH see III:FAG020
DAISHIKI BRILLIANT SCARLET 3R see III:FMU080
DAITO RED BASE TR see II:CLK220
DAITO RED SALT TR see II:CLK235
DAITO SCARLET BASE G see I:NMP500
DAIYA FOIL see III:PKF750
DAL-E-RAD 100 see I:DXE600
DALF see III:MNH000
DALTOGEN see III:TKP500
DAMINOZIDE (USDA) see II:DQD400
2,4-D AMMONIUM SALT see III:DAB020
DAMORAL see II:EOK000
DAN see III:DSU600
DA-2-N see III:DSU800
DANA see I:NJW500
DANABOL see III:DAL300
DANAMID see III:PJY500
DANANTIZOL see III:MCO500
DANAZOL see III:DAB830
DANEX see III:TIQ250
DANIZOL see I:MMN250
DANOCRINE see III:DAB830
DANOL see III:DAB830
DANTAFUR see III:NGE000
DANTEN see I:DKQ000, I:DNU000
DANTHION see III:PAK000
DANTHRON see III:DMH400
DANTINAL see I:DKQ000
DANTOIN see I:DNU000
DANTOINAL KLINOS see I:DKQ000
DANTOINE see I:DKQ000
DANTROLENE see III:DAB845
DANTRON see III:DMH400
DANU see III:DPN400
DANUVIL 70 see III:PKQ059
DAP see III:DCK759, III:DOT000
DAPA see III:DOU600
DAPHENE see III:DSP400

DAPLEN AD see III:PMP500
DAPON 35 see II:DBL200
DAPON R see II:DBL200
DAPRISAL see I:ABG750
DAPSONE see III:SOA500
DARACLOR see III:TGD000
DARAPRAM see III:TGD000
DARAPRIM see III:TGD000
DARAPRIME see III:TGD000
DAR-CHEM 14 see III:SLK000
DARVIC 110 see III:PKQ059
DARVIS CLEAR 025 see III:PKQ059
DARVON COMPOUND see I:ABG750
DAS see III:DOU600
DASIKON see I:ABG750
DASKIL see III:Q900
DATC see III:DBI200
DATRIL see II:HIM000
DAUNAMYCIN see II:DAC000
DAUNOMYCIN see II:DAC000
DAUNORUBICIN see II:DAC000
DAUNORUBICINE see II:DAC000
DAVISON SG-67 see III:SCH000
DAVITAMON PP see III:NCQ900
DAWE'S DESTROL see I:DKA600
DAWSON 100 see III:MHR200
DAWSONITE see III:DAC450
DB-905 see III:TBS000
DBA see I:DCT400, II:DQJ200
DB(a,c)A see III:BDH750
DB(a,h)A see I:DCT400
1,2,5,6-DBA see I:DCT400
DB(a,h)AC see I:DCS400
DB(a,j)AC see I:DCS600
DBA-1,2-DIHYDRODIOL see III:DMK200
trans-DBA-3,4-DIHYDRODIOL see III:DLD400
DBA-5,6-EPOXIDE see III:EBP500
7H-DB(c,g)C see I:DCY000
DBCP see I:DDL800
DBD see III:ASH500, III:DDJ000
DBDPO see III:PAU500
DBE see I:EIY500
DBH see I:BBP750, I:BBQ500
1,1-DBH see III:DEC725
DBM see III:DDP600
DBMP see III:BFW750
DBN see I:BRY500
2,6-DBN see III:DER800
DBN (the herbicide) see III:DER800
DBNA see I:BRY500
DB(a,e)P see II:NAT500
DB(a,i)P see I:BCQ500
DB(a,l)P see II:DCY400
DBPC (technical grade) see III:BFW750
2,4-D BUTYL ESTER see III:BQZ000
DCA see III:DAQ800, III:DEL000
DCB see I:DEQ600, I:DEV000, III:DEP600, III:DER800
1,4-DCB see III:DEV000
D&C BLUE No. 4 see III:FAE000, III:FMU059
DCDD see III:DAC800
2,3-DCDT see III:DBI200
1-1-DCE see II:VPK000
1,2-DCE see I:EIY600
DCEE see III:DFJ050
D&C GREEN No. 4 see III:FAF000
DCM see II:MJP450, III:DFO000
DCMU see III:DXQ500
DCNA see III:RDP300
DCNA (fungicide) see III:RDP300
DCNU see III:CLX000
D&C ORANGE No. 2 see II:TGW000
D&C ORANGE No. 3 see III:FAG010, III:HGC000
DCP see II:DFX800
2,4-DCP see II:DFX800

cis-DCPO see III:DAC975
trans-DCPO see III:DGH500
D&C RED 2 see III:FAG020
D&C RED No. 3 see III:FAG040
D&C RED No. 5 see III:FMU070
D&C RED No. 9 see III:CHP500
D&C RED No. 14 see III:TGX000
D&C RED No. 17 see III:OHA000
D&C RED No. 21 see III:BMO250
D&C RED No. 22 see III:BNH500
D.C.S. see II:BGJ750
D&C YELLOW No. 8 see III:FEW000
DDC see I:DQY950, III:SGJ000
cis-DDCP see III:DAD040
trans(−)-DDCP see III:DAD075
trans(+)-DDCP see III:DAD050
DDD see I:BIM500
2,4'-DDD see III:CDN000
o,p'-DDD see III:CDN000
p,p'-DDD see I:BIM500
DDE see II:BIM750
p,p'-DDE see II:BIM750
DDETA see III:HMQ500
DDM see I:MJQ000
DDOA see I:ABC250
DDP see II:PJD000
cis-DDP see II:PJD000
DDS see III:SOA500
DDT see I:DAD200
p,p'-DDT see I:DAD200
DDT DEHYDROCHLORIDE see II:BIM750
DE 83R see III:PAU500
DEACTIVATOR E see III:DJD600
DEACTIVATOR H see III:DJD600
DEADOPA see III:DNA200
DEAE-D see III:DHW600
3′-DEAMINO-3′-(3-CYANO-4-MORPHOLINYL)DOXORUBI-
    CIN see III:COP765
3′-DEAMINO-3′-MORPHOLINO-ADRIAMYCIN see
    III:MRT100
3′-DEAMINO-3′-(4-MORPHOLINYL)DAUNORUBICIN see
    III:MRT100
DEANOX see III:IHD000
DEASERPYL see III:MEK700
DEB see I:BGA750, I:DKA600
DEBANTIC see III:RAF100
DEBROUSSAILLANT 600 see II:DAA800
DEBROUSSAILLANT CONCENTRE see II:TAA100
DEBROXIDE see III:BDS000
DEC see III:DAE800, III:DIX200
DECABANE see III:DER800
DECABROMOBIPHENYL ETHER see III:PAU500
DECABROMOBIPHENYL OXIDE see III:PAU500
DECABROMODIPHENYL OXIDE see III:PAU500
DECABROMOPHENYL ETHER see III:PAU500
1,2,3,5,6,7,8,9,10,10-DECACHLORO(5.2.1.0$^{(2,6)}$.0$^{(3,9)}$.0$^{(5,8)}$)
    DECANO-4-ONE see I:KEA000
DECACHLOROKETONE see I:KEA000
DECACHLORO-1,3,4-METHENO-2H-CYCLOBUTA(cd)PEN-
    TALEN-2-ONE see I:KEA000
DECACHLOROOCTAHYDROKEPONE-2-ONE see I:KEA000
DECACHLOROOCTAHYDRO-1,3,4-METHENO-2H-CYCLO-
    BUTA(cd)PENTALEN-2-ONE see I:KEA000
1,1a,3,3a,4,5,5,5a,5b,6-DECACHLOROOCTAHYDRO-1,3,4-
    METHENO-2H-CYCLOBUTA(cd)PENTALEN-2-ONE see
    I:KEA000
DECACHLOROPENTACYCLO(5.2.1.0$^{(2,6)}$.0$^{(3,9)}$.0$^{(5,8)}$)
    DECAN-4-ONE see I:KEA000
DECACHLOROPENTACYCLO(5.3.0.0$^{(2,6)}$.0$^{(4,10)}$.0$^{(5,9)}$)
    DECAN-3-ONE see I:KEA000
DECACHLOROTETRACYCLODECANONE see I:KEA000
DECACHLOROTETRAHYDRO-4,7-METHANOINDENEONE
    see I:KEA000
DECAHYDRONAPHTHALENE see III:DAE800

DECALIN see III:DAE800
DECALIN (DOT) see III:DAE800
DECALIN SOLVENT see III:DAE800
DECAMINE see II:DAA800
DECAMINE 4T see II:TAA100
DECANAL DIMETHYL ACETAL see III:DAI600
DECANE see III:DAG400
n-DECANE (DOT) see III:DAG400
DECANOL see III:DAI600
n-DECANOL see III:DAI600
1-DECANOL (FCC) see III:DAI600
DECASERPIL see III:MEK700
DECASERPINE see III:MEK700
DECASERPYL see III:MEK700
DECASERPYL PLUS see III:MEK700
n-DECATYL ALCOHOL see III:DAI600
DECELITH H see III:PKQ059
DECHAN see III:DGU200
DECHLORANE 4070 see I:MQW500
DECHLORANE-A-O see I:AQF000
2,4-DECHLOROPHENYL-p-NITROPHENYL ETHER see
   I:DFT800
DECOFOL see III:BIO750
DECORTANCYL see III:PLZ000
DECORTIN see III:DAQ800, III:PLZ000
DECORTISYL see III:PLZ000
DECORTON see III:DAQ800
DECOSERPYL see III:MEK700
DECOSTERONE see III:DAQ800
DECOSTRATE see III:DAQ800
DECYL ALCOHOL see III:DAI600
n-DECYL ALCOHOL see III:DAI600
DECYLIC ALCOHOL see III:DAI600
DECYL OCTYL ALCOHOL see III:OAX000
DEDC see III:SGJ000
DEDELO see I:DAD200
DEDK see III:SGJ000
DED-WEED see II:CIR250, II:DAA800, II:TIX500
DED-WEED BRUSH KILLER see II:TAA100
DED-WEED LV-69 see II:DAA800
DED-WEED LV-6 BRUSH KIL and T-5 BRUSH KIL see
   II:TAA100
DEEP LEMON YELLOW see I:SMH000
DE-FEND see III:DSP400
DEFLAMON-WIRKSTOFF see I:MMN250
DEFLOGIN see III:HNI500
DEFONIN see III:ILD000
DEG see III:DJD600
DEGALAN S 85 see III:PKB500
DEGALOL see III:DAQ400
DEH see III:HHH000
DEHA see III:AEO000
DEHP see I:DVL700
DEHYDRACETIC ACID see III:MFW500
DEHYDROACETIC ACID (FCC) see III:MFW500
trans-DEHYDROANDROSTERONE see III:AOO450
6-DEHYDRO-6-CHLORO-17-α-ACETOXYPROGESTERONE
   see II:CBF250
7-DEHYDROCHOLESTERIN see III:DAK600
DEHYDROCHOLESTERIN (GERMAN) see III:DAK600
DEHYDROCHOLESTEROL see III:DAK600
7-DEHYDROCHOLESTEROL see III:DAK600
7-DEHYDROCHOLESTEROL ACETATE see III:DAK800
7-DEHYDROCHOLESTERYL ACETATE see III:DAK800
1-DEHYDROCORTISONE see III:PLZ000
Δ-1-DEHYDROCORTISONE see III:PLZ000
DEHYDROEPIANDROSTERONE see III:AOO450
5-DEHYDROEPIANDROSTERONE see III:AOO450
DEHYDROFOLLICULINIC ACID see III:BIT000
11-DEHYDRO-17-HYDROXYCORTICOSTERONE ACETATE
   see III:CNS825
11-DEHYDRO-17-HYDROXYCORTICOSTERONE-21-ACE-
   TATE see III:CNS825
DEHYDROISOANDROSTERONE see III:AOO450

5,6-DEHYDROISOANDROSTERONE see III:AOO450
6-DEHYDRO-6-METHYL-17-α-ACETOXYPROGESTERONE
   see II:VTF000
DEHYDRO-3-METHYLCHOLANTHRENE see III:DAL200
1,2-DEHYDRO-3-METHYLCHOLANTHRENE see III:DAL200
DEHYDROMETHYLTESTERONE see III:DAL300
1-DEHYDRO-17-α-METHYLTESTOSTERONE see
   III:DAL300
DEHYDROMONOCROTALINE see III:DAL350
DEHYDRORETRONECINE see I:DAL400
DEHYDROSTILBESTROL see II:DAL600
DEHYDROSTILBOESTROL see II:DAL600
Δ³-DEHYDRO-3,4-TRIMETHYLENE-ISOBENZANTHRENE-2
   see III:BCI000
DE-KALIN see III:DAE800
DEKALINA (POLISH) see III:DAE800
DEKORTIN see III:PLZ000
DEKSONAL see III:DOU600
DELAC J see III:DWI000
DELADIOL see II:EDS100
DELAGIL see III:CLD000
DELAHORMONE UNIMATIC see II:EDS100
DELALUTIN see III:HNT500
DELATESTRYL see III:MPN500, III:TBF750
DELESTROGEN see II:EDS100
DELESTROGEN 4X see II:EDS100
DELIVA see III:ARQ750
DELMOFULVINA see GKE000
DELPET 50M see III:PKB500
DELTACORTELAN see III:PLZ000
DELTACORTISONE see III:PLZ000
DELTACORTONE see III:PLZ000
DELTA-DOME see III:PLZ000
DELTA-MVE see I:MKB750
DELTAN see III:DUD800
DELTISONE see III:PLZ000
DEMA see I:BIE500
DEMASORB see III:DUD800
DEMAVET see III:DUD800
DEMESO see III:DUD800
11-DEMETHOXYRESERPINE see III:RDF000
DEMETHYLDOPAN see II:BIA250
DEMETRIN see III:DAP700
DEMOS-L40 see III:DSP400
DEMSODROX see III:DUD800
DEN see I:NJW500
DENA see I:NJW500
DENAPON, NITROSATED (JAPANESE) see I:NBJ500
DENDRID see III:DAS000
DENKALAC 61 see II:AAX175
DENKA QP3 see III:SMQ500
DENKA VINYL SS 80 see III:PKQ059
DENSINFLUAT see II:TIO750
DENYL see I:DKQ000, I:DNU000
DENYLSODIUM see I:DNU000
DEODORIZED WINTERIZED COTTONSEED OIL see
   III:CNU000
DEOFED see III:MDT600
DEOVAL see I:DAD200
DEOXYCHOLATIC ACID see III:DAQ400
7-α-DEOXYCHOLIC ACID see III:DAQ400
DEOXYCHOLIC ACID (FCC) see III:DAQ400
11-DEOXYCORTICOSTERONE ACETATE see III:DAQ800
11-DEOXYCORTICOSTERONE-21-ACETATE see
   III:DAQ800
DEOXYCORTONE ACETATE see III:DAQ800
d-DEOXYEPHEDRINE HYDROCHLORIDE see III:MDT600
2'-DEOXY-5-IODOURIDINE see III:DAS000
1-DEOXY-1-(METHYLNITROSAMINO)-d-GLUCITOL see
   III:DAS400
2-DEOXY-2-(((METHYLNITROSOAMINO)CARBONYL)
   AMINO)-d-GLUCOPYRANOSE see I:SMD000
2-DEOXY-2-(3-METHYL-3-NITROSOUREIDO)-d-GLUCOPY-
   RANOSE see I:SMD000

4-β,15-DIACETOXY-8-α-(3-METHYLBUTYRYLOXY)-3-α-HYDROXY-12,13-EPOXYTRICHOTHEC-9-ENE see III:FQS000

3-β,17-β-DIACETOXY-19-NOR-17-α-PREGN-4-EN-20-YNE see II:EQJ500

4,4'-DIACETYLAMINOBIPHENYL see II:BFX000

2-DIACETYLAMINOFLUORENE see II:DBF200

2,7-DIACETYLAMINOFLUORENE see II:BGP250

N-DIACETYL-2-AMINOFLUORENE see II:DBF200

N,N-DIACETYL-2-AMINOFLUORENE see II:DBF200

DI-(p-ACETYLAMINOPHENYL)SULFONE see III:SNY500

4,4'-DIACETYLBENZIDINE see II:BFX000

N,N'-DIACETYL BENZIDINE see II:BFX000

DIACETYLDAPSONE see III:SNY500

N,N'-DIACETYLDAPSONE see III:SNY500

4,4'-DIACETYLDIAMINODIPHENYL SULFONE see III:SNY500

N,N'-DIACETYL-4,4'-DIAMINODIPHENYL SULFONE see III:SNY500

N,N'-DIACETYL-3,3'-DIMETHYLBENZIDINE see III:DRI400

N,N-DIACETYL-2-FLUORENAMINE see II:DBF200

O,O'-DIACETYL 4-HYDROXYAMINOQUINOLINE-1-OXIDE see III:ABN500

DIACETYL PEROXIDE (MAK) see III:ACV500

N,O-DIACETYL-N-(p-STYRYLPHENYL)HYDROXYLAMINE see III:ABW500

trans-N,o-DIACETYL-N-(p-STYRYLPHENYL)HYDROXYLAMINE see III:ABL250

DIACOTTON BLUE BB see I:CMO000

DIACOTTON DEEP BLACK see I:AQP000

DIACRID see III:DBX400

DIADEM CHROME BLUE R see III:HJF500

DIAETHANOLNITROSAMIN (GERMAN) see I:NKM000

DIAETHYLCARBONAT (GERMAN) see III:DIX500

1,2-DIAETHYLHYDRAZINE (GERMAN) see II:DJL400

O,O-DIAETHYL-O-(4-NITROPHENYL)-MONOTHIOPHOSPHAT (GERMAN) see III:PAK000

DIAETHYLNITROSAMIN (GERMAN) see I:NJW500

DIAETHYLSULFAT (GERMAN) see I:DKB110

DIAFURON see III:NGG500

DIAKON see III:MLH750, III:PKB500

DIAL-A-GESIC see II:HIM000

DIALLAAT (DUTCH) see III:DBI200

DIALLAT (GERMAN) see III:DBI200

DIALLATE see III:DBI200

DIALLYINITROSAMIN (GERMAN) see III:NJV500

DIALLYLHYDRAZINE see III:DBK100

1,1-DIALLYLHYDRAZINE see III:DBK100

1,2-DIALLYLHYDRAZINE DIHYDROCHLORIDE see III:DBK120

DIALLYLNITROSAMINE see III:NJV500

2,6-DIALLYLPHENOL see III:DBK800

DIALLYL PHTHALATE see II:DBL200

DIALUMINUM TRIOXIDE see III:AHE250

DIAMIDE see I:HGS000

DIAMINE see I:HGS000

2,4-DIAMINEANISOLE see I:DBO000

DIAMINE BLUE 2B see I:CMO000

DIAMINE BLUE 3B see II:CMO250

DIAMINE DEEP BLACK EC see I:AQP000

cis-DIAMINEDICHLOROPLATINUM see II:PJD000

(4,4'-DIAMINE-3,3'-DIMETHYL(1,1'-BIPHENYL) see I:TGJ750

DIAMINE SKY BLUE FF see III:BGT250

DIAMINE VIOLET N see III:CMP000

DIAMINIDE MALEATE see III:DBM800

3,6-DIAMINOACRIDINE see III:DBN600

3,6-DIAMINOACRIDINE mixture with 3,6-DIAMINO-10-METHYLACRIDINIUM CHLORIDE see III:DBX400

2,8-DIAMINOACRIDINE (EUROPEAN) see III:DBN600

3,6-DIAMINOACRIDINE HEMISULFATE see III:PMH100

3,6-DIAMINOACRIDINE HYDROCHLORIDE HEMIHYDRATE see III:DBN200

3,6-DIAMINOACRIDINE MONOHYDROCHLORIDE see III:PMH250

2,8-DIAMINOACRIDINIUM see III:DBN600

3,6-DIAMINOACRIDINIUM see III:DBN600

3,6-DIAMINOACRIDINIUM CHLORIDE see III:PMH250

3,6-DIAMINOACRIDINIUM CHLORIDE HYDROCHLORIDE see III:PMH250

2,8-DIAMINOACRIDINIUM CHLORIDE MONOHYDROCHLORIDE see III:PMH250

2,4-DIAMINOANISOL see I:DBO000

2,4-DIAMINOANISOLE see I:DBO000

2,4-DIAMINOANISOLE BASE see I:DBO000

m-DIAMINOANISOLE 1,3-DIAMINO-4-METHOXYBENZENE see I:DBO000

2,4-DIAMINOANISOLE SULFATE see I:DBO400

2,4-DIAMINOANISOLE SULPHATE see I:DBO400

2,4-DIAMINO-ANISOL SULPHATE see I:DBO400

3,7-DIAMINO-5-AZAANTHRACENE see III:DBN600

2,4-DIAMINOAZOBENZENE HYDROCHLORIDE see III:PEK000

m-DIAMINOBENZENE see III:PEY000

p-DIAMINOBENZENE see III:PEY500

1,3-DIAMINOBENZENE see III:PEY000

1,4-DIAMINOBENZENE see III:PEY500

m-DIAMINOBENZENE DIHYDROCHLORIDE see III:PEY750

p-DIAMINOBENZENE DIHYDROCHLORIDE see III:PEY650

1,3-DIAMINOBENZENE DIHYDROCHLORIDE see III:PEY750

1,4-DIAMINOBENZENE DIHYDROCHLORIDE see III:PEY650

3,3'-DIAMINOBENZIDENE see III:BGK500

3,3'-DIAMINOBENZIDINE TETRAHYDROCHLORIDE see III:BGK750

6,6'-DIAMINO-m,m'-BIPHENOL see II:DMI400

4,4'-DIAMINOBIPHENYL see I:BBX000

o,p'-DIAMINOBIPHENYL see III:BGF109

p,p'-DIAMINOBIPHENYL see I:BBX000

4,4'-DIAMINO-1,1'-BIPHENYL see I:BBX000

4,4'-DIAMINO-3,3'-BIPHENYLDICARBOXYLIC ACID see III:BFX250

4,4'-DIAMINOBIPHENYL-3,3'-DICARBOXYLIC ACID see III:BFX250

4,4'-DIAMINO-3,3'-BIPHENYLDICARBOXYLIC ACID DISODIUM SALT see III:BBX250

4,4'-DIAMINO-3,3'-BIPHENYLDIOL see II:DMI400

4,4'-((4,4'-DIAMINO-(1,1'-BIPHENYL)-3,3'-DIYL)BIS(OXY) BISBUTANOIC ACID, DIHYDROCHLORIDE see III:DEK000

4,4'-(3,3'-DIAMINO-p,p'-BIPHENYLENEDIOXY)DIBUTYRIC ACID see III:DEK400

4,4'-DIAMINOBIPHENYLOXIDE see I:OPM000

4,4'-DIAMINO-3-BIPHENYL-3-SULFONIC ACID see III:BBY250

3.4-DIAMINOCHLOROBENZENE see I:CFK125

1,2-DIAMINO -4-CHLOROBENZENE see I:CFK125

3,4-DIAMINO-1-CHLOROBENZENE see I:CFK125

2,4-DIAMINO-5-(4-CHLOROPHENYL)-6-ETHYLPYRIMIDINE see III:TGD000

2,4-DIAMINO-5-p-CHLOROPHENYL-6-ETHYLPYRIMIDINE see III:TGD000

DI-(4-AMINO-3-CHLOROPHENYL)METHANE see I:MJM200

DI-(4-AMINO-3-CLOROFENIL)METANO (ITALIAN) see I:MJM200

1,2-DIAMINOCYCLOHEXANEPLATINUM(II) CHLORIDE see III:DAD040

1,4-DIAMINO-2,6-DICHLOROBENZENE see III:DBR400

4,4'-DIAMINO-3,3'-DICHLOROBIPHENYL see I:DEQ600

4,4'-DIAMINO-3,3'-DICHLORODIPHENYL see I:DEQ600

4,4'-DIAMINO-3,3'-DICHLORODIPHENYLMETHANE see I:MJM200

4:4'-DIAMINO-2:2'-DICHLOROSTILBENE see III:DGK400

4:4'-DIAMINO-3:3'-DICHLOROSTILBENE see III:DGK600

DIAMINODIFENILSULFONA (SPANISH) see III:SOA500

p,p'-DIAMINODIFENYLMETHAN (CZECH) see I:MJQ000

4,4'-DIAMINO-3,3'-DIMETHYLBIPHENYL see I:TGJ750

4,4'-DIAMINO-3,3'-DIMETHYLDIPHENYL see I:TGJ750

1:2'-DIAMINO-1':2-DINAPHTHYL see III:BGC000
2,2'-DIAMINO-1,1'-DINAPHTHYL see III:BGB750
p-DIAMINODIPHENYL see I:BBX000
2,4'-DIAMINODIPHENYL see III:BGF109
4,4'-DIAMINODIPHENYL see I:BBX000
DIAMINODIPHENYL ETHER see I:OPM000
4,4-DIAMINODIPHENYL ETHER see I:OPM000
p,p'-DIAMINODIPHENYL ETHER see I:OPM000
4,4'-DIAMINODIPHENYLMETHAN (GERMAN) see
    I:MJQ000
DIAMINODIPHENYLMETHANE see I:MJQ000
4,4'-DIAMINODIPHENYLMETHANE see I:MJQ000
p,p'-DIAMINODIPHENYLMETHANE see I:MJQ000
4,4'-DIAMINODIPHENYL OXIDE see I:OPM000
4,4'-DIAMINODIPHENYL SULFIDE see I:TFI000
p,p'-DIAMINODIPHENYL SULFIDE see I:TFI000
DIAMINO-4,4'-DIPHENYL SULFONE see III:SOA500
4,4'-DIAMINODIPHENYL SULFONE see III:SOA500
p,p'-DIAMINODIPHENYL SULFONE see III:SOA500
p,p'-DIAMINODIPHENYL SULPHIDE see I:TFI000
p,p-DIAMINODIPHENYL SULPHONE see III:SOA500
DIAMINO-4,4'-DIPHENYL SULPHONE see III:SOA500
4:4'-DIAMINO-3-DIPHENYLYL HYDROGEN SULFATE see
    III:BBY250, III:BBY500
DIAMINODITOLYL see I:TGJ750
2,7-DIAMINOFLUORENE see III:FDM000
α,2-DIAMINO-3-HYDROXY-γ-OXOBENZENEBUTANOIC
    ACID see III:HJD000
2,4-DIAMINO-1-METHOXYBENZENE see I:DBO000,
    I:DBO400
1,3-DIAMINO-4-METHOXYBENZENE SULPHATE see
    I:DBO400
2,4-DIAMINO-1-METHOXYBENZENE SULPHATE see
    I:DBO400
3,6-DIAMINO-10-METHYLACRIDINIUM CHLORIDE with 3,6-
    ACRIDINEDIAMINE see III:DBX400
2,8-DIAMINO-10-METHYLACRIDINIUM CHLORIDE mixture
    with 2,8-DIAMINOACRIDINE see III:DBX400
1,3-DIAMINO-4-METHYLBENZENE see I:TGL750
2,4-DIAMINO-1-METHYLBENZENE see I:TGL750
1,5-DIAMINONAPHTHALENE see II:NAM000
1,4-DIAMINO-5-NITRO ANTHRAQUINONE see III:DBY700
1,4-DIAMINO-2-NITROBENZENE see II:ALL750
4,6-DIAMINO-2-(5-NITRO-2-FURYL)-S-TRIAZINE see
    III:DBY800
2,6-DIAMINO-3-PHENYLAZOPYRIDINE see III:PEK250
2,6-DIAMINO-3-PHENYLAZOPYRIDINE HYDROCHLORIDE
    see I:PDC250
2,6-DIAMINO-3-(PHENYLAZO)PYRIDINE MONOHYDRO-
    CHLORIDE see I:PDC250
4,4'-DIAMINOPHENYL ETHER see I:OPM000
DI-(4-AMINOPHENYL)METHANE see I:MJQ000
DI(p-AMINOPHENYL) SULFIDE see I:TFI000
DI(4-AMINOPHENYL)SULFONE see III:SOA500
DI(p-AMINOPHENYL) SULFONE see III:SOA500
DI(p-AMINOPHENYL)SULPHIDE see I:TFI000
DI(4-AMINOPHENYL)SULPHONE see III:SOA500
DI(p-AMINOPHENYL)SULPHONE see III:SOA500
l-(+)-N-(p-(((2,4-DIAMINO-6-PTERIDINYL)METHYL)
    METHYLAMINO)BENZOYL)GLUTAMIC ACID see
    III:MDV500
DIAMINOPYRITAMIN see III:TGD000
2,4-DIAMINOSOLE SULPHATE see I:DBO400
4:4'-DIAMINOSTILBENE see III:SLR500
2,4-DIAMINOTOLUEN (CZECH) see I:TGL750
DIAMINOTOLUENE see I:TGL750
2,4-DIAMINOTOLUENE see I:TGL750
2,5-DIAMINOTOLUENE see III:TGM000
2,4-DIAMINO-1-TOLUENE see I:TGL750
2,4-DIAMINOTOLUENE DIHYDROCHLORIDE see
    III:DCE000
p-DIAMINOTOLUENE SULFATE see III:DCE600
2,5-DIAMINOTOLUENE SULFATE see III:DCE600
2,5-DIAMINOTOLUENE SULPHATE see III:DCE600

2,4-DIAMINOTOLUOL see I:TGL750
(4-((4,6-DIAMINO-m-TOLYL)IMINO)-2,5-CYCLOHEXADIEN-
    1-YLIDENE)DIMETHYLAMMONIUM CHLORIDE H₂O see
    III:TGU500
3,5-DIAMINO-s-TRIAZOLE see III:DCF200
trans-DIAMMINEDICHLOROPLATINUM(II) see III:DEX000
DIAMOND SHAMROCK 40 see III:PKQ059
DIAMOND SHAMROCK 744 see II:AAX175
DIAMYLNITROSAMIN (GERMAN) see III:DCH600
DI-n-AMYLNITROSAMINE see III:DCH600
DIANABOL see III:DAL300, III:MPN500
DIANABOLE see III:DAL300
DIANALINEMETHANE see I:MJQ000
DIANDRON see III:AOO450
DIANDRONE see III:AOO450
1,2·3,4-DIANHYDROERYTHRITOL see II:DHB800
1,2:3,4-DIANHYDRO-dl-THREITOL see II:DHB600
DIANILBLAU see II:CMO250
DIANIL BLUE see II:CMO250
o,p'-DIANILINE see III:BGF109
p,p'-DIANILINE see I:BBX000
o-DIANISIDIN (CZECH, GERMAN) see I:DCJ200
o-DIANISIDINA (ITALIAN) see I:DCJ200
o-DIANISIDINE see I:DCJ200
3,3'-DIANISIDINE see I:DCJ200
O,O'DIANISIDINE see I:DCJ200
o-DIANISIDINE DIHYDROCHLORIDE see II:DOA800
DIANISIDINE DIISOCYANATE see III:DCJ400
3,4-DIANISYL-3-HEXENE see III:DJB200
DIANISYLTRICHLORETHANE see II:MEI450
2,2-DI-p-ANISYL-1,1,1-TRICHLOROETHANE see II:MEI450
DIANTIMONY TRIOXIDE see I:AQF000
DIAPAM see III:DCK759
DIAPHENYLSULFONE see III:SOA500
DIAPHENYLSULPHON see III:SOA500
DIAPHENYLSULPHONE see III:SOA500
DIAPHTAMINE BLACK V see I:AQP000
DIAPHTAMINE BLUE BB see I:CMO000
DIAPHTAMINE VIOLET N see III:CMP000
DIAPP see III:BEN000
DIAQUONE see III:DMH400
DIAREX 43G see III:SMQ500
DIAREX 600 see III:SMR000
DIAREX HF 77 see II:SMQ000
DIARSEN see I:DXE600
DIARSENIC PENTOXIDE see I:ARH500
DIARSENIC TRIOXIDE see I:ARI750
DIARSENIC TRISULFIDE see I:ARI000
DIASTYL see I:DKA600
DIATER see III:DXQ500
DIATO BLUE BASE B see I:DCJ200
6,12-DIAZAANTHANTHRENE see III:ADK250
6,12-DIAZAANTHANTHRENE SULFATE see III:DCK200
6,12-DIAZAANTHANTHRENE SULPHATE see III:DCK200
7,14-DIAZADIBENZ(a,h)ANTHRACENE see III:DDC800
1,12-DIAZADIBENZO(a,i)PYRENE see III:NAU000
4,11-DIAZADIBENZO(a,h)PYRENE see III:NAU500
1,2-DIAZA-3,4:9,10-DIBENZPYRENE see III:APF750
2,3-DIAZAINDOLE see III:BDH250
DIAZALE see III:THE500
DIAZEPAM see III:DCK759
DIAZETARD see III:DCK759
DIAZINE BLACK E see I:AQP000
DIAZINE BLUE 2B see I:CMO000
DIAZINE BLUE 3B see II:CMO250
DIAZINE VIOLET N see III:CMP000
DIAZIRINE see I:DCP800
DI-AZO see I:PDC250
DIAZOACETATE (ESTER)-l-SERINE see II:ASA500
l-DIAZOACETATE (ESTER) SERINE see II:ASA500
DIAZO-ACETIC ACID ESTER with SERINE see II:ASA500
DIAZOACETIC ACID, ETHYL ESTER see III:DCN800
DIAZOACETIC ESTER see III:DCN800
N-DIAZOACETILGLICINA-AMIDE (ITALIAN) see
    III:CBK000

N-DIAZOACETILGLICINA-IDRAZIDE (ITALIAN) see III:DCO800
DIAZOACETYLGLYCINAMIDE see III:CBK000
N-(DIAZOACETYL)GLYCINAMIDE see III:CBK000
DIAZOACETYLGLYCINE AMIDE see III:CBK000
N-DIAZOACETYLGLYCINE AMIDE see III:CBK000
DIAZOACETYLGLYCINE HYDRAZIDE see III:DCO800
N-(DIAZOACETYL)GLYCINE HYDRAZINE see III:DCO800
N-DIAZOACETYL GLYCYLHYDRAZIDE see III:DCO800
o-DIAZOACETYL-l-SERINE see II:ASA500
DIAZOAMINOBENZEN (CZECH) see III:DWO800
DIAZOAMINOBENZENE see III:DWO800
p-DIAZOAMINOBENZENE see III:DWO800
DIAZOAMINOBENZOL (GERMAN) see III:DWO800
DIAZOBENZENE see III:ASL250
DIAZOBLEU see III:BGT250
DIAZOCARD CHRYSOIDINE G see III:PEK000
DIAZOESSIGSAEURE-AETHYLESTER (GERMAN) see III:DCN800
DIAZO FAST RED AL see III:AIA750
DIAZO FAST RED TR see II:CLK235
DIAZO FAST RED TRA see II:CLK220, II:CLK235
DIAZO FAST SCARLET G see I:NMP500
DIAZO-ICA see III:DCP400
DIAZOIMIDAZOLE-4-CARBOXAMIDE see III:DCP400
5-DIAZOIMIDAZOLE-4-CARBOXAMIDE see III:DCP400
5-DIAZOIMIDAZOLE-4-CARBOXAMIDE HYDROCHLORIDE see III:DCP600
DIAZOL BLACK 2V see I:AQP000
DIAZOL BLUE 2B see I:CMO000
DIAZOL-C see III:AKK250
DIAZOL PURE BLUE FF see III:BGT250
DIAZOL VIOLET N see III:CMP000
DIAZOMETHANE see I:DCP800
DIAZO RESIN V see III:DCQ650
DIAZOTIZING SALTS see III:SIQ500
3-DIAZOTYRAMINE HYDROCHLORIDE see III:DCQ575
DIAZO V see III:DCQ650
DIAZYL see III:SNJ000
DIBASIC LEAD ACETATE see I:LCG000
DIBASIC LEAD ARSENATE see I:LCK000
DIBASIC LEAD CARBONATE see III:LCP000
DIBENYLIN see I:PDT250
DIBENYLINE see I:PDT250
DIBENZ(a,e)ACEANTHRYLENE see III:DCR300
DIBENZ(a,j)ACEANTHRYLENE see III:DCR400
13H-DIBENZ(bc,j)ACEANTHRYLENE see III:DCR600
4H-DIBENZ(f,g,j)ACEANTHRYLENE, 5,5a,6,7-TETRAHYDRO- see III:DCR800
DIBENZ(a,d)ACRIDINE see I:DCS400
DIBENZ(a,f)ACRIDINE see I:DCS600
DIBENZ(a,h)ACRIDINE see I:DCS400
DIBENZ(a,j)ACRIDINE see I:DCS600
DIBENZ(c,h)ACRIDINE see III:DCS800
1,2,5,6-DIBENZACRIDINE see I:DCS400
1,2,7,8-DIBENZACRIDINE see I:DCS600
3,4,5,6-DIBENZACRIDINE see I:DCS600
3,4:5,6-DIBENZACRIDINE see III:DCS800
1,2,7,8-DIBENZACRIDINE (FRENCH) see III:DCS800
DIBENZ(a,j)ACRIDINE METHOSULFATE see III:DCT000
3,4:5,6-DIBENZACRIDINE METHOSULFATE see III:DCT000
1,2,5,6-DIBENZANTHRACEEN (DUTCH) see I:DCT400
DIBENZ(a,c)ANTHRACENE see III:BDH750
DIBENZ(a,h)ANTHRACENE see I:DCT400
DIBENZ(a,j)ANTHRACENE see III:DCT600
1,2:3,4-DIBENZANTHRACENE see III:BDH750
1,2:5,6-DIBENZANTHRACENE see I:DCT400
1,2:7,8-DIBENZANTHRACENE see III:DCT600
DIBENZ(de,kl)ANTHRACENE see III:PCQ250
1,2:5,6-DIBENZ(a)ANTHRACENE see I:DCT400
1:2:5:6-DIBENZANTHRACENE-9-CARBAMIDO-ACETIC ACID see III:DCU600
1,2,5,6-DIBENZANTHRACENECHOLEIC ACID see III:DCT800

DIBENZ(a,h)ANTHRACENE-5,6-OXIDE see III:EBP500
1,2:5,6-DIBENZANTHRACENE-9,10-ENDO-α,β-SUCCINIC ACID see III:DCU200
1,2,5,6-DIBENZANTHRACENE-9,10-ENDO-α,β-SUCCINIC ACID, SODIUM SALT see III:SGF000
N-(DIBENZ(a,h)ANTHRACEN-7-YLCARBAMOYL)GLYCINE see III:DCU600
DIBENZANTHRANYL GLYCINE COMPLEX see III:DCU600
3,4,5,6-DIBENZCARBAZOL see I:DCY000
1,2,5,6-DIBENZCARBAZOLE see III:DCX600
1,2,7,8-DIBENZCARBAZOLE see III:DCX800
3,4,5,6-DIBENZCARBAZOLE see I:DCY000
1,2,3,4-DIBENZFLUORENE see III:DCX000
1,2,7,8-DIBENZFLUORENE see III:DDB200
DIBENZ(c,f)INDENO(1,2,3-ij)(2,7)NAPHTHYRIDINE see III:DCX400
1,2,3,4-DIBENZNAPHTHALENE see III:TMS000
DIBENZO(a,j)ACRIDINE see I:DCS600
1,2,5,6-DIBENZOACRIDINE see I:DCS400
DIBENZO(a,c)ANTHRACENE see III:BDH750
DIBENZO(a,h)ANTHRACENE see I:DCT400
1,2:3,4-DIBENZOANTHRACENE see III:BDH750
1,2:5,6-DIBENZOANTHRACENE see I:DCT400
3,4,5,6-DIBENZOCARBAZOLE see I:DCY000
7H-DIBENZO(a,g)CARBAZOLE see III:DCX600
7H-DIBENZO(a,i)CARBAZOLE see III:DCX800
7H-DIBENZO(c,g)CARBAZOLE see I:DCY000
DIBENZO(b,def)CHRYSENE see II:DCY200
DIBENZO(def,p)CHRYSENE see II:DCY400
DIBENZO-(drf,mno)CHRYSENE see III:APE750
DIBENZO(b,def)CHRYSENE-7-CARBOXALDEHYDE see III:DCY600
DIBENZO(def,p)CHRYSENE-10-CARBOXALDEHYDE see III:DCY800
DIBENZO(def,mno)CHRYSENE-12-CARBOXALDEHYDE see III:FNK000
DIBENZO(b,def)CHRYSENE-7,14-DIONE see III:DCZ000
DIBENZODIOXIN see III:DDA800
DIBENZO-p-DIOXIN see III:DDA800
DIBENZO(1,4)DIOXIN see III:DDA800
DIBENZO(b.e)(1,4)DIOXIN see III:DDA800
DIBENZO(a,e)FLUORANTHENE see III:DCR300
2,3,5,6-DIBENZOFLUORANTHENE see III:DCR300
DIBENZO(a,jk)FLUORENE see II:BCJ500
DIBENZO(b,jk)FLUORENE see I:BCJ750
1,2,5,6-DIBENZOFLUORENE see III:DDB000
13H-DIBENZO(a,g)FLUORENE see III:DDB000
13H-DIBENZO(a,i)FLUORENE see III:DDB200
2-DIBENZOFURANAMINE see III:DDB600
3-DIBENZOFURANAMINE see III:DDB800
3-DIBENZOFURANYLACETAMIDE see III:DDC000
N-3-DIBENZOFURANYLACETAMIDE see III:DDC000
DIBENZOFURANYLAMINE see III:DDB800
1,2,5,6-DIBENZONAPHTHALENE see I:CML810
DIBENZOPARADIAZINE see III:PDB500
DIBENZO(h,rst)PENTAPHENE see III:DDC200
DIBENZO(cd,lm)PERYLENE see III:DDC400
DIBENZO(a,i)PHENANTHRENE see III:PIB750
1,2,3,4-DIBENZOPHENANTHRENE see III:BCH000
1,2,6,7-DIBENZOPHENANTHRENE see III:BCG500
1,2:7,8-DIBENZOPHENANTHRENE see III:PIB750
2,3:7,8-DIBENZOPHENANTHRENE see III:BCG500
DIBENZO-2,3,7,8-PHENANTHRENE see III:BCG500
DIBENZO(a,c)PHENAZINE see III:DDC600
DIBENZO(a,h)PHENAZINE see III:DDC800
DIBENZO PQD see III:DVR200
DIBENZOPYRAZINE see III:PDB500
DIBENZO(a,d)PYRENE see II:DCY400
DIBENZO(a,e)PYRENE see II:NAT500
DIBENZO(a,h)PYRENE see II:DCY200
DIBENZO(a,i)PYRENE see I:BCQ500
DIBENZO(a,l)PYRENE see II:DCY400
DIBENZO(b,h)PYRENE see I:BCQ500
1,2:3,4-DIBENZOPYRENE see II:DCY400

1,2,4,5-DIBENZOPYRENE see II:NAT500
1,2,6,7-DIBENZOPYRENE see II:DCY200
1,2,7,8-DIBENZOPYRENE see II:BCQ500
2,3:4,5-DIBENZOPYRENE see II:DCY400
3,4,8,9-DIBENZOPYRENE see II:DCY200
DIBENZO(cd,mk)PYRENE see III:APE750
1,2,9,10-DIBENZOPYRENE see II:DCY400
3,4:9,10-DIBENZOPYRENE see I:BCQ500
DIBENZO(a,b)PYRENE-7,14-DIONE see III:DCZ000
2,3,7,8-DIBENZOPYRENE-1,6-QUINONE see III:DCZ000
DIBENZOPYRROLE see III:CBN000
DIBENZO(b,d)PYRROLE see III:CBN000
DI-2-BENZOTHIAZOLYLDISULFIDE see III:BDE750
DIBENZOTHIAZYL DISULFIDE see III:BDE750
2,2'-DIBENZOTHIAZYLDISULFIDE see III:BDE750
N-2-DIBENZOTHIENYLACETAMIDE see III:DDD400
N-3-DIBENZOTHIENYLACETAMIDE see III:DDD600
N-3-DIBENZOTHIENYLACETAMIDE-5-OXIDE see
    III:DDD800
DIBENZ(b,f)(1,4)OXAZEPINE see III:DDE200
DIBENZOYLPEROXID (GERMAN) see III:BDS000
DIBENZOYL PEROXIDE (MAK) see III:BDS000
DIBENZOYLPEROXYDE (DUTCH) see III:BDS000
DIBENZOYLTHIAZYL DISULFIDE see III:BDE750
1,2,3,4-DIBENZPHENANTHRENE see III:BCH000
1,2,5,6-DIBENZPHENANTHRENE see III:BCG750
DIBENZ(a,h)PHENAZINE see III:DDC800
1,2,3,4-DIBENZPHENAZINE see III:DDC600
1,2:5,6-DIBENZPHENAZINE see III:DDC800
DIBENZ(a,i)PYRENE see I:BCQ500
1,2,3,4-DIBENZPYRENE see II:DCY400
1,2:7,8-DIBENZPYRENE see I:BCQ500
3,4,8,9-DIBENZPYRENE see II:DCY200
4,5,6,7-DIBENZPYRENE see II:DCY400
3,4:9,10-DIBENZPYRENE see I:BCQ500
1',2',6',7'-DIBENZPYRENE-7,14-QUINONE see III:DCZ000
DIBENZTHIAZYL DISULFIDE see III:BDE750
7,14-DIBENZYLDIBENZ(a,h)ANTHRACENE see III:DDF400
9,10-DIBENZYL-1,2,5,6-DIBENZANTHRACENE see
    III:DDF400
DIBENZYLENE see II:DDG800
DIBENZYLIN see II:DDG800
DIBENZYLINE see I:PDT250
DIBENZYLINE HYDROCHLORIDE see II:DDG800
DIBENZYRAN see II:DDG800
DIBESTIL see I:DKB000
DIBESTROL see I:DKA600
DIBOVAN see I:DAD200
1,2-DIBROMAETHAN (GERMAN) see I:EIY500
DIBROMANNIT see III:DDP600
DIBROMANNITOL see III:DDP600
d-DIBROMANNITOL see III:DDP600
DIBROMCHLORPROPAN (GERMAN) see I:DDL800
1,2-DIBROM-3-CHLOR-PROPAN (GERMAN) see I:DDL800
DIBROMDULCITOL see III:DDJ000
DIBROMOACETONITRILE see III:DDJ400
DIBROMOCHLOROPROPANE see I:DDL800
1,2-DIBROMO-3-CHLOROPROPANE see I:DDL800
1,2-DIBROMO-3-CLORO-PROPANO (ITALIAN) see
    I:DDL800
1,6-DIBROMODIDEOXYDULCITOL see III:DDJ000
1,6-DIBROMO-1,6-DIDEOXYDULCITOL see III:DDJ000
1,6-DIBROMO-1,6-DIDEOXYGALACTITOL see III:DDJ000
1,6-DIBROMO-1,6-DIDEOXY-d-GALACTITOL see
    III:DDJ000
1,6-DIBROMO-1,6-DIDEOXY-d-MANNITOL see III:DDP600
1,6-DIBROMO-1,6-d-DIDESOXYMANNITOL see III:DDP600
DIBROMODULCITOL see III:DDJ000
1,6-DIBROMODULCITOL see III:DDJ000
1,2-DIBROMOETANO (ITALIAN) see I:EIY500
1,2-DIBROMOETHANE (MAK) see I:EIY500
α,β-DIBROMOETHANE see I:EIY500
sym-DIBROMOETHANE see I:EIY500
1,6-DIBROMOMANNITOL see III:DDP600

3,4-DIBROMONITROSOPIPERIDINE see III:DDQ800
2,3-DIBROMO-1-PROPANOL PHOSPHATE see I:TNC500
2,3-DIBROMO-1-PROPANOL, PHOSPHATE (3:1) see
    I:TNC500
(2,3-DIBROMOPROPYL) PHOSPHATE see I:TNC500
DIBROMURE d'ETHYLENE (FRENCH) see I:EIY500
1,2-DIBROOM-3-CHLOORPROPAAN (DUTCH) see I:DDL800
1,2-DIBROOMETHAAN (DUTCH) see I:EIY500
DIBUTIN see III:ILD000
DIBUTYLAMINE, 4-HYDROXY-N-NITROSO- see I:HJQ350
DIBUTYLATED HYDROXYTOLUENE see III:BFW750
2,6-DI-tert-BUTYL-p-CRESOL (OSHA, ACGIH) see
    III:BFW750
9,10-DI-n-BUTYL-1,2,5,6-DIBENZANTHRACENE see
    III:DDX200
DIBUTYLDITHIOCARBAMIC ACID, NICKEL SALT see
    III:BIW750
DIBUTYLDITHIO-CARBAMIC ACID ZINC COMPLEX see
    III:BIX000
DIBUTYLDITHIOCARBAMIC ACID ZINC SALT see
    III:BIX000
DIBUTYL ESTER SULFURIC ACID see III:DEC000
1,1-DIBUTYLHYDRAZINE see III:DEC725
N,N-DIBUTYLHYDRAZINE see III:DEC725
1,1-DI-n-BUTYLHYDRAZINE see III:DEC725
1,2-DI-n-BUTYLHYDRAZINE DIHYDROCHLORIDE see
    III:DEC775
2,6-DI-tert-BUTYL-1-HYDROXY-4-METHYLBENZENE see
    III:BFW750
3,5-DI-tert-BUTYL-4-HYDROXYTOLUENE see III:BFW750
2,6-DI-terc. BUTYL-p-KRESOL (CZECH) see III:BFW750
2,6-DI-tert-BUTYL-4-METHYLPHENOL see III:BFW750
2,6-DI-tert-BUTYL-p-METHYLPHENOL see III:BFW750
DI-n-BUTYLNITROSAMIN (GERMAN) see I:BRY500
DI-n-BUTYLNITROSAMINE see I:BRY500
N,N-DI-n-BUTYLNITROSAMINE see I:BRY500
DIBUTYLNITROSOAMINE see I:BRY500
N,N-DIBUTYLNITROSOAMINE see I:BRY500
DI-tert-BUTYLPEROXID (GERMAN) see III:BSC750
DI-tert-BUTYL PEROXIDE (MAK) see III:BSC750
DI-tert-BUTYL PEROXYDE (DUTCH) see III:BSC750
DI-n-BUTYLSULFAT (GERMAN) see III:DEC000
DIBUTYL SULFATE see III:DEC000
DIC see II:DAB600
DICALITE see III:SCH000
S-(1,2-DICARBETHOXYETHYL)-O,O-DIMETHYLDITHIO-
    PHOSPHATE see III:MAK700
DICARBOETHOXYETHYL-O,O-DIMETHYL PHOSPHORO-
    DITHIOATE see III:MAK700
DICARBOXIDINE HYDROCHLORIDE see III:DEK000
3,3'-DICARBOXYBENZIDINE see III:BFX250
DICARBOXYDINE see III:DEK400
DICHAN (CZECH) see III:DGU200
DICHINALEX see III:CLD000
DICHLOBENIL (DOT) see III:DER800
DICHLONE (DOT) see III:DFT000
p-DICHLOORBENZEEN (DUTCH) see II:DEP800
1,4-DICHLOORBENZEEN (DUTCH) see II:DEP800
1,1-DICHLOOR-2,2-BIS(4-CHLOOR FENYL)-ETHAAN
    (DUTCH) see I:BIM500
1,1-DICHLOORETHAAN (DUTCH) see III:DFF809
1,2-DICHLOORETHAAN (DUTCH) see I:EIY600
2,2'-DICHLOORETHYLETHER (DUTCH) see III:DFJ050
(2,4-DICHLOOR-FENOXY)-AZIJNZUUR (DUTCH) see
    II:DAA800
2-(2,4-DICHLOOR-FENOXY)-PROPIONZUUR (DUTCH) see
    II:DGB000
3-(3,4-DICHLOOR-FENYL)-1,1-DIMETHYLUREUM (DUTCH)
    see III:DXQ500
DICHLORACETIC ACID see III:DEL000
DICHLORACETYL CHLORIDE see III:DEN400
1,1-DICHLORAETHAN (GERMAN) see III:DFF809
1,2-DICHLOR-AETHAN (GERMAN) see I:EIY600
p-DI-(2-CHLORAETHYL)-AMINO-dl-PHENYL-ALANIN (GER-
    MAN) see II:BHT750

2',4'-DICHLORO-4-NITROBIPHENYL ETHER see I:DFT800
2,4-DICHLORO-4'-NITRODIPHENYL ETHER see I:DFT800
1,2-DICHLORO-3-NITRONAPHTHALENE see III:DFU400
2,4-DICHLORO-1-(4-NITROPHENOXY)BENZENE see
    I:DFT800
6,7-DICHLORO-4-NITROQUINOLINE-1-OXIDE see
    III:DFV200
2,2'-DICHLORO-N-NITROSODIPROPYLAMINE see
    III:DFW000
3,4-DICHLORONITROSOPIPERIDINE see III:DFW200
3,4-DICHLORO-N-NITROSOPYRROLIDINE see III:DFW600
2,3-DICHLORO-4-OXO-2-BUTENOIC ACID see III:MRU900
4,5-DICHLORO-2-OXO-1,3-DIOXOLANE see III:DFI800
DICHLOROOXOZIRCONIUM see III:ZSJ000
2,4-DICHLOROPHENOL see II:DFX800
2,4-DICHLOROPHENOL BENZENESULFONATE see
    III:DFY400
3-(3,4-DICHLOROPHENOL)-1,1-DIMETHYLUREA see
    III:DXQ500
DICHLOROPHENOXYACETIC ACID see II:DAA800
2,4-DICHLOROPHENOXYACETIC ACID (DOT) see
    II:DAA800
(2,4-DICHLOROPHENOXY)ACETIC ACID, BUTYL ESTER see
    III:BQZ000
2,4-DICHLOROPHENOXYACETIC ACID ISOOCTYL ESTER
    see III:ILO000
(2,4-DICHLOROPHENOXY)ACETIC ACID, ISOPROPYL
    ESTER see III:IOY000
(2-4-DICHLOROPHENOXY)ACETIC ACID-1-METHYLETHYL
    ESTER (9CI) see III:IOY000
4-(2,4-DICHLOROPHENOXY)NITROBENZENE see I:DFT800
2-(2,4-DICHLOROPHENOXY) PROPIONIC ACID see
    II:DGB000
2-(2,5-DICHLOROPHENOXY)PROPIONIC ACID see
    III:DGB200
α-(2,4-DICHLOROPHENOXY) PROPIONIC ACID see
    II:DGB000
α-(2,5-DICHLOROPHENOXY)PROPIONIC ACID see
    III:DGB200
N-(3,4-DICHLOROPHENYL)-1-AZIRIDINECARBOXAMIDE
    see III:DGB800
p-((3,4-DICHLOROPHENYL)AZO)-N,N-DIMETHYLANILINE
    see III:DFD400
2,4-DICHLOROPHENYL BENZENESULFONATE see
    III:DFY400
2,4-DICHLOROPHENYL BENZENESULPHONATE see
    III:DFY400
3,4-DICHLOROPHENYL-N-CARBAMOYLAZIRIDINE see
    III:DGB800
2,4'-DICHLOROPHENYLDICHLOROETHANE see
    III:CDN000
N'-(3,4-DICHLOROPHENYL)-N,N-DIMETHYLUREA see
    III:DXQ500
1-(3,4-DICHLOROPHENYL)-3,3-DIMETHYLUREE (FRENCH)
    see III:DXQ500
2,6-DICHLORO-p-PHENYLENEDIAMINE see III:DBR400
2,4-DICHLOROPHENYL ESTER of BENZENESULFONIC ACID
    see III:DFY400
2,4-DICHLOROPHENYL ESTER BENZENESULPHONIC ACID
    see III:DFY400
2,4-DICHLOROPHENYL-4-NITROPHENYL ETHER see
    I:DFT800
2,4-DICHLOROPHENYL-p-NITROPHENYL ETHER see
    I:DFT800
1-(3,5-DICHLOROPHENYL)-2,5-PYRROLIDINEDIONE see
    III:DGF000
N-(3,5-DICHLOROPHENYL)SUCCINIMIDE see III:DGF000
DI-(p-CHLOROPHENYL)TRICHLOROMETHYLCARBINOL
    see III:BIO750
DICHLOROPROP see II:DGB000
1,2-DICHLOROPROPANE see III:PNJ400
α,β-DICHLOROPROPANE see III:PNJ400
1,3-DICHLORO-2-PROPANOL PHOSPHATE (3:1) see
    III:FQU875

1,3-DICHLOROPROPENE see I:DGG950
1,3-DICHLOROPROPENE-1 see I:DGG950
(Z)-1,3-DICHLOROPROPENE see I:DGH200
cis-1,3-DICHLOROPROPENE see I:DGH200
cis-1,3-DICHLOROPROPENE OXIDE see III:DAC975
trans-1,3-DICHLOROPROPENE OXIDE see III:DGH500
2,3-DICHLORO-2-PROPENE-1-THIOL DIISOPROPYLCARBA-
    MATE see III:DBI200
S-(2,3-DICHLORO-2-PROPENYL)ESTER, BIS(1-METHYLE-
    THYL) CARBAMOTHIOIC ACID see III:DBI200
1,3-DICHLOROPROPYLENE see I:DGG950
α,γ-DICHLOROPROPYLENE see I:DGG950
cis-1,3-DICHLOROPROPYLENE see I:DGH200
2,2'-DICHLORO-4,4'-STILBENAMINE see III:DGK400
2,2'-DICHLORO-4,4'-STILBENEDIAMINE see III:DGK400
3,3'-DICHLORO-4,4'-STILBENEDIAMINE see III:DGK600
2,3-DICHLOROTETRAHYDROFURAN see III:DGL800
DICHLOROTITANOCENE see III:DGW200
α,α-DICHLOROTOLUENE see II:BAY300
4,4'-DICHLORO-α-(TRICHLOROMETHYL)BENZHYDROL
    see III:BIO750
2,4-DICHLORPHENOXYACETIC ACID see II:DAA800
(2,4-DICHLOR-PHENOXY)-ESSIGSAEURE (GERMAN) see
    II:DAA800
2-(2,4-DICHLOR-PHENOXY)-PROPIONSAEURE (GERMAN)
    see II:DGB000
3-(3,4-DICHLOR-PHENYL)-1,1-DIMETHYL-HARNSTOFF
    (GERMAN) see III:DXQ500
2,4,-DICHLORPHENYL-4-NITROPHENYLAETHER (GER-
    MAN) see I:DFT800
DICHLORPROP see II:DGB000
DICHROMIUM TRIOXIDE see II:CMJ900
DICLORAN see III:RDP300
p-DICLOROBENZENE (ITALIAN) see II:DEP800
1,4-DICLOROBENZENE (ITALIAN) see II:DEP800
1,1-DICLORO-2,2-BIS(4-CLORO-FENIL)-ETANO (ITALIAN)
    see I:BIM500
3,3'-DICLORO-4,4'-DIAMINODIFENILMETANO (ITALIAN)
    see I:MJM200
1,1-DICLOROETANO (ITALIAN) see III:DFF809
1,2-DICLOROETANO (ITALIAN) see I:EIY600
2,2'-DICLOROETILETERE (ITALIAN) see III:DFJ050
3-(3,4-DICLORO-FENYL)-1,1-DIMETIL-UREA (ITALIAN) see
    III:DXQ500
DICOFOL see III:BIO750
DICOL see III:DJD600
DICOPHANE see I:DAD200
DICOPUR see II:DAA800
DICOPUR-M see II:CIR250
DICORVIN see I:DKA600
DICOTEX see II:CIR250
DICOTOX see II:DAA800
DICUPRAL see III:DXH250
o-DICYANOBENZENE see III:PHY000
1,2-DICYANOBENZENE see III:PHY000
1,3-DICYANOTETRACHLOROBENZENE see III:TBQ750
N,N-DICYCLOHEXYLAMINE see III:DGT600
DICYCLOHEXYLAMINE (DOT) see III:DGT600
DICYCLOHEXYLAMINE NITRITE see III:DGU200
DICYCLOHEXYLAMINONITRITE see III:DGU200
DICYCLOHEXYLAMMONIUM NITRITE see III:DGU200
DICYCLOPENTADIENYLCOBALT see III:BIR529
DICYCLOPENTADIENYLDICHLOROTITANIUM see
    III:DGW200
DI-2,4-CYCLOPENTADIEN-1-YL IRON see III:FBC000
DICYCLOPENTADIENYL IRON (OSHA, ACGIH) see
    III:FBC000
DI-pi-CYCLOPENTADIENYLNICKEL see I:NDA500
DI-pi-CYCLOPENTADIENYLTITANIUM see III:TGH500
DICYCLOPENTADIENYLTITANIUMDICHLORIDE see
    III:DGW200
DICYCLOPENTA(c,lmn)PHENANTHREN-1(9H)-ONE, 2,3-
    DIHYDRO- see III:DGW300
cis-DICYCLOPENTYLAMMINEDICHLOROPLATINUM(II) see
    III:BIS250

DIETHYLDIPHENYL DICHLOROETHANE see III:DJC000
DIETHYLDITHIOCARBAMATE SODIUM see III:SGJ000
DIETHYLDITHIOCARBAMIC ACID-2-CHLOROALLYL ESTER see CDO250
DIETHYLDITHIOCARBAMIC ACID SODIUM see III:SGJ000
DIETHYLDITHIOCARBAMIC ACID, SODIUM SALT see III:SGJ000
DIETHYLDITHIO CARBAMIC ACID TELLURIUM SALT see III:EPJ000
DIETHYLDITHIOCARBAMIC ACID ZINC SALT see III:BJC000
DIETHYLENE DIOXIDE see I:DVQ000
1,4-DIETHYLENE DIOXIDE see I:DVQ000
DIETHYLENE ETHER see I:DVQ000
DIETHYLENE GLYCOL see III:DJD600
DIETHYLENE GLYCOL BISPHTHALATE see III:DJD700
DIETHYLENEIMIDE OXIDE see III:MRP750
DIETHYLENE IMIDOXIDE see III:MRP750
DI(ETHYLENE OXIDE) see I:DVQ000
DIETHYLENE OXIMIDE see III:MRP750
1,3,-DI(ETHYLENESULPHAMOYL)PROPANE see III:BJP899
DIETHYLENIMIDE OXIDE see III:MRP750
α,α'-DIETHYL-α,α'-EPOXYBIBENZYL-4,4'-DIOL see III:DKB100
DIETHYL-β,γ-EPOXYPROPYLPHOSPHONATE see III:DJH200
DIETHYL ESTER SULFURIC ACID see I:DKB110
(E)-1,1'-(1,2-DIETHYL-1,2-ETHENE-DIYL)BIS(4-METHOXY-BENZENE) see III:DJB200
4,4'-(1,2-DIETHYL-1,2-ETHENEDIYL)BIS-PHENOL see I:DKA600
trans-4,4'-(1,2-DIETHYL-1,2-ETHENEDIYL)BISPHENOL see I:DKA600
trans-4,4'-(1,2-DIETHYL-1,2-ETHENEDIYL)BISPHENOL DI-PROPIONATE see I:DKB000
4,4'-(1,2-DIETHYLETHYLENE)DIPHENOL see III:DLB400
DI-2-ETHYLHEXYL ADIPATE see III:AEO000
DI(2-ETHYLHEXYL)ORTHOPHTHALATE see I:DVL700
DI(2-ETHYLHEXYL)PHTHALATE see I:DVL700
1,2-DIETHYLHYDRAZINE see II:DJL400
N-N'-DIETHYLHYDRAZINE see II:DJL400
sym-DIETHYLHYDRAZINE see II:DJL400
1,2-DIETHYLHYDRAZINE DIHYDROCHLORIDE see III:DJL600
4,4'-(1,2-DIETHYLIDENE-1,2-ETHANEDIYL)BISPHENOL see II:DAL600
4,4'-(DIETHYLIDENEETHYLENE)DIPHENOL see II:DAL600
p,p'-(DIETHYLIDENEETHYLENE)DIPHENOL see II:DAL600
DIETHYL MERCAPTOSUCCINATE-O,O-DIMETHYL DITHIO-PHOSPHATE, S-ESTER see III:MAK700
DIETHYL MERCAPTOSUCCINATE-O,O-DIMETHYL PHOS-PHORODITHIOATE see III:MAK700
DIETHYL MERCAPTOSUCCINATE-O,O-DIMETHYL THIO-PHOSPHATE see III:MAK700
DIETHYL MERCAPTOSUCCINATE-S-ESTER with O,O-DI-METHYLPHOSPHORODITHIOATE see III:MAK700
DIETHYL MERCAPTOSUCCINIC ACID O,O-DIMETHYL PHOSPHORODITHIOATE see III:MAK700
1,1-DIETHYL-3-METHYL-3-NITROSOUREA see III:DJP600
DIETHYLNITRAMINE see III:DJS500
O,O-DIETHYL-O-(4-NITRO-FENIL)-MONOTHIOFOSFAAT (DUTCH) see III:PAK000
O,O-DIETHYL-O-p-NITROFENYLESTER KYSELINYTHIO-FOSFORECNE (CZECH) see III:PAK000
O,O-DIETHYL-O-p-NITROFENYLTIOFOSFAT (CZECH) see III:PAK000
O,O-DIETHYL-O-4-NITROPHENYLPHOSPHOROTHIOATE see III:PAK000
O,O-DIETHYL-O-(4-NITROPHENYL) PHOSPHOROTHIOATE see III:PAK000
O,O-DIETHYL-O-(p-NITROPHENYL) PHOSPHOROTHIOATE see III:PAK000
DIETHYL-4-NITROPHENYL PHOSPHOROTHIONATE see III:PAK000

DIETHYL-p-NITROPHENYLTHIONOPHOSPHATE see III:PAK000
O,O-DIETHYL-O-(p-NITROPHENYL)THIONOPHOSPHATE see III:PAK000
DIETHYL-p-NITROPHENYLTHIOPHOSPHATE see III:PAK000
O,O-DIETHYL-O-4-NITROPHENYL THIOPHOSPHATE see III:PAK000
O,O-DIETHYL-O-p-NITROPHENYL THIOPHOSPHATE see III:PAK000
DIETHYLNITROSAMINE see I:NJW500
N,N-DIETHYLNITROSAMINE see I:NJW500
DIETHYLNITROSOAMINE see I:NJW500
o,N-DIETHYL-N-NITROSOHYDROXYLAMINE see III:NKC500
DIETHYLPARATHION see III:PAK000
p-((3,4-DIETHYLPHENYL)AZO)-N,N-DIMETHYLANILINE see III:DJB400
DI(p-ETHYLPHENYL)DICHLOROETHANE see III:DJC000
3,3-DIETHYL-1-PHENYLTRIAZENE see III:PEU500
N,N-DIETHYL-4-(4'-(PYRIDYL-1'-OXIDE)AZO)ANILINE see III:DIP000
3,3-DIETHYL-1-(m-PYRIDYL)TRIAZENE see III:DJY000
DIETHYL PYROCARBONATE mixed with AMMONIA see III:DJY050
DIETHYL SODIUM DITHIOCARBAMATE see III:SGJ000
N,N-DIETHYL-4-STILBENAMINE see III:DKA000
α,α'-DIETHYLSTILBENEDIOL see I:DKA600
2,2'-DIETHYL-4,4'-STILBENEDIOL see I:DKA600
α,α'-DIETHYL-4,4'-STILBENEDIOL see I:DKA600
α,α'-DIETHYL-(E)-4,4'-STILBENEDIOL see I:DKA600
trans-α,α'-DIETHYL-4,4'-STILBENEDIOL see I:DKA600
α,α'-DIETHYL-4,4'-STILBENEDIOL DIPALMITATE see III:DKA800
α,α'-DIETHYL-4,4'-STILBENEDIOL, DIPROPIONATE see I:DKB000
trans-α,α'-DIETHYL-4,4'-STILBENEDIOL DIPROPIONATE see I:DKB000
α,α'-DIETHYL-4,4'-STILBENEDIOL trans-DIPROPIONATE see I:DKB000
α,α'-DIETHYL-4,4'-STILBENEDIOL DIPROPIONYL ESTER see I:DKB000
α,α'-DIETHYL-4,4'-STILBENEDIOL DISODIUM SALT see III:DKA400
DIETHYLSTILBENE DIPROPIONATE see I:DKB000
DIETHYLSTILBESTEROL see I:DKA600
trans-DIETHYLSTILBESTEROL see I:DKA600
DIETHYLSTILBESTEROL DIPROPIONATE see I:DKB000
DIETHYLSTILBESTROL see I:DKA600
trans-DIETHYLSTILBESTROL see I:DKA600
DIETHYLSTILBESTROL DIMETHYL ETHER see III:DJB200
DIETHYLSTILBESTROL DIPALMITATE see III:DKA800
DIETHYLSTILBESTROL DIPROPIONATE see I:DKB000
DIETHYLSTILBESTROL DISODIUM SALT see III:DKA400
DIETHYLSTILBESTROL and ETHISTERONE see III:EEH900
DIETHYLSTILBESTROL, IODINE DERIVATIVE see III:TDE000
DIETHYLSTILBESTROL and PRANONE see III:EEH900
DIETHYLSTILBESTROL PROPIONATE see I:DKB000
DIETHYLSTILBOESTEROL see I:DKA600
trans-DIETHYLSTILBOESTEROL see I:DKA600
DIETHYLSTILBOESTROL-3,4-OXIDE see III:DKB100
DIETHYLSTILBOESTROL-α,β-OXIDE see III:DKB100
DIETHYL SULFATE see I:DKB110
DIETHYLSULFONMETHYLETHYLMETHANE see III:BJT750
α,α'-DIETHYL-3,3',5,5'-TETRAFLUORO-4,4'-STILBENE-DIOL (E)- see III:TCH325
trans-α,α'-DIETHYL-3,3',5,5'-TETRAFLUORO-4,4'-STILBEN-EDIOL see III:TCH325
N,N'-DIETHYLTHIOCARBAMIDE see III:DKC400
1,3-DIETHYLTHIOUREA see III:DKC400
1,3-DIETHYL-2-THIOUREA see III:DKC400
N,N'-DIETHYLTHIOUREA see III:DKC400

DIETHYL TRIAZENE see III:DKD200
DIETIL see III:CAR000
DIETILESTILBESTROL (SPANISH) see I:DKA600
O,O-DIETIL-O-(4-NITRO-FENIL)-MONOTIOFOSFATO (ITAL-
  IAN) see III:PAK000
DIETREEN see III:RAF100
DIFENILHIDANTOINA (SPANISH) see I:DKQ000
DIFENIL-METAN-DIISOCIANATO (ITALIAN) see III:MJP400
DIFENIN see I:DKQ000, I:DNU000
DIFENSON see III:CJT750
N,N'-DIFENYL-p-FENYLENDIAMIN (CZECH) see
  III:BLE500
DIFENYLIN see III:BGF109
DIFENYLMETHAAN-DISSOCYANAAT (DUTCH) see
  III:MJP400
DIFETOIN see I:DNU000
DIFFOLLISTEROL see I:EDP000
DIFHYDAN see I:DKQ000, I:DNU000
2,10-DIFLUOROBENZO(rst)PENTAPHENE see III:DKG400
DIFLUOROCHLOROMETHANE see III:CFX500
2,10-DIFLUORODIBENZO(a,i)PYRENE see III:DKG400
2',4'-DIFLUORO-4-DIMETHYLAMINOAZOBENZENE see
  III:DKG980
2',5'-DIFLUORO-4-DIMETHYLAMINOAZOBENZENE see
  III:DKH000
3',4'-DIFLUORO-4-DIMETHYLAMINOAZOBENZENE see
  III:DRL000
3',5'-DIFLUORO-4-DIMETHYLAMINOAZOBENZENE see
  III:DKH100
1,1-DIFLUOROETHYLENE (DOT, MAK) see II:VPP000
DIFLUOROMONOCHLOROMETHANE see III:CFX500
p-((3,5-DIFLUOROPHENYL)AZO)-N,N-DIMETHYLANILINE
  see III:DKH100
3,8-DIFLUOROTRICYCLOQUINAZOLINE see III:DKJ200
DIFOLATAN see III:CBF800
DIFOLLICULINE see I:EDP000
DIFORIN see III:ILD000
7,12-DIFORMYLBENZ(a)ANTHRACENE see III:BBD000
1,2-DIFORMYLHYDRAZIN (GERMAN) see III:DKJ600
1,2-DIFORMYLHYDRAZINE see III:DKJ600
DIFOSAN see III:CBF800
DIFURAN see III:PAF500
DIFURAZONE see III:PAF500
DIGERMIN see III:DUV600
DIGIBUTINA see III:BRF500
DIGLYCIDYL BISPHENOL A ETHER see III:BLD750
N,N'-DIGLYCIDYL-5,5-DIMETHYLHYDANTOIN see
  III:DKM130
DIGLYCIDYL ETHER see II:DKM200
DIGLYCIDYL ETHER of N,N-BIS(2-HYDROXYETHOXY-
  ETHYL)ANILINE see III:BJN850
DIGLYCIDYL ETHER of 2,2-BIS(4-HYDROXYPHENYL)PRO-
  PANE see III:BLD750
DIGLYCIDYL ETHER of 2,2-BIS(p-HYDROXYPHENYL)PRO-
  PANE see III:BLD750
DIGLYCIDYL ETHER of N,N-BIS(2-HYDROXYPROPYL)-tert-
  BUTYLAMINE see III:DKM400
DIGLYCIDYL ETHER of BISPHENOL A see III:BLD750
DIGLYCIDYL ETHER of BISPHENOL A mixed with BIS(2,3-
  EPOXYCYCLOPENTYL) ETHER (1:1) see III:OPI200
DIGLYCIDYL ETHER of 4,4'-ISOPROPYLIDENEDIPHENOL
  see III:BLD750
DIGLYCIDYL ETHER of NEOPENTYL GLYCOL see
  III:NCI300
DIGLYCIDYL ETHER of PHENYLDIETHANOLAMINE see
  III:BJN875
1,3-DIGLYCIDYLOXYBENZENE see II:REF000
DIGLYCIDYL RESORCINOL ETHER see II:REF000
N,N-DIGLYCIDYL-p-TOLUENESULFONAMIDE see
  III:DKM800
N,N-DIGLYCIDYL-p-TOLUENESULPHONAMIDE see
  III:DKM800
DIGLYCIDYLTRIETHYLENE GLYCOL see III:TJQ333
DIGLYCOL see III:DJD600

DIHEXYL see III:DXT200
DIHIDROCLORURO de BENZIDINA (SPANISH) see
  II:BBX750
DIHYCON see I:DKQ000
DI-HYDAN see I:DKQ000, I:DNU000
DIHYDANTOIN see I:DKQ000, I:DNU000
1,2-DIHYDRO-5-ACENAPHTHYLENAMINE see III:AAF250
DIHYDROAFLATOXIN B1 see I:AEU750
DIHYDROAZIRENE see EJM900
DIHYDRO-1H-AZIRINE see I:EJM900
1,2-DIHYDROBENZ(1)ACEANTHRYLENE see III:BAW000
1,2-DIHYDROBENZ(e)ACEANTHRYLENE see III:AAE000
1,2-DIHYDRO-BENZ(j)ACEANTHRYLENE see III:CMC000
4,5-DIHYDROBENZ(k)ACEPHENANTHRYLENE see
  III:AAF000
1,2-DIHYDROBENZ(a)ANTHRACENE see III:DKS400
3,4-DIHYDROBENZ(a)ANTHRACENE see III:DKS600
1a,11b-DIHYDROBENZ(3,4)ANTHRA(1,2-b)OXIRENE see
  III:EBP000
5,6-DIHYDROBENZENE(e)ACEANTHRYLENE see
  III:AAE000
1,2-DIHYDROBENZO(a)ANTHRACENE see III:DKS400
3,4-DIHYDROBENZO(a)ANTHRACENE see III:DKS600
6,13-DIHYDROBENZO(e)(1)BENZOTHIOPYRANO(4,3-b)IN-
  DOLE see III:DKS800
2,3-DIHYDRO-1H-BENZO(h,i)CHRYSENE see III:DKT400
6-β,7-α-DIHYDROBENZO(10,11)CHRYSENO(1,2-b)OXIRENE
  see III:BCV750
2,3-DIHYDRO-1H-BENZO(a)CYCLOPENT(b)ANTHRACENE
  see III:CPY750
7,8-DIHYDROBENZO(a)PYRENE see III:DKU000
9,10-DIHYDROBENZO(e)PYRENE see III:DKU400
9,10-DIHYDROBENZO(a)PYRENE-9,10-DIOL see III:DLC000
trans-4,5-DIHYDROBENZO(a)PYRENE-4,5-DIOL see
  III:DLC600
6,12,b-DIHYDROCHOLANTHRENE see III:DKV800
meso-DIHYDROCHOLANTHRENE see III:DKV800
DIHYDROCHOLESTEROL see III:DKW000
DIHYDROCHRYSENE see III:DKW200
1,2-DIHYDROCHRYSENE see III:DKW200
3,4-DIHYDROCHRYSENE see III:DKW400
trans-1,2-DIHYDROCHRYSENE-1,2-DIOL see III:DLD200
(E)-1,2-DIHYDRO-1,2-CHYRSENEDIOL see III:DLD200
trans-1,2-DIHYDRODIBENZ(a,e)ACEANTHRYLENE-1,2-DIOL
  see III:DKX875
trans-10,11-DIHYDRODIBENZ(a,e)ACEANTHRYLENE-10,11-
  DIOL see III:DKX900
5,6-DIHYDRODIBENZ(a,h)ANTHRACENE see III:DKY000
-5,6-DIHYDRODIBENZ(a,j)ANTHRACENE see III:DKY200
7,14-DIHYDRODIBENZ(a,h)ANTHRACENE see III:DKY400
9,10-DIHYDRO-1,2,5,6-DIBENZANTHRACENE see
  III:DKY400
3,4-DIHYDRO-1,2,5,6-DIBENZCARBAZOLE see III:DLA000
12,13-DIHYDRO-7H-DIBENZO(a,g)CARBAZOLE see
  III:DLA000
5,8-DIHYDRODIBENZO(a,def)CHRYSENE see III:DLA100
7,14-DIHYDRODIBENZO(b,def)CHRYSENE see III:DLA120
5,10-DIHYDRO-3,4:8,9-DIBENZOPYRENE see III:DLA120
5,8-DIHYDRO-3,4:9,10-DIBENZOPYRENE see III:DLA100
2,3-DIHYDRODICYCLOPENTA(c,lmn)PHENANTHREN-1(9H)-
  ONE see III:DGW300
DIHYDRODIETHYLSTILBESTROL see III:DLB400
(−)(3R,4R)-trans-3,4-DIHYDRO-3,4-DIHYDROXYBENZ(a)AN-
  THRACENE see III:BBG000
(+)-(3S,4S)-trans-3,4-DIHYDRO-3,4-DIHYDROXYBENZ(a)
  ANTHRACENE see III:BBD750
trans-3,4-DIHYDRO-3,4-DIHYDROXYBENZO(a)ANTHRA-
  CENE see III:BBD500
(−)(3R,4R)trans-3,4-DIHYDRO-3,4-DIHYDROXYBEN-
  ZO(a)ANTHRACENE see III:BBG000
(+)-(3S,4S)-trans-3,4-DIHYDRO-3,4-DIHYDROXYBEN-
  ZO(a)ANTHRACENE see III:BBD750
4,5-DIHYDRO-4,5-DIHYDROXYBENZO(a)PYRENE see
  III:DLB800

1-(2-(4-(3,4-DIHYDRO-6-METHOXY-2-PHENYL-1-NAPHTHALENYL)PHENOXY)ETHYL)PYRROLIDENE see III:NAD500

1-(2-(p-(3,4-DIHYDRO-6-METHOXY-2-PHENYL-1-NAPHTHYL)PHENOXY)ETHYL)PYRROLIDINE see III:NAD500

3,12-DIHYDRO-6-METHOXY-3,3,12-TRIMETHYL-7H-PYRANO(2,3-C)ACRIDIN-7-ONE see III:ADR750

1,2-DIHYDRO-3-METHYL-BENZ(j)ACEANTHRYLENE see II:MIJ750

1,2-DIHYDRO-3-METHYLBENZ(j)ACEANTHRYLENE COMPOUND with 2,4,6-TRINITROPHENOL (1:1) see III:MIL750

9,10-DIHYDRO-7-METHYLBENZO(a)PYRENE see III:DLT000

1':2'-DIHYDRO-4'-METHYL-3:4-BENZPYRENE see III:DLT000

11,12-DIHYDRO-3-METHYLCHOLANTHRENE see III:DLT400

6,12b-DIHYDRO-3-METHYLCHOLANTHRENE see III:DLT200

meso-DIHYDRO-3-METHYLCHOLANTHRENE see III:DLT200

(E)-11,12-DIHYDRO-3-METHYLCHOLANTHRENE-11,12-DIOL see III:DML800

9,10-DIHYDRO-3-METHYLCHOLANTHRENE-1,9,10-TRIOL see III:DLT600

1,2-DIHYDRO-5-METHYL-1,2-CHRYSENEDIOL see III:DLF400

7,8-DIHYDRO-5-METHYL-7,8-CHRYSENEDIOL see III:DLF600

16,17-DIHYDRO-7-METHYL-15H-CYCLOPENTA(a)PHENANTHRENE see III:MIV250

16,17-DIHYDRO-11-METHYL-15H-CYCLOPENTA(a)PHENANTHRENE see III:MJD750

15,16-DIHYDRO-11-METHYL-17H-CYCLOPENTA(a)PHENANTHREN-17-OL see III:DLT800

15,16-DIHYDRO-7-METHYLCYCLOPENTA(a)PHENANTHREN-17-ONE see III:DLU400

15,16-DIHYDRO-11-METHYLCYCLOPENTA(a)PHENANTHREN-17-ONE see II:MJE500

16,17-DIHYDRO-11-METHYLCYCLOPENTA(a)PHENANTHREN-15-ONE see III:DLU200

15,16-DIHYDRO-7-METHYL-17H-CYCLOPENTA(a)PHENANTHREN-17-ONE see III:DLU400

15,16-DIHYDRO-11-METHYL-17H-CYCLOPENTA(a)PHENANTHREN-17-ONE see II:MJE500

16,17-DIHYDRO-17-METHYLENE-15H-CYCLOPENTA(a)PHENANTHRENE see III:DLU600

15,16-DIHYDRO-11-METHYL-15-METHOXYCYCLOPENTA(a)PHENANTHREN-17-ONE see III:DLU700

15,16-DIHYDRO-11-METHYL-6-METHOXY-17H-CYCLOPENTA(a)PHENANTHREN-17-ONE see III:MEV250

1,4-DIHYDRO-1-METHYL-7-(2-(5-NITRO-2-FURYL)VINYL)-4-OXO-1,8-NAPHTHYRIDINE-3-CARBOXYLIC ACID, POTASSIUM SALT see III:DLU800

(S)-(+)-5,6-DIHYDRO-6-METHYL-2H-PYRAN-2-ONE see III:PAJ500

2,3-DIHYDRO-6-METHYL-2-THIOXO-4(1H)-PYRIMIDINONE see II:MPW500

3,4-DIHYDROMORPHOL see III:PCW500

4,5-DIHYDRONAPHTH(1,2-k)ACEPHENANTHRYLENE see III:PCW000

1,2-DIHYDRO-5-NITRO-ACENAPHTHYLENE see I:NEJ500

1,2-DIHYDRO-2-(5'-NITROFURYL)-4-HYDROXY-CHINAZOLIN-3-OXID (GERMAN) see III:DLX800

1,2-DIHYDRO-2-(5'-NITROFURYL)-4-HYDROXYQUINAZOLINE-3-OXIDE see III:DLX800

3,6-DIHYDRO-2-NITROSO-2H-1,2-OXAZINE see III:NJX000

DIHYDRO-1-NITROSO-2,4(1H,3H)-PYRIMIDINEDIONE see III:NJY000

2,5-DIHYDRO-1-NITROSO-1H-PYRROLE see III:NLQ000

5,6-DIHYDRO-1-NITROSOURACIL see III:NJY000

1,2-DIHYDRO-2-(5-NITRO-2-THIENYL)QUINAZOLIN-4(3H)-ONE see III:DLY200

1,2-DIHYDRO-2-(5-NITRO-2-THIENYL)-4(3H)-QUINAZOLINONE see III:DLY200

DIHYDROOXIRENE see I:EJN500

2,3-DIHYDRO-3-OXOBENZISOSULFONAZOLE see II:BCE500

2,3-DIHYDRO-3-OXOBENZISOSULPHONAZOLE see II:BCE500

5,13-DIHYDRO-5-OXOBENZO(e)(2)BENZOPYRANO(4,3-b)INDOLE see III:DLY800

S-(3,4-DIHYDRO-4-OXO-1,2,3-BENZOTRIAZIN-3-YL-METHYL)- O,O-DIMETHYL PHOSPHORODITHIOATE see III:ASH500

S-(3,4-DIHYDRO-4-OXO-BENZO(α)(1,2,3)TRIAZIN-3-YL-METHYL)-O,O-DIMETHYL PHOSPHORODITHIOATE see III:ASH500

1,2-DIHYDROPHENANTHRENE see III:DLZ000

1,2-DIHYDRO-1,2-PHENANTHRENEDIOL see III:DMA000

3,4-DIHYDRO-3,4-PHENANTHRENEDIOL see III:PCW500

1a,9b-DIHYDROPHENANTHRO(9,10-B)OXIRENE (9CI) see III:PCX000

N-(9,10-DIHYDRO-2-PHENANTHRYL)ACETAMIDE see III:DMA400

2,3-DIHYDROPHORBOL ACETATE MYRISTATE see III:DMB200

2,3-DIHYDROPHORBOL MYRISTATE ACETATE see III:DMB200

2,3-DIHYDRO-6-PROPYL-2-THIOXO-4(1H)-PYRIMIDINONE see I:PNX000

3,7-DIHYDRO-1H-PURINE-2,6-DIONE see III:XCA000

1,7-DIHYDRO-6H-PURINE-6-THIONE see III:POK000

1,2-DIHYDROPYRIDAZINE-3,6-DIONE see III:DMC600

1,2-DIHYDRO-3,6-PYRIDAZINEDIONE see III:DMC600

DIHYDROSAFROLE see II:DMD600

DIHYDROSTILBESTROL see III:DLB400

5-β-DIHYDROTESTOSTERONE see III:HJB100

DIHYDRO-5-TETRADECYL-2(3H)-FURANONE see III:SLL400

DIHYDROTHEELIN see I:EDO000

2,3-DIHYDROTHIIRENE see III:EJP500

2,3-DIHYDRO-2-THIOXO-4(1H)-PYRIMIDINONE see III:TFR250

16,17-DIHYDRO-11,12,17-TRIMETHYLCYCLOPENTA(a)PHENANTHRENE see III:DMF600

3,7-DIHYDRO-1,3,7-TRIMETHYL-1H-PURINE-2,6-DIONE see III:CAK500

1,8-DIHYDROXY-10-ACETYL-9-ANTHRONE see III:ACA750

1,8-DIHYDROXY-9,10-ANTHRACENEDIONE see III:DMH400

1,8-DIHYDROXYANTHRACHINON (CZECH) see III:DMH400

DIHYDROXYANTHRANOL see III:APH250

1,8-DIHYDROXYANTHRANOL see III:APH250

1,8-DIHYDROXY-9-ANTHRANOL see III:APH250

1,8-DIHYDROXYANTHRAQUINONE see III:DMH400

1,8-DIHYDROXY-9-ANTHRONE see III:APH250

1,4-DIHYDROXY-BENZEEN (DUTCH) see III:HIH000

1,4-DIHYDROXYBENZEN (CZECH) see III:HIH000

DIHYDROXYBENZENE see III:HIH000

m-DIHYDROXYBENZENE see III:REA000

o-DIHYDROXYBENZENE see III:CCP850

p-DIHYDROXYBENZENE see III:HIH000

1,2-DIHYDROXYBENZENE see III:CCP850

1,3-DIHYDROXYBENZENE see III:REA000

1,4-DIHYDROXYBENZENE see II:HIH000

3,3'-DIHYDROXYBENZIDINE see II:DMI400

1,4-DIHYDROXY-BENZOL (GERMAN) see III:HIH000

2,6-DIHYDROXY-5-BIS(2-CHLOROETHYL)AMINOPYRAMIDINE see II:BIA250

3,12-DIHYDROXYCHOLANIC ACID see III:DAQ400

3-α,7-α-DIHYDROXYCHOLANIC ACID see III:CDL325

3-α,12-α-DIHYDROXYCHOLANIC ACID see III:DAQ400

3-α,12-α-DIHYDROXY-5-β-CHOLANOIC ACID see III:DAQ400

DIMETHACHLON see III:DGF000
1,6-DIMETHANESULFONATE-d-MANNITOL see
  III:BKM500
1,4-DIMETHANESULFONATE THREITOL see I:TFU500
(2s,3s)-1,4-DIMETHANESULFONATE TREITOL see I:TFU500
1,4-DIMETHANESULFONOXYBUTANE see I:BOT250
cis-1,4-DIMETHANE SULFONOXY-2-BUTENE see
  III:DNW800
trans-1,4-DIMETHANE SULFONOXY-2-BUTENE see
  III:DNX000
1,4-DIMETHANESULFONOXY-2-BUTYNE see III:DNX200
1,6-DIMETHANE-SULFONOXY-d-MANNITOL see
  III:BKM500
1,4-DI(METHANESULFONYLOXY)BUTANE see I:BOT250
1,6-DIMETHANESULPHONOXY-1,6-DIDEOXY-d-MANNI-
  TOL see III:BKM500
1,4-DIMETHANESULPHONYLOXYBUTANE see I:BOT250
DIMETHESTERONE see III:DRT200
DIMETHICONE 350 see III:PJR000
DIMETHISTERON see III:DRT200
DIMETHISTERONE see III:DRT200
DIMETHISTERONE and ETHINYL ESTRADIOL see
  II:DNX500
DIMETHOAAT (DUTCH) see III:DSP400
DIMETHOAT (GERMAN) see III:DSP400
DIMETHOATE (USDA) see III:DSP400
DIMETHOAT TECHNISCH 95% see III:DSP400
DIMETHOGEN see III:DSP400
DIMETHOXANE see I:ABC250
3,4-DIMETHOXY-4-AMINOAZOBENZENE see III:DNY400
(trans)-2,5-DIMETHOXY-4'-AMINOSTILBENE see II:DON400
2,3-DIMETHOXYANILINE MUSTARD see III:BIC600
7,12-DIMETHOXYBENZ(a)ANTHRACENE see III:DOA000
2,5-DIMETHOXYBENZENEAZO-β-NAPHTHOL see
  II:DOK200
3,3'-DIMETHOXYBENZIDIN (CZECH) see I:DCJ200
3,3'-DIMETHOXYBENZIDINE see I:DCJ200
3,3'-DIMETHOXYBENZIDINE DIHYDROCHLORIDE see
  II:DOA800
3,3'-DIMETHOXYBENZIDINE-4,4'-DIISOCYANATE see
  III:DCJ400
3,4-DIMETHOXYBENZYL CHLORIDE see III:BKM750
3,3-DIMETHOXY-(1,1'-BIPHENYL)-4,4'-DIAMINE DIHY-
  DROCHLORIDE see II:DOA800
3,3'-DIMETHOXY-4,4'-BIPHENYLENE DIISOCYANATE see
  III:DCJ400
3,4-DIMETHOXY-DBA see III:DOB600
DIMETHOXY-DDT see II:MEI450
5,6-DIMETHOXYDIBENZ(a,h)ANTHRACENE see
  III:DOB600
3,4-DIMETHOXY-1,2:5,6-DIBENZANTHRACENE see
  III:DOB600
4,4'-DIMETHOXY-α,β-DIETHYLSTILBENE see III:DJB200
6,7-DIMETHOXY-2,2-DIMETHYL-2H-BENZO(b)PYRAN see
  III:AEX850
p,p'-DIMETHOXYDIPHENYLTRICHLOROETHANE see
  II:MEI450
DIMETHOXY-DT see II:MEI450
4-(2,5-DIMETHOXYPHENETHYL)ANILINE see II:DON400
1-((2,5-DIMETHOXYPHENYL)AZO)-2-NAPHTHALENOL see
  II:DOK200
1-((2,5-DIMETHOXYPHENYL)AZO)-2-NAPHTHOL see
  II:DOK200
2,5-DIMETHOXY-1-(PHENYLAZO)-2-NAPHTHOL see
  II:DOK200
1-(1-(2,5-DIMETHOXYPHENYL)AZO)-2-NAPHTHOL see
  II:DOK200
4-(2-(2,5-DIMETHOXYPHENYL)ETHYL)BENZENAMINE see
  II:DON400
2,2-DI-(p-METHOXYPHENYL)-1,1,1-TRICHLOROETHANE
  see II:MEI450
DI(p-METHOXYPHENYL)-TRICHLOROMETHYL METHANE
  see II:MEI450
(DIMETHOXYPHOSPHINOTHIOYL)THIO)BUTANEDIOIC
  ACID DIETHYL ESTER see III:MAK700

4-(2,5-DIMETHOXY)STILBENAMINE see II:DON400
2',5'-DIMETHOXYSTILBENAMINE see II:DON400
2,5-DIMETHOXY-4'-STILBENAMINE see II:DON400
DIMETHOXY-2,2,2-TRICHLORO-1-HYDROXY-ETHYL-
  PHOSPHINE OXIDE see III:TIQ250
3,3'-DIMETHOXYTRIPHENYLMETHANE-4,4'-BIS(1''-AZO-
  2''-NAPHTHOL) see III:DOO400
3,4-DIMETHYLACETANILIDE see III:ABP500
3',4'-DIMETHYLACETANILIDE see III:ABP500
DIMETHYLAMINE HYDROCHLORIDE see III:DOR600
4-(DIMETHYLAMINE)-3,5-XYLYL-N-METHYLCARBAMATE
  see III:DOS000
N',N'-DIMETHYL-4'-AMINO-N-ACETYL-N-MONOMETHYL-
  4-AMINOAZOBENZENE see III:DPQ200
DIMETHYLAMINO-ANALGESINE see III:DOT000
DIMETHYLAMINOANTIPYRINE see III:DOT000
4-(DIMETHYLAMINO)ANTIPYRINE see III:DOT000
4-(DIMETHYLAMINO)ANTIPYRINE mixed with SODIUM NI-
  TRITE (1:1) see III:DOT200
p-DIMETHYLAMINOAZOBENZEN (CZECH) see I:DOT300
DIMETHYLAMINOAZOBENZENE see I:DOT300
4-DIMETHYLAMINOAZOBENZENE see I:DOT300
p-DIMETHYLAMINOAZOBENZENE see I:DOT300
4-(N,N-DIMETHYLAMINO)AZOBENZENE see I:DOT300
N,N-DIMETHYL-4-AMINOAZOBENZENE see I:DOT300
N,N-DIMETHYL-p-AMINOAZOBENZENE see I:DOT300
2',3-DIMETHYL-4-AMINOAZOBENZENE see I:AIC250
4-DIMETHYLAMINOAZOBENZENE AMINE-N-OXIDE see
  III:DTK600
p-(DIMETHYLAMINO)AZOBENZENE-o-CARBOXYLIC ACID
  see III:CCE500
4'-DIMETHYLAMINOAZOBENZENE-2-CARBOXYLIC ACID
  see III:CCE500
N,N-DIMETHYLAMINOAZOBENZENE-N-OXIDE see
  III:DTK600
DIMETHYLAMINOAZOBENZOL see I:DOT300
4-DIMETHYLAMINOAZOBENZOL see I:DOT300
p-DIMETHYLAMINO-AZOBENZOL (GERMAN) see
  I:DOT300
DIMETHYLAMINOAZOPHENE see III:DOT000
1-(4-DIMETHYLAMINOBENZAL)INDENE see III:DOT600
p-DIMETHYLAMINOBENZENEAZO-1-NAPHTHALENE see
  III:DSU600
p-DIMETHYLAMINOBENZENE-1-AZO-1-NAPHTHALENE see
  III:DSU600
p-DIMETHYLAMINOBENZENE-1-AZO-2-NAPHTHALENE see
  III:DSU800
p-DIMETHYLAMINOBENZENE DIAZO SODIUM SULFONATE
  see III:DOU600
p-DIMETHYLAMINOBENZENEDIAZOSODIUM SULPHO-
  NATE see III:DOU600
p-(DIMETHYLAMINO)BENZENEDIAZOSULFONATE see
  III:DOU600
4-DIMETHYLAMINOBENZENEDIAZOSULFONIC ACID, SO-
  DIUM SALT see III:DOU600
p-DIMETHYLAMINOBENZENEDIAZOSULFONIC ACID, SO-
  DIUM SALT see III:DOU600
p-(DIMETHYLAMINO)BENZENEDIAZOSULPHONATE see
  III:DOU600
4-DIMETHYLAMINOBENZENEDIAZOSULPHONIC ACID,
  SODIUM SALT see III:DOU600
p-(DIMETHYLAMINO)BENZENEDIAZOSULPHONIC ACID,
  SODIUM SALT see III:DOU600
p-DIMETHYLAMINOBENZOLDIAZOSULFONAT (NATRIUM-
  SALZ) (GERMAN) see III:DOU600
4,4'-DIMETHYLAMINOBENZOPHENONIMIDE see I:IBB000
p-DIMETHYLAMINOBENZYLIDEN-1,2-BENZ-9-METHYL-
  ACRIDINE see III:DQC200
p-DIMETHYLAMINOBENZYLIDEN-3,4-BENZ-9-METHYL-
  ACRIDINE see III:DQC000
p-DIMETHYLAMINOBENZYLIDENE-3,4,5,6-DIBENZ-9-
  METHYLACRIDINE see III:DOV000
(4-DIMETHYLAMINOBENZYLIDENE)INDENE see
  III:DOT600

DIMETHYL DIETHYLAMIDO-1-CHLOROCROTONYL (2) PHOSPHATE see III:FAC025

N,N-DIMETHYL-p-((3,4-DIETHYLPHENYL)AZO)ANILINE see III:DJB400

trans-4,4'-DIMETHYL-α-α'-DIETHYLSTILBENE see III:DRK500

N,N-DIMETHYL-2,5-DIFLUORO-p-(2,5-DIFLUOROPHE-NYLAZO)ANILINE see III:DRK800

N,N-DIMETHYL-p-(2,5-DIFLUOROPHENYLAZO)ANILINE see III:DKH000

N,N-DIMETHYL-p-(3,4-DIFLUOROPHENYLAZO)ANILINE see III:DRL000

N,N-DIMETHYL-p-(3,5-DIFLUOROPHENYLAZO)ANILINE see III:DKH100

N,N-DIMETHYL-3',4'-DIFLUORO-4-(PHENYLAZO)BEN-ZENEAMINE see III:DRL000

9:10-DIMETHYL-9-10-DIHYDRO-1,2-BENZANTHRACENE-9,10-OXIDE see III:DQL800

11,17-DIMETHYL-16,17-DIHYDRO-15H-CYCLOPENTA(a)PHENANTHRENE see III:DLI200

7,11-DIMETHYL-15,16-DIHYDROCYCLOPENTA(a)PHENAN-THREN-17-ONE see III:DLI300

O,O-DIMETHYL-S-(3,4-DIHYDRO-4-KETO-1,2,3-BENZO-TRIAZINYL-3-METHYL) DITHIOPHOSPHATE see III:ASH500

O,O-DIMETHYL-S-1,2-DIKARBETOXYLETHYLDITIOFOS-FAT (CZECH) see III:MAK700

2,4'-DIMETHYL-4-DIMETHYLAMINOAZOBENZENE see III:DRL400

2',3'-DIMETHYL-4-DIMETHYLAMINOAZOBENZENE see III:DUN800

3-keto-1,5-DIMETHYL-4-DIMETHYLAMINO-2-PHENYL-2,3-DIHYDROPYRAZOLE see III:DOT000

1,5-DIMETHYL-4-DIMETHYLAMINO-2-PHENYL-3-PYRAZO-LONE see III:DOT000

2,3-DIMETHYL-4-DIMETHYLAMINO-1-PHENYL-5-PYRAZO-LONE see III:DOT000

6,8-DIMETHYL-(4-p-(DIMETHYLAMINO)STYRYL)QUINO-LINE see III:DQC600

3',4'-DIMETHYL-4-DIMETHYLAMINOZOBENZENE see III:DUO000

N,N-DIMETHYL-p-(2',3'-DIMETHYLPHENYLAZO)ANILINE see III:DUN800

N,N-DIMETHYL-p-(3',4'-DIMETHYLPHENYLAZO)ANILINE see III:DUO000

N,N-DIMETHYL-4-(4'-(2',5'-DIMETHYLPYRIDYL-1'-OX-IDE)AZO)ANILINE see III:DPP600

N,N-DIMETHYL-4-(4'-(2',6'-DIMETHYLPYRIDYL-1'-OX-IDE)AZO)ANILINE see III:DPP800

N,N-DIMETHYL-4-(4'-(3',5'-DIMETHYLPYRIDYL-1'-OX-IDE)AZO)ANILINE see III:DPP709

DIMETHYL-DI-NITROSO-AETHYLENDIAMIN (GERMAN) see III:DVE400

1,6-DIMETHYL-1,6-DINITROSOBIUREA see III:DRN400

DIMETHYLDINITROSOETHYLENEDIAMINE see III:DVE400

N,N'-DIMETHYL-N,N'-DINITROSOETHYLENEDIAMINE see III:DVE400

N,N'-DIMETHYL-N,N'-DINITROSO-1,2-HYDRAZINEDICAR-BOXAMIDE see III:DRN400

2,5-DIMETHYLDINITROSOPIPERAZINE see III:DRN800

2,6-DIMETHYLDINITROSOPIPERAZINE see III:DRO000

2,5-DIMETHYL-1,4-DINITROSOPIPERAZINE see III:DRN800

N,N'-DIMETHYL-N,N'-DINITROSO-1,3-PROPANEDIAMINE see III:DRO200

2,6-DIMETHYL-m-DIOXAN-4-OL ACETATE see I:ABC250

2,6-DIMETHYL-m-DIOXAN-4-YL ACETATE see I:ABC250

3,3'-DIMETHYL-4,4'-DIPHENYLDIAMINE see I:TGJ750

3,3'-DIMETHYLDIPHENYL-4,4'-DIAMINE see I:TGJ750

N,N-DIMETHYL-4-(DIPHENYLMETHYL)ANILINE see III:DRQ000

2,2'-DIMETHYLDIPROPYLINITROSOAMINE see III:DRQ200

DIMETHYLDITHIOCARBAMATE ZINC SALT see III:BJK500

DIMETHYLDITHIOCARBAMIC ACID with DIMETHYLAMINE (II) see III:DRQ600

DIMETHYLDITHIOCARBAMIC ACID DIMETHYL AMINE SALT see III:DRQ600

DIMETHYLDITHIOCARBAMIC ACID DIMETHYLAMMO-NIUM SALT see III:DRQ600

DIMETHYLDITHIOCARBAMIC ACID, IRON SALT see III:FAS000

DIMETHYLDITHIOCARBAMIC ACID, IRON(3+) SALT see III:FAS000

DIMETHYLDITHIOCARBAMIC ACID, LEAD SALT see III:LCW000

DIMETHYLDITHIOCARBAMIC ACID, ZINC SALT see III:BJK500

O,O-DIMETHYLDITHIOPHOSPHATE DIETHYLMERCAPTO-SUCCINATE see III:MAK700

DIMETHYLDITHIOPHOSPHORIC-ACID N-METHYLBENZ-AZIMIDE ESTER see III:ASH500

O,O-DIMETHYLDITHIOPHOSPHORYLACETIC ACID-N-MONOMETHYLAMIDE SALT see III:DSP400

O,O-DIMETHYL-DITHIOPHOSPHORYLESSIGSAEURE MONOMETHYLAMID (GERMAN) see III:DSP400

2,5-DIMETHYL-DNPZ see III:DRN800

2,6-DIMETHYL-DNPZ see III:DRO000

DIMETHYLDODECYLAMINE HYDROCHLORIDE mixed with SODIUM NITRITE (7:8) see III:SIS150

7,8-DIMETHYLENEBENZ(a)ANTHRACENE see III:CMC000

3:4-DIMETHYLENE-1:2-BENZANTHRACENE see III:AAF000

8:9-DIMETHYLENE-1:2-BENZANTHRACENE see III:BAW000

DIMETHYLENEIMINE see I:EJM900

DIMETHYLENE OXIDE see I:EJN500

DIMETHYLENIMINE see I:EJM900

exo-1,2-cis-DIMETHYL-3,6-EPOXYHEXAHYDROPHTHALIC ANHYDRIDE see III:CBE750

DIMETHYLESTER KYSELINY FOSFORITE (CZECH) see III:DSG600

DIMETHYLESTER KYSELINY SIROVE (CZECH) see I:DUD100

7,14-DIMETHYL-7,14-ETHANODIBENZ(a,b)ANTHRACENE-15,16-DICARBOXYLIC ACID see III:DRT000

6-α,21-DIMETHYLETHISTERONE see III:DRT200

N,N-DIMETHYL-p-((3-ETHOXYPHENYL)AZO)ANILINE see III:DRU000

DIMETHYL ETHYL ALLENOLIC ACID METHYL ETHER see III:DRU600

N,N-DIMETHYL-4'-ETHYL-4-AMINOAZOBENZENE see III:EOI500

DI-N-METHYL ETHYL CARBAMATE see III:EII500

N,N-DIMETHYL-p-(3'-ETHYL-4'-METHYLPHENYLAZO)ANILINE see III:EPT500

N,N-DIMETHYL-p-(4'-ETHYL-3'-METHYLPHENYLAZO)ANILINE see III:EPU000

1,1-DIMETHYL-3-ETHYL-3-NITROSOUREA see III:DRV600

4-(1,1-DIMETHYLETHYL)PHENOL see III:BSE500

N,N-DIMETHYL-p((m-ETHYLPHENYL)AZO)ANILINE see III:EOI000

N,N-DIMETHYL-p-((4-ETHYLPHENYL)AZO)ANILINE see III:EOI500

N,N-DIMETHYL-p-((o-ETHYLPHENYL)AZO)ANILINE see III:EIF450

N,N-DIMETHYL-p-(3'-ETHYLPHENYLAZO)ANILINE see III:EOI000

N,N-DIMETHYL-3'-ETHYL-4-(PHENYLAZO)BENZENAMINE see III:EOI000

N,N-DIMETHYL-p-((3-ETHYL-p-TOLYL)AZO)ANILINE see III:EPT500

N,N-DIMETHYL-p-((4-ETHYL-m-TOLYL)AZO) ANILINE see III:EPU000

N,N-DIMETHYL-α-ETHYNYL-α-PHENYLBENZENEACE-TAMIDE see III:DWA700

2,3-DIMETHYLFLUORANTHENE see III:DRX600

O,O-DIMETHYL-S-(4-OXOBENZOTRIAZINO-3-METHYL)
PHOSPHORODITHIOATE see III:ASH500

O,O-DIMETHYL-S-((4-OXO-1,2,3-BENZOTRIAZINO(3)-
METHYL) THIOTHIONOPHOSPHATE see III:ASH500

O,O-DIMETHYL-S-((4-OXO-3H-1,2,3-BENZOTRIAZIN-3-YL)-
METHYL)-DITHIOFOSFAAT (DUTCH) see III:ASH500

O,O-DIMETHYL-S-((4-OXO-3H-1,2,3-BENZOTRIAZIN-3-YL)-
METHYL)-DITHIOPHOSPHAT (GERMAN) see III:ASH500

O,O-DIMETHYL-S-4-OXO-1,2,3-BENZOTRIAZIN-3(4H)-YL-
METHYL PHOSPHORODITHIOATE see III:ASH500

O,O-DIMETHYL-S-(4-OXO-3H-1,2,3-BENZOTRIZIANE-3-
METHYL)PHOSPHORODITHIOATE see III:ASH500

1-(2,5-DIMETHYLOXYPHENYLAZO)-2-NAPHTHOL see
II:DOK200

DIMETHYLOXYQUINAZINE see III:AQN000

O,O-DIMETHYL-1-OXY-2,2,2-TRICHLOROETHYL PHOS-
PHONATE see III:TIQ250

DIMETHYL PARATHION see III:MNH000

1,4-DIMETHYLPHENANTHRENE see III:DTJ200

2,4-DIMETHYLPHENOL see III:XKJ500

2,5-DIMETHYLPHENOL see III:XKS000

2,6-DIMETHYLPHENOL see III:XLA000

3,4-DIMETHYLPHENOL see III:XLJ000

3,5-DIMETHYLPHENOL see III:XLS000

3,6-DIMETHYLPHENOL see III:XKS000

4,5-DIMETHYLPHENOL see III:XLJ000

4,6-DIMETHYLPHENOL see III:XKJ500

5-(2,5-DIMETHYLPHENOXY)-2,2-DIMETHYLPENTANOIC
ACID (9CI) see III:GCK300

2,4-DIMETHYLPHENYLAMINE see II:XMS000

2,5-DIMETHYLPHENYLAMINE see III:XNA000

2,3-DIMETHYL-4-PHENYLAZOANILINE see III:DTL000

N,N-DIMETHYL-p-PHENYLAZOANILINE see I:DOT300

N,N-DIMETHYL-p-PHENYLAZOANILINE-N-OXIDE see
III:DTK600

N,N-DIMETHYL-4-PHENYLAZO-o-ANISIDINE see
III:DTK800

N,N-DIMETHYL-4-(PHENYLAZO)BENZAMINE see
I:DOT300

2,3-DIMETHYL-4-(PHENYLAZO)BENZENAMINE see
III:DTL000

N,N-DIMETHYL-4-(PHENYLAZO)BENZENAMINE see
I:DOT300

4-((2,4-DIMETHYLPHENYL)AZO)-3-HYDROXY-2,7-
NAPHTHALENEDISULFONIC ACID, DISODIUM SALT
see III:FMU070

4-((2,4-DIMETHYLPHENYL)AZO)-3-HYDROXY-2,7-
NAPHTHALENEDISULPHONIC ACID, DISODIUM SALT
see III:FMU070

1-((2,4-DIMETHYLPHENYL)AZO)-2-NAPHTHALENOL see
III:XRA000

N,N-DIMETHYL-4-(PHENYLAZO)-m-TOLUIDINE see
III:TLE750

N,N-DIMETHYL-4-(PHENYLAZO)-o-TOLUIDINE see
III:MJF000

(E)-N,N,-DIMETHYL-4-(2-PHENYLETHENYL)BENZENA-
MINE see III:DUC000

1,3-DIMETHYL-3-PHENYL-1-NITROSOUREA see
III:DTN875

2,3-DIMETHYL-1-PHENYL-3-PYRAZOLIN-5-ONE see
III:AQN000

2,3-DIMETHYL-1-PHENYL-5-PYRAZOLONE see III:AQN000

3,3-DIMETHYL-1-PHENYLTRIAZENE see III:DTP000

3,3-DIMETHYL-1-PHENYL-1-TRIAZENE see III:DTP000

DIMETHYL PHOSPHATE of 2-CHLORO-N,N-DIETHYL-3-HY-
DROXYCROTONAMIDE see III:FAC025

2,2-DIMETHYL-1,3-PROPANEDIOL DIACRYLATE see
III:DUL200

2,2'-((2,2-DIMETHYL-1,3-
PROPANEDIYL)BIS(OXYMETHYLENE))BISOXIRANE see
III:NCI300

2,2-DIMETHYLPROPANOIC ACID see III:PJA500

DIMETHYL PROPIOLACTONE see III:DTH000

3,3-DIMETHYL-β-PROPIOLACTONE see III:DTH000

2,2-DIMETHYLPROPIONIC ACID see III:PJA500

α,α-DIMETHYLPROPIONIC ACID see III:PJA500

7,12-DIMETHYL-8-PROPYL-BENZ(a)ANTHRACENE see
III:PNI500

N,N-DIMETHYL-p-((p-PROPYLPHENYL)AZO)ANILINE see
III:DTT400

N-(1,1-DIMETHYLPROPYNYL)-3,5-DICHLOROBENZAMIDE
see III:DTT600

2,6-DIMETHYLPYRIDINE-1-OXIDE-4-AZO-p-DIMETHYL-
ANILINE see III:DPP800

N,N-DIMETHYL-N'-2-PYRIDINYL-N'-(2-THIENYLMEHTYL)-
1,2-ETHANEDIAMINE MONOHYDROCHLORIDE see
III:DPJ400

1,4-DIMETHYL-5H-PYRIDO(4,3-b)INDOL-3-AMINE see
II:TNX275

1,4-DIMETHYL-5H-PYRIDO(4,3-b)INDOL-3-AMINE ACE-
TATE see II:AJR500

1,4-DIMETHYL-5H-PYRIDO(4,3-b)INDOL-3-AMINE MONO-
ACETATE see II:AJR500

N,N-DIMETHYL-p-(3-PYRIDYLAZO)ANILINE see
III:POP750

N,N-DIMETHYL-4-(3'-PYRIDYLAZO)ANILINE see
III:POP750

(3,3-DIMETHYL-1-(m-PYRIDYL-N-OXIDE))TRIAZENE see
III:DTV200

N,N-DIMETHYL-N'-(2-PYRIDYL)-N'-THENYLETHYLENEDI-
AMINE HYDROCHLORIDE see III:DPJ400

N¹-(4,6-DIMETHYL-2-PYRIMIDINYL)SULFANILAMIDE see
III:SNJ000

N-(4,6-DIMETHYL-2-PYRIMIDYL)SULFANILAMIDE see
III:SNJ000

N,N-DIMETHYL-4-(4'-QUINOLYLAZO)ANILINE see
III:DTY200

N,N-DIMETHYL-4-(5'-QUINOLYLAZO)ANILINE see
III:DPQ800

N,N-DIMETHYL-4-(6'-QUINOLYLAZO)ANILINE see
III:DPR000

N,N-DIMETHYL-p-(5'-QUINOLYLAZO)ANILINE see
III:DPQ800

N,N-DIMETHYL-4-(5'-QUINOLYLAZO)-m-TOLUIDINE see
III:DQE400

N,N-DIMETHYL-4-((5'-QUINOLYL-1'-OXIDE)AZO)ANILINE
see III:DPR200

N,N-DIMETHYL-4-((4'-QUINOLYL-1'-OXIDE)AZO)ANILINE
see III:DTY400

N,N'-DIMETHYL-4-((6'-QUINOLYL-1'-OXIDE)AZO)ANILINE
see III:DPR400

N,N-DIMETHYL-p-(6-QUINOXALINYLAZO)ANILINE see
III:DUA400

N,N-DIMETHYL-p-(6-QUINOXALYAZO)ANILINE see
III:DUA400

N,N-DIMETHYL-p-(5-QUINOXALYLAZO)ANILINE see
III:DUA200

DIMETHYL SILOXANE see III:DUB600

N,N-DIMETHYL-4-STILBENAMINE see III:DUB800

(E)-N,N-DIMETHYL-4-STILBENAMINE see III:DUC000

(Z)-N,N-DIMETHYL-4-STILBENAMINE see III:DUC200

cis-N,N-DIMETHYL-4-STILBENAMINE see III:DUC200

trans-N,N-DIMETHYL-4-STILBENAMINE see III:DUC000

N,N-DIMETHYL-p-STYRYLANILINE see III:DUB800

DIMETHYLSULFAAT (DUTCH) see I:DUD100

3,4-DIMETHYL-5-SULFANILAMIDOISOXAZOLE see
III:SNN500

4,6-DIMETHYL-2-SULFANILAMIDOPYRIMIDINE see
III:SNJ000

DIMETHYLSULFAT (CZECH) see I:DUD100

DIMETHYL SULFATE see I:DUD100

1,4-DIMETHYLSULFONOXYBUTANE see I:BOT250

3-((2,4-DIMETHYL-5-SULFOPHENYL)AZO)-4-HYDROXY-1-
NAPHTHALENESULFONIC ACID, DISODIUM SALT see
III:FAG050

DIMETHYL SULFOXIDE see III:DUD800

3,4-DIMETHYL-5-SULPHANILAMIDOISOXAZOLE see
III:SNN500

as-DIMETHYL SULPHATE see III:MLH500
3,4-DIMETHYL-5-SULPHONAMIDOISOXAZOLE see
 III:SNN500
3-((2,4-DIMETHYL-5-SULPHOPHENYL)AZO)-4-HYDROXY-
 1-NAPHTHALENESULPHONIC ACID, DISODIUM SALT see
 III:FAG050
DIMETHYL SULPHOXIDE see III:DUD800
DIMETHYL TEREPHTHALATE see III:DUE000
7,12-DIMETHYL-1,2,3,4-TETRAHYDROBENZ(a)ANTHRA-
 CENE see III:TCP600
7,12-DIMETHYL-8,9,10,11-TETRAHYDROBENZ(a)ANTHRA-
 CENE see III:DUF000
1,11-DIMETHYL-1,2,3,4-TETRAHYDROCHRYSENE see
 III:DUF200
N,N-DIMETHYL-N'-(2-THENYL)-N'-(2-PYRIDYL-ETHYL-
 ENE-DIAMINE HYDROCHLORIDE) see III:DPJ400
N,N-DIMETHYL-4-(p-TOLYLAZO)ANILINE see III:DUH400
N,N-DIMETHYL-p-(m-TOLYLAZO)ANILINE see III:DUH600
N,N-DIMETHYL-p-((o-TOLYL)AZO)ANILINE see
 III:DUH800
3,3-DIMETHYL-1-(m-TOLYL)TRIAZENE see III:DSR200
3,3-DIMETHYL-1-(o-TOLYL)TRIAZENE see III:MNT500
(DIMETHYLTRIAZENO)IMIDAZOLECARBOXAMIDE see
 II:DAB600
4-(DIMETHYLTRIAZENO)IMIDAZOLE-5-CARBOXAMIDE
 see II:DAB600
5-(DIMETHYLTRIAZENO)IMIDAZOLE-4-CARBOXAMIDE
 see II:DAB600
5-(3,3-DIMETHYLTRIAZENO)IMIDAZOLE-4-CARBOXAM-
 IDE see II:DAB600
4-(3,3-DIMETHYL-1-TRIAZENO)IMIDAZOLE-5-CARBOX-
 AMIDE see II:DAB600
5-(3,3-DIMETHYL-1-TRIAZENO)IMIDAZOLE-4-CARBOX-
 AMIDE see II:DAB600
4-(5)-(3,3-DIMETHYL-1-TRIAZENO)IMIDAZOLE-5(4)-CAR-
 BOXAMIDE see II:DAB600
3-(3',3'-DIMETHYLTRIAZENO)PYRIDINE-N-OXIDE see
 III:DTV200
3-(3',3'-DIMETHYLTRIAZENO)-PYRIDIN-N-OXID (GER-
 MAN) see III:DTV200
5-(3,3-DIMETHYL-1-TRIAZENYL)-1H-IMIDAZOLE-4-CAR-
 BOXAMIDE see II:DAB600
O,O-DIMETHYL-(2,2,2-TRICHLOOR-1-HYDROXY-ETHYL)-
 FOSFONAAT (DUTCH) see III:TIQ250
O,O-DIMETHYL-(2,2,2-TRICHLOR-1-HYDROXY-AETHYL)
 PHOSPHONAT (GERMAN) see III:TIQ250
DIMETHYLTRICHLOROHYDROXYETHYL PHOSPHONATE
 see III:TIQ250
DIMETHYL-2,2,2-TRICHLORO-1-HYDROXYETHYLPHOS-
 PHONATE see III:TIQ250
O,O-DIMETHYL-2,2,2-TRICHLORO-1-HYDROXYETHYL
 PHOSPHONATE see III:TIQ250
1,1-DIMETHYL-3-(3-TRIFLUOROMETHYLPHENYL)UREA
 see III:DUK800
N,N-DIMETHYL-N'-(3-TRIFLUOROMETHYLPHENYL)UREA
 see III:DUK800
N,N-DIMETHYL-p-(2,4,6-TRIFLUOROPHENYLAZO)ANILINE
 see III:DUK200
1,1-DIMETHYL-3-(α,α,α-TRIFLUORO-m-TOLYL) UREA see
 III:DUK800
3,7-DIMETHYL-9-(2,6,6-TRIMETHYL-1-CYCLOHEXEN-1-
 YL-2,4,6,8-NONATETRAENOIC ACID see III:VSK950
2,2-DIMETHYLTRIMETHYLENE ACRYLATE see
 III:DUL200
2,2-DIMETHYLTRIMETHYLENE ESTER ACRYLIC ACID see
 III:DUL200
3,3-DIMETHYLTRIMETHYLENE OXIDE see III:EBQ500
β,β-DIMETHYLTRIMETHYLENE OXIDE see III:EBQ500
N,N-DIMETHYL-4-(3,4,5-TRIMETHYLPHENYL)AZOANI-
 LINE see III:DUL400
N,N-DIMETHYL-4-((3,4,5-TRIMETHYLPHENYL)AZO)
 BENZENAMINE see III:DUL400
DIMETHYLUREA and SODIUM NITRITE see III:DUM400
p-N,N-DIMETHYLUREIDOAZOBENZENE see III:DUM600

β,β-DIMETHYLVINYL CHLORIDE see III:IKE000
N,N-DIMETHYL-p-(2,3,XYLYLAZO)ANILINE see
 III:DUN800
N,N-DIMETHYL-p-(3,4-XYLYLAZO)ANILINE see
 III:DUO000
2,2-DIMETHYL-5-(2,5-XYLYLOXY)VALERIC ACID see
 III:GCK300
DIMETHYL YELLOW see I:DOT300
DIMETHYL YELLOW-N,N-DIMETHYLANILINE see
 I:DOT300
O,O-DIMETIL-S-(N-METIL-CARBAMOIL-METIL)-DITIOFOS-
 FATO (ITALIAN) see III:DSP400
O,O-DIMETIL-O-(3-METIL-4-METILTIO-FENIL)-MONOTIO-
 FOSFATO (ITALIAN) see III:FAQ999
O,O-DIMETIL-O-(4-NITRO-FENIL)-MONOTIOFOSFATO
 (ITALIAN) see III:MNH000
O,O-DIMETIL-S-((4-OXO-3H-1,2,3-BENZOTRIAZIN-3-IL)-
 METIL)-DITIOFOSFATO (ITALIAN) see III:ASH500
DIMETILSOLFATO (ITALIAN) see I:DUD100
O,O-DIMETIL-(2,2,2-TRICLORO-1-IDROSSI-ETIL)-FOSFON-
 ATO (ITALIAN) see III:TIQ250
DIMETON see III:DSP400
3,3'-DIMETOSSIBENZODINA (ITALIAN) see I:DCJ200
DIMETOX see III:TIQ250
DIMETRIDAZOLE see III:DSV800
DIMEVUR see III:DSP400
DIMEXIDE see III:DUD800
DIMEZATHINE see III:SNJ000
DIMITAN see I:BIE500
DIN 2.4602 see I:CNA750
DIN 2.4964 see I:CNA750
DINACRIN see III:ILD000
DINAPHTAZIN (GERMAN) see III:DUP000
3,4,5,6-DINAPHTHACARBAZOLE see III:DCY000
1,2,5,6-DINAPHTHACRIDINE see I:DCS400
3,4,6,7-DINAPHTHACRIDINE see I:DCS600
DINAPHTHAZINE see III:DUP000
DI-β-NAPHTHYLDIIMIDE see III:ASN750
DI-β-NAPHTHYL-p-PHENYLDIAMINE see III:NBL000
DI-β-NAPHTHYL-p-PHENYLENEDIAMINE see III:NBL000
N,N'-DI-β-NAPHTHYL-p-PHENYLENEDIAMINE see
 III:NBL000
sym-DI-β-NAPHTHYL-p-PHENYLENEDIAMINE see
 III:NBL000
DINATE see I:DXE600
DINICKEL TRIOXIDE see II:NDH500
DINITRO see III:BRE500
DINITRO-3 see III:BRE500
DINITROBENZENE see II:DUQ180
m-DINITROBENZENE see II:DUQ200
o-DINITROBENZENE see II:DUQ400
p-DINITROBENZENE see II:DUQ600
1,2-DINITROBENZENE see II:DUQ400
1,3-DINITROBENZENE see II:DUQ200
2,4-DINITROBENZENE see II:DUQ200
DINITROBENZENE, solution (DOT) see II:DUQ180
1,3-DINITROBENZOL see II:DUQ200
DINITROBENZOL SOLID (DOT) see II:DUQ180
4,4'-DINITROBIFENYL (CZECH) see III:DUS000
4,4'-DINITROBIPHENYL see III:DUS000
4,6-DINITRO-2-sec.BUTYLFENOL (CZECH) see III:BRE500
DINITROBUTYLPHENOL see III:BRE500
2,4-DINITRO-6-sec-BUTYLPHENOL see III:BRE500
4,6-DINITRO-2-sec-BUTYLPHENOL see III:BRE500
4,6-DINITRO-o-sec-BUTYLPHENOL see III:BRE500
2,4-DINITRO-6-tert-BUTYLPHENYL METHANESULFONATE
 see III:DUS500
4,6-DINITRO-2-CAPRYLPHENYL CROTONATE see
 III:AQT500
4,6-DINITRO-2-(2-CAPRYL)PHENYL CROTONATE see
 III:AQT500
2,4-DINITRO-1-CHLORO-NAPHTHALENE see III:DUS600
2,6-DINITRO-N,N-DIPROPYL-4-(TRIFLUOROMETHYL)
 BENZENAMINE see III:DUV600

DI-n-PENTYLNITROSAMINE see III:DCH600
DIPEZONA see III:DCK759
DIPHANTOIN see I:DKQ000
DIPHANTOINE SODIUM see I:DNU000
DIPHEBUZOL see II:BRF500
DIPHEDAL see I:DKQ000
DIPHEDAN see I:DNU000
DIPHENATE see I:DNU000
DIPHENATRILE see III:DVX200
DIPHENIN see I:DNU000
DIPHENINE see I:DKQ000
DIPHENINE SODIUM see I:DNU000
o-DIPHENOL see III:CCP850
DIPHENTOIN see I:DKQ000, I:DNU000
DIPHENYL see III:BGE000
DIPHENYLACETONITRILE see III:DVX200
DIPHENYLAN see I:DKQ000
DIPHENYLAN SODIUM see I:DNU000
DIPHENYL BLUE 2B see I:CMO000
DIPHENYL BLUE 3B see II:CMO250
DIPHENYLBUTAZONE see II:BRF500
1,2-DIPHENYL-4-BUTYL-3,5-DIOXOPYRAZOLIDINE see
    II:BRF500
1,2-DIPHENYL-4-BUTYL-3,5-PYRAZOLIDINEDIONE see
    II:BRF500
1,1-DIPHENYL-2-BUTYNYL-N-CYCLOHEXYLCARBAMATE
    see III:DVY900
DIPHENYL CARBONATE see III:DVZ000
α,β-DIPHENYLCINNAMONITRILE see III:TMQ250
DIPHENYL-α-CYANOMETHANE see III:DVX200
DIPHENYL DEEP BLACK G see I:AQP000
2,4′-DIPHENYLDIAMINE see III:BGF109
DIPHENYLDIAZENE see III:ASL250
1,2-DIPHENYLDIAZENE see III:ASL250
DIPHENYLDIIMIDE see III:ASL250
3,3-DIPHENYL-3-DIMETHYLCARBAMOYL-1-PROPYNE see
    III:DWA700
1,2-DIPHENYL-3,5-DIOXO-4-BUTYLPYRAZOLIDINE see
    II:BRF500
1,2-DIPHENYL-2,3-DIOXO-4-N-BUTYLPYRAZOLINE see
    II:BRF500
DIPHENYLE CHLORE, 42% de CHLORE (FRENCH) see
    II:PJM500
DIPHENYLE CHLORE, 54% de CHLORE (FRENCH) see
    II:PJN000
4,4′-DIPHENYLENEDIAMINE see I:BBX000
DIPHENYLENE DIOXIDE see III:DDA800
DIPHENYLENEIMINE see III:CBN000
DIPHENYLENIMIDE see III:CBN000
DIPHENYLENIMINE see III:CBN000
DIPHENYL FAST BROWN BRL see II:CMO750
DIPHENYLGLYOXAL PEROXIDE see III:BDS000
DIPHENYLHYDANTOIN see I:DKQ000
5,5-DIPHENYLHYDANTOIN see I:DKQ000
DIPHENYLHYDANTOINE (FRENCH) see I:DKQ000
DIPHENYLHYDANTOIN SODIUM see I:DNU000
5,5-DIPHENYLHYDANTOIN SODIUM see I:DNU000
1,2-DIPHENYLHYDRAZINE see I:HHG000
sym-DIPHENYLHYDRAZINE see I:HHG000
2,2-DIPHENYL-3-HYDROXYPROPIONIC ACID LACTONE see
    III:DWI400
5,5-DIPHENYLIMIDAZOLIDIN-2,4-DIONE see I:DKQ000
5,5-DIPHENYL-2,4-IMIDAZOLIDINEDIONE see I:DKQ000
5,5-DIPHENYL-2,4-IMIDAZOLIDINE-DIONE, MONOSODIUM
    SALT see I:DNU000
DIPHENYLINE see III:BGF109
DIPHENYLMETHAN-4,4′-DIISOCYANAT (GERMAN) see
    III:MJP400
4,4′-DIPHENYLMETHANEDIAMINE see I:MJQ000
DIPHENYL METHANE DIISOCYANATE see III:MJP400
4,4′-DIPHENYLMETHANE DIISOCYANATE see III:MJP400
p,p′-DIPHENYLMETHANE DIISOCYANATE see III:MJP400
DIPHENYLMETHANE 4,4′-DIISOCYANATE (DOT) see
    III:MJP400

DIPHENYLMETHYLCYANIDE see III:DVX200
α-(DIPHENYLMETHYLENE)BENZENEACETIC ACID see
    III:TMQ250
DIPHENYLNITROSAMIN (GERMAN) see III:DWI000
DIPHENYLNITROSAMINE see III:DWI000
N,N-DIPHENYLNITROSAMINE see III:DWI000
DIPHENYL N-NITROSOAMINE see III:DWI000
o-DIPHENYLOL see III:BGJ250
3,3-DIPHENYL-2-OXETANONE see III:DWI400
DIPHENYL-p-PHENYLENEDIAMINE see III:BLE500
N,N′-DIPHENYL-p-PHENYLENEDIAMINE see III:BLE500
α,α-DIPHENYL-β-PROPIOLACTONE see III:DWI400
1,1-DIPHENYL-2-PROPYN-1-OL CYCLOHEXANECARBA-
    MATE see III:DWL400
1,1-DIPHENYL-2-PROPYNYL-N-CYCLOHEXYLCARBA-
    MATE see III:DWL400
1,1-DIPHENYL-2-PROPYNYL ESTER CYCLOHEXANECAR-
    BAMIC ACID see III:DWL400
1,1-DIPHENYL-2-PROPYNYL-N-ETHYLCARBAMATE see
    III:DWL500
1,1-DIPHENYL-2-PROPYNYL 1-PYRROLIDINECARBOX-
    YLATE see III:DWL525
3,3-DIPHENYL-3-(PYRROLIDINE-CARBONYLOXY)-1-PRO-
    PYNE see III:DWL525
3,3′,4,4′-DIPHENYLTETRAMINE see III:BGK500
5,5-DIPHENYL-2-THIOHYDANTOIN see III:DWN600
1,3-DIPHENYLTRIAZENE see III:DWO800
DIPHENYLTRICHLOROETHANE see I:DAD200
DIPHER see III:EIR000
DI-PHETINE see I:DKQ000, I:DNU000
DIPHONE see III:SOA500
DIPIRARTRIL-TROPICO see III:DUD800
DIPIRIN see III:DOT000
DIPN see II:DNB200
DIPOTASSIUM CHROMATE see III:PLB250
DIPOTASSIUM DICHROMATE see III:PKX250
DIPOTASSIUM MONOCHROMATE see III:PLB250
DIPOTASSIUM NICKEL TETRACYANIDE see II:NDI000
DIPOTASSIUM TETRACYANONICKELATE see II:NDI000
DIPRON see III:SNM500
DI-2-PROPENYL ESTER, 1,2-BENZENEDICARBOXYLIC
    ACID see II:DBL200
DIPROPIONATE d′OESTRADIOL (FRENCH) see I:EDR000
DIPROPIONATO de ESTILBENE (SPANISH) see I:DKB000
p,p′-DIPROPIONOXY-trans-α,β-DIETHYLSTILBENE see
    I:DKB000
4-(DI-N-PROPYLAMINO)-3,5-DINITRO-1-TRIFLUORO-
    METHYLBENZENE see III:DUV600
DIPROPYLCARBAMIC ACID ETHYL ESTER see III:DWT400
DIPROPYLDIAZENE 1-OXIDE see III:ASP500
9,10-DI-n-PROPYL-9-10-DIHYDROXY-9,10-DIHYDRO-1,-
    2,5,6-DIBENZANTHRACENE see III:DLK600
N,N-DI-N-PROPYL-2,6-DINITRO-4-TRIFLUOROMETHYL-
    ANILINE see III:DUV600
N,N-DI-n-PROPYL ETHYL CARBAMATE see III:DWT400
DI-n-PROPYL MALEATE-ISOSAFROLE CONDENSATE see
    III:PNP250
DI-n-PROPYL 6,7-METHYLENEDIOXY-3-METHYL-1,2,3,4-
    TETRAHYDRONAPHTHALENE see III:PNP250
DI-n-PROPYL-3-METHYL-6,7-METHYLENEDIOXY-1,2,3,4-
    TETRAHYDRONAPHTHALENE-1,2-DICARBOXYLATE see
    III:PNP250
DI-n-PROPYLNITROSAMINE see I:NKB700
α-DIPROPYLNITROSAMINE METHYL ETHER see
    III:DWU800
DIPROPYLNITROSOAMINE see I:NKB700
DIPROPYL-5,6,7,8-TETRAHYDRO-7-
    METHYLNAPHTHO(2,3-d)-1,3-DIOXOLE-5,6-DICARBOX-
    YLATE see III:PNP250
N,N-DIPROPYL-4-TRIFLUOROMETHYL-2,6-DINITROANI-
    LINE see III:DUV600
DIPROSTRON see I:EDR000
DIPTERAX see III:TIQ250
DIPTEREX see III:TIQ250

DIPTEREX 50 see III:TIQ250
DIPTEVUR see III:TIQ250
DIPYRIDO(2,3-D,2,3-K)PYRENE see III:NAU500
DIPYRIDO(1,2-a:3′,2′-d)IMIDAZOL-2-AMINE see
  II:DWW700
DIPYRIDO(1,2-a:3′,2′-d)IMIDAZOLE, 2-AMINO-, HYDRO-
  CHLORIDE see III:AJS225
DIPYRIDO(1,2-a:3′,2′-d)IMIDAZOLE, 2-AMINO-6-METHYL-,
  HYDROCHLORIDE see III:AKS275
DIPYRIDO(2,3-d,2,3-1)PYRENE see III:NAU000
2,2′-DIPYRIDYL see III:BGO500
α,α′-DIPYRIDYL see III:BGO500
DIPYRIN see III:DOT000
cis-DIPYRROLIDINEDICHLOROPLATINUM(II) see
  III:DEU200
DIRAX see III:AQN635
DIRECT BLACK A see I:AQP000
DIRECT BLACK META see I:AQP000
DIRECT BLUE 6 see I:CMO000
DIRECT BLUE 14 see II:CMO250
DIRECT BROWN 95 see II:CMO750
DIRECT BROWN BR see III:PEY000
DIRECT FAST VIOLET N see III:CMP000
DIRECT VIOLET C see III:CMP000
DIREKTAN see III:NCQ900
DIREX 4L see III:DXQ500
DIRIDONE see I:PDC250, III:PEK250
DIROX see II:HIM000
DISETIL see III:DXH250
DISFLAMOLL TOF see III:TNI250
DISILYN see III:BEN000
DISODIUM ARSENATE see I:ARC000
DISODIUM ARSENATE, HEPTAHYDRATE see I:ARC250
DISODIUM ARSENIC ACID see I:ARC000
DISODIUM DICHROMATE see I:SGI000
DISODIUM DIFLUORIDE see III:SHF500
DISODIUM (2,4-DIMETHYLPHENYLAZO)-2-HYDROXY-
  NAPHTHALENE-3,6-DISULFONATE see III:FMU070
DISODIUM (2,4-DIMETHYLPHENYLAZO)-2-HYDROXY-
  NAPHTHALENE-3,6-DISULPHONATE see III:FMU070
DISODIUM EOSIN see III:BNH500
DISODIUM HYDROGEN ARSENATE see I:ARC000
DISODIUM HYDROGEN ORTHOARSENATE see I:ARC000
DISODIUM-6-HYDROXY-3-OXO-9-XANTHENE-o-BEN-
  ZOATE see III:FEW000
DISODIUM 3-HYDROXY-4-((2,4,5-TRIMETHYLPHE-
  NYL)AZO)-2,7-NAPHTHALENEDISULFONATE see
  II:FAG018
DISODIUM 3-HYDROXY-4-((2,4,5-TRIMETHYLPHE-
  NYL)AZO)-2,7-NAPHTHALENEDISULFONIC ACID see
  II:FAG018
DISODIUM 3-HYDROXY-4-((2,4,5-TRIMETHYLPHE-
  NYL)AZO)-2,7-NAPHTHALENEDISULPHONATE see
  II:FAG018
DISODIUM 3-HYDROXY-4-((2,4,5-TRIMETHYLPHE-
  NYL)AZO)-2,7-NAPHTHALENEDISULPHONIC ACID see
  II:FAG018
DISODIUM INDIGO-5,5-DISULFONATE see III:FAE100
DISODIUM METHANEARSENATE see I:DXE600
DISODIUM METHANEARSONATE see I:DXE600
DISODIUM METHYLARSENATE see I:DXE600
DISODIUM METHYLARSONATE see I:DXE600
DISODIUM MONOHYDROGEN ARSENATE see I:ARC000
DISODIUM MONOMETHYLARSONATE see I:DXE600
DISODIUM SALT of 1-INDIGOTIN-S,S′-DISULPHONIC ACID
  see III:FAE100
DISODIUM SALT of 2-(4-SULPHO-1-NAPHTHYLAZO)-1-
  NAPHTHOL-4-SULPHONIC ACID see III:HJF500
DISODIUM SALT of 1-(2,4-XYLYLAZO)-2-NAPHTHOL-3,6-DI-
  SULFONIC ACID see III:FMU070
DISODIUM SALT of 1-(2,4-XYLYLAZO)-2-NAPHTHOL-3,6-DI-
  SULPHONIC ACID see III:FMU070
DISODIUM SELENATE see III:DXG000
DISODIUM SELENITE see III:SJT500

DISODIUM 2-(4-SULFO-1-NAPHTHYLAZO)-1-NAPHTHOL-4-
  SULFONATE see III:HJF500
DISODIUM 2-(4-SULPHO-1-NAPHTHYLAZO)-1-NAPHTHOL-
  4-SULPHONATE see III:HJF500
DISOLFURO DI TETRAMETILTIOURAME (ITALIAN) see
  III:TFS350
DISOMAR see I:DXE600
2,4-D ISOOCTYL ESTER see III:ILO000
2,4-D ISOPROPYL ESTER see III:IOY000
DISPAL see III:AHE250
DISPASOL M see III:PKB500
DISPERSE BLUE NO 1 see III:TBG700
DISPERSED BLUE 12195 see III:FAE000
DISPERSED VIOLET 12197 see II:FAG120
DISPERSE ORANGE see I:AKP750
DISPERSOL YELLOW PP see III:PEJ500
DISSOLVANT APV see III:DJD600
DISTAVAL see III:TEH500
DISTAXAL see III:TEH500
DISTHENE see III:AHF500
DISTILBENE see I:DKA600, I:DKB000
DISTILLATES (PETROLEUM), ACID-TREATED HEAVY
  NAPHTHENIC (9CI) see I:MQV760
DISTILLATES (PETROLEUM), ACID-TREATED HEAVY
  PARAFFINIC (9CI) see I:MQV765
DISTILLATES (PETROLEUM), ACID-TREATED LIGHT
  NAPHTHENIC (9CI) see I:MQV770
DISTILLATES (PETROLEUM), ACID-TREATED LIGHT
  PARAFFINIC (9CI) see I:MQV775
DISTILLATES (PETROLEUM), HEAVY NAPHTHENIC (9CI)
  see I:MQV780
DISTILLATES (PETROLEUM), HEAVY PARAFFINIC (9CI) see
  I:MQV785
DISTILLATES (PETROLEUM), HYDROTREATED HEAVY
  NAPHTHENIC (9CI) see I:MQV790
DISTILLATES (PETROLEUM), HYDROTREATED HEAVY
  PARAFFINIC (9CI) see I:MQV795
DISTILLATES (PETROLEUM), HYDROTREATED LIGHT
  NAPHTHENIC (9CI) see I:MQV800
DISTILLATES (PETROLEUM), HYDROTREATED LIGHT
  PARAFFINIC (9CI) see I:MQV805
DISTILLATES (PETROLEUM), LIGHT NAPHTHENIC (9CI) see
  I:MQV810
DISTILLATES (PETROLEUM), LIGHT PARAFFINIC (9CI) see
  I:MQV815
DISTILLATES (PETROLEUM), SOLVENT-DEWAXED HEAVY
  NAPHTHENIC (9CI) see III:MQV820
DISTILLATES (PETROLEUM), SOLVENT-DEWAXED HEAVY
  PARAFFINIC (9CI) see III:MQV825
DISTILLATES (PETROLEUM), SOLVENT-DEWAXED LIGHT
  NAPHTHENIC (9CI) see I:MQV835
DISTILLATES (PETROLEUM), SOLVENT-DEWAXED LIGHT
  PARAFFINIC (9CI) see I:MQV840
DISTILLATES (PETROLEUM), SOLVENT-REFINED HEAVY
  NAPHTHENIC (9CI) see III:MQV845
DISTILLATES (PETROLEUM), SOLVENT-REFINED HEAVY
  PARAFFINIC (9CI) see III:MQV850
DISTILLATES (PETROLEUM), SOLVENT-REFINED LIGHT
  NAPHTHENIC (9CI) see I:MQV852
DISTILLATES (PETROLEUM), SOLVENT-REFINED LIGHT
  PARAFFINIC (9CI) see I:MQV855
DISTILLED LIME OIL see III:OGO000
DISTILLED MUSTARD see I:BIH250
DISTOKAL see III:HCI000
DISTOPAN see III:HCI000
DISTOPIN see III:HCI000
DISTOVAL see III:TEH500
1,3-DI(4-SULFAMOYLPHENYL)TRIAZENE see III:THQ900
DISULFAN see III:DXH250
DISULFIRAM see III:DXH250
DISULFIRAM mixed with SODIUM NITRITE see III:SIS200
DISULFURAM see III:DXH250
DISULFURE de TETRAMETHYLTHIOURAME (FRENCH) see
  III:TFS350

DOLKWAL INDIGO CARMINE see III:FAE100
DOLKWAL ORANGE SS see II:TGW000
DOLKWAL PONCEAU 3R see II:FAG018
DOLKWAL YELLOW AB see III:FAG130
DOLKWAL YELLOW OB see III:FAG135
DOLMIX see I:BBQ750
DOLOCHLOR see III:CKN500
DOLONIL see I:PDC250
DOMALIUM see III:DCK759
DOMATOL see I:AMY050
DOMESTROL see I:DKA600
DOMOSO see III:DUD800
DOP see I:DVL700
(−)-DOPA see III:DNA200
l-DOPA see III:DNA200
DOPAFLEX see III:DNA200
DOPAL see III:DNA200
DOPARKINE see III:DNA200
DOPASOL see III:DNA200
DOPN see II:NJN000
DOPRIN see III:DNA200
DORBANE see III:DMH400
DORBANEX see III:DMH400
DORCOSTRIN see III:DAQ800
DORLYL see III:PKQ059
DORMAL see III:CDO000
DORMINA see II:EOK000
DORMIRAL see II:EOK000
DORMONE see II:DAA800
DORSULFAN see III:SNN500
DORVICIDE A see II:BGJ750
DORVON see III:SMQ500
DOSCALUN see II:EOK000
DOTMENT 324 see III:AHE250
DOUBLE STRENGTH see II:TIX500
DOW 209 see III:SMR000
DOW 860 see III:SMQ500
DOWCHLOR see II:CDR750
DOWCIDE 1 see III:BGJ250
DOWCIDE 7 see II:PAX250
DOWCIDE 1 ANTIMICROBIAL see III:BGJ250
DOWCO 139 see III:DOS000
DOW CORNING 346 see III:PJR000
DOW-CORNING 200 FLUID-LOT No. AA-4163 see
   III:DUB600
DOWFLAKE see III:CAO750
DOWFUME see III:MHR200
DOWFUME 40 see I:EIY500
DOWFUME EDB see I:EIY500
DOWFUME MC-2 SOIL FUMIGANT see III:MHR200
DOWFUME W-8 see I:EIY500
DOW GENERAL see III:BRE500
DOW GENERAL WEED KILLER see III:BRE500
DOWICIDE see II:BGJ750
DOWICIDE 2 see II:TIV750
DOWICIDE 6 see II:TBT000
DOWICIDE 7 see II:PAX250
DOWICIDE 2S see I:TIW000
DOWICIDE B see II:TIV750
DOWICIDE EC-7 see II:PAX250
DOWICIDE G see II:PAX250
DOW LATEX 612 see III:SMR000
DOWLEX see III:PKF750
DOW MCP AMINE WEED KILLER see II:CIR250
DOW PENTACHLOROPHENOL DP-2 ANTIMICROBIAL see
   II:PAX250
DOW-PER see II:PCF275
DOW SEED DISINFECTANT No. 5 see III:TBO500
DOW SELECTIVE WEED KILLER see III:BRE500
DOW SODIUM TCA INHIBITED see III:TII250
DOWTHERM E see III:DEP600
DOW-TRI see II:TIO750
DOX HYDROCHLORIDE see III:HKA300
DOXO see III:DAQ800

DOXORUBICIN see I:AES750, III:HKA300
DOXORUBICIN HYDROCHLORIDE see III:HKA300
DOXYFED see III:MDT600
DOZAR see III:DPJ400
2,4-DP see II:DGB000
2-(2,4-DP) see II:DGB000
DPA see III:HET500
DPBS see III:DFY400
DPH see I:DKQ000, I:DNU000
DPMA see III:DMB200
DPN see I:NKB700
DPNA see I:NKB700
DPP see III:PAK000, III:PEK250
DPPD see III:BLE500
DRAKEOL see III:MQV750
DRALZINE see II:HGP500
DREWMULSE POE-SMO see III:PKL100
DREXEL see III:DXQ500
DREXEL DIURON 4L see III:DXQ500
DREXEL DSMA LIQUID see I:DXE600
DREXEL METHYL PARATHION 4E see III:MNH000
DREXEL PARATHION 8E see III:PAK000
DRI-DIE INSECTICIDE 67 see III:SCH000
DRI-KIL see III:RNZ000
DRILL TOX-SPEZIAL AGLUKON see I:BBQ500
DRINALFA see III:MDT600
DRINOX see II:HAR000, III:AFK250
DROMISOL see III:DUD800
DROPCILLIN see III:BDY669
DROXOLAN see III:DAQ400
DRP 859025 see III:TND500
DRUPINA 90 see III:BJK500
DRY AND CLEAR see III:BDS000
DS-M-1 see III:DBD750
DSMA LIQUID see I:DXE600
DSPT see III:THQ900
DSS see III:SOA500
DST 50 see III:SMR000
DTBP see III:BSC750
DTIC see II:DAB600
DTIC-DOME see II:DAB600
DTMC see III:BIO750
DUATOK see III:TEX250
DUBRONAX see III:SOA500
DUKERON see II:TIO750
DUKSEN see III:DCK759
DULCIDOR see III:GFA000
DULCINE see III:EFE000
DULL 704 see III:PJY500
DULZOR-ETAS see III:SGC000
DUMITONE see III:SOA500
DUMOGRAN see III:MPN500
DUNERYL see II:EOK000
DUNKELGELB see III:PEJ500
DUODECANE see III:DXT200
DUODECYL ALCOHOL see III:DXV600
DUODECYLIC ACID see III:LBL000
DUOLAX see III:DMH400
DUOLUTON see III:NNL500
DURA CLOFIBRAT see III:ARQ750
DURA-ESTRADIOL see II:EDS100
DURAFUR BLACK R see III:PEY500
DURAFUR BLACK RC see III:PEY650
DURAFUR BROWN see II:ALL750
DURAFUR BROWN 2R see II:ALL750
DURAFUR BROWN MN see I:DBO400
DURAFUR DEVELOPER C see III:CCP850
DURAFUR DEVELOPER G see III:REA000
DURALUTON see III:HNT500
DURAN see III:DXQ500
DURANATE EXP-D 101 see III:PKO750
DURANIT see III:SMR000
DURANOL BRILLIANT BLUE CB see III:TBG700
DURANOL ORANGE G see I:AKP750

DURASORB see III:DUD800
DURAX see III:CPI250
DURETHAN BK see III:PJY500
DURETTER see III:FBN100
DURFAX 80 see III:PKL100
DUROFERON see III:FBN100
DUROFOL P see III:PKQ059
DUROID 5870 see III:TAI250
DUROTOX see II:PAX250
DUSICNAN KADEMNATY (CZECH) see I:CAH250
DUSITAN DICYKLOHEXYLAMINU (CZECH) see
    III:DGU200
DUSITAN SODNY (CZECH) see III:SIQ500
DUSOLINE see III:CMD750
DUSORAN see III:CMD750
DU-SPREX see III:DER800
DUST M see III:RAF100
DUTCH LIQUID see I:EIY600
DUTCH OIL see I:EIY600
DUTCH-TREAT see I:HKC500
DUXEN see III:DCK759
DV see II:DAL600
DV 400 see III:PKB500
DWUBROMOETAN (POLISH) see I:EIY500
DWUCHLORODWUETYLOWY ETER (POLISH) see
    III:DFJ050
2,4-DWUCHLOROFENOKSYOCTOSY KWAS (POLISH) see
    II:DAA800
DWUCHLOROPROPAN (POLISH) see III:PNJ400
symetryczna DWUMETYLOHYDRAZYNA (POLISH) see
    I:DSF600
DWUMETYLOWY SIARCZAN (POLISH) see I:DUD100
DWU-β-NAFTYLO-p-FENYLODWUAMINA (POLISH) see
    III:NBL000
DWUNITROBENZEN (POLISH) see II:DUQ200
3,3'-DWUOKSYBENZYDYNA (POLISH) see II:DMI400
DWUSIARCZEK DWUBENZOTIAZYLU (POLISH) see
    III:BDE750
DX see I:AES750
DYE EVANS BLUE see III:BGT250
DYE FD AND C RED No. 4 see III:FAG050
DYE FDC RED 2 see III:FAG020
DYE FD&C RED No. 3 see III:FAG040
DYE FD & C RED No. 4 see III:FAG050
DYE GS see II:ALL750
DYE ORANGE No. 1 see III:FAG010
DYE RED RASPBERRY see III:FAG020
DYESTROL see I:DKA600
DYKANOL see I:PJL750
DYKOL see I:DAD200
DYLENE see III:SMQ500
DYLITE F 40 see III:SMQ500
DYLOX see III:TIQ250
DYLOX-METASYSTOX-R see III:TIQ250
DYMADON see II:HIM000
DYNADUR see III:PKQ059
DYNASTEN see I:PAN100
DYNAZONE see II:NGE500
DYNEL see III:ADY250
DYNERIC see III:CMX700
DYNEX see III:DXQ500
DYP-97 F see III:LBR000
DYREX see III:TIQ250
DYTHOL see III:CMD750
DYTOL S-91 see III:DAI600
DYTOL E-46 see III:OAX000
DYTOL J-68 see III:DXV600
DYVON see III:TIQ250

E^1 see I:EDV000
E^2 see I:EDO000
E6 see I:PKO500
E 62 see III:PKQ059
E 127 see III:FAG040

E 132 see III:FAE100
E 605 see III:PAK000
E 66P see III:PKQ059
E 3314 see II:HAR000
EA 3547 see III:DDE200
EAB see III:EOH500
EAMN see III:ENR500
EARTHCIDE see III:PAX000
EARTHNUT OIL see III:PAO000
EASTBOND M 5 see III:PMP500
EB see III:BGT250
EBIDENE see III:ILD000
EBNA see III:NKD500
EBNS see III:EHC800
EBS see III:FAG040
EBZ see I:EDP000
ECATOX see III:PAK000
ECH see I:EAZ500
ECLORIL see I:CDO500
ECOBUTAZONE see II:BRF500
ECONOCHLOR see III:CDP250
ECPN see III:NKE000
ECTILURAN see III:TEH500
EDA see III:DCN800
EDB see I:EIY500
EDB-85 see I:EIY500
E-D-BEE see I:EIY500
EDC see I:EIY600
EDCO see III:MHR200
EDICOL AMARANTH see III:FAG020
EDICOL BLUE CL 2 see III:FAE000
EDICOL PONCEAU RS see III:FMU070
EDICOL SUPRA BLUE E6 see III:FMU059
EDICOL SUPRA CARMOISINE WS see III:HJF500
EDICOL SUPRA ERYTHROSINE A see III:FAG040
EDICOL SUPRA PONCEAU 4R see III:FMU080
EDICOL SUPRA PONCEAU SX see III:FAG050
EDICOL SUPRA ROSE B see III:FAG070
EDISTIR RB 268 see III:SMR000
EDIWAL see III:NNL500
EDROFURADENE see III:EAE500
EENA see II:ELG500
EFACIN see III:NCQ900
EFFEMOLL DOA see III:AEO000
EFFLUDERM (FREE BASE) see III:FMM000
EFH see III:EKL250
EFLORAN see I:MMN250
EFROXINE see III:MDT600
EFUDEX see III:FMM000
EFUDIX see III:FMM000
EGACID ORANGE GG see III:FAG010
EGITOL see III:HCI000
EH 121 see III:TNX000
EHBN see III:ELE500
EHEN see II:ELG500
EHTYLHEXYL PHTHALATE see I:DVL700
EI see I:EJM900
EI-12880 see III:DSP400
EI 38,555 see III:CMF400
EICOSANOIC ACID see III:EAF000
EINALON S see III:CLY500
EISENDEXTRAN (GERMAN) see I:IGS000
EISENDIMETHYLDITHIOCARBAMAT (GERMAN) see
    III:FAS000
EISEN-III-HYDROXID-POLYMALTOSE (GERMAN) see
    III:IHA000
EISENOXYD see III:IHD000
EISEN(III)-TRIS(N,N-DIMETHYLDITHIOCARBAMAT) (GER-
    MAN) see III:FAS000
EKAGOM TB see III:TFS350
EKAGOM TEDS see III:DXH250
EKATIN WF & WF ULV see III:PAK000
EKATOX see III:PAK000
EKAVYL SD 2 see III:PKQ059

EK 1108GY-A see III:TAI250
EKKO CAPSULES see I:DKQ000
EL 4049 see III:MAK700
ELAIOMYCIN see III:EAG000
ELANCOLAN see III:DUV600
ELASIOMYCIN see III:EAG500
ELASTOPAR see III:MJG750
ELASTOPAX see III:MJG750
ELBANIL see III:CKC000
ELCIDE 75 see III:MDI000
ELCORIL see I:CDO500
ELCOZINE CHRYSOIDINE Y see III:PEK000
ELCOZINE RHODAMINE B see III:FAG070
ELDEZOL see II:NGE500
ELDIATRIC C see III:CAK500
ELDOPAL see III:DNA200
ELDOPAQUE see III:HIH000
ELDOQUIN see III:HIH000
ELDRIN see III:RSU000
ELECTRO-CF 22 see III:CFX500
ELECTROCORUNDUM see III:EAL100
ELEMENTAL SELENIUM see III:SBO500
ELEPSINDON see I:DKQ000
ELESTOL see III:CLD000
ELEUDRON see III:TEX250
ELGACID ORANGE 2G see III:FAG010
ELGETOL see III:BRE500
ELGETOL 318 see III:BRE500
ELICIDE see III:MDI000
ELJON LAKE RED C see III:CHP500
ELMASIL see I:AMY050
ELMEDAL see II:BRF500
ELOBROMOL see III:DDJ000
ELPI see III:ARQ750
ELPON see III:PMP500
ELVACITE see III:PKB500
ELVANOL see III:PKP750
ELYZOL see I:MMN250
EM 923 see III:DFY400
EMANIL see III:DAS000
EMAZOL RED B see III:EAJ500
EMBACETIN see II:CDP250
EMBAFUME see III:MHR200
EMBANOX see II:BQI000
EMBECHINE see I:BIE500
EMBICHIN see I:BIE250, I:BIE500
EMBICHIN HYDROCHLORIDE see I:BIE500
EMBIKHINE see I:BIE500
EMCEPAN see II:CIR250
EMEREST 2301 see III:OHW000
EMEREST 2801 see III:OHW000
EMERSOL 120 see III:SLK000
EMERSOL 140 see III:PAE250
EMERSOL 143 see III:PAE250
EMERSOL 210 see III:OHU000
EMERSOL 213 see III:OHU000
EMERSOL 6321 see III:OHU000
EMERSOL 233LL see III:OHU000
EMERSOL 221 LOW TITER WHITE OLEIC ACID see
  III:OHU000
EMERSOL 220 WHITE OLEIC ACID see III:OHU000
EMERY see III:EAL100
EMERY 2218 see III:MJW000
EMERY 2219 see III:OHW000
EMERY 2310 see III:OHW000
EMERY OLEIC ACID ESTER 2301 see III:OHW000
EMETREN see II:CDP250
EMISOL see I:AMY050
EMMATOS see III:MAK700
EMMATOS EXTRA see III:MAK700
EMPAL see II:CIR250
EMPIRIN COMPOUND see I:ABG750, III:ARP250
EMS see II:EMF500
EMSORB 2515 see III:SKV000

EMSORB 6900 see III:PKL100
EMT 25,299 see III:MDV500
EMTAL 596 see III:TAB750
EMTEXATE see III:MDV500
EMTRYL see III:DSV800
EMTRYLVET see III:DSV800
EMTRYMIX see III:DSV800
EMULSAMINE BK see II:DAA800
EMULSAMINE E-3 see II:DAA800
EMULSION 212 see III:FQU875
EN 237 see III:EAL100
ENAMEL WHITE see III:BAP000
ENARMON see I:TBG000
ENAVID see I:EAP000
ENBU see III:ENT000
ENC see III:ENT500
ENCEPHALARTOS HILDEBRANDTII see III:EAQ000
ENCORTON see III:PLZ000
ENDOCEL see III:EAQ750
ENDOFOLLICOLINA D.P. see I:EDR000
ENDOFOLLICULINA see I:EDV000
ENDOSOL see III:EAQ750
ENDOSULFAN see III:EAQ750
ENDOSULPHAN see III:EAQ750
ENDOXAN see I:EAS500
ENDOXANA see I:CQC675
ENDOXANAL see I:EAS500
ENDOXAN-ASTA see I:CQC675, I:EAS500
ENDOXAN MONOHYDRATE see I:CQC675
ENDOXAN R see I:CQC675, I:EAS500
ENDREX see III:EAT500
ENDRIN see III:EAT500
ENDRINE (FRENCH) see III:EAT500
ENDURONYL see III:RDF000
ENDUXAN see I:CQC675
ENELFA see II:HIM000
ENERIL see II:HIM000
ENFLURANE see III:EAT900
ENGLISH RED see III:IHD000
ENHEPTIN see III:ALQ000
ENIACID BRILLIANT RUBINE 3B see III:HJF500
ENIACID LIGHT ORANGE G see III:HGC000
ENIACID ORANGE I see III:FAG010
ENIAL ORANGE I see III:PEJ500
ENIAL YELLOW 2G see I:DOT300
ENIANIL BLACK CN see I:AQP000
ENIANIL BLUE 2BN see I:CMO000
ENICOL see II:CDP250
ENIDREL see I:EAP000, III:CFZ000
ENJAY CD 460 see III:PMP500
ENKALON see III:NOH000
ENKEFAL see I:DNU000
ENKELFEL see I:DKQ000
ENNG see III:ENU000
ENOVID see I:EAP000
ENOVID-E see I:EAP000
ENPROMATE see III:DWL400
ENS see III:EPI300
ENSOBARB see II:EOK000
ENSODORM see II:EOK000
ENSURE see III:EAQ750
17-ENT see II:ABU000
ENT 54 see I:ADX500
ENT 133 see III:RNZ000
ENT 988 see III:BJK500
ENT 1,122 see III:BRE500
ENT 1,506 see I:DAD200
ENT 1,656 see I:EIY600
ENT 1,716 see II:MEI450
ENT 1,860 see II:PCF275
ENT 3,776 see III:DFT000
ENT 3,797 see III:TBO500
ENT 4,225 see I:BIM500
ENT 4,504 see III:DFJ050

ENT 4,705 see CBY000
ENT 7,796 see I:BBQ500
ENT 8,538 see II:DAA800
ENT 8,601 see I:BBP750
ENT 9,232 see I:BBQ000
ENT 9,233 see I:BBR000
ENT 9,735 see I:CDV100
ENT 9,932 see II:CDR750
ENT 14,250 see III:PIX250
ENT 14,611 see III:ASL250
ENT 14,689 see III:FAS000
ENT 14,874 see III:EIR000
ENT 14,875 see III:MAS500
ENT 15,108 see III:PAK000
ENT 15,152 see II:HAR000
ENT 15,266 see III:PNP250
ENT 15,349 see I:EIY500
ENT 15,406 see III:PNJ400
ENT 15,949 see III:AFK250
ENT 16,225 see III:DHB400
ENT 16,358 see III:CJT750
ENT 16,391 see I:KEA000
ENT 16,436 see III:DXX400
ENT 16,519 see I:SOP500
ENT 16,634 see III:ISA000
ENT 17,034 see III:MAK700
ENT 17,251 see III:EAT500
ENT 17,292 see III:MNH000
ENT 18,060 see III:CKC000
ENT 18,596 see II:DER000
ENT 18,870 see III:DMC600
ENT 19,060 see III:DSK200
ENT 19,442 see III:TBC500
ENT 19,763 see III:TIQ250
ENT 23,233 see III:ASH500
ENT 23,648 see III:BIO750
ENT 23,969 see III:CBM750
ENT 23,979 see III:EAQ750
ENT 24,650 see III:DSP400
ENT 24,727 see III:AQT500
ENT 24,915 see III:TND250
ENT 25,208 see III:ABX250
ENT 25,294 see I:BIE250
ENT 25,296 see III:TND500
ENT 25,445 see I:AMY050
ENT 25,515 see III:FAC025
ENT 25,540 see III:FAQ999
ENT 25,545 see III:OAN000
ENT 25,550 see III:SCH000
ENT 25,584 see II:EBW500
ENT 25,719 see I:MQW500
ENT 25,766 see III:DOS000
ENT 25,841 see III:RAF100
ENT 26,079 see III:AMG750
ENT 26,263 see I:EJN500
ENT 26,396 see II:EMF500
ENT 26,538 see III:CBG000
ENT 26,592 see I:BGA750
ENT 27,335 see III:CJJ250
ENT 27,567 see III:CJJ250
ENT 50,003 see III:TNK250
ENT 50,146 see II:RDK000
ENT 50,324 see I:EJM900
ENT 50,439 see II:BIA250
ENT 50,852 see III:HEJ500
ENT 50,882 see I:HEK000
ENTEROMYCETIN see II:CDP250
ENTEROSEDIV see III:TEH500
ENTEROTOXON see III:NGG500
ENTEX see III:FAQ999
ENTIZOL see I:MMN250
ENTOMOXAN see I:BBQ500
ENTRAMIN see III:ALQ000
ENTUSIL see III:SNN500

ENT 25,545-X see III:OAN000
ENT 25,552-X see II:CDR750
ENU see I:ENV000, III:NKE500
ENVERT 171 see II:DAA800
ENVERT DT see II:DAA800
ENVERT-T see II:TAA100
E.O. see I:EJN500
EOSIN see III:BMO250, III:BNK700
EOSINE see III:BMO250, III:BNH500
EOSINE B see III:BNK700
EOSINE FA see III:BNK700
EOSINE LAKE RED Y see III:BNK700
EOSINE SODIUM SALT see III:BNH500
EOSINE YELLOWISH see III:BNH500
EOSIN GELBLICH (GERMAN) see III:BNH500
EP 30 see II:PAX250
EP 201 see III:ECB000
EP-205 see III:BJN250
EP-206 see I:VOA000
EP-333 see III:CJJ250
EP-411 see III:PFC750
EPAL 10 see III:DAI600
EPAL 12 see III:DXV600
E-PAM see III:DCK759
EPAMIN see I:DKQ000, I:DNU000
EPANAL see II:EOK000
EPANUTIN see I:DKQ000, I:DNU000
EPASMIR '5' see I:DKQ000
EPC (the plant regulator) see III:CBL750
EPDANTOINE SIMPLE see I:DKQ000
EPELIN see I:DKQ000, I:DNU000
EPHIRSULPHONATE see III:CJT750
EPHORRAN see III:DXH250
EPIB see III:ARQ750
EPIBLOC see III:CDT750
EPICHLOORHYDRINE (DUTCH) see I:EAZ500
EPICHLORHYDRIN (GERMAN) see I:EAZ500
EPICHLORHYDRINE (FRENCH) see I:EAZ500
EPICHLOROHYDRIN see I:EAZ500
α-EPICHLOROHYDRIN see I:EAZ500
(dl)-α-EPICHLOROHYDRIN see I:EAZ500
EPICHLOROHYDRYNA (POLISH) see I:EAZ500
EPICHLOROPHYDRIN see I:EAZ500
EPI-CLEAR see III:BDS000
EPICLORIDRINA (ITALIAN) see I:EAZ500
EPICURE DDM see I:MJQ000
3,17-EPIDIHYDROXYESTRATRIENE see I:EDO000
3,17-EPIDIHYDROXYOESTRATRIENE see I:EDO000
EPIDORM see II:EOK000
EPIFENYL see I:DKQ000, I:DNU000
EPIHYDAN see I:DKQ000, I:DNU000
EPIHYDRINALDEHYDE see GGW000
EPIHYDRINE ALDEHYDE see GGW000
EPILAN see I:DKQ000
EPILAN-D see I:DNU000
EPILANTIN see I:DKQ000, I:DNU000
EPILOL see II:EOK000
EPINAT see I:DKQ000, I:DNU000
EPI-REZ 508 see III:BLD750
EPI-REZ 510 see III:BLD750
EPI-REZ 508 mixed with ERR 4205 (1:1) see III:OPI200
EPISED see I:DKQ000
EPISEDAL see II:EOK000
EPODYL see III:TJQ333
EPOLENE M 5K see III:PMP500
EPON 828 see III:BLD750
EPON 828 mixed with ERR 4205 (1:1) see III:OPI200
EPORAL see III:SOA500
EPOXIDE-201 see III:ECB000
EPOXIDE 269 see III:LFV000
EPOXIDE A see III:BLD750
1,2-EPOXYAETHAN (GERMAN) see I:EJN500
(E)-1-α-2-α-EPOXYBENZ(c)ACRIDINE-3-α-4-β-DIOL see
    III:EBH850

(Z)-1-β,2-β-EPOXYBENZ(c)ACRIDINE-3-α-4-β-DIOL see
    III:EBH875
1,2-EPOXYBUTANE see III:BOX750
1,2-EPOXYBUTENE-3 see III:EBJ500
3,4-EPOXY-1-BUTENE see III:EBJ500
2,3-EPOXYBUTYRIC ACID, ETHYL ESTER see III:EJS000
1,2-EPOXYBUTYRONITRILE see III:EBK500
3,4-EPOXYBUTYRONITRILE see III:EBK500
1,2-EPOXY-3-CHLOROPROPANE see I:EAZ500
5-α,6-α-EPOXYCHOLESTANOL see III:EBM000
5,6-α-EPOXY-5-α-CHOLESTAN-3-β-OL see III:EBM000
EPOXYCHOLESTEROL see III:EBM000
1,2-EPOXYCYCLOHEXANE see III:CPD000
5,6-EPOXY-5,6-DIHYDROBENZ(a)ANTHRACENE see
    III:EBP000
7,8-EPOXY-7,8-DIHYDROBENZO(a)PYRENE see III:BCV750
5,6-EPOXY-5,6-DIHYDROCHRYSENE see III:CML815
5,6-EPOXY-5,6-DIHYDRODIBENZ(a,h)ANTHRACENE see
    III:EBP500
15,20-EPOXY-15,30-DIHYDRO-12-HYDROXYSENECIONAN-
    11,16-DIONE see III:JAK000
5,6-EPOXY-5,6-DIHYDRO-7-METHYLBENZ(A) ANTHRA-
    CENE see III:MGZ000
11,12-EPOXY-11,12-DIHYDRO-3-METHYLCHOLANTHRENE
    see III:MIL500
9,10-EPOXY-9,10-DIHYDROPHENANTHRENE see
    III:PCX000
1,3-EPOXY-2,2-DIMETHYLPROPANE see III:EBQ500
1,2-EPOXYDODECANE see III:DXU400
1,2-EPOXY-4-(EPOXYETHYL)CYCLOHEXANE see
    I:VOA000
1,2-EPOXY-7,8-EPOXYOCTANE see III:DHD800
4,5-EPOXY-2-(2,3-EPOXYPROPYL)VALERIC ACID, METHYL
    ESTER see III:MJD000
EPOXYETHANE see I:EJN500
1,2-EPOXYETHANE see I:EJN500
7-(EPOXYETHYL)-BENZ(a)ANTHRACENE see III:ONC000
1,2-EPOXYETHYLBENZENE see II:EBR000
EPOXYETHYLBENZENE (8CI) see II:EBR000
α-EPOXYETHYL-1,3-BENZODIOXOLE-5-METHANOL see
    III:HOE500
1-EPOXYETHYL-3,4-EPOXYCYCLOHEXANE see I:VOA000
α-(EPOXYETHYL)-p-METHOXYBENZYL ALCOHOL see
    III:HKI075
3-(EPOXYETHYL)-7-OXABICYCLO(4.1.0)HEPTANE see
    I:VOA000
4-(EPOXYETHYL)-7-OXABICYCLO(4.1.0)HEPTANE see
    I:VOA000
3-(1,2-EPOXYETHYL)-7-OXABICYCLO(4.1.0)HEPTANE see
    I:VOA000
4-(1,2-EPOXYETHYL)-7-OXABICYCLO(4.1.0)HEPTANE see
    I:VOA000
1-EPOXYETHYLPYRENE see III:ONG000
EPOXYHEPTACHLOR see II:EBW500
1,2-EPOXYHEXADECANE see III:EBX500
4,5-EPOXY-3-HYDROXYVALERIC ACID-β-LACTONE see
    III:ECA000
11,12-EPOXY-3-METHYLCHOLANTHRENE see III:ECA500
3,4-EPOXY-6-METHYLCYCLOHEXENECARBOXYLIC ACID
    (3,4-EPOXY-6-METHYLCYCLOHEXYLMETHYL) ESTER
    see III:ECB000
3,4-EPOXY-6-METHYLCYCLOHEXYLMETHYL-3,4-EPOXY-
    6-METHYLCYCLOHEXANECARBOXYLATE see
    III:ECB000
4,5-EPOXY-2-METHYLCYCLOHEXYLMETHYL-4,5-EPOXY-
    2-METHYLCYCLOHEXANECARBOXYLATE see
    III:ECB000
3,4-EPOXY-6-METHYLCYCLOHEXYLMETHYL-3′,4′-
    EPOXY-6′-METHYLCYCLOHEXANE CARBOXYLATE see
    III:ECB000
4-(1,2-EPOXY-1-METHYLETHYL)-1-METHYL-7-
    OXABICYCLO(4.1.0)HEPTANE see III:LFV000
cis-9,10-EPOXYOCTADECANOATE see III:ECD500
cis-9,10-EPOXYOCTADECANOIC ACID see III:ECD500

9,10-EPOXYOCTADECANOIC ACID BUTYL ESTER see
    III:BRH250
1,2-EPOXYOCTANE see III:ECE000
EPOXYOLEIC ACID see III:ECD500
EPOXYPERCHLOROVINYL see III:TBQ275
1,2-EPOXY-3-PHENOXYPROPANE see II:PFH000
2,3-EPOXYPROPANAL see GGW000
2,3-EPOXY-1-PROPANAL see GGW000
EPOXYPROPANE see I:PNL600
1,2-EPOXYPROPANE see I:PNL600
2,3-EPOXYPROPANE see I:PNL600
2,3-EPOXY-1-PROPANOL OLEATE see III:ECJ000
2,3-EPOXY-1-PROPANOL STEARATE see III:SLK500
2,3-EPOXYPROPIONALDEHYDE see GGW000
2-(N-(2-(2,3-EPOXYPROPOXY)ETHYL)ANILINO)ETHANOL
    see III:MRI500
N-(4-(2,3-EPOXYPROPOXY)PHENYL)BENZYLAMINE see
    III:ECG500
p-(2,3-EPOXYPROPOXY)-N-PHENYLBENZYLAMINE see
    III:ECG500
2,3-EPOXYPROPYL CHLORIDE see I:EAZ500
2,3-EPOXYPROPYL ESTER of OLEIC ACID see III:ECJ000
2,3-EPOXYPROPYL ESTER of STEARIC ACID see III:SLK500
2,3-EPOXYPROPYL OLEATE see III:ECJ000
2,3-EPOXYPROPYLPHENYL ETHER see II:PFH000
2,3-EPOXYPROPYL STEARATE see III:SLK500
9,10-EPOXYSTEARIC ACID see III:ECD500
cis-9,10-EPOXYSTEARIC ACID see III:ECD500
EPOXYSTYRENE see II:EBR000
α,β-EPOXYSTYRENE see II:EBR000
3,4-EPOXYSULFOLANE see III:ECP000
cis-1-β,2-β-EPOXY-1,2,3,4-TETRAHYDROBENZO(c)
    PHENANTHRENE-3-α-4-β-DIOL see III:BCS103
trans-1-α-2-α-EPOXY-1,2,3,4-TETRAHYDROBENZO(c)
    PHENANTHRENE-3-α,4-β-DIOL see III:BCS105
trans-1-β,2-β-EPOXY-1,2,3,4-TETRAHYDROBENZO(c)
    PHENANTHRENE-3-β,4-α-DIOL see III:BCS110
9,10-EPOXY-7,8,9,10-TETRAHYDROBENZO(a)PYRENE see
    III:ECQ100
9,10-EPOXY-9,10,11,12-TETRAHYDROBENZO(e)PYRENE
    see III:ECQ150
3,4-EPOXY-1,2,3,4-TETRAHYDROCHRYSENE see
    III:ECQ200
(+)-(E)-3,4-EPOXY-1,2,3,4-TETRAHYDRO-CHRYSENEDIOL
    see III:DMS000
1,2-EPOXY-1,2,3,4-TETRAHYDROPHENANTHRENE see
    III:ECR259
3,4-EPOXY-1,2,3,4-TETRAHYDROPHENANTHRENE see
    III:ECR500
(±)-3-α,4-α-EPOXY-1,2,3,4-TETRAHYDRO-1-β,2-α-
    PHENANTHRENEDIOL see III:ECS000
2,3-EPOXYTETRAMETHYLENE SULFONE see III:ECP000
EPOXY-1,1,2-TRICHLOROETHANE see III:ECT600
EPRAZIN see III:POL500
EPSYLONE see II:EOK000
EPSYLON KAPROLAKTAM (POLISH) see III:CBF700
EPTAC 1 see III:BJK500
EPTACLORO (ITALIAN) see II:HAR000
1,4,5,6,7,8,8-EPTACLORO-3a,4,7,7a-TETRAIDRO-4,7-endo-
    METANO-INDENE (ITALIAN) see II:HAR000
EPTAL see I:DKQ000
EPTOIN see I:DKQ000, I:DNU000
E-PVC see III:PKQ059
EQUI BUTE see II:BRF500
EQUIGYNE see I:ECU750
EQUILENIN see III:ECV000
EQUILENINA (SPANISH) see III:ECV000
EQUILENIN BENZOATE see III:ECV500
EQUILENINE see III:ECV000
EQUILIN see III:ECW000
EQUILIN BENZOATE see III:ECW500
EQUINO-ACID see III:TIQ250
EQUINO-AID see III:TIQ250
ERALON see III:ILD000

ERASE see III:HKC000
ERASOL see I:BIE500
ERASOL HYDROCHLORIDE see I:BIE500
ERASOL-IDO see I:BIE500
ERBAPLAST see II:CDP250
ERBAPRELINA see III:TGD000
ERE 1359 see II:REF000
ERGOMETRINE ACID MALEATE see III:EDB500
ERGOMETRINE MALEATE see III:EDB500
ERGONOVINE, MALEATE (1:1) (SALT) see III:EDB500
ERGOPLAST AdDO see III:AEO000
ERGOPLAST FDO see I:DVL700
ERGOT see III:EDB500
ERGOTRATE see III:EDB500
ERGOTRATE MALEATE see III:EDB500
ERIBUTAZONE see II:BRF500
ERIDAN see III:DCK759
ERIE BLACK B see I:AQP000
ERIE VIOLET 3R see III:CMP000
ERINITRIT see III:SIQ500
ERIO FAST ORANGE AS see III:HGC000
ERIO FAST YELLOW AEN see III:SGP500
ERIOGLAUCINE see III:FMU059
ERIOGLAUCINE G see III:FAE000
ERIONITE (CaKNa (Al$_2$Si$_7$O$_{18}$)$_2$•14H$_2$O) see I:EDC650
ERIOSIN RHODAMINE B see III:FAG070
ERIOSKY BLUE see III:FMU059
ERL-2774 see III:BLD750
ERLA-2270 see I:VOA000
ERLA-2271 see I:VOA000
ERR 4205 see III:BJN250
ERR 4205 mixed with ARALDITE 6010 (1:1) see III:OPI200
ERR 4205 mixed with EPI-REZ 508 (1:1) see III:OPI200
ERR 4205 mixed with EPON 828 (1:1) see III:OPI200
ERTALON 6SA see III:PJY500
ERTILEN see II:CDP250
ERTUBAN see III:ILD000
ERYSAN see I:BIF250
ERYTHRENE see I:BOP500
ERYTHRITOL ANHYDRIDE see I:BGA750, II:DHB800
ERYTHROSIN see III:FAG040
ERYTHROSINE B-FO (BIOLOGICAL STAIN) see III:FAG040
ESACHLOROBENZENE (ITALIAN) see I:HCC500
ESAMETILENTETRAMINA (ITALIAN) see III:HEI500
ESANITRODIFENILAMINA (ITALIAN) see III:HET500
ESBRITE see III:SMQ500
ESCAMBIA 2160 see III:PKQ059
ESCOREZ 7404 see III:SMQ500
ESDRAGOL see III:AFW750
ESKABARB see II:EOK000
ESKALITH see III:LGZ000
ESKIMON 22 see III:CFX500
E 39 SOLUBLE see III:BDC750
ESOPHOTRAST see III:BAP000
ESPENAL see III:DXH250
ESPERAL see III:DXH250
ESPEROX 10 see III:BSC500
ESSO FUNGICIDE 406 see III:CBG000
ESSO HERBICIDE 10 see III:BQZ000
ESTANE 5703 see I:UVA000
ESTAR see I:CMY800, III:PKF750
ESTERCIDE T-2 and T-245 see II:TAA100
S-ESTER with O,O-DIMETHYL PHOSPHOROTHIOATE see
   III:MAK700
ESTERON see II:DAA800
ESTERON 44 see III:IOY000
ESTERON 99 see II:DAA800
ESTERON 76 BE see II:DAA800
ESTERON 245 BE see II:TAA100
ESTERON BRUSH KILLER see II:DAA800, II:TAA100
ESTERON 99 CONCENTRATE see II:DAA800
ESTERONE see I:EDV000
ESTERONE FOUR see II:DAA800
ESTERON 44 WEED KILLER see II:DAA800

ESTER SULFONATE see III:CJT750
ESTEVE see II:BRF500
ESTILBEN see I:DKA600, I:DKB000
ESTILBIN see I:DKB000
ESTINERVAL see III:PFC750
ESTONATE see I:DAD200
ESTON-B see I:EDP000
ESTONMITE see III:CJT750
ESTONOX see I:CDV100
ESTRADIOL see I:EDO000
d-ESTRADIOL see I:EDO000
α-ESTRADIOL see I:EDO000
β-ESTRADIOL see I:EDO000
17-α-ESTRADIOL see III:EDO500
ESTRADIOL-17-β see I:EDO000
17-β-ESTRADIOL see I:EDO000
cis-ESTRADIOL see I:EDO000
3,17-β-ESTRADIOL see I:EDO000
d-3,17-β-ESTRADIOL see I:EDO000
ESTRADIOL BENZOATE see I:EDP000
ESTRADIOL-3-BENZOATE see I:EDP000
β-ESTRADIOL BENZOATE see I:EDP000
β-ESTRADIOL-3-BENZOATE see I:EDP000
ESTRADIOL-17-β-BENZOATE see I:EDP000
17-β-ESTRADIOL BENZOATE see I:EDP000
ESTRADIOL-17-β-3-BENZOATE see I:EDP000
17-β-ESTRADIOL-3-BENZOATE see I:EDP000
ESTRADIOL-17-BENZOATE-3,n-BUTYRATE see III:EDP500
ESTRADIOL BENZOATE mixed with PROGESTERONE (1:14
   moles) see III:EDQ000
ESTRADIOL-3-BENZOATE mixed with PROGESTERONE
   (1:14 moles) see III:EDQ000
ESTRADIOL-17-CAPRYLATE see III:EDQ500
ESTRADIOL DIPROPIONATE see I:EDR000
β-ESTRADIOL DIPROPIONATE see I:EDR000
17-β-ESTRADIOL DIPROPIONATE see I:EDR000
ESTRADIOL-3,17-DIPROPIONATE see I:EDR000
3,17-β-ESTRADIOL DIPROPIONATE see I:EDR000
β-ESTRADIOL-3,17-DIPROPIONATE see I:EDR000
ESTRADIOL MONOBENZOATE see I:EDP000
17-β-ESTRADIOL MONOBENZOATE see I:EDP000
ESTRADIOL MUSTARD see III:EDR500
ESTRADIOL PHOSPHATE POLYMER see I:EDS000
ESTRADIOL POLYESTER with PHOSPHORIC ACID see
   I:EDS000
ESTRADIOL VALERATE see II:EDS100
ESTRADIOL-17-VALERATE see II:EDS100
ESTRADIOL 17-β-VALERATE see II:EDS100
ESTRADIOL VALERIANATE see II:EDS100
ESTRADURIN see I:EDS000, III:PJR750
ESTRAGARD see II:DAL600
ESTRALDINE see I:EDO000
ESTRALUTIN see III:HNT500
α-ESTRA-1,3,5,7,9-PENTANE-3,17-DIOL see III:EDT500
β-ESTRA-1,3,5,7,9-PENTANE-3,17-DIOL see III:EDU000
ESTRATAB see I:ECU750
1,3,5,7-ESTRATETRAEN-3-OL-17-ONE see III:ECW000
ESTRA-1,3,5(10)-TRIENE-2,4-D2-3,17-DIOL, (17-β)- see
   III:DHA425
1,3,5-ESTRATRIENE-3,17-α-DIOL see III:EDO500
1,3,5-ESTRATRIENE-3,17-β-DIOL see I:EDO000
ESTRA-1,3,5(10)-TRIENE-3,17-α-DIOL see III:EDO500
ESTRA-1,3,5(10)-TRIENE-3,17-β-DIOL see I:EDO000
17-β-ESTRA-1,3,5(10)-TRIENE-3,17-DIOL see I:EDO000
ESTRA-1,3,5(10)-TRIENE-3,17-β-DIOL, 3-BENZOATE see
   I:EDP000
1,3,5(10)-ESTRATRIENE-3,17-β-DIOL 3-BENZOATE see
   I:EDP000
ESTRA-1,3,5(10)-TRIENE-3,17-DIOL (17-β)-3-BENZOATE see
   I:EDP000
ESTRA-1,3,5(10)-TRIENE-3,17-β-DIOL-17-BENZOATE-3-n-
   BUTYRATE see III:EDP500
1,3,5(10)-ESTRATRIENE-3,17-β-DIOL DIPROPIONATE see
   I:EDR000

ETHYLENE TRICHLORIDE see II:TIO750
ETHYLENE UREA see III:IAS000
1,3-ETHYLENE UREA see III:IAS000
ETHYLENIMINE see I:EJM900
ETHYL-2,3-EPOXYBUTYRATE see III:EJS000
ETHYL ESTER of 1,2,5,6-DIBENZANTHRACENE-endo-α,β-
SUCCINO GLYCINE see III:EJT000
ETHYL ESTER of 4,4'-DICHLOROBENZILIC ACID see
II:DER000
ETHYL ESTER of METHANESULFONIC ACID see II:EMF500
ETHYL ESTER of 3-METHYLCHOLANTHRENE-endo-α,β-
SUCCINOGLYCINE see III:EJT500
ETHYL ESTER of METHYLNITROSO-CARBAMIC ACID see
II:MMX250
ETHYL ESTER of METHYLSULFONIC ACID see II:EMF500
ETHYL ESTER of METHYLSULPHONIC ACID see II:EMF500
11-β-ETHYLESTRADIOL see III:EJT575
11-β-ETHYLESTRA-1,3,5(10)-TRIENE-3,17-β-DIOL see
III:EJT575
11-β-ETHYL-17-α-ETHINYLESTRADIOL see III:EJV400
ETHYL-N-ETHYL CARBAMATE see III:EJW500
13-ETHYL-17-α-ETHYNYLGON-4-EN-17-β-OL-3-ONE see
III:NNQ500, III:NNQ520
13-ETHYL-17-α-ETHYNYL-17-β-HYDROXY-4-GONEN-3-
ONE see III:NNQ500, III:NNQ520
(±)-13-ETHYL-17-α-ETHYNYL-17-HYDROXYGON-4-EN-3-
ONE see III:NNQ500
dl-13-β-ETHYL-17-α-ETHYNYL-17-β-HYDROXYGON-4-EN-
3-ONE see III:NNQ500
dl-13-β-ETHYL-17-α-ETHYNYL-19-NORTESTOSTERONE see
III:NNQ500
ETHYL FORMATE see III:EKL000
ETHYLFORMIAAT (DUTCH) see III:EKL000
ETHYL FORMIC ESTER see III:EKL000
1-ETHYL-1-FORMYLHYDRAZINE see III:EKL250
N-ETHYL-N-FORMYLHYDRAZINE see III:EKL250
5-ETHYL-2(5H)-FURANONE see III:EKL500
2-ETHYL-1-HEXANOL PHOSPHATE see III:TNI250
2-ETHYLHEXYL ACRYLATE see III:ADU250
2-ETHYLHEXYL PHTHALATE see I:DVL700
2-ETHYLHEXYL-2-PROPENOATE see III:ADU250
2-ETHYLHEXYL SULFATE see III:ELB400
S-ETHYL-HOMOCYSTEINE see II:EEI000
S-ETHYL-l-HOMOCYSTEINE see III:AKB250
S-ETHYL-dl-HOMOCYSTEINE see II:EEI000
ETHYL HYDRATE see I:EFU000
ETHYLHYDRAZINE HYDROCHLORIDE see III:ELC000
ETHYL HYDROXIDE see I:EFU000
4'-ETHYL-4-HYDROXYAZOBENZENE see III:ELD500
ETHYL-2-HYDROXY-2,2-BIS(4-CHLOROPHENYL)ACETATE
see II:DER000
N-ETHYL-N-(4-HYDROXYBUTYL)NITROSOAMINE see
III:ELE500
ETHYL-N-HYDROXYCARBAMATE see III:HKQ025
(±)-13-ETHYL-17-HYDROXY-18,19-DINOR-17-α-PREGN-4-
EN-20-YN-3-ONE see III:NNQ500
ETHYL-2-HYDROXYETHYLNITROSAMINE see II:ELG500
N-ETHYL-N-HYDROXYETHYLNITROSAMINE see
II:ELG500
1-ETHYL-7-HYDROXY-2-METHYL-1,2,3,4,4a,9,10,10a-OC-
TAHYDROPHENANTHRENE-2-CARBOXYLIC ACID see
III:DYB000
N,N'-ETHYLIDENE-BIS(ETHYL CARBAMATE) see
III:ELO000
ETHYLIDENE CHLORIDE see III:DFF809
ETHYLIDENEDICARBAMIC ACID, DIETHYL ESTER see
III:ELO000
ETHYLIDENE DICHLORIDE see III:DFF809
5-ETHYLIDENEDIHYDRO-2(3H)-FURANONE see III:HLF000
ETHYLIDENE DIURETHAN see III:ELO000
ETHYLIDENE-2(5H)-FURANONE see III:MOW500
ETHYLIDENE GYROMITRIN see III:AAH000
trans-15-ETHYLIDENE-12-β-HYDROXY-4,12-α,13-β-TRI-
METHYL 8-OXO-4,8 SECOSENEC-1-ENINE see
III:DMX200

ETHYLIMINE see I:EJM900
2-ETHYLISONICOTINIC ACID THIOAMIDE see III:EPQ000
α-ETHYLISONICOTINIC ACID THIOAMIDE see III:EPQ000
2-ETHYLISONICOTINIC THIOAMIDE see III:EPQ000
α-ETHYLISONICOTINOYLTHIOAMIDE see III:EPQ000
ETHYLISOPROPYLNITROSOAMINE see III:ELX500
ETHYLISOTHIAMIDE see III:EPQ000
2-ETHYLISOTHIONICOTINAMIDE see III:EPQ000
α-ETHYLISOTHIONICOTINAMIDE see III:EPQ000
o-(ETHYLMERCURITHIO)BENZOIC ACID SODIUM SALT see
III:MDI000
ETHYLMERCURITHIOSALICYLIC ACID SODIUM SALT see
III:MDI000
ETHYL METHANESULFONATE see II:EMF500
ETHYL METHANESULPHONATE see II:EMF500
ETHYL METHANOATE see III:EKL000
ETHYL METHANSULFONATE see II:EMF500
ETHYL METHANSULPHONATE see II:EMF500
7-ETHYL-5-METHOXY-BENZ(a)ANTHRACENE see
III:MEN750
4-ETHYLMETHYLAMINOAZOBENZENE see III:ENB000
p-ETHYLMETHYLAMINOAZOBENZENE see III:ENB000
N-ETHYL-N-METHYL-p-AMINOAZOBENZENE see
III:ENB000
4'-ETHYL-N-METHYL-4-AMINOAZOBENZENE see
III:EOJ000
4-((((4-ETHYL-4-METHYL)AMINO)PHENYL)AZO)PYRIDINE
1-OXIDE see III:MKB500
7-ETHYL-9-METHYLBENZ(c)ACRIDINE see III:EMM000
12-ETHYL-7-METHYLBENZ(a)ANTHRACENE see
III:EMN000
7-ETHYL-12-METHYLBENZ(a)ANTHRACENE see
III:EMM500
ETHYL-p-METHYL BENZENESULFONATE see III:EPW500
ETHYL-N-METHYL CARBAMATE see III:EMQ500
4'-ETHYL-2-METHYL-4-DIMETHYLAMINOAZOBENZENE
see III:EMS000
1-ETHYL-2-METHYL-7-METHOXY-1,2,3,4-TETRAHYDRO-
PHENANTHRYL-2-CARBOXYLIC ACID see III:BIT000
ETHYLMETHYLNITROSAMINE see I:MKB000
N-ETHYL-N-METHYL-p-(PHENYLAZO)ANILINE see
III:ENB000
ETHYL MONOBROMOACETATE see III:EGV000
ETHYL MONOCHLOROACETATE see III:EHG500
ETHYL MONOCHLOROACETATE see III:EHG500
N-ETHYL-N-NITROETHANAMINE (9CI) see III:DJS500
N-ETHYL-N'-NITRO-N-NITROSOGUANIDINE see
III:ENU000
3-ETHYL-4-NITROPYRIDINE-1-OXIDE see III:ENR000
2-(ETHYLNITROSAMINO)ETHANOL see II:ELG500
(ETHYLNITROSAMINO)METHYL ACETATE see III:ENR500
4-((ETHYLNITROSAMINO)METHYL)PYRIDINE see
III:NLH000
4-(ETHYLNITROSOAMINO)-1-BUTANOL see III:ELE500
4-(ETHYLNITROSOAMINO)BUTYRIC ACID see III:NKE000
ETHYLNITROSOANILINE see I:NKD000
N-ETHYL-N-NITROSOBENZENAMINE see I:NKD000
N-ETHYL-N-NITROSOBENZYLAMINE see III:ENS500
ETHYLNITROSOBIURET see III:ENT000
N-ETHYL-N-NITROSOBIURET see III:ENT000
N-ETHYL-N-NITROSO-tert-BUTANAMINE see III:NKD500
N-ETHYL-N-NITROSOBUTYLAMINE see III:EHC000
ETHYLNITROSOCARBAMIC ACID, ETHYL ESTER see
III:NKE500
N-ETHYL-N-NITROSOCARBAMIC ACID ETHYL ESTER see
III:NKE500
N-ETHYL-N-NITROSOCARBAMIDE see I:ENV000
ETHYLNITROSOCYANAMIDE see III:ENT500
N-ETHYL-N-NITROSO-ETHANAMINE see I:NJW500
N-ETHYL-N-NITROSOETHENAMINE see III:NKF000
N-ETHYL-N-NITROSOETHENYLAMINE see III:NKF000
N-ETHYL-N-NITROSO-N'-NITROGUANIDINE see
III:ENU000
ETHYL 4-NITROSO-1-PIPERAZINECARBOXYLATE see
III:NJQ000

17-α-ETHYNYL-17-HYDROXYESTR-5(10)-EN-3-ONE see II:EEH550

17-α-ETHYNYL-17-HYDROXY-5(10)-ESTREN-3-ONE see II:EEH550

17-α-ETHYNYL-17-β-HYDROXY-Δ$^{-5(10)}$-ESTREN-3-ONE see II:EEH550

17-α-ETHYNYL-17-β-HYDROXY-5(10)-ESTREN-3-ONE see II:EEH550

17-α-ETHYNYL-17-β-HYDROXYESTR-5(10)-EN-3-ONE see II:EEH550

17-α-ETHYNYL-17-HYDROXYESTR-4-EN-3-ONE ACETATE see II:ABU000

17-α-ETHYNYL-17-HYDROXYESTREN-3-ONE and ETHYNYLESTRADIOL 3-METHYL ETHER see III:MDL750

(+)-17-α-ETHYNYL-17-β-HYDROXY-3-METHOXY-1,3,5(10)-ESTRATRIENE see I:MKB750

(+)-17-α-ETHYNYL-17-β-HYDROXY-3-METHOXY-1,3,5(10)-OESTRATRIENE see I:MKB750

17-α-ETHYNYL-17-β-HYDROXY-19-NORANDROST-4-EN-3-ONE see I:NNP500

17-α-ETHYNYL-17-β-HYDROXY-3-OXO-Δ$^{5(10)}$-ESTRENE see II:EEH550

α-ETHYNYL-p-METHOXYBENZYL ALCOHOL see III:HKA700

α-ETHYNYL-p-METHOXYBENZYL ALCOHOL ACETATE see III:EQN225

17-ETHYNYL-3-METHOXY-1,3,5(10)-ESTRATRIEN-17-β-OL see I:MKB750

17-α-ETHYNYL-3-METHOXY-1,3,5(10)-ESTRATRIEN-17-β-OL see I:MKB750

17-α-ETHYNYL-3-METHOXY-17-β-HYDROXY-Δ-1,3,5(10)-ESTRATRIENE see I:MKB750

17-α-ETHYNYL-3-METHOXY-17-β-HYDROXY-Δ-1,3,5(10)-OESTRATRIENE see I:MKB750

17-ETHYNYL-3-METHOXY-1,3,5(10)-OESTRATIEN-17-β-OL see I:MKB750

17-ETHYNYL-18-METHYL-19-NORTESTOSTERONE see III:NNQ500, III:NNQ520

17-α-ETHYNYL-19-NORANDROST-4-ENE-3-β,17-β-DIOL DIACETATE see II:EQJ500

17-α-ETHYNYL-19-NORANDROST-4-EN-17-β-OL-3-ONE see I:NNP500

17-α-ETHYNYL-19-NOR-4-ANDROSTEN-17-β-OL-3-ONE see I:NNP500

17-α-ETHYNYL-19-NOR-5(10)-ANDROSTEN-17-β-OL-3-ONE see II:EEH550

17-α-ETHYNYL-19-NORTESTOSTERONE see I:NNP500

17-α-ETHYNYL-19-NORTESTOSTERONE ACETATE see II:ABU000

17-α-ETHYNYL-19-NORTESTOSTERONE and ETHYNYLESTRADIOL 3-METHYL ETHER see III:MDL750

ETHYNYLOESTRADIOL see I:EEH500

17-ETHYNYLOESTRADIOL see I:EEH500

17-α-ETHYNYLOESTRADIOL see I:EEH500

17-α-ETHYNYL-17-β-OESTRADIOL see I:EEH500

17-α-ETHYNYLOESTRADIOL-17-β see I:EEH500

ETHYNYLOESTRADIOL METHYL ETHER see I:MKB750

17-ETHYNYLOESTRADIOL-3-METHYL ETHER see I:MKB750

17-α-ETHYNYLOESTRADIOL METHYL ETHER see I:MKB750

17-α-ETHYNYLOESTRADIOL-3-METHYL ETHER see I:MKB750

17-α-ETHYNYL-1,3,5-OESTRATRIENE-3,17-β-DIOL see I:EEH500

17-ETHYNYLOESTRA-1,3,5(10)-TRIENE-3,17-β-DIOL see I:EEH500

17-α-ETHYNYL-1,3,5(10)-OESTRATRIENE-3,17-β-DIOL see I:EEH500

17-α-ETHYNYLOESTRA-1,3,5(10)-TRIENE-3,17-β-DIOL see I:EEH500

17-α-ETHYNYLOESTRENOL see III:NNV000

17-α-ETHYNYLOESTR-4-EN-17-β-OL see III:NNV000

ETHYONOMIDE see III:EPQ000

ETIL ACRILATO (ITALIAN) see II:EFT000

ETILACRILATULUI (ROMANIAN) see II:EFT000

ETILE (FORMIATO di) (ITALIAN) see III:EKL000

N,N'-ETILEN-BIS(DITIOCARBAMMATO) di MANGANESE (ITALIAN) see III:MAS500

ETILENE (OSSIDO di) (ITALIAN) see I:EJN500

ETILENIMINA (ITALIAN) see I:EJM900

ETILFEN see II:EOK000

ETIMID see III:EPQ000

ETIOCHOLANE-17-β-OL-3-ONE see III:HJB100

ETIOCHOLAN-17-β-OL-3-ONE see III:HJB100

ETIOCIDAN see III:EPQ000

ETIOL see III:MAK700

ETIONAMID see III:EPQ000

ETIONIZINA see III:EPQ000

ETO see I:EJN500

ETOCIL see III:EEM000

ETOGLUCID see III:TJQ333

ETOSALICIL see III:EEM000

ETOSALICYL see III:EEM000

ETP see III:EPQ000

ETRENOL see III:HGO500

ETROZOLIDINA see III:HNI500

ETU see I:IAQ000

ETYLENU TLENEK (POLISH) see I:EJN500

ETYLOWY ALKOHOL (POLISH) see I:EFU000

EUBASIN see III:PPO000

EUBASINUM see III:PPO000

EUCALYPTUS REDUNCA TANNIN see III:MSC000

EUCANINE GB see I:TGL750

EUCHEUMA SPINOSUM GUM see III:CCL250

EUCHRYSINE see III:BJF000

EUCISTIN see I:PDC250

EUFIN see III:DIX200

EUFLAVINE see III:DBX400

EUFODRIANL see III:MDT600

EUGENIC ACID see III:EQR500

EUGENOL see III:EQR500

EUGYON see III:NNL500

EUKYSTOL see III:CLY500

EUMIN see I:MMN250

EUNERYL see II:EOK000

EUPHORBIA ABYSSINICA LATEX see III:EQT500

EUPHORBIA CANARIENSIS LATEX see III:EQU000

EUPHORBIA CANDELABRIUM LATEX see III:EQU500

EUPHORBIA ESULA LATEX see III:EQV000

EUPHORBIA GRANDIDENS LATEX see III:EQV500

EUPHORBIA LATHYRIS LATEX see III:EQW000

EUPHORBIA OBOVALIFOLIA LATEX see III:EQW500

EUPHORBIA SERRATA LATEX see III:EQX500

EUPHORBIA TIRUCALLI LATEX see III:EQY000

EUPHORIA WULFENII LATEX see III:EQY500

EUPHORIN see III:CBL750

EUPHOZID see III:ILE000

EURECEPTOR see III:TAB250

EUROCERT AMARANTH see III:FAG020

EUROCERT AZORUBINE see III:HJF500

EUROCERT COCHINEAL RED A see III:FMU080

EURODOPA see III:DNA200

EUROPHAN see III:PKQ059

EUSAL see III:EEM000

EUSAPRIM see III:SNK000

EUTIZON see III:ILD000

EUVESTIN see I:DKB000

EVABLIN see III:BGT250

EVALON see III:ILD000

EVANS BLUE DYE see III:BGT250

EVEX see I:ECU750

EVIPLAST 80 see I:DVL700

EVIPLAST 81 see I:DVL700

EVOLA see II:DEP800

EWEISS see III:BAP000

EXAGAMA see I:BBQ500

EXAL see III:VLA000

FD&C RED No. 32 see III:FAG080
FD&C RED No. 2-ALUMINIUM LAKE see III:FAG020
FD & C RED No. 4-ALUMINIUM LAKE see III:FAG050
FD&C VIOLET No. 1 see II:FAG120
FD&C YELLOW No. 3 see III:FAG130
FD&C YELLOW No. 4 see III:FAG135
FD&C YELLOW No. 6 see III:FAG150
F-diAA see II:DBF200
FEBRILIX see II:HIM000
FEBRININA see III:DOT000
FEBRO-GESIC see II:HIM000
FEBROLIN see II:HIM000
FEBRON see III:DOT000
FEBUZINA see II:BRF500
FECTRIM see III:SNK000
FEDACIN see II:NGE500
FEDAL-UN see II:PCF275
Fe-DEXTRAN see I:IGS000
FELAZINE see III:PFC750
FELSULES see III:CDO000
FEMACOID see I:ECU750
FEMA No. 2003 see II:AAG250
FEMA No. 2034 see II:AGJ250
FEMA No. 2045 see II:ISV000
FEMA No. 2086 see III:PMQ750
FEMA No. 2135 see III:BDX000
FEMA No. 2179 see III:IIL000
FEMA No. 2183 see II:BQI000
FEMA No. 2184 see III:BFW750
FEMA No. 2223 see III:TIG750
FEMA No. 2224 see III:CAK500
FEMA No. 2295 see II:API750
FEMA No. 2365 see III:DAI600
FEMA No. 2418 see II:EFT000
FEMA No. 2433 see I:EJN500
FEMA No. 2434 see III:EKL000
FEMA No. 2467 see III:EQR500
FEMA No. 2593 see III:ICM000
FEMA No. 2617 see III:DXV600
FEMA No. 2633 see III:LFU000
FEMA No. 3291 see II:BOV000
FEMANTHREN GOLDEN YELLOW see III:DCZ000
FEMEST see I:ECU750
FEMESTRAL see I:EDO000
FEMESTRONE see I:EDP000
FEMESTRONE INJECTION see I:EDV000
FEM H see I:ECU750
FEMIDYN see I:EDV000
FEMOGEN see I:ECU750, I:EDO000
FEMOGEX see II:EDS100
FEMULEN see II:EQJ500
FENACET BLUE G see III:TBG700
FENACETINA see I:ABG750
FENALAN YELLOW E see III:SGP500
FENAMIN see III:ARQ725
FENAMIN BLACK E see I:AQP000
FENAMIN BLUE 2B see I:CMO000
FENAMINE see I:AMY050, III:ARQ725
FENAMINOSULF see III:DOU600
FENANTOIN see I:DKQ000, I:DNU000
FENARSONE see III:CBJ000
FENARTIL see II:BRF500
FENATE see I:IGS000
FENATROL see III:ARQ725
FENAVAR see I:AMY050
FENAZO BLUE XI see III:FAE000
FENAZO BLUE XR see III:FMU059
FENAZO EOSINE XG see III:BNH500, III:BNK700
FENAZO GREEN 7G see III:FAF000
FENAZO RED C see III:HJF500
FENAZO SCARLET 2R see III:FMU070
FENAZO SCARLET 3R see III:FMU080
FENBITAL see II:EOK000
FENCLOR see I:PJL750

FENDON see II:HIM000
FENELZIN see III:PFC750
FENEMAL see II:EOK000
FENESTERIN see II:CME250
FENESTREL see III:FAO200
FENESTRIN see II:CME250
FENIBUTASAN see II:BRF500
FENIBUTAZONA see II:BRF500
FENIBUTOL see II:BRF500
FENICOL see II:CDP250
FENIDANTOIN "S" see I:DKQ000
FENILBUTAZONA see II:BRF500
FENILBUTINE see II:BRF500
FENILIDINA see II:BRF500
FENILIDRAZINA (ITALIAN) see II:PFI000
FENITOIN see I:DNU000
FENNOSAN see III:QPA000
FENOBARBITAL see II:EOK000
FENOCYCLIN see III:BIT000
FENOCYCLINE see III:BIT000
FENOL (DUTCH, POLISH) see III:PDN750
FENOLO (ITALIAN) see III:PDN750
FENOLOVO ACETATE see III:ABX250
FENOPROP see II:TIX500
FENORMONE see II:TIX500
FENOSED see II:EOK000
FENOTONE see II:BRF500
FENOXYBENZAMIN see II:DDG800
FENTAL see III:FMB000
FENTHION see III:FAQ999
FENTIN ACETAAT (DUTCH) see III:ABX250
FENTIN ACETAT (GERMAN) see III:ABX250
FENTIN ACETATE see III:ABX250
FENTINE ACETATE (FRENCH) see III:ABX250
FENYLBUTAZON see II:BRF500
1-FENYL-3,3-DIETHYLTRIAZEN (CZECH) see III:PEU500
1-FENYL-3,3-DIMETHYLTRIAZIN see III:DTP000
m-FENYLENDIAMIN (CZECH) see III:PEY000
FENYLENODWUAMINA (POLISH) see III:PEY500
FENYLEPSIN see I:DKQ000
FENYLETTAE see II:EOK000
FENYL-GLYCIDYLETHER (CZECH) see II:PFH000
FENYLHYDRAZINE (DUTCH) see II:PFI000
FENYTOINE see I:DKQ000, I:DNU000
FENZEN (CZECH) see I:BBL250
FEOJECTIN see I:IHG000
FEOSOL see III:FBN100
FEOSPAN see III:FBN100
FERBAM see III:FAS000
FERBAM 50 see III:FAS000
FERBAM, IRON SALT see III:FAS000
FERBECK see III:FAS000
FERDEX 100 see I:IGS000
FERGON see III:FBK000
FERGON PREPARATIONS see III:FBK000
FER-IN-SOL see III:FBN100
FERKETHION see III:DSP400
FERLUCON see III:FBK000
FERMATE FERBAM FUNGICIDE see III:FAS000
FERMENICIDE LIQUID see III:SOH500
FERMENICIDE POWDER see III:SOH500
FERMENTATION ALCOHOL see I:EFU000
FERMENTATION AMYL ALCOHOL see III:IHP000
FERMENTATION BUTYL ALCOHOL see III:IIL000
FERMIDE see III:TFS350
FERMOCIDE see III:FAS000
FERNACOL see III:TFS350
FERNASAN see III:TFS350
FERNESTA see II:DAA800, III:BQZ000
FERNIDE see III:TFS350
FERNIMINE see II:DAA800
FERNOXONE see II:DAA800
FERO-GRADUMET see III:FBN100
FERRADOW see III:FAS000

FERRALYN see III:FBN100
FERRIAMICIDE see I:MQW500
FERRIC ARSENATE, SOLID (DOT) see I:IGN000
FERRIC ARSENITE, BASIC see I:IGO000
FERRIC ARSENITE, SOLID (DOT) see I:IGO000
FERRIC DEXTRAN see I:IGS000
FERRIC DIMETHYLDITHIOCARBAMATE see III:FAS000
FERRIC HYDROXIDE NITRILOTRIPROPIONIC ACID COM-
   PLEX see III:FAY000
FERRIC NITRILOTRIACETATE see III:IHC100
FERRIC NITROSODIMETHYL DITHIOCARBAMATE and TET-
   RAMETHYL THIURAM DISULFIDE see III:FAZ000
FERRIC OXIDE see III:IHD000
FERRIC OXIDE, SACCHARATED see I:IHG000
FERRIC SACCHARATE IRON OXIDE (MIX.) see I:IHG000
FERRIC SODIUM GLUCONATE COMPLEX see III:IHK000
FERRIDEXTRAN see I:IGS000
FERRIGEN see III:IGU000
FERRITIN see III:FBB000
FERRIVENIN see I:IHG000
FERRLECIT see III:FBB100
FERROACTINOLITE see III:FBG200
FERROANTHOPHYLLITE see I:ARM264
FERROCENE see III:FBC000
FERROCHROME see III:FBD000
FERROCHROME (exothermic) see III:FBD000
FERROCHROME, exothermic (DOT) see III:FBD000
FERROCHROMIUM see III:FBD000
FERRODEXTRAN see I:IGS000
FERROFLUKIN 75 see I:IGS000
FERROGLUCIN see I:IGS000
FERROGLUKIN 75 see I:IGS000
FERRO-GRADUMET see III:FBN100
FERRONICUM see III:FBK000
FERROSULFAT (GERMAN) see III:FBN100
FERROSULFATE see III:FBN100
FERRO-THERON see III:FBN100
FERROTREMOLITE see III:FBG200
FERROUS ARSENATE (DOT) see I:IGM000
FERROUS ARSENATE, SOLID (DOT) see I:IGM000
FERROUS GLUCONATE see III:FBK000
FERROUS GLUTAMATE see III:FBM000
FERROUS LACTATE see III:LAL000
FERROUS SULFATE see III:FBN100
FERRO YELLOW see I:CAJ750
FERRUGO see III:IHD000
FERSOLATE see III:FBN100
FES see III:ZAT000
FETTORANGE B see III:XRA000
FETTORANGE R see III:PEJ500
FETTSCHARLACH see III:OHA000
FF see II:FQN000
F-5-FU see III:FMB000
FH 122-A see III:NNQ500
FHCH see I:BBQ750
F.I 106 see I:AES750
FI 106 see III:HKA300
F.I. 58-30 see III:EPQ000
FI6339 see II:DAC000
FI 6804 see III:HKA300
FIBERGLASS see III:FBQ000
FIBERS, REFRACTORY CERAMIC see III:RCK725
FIBER V see III:PKF750
FIBRALEM see III:ARQ750
FIBRE BLACK VF see I:AQP000
FIBRENE C 400 see III:TAB750
FIBROUS CROCIDOLITE ASBESTOS see I:ARM275
FIBROUS GLASS see III:FBQ000
FIBROUS GLASS DUST (ACGIH) see III:FBQ000
FIBROUS GRUNERITE see I:ARM250
FIBROUS TREMOLITE see I:ARM280
FIDDLE-NECK see III:TAG250
FILMERINE see III:SIQ500
FIMALENE see III:ILD000

FINE GUM HES see III:SFO500
FINEMEAL see III:BAP000
FINIMAL see II:HIM000
FINTIN ACETATO (ITALIAN) see III:ABX250
FIORINAL see I:ABG750
FIREMASTER BP-6 see III:FBU000
FIREMASTER FF-1 see II:FBU509
FIREMASTER T23P-LV see I:TNC500
FISH-TOX see III:RNZ000
FISIOQUENS see III:EEH575
FIXANOL BLACK E see I:AQP000
FIXANOL BLUE 2B see I:CMO000
FIXANOL VIOLET N see III:CMP000
FLACAVON R see I:TNC500
FLAGEMONA see I:MMN250
FLAGESOL see I:MMN250
FLAGIL see I:MMN250
FLAGYL see I:MMN250
FLAMARIL see III:HNI500
FLAMENCO see III:TGG760
FLAMMEX AP see I:TNC500
FLANARIL see III:HNI500
FLANOGEN ELA see III:CCL250
FLAVACRIDINUM HYDROCHLORICUM see III:DBX400
FLAVAZONE see II:NGE500
FLAVINE see III:DBX400
FLAVIOFORM see III:DBX400
FLAVIPIN see III:DBX400
FLAVISEPT see III:DBX400
FLAVOMYCELIN see III:LIV000
FLECK-FLIP see II:TIO750
FLEXAMINE G see III:BLE500
FLEXAZONE see II:BRF500
FLEXIMEL see I:DVL700
FLEXOL A 26 see III:AEO000
FLEXOL DOP see I:DVL700
FLEXOL PLASTICIZER DOP see I:DVL700
FLEXOL TOF see III:TNI250
FLIBOL E see III:TIQ250
FLIEGENTELLER see III:TIQ250
FLINT see I:SCJ500
FLIT 406 see III:CBG000
FLOCOR see III:PKQ059
FLO-GARD see III:SCH000
FLOGHENE see III:HNI500
FLOGISTIN see III:HNI500
FLOGITOLO see III:HNI500
FLOGODIN see III:HNI500
FLOGORIL see III:HNI500
FLOGOSTOP see III:HNI500
FLOPIRINA see III:HNI500
FLO PRO T SEED PROTECTANT see III:TFS350
FLORALTONE see III:GEM000
FLORIDINE see III:SHF500
FLOROCID see III:SHF500
FLOWERS of ANTIMONY see I:AQF000
FLOZENGES see III:SHF500
FLUATE see II:TIO750
FLUE DUST, ARSENIC containing see III:ARE500
FLUIBIL see III:CDL325
FLUKOIDS see CBY000
FLUO-KEM see III:TAI250
FLUOMETURON see III:DUK800
FLUON see III:TAI250
5-FLUORACIL (GERMAN) see III:FMM000
FLUORAL see III:SHF500
FLUORANTHENE see III:FDF000
N-FLUORANTHEN-3-YLACETAMIDE see III:AAK400
N-3-FLUORANTHENYLACETAMIDE see III:AAK400
FLUOREN-2-AMINE see II:FDI000
2-FLUORENAMINE see II:FDI000
2-FLUORENEAMINE see II:FDI000
FLUORENE-2,7-DIAMINE see III:FDM000
2,7-FLUORENEDIAMINE see III:FDM000

2-FLUORO-(1)BENZOTHIOPYRANO(4,3-b)INDOLE see III:FGJ000

4-FLUORO-(1)BENZOTHIOPYRANO(4,3-b)INDOLE see III:FGL000

4-FLUORO-6H-(1)BENZOTHIOPYRANO(4,3-b)QUINOLINE see III:FGO000

1-(3-p-FLUOROBENZOYLPROPYL)-4-p-CHLOROPHENYL-4-HYDROXYPIPERIDINE see III:CLY500

N-4-(4'-FLUORO)BIPHENYLACETAMIDE see III:FKZ000

4'-FLUORO-4-BIPHENYLAMINE see III:AKC500

N-(4'-FLUORO-4-BIPHENYLYL)ACETAMIDE see III:FKZ000

FLUOROBLASTIN see III:FMM000

6-FLUORO-7-BROMOMETHYLBENZ(a)ANTHRACENE see III:BNQ250

FLUOROCARBON-22 see III:CFX500

5-FLUORO-7-CHLOROMETHYL-12-METHYLBENZ(a)AN-THRACENE see III:FHH025

6-FLUORODIBENZ(a,h)ANTHRACENE see III:FHP000

4-FLUORO-1,2:5,6-DIBENZANTHRACENE see III:FHP000

m-FLUORODIMETHYLAMINOAZOBENZENE see III:FHQ100

2-FLUORO-4-DIMETHYLAMINOAZOBENZENE see III:FHQ000

2'-FLUORO-4-DIMETHYLAMINOAZOBENZENE see III:FHQ010

3'-FLUORO-4-DIMETHYLAMINOAZOBENZENE see III:FHQ100

4'-FLUORO-4-DIMETHYLAMINOAZOBENZENE see III:DSA000

4'-FLUORO-p-DIMETHYLAMINOAZOBENZENE see III:DSA000

4'-FLUORO-N,N-DIMETHYL-4-AMINOAZOBENZENE see III:DSA000

2'-FLUORO-4-DIMETHYLAMINOSTILBENE see III:FHU000

4'-FLUORO-4-DIMETHYLAMINOSTILBENE see III:FHV000

10-FLUORO-9,12-DIMETHYLBENZ(a)ACRIDINE see III:FHR000

3-FLUORO-2,10-DIMETHYL-5,6-BENZACRIDINE see III:FHR000

1-FLUORO-7,12-DIMETHYLBENZ(a)ANTHRACENE see III:FHS000

4-FLUORO-7,12-DIMETHYLBENZ(a)ANTHRACENE see III:DRY400

5-FLUORO-7,12-DIMETHYLBENZ(a)ANTHRACENE see III:DRY600

8-FLUORO-7,12-DIMETHYLBENZ(a)ANTHRACENE see III:DRY800

11-FLUORO-7,12-DIMETHYLBENZ(a)ANTHRACENE see III:DRZ000

4'-FLUORO-N,N-DIMETHYL-p-PHENYLAZOANILINE see III:DSA000

2'-FLUORO-N,N-DIMETHYL-4-STILBENAMINE see III:FHU000

4'-FLUORO-N,N-DIMETHYL-4-STILBENAMINE see III:FHV000

2,7-FLUOROENEDIAMINE see III:FDM000

4-FLUOROESTRADIOL see III:FIA500

4-FLUOROESTRA-1,3,5-(10)-TRIENE-3,17-β-DIOL see III:FIA500

1-(2-FLUOROETHYL)-1-NITROSO-UREA see III:NKG000

1-FLUORO-2-FAA see III:FFL000

3-FLUORO-2-FAA see III:FFM000

4-FLUORO-2-FAA see III:FFN000

5-FLUORO-2-FAA see III:FFO000

6-FLUORO-2-FAA see III:FFP000

7-FLUORO-2-FAA see III:FIT200

8-FLUORO-2-FAA see III:FFQ000

FLUOROFLEX see III:TAI250

N-(7-FLUOROFLUORENE-2-YL)ACETAMIDE see III:FFG000

N-(1-FLUOROFLUOREN-2-YL)ACETAMIDE see III:FFL000

N-(3-FLUOROFLUOREN-2-YL)ACETAMIDE see III:FFM000

N-(4-FLUOROFLUOREN-2-YL)ACETAMIDE see III:FFN000

N-(5-FLUOROFLUOREN-2-YL)ACETAMIDE see III:FFO000

N-(6-FLUOROFLUOREN-2-YL)ACETAMIDE see III:FFP000

N-(8-FLUOROFLUOREN-2-YL)ACETAMIDE see III:FFQ000

7-FLUORO-2-N-(FLUORENYL)ACETHYDROXAMIC ACID see III:FIT200

7-FLUORO-N-(FLUOREN-2-YL)ACETOHYDROXAMIC ACID see III:FIT200

N-(7-FLUORO-2-FLUORENYL)ACETOHYDROXAMIC ACID see III:FIT200

FLUOROFUR see III:FMB000

7-FLUORO-N-HYDROXY-N-2-ACETYLAMINOFLUORENE see III:FIT200

4'-FLUORO-4-(4-HYDROXY-4-(4'-CHLOROPHENYL)PIPERIDINO)BUTYROPHENONE see III:CLY500

FLUOROLON 4 see III:TAI250

10-FLUORO-12-METHYL-BENZ(a)ACRIDINE see III:MKD750

1-FLUORO-10-METHYL-7,8-BENZACRIDINE see III:MKD500

3-FLUORO-10-METHYL-5,6-BENZACRIDINE see III:MKD750

3-FLUORO-10-METHYL-7,8-BENZACRIDINE (FRENCH) see III:MKD250

2-FLUORO-7-METHYLBENZ(a)ANTHRACENE see III:FJN000

3-FLUORO-7-METHYLBENZ(a)ANTHRACENE see III:FJO000

6-FLUORO-7-METHYLBENZ(a)ANTHRACENE see III:FJP000

9-FLUORO-7-METHYLBENZ(a)ANTHRACENE see III:FJQ000

10-FLUORO-7-METHYLBENZ(a)ANTHRACENE see III:FJR000

6-FLUORO-10-METHYL-1,2-BENZANTHRACENE see III:FJQ000

7-FLUORO-10-METHYL-1,2-BENZANTHRACENE see III:FJR000

3'-FLUORO-10-METHYL-1,2-BENZANTHRACENE see III:FJO000

4-FLUORO-7-METHYL-6H-(1)BENZOTHIOPYRANO(4,3-b)QUINOLINE see III:FJT000

2-FLUORO-3-METHYLCHOLANTHRENE see III:FJU000

6-FLUORO-3-METHYLCHOLANTHRENE see III:FJV000

9-FLUORO-3-METHYLCHOLANTHRENE see III:FJW000

1-FLUORO-5-METHYLCHRYSENE see III:FJY000

6-FLUORO-5-METHYLCHRYSENE see III:FKA000

7-FLUORO-5-METHYLCHRYSENE see III:FKB000

9-FLUORO-5-METHYLCHRYSENE see III:FKC000

11-FLUORO-5-METHYLCHRYSENE see III:FKD000

12-FLUORO-5-METHYLCHRYSENE see III:FKE000

p-FLUORO-N-METHYL-N-NITROSOANILINE see III:FKF800

3-FLUORO-4-NITROQUINOLINE-1-OXIDE see III:FKO000

8-FLUORO-4-NITROQUINOLINE-1-OXIDE see III:FKP000

FLUOROPAK 80 see III:TAI250

4-FLUOROPHENOL see III:FKV000

4'-(m-FLUOROPHENYL)ACETANILIDE see III:FKY000

4'-(p-FLUOROPHENYL)ACETANILIDE see III:FKZ000

2'-FLUORO-4'-PHENYLACETANILIDE see III:FKX000

p-((p-FLUOROPHENYL)AZO)-N,N-DIMETHYLANILINE see III:DSA000

4-((4-FLUOROPHENYL)AZO)-N,N-DIMETHYLBENZENA-MINE see III:DSA000

FLUOROPLAST 4 see III:TCH500

FLUOROPLEX see III:FMM000

5-FLUORO-2,4-PYRIMIDINEDIONE see III:FMM000

5-FLUORO-2,4(1H,3H)-PYRIMIDINEDIONE see III:FMM000

4'-FLUORO-4-STILBENAMINE see III:FLY000

2-FLUORO-4-STILBENYL-N,N-DIMETHYLAMINE see III:FHU000

4'-FLUORO-4-STILBENYL-N,N-DIMETHYLAMINE see III:FHV000

5-FLUORO-1-(TETRAHYDRO-2-FURANYL)-2,4-PYRIMIDI-NEDIONE see III:FMB000

5-FLUORO-1-(TETRAHYDRO-2-FURANYL)-2,4(1H,3H)-PY-RIMIDINEDIONE see III:FMB000

5-FLUORO-1-(TETRAHYDROFURAN-2-YL)URACIL see III:FMB000

5-FLUORO-1-(TETRAHYDRO-3-FURYL)URACIL see III:FMB000
2-FLUOROTHIOPYRANO(4,3-b)BENZ(e)INDOLE see III:FGJ000
4-FLUOROTHIOPYRANO(4,3-b)BENZ(e)INDOLE see III:FGL000
2-FLUOROTRICYCLOQUINAZOLINE see III:FMF000
3-FLUORO-TRICYCLOQUINAZOLINE see III:FMG000
FLUOROURACIL see III:FMM000
5-FLUOROURACIL see III:FMM000
FLUORPLAST 4 see III:TAI250
5-FLUORPROPYRIMIDINE-2,4-DIONE see III:FMM000
5-FLUORURACIL (GERMAN) see III:FMM000
FLUORURE de SODIUM (FRENCH) see III:SHF500
FLURACIL see III:FMM000
FLURA-GEL see III:SHF500
FLURCARE see III:SHF500
FLURI see III:FMM000
FLURIL see III:FMM000
FMC 5273 see III:PIX250
FMC 5462 see III:EAQ750
F-6-NDBA see III:NJN300
F-NORSTEARANTHRENE see III:TCJ500
FNT see II:NDY500
FOGARD see III:FMR700
FOGARD S see III:FMR700
FOLBEX see II:DER000
FOLBEX SMOKE-STRIPS see II:DER000
FOLCID see III:CBF800
FOLIC ACID, 4-AMINO- see III:AMG750
FOLIDOL see III:PAK000
FOLIDOL E605 see III:PAK000
FOLIDOL E & E 605 see III:PAK000
FOLIDOL M see III:MNH000
FOLIKRIN see I:EDV000
FOLIPEX see I:EDV000
FOLISAN see I:EDV000
FOLLESTRINE see I:EDV000
FOLLICORMON see I:EDP000
FOLLICULAR HORMONE see I:EDV000
FOLLICULAR HORMONE HYDRATE see II:EDU500
FOLLICULIN see I:EDV000
FOLLICULINE BENZOATE see I:EDV000
FOLLICUNODIS see I:EDV000
FOLLICYCLIN P see I:EDR000
FOLLIDIENE see I:DKA600, II:DAL600
FOLLIDRIN see I:EDP000, I:EDV000
FOLLINYL see III:NNL500
FOLLORMON see II:DAL600
FOLOSAN see III:PAX000, III:TBR750
FOLOSAN DB-905 FUMITE see III:TBS000
FOLPAN see III:TIT250
FOLPET see III:TIT250
FOLSAN see III:TBS000
FOMAC see III:HCL000
FOMAC 2 see III:PAX000
FONATOL see I:DKA600
FONOLINE see III:MQV750
FOOD BLUE 1 see III:FMU059
FOOD BLUE 2 see III:FAE000
FOOD BLUE 3 see III:ADE500
FOOD BLUE DYE No. 1 see III:FAE000
FOOD GREEN 2 see III:FAF000
FOOD RED 2 see III:FAG020
FOOD RED 4 see III:FAG050
FOOD RED 5 see III:HJF500
FOOD RED 6 see III:FMU080
FOOD RED 7 see III:FMU080
FOOD RED 9 see III:FAG020
FOOD RED 14 see III:FAG040
FOOD RED 15 see III:FAG070
FOOD RED No. 101 see III:FMU070
FOOD RED No. 102 see III:FMU080
FOREDEX 75 see II:DAA800

FORLIN see I:BBQ500
FORMAL see III:MAK700
FORMALDEHYD (CZECH, POLISH) see I:FMV000
FORMALDEHYDE see I:FMV000
FORMALDEHYDE, solution (DOT) see I:FMV000
FORMAL HYDRAZINE see III:FNN000
FORMALIN see I:FMV000
FORMALIN 40 see I:FMV000
FORMALIN (DOT) see I:FMV000
FORMALINA (ITALIAN) see I:FMV000
FORMALINE (GERMAN) see I:FMV000
FORMALINE BLACK C see I:AQP000
FORMALIN-LOESUNGEN (GERMAN) see I:FMV000
FORMALITH see I:FMV000
FORMAMIDE, N-(1,1'-BIPHENYL)-4-YL-N-HYDROXY- see III:HLE650
FORMAMINE see III:HEI500
FORMATRIX see I:ECU750
FORMHYDRAZID (GERMAN) see III:FNN000
FORMHYDRAZIDE see III:FNN000
FORMIC ACID, 1-BUTYLHYDRAZIDE see III:BRK100
FORMIC ACID, ETHYL ESTER see III:EKL000
FORMIC ACID, 1-ETHYLHYDRAZIDE see III:EKL250
FORMIC ACID, HYDRAZIDE see III:FNN000
FORMIC ACID, METHYLHYDRAZIDE see II:FNW000
FORMIC ACID, METHYLPENTYLIDENEHYDRAZIDE see III:PBJ875
FORMIC ACID (2-(4-METHYL-2-THIAZOLYL)HYDRAZIDE see III:FNB000
FORMIC ACID, 1-PROPYLHYDRAZIDE see III:PNM650
FORMIC ALDEHYDE see I:FMV000
FORMIC BLACK C see I:AQP000
FORMIC ETHER see III:EKL000
FORMIC HYDRAZIDE see III:FNN000
FORMIC 2-(4-(5-NITROFURYL)-2-THIAZOLYL)HYDRAZIDE see II:NDY500
FORMIN see III:HEI500
FORMOHYDRAZIDE see III:FNN000
FORMOL see I:FMV000
FORMOLA 40 see II:DAA800
FORMOSULFATHIAZOLE see III:TEX250
2-FORMYLAMINOFLUORENE see III:FEF000
2-FORMYLAMINO-4-(5-NITRO-2-FURYL)THIAZOLE see II:NGM500
6-FORMYLANTHANTHRENE see III:FNK000
7-FORMYLBENZ(c)ACRIDINE see III:BAX250
7-FORMYLBENZO(c)ACRIDINE see III:BAX250
6-FORMYLBENZO(a)PYRENE see III:BCT250
2-FORMYL-3:4-BENZPHENANTHRENE see III:BCS000
5-FORMYL-1,2:3,4-DIBENZOPYRENE see III:DCY800
5-FORMYL-3,4:8,9-DIBENZOPYRENE see III:DCY600
5-FORMYL-3,4:9,10-DIBENZOPYRENE see III:BCQ750
N-FORMYL-N-2-FLUORENYLHYDROXYLAMINE see III:FEG000
FORMYLHYDRAZIDE see III:FNN000
FORMYLHYDRAZINE see III:FNN000
N-FORMYLHYDRAZINE see III:FNN000
2-(2-FORMYLHYDRAZINO)-4-(5-NITRO-2-FURYL)THIA-ZOLE see II:NDY500
6-FORMYL-12-METHYLANTHANTHRENE see III:FNQ000
7-FORMYL-9-METHYLBENZ(c)ACRIDINE see III:FNR000
7-FORMYL-11-METHYLBENZ(c)ACRIDINE see III:FNS000
12-FORMYL-7-METHYLBENZ(a)ANTHRACENE see III:MGY500
7-FORMYL-12-METHYLBENZ(a)ANTHRACENE see III:FNT000
5-FORMYL-10-METHYL-3,4,:8,9-DIBENZOPYRENE see III:FNV000
5-FORMYL-8-METHYL-3,4:9,10-DIBENZOPYRENE see III:FNU000
1-FORMYL-1-METHYLHYDRAZINE see II:FNW000
N-FORMYL-N-METHYLHYDRAZINE see II:FNW000
N-FORMYL-N-METHYL-p-(PHENYLAZO)ANILINE see III:FNX000

4-FORMYLMONOMETHYLAMINOAZOBENZENE see III:FNX000
1-FORMYL-3-THIOSEMICARBAZIDE see III:FOJ000
FORMYL TRICHLORIDE see I:CHJ500
FORMYL VIOLET S4BN see II:FAG120
FOROTOX see III:TIQ250
FORRON see II:TAA100
FORST U 46 see II:TAA100
FORTEX see II:TAA100
FORTHION see III:MAK700
FORTION NM see III:DSP400
FORTURF see III:TBQ750
FOSCHLOR see III:TIQ250
FOSCHLOREM (POLISH) see III:TIQ250
FOSCHLOR R-50 see III:TIQ250
FOSFAMID see III:DSP400
FOSFAMIDON see III:FAC025
FOSFAMIDONE see III:FAC025
FOSFAZIDE see III:ILE000
FOSFERMO see III:PAK000
FOSFERNO see III:PAK000
FOSFEX see III:PAK000
FOSFIVE see III:PAK000
FOSFORAN TROJ-(1,3-DWUCHLOROIZOPROPYLOWY)
  (POLISH) see III:FQU875
FOSFOTHION see III:MAK700
FOSFOTION see III:MAK700
FOSFOTOX see III:DSP400
FOSOVA see III:PAK000
FOSSIL FLOUR see III:SCH000
FOSTER GRANT 834 see III:SMQ500
FOSTERN see III:PAK000
FOSTEX see III:BDS000
FOSTION MM see III:DSP400
FOSTOX see III:PAK000
FOSTRIL see III:HCL000
FOSZFAMIDON see III:FAC025
FOURAMIEN 2R see II:ALL750
FOURAMINE see I:TGL750
FOURAMINE BA see I:DBO400
FOURAMINE BROWN AP see III:PPQ500
FOURAMINE D see III:PEY500
FOURAMINE PCH see III:CCP850
FOURAMINE RS see III:REA000
FOURAMINE STD see III:TGM400
FOURINE DS see III:PEY650
FOURNEAU 1162 see III:SNM500
FOURRINE 1 see III:PEY500
FOURRINE 36 see II:ALL750
FOURRINE 57 see II:NEM480
FOURRINE 64 see III:PEY650
FOURRINE 68 see III:CCP850
FOURRINE 79 see III:REA000
FOURRINE 81 see III:CEG625
FOURRINE BROWN 2R see II:ALL750
FOURRINE BROWN PR see II:NEM480
FOURRINE BROWN PROPYL see II:NEM480
FOURRINE D see III:PEY500
FOURRINE M see I:TGL750
FOURRINE PG see III:PPQ500
FOURRINE SLA see I:DBO400
FOURRINE SO see III:CEG625
FOUR THOUSAND FORTY-NINE see III:MAK700
FOWLER'S SOLUTION see I:FOM050
F 10 (PESTICIDE) see III:MAS500
FPF 1002 see III:TAB250
FR 300 see III:PAU500
FRABEL see III:HNI500
FRACINE see II:NGE500
FRAMED see III:BJP000
FRANROZE see III:FMB000
FREE BENZYLPENICILLIN see III:BDY669
FRENTIROX see III:MCO500
FREON see III:CFX500

FREON 22 see III:CFX500
FREON 30 see II:MJP450
FREON 31 see I:CHI900
FREON 133a see III:TJY175
FREUDAL see III:DCK759
FRIGEN see III:CFX500
FRP 53 see III:PAU500
FRUCTOSE (FCC) see III:LFI000
FRUITDO see III:BLC250
FRUITONE A see II:TAA100
FRUITONE T see II:TIX500
FRUIT RED A EXTRA YELLOWISH GEIGY see III:HJF500
FRUIT RED A GEIGY see III:FAG020
FRUIT SUGAR see III:LFI000
FRUSTAN see III:DCK759
FRUTABS see III:LFI000
FTA see III:FQQ100
F1-TABS see III:SHF500
FTALAN see III:TIT250
FTIVAZID see III:VEZ925
FTIVAZIDE see III:VEZ925
FTORAFUR see III:FMB000
FTORLON 4 see III:TAI250
FTOROPLAST 4 see III:TAI250
F-2 TOXIN see III:ZAT000
5-FU see III:FMM000
FUCHSIN see III:MAC250
p-FUCHSIN see II:RMK020
FUCHSINE DR-001 see II:RMK020
FUCHSINE SPC see II:RMK020
FUCLASIN see III:BJK500
FUCLASIN ULTRA see III:BJK500
FUEL OIL, pyrolyzate see III:FOP100
FUKI-NO-TOH (JAPANESE) see II:PCR000
FUKINOTOXIN see III:PCQ750
FUKLASIN see III:BJK500
FUKLASIN ULTRA see III:FAS000
FULAID see III:FMB000
FULCIN see GKE000
FULCINE see GKE000
FULFEEL see III:FMB000
FUL-GLO see III:FEW000
FULVICAN GRISACTIN see GKE000
FULVICIN see GKE000
FULVINA see GKE000
FULVISTATIN see GKE000
FUMAGON see I:DDL800
FUMAZONE see I:DDL800
FUMED SILICA see III:SCH000
FUMED SILICON DIOXIDE see III:SCH000
FUMIGANT-1 (OBS.) see III:MHR200
FUMIGRAIN see I:ADX500
FUMO-GAS see I:EIY500
FUNDAL see III:CJJ250
FUNDAL 500 see III:CJJ250
FUNDEX see III:CJJ250
FUNDUSCEIN see III:FEW000
FUNGICLOR see III:PAX000
FUNGIFEN see II:PAX250
FUNGIVIN see GKE000
FUNGOL B see III:SHF500
FUNGOSTOP see III:BJK500
FUNGUS BAN TYPE II see III:CBG000
FURACILLIN see II:NGE500
FURACINETTEN see II:NGE500
FURACOCCID see II:NGE500
FURACORT see II:NGE500
FURACYCLINE see II:NGE500
FURADANTIN see III:NGE000
FURADONIN see III:NGE000
FURAFLUOR see III:FMB000
FURALDON see II:NGE500
1-FURALTADONE HYDROCHLORIDE see II:FPI150
2,5-FURANDIONE see III:MAM000

FURANIUM see III:FEW000
FURAN-OFTENO see II:NGE500
FURANTOIN see III:NGE000
FURAPLAST see II:NGE500
FURASEPTYL see II:NGE500
FURATONE see II:BKH500
FURATONE-S see II:BKH500
FURAXONE see III:NGG500
FURAZOL see III:NGG500
FURAZOLIDON see III:NGG500
FURAZOLIDONE (USDA) see III:NGG500
FURAZON see III:NGG500
FURAZONE see II:NGE500
FUR BLACK 41867 see III:PEY500
FUR BROWN 41866 see III:PEY500
FURESOL see II:NGE500
FURFURIN see II:NGE500
FURIDIAZINE see II:NGI500
FURIDON see III:NGG500
FURLOE see III:CKC000
FURLOE 4EC see III:CKC000
FURMETHONOL see II:FPI150
FURNACE BLACK see III:CBT750
FUROBACTINA see III:NGE000
2H-FURO(2,3-h)(1)BENZOPYRAN-2-ONE see III:FQC000
FURO(5′,4′,7,8)COUMARIN see III:FQC000
FUROFUTRAN see III:FMB000
FUROTHIAZOLE see III:FQJ000
FUROVAG see III:NGG500
FUROX see III:NGG500
FUROXAL see III:NGG500
FUROXANE see III:NGG500
FUROXONE SWINE MIX see III:NGG500
FUROZOLIDINE see III:NGG500
FURRO D see III:PEY500
FURRO L see I:DBO000
FURRO SLA see I:DBO400
FUR YELLOW see III:PEY500
FURYLAMIDE see II:FQN000
FURYLFURAMIDE see II:FQN000
α-2-FURYL-5-NITRO-2-FURANACYRLAMIDE see II:FQN000
2-(2-FURYL)-3-(5-NITRO-2-FURYL)ACRYLAMIDE see
    II:FQN000
2-(2-FURYL)-3-(5-NITRO-2-FURYL)ACRYLIC ACID AMIDE
    see II:FQN000
α-(FURYL)-β-(5-NITRO-2-FURYL)ACRYLIC AMIDE see
    FQN000
N-(4-(2-FURYL)-2-THIAZOLYL)ACETAMIDE see III:FQQ100
N-(4-(2-FURYL)-2-THIAZOLYL)FORMAMIDE see
    III:FQQ400
FUSARENONE X see III:FQR000
FUSAREX see III:TBR750, III:TBS000
FUSARIOTOXIN T 2 see III:FQS000
FUSARIUM TOXIN see III:ZAT000
FUSED QUARTZ see I:SCK600
FUSED SILICA (ACGIH) see I:SCK600
FUTRAFUL see III:FMB000
FUTRAMINE D see III:PEY500
FUVACILLIN see II:NGE500
FW 50 see III:WCJ000
FW 293 see III:BIO750
FW 925 see I:DFT800
FW 200 (mineral) see III:WCJ000
FYDE see I:FMV000
FYFANON see III:MAK700
FYROL FR 2 see III:FQU875
FYROL HB32 see I:TNC500
FYSIOQUENS see III:EEH575

G 1 see II:HIM000
G-11 see III:HCL000
G 338 see II:DER000
G 23992 see II:DER000
G-25804 see III:TBO500

G 27202 see III:HNI500
G 27692 see III:BJP000
G 30027 see III:ARQ725
GA see III:GEM000
GADOLINIUM see III:GAF000
GAFCOTE see III:PKQ059
GALACTICOL see III:DDJ000
d-GALACTOSAMINE HYDROCHLORIDE see III:GAT000
4-(β-d-GALACTOSIDO)-d-GLUCOSE see III:LAR000
GALECRON see III:CJJ250
GALLIC ACID, PROPYL ESTER see III:PNM750
GALLIUM-NICKEL ALLOY see II:NDD500
GALLODESOXYCHOLIC ACID see III:CDL325
GALLOGAMA see I:BBQ500
GALLOTANNIC ACID see III:TAD750
GALLOTANNIN see III:TAD750
GALOFAK see III:BDY669
GALOPERIDOL see III:CLY500
GALOZONE see III:CCL250
GAMACID see I:BBQ500
GAMAPHEX see I:BBQ500
GAMASOL 90 see III:DUD800
GAMENE see I:BBQ500
GAMISO see I:BBQ500
GAMMA-COL see I:BBQ500
GAMMAHEXA see I:BBQ500
GAMMAHEXANE see I:BBQ500
GAMMALIN see I:BBQ500
GAMMEXANE see I:BBP750
GAMMOPAZ see I:BBQ500
GAMOPHENE see III:HCL000
GANEAKE see I:ECU750
GANEX P 804 see III:PKQ250
GANTANOL see III:SNK000
GANTRISINE see III:SNN500
GARANTOSE see II:BCE500
GARDCIDE see III:RAF100
GARDENAL see II:EOK000
GARDENAL SODIUM see I:SID000
GARDEPANYL see II:EOK000
GARDONA see III:RAF100
GAROX see III:BDS000
GAS OIL see III:GBW000
GAS OILS (petroleum), hydrodesulfurized heavy vacuum see
    III:GBW010
GAS OILS (petroleum), light vacuum see III:GBW025
GASOLINE see III:GBY000
GASOLINE ENGINE EXHAUST CONDENSATE see
    III:GCE000
GASOLINE ENGINE EXHAUST "TAR" see III:GCE000
GASOLINE, UNLEADED see GCE100
GASTRACID see III:PEK250
GASTRINIDE see III:TEH500
GASTROMET see III:TAB250
GASTROTEST see III:PEK250
GC 6936 see III:ABX250
GC 3944-3-4 see III:PAX000
GEABOL see III:DAL300
GEARPHOS see III:MNH000, III:PAK000
GEBUTOX see III:BRE500
GECHLOREERDEDIFENYL (DUTCH) see II:PJM500
GEDEX see III:SMQ500
GEIGY 338 see II:DER000
GEIGY 27,692 see III:BJP000
GEIGY 30,027 see III:ARQ725
GEIGY-BLAU 536 see III:BGT250
GEIGY-444E see III:TBO500
GEIGY G-23611 see III:DSK200
GELACILLIN see III:BDY669
GELBIN see I:CAP500
GELBIN YELLOW ULTRAMARINE see I:CAP750
GELBORANGE-S (GERMAN) see III:FAG150
GELCARIN see III:CCL250
GELCARIN HMR see III:CCL250

G-ELEVEN see III:HCL000
GEL II see III:SHF500
GELIOMYCIN see III:HAL000
GELOCATIL see II:HIM000
GELOZONE see III:CCL250
GELUTION see III:SHF500
GELVATOLS see III:PKP750
GEMFIBROZIL see III:GCK300
GENAZO RED KB SOLN see II:CLK225
GENERAL CHEMICALS 1189 see I:KEA000
GENETRON 22 see III:CFX500
GENETRON 133a see III:TJY175
GENIPHENE see I:CDV100
GENISIS see I:ECU750
GENITE see III:DFY400
GENITE 883 see III:CJT750
GENITHION see III:PAK000
GENITOL see III:DFY400
GENITOX see I:DAD200
GENO-CRISTAUZ GREMY see I:TBF500
GENOTHERM see III:PKQ059
GENOXAL see I:CQC675, I:EAS500
GENOZYM see III:CMX700
GENTIAN VIOLET see III:AOR500
GENU see III:CCL250
GENUGEL see III:CCL250
GENUGEL CJ see III:CCL250
GENUGOL RLV see III:CCL250
GENUINE ACETATE CHROME ORANGE see I:LCS000
GENUINE ORANGE CHROME see I:LCS000
GENUVISCO J see III:CCL250
GEON see III:PJR000, III:PKQ059
GEON 135 see II:AAX175
GEON LATEX 151 see III:PKQ059
GERANIUM LAKE N see III:FAG070
GERASTOP see III:ARQ750
GERFIL see III:PMP500
GERISON see III:SNM500
GERMALGENE see II:TIO750
GERMA-MEDICA see III:HCL000
GEROT-EPILAN-D see I:DKQ000
GERVOT see III:MDT600
GESAFID see I:DAD200
GESAMIL see III:PMN850
GESAPON see I:DAD200
GESAPRIM see III:ARQ725
GESARAN see III:BJP000
GESAREX see I:DAD200
GESAROL see I:DAD200
GESATOP see III:BJP000
GESATOP 50 see III:BJP000
GESOPRIM see III:ARQ725
GESTEROL L.A. see III:HNT500
GEVILON see III:GCK300
GIALLO CROMO (ITALIAN) see I:LCR000
GIARDIL see III:NGG500
GIARLAM see III:NGG500
GIATRICOL see I:MMN250
GIBBERELLIC ACID see III:GEM000
GIBBERELLIN see III:GEM000
GIBBREL see III:GEM000
GIB-SOL see III:GEM000
GIB-TABS see III:GEM000
GIGANTIN see III:CMV000
GIHITAN see III:DCK759
GINEFLAVIR see I:MMN250
GINGILLI OIL see III:SCB000
GIRACID see I:PDC250
GIROSTAN see I:TFQ750
GLANDUBOLIN see I:EDV000
GLANDUCORPIN see I:PMH500
GLASS see III:FBQ000
GLASS FIBERS see III:FBQ000
GLAURAMINE see I:IBB000

GLAZD PENTA see II:PAX250
GLEEM see III:SHF500
GLIKOCEL TA see III:SFO500
GLIRICIDIAL SEPIUM see III:RBZ000
GLOBENICOL see II:CDP250
GLOBULARIACITRIN see III:RSU000
GLOGAL see III:HNI500
GLONOIN see III:NGY000
GLOROUS see II:CDP250
GLOSSO STERANDRYL see III:MPN500
GLOVER see II:LCF000
GLU-P-2 see II:DWW700
GLUCID see II:BCE500
GLUCINUM see I:BFO750
GLUCOCHLORAL see III:GFA000
GLUCOCHLORALOSE see III:GFA000
α-d-GLUCOCHLORALOSE see III:GFA000
GLUCO-FERRUM see III:FBK000
GLUCOLIN see III:GFG000
4-(α-d-GLUCOPYRANOSIDO)-α-GLUCOPYRANOSE see
   III:MAO500
β-D-GLUCOPYRANOSIDURONIC ACID, (METHYL-ON-
   N-AZOXY)METHYL- see III:MGS700
(d-GLUCOPYRANOSYLTHIO)GOLD see I:ART250
β-D-GLUCOPYRANURONIC ACID, 1-DEOXY-1-(9H-
   FLUOREN-2-YLHYDROXYAMINO)- see III:HLE750
GLUCOSE see III:GFG000
d-GLUCOSE see III:GFG000
d-GLUCOSE, ANHYDROUS see III:GFG000
GLUCOSE LIQUID see III:GFG000
4-(α-d-GLUCOSIDO)-d-GLUCOSE see III:MAO500
N-d-GLUCOSYL(2)-N'-NITROSOMETHYLHARNSTOFF (GER-
   MAN) see I:SMD000
N-d-GLUCOSYL-(2)-N'-NITROSOMETHYLUREA see
   I:SMD000
β-d-GLUCOSYLOXYAZOXYMETHANE see I:COU000
(1-d-GLUCOSYLTHIO)GOLD see I:ART250
GLUCURONIC ACID, 1-DEOXY-1-(2-FLUORENYLHY-
   DROXYAMINO)- see III:HLE750
N-GLUCURONIDE of N-HYDROXY-2-AMINOFLUORENE see
   III:HLE750
GLU-P-I see II:AKS250
GLUPAN see III:TEH500
GLUSIDE see II:BCE500
l-GLUTAMIC ACID, 5-(2-(4-CARBOXYPHENYL)HYDRA-
   ZIDE) see III:GFO100
GLUTAMIC ACID, IRON (2+) SALT (1:1) see III:FBM000
GLUTAMIC ACID, N-NITROSO-N-PTEROYL-, l- see
   III:NKG450
GLUTANON see III:TEH500
GLYCERIN-α-MONOCHLORHYDRIN see III:CDT750
GLYCERINTRINITRATE (CZECH) see III:NGY000
GLYCERITE see III:TAD750
GLYCEROL CHLOROHYDRIN see III:CDT750
GLYCEROL-α-CHLOROHYDRIN see III:CDT750
GLYCEROL EPICHLORHYDRIN see I:EAZ500
GLYCEROL-α-MONOCHLOROHYDRIN (DOT) see
   III:CDT750
GLYCEROL, NITRIC ACID TRIESTER see III:NGY000
GLYCEROL TRIBUTYRATE see III:TIG750
GLYCEROL (TRI(CHLOROMETHYL))ETHER see GGI000
GLYCEROL TRINITRATE see III:NGY000
GLYCEROL(TRINITRATE de) (FRENCH) see III:NGY000
GLYCEROLTRINTRAAT (DUTCH) see III:NGY000
GLYCERYL-α-CHLOROHYDRIN see III:CDT750
GLYCERYL NITRATE see III:NGY000
GLYCERYL TRINITRATE see III:NGY000
GLYCERYL TRINITRATE, solution up to 1% in alcohol (DOT)
   see III:NGY000
GLYCIDAL see GGW000
GLYCIDALDEHYDE see GGW000
GLYCIDOL OLEATE see III:ECJ000
GLYCIDOL STEARATE see III:SLK500
GLYCIDYLALDEHYDE see GGW000

GLYCIDYL ESTER of DODECANOIC ACID see III:TJI500
GLYCIDYL ESTER of HEXANOIC ACID see III:GGY000
GLYCIDYL LAURATE see III:LBM000
GLYCIDYL OCTADECANOATE see III:SLK500
GLYCIDYL OCTADECENOATE see III:ECJ000
GLYCIDYL OLEATE see III:ECJ000
GLYCIDYL PHENYL ETHER see II:PFH000
GLYCIDYL STEARATE see III:SLK500
GLYCO-FLAVINE see III:DBX400
GLYCOL BROMIDE see I:EIY500
GLYCOL BROMOHYDRIN see III:BNI500
GLYCOL DIBROMIDE see I:EIY500
GLYCOL DICHLORIDE see I:EIY600
GLYCOL ETHER see III:DJD600
GLYCOL ETHYLENE ETHER see I:DVQ000
GLYCOL ETHYL ETHER see III:DJD600
GLYCOL SULFATE see III:EJP000
GLYCOL SULFITE see III:COV750
GLYCON S-70 see III:SLK000
GLYCON DP see III:SLK000
GLYCON RO see III:OHU000
GLYCON TP see III:SLK000
GLYCON WO see III:OHU000
GLYCOSPERSE O-20 see III:PKL100
2-GLYCYLAMINOFLUORENE see III:AKC000
GLYESTRIN see I:ECU750
GLYMOL see III:MQV750
GLYODEX 3722 see III:CBG000
GLYSANOL B see I:ART250
GLYSOLETTEN see II:EOK000
G-M-F see III:DVR200
GOHSENOLS see III:PKP750
GOLD see III:GIS000
1721 GOLD see III:CNI000
GOLD BRONZE see III:CNI000
GOLDEN YELLOW see III:DCZ000
GOLD FLAKE see III:GIS000
GOLD LEAF see III:GIS000
GOLD ORANGE MP see III:DOU600
GOLD POWDER see III:GIS000
GOLD THIOGLUCOSE see I:ART250
GOMBARDOL see III:SNM500
GONACRINE see III:DBX400
GONTOCHIN see III:CLD000
GOOD-RITE see III:PJR000
GOODRITE 1800X73 see III:SMR000
GOOD-RITE GP 264 see I:DVL700
GORDONA see III:RAF100
GORE-TEX see III:TAI250
GOTHNION see III:ASH500
G 2 (OXIDE) see III:AHE250
GP-40-66:120 see II:HCD250
GPKh see II:HAR000
GRAAFINA see I:EDP000
de GRAAFINA see I:EDP000
GRAFESTROL see I:DKA600
GRAIN ALCOHOL see I:EFU000
GRANOX NM see I:HCC500
GRANOX PPM see III:CBG000
GRAPE BLUE A GEIGY see III:FAE100
GRAPEFRUIT OIL see III:GJU000
GRAPEFRUIT OIL, COLDPRESSED see III:GJU000
GRAPEFRUIT OIL, EXPRESSED see III:GJU000
GRAPE SUGAR see III:GFG000
GRASAL BRILLIANT YELLOW see I:DOT300
GRASAL YELLOW see III:FAG130
GRASAN ORANGE 3R see III:XRA000
GRASAN ORANGE R see III:PEJ500
GRASOL BLUE 2GS see III:TBG700
GRAVISTAT see III:NNL500
GREEN 5 see III:ADF000
1724 GREEN see III:FAG000
11661 GREEN see II:CMJ900
GREEN CHROME OXIDE see II:CMJ900

GREEN CHROMIC OXIDE see II:CMJ900
GREEN CINNABAR see II:CMJ900
GREEN CROSS WARBLE POWDER see III:RNZ000
GREEN NICKEL OXIDE see I:NDF500
GREEN No. 203 see III:FAF000
GREENOCKITE see I:CAJ750
GREEN OIL see I:COD750, III:APG500
GREEN ROUGE see II:CMJ900
GREEN VITRIOL see III:FBN100
GREOSIN see GKE000
GRESFEED see GKE000
GREY ARSENIC see ARA750
GRICIN see GKE000
GRIFFEX see III:ARQ725
GRIFFIN MANEX see III:MAS500
GRIFULVIN see GKE000
GRILON see III:NOH000, III:PJY500
GRIPPEX see III:TEH500
GRISACTIN see GKE000
GRISCOFULVIN see GKE000
GRISEFULINE see GKE000
GRISEO see GKE000
(+)-GRISEOFULVIN see GKE000
GRISEOFULVIN-FORTE see GKE000
GRISEOFULVINUM see GKE000
GRISETIN see GKE000
GRISOFULVIN see GKE000
GRISOVIN see GKE000
GRIS-PEG see GKE000
GROCEL see III:GEM000
GROCO 2 see III:OHU000
GROCO 4 see III:OHU000
GROCO 54 see III:SLK000
GROCO 5L see III:OHU000
GROFAS see III:QSA000
GROUNDNUT OIL see III:PAO000
GROWTH HORMONE see III:PJA250
GRUNDIER ARBEZOL see II:PAX250
GRUNERITE see III:GKE900
GRYSIO see GKE000
GT41 see I:BOT250
GT 2041 see I:BOT250
GTG see I:ART250
GTN see III:NGY000
GUANAZOLE see III:DCF200
GUANINE see III:GLI000
GUANINE-7-N-OXIDE see III:GLM000
GUANINE-3-N-OXIDE HEMIHYDROCHLORIDE see
    III:GLO000
GUARANINE see III:CAK500
GUAVA see III:GLW000
GUDAKHU (INDIA) see I:SED400
GUESAPON see I:DAD200
GUESAROL see I:DAD200
GUIGNER'S GREEN see II:CMJ900
GUINEA GREEN B see III:FAE950
GUM see III:PJR000
GUM CARRAGEENAN see III:CCL250
GUM CHON 2 see III:CCL250
GUM CHROND see III:CCL250
GUSATHION see III:ASH500
GUSERVIN see GKE000
GUSTAFSON CAPTAN 30-DD see III:CBG000
GUTHION (DOT) see III:ASH500
GUTHION, liquid (DOT) see III:ASH500
GUTTAGENA see III:PKQ059
GIV GARD DXN see I:ABC250
GYNAESAN see II:EDU500
GYN-ANOVLAR see II:EEH520
GYNECORMONE see I:EDP000
GYNEFOLLIN see II:DAL600
GYNERGON see I:EDO000
GYNESTREL see I:EDO000
GYNFORMONE see I:EDP000

1,4,5,6,7,8,8-HEPTACHLOR-3a,4,7,7,7a-TETRAHYDRO-4,7-endo-METHANO-INDEN (GERMAN) see II:HAR000
1-HEPTADECANECARBOXYLIC ACID see III:SLK000
HEPTAGRAN see II:HAR000
HEPTAMETHYLENEIMINE mixed with SODIUM NITRITE see III:SIT000
HEPTAMUL see II:HAR000
HEPTANOIC ACID, ester with TESTOSTERONE see III:TBF750
17-β-HEPTANOYLOXY-19-NOR-17-α-PREGNEN-20-YNONE see III:NNQ000
8-HEPTYLBENZ(a)ANTHRACENE see III:HBN000
5-n-HEPTYLBENZ(1:2)BENZANTHRACENE see III:HBN000
HEPTYLMETHYLINITROSAMINE see III:HBP000
1-HEPTYL-1-NITROSOUREA see III:HBP250
n-HEPTYL NITROSUREA see III:HBP250
HEPZIDE see II:NV500
HERBATOX see III:DXQ500
HERBAZIN see III:BJP000
HERBAZIN 50 see III:BJP000
HERBEX see III:BJP000
HERBICIDE C-2059 see III:DUK800
HERBICIDE M see II:CIR250
HERBICIDES, MONURON see III:CJX750
HERBICIDES, SILVEX see II:TIX500
HERBICIDE TOTAL see I:AMY050
HERBIDAL see II:DAA800
HERBIZOLE see I:AMY050
HERBOXY see III:BJP000
HERCOFLAT 135 see III:PMP500
HERCOFLEX 260 see I:DVL700
HERCULES 3956 see I:CDV100
HERCULES TOXAPHENE see I:CDV100
HERCULON see III:PMP500
HERMAL see III:TFS350
HERMAT TMT see III:TFS350
HERMAT ZDM see III:BJK500
HERMAT Zn-MBT see III:BHA750
HERMESETAS see II:BCE500
HERPESIL see III:DAS000
HERPIDU see III:DAS000
HERPLEX see III:DAS000
HERPLEX LIQUIFILM see III:DAS000
HERYL see III:TFS350
HETEROAUXIN see III:ICN000
HEV-4 see I:CNA750
HEXA see I:BBP750
HEXABALM see III:HCL000
HEXABENZOBENZENE see III:CNS250
HEXABROMOBIPHENYL (technical grade) see III:FBU000
2,4,5,2',4',5'-HEXABROMOBIPHENYL see II:FBU509
HEXACAP see III:CBG000
HEXACARBONYLCHROMIUM see I:HCB000
HEXACARBONYL CHROMIUM see I:HCB000
HEXA C.B. see I:HCC500
HEXACERT RED No. 2 see III:FAG020
HEXACERT RED No. 3 see III:FAG040
HEXACHLOR see I:BBP750
HEXACHLOR-AETHAN (GERMAN) see III:HCI000
HEXACHLORAN see I:BBP750, I:BBQ500
γ-HEXACHLORAN see I:BBQ500
α-HEXACHLORANE see I:BBQ000
γ-HEXACHLORANE see I:BBQ500
HEXACHLORBENZOL (GERMAN) see I:HCC500
HEXACHLOR-1,3-BUTADIEN (CZECH) see II:HCD250
HEXACHLORBUTADIENE see II:HCD250
HEXACHLORCYCLOHEXAN (GERMAN) see I:BBQ000
HEXACHLOROBENZENE see I:HCC500
β-HEXACHLOROBENZENE see I:BBR000
γ-HEXACHLOROBENZENE see I:BBQ500
1,2,3,4,7,7-HEXACHLOROBICYCLO(2.2.1)HEPTEN-5,6-BI-OXYMETHYLENESULFITE see III:EAQ750
α,β-1,2,3,4,7,7-HEXACHLOROBICYCLO(2.2.1)-2-HEPTENE-5,6-BISOXYMETHYLENE SULFITE see III:EAQ750

2,2',4,4'5,5'-HEXACHLOROBIPHENYL see III:HCD000
2,4,5,2',4',5'-HEXACHLOROBIPHENYL see III:HCD000
2,2',4,4',5'5'-HEXACHLORO-1,1'-BIPHENYL see III:HCD000
1,1,2,3,4,4-HEXACHLORO-1,3-BUTADIENE see II:HCD250
HEXACHLORO-1,3-BUTADIENE (MAK) see II:HCD250
HEXACHLOROCYCLOHEXANE see I:BBP750
α-HEXACHLOROCYCLOHEXANE see I:BBQ000
β-HEXACHLOROCYCLOHEXANE see I:BBR000
γ-HEXACHLOROCYCLOHEXANE (MAK) see I:BBQ500
1,2,3,4,5,6-HEXACHLOROCYCLOHEXANE see I:BBP750
1,2,3,4,5,6-HEXACHLOROCYCLOHEXANE (mixture of isomers) see I:BBQ750
α-1,2,3,4,5,6-HEXACHLOROCYCLOHEXANE (MAK) see I:BBQ000
β-1,2,3,4,5,6-HEXACHLOROCYCLOHEXANE (MAK) see I:BBR000
1-α,2-α,3-β,4-α,5-α,6-β-HEXACHLOROCYCLOHEXANE see I:BBQ500
1-α,2-α,3-β,4-α,5-β,6-β-HEXACHLOROCYCLOHEXANE see I:BBQ000
1-α,2-β,3-α,4-β,5-α,6-β-HEXACHLOROCYCLOHEXANE see I:BBR000
HEXACHLOROCYCLOHEXANE, delta and epsilon mixture see III:HCE400
Δ-HEXACHLOROCYCLOHEXANE mixed with epsilon-HEXA-CHLOROCYCLOHEXANE see III:HCE400
1,2,3,4,5,6-HEXACHLOROCYCLOHEXANE, γ-ISOMER see I:BBQ500
HEXACHLOROCYCLOPENTADIENEDIMER see I:MQW500
1,2,3,4,5,5-HEXACHLORO-1,3-CYCLOPENTADIENE DIMER see I:MQW500
1,2,3,4,7,8-HEXACHLORODIBENZO-p-DIOXIN see III:HCF000
1,2,3,6,7,8-HEXACHLORODIBENZO-p-DIOXIN mixed with 1,2,3,7,8,9-HEXACHLORODIBENZO-p-DIOXIN see II:HCF500
1,2,3,7,8,9-HEXACHLORODIBENZO-p-DIOXIN mixed with 1,2,3,6,7,8-HEXACHLORODIBENZO-p-DIOXIN see II:HCF500
2,2',3,3',5,5'-HEXACHLORO-6,6'-DIHYDROXYDIPHENYL-METHANE see III:HCL000
HEXACHLOROEPOXYOCTAHYDRO-endo,endo-DIMETH-ANONAPHTHALENE see III:EAT500
HEXACHLOROEPOXYOCTAHYDRO-ENDO,EXO-DIMETH-ANONAPHTHALENE see III:DHB400
HEXACHLOROETHANE see III:HCI000
1,1,1,2,2,2-HEXACHLOROETHANE see III:HCI000
HEXACHLOROETHYLENE see III:HCI000
HEXACHLOROFEN (CZECH) see III:HCL000
HEXACHLOROHEXAHYDRO-endo-exo-DIMETHANO-NAPHTHALENE see III:AFK250
1,2,3,4,10,10-HEXACHLORO-1,4,4a,5,8,8a-HEXAHYDRO-1,4,5,8-DIMETHANONAPHTHALENE see III:AFK250
1,2,3,4,10,10-HEXACHLORO-1,4,4a,5,8,8a-HEXAHYDRO-exo-1,4,-endo-5,8-DIMETHANONAPHTHALENE see III:AFK250
1,2,3,4,10,10-HEXACHLORO-1,4,4a,5,8,8a-HEXAHYDRO-1,4-endo-exo-5, 8-DIMETHANONAPHTHALENE see III:AFK250
HEXACHLOROHEXAHYDROMETHANO 2,4,3-BENZODIOX-ATHIEPIN-3-OXIDE see III:EAQ750
6,7,8,9,10,10-HEXACHLORO-1,5,5a,6,9,9a-HEXAHYDRO-6,9-METHANO-2,4,3-BENZODIOXATHIEPIN-3-OXIDE see III:EAQ750
1,4,5,6,7,7-HEXACHLORO-5-NORBORNENE-2,3-DICAR-BOXYLIC ACID see II:CDS000
1,4,5,6,7,7-HEXACHLORO-5-NORBORNENE-2,3-DIMETH-ANOL CYCLIC SULFITE see III:EAQ750
3,4,5,6,9,9-HEXACHLORO-1a,2,2a,3,6,6a,7,7a-OCTAHYDRO-2,7:3,6-DIMETHANONAPHTH(2,3-b)OXIRENE see III:DHB400, III:EAT500
HEXACHLOROPHANE see III:HCL000
HEXACHLOROPHEN see III:HCL000

HEXACHLOROPHENE see III:HCL000
HEXACHLOROPHENE (DOT) see III:HCL000
HEXACOL BRILLIANT BLUE A see III:FAE000
HEXACOL CARMOISINE see III:HJF500
HEXACOL ERYTHROSINE BS see III:FAG040
HEXACOL OIL ORANGE SS see II:TGW000
HEXACOL ORANGE GG CRYSTALS see III:HGC000
HEXACOL PONCEAU 4R see III:FMU080
HEXACOL PONCEAU MX see III:FMU070
HEXACOL PONCEAU SX see III:FAG050
HEXACOL RHODAMINE B EXTRA see III:FAG070
HEXADECANOIC ACID see III:PAE250
HEXADECENE EPOXIDE see III:EBX500
n-HEXADECOIC ACID see III:PAE250
HEXADECYLIC ACID see III:PAE250
HEXADIENIC ACID see III:SKU000
HEXADIENOIC ACID see III:SKU000
2,4-HEXADIENOIC ACID see III:SKU000
trans-trans-2,4-HEXADIENOIC ACID see III:SKU000
HEXADRIN see I:EAS500, III:EAT500
HEXAETHYLBENZENE see III:HCX000
HEXAFEN see III:HCL000
HEXAFERB see III:FAS000
4,4,4,4′,4′,4′-HEXAFLUORO-N-NITROSODIBUTYLAMINE
    see III:NJN300
HEXAFLUOROSILICATE (2−), NICKEL see II:NDD000
HEXAFORM see III:HEI500
HEXAHYDROANILINE see III:CPF500
HEXAHYDRO-2-AZEPINONE see III:CBF700
HEXAHYDRO-2H-AZEPIN-2-ONE see III:CBF700
HEXAHYDRO-2H-AZEPIN-2-ONE HOMOPOLYMER see
    III:PJY500
1,2,4,5,6,7-HEXAHYDROBENZ(e)ACEANTHRYLENE see
    III:HDH000
HEXAHYDROBENZENAMINE see III:CPF500
1,2,3,4,12,13-HEXAHYDRODIBENZ(a,h)ANTHRACENE see
    III:HDK000
HEXAHYDRO-3A,7A-DIMETHYL-4,7-EPOXYISOBENZOFU-
    RAN-1,3-DIONE see III:CBE750
HEXAHYDRO-1,4-DINITROSO-1H-1,4-DIAZEPINE see
    III:DVE600
exo-HEXAHYDRO-4,7-METHANOINDAN see III:TLR675
6,7,8,9,10,12b-HEXAHYDRO-3-METHYL CHOLANTHRENE
    see III:HDR500
HEXAHYDRO-1-NITROSO-1H-AZEPINE see II:NKI000
HEXAHYDRO-N-NITROSOPYRIDINE see I:NLJ500
HEXAHYDRO-1,3,5-s-TRIAZINE see III:HDV500
HEXAHYDRO-1,3,5-TRINITROSO-s-TRIAZINE see
    III:HDV500
HEXAHYDRO-1,3,5-TRINITROSO-1,3,5-TRIAZINE see
    III:HDV500
HEXAKIS(μ-ACETATO-O:O′))-μ(^{4})-OXOTETRABERYLLIUM
    see I:BFT500
HEXAKIS(μ-ACETATO)-μ(^{4})-OXOTETRABERYLLIUM see
    I:BFT500
HEXAMETAPOL see I:HEK000
HEXAMETHYLBENZENE see III:HEC000
HEXAMETHYL-BICYCLO(2.2.0)HEXA-2,5-DIEN (GERMAN)
    see III:HEC500
HEXAMETHYLBICYCLO(2.2.0)HEXA-2,5-DIENE see
    III:HEC500
HEXAMETHYLDISILAZANE see III:HED500
HEXAMETHYLENAMINE see III:HEI500
HEXAMETHYLENEAMINE see III:HEI500
HEXAMETHYLENETETRAAMINE see III:HEI500
HEXAMETHYLENETETRAMINE see III:HEI500
HEXAMETHYLENTETRAMIN (GERMAN) see III:HEI500
HEXAMETHYLMELAMINE see III:HEJ500
HEXAMETHYL PHOSPHORAMIDE see I:HEK000
HEXAMETHYLPHOSPHORIC ACID TRIAMIDE (MAK) see
    I:HEK000
HEXAMETHYLPHOSPHORIC TRIAMIDE see I:HEK000
N,N,N,N,N,N-HEXAMETHYLPHOSPHORIC TRIAMIDE see
    I:HEK000

HEXAMETHYLPHOSPHOROTRIAMIDE see I:HEK000
HEXAMETHYLPHOSPHOTRIAMIDE see I:HEK000
HEXAMETHYL-p-ROSANILINE HYDROCHLORIDE see
    III:AOR500
HEXAMETHYLSILAZANE see III:HED500
N,N,N′,N′,N′′,N′′-HEXAMETHYL-1,3,5-TRIAZINE-2,4,6-TRI-
    AMINE see III:HEJ500
HEXAMETHYL VIOLET see III:AOR500
HEXAMIC ACID see II:CPQ625
HEXAMINE (DOT) see III:HEI500
HEXANAMIDE see III:HEM500
HEXANEDIAMIDE (9CI) see III:AEN000
HEXANEDIOIC ACID, BIS(2-ETHYLHEXYL) ESTER see
    III:AEO000
HEXANEDIOIC ACID, DIOCTYL ESTER see III:AEO000
HEXANEDIOIC ACID, POLYMER with 1,4-BUTANEDIOL and
    1,1′-METHYLENEBIS(4-ISOCYANATOBENZENE) see
    I:PKM250
HEXANEDIOIC ACID, POLYMER with 1,3-ETHANEDIOL and
    1,1′-METHYLENEBIS(4-ISOCYANATOBENZENE) see
    I:PKL750
6-HEXANELACTAM see III:CBF700
HEXANITRODIFENYLAMINE (DUTCH) see III:HET500
HEXANITRODIPHENYLAMINE see III:HET500
HEXANITRODIPHENYLAMINE (FRENCH) see III:HET500
2,2′,4,4′,6,6′-HEXANITRODIPHENYLAMINE see III:HET500
2,4,6,2′,4′,6′-HEXANITRODIPHENYLAMINE see III:HET500
HEXANOESTROL see III:DLB400
HEXANONE ISOXIME see III:CBF700
HEXANONISOXIM (GERMAN) see III:CBF700
1-HEXANOYLAZIRIDINE see III:HEW000
HEXANOYLETHYLENEIMINE see III:HEW000
17-α-HEXANOYLOXYPREGN-4-ENE-3,20-DIONE see
    III:HNT500
HEXASTAT see III:HEJ500
HEXATHANE see III:EIR000
HEXATHIR see III:TFS350
HEXATOX see I:BBQ500
HEXATYPE CARMINE B see III:EOJ500
HEXAZIR see III:BJK500
γ-HEXENOLACTONE see III:PAJ500
2-HEXEN-5,1-OLIDE see III:PAJ500
HEXESTROL see III:DLB400
meso-HEXESTROL see III:DLB400
HEXICIDE see I:BBQ500
HEXIDE see III:HCL000
HEXILMETHYLENAMINE see III:HEI500
HEXMETHYLPHOSPHORAMIDE see I:HEK000
HEXOESTROL see III:DLB400
1,6-HEXOLACTAM see III:CBF700
HEXOPHENE see III:HCL000
HEXOSAN see III:HCL000
HEXYCLAN see I:BBQ500
HEXYL (GERMAN, DUTCH) see III:HET500
HEXYLAN see I:BBP750
8-HEXYL-BENZ(a)ANTHRACENE see III:HFL000
5-n-HEXYL-1,2-BENZANTHRACENE see III:HFL000
4-HEXYL-1,3-BENZENEDIOL see III:HFV500
2-HEXYL-4-CHLOROPHENOL see III:CHL500
4-HEXYL-1,3-DIHYDROXYBENZENE see III:HFV500
1-HEXYL-1-NITROSOUREA see III:HFS500
HEXYLRESORCIN (GERMAN) see III:HFV500
4-HEXYLRESORCINE see III:HFV500
HEXYLRESORCINOL see III:HFV500
4-HEXYLRESORCINOL see III:HFV500
p-HEXYLRESORCINOL see III:HFV500
4-n-HEXYLRESORCINOL see III:HFV500
HEYDEFLON see III:TAI250
HGI see I:BBQ500
HHDN see III:AFK250
HIBESTROL see I:DKA600
HICO CCC see III:CMF400
HIDACID AMARANTH see III:FAG020
HIDACID AZO RUBINE see III:HJF500

HIDACID AZURE BLUE see III:FMU059
HIDACID BROMO ACID REGULAR see III:BNK700
HIDACID DIBROMO FLUORESCEIN see III:BNH500, III:BNK700
HIDACID FAST ORANGE G see III:HGC000
HIDACID FAST SCARLET 3R see III:FMU080
HIDACID SCARLET 2R see III:FMU070
HIDACID URANINE see III:FEW000
HIDACO OIL ORANGE see III:PEJ500
HIDACO OIL YELLOW see I:AIC250
HIDACO VICTORIA BLUE R see III:VKA600
HIDAN see I:DKQ000
HIDANTILO see I:DKQ000
HIDANTINA SENOSIAN see I:DKQ000
HIDANTINA VITORIA see I:DKQ000
HIDANTOMIN see I:DKQ000
HIDRALAZIN see II:HGP500, III:PHW000
HIDRANIZIL see III:ILD000
HIDRASONIL see III:ILD000
HIDRIX see III:HOO500
HIDROESTRON see I:EDP000
HIDRULTA see III:ILD000
HIDRUN see III:ILD000
HIESTRONE see I:EDV000
HIFOL see III:BIO750
HI-JEL see III:BAV750
HILDAN see III:EAQ750
HILDIT see I:DAD200
HILONG see III:CFZ000
HILTHION see III:MAK700
HILTHION 25WDP see III:MAK700
HILTONIL FAST BLUE B BASE see I:DCJ200
HILTONIL FAST RED KB BASE see II:CLK225
HILTONIL FAST SCARLET G BASE see I:NMP500
HILTOSAL FAST BLUE B SALT see I:DCJ200
HINDASOL BLUE B SALT see I:DCJ200
HINDASOL RED TR SALT see II:CLK235
HIOXYL see III:HIB000
HIPOFTALIN see II:HGP500, III:PHW000
HI-POINT 90 see III:MKA500
HIPPUZON see III:TEH500
HIPTAGENIC ACID see III:NIY500
HI-SEL see III:SCH000
HISHIREX 502 see III:PKQ059
HISPACID BRILLIANT SCARLET 3RF see III:FMU080
HISPACID FAST ORANGE 2G see III:HGC000
HISPACID GREEN GB see III:FAE950
HISPACID ORANGE 1 see III:FAG010
HISPAMIN BLACK EF see I:AQP000
HISPAMIN BLUE 2B see I:CMO000
HISPAMIN BLUE 3BX see II:CMO250
HISPAMIN VIOLET 3R see III:CMP000
HISPAVIC 229 see III:PKQ059
HISPERSE YELLOW G see II:AAQ250
HISTADYL HYDROCHLORIDE see III:DPJ400
HISTAFED see III:DPJ400
HISTAMINE HYDROCHLORIDE see III:HGE500
HISTATEX see III:DBM800
HISTIDYL see III:DPJ400
HISTOCARB see III:CBJ000
HISTYRENE S 6F see III:SMR000
HI-STYROL see III:SMQ500
HI-YIELD DESSICANT H-10 see I:ARB250
H.K. FORMULA No. K. 7117 see III:FMU059
7-HMBA see III:BBH250
HMBD see II:HLX925, III:HLX900
HMD see I:PAN100
HMDS see III:HED500
HMF see III:ORG000
HMM see III:HEJ500
12-HM-7-MBA see III:HMF500
7-HM-12-MBA see III:HMF000
HMPA see I:HEK000
HMPT see I:HEK000

HMT see III:HEI500
HN2 see I:BIE250
HN2.HCl see I:BIE500
HN2 HYDROCHLORIDE see I:BIE500
HN$_2$ OXIDE HYDROCHLORIDE see II:CFA750
HNT see III:HHD500
HNU see II:HKW500
3-HO-AAF see III:HIO875
HOCA see III:DXH250
HOCH see I:FMV000
HODAG SVO 9 see III:PKL100
HOE 2,671 see III:EAQ750
HOE-2824 see III:ABX250
HOECHST PA 190 see III:PJS750
HOKMATE see III:FAS000
HOLIN see II:EDU500
HOLOXAN see II:IMH000
HOMANDREN (amps) see I:TBG000
HOMANDREN see III:MPN500
HOMBITAN see III:TGG760
HOMOANISIC ACID see III:MFE250
HOMOOLAN see II:HIM000
HOMOSTERONE see I:TBF500
HOOKER No. 1 CHRYSOTILE ASBESTOS see I:ARM268
HORFEMINE see I:DKB000
HORIZON see III:DCK759
HORMALE see III:MPN500
HORMATOX see II:DGB000
HORMOCEL-2CCC see III:CMF400
HORMOESTROL see III:DLB400
HORMOFEMIN see II:DAL600
HORMOFLAVEINE see I:PMH500
HORMOFOLLIN see I:EDV000
17-HORMOFORIN see III:AOO450
HORMOFORT see III:HNT500
HORMOGYNON see I:EDP000
HORMOLUTON see I:PMH500
HORMOMED see II:EDU500
HORMONE SOMATOTROPE (FRENCH) see III:PJA250
HORMONIN see II:EDU500
HORMONISENE see II:CLO750
HORMOTESTON see I:TBG000
HORMOTUHO see II:CIR250
HORMOVARINE see I:EDV000
HORSE HEAD A-410 see III:TGG760
HORTFENICOL see II:CDP250
HOSTACORTIN see III:PLZ000
HOSTADUR see III:PKF750
HOSTAFLEX VP 150 see II:AAX175
HOSTAFLON see III:TAI250
HOSTALEN PP see III:PMP500
HOSTALIT see III:PKQ059
HOSTAPHAN see III:PKF750
HOSTAVAT GOLDEN YELLOW see III:DCZ000
HOSTYREN S see III:SMQ500
HOWFLEX GBP see III:DJD700
H.P. 209 see III:EEM000
HPA see III:EPI300
HPC see III:HNT500
HPOP see II:HNX500
HPT see I:HEK000
HRS 1276 see I:MQW500
HS see I:HGW500
H. TERNATUM see III:SAF500
HT-F 76 see III:SMQ500
HUILE d'ANILINE (FRENCH) see II:AOQ000
HULS P 6500 see III:PMP500
HUMAN SPERM see III:HGM000
HUNGAZIN see III:ARQ725
HUNGAZIN DT see III:BJP000
HUNGAZIN PK see III:ARQ725
HW 920 see III:DXQ500
HYADUR see III:DUD800
HYAMINE see III:BEN000

HYAMINE 1622 see III:BEN000
HYBAR X see III:UNJ800
HYCANTHON see III:LIM000
HYCANTHONE see III:LIM000
HYCANTHONE MESYLATE see III:HGO500
HYCANTHONE METHANESULFONATE see III:HGO500
HYCANTHONE METHANESULPHONATE see III:HGO500
HYCANTHONE MONOMETHANESULPHONATE see
   III:HGO500
HYCAR see III:PJR000
HYCAR LX 407 see III:SMR000
HYCLORATE see III:ARQ750
HYCOZID see III:ILD000
HYDANTAL see I:DKQ000
HYDANTIN SODIUM see I:DNU000
HYDANTOIN see I:DKQ000
HYDANTOIN, 1-((5-(p-NITROPHENYL)FURFURYL-
   IDENE)AMINO)- see III:DAB845
HYDANTOIN SODIUM see I:DNU000
HYDRACETIN see III:ACX750
HYDRACRYLIC ACID β-LACTONE see I:PMT100
HYDRAL see III:CDO000
HYDRALAZINE see III:PHW000
HYDRALAZINE CHLORIDE see II:HGP500
HYDRALAZINE HYDROCHLORIDE see II:HGP500
HYDRALAZINE MONOHYDROCHLORIDE see II:HGP500
HYDRAL de CHLORAL see III:CDO000
HYDRALLAZINE see III:PHW000
HYDRALLAZINE HYDROCHLORIDE see II:HGP500
HYDRAPRESS see II:HGP500
HYDRAZID see III:ILD000
HYDRAZIDE see III:ILD000
HYDRAZINE see I:HGS000
HYDRAZINE, ANHYDROUS (DOT) see I:HGS000
HYDRAZINE, AQUEOUS SOLUTION (DOT) see I:HGS000
HYDRAZINE BASE see I:HGS000
HYDRAZINE-BENZENE see II:PFI000
HYDRAZINE-BENZENE and BENZIDINE SULFATE see
   II:BBY300
HYDRAZINECARBOTHIOAMIDE see III:TFQ000
HYDRAZINECARBOXALDEHYDE see III:FNN000
HYDRAZINECARBOXAMIDE see III:HGU000
HYDRAZINECARBOXAMIDE MONOHYDROCHLORIDE see
   III:SBW500
1,2-HYDRAZINEDICARBOTHIOAMIDE see III:BLJ250
HYDRAZINE, 1,1-DI-2-PROPENYL-(9CI) see III:DBK100
HYDRAZINE HYDRATE see III:HGU500
HYDRAZINE HYDROGEN SULFATE see I:HGW500
HYDRAZINE MONOHYDRATE see III:HGU500
HYDRAZINE MONOSULFATE see I:HGW500
HYDRAZINE SULFATE (1:1) see I:HGW500
HYDRAZINE SULPHATE see I:HGW500
HYDRAZINIUM SULFATE see I:HGW500
2-HYDRAZINO-4-(4-AMINOPHENYL)THIAZOLE see
   III:HHB000
2-HYDRAZINO-4-(p-AMINOPHENYL)THIAZOLE see
   III:HHB000
HYDRAZINOBENEZENE see II:PFI000
2-HYDRAZINOETHANOL see III:HHC000
2-HYDRAZINO-4-(5-NITRO-2-FURANYL)THIAZOLE see
   III:HHD500
2-HYDRAZINO-4-(5-NITRO-2-FURYL)THIAZOLE see
   III:HHD500
2-HYDRAZINO-4-(4-NITROPHENYL)THIAZOLE see
   III:HHE000
1-HYDRAZINO-2-PHENYLETHANE HYDROGEN SULPHATE
   see III:PFC750
HYDRAZINOPHTHALAZINE see III:PHW000
1-HYDRAZINOPHTHALAZINE see III:PHW000
1-HYDRAZINOPHTHALAZINE HYDROCHLORIDE see
   II:HGP500
1-HYDRAZINOPHTHLAZINE MONOHYDROCHLORIDE see
   II:HGP500
HYDRAZOBENZEN (CZECH) see I:HHG000

HYDRAZOBENZENE see I:HHG000
HYDRAZODIBENZENE see I:HHG000
HYDRAZODICARBONSAEUREABIS(METHYLNITROSAMID)
   (GERMAN) see III:DRN400
HYDRAZODICARBOXYLIC ACID BIS(METHYLNITROS-
   AMIDE) see III:DRN400
HYDRAZODIFORMIC ACID see III:DKJ600
HYDRAZOETHANE see II:DJL400
HYDRAZOMETHANE see I:DSF600, II:MKN000
HYDRAZONIUM SULFATE see I:HGW500
2,2'-HYDRAZONODIETHANOL see III:HHH000
HYDRAZYNA (POLISH) see I:HGS000
HYDREA see III:HOO500
HYDROAZODICARBOXYBIS(METHYLNITROSAMIDE) see
   III:DRN400
HYDROAZOETHANE see II:DJL400
HYDROCELLULOSE see III:HHK000
HYDROCERIN see III:CMD750
HYDROCHINON (CZECH, POLISH) see III:HIH000
HYDROCHLORIC ACID DICARBOXIDE see III:DEK000
HYDROCHLORIC ACID DIMETHYLAMINE see III:DOR600
HYDROCYCLIN see III:HOI000
HYDRODESULFURIZED HEAVY VACUUM GAS OIL see
   III:GBW010
HYDROFOL see III:PAE250
HYDROFOL ACID 1255 see III:LBL000
HYDROFOL ACID 1655 see III:SLK000
HYDROGEN ARSENIDE see I:ARK250
HYDROGENATED COAL OIL FRACTION 1 see III:HHW509
HYDROGENATED COAL OIL FRACTION 3 see III:HHW519
HYDROGENATED COAL OIL FRACTION 4 see III:HHW529
HYDROGENATED COAL OIL FRACTION 7 see III:HHW539
HYDROGENATED COAL OIL FRACTION 9 see III:HHW549
HYDROGEN DIOXIDE see III:HIB000
HYDROGEN PEROXIDE see III:HIB000
HYDROGEN PEROXIDE, 30% see III:HIB010
HYDROGEN PEROXIDE SOLUTION 30% see III:HIB010
HYDROGEN PEROXIDE SOLUTION (8% to 40% PEROXIDE)
   (DOT) see III:HIB010
HYDROGEN PEROXIDE, SOLUTION (over 52% peroxide) (DOT)
   see III:HIB000
HYDROGEN PEROXIDE, STABILIZED (over 60% peroxide)
   (DOT) see III:HIB000
HYDROMIREX see III:MRI750
HYDROPEROXIDE see III:HIB000
HYDROPEROXIDE, ACETYL see III:PCL500
6-HYDROPEROXY-4-CHOLESTEN-3-ONE see III:HID500
6-β-HYDROPEROXYCHOLEST-4-EN-3-ONE see III:HID500
1-HYDROPEROXYCYCLOHEX-3-ENE see III:HIE000
1-HYDROPEROXY-3-CYCLOHEXENE see III:HIE000
HYDROPEROXYDE de CUMENE (FRENCH) see III:IOB000
HYDROPEROXYDE de CUMYLE (FRENCH) see III:IOB000
6-β-HYDROPEROXY-Δ⁴CHOLESTEN-3-ONE see III:HID500
N-(HYDROPEROXYMETHYL)-N-NITROSOPROPYLAMINE
   see III:HIE570
HYDROPEROXY-N-NITROSODIBUTYLAMINE see
   III:HIE600
1-(HYDROPEROXY)-N-NITROSODIMETHYLAMINE see
   III:HIE700
1-HYDROPEROXY-1-VINYLCYCLOHEX-3-ENE see
   III:HIF575
4-HYDROPEROXY-4-VINYL-1-CYCLOHEXENE see
   III:HIF575
HYDROQUINOL see III:HIH000
HYDROQUINONE see III:HIH000
m-HYDROQUINONE see III:REA000
o-HYDROQUINONE see III:CCP850
p-HYDROQUINONE see III:HIH000
α-HYDROQUINONE see III:HIH000
HYDROQUINONE BENZYL ETHER see III:AEY000
HYDROQUINONE MONOBENZYL ETHER see III:AEY000
HYDROQUINONE MUSTARD see III:BHB750
HYDROTREATED HEAVY NAPHTHENIC DISTILLATE see
   I:MQV790

3-HYDROXYPURIN-2(3H)-ONE see III:HOB000
6-HYDROXY-3(2H)-PYRIDAZINONE see III:DMC600
6-HYDROXY-3-(2H)-PYRIDAZINONE DIETHANOLAMINE
  see III:DHF200
4-HYDROXY-2(1H)-PYRIMIDINETHIONE see III:TFR250
8-HYDROXYQUINALDIC ACID see III:HOE000
4-HYDROXYQUINOLINAMINE-1-OXIDE MONOHYDRO-
  CHLORIDE see III:HIZ000
N-HYDROXY-4-QUINOLINAMINE-1-OXIDE MONOHYDRO-
  CHLORIDE see III:HIZ000
8-HYDROXYQUINOLINE see III:QPA000
8-HYDROXYQUINOLINE COPPER COMPLEX see
  III:BLC250
1′-HYDROXYSAFROLE see II:BCJ000
1′-HYDROXYSAFROLE-2′,3′-OXIDE see III:HOE500
3-HYDROXY-16,7-SECOESTRA-1,3,5(10)-TRIEN-17-OIC
  ACID see III:DYB000
HYDROXYSENKIRKINE see III:HOF000
12-HYDROXYSTEARIC ACID see III:HOG000
12-HYDROXYSTEARIC ACID, METHYL ESTER see
  III:HOG500
(E)-4′-(p-HYDROXYSTYRYL) ACETANILIDE see III:HIK000
4-HYDROXY-3-((4-SULFO-1-NAPHTHALENYL)AZO)-1-
  NAPHTHALENESULFONIC ACID, DISODIUM SALT see
  III:HJF500
3-HYDROXY-4-((4-SULFO-1-NAPHTHALENYL)AZO)-2,7-
  NAPHTHLENEDISULFONIC ACID, TRISODIUM SALT see
  III:FAG020
3-HYDROXY-4-((4-SULFO-1-NAPHTHYL)AZO)-2,7-
  NAPHTHALENEDISULFONIC ACID, TRISODIUM SALT see
  III:FAG020
4-HYDROXY-3-((5-SULFO-2,4-XYLYL)AZO)-1-NAPHTHA-
  LENESULFONIC ACID, DISODIUM SALT see III:FAG050
3-HYDROXY-4-((4-SULPHO-1-NAPHTHALENYL)AZO)-2,7-
  NAPHTHALENEDISULPHONIC ACID, TRISODIUM SALT
  see III:FAG020
3-HYDROXY-4-((4-SULPHO-1-NAPHTHYL)AZO)-2,7-
  NAPHTHALENEDISULPHONIC ACID, TRISODIUM SALT
  see III:FAG020
4-HYDROXY-3-((5-SULPHO-2,4-XYLYL)AZO)-1-NAPHTHA-
  LENESULPHONIC ACID, DISODIUM SALT see III:FAG050
5-HYDROXYTETRACYCLINE HYDROCHLORIDE see
  III:HOI000
N-HYDROXY-N-TETRADECANOYL-2-AMINOFLUORENE
  see III:HMU000
7-HYDROXYTHEOPHYLLIN (GERMAN) see III:HOJ000
7-HYDROXYTHEOPHYLLINE see III:HOJ000
4-HYDROXYTOLUENE see III:CNX250
m-HYDROXYTOLUENE see III:CNW750
o-HYDROXYTOLUENE see III:CNX000
p-HYDROXYTOLUENE see III:CNX250
4′-((6-HYDROXY-m-TOLYL)AZO)ACETANILIDE see
  II:AAQ250
4-HYDROXY-3H-o-TRIAZOLO(4,5-d)PYRIMIDINE-5,7(4H-
  6H)-DIONE see III:HJE575
1-HYDROXY-2,2,2-TRICHLOROETHYLPHOSPHONIC ACID
  DIMETHYL ESTER see III:TIQ250
3-HYDROXY-2,2,4-TRIMETHYL-3-PENTENOIC ACID,
  β-LACTONE see III:IPL000
3-HYDROXY-4-((2,4,5-TRIMETHYLPHENYL)AZO)-2,7-
  NAPHTHALENEDISULFONIC ACID, DISODIUM SALT see
  II:FAG018
3-HYDROXY-4-((2,4,5-TRIMETHYLPHENYL)AZO)-2,7-
  NAPHTHALENEDISULPHONIC ACID, DISODIUM SALT
  see II:FAG018
3-HYDROXY-l-TYROSINE see III:DNA200
l-o-HYDROXYTYROSINE see III:DNA200
HYDROXYUREA see III:HOO500
N-HYDROXYUREA see III:HOO500
N-HYDROXYURETHAN see III:HKQ025
N-HYDROXYURETHANE see III:HKQ025
3-HYDROXYURIC ACID see III:HOO875
3-HYDROXYXANTHINE see III:HOP000, III:HOQ500
7-HYDROXYXANTHINE see III:HOP259

1-HYDROXYXANTHINE DIHYDRATE see III:HOQ000
3-HYDROXYXANTHINE HYDRATE see III:HOQ500
3-HYDROXY-4-(2,4-XYLYLAZO)-3,7-NAPHTHALENEDISUL-
  FONIC ACID, DISODIUM SALT see III:FMU070
3-HYDROXY-4-(2,4-XYLYLAZO)-3,7-NAPHTHALENEDISUL-
  PHONIC ACID, DISODIUM SALT see III:FMU070
o-HYDROXYZIMTSAURE-LACTON (GERMAN) see
  III:CNV000
HYDURA see III:HOO500
HYLENE M50 see III:MJP400
HYLENE-T see I:TGM740, I:TGM750
HYLENE TCPA see I:TGM750
HYLENE TLC see I:TGM750
HYLENE TM see I:TGM750, II:TGM800
HYLENE TM-65 see I:TGM750
HYLENE TRF see I:TGM750
HYLUTIN see III:HNT500
HYOZID see III:ILD000
HYPERAZIN see II:HGP500
HY-PHI 1055 see III:OHU000
HY-PHI 1088 see III:OHU000
HY-PHI 1199 see III:SLK000
HY-PHI 2066 see III:OHU000
HY-PHI 2088 see III:OHU000
HY-PHI 2102 see III:OHU000
HYPNALETTEN see II:EOK000
HYPNOGEN see II:EOK000
HYPNOLONE see II:EOK000
HYPNOREX see III:LGZ000
HYPNO-TABLINETTEN see II:EOK000
HYPODERMACID see III:TIQ250
HYPOPHTHALIN see II:HGP500, III:PHW000
HYPOPHYSEAL GROWTH HORMONE see III:PJA250
HYPOS see II:HGP500
HYPROVAL-PA see III:HNT500
HYSTEPS see II:EOK000
HYSTRENE 80 see III:SLK000
HYSTRENE 8016 see III:PAE250
HYSTRENE 9512 see III:LBL000
HYZYD see III:ILD000

I 337A see II:CDP250
IA see III:IDZ000
IAA see III:ICN000
IA-BUT see II:BRF500
IAMBOLEN see III:PKF750
IBDU see III:IIV000
IBENZMETHYZINE see I:PME250
IBENZMETHYZINE HYDROCHLORIDE see I:PME500
IBENZMETHYZIN HYDROCHLORIDE see I:PME500
IBIOFURAL see II:NGE500
IBIOSUC see III:SGC000
IBZ see I:PME500
ICI 543 see III:PMP500
ICI 28257 see III:ARQ750
ICI-32865 see III:TJQ333
ICI 38174 see III:INT000
ICI 42464 see III:CHT500
ICI 43823 see III:BPI300
ICI 59118 see II:RCA375
ICIG 1109 see I:CGV250
I.C.I. HYDROCHLORIDE see III:INT000
ICI 54856 METHYL ESTER see III:MIO975
ICR 10 see III:QDS000
ICR-48b see III:DFH000
ICR-125 see III:QCS875
ICR 170 see III:ADJ875
ICR-25A see III:CLD500
ICR 292 see III:EHJ000
ICR 311 see III:EHI500
ICR 340 see III:IAE000
ICR 342 see III:CFA250
ICR 377 see III:EHJ500
ICR 394 see III:CHH000

ICR 433 see III:CIN500
ICR-450 see III:BIJ750
ICR 451 see III:CIG250
ICR 486 see III:CFB500
ICR 498 see III:BNO750
ICR 502 see III:BNR000
ICR 506 see III:BNO500
ICRF-159 see II:PIK250, II:RCA375
ICTALIS SIMPLE see I:DKQ000
IDANTOIL see I:DNU000
IDANTOIN see I:DKQ000
IDANTOINAL see I:DNU000
IDEXUR see III:DAS000
IDOXENE see III:DAS000
IDOXURIDIN see III:DAS000
IDOXURIDINE see III:DAS000
IDRALAZINA (ITALIAN) see III:PHW000
IDRAZIDE DELL'ACIDO ISONICOTINICO see III:ILD000
IDRAZIL see III:ILD000
IDRAZINA IDRATA (ITALIAN) see III:HGU500
IDRAZINA SOLFATO (ITALIAN) see I:HGW500
IDROBUTAZINA see III:HNI500
IDROCHINONE (ITALIAN) see III:HIH000
IDROESTRIL see I:DKA600
IDROGESTENE see III:HNT500
IDROPEROSSIDO di CUMENE (ITALIAN) see III:IOB000
IDROPEROSSIDO di CUMOLO (ITALIAN) see III:IOB000
d-N,N'-(1-IDROSSIMETIL PROPIL)-ETILENDINITROSAMINA
    (ITALIAN) see III:HMQ500
IDRYL see III:FDF000
IDU see III:DAS000
IDUCHER see III:DAS000
IDULEA see III:DAS000
IDUOCULOS see III:DAS000
IDUR see III:DAS000
IDURIDIN see III:DAS000
IFC see III:CBM000
IFOSFAMID see II:IMH000
IFOSFAMIDE see II:IMH000
IGELITE F see III:PKQ059
IIH see III:ILE000
IKACLOMIN see III:CMX700
IKADA RHODAMINE B see III:FAG070
ILIXATHIN see III:RSU000
ILLOXOL see III:DHB400
IMAGON see III:CLD000
IMET 3393 see III:CQM750
IMFERON see I:IGS000
IMI 115 see III:TGF250
IMIDA-LAB see III:TEH500
IMIDAN (PEYTA) see III:TEH500
IMIDAZOLE MUSTARD see II:IAN000
2-IMIDAZOLIDINETHIONE see I:IAQ000
2-IMIDAZOLIDINETHIONE mixed with SODIUM NITRITE see
    II:IAR000
2-IMIDAZOLIDINONE see III:IAS000
2-IMIDAZOLIDONE see III:IAS000
7H-IMIDAZO(4,5-D)PYRIMIDINE see III:POJ250
IMIDENE see III:TEH500
4,4'-(IMIDOCARBONYL)BIS(N,N-DIMETHYLAMINE)
    MONOHYDROCHLORIDE see I:IBA000
4,4'-(IMIDOCARBONYL)BIS(N,N-DIMETHYLANILINE) see
    I:IBB000
3,3'-IMIDODI-1-PROPANOL, DIMETHANESULFONATE (es-
    ter), HYDROCHLORIDE see III:YCJ000
4,4'-((4-IMINO-2,5-CYCLOHEXADIEN-1-YLIDENE)METHY-
    LENE)DIANILINE MONOHYDROCHLORIDE-o-TOLUI-
    DINE see II:RMK020
2,2'-IMINODI-ETHANOL with 1,2-DIHYDRO-3,6-PYRIDAZI-
    NEDIONE (1:1) see III:DHF200
2,2'-IMINODI-N-NITROSOETHANOL see I:NKM000
IMPERON FIXER T see III:TND250
IMPERVOTAR see I:CMY800
IMPOSIL see I:IGS000

IMPROVED WILT PRUF see III:PKQ059
IMPRUVOL see III:BFW750
IMURAN see I:ASB250
IMUREK see I:ASB250
IMUREL see I:ASB250
IMVITE I.G.B.A. see III:BAV750
INAKOR see III:ARQ725
INCIDOL see III:BDS000
INCORTIN see III:CNS825
INCRECEL see III:CMF400
INDANTHRENE GOLDEN YELLOW see III:DCZ000
13H-INDENO(1,2-1)PHENANTHRENE see III:DCX000
INDENO(1,2,3-cd)PYRENE see I:IBZ000
INDENO(1,2,3-cd)PYRENE-1,2-OXIDE see III:DLK750
INDENO(1,2,3-cd)PYREN-8-OL see III:IBZ100
4-(1H-INDEN-1-YLIDENEMETHYL)-N,N-DIMETHYLBEN-
    ZENAMINE see III:DOT600
4-(1-H-INDEN-1-YLIDENEMETHYL)-N-METHYL-N-NI-
    TROSOBENZENAMINE see III:MMR750
INDIAN RED see I:LCS000, III:IHD000
INDICAN (POTASSIUM SALT) see III:ICD000
INDIGENOUS PEANUT OIL see III:PAO000
INDIGO BLUE 2B see I:CMO000
INDIGO CARMINE see III:FAE100
INDIGO CARMINE (BIOLOGICAL STAIN) see III:FAE100
INDIGO CARMINE DISODIUM SALT see III:FAE100
INDIGO EXTRACT see III:FAE100
INDIGO-KARMIN (GERMAN) see III:FAE100
5,5'-INDIGOTIN DISULFONIC ACID see III:FAE100
INDIGOTINE see III:FAE100
INDIGOTINE DISODIUM SALT see III:FAE100
INDIGO YELLOW see III:ICE000
INDOL (GERMAN) see III:ICM000
INDOLE see III:ICM000
3-INDOLEACETIC ACID see III:ICN000
β-INDOLEACETIC ACID see III:ICN000
β-INDOLE-3-ACETIC ACID see III:ICN000
1H-INDOLE-3-ACETIC ACID see III:ICN000
INDOLE-3-ACRYLIC ACID see III:ICO000
INDOLE-3-ALANINE see III:TNX000
INDOL-3-OL, HYDROGEN SULFATE (ESTER), POTASSIUM-
    SALT see III:ICD000
INDOL-3-OL, POTASSIUM SULFATE see III:ICD000
INDOLYACETIC ACID see III:ICN000
INDOLYL-3-ACETIC ACID see III:ICN000
3-INDOLYLACETIC ACID see III:ICN000
β-INDOLYLACETIC ACID see III:ICN000
α-INDOL-3-YL-ACETIC ACID see III:ICN000
3-INDOLYLACRYLIC ACID see III:ICO000
1-β-3-INDOLYLALANINE see III:TNX000
INDOL-3-YL POTASSIUM SULFATE see III:ICD000
3-(1-H-INDOL-3-YL)-2-PROPENOIC ACID see III:ICO000
INDOL-3-YL SULFATE, POTASSIUM SALT see III:ICD000
INDUSTRENE 105 see III:OHU000
INDUSTRENE 205 see III:OHU000
INDUSTRENE 206 see III:OHU000
INDUSTRENE 4516 see III:PAE250
INDUSTRENE 5016 see III:SLK000
INERTEEN see I:PJL750
INETOL see III:INS000, III:INT000
INEXIT see I:BBQ500
INFAMIL see III:HNI500
INFILTRINA see III:DUD800
INGENANE HEXADECANOATE see III:OBW509
INHIBINE see III:HIB000
INHIBISOL see III:MIH275
INK ORANGE JSN see III:HGC000
INSARIOTOXIN see III:FQS000
INSECTICIDE No. 497 see III:DHB400
INSECTICIDE No. 4049 see III:MAK700
INSECTOPHENE see III:EAQ750
INSOLUBLE SACCHARINE see II:BCE500
IN-SONE see III:PLZ000
INSULAMINA see III:DNA200

INTALBUT see II:BRF500
INTENSE BLUE see III:FAE100
INTERCHEM DIRECT BLACK Z see I:AQP000
INTERNATIONAL ORANGE 2221 see I:LCS000
INTEROX see III:HIB010
INTRABUTAZONE see II:BRF500
INTRACID FAST ORANGE G see III:HGC000
INTRACID PURE BLUE L see III:FAE000
INTRAMYCETIN see II:CDP250
INTRASPERSE YELLOW GBA EXTRA see II:AAQ250
INVERTON 245 see II:TAA100
IODOACETAMIDE see III:IDW000
2-IODOACETAMIDE see III:IDW000
α-IODOACETAMIDE see III:IDW000
IODOACETATE see III:IDZ000
IODOACETIC ACID see III:IDZ000
1-IODOBUTANE see III:BRQ250
2-IODOBUTANE see III:IEH000
5-IODODEOXYURIDINE see III:DAS000
5-IODO-2'-DEOXYURIDINE see III:DAS000
3-IODO-2-FAA see III:IEO000
N-(3-IODO-2-FLUORENYL)ACETAMIDE see III:IEO000
IODOMETANO (ITALIAN) see I:MKW200
IODOMETHANE see I:MKW200
7-IODOMETHYL-12-METHYLBENZ(a)ANTHRACENE see
  III:IER000
4-IODOPHENOL see III:IEW000
p-IODOPHENOL see III:IEW000
1-IODOPROPANE see III:PNO750
2-IODOPROPANE see III:IPS000
3-IODOPROPIONIC ACID see III:IEY000
5-IODO-2-THIOURACIL, SODIUM SALT see III:SHX500
5-IODOURACIL DEOXYRIBOSIDE see III:DAS000
IODURE de METHYLE (FRENCH) see I:MKW200
IONOL see III:BFW750
IONOL (antioxidant) see III:BFW750
IOPEZITE see III:PKX250
IPABUTONA see III:HNI500
IPANER see II:DAA800
IPD see III:YCJ000
IP-1,2-DIOL see III:DLE400
IPHOSPHAMIDE see II:IMH000
IPN see III:ILE000
IPO 8 see II:TBW100
IPOLINA see II:HGP500
IPPC see III:CBM000
IPRAZID see III:ILE000
IPRONIAZID see III:ILE000
IPRONID see III:ILE000
IPRONIN see III:ILE000
IPSOFLAME see II:BRF500
IQ DIHYDROCHLORIDE see III:AKT620
IRADICAV see III:SHF500
IRAGEN RED L-U see III:FAG070
IRC 453 see III:CIN750
IRGACHROME ORANGE OS see I:LCS000
IRGALITE BRONZE RED CL see III:BNH500, III:BNK700
IRGALITE RED CBN see III:CHP500
IRIDIL see III:HNI500
IRIDOCIN see III:EPQ000
IRIDOZIN see III:EPQ000
IRISH GUM see III:CCL250
IRISH MOSS EXTRACT see III:CCL250
IRISH MOSS GELOSE see III:CCL250
IRISONE ACETATE see III:CNS825
IRO-JEX see I:IGS000
IROMIN see III:FBK000
IRON see III:IGK800
IRON ARSENATE (DOT) see I:IGM000
IRON(II) ARSENATE (3:2) see I:IGM000
IRON(III) ARSENATE (1:1) see I:IGN000
IRON(III)-o-ARSENITE PENTAHYDRATE see I:IGO000
IRON, (N,N-BIS(CARBOXYMETHYL)GLYCINATO(3-)-
  N,O,O',O'')-, (T-4)-(9CI) see III:IHC100

IRON BIS(CYCLOPENTADIENE) see III:FBC000
IRON CARBOHYDRATE COMPLEX see III:IGU000
IRON, CARBONYL (FCC) see III:IGK800
IRON CHROMITE see I:CMI500
IRON DEXTRAN see I:IGS000
IRON-DEXTRAN COMPLEX see I:IGS000
IRON DEXTRAN GLYCEROL GLYCOSIDE see III:IGT000
IRON DEXTRAN INJECTION see I:IGS000
IRON-DEXTRIN COMPLEX see III:IGU000
IRON DEXTRIN INJECTION see III:IGU000
IRON DICYCLOPENTADIENYL see III:FBC000
IRON DIMETHYLDITHIOCARBAMATE see III:FAS000
IRON DUST see II:IGW000
α-IRONE see III:IGW500
IRON, ELECTROLYTIC see III:IGK800
IRON, ELEMENTAL see III:IGK800
IRON complex with N-FLUOREN-2-YL ACETOHYDROXAMIC
  ACID see III:HIQ000
IRON GLUCONATE see III:FBK000
IRON HYDROGENATED DEXTRAN see I:IGS000
IRON(+3) HYDROXIDE COMPLEX with NITRILO-TRI-PRO-
  PIONIC ACID see III:FAY000
IRON(III)HYDROXIDE-POLYMALTOSE see III:IHA000
IRON(2+) LACTATE see III:LAL000
IRON MONOSULFATE see III:FBN100
IRON NICKEL SULFIDE see II:NDE500
IRON NITRILOTRIACETATE see III:IHC100
IRON-NITRILOTRIACETATE CHELATE see III:IHC100
IRON(3+) NTA see III:IHC100
IRON ORE see I:HAO875
IRONORM INJECTION see I:IGS000
IRON OXIDE see III:IHD000
IRON(III) OXIDE see III:IHD000
IRON OXIDE, CHROMIUM OXIDE, and NICKEL OXIDE FUME
  see I:IHE000
IRON OXIDE FUME see II:IHF000
IRON OXIDE RED see III:IHD000
IRON OXIDE, SACCHARATED see I:IHG000
IRON-POLYSACCHARIDE COMPLEX see III:IHH000
IRON PROTOSULFATE see III:FBN100
IRON, REDUCED (FCC) see III:IGK800
IRON SACCHARATE see I:IHG000
IRON SESQUIOXIDE see III:IHD000
IRON SODIUM GLUCONATE see III:IHK000
IRON SORBITEX see III:IHL000
IRON SORBITOL CITRATE see III:IHL000
IRON-SORBITOL-CITRIC ACID see III:IHL000
IRON SUGAR see I:IHG000
IRON(II) SULFATE (1:1) see III:FBN100
IRON VITRIOL see III:FBN100
IROQUINE see III:CLD000
IROSPAN see III:FBN100
IROSUL see III:FBN100
IROX (GADOR) see III:FBK000
ISATIDINE see III:RFU000
ISCEON 22 see III:CFX500
ISCOBROME see III:MHR200
ISCOBROME D see I:EIY500
ISCOTIN see III:ILD000
ISCOVESCO see I:DKA600
ISIDRINA see III:ILD000
ISLANDITOXIN see III:COW750
ISMAZIDE see III:ILD000
ISMICETINA see II:CDP250
ISMIPUR see III:POK000
ISOACETOPHORONE see III:IMF400
ISOAMYL ALCOHOL see III:IHP000
ISOAMYL ALKOHOL (CZECH) see III:IHP000
ISO-AMYLALKOHOL (GERMAN) see III:IHP000
ISOAMYLOL see III:IHP000
ISOANETHOLE see III:AFW750
trans-ISOASARONE see III:IHX400
ISOBAC 20 see III:HCL000
ISOBENZAN see III:OAN000

ISOBICINA see III:ILD000
ISO-BNU see III:IJF000
ISOBUTANOL (DOT) see III:IIL000
ISOBUTAZINA see III:HNI500
ISOBUTENYL CHLORIDE see II:CIU750
ISOBUTIL see III:HNI500
N-ISOBUTYL-N-(ACETOXYMETHYL)NITROSAMINE see
   III:ABR125
ISOBUTYL ALCOHOL see III:IIL000
ISOBUTYLALKOHOL (CZECH) see III:IIL000
ISOBUTYL BROMIDE see III:BNR750
ISOBUTYLCARBINOL see III:IHP000
ISOBUTYLDIUREA see III:IIV000
ISOBUTYLENEDIUREA see III:IIV000
1,1'-ISOBUTYLIDENEBISUREA see III:IIV000
ISOBUTYLIDENEDIUREA see III:IIV000
1-ISO-BUTYL-1-NITROSOUREA see III:IJF000
N-ISOBUTYL-N-NITROSOUREA see III:IJF000
ISOCHRYSENE see III:TMS000
ISOCID see III:ILD000
ISOCIDENE see III:ILD000
ISO-CORNOX see II:CIR500
ISOCOTIN see III:ILD000
ISOCROTYL CHLORIDE see III:IKE000
ISOCYANIC ACID, BENZ(a)ANTHRACEN-7-YL ESTER see
   III:BBJ250
ISOCYANIC ACID, HEXAMETHYLENE ESTER, POLYMER
   with 1,4-BUTANEDIOL see III:PKO750
ISOCYANIC ACID, METHYLENEDI-p-PHENYLENE ESTER,
   POLYMER with 1,4-BUTANEDIOL see I:PKP000
ISOCYANIC ACID, METHYLPHENYLENE ESTER see
   I:TGM740, I:TGM750
ISOCYANIC ACID, 4-METHYL-m-PHENYLENE ESTER see
   I:TGM750
ISOCYANIC ACID-1,5-NAPHTHYLENE ESTER see
   III:NAM500
ISOCYANURIC ACID see III:THS000
ISODIENESTROL see II:DAL600
ISODIN see III:CFZ000
ISODUR see III:IIV000
ISOENDOXAN see II:IMH000
ISOESTRAGOLE see III:PMQ750
ISOFLAV BASE see III:DBN600
ISOFORON see III:IMF400
ISOFORONE (ITALIAN) see III:IMF400
ISOFOSFAMIDE see II:IMH000
ISOHOL see III:INJ000
ISOLAN see III:DSK200
ISOLANE (FRENCH) see III:DSK200
ISOL LAKE RED LCS 12527 see III:CHP500
ISOLYN see III:ILD000
β-ISOMER see I:BBR000
ISOMIN see III:TEH500
ISONATE see III:MJP400
ISONERIT see III:ILD000
ISONEX see III:ILD000
ISONIACID see III:ILD000
ISONIAZID see III:ILD000
ISONIAZIDE see III:ILD000
ISONIAZID SODIUM METHANESULFONATE see III:SIJ000
ISONICAZIDE see III:ILD000
ISONICID see III:ILD000
ISONICO see III:ILD000
ISONICOTAN see III:ILD000
ISONICOTIL see III:ILD000
ISONICOTINHYDRAZID see III:ILD000
ISONICOTINIC ACID HYDRAZIDE see III:ILD000
ISONICOTINIC ACID-2-ISOPROPYLHYDRAZIDE see
   III:ILE000
ISONICOTINIC ACID, SODIUM SALT see III:ILF000
ISONICOTINIC ACID, VANILLYLIDENEHYDRAZIDE see
   III:VEZ925
ISONICOTINOYL HYDRAZIDE see III:ILD000
ISONICOTINOYLHYDRAZINE see III:ILD000

4-(ISONICOTINOYLHYDRAZONE)PIMELIC ACID see
   III:ILG000
1-ISONICOTINOYL-2-ISOPROPYLHYDRAZINE see
   III:ILE000
ISONICOTINSAEUREHYDRAZID see III:ILD000
ISONICOTINYL HYDRAZIDE see III:ILD000
1-ISONICOTINYL-2-ISOPROPYLHYDRAZINE see III:ILE000
ISONIDE see III:ILD000
ISONIDRIN see III:ILD000
ISONIKAZID see III:ILD000
ISONILEX see III:ILD000
ISONIN see III:ILD000
ISONINDON see III:ILD000
ISONIRIT see III:ILD000
ISONITON see III:ILD000
ISONITROPROPANE see I:NIY000
ISONIZIDE see III:ILD000
ISOOCTYL ALCOHOL (2,4-DICHLOROPHENOXY)ACETATE
   see III:ILO000
ISOOCTYL-2,4-DICHLOROPHENOXYACETATE see
   III:ILO000
ISOPENTANOL see III:IHP000
ISOPENTYL ALCOHOL see III:IHP000
3-((ISOPENTYL)NITROSOAMINO)-2-BUTANONE see
   II:MHW350
ISOPHEN see III:MDT600
ISOPHENICOL see II:CDP250
ISOPHORONE see III:IMF400
ISOPHOSPHAMIDE see II:IMH000
ISOPROPANOL (DOT) see III:INJ000
ISOPROPANOLAMINE see III:AMA500
(+)-4-ISOPROPENYL-1-METHYLCYCLOHEXENE see
   III:LFU000
ISOPROPIL-N-FENIL-CARBAMMATO (ITALIAN) see
   III:CBM000
(1-ISOPROPIL-3-METIL-1H-PIRAZOL-5-IL)-N,N-DIMETIL-
   CARBAMMATO (ITALIAN) see III:DSK200
11-ISOPROPOXY-15,16-DIHYDRO-17-CYCLOPENTA(a)
   PHENANTHREN-17-ONE see III:INA400
4-ISOPROPOXYDIPHENYLAMINE see III:HKF000
p-ISOPROPOXYDIPHENYLAMINE see III:HKF000
N-(4-ISOPROPOXYPHENYL)ANILINE see III:HKF000
2-ISOPROPOXYPHENYL N-METHYLCARBAMATE, nitrosated
   see III:PMY310
o-ISOPROPOXYPHENYL METHYLNITROSOCARBAMATE
   see III:PMY310
o-ISOPROPOXYPHENYL N-METHYL-N-NITROSOCARBA-
   MATE see III:PMY310
ISOPROPYL ALCOHOL see III:INJ000
ISO-PROPYLALKOHOL (GERMAN) see III:INJ000
α-((ISOPROPYLAMINO)METHYL)-2-NAPHTHALENEMETH-
   ANOL see III:INS000
α-((ISOPROPYLAMINO)METHYL)NAPHTHALENEMETH-
   ANOL, HYDROCHLORIDE see III:INT000
2-ISOPROPYLAMINO-1-(NAPHTH-2-YL)ETHANOL see
   III:INS000
2-ISOPROPYLAMINO-1-(2-NAPHTHYL)ETHANOL see
   III:INS000
2-ISOPROPYLAMINO-1-(2-NAPHTHYL)ETHANOL HYDRO-
   CHLORIDE see III:INT000
8-ISOPROPYLBENZ(a)ANTHRACENE see III:INZ000
9-ISOPROPYLBENZ(a)ANTHRACENE see III:IOA000
5-ISOPROPYL-1:2-BENZANTHRACENE see III:INZ000
6-ISOPROPYL-1:2-BENZANTHRACENE see III:IOA000
ISOPROPYLBENZENE HYDROPEROXIDE see III:IOB000
2-ISOPROPYL-3:4-BENZPHENANTHRENE see III:IOF000
ISOPROPYL CARBAMATE see III:IOJ000
ISOPROPYLCARBAMIC ACID, ETHYL ESTER see III:IPA000
2-(p-ISOPROPYL CARBAMOYL BENZYL)-1-METHYLHY-
   DRAZINE see I:PME250
1-(p-ISOPROPYLCARBAMOYLBENZYL)-2-METHYLHYDRA-
   ZINE HYDROCHLORIDE see I:PME500

K25 (polymer) see III:PKQ250
KADMIUM (GERMAN) see I:CAD000
KADMIUMCHLORID (GERMAN) see I:CAE250
KADMIUMSTEARAT (GERMAN) see I:OAT000
KADMU TLENEK (POLISH) see I:CAH500
KADOL see II:BRF500
KAERGONA see III:MMD500
KAFAR COPPER see III:CNI000
KAKO BLUE B SALT see I:DCJ200
KAKO RED TR BASE see II:CLK220
KALGAN see III:PFC750
KALIUMARSENIT (GERMAN) see I:PKV500
KALIUMDICHROMAT (GERMAN) see III:PKX250
KALLOCRYL K see III:PKB500
KALLODENT CLEAR see III:PKB500
KALMETTUMSOMNIFERUM see III:GFA000
KALMUS OEL (GERMAN) see III:OGK000
KALZIUMARSENIAT (GERMAN) see I:ARB750
KALZIUMZYKLAMATE (GERMAN) see III:CAR000
KAM 1000 see III:SLK000
KAM 2000 see III:SLK000
KAM 3000 see III:SLK000
KAMAVER see II:CDP250
KAMBAMINE RED TR see II:CLK220
KAMFOCHLOR see I:CDV100
KAMPSTOFF "LOST" see I:BIH250
KANDISET see II:BCE500
KANECHLOR see I:PJL750
KANECHLOR 300 see II:PJO500
KANECHLOR 400 see II:PJO750
KANECHLOR 500 see II:PJP000, III:PJP250
KANEKALON see III:ADY250
KANONE see III:MMD500
KAN-TO-KA (JAPANESE) see III:CNH250
KAPPAXAN see III:MMD500
e-KAPROLAKTAM (CZECH) see III:CBF700
KAPROLIT see III:PJY500
KAPROLON see III:PJY500
KAPROMIN see III:PJY500
KAPRON see III:NOH000, III:PJY500
KAPTAN see III:CBG000
KARBAM BLACK see III:FAS000
KARBAM WHITE see III:BJK500
KARBARYL (POLISH) see III:CBM750
KARBOFOS see III:MAK700
KARCON see III:MMD500
KAREON see III:MMD500
KARIDIUM see III:SHF500
KARIGEL see III:SHF500
KARI-RINSE see III:SHF500
KARMESIN see III:HJF500
KARMEX see III:DXQ500
KARMEX DIURON HERBICIDE see III:DXQ500
KARMEX DW see III:DXQ500
KARMEX MONURON HERBICIDE see III:CJX750
KARMEX W. MONURON HERBICIDE see III:CJX750
KARSAN see I:FMV000
KASTONE see III:HIB010
KATAGRIPPE see III:EEM000
KATCHUNG OIL see III:PAO000
KATHRO see III:CMD750
KATIV-G see III:MMD500
KAYAFUME see III:MHR200
KAYAKU ACID BRILLIANT SCARLET 3R see III:FMU080
KAYAKU AMARANTH see III:FAG020
KAYAKU BLUE B BASE see I:DCJ200
KAYAKU DIRECT see I:CMO000
KAYAKU DIRECT DEEP BLACK EX see I:AQP000
KAYAKU SCARLET G BASE see I:NMP500
KAYALON FAST BLUE BR see III:TBG700
KAYDOL see III:MQV750
KAYKLOT see III:MMD500
KAYLITE see III:PKQ059
KAYQUINONE see III:MMD500

KAZOE see III:SFA000
KB (POLYMER) see III:SMQ500
KC-400 see II:PJO750
KC-500 see II:PJP000
KCA FOODCOL AMARANTH A see III:FAG020
KEBILIS see III:CDL325
KEDAVON see III:TEH500
KEIMSTOP see III:CBL750
KEL-F see III:KDK000
KELTANE see III:BIO750
KELTHANE (DOT) see III:BIO750
p,p'-KELTHANE see III:BIO750
KELTHANE DUST BASE see III:BIO750
KELTHANETHANOL see III:BIO750
KEMAMIDE S see III:OAR000
KEMESTER 103 scc III:OHW000
KEMESTER 115 see III:OHW000
KEMESTER 205 see III:OHW000
KEMESTER 213 see III:OHW000
KEMICETINE see II:CDP250
KENACHROME BLUE 2R see III:HJF500
KEPONE see I:KEA000
KER 710 see III:EAL100
KERB see III:DTT600
KERECID see III:DAS000
KESELAN see III:CLY500
KESSODANTEN see I:DKQ000
KESSODRATE see III:CDO000
KESTRIN see I:ECU750
KESTRONE see I:EDV000
3-(3-KETO-7-α-ACETYLTHIO-17-β-HYDROXY-4-ANDRO-
     STEN-17-α-YL)PROPIONIC ACID LACTONE see
     III:AFJ500
7-KETOCHOLESTEROL see III:ONO000
KETODESTRIN see I:EDV000
2-KETOHEXAMETHYLENIMINE see III:CBF700
KETOHYDROXY-ESTRATRIENE see I:EDV000
KETOHYDROXYESTRIN see I:EDV000
KETOHYDROXYESTRIN BENZOATE see II:EDV500
KETOHYDROXYOESTRIN see I:EDV000
KETOLE see III:ICM000
KETOLIN-H see III:CJU250
γ-KETO-β-METHOXY-Δ-METHYLENE-Δα-HEXENOIC ACID
     see III:PAP750
15-KETO-20-METHYLCHOLANTHRENE see III:MIM250
KETONE, 5-AMINO-1,3-DIMETHYLPYRAZOL-4-YL o-FLUO-
     ROPHENYL see III:AJR400
4-KETOSTEARIC ACID see III:KGK150
KEVADON see III:TEH500
KH 360 see III:TGG760
KHAINI (INDIA) see I:SED400
KHLORIDIN see III:TGD000
KHLORTRIANIZEN see II:CLO750
KHP 2 see III:AHE250
KIATRIUM see III:DCK759
KIESELSAURE (GERMAN) see III:SCL000
KILDIP see II:DGB000
KILL-ALL see I:SEY500
KILLEEN see III:CCL250
KILL KANTZ see III:AQN635
KILOSEB see III:BRE500
KILPROP see II:CIR500
KILSEM see II:CIR250
KING'S YELLOW see I:ARI000, I:LCR000
KIPCA see III:MMD500
KITON CRIMSON 2R see III:HJF500
KITON FAST ORANGE G see III:HGC000
KITON FAST YELLOW A see III:SGP500
KITON PONCEAU R see III:FMU070
KITON PURE BLUE L see III:FMU059
KITON RUBINE S see III:FAG020
KITON SCARLET 4R see III:FMU080
KIWAM (INDIA) see I:SED400
KIWI LUSTR 277 see III:BGJ250

K. IXINA see III:CAC500
KLAVI KORDAL see III:NGY000
KLEER-LOT see I:AMY050
KLEGECELL see III:PKQ059
KLIMORAL see II:EDU500
KLINOSORB see III:CMV850
KLION see I:MMN250
KLOFIRAN see III:ARQ750
KLORAMIN see I:BIE500
KLORINOL see III:TIX000
KLOROKIN see III:CLD000
KLOTTONE see III:MMD500
KLT 40 see III:PKF750
4K-2M see II:CIR250
KMTS 212 see III:SFO500
KNOCKMATE see III:FAS000
KO 7 see III:EAL100
KOAXIN see III:MMD500
KOBALT (GERMAN, POLISH) see I:CNA250
KOBALT CHLORID (GERMAN) see III:CNB599
KOBU see III:PAX000
KOBUTOL see III:PAX000
KOCHINEAL RED A FOR FOOD see III:FMU080
KODAFLEX see III:TIG750
KODAFLEX DOA see III:AEO000
KODAFLEX DOP see I:DVL700
KOFFEIN (GERMAN) see III:CAK500
KOKOTINE see I:BBQ500
KOLKLOT see III:MMD500
KOLLIDON see III:PKQ250
KOLPHOS see III:PAK000
KOLPON see I:EDV000
KONDREMUL see III:MQV750
KONESTA see III:TII250
KOPFUME see I:EIY500
KOP MITE see II:DER000
KOPOLYMER BUTADIEN STYRENOVY (CZECH) see
     III:SMR000
KOPROSTERIN (GERMAN) see III:DKW000
KOPSOL see I:DAD200
KOP-THIODAN see III:EAQ750
KOP-THION see III:MAK700
KORAD see III:PKB500
KOREON see III:NBW000
KOROSEAL see III:PKQ059
KORO-SULF see III:SNN500
KORUM see II:HIM000
KORUND see III:EAL100
KOTOL see I:BBQ750
KP 2 see III:PAX000
K-PIN see III:PIB900
KRAMERIA IXINA see III:CAC500
KRAMERIA TRIANDRA see III:RGA000
KRASTEN 1.4 see III:SMQ500
KREGASAN see III:TFS350
KRESIDIN see I:MGO750
m-KRESOL see III:CNW750
p-KRESOL see III:CNX250
o-KRESOL (GERMAN) see III:CNX000
KREZIDINE see I:MGO750
KREZONE see II:CIR250
KRINOCORTS see III:DAQ800
KRISTALLOSE see II:SJN700
KRO 1 see III:SMR000
KROKYDOLITH (GERMAN) see I:ARM275
KROMAD see I:KHU000
KROMON GREEN B see II:CLK235
KRONITEX TOF see III:TNI250
KRONOS TITANIUM DIOXIDE see III:TGG760
KROTENAL see III:DXH250
KROTILINE see II:DAA800
KROTONALDEHYD (CZECH) see II:COB250
KRYOGENIN see III:CBL000
KRYSID see III:AQN635

K-THROMBYL see III:MMD500
KU 5-3 see III:EAL100
KUPFERRON (CZECH) see I:ANO500
KUPPERSULFAT (GERMAN) see III:CNP250
KUPRATSIN see III:EIR000
KURAN see II:TIX500
KURON see II:TIX500
KUROSAL see II:TIX500
K-VITAN see III:MMD500
KW-125 see I:AES750
KWAS BENZYDYNODWUKAROKSYLOWY (POLISH) see
     III:BFX250
KWELL see I:BBQ500
KWIK (DUTCH) see III:MCW250
KYANITE see III:AHF500
KYANURCHLORID (CZECH) see III:TJD750
KYLAR see II:DQD400
KYOCRISTINE see III:LEZ000
KYPCHLOR see II:CDR750
KYPFOS see III:MAK700
KYPMAN 80 see III:MAS500
KYPTHION see III:PAK000
KYPZIN see III:EIR000
KYSELINA 3,6-ENDOMETHYLEN-3,4,5,6,7,7-HEXACHLOR-
     Δ^4-TETRAHYDROFTALOVA (CZECH) see II:CDS000
KYSELINA HET (CZECH) see II:CDS000
KYSELINA KYANUROVA (CZECH) see III:THS000
KYSELINA MUKOCHLOROVA see III:MRU900
KZ 3M see III:SCQ000
KZ 5M see III:SCQ000
KZ 7M see III:SCQ000

L-395 see III:DSP400
L-5103 see II:RKP000
L-36352 see III:DUV600
LABOPAL see I:DKQ000
LAC LSP-1 see III:LIJ000
LACQREN 550 see III:SMQ500
LACQUER ORANGE V see II:TGW000
LACQUER ORANGE VG see III:PEJ500
LACQUER ORANGE VR see III:XRA000
LACQUER RED V3B see III:EOJ500
LACTIC ACID, BERYLLIUM SALT see I:LAH000
LACTIC ACID, CADMIUM SALT see I:CAG750
LACTIC ACID, IRON(2+) SALT (2:1) see III:LAL000
LACTIN see III:LAR000
LACTOBARYT see III:BAP000
LACTOBIOSE see III:LAR000
LACTOSE see III:LAR000
d-LACTOSE see III:LAR000
LADAKAMYCIN see III:ARY000
LADOGAL see III:DAB830
LAEVORAL see III:LFI000
LAEVOSAN see III:LFI000
LA-III see III:DCK759
LAKE BLUE B BASE see I:DCJ200
LAKE PONCEAU see III:FMU070
LAKE RED C see III:CHP500
LAKE RED KB BASE see II:CLK225
LAKE SCARLET G BASE see I:NMP500
LAMAR see III:FMB000
LAMBETH see III:PMP500
LAMDIOL see I:EDO000
LAMORYL see GKE000
LAMP BLACK see III:CBT750
LAMPIT see III:NGG000
LANADIN see II:TIO750
LAND PLASTER see III:CAX750
LANDRIN, NITROSO DERIVATIVE see III:NLY500
LANEX see III:DUK800
LANIAZID see III:ILD000
LANIOZID see III:ILD000
LANOL see III:CMD750
LAPAQUIN see III:CLD000

LARAHA see III:LBE000
LARODOPA see III:DNA200
LARVACIDE see III:CKN500
LASIOCARPINE see II:LBG000
LATEX see III:PJR000
LATEXOL SCARLET R see III:CHP500
LATHOSTEROL see III:CMD000
LAURIC ACID see III:LBL000
LAURIC ACID-2,3-EPOXYPROPYL ESTER see III:LBM000
LAURIC ALCOHOL see III:DXV600
LAURINIC ALCOHOL see III:DXV600
LAUROSTEARIC ACID see III:LBL000
LAUROX see III:LBR000
1-LAUROYLAZIRIDINE see III:LBQ000
LAUROYLETHYI ENEIMINE see III:LBQ000
LAUROYL PEROXIDE see III:LBR000
LAUROYL PEROXIDE, TECHNICALLY PURE (DOT) see
   III:LBR000
LAURYDOL see III:LBR000
LAURYL 24 see III:DXV600
LAURYL ALCOHOL (FCC) see III:DXV600
n-LAURYL ALCOHOL, PRIMARY see III:DXV600
LAURYLGUANIDINE ACETATE see III:DXX400
LAUXTOL see II:PAX250
LAUXTOL A see II:PAX250
LAV see I:CMY800
LAVATAR see I:CMY800
LAVSAN see III:PKF750
LAWN-KEEP see II:DAA800
LAWSONITE see III:PKF750
LAXANORM see III:DMH400
LAXANTHREEN see III:DMH400
LAXIPUR see III:DMH400
LAXIPURIN see III:DMH400
LB-ROT 1 see III:FAG040
LCR see III:LEY000
LD-813 see III:LCE000
LD NORGESTREL (FRENCH) see III:NNQ500
LD RUBBER RED 16913 see III:CHP500
29060 LE see III:VLA000
LEA-COV see III:SHF500
LEAD see II:LCF000
LEAD ACETATE see I:LCG000
LEAD (2+) ACETATE see I:LCG000
LEAD(II) ACETATE see I:LCG000
LEAD ACETATE, BASIC see III:LCH000
LEAD ACETATE TRIHYDRATE see I:LCJ000
LEAD ACETATE(II), TRIHYDRATE see I:LCJ000
LEAD ACID ARSENATE see I:LCK000
LEAD ARSENATE see I:ARC750, I:LCK000
LEAD ARSENATE, SOLID (DOT) see I:LCK000
LEAD ARSENATE (STANDARD) see I:LCK000
LEAD(II) ARSENITE see I:LCL000
LEAD ARSENITE, SOLID (DOT) see I:LCL000
LEAD CARBONATE see III:LCP000
LEAD(2+) CARBONATE see III:LCP000
LEAD CHLORIDE see III:LCQ000
LEAD (2+) CHLORIDE see III:LCQ000
LEAD (II) CHLORIDE see III:LCQ000
LEAD CHROMATE see I:LCR000
LEAD CHROMATE(VI) see I:LCR000
LEAD CHROMATE, BASIC see I:LCS000
LEAD CHROMATE OXIDE (MAK) see I:LCS000
LEAD CHROMATE, RED see I:LCS000
LEAD CHROMATE, SULPHATE and MOLYBDATE see
   III:LDM000
LEAD DIACETATE see I:LCG000
LEAD DIACETATE TRIHYDRATE see I:LCJ000
LEAD DIBASIC ACETATE see I:LCG000
LEAD DICHLORIDE see III:LCQ000
LEAD DIMETHYLDITHOCARBAMATE see III:LCW000
LEAD DINITRATE see III:LDO000
LEAD FLAKE see II:LCF000
LEAD-MOLYBDENUM CHROMATE see III:LDM000

LEAD MONOSUBACETATE see III:LCH000
LEAD MONOXIDE see III:LDN000
LEAD NAPHTHENATE see III:NAS500
LEAD NITRATE see III:LDO000
LEAD (2+) NITRATE see III:LDO000
LEAD(II) NITRATE see III:LDO000
LEAD(II) NITRATE (1:2) see III:LDO000
LEAD ORTHOPHOSPHATE see I:LDU000
LEAD OXIDE see III:LDN000
LEAD(II) OXIDE see III:LDN000
LEAD OXIDE YELLOW see III:LDN000
LEAD PHOSPHATE see I:LDU000
LEAD (2+) PHOSPHATE see I:LDU000
LEAD PHOSPHATE (3:2) see I:LDU000
LEAD(II) PHOSPHATE (3:2) see I:LDU000
LEAD PROTOXIDE see III:LDN000
LEAD S2 see II:LCF000
LEAD SUBACETATE see III:LCH000
LEAF GREEN see II:CMJ900
LEALGIN COMPOSITUM see III:CLY500
LEATHER BLUE G see III:ADE500
LEATHER GREEN B see III:FAE950
LEATHER GREEN SF see III:FAF000
LEATHER ORANGE HR see III:PEK000
LEBAYCID see III:FAQ999
LE CAPTANE (FRENCH) see III:CBG000
LEFEBAR see II:EOK000
LEGUMEX DB see II:CIR250
LEHYDAN see I:DKQ000
LEIPZIG YELLOW see I:LCR000
LEIVASOM see III:TIQ250
LEKAMIN see III:TNF500
LEMBROL see III:DCK759
LEMOFLUR see III:SHF500
LEMON CHROME see I:BAK250
LEMONENE see III:BGE000
LEMON OIL see III:LEI000
LEMON OIL, COLDPRESSED (FCC) see III:LEI000
LEMON OIL, EXPRESSED see III:LEI000
LEMON YELLOW see I:BAK250, I:LCR000
LENDINE see I:BBQ500
LENTOX see I:BBQ500
LEONAL see II:EOK000
LEPHEBAR see II:EOK000
LEPINAL see II:EOK000
LEPINALETTEN see II:EOK000
LEPITOIN see I:DKQ000, I:DNU000
LEPITOIN SODIUM see I:DNU000
LEPSIN see I:DKQ000
LESAN see III:DOU600
LESTEMP see II:HIM000
LETHALAIRE G-54 see III:PAK000
LETHALAIRE G-58 see III:CJT750
LETHURIN see II:TIO750
LEUCARSONE see III:CBJ000
LEUCETHANE see I:UVA000
LEUCOGEN see III:ARN800
LEUCOL see III:QMJ000
LEUCOLINE see III:QMJ000
LEUCOPARAFUCHSIN see III:THP000
LEUCOPARAFUCHSINE see III:THP000
LEUCOPIN see III:CMV000
LEUCOSOL GOLDEN YELLOW see III:DCZ000
LEUCOSULFAN see I:BOT250
LEUCOTHANE see I:UVA000
LEUCOVYL PA 1302 see II:AAX175
LEUKAEMOMYCIN C see II:DAC000
LEUKERAN see I:CDO500, III:POK000
LEUKERSAN see I:CDO500
LEUKOL see III:QMJ000
LEUKOMYAN see II:CDP250
LEUKORAN see I:CDO500
LEUNA M see II:CIR250
LEUPURIN see III:POK000

LEUROCRISTINE see III:LEY000
LEUROCRISTINE SULFATE (1:1) see III:LEZ000
LEVANOX GREEN GA see II:CMJ900
LEVANOX RED 130A see III:IHD000
LEVANOX WHITE RKB see III:TGG760
LEVATROM see III:ARQ750
LEVIUM see III:DCK759
LEVOMYCETIN see II:CDP250
LEVUGEN see III:LFI000
LEVULOSE see III:LFI000
LEYSPRAY see II:CIR250
LGYCOSPERSE S-20 see III:PKL030
LH see III:ILE000
LIBERETAS see III:DCK759
LICHTGRUEN (GERMAN) see III:FAF000
LIDENAL see I:BBQ500
LIFRIL see III:FMB000
LIGHT FAST YELLOW ES see III:SGP500
LIGHT GAS OIL see III:GBW025
LIGHT GREEN FCF YELLOWISH see III:FAF000
LIGHT GREEN LAKE see III:FAF000
LIGHTHOUSE CHROME BLUE 2R see III:HJF500
LIGHT NAPHTHENIC DISTILLATE see I:MQV810
LIGHT NAPHTHENIC DISTILLATE, SOLVENT EXTRACT see
   I:MQV860
LIGHT NAPHTHENIC DISTILLATES (PETROLEUM) see
   I:MQV810
LIGHT ORANGE CHROME see I:LCS000
LIGHT PARAFFINIC DISTILLATE see I:MQV815
LIGHT PARAFFINIC DISTILLATE, SOLVENT EXTRACT see
   I:MQV862
LIGHT RED see III:IHD000
LIGHT SF YELLOWISH (BIOLOGICAL STAIN) see
   III:FAF000
LIGHT SPAR see III:CAX750
LIHOCIN see III:CMF400
LIKUDEN see GKE000
LILLY 22641 see III:RDF000
LILLY 36,352 see III:DUV600
LILLY 37231 see III:LEZ000
LIMAS see III:LGZ000
LIMBIAL see III:CFZ000
LIME-NITROGEN (DOT) see III:CAQ250
LIME OIL see III:OGO000
LIME OIL, DISTILLED (FCC) see III:OGO000
d-LIMONENE see III:LFU000
(+)-R-LIMONENE see III:LFU000
d-(+)-LIMONENE see III:LFU000
LIMONENE DIOXIDE see III:LFV000
LIMONIUM NASHII see III:MBU750
LINASEN see II:EOK000
LINDAGRAIN see I:BBQ500
α-LINDANE see I:BBQ000
β-LINDANE see I:BBR000
LINDANE (ACGIH, DOT, USDA) see I:BBQ500
LINDATOX see III:EEM000
LINE RIDER see II:TAA100
LINESTRENOL see III:NNV000
LINFOLIZIN see I:CDO500
LINFOLYSIN see I:CDO500
LINGEL see II:BRF500
LINGUSORBS see I:PMH500
LINOLEIC ACID mixed with OLEIC ACID see III:LGI000
LINOLENATE HYDROPEROXIDE see III:PCN000
LINOLENIC HYDROPEROXIDE see III:PCN000
LINORMONE see II:CIR250
LINTON see III:CLY500
LINTOX see I:BBQ500
LIPAMID see III:ARQ750
LIPAVIL see III:ARQ750
LIPAVLON see III:ARQ750
LIPIDE 500 see III:ARQ750
LIPIDSENKER see III:ARQ750
LIPOFACTON see III:ARQ750

LIPO-LUTIN see I:PMH500
LIPOMID see III:ARQ750
LIPONORM see III:ARQ750
LIPOREDUCT see III:ARQ750
LIPORIL see III:ARQ750
LIPOSID see III:ARQ750
LIPOSORB O-20 see III:PKL100
LIPOSORB S-20 see III:PKL030
LIPRIN see III:ARQ750
LIPRINAL see III:ARQ750
LIPUR see III:GCK300
LIQUACILLIN see III:BDY669
LIQUAGESIC see II:HIM000
LIQUAMYCIN INJECTABLE see III:HOI000
LIQUIBARINE see III:BAP000
LIQUIDAMBAR STYRACIFLUA see III:SOY500
LIQUID BRIGHT PLATINUM see III:PJD500
LIQUID DERRIS see III:RNZ000
LIQUIDOW see III:CAO750
LIQUID PITCH OIL see I:CMY825
LIQUIPRON see III:LGM200
LIQUITAL see II:EOK000
LIRANOX see II:CIR500
LIROBETAREX see III:CJX750
LIRO CIPC see III:CKC000
LIROMATIN see III:ABX250
LIRONOX see III:BQZ000
LIROPREM see II:PAX250
LIROSTANOL see III:ABX250
LIROTAN see III:EIR000
LIROTHION see III:PAK000
LISACORT see III:PLZ000
LISKONUM see III:LGZ000
LISSAMINE AMARANTH AC see III:FAG020
LISSAMINE FAST YELLOW AE see III:SGP500
LISSAMINE LAKE GREEN SF see III:FAF000
LITALER see III:HOO500
LITEX CA see III:SMR000
LITHANE see III:LGZ000
LITHARGE see III:LDN000
LITHARGE YELLOW L-28 see III:LDN000
LITHICARB see III:LGZ000
LITHINATE see III:LGZ000
LITHIUM CARBONATE see III:LGZ000
LITHIUM CARBONATE (2:1) see III:LGZ000
LITHIUM CHLORIDE see III:LHB000
LITHOBID see III:LGZ000
LITHONATE see III:LGZ000
LITHOSOL ORANGE R BASE see I:NMP500
LITHOTABS see III:LGZ000
LIXOPHEN see II:EOK000
LOBETRIN see III:ARQ750
LOISOL see III:TIQ250
LO MICRON TALC 1 see III:TAB750
LO MICRON TALC, BC 1621 see III:TAB750
LO MICRON TALC USP, BC 2755 see III:TAB750
LOMUSTINE see I:CGV250
S-LON see III:PKQ059
LONACOL see III:EIR000
LONARID see II:HIM000
β-LONGILOBINE see III:RFP000
LONOCOL M see III:MAS500
LONZA G see III:PKQ059
LO/OVRAL see III:NNL500
LOPID see III:GCK300
LOPRESS see II:HGP500
LORINAL see III:CDO000
LORMIN see II:CBF250
LOROL see III:DXV600
LOROL 22 see III:DAI600
LOROL 28 see III:OAX000
LOROMISIN see II:CDP250
LOROTHIDOL see III:TFD250
LOROXIDE see III:BDS000

N-LOST see I:BIE500
N-LOST (GERMAN) see I:BIE250
S-LOST see I:BIH250
LO-VEL see III:SCH000
LOVOSA see III:SFO500
LPT see III:PKB500
LSP 1 see III:LIJ000
LTAN see III:DMH400
LUBERGAL see II:EOK000
LUBROKAL see II:EOK000
LUCALOX see III:AHE250
LUCAMIDE see III:EEM000
LUCANTHONE METABOLITE see III:LIM000
LUCEL (polysaccharide) see III:SFO500
LUCIDOL see III:BDS000
LUCITE see III:PKB500
LUCOFLEX see III:PKQ059
LUCORTEUM SOL see I:PMH500
LUCOVYL PE see III:PKQ059
LUDOX see III:SCH000
LUETOCRIN DEPOT see III:HNT500
LULAMIN see III:TEH500
LULLAMIN see III:DPJ400
LUMEN see II:EOK000
LUMESETTES see II:EOK000
LUMESYN see II:EOK000
LUMILAR 100 see III:PKF750
LUMINAL see II:EOK000
LUMINAL SODIUM see I:SID000
LUMIRROR see III:PKF750
LUMOFRIDETTEN see II:EOK000
LUNAR CAUSTIC see III:SDS000
LUPAREEN see III:PMP500
LUPERCO see III:BDS000
LUPEROX FL see III:BDS000
LUPERSOL see III:MKA500
LUPHENIL see II:EOK000
LURAMIN see II:EOK000
LURAZOL BLACK BA see I:AQP000
LURGO see III:DSP400
LURIDE see III:SHF500
LUSIL see III:SNM500
LUSTREX see III:SMQ500
LUTATE see III:HNT500
LUTEAL HORMONE see I:PMH500
LUTEOCRIN see III:HNT500
LUTEOHORMONE see I:PMH500
LUTEOSAN see I:PMH500
LUTEOSKYRIN see III:LIV000
(−)-LUTEOSKYRIN see III:LIV000
LUTESTRAL (FRENCH) see III:CNV750
LUTETIA RED CLN see III:CHP500
LUTEX see I:PMH500
LUTINYL see II:CBF250
LUTOCYCLIN see I:PMH500
LUTOFAN see III:PKQ059
LUTOGAN see III:DRT200
LUTO-METRODIOL see II:EQJ500
LUTOPRON see III:HNT500
LUTOSAN see III:DRT200
LUTOSOL see III:INJ000
LUTROL see III:PJT000
LUTROMONE see I:PMH500
LUVISKOL see III:PKQ250
LYGOMME CDS see III:CCL250
LYNDIOL see II:LJE000
LYNENOL see III:NNV000
LYNESTRENOL see III:NNV000
LYNESTRENOL mixed with MESTRANOL see II:LJE000
LYNESTROL see II:EEH550
LYNESTROL mixed with MESTRANOL see II:LJE000
LYNOESTRENOL see III:NNV000
LYNOESTRENOL mixed with ETHINYLOESTRADIOL see
  III:EEH575

LYNOESTRENOL mixed with MESTRANOL see II:LJE000
LYOVAC COSMEGEN see III:AEB000
LYP 97 see III:LBR000
LYSANXIA see III:DAP700
LYSOCOCCINE see III:SNM500
LYSOFORM see I:FMV000
LYTECA SYRUP see II:HIM000
LYTRON 5202 see III:SMR000

M 40 see II:CIR250
M 140 see II:CDR750
M 176 see III:DUD800
M 410 see II:CDR750
M 5055 see I:CDV100
M-9500 see III:TND500
M1 (COPPER) see III:CNI000
M2 (COPPER) see III:CNI000
MA see III:DAL300
MA-1214 see III:DXV600
1-N-2-MA (RUSSIAN) see II:MMG000
MAA SODIUM SALT see I:DXE600
MAB see III:MNR500
MABLIN see I:BOT250
MACE (lacrimator) see III:CEA750
MACQUER'S SALT see I:ARD250
MACRODANTIN see III:NGE000
MACRODIOL see I:EDO000
MACROGOL 1000 see III:PJT250
MACROL see I:EDO000
MACRONDRAY see II:DAA800
MACROPAQUE see III:BAP000
MADECASSOL see III:ARN500
MADHURIN see II:SJN700
MAGBOND see III:BAV750
MAGENTA see III:MAC250
MAGNACAT see III:MAP750
MAGNACIDE H see III:ADR000
MAGNESIA see III:MAH500
MAGNESIA USTA see III:MAH500
MAGNESIA WHITE see III:CAX750
MAGNESIUM ARSENATE see I:ARD000
MAGNESIUM ARSENATE PHOSPHOR see I:ARD000
MAGNESIUM GOLD PURPLE see III:GIS000
MAGNESIUM OXIDE see III:MAH500
MAGNESIUM PHTHALOCYANINE see III:MAI250
MAGNESIUM SULFATE and CALOMEL (8:5) see III:CAZ000
MAGNEZU TLENEK (POLISH) see III:MAH500
MAIPEDOPA see III:DNA200
MAJOL PLX see III:SFO500
MAKAROL see I:DKA600
MALACID see III:TGD000
MALACIDE see III:MAK700
MALAFOR see III:MAK700
MALAGRAN see III:MAK700
MALAKILL see III:MAK700
MALAMAR see III:MAK700
MALAMAR 50 see III:MAK700
MALAPHELE see III:MAK700
MALAPHOS see III:MAK700
MALAQUIN see III:CLD000
MALAREN see III:CLD000
MALAREX see III:CLD000
MALASOL see III:MAK700
MALASPRAY see III:MAK700
MALATHION see III:MAK700, III:MAK700
MALATHION ULV CONCENTRATE see III:MAK700
MALATHIOZOO see III:MAK700
MALATHON see III:MAK700
MALATHYL LV CONCENTRATE & ULV CONCENTRATE see
  III:MAK700
MALATION (POLISH) see III:MAK700
MALATOL see III:MAK700
MALATOX see III:MAK700
MALDISON see III:MAK700

MALEALDEHYDIC ACID, DICHLORO-4-OXO-, (Z)-(9CI) see III:MRU900
MALEIC ACID ANHYDRIDE (MAK) see III:MAM000
MALEIC ACID HYDRAZIDE see III:DMC600
MALEIC ANHYDRIDE see III:MAM000
MALEIC HYDRAZIDE see III:DMC600
MALEIC HYDRAZIDE DIETHANOLAMINE SALT see III:DHF200
N,N-MALEOYLHYDRAZINE see III:DMC600
MALESTRONE see III:MPN500
MALESTRONE (AMPS) see I:TBF500
MALGESIC see II:BRF500
MALIPUR see III:CBG000
MALIX see III:EAQ750
MALLOFEEN see I:PDC250
MALLOPHENE see I:PDC250, III:PEK250
MALMED see III:MAK700
MALOCID see III:TGD000
MALOCIDE see III:TGD000
MALOGEN see III:MPN500
MALOGEN L.A.200 see III:TBF750
MALONALDEHYDE see III:PMK000
MALONALDEHYDE, ION(1-), SODIUM see III:MAN700
MALONALDEHYDE SODIUM SALT see III:MAN700
MALONDIALDEHYDE see III:PMK000
MALONIC ALDEHYDE see III:PMK000
MALONIC DIALDEHYDE see III:PMK000
MALONODIALDEHYDE see III:PMK000
MALONYLDIALDEHYDE see III:PMK000
MALOPRIM see III:SOA500, III:TGD000
MALPHOS see III:MAK700
MALTOBIOSE see III:MAO500
MALTOSE see III:MAO500
d-MALTOSE see III:MAO500
MALTOX see III:MAK700
MALTOX MLT see III:MAK700
MALT SUGAR see III:MAO500
α-MALT SUGAR see III:MAO500
MAM see II:HMG000
MAM AC see II:MGS750
MAM ACETATE see II:MGS750
MAMALLET-A see III:DOT000
MAMBNA see II:MHW350
MAMMEX see II:NGE500
MAMN see II:AAW000
MANAM see III:MAS500
MANEB see III:MAS500
MANEB, stabilized against self-heating (DOT) see III:MAS500
MANEBE (FRENCH) see III:MAS500
MANEB, with not less than 60% maneb (DOT) see III:MAS500
MANGAAN(II)-(N,N'-ETHYLEEN-BIS(DITHIOCARBA-MAAT)) (DUTCH) see III:MAS500
MANGAN (POLISH) see III:MAP750
MANGAN(II)-(N,N'-AETHYLEN-BIS(DITHIOCARBAMATE)) (GERMAN) see III:MAS500
MANGANESE see III:MAP750
MANGANESE ACETYLACETONATE see III:MAQ500
MANGANESE(II) CHLORIDE (1:2) see III:MAR000
MANGANESE DICHLORIDE see III:MAR000
MANGANESE ETHYLENE-1,2-BISDITHIOCARBAMATE see III:MAS500
MANGANESE(II) ETHYLENEBIS(DITHIOCARBAMATE) see III:MAS500
MANGANESE(II) ETHYLENE DI(DITHIOCARBAMATE) see III:MAS500
MANGANESE complex with N-FLUOREN-2-YL ACETOHY-DROXAMIC ACID see III:HIR000
MANGANESE(II) SULFATE (1:1) see III:MAU250
MANGANESE ZINC BERYLLIUM SILICATE see I:BFS750
MANGAN NITRIDOVANY (CZECH) see III:MAP750
MANGANOUS ACETYLACETONATE see III:MAQ500
MANGANOUS CHLORIDE see III:MAR000
MANGANOUS SULFATE see III:MAU250
MAN-GRO see III:MAU250

d-MANNITOL BUSULFAN see III:BKM500
MANNITOL MUSTARD DIHYDROCHLORIDE see III:MAW750
MANNITOL MYLERAN see III:BKM500
MANNOGRANOL see III:BKM500
MANNOMUSTINE DIHYDROCHLORIDE see III:MAW750
MANUFACTURED IRON OXIDES see III:IHD000
MANZATE see III:MAS500
MANZATE MANEB FUNGICIDE see III:MAS500
MAO-REM see III:PFC750
MAPLE AMARANTH see III:FAG020
MAPLE BRILLIANT BLUE FCF see III:FMU059
MAPLE ERYTHROSINE see III:FAG040
MAPLE INDIGO CARMINE see III:FAE100
MAPLE PONCEAU 3R see II:FAG018
MAPO see III:250
MARALATE see II:MEI450
MARANYL F 114 see III:PJY500
MARBON 9200 see III:SMR000
MARCELLOMYCIN see III:MAX000
MARIJUANA, SMOKE RESIDUE see III:CBD760
MARLATE see II:MEI450
MARLEX 9400 see III:PMP500
MARMER see III:DXQ500
MARSALID see III:ILE000
MARS BROWN see III:IHD000
MARSH ROSEMARY EXTRACT see III:MBU750
MARSILID see III:ILE000
MARS RED see III:IHD000
MARVINAL see III:PKQ059
MASENATE see I:TBG000
MASENONE see III:MPN500
MASHERI (INDIA) see I:SED400
MASOTEN see III:TIQ250
MASSICOT see III:LDN000
MASSICOTITE see III:LDN000
MASTESTONA see III:MPN500
MASTIPHEN see II:CDP250
MATENON see III:MQS225
MATULANE see I:PME250, I:PME500
MAURYLENE see III:PMP500
MAYVAT GOLDEN YELLOW see III:DCZ000
MAZOTEN see III:TIQ250
MB see III:MHR200
M+B 695 see III:PPO000
M+B 760 see III:TEX250
MBA see I:BIE250
7-MBA see III:MGW750
7-MBA-3,4-DIHYDRODIOL see III:MBV500
MBA HYDROCHLORIDE see I:BIE500
MBAO HYDROCHLORIDE see II:CFA750
MBH see I:PME500
MBMA see III:MJQ250
MBNA see III:MHW500
MBOCA see I:MJM200
MBOT see I:MJO250
MBT see II:BDF000
MBTS see III:BDE750
MBTS RUBBER ACCELERATOR see III:BDE750
MBX see III:MHR200
2M-4C see II:CIR250
MCA see III:CEA000
3-MCA see II:MIJ750
MCA-11,12-EPOXIDE see III:ECA500
MCA-11,12-OXIDE see III:ECA500
(E)-MC 11,12-DIHYDRODIOL see III:DML800
MCP see II:CIR250
2M-4CP see II:CIR500
MCPA see II:CIR250
MCPP see III:CIR500
2-MCPP see II:CIR500
MCPP-D-4 see II:CIR500
MCPP 2,4-D see II:CIR500
MCPP-K-4 see II:CIR500

10-MD see III:MEK700
MDA see I:MJQ000
MDAB see III:DUH600
3'-MDAB see III:DUH600
MDI see III:MJP400
MDS see III:DBD750
ME-1700 see I:BIM500
MEARLMAID see III:GLI000
MEB see III:MAS500
MEBICHLORAMINE see I:BIE500
MEBR see III:MHR200
ME-CCNU see II:CHD250
MECHLORETHAMINE see I:BIE250
MECHLORETHAMINE HYDROCHLORIDE see I:BIE500
MECHLORETHAMINE OXIDE see III:CFA500
MECHLORETHAMINE OXIDE HYDROCHLORIDE see
   II:CFA750
MECOBALAMIN see III:VSZ050
MECOMEC see II:CIR500
MECOPEOP see II:CIR500
MECOPER see II:CIR500
MECOPEX see II:CIR500
MECOPROP see II:CIR500
MECOTURF see II:CIR500
MECPROP see II:CIR500
2-MeDAB see III:TLE750
MEDARON see III:NGG500
MEDFALAN see III:SAX200
MEDIAMYCETINE see II:CDP250
MEDIFLAVIN see III:DBX400
MEDPHALAN see III:SAX200
MEDROXYPROGESTERONE ACETATE see II:MCA000
MEE see I:EDP000
MEGACE see II:VTF000
MEGESTROL ACETATE see II:VTF000
MEGESTROL ACETATE + ETHINYLOESTRADIOL see
   III:MCA500
MEGESTROL ACETATE 4 MG., ETHINYLOESTRADIOL 50
   μg see III:MCA500
MEGESTRYL ACETATE see II:VTF000
6-ME-GLU-P-2 see II:AKS250
MEISEI TERYL DIAZO BLUE HR see I:DCJ200
MEKP see III:MKA500
MEK PEROXIDE see III:MKA500
MELABON see I:ABG750
MELADININ see I:XDJ000
MELADININE see I:XDJ000
MELAMINE see III:MCB000
MELATONIN see III:MCB350
MELATONINE see III:MCB350
MELETIN see III:QCA000
MELIFORM see III:PKF750
MELIN see III:RSU000
MELINEX see III:PKF750
MELIPAN see II:MCB500
MELIPAX see I:CDV100
MELOCHIA TOMENTOSA see III:BAR500
MELOXINE see I:XDJ000
MELPHALAN see I:PED750
MELPHALAN HYDROCHLORIDE see III:BHV250
MELPREX see III:DXX400
ME-MDA see I:MJO250
MEMPA see I:HEK000
MENADION see III:MMD500
MENADIONE see III:MMD500
MENAGEN see I:EDV000
MENAPHTHON see III:MMD500
MENAPHTONE see III:MMD500
MENDRIN see III:EAT500
MENEST see I:ECU750
MENFORMON see I:EDV000
Me2NMOR see II:DTA000
MENOGEN see I:ECU750
MENOQUENS see III:MCA500

MENOSTILBEEN see I:DKA600
MENOTAB see I:ECU750
MENOTROL see I:ECU750
p-MENTHA-1,8-DIENE see III:LFU000
d-p-MENTHA-1,8-DIENE see III:LFU000
p-MENTHANE HYDROPEROXIDE see III:MCE000
p-MENTHANE-8-HYDROPEROXIDE see III:MCE000
ME-PARATHION see III:MNH000
MEPATON see III:MNH000
MEPHABUTAZONE see II:BRF500
MEPHANAC see II:CIR250
2'-MePO₄' see III:DSS200
MEPRO see II:CIR500
MEPTOX see III:MNH000
MEPYRAMINE MALEATE see III:DBM800
MER 25 see III:DIIS000
MER-41 see III:CMX700
MERACTINOMYCIN see III:AEB000
MERAKLON see III:PMP500
MERANTINE BLUE EG see III:FAE000
MERANTINE GREEN SF see III:FAF000
MERBENTUL see II:CLO750
MERCALEUKIN see III:POK000
MERCAPTAZOLE see III:MCO500
7-MERCAPTOBENZ(a)ANTHRACENE see III:BBH750
MERCAPTOBENZOTHIAZOLE see II:BDF000
2-MERCAPTOBENZOTHIAZOLE see II:BDF000
2-MERCAPTOBENZOTHIAZOLEDISULFIDE see III:BDE750
2-MERCAPTOBENZOTHIAZOLE ZINC SALT see III:BHA750
2-MERCAPTOBENZOTHIAZYLDISULFIDE see III:BDE750
2-MERCAPTO-4-HYDROXY-6-METHYLPYRIMIDINE see
   II:MPW500
2-MERCAPTO-4-HYDROXY-6-N-PROPYLPYRIMIDINE see
   I:PNX000
2-MERCAPTO-4-HYDROXYPYRIMIDINE see III:TFR250
2-MERCAPTOIMIDAZOLINE see I:IAQ000
(MERCAPTOMETHYL)BENZENE see III:TGO750
3-(MERCAPTOMETHYL)-1,2,3-BENZOTRIAZIN-4(3H)-ONE-
   O,O-DIMETHYL PHOSPHORODITHIOATE see III:ASH500
3-(MERCAPTOMETHYL)-1,2,3-BENZOTRIAZIN-4(3H)-ONE-
   O,O-DIMETHYL PHOSPHORODITHIOATE-S-ESTER see
   III:ASH500
2-MERCAPTO-1-METHYLIMIDAZOLE see III:MCO500
2-MERCAPTO-6-METHYLPYRIMID-4-ONE see II:MPW500
2-MERCAPTO-6-METHYL-4-PYRIMIDONE see II:MPW500
MERCAPTOPHOS see III:FAQ999
2-MERCAPTO-6-PROPYL-4-PYRIMIDONE see I:PNX000
2-MERCAPTO-6-PROPYLPYRIMID-4-ONE see I:PNX000
6-MERCAPTOPURIN see III:POK000
MERCAPTOPURIN (GERMAN) see III:POK000
6-MERCAPTOPURINE see III:POK000
6-MERCAPTOPURINE 3-N-OXIDE MONOHYDRATE see
   III:OMY800
2-MERCAPTO-4-PYRIMIDINOL see III:TFR250
2-MERCAPTO-4-PYRIMIDONE see III:TFR250
2-MERCAPTOPYRIMID-4-ONE see III:TFR250
MERCAPTOSUCCINIC ACID DIETHYL ESTER see
   III:MAK700
7-MERCAPTO-1,3,4,6-TETRAZAINDENE see III:POK000
MERCAPTOTHION see III:MAK700
MERCAPTOTION (SPANISH) see III:MAK700
α-MERCAPTOTOLUENE see III:TGO750
d-MERCAPTOVALINE see III:MCR750
d,3-MERCAPTOVALINE see III:MCR750
MERCAPURIN see III:POK000
MERCAZOLYL see III:MCO500
MERCHLORETHANAMINE see I:BIE500
MERCURAM see III:TFS350
MERCURE (FRENCH) see III:MCW250
MERCURIC ARSENATE see I:MDF350
MERCURIO (ITALIAN) see III:MCW250
MERCUROTHIOLATE see III:MDI000
MERCURY see III:MCW250
MERCURY, METALLIC (DOT) see III:MCW250

MERCURY METHYLCHLORIDE see III:MDD750
MERCURY(II) ORTHOARSENATE see I:MDF350
MERCURY ZINC CHROMATE COMPLEX see I:ZJA000
MEREX see I:KEA000
MERFALAN see II:BHT750
MERFAMIN see III:MDI000
MERIZONE see II:BRF500
2-MERKAPTOBENZOTIAZOL (POLISH) see II:BDF000
2-MERKAPTOIMIDAZOLIN (CZECH) see I:IAQ000
MERMETH see III:SNJ000
MERN see III:POK000
MERONIDAL see I:MMN250
MERPAN see III:CBG000
MERPHALAN see II:BHT750
o-MERPHALAN see II:BHT750
MERPOL see I:EJN500
MERTESTATE see I:TBF500
MERTHIOLATE see III:MDI000
MERTHIOLATE SALT see III:MDI000
MERTHIOLATE SODIUM see III:MDI000
MERTORGAN see III:MDI000
MERZONIN SODIUM see III:MDI000
MESEREIN see III:MDJ250
MESIDIN (CZECH) see III:TLG500
MESIDINE see III:TLG500
MESIDINE HYDROCHLORIDE see II:TLH000
MESITYLAMINE see III:TLG500
MESITYLAMINE HYDROCHLORIDE see II:TLH000
MESTERONE see III:MPN500
MESTRANOL see I:MKB750
MESTRANOL mixed with ANAGESTONE ACETATE (1:10) see
    III:AOO000
MESTRANOL mixed with CHLORMADINONE ACETATE see
    III:CNV750
MESTRANOL mixed with 6-CHLORO-6-DEHYDRO-17-α-
    ACETOXYPROGESTERONE see III:CNV750
MESTRANOL mixed with CHLOROETHYNYL NORGESTREL
    (1:20) see III:CHI750
MESTRANOL mixed with ETHYNERONE (1:20) see
    III:EQJ000
MESTRANOL mixed with ETHYNODIOL see III:EQK100
MESTRANOL mixed with ETHYNODIOL DIACETATE see
    III:EQK010
MESTRANOL mixed with LYNESTRENOL see II:LJE000
MESTRANOL mixed with LYNESTROL see II:LJE000
MESTRANOL mixed with NORETHINDRONE see III:MDL750
MESTRANOL mixed with NORETHISTERONE see III:MDL750
MESTRANOL mixed with NORETHYNODREL see I:EAP000
MESTRANOL mixed with NORGESTREL see III:NNR000
MESTRENOL see I:MKB750
MESTRENOL mixed with 6-CHLORO-6-DEHYDRO-17-α-
    ACETOXYPROGESTERONE see III:CNV750
MESUPRINE HYDROCHLORIDE see III:MDM000
MESYLITH see III:CLD000
METAARSENIC ACID see ARB000
META BLACK see I:AQP000
METABOLITE C see III:SOA500
METABOLITE I see III:HNI500
METACE see II:CLO750
METACIDE see III:MNH000
METACIL see II:MPW500
METACORTANDRACIN see III:PLZ000
METAFOS see III:MNH000
METAFUME see III:MHR200
METAKRYLAN METYLU (POLISH) see III:MLH750
METALCAPTASE see III:MCR750
METALLIC ARSENIC see ARA750
METAMID see III:PJY500
METAMPHETAMINE HYDROCHLORIDE see III:MDT600
METANABOL see III:DAL300
METANDIENON see III:DAL300
METANDIENONE see III:DAL300
METANDIENONUM see III:DAL300
METANDREN see III:MPN500

METANDROSTENOLON see III:DAL300
METANDROSTENOLONE see III:DAL300
METANICOTINE see III:MDM750
METAPHENYLENEDIAMINE see III:PEY000
METAPHOR see III:MNH000
METAPHOS see III:MNH000
METAPHOSPHORIC ACID, CALCIUM SODIUM SALT see
    III:CAX260
METAPLEX NO see III:PKB500
METASILICIC ACID see III:SCL000
METASTENOL see III:DAL300
META TOLUYLENE DIAMINE see I:TGL750
METATOLYLENEDIAMINE DIHYDROCHLORIDE see
    III:DCE000
METAUPON see III:OHU000
METAXITE see I:ARM268
METAXON see II:CIR250
METAZIN see III:SNJ000
METAZOLO see III:MCO500
METEPA see III:TNK250
METHABOL see I:PAN100
METHACON see III:DPJ400
METHACRYLATE de METHYLE (FRENCH) see III:MLH750
METHACRYLIC ACID, METHYL ESTER (MAK) see
    III:MLH750
METHACRYLIC ACID METHYL ESTER POLYMERS see
    III:PKB500
METHACRYLSAEUREMETHYL ESTER (GERMAN) see
    III:MLH750
METHALLYL CHLORIDE see II:CIU750
α-METHALLYL CHLORIDE see II:CIU750
METHAMIN see III:HEI500
(+)-METHAMPHETAMINE CHLORIDE see III:MDT600
METHAMPHETAMINE HYDROCHLORIDE see III:MDT600
(+)-METHAMPHETAMINE HYDROCHLORIDE see
    III:MDT600
d-METHAMPHETAMINE HYDROCHLORIDE see III:MDT600
METHAMPHETAMINIUM CHLORIDE see III:MDT600
METHANAL see I:FMV000
METHANDIENONE see III:DAL300
METHANDROLONE see III:DAL300
METHANDROSTENOLONE see III:DAL300
METHANE BASE see I:MJN000
METHANECARBOXAMIDE see II:AAI000
METHANE DICHLORIDE see II:MJP450
METHANESULFONIC ACID, 2-PROPENYL ESTER (9CI) see
    III:AGK750
METHANESULFONIC ACID TETRAMETHYLENE ESTER see
    I:BOT250
METHANESULPHONIC ACID ETHYL ESTER see II:EMF500
METHANESULPHONIC ACID METHYL ESTER see
    III:MLH500
METHANE TETRACHLORIDE see CBY000
1,1′,1″,1‴-METHANETHETRAYLTETRAKISBENZENE see
    III:TEA750
METHANE TRICHLORIDE see I:CHJ500
METHANOL, (METHYL-ONN-AZOXY)-, BENZOATE (ester)
    (9CI) see III:MGS925
4,7-METHANO-2,3,8-METHENOCYCLOPENT(a)INDENE, DO-
    DECAHYDRO-, stereoisomer see III:DLJ500
METHANONE, (5-AMINO-1,3-DIMETHYL-1H-PYRAZOL-4-
    YL)(2-FLUOROPHENYL)- see III:AJR400
METHAPHOXIDE see III:TNK250
METHAPYRILENE HYDROCHLORIDE see III:DPJ400
METHAPYRILENE HYDROCHLORIDE (L.A.) see III:DPJ400
METHAPYRILENE HYDROCHLORIDE (S.A.) see III:DPJ400
METHAPYRILENE mixed with SODIUM NITRITE (1:2) see
    III:MDT000
METHAR see I:DXE600
METHARSINAT see I:DXE600
METHASAN see III:BJK500
METHAZATE see III:BJK500
METHEDRINE see III:MDT600
METHEDRINE HYDROCHLORIDE see III:MDT600

7-METHOXY-N-2-FLUORENYLACETAMIDE see III:MER250
N-(1-METHOXYFLUOREN-2-YL)ACETAMIDE see
  III:MER000
N-(1-METHOXY-2-FLUORENYL)ACETAMIDE see
  III:MER000
N-(7-METHOXY-2-FLUORENYL)ACETAMIDE see
  III:MER250
N-(7-METHOXYFLUOREN-2-YL)ACETAMIDE see
  III:MER250
8-METHOXY-(FURANO-3'.2':6.7-COUMARIN) see I:XDJ000
9-METHOXY-7H-FURO(3,2-g)BENZOPYRAN-7-ONE see
  I:XDJ000
4-METHOXY-7H-FURO(3,2-g)(1)BENZOPYRAN-7-ONE see
  II:MFN275
8-METHOXY-2',3',6,7-FUROCOUMARIN see I:XDJ000
8-METHOXY-4',5',6,7-FUROCOUMARIN see I:XDJ000
8-METHOXY-4-HYDROXYQUINOLINE-2-CARBOXYLIC
  ACID see III:HLT500
METHOXYINDOLEACETIC ACID see III:MES850
5-METHOXYINDOLEACETIC ACID see III:MES850
5-METHOXYINDOLE-3-ACETIC ACID see III:MES850
METHOXYLENE see III:DPJ400
METHOXYMETHYL-AETHYLNITROSAMINE (GERMAN) see
  III:MEV750
3-METHOXYMETHYLAMINOAZOBENZENE see
  III:MNS000
2-METHOXY-5-METHYLANILINE see I:MGO750
4-METHOXY-2-METHYLANILINE see II:MGO500
3-METHOXY-7-METHYLBENZ(c)ACRIDINE see III:MET875
5-METHOXY-7-METHYL-BENZ(a)ANTHRACENE see
  III:MEU000
8-METHOXY-7-METHYL-BENZ(a)ANTHRACENE see
  III:MEU250
7-METHOXY-12-METHYLBENZ(a)ANTHRACENE see
  III:MEU500
3-METHOXY-10-METHYL-1,2-BENZANTHRACENE see
  III:MEU000
5-METHOXY-10-METHYL-1,2-BENZANTHRACENE see
  III:MEU250
4-METHOXY-2-METHYLBENZENAMINE see II:MGO500
2-METHOXY-5-METHYL-BENZENAMINE (9CI) see
  I:MGO750
3-METHOXY-17-METHYL-15H-CYCLOPENTAPHENAN-
  THRENE see III:MEU750
3-METHOXY-17-METHYL 15H-CYCLOPENTA(a)PHENAN-
  THRENE see III:MEU750
11-METHOXY-17-METHYL-15H-CYCLOPENTA(a)PHENAN-
  THRENE see III:MEV000
6-METHOXY-11-METHYL-15,16-DIHYDRO-17H-CYCLOPEN-
  TA(a) PHENANTHREN-17-ONE see III:MEV250
METHOXYMETHYL ETHYL NITROSAMINE see III:MEV750
7-METHOXYMETHYL-12-METHYLBENZ(a)ANTHRACENE
  see III:MEW000
METHOXYMETHYL-METHYLNITROSAMIN (GERMAN) see
  III:MEW250
METHOXYMETHYL METHYLNITROSAMINE see
  III:MEW250
7-METHOXYMETHYL-1-METHYL-2-NITRONAPHTHO(2,1-b)FURAN
  see III:MEW975
3-METHOXY-5-METHYL-4-OXO-2,5-HEXADIENOIC ACID
  see III:PAP750
p-METHOXY-β-METHYLSTYRENE see III:PMQ750
3-METHOXY-4-MONOMETHYLAMINOAZOBENZENE see
  III:MNS000
1-METHOXY-2-NAPHTHYLAMINE see III:MFA000
1-METHOXY-2-NAPHTHYLAMINE HYDROCHLORIDE see
  III:MFA250
2-METHOXY-5-NITROANILINE see II:NEQ500
2-METHOXY-5-NITROBENZENAMINE see II:NEQ500
7-METHOXY-2-NITRONAPHTHO(2,1-b)FURAN see
  II:MFB400
8-METHOXY-6-NITROPHENANTHOL-(3,4-d)-1,3-DIOXOLE-
  5-CARBOXYLIC ACID see AQY250
8-METHOXY-6-NITROPHENANTHRO(3,4-d)-1,3-DIOXOLE-5-
  CARBOXYLIC ACID SODIUM SALT see III:AQY125

N-METHOXY-N-NITROSOMETHYLAMINE see III:DSZ000
1-METHOXY-N-NITROSO-N-PROPYLPROPYLAMINE see
  III:DWU800
3-METHOXY-17-α-19-NORPREGNA-K,3,5(10)-TRIEN-20-YN-
  17-OL see I:MKB750
11-β-METHOXY-19-NOR-17-α-PREGNA-1,3,5(10)-TRIEN-20-
  YNE-3,17-DIOL see III:MRU600
3-METHOXY-19-NOR-17-α-PREGNA-1,3,5(10)-TRIEN-10-YN-
  17-OL see I:MKB750
(17-α)-3-METHOXY-19-NORPREGN-1,3,5(10)-TRIEN-20-YN-
  17-OL see I:MKB750
d-threo-METHOXY-3-(1-OCTENYL-ONN-AZOXY)-2-BUTA-
  NOL see III:EAG000
4-METHOXYPHENYLACETIC ACID see III:MFE250
p-METHOXYPHENYLACETIC ACID see III:MFE250
o-METHOXYPHENYLAMINE see II:AOV900
N-(p-METHOXYPHENYL)-1-AZIRIDINECARBOXAMIDE see
  III:MFF250
2-METHOXY-4-PHENYLAZOANILINE see III:MFF500
4-((p-METHOXYPHENYL)AZO)-o-ANISIDINE see
  III:DNY400
N-(2-METHOXY-4-(PHENYLAZO)PHENYL)HYDROXYLA-
  MINE see III:HLR000
p-METHOXYPHENYL-N-CARBAMOYLAZIRIDINE see
  III:MFF250
1-(p-METHOXYPHENYL)-3,3-DIMETHYLTRIAZENE see
  III:DSN600
2-(p-METHOXYPHENYL)-3,3-DIPHENYLACRYLONITRILE
  see III:MFF750
α-(p-METHOXYPHENYL)-β,β-DIPHENYLACRYLONITRILE
  see III:MFF750
4-METHOXY-m-PHENYLENEDIAMINE see I:DBO000
p-METHOXY-m-PHENYLENEDIAMINE see I:DBO000
4-METHOXY-m-PHENYLENEDIAMINE SULFATE see
  I:DBO400
4-METHOXY-m-PHENYLENEDIAMINE SULPHATE see
  I:DBO400
p-METHOXY-m-PHENYLENEDIAMINE SULPHATE see
  I:DBO400
1-(p-METHOXYPHENYL)-3-METHYL-3-NITROSOUREA see
  III:MFG400
1-(p-METHOXYPHENYL)PROPENE see III:PMQ750
4-METHOXYPROPENYLBENZENE see III:PMQ750
1-METHOXY-4-PROPENYLBENZENE see III:PMQ750
1-METHOXY-4-(2-PROPENYL)BENZENE see III:AFW750
2-METHOXY-4-PROP-2-ENYLPHENOL see III:EQR500
2-METHOXY-4-(2-PROPENYL)PHENOL see III:EQR500
1-METHOXYPROPYLPROPYLNITROSAMIN (GERMAN) see
  III:DWU800
1-METHOXYPROPYLPROPYLNITROSAMINE see
  III:DWU800
5-METHOXY PSORALEN see II:MFN275
8-METHOXYPSORALEN see I:XDJ000
9-METHOXYPSORALEN see I:XDJ000
3-METHOXY-4-STILBENAMINE see III:MFP500
4-METHOXY-m-TOLUIDINE see I:MGO750
2-METHOXYTRICYCLOQUINAZOLINE see III:MFQ750
3-METHOXYTRICYCLOQUINAZOLINE see III:MFR000
N-METHOXYURETHANE see III:MEO000
p-METHOXY-α-VINYLBENZYL ALCOHOL see III:HKI000
p-METHOXY-α-VINYLBENZYL ALCOHOL ACETATE (ES-
  TER) see III:ABN725
12-METHYBENZ(a)ANTHRACENE-7-METHANOL see
  III:HMF000
METHYCOBAL see III:VSZ050
METHYLACETOPYRONONE see III:MFW500
METHYL(ACETOXYMETHYL)NITROSAMINE see
  II:AAW000
6-METHYL-17-α-ACETOXYPREGNA-4,6-DIENE-3,20-DIONE
  see II:VTF000
6-α-METHYL-17-α-ACETOXYPREGN-4-ENE-3,20-DIONE see
  II:MCA000
6-α-METHYL-17-α-ACETOXYPROGESTERONE see
  II:MCA000

12-METHYLBENZ(a)ANTHRACENE-7-CARBOXALDEHYDE
see III:FNT000
7-METHYLBENZ(a)ANTHRACENE-12-CARBOXALDEHYDE
see III:MGY500
12-METHYL BENZ(A)ANTHRACENE-7-ETHANOL see
III:HKU000
7-METHYLBENZ(a)ANTHRACENE-12-METHANOL see
III:HMF500
12-METHYLBENZ(a)ANTHRACENE-7-METHANOL ACE-
TATE (ESTER) see III:ABR250
12-METHYLBENZ(a)ANTHRACENE-7-METHANOL BEN-
ZOATE (ESTER) see III:BDQ250
7-METHYLBENZ(a)ANTHRACENE-5,6-OXIDE see
III:MGZ000
7-METHYLBENZ(a)ANTHRACEN-8-YL CARBAMIDE see
III:MGX750
S-(12-METHYL-7-BENZ(a)ANTHRYLMETHYL)HOMO-
CYSTEINE see III:MHA000
N-METHYLBENZAZIMIDE, DIMETHYLDITHIOPHOS-
PHORIC ACID ESTER see III:ASH500
2-METHYLBENZENAMINE see I:TGQ750
o-METHYLBENZENAMINE see I:TGQ750
2-METHYLBENZENAMINE HYDROCHLORIDE see I:TGS500
4-METHYLBENZENAMINE HYDROCHLORIDE see
III:TGS750
o-METHYLBENZENAMINE HYDROCHLORIDE see I:TGS500
2-METHYL-1,4-BENZENEDIAMINE see III:TGM000,
III:TGM400
4-METHYL-1,3-BENZENEDIAMINE see I:TGL750
2-METHYL-1,4-BENZENEDIAMINE SULFATE see
III:DCE600
2-METHYLBENZENESULFONAMIDE see II:TGN250
o-METHYLBENZENESULFONAMIDE see II:TGN250
METHYL-2-BENZIMIDAZOLE CARBAMATE and SODIUM NI-
TRITE see II:CBN375
7-METHYLBENZO(c)ACRIDINE see III:MGT500
6-METHYL-3,4-BENZOCARBAZOLE see III:MHD000
9-METHYL-1:2-BENZOCARBAZOLE see III:MHD250
10-METHYL-7H-BENZO(c)CARBAZOLE see III:MHD000
11-METHYL-11H-BENZO(a)CARBAZOLE see III:MHD250
3-METHYLBENZO(b)FLUORANTHENE see III:MGT400
7-METHYLBENZO(b)FLUORANTHENE see III:MGT410
8-METHYLBENZO(b)FLUORANTHENE see III:MGT415
12-METHYLBENZO(b)FLUORANTHENE see III:MGT420
5-METHYLBENZO(rat)PENTAPHENE see III:MHE250
8-METHYLBENZO(rst)PENTAPHENE-5-CARBOXALDEHYDE
see III:FNU000
METHYL-1,12-BENZOPERYLENE see III:MHE500
7-METHYLBENZO(h)PHENALENO(1,9-bc)ACRIDINE see
III:MHF000
7-METHYLBENZO(a)PHENALENO(1,9-hi)ACRIDINE see
III:MHE750
4-METHYLBENZO(c)PHENANTHRENE see III:MHL750
5-METHYLBENZO(c)PHENANTHRENE see III:MHF250
6-METHYLBENZO(c)PHENANTHRENE see III:MHF500
1-METHYLBENZO(a)PYRENE see III:MHG250
2-METHYLBENZO(a)PYRENE see III:MHG500
3-METHYLBENZO(a)PYRENE see III:MHM250
4-METHYLBENZO(a)PYRENE see III:MHG750
5-METHYLBENZO(a)PYRENE see III:MHH200
6-METHYLBENZO(a)PYRENE see III:MHM000
7-METHYLBENZO(a)PYRENE see III:MHH000
10-METHYLBENZO(a)PYRENE see III:MHH500
11-METHYLBENZO(a)PYRENE see III:MHH750
12-METHYLBENZO(a)PYRENE see III:MHI000
4'-METHYLBENZO(a)PYRENE see III:MHH000
5-METHYL-3,4-BENZOPYRENE see III:MHM000
7-METHYL-6H-(1)BENZOTHIOPYRANO(4,3-b)QUINOLINE
see III:MHJ750
1-METHYL-3,4-BENZPHENANTHRENE see III:MHF500
2-METHYL-3,4-BENZPHENANTHRENE see III:MHF250
6-METHYL-3:4-BENZPHENANTHRENE see III:MHL250
7-METHYL-3,4-BENZPHENANTHRENE see III:MHL500

8-METHYL-3:4-BENZPHENANTHRENE see III:MHL750
5-METHYL-3,4-BENZPYRENE see III:MHM000
6-METHYL-3,4-BENZPYRENE see III:MHH750
8-METHYL-3,4-BENZPYRENE see III:MHM250
9-METHYL-3,4-BENZPYRENE see III:MHG500
4'-METHYL-3:4-BENZPYRENE see III:MHH000
METHYLBENZYLAMINE mixed with SODIUM NITRITE
(2:3) see III:MHN250
N-METHYLBENZYLAMINE mixed with SODIUM NITRITE
(1:1) see III:MHN000
N-METHYLBENZYLAMINE mixed with SODIUM NITRITE
(2:3) see III:MHN250
1-METHYL-2-BENZYLHYDRAZINE see III:MHN750
N-METHYL-N-BENZYLNITROSAMINE see III:MHP250
METHYL-BENZYL-NITROSOAMIN (GERMAN) see
III:MHP250
2-METHYL-2,2'-BIOXIRANE (9CI) see III:DHD200
4'-METHYLBIPHENYLAMINE see III:MGF750
N-METHYL-BIS-CHLORAETHYLAMIN (GERMAN) see
I:BIE250
γ(1-METHYL-5-BIS(β-CHLORAETHYL)AMINOBENZIMID-
AZOLYL)BUTTERSAEUREHYDROCHLORID(GERMAN)
see III:CQM750
METHYL-BIS-(β-CHLORAETHYL)-AMIN-N-OXYD-HYDRO-
CHLORID (GERMAN) see II:CFA750
N-METHYL-BIS-β-CHLORETHYLAMINE HYDROCHLORIDE
see I:BIE500
γ-(1-METHYL-5-BIS(β-CHLOROAETHYL) AMINOBENZI-
MIDAZOYL) BUTTERSAUERHYDROCHLORID(GERMAN)
see III:CQM750
METHYLBIS(β-CHLOROETHYL)AMINE see I:BIE250
N-METHYL-BIS(β-CHLOROETHYL)AMINE see I:BIE250
METHYLBIS(2-CHLOROETHYL)AMINE HYDROCHLORIDE
see I:BIE500
METHYLBIS(β-CHLOROETHYL)AMINE HYDROCHLORIDE
see I:BIE500
N-METHYLBIS(2-CHLOROETHYL)AMINE HYDROCHLO-
RIDE see I:BIE500
N-METHYL-BIS-(2-CHLOROETHYL)AMINE (MAK) see
I:BIE250
METHYLBIS(β-CHLOROETHYL)AMINE-N-OXIDE see
III:CFA500
METHYLBIS(β-CHLOROETHYL)AMINE-N-OXIDE HYDRO-
CHLORIDE see II:CFA750
N-METHYLBIS(2-CHLOROETHYL)AMINE-N-OXIDE HY-
DROCHLORIDE see II:CFA750
7-METHYLBISDEHYDRODOISYNOLIC ACID see III:BIT000
1-METHYL-BP see III:MHG250
5-METHYL-BP see III:MHH200
METHYLBROMID (GERMAN) see III:MHR200
METHYL BROMIDE see III:MHR200
1-METHYL-7-BROMOMETHYLBENZ(a)ANTHRACENE see
III:BNQ750
1-METHYL-3-(p-BROMOPHENYL)-1-NITROSOUREA see
III:BNX125
1-METHYL-3-(p-BROMOPHENYL)UREA see III:MHS375
1-METHYL-3-(p-BROMOPHENYL)UREA mixed with SODIUM
NITRITE see III:SIQ675
1-METHYL-3-(p-BROMPHENYL)HARNSTOFF see
III:MHS375
1-METHYL-3-(p-BROMPHENYL)-1-NITROSOHARNSTOFF
(GERMAN) see III:BNX125
3-METHYLBUTANOIC ACID, 2-PROPENYL ESTER see
II:ISV000
3-METHYL BUTANOL see III:IHP000
2-METHYL-4-BUTANOL see III:IHP000
3-METHYLBUTAN-1-OL see III:IHP000
3-METHYL-1-BUTANOL (CZECH) see III:IHP000
2-METHYLBUTENOIC ACID-7-((2,3-DIHYDROXY-2-(1-
METHYLETHYL)-1-OXOBUTOXY)METHYL-2,3,5,7a-TET-
RAHYDRO-1H-PYRROLIZIN-1-YL ESTER see III:SPB500
3'-METHYLBUTTERGELB (GERMAN) see III:DUH600
METHYLBUTYL HYDRAZINE see III:MHW000
1-METHYL-2-BUTYL-HYDRAZINE DIHYDROCHLORIDE see
III:MHW250

N-3-METHYLBUTYL-N-1-METHYL ACETONYLNITROSA-
MINE see II:MHW350
METHYL-BUTYL-NITROSAMIN (GERMAN) see
III:MHW500
METHYLBUTYLNITROSAMINE see III:MHW500
METHYL-N-BUTYLNITROSAMINE see III:MHW500
3-METHYLBUTYRIC ACID, ALLYL ESTER see II:ISV000
8-(3-METHYLBUTYRYLOXY)-DIACETOXYSCIRPENOL see
III:FQS000
METHYL CADMIUM AZIDE see I:MHY550
METHYL CARBAMATE see III:MHZ000
METHYLCARBAMATE-1-NAPHTHALENOL see III:CBM750
METHYLCARBAMATE-1-NAPHTHOL see III:CBM750
N-METHYLCARBAMATE de 1-NAPHTYLE (FRENCH) see
III·CBM750
METHYLCARBAMIC ACID, ETHYL ESTER see III:EMQ500
METHYLCARBAMIC ACID-1-NAPHTHYL ESTER see
III:CBM750
S-METHYLCARBAMOYLMETHYL-O,O-DIMETHYL PHOS-
PHORODITHIOATE see III:DSP400
METHYLCARBINOL see I:EFU000
METHYL-4-CARBOMETHOXY BENZOATE see III:DUE000
17-β-(1-METHYL-3-CARBOXYPROPYL)-ETIOCHOLANE-3-
α,12-α-DIOL see III:DAQ400
N-METHYL-N-(3-CARBOXYPROPYL)NITROSAMINE see
III:MIF250
METHYL-CCNU see II:CHD250
trans-METHYL-CCNU see II:CHD250
METHYL CHAVICOL see III:AFW750
METHYL-2-CHLORAETHYLNITROSAMIN (GERMAN) see
III:CIQ500
METHYLCHLORID (GERMAN) see II:MIF765
METHYL CHLORIDE see II:MIF765
2-METHYL-4-CHLOROANILINE see II:CLK220
2-METHYL-4-CHLOROANILINE HYDROCHLORIDE see
II:CLK235
METHYL(2-CHLOROETHYL)NITROSAMINE see III:CIQ500
METHYL CHLOROFORM see III:MIH275
METHYLCHLOROFORM see III:MIH275
METHYLCHLOROMETHYL ETHER see I:CIO250
METHYLCHLOROMETHYL ETHER (DOT) see I:CIO250
METHYL CHLOROMETHYL ETHER, ANHYDROUS (DOT) see
I:CIO250
4-METHYL-6-(((2-CHLORO-4-NITRO)PHENYL)AZO)-m-ANI-
SIDINE see III:MIH500
2-METHYL-4-CHLOROPHENOXYACETIC ACID see
II:CIR250
2-(2-METHYL-4-CHLOROPHENOXY)PROPIONIC ACID see
II:CIR500
2-METHYL-4-CHLOROPHENOXY-α-PROPIONIC ACID see
II:CIR500
α-(2-METHYL-4-CHLOROPHENOXY)PROPIONIC ACID see
II:CIR500
N'-(2-METHYL-4-CHLOROPHENYL)-N,N-DIMETHYL-
FORMAMIDINE see III:CJJ250
N-METHYL-N'-(p-CHLOROPHENYL)-N-NITROSOUREA see
II:MMW775
METHYL-2-(4-(p-CHLOROPHENYL)PHENOXY)-2-METHYL-
PROPIONATE see III:MIO975
METHYL CHLOROPHOS see III:TIQ250
2-METHYL-4-CHLORPHENOXYESSIGSAEURE (GERMAN)
see II:CIR250
2-(2-METHYL-4-CHLORPHENOXY)-PROPIONSAEURE (GER-
MAN) see II:CIR500
N'-(2-METHYL-4-CHLORPHENYL)-FORMAMIDIN-HYDRO-
CHLORID (GERMAN) see III:CJJ250
METHYLCHOLANTHRENE see II:MIJ750
3-METHYLCHOLANTHRENE see II:MIJ750
4-METHYLCHOLANTHRENE see III:MIK250
5-METHYLCHOLANTHRENE see III:MIK000
20-METHYLCHOLANTHRENE see II:MIJ750
22-METHYLCHOLANTHRENE see III:MIK250
20-METHYLCHOLANTHRENE CHOLEIC ACID see
III:MIK500

3-METHYLCHOLANTHRENE COMPOUND with PICRIC ACID
(1:1) see III:MIL750
3-METHYLCHOLANTHRENE COMPOUND with 1,3,5-TRINI-
TROBENZENE (1:1) see III:MIM000
(E)-3-METHYLCHOLANTHRENE-11,12-DIHYDRODIOL see
III:DML800
cis-3-METHYLCHOLANTHRENE-1,2-DIOL see III:MIK750
3-METHYLCHOLANTHRENE-11,12-EPOXIDE see
III:ECA500
3-METHYLCHOLANTHRENE-2-ONE see III:MIL250
3-METHYLCHOLANTHRENE-11,12-OXIDE see III:MIL500
20-METHYLCHOLANTHRENE PICRATE see III:MIL750
20-METHYLCHOLANTHRENE-TRINITROBENZENE see
III:MIM000
3-METHYLCHOLANTHREN-1-OL see III:HMA000
3-METHYL-1-CHOLANTHRENOL see III:HMA000
3-METHYLCHOLANTHREN-2-OL see III:HMA500
3-METHYLCHOLANTHREN-1-ONE see III:MIM250
3-METHYLCHOLANTHREN-2-ONE see III:MIL250
20-METHYLCHOLANTHREN-15-ONE see III:MIM250
3-METHYLCHOLANTHRYLENE see III:DAL200
20-METHYLCHOLANTHRYLENE see III:DAL200
1-METHYLCHRYSENE see III:MIM500
2-METHYLCHRYSENE see III:MIM750
3-METHYLCHRYSENE see III:MIN000
4-METHYLCHRYSENE see III:MIN250
5-METHYLCHRYSENE see III:MIN500
6-METHYLCHRYSENE see III:MIO975
METHYL CLOFENAPATE see III:MIO975
METHYLCOBALAMIN see III:VSZ050
METHYL COBALAMINE see III:VSZ050
6-METHYL-m-CRESOL see III:XKS000
γ-METHYL-α,β-CROTONOLACTONE see III:MKH500
9-METHYL-10-CYANO-1,2-BENZANTHRACENE see
III:MIQ250
METHYLCYCLOHEXYLNITROSAMIN (GERMAN) see
III:NKT500
METHYLCYCLOHEXYLNITROSAMINE see III:NKT500
17-METHYL-15H-CYCLOPENTA(a)PHENANTHRENE see
III:MIU750
10-METHYL-1,2-CYCLOPENTENOPHENANTHRENE see
III:MIV250
2-METHYL-DAB see III:TLE750
3'-METHYL-DAB see III:DUH600
3-METHYL-4-DAB see III:MJF000
6-METHYL-6-DEHYDRO-17-α-ACETOXYPROGESTERONE
see II:VTF000
6-METHYL-6-DEHYDRO-17-α-ACETYLPROGESTERONE see
II:VTF000
2-METHYLDIACETYLBENZIDINE see III:MIX000
2-METHYL-N,N'-DIACETYLBENZIDINE see III:MIX000
METHYL DIAZEPINONE see III:DCK759
7-METHYLDIBENZ(c,h)ACRIDINE see III:MIY000
14-METHYLDIBENZ(a,h)ACRIDINE see III:MIY200
14-METHYLDIBENZ(a,j)ACRIDINE see III:MIY250
9-METHYL-3,4,5,6-DIBENZACRIDINE see III:MIY000
10-METHYL-1,2:5,6-DIBENZACRIDINE see III:MIY200
10-METHYL-3,4,5,6-DIBENZACRIDINE see III:MIY250
2-METHYLDIBENZ(a,h)ANTHRACENE see III:MIY500
3-METHYLDIBENZ(a,h)ANTHRACENE see III:MIY750
6-METHYL DIBENZ(a,h)ANTHRACENE see III:MIZ000
10-METHYLDIBENZ(a,c)ANTHRACENE see III:MJA000
4-METHYL-1,2,5,6-DIBENZANTHRACENE see III:MIZ000
2'-METHYL-1:2:5:6-DIBENZANTHRACENE see III:MIY500
3'-METHYL-1:2:5:6-DIBENZANTHRACENE see III:MIY750
N-METHYL-3:4:5:6-DIBENZCARBAZOLE see III:MJA250
N-METHYL-7H-DIBENZO(c,g)CARBAZOLE see III:MJA250
5-METHYL-DIBENZO(b,def)CHRYSENE see III:MJA500
10-METHYLDIBENZO(def,p)CHRYSENE see III:MJB000
12-METHYL DIBENZO(def,mno)CHRYSENE see III:MGP250
14-METHYLDIBENZO(b,def)CHRYSENE-7-CARBOXALDE-
HYDE see III:FNV000
6-METHYLDIBENZO(def,mno)CHRYSENE-12-CARBOXAL-
DEHYDE see III:FNQ000

7-METHYLDIBENZO(h,rst)PENTAPHENE see III:MJA750
5-METHYL-1,2,3,4-DIBENZOPYRENE see III:MJB000
2'-METHYL-1,2:4,5-DIBENZOPYRENE see III:MMD000
3'-METHYL-1,2:4,5-DIBENZOPYRENE see III:MMD250
5-METHYL-3,4:8,9-DIBENZOPYRENE (FRENCH) see
  III:MJA500
7-METHYL-1:2:3:4-DIBENZPYRENE see III:MJB250
5-METHYL-3,4,9,10-DIBENZPYRENE (FRENCH) see
  III:MHE250
4-METHYL-2,6-DI-terc. BUTYLFENOL (CZECH) see
  III:BFW750
METHYL DI-tert-BUTYLPHENOL see III:BFW750
4-METHYL-2,6-DI-tert-BUTYLPHENOL see III:BFW750
N-METHYL-2,2'-DICHLORODIETHYLAMINE see
  I:BIE250
N-METHYL-2,2'-DICHLORODIETHYLAMINE HYDROCHLO-
  RIDE see I:BIE500
N-METHYL-2,2'-DICHLORODIETHYLAMINE-N-OXIDE HY-
  DROCHLORIDE see II:CFA750
METHYLDI(2-CHLOROETHYL)AMINE see I:BIE250
METHYLDI(2-CHLOROETHYL)AMINE HYDROCHLORIDE
  see I:BIE500
METHYLDI(β-CHLOROETHYL)AMINE HYDROCHLORIDE
  see I:BIE500
N-METHYL-DI-2-CHLOROETHYLAMINE HYDROCHLORIDE
  see I:BIE500
N-METHYL-DI-2-CHLOROETHYLAMINE-N-OXIDE see
  III:CFA500
METHYLDI(2-CHLOROETHYL)AMINE-N-OXIDE HYDRO-
  CHLORIDE see II:CFA750
METHYL DIEPOXYDIALLYLACETATE see III:MJD000
trans-3-METHYL-9,10-DIHYDROCHOLANTHRENE-9,10-DIOL
  see III:MJD610
trans-3-METHYL-11,12-DIHYDROCHOLANTHRENE-11,12-
  DIOL see III:DML800
11-METHYL-15,16-DIHYDRO-17H-CYCLOPENTA(a)PHEN-
  ANTHRENE see III:MJD750
11-METHYL-15,16-DIHYDRO-17H-CYCLOPENTA(a)PHEN-
  ANTHREN-17-ONE see II:MJE500
11-METHYL-15,16-DIHYDRO-17-OXOCYCLOPENTA(a)
  PHENANTHRENE see II:MJE500
3'-METHYL-4-DIMETHYLAMINOAZOBENZEN (CZECH) see
  III:DUH600
2-METHYL-4-DIMETHYLAMINOAZOBENZENE see
  III:TLE750
3-METHYL-4-DIMETHYLAMINOAZOBENZENE see
  III:MJF000
2'-METHYL-4-DIMETHYLAMINOAZOBENZENE see
  III:DUH800
3'-METHYL-4-DIMETHYLAMINOAZOBENZENE see
  III:DUH600
4'-METHYL-4-DIMETHYLAMINOAZOBENZENE see
  III:DUH400
M'-METHYL-p-DIMETHYLAMINOAZOBENZENE see
  III:DUH600
o'-METHYL-p-DIMETHYLAMINOAZOBENZENE see
  III:DUH800
p'-METHYL-p-DIMETHYLAMINOAZOBENZENE see
  III:DUH400
2-METHYL-N,N-DIMETHYL-4-AMINOAZOBENZENE see
  III:DUH800, III:TLE750
3'-METHYL-N,N-DIMETHYL-4-AMINOAZOBENZENE see
  III:DUH600
3'-METHYLDIMETHYLAMINOAZOBENZOL (GERMAN) see
  III:DUH600
2-METHYL-5'-(p-DIMETHYLAMINOPHENYLAZO)QUIN-
  OLINE see III:DQE600
3-METHYL-5'-(p-DIMETHYLAMINOPHENYLAZO)QUIN-
  OLINE see III:DQE400
2'-METHYL-5'-(p-DIMETHYLAMINOPHENYLAZO)QUIN-
  OLINE see III:DPQ600
3'-METHYL-5'-(p-DIMETHYLAMINOPHENYLAZO)QUIN-
  OLINE see III:MJF500

6'-METHYL-5'-(p-DIMETHYLAMINOPHENYLAZO)QUIN-
  OLINE see III:MJF750
7'-METHYL-5'-(p-DIMETHYLAMINOPHENYLAZO)QUIN-
  OLINE see III:DPQ400
8'-METHYL-5'-(p-DIMETHYLAMINOPHENYLAZO)QUIN-
  OLINE see III:MJG000
2'-METHYL-4-DIMETHYLAMINOSTILBENE see III:TMF750
3'-METHYL-4-DIMETHYLAMINOSTILBENE see III:TMG000
4'-METHYL-4-DIMETHYLAMINOSTILBENE see III:TMG250
METHYL-4-DIMETHYLAMINO-3,5-XYLYL CARBAMATE
  see III:DOS000
METHYL-4-DIMETHYLAMINO-3,5-XYLYL ESTER of CAR-
  BAMIC ACID see III:DOS000
METHYL-1,1-DIMETHYLBUTANON(3)-NITROSAMIN (GER-
  MAN) see III:MMX750
METHYLDINITROBENZENE see I:DVG600
1-METHYL-2,4-DINITROBENZENE see II:DVH000
2-METHYL-1,3-DINITROBENZENE see III:DVH400
N-METHYL-N,4-DINITROSOANILINE see III:MJG750
N-METHYL-N,p-DINITROSOANILINE see III:MJG750
N-METHYL-N,4-DINITROSOBENZENAMINE see
  III:MJG750
2-METHYLDINITROSOPIPERAZINE see III:MJH000
6-METHYL DIPYRIDO(1,2-a:3',2'-d)IMIDAZOL-2-AMINE see
  II:AKS250
2-METHYL-DNPZ see III:MJH000
METHYL-E 605 see III:MNH000
3,4-METHYLENDIOXY-6-PROPYLBENZYL-n-BUTYL-DI-
  AETHYLENGLYKOLAETHER (GERMAN) see
  III:PIX250
METHYLENE BICHLORIDE see II:MJP450
METHYLENEBIS(2-AMINO-BENZOIC ACID) DIMETHYL ES-
  TER (9CI) see III:MJQ250
METHYLENEBIS(ANILINE) see I:MJQ000
4,4'-METHYLENEBISANILINE see I:MJQ000
4,4'-METHYLENEBIS(2-CARBOMETHOXYANILINE) see
  III:MJQ250
4,4'-METHYLENE(BIS)-CHLOROANILINE see I:MJM200
4,4'-METHYLENE BIS(2-CHLOROANILINE) see I:MJM200
METHYLENE-4,4'-BIS(o-CHLOROANILINE) see I:MJM200
4,4'-METHYLENEBIS(o-CHLOROANILINE) see I:MJM200
p,p'-METHYLENEBIS(o-CHLOROANILINE) see I:MJM200
p,p'-METHYLENEBIS(α-CHLOROANILINE) see I:MJM200
4,4'-METHYLENE-BIS(2-CHLOROANILINE) HYDROCHLO-
  RIDE see III:MJM250
4,4'-METHYLENEBIS-2-CHLOROBENZENAMINE see
  I:MJM200
4,4'-METHYLENE BIS(N,N'-DIMETHYLANILINE) see
  I:MJN000
4,4'-METHYLENEBIS(N,N-DIMETHYL)BENZENAMINE see
  I:MJN000
N,N-METHYLENE-BIS(ETHYL CARBAMATE) see
  III:MJT750
4,4'-METHYLENEBIS(3-HYDROXY-2-NAPHTHOIC ACID)
  with TRIS-(p-AMINOPHENYL)CARBONIUM SALT (1:2) see
  III:TNC725, III:TNC750
4,4'-METHYLENEBIS(3-HYDROXY-2-NAPHTHOIC ACID)
  with TRIS-(p-AMINOPHENYL)METHYLIUM SALT (1:2) see
  III:TNC725, III:TNC750
METHYLENEBIS(4-ISOCYANATOBENZENE) see III:MJP400
1,1-METHYLENEBIS(4-ISOCYANATOBENZENE) see
  III:MJP400
4,4'-METHYLENEBIS(2-METHYLANILINE) see I:MJO250
4,4'-METHYLENEBIS(N-METHYLANILINE) see
  III:MJO000
METHYLENE-BIS(METHYL ANTHRANILATE) see
  III:MJQ250
4,4'-METHYLENEBIS(2-METHYLBENZENAMINE) see
  I:MJO250
METHYLENE-BIS-ORTHOCHLOROANILINE see I:MJM200
2,2'-METHYLENEBIS OXIRANE (9CI) see III:DHE000
METHYLENEBIS(4-PHENYLENE ISOCYANATE) see
  III:MJP400

METHYLENEBIS(p-PHENYLENE ISOCYANATE) see III:MJP400

METHYLENE BISPHENYL ISOCYANATE see III:MJP400

METHYLENEBIS(4-PHENYL ISOCYANATE) see III:MJP400

METHYLENEBIS(p-PHENYL ISOCYANATE) see III:MJP400

4,4'-METHYLENEBIS(PHENYL ISOCYANATE) see III:MJP400

p,p'-METHYLENEBIS(PHENYL ISOCYANATE) see III:MJP400

2,2'-METHYLENEBIS(3,4,6-TRICHLOROPHENOL) see III:HCL000

METHYLENE CHLORIDE see II:MJP450

1,2-α-METHYLENE-6-CHLORO-Δ⁶-17-α-HYDROXYPRO-GESTERONE ACETATE see III:CQJ500

1,2 α-METHYLENE-6-CHLORO-PREGNA-4,6-DIENE-3,20-DIONE 17-α-ACETATE see III:CQJ500

1,2-α-METHYLENE-6-CHLORO-Δ⁻⁴,⁶-PREGNADIENE-17-α-OL-3,20-DIONE 17-α-ACETATE see III:CQJ500

1,2-α-METHYLENE-6-CHLORO-Δ⁻⁴,⁶-PREGNADIENE-17-α-OL-3,20-DIONE ACETATE see III:CQJ500

4,5-METHYLENECHRYSENE see III:CPU000

METHYLENEDIANILINE see I:MJQ000

4,4'-METHYLENEDIANILINE see I:MJQ000

p,p'-METHYLENEDIANILINE see I:MJQ000

4,4'-METHYLENEDIANILINE DIHYDROCHLORIDE see I:MJQ100

METHYLENEDIANTHRANILIC ACID DIMETHYL ESTER see III:MJQ250

1',9-METHYLENE-1,2:5,6-DIBENZANTHRACENE see III:DCR600

METHYLENE DICHLORIDE see II:MJP450

4,4'-METHYLENEDIMORPHOLINE see III:MJQ750

1,5-METHYLENE-3,7-DINITROSO-1,3,5,7-TETRAAZACY-CLOOCTAINE see III:DVF400

1,5-METHYLENE-3,7-DINITROSO-1,3,5,7-TETRAAZACY-CLOOCTANE see III:DVF400

3,4-METHYLENEDIOXY-ALLYBENZENE see I:SAD000

1,2-METHYLENEDIOXY-4-ALLYLBENZENE see I:SAD000

1,2-(METHYLENEDIOXY)-4-(3-BROMO-1-PROPENYL)BEN-ZENE see III:BOA750

1,2-METHYLENEDIOXY-4-(1-HYDROXYALLYL)BENZENE see II:BCJ000

1,2-(METHYLENEDIOXY)-4-(2-(OCTYLSULFINYL)PROPYL)BENZENE see III:ISA000

1,2-METHYLENEDIOXY-4-PROPENYLBENZENE see III:IRZ000

3,4-METHYLENEDIOXY-1-PROPENYL BENZENE see III:IRZ000

1,2-(METHYLENEDIOXY)-4-PROPYLBENZENE see II:DMD600

(3,4-METHYLENEDIOXY-6-PROPYLBENZYL) (BUTYL) DI-ETHYLENE GLICOL ETHER see III:PIX250

3,4-METHYLENEDIOXY-6-PROPYLBENZYL n-BUTYL DI-ETHYLENEGLYCOL ETHER see III:PIX250

4,4'-METHYLENEDIPHENYL DIISOCYANATE see III:MJP400

METHYLENEDI-p-PHENYLENE DIISOCYANATE see III:MJP400

METHYLENEDI-p-PHENYLENE ISOCYANATE see III:MJP400

4,4'-METHYLENEDIPHENYLENE ISOCYANATE see III:MJP400

METHYLENE DI(PHENYLENE ISOCYANATE) (DOT) see III:MJP400

4,4'-METHYLENEDIPHENYL ISOCYANATE see III:MJP400

4,4'-METHYLENE DI-o-TOLUIDINE see I:MJO250

METHYLENE DIURETHAN see III:MJT750

METHYLENE ETHER of OXYHYDROQUINONE see III:MJU000

METHYLENE GLYCOL see I:FMV000

METHYLENE OXIDE see I:FMV000

2-METHYLENE-3-OXO-CYCLOPENTANECARBOXYLIC ACID see III:SAX500

2-METHYLENE-3-OXOCYCLOPENTANECARBOXYLIC ACID, SODIUM SALT see III:SJS500

3-METHYL-11,12-EPOXYCHOLANTHRENE see III:ECA500

6-METHYL-3,4-EPOXYCYCLOHEXYLMETHYL-6-METHYL-3,4-EPOXYCYCLOHEXANE CARBOXYLATE see III:ECB000

METHYLESTER KYSELINY p-TOLUENSULFONOVE (CZECH) see III:MLL250

METHYL ESTER of METHANESULFONIC ACID see III:MLH500

METHYL ESTER of METHANESULPHONIC ACID see III:MLH500

METHYL ESTER STEARIC ACID see III:MJW000

METHYLE (SULFATE de) (FRENCH) see I:DUD100

1,1'-(METHYLETHANEDILIDENEDINITRILO)BIGUANIDINE DIHYDROCHLORIDE DIHYDRATE see III:MKI000

4,4'-(1-METHYL-1,2-ETHANEDIYL)BIS-2,6-PIPERAZINE-DIONE see II:PIK250

METHYLETHENE see III:PMO500

8-METHYL ETHER of XANTHURENIC ACID see III:HLT500

11-β-METHYL-17-α-ETHINYLESTRADIOL see III:MJW875

9-METHYL-10-ETHOXYMETHYL-1,2-BENZANTHRACENE see III:EEX000, III:MJX000

4-(METHYLETHYL)AMINOAZOBENZENE see III:ENB000

N-METHYL-N-ETHYL-p-AMINOAZOBENZENE see III:ENB000

N-METHYL-4'-ETHYL-p-AMINOAZOBENZENE see III:EOJ000

4-(((1-METHYLETHYL)AMINO)CARBONYL)-BENZOIC ACID (9CI) see III:IRN000

α-(((1-METHYLETHYL)AMINO)METHYL)-2-NAPHTHA-LENEMETHANOL, HYDROCHLORIDE see III:INT000

7-METHYL-9-ETHYLBENZ(c)ACRIDINE see III:MJY250

3-METHYL-10-ETHYLBENZ(c)ACRIDINE see III:EMM000

10-METHYL-3-ETHYL-7,8-BENZACRIDINE (FRENCH) see III:MJY250

3-METHYL-10-ETHYL-7,8-BENZACRIDINE (FRENCH) see III:EMM000

METHYLETHYLBROMOMETHANE see III:BMX750

METHYLETHYLENE see III:PMO500

METHYL ETHYLENE OXIDE see I:PNL600

METHYLETHYLENIMINE see I:PNL400

2-METHYLETHYLENIMINE see I:PNL400

2,2'-((1-METHYLETHYLIDENE)BIS(4,1-PHENYLENEOXYMETHYLENE))BISOXIRANE see III:BLD750

METHYL ETHYL KETONE PEROXIDE see III:MKA500

METHYLETHYLKETONHYDROPEROXIDE see III:MKA500

N-(1-METHYLETHYL)-4-((2-METHYLHYDRAZINO)METHYL)BENZAMIDE MONOHYDROCHLORIDE see I:PME500

METHYLETHYLNITROSAMINE see I:MKB000

N,N-METHYLETHYLNITROSAMINE see I:MKB000

N-(1-METHYLETHYL)-N-NITROSO-UREA (9CI) see III:NKO425

2-METHYL-3-ETHYL-4-PHENYL-4-CYCLOHEXENE CAR-BOXYLIC ACID see III:FAO200

2-METHYL-3-ETHYL-4-PHENYL-Δ⁴-CYCLOHEXENECAR-BOXYLIC ACID see III:FAO200

N-METHYL-N-ETHYL-4-(4'-(PYRIDYL-1'OXIDE)AZO)ANILINE see III:MKB500

1-(METHYLETHYL)UREA and SODIUM NITRITE see III:SIS675

3-METHYLETHYNYLESTRADIOL see I:MKB750

18-METHYL-17-α-ETHYNYL-19-NORTESTOSTERONE see III:NNQ500, III:NNQ520

3-METHYLETHYNYLOESTRADIOL see I:MKB750

2-METHYLFLUORANTHENE see III:MKC500

3-METHYLFLUORANTHENE see III:MKC750

7-METHYL-9-FLUOROBENZ(c)ACRIDINE see III:MKD250

7-METHYL-11-FLUOROBENZ(c)ACRIDINE see III:MKD500

10-METHYL-3-FLUORO-5,6-BENZACRIDINE see III:MKD750

7-METHYL-2-FLUOROBENZ(a)ANTHRACENE see III:FJN000

METHYLFLURETHER see III:EAT900
N-METHYL-N-FORMLYHYDRAZINE see II:FNW000
N-METHYL-N-FORMYL HYDRAZONE of ACETALDEHYDE see III:AAH000
METHYL FOSFERNO see III:MNH000
5-METHYL-2(5H)-FURANONE see III:MKH500
METHYL GAG see III:MKI000
METHYLGUANIDINE mixed with SODIUM NITRITE (1:1) see III:MKJ000
METHYL GUTHION see III:ASH500
METHYLHARNSTOFF and NATRIUMNITRIT (GERMAN) see III:MQJ250
(6-(1-METHYL-HEPTYL)-2,4-DINITRO-FENYL)-CROTO-NAAT (DUTCH) see III:AQT500
(6-(1-METHYL-HEPTYL)-2,3-DINITRO-PHENYL)-CROTO-NAT (GERMAN) see III:AQT500
2-(1-METHYLHEPTYL)-4,6-DINITROPHENYL CROTONATE see III:AQT500
METHYLHEPTYLNITROSAMIN (GERMAN) see III:HBP000
3-β-14-METHYLHEXADECANOATE-CHOLEST-5-EN-3-OL see III:CCJ500
METHYL HYDRAZINE see II:MKN000
1-METHYL HYDRAZINE see II:MKN000
METHYLHYDRAZINE (DOT) see II:MKN000
METHYL HYDRAZINE SULFATE see III:MKN500
4-((2-METHYLHYDRAZINO)METHYL)-N-ISOPROPYLBENZ-AMIDE see I:PME250
(α-(2-METHYLHYDRAZINO)-p-TOLUOYL)UREA, MONOHY-DROBROMIDE see III:MKN750
N-METHYL-N-(HYDROPEROXYMETHYL)NITROSAMINE see III:HIE700
4-(N-METHYLHYDROXYAMINO)-QUINOLINE-1-OXIDE see III:HLX550
17-α-METHYL-17-β-HYDROXY-1,4-ANDROSTADIEN-3-ONE see III:DAL300
METHYL-3-HYDROXYANTHRANILATE see III:HJC500
1-METHYL-4-HYDROXYBENZENE see III:CNX250
N-METHYL-N-(4-HYDROXYBUTYL)NITROSAMINE see III:MKP000
2-METHYL-1-(2-HYDROXYETHYL)-5-NITROIMIDAZOLE see I:MMN250
2-METHYL-3-(2-HYDROXYETHYL)-4-NITROIMIDAZOLE see I:MMN250
METHYL-2-HYDROXYETHYLNITROSAMINE see III:NKU350
METHYL-2-HYDROXYETHYLNITROSOAMINE see III:NKU350
2-METHYL-4-HYDROXYLAMINOQUINOLINE 1-OXIDE see III:MKR000
5-METHYL-4-HYDROXYLAMINOQUINOLINE-1-OXIDE see III:HIV000
6-METHYL-4-HYDROXYLAMINOQUINOLINE-1-OXIDE see III:HIV500
7-METHYL-4-HYDROXYLAMINOQUINOLINE-1-OXIDE see III:HIW000
8-METHYL-4-HYDROXYLAMINOQUINOLINE-1-OXIDE see III:HIW500
7-METHYL-12-HYDROXYMETHYLBENZ(a)ANTHRACENE see III:HMF500
17-α-METHYL-2-HYDROXYMETHYLENE-17-HYDROXY-5-α-ANDROSTAN-3-ONE see I:PAN100
METHYL HYDROXYOCTADECADIENOATE see III:MKR500
6-α-METHYL-17-α-HYDROXYPROGESTERONE ACETATE see II:MCA000
6-METHYL-17-α-HYDROXY-Δ⁶-PROGESTERONE ACETATE see II:VTF000
METHYL-12-HYDROXYSTEARATE see III:HOG500
4,4′,4″-METHYLIDYNETRIANILINE see III:THP000
4,4′,4″-METHYLIDYNETRISBENZENEAMINE see III:THP000
1-METHYLIMIDAZOLE-2-THIOL see III:MCO500
METHYL IODIDE see I:MKW200

METHYLISOMYN see III:MDT600
1-METHYL-2-p-(ISOPROPYLCARBAMOYL)BENZOHY-DRAZINE HYDROCHLORIDE see I:PME500
1-METHYL-2-(-ISOPROPYLCARBAMOYL)BENZYL)HY-DRAZINE see I:PME250
1-METHYL-2-(p-ISOPROPYLCARBAMOYLBENZYL)HY-DRAZINE HYDROCHLORIDE see I:PME500
5-METHYL-2-ISOPROPYL-3-PYRAZOLYL DIMETHYLCAR-BAMATE see III:DSK200
N′-(5-METHYL-3-ISOXAZOLE)SULFANILAMIDE see III:SNK000
N′-(5-METHYL-3-ISOXAZOLYL)SULFANILAMIDE see III:SNK000
N′-(5-METHYLISOXAZOL-3-YL)SULPHANILAMIDE see III:SNK000
N¹-(5-METHYL-3-ISOXAZOLYL)SULPHANILAMIDE see III:SNK000
METHYLIUM, TRIS(4-AMINOPHENYL)-, 4,4′-METHYLENEBIS(3-HYDROXY-NAPHTHOATE) (2:1) see III:TNC725
METHYLJODID (GERMAN) see I:MKW200
METHYLJODIDE (DUTCH) see I:MKW200
METHYL LEDATE see III:LCW000
METHYL-LOMUSTINE see II:CHD250
N-METHYL-LOST see I:BIE250
1-METHYL-2-MERCAPTOIMIDAZOLE see III:MCO500
4-METHYLMERCAPTO-3-METHYLPHENYL DIMETHYL THIOPHOSPHATE see III:FAQ999
6-METHYLMERCAPTOPURINE RIBONUCLEOSIDE see III:MPU000
6-METHYLMERCAPTOPURINE RIBOSIDE see III:MPU000
METHYLMERCURIC CHLORIDE see III:MDD750
METHYLMERCURY CHLORIDE see III:MDD750
METHYL MESYLATE see III:MLH500
METHYLMETHACRYLAAT (DUTCH) see III:MLH750
METHYL-METHACRYLAT (GERMAN) see III:MLH750
METHYL METHACRYLATE see III:MLH750
METHYL METHACRYLATE HOMOPOLYMER see III:PKB500
METHYL METHACRYLATE MONOMER, INHIBITED (DOT) see III:MLH750
METHYL METHACRYLATE POLYMER see III:PKB500
METHYL METHACRYLATE RESIN see III:PKB500
N-METHYLMETHANAMINE HYDROCHLORIDE see III:DOR600
METHYL METHANESULFONATE see III:MLH500
METHYL METHANESULPHONATE see III:MLH500
METHYLMETHANSULFONAT (GERMAN) see III:MLH500
METHYL METHANSULFONATE see III:MLH500
METHYL METHANSULPHONATE see III:MLH500
2-METHYL-4-METHOXYANILINE see II:MGO500
9-METHYL-10-METHOXYMETHYL-1,2-BENZANTHRACENE see III:MEW000
METHYL(METHOXYMETHYL)NITROSAMINE see III:MEW250
N-METHYL-N′-(p-METHOXYPHENYL)-N-NITROSOUREA see III:MFG400
METHYL-α-METHYLACRYLATE see III:MLH750
N-METHYL-3-METHYL-p-AMINOAZOBENZENE see III:MLY250
N-METHYL-2′-METHYL-4-AMINOAZOBENZENE see III:MPY250
N-METHYL-2′-METHYL-p-AMINOAZOBENZENE see III:MPY250
N-METHYL-3′-METHYL-4-AMINOAZOBENZENE see III:MPY000
N-METHYL-3′-METHYL-p-AMINOAZOBENZENE see III:MPY000
N-METHYL-4′-METHYL-4-AMINOAZOBENZENE see III:MPY500
N-METHYL-4′-METHYL-p-AMINOAZOBENZENE see III:MPY500

METHYLSULFINYLMETHANE see III:DUD800
METHYLSULFONAL see III:BJT750
METHYLSULFONIC ACID, ETHYL ESTER see II:EMF500
METHYL SULFOXIDE see III:DUD800
5-METHYL-3-SULPHANIL-AMIDOISOXAZOLE see
  III:SNK000
METHYLSULPHONAL see III:BJT750
17-METHYLTESTOSTERON see III:MPN500
METHYLTESTOSTERONE see III:MPN500
17-METHYLTESTOSTERONE see III:MPN500
17-α-METHYLTESTOSTERONE see III:MPN500
Δ'-17-METHYLTESTOSTERONE see III:DAL300
Δ(^{1})-17-α-METHYLTESTOSTERONE see III:DAL300
10-METHYL-1,2-TETRAHYDRO-1,2:5,6-BENZACRIDINE see
  III:MPO400
10-METHYL-1,2-TETRAHYDRO-1,2:7,8-BENZACRIDINE see
  III:MPO390
6-METHYL-1,2,3,4-TETRAHYDROBENZ(a)ANTHRACENE
  see III:MPO250
4-METHYL-1',2',3',4'-TETRAHYDRO-1,2-BENZANTHRA-
  CENE see III:MPO250
7-METHYL-1,2,3,4-TETRAHYDRODIBENZ(c,h)ACRIDINE
  see III:MPO390
14-METHYL-8,9,10,11-TETRAHYDRODIBENZ(a,h)ACRIDINE
  see III:MPO400
METHYL-1,2,5,6-TETRAHYDRO-1-METHYLNICOTINATE
  see III:AQT750
2-METHYL-2-(4-(1,2,3,4-TETRAHYDRO-1-NAPHTHA-
  LENYL)PHENOXY)PROPANOIC ACID see II:MCB500
2-METHYL-2-(4-(1,2,3,4-TETRAHYDRO-1-NAPHTHYL)
  PHENOXY)PROPANOIC ACID see II:MCB500
2-METHYL-2-(p-(1,2,3,4-TETRAHYDRO-1-NAPHTHYL)
  PHENOXY)PROPIONIC ACID see II:MCB500
α-METHYL-α-(p-1,2,3,4-TETRAHYDRONAPHTH-1-
  YLPHENOXY)PROPIONIC ACID see II:MCB500
N-METHYL-Δ-TETRAHYDRONICOTINIC ACID METHYL ES-
  TER see III:AQT750
N-METHYLTETRAHYDROPYRIDINE-β-CARBOXYLIC ACID
  METHYL ESTER see III:AQT750
α-METHYL TETRONIC ACID see III:MPQ500
METHYLTHEOBROMIDE see III:CAK500
1-METHYLTHEOBROMINE see III:CAK500
7-METHYLTHEOPHYLLINE see III:CAK500
N^1-(5-METHYL-1,3,4-THIADIAZOL-2-YL)-SULFANILAMIDE
  see III:MPQ750
METHYLTHIOINOSINE see III:MPU000
6-METHYLTHIOINOSINE see III:MPU000
METHYLTHIOPHOS see III:MNH000
6-(METHYLTHIO)PURINE RIBONUCLEOSIDE see
  III:MPU000
6-METHYLTHIOPURINE RIBOSIDE see III:MPU000
6-METHYL-2-THIO-2,4-(1H3H)PYRIMIDINEDIONE see
  II:MPW500
METHYLTHIOURACIL see II:MPW500
6-METHYLTHIOURACIL see II:MPW500
4-METHYL-2-THIOURACIL see II:MPW500
6-METHYL-2-THIOURACIL see II:MPW500
METHYL THIRAM see III:TFS350
METHYL THIURAMDISULFIDE see III:TFS350
METHYL TOLUENE-4-SULFONATE see III:MLL250
METHYL-p-TOLUENESULFONATE see III:MLL250
2-METHYL-p-TOLUIDINE see II:XMS000
4-METHYL-o-TOLUIDINE see II:XMS000
5-METHYL-o-TOLUIDINE see III:XNA000
6-METHYL-m-TOLUIDINE see III:XNA000
2-METHYL-p-TOLUIDINE HYDROCHLORIDE see
  III:XOJ000
4-METHYL-o-TOLUIDINE HYDROCHLORIDE see
  III:XOJ000
5-METHYL-o-TOLUIDINE HYDROCHLORIDE see
  III:XOS000
6-METHYL-m-TOLUIDINE HYDROCHLORIDE see
  III:XOS000
N-METHYL-p-(m-TOLYLAZO)ANILINE see III:MPY000

N-METHYL-p-(o-TOLYLAZO)ANILINE see III:MPY250
N-METHYL-p-(p-TOLYLAZO)ANILINE see III:MPY500
2'-METHYL-4'-(o-TOLYLAZO)OXANILIC ACID see
  III:OLG000
METHYL TOSYLATE see III:MLL250
METHYL-p-TOSYLATE see III:MLL250
5-(3-METHYL-1-TRIAZENO)IMIDAZOLE-4-CARBOXAMIDE
  see III:MQB750
2'-METHYL-1,2:4,5:8,9-TRIBENZOPYRENE see III:MJA750
METHYL TRICHLORIDE see I:CHJ500
METHYLTRICHLOROMETHANE see III:MIH275
1-METHYLTRICYCLOQUINAZOLINE see III:MQD000
3-METHYLTRICYCLOQUINAZOLINE see III:MQD250
4-METHYLTRICYCLOQUINAZOLINE see III:MQD500
1-5-METHYLTRYPTOPHAN see III:MQI250
METHYL TUADS see III:TFS350
4-METHYLURACIL see II:MPW500, III:MQI750
6-METHYLURACIL see III:MQI750
METHYL UREA and SODIUM NITRITE see III:MQJ250
METHYLURETHAN see III:MHZ000
N-METHYL URETHAN see III:EMQ500
METHYLURETHANE see III:MHZ000
METHYL VINYL CARBINOL see III:MQL250
METHYLVINYLNITROSAMIN (GERMAN) see II:NKY000
METHYLVINYLNITROSAMINE see II:NKY000
METHYL YELLOW see I:DOT300
METHYL ZIMATE see III:BJK500
METHYL ZINEB see III:BJK500
METHYL ZIRAM see III:BJK500
METIFONATE see III:TIQ250
METILACRILATO (ITALIAN) see III:MGA500
3-METIL-BUTANOLO (ITALIAN) see III:IHP000
4,4-METILENE-BIS-o-CLOROANILINA (ITALIAN) see
  I:MJM200
(6-(1-METIL-EPITL)-2,4-DINITRO-FENIL)-CROTONATO
  (ITALIAN) see III:AQT500
METILESTER del ACIDO BISDEHIDROISYNOLICO (SPAN-
  ISH) see III:BIT000
7-METILETER del ACIDO BISDEHIDRODOISYNOLICO see
  III:BIT030
METIL METACRILATO (ITALIAN) see III:MLH750
N-METIL-1-NAFTIL-CARBAMMATO (ITALIAN) see
  III:CBM750
METILPARATION (HUNGARIAN) see III:MNH000
6-(1-METIL-PROPIL)-2,4-DINITRO-FENOLO (ITALIAN) see
  III:BRE500
6-METIL-TIOURACILE (ITALIAN) see II:MPW500
METILTRIAZOTION see III:ASH500
METIPREGNONE see II:MCA000
METIZOL see III:MCO500
2-METOKSY-4-ALLILOFENOL (POLISH) see III:EQR500
METOKSYCHLOR (POLISH) see II:MEI450
METOTHYRINE see III:MCO500
METOX see II:MEI450
METOXAL see III:SNK000
METOXON see III:CKC000
4-o-METPA see III:MQR250
METRIFONATE see III:TIQ250
METRIPHONATE see III:TIQ250
METRODIOL see II:EQJ500
METRODIOL DIACETATE see II:EQJ500
METROGEN RED FORMER KB SOLN see II:CLK225
METRON see III:MNH000
METRONE see III:MPN500
METRONIDAZ see I:MMN250
METRONIDAZOL see I:MMN250
METRONIDAZOLO see I:MMN250
METRO TALC 4604 see III:TAB750
METRO TALC 4608 see III:TAB750
METRO TALC 4609 see III:TAB750
METYLENU CHLOREK (POLISH) see II:MJP450
METYLOHYDRAZYNA (POLISH) see II:MKN000
niesymetryczna DWU METYLOHYDRAZYNA (POLISH) see
  I:DSF400

1-METYLO-2-MERKAPTOIMIDAZOLEM (POLISH) see
  III:MCO500
N-METYLO-N′-NITRO-N-NITROZOGOUANIDYNY (POLISH)
  see II:MMP000
METYLOPARATION (POLISH) see III:MNH000
METYLPARATION (CZECH) see III:MNH000
METYLU BROMEK (POLISH) see III:MHR200
METYLU CHLOREK (POLISH) see II:MIF765
METYLU JODEK (POLISH) see I:MKW200
MEXACARBATE (DOT) see III:DOS000
MEXENE see III:BJK500
MEXIDE see III:RNZ000
MEZENE see III:BJK500
MEZEREIN see III:MDJ250
MEZIDINE see III:TLG500
MEZOTOX see I:DFT800
MFH see II:FNW000
MH-30 see III:DHF200
MHP see III:NKU500
MIA see III:IDZ000
MIBOLERON see III:MQS225
MIBOLERONE see III:MQS225
MICHLER'S BASE see I:MJN000
MICHLER'S HYDRIDE see I:MJN000
MICHLER'S KETONE see I:MQS500
p,p′-MICHLER'S KETONE see I:MQS500
MICHLER'S METHANE see I:MJN000
MICIDE see III:EIR000
MICOCHLORINE see II:CDP250
MICREST see I:DKA600
MICROCETINA see II:CDP250
MICRO-CHECK 12 see III:CBG000
MICRO DDT 75 see I:DAD200
MICRODIOL see I:EDO000
MICROEST see I:DKA600
MICROGRIT WCA see III:AHE250
MICROGYNON see III:NNL500
MICROLYSIN see III:CKN500
MICROSETILE BLUE EB see III:TBG700
MICROSETILE ORANGE RA see I:AKP750
MICROSETILE YELLOW GR see II:AAQ250
MICROTEX LAKE RED CR see III:CHP500
MICROTHENE see III:PJS750
MIELUCIN see I:BOT250
MIEOBROMOL see III:DDP600
MIGHTY 150 see III:NAJ500
MIH see I:PME250
MIH HYDROCHLORIDE see I:PME500
MIKETHRENE GOLD YELLOW see III:DCZ000
MIKETON FAST BLUE see III:TBG700
MILBAM see III:BJK500
MILBAN see III:BJK500
MILBOL see III:BIO750
MILBOL 49 see I:BBQ500
MIL-DU-RID see II:BGJ750
MILESTROL see I:DKA600
MILK SUGAR see III:LAR000
MILLER NU SET see II:TIX500
MILMER see III:BLC250
MILOGARD see III:PMN850
MILPREM see I:ECU750
MILPREX see III:DXX400
MILTOX see III:EIR000
MILTOX SPECIAL see III:EIR000
MIMOSA TANNIN see III:MQV250
MINERAL NAPHTHA see I:BBL250
MINERAL OIL see III:MQV750
MINERAL OIL, PETROLEUM CONDENSATES, VACUUM
  TOWER see I:MQV755
MINERAL OIL, PETROLEUM DISTILLATES, ACID-TREATED
  HEAVY NAPHTHENIC see I:MQV760
MINERAL OIL, PETROLEUM DISTILLATES, ACID-TREATED
  HEAVY PARAFFINIC see I:MQV765
MINERAL OIL, PETROLEUM DISTILLATES, ACID-TREATED
  LIGHT NAPHTHENIC see I:MQV770

MINERAL OIL, PETROLEUM DISTILLATES, ACID-TREATED
  LIGHT PARAFFINIC see I:MQV775
MINERAL OIL, PETROLEUM DISTILLATES, HEAVY
  NAPHTHENIC see I:MQV780
MINERAL OIL, PETROLEUM DISTILLATES, HEAVY PARAF-
  FINIC see I:MQV785
MINERAL OIL, PETROLEUM DISTILLATES, HYDRO-
  TREATED HEAVY NAPHTHENIC see I:MQV790
MINERAL OIL, PETROLEUM DISTILLATES, HYDRO-
  TREATED HEAVY PARAFFINIC see I:MQV795
MINERAL OIL, PETROLEUM DISTILLATES, HYDRO-
  TREATED LIGHT NAPHTHENIC see I:MQV800
MINERAL OIL, PETROLEUM DISTILLATES, HYDRO-
  TREATED LIGHT PARAFFINIC see I:MQV805
MINERAL OIL, PETROLEUM DISTILLATES, LIGHT
  NAPHTHENIC see I.MQV810
MINERAL OIL, PETROLEUM DISTILLATES, LIGHT PARAF-
  FINIC see I:MQV815
MINERAL OIL, PETROLEUM DISTILLATES, SOLVENT-DE-
  WAXED HEAVY NAPHTHENIC see III:MQV820
MINERAL OIL, PETROLEUM DISTILLATES, SOLVENT-DE-
  WAXED HEAVY PARAFFINIC see III:MQV825
MINERAL OIL, PETROLEUM DISTILLATES, SOLVENT-DE-
  WAXED LIGHT NAPHTHENIC see I:MQV835
MINERAL OIL, PETROLEUM DISTILLATES, SOLVENT-DE-
  WAXED LIGHT PARAFFINIC see I:MQV840
MINERAL OIL, PETROLEUM DISTILLATES, SOLVENT-RE-
  FINED HEAVY NAPHTHENIC see III:MQV845
MINERAL OIL, PETROLEUM DISTILLATES, SOLVENT-RE-
  FINED HEAVY PARAFFINIC see III:MQV850
MINERAL OIL, PETROLEUM DISTILLATES, SOLVENT-RE-
  FINED LIGHT NAPHTHENIC see I:MQV852
MINERAL OIL, PETROLEUM DISTILLATES, SOLVENT-RE-
  FINED LIGHT PARAFFINIC see I:MQV855
MINERAL OIL, PETROLEUM EXTRACTS, HEAVY
  NAPHTHENIC DISTILLATE SOLVENT see I:MQV857
MINERAL OIL, PETROLEUM EXTRACTS, HEAVY PARAF-
  FINIC DISTILLATE SOLVENT see I:MQV859
MINERAL OIL, PETROLEUM EXTRACTS, LIGHT
  NAPHTHENIC DISTILLATE SOLVENT see I:MQV860
MINERAL OIL, PETROLEUM EXTRACTS, LIGHT PARAF-
  FINIC DISTILLATE SOLVENT see I:MQV862
MINERAL OIL, PETROLEUM EXTRACTS, RESIDUAL OIL
  SOLVENT see I:MQV863
MINERAL OIL, PETROLEUM NAPHTHENIC OILS, CATA-
  LYTIC DEWAXED HEAVY see I:MQV865
MINERAL OIL, PETROLEUM NAPHTHENIC OILS, CATA-
  LYTIC DEWAXED LIGHT see I:MQV867
MINERAL OIL, PETROLEUM PARAFFIN OILS, CATALYTIC
  DEWAXED HEAVY see I:MQV868
MINERAL OIL, PETROLEUM PARAFFIN OILS, CATALYTIC
  DEWAXED LIGHT see I:MQV870
MINERAL OIL, PETROLEUM RESIDUAL OILS, ACID-
  TREATED see I:MQV872
MINERAL OIL, SLAB OIL see I:MQV875
MINERAL OIL, WHITE (FCC) see III:MQV750
MINERAL PITCH see II:ARO500
MINERAL WHITE see III:CAX750
MINETOIN see I:DKQ000, I:DNU000
MINIDRIL see III:NNL500
MINIHIST see III:DBM800
MINILYN see III:EEH575
MINORAN see III:MEK700
MINORLAR see II:EEH520
MINOVLAR see II:EEH520
MIRACLE see II:DAA800
MIRAMID WM 55 see III:PJY500
MIREX see I:MQW500
MIRLON see III:NOH000
MIRREX MCFD 1025 see III:PKQ059
MISCLERON see III:ARQ750
MISHERI (INDIA) see I:SED400
MISHRI (INDIA) see I:SED400
MISTRON 2SC see III:TAB750

MISTRON FROST P see III:TAB750
MISTRON RCS see III:TAB750
MISTRON STAR see III:TAB750
MISTRON SUPER FROST see III:TAB750
MISTRON VAPOR see III:TAB750
MISULBAN see I:BOT250
MIT-C see II:AHK500
MITENON see III:MMD500
MITICIDE K-101 see III:CJT750
MITIGAN see III:BIO750
MITOBRONITOL see III:DDP600
MITO-C see II:AHK500
MITOCIN-C see II:AHK500
MITOLAC see III:DDJ000
MITOLACTOL see III:DDJ000
MITOMEN see II:CFA750
MITOMYCIN see II:AHK500
MITOMYCIN-C see II:AHK500
MITOMYCINUM see II:AHK500
MITOSTAN see I:BOT250
MITOTANE see III:CDN000
MITOXAN see I:CQC675, I:EAS500
MITOXANA see II:IMH000
MITOXINE see I:BIE500
MITSUI AURAMINE O see I:IBA000
MITSUI BLUE B BASE see I:DCJ200
MITSUI DIRECT BLACK EX see I:AQP000
MITSUI DIRECT BLUE 2BN see I:CMO000
MITSUI RED TR BASE see II:CLK220
MITSUI RHODAMINE BX see III:FAG070
MITSUI SCARLET G BASE see I:NMP500
MJ 1992 see III:SKW500
MJF 9325 see II:IMH000
MJF-12264 see III:FMB000
MK 56 see III:POL500
MK 665 see III:CHP750
2M 4KHP see II:CIR500
ML 97 see III:FAC025
MLT see III:MAK700
MM see III:BKM500
MMC see II:AHK500, III:MDD750
MME see III:MLH750
MMH see II:MKN000
4-MMPD see I:DBO000
4-MMPD SULPHATE see I:DBO400
MMS see III:MLH500
MNA see I:MMU250
6-MNA see III:MMT250
MNB see III:MMU500
MNC see III:MMX000
MNCO see II:MQY325
MNG see II:MMP000
MNNG see II:MMP000
MNPN see II:MMS200
MNQ see III:MMD500
MNU see I:MNA750, II:MMX250
M-2-OB see III:MMR800
M-3-OB see III:MMR810
MOCA see I:MJM200
MODANE see III:DMH400
MODOCOLL 1200 see III:SFO500
MODR FRALOSTANOVA 3G (CZECH) see III:DNE400
MOHICAN RED A-8008 see III:CHP500
MOLASSES ALCOHOL see I:EFU000
MOLINAL see II:EOK000
MOLLAN O see I:DVL700
MOLOL see III:MQV750
MOLURAME see III:BJK500
MOLYBDENUM-COBALT-CHROMIUM ALLOY see
    III:VSK000
MOLYBDENUM-LEAD CHROMATE see III:LDM000
MOLYBDENUM ORANGE see III:LDM000
MOLYBDENUM(VI) OXIDE see III:MRE000
MOLYBDENUM TRIOXIDE see III:MRE000

MOLYBDIC ANHYDRIDE see III:MRE000
MOLYBDIC TRIOXIDE see III:MRE000
MOLYKOTE 522 see III:TAI250
MOMENTUM see II:HIM000
MONAGYL see I:MMN250
MONASIRUP see III:PMQ750
MONDUR-TD see I:TGM740, I:TGM750
MONDUR-TD-80 see I:TGM740, I:TGM750
MONDUR TDS see I:TGM750
MONEX see III:BJL600
MONITAN see III:PKL100
MONOACETYL 4-HYDROXYAMINOQUINOLINE see
    III:QQA000
MONOBASIC CHROMIUM SULFATE see III:NBW000
MONOBASIC CHROMIUM SULPHATE see III:NBW000
MONOBASIC LEAD ACETATE see III:LCH000
MONOBENZONE see III:AEY000
MONOBENZYL ETHER HYDROQUINONE see III:AEY000
MONOBENZYL HYDROQUINONE see III:AEY000
MONOBROMOMETHANE see III:MHR200
MONO-n-BUTYLAMINE see III:BPX750
MONOCHLOORAZIJNZUUR (DUTCH) see III:CEA000
MONOCHLORACETIC ACID see III:CEA000
MONOCHLORESSIGSAEURE (GERMAN) see III:CEA000
MONOCHLORHYDRIN see III:CDT750
MONOCHLOROACETIC ACID see III:CEA000
MONOCHLOROACETONITRILE see III:CDN500
MONOCHLORODIFLUOROMETHANE see III:CFX500
MONOCHLORODIMETHYL ETHER (MAK) see I:CIO250
MONOCHLOROETHANOIC ACID see III:CEA000
MONOCHLOROETHENE see I:VNP000
MONOCHLOROETHYLENE (DOT) see I:VNP000
MONOCHLOROETHYLENE OXIDE see III:CGX000
MONOCHLOROHYDRIN see III:CDT750
α-MONOCHLOROHYDRIN see III:CDT750
MONOCHLOROMETHANE see II:MIF765
MONOCHLOROMETHYL CYANIDE see III:CDN500
MONOCHLOROMONOFLUOROMETHANE see I:CHI900
β-MONOCHLOROPROPIONIC ACID see III:CKS500
MONOCHROMIUM OXIDE) see I:CMK000
MONOCHROMIUM TRIOXIDE see I:CMK000
''MONOCITE'' METHACRYLATE MONOMER see
    III:MLH750
MONOCOBALT OXIDE see III:CND125
MONOCRATILIN see III:MRH000
MONOCROTALINE see II:MRH000
MONOCROTALINE, 3,8-DIDEHYDRO- see III:DAL350
MONOFURACIN see II:NGE500
MONOGLYCIDYL ETHER of N-PHENYLDIETHANOLAMINE
    see III:MRI500
8-MONOHYDRO MIREX see III:MRI750
MONOHYDROXYBENZENE see III:PDN750
MONOIODOACETAMIDE see III:IDW000
MONOIODOACETATE see III:IDZ000
MONOIODOACETIC ACID see III:IDZ000
MONOIODURO di METILE (ITALIAN) see I:MKW200
MONO-ISO-PROPANOLAMINE see III:AMA500
N-MONOMETHYLAMIDE of O,O-DIMETHYLDITHIO-
    PHOSPHORYLACETIC ACID see III:DSP400
4-MONOMETHYLAMINOAZOBENZENE see III:MNR500
p-MONOMETHYLAMINOAZOBENZENE see III:MNR500
2-MONOMETHYLAMINOFLUORENE see III:FEI500
N-MONOMETHYL-2-AMINOFLUORENE see III:FEI500
10-MONOMETHYLBENZO(a)PYRENE see III:MHH500
MONOMETHYL HYDRAZINE see II:MKN000
MONOMETHYL MERCURY CHLORIDE see III:MDD750
MONONITROSOPIPERAZINE see III:MRJ750
MONOPHEN see III:PFC750
MONOPHENOL see III:PDN750
MONOPLEX DOA see III:AEO000
MONOPOTASSIUM ARSENATE see I:ARD250
MONOPOTASSIUM DIHYDROGEN ARSENATE see
    I:ARD250
MONOSAN see II:DAA800

MONOSODIUM ARSENATE see I:ARD600
MONOSODIUM BARBITURATE see III:MRK750
MONOTEN see III:PFC750
MONOTHIOSUCCINIMIDE see III:MRN000
MONO-THIURAD see III:BJL600
MONOTHIURAM see III:BJL600
MONOTRICHLOR-AETHYLIDEN-α-GLUCOSE (GERMAN)
  see III:GFA000
MONOVAR see III:NNQ500
MONTANOX 80 see III:PKL100
MONTAR see I:PJL750
MONTMORILLONITE see III:BAV750
MONUREX see III:CJX750
MONURON see III:CJX750
MONUROX see III:CJX750
MONURUON see III:CJX750
MONUURON see III:CJX750
MOP see II:NKV000
8-MOP see I:XDJ000
MOPA see III:MFE250
MOPLEN see III:PMP500
MORBOCID see I:FMV000
MOROSAN see III:DCK759
MORPHOLINE see III:MRP750
MORPHOLINE, AQUEOUS MIXTURE (DOT) see III:MRP750
MORPHOLINE, 2,6-DIMETHYL-4-NITROSO-, (Z)- see
  III:NKA695
MORPHOLINE, 2,6-DIMETHYL-N-NITROSO-, (cis)- see
  III:NKA695
MORPHOLINE and SODIUM NITRITE (1:1) see III:SIN675
MORPHOLINO-CNU see III:MRR775
MORPHOLINODAUNOMYCIN see III:MRR850
3′-MORPHOLINO-3′-DEAMINODAUNORUBICIN see
  III:MRT100
1-5-(MORPHOLINOMETHYL)-3-((5-NITROFURFURYLI-
  DENE)AMINO)-2-OXAZOLIDINONEHYDROCHLORIDE
  see II:FPI150
4-MORPHOLINO-2-(5-NITRO-2-THIENYL)QUINAZOLINE see
  III:MRU000
MORPHOLINOPHOSPHONIC ACID DIMETHYL ESTER see
  III:DST800
2-(MORPHOLINOTHIO)BENZOTHIAZOLE see III:BDG000
MORPHOLINYLMERCAPTOBENZOTHIAZOLE see
  III:BDG000
4-MORPHOLINYLPHOSPHONIC ACID DIMETHYL ESTER see
  III:DST800
2-(4-MORPHOLINYLTHIO)BENZOTHIAZOLE see
  III:BDG000
MOSCARDA see III:MAK700
MOSTEN see III:PMP500
MOTH BALLS see III:NAJ500
MOTH FLAKES see III:NAJ500
MOTIORANGE R see III:PEJ500
MOTIROT G see III:XRA000
MOTOR BENZOL see I:BBL250
MOTOR FUEL (DOT) see III:GBY000
MOTOR SPIRIT (DOT) see III:GBY000
MOTOX see I:CDV100
MOTTENHEXE see III:HCI000
MOVINYL 100 see III:PKQ059
MOXESTROL see III:MRU600
MOXIE see II:MEI450
MOXONE see II:DAA800
MP see III:POK000
8-MP see I:XDJ000
MP 12-50 see III:TAB750
MP 25-38 see III:TAB750
MP 45-26 see III:TAB750
MP 1 (refractory) see III:EAL100
MPK 90 see III:PKQ250
MPN see II:MNA000, III:NKV100
MPNU see II:MMY500
MPP see III:FAQ999
1-MPPN see III:DWU800

MRA-CN see III:COP765
MRL 41 see III:CMX700
MROWCZAN ETYLU (POLISH) see III:EKL000
MS 53 see III:SNK000
MSMED see I:ECU750
MSZYCOL see I:BBQ500
MTD see I:TGL750
MTIC see III:MQB750
M.T. MUCORETTES see III:MPN500
MTU see II:MPW500
MTX see III:MDV500
MUCOCHLORIC ACID see III:MRU900
MUL F 66 see I:PKL750
MULTIN see II:HIM000
MURACIL see II:MPW500
MUREX see III:GFA000
MURFOS see III:PAK000
MURFULVIN see GKE000
MUSCULARON see III:IHH000
MUSTARD GAS see I:BIH250
MUSTARD HD see I:BIH250
MUSTARD OIL see II:AGJ250
MUSTARD VAPOR see I:BIH250
MUSTARGEN see I:BIE250, I:BIE500
MUSTARGEN HYDROCHLORIDE see I:BIE500
MUSTINE see I:BIE250
MUSTINE HYDROCHLOR see I:BIE500
MUSTINE HYDROCHLORIDE see I:BIE500
MUSTRON see II:CFA750
MUTAGEN see I:BIE250
MUTAMYCIN see II:AHK500
MUTAMYCIN (MITOMYCIN for INJECTION) see II:AHK500
MUTHMANN'S LIQUID see III:ACK250
MUTOXIN see I:DAD200
MVNA see II:NKY000
MX 5517-02 see III:SMQ500
MY/68 see III:FAF000
MYBASAN see III:ILD000
MYCHEL see II:CDP250
MYCINOL see II:CDP250
MYCOFARM see III:BFD250
MYCOIN see III:CMV000
MYCOTOXIN F2 see III:ZAT000
MYCRONIL see III:BJK500
MYEBROL see III:DDP600
MYELOBROMOL see III:DDP600
MYELOLEUKON see I:BOT250
MYLAR see III:PKF750
MYLERAN see I:BOT250
MYLOSAR see III:ARY000
MYOCON see III:NGY000
MYOFER 100 see I:IGS000
MYRAFORM see III:PKQ059
MYRICA CERIFERA see III:WBA000
MYRISIIC ALCOHOL see III:TBY500
9-MYRISTOYL-1,7,8-ANTHRACENETRIOL see III:MSA750
10-MYRISTOYL-1,8,9-ANTHRACENETRIOL see III:MSA750
1-MYRISTOYLAZIRIDINE see III:MSB000
MYRISTOYLETHYLENEIMINE see III:MSB000
N-MYRISTOYLOXY-AAF see III:ACS000
N-MYRISTOYLOXY-AAIF see III:MSB100
N-MYRISTOYLOXY-N-ACETYL-2-AMINOFLUORENE see
  III:ACS000
N-MYRISTOYLOXY-N-ACETYL-2-AMINO-7-IODOFLUOR-
  ENE see III:MSB100
N-MYRISTOYLOXY-N-MYRISTOYL-2-AMINOFLUORENE
  see III:MSB250
MYRITICALORIN see III:RSU000
MYRITICOALORIN see III:RSU000
MYROBALANS TANNIN see III:MSB750
MYRTAN TANNIN see III:MSC000
MYSORITE see I:ARM262
MYSTOX WFA see II:BGJ750
MYTOMYCIN see II:AHK500

MYVAK see III:VSK900
MYVAX see III:VSK900
N-6-MI see II:NKI000

NA see I:NBE500
NA-22 see I:IAQ000
NA-101 see III:TDX000
N-1544A see III:PFC750
NAB see III:NJK150
NABAC see III:HCL000
NABOLIN see III:MPN500
NACARAT A EXPORT see III:HJF500
NACCONATE-100 see I:TGM740, I:TGM750
NACCONATE 300 see III:MJP400
NACELAN BLUE G see III:TBG700
NACELAN FAST YELLOW CG see II:AAQ250
NACM-CELLULOSE SALT see III:SFO500
NACYCLYL see I:EDR000
NADAZONE see II:BRF500
NADOZONE see II:BRF500
NAFEEN see III:SHF500
NAFENOIC ACID see II:MCB500
NAFENOPIN see II:MCB500
NAFOXIDINE see III:NAD500
NaFPAK see III:SHF500
Na FRINSE see III:SHF500
NAFTALEN (POLISH) see III:NAJ500
1-NAFTILAMINA (SPANISH) see I:NBE000
β-NAFTILAMINA (ITALIAN) see I:NBE500
1-NAFTIL-TIOUREA (ITALIAN) see III:AQN635
α-NAFTYLAMIN (CZECH) see I:NBE000
β-NAFTYLAMIN (CZECH) see I:NBE500
1-NAFTYLAMINE (DUTCH) see I:NBE000
2-NAFTYLAMINE (DUTCH) see I:NBE500
α-NAFTYL-N-METHYLKARBAMAT (CZECH) see
    III:CBM750
β-NAFTYLOAMINA (POLISH) see I:NBE500
1-NAFTYLTHIOUREUM (DUTCH) see III:AQN635
NAH see III:NCQ900
NAHP see III:NJJ950
NAKO H see III:PEY500
NAKO TGG see III:REA000
NAKO TMT see I:TGL750
NAKO TSA see I:DBO400
NALCOAG see III:SCH000
NALOX see I:MMN250
NALUTRON see I:PMH500
NAMATE see I:DXE600
5-NAN see I:NEJ500
NANKAI ACID ORANGE I see III:FAG010
NAOP see III:AGM125
NAOTIN see III:NCQ900
NAPA see II:HIM000
NAPHTAMINE BLUE 2B see I:CMO000, II:CMO250
NAPHTAMINE VIOLET N see III:CMP000
5,12-NAPHTHACENEDIONE, 7,8,9,10-TETRAHYDRO-8-
    ACETYL-1-METHOXY-10-((2,3,6-TRIDEOXY-3-(4-MOR-
    PHOLINYL)-α-L-lyxo-HEXOPYRANOSYL)OXY)-6,8,11-
    TRIHYDROXY-, (8S-cis)- see III:MRR850
5,12-NAPHTHACENEDIONE, 7,8,9,10-TETRAHYDRO-10--
    ((3-(3-CYANOMORPHOLINO)-2,3,6-TRIDEOXY-α-L-lyxo-
    HEXOPYRANOSYL)OXY)-8-(HYDROXYACETYL)-1-
    METHOXY-6,8,11-TRIHYDR OXY-, (8s-cis)- see
    III:COP765
5,12-NAPHTHACENEDIONE, 7,8,9,10-TETRAHYDRO-8-(HY-
    DROXYACETYL)-1-METHOXY-10-((2,3,6-TRIDEOXY-
    MORPHOLINO-α-L-lyxo-HEXOPYRANOSYL)OXY)-6,8,11-
    TRIHYDROXY- see III:MRT100
α-NAPHTHACRIDINE see III:BAW750
2-NAPHTHALAMINE see I:NBE500
NAPHTHALANE see III:DAE800
2-NAPHTHALENAMINE see I:NBE500
1-NAPHTHALENAZO-2',4'-DIAMINOBENZENE see
    III:NBG500

NAPHTHALENE see III:NAJ500
NAPHTHALENE, CRUDE or REFINED (DOT) see III:NAJ500
1,5-NAPHTHALENEDIAMINE see II:NAM000
1,5-NAPHTHALENE DIISOCYANATE see III:NAM500
1,4-NAPHTHALENEDIONE see III:NBA500
1,3-NAPHTHALENEDISULFONIC ACID, 7-HYDROXY-8-((4-
    SULFO-1-NAPHTHYL)AZO)-, TRISODIUM SALT see
    III:FMU080
1,2-(1,8-NAPHTHALENEDIYL)BENZENE see III:FDF000
NAPHTHALENE FAST ORANGE 2GS see III:HGC000
NAPHTHALENE GREEN G see III:FAE950
NAPHTHALENE INK SCARLET 4R see III:FMU080
NAPHTHALENE LAKE SCARLET R see III:FMU070
NAPHTHALENE, MOLTEN (DOT) see III:NAJ500
NAPHTHALENE OIL see I:CMY825
NAPHTHALENE ORANGE I see III:FAG010
4-(1-NAPHTHALENYLAZO)-1,3-PHENYLENEDIAMINE see
    III:NBG500
1-NAPHTHALENYLTHIOUREA see III:AQN635
NAPHTHALIDINE see I:NBE000
NAPHTHALIN (DOT) see III:NAJ500
NAPHTHALINE see III:NAJ500
α-NAPHTHALTHIOHARNSTOFF (GERMAN) see III:AQN635
NAPHTHANE see III:DAE800
NAPHTHANIL BLUE B BASE see I:DCJ200
NAPHTHANIL SCARLET G BASE see I:NMP500
NAPHTHANTHRACENE see I:BBC250
NAPHTHENE see III:NAJ500
NAPHTHENIC ACID, LEAD SALT see III:NAS500
NAPHTHENIC OILS (PETROLEUM), CATALYTIC DEWAXED
    HEAVY(9CI) see I:MQV865
NAPHTHENIC OILS (PETROLEUM), CATALYTIC DEWAXED
    LIGHT (9CI) see I:MQV867
NAPHTHO(1,2,3,4-def)CHRYSENE see II:NAT500
NAPHTHO(1,8-gh:4,5-g'h')DIQUINOLINE see III:NAU000
NAPHTHO(1,8-gh:5,4-g'h')DIQUINOLINE see III:NAU500
1-NAPHTHOL-N-METHYLCARBAMATE see III:CBM750
NAPHTHOL ORANGE see III:FAG010
α-NAPHTHOL ORANGE see III:FAG010
NAPHTHOL RED B see III:FAG020
NAPHTHO(2,3-f)QUINOLINE see III:NAZ000
α-NAPHTHOQUINONE see III:NBA500
1,4-NAPHTHOQUINONE see III:NBA500
NAPHTHOSOL FAST RED KB BASE see II:CLK225
NAPHTHO(1,2-e)THIANAPHTHENO(3,2-b)PYRIDINE see
    III:BCF500
NAPHTHO(2,1-e)THIANAPHTHENO(3,2-b)PYRIDINE see
    III:BCF750
α-NAPHTHOTHIOUREA see III:AQN635
1-(2-NAPHTHOYL)-AZIRIDINE see III:NBC000
β-NAPHTHOYLETHYLENEIMINE see III:NBC000
N-2-NAPHTHYLACETOHYDROXAMIC ACID see
    III:NBD000
1-NAPHTHYLAMIN (GERMAN) see I:NBE000
2-NAPHTHYLAMIN (GERMAN) see I:NBE500
β-NAPHTHYLAMIN (GERMAN) see I:NBE500
1-NAPHTHYLAMINE see I:NBE000
2-NAPHTHYLAMINE see I:NBE500
6-NAPHTHYLAMINE see I:NBE500
α-NAPHTHYLAMINE see I:NBE000
β-NAPHTHYLAMINE see I:NBE500
NAPHTHYLAMINE BLUE see II:CMO250
2-NAPHTHYLAMINE-6,8-DISULFONIC ACID see III:NBE850
2-NAPHTHYLAMINE-1-d-GLUCOSIDURONIC ACID see
    III:ALL000
NAPHTHYLAMINE MUSTARD see I:BIF250
2-NAPHTHYLAMINE MUSTARD see I:NBE500
2-NAPHTHYLAMINE-8-SULFONIC ACID see III:ALI300
N-(1-NAPHTHYL)ANILINE see III:PFT250
N-(2-NAPHTHYL)ANILINE see II:PFT500
4-(1-NAPHTHYLAZO)-2-NAPHTHYLAMINE see III:NBG000
4-(1-NAPHTHYLAZO)-m-PHENYLENEDIAMINE see
    III:NBG500

5-(β-NAPHTHYLAZO)-2,4,6-TRIAMINOPYRIMIDINE see
  III:NBO500
2-NAPHTHYLBIS(2-CHLOROETHYL)AMINE see I:BIF250
β-NAPHTHYL-BIS-(β-CHLOROETHYL)AMINE see I:BIF250
β-NAPHTHYL-DI-(2-CHLOROETHYL)AMINE see I:BIF250
1,2-(1,8-NAPHTHYLENE)BENZENE see III:FDF000
1,5-NAPHTHYLENEDIAMINE see II:NAM000
1-NAPHTHYLHYDROXYLAMINE see III:HIX000
2-NAPHTHYLHYDROXYLAMINE see III:NBI500
N-1-NAPHTHYLHYDROXYLAMINE see III:HIX000
(2-NAPHTHYL)-1-ISOPROPYLAMINOETHANOL see
  III:INS000
NAPHTHYLISOPROTERENOL see III:INS000
NAPHTHYLISOPROTERENOL HYDROCHLORIDE see
  III:INT000
1-NAPHTHYL METHYLCARBAMATE see III:CBM750
1-NAPHTHYL-N-METHYLCARBAMATE see III:CBM750
α-NAPHTHYL N-METHYLCARBAMATE see III:CBM750
1-NAPHTHYL METHYLNITROSOCARBAMATE see
  I:NBJ500
1-NAPHTHYL-N-METHYL-N-NITROSOCARBAMATE see
  I:NBJ500
2-NAPHTHYLPHENYLAMINE see II:PFT500
β-NAPHTHYLPHENYLAMINE see II:PFT500
2-NAPHTHYL-p-PHENYLENEDIAMINE see III:NBL000
α-NAPHTHYLTHIOCARBAMIDE see III:AQN635
1-NAPHTHYL-THIOHARNSTOFF (GERMAN) see
  III:AQN635
α-NAPHTHYLTHIOUREA see III:AQN635
1-(1-NAPHTHYL)-2-THIOUREA see III:AQN635
N-(1-NAPHTHYL)-2-THIOUREA see III:AQN635
α-NAPHTHYLTHIOUREA (DOT) see III:AQN635
1-NAPHTHYL THIOUREA (MAK) see III:AQN635
1-NAPHTHYL-THIOUREE (FRENCH) see III:AQN635
5-β-NAPHTHYL-2:4:6-TRIAMINOAZOPYRIMIDINE see
  III:NBO500
NAPHTOELAN FAST SCARLET G SALT see I:NMP500
NAPHTO(1,2-c-d-e)NAPHTACENE (FRENCH) see III:BCP750
NAPHTOX see III:AQN635
NAPRINOL see II:HIM000
NAPTHOLROT S see III:FAG020
NARCOGEN see II:TIO750
NARDELZINE see III:PFC750
NARDIL see III:PFC750
NARKOSOID see II:TIO750
NASDOL see I:TBG000
NASS (IRAN) see I:SED400
NASTENON see I:PAN100
NASWAR (PAKISTAN and AFGHANISTAN) see I:SED400
NATASOL FAST RED TR SALT see II:CLK235
NATHULANE see I:PME500
NATIVE CALCIUM SULFATE see III:CAX750
NATREEN see II:BCE500, III:SGC000
NATRIPHENE see II:BGJ750
NATRIUMARSENIT (GERMAN) see I:ARJ500
NATRIUMAZID (GERMAN) see III:SFA000
NATRIUMBICHROMAAT (DUTCH) see I:SGI000
NATRIUMDICHROMAAT (DUTCH) see I:SGI000
NATRIUMDICHROMAT (GERMAN) see I:SGI000
NATRIUM FLUORIDE see III:SHF500
NATRIUMMAZIDE (DUTCH) see III:SFA000
NATRIUMNITRAT UND N-METHYLANILIN (GERMAN) see
  III:MGO250
NATRIUM NITRIT (GERMAN) see III:SIQ500
NATRIUMSELENIAT (GERMAN) see III:DXG000
NATRIUMSELENIT (GERMAN) see III:SJT500
NATRIUMZYKLAMATE (GERMAN) see III:SGC000
NATULAN see I:PME250, I:PME500
NATULANAR see I:PME500
NATULAN HYDROCHLORIDE see I:PME500
NATURAL GASOLINE (DOT) see III:GBY000
NATURAL IRON OXIDES see III:IHD000
NATURAL RED OXIDE see III:IHD000
NAUGARD TJB see III:DWI000

NAUGARD TKB see I:NKB500
NAULI "GUM" see III:PMQ750
NAXAMIDE see II:IMH000
NAYPER B and BO see III:BDS000
NB2B see I:CMO000
NBBA see III:NJO150
NBHA see I:HJQ350
N.B. MECOPROP see II:CIR500
NBS 706 see III:SMQ500
NC 150 see I:PDC250, III:PEK250
NC-262 see III:DSP400
NCI-C00044 see III:AFK250
NCI-C00055 see III:AJM000
NCI-C00066 see III:ASH500
NCI-C00077 see III:CBG000
NCI-C00099 see II:CDR750
NCI-C00102 see III:TBQ750
NCI-C00124 see III:DHB400
NCI-C00135 see III:DSP400
NCI-C00157 see III:EAT500
NCI C00168 see II:TBW100
NCI-C00180 see II:HAR000
NCI-C00191 see I:KEA000
NCI-C00204 see I:BBQ500
NCI-C00215 see III:MAK700
NCI-C00226 see III:PAK000
NCI-C00237 see III:PIB900
NCI-C00259 see I:CDV100
NCI-C00408 see I:DER000
NCI-C00419 see III:PAX000
NCI-C00420 see I:DFT800
NCI-C00442 see III:DUV600
NCI-C00453 see CDO250
NCI-C00464 see I:DAD200
NCI-C00475 see I:BIM500
NCI-C00486 see III:BIO750
NCI-C00497 see II:MEI450
NCI-C00500 see I:DDL800
NCI-C00511 see I:EIY600
NCI-C00522 see I:EIY500
NCI-C00533 see III:CKN500
NCI-C00544 see III:DOS000
NCI-C00555 see II:BIM750
NCI-C00566 see III:EAQ750
NCI-C00588 see III:FAC025
NCI-C01445 see II:NEI000
NCI-C01478 see II:LBG000
NCI-C01514 see I:AES750
NCI-C01536 see III:ADR750
NCI-C01547 see III:YCJ000
NCI-C01558 see II:CME250
NCI-C01569 see III:ARY000
NCI-C01570 see III:EDR500
NCI-C01592 see I:BOT250
NCI-C01616 see II:IAN000
NCI-C01627 see II:PIK250
NCI-C01638 see II:IMH000
NCI-C01649 see I:TFQ750
NCI-C01661 see II:DDG800
NCI-C01672 see I:PDC250
NCI-C01683 see III:TGD000
NCI-C01694 see III:EPQ000
NCI-C01707 see I:TFI000
NCI-C01718 see III:SOA500
NCI-C01729 see III:TNX000
NCI-C01730 see III:API500
NCI-C01785 see III:POL500
NCI-C01810 see I:PME500
NCI-C01821 see III:DSY600
NCI-C01832 see III:DCE600, III:TGM400
NCI-C01843 see I:NMP500
NCI-C01854 see I:HHG000
NCI-C01865 see II:DVH000
NCI-C01876 see I:AIB000

NCI-C01887 see III:AJT750
NCI-C01901 see I:AKP750
NCI-C01912 see III:NFD500
NCI-C01923 see II:MMG000
NCI-C01934 see II:NEQ500
NCI-C01967 see I:NEJ500
NCI C01978 see III:NEL000
NCI-C01989 see I:DBO400
NCI-C01990 see I:MJN000
NCI-C02006 see I:MQS500
NCI-C02039 see III:CEH680
NCI-C02051 see II:CLK225
NCI-C02073 see III:EFE000
NCI-C02084 see III:SIQ500
NCI-C02095 see III:AEN000
NCI-C02108 see II:AAI000
NCI-C02119 see III:USS000
NCI-C02142 see III:HEM500
NCI-C02153 see III:THG000
NCI-C02175 see III:DCJ400
NCI-C02186 see III:TMH750
NCI-C02200 see II:SMQ000
NCI-C02222 see II:ALL750
NCI-C02244 see I:NKB500
NCI-C02299 see I:TLG250
NCI-C02302 see I:TGL750
NCI-C02335 see I:TGS500
NCI-C02368 see II:CLK235
NCI-C02551 see I:CAH500
NCI-C02653 see III:HCL000
NCI-C02664 see II:PJN000
NCI-C02686 see I:CHJ500
NCI-C02697 see III:ARP250
NCI-C02711 see I:CAJ750
NCI-C02733 see III:CAK500
NCI-C02766 see I:AMT500
NCI-C02799 see I:FMV000
NCI-C02813 see III:PIX250
NCI-C02824 see III:ISA000
NCI-C02835 see III:SGJ000
NCI-C02846 see III:CJX750
NCI-C02857 see III:EPJ000
NCI-C02868 see III:DJC000
NCI-C02880 see III:DWI000
NCI-C02891 see III:LCW000
NCI-C02904 see I:TIW000
NCI-C02915 see II:PFT500
NCI-C02926 see III:ASL250
NCI-C02937 see III:CAQ250
NCI-C02959 see III:DXH250
NCI-C02960 see III:CMF400
NCI-C02971 see III:MNH000
NCI-C02982 see I:MGO750
NCI-C02993 see II:MGO500
NCI-C03009 see III:BLJ250
NCI-C03010 see III:DOU600
NCI-C03021 see II:NAM000
NCI-C03043 see II:AJV250
NCI-C03065 see III:ALQ000
NCI-C03076 see III:NIY500
NCI-C03134 see I:EFU000
NCI-C03167 see I:SMD000
NCI-C03258 see I:ANO500
NCI-C03270 see I:TNC500
NCI-C03292 see I:CFK125
NCI-C03305 see II:CJS125
NCI-C03316 see III:CEG625
NCI-C03361 see I:BBX000
NCI-C03372 see I:IAQ000
NCI-C03474 see I:ASB250
NCI-C03485 see I:CDO500
NCI-C03510 see II:API750
NCI-C03521 see III:BDH250
NCI-C03554 see III:TBQ100

NCI-C03565 see III:DCZ000
NCI-C03598 see III:BFW750
NCI-C03656 see III:DDA800
NCI-C03667 see III:DAC800
NCI-C03678 see III:OAJ000
NCI-C03689 see I:DVQ000
NCI-C03703 see II:HCF500
NCI-C03714 see I:TAI000
NCI-C03736 see II:AOQ000, II:BBL000
NCI-C03747 see I:AOX250
NCI-C03758 see III:AOX500
NCI-C03781 see II:TMD250
NCI-C03792 see II:ENV500
NCI-C03816 see III:DKC400
NCI-C03827 see II:DQD400
NCI-C03838 see II:CIV000
NCI-C03850 see III:DVR200
NCI-C03918 see II:DQJ200
NCI-C03930 see III:PEY650
NCI-C03963 see II:NEM480
NCI-C03985 see I:DGG950
NCI-C04126 see III:DTH000
NCI-C04137 see III:DBN200
NCI-C04159 see II:BKF250
NCI-C04240 see III:TGG760
NCI-C04251 see III:TGF250
NCI-C04502 see III:DGW200
NCI-C04535 see III:DFF809
NCI-C04546 see I:TIO750
NCI-C04579 see II:TIN000
NCI-C04580 see II:PCF275
NCI-C04604 see III:HCI000
NCI-C04615 see II:AGB250
NCI-C04626 see III:MIH275
NCI-C04671 see III:MDV500
NCI-C04682 see III:AEB000
NCI-C04693 see II:DAC000
NCI-C04706 see II:AHK500
NCI-C04717 see II:DAB600
NCI-C04728 see III:AQQ750
NCI-C04739 see III:ADA000
NCI-C04740 see I:CGV250
NCI-C04762 see III:DDP600
NCI-C04773 see I:BIF750
NCI-C04784 see III:MPU000
NCI-C04795 see III:DDJ000
NCI-C04819 see III:DCF200
NCI-C04820 see II:BIA250
NCI-C04831 see III:HOO500
NCI-C04842 see III:VKZ000
NCI-C04853 see I:PED750
NCI-C04864 see III:LEY000
NCI-C04875 see III:DFO000
NCI-C04886 see III:POK000
NCI-C04897 see III:PLZ000
NCI-C04900 see I:EAS500
NCI-C04922 see I:CQN000
NCI-C04933 see III:CDN000
NCI-C04944 see II:BHT750
NCI-C04955 see II:CHD250
NCI-C05970 see III:REA000
NCI-C06008 see III:TAB750
NCI-C06360 see II:BEE375
NCI-C06428 see I:MQW500
NCI-C06462 see III:SFA000
NCI-C06508 see III:BDX000
NCI-C08651 see III:FAQ999
NCI-C08695 see III:DUK800
NCI-C08991 see I:ARM280
NCI-C08991 see I:ARM250
NCI C09007 see I:ARM275
NCI-C50033 see I:SBT000
NCI-C50044 see III:BII250
NCI-C50055 see III:DUE000

NCI-C50077 see III:PMO500
NCI-C50088 see I:EJN500
NCI-C50099 see I:PNL600
NCI-C50102 see II:MJP450
NCI-C50124 see III:PDN750
NCI-C50146 see I:OPM000
NCI-C50157 see II:RDK000
NCI-C50168 see III:CNU000
NCI-C50226 see III:ZAT000
NCI-C50259 see III:HEJ500
NCI-C50260 see III:DBR400
NCI-C50282 see III:BGE325
NCI-C50351 see III:BGJ250
NCI-C50384 see II:EFT000
NCI-C50442 see III:BJK500
NCI-C50453 see III:EQR500
NCI-C50464 see II:AGJ250
NCI-C50533 see I:TGM750
NCI-C50544 see III:WCB000
NCI-C50602 see I:BOP500
NCI-C50613 see III:AMW000
NCI-C50646 see III:CBF700
NCI-C50657 see II:DBL200
NCI-C50668 see III:MJP400
NCI-C50680 see III:MLH750
NCI-C50715 see III:MCB000
NCI-C52459 see III:TBQ000
NCI-C52733 see I:DVL700
NCI-C52904 see III:NAJ500
NCI-C53781 see II:AAQ250
NCI-C53792 see III:CHP500
NCI-C53838 see III:HGC000
NCI-C53849 see III:HJF500
NCI-C53894 see III:PAW500
NCI-C53929 see III:PEJ500
NCI-C54262 see II:VPK000
NCI-C54375 see III:BEC500
NCI-C54386 see III:AEO000
NCI-C54557 see I:AQP000
NCI-C54568 see II:CMO750
NCI-C54579 see I:CMO000
NCI-C54604 see I:MJQ000, I:MJQ100
NCI-C54660 see III:DHF200
NCI-C54706 see III:FEW000
NCI-C54717 see II:ISV000
NCI-C54739 see II:RMK020
NCI-C54740 see III:DST800
NCI-C54751 see III:TNI250
NCI-C54773 see III:DSG600
NCI-C54819 see III:IKE000
NCI-C54820 see II:CIU750
NCI-C54831 see III:TIQ250
NCI-C54842 see III:PMK000
NCI-C54900 see III:TBG700
NCI-C54911 see III:SGP500
NCI-C54922 see III:ALO750
NCI-C54933 see II:PAX250
NCI-C54944 see III:DEP600
NCI-C54955 see II:DEP800
NCI-C54966 see II:REF000
NCI-C54977 see II:EBR000
NCI-C54988 see III:TCF000
NCI-C54999 see III:CPD750
NCI-C55072 see II:CDS000
NCI-C55107 see III:CEA750
NCI-C55130 see III:BNL000
NCI-C55141 see III:PNJ400
NCI-C55152 see I:AQF000
NCI-C55196 see III:NGE000
NCI-C55210 see III:RNZ000
NCI-C55221 see III:SHF500
NCI-C55243 see II:BND500
NCI-C55276 see I:BBL250
NCI-C55287 see III:PAU500

NCI-C55298 see III:QPA000
NCI-C55345 see II:DFX800
NCI-C55378 see II:PAX250
NCI-C55447 see III:MKA500
NCI-C55470 see III:WCJ000
NCI-C55527 see III:BOX750
NCI-C55538 see III:EBX500
NCI-C55572 see III:LFU000
NCI-C55583 see I:NKM000
NCI-C55594 see III:MHZ000
NCI-C55618 see III:IMF400
NCI-C55696 see III:SNC000
NCI-C55709 see II:CDP250
NCI-C55765 see I:DKQ000
NCI-C55776 see II:PJD000
NCI-C55787 see III:HFV500
NCI-C55801 see II:HIM000
NCI-C55823 see III:GEM000
NCI-C55834 see III:HIH000
NCI-C55845 see III:QQS200
NCI-C55856 see III:CCP850
NCI-C55878 see III:BOV000
NCI-C55889 see III:HAP500
NCI-C55903 see I:XDJ000
NCI-C55958 see III:NEM500
NCI-C55969 see III:AOR500
NCI C55970 see III:ALO000
NCI-C56064 see II:NGE500
NCI-C56122 see III:RGW000
NCI-C56213 see I:ABC250
NCI-C56326 see II:AAG250
NCI-C56382 see I:BIE500
NCI-C56451 see III:PKL500
NCI-C56462 see II:MRH000
NCI-C56519 see II:BDF000
NCI-C56531 see II:BRF500
NCI-C56586 see III:CHP250
NCI-C56600 see III:SNJ000
NCI-C56655 see II:PAX250
NCI-C60106 see III:QCA000
NCI-C60139 see I:VOA000
NCI-C60184 see III:PAD500
NCI-C60208 see II:VPP000
NCI-C60231 see III:CEA000
NCI-C60253A see I:ARM262
NCI-C60286 see III:PKL100
NCI-C60297 see III:CNV000
NCI-C60311 see I:CNA250
NCI-C60344 see II:NDK500
NCI-C60399 see III:MCW250
NCI-C60413 see II:DER000
NCI-C60582 see II:PKQ500, II:PKQ750, II:PKR000,
    II:PKR250, II:PKR750, II:PKS000, III:PKQ250
NCI-C60628 see III:TFD250
NCI-C60797 see III:PKQ059
NCI-C60811 see III:ZSJ000
NCI-C60899 see III:DIX200
NCI-C60946 see III:AFW750
NCI-C61143 see III:MAU250
NCI-C61187 see II:TIV750
NCI-C61201 see III:CJU250
NCI-C61223A see I:ARM268
NCI-C61289 see II:CMO250
NCI-C61494 see III:BEN000
NDBA see I:BRY500
NDC 002-1452-01 see III:VKZ000
NDEA see I:NJW500
NDELA see I:NKM000
NDHU see III:NJY000
NDMA see I:NKA600, III:DSY600
NDMI see III:NJK500
NDPA see I:NKB700, III:DWI000
NDPEA see III:NBR100
NDPhA see III:DWI000

NEA see I:NKD000
NEASINA see III:SNJ000
NEATHALIDE see III:INS000
NEAT OIL of SWEET ORANGE see III:OGY000
NEAUFATIN see III:TEH500
NEBERK see III:FMB000
NECATORINA see CBY000
NECATORINE see CBY000
NEFCO see II:NGE500
NEFRECIL see I:PDC250
NEFTIN see III:NGG500
NEFURTHIAZOLE see II:NDY500
NEGALIP see III:ARQ750
NEGUVON see III:TIQ250
NEGUVON A see III:TIQ250
NEKLACID FAST ORANGE 2G see III:HGC000
NEKLACID ORANGE 1 see III:FAG010
NEKLACID RED 3R see III:FMU080
NEKLACID RED A see III:FAG020
NEKLACID RED RR see III:FMU070
NEKLACID RUBINE W see III:HJF500
NEMA see I:MKB000, II:PCF275
NEMABROM see I:DDL800
NEMAFUME see I:DDL800
NEMAGON see I:DDL800
NEMAGONE see I:DDL800
NEMAGON SOIL FUMIGANT see I:DDL800
NEMALITE see III:NBT000
NEMALITH (GERMAN) see III:NBT000
NEMANAX see I:DDL800
NEMAPAZ see I:DDL800
NEMASET see I:DDL800
NEMATOCIDE see I:DDL800
NEMATOX see I:DDL800
NEMAZON see I:DDL800
NENDRIN see III:EAT500
NEO see III:TEH500
NEOANTERGAN MALEATE see III:DBM800
NEOASYCODILE see I:DXE600
NEO-ATOMID see III:ARQ750
NEOBAR see III:BAP000
NEOCHIN see III:CLD000
NEOCHROMIUM see III:NBW000
NEOCID see I:DAD200
NEOCOCCYL see III:SNM500
NEOCOMPENSAN see III:PKQ250
NEO-CULTOL see III:MQV750
NEODELPREGNIN see III:MCA500
NEO-ESTRONE see I:ECU750
NEO-FARMADOL see III:HNI500
NEO-FAT 12 see III:LBL000
NEO-FAT 18-61 see III:SLK000
NEO-FAT 90-04 see III:OHU000
NEO-FAT 92-04 see III:OHU000
NEO-FAT 18-S see III:SLK000
NEOFEN see III:HNI500
NEO-FERRUM see I:IHG000
NEOFOLLIN see II:EDS100
NEO-FULCIN see GKE000
NEOGYNON see III:NNL500
NEO-HOMBREOL see I:TBG000
NEO-HOMBREOL-M see III:MPN500
NEOISCOTIN see III:SIJ000
NEOLUTIN see III:HNT500
NEO-OESTRANOL 1 see I:DKA600
NEO-OESTRANOL II see I:DKB000
NEOPELLIS see III:TFD250
NEOPENTANOIC ACID see III:PJA500
NEOPENTYL GLYCOL DIACRYLATE see III:DUL200
NEOPENTYL GLYCOL DIGLYCIDYL ETHER see III:NCI300
NEOPLATIN see II:PJD000
NEOPRENE see III:NCI500
NEOSABENYL see III:CJU250
NEOSAR see I:EAS500

NEO-SCABICIDOL see I:BBQ500
NEOSEDYN see III:TEH500
NEOSEPT see III:HCL000
NEOSETILE BLUE EB see III:TBG700
NEOS-HIDANTOINA see I:DKQ000
NEOSONE D see III:MFA250
NEOSTREPSAN see III:TEX250
NEOSYDYN see III:TEH500
NEOTEBEN see III:ILD000
NEO-TESTIS see I:TBF500
NEOTIZIDE see III:SIJ000
NEO-TIZIDE SODIUM SALT see III:SIJ000
NEO-TRIC see I:MMN250
NEOVLETTA see III:NNL500
NEOXAZOL see III:SNN500
NEOXIN see HI:ILD000
NEO-ZOLINE see II:BRF500
NEOZONE A see III:PFT250
NEOZONE D see II:PFT500
NEPHIS see I:EIY500
NEPTUNE BLUE BRA CONCENTRATION see III:FMU059
NERACID see III:CBG000
NEROBOL see III:DAL300
NEROBOLETTES see III:DAL300
NESONTIL see III:CFZ000
NESPOR see III:MAS500
NETAGRONE 600 see II:DAA800
NETALID see III:INS000
NETAZOL see II:CIR250
NETH see III:INS000
NETHALIDE see III:INS000
NETHALIDE HYDROCHLORIDE see III:INT000
NETSUSARIN see III:DOT000
NEU see I:ENV000, III:NKE500
NEUCOCCIN see III:FMU080
NEUMANDIN see III:ILD000
NEUROBARB see III:EOK000
NEURODYN see III:TEH500
NEUROSEDIN see III:TEH500
NEUTRAL ACRIFLAVINE see III:DBX400
NEUTRAL POTASSIUM CHROMATE see II:PLB250
NEUTROSEL NAVY BN see I:DCJ200
NEUTROSEL RED TRVA see II:CLK235
NEVIN see III:ILD000
NEVRODYN see III:TEH500
NEW COCCIN see III:FMU080
NEW PINK BLUISH GEIGY see III:FAG040
NEW PONCEAU 4R see III:FMU070
NEXIT see I:BBQ500
NEXOVAL see III:CKC000
NF see II:NGE500
NF 246 see II:NDY000
NF 1010 see III:EAE500
NFIP see II:NGI800
NFN see III:DLU800
NG see III:NGY000
NG-180 see III:NGG500
N^2-(γ-l-(+)-GLUTAMYL)-4-CARBOXYPHENYLHYDRAZINE
see III:GFO100
NHA see III:NBI500
NHMI see III:OBY000
NHU see III:HKQ025
NHYD see III:NKJ000
Ni 270 see I:NCW500
Ni 0901-S see I:NCW500
Ni 4303T see I:NCW500
NIA 5273 see III:PIX250
NIA 5462 see III:EAQ750
NIA 5996 see III:DER800
NIACIDE see III:FAS000
NIACIN see III:NCQ900
NIADRIN see III:ILD000
NIAGARA 5006 see III:DER800
NIAGARA 5,462 see III:EAQ750

NIAGARA 5,996 see III:DER800
NIAGARA BLUE see II:CMO250
NIAGARA BLUE 2B see I:CMO000
NIAGARAMITE see I:SOP500
NIAGARATRAN see III:CJT750
NIALK see II:TIO750
NIAX ISOCYANATE TDI see I:TGM740
NIAX TDI see I:TGM750, II:TGM800
NIAX TDI-P see I:TGM750
NIBROL see III:TEH500
NICACID see III:NCQ900
NICAMIN see III:NCQ900
NICANGIN see III:NCQ900
NICAZIDE see III:ILD000
NICETAL see III:ILD000
NICHEL TETRACARBONILE (ITALIAN) see I:NCZ000
NICIZINA see III:ILD000
NICKEL see I:NCW500
NICKEL 270 see I:NCW500
NICKEL (ITALIAN) see I:NCW500
NICKEL(II) ACETATE (1:2) see I:NCX000
NICKEL ACETATE TETRAHYDRATE see II:NCX500
NICKEL ANTIMONIDE see III:NCY100
NICKEL ARSENIDE (As$_2$-Ni$_5$) see I:NDJ399
NICKEL ARSENIDE (As$_8$-Ni$_{11}$) see I:NDJ400
NICKEL ARSENIDE SULFIDE see I:NCY125
NICKEL BISCYCLOPENTADIENE see I:NDA500
NICKEL BOROFLUORIDE see II:NDC000
NICKEL(II) CARBONATE (1:1) see I:NCY500
NICKEL CARBONYL see I:NCZ000
NICKEL CARBONYLE (FRENCH) see I:NCZ000
NICKEL CHLORIDE (DOT) see II:NDH000
NICKEL(II) CHLORIDE (1:2) see II:NDH000
NICKEL(II) CHLORIDE HEXAHYDRATE (1:2:6) see
  II:NDA000
NICKEL COMPLEX with N-FLUOREN-2-YL ACETOHYDROX-
  AMIC ACID see III:HIR500
NICKEL, COMPOUND with pi-CYCLOPENTADIENYL
  (1:2) see I:NDA500
NICKEL COMPOUNDS see I:NDB000
NICKEL CYANIDE (solid) see II:NDB500
NICKEL CYANIDE (DOT) see II:NDB500
NICKEL DIBUTYLDITHIOCARBAMATE see III:BIW750
NICKEL DIFLUORIDE see II:NDC500
NICKEL DISULFIDE see III:NDB875
NICKEL (DUST) see I:NCW500
NICKEL(II) FLUOBORATE see II:NDC000
NICKEL(II) FLUORIDE (1:2) see II:NDC500
NICKEL FLUOROBORATE see II:NDC000
NICKEL(II) FLUOSILICATE (1:1) see II:NDD000
NICKEL-GALLIUM ALLOY see II:NDD500
NICKEL(II) HYDROXIDE see I:NDE000
NICKEL HYDROXIDE (DOT) see I:NDE000
NICKELIC OXIDE see II:NDH500
NICKEL IRON SULFIDE see II:NDE500
NICKEL-IRON SULFIDE MATTE see II:NDE500
NICKEL(II) ISODECYL ORTHOPHOSPHATE (3:2) see
  III:NDF000
NICKEL MONOANTIMONIDE see III:NCY100
NICKEL MONOSELENIDE see III:NDF400
NICKEL MONOSULFATE HEXAHYDRATE see II:NDL000
NICKEL MONOSULFIDE see I:NDL100
NICKEL MONOXIDE see I:NDF500
NICKEL NITRATE (DOT) see II:NDG000
NICKEL(II) NITRATE (1:2) see II:NDG000
NICKEL(2+) NITRATE, HEXAHYDRATE see II:NDG500
NICKEL(II) NITRATE, HEXAHYDRATE (1:2:6) see
  II:NDG500
NICKELOCENE see I:NDA500
NICKELOUS ACETATE see I:NCX000
NICKELOUS CARBONATE see I:NCY500
NICKELOUS CHLORIDE see II:NDH000
NICKELOUS FLUORIDE see II:NDC500
NICKELOUS HYDROXIDE see I:NDE000

NICKELOUS OXIDE see I:NDF500
NICKELOUS SULFATE see II:NDK500
NICKELOUS SULFIDE see I:NDL100
NICKELOUS TETRAFLUOROBORATE see II:NDC000
NICKEL OXIDE see II:NDH500
NICKEL OXIDE (MAK) see I:NDF500
NICKEL(II) OXIDE (1:1) see I:NDF500
NICKEL OXIDE, IRON OXIDE, and CHROMIUM OXIDE FUME
  see I:IHE000
NICKEL OXIDE PEROXIDE see II:NDH500
NICKEL PARTICLES see I:NCW500
NICKEL(2+) PERCHLORATE, HEXAHYDRATE see
  II:NDJ000
NICKEL PEROXIDE see II:NDH500
NICKEL POTASSIUM CYANIDE see II:NDI000
NICKEL PROTOXIDE see I:NDF500
NICKEL REFINERY DUST see I:NDI500
NICKEL(2+) SALT PERCHLORIC ACID HEXAHYDRATE see
  II:NDJ000
NICKEL SELENIDE see I:NDJ475, III:NDF400
NICKEL SELENIDE (3:2) CRYSTALLINE see I:NDJ475
NICKEL SISQUIOXIDE see II:NDH500
NICKEL SPONGE see I:NCW500
NICKEL SUBARSENIDE see I:NDJ399, I:NDJ400
NICKEL SUBSELENIDE see I:NDJ475
NICKEL SUBSULFIDE see I:NDJ500
NICKEL SUBSULPHIDE see I:NDJ500
NICKEL (II) SULFAMATE see II:NDK000
NICKEL SULFARSENIDE see I:NCY125
NICKEL SULFATE see II:NDK500
NICKEL SULFATE(1:1) see II:NDK500
NICKEL(II) SULFATE see II:NDK500
NICKEL(2+)SULFATE(1:1) see II:NDK500
NICKEL(II) SULFATE (1:1) see II:NDK500
NICKEL SULFATE HEXAHYDRATE see II:NDL000
NICKEL (II) SULFATE HEXAHYDRATE see II:NDL000
NICKEL(II) SULFATE HEXAHYDRATE (1:1:6) see
  II:NDL000
NICKEL SULFIDE see I:NDJ500, I:NDL100, III:NDB875
NICKEL(II) SULFIDE see I:NDL100
α-NICKEL SULFIDE (1:1) CRYSTALLINE see I:NDL100
α-NICKEL SULFIDE (3:2) CRYSTALLINE see I:NDJ500
NICKEL SULPHATE HEXAHYDRATE see II:NDL000
NICKEL SULPHIDE see I:NDJ500
NICKEL TELLURIDE see II:NDL425
NICKEL TETRACARBONYL see I:NCZ000
NICKEL TETRACARBONYLE (FRENCH) see I:NCZ000
NICKEL(II) TETRAFLUOROBORATE see II:NDC000
NICKEL-TITANATE see II:NDL500
NICKEL TITANIUM OXIDE see II:NDL500
NICKEL TRIOXIDE see II:NDH500
NICKEL TRITADISULPHIDE see I:NDJ500
NICLOFEN see I:DFT800
NICO see III:NCQ900
NICO-400 see III:NCQ900
NICOBID see III:NCQ900
NICOCAP see III:NCQ900
NICOCIDIN see III:NCQ900
NICOCRISINA see III:NCQ900
NICODAN see III:NCQ900
NICODELMINE see III:NCQ900
NICOLAR see III:NCQ900
NICOLEN see III:NGG500
NICONACID see III:NCQ900
NICONAT see III:NCQ900
NICONAZID see III:NCQ900
NICONYL see III:ILD000
NICOROL see III:NCQ900
NICOSIDE see III:NCQ900
NICO-SPAN see III:NCQ900
NICOSYL see III:NCQ900
NICOTAMIN see III:NCQ900
NICOTENE see III:NCQ900
NICOTIANA ATTENUATA see I:TGI100

NICOTIANA GLAUCA see I:TGI100
NICOTIANA LONGIFLORA see I:TGI100
NICOTIANA RUSTICA see I:TGI100
NICOTIANA TABACUM see I:TGI100
NICOTIBINA see III:ILD000
NICOTIBINE see III:ILD000
NICOTIL see III:NCQ900
NICOTINE ACID see III:NCQ900
NICOTINE, COMPOUND, with NICKEL(II)-o-BENZOYL BEN-
    ZOATE TRIHYDRATE (2:1) see II:BHB000
NICOTINE, 1'-DEMETHYL-1'-NITROSO-, 1-OXIDE see
    III:NLD525
NICOTINIC ACID see III:NCQ900
NICOTINIC ACID, HYDRAZIDE see III:NDU500
NICOTINIC ACID-1,2,5,6-TETRAHYDRO-1-METHYL-,
    METHYL ESTER, HYDROCHLORIDE see III:AQU250
NICOTINIPCA see III:NCQ900
NICOTINOYL HYDRAZINE see III:NCQ900, III:NDU500
NICOTINSAURE (GERMAN) see III:NCQ900
NICOTINYLHYDRAZIDE see III:NDU500
NICOTION see III:EPQ000
NICOULINE see III:RNZ000
NICOVASAN see III:NCQ900
NICOVASEN see III:NCQ900
NICOVEL see III:NCQ900
NICOZIDE see III:ILD000
NICYL see III:NCQ900
NIDA see I:MMN250
NIDATON see III:ILD000
NIDRAZID see III:ILD000
NIEA see III:HKW475
NIFULIDONE see III:NGG500
NIFURADENE see II:NDY000
NIFURAN see III:NGG500
NIFURATRONE see III:HKW450
NIFURDAZIL see III:EAE500
NIFURTHIAZOLE see II:NDY500
NIFURTIMOX see III:NGG000
NIFUZON see II:NGE500
NIGLYCON see III:NGY000
NIHONTHRENE GOLDEN YELLOW see III:DCZ000
NIKA-TEMP see III:PKQ059
NIKAVINYL SG 700 see III:PKQ059
NIKKELTETRACARBONYL (DUTCH) see I:NCZ000
NIKKOL TO see III:PKL100
NIKOZID see III:ILD000
NILOX PBNA see II:PFT500
NIMCO CHOLESTEROL BASE H see III:CMD750
NINCALUICOLFLASTINE see III:VKZ000
NINOL AA62 EXTRA see III:LBL000
NIONATE see III:FBK000
NIONG see III:NGY000
NIP see I:DFT800
NIPA 49 see III:PNM750
NIPAGALLIN P see III:PNM750
NIPANTIOX 1-F see II:BQI000
NIPAR S-20 see I:NIY000
NIPAR S-20 SOLVENT see I:NIY000
NIPAR S-30 SOLVENT see I:NIY000
NIPELLEN see III:NCQ900
NIPEON A 21 see III:PKQ059
NIPLEN see III:ILD000
NIPOL 407 see III:SMR000
NIPOL 576 see III:PKQ059
NIPPON BLUE BB see I:CMO000
NIPPON DEEP BLACK see I:AQP000
NIRAN see II:CDR750, III:PAK000
NIRAN E-4 see III:PAK000
NIRIDAZOLE see II:NML000
NIRVONAL see II:EOK000
NISOTIN see III:EPQ000
NITADON see III:ILD000
NITEBAN see III:ILD000
NITHIAZID see II:ENV500

NITHIAZIDE see II:ENV500
NITOBANIL see III:FMB000
NITOFEN see I:DFT800
NITOL see I:BIE500
NITOL "TAKEDA" see I:BIE500
NITRAFEN see I:DFT800
NITRAMIN see III:ALQ000
NITRAMINE see III:ALQ000
NITRAN see III:DUV600
NITRAPHEN see I:DFT800
NITRATE d'ARGENT (FRENCH) see III:SDS000
NITRATE de PLOMB (FRENCH) see III:LDO000
NITRATE de SODIUM (FRENCH) see III:SIO900
NITRATINE see III:SIO900
NITRATION BENZENE see I:BBL250
NITRIC ACID, BERYLLIUM SALT see I:BFT000
NITRIC ACID, CADMIUM SALT see I:CAH000
NITRIC ACID, CADMIUM SALT, TETRAHYDRATE see
    I:CAH250
NITRIC ACID, COBALT (2+) SALT see III:CNC500
NITRIC ACID, LEAD (2+) SALT see III:LDO000
NITRIC ACID, NICKEL(II) SALT see II:NDG000
NITRIC ACID, NICKEL(2+) SALT, HEXAHYDRATE see
    II:NDG500
NITRIC ACID, SILVER(1+) SALT see III:SDS000
NITRIC ACID, SODIUM SALT see III:SIO900
NITRIC ACID TRIESTER of GLYCEROL see III:NGY000
NITRIC ACID, YTTRIUM(3+) SALT see III:YFJ000
NITRIDAZOLE see II:NML000
NITRILE ACRILICO (ITALIAN) see I:ADX500
NITRILE ACRYLIQUE (FRENCH) see I:ADX500
NITRILOACETIC ACID TRISODIUM SALT MONOHYDRATE
    see II:NEI000
NITRILOTRIACETIC ACID see I:AMT500
NITRILOTRIACETIC ACID, TRISODIUM SALT see III:SIP500
NITRILOTRIACETIC ACID TRISODIUM SALT MONOHY-
    DRATE see II:NEI000
NITRILO-2,2',2''-TRIETHANOL see III:TKP500
2,2',2''-NITRILOTRIETHANOL see III:TKP500
NITRINE-TDC see III:NGY000
N-NITROSO-N-(2,3-DIHYDROXYPROPYL)-N-(2-HYDROXY-
    ETHYL)AMINE see III:NBR100
NITRITE de SODIUM (FRENCH) see III:SIQ500
5-NITROACENAPHTHENE see I:NEJ500
5-NITROACENAPHTHYLENE see I:NEJ500
5-NITROACENAPTHENE see I:NEJ500
2-NITRO-4-ACETAMINOFENETOL (CZECH) see III:NEL000
3-NITRO-p-ACETOPHENETIDE see III:NEL000
3-NITRO-p-ACETOPHENETIDIDE see III:NEL000
5-NITRO-p-ACETOPHENETIDIDE see III:NEL000
3'-NITRO-p-ACETOPHENETIDIN see III:NEL000
4-NITRO-2-AMINOFENOL (CZECH) see III:NEM500
p-NITROAMINOFENOL (POLISH) see III:NEM500
4'-NITRO-4-AMINO-3-HYDROXYDIPHENYL HYDROCHLO-
    RIDE see III:AKI500
4'-NITRO-4-AMINO-3-HYDROXYDIPHENYL HYDROGEN
    CHLORIDE see III:AKI500
2-NITRO-4-AMINOPHENOL see II:NEM480
o-NITRO-p-AMINOPHENOL see II:NEM480
p-NITRO-o-AMINOPHENOL see III:NEM500
5-NITRO-2-AMINOTHIAZOLE see III:ALQ000
4-NITRO-2-AMINOTOLUENE (MAK) see I:NMP500
4-NITROANILINE, 2,6-DICHLORO- see III:RDP300
5-NITRO-o-ANISIDINE see II:NEQ500
2-NITRO-1,4-BENZENEDIAMINE see II:ALL750
6-NITRO-BENZIMIDAZOLE see III:NFD500
5-NITRO-1H-BENZIMIDAZOLE see III:NFD500
p-NITROBENZOIC ACID, PIPERIDINO ESTER see III:NFL500
N-(4-NITRO)BENZOYLOXYPIPERIDINE see III:NFL500
6-NITROBENZ(a)PYRENE see III:NFM500
2-((m-NITROBENZYLIDENE)AMINO)ETHANOL N-OXIDE see
    III:HKW345
2-((p-NITROBENZYLIDENE)AMINO)ETHANOL N-OXIDE see
    III:HKW350

NITROGEN LIME see III:CAQ250
NITROGEN MUSTARD see I:BIE250
NITROGEN MUSTARD AMINE OXIDE see III:CFA500
NITROGEN MUSTARD HYDROCHLORIDE see I:BIE500
NITROGEN MUSTARD OXIDE see II:CFA750
NITROGEN MUSTARD-N-OXIDE see II:CFA750,
  III:CFA500
NITROGEN MUSTARD-N-OXIDE HYDROCHLORIDE see
  II:CFA750
NITROGLICERINA (ITALIAN) see III:NGY000
NITROGLICERYNA (POLISH) see III:NGY000
NITROGLYCERIN see III:NGY000
NITROGLYCERINE see III:NGY000
NITROGLYCERIN, LIQUID, DESENSITIZED (DOT) see
  III:NGY000
NITROGLYCERIN, LIQUID, NOT DESENSITIZED (DOT) see
  III:NGY000
NITROGLYCEROL see III:NGY000
NITROGLYN see III:NGY000
NITROGRANULOGEN see I:BIE500
NITROGRANULOGEN HYDROCHLORIDE see I:BIE500
3-NITRO-3-HEXENE see III:NHE000
6-NITRO-4-HYDROXYLAMINOQUINOLINE-1-OXIDE see
  III:HIX500
7-NITRO-4-HYDROXYLAMINOQUINOLINE-1-OXIDE see
  III:HIY000
5-NITRO-8-HYDROXYQUINOLINE see III:NHF500
1-NITRO-2-IMIDAZOLIDONE see III:NKL000
N-NITRO-2-IMIDAZOLIDONE see III:NKL000
NITROISOPROPANE see I:NIY000
NITROL see III:NGY000, III:NHK800
NITROLIME see III:CAQ250
NITROLINGUAL see III:NGY000
NITROLOWE see III:NGY000
NITROL (PROMOTER) see III:NHK800
3-NITRO-6-METHOXYANILINE see II:NEQ500
5-NITRO-2-METHOXYANILINE see II:NEQ500
2-NITRO-7-METHOXYNAPHTHO(2,1-b)FURAN see
  II:MFB400
1-NITRO-2-METHYLANTHRAQUINONE see II:MMG000
NITROMIM see II:CFA750
NITROMIN HYDROCHLORIDE see II:CFA750
NITROMIN IDO see III:ALQ000
2-NITRONAPHTHALENE see I:NHQ500
β-NITRONAPHTHALENE see I:NHQ500
5-NITRONAPHTHALENE ETHYLENE see I:NEJ500
2-NITRONAPHTHO(2,1-b)FURAN see III:NHQ950
3-NITRO-2-NAPHTHYLAMINE see III:NHR500
NITRONET see III:NGY000
NITRONG see III:NGY000
N'-NITRO-N-NITROSO-N-METHYLGUANIDINE see
  II:MMP000
3-NITRO-1-NITROSO-1-PENTYLGUANIDINE see III:NLC500
NITRON LAVSAN see III:PKF750
NITRON (POLYESTER) see III:PKF750
5-NITRO-N-(2-OXO-3-OXAZOLIDINYL)-2-FURANMETHANI-
  MINE see III:NGG500
p-NITROPEROXYBENZOIC ACID see III:NIB000
NITROPHEN see I:DFT800
NITROPHENE see I:DFT800
p-NITROPHENOL, O-ESTER with O,O-DIETHYLPHOSPHO-
  ROTHIOATE see III:PAK000
4-((p-NITROPHENYL)AZO)DIPHENYLAMINE see III:NIK000
7-((NITROPHENYL)AZO)METHYLBENZ(c)ACRIDINE see
  III:NIK500
d-(−)-threo-1-p-NITROPHENYL-2-DICHLORACETAMIDO-1,3-
  PROPANEDIOL see II:CDP250
d-threo-1-(p-NITROPHENYL)-2-(DICHLOROACETYLAMINO)-
  1,3-PROPANEDIOL see II:CDP250
p-NITROPHENYLDIMETHYLTHIONOPHOSPHATE see
  III:MNH000
1-(p-NITROPHENYL-3,3-DIMETHYL-TRIAZEN (GERMAN)
  see III:DSX400
1-(4-NITROPHENYL)-3,3-DIMETHYLTRIAZENE see
  III:DSX400

1-(p-NITROPHENYL)-3,3-DIMETHYL-TRIAZENE see
  III:DSX400
NITRO-p-PHENYLENEDIAMINE see II:ALL750
2-NITRO-p-PHENYLENEDIAMINE see II:ALL750
2-NITRO-1,4-PHENYLENEDIAMINE see II:ALL750
o-NITRO-p-PHENYLENEDIAMINE (MAK) see II:ALL750
4-(4-NITROPHENYL)THIAZOLE see III:NIW400
NITROPONE C see III:BRE500
2-NITROPROPANE see I:NIY000
β-NITROPROPANE see I:NIY000
3-NITROPROPIONIC ACID see III:NIY500
β-NITROPROPIONIC ACID see III:NIY500
1-NITROPYRENE see I:NJA000
3-NITROPYRENE see II:NJA000
4-NITROPYRENE see III:NJA100
4-NITROPYRIDINE-1-OXIDE see III:NJA500
4-NITROPYRIDINE-N-OXIDE see III:NJA500
4-NITROQUINALDINE-N-OXIDE see III:MMQ250
2-NITROQUINOLINE see III:NJB500
8-NITROQUINOLINE see III:NJD500
4-NITROQUINOLINE-6-CARBOXYLIC ACID-1-OXIDE see
  III:CCG000
4-NITRO-6-QUINOLINECARBOXYLIC ACID-1-OXIDE see
  III:CCG000
4-NITROQUINOLINE-1-OXIDE see II:NJF000
4-NITROQUINOLINE-N-OXIDE see II:NJF000
5-NITRO-8-QUINOLINOL see III:NHF500
NITROSAMINES see I:NJH000
N-NITROSAMINO DIACETONITRIL (GERMAN) see
  III:NKL500
N-NITROSAZETIDINE see III:NJL000
NITROSIMINODIACETONITRILE see III:NKL500
N-NITROSO-N-(1-ACETOXYMETHYL)BUTYLAMINE see
  III:BRX500
N-NITROSO-N-(ACETOXYMETHYL)-N-ISOBUTYLAMINE
  see III:ABR125
N-NITROSO-N-(ACETOXY)METHYL-N-METHYLAMINE see
  II:AAW000
N-NITROSO-N-(1-ACETOXYMETHYL)PROPYL AMINE see
  III:PNR250
NITROSO-N-(1-
  ACETOXYMETHYL)TRIDEUTEROMETHYLAMINE see
  III:MMS000
1-NITROSO-4-ACETYL-3,5-DIMETHYLPIPERAZINE see
  III:NJI850
N-NITROSOAETHYLAETHANOLAMIN (GERMAN) see
  II:ELG500
NITROSOAETHYLDIMETHYLHARNSTOFF see III:DRV600
NITROSOALDICARB see III:NJJ500
N-NITROSOALLYL-2,3-DIHYDROXYPROPYLAMINE see
  III:NJY500
N-NITROSOALLYLETHANOLAMINE see III:NJJ875
NITROSO-ALLYL-2-HYDROXYPROPYLAMINE see
  III:NJJ950
N-NITROSOALLYL-2-HYDROXYPROPYLAMINE see
  III:NJJ950
N-NITROSO-N-ALLYL-N-(2-HYDROXYPROPYL)AMINE see
  III:NJJ950
N-NITROSOALLYLMETHYLAMINE see III:MMT500
N-NITROSOALLYL-2-OXOPROPYLAMINE see III:AGM125
N-NITROSOAMINODIETHANOL see I:NKM000
4-(NITROSOAMINO-N-METHYL)-1-(3-PYRIDYL)-1-BUTA-
  NONE see II:MMS500
1-NITROSOANABASINE see III:NJK150
N-NITROSOANABASINE see III:NJK150
N'-NITROSOANABASINE see III:NJK150
N-(p-NITROSOANILINOMETHYL)-2-NITROPROPANE see
  III:NHK800
N-NITROSOAZACYCLOHEPTANE see II:NKI000
N-NITROSOAZACYCLONONANE see III:OCA000
N-NITROSOAZACYCLOOCTANE see III:OBY000
1-NITROSOAZACYCLOTRIDECANE see III:NJK500
NITROSO-AZETIDIN (GERMAN) see III:NJL000
NITROSOAZETIDINE see III:NJL000

NITROSOTRIS(CHLOROETHYL)UREA see III:NLZ000
1-NITROSO-1,3,3-TRIS-(2-CHLOROETHYL)UREA see III:NLZ000
NITROSOUNDECYLUREA see III:NMA000
N-NITROSO-N-UNDECYLUREA see III:NMA000
NITRO-SPAN see III:NGY000
NITROSTAT see III:NGY000
NITROSTIGMIN (GERMAN) see III:PAK000
NITROSTIGMINE see III:PAK000
4-NITROSTILBEN (GERMAN) see III:NMC000
4-NITROSTILBENE see III:NMC000
7-(m-NITROSTYRYL)BENZ(c)ACRIDINE see III:NMD500
7-(o-NITROSTYRYL)BENZ(c)ACRIDINE see III:NME000
7-(p-NITROSTYRYL)BENZ(c)ACRIDINE see III:NME500
12-(m-NITROSTYRYL)BENZ(a)ACRIDINE see III:NMF000
12-(o-NITROSTYRYL)BENZ(a)ACRIDINE see III:NMF500
12-(p-NITROSTYRYL)BENZ(a)ACRIDINE see III:NMG000
3-NITRO-1,2,4,5-TETRACHLOROBENZENE see III:TBR750
4-NITRO-1,2,3,5-TETRACHLORO-BENZENE see III:TBR500
NITROTHIAMIDAZOL see II:NML000
NITROTHIAMIDAZOLE see II:NML000
NITROTHIAZOLE see II:NML000
5-NITRO-2-THIAZOLYLAMINE see III:ALQ000
1-(5-NITRO-2-THIAZOLYL)IMIDAZOLIDIN-2-ONE see II:NML000
1-(5-NITRO-2-THIAZOLYL)-2-IMIDAZOLIDINONE see II:NML000
1-(5-NITRO-2-THIAZOLYL)-2-IMIDAZOLINONE see II:NML000
1-(5-NITRO-2-THIAZOLYL)-2-OXOTETRAHYDROIMIDAZOL see II:NML000
1-(5-NITRO-2-THIAZOLYL)-2-OXOTETRAHYDROIMIDA-ZOLE see II:NML000
5-NITRO-o-TOLUIDINE see I:NMP500
NITROTRICHLOROMETHANE see III:CKN500
NITROUS ACID, SODIUM SALT see III:SIQ500
NITROUS DIPHENYLAMIDE see III:DWI000
NITROX see III:MNH000
NITROZAN K see III:MJG750
NITROZONE see II:NGE500
NITRUMON see I:BIF750
NIUIF-100 see III:PAK000
NIVACHINE see III:CLD000
NIVALENOL-4-O-ACETATE see III:FQR000
NIVAQUINE B see III:CLD000
NIZOTIN see III:EPQ000
NK 631 see III:PCB000
NK-843 see III:NGY000
NMA see I:MMU250
NMBA see III:MHW500
NMBA-d2 see III:NKT100
NMBA-d3 see III:NKT105
NMDDA see III:NKU000
NMDHP see III:NMV450
NMEA see I:MKB000
p-(N'-METHYLHYDRAZINOMETHYL)-N-ISOPROPYL) BENZAMIDE see I:PME500
p-(N'-METHYLHYDRAZINOMETHYL)-N-ISOPROPYL-BENZAMIDE HYDROCHLORIDE see I:PME500
NMH see I:MNA750
NMHP see III:NKU500
NMNA see III:NKU570
NMOP see II:NKV000
NMOR see I:NKZ000
NMU see I:MNA750
NMUM see II:MMX250
N-MUSTARD (GERMAN) see I:BIE500
NMUT see II:MMX250
NMVA see II:NKY000
NNA see III:MMS250
NNK see II:MMS500
NNN see I:NLD500
NOAN see III:DCK759
NOBECUTAN see III:TFS350

NOBEDON see II:HIM000
NOBILEN see III:TFR250
NOBLEN see III:PMP500
NO BUNT LIQUID see I:HCC500
NOCBIN see III:DXH250
No. 3 CONC. SCARLET see III:CHP500
NOCTAZEPAM see III:CFZ000
NOCTEC see III:CDO000
NOCTOSEDIV see III:TEH500
NO-DHU see III:NJY000
NO-DOZ see III:CAK500
NO-ETU see III:NKK500
NOFLAMOL see I:PJL750
NOGEST see II:MCA000
NOHDABZ see III:HKB000
NOHFAA see II:HIP000
NOMERSAN see III:TFS350
No. 907 METRO TALC see III:TAB750
NONABROMOBIPHENYL see III:NMV735
1-NONANOYLAZIRIDINE see III:NNA000
NONANOYLETHYLENEIMINE see III:NNA000
NONOX CL see III:NBL000
NONOX D see II:PFT500
NONOX DPPD see III:BLE500
NONOX TBC see III:BFW750
1-NONYLAMINE, N-METHYL-N-NITROSO- see III:NKU580
NONYLCARBINOL see III:DAI600
No. 156 ORANGE CHROME see I:LCS000
NOPCOCIDE see III:TBQ750
NO-PIP see I:NLJ500
NO-Pro see III:NLL500
NOPTIL see II:EOK000
NO-PYR see I:NLP500
NORACYCLINE see II:LJE000
20-NORCROTALANAN-11,15-DIONE, 3,8-DIDEHYDRO-14,19-DIHYDRO-12,13-DIHYDROXY-, (13-α-14-α)- see III:DAL350
NORDETTE see III:NNL500
NORDICOL see I:EDO000
NORDIOL see III:NNL500
NORDIOL-28 see III:NNL500
NORDOPAN see II:BIA250
NORETHANDROL see I:EAP000
NORETHINDRONE-17-ACETATE see II:ABU000
NORETHINDRONE ACETATE and ETHINYLESTRADIOL see II:EEH520
NORETHINDRONE mixed with ETHYNYLESTRADIOL see III:EQM500
NORETHINDRONE mixed with MESTRANOL see III:MDL750
NORETHINODREL see II:EEH550
19-NOR-ETHINYL-4,5-TESTOSTERONE see I:NNP500
19-NOR-ETHINYL-5,10-TESTOSTERONE see II:EEH550
NORETHINYNODREL see II:EEH550
19-NORETHISTERONE see I:NNP500
19-NORETHISTERONE ACETATE see II:ABU000
NORETHISTERONE ACETATE mixed with ETHINYL OESTRA-DIOL see II:EEH520
NORETHISTERONE ENANTHATE see III:NNQ000
NORETHISTERONE mixed with ETHINYL OESTRADIOL (60:1) see III:EQM500
NORETHISTERONE mixed with MESTRANOL see III:MDL750
NORETHISTERONE OENANTHATE see III:NNQ000
NORETHYNODRAL see II:EEH550
NORETHYNODREL see II:EEH550
19-NORETHYNODREL see II:EEH550
NORETHYNODREL and ETHINYLESTRADIOL-3-METHYL ETHER (50:1) see I:EAP000
NORETHYNODREL mixed with MESTRANOL see I:EAP000
19-NOR-17-α-ETHYNYLANDROSTEN-17-β-OL-3-ONE see I:NNP500
19-NOR-17-α-ETHYNYL-17-β-HYDROXY-4-ANDROSTEN-3-ONE see I:NNP500
19-NOR-17-α-ETHYNYLTESTOSTERONE see I:NNP500
19-NORETHYNYLTESTOSTERONE ACETATE see II:ABU000

1,2,4,5,6,7,8,8-OCTACHLORO-2,3,3a,4,7,7a-HEXAHYDRO-4,7-METHANOINDENE see II:CDR750

1,2,4,5,6,7,8,8-OCTACHLORO-2,3,3a,4,7,7a-HEXAHYDRO-4,7-METHANO-1H-INDENE see II:CDR750

OCTACHLORO-HEXAHYDRO-METHANOISOBENZOFURAN see III:OAN000

1,3,4,5,6,8,8-OCTACHLORO-1,3,3a,4,7,7a-HEXAHYDRO-4,7-METHANO ISOBENZOFURAN see III:OAN000

1,2,4,5,6,7,8,8-OCTACHLORO-3a,4,7,7a-HEXAHYDRO-4,7-METHYLENE INDANE see II:CDR750

OCTACHLORO-4,7-METHANOHYDROINDANE see II:CDR750

OCTACHLORO-4,7-METHANOTETRAHYDROINDANE see II:CDR750

1,2,4,5,6,7,8,8-OCTACHLORO-4,7-METHANO-3a,4,7,7a-TETRAHYDROINDANE see II:CDR750

1,3,4,5,6,7,10,10-OCTACHLORO-4,7-endo-METHYLENE-4,7,8,9-TETRAHYDROPHTHALAN see III:OAN000

1,3,4,5,6,7,8,8-OCTACHLORO-2-OXA-3a,4,7,7a-TETRAHYDRO-4,7-METHANOINDENE see III:OAN000

1,2,4,5,6,7,8,8-OCTACHLORO-3a,4,7,7a-TETRAHYDRO-4,7-METHANOINDAN see II:CDR750

1,2,4,5,6,7,8,8-OCTACHLORO-3a,4,7,7a-TETRAHYDRO-4,7-METHANOINDENE see II:CDR750

1,2,4,5,6,7,10,10-OCTACHLORO-4,7,8,9-TETRAHYDRO-4,7-METHYLENEINDANE see II:CDR750

1,2,4,5,6,7,8,8-OCTACHLOR-3a,4,7,7a-TETRAHYDRO-4,7-endo-METHANO-INDAN (GERMAN) see II:CDR750

OCTADECANNAMIDE see III:OAR000

OCTADECANOIC ACID see III:SLK000

OCTADECANOIC ACID, CADMIUM SALT see I:OAT000

OCTADECANOIC ACID, METHYL ESTER see III:MJW000

OCTADECANOL see III:OAX000

1-OCTADECANOL see III:OAX000

n-OCTADECANOL see III:OAX000

9,12,15-OCTADECATRIENEPEROXOIC ACID (Z,Z,Z) (9CI) see III:PCN000

9,10-OCTADECENOIC ACID see III:OHU000

cis-OCTADEC-9-ENOIC ACID see III:OHU000

cis-9-OCTADECENOIC ACID see III:OHU000

cis-Δ⁹-OCTADECENOIC ACID see III:OHU000

(Z)-9-OCTADECENOIC ACID METHYL ESTER see III:OHW000

(Z)-9-OCTADECENOIC ACID mixed with (Z,Z)-9,12-OCTADECADIENOIC ACID see III:LGI000

OCTA DECYL ALCOHOL see III:OAX000

n-OCTADECYL ALCOHOL see III:OAX000

OCTAHYDROAZOCINE HYDROCHLORIDE mixed with SODIUM NITRITE (1:1) see III:SIT000

OCTAHYDRODIBENZ(a,h)ANTHRACENE see III:OBW000

OCTAHYDRO-1:2:5:6-DIBENZANTHRACENE see III:OBW000

2,5,5a,6,9,10,10a,1a-OCTAHYDRO-4-HYDROXYMETHYL-1,1,7,9-TETRAMETHYL-5,5a-6-TRIHYDROXY-1H-2,8a-METHANOCYCLOPENTA(a)CYCLOPROPA(e)CYCLODECEN-11-ONE-5-HEXADECANOATE see III:OBW509

1,2,6,7,8,9,10,12b-OCTAHYDRO-3-METHYLBENZ(j)ACEANTHRYLENE see III:HDR500

OCTAHYDRO-1-NITROSOAZOCINE see III:OBY000

OCTAHYDRO-1-NITROSO-1H-AZONINE see III:OCA000

OCTA-KLOR see II:CDR750

OCTALENE see III:AFK250

OCTALOX see III:DHB400

OCTANE-1-NNO-AZOXYMETHANE see III:MGT000

OCTANOIC ACID, CADMIUM SALT (2:1) see I:CAD750

OCTAN WINYLU (POLISH) see III:VLU250

OCTOIL see I:DVL700

OCTOWY ALDEHYD (POLISH) see II:AAG250

OCTYL ACRYLATE see III:ADU250

OCTYL ADIPATE see III:AEO000

1-OCTYLAMINE, N-METHYL-N-NITROSO- see III:NKU590

OCTYLENE EPOXIDE see III:ECE000

n-OCTYLISOSAFROLE SULFOXIDE see III:ISA000

n-OCTYL NITROSOUREA see III:NLD800

cis-3-OCTYL-OXIRANEOCTANOIC ACID see III:ECD500

p-tert-OCTYLPHENOL see III:TDN500

p-tert-OCTYLPHENOXYETHOXYETHYLDIMETHYLBENZYL AMMONIUM CHLORIDE see III:BEN000

OCTYL PHTHALATE see I:DVL700

ODA see II:SJN700

ODB see I:EDP000, III:DEP600

ODCB see III:DEP600

OE3 see II:EDU500

OEKOLP see I:DKA600

OESTERGON see I:EDO000

OESTRADIOL see I:EDO000

d-OESTRADIOL see I:EDO000

α-OESTRADIOL see I:EDO000

β-OESTRADIOL see I:EDO000

OESTRADIOL-17-α see III:EDO500

OESTRADIOL-17-β see I:EDO000

cis-OESTRADIOL see I:EDO000

3,17-β-OESTRADIOL see I:EDO000

d-3,17-β-OESTRADIOL see I:EDO000

OESTRADIOL BENZOATE see I:EDP000

OESTRADIOL-3-BENZOATE see I:EDP000

β-OESTRADIOL BENZOATE see I:EDP000

β-OESTRADIOL-3-BENZOATE see I:EDP000

17-β-OESTRADIOL-3-BENZOATE see I:EDP000

OESTRADIOL DIPROPIONATE see I:EDR000

β-OESTRADIOL DIPROPIONATE see I:EDR000

17-β-OESTRADIOL DIPROPIONATE see I:EDR000

OESTRADIOL-3,17-DIPROPIONATE see I:EDR000

3,17-β-OESTRADIOL DIPROPIONATE see I:EDR000

OESTRADIOL MONOBENZOATE see I:EDP000

OESTRADIOL MUSTARD see III:EDR500

OESTRADIOL PHOSPHATE POLYMER see I:EDS000

OESTRADIOL POLYESTER with PHOSPHORIC ACID see I:EDS000

OESTRADIOL R see I:EDO000

OESTRAFORM (BDH) see I:EDP000

OESTRASID see II:DAL600

OESTRA-1,3,5(10)-TRIENE-3,17-β-DIOL see I:EDO000

17-β-OESTRA-1,3,5(10)-TRIENE-3,17-DIOL see I:EDO000

1,3,5(10)-OESTRATRIENE-3,17-β-DIOL 3-BENZOATE see I:EDP000

OESTRA-1,3,5(10)-TRIENE-3,16-α,17-β-TRIOL see II:EDU500

1,3,5-OESTRATRIENE-3-β-3,16-α,17-β-TRIOL see II:EDU500

(16-α,17-β)-OESTRA-1,3,5(10)-TRIENE-3,16,17-TRIOL see II:EDU500

1,3,5-OESTRATRIEN-3-OL-17-ONE see I:EDV000

1,3,5(10)-OESTRATRIEN-3-OL-17-ONE see I:EDV000

Δ-1,3,5-OESTRATRIEN-3-β-OL-17-ONE see I:EDV000

OESTRATRIOL see II:EDU500

OESTRILIN see I:ECU750

OESTRIN see I:EDV000

OESTRIOL see II:EDU500

16-α,17-β-OESTRIOL see II:EDU500

3,16-α,17-β-OESTRIOL see II:EDU500

OESTRODIENE see II:DAL600

OESTRODIENOL see II:DAL600

OESTRO-FEMINAL see I:ECU750

OESTROFORM see I:EDV000

OESTROGENINE see I:DKA600

OESTROGLANDOL see I:EDO000

OESTROGYNAEDRON see I:DKB000

OESTROGYNAL see I:EDO000

OESTROL VETAG see I:DKA600

OESTROMENIN see I:DKA600

OESTROMENSIL see I:DKA600

OESTROMENSYL see I:DKA600

OESTROMIENIN see I:DKA600

OESTROMON see I:DKA600

OESTRONBENZOAT (GERMAN) see II:EDV500

OESTRONE see I:EDV000

OESTROPAK MORNING see I:ECU750

OESTROPEROS see I:EDV000

OESTRORAL see II:DAL600
OFFITRIL see III:HNI500
OFHC Cu see III:CNI000
OFNA-PERL SALT RRA see II:CLK235
OFTALENT see II:CDP250
3-OHAA see III:AKE750
OH-BBN see I:HJQ350
4-OH-E2 see III:HKH850
4-OH-ESTRADIOL see III:HKH850
17-β-OH-ESTRADIOL see I:EDO000
OHIO 347 see III:EAT900
7-OHM-MBA see III:HMF000
7-OHM-12-MBA see III:HMF000
17-β-OH-OESTRADIOL see I:EDO000
OHRIC see III:DGF000
OIL of ANISEED see III:PMQ750
OIL of ARGEMONE mixed with OIL of MUSTARD see
    III:OGS000
OIL of CALAMUS, GERMAN see III:OGK000
OIL-DRI see III:AHF500
OIL of GRAPEFRUIT see III:GJU000
OIL GREEN see II:CMJ900
OIL of LEMON see III:LEI000
OIL of LIME, DISTILLED see III:OGO000
OIL MIST, MINERAL (OSHA, ACGIH) see III:MQV750
OIL of MUSTARD, ARTIFICIAL see II:AGJ250
OIL of MUSTARD, EXPRESSED mixed with OIL of ARGEMONE
    see III:OGS000
OIL ORANGE see III:PEJ500
OIL of ORANGE see III:OGY000
OIL ORANGE 2R see III:XRA000
OIL ORANGE KB see III:XRA000
OIL ORANGE N EXTRA see III:XRA000
OIL ORANGE O'PEL see II:TGW000
OIL ORANGE R see III:XRA000
OIL ORANGE SS see II:TGW000
OIL ORANGE X see III:XRA000
OIL ORANGE XO see III:XRA000
OIL RED see III:OHA000
OIL RED GRO see III:XRA000
OIL RED O see III:XRA000
OIL RED RO see III:XRA000
OIL RED XO see III:FAG080, III:XRA000
OIL SCARLET see III:OHA000, III:XRA000
OIL SCARLET 6G see III:XRA000
OIL SCARLET 371 see III:XRA000
OIL SCARLET APYO see III:XRA000
OIL SCARLET BL see III:XRA000
OIL SCARLET L see III:XRA000
OIL SCARLET YS see III:XRA000
OIL of SHADDOCK see III:GJU000
OIL-SHALE PYROLYSE LAC LSP-1 see III:LIJ000
OILS, LIME see III:OGO000
OIL SOLUBLE ANILINE YELLOW see II:PEI000
OIL of SWEET FLAG see III:OGK000
OIL of SWEET ORANGE see III:OGY000
OIL of TURPENTINE see III:TOD750
OIL of TURPENTINE, RECTIFIED see III:TOD750
OIL VIOLET see III:EOJ500
OIL YELLOW see I:AIC250, I:DOT300
OIL YELLOW 21 see I:AIC250
OIL YELLOW 2R see I:AIC250
OIL YELLOW 2681 see I:AIC250
OIL YELLOW A see I:AIC250, III:FAG130
OIL YELLOW AAB see II:PEI000
OIL YELLOW AT see I:AIC250
OIL YELLOW C see I:AIC250
OIL YELLOW HA see III:OHK000
OIL YELLOW I see I:AIC250
OIL YELLOW OB see III:FAG135
OIL YELLOW OPS see III:OHK000
OIL YELLOW T see I:AIC250
OKASA-MASCUL see I:TBG000
OKTATERR see II:CDR750

p-terc.OKTYLFENOL (CZECH) see III:TDN500
OKULTIN M see II:CIR250
OL 27-400 see III:CQH100
OLEAL ORANGE R see III:PEJ500
OLEAL ORANGE SS see II:TGW000
OLEAL YELLOW 2G see I:DOT300
OLEAL YELLOW RE see III:OHK000
OLEIC ACID see III:OHU000
OLEIC ACID GLYCIDYL ESTER see III:ECJ000
OLEIC ACID mixed with LINOLEIC ACID see III:LGI000
cis-OLEIC ACID, METHYL ESTER see III:OHW000
OLEIC ACID, ZINC SALT see III:ZJS000
OLEOFOS 20 see III:PAK000
OLEOGESAPRIM see III:ARQ725
OLEOMYCETIN see II:CDP250
OLEOPARAPHENE see III:PAK000
OLEOPARATHION see III:PAK000
OLEOPHOSPHOTHION see III:MAK700
OLEOVOFOTOX see III:MNH000
1-OLEOYLAZIRIDINE see III:OIC000
OLEOYLETHYLENEIMINE see III:OIC000
OLETAC 100 see III:PMP500
OLEUM SINAPIS VOLATILE see II:AGJ250
OLEUM TIGLII see III:COC250
OLIO DI CROTON (ITALIAN) see III:COC250
OLITREF see III:DUV600
OLOTHORB see III:PKL100
OLOW (POLISH) see II:LCF000
OLPISAN see III:PAX000
OMAHA see II:LCF000
OMAHA & GRANT see II:LCF000
OMAL see I:TIW000
OMEGA CHROME BLUE FB see III:HJF500
OM-HYDANTOINE see I:DKQ000
OM-HYDANTOINE SODIUM see I:DNU000
OMIFIN see III:CMX700
OMS 2 see III:FAQ999
OMS-47 see III:DOS000
OMS 570 see III:EAQ750
OMS 1325 see III:FAC025
OMTAN see III:OAN000
ONCB see III:CJB750
ONCO-CARBIDE see II:TGN250, III:HOO500
ONCOSTATIN K see III:AEB000
ONCOTEPA see I:TFQ750
ONCOTIOTEPA see I:TFQ750
ONCOVEDEX see III:TND000
ONCOVIN see III:LEY000, III:LEZ000
ONEX see III:CJT750
ONGROVIL S 165 see III:PKQ059
ONYX see I:SCJ500
OOS see III:TAB750
OPALON see III:PKQ059
OPALON 400 see II:AAX175
OPHTHALMADINE see III:DAS000
OPLOSSINGEN (DUTCH) see I:FMV000
OPP see III:BGJ250
OPP-Na see II:BGJ750
OPTAL see III:PND000
OP-THAL-ZIN see III:ZNA000
OPTHOCHLOR see II:CDP250
8-OQ see III:QPA000
OR 1191 see III:FAC025
ORACET SAPPHIRE BLUE G see III:TBG700
ORACON see III:DNX500
ORACONAL see III:MCA500
ORAFURAN see III:NGE000
ORAGEST see II:MCA000
ORANGE #10 see III:HGC000
1333 ORANGE see III:FAG010
ORANGE A L'HUILE see III:PEJ500
ORANGE CHROME see I:LCS000
ORANGE G (BIOLOGICAL STAIN) see III:HGC000
ORANGE G DYE see III:HGC000

ORANGE G (INDICATOR) see III:HGC000
ORANGE I see III:FAG010
ORANGE INSOLUBLE OLG see III:PEJ500, III:XRA000
ORANGE INSOLUBLE RR see III:XRA000
ORANGE NITRATE CHROME see I:LCS000
ORANGE OIL see III:OGY000
ORANGE OIL, COLDPRESSED (FCC) see III:OGY000
ORANGE OIL KB see III:XRA000
ORANGE PEL see III:PEJ500
ORANGE RESENOLE No. 3 see III:PEJ500
ORANGE SOLUBLE A l'HUILE see III:PEJ500
ORANGE 3R SOLUBLE IN GREASE see II:TGW000
ORANZ G (POLISH) see III:HGC000
ORASECRON see III:NNL500
ORASONE see III:PLZ000
ORATRAST see III:BAP000
ORAVIRON see III:MPN500
ORCANON see II:MPW500
ORCHARD BRAND ZIRAM see III:BJK500
ORCHIOL see I:TBG000
ORCHISTIN see I:TBG000
OREMET see III:TGF250
ORESTOL see I:DKB000
ORETON see I:TBG000
ORETON-F see I:TBF500
ORETON-M see III:MPN500
ORETON METHYL see III:MPN500
ORETON PROPIONATE see I:TBG000
ORF 3858 see III:FAO200
ORG 485-50 see III:NNV000
ORGA-414 see I:AMY050
ORGAMETIL see III:NNV000
ORGAMETRIL see III:NNV000
ORGAMETROL see III:NNV000
ORGAMIDE see III:PJY500
ORGANEX see III:CAK500
ORGANIC GLASS E 2 see III:PKB500
ORGANOL BORDEAUX B see III:EOJ500
ORGANOL BROWN 2R see III:NBG500
ORGANOL ORANGE see III:PEJ500
ORGANOL ORANGE 2R see II:TGW000
ORGANOL SCARLET see III:OHA000
ORGANOL YELLOW see II:PEI000
ORGANOL YELLOW 25 see I:AIC250
ORGANOL YELLOW ADM see I:DOT300
ORGANON'S DOCA ACETATE see III:DAQ800
ORGASEPTINE see III:SNM500
ORGASTYPTIN see II:EDU500
ORIENT BASIC MAGENTA see III:MAC250
ORIENT OIL ORANGE PS see III:PEJ500
ORIENT OIL YELLOW GG see I:DOT300
ORION BLUE 3B see II:CMO250
ORLUTATE see II:ABU000
ORNAMENTAL WEED see III:AJM000
ORONOL see I:ART250
OROTIC ACID mixed with CHOLESTEROL and CHOLIC ACID
    (2:2:1) see III:OJV525
ORPHENOL see II:BGJ750
ORPIMENT see I:ARI000
ORQUISTERONE see I:TBF500
ORSIN see III:PEY500
ORTHO 5865 see III:CBF800
ORTHOARSENIC ACID see I:ARB250
ORTHOARSENIC ACID HEMIHYDRATE see I:ARC500
ORTHOCIDE see III:CBG000
ORTHOCRESOL see III:CNX000
ORTHODICHLOROBENZENE see III:DEP600
ORTHODICHLOROBENZOL see III:DEP600
ORTHO GRASS KILLER see III:CBM000
ORTHOHYDROXYDIPHENYL see III:BGJ250
ORTHO-KLOR see II:CDR750
ORTHO L10 DUST see I:LCK000
ORTHO L40 DUST see I:LCK000
ORTHO MALATHION see III:MAK700

ORTHO-MITE see I:SOP500
ORTHO-NOVUM see III:MDL750
ORTHOPHALTAN see III:TIT250
ORTHOPHENYLPHENOL see III:BGJ250
ORTHOPHOS see III:PAK000
ORTHOSILICATE see II:SCN500
ORTHOTRAN see III:CJT750
ORTHOXENOL see III:BGJ250
ORTUDUR see III:PKQ059
ORVAGIL see I:MMN250
OS 1897 see I:DDL800
OSCOPHEN see III:ARP250
OSIREN see III:AFJ500
OSMOFERRIN see III:IHK000
OSMOSOL EXTRA see III:PND000
OSOCIDE see III:CBG000
OSSALIN see III:SHF500
OSSIAMINA see II:CFA750
OSSICHLORIN see II:CFA750
OSSIN see III:SHF500
OSTAMER see I:CDV625
OSTEOBOND SURGICAL BONE CEMENT see III:PKB500
OSYRITRIN see III:RSU000
OSYROL see III:AFJ500
OTETRYN see III:HOI000
OTOFURAN see II:NGE500
OTOPHEN see II:CDP250
OTRACID see III:CJT750
OTS see II:TGN250
1,2,4,5,6,7,8,8-OTTOCHLORO-3A,4,7,7A-TETRAIDRO-4,7-
    endo-METANO-INDANO (ITALIAN) see II:CDR750
OVABAN see II:VTF000
OVADZIAK see I:BBQ500
OVAHORMON see I:EDO000
OVAHORMON BENZOATE see I:EDP000
OVANON see II:LJE000
OVARIOSTAT (FRENCH) see II:LJE000
OVASTEROL see I:EDO000
OVASTEROL-B see I:EDP000
OVASTEVOL see I:EDO000
OVATRAN see III:CJT750
OVEST see I:ECU750
OVESTERIN see II:EDU500
OVESTIN see II:EDU500
OVESTINON see II:EDU500
OVESTRION see II:EDU500
OVEX see I:EDP000, I:EDV000, III:CJT750
OVIDON see III:NNL500
OVIFOLLIN see I:EDV000
OVIN see II:DNX500
OVOCHLOR see III:CJT750
OVOCICLINA see I:EDO000
OVOCYCLIN see I:EDO000
OVOCYCLIN BENZOATE see I:EDP000
OVOCYCLIN DIPROPIONATE see I:EDR000
OVOCYCLINE see I:EDO000
OVOCYCLIN M see I:EDP000
OVOCYCLIN-MB see I:EDP000
OVOCYCLIN-P see I:EDR000
OVOCYLIN see I:EDO000
OVOSTAT see III:EEH575
OVOSTAT 1375 see III:EEH575
OVOSTAT E see III:EEH575
OVOTOX see III:CJT750
OVOTRAN see III:CJT750
OVRAL see III:NNL500
OVRAL 21 see III:NNL500
OVRAL 28 see III:NNL500
OVRAN see III:NNL500
OVRANETT see III:NNL500
OVULEN see III:EQK100
OVULEN 50 see II:EQJ500
OWISPOL GF see III:SMQ500
OX see III:CFZ000

OXYFUME see I:EJN500
OXYFUME 12 see I:EJN500
OXYFURADENE see II:NDY000
OXYJECT 100 see III:HOI000
OXYLAN see I:DKQ000
OXYLITE see III:BDS000
OXYMETHALONE see I:PAN100
OXYMETHENOLONE see I:PAN100
OXYMETHOLONE see I:PAN100
OXYMETHYLENE see I:FMV000
5-OXYMETHYLFURFUROLE see III:ORG000
OXYPHENBUTAZONE see III:HNI500
OXYPHENIC ACID see III:CCP850
OXYPHENYLBUTAZONE see III:HNI500
β-OXYPROPYLPROPYLNITROSAMINE see II:ORS000
OXYPSORALEN see I:XDJ000
OXYQUINOLINE see III:QPA000
8-OXYQUINOLINE see III:QPA000
OXYQUINOLINOLEATE de CUIVRE (FRENCH) see
     III:BLC250
OXYRITIN see III:RSU000
OXYTETRACYCLINE HYDROCHLORIDE see III:HOI000
OXYTOCIC see III:EDB500
m-OXYTOLUENE see III:CNW750
o-OXYTOLUENE see III:CNX000
p-OXYTOLUENE see III:CNX250
OXYUREA see II:TGN250, III:HOO500
OXY WASH see III:BDS000
OZON (POLISH) see III:ORW000
OZONE see III:ORW000

P07 see I:PKO500
P-40 see III:DXG000
P-165 see II:ASA500
P 887 see III:ILE000
P 1531 see III:PFC750
P-2292 see III:ADA000
P-5048 see III:DRT200
PA see III:PAP750
PA 6 (polymer) see III:PJY500
PABESTROL see I:DKA600, I:DKB000
PABS see III:SNM500
PAC see III:PAK000
PACEMO see II:HIM000
PACIENX see III:CFZ000
PACITRAN see III:DCK759
PAISLEY POLYMER see III:PMP500
PAKA (HAWAII) see I:TGI100
PAKHTARAN see III:DUK800
PALACOS see III:PKB500
PALANTHRENE GOLDEN YELLOW see III:DCZ000
PALATINOL AH see I:DVL700
PALATINOL BB see III:BEC500
PALE ORANGE CHROME see I:LCS000
PALESTROL see I:DKA600
PALIUROSIDE see III:RSU000
PALLADIUM CHLORIDE see III:PAD500
PALLADIUM(2+) CHLORIDE see III:PAD500
PALLADOUS CHLORIDE see III:PAD500
PALMITIC ACID see III:PAE250
PALOPAUSE see I:ECU750
PALYGORSCITE see III:PAE750
PALYGORSKIT (GERMAN) see III:PAE750
l-PAM see I:PED750
PAMA see III:PGV250
PAMN see III:PNR250
PAMOLYN see III:OHU000
PAMOSOL 2 FORTE see III:EIR000
PANA see III:PFT250
PANADOL see II:HIM000
PANAZONE see III:PAF500
PANCID see III:SNN500
PANDEX see I:PKM250
PANESTIN see I:TBG000

PANETS see II:HIM000
PANEX see II:HIM000
PANFLAVIN see III:DBX400
PANFURAN-S see II:BKH500
PANGUL see III:TEH500
PANOFEN see II:HIM000
PANORAM 75 see III:TFS350
PANORAM D-31 see III:DHB400
PANOSINE see III:MMD500
PANOXYL see III:BDS000
PANTASOTE R 873 see III:PKQ059
PANTHER CREEK BENTONITE see III:BAV750
PANTHION see III:PAK000
PANTONSILETTEN see III:DBX400
PANTOSEDIV see III:TEH500
PANTOVERNIL see II:CDP250
PAP see I:PDC250
PAPER BLACK BA see I:AQP000
PAPER RED HRR see III:FMU070
PARA see III:PEY500
PARAAMINODIPHENYL see I:AJS100
PARABAR 441 see III:BFW750
PARACETAMOLE see II:HIM000
PARACETAMOLO (ITALIAN) see II:HIM000
PARACETANOL see II:HIM000
PARACETOPHENETIDIN see I:ABG750
PARACHLOROCIDUM see I:DAD200
PARACIDE see II:DEP800
PARACORT see III:PLZ000
PARA CRYSTALS see II:DEP800
PARADERIL see III:RNZ000
PARADI see II:DEP800
PARADICHLORBENZOL (GERMAN) see II:DEP800
PARADICHLOROBENZENE see II:DEP800
PARADICHLOROBENZOL see II:DEP800
PARA-DIEN see II:DAL600
PARADONE GOLDEN YELLOW see III:DCZ000
PARADOW see II:DEP800
PARADUST see III:PAK000
PARAFFIN see III:PAH750
PARAFFIN OILS (PETROLEUM), CATALYTIC DEWAXED
     HEAVY (9CI) see I:MQV868
PARAFFIN OILS (PETROLEUM), CATALYTIC DEWAXED
     LIGHT (9CI) see I:MQV870
PARAFFIN WAX see III:PAH750
PARAFFIN WAXES and HYDROCARBON WAXES, CHLORI-
     NATED (C12, 60% CHLORINE) see II:PAH800
PARAFFIN WAXES and HYDROCARBON WAXES, CHLORI-
     NATED (C23, 43% CHLORINE) see III:PAH810
PARAFFIN WAX FUME (ACGIH) see III:PAH750
PARAFORM see I:FMV000
PARAFUCHSIN (GERMAN) see II:RMK020
PARAGLAS see III:PKB500
PARA-MAGENTA see II:RMK020
PARAMAL see III:DBM800
PARAMAR see III:PAK000
PARAMAR 50 see III:PAK000
PARAMETHYL PHENOL see III:CNX250
PARAMINE BLACK B see AQP000
PARAMINE BLUE 2B see I:CMO000
PARAMINE BLUE 3B see II:CMO250
PARAMINE FAST VIOLET N see III:CMP000
PARAMINYL MALEATE see III:DBM800
PARAMOTH see II:DEP800
PARANAPHTHALENE see III:APG500
PARANITROSODIMETHYLANILIDE see III:DSY600
PARANTEN see III:DCK759
PARANUGGETS see II:DEP800
PARAPAN see II:HIM000
PARAPEST M-50 see III:MNH000
PARAPHENOLAZO ANILINE see II:PEI000
PARAPHENYLEN-DIAMINE see III:PEY500
PARAPHOS see III:PAK000
PARAPLEX P 543 see III:PKB500

PARAROSANILINE see II:RMK020
PARAROSANILINE CHLORIDE see II:RMK020
PARAROSANILINE HYDROCHLORIDE see II:RMK020
PARASCORBIC ACID see III:PAJ500
PARASORBIC ACID see III:PAJ500
(+)-PARASORBINSAEURE (GERMAN) see III:PAJ500
PARASPEN see II:HIM000
PARATAF see III:MNH000
PARATHENE see III:PAK000
PARATHION see III:PAK000
M-PARATHION see III:MNH000
PARATHION-ETHYL see III:PAK000
PARATHION, LIQUID (DOT) see III:PAK000
PARATHION METHYL see III:MNH000
PARATHION-METILE (ITALIAN) see III:MNH000
PARATOX see III:MNH000
PARAWET see III:PAK000
PARAXENOL see III:BGJ500
PARAXIN see II:CDP250
PARAZENE see II:DEP800
PARCLOID see III:PKQ059
PARDA see III:DNA200
PARDROYD see I:PAN100
PAR ESTRO see I:ECU750
PARFURAN see II:NGE000
PARIDINE RED LCL see III:CHP500
PARIS YELLOW see I:LCR000
PARKIBLEU see II:CMO250
PARKIPAN see II:CMO250
PARKOTAL see II:EOK000
PARMOL see II:HIM000
PAROL see III:MQV750
PAROLEINE see III:MQV750
PARRAFIN OIL see III:MQV750
PARZATE see III:EIR000
PATENTBLAU V (GERMAN) see III:ADE500
PATENT BLUE AE see III:FMU059
PATTINA V 82 see III:PKQ059
PATULIN see III:CMV000
PAVISOID see I:PAN100
PAXATE see III:DCK759
PAXEL see III:DCK759
PAYZONE see III:PAF500
PB see III:PIX250
PBB see II:FBU509, III:FBU000
PBNA see II:PFT500
PB-1,6-QUINONE see III:BCU500
PBS see I:SID000
PBZ see II:BRF500
PCA see III:MCR750
PCB see I:PME250
PCB (DOT, USDA) see I:PJL750
PCB HYDROCHLORIDE see I:PME500
PCB's see I:PJM500, II:PJN000
PCC see I:CDV100
PCEO see III:TBQ275
PCNB see III:PAX000
PCP see II:PAX250
PCPCBS see III:CJT750
PD 71627 see III:AJR400
PD 109394 see III:AAI100
2-N-p-PDA see II:ALL750
P.D.A.B. see I:DOT300
p-PDA HCl see III:PEY650
PDB see II:DEP800
PDCB see II:DEP800
PDD see III:PGT250
p-PD HCl see III:PEY650
PDMT see III:DTP000
PDP see I:PDC250
PDT see III:DTP000
PEACOCK BLUE X-1756 see III:FMU059
PEANUT OIL see III:PAO000
PEARLPUSS see III:CCL250

PEARL STEARIC see III:SLK000
PEB1 see I:DAD200
PEBC see III:PNF500
PEBULATE see III:PNF500
PECAN SHELL POWDER see III:PAO000
PEDIAFLOR see III:SHF500
PEDIDENT see III:SHF500
PEDRACZAK see I:BBQ500
PEDRIC see II:HIM000
PEERAMINE BLACK E see AQP000
PEG see III:PJT000
PEG 1000 see III:PJT250
PEGOTERATE see III:PKF750
PELADOW see III:CAO750
PELAGOL CD see III:PEY650
PELAGOL D see III:PEY500
PELAGOL DA see I:DBO000
PELAGOL DR see III:PEY500
PELAGOL GREY see I:DBO400
PELAGOL GREY C see III:CCP850
PELAGOL GREY CD see III:PEY650
PELAGOL GREY D see III:PEY500
PELAGOL GREY J see I:TGL750
PELAGOL GREY L see I:DBO000
PELAGOL GREY RS see III:REA000
PELAGOL L see I:DBO000
PELARGIDENOLON see III:ICE000
PELAZID see III:ILD000
PELLAGRAMIN see III:NCQ900
PELLAGRA PREVENTIVE FACTOR see III:NCQ900
ANTI-PELLAGRA VITAMIN see III:NCQ900
PELLAGRIN see III:NCQ900
PELLON 2506 see III:PMP500
PELLUGEL see III:CCL250
PELONIN see III:NCQ900
PELTOL D see III:PEY500
PELUCES see III:CLY500
PEN-A-BRASIVE see III:BFD250
d-PENAMINE see III:MCR750
PENATIN see III:CMV000
PENCHLOROL see II:PAX250
PENCIL GREEN SF see III:FAF000
PENCILLIC ACID see III:PAP750
PENCOGEL see III:CCL250
PENETECK see III:MQV750
PENICIDIN see III:CMV000
PENICILLAMIN see III:MCR750
(S)-PENICILLAMIN see III:MCR750
PENICILLAMINE see III:MCR750
d-PENICILLAMINE see III:MCR750
PENICILLIC ACID see III:PAP750
PENICILLIN G see III:BDY669
PENICILLIN-G, MONOSODIUM SALT see III:BFD250
PENICILLIN G, SODIUM see III:BFD250
PENICILLIN G, SODIUM SALT see III:BFD250
PENICILLIUM ROQUEFORTI TOXIN see III:PAQ875
PENICIN see III:PCU500
PENILARYN see III:BFD250
PENITE see I:SEY500
PENNAC CBS see III:CPI250
PENNAC CRA see I:IAQ000
PENNAC MBT POWDER see II:BDF000
PENNAC MS see III:BJL600
PENNAC ZT see III:BHA750
PENNAMINE see II:DAA800
PENNCAP-M see III:MNH000
PENNWHITE see III:SHF500
PENNZONE E see III:DKC400
PENPHENE see I:CDV100
PENRECO see III:MQV750
PENTA see II:PAX250
PENTABROMOPHENYL ETHER see III:PAU500
PENTACHLOORETHAAN (DUTCH) see III:PAW500
PENTACHLOORFENOL (DUTCH) see II:PAX250

PENTACHLORAETHAN (GERMAN) see III:PAW500
PENTACHLORETHANE (FRENCH) see III:PAW500
PENTACHLORIN see I:DAD200
PENTACHLORNITROBENZOL (GERMAN) see III:PAX000
1,2,3,7,8-PENTACHLORODIBENZO-p-DIOXIN see III:PAW000
PENTACHLOROETHANE see III:PAW500
PENTACHLOROFENOL see II:PAX250
PENTACHLORONITROBENZENE see III:PAX000
PENTACHLOROPHENATE see II:PAX250
PENTACHLOROPHENOL see II:PAX250
2,3,4,5,6-PENTACHLOROPHENOL see II:PAX250
PENTACHLOROPHENOL (GERMAN) see II:PAX250
PENTACHLOROPHENOL, DOWICIDE EC-7 see II:PAX250
PENTACHLOROPHENOL, DP-2 see II:PAX250
PENTACHLOROPHENOL, TECHNICAL see II:PAX250
PENTACHLOROPHENYL CHLORIDE see I:HCC500
PENTACLOROETANO (ITALIAN) see III:PAW500
PENTACLOROFENOLO (ITALIAN) see II:PAX250
PENTACON see II:PAX250
1-PENTADECANECARBOXYLIC ACID see III:PAE250
1,3-PENTADIENE-1-CARBOXYLIC ACID see III:SKU000
1:4-PENTADIENE DIOXIDE see III:DHE000
PENTAERYTHRITOL TRIACRYLATE see III:PBC750
PENTAGEN see III:PAX000
3,5,7,3',4'-PENTAHYDROXYFLAVONE see III:QCA000
3,3',4',5,7-PENTAHYDROXYFLAVONE-3-(o-RHAMNOSYL-GLUCOSIDE) see III:RSU000
3,3',4',5,7-PENTAHYDROXYFLAVONE-3-RUTINOSIDE see III:RSU000
PENTAHYDROXY-TIGLIADIENONE-MONOACETATE(C) MONOMYRISTATE(B) see III:PGV000
PENTA-KIL see II:PAX250
PENTALIN see III:PAW500
N,N-3',4',5'-PENTAMETHYLAMINOAZOBENZENE see III:DUL400
PENTANAL, N-FORMYL-N-METHYLHYDRAZONE see III:PBJ875
PENTANAL METHYLFORMYLHYDRAZONE see III:PBJ875
tert-PENTANOIC ACID see III:PJA500
PENTANOL-1 see III:AOE000
PENTAN-1-OL see III:AOE000
N-PENTANOL see III:AOE000
PENTASOL see II:PAX250, III:AOE000
PENTECH see I:DAD200
PENTYL ALCOHOL see III:AOE000
8-PENTYLBENZ(a)ANTHRACENE see III:AOE750
n-PENTYLHYDRAZINE HYDROCHLORIDE see III:PBX250
N-PENTYL-N-(4-HYDROXYBUTYL)NITROSAMINE see III:NLE500
PENTYLIDENE GYROMITRIN see III:PBJ875
1-PENTYL-3-NITRO-1-NITROSOGUANIDINE see III:NLC500
4-(PENTYLNITROSAMINO)-1-BUTANOL see III:NLE500
n-PENTYLNITROSOUREA see III:PBX500
p-PENTYLPHENOL see III:AOM250
o-(sec-PENTYL) PHENOL see III:AOM500
p-(sec-PENTYL) PHENOL see III:AOM750
m-(3-PENTYL)PHENYL-N-METHYL-N-NITROSOCARBA-MATE see III:PBX750
3-PENTYL-6,6,9-TRIMETHYL-6a,7,8,10a-TETRAHYDRO-6H-DIBENZO(b,d)PYRAN-1-OL see III:TCM250
PENWAR see II:PAX250
PENZYLPENICILLIN SODIUM SALT see III:BFD250
PEP see I:EDS000, III:PJR750
PEPLEOMYCIN SULFATE see III:PCB000
PERACETIC ACID (MAK) see III:PCL500
PERACETIC ACID SOLUTION (DOT) see III:PCL500
PERAGAL ST see III:PKQ250
PERANDREN see I:TBF500, I:TBG000
PERATOX see II:PAX250
PERAWIN see II:PCF275
PERBENZOATE de BUTYLE TERTIAIRE (FRENCH) see III:BSC500
PERBENZOIC ACID see III:PCM000

PERCHLOORETHYLEEN, PER (DUTCH) see II:PCF275
PERCHLOR see II:PCF275
PERCHLORAETHYLEN, PER (GERMAN) see II:PCF275
PERCHLORETHYLENE see II:PCF275
PERCHLORETHYLENE, PER (FRENCH) see II:PCF275
PERCHLOROBENZENE see I:HCC500
PERCHLOROBUTADIENE see II:HCD250
PERCHLORO-2-CYCLOBUTENE-1-ONE see III:PCF250
PERCHLORODIHOMOCUBANE see I:MQW500
PERCHLOROETHANE see III:HCI000
PERCHLOROETHYLENE see II:PCF275
PERCHLOROMETHANE see CBY000
PERCHLOROPENTACYCLODECANE see I:MQW500
PERCHLOROPENTACYCLO(5.2.1.0^{2,6}.0^{3,9}.0^{5,8})DECANE see I:MQW500
PERCIN see III:ILD000
PERCLENE see II:PCF275
PERCLOROETILENE (ITALIAN) see II:PCF275
PERCOBARB see I:ABG750
PERCODAN see I:ABG750
PERCORTEN see III:DAQ800
PERCOSOLVE see II:PCF275
PERCOTOL see III:DAQ800
PERCUTACRINE see I:PMH500
PERCUTACRINE ANDROGENIQUE see I:TBF500
PERCUTATRINE OESTROGENIQUE ISCOVESCO see I:DKA600
PERFECTA see III:MQV750
PERFECTHION see III:DSP400
PERFLUOROETHENE see III:TCH500
PERFLUOROETHYLENE see III:TCH500
PERGACID VIOLET 2B see II:FAG120
PERGANTENE see III:SHF500
PERGLOTTAL see III:NGY000
2-PERHYDROAZEPINONE see III:CBF700
PERHYDROL see III:HIB000
PERHYDRONAPHTHALENE see III:DAE800
PERI-DINAPHTHALENE see III:PCQ250
PERILENE see III:PCQ250
PERISTON see III:PKQ250
PERK see II:PCF275
PERKLONE see II:PCF275
PERLATAN see I:EDV000
PERLITON BLUE B see III:TBG700
PERLITON ORANGE 3R see I:AKP750
PERLON see III:NOH000
PERLUTEX see II:MCA000
PERM-A-CHLOR see II:TIO750
PERMACIDE see II:PAX250
PERMAGARD see II:PAX250
PERMASAN see II:PAX250
PERMASEAL see III:PJH500
PERMATOX DP-2 see II:PAX250
PERMATOX PENTA see II:PAX250
PERMITE see II:PAX250
PERNOX see III:CLY500
PERONE see III:HIB000
PERONE 30 see III:HIB010
PERONE 35 see III:HIB010
PERONE 50 see III:HIB010
PEROPYRENE see III:DDC400
PEROSIN see III:EIR000
PEROSSIDO di BENZOILE(ITALIAN) see III:BDS000
PEROSSIDO di BUTILE TERZIARIO (ITALIAN) see III:BSC750
PEROSSIDO di IDROGENO (ITALIAN) see III:HIB000
PEROXAN see III:HIB000
PEROXIDE see III:HIB000
1,4-PEROXIDO-p-MENTHENE-2 see III:ARM500
PEROXYACETIC ACID see III:PCL500
PEROXYACETIC ACID, maximum concentration 43% in acetic acid (DOT) see III:PCL500

PEROXYBENZOIC ACID see III:PCM000
PEROXYDE de BENZOYLE (FRENCH) see III:BDS000
PEROXYDE de BUTYLE TERTIAIRE (FRENCH) see
    III:BSC750
PEROXYDE d'HYDROGENE (FRENCH) see III:HIB000
PEROXYDE de LAUROYLE (FRENCH) see III:LBR000
PEROXYLINOLEIC ACID, SODIUM SALT see III:SIC250
PEROXYLINOLENIC ACID see III:PCN000
PERSADOX see III:BDS000
PERSANTINAT see III:ARQ750
PERSEC see II:PCF275
PERSIAN RED see I:LCS000
PERSIA-PERAZOL see II:DEP800
PERSIMMON see III:PCP500
PERSISTOL see III:TND500
PERSPEX see III:PKB500
PERTHANE see III:DJC000
PERVITIN see III:MDT600
PERYLENE see III:PCQ250
PESTMASTER see I:EIY500
PESTMASTER EDB-85 see I:EIY500
PESTMASTER (OBS.) see III:MHR200
PESTOX PLUS see III:PAK000
PETA see III:PBC750
PETASITENINE see III:PCQ750
PETASITES JAPONICUS MAXIM see II:PCR000
PETHION see III:PAK000
PETNAMYCETIN see II:CDP250
PETROGALAR see III:MQV750
PETROHOL see III:INJ000
PETROL (DOT) see III:GBY000
PETROLATUM, LIQUID see III:MQV750
PETROLEUM see III:PCR250
PETROLEUM ASPHALT see III:PCR500
PETROLEUM CRUDE see III:PCR250
PETROLEUM DISTILLATES, CLAY-TREATED HEAVY
    NAPHTHENIC see III:PCS260
PETROLEUM DISTILLATES, CLAY-TREATED LIGHT
    NAPHTHENIC see III:PCS270
PETROLEUM DISTILLATES, HYDROTREATED HEAVY
    NAPHTHENIC see I:MQV790
PETROLEUM DISTILLATES, SOLVENT-DEWAXED HEAVY
    PARAFFINIC see III:MQV825
PETROLEUM PITCH see II:ARO500
PETROLEUM ROOFING TAR see III:PCR500
PETROL ORANGE Y see III:PEJ500
PETROL YELLOW WT see I:DOT300
PETZINOL see II:TIO750
PEVIKON D 61 see III:PKQ059
PEVITON see III:NCQ900
PEYRONE'S CHLORIDE see II:PJD000
PF 38 see III:FQU875
PFH see III:PNM650
PGE see II:PFH000
PHALDRONE see III:CDO000
PHALTAN see III:TIT250
PHANANTIN see I:DKQ000
PHARLON see II:EDS100
PHARMANTHRENE GOLDEN YELLOW see III:DCZ000
PHARMAZOID RED KB see II:CLK225
PHARMETTEN see II:EOK000
PHAROS 100.1 see III:SMR000
PHBN see III:NLN000
PHEBUZIN see II:BRF500
PHEBUZINE see II:BRF500
PHEMERIDE see III:BEN000
PHEMEROL CHLORIDE see III:BEN000
PHEMITHYN see III:BEN000
p-PHENACETIN see I:ABG750
PHENACHLOR see I:TIW000
PHENACIDE see I:CDV100
PHENACITE see II:SCN500
PHENACYLAMINE see III:AHR250
PHENACYL-6-AMINOPENICILLINATE see III:PCU500

PHENACYL CHLORIDE see III:CEA750
PHENADOR-X see III:BGE000
PHENAEMAL see II:EOK000
PHENAKITE see II:SCN500
PHENALENO(1,9-gh)QUINOLINE see III:PCV500
PHENALZINE see III:PFC750
PHENALZINE DIHYDROGEN SULFATE see III:PFC750
PHENALZINE HYDROGEN SULPHATE see III:PFC750
PHENAMINE BLUE BB see I:CMO000
PHENANTHRA-ACENAPHTHENE see III:PCW000
9,10-PHENANTHRAQUINONE see III:PCX250
PHENANTHREN (GERMAN) see III:PCW250
PHENANTHRENE see III:PCW250
PHENANTHRENE-1,2-DIHYDRODIOL see III:DMA000
PHENANTHRENE-3,4-DIHYDRODIOL see III:PCW500
9,10-PHENANTHRENEDIONE see III:PCX250
PHENANTHRENE-9,10-EPOXIDE see III:PCX000
9,10-PHENANTHRENE OXIDE see III:PCX000
PHENANTHRENEQUINONE see III:PCX250
9,10-PHENANTHRENEQUINONE see III:PCX250
PHENANTHRENETETRAHYDRO-3,4-EPOXIDE see
    III:ECR500
PHENANTHRO(2,1-d)THIAZOLE see III:PCY400
2-PHENANTHRYLACETAMIDE see III:AAM250
9-PHENANTHRYLACETAMIDE see III:PCY750
N-2-PHENANTHRYLACETAMIDE see III:AAM250
N-(2-PHENANTHRYL)ACETAMIDE see III:AAM250
N-3-PHENANTHRYLACETAMIDE see III:PCY500
N-9-PHENANTHRYLACETAMIDE see III:PCY750
2-PHENANTHRYLACETHYDROXAMIC ACID see
    III:PCZ000
N-(2-PHENANTHRYL)ACETOHYDROXAMIC ACETATE see
    III:ABK250
N-2-PHENANTHRYLACETOHYDROXAMIC ACID see
    III:PCZ000
2-PHENANTHRYLAMINE see III:PDA250
3-PHENANTHRYLAMINE see III:PDA500
9-PHENANTHRYLAMINE see III:PDA750
PHENANTRIN see III:PCW250
PHENATOINE see I:DKQ000
PHENATOX see I:CDV100
PHENAZINE see III:PDB500
PHENAZITE see II:SCN500
PHENAZO see I:PDC250
PHENAZODINE see I:PDC250, III:PEK250
PHENAZONE (PHARMACEUTICAL) see III:AQN000
PHENAZOPYRIDINE see III:PEK250
PHENAZOPYRIDINE HYDROCHLORIDE see I:PDC250
PHENAZOPYRIDINIUM CHLORIDE see I:PDC250
PHEN-BUTA-VET see II:BRF500
PHENBUTAZOL see II:BRF500
PHENE see I:BBL250
PHENELZIN see III:PFC750
PHENELZINE ACID SULFATE see III:PFC750
PHENELZINE BISULPHATE see III:PFC750
PHENELZINE SULFATE see III:PFC750
PHENEMALUM see I:SID000
PHENESTERINE see II:CME250
PHENESTRIN see II:CME250
PHENETHYLCARBAMID (GERMAN) see III:EFE000
PHENETHYLENE see II:SMQ000
PHENETHYLENE OXIDE see II:EBR000
PHENETHYLHYDRAZINE SULFATE (1:1) see III:PFC750
N-(p-PHENETHYL)PHENYLACETOHYDROXAMIC ACID see
    III:PDI250
p-PHENETOLCARBAMID (GERMAN) see III:EFE000
p-PHENETOLCARBAMIDE see III:EFE000
p-PHENETOLECARBAMIDE see III:EFE000
p-PHENETYLUREA see III:EFE000
PHENIC ACID see III:PDN750
PHENLINE see III:PFC750
PHENOBAL see II:EOK000
PHENOBAL SODIUM see I:SID000
PHENOBARBITAL see II:EOK000

PHENOBARBITAL ELIXIR see I:SID000
PHENOBARBITAL Na see I:SID000
PHENOBARBITAL SODIUM see I:SID000
PHENOBARBITAL SODIUM SALT see I:SID000
PHENOBARBITONE see II:EOK000
PHENOBARBITONE SODIUM see I:SID000
PHENOBARBITONE SODIUM SALT see I:SID000
PHENOBARBITURIC ACID see II:EOK000
PHENO BLACK EP see AQP000
PHENO BLUE 2B see I:CMO000
PHENOCHLOR see I:PJL750
PHENOCLOR DP6 see II:PJN250
PHENODIOXIN see III:DDA800
PHENODYNE see III:PFC750
PHENOHEP see III:HCI000
PHENOL see III:PDN750
PHENOL ALCOHOL see III:PDN750
PHENOL, 4,4'-(1,2-DIETHYLIDENE-1,2-ETHANEDIYL)BIS-,
    (E,E)-(9CI) see III:DHB550
PHENOLE (GERMAN) see III:PDN750
PHENOL-GLYCIDAETHER (GERMAN) see II:PFH000
PHENOL GLYCIDYL ETHER (MAK) see II:PFH000
PHENOL, MOLTEN (DOT) see III:PDN750
PHENOLURIC see II:EOK000
PHENOMET see II:EOK000
PHENONYL see II:EOK000
PHENOTAN see III:BRE500
PHENOTURIC see II:EOK000
PHENO VIOLET N see III:CMP000
PHENOX see II:DAA800
PHENOXYBENZAMIDE HYDROCHLORIDE see II:DDG800
PHENOXYBENZAMINE see I:PDT250
3-PHENOXY-1,2-EPOXYPROPANE see II:PFH000
N-PHENOXYISOPROPYL-N-BENZYL-β-CHLOROETHYL-
    AMINE see I:PDT250
N-2-PHENOXYISOPROPYL-N-BENZYL-CHLOROETHYL-
    AMINE HYDROCHLORIDE see II:DDG800
N-PHENOXYISOPROPYL-N-BENZYL-β-CHLOROETHYL-
    AMINE HYDROCHLORIDE see II:DDG800
PHENOXYLENE SUPER see II:CIR250
PHENOXYPROPENE OXIDE see II:PFH000
PHENOXYPROPYLENE OXIDE see II:PFH000
PHENTIN ACETATE see III:ABX250
PHENTINOACETATE see III:ABX250
PHENYLACETAMIDOPENICILLANIC ACID see III:BDY669
p-PHENYLACETANILIDE see III:PDY500
2'-PHENYLACETANILIDE see III:PDY000
3'-PHENYLACETANILIDE see III:PDY250
4'-PHENYLACETANILIDE see III:PDY500
N'-PHENYLACETHYDRAZIDE see III:ACX750
4'-PHENYL-o-ACETOTOLUIDE see II:PEB250
PHENYLAETHYL-HYDRAZIN see III:PFC750
d-PHENYLALANINE MUSTARD see III:SAX200
l-PHENYLALANINE MUSTARD see I:PED750
dl-PHENYLALANINE MUSTARD see III:BHT750
l-PHENYLALANINE MUSTARD HYDROCHLORIDE see
    III:BHV250
PHENYLALANINE NITROGEN MUSTARD see I:PED750
PHENYLALANIN-LOST (GERMAN) see II:BHT750
PHENYLAMINE see II:AOQ000
PHENYLAMINE HYDROCHLORIDE see II:BBL000
N-PHENYLAMINOCARBONYL)AZIRIDINE see III:PEH250
17-β-PHENYLAMINOCARBONYLOXYOESTRA-1,3,5(10)-
    TRIENE-3-METHYL ETHER see III:PEE600
4-PHENYLAMINODIPHENYLAMINE see III:BLE500
p-PHENYLAMINODIPHENYLAMINE see III:BLE500
p-PHENYLANILINE see I:AJS100
p-PHENYLANISOLE see III:PEG250
N-PHENYL-1-AZIRIDINECARBOXAMIDE see III:PEH250
p-PHENYLAZOACETANILIDE see III:PEH750
4'-PHENYLAZOACETANILIDE see III:PEH750

4-(PHENYLAZO)ANILINE see II:PEI000
N-(PHENYLAZO)ANILINE see III:DWO800
p-(PHENYLAZO)ANILINE see II:PEI000
4-(PHENYLAZO)-o-ANISIDINE see III:MFF500
1-PHENYLAZO-2-ANTHROL see III:PEI750
4-(PHENYLAZO)BENZENAMINE see II:PEI000
4-(PHENYLAZO)-1,3-BENZENEDIAMINE MONOHYDRO-
    CHLORIDE see III:PEK000
PHENYLAZODIAMINOPYRIDINE HYDROCHLORIDE see
    I:PDC250
3-PHENYLAZO-2,6-DIAMINOPYRIDINE HYDROCHLORIDE
    see I:PDC250
β-PHENYLAZO-α,α'-DIAMINOPYRIDINE HYDROCHLORIDE
    see I:PDC250
PHENYLAZO-α,α'-DIAMINOPYRIDINE MONOHYDRO-
    CHLORIDE see I:PDC250
N-PHENYLAZO-N-METHYLTAURINE SODIUM SALT see
    III:PEJ250
1-(PHENYLAZO)-2-NAPHTHALENAMINE see III:FAG130
1-(PHENYLAZO)-2-NAPHTHALENOL see III:PEJ500
1-(PHENYLAZO)-2-NAPHTHOL see III:PEJ500
1-PHENYLAZO-β-NAPHTHOL see III:PEJ500
1-PHENYLAZO-2-NAPHTHOL-6,8-DISULFONIC ACID, DISO-
    DIUM SALT see III:HGC000
1-PHENYLAZO-2-NAPHTHOL-6,8-DISULPHONIC ACID, DI-
    SODIUM SALT see III:HGC000
1-(PHENYLAZO)-2-NAPHTHYLAMINE see III:FAG130
4-PHENYLAZOPHENOL see III:HJF000
p-PHENYLAZOPHENOL see III:HJF000
p-PHENYLAZOPHENYLAMINE see II:PEI000
1-(4-PHENYLAZO-PHENYLAZO)-2-ETHYLAMINO-
    NAPHTHALENE see III:EOJ500
(PHENYLAZO-4-PHENYLAZO)-1-ETHYLAMINO-2-
    NAPHTHALENE see III:EOJ500
1-((4-(PHENYLAZO)PHENYL)AZO)-2-NAPHTHALENOL see
    III:OHA000
1-(p-PHENYLAZOPHENYLAZO)-2-NAPHTHOL see
    III:OHA000
4-PHENYLAZO-m-PHENYLENEDIAMINE see III:PEK000
4-(PHENYLAZO)-m-PHENYLENEDIAMINE MONOHYDRO-
    CHLORIDE see III:PEK000
3-(PHENYLAZO)-2,6-PYRIDINEDIAMINE see III:PEK250
3-(PHENYLAZO)-2,6-PYRIDINEDIAMINE, HYDROCHLO-
    RIDE see I:PDC250
PHENYLAZOPYRIDINE HYDROCHLORIDE see I:PDC250
PHENYLAZO TABLET see III:PEK250
PHENYLAZO TABLETS see I:PDC250
4'-PHENYLBENZANILIDE see III:BGF000
5-PHENYL-1:2-BENZANTHRACENE see III:PEK750
PHENYLBENZENE see III:BGE000
α-PHENYLBENZYLCYANIDE see III:DVX200
PHENYLBUTAZ see II:BRF500
PHENYLBUTAZON (GERMAN) see II:BRF500
PHENYLBUTAZONE see II:BRF500
PHENYLBUTAZONUM see II:BRF500
PHENYLBUTYRIC ACID NITROGEN MUSTARD see
    I:CDO500
N-PHENYLCARBAMATE D'ISOPROPYLE (FRENCH) see
    III:CBM000
PHENYLCARBAMIC ACID-1-METHYLETHEL ESTER see
    III:CBM000
1-PHENYLCARBAMOYLAZIRIDINE see III:PEH250
PHENYL-N-CARBAMOYLAZIRIDINE see III:PEH250
PHENYL CARBONATE see III:DVZ000
PHENYL CHLOROFORM see I:BFL250
PHENYLCHLOROMETHYLKETONE see III:CEA750
1-PHENYL-3,3-DIAETHYLTRIAZEN (GERMAN) see
    III:PEU500
2-PHENYLDIAZENECARBOXAMIDE see III:CBL000
PHENYLDIAZONIUM FLUOROBORATE (SALT) see
    III:BBO325
PHENYLDIAZONIUM TETRAFLUOROBORATE see
    III:BBO325
3-PHENYL-5-(β-(DIETHYLAMINO)ETHYL)-1,2,4-OXADIA-
    ZOLE CITRATE see III:OOE000

1-PHENYL-3,3-DIETHYLTRIAZENE see III:PEU500
1-PHENYL-2,3-DIMETHYL-4-DIMETHYLAMINOPYRAZOL-5-ONE see III:DOT000
1-PHENYL-2,3-DIMETHYL-4-DIMETHYLAMINOPYRAZO-LONE-5 see III:DOT000
1-PHENYL-2,3-DIMETHYLPYRAZOLE-5-ONE see III:AQN000
1-PHENYL-2,3-DIMETHYL-5-PYRAZOLONE see III:AQN000
1-PHENYL-2,3-DIMETHYL-5-PYRAZOLONE-4-METHYLAMINOMETHANESULFONATESODIUM see III:AMK500
1-PHENYL-2,3-DIMETHYLPYRAZOLONE-(5)-4-METHYLAMINOMETHANESULFONICACID SODIUM see III:AMK500
PHENYL DIMETHYL PYRAZOLON METHYL AMINOMETH-ANE SODIUM SULFONATE see III:AMK500
1-PHENYL-3,3-DIMETHYLTRIAZENE see III:DTP000
PHENYLDIMETHYLTRIAZINE see III:DTP000
2,2'-(1,3-PHENYLENEBIS(OXYMETHYLENE))BISOXIRANE see II:REF000
m-PHENYLENEDIAMINE see III:PEY000
p-PHENYLENEDIAMINE see III:PEY500
1,3-PHENYLENEDIAMINE see III:PEY000
1,4-PHENYLENEDIAMINE see III:PEY500
m-PHENYLENEDIAMINE (DOT) see III:PEY000
o-PHENYLENEDIAMINE, DIHYDROCHLORIDE see III:PEY600
p-PHENYLENEDIAMINE DIHYDROCHLORIDE see III:PEY650
1,3-PHENYLENEDIAMINE DIHYDROCHLORIDE see III:PEY750
1,4-PHENYLENEDIAMINE DIHYDROCHLORIDE see III:PEY650
m-PHENYLENEDIAMINE HYDROCHLORIDE see III:PEY750
p-PHENYLENEDIAMINE HYDROCHLORIDE see III:PEY650
PHENYLENEDIAMINE, META, SOLID (DOT) see III:PEY000
PHENYLENEDIAMINE, PARA, SOLID (DOT) see III:PEY500
o-PHENYLENEDIOL see III:CCP850
2,3-PHENYLENEPYRENE see I:IBZ000
2,3-o-PHENYLENEPYRENE see I:IBZ000
1,10-(o-PHENYLENE)PYRENE see I:IBZ000
1,10-(1,2-PHENYLENE)PYRENE see I:IBZ000
1-PHENYL-1,2-EPOXYETHANE see II:EBR000
PHENYL-2,3-EPOXYPROPYL ETHER see II:PFH000
PHENYLETHENE see II:SMQ000
4-(2-PHENYLETHENYL)BENZENAMINE see III:SLQ900
4-(2-PHENYLETHENYL)BENZENAMINE,(E) see III:AMO000
N-(4-(2-PHENYLETHENYL)PHENYL)ACETAMIDE see III:SMR500
PHENYLETHYLBARBITURATE see II:EOK000
PHENYL-ETHYL-BARBITURIC ACID see II:EOK000
5-PHENYL-5-ETHYLBARBITURIC ACID see II:EOK000
PHENYLETHYLBARBITURIC ACID, SODIUM SALT see I:SID000
PHENYLETHYL CARBAMATE see III:CBL750
PHENYLETHYLENE see II:SMQ000
PHENYLETHYLENE OXIDE see II:EBR000
β-PHENYLETHYLHYDRAZINE DIHYDROGEN SULFATE see III:PFC750
2-PHENYLETHYLHYDRAZINE DIHYDROGEN SULPHATE see III:PFC750
β-PHENYLETHYLHYDRAZINE HYDROGEN SULPHATE see III:PFC750
β-PHENYLETHYLHYDRAZINE SULFATE see III:PFC750
PHENYLETHYLHYDRAZINE SULPHATE see III:PFC750
PHENYLETHYLMALONYLUREA see II:EOK000
PHENYLETTEN see II:EOK000
N-PHENYL-2-FLUORENAMINE see III:PFE900
N-PHENYL-9H-FLUORENAMINE see III:PFE900
N-PHENYL-2-FLUORENYLHYDROXYLAMINE see III:PFF000
N-PHENYL-N-9H-FLUOREN-2-YLHYDROXYLAMINE see III:PFF000
PHENYL GLYCYDYL ETHER see II:PFH000

PHENYL HYDRATE see III:PDN750
2-PHENYLHYDRAZIDE, CARBAMIC ACID see III:CBL000
PHENYLHYDRAZIN (GERMAN) see II:PFI000
PHENYLHYDRAZINE see II:PFI000
1-PHENYLHYDRAZINE CARBOXAMIDE see III:CBL000
2-PHENYLHYDRAZINECARBOXAMIDE see III:CBL000
PHENYLHYDRAZINE HYDROCHLORIDE see III:PFI250
PHENYLHYDRAZINE MONOHYDROCHLORIDE see III:PFI250
PHENYLHYDRAZIN HYDROCHLORID (GERMAN) see III:PFI250
PHENYLHYDRAZINIUM CHLORIDE see III:PFI250
PHENYL HYDRIDE see I:BBL250
PHENYL HYDROXIDE see III:PDN750
1-PHENYL-2-(p-HYDROXYPHENYL)-3,5-DIOXO-4-BUTYL-PYRAZOLIDINE see III:HNI500
PHENYLIC ACID see III:PDN750
PHENYLIC ALCOHOL see III:PDN750
PHENYL-IDIUM see I:PDC250
PHENYL-IDIUM 200 see I:PDC250
N-PHENYL ISOPROPYL CARBAMATE see III:CBM000
PHENYLMETHANAL see III:BBM500
PHENYLMETHANETHIOL see III:TGO750
4-(PHENYLMETHOXY)PHENOL see III:AEY000
3-PHENYL-10-METHYL-7:8 BENZACRIDINE (FRENCH) see III:MNS250
1-PHENYL-3-METHYL-3-(2-HYDROXYAETHYL)-TRIAZEN (GERMAN) see III:HKV000
1-PHENYL-3-METHYL-3-(2-HYDROXYETHYL)TRIAZENE see III:HKV000
1-PHENYL-3-METHYL-3-HYDROXY-TRIAZEN (GERMAN) see III:HMP000
1-PHENYL-3-METHYL-3-HYDROXY-TRIAZENE see III:HMP000
PHENYLMETHYL MERCAPTAN see III:TGO750
PHENYLMETHYLNITROSAMINE see I:MMU250
PHENYL METHYLNITROSOCARBAMATE see III:NKV500
3-PHENYL-1-METHYL-1-NITROSOHARNSTOFF (GERMAN) see II:MMY500
(PHENYLMETHYL) PENICILLINIC ACID see III:BDY669
1-PHENYL-3-METHYL-3-(2-SULFOAETHYL) NATRIUM SALZ (GERMAN) see III:PEJ250
1-PHENYL-3-METHYL-3-(2-SULFOETHYL)TRIAZENE, SO-DIUM SALT see III:PEJ250
1-PHENYL-3-METHYLTRIAZINE see III:MOA725
PHENYL-MOBUZON see II:BRF500
1-PHENYL-3-MONOMETHYLTRIAZENE see III:MOA725, III:PFS500
PHENYL-β-NAPHTHALAMINE see III:MFA250
PHENYLNAPHTHYLAMINE see III:PFT250
PHENYL-2-NAPHTHYLAMINE see II:PFT500
PHENYL-α-NAPHTHYLAMINE see III:PFT250
α-PHENYLNAPHTHYLAMINE see III:PFT250
PHENYL-β-NAPHTHYLAMINE see II:PFT500
N-PHENYL-1-NAPHTHYLAMINE see III:PFT250
N-PHENYL-2-NAPHTHYLAMINE see II:PFT500
N-PHENYL-α-NAPHTHYLAMINE see III:PFT250
N-PHENYL-β-NAPHTHYLAMINE see II:PFT500
4-PHENYL-NITROBENZENE see I:NFQ000
p-PHENYL-NITROBENZENE see I:NFQ000
N-PHENYL-p-NITROSOANILINE see III:NKB500
PHENYL-NITROSO-HANRSTOFF (GERMAN) see III:NLG500
4-PHENYLNITROSOPIPERIDINE see III:PFT600
N-PHENYL-N-NITROSOUREA see III:NLG500
PHENYLOXIRANE see II:EBR000
1-PHENYLOXIRANE see II:EBR000
2-PHENYLOXIRANE see II:EBR000
PHENYL PERCHLORYL see I:HCC500
2-PHENYLPHENOL see III:BGJ250
4-PHENYLPHENOL see III:BGJ500
o-PHENYLPHENOL see III:BGJ250
p-PHENYLPHENOL see III:BGJ500
2-PHENYLPHENOL SODIUM SALT see II:BGJ750
o-PHENYLPHENOL SODIUM SALT see II:BGJ750

α-PHENYLPHENYLACETONITRILE see III:DVX200
3-PHENYL-2-PROPENYLANTHRANILATE see II:API750
3-PHENYL-2-PROPEN-1-YL ANTHRANILATE see II:API750
PHENYLSEMICARBAZIDE see III:CBL000
1-PHENYLSEMICARBAZIDE see III:CBL000
5'-PHENYL-m-TERPHENYL see III:TMR000
PHENYLTRICHLOROMETHANE see I:BFL250
PHENYLURETHAN see III:CBL750
PHENYLURETHAN(E) see III:CBL750
N-PHENYLURETHANE see III:CBL750
PHENYLVINYL KETONE see III:PMQ250
1-PHENYL-1-(3,4-XYLYL)-2-PROPYNYL N-CYCLOHEXYL-
    CARBAMATE see III:PGQ000
PHENYRAL see II:EOK000
PHENYTOIN SODIUM see I:DNU000
PHILOPON see III:MDT600
PHISODANV see III:HCL000
PHISOHEX see III:HCL000
PHLOROL see III:PGR250
PHLOXINE RED 20-7600 see III:BNK700
PHLOXINE TONER B see III:BNH500
PHLOX RED TONER X-1354 see III:BNH500
PHOB see II:EOK000
PHORBOL see III:PGS250
PHORBOL ACETATE, CAPRATE see III:ACZ000
PHORBOL ACETATE, LAURATE see III:PGS500,
    III:PGU250
PHORBOL ACETATE, MYRISTATE see III:PGV000
PHORBOL-12-o-BUTYROYL-13-DODECANOATE see
    III:BSX750
PHORBOL CAPRATE, (+)-(S)-2-METHYLBUTYRATE see
    III:PGU500
PHORBOL CAPRATE, TIGLATE see III:PGU750
PHORBOL-12,13-DIACETATE see III:PGS750
PHORBOL-12,13-DIBENZOATE see III:PGT000
PHORBOL-12,13-DIDECANOATE see III:PGT250
PHORBOL-12,13-DIHEXA(Δ-2,4)-DIENOATE see III:PGT500
PHORBOL-12,13-DIHEXANOATE see III:PGT750
PHORBOL LAURATE, (+)-S-2-METHYLBUTYRATE see
    III:PGU000
PHORBOL MONOACETATE MONOLAURATE see
    III:PGS500
PHORBOL MONOACETATE MONOLAURATE see
    III:PGU250
PHORBOL MONOACETATE MONOMYRISTATE see
    III:PGV000
PHORBOL MONODECANOATE (S)-(+)-MONO(2-METHYL-
    BUTYRATE) see III:PGU500
(E)-PHORBOL MONODECANOATE MONO(2-METHYLCRO-
    TONATE) see III:PGU750
PHORBOL MONOLAURATE MONO(S)-(+)-2-METHYLBUTY-
    RATE see III:PGU000
PHORBOL MYRISTATE ACETATE see III:PGV000
PHORBOL-9-MYRISTATE-9a-ACETATE-3-ALDEHYDE see
    III:PGV250
PHORBOL-12-o-TIGLYL-13-BUTYRATE see III:PGV750
PHORBOL-12-o-TIGLYL-13-DODECANOATE see
    III:PGW000
PHORTOX see II:TAA100
PHOSCHLOR R50 see III:TIQ250
PHOS-FLUR see III:SHF500
PHOSKIL see III:PAK000
PHOSPHAMID see III:DSP400
PHOSPHAMIDON see III:FAC025
PHOSPHATE de DIMETHYLE et de (2-CHLORO-2-DIETHYL-
    CARBAMOYL-1-METHYL-VINYLE) see III:FAC025
PHOSPHEMOL see III:PAK000
PHOSPHENOL see III:PAK000
1,1',1''-PHOSPHINOTHIOYLIDYNETRISAZIRIDINE see
    I:TFQ750
1,1',1''-PHOSPHINYLIDYNETRISAZIRIDINE see III:TND250
1,1',1''-PHOSPHINYLIDYNETRIS(2-METHYL)AZIRIDINE see
    III:TNK250
PHOSPHONIC ACID, DIMETHYL ESTER see III:DSG600

PHOSPHORIC ACID, BERYLLIUM SALT (1:1) see I:BFS000
PHOSPHORIC ACID, 2-CHLORO-1-(2,4,5-TRICHLOROPHE-
    NYL)ETHENYL DIMETHYL ESTER see II:TBW100
(Z)-PHOSPHORIC ACID-2-CHLORO-1-(2,4,5-TRICHLORO-
    PHENYL)ETHENYL DIMETHYL ESTER see III:RAF100
PHOSPHORIC ACID, ISODECYL NICKEL(2+) SALT (2:3) see
    III:NDF000
PHOSPHORIC ACID, LEAD (2+) SALT (2:3) see I:LDU000
PHOSPHORIC ACID TRIETHYLENE IMIDE see III:TND250
PHOSPHORIC ACID TRIETHYLENEIMINE (DOT) see
    III:TND250
PHOSPHORIC ACID, TRIMETHYL ESTER see II:TMD250
PHOSPHORIC ACID, TRIS(2,3-DIBROMOPROPYL) ESTER see
    I:TNC500
PHOSPHORIC ACID TRIS(1,3-DICHLORO-2-PROPYL)ESTER
    see III:FQU875
PHOSPHORIC ACID, TRIS(2-ETHYLHEXYL) ESTER see
    III:TNI250
PHOSPHORIC TRIS(DIMETHYLAMIDE) see I:HEK000
PHOSPHORODITHIOIC ACID-O,O-DIMETHYL ESTER-S-ES-
    TER with DIETHYL MERCAPTOSUCCINATE see
    III:MAK700
PHOSPHORODITHIOIC ACID-O,O-DIMETHYL-S-(2-(METH-
    YLAMINO)-2-OXOETHYL) ESTER see III:DSP400
PHOSPHOROTHIOIC ACID, O,O-DIETHYL-O-(4-NITROPHE-
    NYL) ESTER see III:PAK000
PHOSPHOROTHIOIC ACID-O,O-DIMETHYL-O-(3-METHYL-
    4-METHYLTHIOPHENYLE) (FRENCH) see III:FAQ999
PHOSPHOROTHIOIC ACID TRIETHYLENETRIAMIDE see
    I:TFQ750
PHOSPHOROUS ACID, BERYLLIUM SALT see I:BFS000
PHOSPHORYL HEXAMETHYLTRIAMIDE see I:HEK000
PHOSPHOSTIGMINE see III:PAK000
PHOSPHOTHION see III:MAK700
PHOTOMIREX see III:MRI750
PHPH see III:BGE000
PHRILON see III:NOH000
1(2H)-PHTHALAZINONE HYDRAZONE see III:PHW000
1(2H)-PHTHALAZINONE HYDRAZONE HYDROCHLORIDE
    see II:HGP500
PHTHALIC ACID, DIALLYL ESTER see II:DBL200
o-PHTHALIC ACID, DIALLYL ESTER see II:DBL200
PHTHALIC ACID DINITRILE see III:PHY000
PHTHALIC ACID DIOCTYL ESTER see I:DVL700
PHTHALIMIDIMIDE see III:DNE400
2-PHTHALIMIDOGLUTARIMIDE see III:TEH500
3-PHTHALIMIDOGLUTARIMIDE see III:TEH500
α-PHTHALIMIDOGLUTARIMIDE see III:TEH500
α-(N-PHTHALIMIDO)GLUTARIMIDE see III:TEH500
(PHTHALOCYANINATO(2−))MAGNESIUM see III:MAI250
PHTHALOCYANINE BLUE 01206 see III:DNE400
PHTHALODINITRILE see III:PHY000
o-PHTHALODINITRILE see III:PHY000
PHTHALOGEN see III:DNE400
PHTHALONITRILE see III:PHY000
N-PHTHALOYLGLUTAMIMIDE see III:TEH500
PHTHALTAN see III:TIT250
N-PHTHALYLGLUTAMIC ACID IMIDE see III:TEH500
N-PHTHALYL-GLUTAMINSAEURE-IMID (GERMAN) see
    III:TEH500
α-N-PHTHALYLGLUTARAMIDE see III:TEH500
PHTHISEN see III:ILD000
1(2H)-PHTHLAZINONE, HYDRAZONE, MONOHYDROCHLO-
    RIDE see II:HGP500
PHTIVAZID see III:VEZ925
PHTIVAZIDE see III:VEZ925
PHYGON see III:DFT000
PHYGON PASTE see III:DFT000
PHYGON SEED PROTECTANT see III:DFT000
PHYGON XL see III:DFT000
PHYOL see III:PJA250
PHYONE see III:PJA250
PHYTAR see III:HKC000
PHYTAR 560 see I:HKC500

PHYTOMELIN see III:RSU000
PIAPONON see I:PMH500
PIC-CLOR see III:CKN500
PICCOLASTIC see III:SMQ500
PICENE see III:PIB750
PICFUME see III:CKN500
PICLORAM see III:PIB900
PICRIDE see III:CKN500
PIELIK see II:DAA800
PIGMENT GREEN 15 see I:LCR000
PIGMENT PONCEAU R see III:FMU070
PIGMENT RED CD see III:CHP500
PIGMENT YELLOW 33 see CAP750
PIGMEX see III:AEY000
PIG-WRACK see III:CCL250
PILLS (INDIA) see I:SED400
PINANG see II:BFW000
N-N-PIP see I:NLJ500
PIPERAZINE, 1-BENZOYL-2,6-DIMETHYL-4-NITROSO-(9CI)
    see III:NJL850
2,6-PIPERAZINEDIONE-4,4'-PROPYLENE DIOXOPIPERA-
    ZINE see II:PIK250
PIPERAZINE and SODIUM NITRITE (4:1) see III:PIJ250
PIPERIDINE, 4-tert-BUTYL-1-NITROSO see III:NJO300
PIPERIDINE, 3,5-DIMETHYL-1-NITROSO-, (E)- see
    III:DTA700
PIPERIDINE, 3,5-DIMETHYL-1-NITROSO-, (Z)- see
    III:DTA690
PIPERONYL BUTOXIDE see III:PIX250
PIPERONYL SULFOXIDE see III:ISA000
PIRABUTINA see III:HNI500
PIRAFLOGIN see III:HNI500
PIRAMIDON see III:DOT000
PIRARREUMOL 'B'' see II:BRF500
PIRID see I:PDC250, III:PEK250
PIRIDACIL see I:PDC250
PIRIDOL see III:DOT000
PIRIMECIDAN see III:TGD000
PIRIMETAMINA (SPANISH) see III:TGD000
PIRINIXIL see II:CLW500
PIRMAZIN see III:SNJ000
PIROD see III:UNJ800
PIROMIDINA see III:DOT000
PIROSOLVINA see III:EEM000
PITCH see I:CMZ100
PITCH, COAL TAR see I:CMZ100
PITTSBURGH PX-138 see I:DVL700
PITUITARY GROWTH HORMONE see III:PJA250
PIVALIC ACID see III:PJA500
PIVALIC ACID LACTONE see III:DTH000
PIVALOLACTONE see III:DTH000
PIXALBOL see I:CMY800
PIX CARBONIS see I:CMY800
PKhNB see III:PAX000
PLANOMIDE see III:TEX250
PLANOTOX see II:DAA800
PLANTGARD see II:DAA800
PLANTIFOG 160M see III:MAS500
PLANTULIN see III:PMN850
PLASDONE see III:PKQ250
PLASKON 201 see III:PJY500
PLASTIBEST 20 see I:ARM268
PLASTOMOLL DOA see III:AEO000
PLASTORESIN ORANGE F4A see III:PEJ500
PLATIBLASTIN see II:PJD000
cis-PLATIN see II:PJD000
PLATIN (GERMAN) see III:PJD500
PLATINEX see II:PJD000
PLATINOL see II:PJD000
PLATINOL AH see I:DVL700
PLATINOL DOP see I:DVL700
cis-PLATINOUS DIAMMINE DICHLORIDE see II:PJD000
PLATINUM see III:PJD500
PLATINUM BLACK see III:PJD500

cis-PLATINUM(II) DIAMINEDICHLORIDE see II:PJD000
trans-PLATINUM(II)DIAMMINEDICHLORIDE see
    III:DEX000
PLATINUM SPONGE see III:PJD500
PLENASTRIL see I:PAN100
PLENUR see III:LGZ000
PLEXIGLAS see III:PKB500
PLEXIGUM M 920 see III:PKB500
PLIDAN see III:DCK759
PLIOFILM see III:PJH500
PLIOFLEX see III:SMR000
PLIOLITE S5 see III:SMR000
PLIOVAC AO see II:AAX175
PLIOVIC see III:PKQ059
PLIVA see I:BIE500
PLUMBOUS ACETATE see I:LCG000, I:LCJ000
PLUMBOUS CHLORIDE see III:LCQ000
PLUMBOUS CHROMATE see I:LCR000
PLUMBOUS OXIDE see III:LDN000
PLUMBOUS PHOSPHATE see I:LDU000
PLURACOL P-410 see III:PJT000
PMA see III:PGV000
PMB see I:ECU750
PMMA see III:PKB500
PMT see III:MOA725, III:PFS500
PNB see I:NFQ000
PNCB see III:NFS525
PNNG see III:NLD000
PNOT see I:NMP500
PNU see II:NLO500
PODOPHYLLIN see III:PJJ000
PODOPHYLLUM see III:PJJ000
PODOPHYLLUM RESIN see III:PJJ000
POINT TWO see III:SHF500
POLAAX see III:OAX000
POLCOMINAL see II:EOK000
POLFOSCHLOR see III:TIQ250
POLICAPRAN see III:PJY500
POLIFEN see III:TAI250
POLIFLOGIL see III:HNI500
POLIGOSTYRENE see III:SMQ500
POLINALIN see III:DOT000
POLISEPTIL see III:TEX250
POLITEF see III:TAI250
POLIVINIT see III:PKQ059
POLONIUM see II:PJJ750
POLONIUM CARBONYL see II:PJK000
POLOXAL RED 2B see III:HJF500
POLYAETHYLENGLYKOLE 1000 (GERMAN) see III:PJT250
POLYAMID (GERMAN) see III:NOH000
POLYAMIDE 6 see III:PJY500
POLY(epsilon-AMINOCAPROIC ACID) see III:PJY500
POLYBROMINATED BIPHENYL see II:FBU509
POLYBROMINATED BIPHENYL (FF-1) see II:FBU509
POLYBROMINATED BIPHENYLS see III:FBU000
POLYBROMOETHYLENE see III:PKQ000
POLYBUTADIENE-POLYSTYRENE COPOLYMER see
    III:SMR000
POLYCAPROAMIDE see III:PJY500
POLY(epsilon-CAPROAMIDE) see III:PJY500
POLYCAPROLACTAM see III:PJY500
POLY(epsilon-CAPROLACTAM) see III:PJY500
POLYCHLORCAMPHENE see I:CDV100
POLYCHLORINATED BIPHENYL see I:PJL750
POLYCHLORINATED BIPHENYL (AROCLOR 1221) see
    II:PJM000
POLYCHLORINATED BIPHENYL (AROCLOR 1232) see
    II:PJM250
POLYCHLORINATED BIPHENYL (AROCLOR 1242) see
    II:PJM500
POLYCHLORINATED BIPHENYL (AROCLOR 1248) see
    II:PJM750
POLYCHLORINATED BIPHENYL (AROCLOR 1254) see
    II:PJN000

POLYCHLORINATED BIPHENYL (AROCLOR 1260) see II:PJN250

POLYCHLORINATED BIPHENYL (AROCLOR 1262) see II:PJN500

POLYCHLORINATED BIPHENYL (AROCLOR 1268) see II:PJN750

POLYCHLORINATED BIPHENYL (AROCLOR 2565) see II:PJO000

POLYCHLORINATED BIPHENYL (AROCLOR 4465) see II:PJO250

POLYCHLORINATED BIPHENYL (KANECHLOR 300) see II:PJO500

POLYCHLORINATED BIPHENYL (KANECHLOR 400) see II:PJO750

POLYCHLORINATED BIPHENYL (KANECHLOR 500) see II:PJP000

POLYCHLORINATED BIPHENYLS see I:PJL750

POLYCHLORINATED CAMPHENES see I:CDV100

POLYCHLORINATED TERPHENYL see III:PJP250

POLYCHLOROBIPHENYL see I:PJL750

POLYCHLOROCAMPHENE see I:CDV100

POLY(CHLOROETHYLENE) see III:PKQ059

POLYCLAR L see III:PKQ250

POLYCLENE see II:DGB000

POLYCO 2410 see III:SMR000

POLY(1,2-DIHYDRO-2,2,4-TRIMETHYLQUINOLINE) see III:PJQ750

POLYDIMETHYL SILOXANE see III:PJR000

POLYDIMETHYLSILOXANE RUBBER see III:PJR250

POLY(ESTRADIOL PHOSPHATE) see I:EDS000

POLYESTRADIOL PHOSPHATE see III:PJR750

POLYETHYLENE see III:PJS750

POLYETHYLENE AS see III:PJS750

POLYETHYLENE GLYCOL see III:PJT000

POLYETHYLENE GLYCOL 1000 see III:PJT250

POLYETHYLENE GLYCOL MONOSTEARATE see III:PJV250

POLY(ETHYLENE OXIDE) see III:PJT000

POLYETHYLENE TEREPHTHALATE see III:PKF750

POLYETHYLENE TEREPHTHALATE FILM see III:PKF750

POLY(ETHYLENE TETRAFLUORIDE) see III:TAI250

POLYETHYLENE Y-141-A see III:PJX750

POLYFENE see III:TAI250

POLYFER see I:IGS000

POLYFIBRON 120 see III:SFO500

POLYFLON see III:TAI250

POLYFOAM PLASTIC SPONGE see III:PKL500

POLYFOAM SPONGE see III:PKL500

POLY-GIRON see III:TEH500

POLYGLYCOL 1000 see III:PJT250

POLYGLYCOL E1000 see III:PJT250

POLYGRIPAN see III:TEH500

POLY-G SERIES see III:PJT000

POLY(IMINOCARBONYLPENTAMETHYLENE) see III:PJY500

POLY(IMINO(1-OXO-1,6-HEXANEDIYL)) see III:PJY500

POLYMERIC DIALDEHYDE see III:PKA000

POLYMERS, WATER INSOLUBLE see III:PKA850

POLYMERS, WATER SOLUBLE see III:PKA860

POLYMETHYLMETHACRYLATE see III:PKB500

POLYMINE D see III:BEN000

POLYMONE see II:DGB000

POLYOESTRADIOL PHOSPHATE see I:EDS000

POLYOX see III:PJT000

POLY(1-(2-OXO-1-PYRROLIDINYL)ETHYLENE) see III:PKQ250

POLY(OXY(DIMETHYLSILYLENE)) see III:PJR000

POLY(OXY-1,2-ETHANEDIYLOXYCARBONYL-1,4-PHE-NYLENECARBONYL) see III:PKF750

POLYOXYETHYLENE-8-MONOSTEARATE see III:PJV250

POLY(OXYETHYLENEOXYTEREPHTHALOYL) see III:PKF750

POLYOXYETHYLENE SORBITAN MONOOLEATE see III:PKL100

POLYOXYETHYLENE SORBITAN MONOSTEARATE see III:PKL030

POLYOXYETHYLENE 20 SORBITAN MONOSTEARATE see III:PKL030

POLYOXYETHYLENE SORBITAN OLEATE see III:PKL100

POLYOXYETHYLENE(8)STEARATE see III:PJV250

POLYOXYMETHYLENE GLYCOLS see I:FMV000

POLYPHENOL FRACTION of BETEL NUT see III:PKH500

POLY p-PHENYLENE TEREPTHALAMIDE ARAMID FIBER see III:PKH850

POLYPRO 1014 see III:PMP500

POLYPROPENE see III:PMP500

POLYPROPYLENE see III:PMP500

POLYRAM M see III:MAS500

POLYRAM ULTRA see III:TFS350

POLYRAM Z see III:EIR000

POLYSILICONE see III:PJR250

POLYSORBAN 80 see III:PKL100

POLYSORBATE 60 see III:PKL030

POLYSORBATE 80 see III:PKL100

POLYSORBATE 80, U.S.P. see III:PKL100

POLYSTROL D see III:SMQ500

POLYSTYRENE see III:SMQ500

POLYSTYRENE BEADS (DOT) see III:SMQ500

POLYSTYRENE LATEX see III:SMQ500

POLYSTYROL see III:SMQ500

POLYTAC see III:PMP500

POLYTAR BATH see I:CMY800

POLYTEF see III:TAI250

POLYTETRAFLUOROETHENE see III:TAI250

POLYTETRAFLUOROETHYLENE see III:TAI250

POLYTHERM see III:PKQ059

POLYTOX see II:DGB000

POLYURETHANE ESTER FOAM see III:PKL500

POLYURETHANE ETHER FOAM see III:PKL500

POLYURETHANE FOAM see III:PKL500

POLYURETHANE SPONGE see III:PKL500

POLYURETHANE Y-195 see I:PKL750

POLYURETHANE Y-217 see I:PKM000

POLYURETHANE Y-218 see I:PKM250

POLYURETHANE Y-221 see I:PKM500

POLYURETHANE Y-222 see I:PKM750

POLYURETHANE Y-223 see I:PKN000

POLYURETHANE Y-224 see I:PKN250

POLYURETHANE Y-225 see I:PKN500

POLYURETHANE Y-226 see I:PKN750

POLYURETHANE Y-227 see I:PKO000

POLYURETHANE Y-238 see I:CDV625

POLYURETHANE Y-290 see I:PKO500

POLYURETHANE Y-299 see III:PKO750

POLYURETHANE Y-302 see I:PKP000

POLYURETHANE Y-304 see I:PKP250

POLYVIDONE see III:PKQ250

POLYVINYL ACETATE CHLORIDE see III:PKP500

POLYVINYL ALCOHOL see III:PKP750

POLY(VINYL ALCOHOL) see III:PKP750

POLYVINYLBROMIDE see III:PKQ000

POLY(n-VINYLBUTYROLACTAM) see III:PKQ250

POLYVINYLCHLORID (GERMAN) see III:PKQ059

POLYVINYL CHLORIDE see III:PKQ059

POLYVINYLCHLORIDE ACETATE see III:PKP500

POLYVINYL CHLORIDE-POLYVINYL ACETATE see II:AAX175

POLY(1-VINYL-2-PYRROLIDINONE) HOMOPOLYMER see III:PKQ250

POLY(1-VINYL-2-PYRROLIDINONE) HUEPER'S POLYMER No. 1 see II:PKQ500

POLY(1-VINYL-2-PYRROLIDINONE) HUEPER'S POLYMER No. 2 see II:PKQ750

POLY(1-VINYL-2-PYRROLIDINONE) HUEPER'S POLYMER No. 3 see II:PKR000

POLY(1-VINYL-2-PYRROLIDINONE) HUEPER'S POLYMER No. 4 see II:PKR250

POLY(1-VINYL-2-PYRROLIDINONE) HUEPER'S POLYMER No. 5 see II:PKR500

POLY(1-VINYL-2-PYRROLIDINONE) HUEPER'S POLYMER No. 6 see II:PKR750

POLY(1-VINYL-2-PYRROLIDINONE) HUEPER'S POLYMER
   No. 7 see II:PKS000
POLYVINYLPYRROLIDONE see III:PKQ250
POLYWAX 1000 see III:PJS750
POMARSOL see III:TFS350
POMARSOL Z FORTE see III:BJK500
POMASOL see III:TFS350
PONCEAU 3R see II:FAG018
PONCEAU 4R see III:FMU080
PONCEAU 4R ALUMINUM LAKE see III:FMU080
PONCEAU BNA see III:FMU070
PONCEAU INSOLUBLE OLG see III:XRA000
PONCEAU R (BIOLOGICAL STAIN) see III:FMU070
PONCEAU SX see III:FAG050
PONCEAU XYLIDINE (BIOLOGICAL STAIN) see III:FMU070
PONCYL see GKE000
PONTACYL GREEN BL see III:FAE950
PONTACYL RUBINE R see III:HJF500
PONTACYL SCARLET RR see III:FMU080
PONTALITE see III:PKB500
PONTAMINE BLACK E see AQP000
PONTAMINE BLUE BB see I:CMO000
PONTAMINE BLUE 3BX see II:CMO250
PONTAMINE DEVELOPER TN see I:TGL750
PONTAMINE VIOLET N see III:CMP000
POOGIPHALAM, nut extract see II:BFW000
POPROLIN see III:PMP500
POROFOR CHKHC-18 see III:DVF400
POROPHOR B see III:DVF400
POSTINOR see III:NNQ500, III:NNQ520
POTASSIUM ACID ARSENATE see I:ARD250
POTASSIUM ARSENATE see I:ARD250
POTASSIUM ARSENITE see I:PKV500
POTASSIUM ARSENITE SOLUTION see I:FOM050
POTASSIUM BICHROMATE see III:PKX250
POTASSIUM BIS(2-HYDROXYETHYL)DITHIOCARBAMATE
   see III:PKX500
POTASSIUM BROMATE see II:PKY300
POTASSIUM CHROMATE(VI) see III:PLB250
POTASSIUM CHROMIUM ALUM see III:CMG850
POTASSIUM CYANONICKELATE HYDRATE see II:TBW250
POTASSIUM DICHROMATE(VI) see III:PKX250
POTASSIUM DICHROMATE, ZINC CHROMATE and ZINC HY-
   DROXIDE (1:3:1) see I:ZFJ150
POTASSIUM DIHYDROGEN ARSENATE see I:ARD250
POTASSIUM N-FLUOREN-2-YL ACETOHYDROXAMATE see
   III:HIS000
POTASSIUM HYDROGEN ARSENATE see I:ARD250
POTASSIUM INDOL-3-YL SULFATE see III:ICD000
POTASSIUM METAARSENITE see I:PKV500
POTASSIUM METABISULFITE (DOT, FCC) see III:PLR250
POTASSIUM OCTATITANATE see III:PLW150
POTASSIUM PYROSULFITE see III:PLR250
POTASSIUM TETRACYANONICKELATE see II:NDI000
POTASSIUM TETRACYANONICKELATE(II) see II:NDI000
POTASSIUM TITANIUM OXIDE see III:PLW150
POTASSIUM ZINC CHROMATE see I:CMK400, I:PLW500
POTASSIUM ZINC CHROMATE HYDROXIDE see I:PLW500
POTATO ALCOHOL see I:EFU000
POTATO, GREEN PARTS see III:PLW750
POTOMAC RED see III:CHP500
POVIDONE (USP XIX) see III:PKQ250
POWDER and ROOT see III:RNZ000
PPD see III:PEY500
PPE201 see I:PKO500
PP FACTOR see III:NCQ900
P.P. FACTOR-PELLAGRA PREVENTIVE FACTOR see
   III:NCQ900
PPZEIDAN see I:DAD200
PQD see III:DVR200
PRACARBAMIN see I:UVA000
PRACARBAMINE see I:UVA000
PRADUPEN see III:BDY669
PRAECIRHEUMIN see II:BRF500

PRANONE and DIETHYLSTILBESTROL see III:EEH900
PRANONE and STILBESTROL see III:EEH900
PRAPARAT 5968 see II:HGP500
PRASTERONE see III:AOO450
PRAXITEN see III:CFZ000
PRAZEPAM see III:DAP700
PRECIPITATED BARIUM SULPHATE see III:BAP000
PRECIPITATED CALCIUM SULFATE see III:CAX750
PRECIPITATED SILICA see III:SCL000
PRECOCENE 2 see III:AEX850
PRECOCENE II see III:AEX850
PRECORT see III:PLZ000
PREDENT see III:SHF500
PREDNICEN-M see III:PLZ000
PREDNILONGA see III:PLZ000
PREDNI-SEDIV see III:TEH500
PREDNISON see III:PLZ000
PREDNISONE see III:PLZ000
PREDNIZON see III:PLZ000
1,4-PREGNADIENE-17-α,21-DIOL-3,11,20-TRIONE see
   III:PLZ000
PREGNA-4,6-DIENE-3,20-DIONE, 6-CHLORO-17-HYDROXY-
   1-α,2-α-METHYLENE-, ACETATE see III:CQJ500
17-α-2,4-PREGNADIEN-20-YNO(2,3-d)ISOXAZOL-17-OL see
   III:DAB830
17-α-PREGNA-2,4-DIEN-20-YNO(2,3-d)ISOXAZOL-17-OL see
   III:DAB830
3,20-PREGNENE-4 see I:PMH500
17-α-PREGN-4-ENE-21-CARBOXYLIC ACID, 1-HYDROXY-7-
   α-MERCAPTO-3-OXO-α-LACTONE see III:AFJ500
4-PREGNENE-17,α,21-DIOL-3,11,20-TRIONE 21-ACETATE
   see III:CNS825
PREGNENEDIONE see I:PMH500
PREGNENE-3,20-DIONE see I:PMH500
PREGN-4-ENE-3,20-DIONE see I:PMH500
4-PREGNENE-3,20-DIONE see I:PMH500
Δ^4-PREGNENE-3,20-DIONE see I:PMH500
4-PREGNENE-3,20-DIONE-21-OL ACETATE see III:DAQ800
17-α-PREGN-4-EN-20-YNO(2,3-d)ISOXAZOL-17-OL see
   III:DAB830
17-α-PREGN-4-EN-20-YN-3-ONE, 17-HYDROXY-, and trans-α-
   α'-DIETHYL-4,4'-STILBENEDIOL see III:EEH900
PREMALOX see III:CBM000
PREMARIN see I:ECU750, I:PMB000
PREMAZINE see III:BJP000
PREMERGE see III:BRE500
PREMERGE 3 see III:BRE500
PREMERGE PLUS see II:BQI000
PRENIMON see III:TND000
PRENTOX see III:PIX250, III:RNZ000
PREPARATION 125 see I:DFT800
PREPARATION AF see III:HEI500
PREPARATION HE 166 see III:DUS500
PRESERV-O-SOTE see I:CMY825
PRESOMEN see I:ECU750
PRESPERSION, 75 UREA see III:USS000
PREVENOL see III:CKC000
PREVENOL 56 see III:CKC000
PREVENTOL see III:CKC000
PREVENTOL 56 see III:CKC000
PREVENTOL I see II:TIV750
PREVENTOL O EXTRA see III:BGJ250
PREVENTOL-ON see II:BGJ750
PREWEED see III:CKC000
PRIADEL see III:LGZ000
PRILTOX see II:PAX250
PRIMARY AMYL ALCOHOL see III:AOE000
PRIMARY DECYL ALCOHOL see III:DAI600
PRIMATOL see III:ARQ725
PRIMATOL P see III:PMN850
PRIMATOL S see III:BJP000
PRIMAZE see III:ARQ725
PRIMAZIN see III:SNJ000
PRIMIDOLOL HYDROCHLORIDE see III:PMC600

PRIMIN see III:DSK200
PRIMOCORT see III:DAQ800
PRIMOCORTAN see III:DAQ800
PRIMODOS see II:EEH520
PRIMOFOL see I:EDO000
PRIMOGYN B see I:EDP000
PRIMOGYN BOLEOSUM see I:EDP000
PRIMOGYN I see I:EDP000
PRIMOL 335 see III:MQV750
PRIMOLUT DEPOT see III:HNT500
PRIMOTEST see I:TBF500
PRIMOVLAR see III:NNL500
PRIMROSE YELLOW see I:ZFJ100
PRINCEP see III:BJP000
PRINTEL'S see III:SMQ500
PRINTOP see III:BJP000
PRIODERM see III:MAK700
PRISTANE see III:PMD500
PRO-BAN M see III:TEH500
PROCARBAZIN (GERMAN) see I:PME500
PROCARBAZINE see I:PME250
PROCARBAZINE HYDROCHLORIDE see I:PME500
PROCASIL see I:PNX000
PROCION YELLOW MX 4R see III:RCZ000
PROCYTOX see I:CQC675, I:EAS500
PRODALUMNOL see I:SEY500
PRODALUMNOL DOUBLE see I:SEY500
PRODARAM see III:BJK500
PRO-DUOSTERONE see III:NNL500
PROFAM see III:CBM000
PROFARMIL see III:TEH500
PROFAX see III:PMP500
PROFERRIN see I:IHG000
PROFLAVIN see III:DBN600
PROFLAVINE see III:DBN600, III:PMH100
PROFLAVINE HEMISULPHATE see III:PMH100
PROFLAVINE HYDROCHLORIDE see III:PMH250
PROFLAVINE MONOHYDROCHLORIDE see III:PMH250
PROFLAVINE MONOHYDROCHLORIDE HEMIHYDRATE see
  III:DBN200
PROFOLIOL see I:EDO000, III:DBN600
PROFORMIPHEN see III:DBN600
PROFUME A see III:CKN500
PROFUME (OBS.) see III:MHR200
PROFUNDOL see III:DBN600
PROFURA see III:DBN600
PROGALLIN P see III:PNM750
PROGARMED see III:DBN600
PROGEKAN see I:PMH500
PRO-GEN see III:DBN600
PROGESIC see III:DBN600
PROGESTEROL see I:PMH500
PROGESTERONE see I:PMH500
β-PROGESTERONE see I:PMH500
PROGESTERONE CAPROATE see III:HNT500
PROGESTERONE mixed with ESTRADIOL BENZOATE (14:1
  moles) see III:EDQ000
PROGESTERONE mixed with ESTRA-1,3,5(10)-TRIENE-3,17-β-
  DIOL-3-BENZOATE (14:1 moles) see III:EDQ000
PROGESTERONE RETARD PHARLON see III:HNT500
PROGESTERONUM see I:PMH500
PROGESTIN see I:PMH500
PROGESTONE see I:PMH500
PRO-GIBB see III:GEM000
PROGYNON see I:EDO000, II:EDS100
PROGYNON B see I:EDP000
PROGYNON BENZOATE see I:EDP000
PROGYNON-DEPOT see II:EDS100
PROGYNON-DH see I:EDO000
PROGYNON-DP see I:EDR000
PROGYNOVA see II:EDS100
PROKAYVIT see III:MMD500
PROLIDON see I:PMH500
PROLONGAL see I:IGS000

PROLUTON DEPOT see III:HNT500
PROMAMIDE see III:DTT600
PROMARIT see I:ECU750
PROMOTESTON see I:TBF500
PROMPTONAL see II:EOK000
PRONAMIDE see III:DTT600
PRONETALOL see III:INS000
PRONETHALOL see III:INS000, III:INT000
PRONETHALOL HYDROCHLORIDE see III:INT000
PRONTALBIN see III:SNM500
PRONTOSIL I see III:SNM500
PROPACIL see I:PNX000
PROPAL see II:CIR500
PROPANAL, 2-CHLORO-(9CI) see III:CKR100
PROPANE, 1-CHLORO-1,2-EPOXY-, (E)- see III:CKS100
PROPANE, 1-CHLORO-1,2-EPOXY-, (Z)- see III:CKS099
PROPANEDIAL see III:PMK000
1,3-PROPANEDIAL see III:PMK000
1,3-PROPANEDIALDEHYDE see III:PMK000
PROPANEDIAL, ION(1-), SODIUM (9CI) see III:MAN700
1,2-PROPANEDIOL, 3-(NITROSO-2-PROPENYLAMINO)- see
  III:NJY500
1,3-PROPANEDIONE see III:PMK000
PROPANENITRILE, 3-(METHYLNITROSOAMINO)- see
  II:MMS200
1-PROPANESULFONIC ACID-3-HYDROXY-γ-SULTONE see
  I:PML400
PROPANE SULTONE see I:PML400
1,3-PROPANE SULTONE (MAK) see I:PML400
1,2,3-PROPANETRIOL, TRINITRATE see III:NGY000
1,2,3-PROPANETRIYL NITRATE see III:NGY000
PROPANOIC ACID see III:PJA500
PROPANOIC ACID, 2-((4'-CHLORO(1,1'-BIPHENYL)-4-
  YL)OXY)-2-METHYL-, METHYL ESTER (9CI) see
  III:MIO975
PROPANOIC ACID, 2-(4-(2,2-DICHLOROCYCLOPROPYL)
  PHENOXY)-2-METHYL- see III:CMS210
PROPANOL-1 see III:PND000
1-PROPANOL see III:PND000
PROPAN-2-OL see III:INJ000
2-PROPANOL see III:INJ000
n-PROPANOL see III:PND000
i-PROPANOL (GERMAN) see III:INJ000
PROPANOLE (GERMAN) see III:PND000
PROPANOLEN (DUTCH) see III:PND000
PROPANOLI (ITALIAN) see III:PND000
PROPANOLIDE see I:PMT100
PROPASIN see III:PMN850
PROPATHENE see III:PMP500
PROPAX see III:CFZ000
PROPAZINE see III:PMN850
PROPELLANT 22 see III:CFX500
PROPENAL (CZECH) see III:ADR000
2-PROPENAL see III:ADR000
PROP-2-EN-1-AL see III:ADR000
PROPENAMIDE see I:ADS250
2-PROPENAMIDE see I:ADS250
PROPENE see III:PMO500
1-PROPENE see III:PMO500
PROPENE ACID see III:ADS750
1-PROPENE HOMOPOLYMER (9CI) see III:PMP500
PROPENENITRILE see I:ADX500
2-PROPENENITRILE see I:ADX500
2-PROPENENITRILE, POLYMER with CHLOROETHENE see
  III:ADY250
PROPENE OXIDE see I:PNL600
PROPENE POLYMERS see III:PMP500
2-PROPENOIC ACID see III:ADS750
2-PROPENOIC ACID-2,2-DIMETHYL-1,3-PROPANEDIYL ES-
  TER see III:DUL200
2-PROPENOIC ACID, 1,2-ETHANEDIYLBIS(OXY-2,1-ETHAN-
  EDIYL) ESTER (9CI) see III:TJQ100
2-PROPENOIC ACID, ETHYL ESTER (MAK) see II:EFT000
2-PROPENOIC ACID-2-ETHYLHEXYL ESTER see
  III:ADU250

2-PROPENOIC ACID, HOMOPOLYMER, ZINC SALT see III:ADW250
2-PROPENOIC ACID-2-(HYDROXYMETHYL)-2-(((1-OXO-2-PROPENYL)OXY)METHYL)-1,3-PROPANEDIYL ESTER see III:PBC750
PROPENOIC ACID METHYL ESTER see III:MGA500
2-PROPENOIC ACID METHYL ESTER see III:MGA500
2-PROPENOIC ACID, OXYBIS(2,1-ETHANEDIYLOXY-2,1-ETHANEDIYL)ESTER see III:ADT050
2-PROPEN-1-ONE see III:ADR000
2-PROPENOPHENONE see III:PMQ250
2-PROPENYLACRYLIC ACID see III:SKU000
4-PROPENYLANISOLE see III:PMQ750
p-PROPENYLANISOLE see III:PMQ750
p-1-PROPENYLANISOLE see III:PMQ750
5-(1-PROPENYL)-1,3-BENZODIOXOLE see III:IRZ000
5-(2-PROPENYL)-1,3-BENZODIOXOLE see I:SAD000
4-PROPENYLCATECHOL METHYLENE ETHER see III:IRZ000
PROPENYL CHLORIDE see III:PMR750
2-PROPENYL CHLORIDE see II:AGB250
2-PROPENYL ISOTHIOCYANATE see II:AGJ250
2-PROPENYL ISOVALERATE see II:ISV000
2-PROPENYL 3-METHYLBUTANOATE see II:ISV000
4-PROPENYL-1,2-METHYLENEDIOXYBENZENE see III:IRZ000
2-PROPENYLPHENOL see III:PMS250
o-PROPENYLPHENOL see III:PMS250
2-(1-PROPENYL)PHENOL see III:PMS250
p-PROPENYLPHENYL METHYL ETHER see III:PMQ750
PROPHAM see III:CBM000
PROPILTHIOURACIL see I:PNX000
6-PROPIL-TIOURACILE (ITALIAN) see I:PNX000
PROPIOKAN see I:TBG000
PROPIOLACTONE see I:PMT100
3-PROPIOLACTONE see I:PMT100
β-PROPIOLACTONE see I:PMT100
1,3-PROPIOLACTONE see I:PMT100
β-PROPIONOLACTONE see I:PMT100
10-PROPIONYL DITHRANOL see III:PMW760
N-PROPIONYL-N-2-FLUORENYLHYDROXYLAMINE see III:FEO000
PROPOLIN see III:PMP500
PROPON see II:TIX500
PROPONEX-PLUS see II:CIR500
PROPOPHANE see III:PMP500
PROPOXUR NITROSO see III:PMY310
β-PROPRIOLACTONE (OSHA) see I:PMT100
β-PROPROLACTONE see I:PMT100
PROPYCIL see I:PNX000
PROPYL ACETOXYMETHYLNITROSAMINE see III:PNR250
N-PROPYL-N-(ACETOXYMETHYL)NITROSAMINE see III:PNR250
S-PROPYL-N-AETHYL-N-BUTYL-THIOCARBAMAT (GERMAN) see III:PNF500
PROPYL ALCOHOL see III:PND000
1-PROPYL ALCOHOL see III:PND000
n-PROPYL ALCOHOL see III:PND000
sec-PROPYL ALCOHOL (DOT) see III:INJ000
i-PROPYLALKOHOL (GERMAN) see III:INJ000
n-PROPYL ALKOHOL (GERMAN) see III:PND000
8-PROPYLBENZ(a)ANTHRACENE see III:PNE750
5-n-PROPYL-1,2-BENZANTHRACENE see III:PNE750
5-PROPYL-1,3-BENZODIOXOLE see II:DMD600
5-PROPYLBENZO(c)PHENANTHRENE see III:PNF000
2-n-PROPYL-3:4-BENZPHENANTHRENE see III:PNF000
S-PROPYL BUTYLETHYLTHIOCARBAMATE see III:PNF500
N-PROPYL-N-BUTYLNITROSAMINE see III:PNF750
PROPYL CARBAMATE see III:PNG250
N-PROPYL CARBAMATE see III:PNG250
4'-N-PROPYL-4-DIMETHYLAMINOAZOBENZENE see III:DTT400
5-n-PROPYL-9,10-DIMETHYL-1,2-BENZANTHRACENE see III:PNI500

PROPYLENE (DOT) see III:PMO500
PROPYLENE ALDEHYDE see III:ADR000
PROPYLENE CHLORIDE see III:PNJ400
PROPYLENE DICHLORIDE see III:PNJ400
α,β-PROPYLENE DICHLORIDE see III:PNJ400
4,4'-PROPYLENEDI-2,6-PIPERAZINEDIONE see II:RCA375
PROPYLENE EPOXIDE see I:PNL600
PROPYLENE IMINE see I:PNL400
1,2-PROPYLENEIMINE see I:PNL400
PROPYLENE IMINE, INHIBITED (DOT) see I:PNL400
PROPYLENE OXIDE see I:PNL600
1,2-PROPYLENE OXIDE see I:PNL600
1,3-PROPYLENE OXIDE see III:OMW000
PROPYLENE POLYMER see III:PMP500
n-PROPYL ESTER of 3,4,5-TRIHYDROXYBENZOIC ACID see III:PNM750
PROPYL-ETHYLBUTYLTHIOCARBAMATE see III:PNF500
PROPYLETHYL-N-BUTYLTHIOCARBAMATE see III:PNF500
PROPYL N-ETHYL-N-BUTYLTHIOCARBAMATE see III:PNF500
N-PROPYL-N-ETHYL-N-(N-BUTYL)THIOCARBAMATE see III:PNF500
S-(N-PROPYL)-N-ETHYL-N-N-BUTYLTHIOCARBAMATE see III:PNF500
PROPYL ETHYLBUTYLTHIOLCARBAMATE see III:PNF500
N-PROPYL-N-ETHYL-N-(N-BUTYL)THIOLCARBAMATE see III:PNF500
N,N-PROPYL ETHYL CARBAMATE see III:EPC050
N-n-PROPYL-N-FORMYLHYDRAZINE see III:PNM650
PROPYL GALLATE see III:PNM750
n-PROPYL GALLATE see III:PNM750
N-PROPYLHYDRAZINE HYDROCHLORIDE see III:PNO000
N-PROPYL-N-(HYDROPEROXYMETHYL)NITROSAMINE see III:HIE570
PROPYL(4-HYDROXYBUTYL)NITROSAMINE see III:NLN000
PROPYLIC ALCOHOL see III:PND000
i-PROPYL IODIDE see III:IPS000
n-PROPYL IODIDE see III:PNO750
PROPYL ISOMER see III:PNP250
n-PROPYL ISOMER see III:PNP250
4-PROPYL-1,2-METHYLENEDIOXYBENZENE see II:DMD600
N-PROPYL-N'-NITRO-N-NITROSOGUANIDINE see III:NLD000
4-(PROPYLNITROSAMINO)-1-BUTANOL see III:NLN000
PROPYLNITROSAMINOMETHYL ACETATE see III:PNR250
1-(PROPYLNITROSAMINO)PROPYL ACETATE see III:ABT750
N-PROPYLNITROSOHARNSTOFF (GERMAN) see II:NLO500
1-PROPYL-1-NITROSOUREA see II:NLO500
N-PROPYL-N-NITROSOURETHANE see III:PNR500
N-PROPYLNITROSUREA see II:NLO500
PROPYLOWY ALKOHOL (POLISH) see III:PND000
PROPYL OXIRANE see III:BOX750
6-(PROPYLPIPERONYL)-BUTYL CARBITYL ETHER see III:PIX250
6-PROPYLPIPERONYL BUTYL DIETHYLENE GLYCOL ETHER see III:PIX250
6-PROPYL-2-THIO-2,4(1H,3H)PYRIMIDINEDIONE see I:PNX000
PROPYL-THIORIST see I:PNX000
PROPYLTHIOURACIL see I:PNX000
4-PROPYL-2-THIOURACIL see I:PNX000
6-PROPYL-2-THIOURACIL see I:PNX000
6-N-PROPYLTHIOURACIL see I:PNX000
6-N-PROPYL-2-THIOURACIL see I:PNX000
PROPYL-THYRACIL see I:PNX000
n-PROPYL-3,4,5-TRIHYDROXYBENZOATE see III:PNM750
5-PROPYL-4-(2,5,8-TRIOXA-DODECYL)-1,3-BENZODIOXOL (GERMAN) see III:PIX250
1-PROPYLUREA and SODIUM NITRITE see III:SIT750
n-PROPYLUREA and SODIUM NITRITE see III:SIT750

PROPYL URETHANE see III:PNG250
PROPYTHIOURACIL see I:PNX000
PROPYZAMIDE see III:DTT600
P. ROQUEFORTI TOXIN see III:PAQ875
PRORALONE-MOP see I:XDJ000
PROSEPTINE see III:SNM500
PROSEPTOL see III:SNM500
PROSTRUMYL see II:MPW500
PROTACTINIUM see I:POD500
PROTAGENT see III:PKQ250
PROTANABOL see I:PAN100
PROTASORB O-20 see III:PKL100
PROTECTONA see I:DKA600
PROTHIUCIL see I:PNX000
PROTHIURONE see I:PNX000
PROTHYCIL see I:PNX000
PROTHYRAN see I:PNX000
PROTIURAL see I:PNX000
PROTOBOLIN see III:DAL300
PROTOPET see III:MQV750
PROTOPYRIN see III:EEM000
PROTOTYPE III SOFT see III:PKQ059
PROVITAMIN D see III:CMD750
PROVITAMIN D₃ see III:DAK600
PROXOL see III:TIQ250
PROZINEX see III:PMN850
PRT see III:POF800
PR TOXIN see III:PAQ875, III:POF800
PR TOXINE see III:POF800
PRUSSIAN BROWN see III:IHD000
PS see III:CKN500
PS 1 see III:AHE250
PSEUDOCUMIDINE see I:TLG250
PSEUDOCUMIDINE HYDROCHLORIDE see III:TLG750
PSEUDOCYANURIC ACID see III:THS000
PSEUDOTHIOUREA see I:ISR000
PSEUDOTHYMINE see III:MQI750
PSEUDOUREA see III:USS000
PSEUDOXANTHINE see III:XCA000
PSICOPAX see III:CFZ000
PSICOSTERONE see III:AOO450
PSIDIUM GUAJAVA see III:GLW000
PSORADERM see II:MFN275
PSYCHOLIQUID see III:TEH500
PSYCHOTABLETS see III:TEH500
PT 155 see III:DAD040
PTAQUILOSIDE see III:POI100
PTERIDIUM AQUILINUM see I:BML000
PTERIDIUM AQUILINUM TANNIN see III:BML250
PTERIS AQUALINA see I:BML000
PTFE see III:TAI250
PTU (THYREOSTATIC) see I:PNX000
PURADIN see III:NGG500
PURALIN see III:TFS350
PURATRONIC CHROMIUM TRIOXIDE see I:CMK000
PURE CHRYSOIDINE YBH see III:PEK000
PURE CHRYSOIDINE YD see III:PEK000
PURE EOSINE YY see III:BNH500
PURE LEMON CHROME L3GS see I:LCR000
PURE ORANGE CHROME M see I:LCS000
PURE QUARTZ see I:SCJ500
PURE ZINC CHROME see I:ZFJ100
PURIMETHOL see III:POK000
PURINE see III:POJ250
7H-PURINE see III:POJ250
9H-PURINE see III:POJ250
PURINE-2,6-DIOL see III:XCA000
9H-PURINE-2,6-DIOL see III:XCA000
2,6(1,3)-PURINEDION see III:XCA000
PURINE-2,6-(1H,3H)-DIONE see III:XCA000
PURINE-3-OXIDE see III:POJ750
PURINE-6-THIOL see III:POK000
6-PURINETHIOL see III:POK000
3H-PURINE-6-THIOL see III:POK000

PURINETHOL see III:POK000
PURPLE 4R see III:FAG050
PURPLE RED see III:FMU080
PURTALC USP see III:TAB750
PVBR see III:PKQ000
PVC CORDO see II:AAX175
PVC (MAK) see III:PKQ059
PVP 1 see II:PKQ500
PVP 2 see II:PKQ750
PVP 3 see II:PKR000
PVP 4 see II:PKR250
PVP 5 see II:PKR500
PVP 6 see II:PKR750
PVP 7 see II:PKS000
PVP (FCC) see III:PKQ250
PX-238 see III:AEO000
PYBUTHRIN see III:PIX250
PYCAZIDE see III:ILD000
PYDT see III:DJY000
PYMAFED see III:DBM800
PYNDT see III:DTV200
N-N-PYR see I:NLP500
PYRABUTOL see II:BRF500
PYRACRYL ORANGE Y see III:PEK000
PYRADEX see III:DBI200
PYRADONE see III:DOT000
PYRALENE see I:PJL750
PYRA MALEATE see III:DBM800
PYRAMIDON see III:DOT000
PYRAMIDONE see III:DOT000
PYRANILAMINE MALEATE see III:DBM800
PYRANINYL see III:DBM800
PYRANISAMINE MALEATE see III:DBM800
PYRANOL see I:PJL750
PYRATHYN see III:DPJ400
PYRAZAPON see III:POL475
PYRAZINAMIDE see III:POL500
PYRAZINEAMIDE see III:POL500
PYRAZINECARBOXAMIDE see III:POL500
PYRAZINE CARBOXYLAMIDE see III:POL500
PYRAZINOIC ACID AMIDE see III:POL500
PYRAZODINE see I:PDC250
PYRAZOFEN see I:PDC250, III:PEK250
PYRAZOL BLUE 3B see II:CMO250
PYRAZOLIDIN see II:BRF500
PYREAZID see III:ILD000
PYREDAL see I:PDC250
PYREN (GERMAN) see III:PON250
PYRENE see III:PON250
PYRENOLINE see III:PCV500
PYRENONE 606 see III:PIX250
N-PYREN-2-YLACETAMIDE see III:PON500
1-PYRENYLOXIRANE see III:ONG000
PYRICIDIN see III:ILD000
PYRIDACIL see I:PDC250, III:PEK250
PYRIDENAL see I:PDC250
PYRIDENE see I:PDC250
PYRIDIATE see I:PDC250
PYRIDICIN see III:ILD000
PYRIDINE-3-AZO-p-DIMETHYLANILINE see III:POP750
PYRIDINE-4-AZO-p-DIMETHYLANILINE see III:POQ000
PYRIDINE-3-CARBONIC ACID see III:NCQ900
PYRIDINE-3-CARBOXYLIC ACID see III:NCQ900
3-PYRIDINECARBOXYLIC ACID see III:NCQ900
PYRIDINE-β-CARBOXYLIC ACID see III:NCQ900
4-PYRIDINECARBOXYLIC ACID-2-ACETYLHYDRAZIDE see III:ACO750
2-PYRIDINECARBOXYLIC ACID-2-ACETYLHYDRAZIDE (9CI) see III:ADA000
4-PYRIDINECARBOXYLIC ACID, HYDRAZIDE see III:ILD000
4-PYRIDINECARBOXYLIC ACID, ((4-HYDROXY-3-METHOXYPHENYL)METHYLENE)HYDRAZIDE see III:VEZ925

3-PYRIDINECARBOXYLIC ACID-1,2,5,6-TETRAHYDRO-1-
  METHYL ESTER, HYDROCHLORIDE see III:AQU250
PYRIDINE-CARBOXYLIQUE-3 (FRENCH) see III:NCQ900
PYRIDINE, 3-(1-NITROSO-2-PIPERIDINYL)-, (S)-(9CI) see
  III:NJK150
PYRIDINE-1-OXIDE-3-AZO-p-DIMETHYLANILINE see
  III:POS250
PYRIDINE-1-OXIDE-4-AZO-p-DIMETHYLANILINE see
  III:POS500
PYRIDIUM see I:PDC250, III:PEK250
PYRIDIVITE see I:PDC250
PYRIDO(3′,2′:5,6)CHRYSENE see III:BCQ000
PYRIDO(3′,2′:3,4)FLUORANTHENE see III:FDP000
5H-PYRIDO(4,3-b)INDOL-3-AMINE, 1-METHYL-1, MONO-
  ACETATE see III:ALE750
PYRIDO(2′,3′:4)PYRENE see III:PCV500
12H-PYRIDO(2,3-a)THIENO(2,3-i)CARBAZOLE see
  III:PPI815
3-PYRIDOYL HYDRAZINE see III:NDU500
1-(PYRIDYL-3-)-3,3-DIAETHYL-TRIAZEN (GERMAN) see
  III:DJY000
m-PYRIDYL-DIETHYL-TRIAZENE see III:DJY000
1-PYRIDYL-3,3-DIETHYLTRIAZENE see III:DJY000
1-(PYRIDYL-3)-3,3-DIETHYLTRIAZENE see III:DJY000
1-(3-PYRIDYL)-3,3-DIETHYLTRIAZENE see III:DJY000
1-(PYRIDYL-3)-3,3-DIMETHYL-TRIAZEN (GERMAN) see
  III:PPL500
1-(PYRIDYL-3)-3,3-DIMETHYL TRIAZENE see III:PPL500
1-(m-PYRIDYL)-3,3-DIMETHYL-TRIAZENE see III:PPL500
1-(PYRIDYL-3-N-OXID)-3,3-DIMETHYL-TRIAZEN (GER-
  MAN) see III:DTV200
1-(PYRIDYL-3-N-OXIDE)-3,3-DIMETHYLTRIAZENE see
  III:DTV200
N-2-PYRIDYLSULFANILAMIDE see III:PPO000
N¹-2-PYRIDYLSULFANILAMIDE see III:PPO000
N-(2-PYRIDYL)-N-(2-THIENYL)-N,N′-DIMETHYL-ETHYL-
  ENEDIAMINE HYDROCHLORIDE see III:DPJ400
PYRILAMINE MALEATE see III:DBM800
PYRIMIDINE-DEOXYRIBOSE N1-2′-FURANIDYL-5-FLUO-
  ROURACIL see III:FMB000
2,4-PYRIMIDINEDIOL see III:UNJ800
2,4-PYRIMIDINEDIONE see III:UNJ800
2,4(1H,3H)-PYRIMIDINEDIONE (9CI) see III:UNJ800
2,4,6(1H,3H,5H)-PYRIMIDINETRIONE, MONOSODIUM SALT
  (9CI) see III:MRK750
PYRINAZINE see II:HIM000
β-PYRINE see III:PON250
PYRIPYRIDIUM see I:PDC250, III:PEK250
PYRIZIDIN see III:ILD000
PYRIZIN see I:PDC250
PYROBENZOL see I:BBL250
PYROBENZOLE see I:BBL250
PYROCATECHIN see III:CCP850
PYROCATECHINIC ACID see III:CCP850
PYROCATECHOL see III:CCP850
PYROCATECHUIC ACID see III:CCP850
PYROCHOL see III:DAQ400
PYROD see III:UNJ800
PYRODINE see III:ACX750
PYROGALLIC ACID see III:PPQ500
PYROGALLOL see III:PPQ500
PYRONALORANGE see III:PEJ500
PYRONALROT R see III:XRA000
PYROSET FLAME RETARDANT TKP see III:TDH500
PYROSET TKP see III:TDH500
PYROSULFUROUS ACID, DIPOTASSIUM SALT see
  III:PLR250
PYROTROPBLAU see II:CMO250
PYRROLIDINE, 1-(p-((p-ETHYLPHENYL)AZO)PHENYL)- see
  III:EPC950
PYRROLIDINE, NITROSO- see III:NLP480
PYRROLYLENE see I:BOP500
3-PYRROL-2-YLPYRIDINE see III:PQB500
PYSOCOCCINE see III:SNM500

Q-137 see III:DJC000
QDO see III:DVR200
QSAH 7 see III:PKQ059
QUADRATIC ACID see III:DMJ600
QUANTALAN see III:CME400
QUARTZ see I:SCJ500
QUARTZ GLASS see I:SCK600
QUATRACHLOR see III:BEN000
QUAZO PURO (ITALIAN) see I:SCJ500
QUEBRACHO TANNIN see III:QBJ000
QUECKSILBER (GERMAN) see III:MCW250
QUELETOX see III:FAQ999
QUELLADA see I:BBQ500
QUEMICETINA see II:CDP250
QUEN see III:CFZ000
QUERCETIN see III:QCA000
QUERCETIN-3-(6-o-(6-DEOXY-α-l-MANNOPYRANOSYL-β-d-
  GLUCOPYRANOSIDE) see III:RSU000
QUERCETIN DIHYDRATE see III:QCA175
QUERCETINE see III:QCA000
QUERCETIN RHAMNOGLUCOSIDE see III:RSU000
QUERCETIN-3-RHAMNOGLUCOSINE see III:RSU000
QUERCETIN-3-(6-o-α-l-RHAMNOPYRANOSYL-β-d-GLUCO-
  PYRANOSIDE) see III:RSU000
QUERCETIN-3-RUTINOSIDE see III:RSU000
QUERCETOL see III:QCA000
QUERCITIN see III:QCA000
QUERCUS AEGILOPS L. TANNIN see III:VCK000
QUERCUS FALCATA PAGODAEFOLIA see III:CDL750
QUERTINE see III:QCA000
QUESTRAN see III:CME400
QUETIMID see III:TEH500
QUETINIL see III:DCK759
QUIATRIL see III:DCK759
QUICKSET EXTRA see III:MKA500
QUICK SILVER see III:MCW250
QUIETOPLEX see III:TEH500
QUIEVITA see III:DCK759
QUILIBREX see III:CFZ000
QUILONUM RETARD see III:LGZ000
QUINACHLOR see III:CLD000
QUINACRINE ETHYL M/2 see III:QCS875
QUINACRINE ETHYL MUSTARD see III:DFH000
QUINACRINE MUSTARD see III:QDS000
QUINACRINE MUSTARD DIHYDROCHLORIDE see
  III:QDS000
QUINAGAMINE see III:CLD000
QUINDOXIN see III:QSA000
QUINERCYL see III:CLD000
QUINILON see III:CLD000
8-QUINOL see III:QPA000
β-QUINOL see III:HIH000
4-QUINOLINAMINE, N-HYDROXY-N-METHYL-, 1-OXIDE
  see III:HLX550
QUINOLINE see III:QMJ000
QUINOLINE-6-AZO-p-DIMETHYLANILINE see III:DPR000
8-QUINOLINOL see III:QPA000
QUINOLOR COMPOUND see III:BDS000
N-(4-QUINOLYL)ACETOHYDROXAMIC ACID see
  III:QQA000
N-(4-QUINOLYL)HYDROXYLAMINE-1′-OXIDE see
  III:HIY500
QUINONDO see III:BLC250
QUINONE see III:QQS200
p-QUINONE see III:QQS200
QUINONE DIOXIME see III:DVR200
p-QUINONE DIOXIME see III:DVR200
p-QUINONE OXIME see III:DVR200
QUINOPHENOL see III:QPA000
QUINOSCAN see III:CLD000
QUINOXALINE DIOXIDE see III:QSA000
QUINOXALINE DI-N-OXIDE see III:QSA000
QUINOXALINE 1,4-DIOXIDE see III:QSA000
QUINOXALINE-1,4-DI-N-OXIDE see III:QSA000

QUINTAR see III:DFT000
QUINTAR 540F see III:DFT000
QUINTOCENE see III:PAX000
QUINTOX see III:DHB400
QUINTOZEN see III:PAX000
QUINTOZENE see III:PAX000
QUIRVIL see III:PKQ059
QYSA see III:PKQ059

R 10 see CBY000
R 14 see I:PKL750
R 22 (DOT) see III:CFX500
R-47 see III:TNF500
R48 see I:BIF250
R50 see I:DAD200
R 54 see III:DDP600
88-R see I:SOP500
R-246 see III:TND500
R 694 see III:MEK700
R 133a see III:TJY175
R 1625 see III:CLY500
R-2061 see III:PNF500
R 2858 see III:MRU600
R 40B1 see III:MHR200
R6597 see III:NHQ950
R 6700 see III:OAN000
R7000 see II:MFB400
R 7372 see III:MEW975
R 9985 see III:MDV500
β-RA see III:VSK950
RABON see III:RAF100
RABOND see III:RAF100
RACUSAN see III:DSP400
RADAZIN see III:ARQ725
RADDLE see III:IHD000
RAD-E CATE 16 see I:HKC500
RAD-E-CATE 25 see III:HKC000
RADIASURF 7125 see III:SKV000
RADICALISIN see III:RRA000
RADIUM F see II:PJJ750
RADIZINE see III:ARQ725
RADOCON see III:BJP000
RADOKOR see III:BJP000
RADONIL see III:SNK000
RADOXONE TL see I:AMY050
RAFLUOR see III:SHF500
RAKUTO AMARANTH see III:FAG020
RAMIZOL see I:AMY050
R/AMP see II:RKP000
RANEY ALLOY see I:NCW500
RANEY COPPER see III:CNI000
RANEY NICKEL see I:NCW500
RANKOTEX see II:CIR500
RAPHONE see II:CIR250
RASPBERRY RED for JELLIES see III:FAG020
RATON see III:RBZ000
RATTEX see III:CNV000
RATTRACK see III:AQN635
RAUMANON see III:ILD000
RAUNORINE see III:RDF000
RAUSERPIN see II:RDK000
RAUTRAX see III:RCA275
RAUWOLEAF see II:RDK000
RAVINYL see III:PKQ059
RAW SHALE OIL see I:COD750
RAYBAR see III:BAP000
RAY-GLUCIRON see III:FBK000
RAYOX see III:TGG760
RAZIDE see III:ILD000
RAZOL DOCK KILLER see II:CIR250
RAZOXANE see II:RCA375
RAZOXIN see II:PIK250, II:RCA375
RB see III:PAK000
RB 1509 see I:CGV250

RCA WASTE NUMBER P105 see III:SFA000
RCA WASTE NUMBER U203 see I:SAD000
RC 172DBM see III:AHE250
RC PLASTICIZER DOP see I:DVL700
RCRA WASTE NUMBER 7066 see I:DDL800
RCRA WASTE NUMBER P003 see III:ADR000
RCRA WASTE NUMBER P004 see III:AFK250
RCRA WASTE NUMBER P010 see I:ARB250
RCRA WASTE NUMBER P015 see I:BFO750
RCRA WASTE NUMBER P016 see I:BIK000
RCRA WASTE NUMBER P020 see III:BRE500
RCRA WASTE NUMBER P024 see III:CEH680
RCRA WASTE NUMBER P028 see II:BEE375
RCRA WASTE NUMBER P037 see III:DHB400
RCRA WASTE NUMBER P044 see III:DSP400
RCRA WASTE NUMBER P050 see III:EAQ750
RCRA WASTE NUMBER P051 see III:EAT500
RCRA WASTE NUMBER P054 see III:EJM900
RCRA WASTE NUMBER P059 see II:HAR000
RCRA WASTE NUMBER P067 see I:PNL400
RCRA WASTE NUMBER P068 see II:MKN000
RCRA WASTE NUMBER P071 see III:MNH000
RCRA WASTE NUMBER P072 see III:AQN635
RCRA WASTE NUMBER P073 see I:NCZ000
RCRA WASTE NUMBER P074 see II:NDB500
RCRA WASTE NUMBER P081 see III:NGY000
RCRA WASTE NUMBER P082 see I:NKA600
RCRA WASTE NUMBER P084 see II:NKY000
RCRA WASTE NUMBER P089 see III:PAK000
RCRA WASTE NUMBER P110 see III:TCF000
RCRA WASTE NUMBER P116 see III:TFQ000
RCRA WASTE NUMBER P123 see I:CDV100
RCRA WASTE NUMBER U001 see II:AAG250
RCRA WASTE NUMBER U005 see I:FDR000
RCRA WASTE NUMBER U007 see I:ADS250
RCRA WASTE NUMBER U008 see III:ADS750
RCRA WASTE NUMBER U009 see I:ADX500
RCRA WASTE NUMBER U010 see II:AHK500
RCRA WASTE NUMBER U011 see I:AMY050
RCRA WASTE NUMBER U014 see I:IBB000
RCRA WASTE NUMBER U015 see II:ASA500
RCRA WASTE NUMBER U016 see III:BAW750
RCRA WASTE NUMBER U017 see II:BAY300
RCRA WASTE NUMBER U018 see I:BBC250
RCRA WASTE NUMBER U019 see I:BBL250
RCRA WASTE NUMBER U021 see I:BBX000
RCRA WASTE NUMBER U023 see I:BFL250
RCRA WASTE NUMBER U025 see III:DFJ050
RCRA WASTE NUMBER U026 see I:BIF250
RCRA WASTE NUMBER U027 see III:BII250
RCRA WASTE NUMBER U028 see I:DVL700
RCRA WASTE NUMBER U029 see III:MHR200
RCRA WASTE NUMBER U032 see I:CAP500
RCRA WASTE NUMBER U035 see I:CDO500
RCRA WASTE NUMBER U036 see II:CDR750
RCRA WASTE NUMBER U038 see II:DER000
RCRA WASTE NUMBER U041 see I:EAZ500
RCRA WASTE NUMBER U043 see I:VNP000
RCRA WASTE NUMBER U044 see I:CHJ500
RCRA WASTE NUMBER U045 see II:MIF765
RCRA WASTE NUMBER U046 see I:CIO250
RCRA WASTE NUMBER U048 see III:CJK250
RCRA WASTE NUMBER U049 see II:CLK235
RCRA WASTE NUMBER U050 see I:CML810
RCRA WASTE NUMBER U051 see I:CMY825
RCRA WASTE NUMBER U052 see III:CNW750, III:CNX000,
  III:CNX250
RCRA WASTE NUMBER U053 see II:COB250
RCRA WASTE NUMBER U058 see I:EAS500
RCRA WASTE NUMBER U059 see II:DAC000
RCRA WASTE NUMBER U060 see I:BIM500
RCRA WASTE NUMBER U-061 see I:DAD200
RCRA WASTE NUMBER U062 see III:DBI200
RCRA WASTE NUMBER U063 see I:DCT400

RCRA WASTE NUMBER U064 see I:BCQ500
RCRA WASTE NUMBER U067 see I:EIY500
RCRA WASTE NUMBER U070 see II:DEP800, III:DEP600
RCRA WASTE NUMBER U071 see II:DEP800
RCRA WASTE NUMBER U072 see II:DEP800
RCRA WASTE NUMBER U073 see I:DEQ600
RCRA WASTE NUMBER U074 see I:DEV000
RCRA WASTE NUMBER U076 see III:DFF809
RCRA WASTE NUMBER U077 see I:EIY600
RCRA WASTE NUMBER U078 see II:VPK000
RCRA WASTE NUMBER U080 see II:MJP450
RCRA WASTE NUMBER U081 see II:DFX800
RCRA WASTE NUMBER U083 see III:PNJ400
RCRA WASTE NUMBER U084 see I:DGG950
RCRA WASTE NUMBER U085 see I:BGA750
RCRA WASTE NUMBER U086 see II:DJL400
RCRA WASTE NUMBER U089 see I:DKA600
RCRA WASTE NUMBER U090 see II:DMD600
RCRA WASTE NUMBER U091 see I:DCJ200
RCRA WASTE NUMBER U093 see I:DOT300
RCRA WASTE NUMBER U094 see II:DQJ200
RCRA WASTE NUMBER U095 see I:TGJ750
RCRA WASTE NUMBER U096 see III:IOB000
RCRA WASTE NUMBER U097 see I:DQY950
RCRA WASTE NUMBER U098 see I:DSF400
RCRA WASTE NUMBER U099 see I:DSF600
RCRA WASTE NUMBER U101 see III:XKJ500
RCRA WASTE NUMBER U103 see I:DUD100
RCRA WASTE NUMBER U105 see II:DVH000
RCRA WASTE NUMBER U106 see III:DVH400
RCRA WASTE NUMBER U108 see I:DVQ000
RCRA WASTE NUMBER U109 see I:HHG000
RCRA WASTE NUMBER U111 see I:NKB700
RCRA WASTE NUMBER U113 see II:EFT000
RCRA WASTE NUMBER U115 see I:EJN500
RCRA WASTE NUMBER U116 see I:IAQ000
RCRA WASTE NUMBER U119 see II:EMF500
RCRA WASTE NUMBER U120 see III:FDF000
RCRA WASTE NUMBER U122 see I:FMV000
RCRA WASTE NUMBER U126 see GGW000
RCRA WASTE NUMBER U127 see I:HCC500
RCRA WASTE NUMBER U128 see II:HCD250
RCRA WASTE NUMBER U129 see I:BBQ500
RCRA WASTE NUMBER U131 see III:HCI000
RCRA WASTE NUMBER U132 see III:HCL000
RCRA WASTE NUMBER U133 see I:HGS000
RCRA WASTE NUMBER U136 see III:HKC000
RCRA WASTE NUMBER U137 see I:IBZ000
RCRA WASTE NUMBER U138 see I:MKW200
RCRA WASTE NUMBER U139 see I:IGS000
RCRA WASTE NUMBER U140 see III:IIL000
RCRA WASTE NUMBER U141 see III:IRZ000
RCRA WASTE NUMBER U142 see I:KEA000
RCRA WASTE NUMBER U143 see I:LBG000
RCRA WASTE NUMBER U144 see I:LCG000
RCRA WASTE NUMBER U146 see III:LCH000
RCRA WASTE NUMBER U147 see III:MAM000
RCRA WASTE NUMBER U150 see I:PED750
RCRA WASTE NUMBER U151 see III:MCW250
RCRA WASTE NUMBER U157 see II:MIJ750
RCRA WASTE NUMBER U158 see I:MJM200
RCRA WASTE NUMBER U160 see III:MKA500
RCRA WASTE NUMBER U162 see III:MLH750
RCRA WASTE NUMBER U163 see II:MMP000
RCRA WASTE NUMBER U164 see II:MPW500
RCRA WASTE NUMBER U165 see III:NAJ500
RCRA WASTE NUMBER U166 see III:NBA500
RCRA WASTE NUMBER U167 see I:NBE000
RCRA WASTE NUMBER U168 see I:NBE500
RCRA WASTE NUMBER U171 see I:NIY000
RCRA WASTE NUMBER U172 see I:BRY500
RCRA WASTE NUMBER U173 see I:NKM000
RCRA WASTE NUMBER U174 see I:NJW500
RCRA WASTE NUMBER U176 see I:ENV000

RCRA WASTE NUMBER U177 see I:MNA750
RCRA WASTE NUMBER U178 see II:MMX250
RCRA WASTE NUMBER U179 see I:NLJ500
RCRA WASTE NUMBER U180 see I:NLP500
RCRA WASTE NUMBER U181 see I:NMP500
RCRA WASTE NUMBER U184 see III:PAW500
RCRA WASTE NUMBER U185 see III:PAX000
RCRA WASTE NUMBER U187 see I:ABG750
RCRA WASTE NUMBER U188 see III:PDN750
RCRA WASTE NUMBER U192 see III:DTT600
RCRA WASTE NUMBER U193 see I:PML400
RCRA WASTE NUMBER U197 see III:QQS200
RCRA WASTE NUMBER U201 see III:REA000
RCRA WASTE NUMBER U202 see II:BCE500
RCRA WASTE NUMBER U206 see I:SMD000
RCRA WASTE NUMBER U208 see III:TBQ000
RCRA WASTE NUMBER U209 see III:TBQ100
RCRA WASTE NUMBER U210 see II:PCF275
RCRA WASTE NUMBER U211 see CBY000
RCRA WASTE NUMBER U212 see II:TBT000
RCRA WASTE NUMBER U218 see I:TFA000
RCRA WASTE NUMBER U219 see I:ISR000
RCRA WASTE NUMBER U221 see I:TGL750
RCRA WASTE NUMBER U222 see I:TGS500
RCRA WASTE NUMBER U223 see I:TGM740, I:TGM750
RCRA WASTE NUMBER U225 see III:BNL000
RCRA WASTE NUMBER U226 see III:MIH275
RCRA WASTE NUMBER U227 see II:TIN000
RCRA WASTE NUMBER U228 see II:TIO750
RCRA WASTE NUMBER U230 see II:TIV750
RCRA WASTE NUMBER U231 see I:TIW000
RCRA WASTE NUMBER U232 see II:TAA100
RCRA WASTE NUMBER U233 see II:TIX500
RCRA WASTE NUMBER U235 see I:TNC500
RCRA WASTE NUMBER U236 see II:CMO250
RCRA WASTE NUMBER U237 see II:BIA250
RCRA WASTE NUMBER U238 see I:UVA000
RCRA WASTE NUMBER U240 see II:DAA800
RCRA WASTE NUMBER U242 see II:PAX250
RCRA WASTE NUMBER U244 see III:TFS350
RCRA WASTE NUMBER U247 see II:MEI450
RD 406 see II:DGB000
RD 4593 see II:CIR500
RD-6584 see III:RDP300
RDGE see II:REF000
REACTIVE BLUE 19 see III:BMM500
REBELATE see III:DSP400
RECANESCIN see III:RDF000
RECOLIP see III:ARQ750
RECOLITE RED LAKE C see III:CHP500
RECTHORMONE OESTRADIOL see I:EDP000
RECTHORMONE TESTOSTERONE see I:TBG000
RECTODELT see III:PLZ000
RECTOFASA see II:BRF500
RECTULES see III:CDO000
RED #14 see III:HJF500
1306 RED see III:FAG050
1427 RED see III:FAG040
1671 RED see III:FAG040
1695 RED see III:FMU070
1860 RED see III:CHP500
11411 RED see III:FAG070
11445 RED see III:BNH500
11554 RED see III:IHD000
11959 RED see III:HJF500
12101 RED see III:FAG050
REDAX see III:DWI000
RED B see III:XRA000
RED BASE CIBA IX see II:CLK220, II:CLK235
RED BASE IRGA IX see II:CLK220, II:CLK235
RED BASE NTR see II:CLK220
REDDON see II:TAA100
REDDOX see II:TAA100
RED DYE No. 2 see III:FAG020

REDI-FLOW see III:BAP000
RED IRON ORE see I:HAO875
RED IRON OXIDE see III:IHD000
RED KB BASE see II:CLK225
RED LEAD CHROMATE see I:LCS000
RED No. 1 see III:FAG050
RED No. 2 see III:FAG020
RED No. 4 see III:FAG050
RED No. 5 see III:XRA000
RED No. 213 see III:FAG070
RED OCHRE see III:IHD000
RED OIL see III:OHU000
RED R see III:FMU070
RED SALT CIBA IX see II:CLK235
RED SALT IRGA IX see II:CLK235
RED SCARLET see III:CHP500
REDSKIN see II:AGJ250
RED TR BASE see II:CLK220
RED TRS SALT see II:CLK235
REDUCED-d-PENICILLAMINE see III:MCR750
REED LV 2,4-D see III:ILO000
REED LV 400 2,4-D see III:ILO000
REED LV 600 2,4-D see III:ILO000
REFRACTORY CERAMIC FIBERS see III:RCK725
REFRIGERANT 22 see III:CFX500
REFUSAL see III:DXH250
REGARDIN see III:ARQ750
REGELAN see III:ARQ750
REGENERATED CELLULOSE see III:HHK000
RELAMINAL see III:DCK759
RELANIUM see III:DCK759
RELAX see III:DCK759
RELBAPIRIDINA see III:PPO000
RELON P see III:PJY500
RELUTIN see III:HNT500
REMALAN BRILLIANT BLUE R see III:BMM500
REMASAN CHLOROBLE M see III:MAS500
REMAZIN see III:HNI500
REMAZOL BLACK B see III:RCU000
REMAZOL BRILLIANT BLUE R see III:BMM500
REMAZOL YELLOW G see III:RCZ000
REMOL TRF see III:BGJ250
RENAFUR see II:NDY000
RENAL MD see I:TGL750
RENAL PF see III:PEY500
RENAL SLA see I:DBO400
RENAL SO see III:CEG625
RENARDIN see III:DMX200
RENARDINE see III:DMX200
RENBORIN see III:DCK759
RENOLBLAU 3B see II:CMO250
RENOSULFAN see III:SNN500
RENSTAMIN see III:DBM800
REOMOL D 79P see I:DVL700
REOMOL DOA see III:AEO000
REOMOL DOP see I:DVL700
REPAIRSIN see III:PKB500
REPOSO-TMD see III:TBF750
REPROMIX see II:MCA000
RERANIL see III:TBO500
RESARIT 4000 see III:PKB500
RESCUE SQUAD see III:SHF500
RESERPIDINE see III:RDF000
RESERPINE see II:RDK000
RESIDUAL OIL SOLVENT EXTRACT see I:MQV863
RESIDUAL OILS (PETROLEUM), ACID-TREATED (9CI) see
    I:MQV872
RESINOL BROWN RRN see III:NBG500
RESINOL ORANGE R see III:PEJ500
RESINOL YELLOW GR see I:DOT300
RESIN SCARLET 2R see III:XRA000
RESISAN see III:RDP300
RESISTOMYCIN see III:HAL000
RESOCHIN see III:CLD000

RESOFORM ORANGE G see III:PEJ500
RESOFORM ORANGE R see III:XRA000
RESOFORM YELLOW GGA see I:DOT300
RESOQUINA see III:CLD000
RESOQUINE see III:CLD000
RESORCIN see III:REA000
RESORCINE see III:REA000
RESORCINOL see III:REA000
RESORCINOL BIS(2,3-EPOXYPROPYL)ETHER see
    II:REF000
RESORCINOL DIGLYCIDYL ETHER see II:REF000
RESORCINOL PHTHALEIN SODIUM see III:FEW000
RESORCINYL DIGLYCIDYL ETHER see II:REF000
RESOTROPIN see III:HEI500
RESOXOL see III:SNN500
RESTOVAR see II:LJE000
RESTROL see II:DAL600
RETACEL see III:CMF400
RETALON see II:DAL600
RETARDER J see III:DWI000
RETIN-A see III:VSK950
RETINOIC ACID see III:VSK950
β-RETINOIC ACID see III:VSK950
all-trans-RETINOIC ACID see III:VSK950
RETINOL ACETATE see III:VSK900
RETINYL ACETATE see III:VSK900
all-trans-RETINYL ACETATE see III:VSK900
RETOZIDE see III:ILD000
cis-RETRONECIC ACID ESTER of RETRONECINE see
    III:RFP000
cis-RETRONECIC ACID ESTER of RETRONECINE-N-OXIDE
    see III:RFU000
RETRONECINE HYDROCHLORIDE see III:RFK000
RETRORSINE see III:RFP000
RETRORSINE-N-OXIDE see III:RFU000
REUDO see II:BRF500
REUDOX see II:BRF500
REUMACHLOR see III:CLD000
REUMAQUIN see III:CLD000
REUMASYL see II:BRF500
REUMAZIN see II:BRF500
REUMAZOL see II:BRF500
REUMOX see III:HNI500
REUPOLAR see II:BRF500
REXALL 413S see III:PMP500
REXENE see III:PMP500
REXOLITE 1422 see III:SMQ500
REZIFILM see III:TFS350
RH 315 see III:DTT600
RHAMNOLUTEIN see III:ICE000
RHAMNOLUTIN see III:ICE000
RHATHANI see III:RGA000
RHEONINE B see III:FAG070
RHIZOPIN see III:ICN000
RHODAMINE see III:FAG070
RHODAMINE 6G (biological stain) see III:RGW000
RHODAMINE 6GEX ETHYL ESTER see III:RGW000
RHODAMINE 6G EXTRA BASE see III:RGW000
RHODAMINE S (RUSSIAN) see III:FAG070
RHODIA see II:DAA800
RHODIACHLOR see II:HAR000
RHODIACID see III:BJK500
RHODIASOL see III:PAK000
RHODIATOX see III:PAK000
RHODIATROX see III:PAK000
RHODIUM CHLORIDE see III:RHK000
RHODIUM(III) CHLORIDE (1:3) see III:RHK000
RHODIUM TRICHLORIDE see III:RHK000
RHODOLNE see III:SMQ500
RHODOPAS 6000 see II:AAX175
RHODULINE ORANGE see III:BJF000
RHOMENE see II:CIR250
RHONOX see II:CIR250
RHOPLEX B 85 see III:PKB500

RHOTHANE see I:BIM500
RHOTHANE D-3 see I:BIM500
RHUS COPALLINA see III:SCF000
RHYUNO OIL see I:SAD000
RIANIL see II:CLO750
β-d-RIBOSYL-6-METHYLTHIOPURINE see III:MPU000
RICIFON see III:TIQ250
RICINIC ACID see III:RJP000
RICINOLEIC ACID see III:RJP000
RICINOLIC ACID see III:RJP000
RICON 100 see III:SMR000
RICORTEX see III:CNS825
RIDDELLINE see III:RJZ000
RIFA see II:RKP000
RIFADINE 3cc II:RKP000
RIFAGEN see II:RKP000
RIFALDAZINE see II:RKP000
RIFALDIN see II:RKP000
RIFAMATE see II:RKP000, III:ILD000
RIFAMPICIN see II:RKP000
RIFAMPICINE (FRENCH) see II:RKP000
RIFAMPICINUM see II:RKP000
RIFAMPIN see II:RKP000
RIFAMYCIN AMP see II:RKP000
RIFAPRODIN see II:RKP000
RIFINAH see II:RKP000
RIFOBAC see II:RKP000
RIFOLDIN see II:RKP000
RIFORAL see II:RKP000
RIGENICID see III:EPQ000
RIGEVIDON see III:NNL500
RIKER 601 see III:TND000
RIMACTAN see II:RKP000
RIMACTAZID see II:RKP000
RIMICID see III:ILD000
RIMIFON see III:ILD000
RIMITSID see III:ILD000
RIMSO-50 see III:DUD800
RIOL see III:FMB000
RIPAZEPAM see III:POL475
RITMENAL see I:DKQ000
RITOSEPT see III:HCL000
RITSIFON see III:TIQ250
RIVIVOL see III:ILE000
RIVOMYCIN see II:CDP250
RJ 5 see III:DLJ500
RO 2-4572 see III:ILE000
RO 2-9757 see III:FMM000
RO 4-2130 see III:SNK000
RO 4-6316 see III:DNA200
RO 4-6467 see I:PME250, I:PME500
RO 5-2807 see III:DCK759
RO 5-6789 see III:CFZ000
ROACH SALT see III:SHF500
ROAD ASPHALT see III:PCR500
ROAD ASPHALT (DOT) see II:ARO500
ROAD TAR (DOT) see II:ARO500
ROBIGRAM see III:ARQ750
ROBISELIN see III:ILD000
ROBISELLIN see III:ILD000
ROBIZON-V see II:BRF500
ROBORAL see I:PAN100
ROCK OIL see III:PCR250
RODANIN S-62 (CZECH) see I:IAQ000
RODILONE see III:SNY500
ROGODIAL see III:DSP400
ROGOR see III:DSP400
RO-KO see III:RNZ000
ROKON see II:BDF000
ROL see III:RAF100
ROLAZINE see II:HGP500
ROMACRYL see III:PKB500
ROMANTRENE GOLDEN YELLOW see III:DCZ000
ROMAN VITRIOL see III:CNP250

ROMOSOL see I:ART250
ROMPHENIL see II:CDP250
ROMULGIN O see III:PKL100
RONDAR see III:CFZ000
RONIN see III:PPO000
RONONE see III:RNZ000
ROPTAZOL see III:NGG500
ROQUINE see III:CLD000
RORASUL see I:ASB250
ROSANILINE CHLORIDE see III:MAC250
p-ROSANILINE HCL see II:RMK020
ROSANILINE HYDROCHLORIDE see III:MAC250
p-ROSANILINE HYDROCHLORIDE see II:RMK020
ROSANILINIUM CHLORIDE see III:MAC250
ROSE QUARTZ see I:SCJ500
RO-SULFIRAM see III:DXH250
ROTAX see II:BDF000
ROT B see III:XRA000
ROTEFIVE see III:RNZ000
ROTEFOUR see III:RNZ000
ROTENONA (SPANISH) see III:RNZ000
ROTENONE see III:RNZ000
ROTESSENOL see III:RNZ000
ROT GG FETTLOESLICH see III:XRA000
ROTHANE see I:BIM500
ROTOCIDE see III:RNZ000
ROTOX see III:MHR200
ROUGE see III:IHD000
ROUGE CERASINE see III:OHA000
ROUGE de COCHENILLE A see III:FMU080
ROXIFEN see III:ILD000
ROXION U.A. see III:DSP400
ROXOSUL TABLETS see III:SNN500
ROYAL MBTS see III:BDE750
ROYALTAC see III:DAI600
ROYAL TMTD see III:TFS350
RP 2990 see III:TEX250
RP 3377 see III:CLD000
4753 R.P. see III:TGD000
8595 R.P. see III:DSV800
RP 8823 see I:MMN250
10257 R.P. see III:TND000
RP 13057 see II:DAC000
13,057 R.P. see II:DAC000
2786 R.P. MALEATE see III:DBM800
R 20 (REFRIGERANT) see I:CHJ500
RS 141 see III:CJJ250
RS 1280 see II:CBF250
RTEC (POLISH) see III:MCW250
RU 2858 see III:MRU600
RUBATONE see III:BRF500
RUBBER HYDROCHLORIDE see III:PJH500
RUBBER HYDROCHLORIDE POLYMER see III:PJH500
RUBIAZOL A see III:SNM500
RUBIDIUM DICHROMATE see II:RPK000
RUBIDOMYCIN see II:DAC000
RUBIDOMYCINE see II:DAC000
RUBIGO see III:IHD000
RUBINATE 44 see III:MJP400
RUBINATE TDI see I:TGM740
RUBINATE TDI 80/20 see I:TGM740, I:TGM750
RUBOMYCIN C see II:DAC000
RUBOMYCIN C 1 see II:DAC000
RUBRUM SCARLATINUM see III:SBC500
RUCOFLEX PLASTICIZER DOA see III:AEO000
RUCON B 20 see III:PKQ059
RUGULOSIN see III:RRA000
(+)-RUGULOSIN see III:RRA000
RUKSEAM see I:DAD200
RUMAPAX see III:HNI500
RUMESTROL 1 see I:DKA600
RUMESTROL 2 see I:DKA600
RUNA RH20 see III:TGG760
RUNCATEX see II:CIR500

RUSSIAN COMFREY LEAVES see III:RRK000
RUSSIAN COMFREY ROOTS see II:RRP000
RUTHENIUM SALT of TETRAMETHYLPHENANTHRENE see III:RSP000
RUTILE see III:TGG760
RUTIN see III:RSU000
RUTINIC ACID see III:RSU000
RUTOSIDE see III:RSU000
R-3-ZON see II:BRF500

S 65 (polymer) see III:PKQ059
S115 see III:NCQ900
S 75M see III:SFO500
S 1544 see III:PFC750
S 1752 see III:FAQ999
S 7481F1 see III:CQH100
SA 111 see III:SNJ000
SAATBEIZFUNGIZID (GERMAN) see I:HCC500
SACARINA see II:BCE500
SACCAHARIMIDE see II:BCE500
SACCHARATED FERRIC OXIDE see I:IHG000
SACCHARATED IRON see I:IHG000
SACCHARIN see II:SJN700
SACCHARINA see II:BCE500
SACCHARIN ACID see II:BCE500
SACCHARINE see II:BCE500
SACCHARINE SOLUBLE see II:SJN700
SACCHARINNATRIUM see II:SJN700
SACCHARINOL see II:BCE500
SACCHARINOSE see II:BCE500
SACCHARIN, SODIUM see II:SJN700
SACCHARIN, SODIUM SALT see II:SJN700
SACCHARIN SOLUBLE see II:SJN700
SACCHAROIDUM NATRICUM see II:SJN700
SACCHAROL see II:BCE500
SACCHARUM LACTIN see III:LAR000
SACERIL see I:DKQ000, I:DNU000
SACHSISCHBLAU see III:FAE100
SADH see II:DQD400
SADOFOS see III:MAK700
SADOPHOS see III:MAK700
SADOPLON see III:TFS350
SAFE-N-DRI see III:AHF500
SAFROL see I:SAD000
SAFROLE see I:SAD000
SAFROLE MF see I:SAD000
SAGRADO see III:SAF000
SAKOLYSIN (GERMAN) see II:BHT750
SAKURAI No. 864 see III:YCJ000
SALI see III:SAF500
SALT of SATURN see I:LCG000
SALVO see II:DAA800, III:HKC000
SANATRICHOM see I:MMN250
SAND see I:SCJ500
SANDIMMUN see III:CQH100
SANDIMMUNE see III:CQH100
SANDOPEL BLACK EX see AQP000
SANDORMIN see III:TEH500
SANDOTHRENE PRINTING YELLOW see III:DCZ000
SAN-EI BRILLIANT SCARLET 3R see III:FMU080
SANEPIL see I:DKQ000
SANFURAN see II:NGE500
SANG gamma see I:BBQ500
SANICLOR 30 see III:PAX000
SANLOSE SN 20A see III:SFO500
SANOCIDE see I:HCC500
SANOHIDRAZINA see III:ILD000
SANOQUIN see III:CLD000
SANPRENE LQX 31 see I:PKP000
SANQUINON see III:DFT000
SANSEL ORANGE G see III:PEJ500
SANSPOR see III:CBF800
SANTICIZER 160 see III:BEC500
SANTOBANE see I:DAD200

SANTOBRITE see II:PAX250
SANTOCEL see III:SCH000
SANTOCHLOR see II:DEP800
SANTOCURE see III:CPI250
SANTOCURE MOR see III:BDG000
SANTOFLEX IC see III:PEY500
SANTOPHEN see II:PAX250, III:CJU250
SANTOPHEN 20 see II:PAX250
SANTOPHEN I GERMICIDE see III:CJU250
SANTOTHERM see I:PJL750
SANYO FAST BLUE SALT B see I:DCJ200
SANYO FAST RED SALT TR see II:CLK235
SANYO FAST RED TR BASE see II:CLK220
SANYO LAKE RED C see III:CHP500
SAOLAN see III:DSK200
SAPPILAN see III:CJT750
SAPPIRAN see III:CJT750
SARAN see III:SAX000
SARCELL TEL see III:SFO500
SARCOCLORIN see II:BHT750
l-SARCOLYSIN see I:PED750
dl-SARCOLYSIN see II:BHT750
p-l-SARCOLYSIN see I:PED750
d-SARCOLYSINE see III:SAX200
dl-SARCOLYSINE see II:BHT750
l-SARCOLYSINE HYDROCHLORIDE see III:BHV250
SARCOMYCIN see III:SAX500
SARKOMYCIN see III:SAX500
SARKOMYCIN B*, SODIUM SALT see III:SJS500
SARKOMYCIN, SODIUM SALT see III:SJS500
S.A. R.L. see III:DCK759
SAROMET see III:DCK759
SARPIFAN HP 1 see II:AAX175
SASSAFRAS see III:SAY900
SASSAFRAS ALBIDUM see III:SAY900
SATIAGEL GS 350 see III:CCL250, III:CCL350
SATIAGUM 3 see III:CCL250
SATIAGUM STANDARD see III:CCL250
SATINITE see III:CAX750
SATIN SPAR see III:CAX750
SATOX 20WSC see III:TIQ250
SATURN BROWN LBR see II:CMO750
SAUTERAZID see III:ILD000
SAUTERZID see III:ILD000
SAXIN see II:BCE500, II:SJN700
SAXOL see III:MQV750
SAXOSOZINE see III:SNN500
SAYTEX 102 see III:PAU500
SAYTEX 102E see III:PAU500
SBS see III:SMR000
SC-4642 see II:EEH550
SC 4722 see III:ONO000
SC 10295 see I:MMN250
SC10363 see II:VTF000
SCANBUTAZONE see II:BRF500
SCARLET BASE CIBA II see I:NMP500
SCARLET R see III:FMU070
SCARLET RED see III:SBC500
SCHARLACH B see III:PEJ500
SCHEMERGIN see II:BRF500
SCHERING 36268 see III:CJJ250
SCHEROSON see III:CNS825
SCHINOPSIS LORENTZII TANNIN see III:QBJ000
SCHULTENITE see I:LCK000
SCHULTZ No. 39 see III:HGC000
SCHULTZ No. 95 see III:FMU070
SCHULTZ No. 770 see III:FMU059
SCHULTZ Nr. 208 (GERMAN) see III:HJF500
SCHULTZ Nr. 826 (GERMAN) see III:ADE500
SCHULTZ Nr. 836 (GERMAN) see III:ADF000
SCHULTZ Nr. 1309 (GERMAN) see III:FAE100
SCHULTZ-TAB No. 779 (GERMAN) see II:RMK020
SCHWEFELDIOXYD (GERMAN) see III:SOH500
SCHWEFEL-LOST see I:BIH250

SCLAVENTEROL see III:NGG500
SCON 5300 see III:PKQ059
SCONATEX see II:AAX175, II:VPK000
SCOTCH PAR see III:PKF750
SCROBIN see III:ARQ750
SD 354 see III:SMR000
SD 1897 see I:DDL800
SD 4402 see III:OAN000
SD 5532 see II:CDR750
SD 8447 see III:RAF100
SD ALCOHOL 23-HYDROGEN see I:EFU000
SDEH see II:DJL400
SDMH see I:DSF600
SDPH see I:DNU000
SEA COAL see III:CMY635
SEAKEM CARRAGEENIN see III:CCL250
SEATREM see III:CCL250
SEAWATER MAGNESIA see III:MAH500
SEAZINA see III:SNJ000
16,17-SECOESTRA-1,3,5(10),6,8-PENTAEN-17-OIC ACID, 3-
    METHOXY- see III:BIT030
16,17-SECO-13-α-ESTRA-1,3,5,6,7,9-PENTAEN-17-OIC ACID,
    METHYL ESTER see III:BIT000
SECROSTERON see III:DRT200
SECROVIN see II:DNX500
SECURITY see I:LCK000
SEDABAR see II:EOK000
SEDALIS SEDI-LAB see III:TEH500
SEDAPRAN see III:DAP700
SEDA-TABLINEN see II:EOK000
SEDESTRAN see I:DKA600
SEDICAT see II:EOK000
SEDIMIDE see III:TEH500
SEDIN see III:TEH500
SEDIPAM see III:DCK759
SEDISPERIL see III:TEH500
SEDIZORIN see II:EOK000
SEDLYN see II:EOK000
SEDOFEN see II:EOK000
SEDONAL see II:EOK000
SEDONETTES see II:EOK000
SEDOPHEN see II:EOK000
SEDOVAL see III:TEH500
SEDUKSEN see III:DCK759
SEDURAL see I:PDC250, III:PEK250
SEDUXEN see III:DCK759
SEED of FIDDLENECK see III:TAG250
SEEDRIN see III:AFK250
SEGNALE RED LC see III:CHP500
S. EGRELTRI ATUNUN (TURKISH) see I:BML000
SELEN (POLISH) see III:SBO500
SELENIOUS ACID, DISODIUM SALT see III:SJT500
SELENIUM see III:SBO500
SELENIUM ALLOY see III:SBO500
SELENIUM BASE see III:SBO500
SELENIUM DIETHYLDITHIOCARBAMATE see III:SBP900
SELENIUM DIMETHYLDITHIOCARBAMATE see II:SBQ000
SELENIUM DUST see III:SBO500
SELENIUM ELEMENTAL see III:SBO500
SELENIUM HOMOPOLYMER see III:SBO500
SELENIUM METAL POWDER, NON-PYROPHORIC (DOT) see
    III:SBO500
SELENIUM MONOSULFIDE see I:SBT000
SELENIUM SULFIDE see I:SBT000
SELENIUM SULPHIDE see I:SBT000
SELENSULFID (GERMAN) see I:SBT000
SELEPHOS see III:PAK000
SELF ROCK MOSS see III:CCL250
SEL-TOX SSO2 and SS-20 see III:DXG000
SEM (CYTOSTATIC) see III:TND500
SEMDOXAN see I:CQC675, I:EAS500
SEMICARBAZIDE see III:HGU000
SEMICARBAZIDE HYDROCHLORIDE see III:SBW500
SEMIKON see III:DPJ400

SEMIKON HYDROCHLORIDE see III:DPJ400
SEMUSTINE see II:CHD250
SENAQUIN see III:CLD000
SENDOXAN see I:CQC675
SENDUXAN see I:CQC675, I:EAS500
SENECA OIL see III:PCR250
SENECIO CANNABIFOLIUS, leaves and stalks see III:SBW950
SENECIO LONGILOBUS see III:SBX000
SENECIONANIUM, 12-(ACETYLOXY)-14,15,20,21-TETRA-
    DEHYDRO-15,20-DIHYDRO-8-HYDROXY-4-METHYL-
    11,16-DIOXO-, (8-xi,12-β,14-Z)- see III:CMV950
SENECIO NEMORENSIS FUCHSII, alkaloidal extract see
    III:SBX200
SENECIPHYLLIN see III:SBX500
SENECIPHYLLINE see III:SBX500
SENF OEL (GERMAN) see II:AGJ250
SENKIRKIN see III:DMX200
SENKIRKINE see III:DMX200
SENTIPHENE see III:CJU250
SEPPIC MMD see II:CIR250
SEPTAMIDE ALBUM see III:SNM500
SEPTICOL see II:CDP250
SEPTINAL see III:SNM500
SEPTIPULMON see III:PPO000
SEPTISOL see III:HCL000
SEPTOCHOL see III:DAQ400
SEPTOFEN see III:HCL000
SEPTOPLEX see III:SNM500
SEPTRA see III:SNK000
SEPTRAN see III:SNK000
SEQUILAR see III:NNL500
SEQUOSTAT see III:NNL500
SERAX see III:CFZ000
SERENACE see III:CLY500
SERENACK see III:DCK759
SERENAL see III:CFZ000
SERENAMIN see III:DCK759
SERENID see III:CFZ000
SERENID-D see III:CFZ000
SERENZIN see III:DCK759
SEREPAX see III:CFZ000
SERESTA see III:CFZ000
SERIAL see III:MCA500
l-SERINE DIAZOACETATE see II:ASA500
l-SERINE DIAZOACETATE (ester) see II:ASA500
SERINYL BLUE 2G see III:TBG700
SERISOL ORANGE YL see I:AKP750
SERISTAN BLACK B see AQP000
SERITOX 50 see II:DGB000
SERNAS see III:CLY500
SERNEL see III:CLY500
SEROFINEX see III:ARQ750
SEROTINEX see III:ARQ750
SERPASIL see II:RDK000
SERPASIL APRESOLINE see II:RDK000
SERPASIL APRESOLINE No. 2 see II:HGP500
SERPAX see III:CFZ000
SERPENTINE see I:ARM250, I:ARM268
SERPENTINE CHRYSOTILE see I:ARM268
SERRAL see I:DKA600
SERTINON see III:EPQ000
SERVISONE see III:PLZ000
SESAME OIL see III:SCB000
SESAMOL see III:MJU000
SET see III:MDI000
SETACYL DIAZO NAVY R see I:DCJ200
SETONIL see III:DCK759
SETTIMA see III:DAP700
SEVENAL see II:EOK000
SEVIN see III:CBM750
SEXADIEN see II:DAL600
SEXOCRETIN see I:DKA600
SEXTRA see III:SCB000
SF 60 see III:MAK700

S6F HISTYRENE RESIN see III:SMR000
SG-67 see III:SCH000
SH 393 see III:NNQ000
SH 714 see III:CQJ500
SH 850 see III:NNQ500
SH 70850 see III:NNQ500
SH 71121 see III:NNL500
SHALE OIL (DOT) see I:COD750
SHAMMAH (SAUDI ARABIA) see I:SED400
SHAMROX see II:CIR250
SHB 261AB see III:NNL500
SHB 264AB see III:NNL500
SHELL 40 see III:BQZ000
SHELL 300 see III:SMQ500
SHELL 4402 see III:OAN000
SHELL 5520 see III:PMP500
SHELL ATRAZINE HERBICIDE see III:ARQ725
SHELL GOLD see III:GIS000
SHELLOYNE H see III:DLJ500
SHELL SD-5532 see II:CDR750
SHELL SILVER see III:SDI500
SHELL WL 1650 see III:OAN000
SHIGRODIN see II:BRF500
SHIKIMATE see III:SCE000
SHIKIMIC ACID see III:SCE000
SHIKIMOLE see I:SAD000
SHIKISO AMARANTH see III:FAG020
SHIKOMOL see I:SAD000
SHINING SUMAC see III:SCF000
SHINKOLITE see III:PKB500
SHIN-NAITO S see III:TEH500
SHINNIBROL see III:TEH500
SHOALLOMER see III:PMP500
cis-SHP see III:SCF025
trans(−)-SHP see III:SCF050
trans(+)-SHP see III:SCF075
SI see II:LCF000
SIARKI DWUTLENEK (POLISH) see III:SOH500
SIBAZON see III:DCK759
SIBOL see I:DKA600
SICILIAN CERISE TONER A-7127 see III:FAG070
SICOL 150 see I:DVL700
SICOL 160 see III:BEC500
SICOL 250 see III:AEO000
SICO LAKE RED 2L see III:CHP500
SICRON see III:PKQ059
SIENNA see III:IHD000
SIERRA C-400 see III:TAB750
SIGACALM see III:CFZ000
SILANTIN see I:DKQ000
SILASTIC see III:PJR250
SILBER (GERMAN) see III:SDI500
SILBERNITRAT see III:SDS000
SILBESAN see III:CLD000
SILICA AEROGEL see III:SCH000
SILICA, AMORPHOUS see III:SCH000
SILICA, AMORPHOUS FUMED see III:SCH000
SILICA, AMORPHOUS FUSED see I:SCK600
SILICA, CRYSTALLINE-CRISTOBALITE see I:SCJ000
SILICA, CRYSTALLINE-QUARTZ see I:SCJ500
SILICA, CRYSTALLINE-TRIDYMITE see I:SCK000
SILICA FLOUR (powdered crystalline silica) see I:SCJ500
SILICA, FUSED see I:SCK600
SILICA GEL see III:SCL000
SILICA, GEL and AMORPHOUS-PRECIPITATED see
  III:SCL000
SILICA, VITREOUS see I:SCK600
SILICIC ACID see III:SCL000
SILICIC ACID ALUMINUM SALT see III:AHF500
SILICIC ACID, BERYLLIUM SALT see II:SCN000
SILICIC ANHYDRIDE see I:SCJ500, III:SCH000
SILICON CARBIDE see III:SCQ000
SILICON DIOXIDE see I:SCK600
SILICON DIOXIDE (FCC) see III:SCH000

SILICONE RUBBER see III:PJR250
SILICON MONOCARBIDE see III:SCQ000
SILIKILL see III:SCH000
SILK see III:SDI000
SILON see III:NOH000
SILOTRAS ORANGE TR see III:PEJ500
SILOTRAS YELLOW T2G see I:DOT300
SILUNDUM see III:SCQ000
SILVER see III:SDI500
SILVER ATOM see III:SDI500
SILVER MATT POWDER see III:TGB250
SILVER(1+) NITRATE see III:SDS000
SILVER NITRATE (DOT) see III:SDS000
SILVER(I) NITRATE (1:1) see III:SDS000
SILVER PEROXYCHROMATE see I:SDW000
SILVEX (USDA) see II:TIX500
SILVI-RHAP see II:TIX500
SILVISAR see I:HKC500
SILVISAR 510 see III:HKC000
SIM see III:SNK000
SIMADEX see III:BJP000
SIMANEX see III:BJP000
SIMAZIN see III:BJP000
SIMAZINE 80W see III:BJP000
SIMAZINE (USDA) see III:BJP000
SIMAZOL see I:AMY050
SINAFID M-48 see III:MNH000
SINALOST see III:TNF500
SINCICLAN see I:DKB000
SINCORTEX see III:DAQ800
SINESTROL see III:DLB400
SINITUHO see II:PAX250
SINOFLUROL see III:FMB000
SINOMIN see III:SNK000
SINORATOX see III:DSP400
SINOX GENERAL see III:BRE500
SINTESTROL see I:DKA600
SINTOMICETINA see II:CDP250
SINUTAB see I:ABG750
SIPOL L10 see III:DAI600
SIPOL L12 see III:DXV600
SIPOL S see III:OAX000
SIPONOL S see III:OAX000
SIPTOX I see III:MAK700
SIRAGAN see III:CLD000
SIRAN HYDRAZINU (CZECH) see I:HGW500
SIRUP see III:GFG000
SISTOMETRENOL see II:LJE000
SIXTY-THREE SPECIAL E.C. INSECTICIDE see III:MNH000,
  III:PAK000
SK-100 see III:TNF500
SK-598 see II:CFA750
SK-106N see III:NGY000
SK1133 see III:TND500
SK-3818 see III:TND250
SK 6882 see I:TFQ750
SK-15673 see I:PED750
SK-19849 see II:BIA250
SK 20501 see I:EAS500
SK 22591 see III:HOO500
SK 27702 see I:BIF750
SK-Apap see II:HIM000
φ-SKATOLE CARBOXYLIC ACID see III:ICN000
SK-CHORAL HYDRATE see III:CDO000
SKEDULE see II:CBF250
SKEKhG see I:EAZ500
SKEROLIP see III:ARQ750
SK-ESTROGENS see I:ECU750
SKF 2170 see III:AOO425
SKF 688A see II:DDG800
SKF 92334 see III:TAB250
SK&F 14287 see III:DAS000
SKI 24464 see I:MNA750
SKLEROMEX see III:ARQ750

SODIUM MALONDIALDEHYDE see III:MAN700
SODIUM MERTHIOLATE see III:MDI000
SODIUM METAARSENATE see I:ARD500
SODIUM METAARSENITE see I:SEY500
SODIUM METHANEARSONATE see I:DXE600
SODIUM METHANESULFONATE see III:SIJ000
4-SODIUM METHANESULFONATE METHYLAMINE-ANTI-
PYRINE see III:AMK500
SODIUM METHARSONATE see I:DXE600
SODIUM METHYLAMINOANTIPYRINE METHANESULFO-
NATE see III:AMK500
SODIUM-4-METHYLAMINO-1,5-DIMETHYL-2-PHENYL-3-
PYRAZOLONE 4-METHANESULFONATE see III:AMK500
SODIUM METHYLARSONATE see I:DXE600
SODIUM MONOFLUORIDE see III:SHF500
SODIUM MONOHYDROGEN ARSENATE see I:ARD500
SODIUM MORPHOLINE and NITRITE (1:1) see III:SIN675
SODIUM-22 NEOPRENE ACCELERATOR see I:IAQ000
SODIUM NITRATE (DOT) see III:SIO900
SODIUM(I) NITRATE (1:1) see III:SIO900
SODIUM NITRILOTRIACETATE see III:SIP500
SODIUM NITRITE see III:SIQ500
SODIUM NITRITE mixed with AMINOPYRINE (1:1) see
III:DOT200
SODIUM NITRITE and BENLATE see III:BAV500
SODIUM NITRITE mixed with
BIS(DIETHYLTHIOCARBAMOYL)DISULFIDE see
III:SIS200
SODIUM NITRITE mixed with 1-(p-BROMOPHENYL)-3-
METHYLUREA see III:SIQ675
SODIUM NITRITE and CARBENDAZIM (1:5) see II:CBN375
SODIUM NITRITE and CARBENDAZIME (1:1) see III:SIQ700
SODIUM NITRITE mixed with CHLORDIAZEPOXIDE (1:1) see
III:SIS000
SODIUM NITRITE and l-CITRULLINE (1:2) see III:SIS100
SODIUM NITRITE mixed with 4-(DIMETHYLAMINO)ANTIPY-
RINE (1:1) see III:DOT200
SODIUM NITRITE mixed with DIMETHYLDODECYLAMINE
(8:7) see III:SIS150
SODIUM NITRITE and DIMETHYLUREA see III:DUM400
SODIUM NITRITE mixed with DISULFIRAM see III:SIS200
SODIUM NITRITE with DODECYL GUANIDINE ACETATE (5:
3) see III:DXX600
SODIUM NITRITE mixed with ETHAMBUTOL (1:1) see
III:SIS500
SODIUM NITRITE mixed with ETHYLENETHIOUREA see
II:IAR000
SODIUM NITRITE and ETHYLUREA (1:2) see II:EQE000
SODIUM NITRITE mixed with HEPTAMETHYLENEIMINE see
III:SIT000
SODIUM NITRITE and ISOPROPYLUREA see III:SIS675
SODIUM NITRITE mixed with METHAPYRILENE (2:1) see
III:MDT000
SODIUM NITRITE mixed with N-METHYLADENOSINE (4:1)
see III:SIS650
SODIUM NITRITE and METHYLANILINE (1:1.2) see
III:MGO000
SODIUM NITRITE mixed with N-METHYLANILINE (35:1) see
III:MGO250
SODIUM NITRITE and METHYL-2-BENZIMIDAZOLE CARBA-
MATE see II:CBN375
SODIUM NITRITE mixed with METHYLBENZYLAMINE (3:2)
see III:MHN250
SODIUM NITRITE mixed with N-METHYLBENZYLAMINE
(1:1) see III:MHN000
SODIUM NITRITE mixed with 1-METHYL-3-(p-BROMOPHE-
NYL)UREA see III:SIQ675
SODIUM NITRITE and 1-(METHYLETHYL)UREA see
III:SIS675
SODIUM NITRITE mixed with METHYLGUANIDINE (1:1) see
III:MKJ000
SODIUM NITRITE mixed with 1-METHYL-3-NITROGUANI-
DINE (1:1) see III:MML500

SODIUM NITRITE and 2-METHYL-N-NITROSO-BENZIMIDA-
ZOLE CARBAMATE (1:1) see III:SIQ700
SODIUM NITRITE and 1-METHYL-1-NITROSO-3-PHENYL-
UREA see III:SIS700
SODIUM NITRITE and METHYL UREA see III:MQJ250
SODIUM NITRITE mixed with OCTAHYDROAZOCINE HY-
DROCHLORIDE (1:1) see III:SIT000
SODIUM NITRITE and PIPERAZINE (1:4) see III:PIJ250
SODIUM NITRITE and 1-PROPYLUREA see III:SIT750
SODIUM NITRITE and n-PROPYLUREA see III:SIT750
SODIUM NITRITE and TRIFORINE see III:SIT800
SODIUM NORAMIDOPYRINE METHANESULFONATE see
III:AMK500
SODIUM ORTHOARSENATE see I:ARD750
SODIUM ORTHOARSENITE see I:ARJ500
SODIUM PATENT BLUE V see III:ADE500
SODIUM PENICILLIN see III:BFD250
SODIUM PENICILLIN G see III:BFD250
SODIUM PENICILLIN II see III:BFD250
SODIUM PERACETATE see III:SJB000
SODIUM PEROXYACETATE see III:SJB000
SODIUM PHENOBARBITAL see I:SID000
SODIUM PHENOBARBITONE see I:SID000
SODIUM-1-PHENYL-2,3-DIMETHYL-4-METHYLAMINOPY-
RAZOLON-N-METHANESULFONATE see III:AMK500
SODIUM-1-PHENYL-2,3-DIMETHYL-5-PYRAZOLONE-4-
METHYLAMINO METHANESULFONATE see III:AMK500
SODIUM PHENYLDIMETHYLPYRAZOLONMETHYLAMINO-
METHANE SULFONATE see III:AMK500
SODIUM PHENYLETHYLBARBITURATE see I:SID000
SODIUM PHENYLETHYLMALONYLUREA see I:SID000
SODIUM-2-PHENYLPHENATE see II:BGJ750
SODIUM-o-PHENYLPHENATE see II:BGJ750
SODIUM-o-PHENYLPHENOLATE see II:BGJ750
SODIUM-o-PHENYLPHENOXIDE see II:BGJ750
SODIUM SACCHARIDE see II:SJN700
SODIUM SACCHARIN see II:SJN700
SODIUM SACCHARINATE see II:SJN700
SODIUM SACCHARINE see II:SJN700
SODIUM SALT of CACODYLIC ACID see I:HKC500
SODIUM SALT of CARBOXYMETHYLCELLULOSE see
III:SFO500
SODIUM SALT of N,N-DIETHYLDITHIOCARBAMIC ACID see
III:SGJ000
SODIUM SALT of HYDROXY-o-CARBOXY-PHENYL-FLUO-
RONE see III:FEW000
SODIUM SALT of ISONICOTINIC ACID see III:ILF000
SODIUM SARKOMYCIN see III:SJS500
SODIUM SELENATE see III:DXG000
SODIUM SELENITE see III:SJT500
SODIUM SUCARYL see III:SGC000
SODIUM TCA SOLUTION see III:TII250
SODIUM TETRAPEROXYCHROMATE see I:SKF000
SODIZOLE see III:SNN500
SO-FLO see III:SHF500
SOFTENIL see III:TEH500
SOFTENON see III:TEH500
SOILBROM-40 see I:EIY500
SOILBROM-85 see I:EIY500
SOILFUME see I:EIY500
SOIL STABILIZER 661 see III:SMR000
SOL see III:PKB500
SOLAMINE see III:BEN000
SOLANTHRENE BRILLIANT YELLOW see III:DCZ000
SOLANTIN see I:DKQ000
SOLANTOIN see I:DNU000
SOLANTYL see I:DNU000
SOLANUM TUBEROSUM L see III:PLW750
SOLAR BROWN PL see II:CMO750
SOLAR LIGHT ORANGE GX see III:HGC000
SOLAR RUBINE see III:HJF500
SOLAR VIOLET 5BN see II:FAG120
SOLBAR see III:BAP000
SOLDEP see III:TIQ250

SOLESTRO see I:EDP000
SOLFOTON see II:EOK000
SOLGANAL see I:ART250
SOLGANAL B see I:ART250
SOLID GREEN FCF see III:FAG000
SOLLICULIN see I:EDV000
SOLMETHINE see II:MJP450
SOLOCHROME BLUE FB see III:HJF500
SOL PHENOBARBITAL see I:SID000
SOL PHENOBARBITONE see I:SID000
SOLPRENE 300 see III:SMR000
SOLPRINA see III:CLD000
SOLUBLE FLUORESCEIN see III:FEW000
SOLUBLE GLUSIDE see II:SJN700
SOLUBLE INDIGO see III:FAE100
SOLUBLE PHENOBARBITAL see I:SID000
SOLUBLE PHENOBARBITONE see I:SID000
SOLUBLE PHENYTOIN see I:DNU000
SOLUBLE SACCHARIN see II:SJN700
SOLUTION CONCENTREE T271 see I:AMY050
SOLVENT 111 see III:MIH275
SOLVENT-DEWAXED HEAVY NAPHTHENIC DISTILLATE
    see III:MQV820
SOLVENT-DEWAXED HEAVY PARAFFINIC DISTILLATE see
    III:MQV825
SOLVENT-DEWAXED LIGHT NAPHTHENIC DISTILLATE see
    I:MQV835
SOLVENT-DEWAXED LIGHT PARAFFINIC DISTILLATE see
    I:MQV840
SOLVENT ORANGE 15 see III:BJF000
SOLVENT RED 19 see III:EOJ500
SOLVENT-REFINED HEAVY NAPHTHENIC DISTILLATE see
    III:MQV845
SOLVENT-REFINED HEAVY PARAFFINIC DISTILLATE see
    III:MQV850
SOLVENT-REFINED LIGHT NAPHTHENIC DISTILLATE see
    I:MQV852
SOLVENT-REFINED LIGHT PARAFFINIC DISTILLATE see
    I:MQV855
SOLVENT YELLOW 1 see II:PEI000
SOLVENT YELLOW 14 see III:PEJ500
SOLVIC see III:PKQ059
SOLVIC 523KC see II:AAX175
SOMACTON see III:PJA250
SOMALIA ORANGE 2R see III:XRA000
SOMALIA ORANGE A2R see III:XRA000
SOMALIA ORANGE I see III:PEJ500
SOMALIA RED III see III:OHA000
SOMALIA YELLOW A see I:DOT300
SOMALIA YELLOW R see I:AIC250
SOMAR see I:DXE600
SOMATOTROPIC HORMONE see III:PJA250
SOMATOTROPIN see III:PJA250
SOMBUTOL see II:EOK000
SOMIO see III:GFA000
SOMIPRONT see III:DUD800
SOMNICAPS see III:DPJ400
SOMNI SED see III:CDO000
SOMNOLENS see II:EOK000
SOMNOLETTEN see II:EOK000
SOMNOS see III:CDO000
SOMNOSAN see II:EOK000
SOMONAL see II:EOK000
SONACON see III:DCK759
SONTEC see III:CDO000
SOOT see I:SKS750
SOPAQUIN see III:CLD000
SOPHIA see III:MDL750
SOPHORETIN see III:QCA000
SOPHORIN see III:RSU000
SOPP see II:BGJ750
SOPRABEL see I:LCK000
SOPRATHION see III:PAK000
SOPROCIDE see I:BBQ750

SORBA-SPRAY Mn see III:MAU250
SORBIC ACID see III:SKU000
SORBIC OIL see III:PAJ500
SORBIMACROGOL OLEATE see III:PKL100
SORBISTAT see III:SKU000
SORBITAL O 20 see III:PKL100
SORBITAN MONODODECANOATE see III:SKV000
SORBITAN MONOLAURATE see III:SKV000
SORBITAN, MONOOCTADECANOATE, POLY(OXY-1,2-ETH-
    ANEDIYL) DERIVATIVES see III:PKL030
SOREFLON 604 see III:TAI250
SORETHYTAN (20) MONOOLEATE see III:PKL100
SORLATE see III:PKL100
SORSAKA see III:SKV500
l-SORSAKA, LEAF and STEM EXTRACT see III:SKV500
3OTERENOL HYDROCHLORIDE 3cc III:SKW500
SOTIPOX see III:TIQ250
SOUDAN I see III:PEJ500
SOUDAN II see III:XRA000
SOUP see III:NGY000
SOUTHERN BAYBERRY see III:WBA000
SOUTHERN BENTONITE see III:BAV750
SOVIET TECHNICAL HERBICIDE 2M-4C see II:CIR250
SOVOL see I:PJL750
SOXINAL PZ see III:BJK500
SOXINOL PZ see III:BJK500
SOXISOL see III:SNN500
SOXYSYMPAMINE see III:MDT600
SP 104 see III:TCM250
SPAN 20 see III:SKV000
SPANBOLET see III:SNJ000
SPANON see III:CJJ250
SPANONE see III:CJJ250
SPARIC see III:BRE500
SPASEPILIN see II:EOK000
SP 60 (CHLOROCARBON) see III:PKQ059
SPECIAL BLUE X 2137 see III:EOJ500
SPECIAL TERMITE FLUID see III:DEP600
SPECILLINE G see III:BDY669
SPECTRAR see III:INJ000
SPECTROLENE BLUE B see I:DCJ200
SPECTROLENE RED KB see II:CLK225
SPECULAR IRON see III:IHD000
SPENCER 401 see III:PJY500
SPERGON I see III:TBO500
SPERGON TECHNICAL see III:TBO500
SPERLOX-Z see III:EIR000
SPIRESIS see III:AFJ500
SPIRIDON see III:AFJ500
SPIRIT ORANGE see III:PEJ500
SPIRITS of TURPENTINE see III:TOD750
SPIRITS of WINE see I:EFU000
SPIRIT of TURPENTINE see III:TOD750
SPIRIT YELLOW I see III:PEJ500
SPIROCTANIE see III:AFJ500
SPIROFULVIN see GKE000
SPIRO(ISOBENZOFURAN-1(3H),9'-(9H)XANTHENE-3-ONE,
    3',6'-DIHYDROXY-DISODIUM SALT see III:FEW000
SPIROLACTONE see III:AFJ500
SPIRO(NAPHTHALENE-2(1H),2'-OXIRANE)-3'-CARBOXAL-
    DEHYDE, 3,5,6,7,8,8a-HEXAHYDRO-7-ACETOXY-5,6-
    EPOXY-3',8,8a-TRIMETHYL-3-OXO- see III:POF800
SPIRONOLACTONE see III:AFJ500
SPIRT see I:EFU000
SPONTOX see II:TAA100
SPOROSTATIN see GKE000
SPOTRETE see III:TFS350
SPOTTED ALDER see III:WCB000
SPOTTON see III:FAQ999
SPRAY-DERMIS see II:NGE500
SPRAY-FORAL see II:NGE500
SPRAYSET MEKP see III:MKA500
SPRITZ-HORMIN/2,4-D see II:DAA800
SPROUT NIP see III:CKC000

SPROUT-NIP EC see III:CKC000
SPUD-NIC see III:CKC000
SPUD-NIE see III:CKC000
SPURGE see III:BRE500
SQ 1089 see III:HOO500
SQ 1489 see III:TFS350
SQ 9453 see III:DUD800
SQ 16819 see III:HKQ025
SQ 21977 see III:MPU000
SQUARIC ACID see III:DMJ600
SQUIBB see III:HNT500
SR 247 see III:DUL200
SR406 see III:CBG000
SRC-II HEAVY DISTILLATE see II:CMY625
SRI 859 see I:MNA750
SRI 1666 see III:DRN400
SRI 1720 see I:BIF750
SRI 1869 see III:NKL000
SRI 2200 see I:CGV250
SRI 2489 see II:IAN000
S.T. 37 see III:HFV500
ST 155 see II:CBF250
STABILAN see III:CMF400
STABILIZATOR AR see I:PFT500
STABILIZED ETHYL PARATHION see III:PAK000
STABLE RED KB BASE see II:CLK225
STA-FAST see II:TIX500
STAFLEX DOP see I:DVL700
STANDACOL CARMOISINE see III:HJF500
STANDACOL ORANGE G see III:HGC000
STANDARD LEAD ARSENATE see I:LCK000
STANGEN MALEATE see III:DBM800
STANNOUS FLUORIDE see III:TGD100
STANOMYCETIN see II:CDP250
STANOZIDE see III:ILD000
STANSIN see III:SNN500
STARIFEN see II:EOK000
STARILETTAE see II:EOK000
STATHION see III:PAK000
STATOMIN MALEATE see III:DBM800
STAUFFER CAPTAN see III:CBG000
STAUFFER R-2061 see III:PNF500
STAY-FLO see III:SHF500
STEARAMIDE see III:OAR000
STEAREX BEADS see III:SLK000
STEARIC ACID see III:SLK000
STEARIC ACID ALUMINUM DIHYDROXIDE SALT see
   III:AHA250
STEARIC ACID, CADMIUM SALT see I:OAT000
STEARIC ACID-2,3-EPOXYPROPYL ESTER see III:SLK500
STEARIX ORANGE see III:PEJ500
STEAROL see III:OAX000
γ-STEAROLACTONE see III:SLL400
STEAROPHANIC ACID see III:SLK000
1-STEAROYLAZIRIDINE see III:SLM000
STEAROYL ETHYLENEIMINE see III:SLM000
STEAR YELLOW JB see I:DOT300
STEARYL ALCOHOL see III:OAX000
STEAWHITE see III:TAB750
STEDIRIL see III:NNL500
STEDIRIL D see III:NNL500
STEINBUHL YELLOW see I:BAK250
STEINBUHL YELLOW see CAP750
STELLITE see III:VSK000
STELLON PINK see III:PKB500
STENOLON see III:DAL300, III:MPN500
STENOLONE see III:DAL300
STENOSINE see I:DXE600
STENTAL EXTENTABS see II:EOK000
STERAFFINE see III:OAX000
STERAL see III:HCL000
STERANDRYL see I:TBG000
STERAQ see III:DAQ800
STERASKIN see III:HCL000

STERCORIN see III:DKW000
STERIGMATOCYSTIN see II:SLP000
STERILIZING GAS ETHYLENE OXIDE 100% see I:EJN500
STEROLAMIDE see III:TKP500
STERONYL see III:MPN500
STESOLID see III:DCK759
STESOLIN see III:DCK759
STEVIA REBAUDIANA Bertoni, extract see III:SLP350
STIBILIUM see I:DKA600
STIBIUM see III:AQB750
STICKSTOFFLOST see I:BIE500
STIL see I:DKA600
4-STILBENAMINE see III:SLQ900
4-N-STILBENAMINE see III:SLQ900
trans-4-N-STILBENAMINE see III:AMO000
trans-4-STILBENE see III:AMO000
4,4'-STILBENEDIAMINE see III:SLR500
STILBENE, α-α'-DIETHYL-4,4'-DIMETHYL-, (E)- see
   III:DRK500
4-STILBENYL-N,N-DIETHYLAMINE see III:DKA000
STILBENYL-N,N-DIMETHYLAMINE see III:DUB800
STILBESTROL see I:DKA600
STILBESTROL DIETHYL DIPROPIONATE see I:DKB000
STILBESTROL DIMETHYL ETHER see III:DJB200
STILBESTROL DIPROPIONATE see I:DKB000
STILBESTROL and PRANONE see III:EEH900
STILBESTROL PROPIONATE see I:DKB000
STILBESTRONATE see I:DKB000
STILBESTRONE see I:DKA600
STILBETIN see I:DKA600
STILBOEFRAL see I:DKA600
STILBOESTROFORM see I:DKA600
STILBOESTROL see I:DKA600
STILBOESTROL DIPROPIONATE see I:DKB000
STILBOFAX see I:DKB000
STILBOFOLLIN see I:DKA600
STILBOL see I:DKA600
STILKAP see I:DKA600
STILON see III:PJY500
STIL-ROL see I:DKA600
STILRONATE see I:DKB000
STINERVAL see III:PFC750
STIPTANON see II:EDU500
STIROFOS see III:RAF100
STIROLO (ITALIAN) see II:SMQ000
STIROPHOS see III:RAF100
STOMOLD B see II:BGJ750
STONE RED see III:IHD000
STOPAETHYL see III:DXH250
STOPETHYL see III:DXH250
STOPETYL see III:DXH250
STOPGERME-S see III:CKC000
STOPTON ALBUM see III:SNM500
STOXIL see III:DAS000
STR see I:SMD000
STRATHION see III:PAK000
STRAWBERRY RED A GEIGY see III:FMU080
STRAZINE see III:ARQ725
STREPAMIDE see III:SNM500
STREPTAGOL see III:SNM500
STREPTOCLASE see III:SNM500
STREPTOL see III:SNM500
STREPTOMYCES PEUCETIUS see II:DAC000
STREPTOSIL see III:SNM500
STREPTOSILTHIAZOLE see III:TEX250
STREPTOZOCIN see I:SMD000
STREPTOZONE see III:SNM500
STREPTOZOTICIN see I:SMD000
STREPTROCIDE see III:SNM500
STREUNEX see I:BBQ500
STRIPED ALDER see III:WCB000
STROBANE see III:MIH275, III:TBC500
STROBANE-T-90 see I:CDV100
STRONTIUM ARSENITE see I:SME500

STRONTIUM ARSENITE, SOLID (DOT) see I:SME500
STRONTIUM CHROMATE (1:1) see I:SMH000
STRONTIUM CHROMATE (VI) see I:SMH000
STRONTIUM CHROMATE 12170 see I:SMH000
STRONTIUM YELLOW see I:SMH000
STRUMACIL see II:MPW500
STRUMAZOLE see III:MCO500
STRZ see I:SMD000
STS 153 see III:PEE600
STUDAFLUOR see III:SHF500
STYRAFOIL see III:SMQ500
STYRAGEL see III:SMQ500
STYREEN (DUTCH) see II:SMQ000
STYREN (CZECH) see II:SMQ000
STYRENE see II:SMQ000
STYRENE-BUTADIENE COPOLYMER see III:SMR000
STYRENE-1,3-BUTADIENE COPOLYMER see III:SMR000
STYRENE-BUTADIENE POLYMER see III:SMR000
STYRENE EPOXIDE see II:EBR000
STYRENE MONOMER (ACGIH) see II:SMQ000
STYRENE MONOMER, inhibited (DOT) see II:SMQ000
STYRENE OXIDE see II:EBR000
STYRENE-7,8-OXIDE see II:EBR000
STYRENE POLYMER see III:SMQ500
STYRENE POLYMER with 1,3-BUTADIENE see III:SMR000
STYRENE POLYMERS see III:SMQ500
STYROFOAM see III:SMQ500
STYROL (GERMAN) see II:SMQ000
STYROLE see II:SMQ000
STYROLENE see II:SMQ000
STYROLUX see III:SMQ500
STYRON see II:SMQ000, III:SMQ500
STYROPOR see II:SMQ000
STYRYL 430 see III:AMO250
trans-4'-STYRYLACETANILIDE see III:SMR500
p-STYRYLANILINE see III:SLQ900
6-STYRYL-BENZO(a)PYRENE see III:SMS000
5-STYRYL-3,4-BENZOPYRENE see III:SMS000
STYRYL OXIDE see II:EBR000
N-(p-STYRYLPHENYL)ACETOHYDROXAMIC ACETATE see
  III:ABW500
trans-N-(p-STYRYLPHENYL)ACETOHYDROXAMIC ACID see
  III:SMT500
N-(p-STYRYLPHENYL)ACETOHYDROXAMIC ACID ACE-
  TATE see III:ABW500
trans-N-(p-STYRYLPHENYL)ACETOHYDROXAMIC ACID,
  COPPER(2+) COMPLEX see III:SMU000
(E)-N-(p-STYRYLPHENYL)HYDROXYLAMINE see
  III:HJA000
trans-N-(4-STYRYLPHENYL)HYDROXYLAMINE see
  III:HJA000
trans-N-(p-STYRYLPHENYL)HYDROXYLAMINE see
  III:HJA000
STZ see I:SMD000
SU-13437 see II:MCB500
SUBACETATE LEAD see III:LCH000
SUBITEX see III:BRE500
SUBTOSAN see III:PKQ250
SUCARYL see II:CPQ625
SUCARYL ACID see II:CPQ625
SUCARYL CALCIUM see III:CAR000
SUCARYL SODIUM see III:SGC000
SUCCARIL see II:SJN700, III:SGC000
SUCCINCHLORIMIDE see III:SND500
SUCCINIC ACID ANHYDRIDE see III:SNC000
SUCCINIC ACID, CADMIUM SALT (1:1) see I:CAI750
SUCCINIC ACID-2,2-DIMETHYLHYDRAZIDE see
  II:DQD400
SUCCINIC ANHYDRIDE see III:SNC000
SUCCINIC-1,1-DIMETHYL HYDRAZIDE see II:DQD400
SUCCINOCHLORIMIDE see III:SND500
4'-SUCCINOYLAMINO-2,3'-DIMETHYLAZOBENZENE see
  III:SNF500
4'-SUCCINYLAMINO-2,3'-DIMETHYLAZOBENZOL see
  III:SNF500

SUCCINYL OXIDE see III:SNC000
SUCRA see II:SJN700
SUCRE EDULCOR see II:BCE500
SUCRETS see III:HFV500
SUCRETTE see II:BCE500
SUCROFER see I:IHG000
SUCROL see III:EFE000
SUCROSA see III:SGC000
SUDAN AX see III:XRA000
SUDAN BROWN RR see III:NBG500
SUDAN III see III:OHA000
SUDAN ORANGE see III:XRA000
SUDAN ORANGE R see III:PEJ500
SUDAN ORANGE RPA see III:XRA000
SUDAN ORANGE RRA see III:XRA000
SUDAN RED see III:XRA000
SUDAN RED 7B see III:EOJ500
SUDANROT 7B see III:EOJ500
SUDAN SCARLET 6G see III:XRA000
SUDAN X see III:XRA000
SUDAN YELLOW see I:DOT300
SUDAN YELLOW R see II:PEI000
SUDAN YELLOW RRA see I:AIC250
SUESSETTE see III:SGC000
SUESSTOFF see III:EFE000
SUESTAMIN see III:SGC000
SUGAI CHRYSOIDINE see III:PEK000
SUGAI FAST SCARLET G BASE see I:NMP500
SUGARIN see III:SGC000
SUGAR of LEAD see I:LCG000
SUGARON see III:SGC000
SULADYNE see I:PDC250
SUL ANILINOVA (CZECH) see II:BBL000
SULFACID BRILLIANT GREEN 1B see III:FAE950
SULFACID LIGHT ORANGE J see III:HGC000
SULFACOMBIN see III:SNI000
SULFADENE see II:BDF000
SULFADIAMINE see III:SNY500
SULFADIMERAZINE see III:SNJ000
SULFADIMETHYLDIAZINE see III:SNJ000
SULFADIMETHYLISOXAZOLE see III:SNN500
SULFADIMETHYLPYRIMIDINE see III:SNJ000
SULFADIMETINE see III:SNJ000
SULFADIMEZINE see III:SNJ000
SULFADIMIDINE see III:SNJ000
SULFADINE see III:SNJ000
SULFADSIMESINE see III:SNJ000
SULFAFURAZOL see III:SNN500
SULFAGAN see III:SNN500
SULFA-ISODIMERAZINE see III:SNJ000
SULFAISODIMIDINE see III:SNJ000
SULFALLATE see CDO250
SULFAMETHALAZOLE see III:SNK000
SULFAMETHIAZINE see III:SNJ000
SULFAMETHIN see III:SNJ000
SULFAMETHIZOLE see III:MPQ750
SULFAMETHOXAZOL see III:SNK000
SULFAMETHOXAZOLE see III:SNK000
SULFAMETHYLISOXAZOLE see III:SNK000
SULFAMETHYLTHIADIAZOLE see III:MPQ750
SULFAMEZATHINE see III:SNJ000
p-SULFAMIDOANILINE see III:SNM500
SULFAMIDYL see III:SNM500
SULFAMUL see III:TEX250
SULFANA see III:SNM500
SULFANALONE see III:SNM500
SULFANIL see III:SNM500
SULFANILAMIDE see III:SNM500
5-SULFANILAMIDO-3,4-DIMETHYL-ISOXAZOLE see
  III:SNN500
2-SULFANILAMIDO-4,6-DIMETHYLPYRIMIDINE see
  III:SNJ000
3-SULFANILAMIDO-5-METHYLISOXAZOLE see III:SNK000
2-SULFANILAMIDO-5-METHYL-1,3,4-THIADIAZOLE see
  III:MPQ750

2-SULFANILAMIDOTHIAZOLE see III:TEX250
2-SULFANILYL AMINOPYRIDINE see III:PPO000
2-(SULFANILYLAMINO)THIAZOLE see III:TEX250
SULFAPYRIDINE see III:PPO000
2-SULFAPYRIDINE see III:PPO000
SULFASOXAZOLE see III:SNN500
SULFATE de CUIVRE (FRENCH) see III:CNP250
SULFATED AMYLOPECTIN see III:AOM150
SULFATE DIMETHYLIQUE (FRENCH) see I:DUD100
SULFATE ESTER of N-HYDROXY-N-2-FLUORENYL ACET-
    AMIDE see III:FDV000
SULFATE de METHYLE (FRENCH) see I:DUD100
SULFATE de ZINC (FRENCH) see III:ZNA000
SULFATHIAZOL see III:TEX250
SULFATHIAZOLE (USDA) see III:TEX250
cis-SULFATO-1,2-DIAMINOCYCLOHEXANEPLATINUM(II)
    see III:SCF025
trans(−)-SULFATO-1,2-DIAMINOCYCLOHEXANEPLATI-
    NUM(II) see III:SCF050
trans(+)-SULFATO-1,2-DIAMINOCYCLOHEXANEPLATI-
    NUM(II) see III:SCF075
SULFAZOLE see III:SNN500
SULFENAMIDE M see III:BDG000
SULFENAMIDE TS see III:CPI250
SULFERROUS see III:FBN100
SULFIDINE see III:PPO000
SULFINYLBIS(METHANE) see III:DUD800
SULFISIN see III:SNN500
SULFISOMEZOLE see III:SNK000
SULFISOMIDIN see III:SNJ000
SULFISOMIDINE see III:SNJ000
SULFISOXAZOLE see III:SNN500
SULFIZOLE see III:SNN500
3-SULFOBENZIDINE see III:BBY250
o-SULFOBENZIMIDE see II:BCE500
o-SULFOBENZOIC ACID IMIDE see II:BCE500
SULFOCIDINE see III:SNM500
SULFODIAMINE see III:SNY500
SULFODIMESIN see III:SNJ000
SULFODIMEZINE see III:SNJ000
SULFO GREEN J see III:FAF000
SULFONA see III:SOA500
SULFONAMIDE see III:SNM500
4-SULFONAMIDE-4′-DIMETHYLAMINOAZOBENZENE see
    III:SNW800
SULFONAMIDE P see III:SNM500
4-SULFONAMIDO-3′-METHYL-4′-AMINOAZOBENZENE see
    III:SNX000
2-SULFONAMIDOTHIAZOLE see III:TEX250
2-(4-SULFO-1-NAPHTHYLAZO)-1-NAPHTHOL-4-SULFONIC
    ACID, DISODIUM SALT see III:HJF500
o-SULFONBENZOIC ACID IMIDE SODIUM SALT see
    II:SJN700
SULFONETHYLMETHANE see III:BJT750
SULFONIMIDE see III:CBF800
N-SULFONOXY-AAF see III:FDV000
N-SULFONOXY-N-ACETYL-2-AMINOFLUORENE see
    III:FDV000
4,4′-SULFONYLBISACETANILIDE see III:SNY500
p,p′-SULFONYLBISACETANILIDE see III:SNY500
4′,4′′′-SULFONYLBIS(ACETANILIDE) see III:SNY500
1,1′-SULFONYLBIS(4-AMINOBENZENE) see III:SOA500
4,4′-SULFONYLBISANILINE see III:SOA500
p,p-SULFONYLBISBENZAMINE see III:SOA500
4,4′-SULFONYLBISBENZAMINE see III:SOA500
p,p-SULFONYLBISBENZENAMINE see III:SOA500
SULFONYL CHLORIDE see III:SOT000
4,4′-SULFONYLDIANILINE see III:SOA500
p,p′-SULFONYLDIANILINE see III:SOA500
4-p-SULFOPHENYLAZO-1-NAPHTHOL MONOSODIUM SALT
    see III:FAG010
SULFOTRINAPHTHYLENOFURAN, SODIUM SALT see
    III:SOD200
SULFOX-CIDE see III:ISA000

SULFOXIDE see III:ISA000
SULFOXYL see III:BDS000, III:ISA000
2-(6-SULFO-2,4-XYLYLAZO)-1-NAPHTHOL-4-SULFONIC
    ACID, DISODIUM SALT see III:FAG050
SULFUR DIOXIDE see III:SOH500
SULFURIC ACID, BARIUM SALT (1:1) see III:BAP000
SULFURIC ACID, BERYLLIUM SALT (1:1) see I:BFU250
SULFURIC ACID, BERYLLIUM SALT (1:1), TETRAHYDRATE
    see I:BFU500
SULFURIC ACID, CADMIUM(2+) SALT see I:CAJ000
SULFURIC ACID, CADMIUM SALT, HYDRATE see I:CAJ250
SULFURIC ACID, CADMIUM SALT, TETRAHYDRATE see
    I:CAJ500
SULFURIC ACID, CALCIUM(2+) SALT, DIHYDRATE see
    III:CAX750
SULFURIC ACID, CHROMIUM(3+)POTASSIUM SALT(2:1:1),
    DODECAHYDRATE see III:CMG850
SULFURIC ACID, CHROMIUM SALT, BASIC see III:NBW000
SULFURIC ACID, COPPER(2+) SALT (1:1) see III:CNP250
SULFURIC ACID, CYCLIC ETHYLENE ESTER see III:EJP000
SULFURIC ACID, DIMETHYL ESTER see I:DUD100
SULFURIC ACID, IRON(2+) SALT (1:1) see III:FBN100
SULFURIC ACID, MANGANESE(2+) SALT see III:MAU250
SULFURIC ACID, MONO(2-ETHYLHEXYL)ESTER see
    III:ELB400
SULFURIC ACID, NICKEL(2+)SALT see II:NDK500
SULFURIC ACID, NICKEL(2+) SALT (1:1) see II:NDK500
SULFURIC ACID, NICKEL(2+) SALT, HEXAHYDRATE see
    II:NDL000
SULFURIC ACID, ZINC SALT (1:1) see III:ZNA000
SULFURIC OXYCHLORIDE see III:SOT000
SULFUR MUSTARD see I:BIH250
SULFUR MUSTARD GAS see I:BIH250
SULFUROUS ACID ANHYDRIDE see III:SOH500
SULFUROUS ACID, 2-(p-tert-BUTYLPHENOXY)-1-METHYL-
    ETHYL-2-CHLOROETHYL ESTER see I:SOP500
SULFUROUS ACID, cyclic ester with 1,4,5,6,7,7-HEXA-
    CHLORO-5-NORBORNENE-2,3-DIMETHANOL see
    III:EAQ750
SULFUROUS ANHYDRIDE see III:SOH500
SULFUROUS OXIDE see III:SOH500
SULFUR OXIDE see III:SOH500
SULFUR SELENIDE see I:SBT000
SULFURYL CHLORIDE see III:SOT000
SULMET see III:SNJ000
SULODYNE see I:PDC250
SULOUREA see I:ISR000
SULPHABUTIN see I:BOT250
SULPHADIMETHYLISOXAZOLE see III:SNN500
SULPHADIMETHYLPYRIMIDINE see III:SNJ000
SULPHADIMIDINE see III:SNJ000
SULPHADIONE see III:SOA500
SULPHAFURAZ see III:SNN500
SULPHAMETHALAZOLE see III:SNK000
SULPHAMETHOXAZOL see III:SNK000
SULPHAMETHOXAZOLE see III:SNK000
SULPHAMETHYLISOXAZOLE see III:SNK000
SULPHANILAMIDE see III:SNM500
5-SULPHANILAMIDO-3,4-DIMETHYL-ISOXAZOLE see
    III:SNN500
3-SULPHANILAMIDO-5-METHYLISOXAZOLE see
    III:SNK000
SULPHATHIAZOLE see III:TEX250
SULPHEIMIDE see III:CBF800
SULPHISOMEZOLE see III:SNK000
SULPHISOXAZOL see III:SNN500
2-SULPHOBENZOIC IMIDE see II:BCE500
SULPHOBENZOIC IMIDE, SODIUM SALT see II:SJN700
SULPHOFURAZOLE see III:SNN500
1-(4-SULPHO-1-NAPHTHYLAZO)-2-NAPHTHOL-3,6-DISUL-
    PHONIC ACID, TRISODIUM SALT see III:FAG020
SULPHON-MERE see III:SOA500
1,1′-SULPHONYLBIS(4-AMINOBENZENE) see III:SOA500
p,p-SULPHONYLBISBENZAMINE see III:SOA500

4,4'-SULPHONYLBISBENZAMINE see III:SOA500
p,p-SULPHONYLBISBENZENAMINE see III:SOA500
4,4'-SULPHONYLBISBENZENAMINE see III:SOA500
SULPHONYLDIANILINE see III:SOA500
p,p-SULPHONYLDIANILINE see III:SOA500
SULPHOS see III:PAK000
SULPHOXIDE see III:ISA000
SULPHUR DIOXIDE, LIQUEFIED (DOT) see III:SOH500
SULPHURIC ACID, CADMIUM SALT (1:1) see I:CAJ000
SULPHUR MUSTARD GAS see I:BIH250
SULZOL see III:TEX250
SUMILIT EXA 13 see III:PKQ059
SUMILIT PCX see II:AAX175
SUMIPLEX LG see III:PKB500
SUMITOMO LIGHT GREEN SF YELLOWISH see III:FAF000
SUMITOMO PX 11 see III:PKQ059
SUMITOX see III:MAK700
SUNCIDE, nitrosated see III:PMY310
SUNFRAL see III:FMB000
SUNSET YELLOW FCF see III:FAG150
SUPARI, nut extract see II:BFW000
SUPARI (INDIA) see III:AQT650
SUPERACRYL AE see III:PKB500
SUPERCEL 3000 see III:USS000
SUPER COBALT see I:CNA250
SUPERCORTIL see III:PLZ000
SUPER-DENT see III:SHF500
SUPER D WEEDONE see II:DAA800, II:TAA100
SUPERFLAKE ANHYDROUS see III:CAO750
SUPERFLOC see III:PKF750
SUPER HARTOLAN see III:CMD750
SUPERIAN YELLOW R see III:SGP500
SUPERLYSOFORM see I:FMV000
SUPEROL RED C RT-265 see III:CHP500
SUPERORMONE CONCENTRE see II:DAA800
SUPEROX see III:BDS000
SUPEROXOL see III:HIB000
SUPER RODIATOX see III:PAK000
SUPERSEPTIL see III:SNJ000
SUPERTAH see I:CMY800
SUPRA see III:IHD000
SUPRACET BRILLIANT BLUE 2GN see III:TBG700
SUPRACET ORANGE R see I:AKP750
SUPRAMIKE see III:BAP000
SUPREME DENSE see III:TAB750
SUP'R FLO see III:DXQ500
SUP'R FLO FERBAM FLOWABLE see III:FAS000
SURAUTO see III:IDW000
SURESTRINE see III:BIT000
SURESTRYL see III:BIT000, III:MRU600
SURGICAL SIMPLEX see III:PKB500
SURGI-CEN see III:HCL000
SUROFENE see III:HCL000
SU SEGURO CARPIDOR see III:DUV600
SUSTANE see II:BQI000, III:BFW750
SUSTANE 1-F see II:BQI000
SUSTANONE see I:TBF500
SUZU see III:ABX250
SVO 9 see III:PKL100
SWEEP see III:TBQ750
SWEETA see II:SJN700
SWEET GUM see III:SOY500
SWEET MYRTLE see III:WBA000
SWEET ORANGE OIL see III:OGY000
SYKOSE see II:BCE500, II:SJN700
SYLANTOIC see I:DKQ000, I:DNU000
SYLLIT see III:DXX400
SYLODEX see I:ARM268
SYMAZINE see III:BJP000
SYMPHYTINE see III:SPB500
SYMPHYTUM OFFICINALE L see II:RRP000, III:RRK000
SYMULER EOSIN TONER see III:BNH500
SYMULER LAKE RED C see III:CHP500
SYMULEX MAGENTA F see III:FAG070

SYMULEX PINK F see III:FAG070
SYMULON ACID BRILLIANT SCARLET 3R see III:FMU080
SYMULON SCARLET G BASE see I:NMP500
SYNANDRETS see III:MPN500
SYNANDROL see I:TBG000
SYNANDROL F see I:TBF500
SYNANDROTABS see III:MPN500
SYNAPAUSE see II:EDU500
SYNASTERON see I:PAN100
SYNCAL see II:BCE500
SYNCORT see III:DAQ800
SYNCORTA see III:DAQ800
SYNCORTYL see III:DAQ800
SYNDIOL see I:EDO000
SYNDIOTACTIC POLYPROPYLENE see III:PMP500
SYNDROX see III:MDT600
SYNERONE see I:TBG000
SYNESTRIN see I:DKA600, I:DKB000
SYNESTROL see II:DAL600, III:DLB400
SYNGESTERONE see I:PMH500
SYNGYNON see III:HNT500
SYNKAY see III:MMD500
SYNKLOR see II:CDR750
SYNMIOL see III:DAS000
SYNOESTRON see I:DKB000
SYNOVEX S see I:PMH500
SYNPOL 1500 see III:SMR000
SYNPREN-FISH see III:PIX250
SYNTAR see I:CMY800
SYNTESTRIN see I:DKB000
SYNTESTRINE see I:DKB000
SYNTEXAN see III:DUD800
SYNTHETIC 3956 see I:CDV100
SYNTHETIC AMORPHOUS SILICA see III:SCH000
SYNTHETIC EUGENOL see III:EQR500
SYNTHETIC IRON OXIDE see III:IHD000
SYNTHETIC MUSTARD OIL see II:AGJ250
SYNTHILA see III:DJB200
SYNTHOESTRIN see I:DKA600
SYNTHOFOLIN see I:DKA600
SYNTHOMYCINE see II:CDP250
SYNTHOVO see III:DLB400
SYNTOFOLIN see I:DKA600
SYNTOLUTAN see I:PMH500
SYNTROGENE see III:DLB400

α-T see III:MIH275
β-T see II:TIN000
T-47 see III:PAK000
T 72 see I:PNX000
T 100 see I:TGM740
2,4,5-T see II:TAA100
T 1824 see III:BGT250
TAA see I:TFA000
TABAC (FRENCH) see I:TGI100
TABACO (SPANISH) see I:TGI100
TABALGIN see II:HIM000
TACE see II:CLO750
TACE-FN see II:CLO750
TACOSAL see I:DKQ000, I:DNU000
TACP see III:TNC725
TAFAZINE see III:BJP000
TAFAZINE 50-W see III:BJP000
TAG-39 see I:ECU750
TAGAMET see III:TAB250
TAK see III:MAK700
TAKAOKA AMARANTH see III:FAG020
TAKAOKA BRILLIANT SCARLET 3R see III:FMU080
TAKAOKA RHODAMINE B see III:FAG070
TAKILON see III:PKQ059
TALARGAN see III:TEH500
TALBOT see I:LCK000
TALC (powder) see III:TAB750
TALC, containing asbestos fibers see I:TAB775

TALCUM see III:TAB750
TALIMOL see III:TEH500
TALODEX see III:FAQ999
TALPHENO see II:EOK000
TAMETIN see III:TAB250
TAMPOVAGAN STILBOESTROL see I:DKA600
TANAKAN see III:CLD000
TANDACOTE see III:HNI500
TANDALGESIC see III:HNI500
TANDEARIL see III:HNI500
TANDERAL see III:HNI500
TANNIC ACID see III:TAD750
TANNIN see III:TAD750
TANNIN from BETEL NUT see III:BFW050
TANNIN from BRACKEN FERN see III:BML250
TANNIN from CHERRY BARK OAK see III:CDL750
TANNIN from CHESTNUT see III:CDM250
TANNIN-FREE FRACTION of BRACKEN FERN see
   III:TAE250
TANNIN from LIMONIUM NASHII see III:MBU750
TANNIN from MARSH ROSEMARY see III:MBU750
TANNIN from MIMOSA see III:MQV250
TANNIN from MYROBALANS see III:MSB750
TANNIN from MYRTAN see III:MSC000
TANNIN from PERSIMMON see III:PCP500
TANNIN from QUEBRACHO see III:QBJ000
TANNIN from SWEET GUM see III:SOY500
TANNIN from VALONEA see III:VCK000
TANNIN from WAX MYRTLE see III:WBA000
TANRUTIN see III:RSU000
TANTALUM see III:TAE750
TANTALUM-181 see III:TAE750
TAP 85 see I:BBQ500
TAPAR see II:HIM000
TAPAZOLE see III:MCO500
TAPHAZINE see III:BJP000
TAR see I:CMY800
TAR, from tobacco see II:CMP800
TARAPACAITE see III:PLB250
TAR CAMPHOR see III:NAJ500
TAR, COAL see I:CMY800
TARDEX 100 see III:PAU500
TARFLEN see III:TAI250
TARIMYL see III:SOA500
TAR, LIQUID (DOT) see I:CMY800
TARLON XB see III:PJY500
TARNAMID T see III:PJY500
TAR OIL see I:CMY825
TARRAGON see III:AFW750
TARWEED see III:TAG250
TAT CHLOR 4 see II:CDR750
TATD see III:DXH250
TATERPEX see III:CKC000
TAZEPAM see III:CFZ000
TAZONE see II:BRF500
TB see II:CMO250
TBE see III:ACK250
TBP see III:TFD250
2,4,5-TC see II:TIX500
TCA see III:TII250
TCBN see III:TBS000
TCDBD see I:TAI000
TCDD see I:TAI000
2,3,7,8-TCDD see I:TAI000
TCE see III:TBQ100
1,1,1-TCE see III:MIH275
TCEO see III:ECT600
TCIN see III:TBQ750
TCM see I:CHJ500
TCNB see III:TBR750
TCPE see III:TIX000
m-TCPN see III:TBQ750
TCPP see III:FQU875
2,4,5-TCPPA see II:TIX500

TCT see III:TFZ000
TDA see I:TGL750
TDBP (CZECH) see I:TNC500
TDCPP see III:FQU875
TDE see I:BIM500, III:TJQ333
o,p-TDE see III:CDN000
TDE (DOT) see I:BIM500
o,p'-TDE see III:CDN000
p,p'-TDE see I:BIM500
TDI see I:TGM740, I:TGM750
2,4-TDI see I:TGM750
2,6-TDI see II:TGM800
TDI-80 see I:TGM740, I:TGM750
TDI 80-20 see I:TGM740
TDI (OSHA) see I:TGM750
2,5-TDS see III:TGM400
TE see III:TBF750
TEBECID see III:ILD000
TEBENIC see III:ILD000
TEBERUS see III:EPQ000
TEBEXIN see III:ILD000
TEBOS see III:ILD000
TEBRAZID see III:POL500
TECH DDT see I:DAD200
TECHNICAL BHC see I:BBQ750
TECHNICAL HCH see I:BBQ750
TECHNOPOR see III:PKQ059
TECH PET F see III:MQV750
TECNAZEN (GERMAN) see III:TBR750
TECNAZENE see III:TBR750
TECOFLEX HR see I:PKN000
TECQUINOL see III:HIH000
TECSOL see I:EFU000
TECTILON ORANGE 3GT see III:SGP500
TEEBACONIN see III:ILD000
TEF see III:TND250
TEFLON see III:TAI250
TEFLON (various) see III:TAI250
TEFSIEL C see III:FMB000
TEGAFUR see III:FMB000
TEGOLAN see III:CMD750
TEGO-OLEIC 130 see III:OHU000
TEGOSTEARIC 254 see III:SLK000
TEIB see III:TND000
TEKAZIN see III:ILD000
TEKWAISA see III:MNH000
TEL see III:TCF000
TELAGAN see III:TEH500
TELARGAN see III:TEH500
TELARGEAN see III:TEH500
TELIDAL see III:HNI500
TELIPEX see I:TBG000
TELLURIUM DIETHYLDITHIOCARBAMATE see III:EPJ000
TELODRIN see III:OAN000
TELONE see I:DGG950
TELONE II SOIL FUMIGANT see I:DGG950
TELON FAST BLACK E see AQP000
TELVAR see III:CJX750, III:DXQ500
TELVAR DIURON WEED KILLER see III:DXQ500
TELVAR MONURON WEEDKILLER see III:CJX750
TEM-HISTINE see III:DPJ400
TEMLO see II:HIM000
TEMPANAL see II:HIM000
TEMPRA see II:HIM000
TENDEARIL see III:HNI500
TENITE 423 see III:PMP500
TENITE 800 see III:PJS750
TENNECO 1742 see III:PKQ059
TENNUS 0565 see II:AAX175
TENOX BHA see II:BQI000
TENOX BHT see III:BFW750
TENOX HQ see III:HIH000
TENOX PG see III:PNM750
TENSIVAL see III:TEH500

TENSOL 7 see III:PKB500
TENSOPAM see III:DCK759
TENURID see III:DXH250
TENUTEX see III:DXH250
TEOLAXIN see II:EOK000
TEPA see III:TND250
TERABOL see III:MHR200
TERALIN see III:DPJ400
TERALUTIL see III:HNT500
TERAMETHYL THIURAM DISULFIDE see III:TFS350
TERAMYCIN HYDROCHLORIDE see III:HOI000
TERCININ see III:CMV000
TEREBENTHINE (FRENCH) see III:TOD750
TEREPHTAHLIC ACID-ETHYLENE GLYCOL POLYESTER see III:PKF750
TEREPHTHALIC ACID ISOPROPYLAMIDE see III:IRN000
TEREPHTHALIC ACID METHYL ESTER see III:DUE000
TERFAN see III:PKF750
TERGAL see III:PKF750
TERININ see III:CMV000
TERMIL see III:TBQ750
TERMINALIA CHEBULA RETZ TANNING see III:MSB750
TERMITKIL see III:DEP600
TERM-I-TROL see II:PAX250
TERMOSOLIDO RED LCG see III:CHP500
TEROM see III:PKF750
TERPENE POLYCHLORINATES see III:TBC500
TERPENTIN OEL (GERMAN) see III:TOD750
TERPHAN see III:PKF750
p-TERPHENYL-4-YLACETAMIDE see III:TBD250
TERRA ALBA see III:CAX750
TERRACHLOR see III:PAX000
TERRAFUN see III:PAX000
TERR-O-GAS 100 see III:MHR200
TERSAN see III:TFS350
TERSASEPTIC see III:HCL000
TERTRACID LIGHT ORANGE G see III:HGC000
TERTRACID LIGHT YELLOW 2R see III:SGP500
TERTRACID ORANGE I see III:FAG010
TERTRACID PONCEAU 2R see III:FMU070
TERTRACID RED A see III:FAG020
TERTRACID RED CA see III:HJF500
TERTRAL D see III:PEY500
TERTROCHROME BLUE FB see III:HJF500
TERTRODIRECT BLACK E see AQP000
TERTRODIRECT BLUE 2B see I:CMO000
TERTRODIRECT VIOLET N see III:CMP000
TERTROGRAS ORANGE SV see III:PEJ500
TERTROPHENE BROWN CG see III:PEK000
TESERENE see II:DAL600
TESLEN see I:TBF500
TESPAMINE see I:TFQ750
TESTAFORM see I:TBG000
TESTANDRONE see I:TBF500
TESTATE see III:TBF750
TESTEX see I:TBG000
TESTHORMONE see III:MPN500
TESTICULOSTERONE see I:TBF500
TESTOBASE see I:TBF500
TESTODET see I:TBG000
TESTODRIN see I:TBG000
TESTOGEN see I:TBG000
TESTONIQUE see I:TBG000
TESTOPROPON see I:TBF500
TESTORA see III:MPN500
TESTORMOL see I:TBG000
TESTOSTEROID see I:TBF500
TESTOSTERONE see I:TBF500
trans-TESTOSTERONE see I:TBF500
TESTOSTERONE ENANTHATE see III:TBF750
TESTOSTERONE ETHANATE see III:TBF750
TESTOSTERONE HEPTANOATE see III:TBF750
TESTOSTERONE HEPTOATE see III:TBF750
TESTOSTERONE HEPTYLATE see III:TBF750

TESTOSTERONE HYDRATE see I:TBF500
TESTOSTERONE OENANTHATE see III:TBF750
TESTOSTERONE PROPIONATE see I:TBG000
TESTOSTERONE-17-PROPIONATE see I:TBG000
TESTOSTERONE-17-β-PROPIONATE see I:TBG000
TESTOSTERON PROPIONATE see I:TBG000
TESTOSTSTERONE see I:TBF500
TESTOSTROVAL see III:TBF750
TESTOVIRON see I:TBG000, III:MPN500
TESTOVIRON SCHERING see I:TBF500
TESTOVIRON T see I:TBF500
TESTOXYL see I:TBG000
TESTRED see III:MPN500
TESTREX see I:TBG000
TESTRONE see I:TBF500
TESTRYL see I:TBF500
TETD see III:DXH250
TETIDIS see III:DXH250
TETLEN see II:PCF275
TETNOR see II:BRF500
1,4,5,8-TETRAAMINO-9,10-ANTHRACENEDIONE see III:TBG700
1,4,5,8-TETRAAMINOANTHRAQUINONE see III:TBG700
3,3′,4,4′-TETRAAMINOBIPHENYL see III:BGK500
3,3′,4,4′-TETRAAMINOBIPHENYL TETRAHYDROCHLO-RIDE see III:BGK750
1,3,5,7-TETRAAZAADAMANTANE see III:HEI500
9,10,14c-15-TETRAAZANAPHTHO(1,2,-3-fg)NAPHTHACENE NITRATE see III:TBI750
TETRA-BASE see I:MJN000
1,1,2,2-TETRABROMAETHAN (GERMAN) see III:ACK250
TETRABROMOACETYLENE see III:ACK250
2,4,5,7-TETRABROMO-9-o-CARBOXYPHENYL-6-HY-DROXY-3-ISOXANTHONE, DISODIUM SALT see III:BNH500
1,1,2,2-TETRABROMOETANO (ITALIAN) see III:ACK250
S-TETRABROMOETHANE see III:ACK250
1,1,2,2-TETRABROMOETHANE see III:ACK250
2,4,5,7-TETRABROMO-3,6-FLUORANDIOL see III:BMO250, III:BNH500
TETRABROMOFLUORESCEIN see III:BMO250, III:BNH500
2′,4′,5′,7′-TETRABROMOFLUORESCEIN see III:BMO250
2′,4′,5′,7′-TETRABROMOFLUORESCEIN DISODIUM SALT see III:BNH500
TETRABROMOFLUORESCEIN S see III:BNH500
TETRABROMOFLUORESCEIN SOLUBLE see III:BNH500
2-(2,4,5,7-TETRABROMO-6-HYDROXY-3-OXO-3H-XAN-THENE-9-YL)BENZOIC ACID, DISODIUM SALT see III:BNH500
1,1,2,2-TETRABROOMETHAAN (DUTCH) see III:ACK250
TETRACAP see II:PCF275
1,1,2,2-TETRACHLOORETHAAN (DUTCH) see III:TBQ100
TETRACHLOORETHEEN (DUTCH) see II:PCF275
TETRACHLOORKOOLSTOF (DUTCH) see CBY000
TETRACHLOORMETAAN see CBY000
1,1,2,2-TETRACHLORAETHAN (GERMAN) see III:TBQ100
TETRACHLORAETHEN (GERMAN) see II:PCF275
N-(1,1,2,2-TETRACHLORAETHYLTHIO)CYCLOHEX-4-EN-1,4-DIACARBOXIMID (GERMAN) see III:CBF800
N-(1,1,2,2-TETRACHLORAETHYLTHIO)TETRAHYDROPHTHALAMID (GERMAN) see III:CBF800
TETRACHLORETHANE see III:TBQ100
1,1,2,2-TETRACHLORETHANE (FRENCH) see III:TBQ100
TETRACHLORKOHLENSTOFF, TETRA (GERMAN) see CBY000
TETRACHLORMETHAN (GERMAN) see CBY000
2,3,5,6-TETRACHLOR-3-NITROBENZOL (GERMAN) see III:TBR750
TETRACHLOROBENZIDINE see II:TBO000
2,2′,5,5′-TETRACHLOROBENZIDINE see II:TBO000
3,3′,6,6′-TETRACHLOROBENZIDINE see II:TBO000
TETRACHLOROBENZOQUINONE see III:TBO500

TETRACHLORO-p-BENZOQUINONE see III:TBO500
TETRACHLORO-1,4-BENZOQUINONE see III:TBO500
2,3,5,6-TETRACHLORO-p-BENZOQUINONE see III:TBO500
2,3,5,6-TETRACHLORO-1,4-BENZOQUINONE see III:TBO500
2,2′,5,5′-TETRACHLORO-(1,1′-BIPHENYL)-4,4′-DIAMINE, (9CI) see II:TBO000
TETRACHLOROCARBON see CBY000
2,4,5,6-TETRACHLORO-3-CYANOBENZONITRILE see III:TBQ750
2,3,4,5-TETRACHLORO-2-CYCLOBUTEN-1-ONE see III:PCF250
2,3,5,6-TETRACHLORO-2,5-CYCLOHEXADIENE-1,4-DIONE see III:TBO500
2,2′,5,5′-TETRACHLORO-4,4′-DIAMINODIPHENYL see II:TBO000
2,3,7,8-TETRACHLORODIBENZO(b,e)(1,4)DIOXAN see I:TAI000
2,3,6,7-TETRACHLORODIBENZO-p-DIOXIN see I:TAI000
2,3,7,8-TETRACHLORODIBENZO-p-DIOXIN see I:TAI000
2,3,7,8-TETRACHLORODIBENZO-1,4-DIOXIN see I:TAI000
TETRACHLORODIPHENYLETHANE see I:BIM500
TETRACHLOROEPOXYETHANE see III:TBQ275
sym-TETRACHLOROETHANE see III:TBQ100
1,1,1,2-TETRACHLOROETHANE see III:TBQ000
1,1,2,2-TETRACHLOROETHANE see III:TBQ100
TETRACHLOROETHENE see II:PCF275
TETRACHLOROETHYLENE (DOT) see II:PCF275
1,1,2,2-TETRACHLOROETHYLENE see II:PCF275
TETRACHLOROETHYLENE OXIDE see III:TBQ275
N-1,1,2,2-TETRACHLOROETHYLMERCAPTO-4-CYCLOHEXENE-1,2-CARBOXIMIDE see III:CBF800
N-((1,1,2,2-TETRACHLOROETHYL)SULFENYL)-cis-4-CYCLOHEXENE-1,2-DICARBOXIMIDE see III:CBF800
N-(1,1,2,2-TETRACHLOROETHYLTHIO)-4-CYCLOHEXENE-1,2-DICARBOXIMIDE see III:CBF800
TETRACHLOROISOPHTHALONITRILE see III:TBQ750
TETRACHLOROMETHANE see CBY000
2,3,4,5-TETRACHLORONITROBENZENE see III:TBS000
2,3,4,6-TETRACHLORONITROBENZENE see III:TBR500
2,3,5,6-TETRACHLORONITROBENZENE see III:TBR750
1,2,3,4-TETRACHLORO-5-NITROBENZENE see III:TBS000
1,2,3,5-TETRACHLORO-4-NITROBENZENE see III:TBR500
1,2,4,5-TETRACHLORO-3-NITROBENZENE see III:TBR750
2,3,4,6-TETRACHLOROPHENOL see II:TBT000
2,4,5,6-TETRACHLOROPHENOL see II:TBT000
m-TETRACHLOROPHTHALONITRILE see III:TBQ750
TETRACHLOROQUINONE see III:TBO500
TETRACHLORO-p-QUINONE see III:TBO500
TETRACHLORURE de CARBONE (FRENCH) see CBY000
TETRACHLORURE D'ACETYLENE (FRENCH) see III:TBQ100
TETRACHLORVINPHOS see II:TBW100
1,1,2,2-TETRACLOROETANO (ITALIAN) see III:TBQ100
TETRACLOROETENE (ITALIAN) see II:PCF275
TETRACLOROMETANO (ITALIAN) see CBY000
TETRACLORURO di CARBONIO (ITALIAN) see CBY000
TETRACYANONICKELATE(2−) DIPOTASSIUM, HYDRATE see II:TBW250
TETRACYDIN see I:ABG750
TETRADECANE see III:TBX750
1-TETRADECANOL see III:TBY500
N-TETRADECANOL-1 see III:TBY500
TETRADECANOYLETHYLENEIMINE see III:MSB000
12-TETRADECANOYLPHORBOL-13-ACETATE see III:PGV000
N-TETRADECANOYL-N-TETRADECANOYLOXY-2-AMINO-FLUORENE see III:MSB250
12-o-TETRADECA-2-cis-4-trans,6,8-TETRAENOYLPHORBOL-13-ACETATE see III:TCA250
TETRADECYL ALCOHOL see III:TBY500
N-TETRADECYL ALCOHOL see III:TBY500
TETRADEHYDRODOISYNOLIC ACID METHYL ETHER see III:BIT000

12-o-TETRADEKANOYLPHORBOL-13-ACETAT (GERMAN) see III:PGV000
TETRADIN see III:DXH250
TETRADINE see III:DXH250
TETRADIOXIN see I:TAI000
TETRAETHYLDIAMINO-o-CARBOXY-PHENYL-XANTHE-NYL CHLORIDE see III:FAG070
TETRAETHYLENE GLYCOL DIACRYLATE see III:ADT050
TETRAETHYL LEAD see III:TCF000
TETRAETHYLPLUMBANE see III:TCF000
TETRAETHYLRHODAMINE see III:FAG070
TETRAETHYLTHIOPEROXYDICARBONIC DIAMIDE see III:DXH250
TETRAETHYLTHIRAM DISULPHIDE see III:DXH250
TETRAETHYLTHIURAM see III:DXH250
TETRAETHYLTHIURAM DISULFIDE see III:DXH250
TETRAETHYLTHIURAM DISULPHIDE see III:DXH250
N,N,N′,N′-TETRAETHYLTHIURAM DISULPHIDE see III:DXH250
TETRAETIL see III:DXH250
TETRAFINOL see CBY000
TETRAFLUORETHYLENE see III:TCH500
3,5,3′,5′-TETRAFLUORODIETHYLSTILBESTROL see III:TCH325
2,5,2′,5′-TETRAFLUORO-4-DIMETHYLAMINOAZOBEN-ZENE see III:DRK800
TETRAFLUOROETHENE see III:TCH500
TETRAFLUOROETHENE HOMOPOLYMER see III:TAI250
TETRAFLUOROETHENE POLYMER see III:TAI250
TETRAFLUOROETHYLENE see III:TCH500
TETRAFLUOROETHYLENE, inhibited (DOT) see III:TCH500
TETRAFLUOROETHYLENE HOMOPOLYMER see III:TAI250
TETRAFLUOROETHYLENE POLYMERS see III:TAI250
TETRAFLUORO-m-PHENYLENE DIAMINE DIHYDROCHLO-RIDE see III:TCI250
TETRAFORM see CBY000
TETRAHELICENE see III:BCR750
1′,2′,3′,4′-TETRAHYDRO-4,10-ACE-1,2-BENZANTHRA-CENE see III:HDH000
(±)-7,8,8a,9a-TETRAHYDROBENZO(10,11)CHYRSENO(3,4-b)OXIRENE-7,8-DIOL see III:DMR000
1,2,5,6-TETRAHYDROBENZO(j)CYCLOPENT(fg)ACEANTHRYLENE see III:TCJ500
7,8,9,10-TETRAHYDROBENZO(a)PYRENE see III:TCJ775
1′,2′,3′,4′-TETRAHYDRO-3,4-BENZOPYRENE see III:TCJ775
7,8,9,10-TETRAHYDRO-BENZO(a)PYRENE-9,10-EPOXIDE see III:ECQ100
7,8,9,10-TETRAHYDRO-BENZO(a)PYRENE-9,10-EPOXYIDE see III:ECQ100
exo-TETRAHYDROBICYCLOPENTADIENE see III:TLR675
Δ¹-TETRAHYDROCANNABINOL see III:TCM250
(1)-Δ¹-TETRAHYDROCANNABINOL see III:TCM250
(−)-Δ⁹-trans-TETRAHYDROCANNABINOL see III:TCM250
trans-Δ⁹-TETRAHYDROCANNABINOL see III:TCM250
1-trans-Δ⁹-TETRAHYDROCANNABINOL see III:TCM250
(−)-Δ¹-3,4-trans-TETRAHYDROCANNABINOL see III:TCM250
Δ⁹-TETRAHYDROCANNABINON see III:TCM250
trans-1,2,3,4-TETRAHYDROCHRYSENE-1,2,-DIOL see III:DNC600
2,7,8,9-TETRAHYDRO-1H-CYCLOPENT(j)ACEANTHRYL-ENE see III:CPY500
1,2,3,4-TETRAHYDRODIBENZ(a,h)ANTHRACENE see III:TCN750
1,2,3,4-TETRAHYDRODIBENZ(a,j)ANTHRACENE see III:TCO000
exo-TETRAHYDRODI(CYCLOPENTADIENE) see III:TLR675
(+)-Z-7,8,9,10-TETRAHYDRO-7-α,8-β-DIHDYROXY-9-α,10-α-EPOXYBENZO(a)PYRENE see III:DMP600
(−)-Z-7,8,9,10-TETRAHYDRO-7-α,8-β-DIHDYROXY-9-α,10-α-EPOXYBENZO(a)PYRENE see III:DMP800
(E)-8,9,10,11-TETRAHYDRO-8-β,9-α-DIHYDROXY-10-α,11-α-BENZ(a)ANTHRACENE see III:DMO600

2,2,6,6-TETRAMETHYLNITROSOPIPERIDINE see
    III:TDS000
2,6,10,14-TETRAMETHYLPENTADECANE see III:PMD500
1:2:3:4-TETRAMETHYLPHENANTHRENE see III:TDS750
N,N,2,3-TETRAMETHYL-4-(4'-(PYRIDYL-1'-OXIDE)AZO)
    ANILINE see III:DQF200
N,N,2,5-TETRAMETHYL-4-(4'-(PYRIDYL-1'-OXIDE)AZO)
    ANILINE see III:DQF400
N,N,2,6-TETRAMETHYL-4-(4'-(PYRIDYL-1'-OXIDE)AZO)
    ANILINE see III:DQF600
TETRAMETHYLTHIOCARBAMOYLDISULPHIDE see
    III:TFS350
TETRAMETHYLTHIORAMDISULFIDE (DUTCH) see
    III:TFS350
TETRAMETHYLTHIOUREA see III:TDX000
1,1,3,3-TETRAMETHYLTHIOUREA see III:TDX000
TETRAMETHYL-THIRAM DISULFID (GERMAN) see
    III:TFS350
TETRAMETHYLTHIURAM BISULFIDE see III:TFS350
TETRAMETHYLTHIURAM DISULFIDE see III:TFS350
N,N,N',N'-TETRAMETHYLTHIURAM DISULFIDE see
    III:TFS350
TETRAMETHYLTHIURAM DISULFIDE mixed with FERRIC
    NITROSODIMETHYLDITHIOCARBAMATE see
    III:FAZ000
N,N-TETRAMETHYLTHIURAM DISULPHIDE see III:TFS350
TETRAMETHYLTHIURAMMONIUM SULFIDE see
    III:BJL600
TETRAMETHYLTHIURAM MONOSULFIDE see III:BJL600
TETRAMETHYLTHIURAMONOSULFIDE see III:BJL600
TETRAMETHYLTHIURAM SULFIDE see III:BJL600
TETRAMETHYL THIURANE DISULFIDE see III:TFS350
TETRAMETHYLTHIURUM DISULFIDE see III:TFS350
TETRAMETHYLTRITHIO CARBAMIC ANHYDRIDE see
    III:BJL600
TETRAMINE see III:HOI000
TETRAMINE FAST BROWN BRS see II:CMO750
1,4,5,8-TETRAMINOANTHRAQUINONE see III:TBG700
TETRAN HYDROCHLORIDE see III:HOI000
TETRAN PTFE see III:TAI250
TETRA OLIVE N2G see III:APG500
2,2'-(2,5,8,11-TETRAOXA-1,2-DODECANEDIYL)BISOXI-
    RANE see III:TJQ333
2,2'-(2,5,8,11-TETRAOXA-1,12-DODECANE DIYL)BISOXI-
    RANE see III:TJQ333
(±)-(3,5,3',5'-TETRAOXO)-1,2-DIPIPERAZINOPROPANE see
    II:PIK250
TETRAPHENE see I:BBC250
TETRAPHENYL METHANE see III:TEA750
TETRAPOM see III:TFS350
TETRASIPTON see III:TFS350
TETRASOL see CBY000
TETRATHIURAM DISULFIDE see III:TFS350
TETRATHIURAM DISULPHIDE see III:TFS350
TETRAVEC see II:PCF275
TETRAZOBENZENE-β-NAPHTHOL see III:OHA000
TETRAZO DEEP BLACK G see AQP000
TETRODIRECT BLACK EFD see AQP000
TETROGUER see II:PCF275
TETROPIL see II:PCF275
TETROSIN OE see III:BGJ250
TETURAM see III:DXH250
TETURAMIN see III:DXH250
TEVCOCIN see II:CDP250
TEVCODYNE see II:BRF500
TEXAN RED TONER D see III:CHP500
TEXIN 192A see I:PKO500
TEXIN 445D see I:PKM250
TEXTILE see III:SFT500
T-FLUORIDE see III:SHF500
T-GAS see I:EJN500
β-TGDR see III:TFJ250
T-GELB BZW, GRUN 1 see III:QCA000

TH 1314 see III:EPQ000
THACAPZOL see III:MCO500
THALIDOMIDE see III:TEH500
THALIN see III:TEH500
THALINETTE see III:TEH500
THC see III:TCM250
Δ^1-THC see III:TCM250
Δ^9-THC see III:TCM250
TH-DMBA see III:TCP600
THEELIN see I:EDV000
THEELOL see II:EDU500
THEIN see III:CAK500
THEINE see III:CAK500
THELESTRIN see I:EDV000
THELYKININ see I:EDV000
THENOBARBITAL see II:EOK000
THENYLENE see III:DPJ400
THENYLENE HYDROCHLORIDE see III:DPJ400
THENYLPYRAMINE HYDROCHLORIDE see III:DPJ400
THEOGEN see I:ECU750
THEOLOXIN see II:EOK000
THEOMINAL see II:EOK000
THEOPHILCHOLINE see III:TEH500
THERADERM see III:BDS000
THERA-FLUR-N see III:SHF500
THERAPOL see III:SNM500
THERAZONE see II:BRF500
THERMACURE see III:MKA500
THERMALOX see I:BFT250
THERMINOL FR-1 see I:PJL750
THERMOPLASTIC 125 see III:SMR000
THFU see III:FMB000
THIACETAMIDE see I:TFA000
THIACOCCINE see III:TEX250
THIACYCLOPROPANE see III:EJP500
THIAMAZOLE see III:MCO500
THIANIDE see III:EPQ000
THIASIN see III:SNN500
THIATE H see III:DKC400
THIAZAMIDE see III:TEX250
N^1-2-THIAZOLYLSULFANILAMIDE see III:TEX250
THIFOR see III:EAQ750
THIIRANE see III:EJP500
THILLATE see III:TFS350
THILOPHENYL see I:DKQ000
THILOPHENYT see I:DNU000
THIMECIL see II:MPW500
THIMER see III:TFS350
THIMEROSALATE see III:MDI000
THIMEROSOL see III:MDI000
THIMUL see III:EAQ750
THIOACETAMIDE see I:TFA000
THIOALLATE see CDO250
THIOAMIDE see III:EPQ000
THIOANILINE see I:TFI000
4,4'-THIOANILINE see I:TFI000
THIOBENZAMIDE see III:BBM250
THIOBENZYL ALCOHOL see III:TGO750
4,4'-THIOBIS(ANILINE) see I:TFI000
4,4'-THIOBISBENZENAMINE see I:TFI000
1,1'-THIOBIS(2-CHLOROETHANE) see I:BIH250
2,2'-THIOBIS(4,6-DICHLOROPHENOL) see III:TFD250
1,1'-THIOBIS(N,N-DIMETHYLTHIO)FORMAMIDE see
    III:BJL600
THIOCARB see III:SGJ000
THIOCARBAMATE see I:ISR000
THIOCARBAMIDE see I:ISR000
THIOCARBAMYLHYDRAZINE see III:TFQ000
THIODAN see III:EAQ750
p,p-THIODIANILINE see I:TFI000
4,4'-THIODIANILINE see I:TFI000
THIODI-p-PHENYLENEDIAMINE see I:TFI000
THIODOW see III:EIR000
THIOFACO T-35 see III:TKP500

THIOFIDE see III:BDE750
THIOFOR see III:EAQ750
THIOFOZIL see I:TFQ750
(1-THIO-d-GLUCOPYRANOSATO)GOLD see I:ART250
1-THIO-GLUCOPYRANOSE, MONOGOLD(1+) SALT see I:ART250
THIOGLUCOSE d'OR (FRENCH) see I:ART250
β-THIOGUANINE DEOXYRIBOSIDE see III:TFJ250
THIOHYPOXANTHINE see III:POK000
2-THIOL-DIHYDROGLYOXALINE see I:IAQ000
THIOMECIL see II:MPW500
THIOMERSALATE see III:MDI000
2-THIO-6-METHYL-1,3-PYRIMIDIN-4-ONE see II:MPW500
6-THIO-4-METHYLURACIL see II:MPW500
THIOMIDIL see II:MPW500
THIOMUL see III:EAQ750
THIONEX see III:BJL600, III:EAQ750
THIONEX RUBBER ACCELERATOR see III:BJL600
THIONIDEN see III:EPQ000
2-THIO-4-OXO-6-METHYL-1,3-PYRIMIDINE see II:MPW500
2-THIO-4-OXO-6-PROPYL-1,3-PYRIMIDINE see I:PNX000
2-THIO-6-OXYPYRIMIDINE see III:TFR250
THIOPHAL see III:TIT250
THIOPHENIT see III:MNH000
THIOPHOS see III:PAK000
THIOPHOS 3422 see III:PAK000
THIOPHOSPHAMIDE see I:TFQ750
THIOPHOSPHATE de O,O-DIETHYLE et de O-(4-NITROPHE-
    NYLE) (FRENCH) see III:PAK000
THIOPHOSPHATE de O,O-DIMETHYLE et de O-(3-METHYL-
    4-METHYLTHIOPHENYLE) (FRENCH) see III:FAQ999
THIOPHOSPHATE de O,O-DIMETHYLE et de O-(4-NITROPHE-
    NYLE) (FRENCH) see III:MNH000
2-THIO-6-PROPYL-1,3-PYRIMIDIN-4-ONE see I:PNX000
6-THIO-4-PROPYLURACIL see I:PNX000
β-THIOPSEUDOUREA see I:ISR000
2-THIO-1,3-PYRIMIDIN-4-ONE see III:TFR250
THIORYL see II:MPW500
THIOSAN see III:DXH250, III:TFS350
THIOSCABIN see III:DXH250
THIOSEMICARBAZIDE see III:TFQ000
3-THIOSEMICARBAZIDE see III:TFQ000
THIOSEPTAL see III:PPO000
THIOSUCCINIMIDE see III:MRN000
THIOSULFAN see III:EAQ750
THIOSULFAN TIONEL see III:EAQ750
THIOSULFIL-A FORTE see I:PDC250
THIO-TEP see I:TFQ750
THIOTEX see III:TFS350
THIOTHYMIN see II:MPW500
THIOTHYRON see II:MPW500
THIOTOX see III:TFS350
THIOTRIETHYLENEPHOSPHORAMIDE see I:TFQ750
THIOURACIL see III:TFR250
2-THIOURACIL see III:TFR250
6-THIOURACIL see III:TFR250
2-THIOUREA see I:ISR000
THIOUREA (DOT) see I:ISR000
6-THIOXOPURINE see III:POK000
THIOZAMIDE see III:TEX250
THIRAM see III:TFS350
THIRAMAD see III:TFS350
THIRAME (FRENCH) see III:TFS350
THIRASAN see III:TFS350
THIRERANIDE see III:DXH250
THIULIX see III:TFS350
THIURAD see III:TFS350
THIURAGYL see I:PNX000
THIURAM see III:TFS350
THIURAM E see III:DXH250
THIURAMIN see III:TFS350
THIURAMYL see III:TFS350
THIURANIDE see III:DXH250
THIURYL see II:MPW500

THOMAPYRIN see III:ARP250
THOMPSON'S WOOD FIX see II:PAX250
THORIA see I:TFT750
THORIUM see II:TFS750
THORIUM-232 see II:TFS750
THORIUM DIOXIDE see I:TFT750
THORIUM HYDRIDE see II:TFT250
THORIUM METAL, PYROPHORIC (DOT) see II:TFS750
THORIUM OXIDE see I:TFT750
THOROTRAST see I:TFT750
THORTRAST see I:TFT750
THREAMINE see III:AMA500
1-THREITOL-1,4-BISMETHANESULFONATE see I:TFU500
THRETHYLENE see II:TIO750
THU see I:ISR000
THULOL see II:EDU500
THYCAPSOL see III:MCO500
THYLATE see III:TFS350
THYLFAR M-50 see III:MNH000
THYLOGEN MALEATE see III:DBM800
THYLOQUINONE see III:MMD500
THYNESTRON see I:EDV000
THYREONORM see II:MPW500
THYREOSTAT see II:MPW500
THYREOSTAT II see I:PNX000
THYRIL see II:MPW500
THYROCALCITONIN see III:TFZ000
TI-8 see III:TCA250
TIBAZIDE see III:ILD000
TIBEMID see III:ILD000
TIBINIDE see III:ILD000
TIBISON see III:ILD000
TIBIVIS see III:ILD000
TIBIZIDE see III:ILD000
TIBRIC ACID see III:CGJ250
TIBUSAN see III:ILD000
TICINIL see II:BRF500
TICLOBRAN see III:ARQ750
TIC MUSTARD see II:IAN000
TIEZENE see III:EIR000
TIFOMYCINE see II:CDP250
12-o-TIGLYL-PHORBOL-13-BUTYRATE see III:PGV750
12-o-TIGLYL-PHORBOL-13-DODECANOATE see III:PGW000
7-TIGLYLRETRONECINE VIRIDIFLORATE see III:SPB500
7-TIGLYL-9-VIRIDIFLORYLRETRONECINE see III:SPB500
TIGUVON see III:FAQ999
TIKOFURAN see III:NGG500
TILCAREX see III:PAX000
TILLAM (RUSSIAN) see III:PNF500
TILLAM-6-E see III:PNF500
TILLRAM see III:DXH250
TIMAZIN see III:FMM000
TIN see III:TGB250
TIN (α) see III:TGB250
TIN BIFLUORIDE see III:TGD100
TIN DIFLUORIDE see III:TGD100
TINDURIN see III:TGD000
TINESTAN see III:ABX250
TINESTAN 60 WP see III:ABX250
TIN FLAKE see III:TGB250
TIN FLUORIDE see III:TGD100
TINIC see III:NCQ900
TINNING GLUX (DOT) see III:ZFA000
TINON GOLDEN YELLOW see III:DCZ000
TIN POWDER see III:TGB250
TIN TRIPHENYL ACETATE see III:ABX250
TIOBENZAMIDE (ITALIAN) see III:BBM250
TIOFINE see III:TGG760
TIOFOS see III:PAK000
TIOFOSFAMID see I:TFQ750
TIOFOZIL see I:TFQ750
TIOMERACIL see II:MPW500
TIONAL see III:BJT750

TIORALE M see II:MPW500
TIOTIRON see II:MPW500
TIOURACYL (POLISH) see III:TFR250
TIOVEL see III:EAQ750
TIOXIDE see III:TGG760
TIPPON see II:TAA100
TIRAMPA see III:TFS350
TISIN see III:ILD000
TISIODRAZIDA see III:ILD000
TISPERSE MB-2X see III:NBL000
TISPERSE MB-58 see III:BHA750
TITANDIOXID (SWEDEN) see III:TGG760
TITANIUM see III:TGF250
TITANIUM ACETONYL ACETONATE see III:BGQ750
TITANIUM ALLOY see III:TGF250
TITANIUM compounded with BERYLLIUM (1:12) see
  I:BFR000, I:BFR250
TITANIUM DIOXIDE see III:TGG760
TITANIUM FERROCENE see III:DGW200
TITANIUM METAL POWDER, DRY (DOT) see III:TGF250
TITANIUM NICKEL OXIDE see II:NDL500
TITANIUM OXIDE see III:TGG760
TITANIUM OXIDE BIS(ACETYLACETONATE) see
  III:BGQ750
TITANIUM, OXOBIS(2,4-PENTANEDIONATO-O,O') see
  III:BGQ750
TITANIUM SPONGE GRANULES (DOT) see III:TGF250
TITANIUM SPONGE POWDERS (DOT) see III:TGF250
TITANOCENE see III:DGW200, III:TGH500
TITANOCENE, DICHLORIDE see III:DGW200
TITANYL BIS(ACETYLACETONATE) see III:BGQ750
TIURAM see III:DXH250
TIURAM (POLISH) see III:TFS350
TIURAMYL see III:TFS350
TIXOTON see III:BAV750
TIZIDE see III:ILD000
TJB see III:DWI000
TK 1000 see III:PKQ059
TKB see I:NKB500
TL4N see III:DJD600
TL 145 see III:TNF250
TL 146 see I:BIE250
TL 154 see III:CHF500
TL 314 see I:ADX500
TL 337 see I:EJM900
TL 389 see I:DQY950
TL 478 see III:BRZ000
TL 1026 see I:CAG000
TL 1070 see I:CAG500
TL 1091 see II:NDC000
TL 1163 see III:TLN250
TL 1182 see I:CAI000
TM-4049 see III:MAK700
7,8,12-TMBA see III:TLK750
TMCA see III:TLA250
TMP see II:TMD250
TMTD see III:TFS350
TMTDS see III:TFS350
TMTM see III:BJL600
TMTMS see III:BJL600
TMTU see III:TDX000
T-2 MYCOTOXIN see III:FQS000
TNCS 53 see III:CNP250
TNG see III:NGY000
TOBACCO LEAF ABSOLUTE see III:TGH750
TOBACCO PLANT see I:TGI100
TOBACCO REFINED TAR see II:CMP800
TOBACCO SMOKE CONDENSATE see I:SEC000
TOBACCO TAR see I:SEC000, II:CMP800
TOBACCO WOOD see III:WCB000
TODALGIL see II:BRF500
TOF see III:TNI250
TOFURON see FQN000
N-TOIN see III:NGE000

TOIN UNICELLES see I:DKQ000
TOK see I:DFT800
TOK-2 see I:DFT800
TOK E see I:DFT800
TOK E-25 see I:DFT800
TOK E 40 see I:DFT800
TOKKORN see I:DFT800
TOKOKIN see I:EDV000
TOK WP-50 see I:DFT800
2,4-TOLAMINE see I:TGL750
o-TOLIDIN see I:TGJ750
2-TOLIDIN (GERMAN) see I:TGJ750
2-TOLIDINA (ITALIAN) see I:TGJ750
TOLIDINE see I:TGJ750
2-TOLIDINE see I:TGJ750
o-TOLIDINE see I:TGJ750
3,3'-TOLIDINE see I:TGJ750
o,o'-TOLIDINE see I:TGJ750
TOLL see III:MNH000
TOLUEEN-DIISOCYANAAT see I:TGM750
TOLUEN-DISOCIANATO see I:TGM750
TOLUENE-2-AZONAPHTHOL-2 see II:TGW000
o-TOLUENE-1-AZO-2-NAPHTHYLAMINE see III:FAG135
o-TOLUENEAZO-o-TOLUENEAZO-β-NAPHTHOL see
  III:SBC500
o-TOLUENEAZO-o-TOLUENE-β-NAPHTHOL see III:SBC500
o-TOLUENEAZO-o-TOLUIDINE see I:AIC250
m-TOLUENEDIAMINE see I:TGL750
p-TOLUENEDIAMINE see III:TGM000
TOLUENE-2,4-DIAMINE see I:TGL750
2,4-TOLUENEDIAMINE see I:TGL750
TOLUENE-2,5-DIAMINE see III:TGM000
2,4-TOLUENEDIAMINE DIHYDROCHLORIDE see
  III:DCE000
p-TOLUENEDIAMINE SULFATE see III:DCE600,
  III:TGM400
2,5-TOLUENEDIAMINE SULFATE see III:DCE600
TOLUENE-2,5-DIAMINE, SULFATE (1:1) (8CI) see
  III:DCE600
p-TOLUENEDIAMINE SULPHATE see III:DCE600
TOLUENE-2,5-DIAMINE SULPHATE see III:DCE600
TOLUENE DIISOCYANATE see I:TGM740, I:TGM750
TOLUENE-1,3-DIISOCYANATE see I:TGM740
TOLUENE-2,4-DIISOCYANATE see I:TGM750
2,4-TOLUENEDIISOCYANATE see I:TGM750
TOLUENE-2,6-DIISOCYANATE see II:TGM800
2,6-TOLUENE DIISOCYANATE see II:TGM800
TOLUENE-2-SULFONAMIDE see II:TGN250
o-TOLUENESULFONAMIDE see II:TGN250
TOLUENE-p-SULFONYLMETHYLNITROSAMIDE see
  III:THE500
α-TOLUENETHIOL see III:TGO750
TOLUENE TRICHLORIDE see I:BFL250
o-TOLUENO-AZO-β-NAPHTHOL see II:TGW000
o-TOLUIDIN (CZECH) see I:TGQ750
2-TOLUIDINE see I:TGQ750
o-TOLUIDINE see I:TGQ750
2-TOLUIDINE HYDROCHLORIDE see I:TGS500
m-TOLUIDINE HYDROCHLORIDE see III:TGS250
o-TOLUIDINE HYDROCHLORIDE see I:TGS500
p-TOLUIDINE HYDROCHLORIDE see III:TGS750
p-TOLUIDINIUM CHLORIDE see III:TGS750
o-TOLUIDYNA (POLISH) see I:TGQ750
TOLUILENODWUIZOCYJANIAN see I:TGM750
m-TOLUOL see III:CNW750
o-TOLUOL see III:CNX000
p-TOLUOL see III:CNX250
o-TOLUOL-AZO-o-TOLUIDIN (GERMAN) see I:AIC250
ORTHO-TOLUOL-SULFONAMID (GERMAN) see II:TGN250
p-TOLUOLSULFONSAEUREAETHYL ESTER (GERMAN) see
  III:EPW500
p-TOLUOLSULFONSAEURE METHYL ESTER (GERMAN) see
  III:MLL250
α-TOLUOLTHIOL see III:TGO750

m-TOLUYLENDIAMIN (CZECH) see I:TGL750
p-TOLUYLENDIAMINE see III:TGM000
TOLUYLENE BLUE MONOHYDRATE see III:TGU500
m-TOLUYLENEDIAMINE see I:TGL750
TOLUYLENE-2,5-DIAMINE see III:TGM000
2,4-TOLUYLENEDIAMINE (DOT) see I:TGL750
p-TOLUYLENEDIAMINE SULPHATE see III:DCE600
TOLUYLENE-2,5-DIAMINE SULPHATE see III:DCE600
TOLUYLENE-2,4-DIISOCYANATE see I:TGM750
p-TOLYCARBAMIDE see III:THG000
m-TOLYENEDIAMINE see I:TGL750
TOLYENE 2,4-DIISOCYANATE see I:TGM750
p-TOLYL ALCOHOL see III:CNX250
o-TOLYLAMINE see I:TGQ750
o-TOLYLAMINE HYDROCHLORIDE see I:TGS500
N-(p-TOLYL)-1-AZIRIDINECARBOXAMIDE see III.TGV250
m-TOLYLAZOACETANILIDE see III:TGV500
5-(o-TOLYLAZO)-2-AMINOTOLUENE see I:AIC250
p-(o-TOLYLAZO)-ANILINE see III:TGV750
p-(o-TOLYLAZO)-o-CRESOL see III:HJG000
1-(o-TOLYLAZO)-2-NAPHTHOL see II:TGW000
1-(o-TOLYLAZO)-β-NAPHTHOL see II:TGW000
1-(o-TOLYLAZO)-2-NAPHTHYLAMINE see III:FAG135
2-(o-TOLYLAZO)-p-TOLUIDINE see III:TGW500
4-(o-TOLYLAZO)-o-TOLUIDINE see I:AIC250
4-(p-TOLYLAZO)-m-TOLUIDINE see III:AIC500
4-(p-TOLYLAZO)-o-TOLUIDINE see III:TGW750
1-((4-TOLYLAZO)TOLYLAZO)-2-NAPHTHOL see III:TGX000
o-TOLYLAZO-o-TOLYLAZO-2-NAPHTHOL see III:SBC500
o-TOLYLAZO-o-TOLYLAZO-β-NAPHTHOL see III:SBC500
1-((4-(o-TOLYLAZO)-o-TOLYL)AZO)-2-NAPHTHOL) see III:SBC500
p-TOLYL-N-CARBAMOYLAZIRIDINE see III:TGV250
TOLYL CHLORIDE see II:BEE375
m-TOLYLENEDIAMINE see I:TGL750
TOLYLENE-2,4-DIAMINE see I:TGL750
2,4-TOLYLENEDIAMINE see I:TGL750
4-m-TOLYLENEDIAMINE see I:TGL750
p,m-TOLYLENEDIAMINE see III:TGM000
p-TOLYLENEDIAMINE SULPHATE see III:DCE600
TOLYLENE DIISOCYANATE see I:TGM740
m-TOLYLENE DIISOCYANATE see I:TGM750, II:TGM800
TOLYLENE-2,4-DIISOCYANATE see I:TGM750
2,4-TOLYLENEDIISOCYANATE see I:TGM750
TOLYLENE-2,6-DIISOCYANATE see II:TGM800
TOLYLENE ISOCYANATE see I:TGM740
α-TOLYL MERCAPTAN see III:TGO750
p-TOLYLSULFONYL-METHYL-NITROSAMID (GERMAN) see III:THE500
p-TOLYLSULFONYLMETHYLNITROSAMIDE see III:THE500
N-(4'-o-TOLYL-o-TOLYLAZOSUCCINAMIC ACID see III:SNF500
p-TOLYLUREA see III:THG000
p-TOLYUREA see III:THG000
TONARSEN see I:DXE600
TONEDRON see III:MDT600
TONER LAKE RED C see III:CHP500
TONKA BEAN CAMPHOR see III:CNV000
TONOX see I:MJQ000
TONY RED see III:OHA000
TOPANE see II:BGJ750
TOPANOL see III:BFW750
TOPAZONE see III:NGG500
TOPEX see III:BDS000
TOPICHLOR 20 see II:CDR750
TOPICLOR see II:CDR750
TOPICLOR 20 see II:CDR750
TOPOREX 855-51 see III:SMQ500
TOPSYM see III:DUD800
TORDON see III:PIB900
TORDON 10K see III:PIB900
TORDON 22K see III:PIB900

TORDON 101 MIXTURE see III:PIB900
TORMONA see II:TAA100
TORSITE see III:BGJ250
TOSTRIN see I:TBG000
TOSYL see III:CDO000
2,5-TOULENEDIAMINE SULFATE see III:TGM400
TOX 47 see III:PAK000
TOXADUST see I:CDV100
TOXAFEEN (DUTCH) see I:CDV100
TOXAKIL see I:CDV100
TOXAPHEN (GERMAN) see I:CDV100
TOXAPHENE see I:CDV100
TOXICHLOR see II:CDR750
TOXILIC ANHYDRIDE see III:MAM000
TOXIN, PENICILLIUM ROQUEFORTI see III:PAQ875
TOXIN (PENICILLIUM ROQUEFORTII) see III:POF800
TOXIN PR see III:POF800
TOXIN T2 see III:FQS000
TOXON 63 see I:CDV100
TOXYPHEN see I:CDV100
TOYO AMARANTH see III:FAG020
TOYO EOSINE G see III:BNH500
TOYO OIL ORANGE see III:PEJ500
TOYO OIL YELLOW G see I:DOT300
TP see I:TBG000
2,4,5-TP see II:TIX500
TPA see III:PGV000
TPN (pesticide) see III:TBQ750
TPTA see III:ABX250
TPU 2T see I:PKO500
TPU 10M see I:PKM250
TPZA see III:ABX250
TR 201 see III:SMR000
TRACHOSEPT see III:DBX400
TRALGON see II:HIM000
TRAMETAN see III:TFS350
TRANCALGYL see III:EEM000
TRANIMUL see III:DCK759
TRANQDYN see III:DCK759
TRANQUINIL see III:RDF000
TRANQUIRIT see III:DCK759
TRANQUO-BUSCOPAN-WIRKSTOFF see III:CFZ000
TRANSAMINE see II:DAA800, II:TAA100
TRANSANNON see I:ECU750
TRANSPARENT BRONZE SCARLET see III:CHP500
TRASAN see II:CIR250
TRATUL see III:TAB250
TRAVAD see III:BAP000
TRAWOTOX see III:CDO000
TRECATOR see III:EPQ000
TREFANOCIDE see III:DUV600
TREFICON see III:DUV600
TREFLAM see III:DUV600
TREFLAN see III:DUV600
TREFLANOCIDE ELANCOLAN see III:DUV600
TREMOLITE ASBESTOS see I:ARM280
TRENIMON see III:TND000
TREOMICETINA see III:CDP250
TREOSULFAN see I:TFU500
TREPIDAN see III:DAP700
TRESCATYL see III:EPQ000
TRESCAZIDE see III:EPQ000
TRESOCHIN see III:CLD000
TRESPAPHAN see III:PMP500
TRESULFAN see I:TFU500
TRETAMINE see III:TND500
TRETINOIN see III:VSK950
TRIABARB see II:EOK000
TRIAD see II:TIO750
TRIAETHANOLAMIN-NG see III:TKP500
TRIAETHYLENMELAMIN (GERMAN) see III:TND500
TRIAETHYLENPHOSPHORSAEUREAMID (GERMAN) see III:TND250
TRIAMELIN see III:TND500

TRIETHYLENEMELAMINE see III:TND500
N,N',N''-TRIETHYLENEPHOSPHOROTHIOIC TRIAMIDE see I:TFQ750
TRIETHYLENEPHOSPHOROTRIAMIDE see III:TND250
N,N',N''-TRIETHYLENETHIOPHOSPHAMIDE see I:TFQ750
N,N',N''-TRIETHYLENETHIOPHOSPHORAMIDE see I:TFQ750
TRIETHYLENETHIOPHOSPHOROTRIAMIDE see I:TFQ750
TRIETHYLENIMINOBENZOQUINONE see III:TND000
2,4,6-TRIETHYLENIMINO-s-TRIAZINE see III:TND500
2,4,6-TRIETHYLENIMINO-1,3,5-TRIAZINE see III:TND500
TRIETHYLHEXYL PHOSPHATE see III:TNI250
TRI(2-ETHYLHEXYL)PHOSPHATE see III:TNI250
1,1,3-TRIETHYL-3-NITROSOUREA see III:NLX500
TRIETHYLOLAMINE see III:TKP500
TRIFENYLTINACETAAT (DUTCH) see III:ABX250
TRIFLUORALIN (USDA) see III:DUV600
3-(5-TRIFLUORMETHYLPHENYL)-,1-DIMETHYLHARN-STOFF (GERMAN) see III:DUK800
2-(2,2,2-TRIFLUOROACETAMIDO)-4-(5-NITRO-2-FURYL-)THIAZOLE see II:NGN500
2-TRIFLUOROACETYLAMINOFLUORENE see III:FER000
2-TRIFLUOROACETYLAMINOFLUOREN-9-ONE see III:TKH000
TRIFLUOROARSINE see I:ARI250
2,2,2-TRIFLUOROCHLOROETHANE see III:TJY175
1,1,1-TRIFLUORO-2-CHLOROETHANE see III:TJY175
2',4',6'-TRIFLUORO-4-DIMETHYLAMINOAZOBENZENE see III:DUK200
α,α,α-TRIFLUORO-2,6-DINITRO-N,N-DIPROPYL-p-TOLUI-DINE see III:DUV600
1,1,1-TRIFLUOROETHYL CHLORIDE see III:TJY175
2,2,2-TRIFLUORO-N-(FLUOREN-2-YL)ACETAMIDE see III:FER000
4-TRIFLUOROMETHYL-6H-BENZO(e)(1)BENZOTHIOPYRANO(4,3-b)INDOLE see III:TKC000
3-(m-TRIFLUOROMETHYLPHENYL)-1,1-DIMETHYLUREA see III:DUK800
N-(3-TRIFLUOROMETHYLPHENYL)-N'-N'-DIMETHYLUREA see III:DUK800
N-(m-TRIFLUOROMETHYLPHENYL)-N',N'-DIMETHYL-UREA see III:DUK800
2,2,2-TRIFLUORO-N-(4-(5-NITRO-2-FURYL)-2-THIAZOL-YL)ACETAMIDE see II:NGN500
2,2,2-TRIFLUORO-N-(9-OXOFLUOREN-2-YL)ACETAMIDE see III:TKH000
2,4,6-TRIFLUORO-s-TRIAZINE see III:TKK000
TRIFLURALIN see III:DUV600
TRIFLURALINE see III:DUV600
TRIFORINE and SODIUM NITRITE see III:SIT800
TRIFUNGOL see III:FAS000
TRIFUREX see III:DUV600
TRIGLYCINE see I:AMT500
TRIGLYCOLLAMIC ACID see I:AMT500
TRIGONOX C see III:BSC500
TRIHERBICIDE CIPC see III:CKC000
TRIHERBIDE see III:CBM000
TRIHERBIDE-IPC see III:CBM000
3,7,15-TRIHYDROXY-4-ACETOXY-8-OXO-12,13-EPOXY-Δ⁹-TRICHOTHECENE see III:FQR000
1,8,9-TRIHYDROXYANTHRACENE see III:APH250
1,2,3-TRIHYDROXYBENZEN (CZECH) see III:PPQ500
1,2,3-TRIHYDROXYBENZENE see III:PPQ500
3,4,5-TRIHYDROXYBENZENE-1-PROPYLCARBOXYLATE see III:PNM750
3,4,5-TRIHYDROXYBENZOIC ACID, n-PROPYL ESTER see III:PNM750
TRIHYDROXYCYANIDINE see III:THS000
3,4,5-TRIHYDROXY-1-CYCLOHEXENE-1-CARBOXYLIC ACID see III:SCE000
3,16-α,17-β-TRIHYDROXYESTRA-1,3,5(10)-TRIENE see II:EDU500
3,16-α,17-β-TRIHYDROXY-Δ-1,3,5-ESTRATRIENE see II:EDU500

TRIHYDROXYESTRIN see II:EDU500
TRI(HYDROXYETHYL)AMINE see III:TKP500
5,7,4'-TRIHYDROXYFLAVONOL see III:ICE000
8,12,18-TRIHYDROXY-4-METHYL-11,16-DIOXOSENECIO-NANIUM see III:HOF000
2,4a,7-TRIHYDROXY-1-METHYL-8-METHYLENEGIBB-3-ENE-1,10-CARBOXYLIC ACID 1-4-LACTONE see III:GEM000
3,16-α,17-β-TRIHYDROXYOESTRA-1,3,5(10)-TRIENE see II:EDU500
3,16-α,17-β-TRIHYDROXY-Δ-1,3,5-OESTRATRIENE see II:EDU500
TRIHYDROXYOESTRIN see II:EDU500
3,4,5-TRIHYDROXYPHENETHYLAMINE HYDROCHLORIDE see III:HKG000
3,7,15-TRIHYDROXYSCIRP-4-ACETOXY-9-EN-8-ONE see III:FQR000
2,4,6-TRIHYDROXY-1,3,5-TRIAZINE see III:THS000
TRIHYDROXYTRIETHYLAMINE see III:TKP500
2,2',2''-TRIHYDROXYTRIETHYLAMINE see III:TKP500
TRIKEPIN see III:DUV600
TRIKOJOL see I:MMN250
TRILEAD PHOSPHATE see I:LDU000
TRILENE see II:TIO750
TRILLEKAMIN see III:TNF500
TRIM see III:DUV600
TRIMANGOL see III:MAS500
TRIMAR see II:TIO750
TRIMEKS see I:MMN250
3,4,5-TRIMETHOXYBENZOYL METHYL RESERPATE see II:RDK000
3,4,5-TRIMETHOXYCINNAMALDEHYDE see III:TLA250
3-(3,4,5-TRIMETHOXYPHENYL)-2-PROPENAL see III:TLA250
3,4,5-TRIMETHOXY-α-VINYLBENZYL ALCOHOL ACETATE see III:TLC850
2,4,6-TRIMETHYLACETANILIDE see III:TLD250
2',4',6'-TRIMETHYLACETANILIDE see III:TLD250
TRIMETHYLACETIC ACID see III:PJA500
2,N,N-TRIMETHYL-4-AMINOAZOBENZENE see III:TLE750
1,2,4-TRIMETHYL-5-AMINOBENZENE see I:TLG250
1,2,4-TRIMETHYL-5-AMINOBENZENE HYDROCHLORIDE see III:TLG750
3,2',5'-TRIMETHYL-4-AMINODIPHENYL see III:TLF000
2,4,5-TRIMETHYLANILIN (CZECH) see I:TLG250
2,4,5-TRIMETHYLANILINE see I:TLG250
2,4,6-TRIMETHYLANILINE see III:TLG500
2,4,5-TRIMETHYLANILINE HYDROCHLORIDE see III:TLG750
2,4,6-TRIMETHYLANILINE HYDROCHLORIDE see II:TLH000
2,9,10-TRIMETHYLANTHRACENE see III:TLH100
3,5,9-TRIMETHYL-1:2-BENZACRIDINE see III:TLH350
3,8,12-TRIMETHYLBENZ(a)ACRIDINE see III:TLH500
5,6,9-TRIMETHYL-1:2-BENZACRIDINE see III:TLI000
5,7,11-TRIMETHYLBENZ(c)ACRIDINE see III:TLH350
5,7,8-TRIMETHYL-3:4-BENZACRIDINE see III:TLH750
7,8,11-TRIMETHYLBENZ(c)ACRIDINE see III:TLI000
7,9,10-TRIMETHYLBENZ(c)ACRIDINE see III:TLI250
7,9,11-TRIMETHYLBENZ(c)ACRIDINE see III:TLI500
8,10,12-TRIMETHYLBENZ(a)ACRIDINE see III:TLI750
1,3,10-TRIMETHYL-5,6-BENZACRIDINE (FRENCH) see III:TLI750
1,3,10-TRIMETHYL-7,8-BENZACRIDINE (FRENCH) see III:TLI500
1,4,10 TRIMETHYL-7:8 BENZACRIDINE (FRENCH) see III:TLI000
1,6,10-TRIMETHYL-7:8 BENZACRIDINE (FRENCH) see III:TLH350
2,3,10 TRIMETHYL-5:6 BENZACRIDINE (FRENCH) see III:TLH750
2,3,10-TRIMETHYL-7:8 BENZACRIDINE (FRENCH) see III:TLI250
1,10,3'-TRIMETHYL-5,6-BENZACRIDINE (FRENCH) see III:TLH500

TRIS(p-AMINOPHENYL)METHYLIUM SALT with 4,4'-METHYLENEBIS(3-HYDROXY-2-NAPHTHOIC ACID) (2:1) see III:TNC750

TRIS(1-AZIRIDINE)PHOSPHINE OXIDE see III:TND250

2,3,5-TRIS(AZIRIDINO)-1,4-BENZOQUINONE see III:TND000

2,3,5-TRIS(1-AZIRIDINO)-p-BENZOQUINONE see III:TND000

TRIS(AZIRIDINYL)-p-BENZOQUINONE see III:TND000

TRIS(1-AZIRIDINYL)-p-BENZOQUINONE see III:TND000

2,3,5-TRIS(AZIRIDINYL)-1,4-BENZOQUINONE see III:TND000

2,3,5-TRIS(1-AZIRIDINYL)-p-BENZOQUINONE see III:TND000

2,3,5-TRIS(1-AZIRIDINYL)-2,5-CYLOHEXADIENE-1,4-DIONE see III:TND000

TRIS-(1-AZIRIDINYL)PHOSPHINE OXIDE see III:TND250

TRIS(1-AZIRIDINYL)PHOSPHINE SULFIDE see I:TFQ750

TRISAZIRIDINYLTRIAZINE see III:TND500

2,4,6-TRIS(1-AZIRIDINYL)-s-TRIAZINE see III:TND500

2,4,6-TRIS(1'-AZIRIDINYL)-1,3,5-TRIAZINE see III:TND500

TRIS(2-CHLOROETHYL)AMINE see III:TNF250

TRIS(β-CHLOROETHYL)AMINE see III:TNF250

TRIS(2-CHLOROETHYL)AMINE HYDROCHLORIDE see III:TNF500

TRIS(β-CHLOROETHYL)AMINE HYDROCHLORIDE see III:TNF500

TRIS(2-CHLOROETHYL)AMINE MONOHYDROCHLORIDE see III:TNF500

TRIS(2-CHLOROETHYL)AMMONIUM CHLORIDE see III:TNF500

TRIS-1,2,3-(CHLOROMETHOXY)PROPANE see GGI000

TRIS(1-CHLOROMETHYL-2-CHLOROETHYL)PHOSPHATE see III:FQU875

TRIS(DIBROMOPROPYL)PHOSPHATE see I:TNC500

TRIS(2,3-DIBROMOPROPYL) PHOSPHATE see I:TNC500

TRIS(2,3-DIBROMOPROPYL) PHOSPHORIC ACID ESTER see I:TNC500

TRIS-2,3-DIBROMPROPYL ESTER KYSELINY FOSFORECNE (CZECH) see I:TNC500

TRIS(1,3-DICHLOROISOPROPYL)PHOSPHATE see III:FQU875

TRIS-(1,3-DICHLORO-2-PROPYL)-PHOSPHATE see III:FQU875

TRIS(DIMETHYLAMINO)PHOSPHINE OXIDE see I:HEK000

TRIS(DIMETHYLAMINO)PHOSPHORUS OXIDE see I:HEK000

2,4,6-TRIS(DIMETHYLAMINO)-s-TRIAZINE see III:HEJ500

2,4,6-TRIS(DIMETHYLAMINO)-1,3,5-TRIAZINE see III:HEJ500

TRIS(DIMETHYLCARBAMODITHIOATO-S,S')IRON see III:FAS000

TRIS(DIMETHYLDITHIOCARBAMATO)BISMUTH see III:BKW000

TRIS)DIMETHYLDITHIOCARBAMATO)IRON see III:FAS000

TRIS(N,N-DIMETHYLDITHIOCARBAMATO) IRON(111) see III:FAS000

2,3,5-TRISETHYLENEIMINOBENZOQUINONE see III:TND000

TRISETHYLENEIMINOQUINONE see III:TND000

TRIS(ETHYLENEIMINO)TRIAZINE see III:TND500

TRISETHYLENEIMINO-1,3,5-TRIAZINE see III:TND500

2,4,6-TRIS(ETHYLENEIMINO)-s-TRIAZINE see III:TND500

TRIS(N-ETHYLENE)PHOSPHOROTRIAMIDATE see III:TND250

2,3,5-TRIS(ETHYLENIMINO)BENZOQUINONE see III:TND000

2,3,5-TRIS(ETHYLENIMINO)-p-BENZOQUINONE see III:TND000

2,3,5-TRIS(ETHYLENIMINO)-1,4-BENZOQUINONE see III:TND000

TRIS(ETHYLENIMINO)THIOPHOSPHATE see I:TFQ750

2,4,6-TRIS(ETHYLENIMINO)-s-TRIAZINE see III:TND500

TRIS(2-ETHYLHEXYL)PHOSPHATE see III:TNI250

TRIS(2-HYDROXYETHYL)AMINE see III:TKP500

TRIS-N-LOST see III:TNF500

TRIS(p-METHOXYPHENYL)CHLOROETHYLENE see II:CLO750

TRIS(2-METHYL-1-AZIRIDINYL)PHOSPHINE OXIDE see III:TNK250

TRIS(2-METHYLAZIRIDIN-1-YL)PHOSPHINE OXIDE see III:TNK250

N,N',N''-TRIS(1-METHYLETHYLENE)PHOSPHORAMIDE see III:TNK250

TRIS(1-METHYLETHYLENE)PHOSPHORIC TRIAMIDE see III:TNK250

TRISODIUM ARSENATE, HEPTAHYDRATE see I:ARE000

TRISODIUM NITRILOTRIACETATE see III:SIP500

TRISODIUM NITRILOTRIACETATE MONOHYDRATE see II:NEI000

TRISODIUM NITRILOTRIACETIC ACID see III:SIP500

TRISODIUM SALT of 1-(4-SULFO-1-NAPHTHYLAZO)-2-NAPHTHOL-3,6-DISULFONIC ACID see III:FAG020

TRISODIUM TRIFLUORIDE see III:SHF500

TRISULFON VIOLET N see III:CMP000

TRITISAN see III:PAX000

TRITOFTOROL see III:EIR000

TRIVAZOL see I:MMN250

TRIZILIN see I:DFT800

TROCHIN see III:CLD000

TROCOSONE see I:ECU750

TROGAMID T see III:NOH000

TROJCHLOROETAN(1,1,2) (POLISH) see II:TIN000

TROLAMINE see III:TKP500

TROLITUL see III:SMQ500

TROLOVOL see III:MCR750

TRONAMANG see III:MAP750

TRONOX see III:TGG760

TROPAEOLIN 1 see III:FAG010

TROPAEOLIN D see III:DOU600

TROVIDUR see I:VNP000, III:PKQ059

TROVITHERN HTL see III:PKQ059

TROYSAN ANTI-MILDEW O see III:TIT250

TRP-P-1 see II:TNX275

TRP-P-2 see II:ALD500

TRP-P-1 (ACETATE) see II:AJR500

TRP-P-2(ACETATE) see III:ALE750

TRUFLEX DOA see III:AEO000

TRUFLEX DOP see I:DVL700

TRYPAFLAVINE see III:DBX400

TRYPANBLAU (GERMAN) see II:CMO250

TRYPAN BLUE see II:CMO250

TRYPAN BLUE SODIUM SALT see II:CMO250

(−)-TRYPTOPHAN see III:TNX000

dl-TRYPTOPHAN see III:TNW500

l-TRYPTOPHAN (FCC) see III:TNX000

l-TRYPTOPHAN, pyrolyzate see III:TNW950

dl-TRYPTOPHAN, pyrolyzate 1 see II:TNX275

TRYPTOPHANE see III:TNX000

l-TRYPTOPHANE see III:TNX000

TRYPTOPHAN P1 see II:TNX275

TRYPTOPHAN P2 see II:ALD500

TS 160 see III:TNF250, III:TNF500

TSC see III:TFQ000

TSIM see III:TMF250

TSIMAT see III:BJK500

TSINEB (RUSSIAN) see III:EIR000

TSIRAM (RUSSIAN) see III:BJK500

TSITREX see III:DXX400

TSIZP 34 see I:ISR000

TSPA see I:TFQ750

T-STUFF see III:HIB000

TTD see III:DXH250, III:TFS350

T (²)-TRICHOTHECENE see III:FQS000

TTS see III:DXH250

TTT see III:HDV500

TU see III:TFR250

2-TU see III:TFR250
TUADS see III:TFS350
TUBATOXIN see III:RNZ000
TUBAZID see III:ILD000
TUBAZIDE see III:ILD000
TUBECO see III:ILD000
TUBERCID see III:ILD000
TUBERIAN see III:ILD000
TUBERIT see III:CBM000
TUBERITE see III:CBM000
TUBERMIN see III:EPQ000
TUBEROID see III:EPQ000
TUBEROSON see III:EPQ000
TUBICON see III:ILD000
TUBOCIN see II:RKP000
TUBOMEL see III:ILD000
TUBOTIN see III:ABX250
TUEX see III:TFS350
TUFF-LITE see III:PMP500
TUGON see III:TIQ250
TUGON FLY BAIT see III:TIQ250
TUGON STABLE SPRAY see III:TIQ250
TULABASE FAST GARNET GB see I:AIC250
TULABASE FAST GARNET GBC see I:AIC250
TULABASE FAST RED TR see II:CLK220
TULISAN see III:TFS350
TULUYLENDIISOCYANAT see I:TGM750
TUMESCAL OPE see III:BGJ250
TUMEX see III:QPA000
TUR see III:CMF400
TURGEX see III:HCL000
TURPENTINE see III:TOD750
TURPENTINE OIL, RECTIFIER see III:TOD750
TURPENTINE STEAM DISTILLED see III:TOD750
TUSSAPAP see II:HIM000
TUSSILAGO FARFARA L see III:CNH250
TWEEN 60 see III:PKL030
TWEEN 80 see III:PKL100
TYGON see II:AAX175
TYLENOL see II:HIM000
TYLOSE 666 see III:SFO500
TYLOSTERONE see I:DKA600
TYPOGEN CARMINE see III:EOJ500
TYRAMINE, 3-DIAZO-, HYDROCHLORIDE see III:DCQ575
TYRION YELLOW see III:DCZ000
TYVID see III:ILD000

U 46 see II:CIR500, II:DAA800, II:DGB000, II:TAA100
U-1434 see II:EEI000
U-2069 see III:RDP300
U-3886 see III:SFA000
U-4748 see III:POK000
U-5043 see II:DAA800
U-5227 see III:AQN635
U-5897 see III:CDT750
U 6020 see III:PLZ000
U-6062 see II:CDP250
U-6233 see III:BDH250
U-6421 see II:NGE500
U-8344 see II:BIA250
U-8953 see III:FMM000
U-9889 see I:SMD000
U 10997 see III:MQS225
U 15030 see III:DKC400
U 18496 see III:ARY000
U 1 (polymer) see III:PKQ059
UBATOL U 2001 see III:SMQ500
UCAR BUTYLPHENOL 4-T see III:BSE500
UCET TEXTILE FINISH 11-74 (OBS.) see I:VOA000
U-COMPOUND see I:UVA000
UCON 22/HALOCARBON 22 see III:CFX500
UDMH (DOT) see I:DSF400
UDOLAC see III:SOA500
U 46DP see II:DAA800

U46 DP-FLUID see II:DGB000
U 46 M-FLUID see II:CIR250
U 46 KV-ESTER see II:CIR500
U 46 KV-FLUID see II:CIR500
ULCEDINE see III:TAB250
ULCERFEN see III:TEH500
ULCIMET see III:TAB250
ULCOLIND see III:CLY500
ULCOMET see III:TAB250
ULIOLIND see III:CLY500
ULMENIDE see III:CDL325
ULSTRON see III:PMP500
ULTRA BRILLIANT BLUE P see III:DSY600
ULTRACORTEN see III:PLZ000
ULTRAMARINE GREEN see II:CMJ900
ULTRAMARINE YELLOW see I.BAK250
ULTRAMID BMK see III:PJY500
ULTRON see III:PKQ059
ULUP see III:FMM000
UMBRATHOR see I:TFT750
UMBRIUM see III:DCK759
UNADS see III:BJL600
1,2,3,4,5,5,6,7,9,10,10-UNDECACHLOROPENTACYCLO
    (5.3.O.O^{2,6}.0^{3,9}.0^{4,8})DECANE see III:MRI750
1-UNDECANECARBOXYLIC ACID see III:LBL000
UNDEN see I:EDV000
UNFINISHED LUBRICATING OIL see I:COD750
UNIBARYT see III:BAP000
UNICEL-ND see III:DVF400
UNICEL NDX see III:DVF400
UNICHEM see III:PKQ059
UNICOCYDE see III:ILD000
UNICROP CIPC see III:CKC000
UNICROP DNBP see III:BRE500
UNICROP MANEB see III:MAS500
UNIDOCAN see III:DAQ800
UNIDRON see III:DXQ500
UNIFUME see I:EIY500
UNIMOLL BB see III:BEC500
UNIMYCETIN see III:CDP250
UNION BLACK EM see AQP000
UNIROYAL see III:DFT000
UNISEDIL see III:DCK759
UNISOL RH see III:SFO500
UNISTRADIOL see I:EDP000
UNISULF see III:SNN500
UNITANE O-110 see III:TGG760
UNITERTRACID LIGHT ORANGE G see III:HGC000
UNITESTON see I:TBG000
UNIVERM see CBY000
UNLEADED GASOLINE see GCE100
UNLEADED MOTOR GASOLINE see GCE100
UNON P see III:TAI250
UNOX 201 see III:ECB000
UNOXAT EPOXIDE 269 see III:LFV000
UNOX EPOXIDE 201 see III:ECB000
UNOX EPOXIDE 206 see I:VOA000
UP 1E see III:SMR000
URACIL see III:UNJ800
URACILLOST see II:BIA250
URACILMOSTAZA see II:BIA250
URACIL MUSTARD see II:BIA250
URACTONE see III:AFJ500
URAMUSTIN see II:BIA250
URAMUSTINE see II:BIA250
URANIN see III:FEW000
URANIN A EXTRA see III:FEW000
URANINE USP XII see III:FEW000
URANINE YELLOW see III:FEW000
URAZIUM see I:PDC250
UREA see III:USS000
UREA, N-(4-BROMOPHENYL)-N'-METHYL-(9CI) see
    III:MHS375
UREA, N-(2-METHOXYETHYL)-N-NITROSO- see
    III:NKO900

UREAPHIL see III:USS000
p-UREIDOBENZENEARSONIC ACID see III:CBJ000
4-UREIDO-1-PHENYLARSONIC ACID see III:CBJ000
UREOPHIL see III:USS000
URETAN ETYLOWY (POLISH) see I:UVA000
URETHAN see I:UVA000
URETHANE see I:UVA000
URETHYLANE see III:MHZ000
UREVERT see III:USS000
URIDINAL see I:PDC250, III:PEK250
URINARY INDICAN see III:ICD000
URIPLEX see I:PDC250
URISOXIN see III:SNN500
URITONE see III:HEI500
URITRISIN see III:SNN500
URIZEPT see III:NGE000
URNER'S LIQUID see III:DEL000
UROBIOTIC-250 see I:PDC250
URODINE see I:PDC250, III:PEK250
UROFEEN see I:PDC250
UROGAN see III:SNN500
UROMIDE see I:PDC250
UROPHENYL see I:PDC250
UROPYRIDIN see I:PDC250
UROPYRINE see I:PDC250
UROTROPIN see III:HEI500
UROTROPINE see III:HEI500
URSOFERRAN see I:IGS000
URSOL BROWN RR see II:ALL750
URSOL D see III:PEY500
URSOL OLIVE 6G see I:CFK125
URSOL SLA see I:DBO400
URSOL YELLOW BROWN A see III:ALO000
USACERT BLUE No. 1 see III:FAE000
USACERT BLUE No.2 see III:FAE100
USACERT FD & C RED No. 4 see III:FAG050
USACERT RED No. 1 see II:FAG018
USACERT RED No. 3 see III:FAG040
USAF B-22 see III:TFD250
USAF B-30 see III:TFS350
USAF B-32 see III:BJL600
USAF B-33 see III:BDE750, III:DXH250
USAF B-44 see III:BLJ250
USAF CB-2 see III:ILD000
USAF CB-17 see III:XCA000
USAF CB-21 see I:TFA000
USAF CB-22 see I:NBE500
USAF CB-27 see II:RDK000
USAF CB-30 see III:THR750
USAF CF-5 see III:RSU000
USAF CY-2 see III:CAQ250
USAF CY-5 see III:BDE750
USAF CY-7 see III:BDG000
USAF CY-10 see III:NBA500
USAF D-1 see III:IDW000
USAF D-9 see III:CBM000
USAF DO-36 see II:DVF200
USAF DO-41 see I:TNC500
USAF EA-1 see III:NGG500
USAF EA-2 see III:NGE000
USAF EA-4 see II:NGE500
USAF EK-206 see III:PEY750
USAF EK-218 see III:QMJ000
USAF EK-338 see I:DOT300
USAF EK-356 see III:HIH000
USAF EK-394 see III:PEY500
USAF EK-442 see II:BBL000
USAF EK-497 see I:ISR000
USAF EK-600 see III:CBN000
USAF EK-678 see III:PEY600
USAF EK-704 see III:ASL250
USAF EK-794 see III:QPA000
USAF EK-1275 see III:TFQ000
USAF EK-1375 see II:PEI000

USAF EK-1509 see III:TGO750
USAF EK-1719 see I:TFA000
USAF EK-1803 see III:DKC400
USAF EK-2089 see III:TFS350
USAF EK-2219 see III:BGJ250
USAF EK-2596 see III:SGJ000
USAF EK-5185 see III:MMD500
USAF EK-5432 see III:BDE750
USAF EK-6454 see II:MPW500
USAF EK-6561 see III:ALQ000
USAF EK-P-5976 see III:AQN635
USAF EK-P-6255 see III:BJL600
USAF EK-P-6281 see III:BLJ250
USAF EL-30 see III:MCO500
USAF EL-62 see I:IAQ000
USAF EL-101 see III:BQP250
USAF FO-1 see III:BQP250
USAF GE-14 see III:HNI500
USAF GE-15 see II:BRF500
USAF GY-2 see III:BLE500
USAF GY-3 see II:BDF000
USAF GY-5 see III:BIX000
USAF GY-7 see III:BHA750
USAF H-1 see III:QSA000
USAF KF-5 see III:CDN500
USAF KF-13 see III:DVX200
USAF ND-09 see III:PHY000
USAF ND-59 see III:DMH400
USAF P-2 see III:BJK500
USAF P-5 see III:TFS350
USAF P-7 see III:DXQ500
USAF P-8 see III:CJX750
USAF P-220 see III:QQS200
USAF SC-2 see GKE000
USAF SN-9 see III:TEX250
USAF WI-1 see III:MRN000
USAF XR-22 see I:AMY050
USAF XR-29 see II:BDF000
USAF XR-41 see III:CJX750
USAF XR-42 see III:DXQ500
U.S. BLENDED LIGHT TOBACCO CIGARETTE REFINED TAR
   see II:CMP800
USEMPAX AP see III:DCK759
USP XIII STEARYL ALCOHOL see III:OAX000
USR 604 see III:DFT000
U.S. RUBBER 604 see III:DFT000
USTINEX see II:CIR250
UTOSTAN see I:PDC250
UV CHEK AM 104 see III:BIW750
UZONE see II:BRF500

VABEN see III:CFZ000
VABROCID see II:NGE500
VAC see III:VLU250
VAC-10 see II:BRF500
VACATE see II:CIR250
VACUUM RESIDUUM see I:MQV755
VADROCID see II:NGE500
VAGD see II:AAX175
VAGESTROL see I:DKA600
VAGILEN see I:MMN250
VAGILIA see III:SNN500
VAGIMID see I:MMN250
VALADOL see II:HIM000
VALEO see III:DCK759
VALERAMIDE, 2-(2-ACETAMIDO-4-METHYLVALER-
   AMIDO)-N-(1-FORMYL-4-GUANIDINOBUTYL)-4-
   METHYL-(S)- see III:AAL300
Δ-VALEROSULTONE see II:BOU250
VALFLON see III:TAI250
VALFOR see III:AHF500
VALGESIC see II:HIM000
VALGIS see III:TEH500
VALGRAINE see III:TEH500

VALIOIL see III:HNI500
VALITRAN see III:DCK759
VALIUM see III:DCK759
VALONEA TANNIN see III:VCK000
VALZIN see III:EFE000
VANADIUM see III:VCP000
VANCIDA TM-95 see III:TFS350
VANCIDE see III:MAS500, III:VEZ925
VANCIDE 89 see III:CBG000
VANCIDE BL see III:TFD250
VANCIDE FE95 see III:FAS000
VANCIDE MZ-96 see III:BJK500
VANCIDE PB see III:DVI600
VANCIDE TM see III:TFS350
VANDEX see III:SBO500
VANGARD K see III:CBG000
VANGUARD GF see III:FAZ000
VANGUARD N see III:BIW750
VANICID see III:VEZ925
VANICIDE see III:CBG000
VANILLABERON see III:VEZ925
VANIZIDE see III:VEZ925
VANLUBE PCX see III:BFW750
VANOXIDE see III:BDS000
VANSIL W 10 see III:WCJ000
VANSIL W 20 see III:WCJ000
VANSIL W 30 see III:WCJ000
VAPOPHOS see III:PAK000
VARIOFORM II see III:USS000
VARITOX see III:TII250
VAT GOLDEN YELLOW see III:DCZ000
VATRAN see III:DCK759
VAZADRINE see III:ILD000
VC see I:VNP000
VCM see I:VNP000
VCR see III:LEY000
VCR SULFATE see III:LEZ000
VDC see II:VPK000
VDF see II:VPP000
VECTAL see III:ARQ725
VECTAL SC see III:ARQ725
VEDERON see III:ILD000
VEDRIL see III:PKB500
VEGABEN see III:AJM000
VEGADEX see CDO250
VEGADEX SUPER see CDO250
VEGFRU MALATOX see III:MAK700
VELBAN see III:VLA000
VELBE see III:VLA000
VELDOPA see III:DNA200
VELFLON see III:TAI250
VELIUM see III:DCK759
VELSICOL 104 see II:HAR000
VELSICOL 1068 see II:CDR750
VELSICOL 53-CS-17 see II:EBW500
VENDACID LIGHT ORANGE 2G see III:HGC000
VENETIAN RED see III:IHD000
VENTOX see I:ADX500
VENTUROL see III:DXX400
VEON 245 see II:TAA100
VERATRYL CHLORID (GERMAN) see III:BKM750
VERATRYL CHLORIDE see III:BKM750
VERAZINC see III:ZNA000
VERDONE see II:CIR250
VERGEMASTER see II:DAA800
VERMICIDE BAYER 2349 see III:TIQ250
VERMOESTRICID see CBY000
VERON P 130/1 see III:PKQ059
VEROSPIRON see III:AFJ500
VEROSPIRONE see III:AFJ500
VERSAR DSMA LQ see I:DXE600
VERSENE NTA ACID see I:AMT500
VERSOMNAL see II:EOK000
VERSTRAN see III:DAP700

VERTAC see II:BQI000
VERTAC 90% see I:CDV100
VERTAC DINITRO WEED KILLER see III:BRE500
VERTAC GENERAL WEED KILLER see III:BRE500
VERTAC METHYL PARATHION TECHNISCH 80% see
    III:MNH000
VERTAC SELECTIVE WEED KILLER see III:BRE500
VERTAC TOXAPHENE 90 see I:CDV100
VERTISAL see I:MMN250
VERTOLAN see III:SNJ000
VERTON 2T see II:TAA100
VERTON D see II:DAA800
VESAKONTUHO MCPA see II:CIR250
VESALIUM see III:CLY500
VESTIN see I:PDC250
VESTINOL AH see I:DVL700
VESTINOL OA see III:AEO000
VESTOLIT B 7021 see III:PKQ059
VESTROL see II:TIO750
VESTYRON see III:SMQ500
VESTYRON HI see III:SMR000
VETAFLAVIN see III:DBX400
VETERINARY NITROFURAZONE see II:NGE500
VETICILLIN see III:BFD250
VETICOL see II:CDP250
VETIOL see III:MAK700
VFR 3801 see III:PKF750
VI-CAD see I:CAE250
VICTORIA BLUE R see III:VKA600
VICTORIA BLUE RS see III:VKA600
VICTORIA LAKE BLUE R see III:VKA600
VICTORIA RUBINE O see III:FAG020
VICTORIA SCARLET 3R see III:FMU080
VIDDEN D see I:DGG950
VIDLON see III:PJY500
VIDON 638 see II:DAA800
VILLIAUMITE see III:SHF500
VINBLASTIN see III:VKZ000
VINBLASTINE see III:VKZ000
VINBLASTINE SULFATE see III:VLA000
VINCALEUCOBLASTIN see III:VKZ000
VINCALEUKOBLASTINE see III:VKZ000
VINCALEUKOBLASTINE SULFATE see III:VLA000
VINCALEUKOBLASTINE SULFATE (1:1) (SALT) see
    III:VLA000
VINCAMIN COMPOSITUM see III:ARQ750
VINCOBLASTINE see III:VKZ000
VINCRISTINE see III:LEY000
VINCRISTINE SULFATE ONCORIN see III:LEZ000
VINCRISTINSULFAT (GERMAN) see III:LEZ000
VINCRISUL see III:LEZ000
VINCRYSTINE see III:LEY000
VINICIZER 80 see I:DVL700
VINIKA KR 600 see III:PKQ059
VINIKULON see III:PKQ059
VINILE (ACETATO di) (ITALIAN) see III:VLU250
VINILE (BROMURO di) (ITALIAN) see I:VMP000
VINILE (CLORURO di) (ITALIAN) see I:VNP000
VINIPLAST see III:PKQ059
VINIPLEN P 73 see III:PKQ059
VINISIL see III:PKQ250
VINKRISTIN see III:LEY000
4-VINLYCYCLOHEXENE DIOXIDE see I:VOA000
VINNOL E 75 see III:PKQ059
VINNOL H 10/60 see II:AAX175
VINOFLEX see III:PKQ059
VINTHIONINE see II:VLU200
VINYLACETAAT (DUTCH) see III:VLU250
VINYLACETAT (GERMAN) see III:VLU250
VINYL ACETATE see III:VLU250
VINYL ACETATE-VINYL CHLORIDE COPOLYMER see
    II:AAX175
VINYL ACETATE-VINYL CHLORIDE POLYMER see
    II:AAX175

VINYL ALCOHOL POLYMER see III:PKP750
VINYL A MONOMER see III:VLU250
7-VINYLBENZ(a)ANTHRACENE see III:VMF000
VINYLBENZEN (CZECH) see II:SMQ000
VINYLBENZENE see II:SMQ000
VINYLBENZENE POLYMER see III:SMQ500
VINYLBENZOL see II:SMQ000
VINYLBROMID (GERMAN) see I:VMP000
VINYL BROMIDE see I:VMP000
VINYL BROMIDE, inhibited (DOT) see I:VMP000
VINYLBUTYROLACTAM see III:EEG000
N-VINYLBUTYROLACTAM POLYMER see III:PKQ250
VINYL CARBAMATE see III:VNK000
VINYLCHLON 4000LL see III:PKQ059
VINYLCHLORID (GERMAN) see I:VNP000
VINYL CHLORIDE see I:VNP000
VINYL CHLORIDE ACETATE COPOLYMER see III:PKP500
VINYL CHLORIDE HOMOPOLYMER see III:PKQ059
VINYL CHLORIDE MONOMER see I:VNP000
VINYL CHLORIDE POLYMER see III:PKQ059
VINYL CHLORIDE VINYL ACETATE COPOLYMER see III:PKP500
VINYL CHLORIDE-VINYL ACETATE POLYMER see II:AAX175
VINYL C MONOMER see I:VNP000
VINYL CYANIDE see I:ADX500
1-VINYLCYCLOHEXENE-3 see III:CPD750
1-VINYLCYCLOHEX-3-ENE see III:CPD750
4-VINYLCYCLOHEXENE-1 see III:CPD750
4-VINYL-1-CYCLOHEXENE see III:CPD750
VINYL CYCLOHEXENE DIEPOXIDE see I:VOA000
4-VINYLCYCLOHEXENE DIEPOXIDE see I:VOA000
4-VINYL-1-CYCLOHEXENE DIEPOXIDE see I:VOA000
4-VINYL-1,2-CYCLOHEXENE DIEPOXIDE see I:VOA000
VINYL CYCLOHEXENE DIOXIDE see I:VOA000
1-VINYL-3-CYCLOHEXENE DIOXIDE see I:VOA000
4-VINYL-1-CYCLOHEXENE DIOXIDE (MAK) see I:VOA000
VINYLE (ACETATE de) (FRENCH) see III:VLU250
VINYLE (BROMURE de) (FRENCH) see I:VMP000
VINYLE(CHLORURE de) (FRENCH) see I:VNP000
VINYLENE CARBONATE see III:VOK000
4,4'-VINYLENEDIANILINE see III:SLR500
VINYLETHYLENE see I:BOP500
VINYLETHYLNITROSAMIN (GERMAN) see III:NKF000
VINYLETHYLNITROSAMINE see III:NKF000
VINYLFORMIC ACID see III:ADS750
S-VINYL-dl-HOMOCYSTEINE see II:VLU200
VINYLIDENE CHLORIDE see II:VPK000
VINYLIDENE CHLORIDE (II) see II:VPK000
VINYLIDENE DICHLORIDE see II:VPK000
VINYLIDENE FLUORIDE see II:VPP000
VINYLIDINE CHLORIDE see II:VPK000
VINYLITE VYDR 21 see II:AAX175
α-VINYLPIPERONYL ALCOHOL see II:BCJ000
VINYL PRODUCTS R 3612 see III:SMQ500
1-VINYLPYRENE see III:EEF000
3-VINYLPYRENE see III:EEF000
4-VINYLPYRENE see III:EEF500
N-VINYLPYRROLIDINONE see III:EEG000
1-VINYL-2-PYRROLIDINONE see III:EEG000
N-VINYL-2-PYRROLIDINONE see III:EEG000
VINYLPYRROLIDONE see III:EEG000
N-VINYLPYRROLIDONE see III:EEG000
1-VINYL-2-PYRROLIDONE see III:EEG000
N-VINYL-2-PYRROLIDONE see III:EEG000
N-VINYLPYRROLIDONE POLYMER see III:PKQ250
VINYL TRICHLORIDE see II:TIN000
VINYON N see III:ADY250
VIOFURAGYN see III:NGG500
VIOLAQUERCITRIN see III:RSU000
VI-PAR see II:CIR500
VI-PEX see II:CIR500
VIRORMONE see I:TBF500
VIROSTERONE see I:TBF500

VISCARIN see III:CCL250
VISCOL 350P see III:PMP500
VISKING CELLOPHANE see III:CCT250
VISKO-RHAP see II:DGB000
VISKO-RHAP DRIFT HERBICIDES see II:DAA800
VISKO RHAP LOW VOLATILE ESTER see II:TAA100
VISUBUTINA see III:HNI500
VITALLIUM see I:CNA750, III:VSK000
VITAMIN A ACETATE see III:VSK900
trans-VITAMIN A ACETATE see III:VSK900
VITAMIN A ACID see III:VSK950
VITAMIN A ALCOHOL ACETATE see III:VSK900
VITAMIN B12, METHYL see III:VSZ050
VITAMIN K2(O) see III:MMD500
VITAMIN K3 see III:MMD500
VITAMIN L see III:API500
VITAMIN P see III:RSU000
VITAPLEX N see III:NCQ900
VITESTROL see III:DLB400
VITON see I:BBQ500
VITRAN see II:TIO750
VITREOUS QUARTZ see I:SCK600
VITREX see III:PAK000
VITRIOL RED see III:IHD000
VITUF see III:PKF750
VIVAL see III:DCK759
VIVOL see III:DCK759
VLB see III:VKZ000
VLB MONOSULFATE see III:VLA000
VLVF see II:AAX175
VMCC see II:AAX175
VOFATOX see III:MNH000
VOGEL'S IRON RED see III:IHD000
VOLATILE OIL of MUSTARD see II:AGJ250
VOLCLAY see III:BAV750
VOLCLAY BENTONITE BC see III:BAV750
VOLDYS see III:MCA500
VOLFARTOL see III:TIQ250
VOLIDAN see II:VTF000, III:MCA500
VOLTALEF 10 see III:KDK000
VOLUNTAL see III:TIO500
VONDACEL BLACK N see AQP000
VONDACEL BLUE 2B see I:CMO000
VONDACID FAST YELLOW AE see III:SGP500
VONDCAPTAN see III:CBG000
VONDODINE see III:DXX400
VONDURON see III:DXQ500
VOPCOLENE 27 see III:OHU000
VOROX see I:AMY050
VOTEXIT see III:TIQ250
VP 1940 see III:ABX250
V-PYROL see III:EEG000
VUAGT-I-4 see III:TFS350
VULCACEL B-40 see III:DVF400
VULCACEL BN see III:DVF400
VULCACURE see III:BIX000, III:BJC000, III:BJK500
VULCAFIX SCARLET R see III:CHP500
VULCAFOR BSM see III:BDG000
VULCAFOR TMTD see III:TFS350
VULCALENT A see III:DWI000
VULCAN RED LC see III:CHP500
VULCATARD see III:DWI000
VULCOL FAST RED L see III:CHP500
VULKACIT DM see III:BDE750
VULKACIT DM/MGC see III:BDE750
VULKACITE L see III:BJK500
VULKACIT LDA see III:BJC000
VULKACIT LDB/C see III:BIX000
VULKACIT MTIC see III:TFS350
VULKACIT NPV/C2 see I:IAQ000
VULKACIT THIURAM see III:TFS350
VULKACIT THIURAM/C see III:TFS350
VULKACIT THIURAM MS/C see III:BJL600
VULKACIT ZM see III:BHA750

VULKALENT A (CZECH) see III:DWI000
VULKANOX 4020 see III:PEY500
VULKANOX PAN see III:PFT250
VULKASIL see III:SCH000
VULKLOR see III:TBO500
VULTROL see III:DWI000
VULVAN see I:TBG000
VYAC see III:VLU250
VYDYNE see III:NOH000
VYGEN 85 see III:PKQ059
VYNAMON ORANGE CR see I:LCS000
VYNW see II:AAX175

W 101 see III:PMP500
W 1655 see I:PDC250, III:PEK250
W 6658 see III:BJP000
W 7618 see III:CLD000
WALNUT EXTRACT see III:WAT000
WAMPOCAP see III:NCQ900
WARECURE C see I:IAQ000
WASH OIL see I:CMY825
WASSERSTOFFPEROXID (GERMAN) see III:HIB000
WATAPANA SHIMARON see III:AAD750
WATER QUENCH PYROLYSIS FUEL OIL see III:FOP100
WATERSTOFPEROXYDE (DUTCH) see III:HIB000
WAXAKOL ORANGE GL see III:PEJ500
WAXAKOL VERMILION L see III:XRA000
WAXAKOL YELLOW NL see I:AIC250
WAX MYRTLE see III:WBA000
WAXOLINE ORANGE A see III:BJF000
WAXOLINE YELLOW AD see I:DOT300
WAXOLINE YELLOW I see III:PEJ500
WAXOLINE YELLOW O see I:IBB000
WAYNE RED X-2486 see III:CHP500
WEATHERBEE MUSTARD see III:BHB750
WEC 50 see III:TIQ250
WECOLINE 1295 see III:LBL000
WECOLINE OO see III:OHU000
WEED-AG-BAR see II:DAA800
WEEDAR see I:TAA100
WEEDAR-64 see II:DAA800
WEEDAR ADS see I:AMY050
WEEDAR MCPA CONCENTRATE see II:CIR250
WEEDAZIN see I:AMY050
WEEDAZOL see I:AMY050
WEED-B-GON see II:DAA800, II:TIX500
WEED BROOM see I:DXE600
WEED-E-RAD see I:DXE600
WEEDEX A see III:ARQ725
WEEDEX GRANULAT see I:AMY050
WEEDEZ WONDER BAR see II:DAA800
WEED-HOE see I:DXE600
WEEDOCLOR see I:AMY050
WEEDONE see II:PAX250, II:TAA100
WEEDONE 128 see III:IOY000
WEEDONE 170 see II:DGB000
WEEDONE DP see II:DGB000
WEEDONE LV4 see II:DAA800
WEEDONE MCPA ESTER see II:CIR250
WEED-RHAP see II:CIR250
WEED TOX see II:DAA800
WEEDTRINE-II see III:ILO000
WEEDTROL see II:DAA800
WELFURIN see III:NGE000
WELVIC G 2/5 see III:PKQ059
WESCOZONE see II:BRF500
WESTRON see III:TBQ100
WESTROSOL see II:TIO750
WEX 1242 see III:PMP500
WHISKEY see III:WBS000
1700 WHITE see III:TGG760
WHITE ARSENIC see I:ARI750
WHITE ASBESTOS see I:ARM268
WHITE COPPERAS see III:ZNA000

WHITE LEAD see III:LCP000
WHITE MINERAL OIL see I:MQV875, III:MQV750
WHITE STREPTOCIDE see III:SNM500
WHITE TAR see III:NAJ500
WHITE VITRIOL see III:ZNA000
WHORTLEBERRY RED see III:FAG020
W-53 HYDROCHLORIDE see III:DPJ400
WICKENOL 158 see III:AEO000
WIDLON see III:PJY500
WILKINITE see III:BAV750
WILLESTROL see I:DKB000
WILLNESTROL see II:DAL600
WILLOSETTEN see II:SJN700
WILT PRUF see III:PKQ059
WIN 244 see III:CLD000
WIN 17757 see III:DAB830
WIN 24933 see III:LIM000
WIN 35833 see III:CMS210
WINE see III:WCA000
WIN 2848 HYDROCHLORIDE SALT see III:DPJ400
WINIDUR see III:PKQ059
WINOBANIN see III:DAB830
WINTER BLOOM see III:WCB000
WINYLU CHLOREK (POLISH) see I:VNP000
WITAMOL 320 see III:AEO000
WITCH HAZEL see III:WCB000
WITCIZER 312 see I:DVL700
WL 20 see III:NNL500
WL 33 see III:NNL500
WL 1650 see III:OAN000
WNYESTRON see I:EDV000
WOCHEM No. 320 see III:OHU000
WOFATOS see III:MNH000
WOFATOX see III:MNH000
WOFOTOX see III:MNH000
WOJTAB see III:PLZ000
WOLLASTOKUP see III:WCJ000
WOLLASTONITE see III:WCJ000
WONUK see III:ARQ725
WOOL BORDEAUX 6RK see III:FAG020
WOOL BRILLIANT GREEN SF see III:FAF000
WOOL GREEN S (BIOLOGICAL STAIN) see III:ADF000
WOOL ORANGE 2G see III:HGC000
WOOL RED see III:FAG020
WOOL VIOLET see II:FAG120
WORM-AGEN see III:HFV500
WORMWOOD PLANT see III:SAF000
WOTEXIT see III:TIQ250
WR 448 see III:SOA500
WR 2978 see III:TGD000
WS 102 see III:NDU500
WY-3467 see III:DCK759
WY-3498 see III:CFZ000
WY 3707 see III:NNQ500
WY-14,643 see II:CLW250
WY-E 104 see III:NNL500
WY-4355 mixed with MESTRANOL (20:1) see III:CHI750

X 119 see III:DTP000
X 149 see I:BOT250
X-340 see III:HAL000
XA 2 see II:CFA750
X-AB see III:PKQ059
X-ALL LIQUID see I:AMY050
XAN see III:XCA000
XANTHACRIDINUM see III:DBX400
XANTHAURINE see III:QCA000
XANTHIC OXIDE see III:XCA000
XANTHINE see III:XCA000
XANTHINE-3-N-OXIDE see III:HOP000
XANTHINE-7-N-OXIDE see III:HOP259
XANTHINE-x-N-OXIDE see III:HOP000
XANTHOTOXIN see I:XDJ000
XANTHURENIC ACID see III:DNC200

XANTHURENIC ACID-8-METHYL ETHER see III:HLT500
XARIL see I:ABG750
XB 2793 see III:DKM130
XENENE see III:BGE000
o-XENOL see III:BGJ250
XENYLAMIN (CZECH) see I:AJS100
XENYLAMINE see I:AJS100
XERAC see III:BDS000
XL 7 see III:TFD250
XP-470 see III:CJI000
XX 212 see III:DAD050
XYDURIL see III:ARQ750
XYLENE BLUE VS see III:ADE500
XYLENE BLUE VSG see III:FMU059
XYLENE FAST ORANGE G see III:HGC000
XYLENE FAST YELLOW ES see III:SGP500
m-XYLENOL see III:XKJ500
2,4-XYLENOL see III:XKJ500
2,5-XYLENOL see III:XKS000
2,6-XYLENOL see III:XLA000
3,4-XYLENOL see III:XLJ000
3,5-XYLENOL see III:XLS000
1,2,5-XYLENOL see III:XKS000
1,3,4-XYLENOL see III:XLJ000
1,3,5-XYLENOL see III:XLS000
m-XYLENOL (DOT) see III:XKJ500
p-XYLENOL (DOT) see III:XKS000
2,4-XYLIDENE (MAK) see II:XMS000
2,5-XYLIDINE see III:XNA000
m-4-XYLIDINE see II:XMS000
m-XYLIDINE (DOT) see II:XMS000
p-XYLIDINE (DOT) see III:XNA000
m-XYLIDINE HYDROCHLORIDE see III:XOJ000
p-XYLIDINE HYDROCHLORIDE see III:XOS000
2,4-XYLIDINE HYDROCHLORIDE see III:XOJ000
2,5-XYLIDINE HYDROCHLORIDE see III:XOS000
XYLIDINE PONCEAU see III:FMU070
1-XYLYLAZO-2-NAPHTHOL see III:FAG080, III:XRA000
1-(o-XYLYLAZO)-2-NAPHTHOL see III:XRA000
1-(2,4-XYLYLAZO)-2-NAPHTHOL see III:XRA000
1-(2,5-XYLYLAZO)-2-NAPHTHOL see III:FAG080
1-XYLYLAZO-2-NAPHTHOL-3,6-DISULFONIC ACID, DISO-
    DIUM SALT see III:FMU070
1-XYLYLAZO-2-NAPHTHOL-3,6-DISULPHONIC ACID, DISO-
    DIUM SALT see III:FMU070
1-(2,4-XYLYLAZO)-2-NAPHTHOL-3,6-DISULPHONIC ACID,
    DISODIUM SALT see III:FMU070
1-(2,4-XYLYLAZO)-2-NAPHTHOL-3,6-DISULPHONIC ACID,
    DISODIUM SALT see III:FMU070
XYMOSTANOL see III:DKW000

Y 2 see III:CBM000
Y 3 see III:CKC000
Y 195 see I:PKL750
Y 218 see I:PKM250
Y 221 see I:PKM500
Y-223 see I:PKN000
Y-238 see I:CDV625
Y 299 see III:PKO750
Y 302 see I:PKP000
YATROCIN see II:NGE500
YATROZIDE see III:ILE000
YELLOW see III:DCZ000
11824 YELLOW see III:FEW000
12417 YELLOW see III:FEW000
YELLOW AB see III:FAG130
YELLOW CROSS LIQUID see I:BIH250
YELLOW FERRIC OXIDE see III:IHD000
YELLOW G SOLUBLE in GREASE see I:DOT300
YELLOW LEAD OCHER see III:LDN000
YELLOW No. 2 see III:FAG130
YELLOW OB see III:FAG135
YELLOW OXIDE of IRON see III:IHD000
1903 YELLOW PINK see III:BNH500

YELLOW PYOCTANINE see I:IBB000
YELLOW ULTRAMARINE see I:CAP500
YELLOW Z see II:AAQ250
YERMONIL see III:EEH575
YOCLO see III:ARQ750
YODOMIN see III:TEH500
YOHIMBAN-16-CARBOXYLIC ACID DERIVATIVE of
    BENZ(G)INDOLO(2,3-A)QUINOLIZINE see II:RDK000
3-β,20-α-YOHIMBAN-16-β-CARBOXYLIC ACID, 18-β-HY-
    DROXY-10,17-α-DIMETHOXY-, METHYL ESTER, 3,4,5-
    TRIMETHOXYBENZOATE (ester) see III:MEK700
YOSHI 864 see III:YCJ000
YPERITE see I:BIH250
YTTERBIUM see III:YDA000
YTTRIUM CITRATE see III:YFA000
YTTRIUM(III) NITRATE (1:3) see III:YFJ000
YUGOVINYL see III:PKQ059

Z 75 see III:BJK500
Z-78 see III:EIR000
Z 4942 see II:IMH000
ZACTIRIN COMPOUND see I:ABG750
ZACTRAN see III:DOS000
ZADOLETTEN see II:EOK000
ZADONAL see II:EOK000
ZAFFRE see III:CND125
ZAGREB see I:BIE500
ZAHARINA see II:BCE500
ZAMI 1305 see III:BQF750
dl-ZAMI 1305 see III:BQF750
ZAMIA DEBILIS see III:ZAK000
ZANOSAR see I:SMD000
ZARDA (INDIA) see I:SED400
ZARLATE see III:BJK500
Z-C SPRAY see III:BJK500
ZEAPUR see III:BJP000
ZEARALENONE see III:ZAT000
(−)-ZEARALENONE see III:ZAT000
(s)-ZEARALENONE see III:ZAT000
(10s)-ZEARALENONE see III:ZAT000
trans-ZEARALENONE see III:ZAT000
ZEAZIN see III:ARQ725
ZEAZINE see III:ARQ725
ZEBENIDE see III:EIR000
ZEBTOX see III:EIR000
ZECTANE see III:DOS000
ZECTRAN see III:DOS000
ZEIDANE see I:DAD200
ZELAN see II:CIR250
ZELAZA TLENKI (POLISH) see II:IHF000
ZENADRID (VETERINARY) see III:PLZ000
ZENALOSYN see I:PAN100
ZENITE see III:BHA750
ZENITE SPECIAL see III:BHA750
ZENTRONAL see I:DKQ000
ZENTROPIL see I:DKQ000, I:DNU000
ZERDANE see I:DAD200
ZERLATE see III:BJK500
ZESET T see III:VLU250
ZESTE see I:ECU750
ZETAR see I:CMY800
ZETAX see III:BHA750
ZETIFEX ZN see I:TNC500
ZEXTRAN see III:DOS000
ZIDAN see III:EIR000
ZIMALLOY see I:CNA750
ZIMATE see III:BJK500, III:EIR000
ZIMATE METHYL see III:BJK500
ZINADON see III:ILD000
ZINC ARSENATE see I:ZDJ000
ZINC ARSENATE, BASIC see I:ZDJ000
ZINC ARSENATE, SOLID (DOT) see I:ZDJ000
ZINC-m-ARSENITE see I:ZDS000
ZINC ARSENITE, SOLID (DOT) see I:ZDS000

ZINC-2-BENZOTHIAZOLETHIOLATE see III:BHA750
ZINC BENZOTHIAZOLYL MERCAPTIDE see III:BHA750
ZINC BENZOTHIAZOL-2-YLTHIOLATE see III:BHA750
ZINC BENZOTHIAZYL-2-MERCAPTIDE see III:BHA750
ZINC BERYLLIUM SILICATE see I:BFV250
ZINC-BIBUTYLDITHIOCARBAMATE see III:BIX000
ZINC BIS(DIMETHYLDITHIOCARBAMATE) see
  III:BJK500
ZINC BIS(DIMETHYLDITHIOCARBAMOYL)DISULPHIDE see
  III:BJK500
ZINC BIS(DIMETHYLTHIOCARBAMOYL)DISULFIDE see
  III:BJK500
ZINC CHLORIDE see III:ZFA000
ZINC CHLORIDE, ANHYDROUS (DOT) see III:ZFA000
ZINC CHLORIDE, SOLID (DOT) see III:ZFA000
ZINC CHLORIDE, SOLUTION (DOT) see III:ZFA000
ZINC (CHLORURE de) (FRENCH) see III:ZFA000
ZINC CHROMATE see I:ZFJ100
ZINC CHROMATE HYDROXIDE see I:CMK500
ZINC CHROMATE(VI) HYDROXIDE see I:CMK500,
  I:ZFJ100
ZINC CHROMATE, POTASSIUM DICHROMATE and ZINC HY-
  DROXIDE (3:1:1) see I:ZFJ150
ZINC CHROMATE with ZINC HYDROXIDE and CHROMIUM
  OXIDE (9:1) see I:ZFJ120
ZINC CHROME see I:PLW500
ZINC CHROME YELLOW see I:ZFJ100
ZINC CHROMIUM OXIDE see I:ZFJ100
ZINC-DIBUTYLDITHIOCARBAMATE see III:BIX000
ZINC-N,N-DIBUTYLDITHIOCARBAMATE see III:BIX000
ZINC DICHLORIDE see III:ZFA000
ZINC DIETHYLDITHIOCARBAMATE see III:BJC000
ZINC-N,N-DIETHYLDITHIOCARBAMATE see III:BJC000
ZINC DIMETHYLDITHIOCARBAMATE see III:BJK500
ZINC N,N-DIMETHYLDITHIOCARBAMATE see III:BJK500
ZINC ETHYLENEBISDITHIOCARBAMATE see III:EIR000
ZINC ETHYLENE-1,2-BISDITHIOCARBAMATE see
  III:EIR000
ZINC-N-FLUOREN-2-YLACETOHYDROXAMATE see
  III:ZHJ000
ZINC HYDROXYCHROMATE see I:CMK500, I:ZFJ100
ZINC MANGANESE BERYLLIUM SILICATE see I:BFS750
ZINCMATE see III:BJK500
ZINC MERCAPTOBENZOTHIAZOLATE see III:BHA750
ZINC-2-MERCAPTOBENZOTHIAZOLE see III:BHA750
ZINC MERCAPTOBENZOTHIAZOLE SALT see III:BHA750
ZINC MERCURY CHROMATE COMPLEX see I:ZJA000
ZINC METAARSENITE see I:ZDS000
ZINC METHARSENITE see I:ZDS000
ZINC MURIATE, SOLUTION (DOT) see III:ZFA000
ZINCO (CLORURO di) (ITALIAN) see III:ZFA000
ZINC OLEATE (1:2) see III:ZJS000
ZINC POLYACRYLATE see III:ADW250
ZINC POLYCARBOXYLATE see III:ADW250
ZINC POTASSIUM CHROMATE see I:CMK400
ZINC SULFATE see III:ZNA000
ZINC SULPHATE see III:ZNA000
ZINC TETRAOXYCHROMATE 76A see I:ZFJ100
ZINC VITRIOL see III:ZNA000

ZINC YELLOW see I:CMK500, I:PLW500, I:ZFJ100,
  I:ZFJ120
ZINEB see III:EIR000
ZINK-(N,N'-AETHYLEN-BIS(DITHIOCARBAMAT)) (GER-
  MAN) see III:EIR000
ZINK-BIS(N,N-DIMETHYL-DITHIOCARBAMAAT) (DUTCH)
  see III:BJK500
ZINK-BIS(N,N-DIMETHYL-DITHIOCARBAMAT) (GERMAN)
  see III:BJK500
ZINKCARBAMATE see III:BJK500
ZINKCHLORID (GERMAN) see III:ZFA000
ZINKCHLORIDE (DUTCH) see III:ZFA000
ZINK-(N,N-DIMETHYL-DITHIOCARBAMAT) (GERMAN) see
  III:BJK500
ZINKOSITE see III:ZNA000
ZINN (GERMAN) see III:TGB250
ZINOSAN see III:EIR000
ZIPAN see III:DCK759
ZIRAM see III:BJK500
ZIRAM TECHNICAL see III:BJK500
ZIRAMVIS see III:BJK500
ZIRASAN see III:BJK500
ZIRBERK see III:BJK500
ZIRCONIUM CHLORIDE OXIDE OCTAHYDRATE see
  III:ZPS000
ZIRCONIUM OXYCHLORIDE see III:ZSJ000
ZIRCONIUM SODIUM LACTATE see III:ZTA000
ZIRCONYL CHLORIDE see III:ZSJ000
ZIRCONYL CHLORIDE OCTAHYDRATE see III:ZPS000
ZIREX 90 see III:BJK500
ZIRIDE see III:BJK500
ZIRTHANE see III:BJK500
ZITEX H 662-124 see III:TAI250
ZITHIOL see III:MAK700
ZITOX see III:BJK500
ZITRONEN OEL (GERMAN) see III:LEI000
ZLUT MASELNA (CZECH) see I:DOT300
ZMA see I:ZDS000
ZMBT see III:BHA750
ZnMB see III:BHA750
ZOBA BLACK D see III:PEY500
ZOBA BROWN RR see II:ALL750
ZOBA GKE see I:TGL750
ZOBA SLE see I:DBO400
ZOGEN DEVELOPER H see I:TGL750
ZOLAPHEN see II:BRF500
ZOLIDINUM see II:BRF500
ZONAZIDE see III:ILD000
ZOOFURIN see III:NGE000
ZOPAQUE see III:TGG760
ZORANE see II:BRF500
ZORIFLAVIN see III:DBX400
ZOTOX see I:ARB250
ZOTOX CRAB GRASS KILLER see I:ARB250
Z10-TR see III:CFZ000
ZWITSALAX see III:DMH400
ZYKLOPHOSPHAMID (GERMAN) see I:EAS500
ZYTEL 211 see III:PJY500
ZYTOX see III:MHR200

IV.   Reference List

AAATAP Annali dell'Accademia di Agricoltura di Torino Academia de Agricoltura, Via Andrea Doria 10, Turin, Italy) V.119- 1976/77-

AABIAV Annals of Applied Biology. (Biochemical Society, P.O. Box 32, Commerce Way, Whitehall Industrial Estate, Colchester CO2 8HP, Essex, England) V.1- 1914-

AAJRDX AJR, American Journal of Roentgenology. (Charles C. Thomas Publisher, 301-327 E. Lawrence Ave., Springfield, IL 62717) V.126- 1976-

AANLAW Atti della Accademia Nazionale dei Lincei, Rendiconti della Classe di Scienze Fisiche, Matematiche e Naturali. (Academia Nazionale dei Lincei, Ufficio Pubblicazioni, Via della Lungara, 10, I-00165 Rome, Italy) V.1- 1946-

ABCHA6 Agricultural and Biological Chemistry. (Maruzen Co. Ltd., P.O.Box 5050 Tokyo International, Tokyo 100-31, Japan) V.25- 1961-

ABMGAJ Acta Biologica et Medica Germanica. (Berlin, Ger. Dem. Rep.) V.1-41, 1958-82. For publisher information, see BBIADT

ACCBAT Acta Clinica Belgica. (Association des Societes Scientifiques Medicales Belges, rue des Champs-Elysees, 43, 1050 Brussels 5, Belgium) V.1- 1946-

ACGHD2 Annals of the American Conference of Governmental Industrial Hygienists. (American Conference of Governmental Industrial Hygienists, Inc., 6500 Glenway Ave., Bldg. D-5, Cincinnati, Ohio, 54211) V.1- 1981-

ACHAAH Acta Haematologica. (S. Karger AG, Arnold-Boecklin-St 25, CH-4000 Basel 11, Switzerland) V.1- 1948-

ACHCBO Acta Histochemica et Cytochemica. (Japan Society of Histochemistry and Cytochemistry, Dept. Anatomy, Faculty of Medicine, Kyoto University, Konoecho, Yoshida, Sakyo-ku, Kyoto, 606, Japan) V.1- 1968-

ACLRBL Annals of Clinical Research. (Finnish Medical Society, Duodecim Runeberginkatu 47A, SF-00260 Helsinki 26, Finland) V.1- 1969-

ACLSCP Annals of Clinical Laboratory Science. (1833 Delancey Pl., Philadelphia, PA 19103) V.1- 1971-

ACPADQ Acta Pathologica, Microbiologica et Immunologica Scandinavica, Section A: Pathology. (Munksgaard, 35 Noerre Soegade, DK-1370, Copenhagen K, Denmark) V.90- 1982-

ACRAAX Acta Radiologica. (Stockholm, Sweden) V.1-58, 1921-62. For publisher information, see ACRDA8

ACRSAJ Advances in Cancer Research. (Academic Press, 111 5th Ave., New York, NY 10003) V.1- 1953-

ACYTAN Acta Cytologica. (Williams & Wilkins Co., 428 E. Preston St., Baltimore, MD 21202) V.1- 1957-

ADIRDF Advances in Inflammation Research. (Raven Press, 1140 Avenue of the Americas, New York, N Y 10036) V.1- 1979-

ADMFAU Archiv fuer Dermatologische Forschung. (Secaucus, NJ) V.240-252, No.4, 1971-75. For publisher information, see ADREDL

ADRCAC Annali Italiani di Dermatologia Clinica e Sperimentale. (Clinica Dermosifilopatica Universita degli Studi, Policlinica Monteluce, 06100 Perugia, Italy) V.16- 1962-

ADREDL Archives of Dermatological Research. (Springer-Verlag New York, Inc., Service Center, 44 Hartz Way, Secaucus, NJ 07094) V.253- 1975-

ADVEA4 Acta Dermato-Venereologica. (Almqvist & Wiksell International, Box 62, S-101 20 Stockholm, Sweden) V.1- 1920-

ADVED7 Annales de Dermatologie et de Venereologie. (Masson Publishing USA Inc., 133 E. 58th St., New York, NY 10022) V.104- 1977-

ADWMAX Abhandlungen der Deutschen Akademie der Wissenschaften zu Berlin, Klasse fuer Medizin. (Akademie-Verlag GmbH, Leipziger Str. 3-4, DDR-108 Berlin, German Democratic Republic) 1950-

AEHLAU Archives of Environmental Health. (Heldreff Publications, 4000 Albemarle St., N.W., Washington, D.C. 20016) V.1- 1960-

AEMBAP Advances in Experimental Medicine and Biology. (Plenum Publishing Corp., 233 Spring St., New York, NY 10013) V.1- 1967-

AEMIDF Applied and Environmental Microbiology. (American Society for Microbiology, 1913 I St., N.W., Washington, DC 20006) V.31- 1976-

AETODY Advances in Modern Environmental Toxicology. (Senate Press, Inc., P.O. Box 252, Princeton Junction, NJ 08550) V.1- 1980-

AFCPDR Annual Symposium on Fundamental Cancer Research, Proceedings. (University of Texas System Cancer Center, M.D. Anderson Hospital and Tumor Institute, Houston, TX 77030) V.30- 1978-

AFPEAM Archives Francaises de Pediatrie. (Doin Editeurs 8, Place de l'Odeon, F-75006 Paris, France) V.1- 1942-

AGACBH Agents & Actions, A Swiss Journal of Pharmacology. (Birkhaeuser Verlag, P.O. Box 34, Elisabethenst 19, CH-4010, Basel, Switzerland) V.1 ˙ ᵕ ᵕ᷍ᵔ0-

AGGHAR Archiv fuer Gewerbepathologie und Gewerbehygiene. (Berlin, Germany) V.1-18, 1930-61. For publisher information, see IAEHDW

AGMGAK Acta Geneticae Medicae et Gemellologiae. (Cappelli Editore, Via Marsili 9, I-40124 Bologna, Italy) V.1- 1952-

AGTQAH Annales de Genetique. (Expansion Scientifique

Francaise, 5 rue Saint- Benoit, F-75278, Paris 06, France)
V.1- 1958-

AICCA6 Acta Unio Internationalis Contra Cancrum. (Louvain, Belgium) V.1-20, 1936-64. For publisher information, see IJCNAW

AIDZAC Aichi Ika Daigaku Igakkai Zasshi. Journal of the Aichi Medical Univ. Assoc. (Aichi Ika Daigaku, Yazako, Nagakute-machi, Aichi-gun, Aichi- Ken 480-11, Japan) V.1- 1973-

AIHAAP American Industrial Hygiene Association Journal. (AIHA, 475 Wolf Ledges Pkwy., Akron, OH 44311) V.19- 1958-

AIHAM* Annual Meeting of American Industrial Hygiene Association. For publisher information, see AIHAAP

AIMDAP Archives of Internal Medicine. (American Medical Association, 535 N. Dearborn St., Chicago, IL 60610) V.1- 1908-

AIMEAS Annals of Internal Medicine. (American College of Physicians, 4200 Pine St., Philadelphia, PA 19104) V.1- 1927-

AIPTAK Archives Internationales de Pharmacodynamie et de Therapie. (Editeurs, Institut Heymans de Pharmacologie, De Pintelaan 135, B-9000 Ghent, Belgium) V.4-1898-

AIPUAN Archivio Italiano di Patologia e Clinica dei Tumori. (Istituto di Farmacologia della Universita, Via Vanvitelli 32, 20129 Milan, Italy) V.1-15, 1957-72, Discontinued

AISSAW Annali dell'Istituto Superiore di Sanita. (Istituto Poligrafico dello Stato, Libreria dello Stato, Piazza Verdi, 10 Rome, Italy) V.1- 1965-

AJBSAM Australian Journal of Biological Sciences. (Commonwealth Scientific and Industrial Research Organization, POB 89, E. Melbourne, Vic 3002, Australia) V.6-1953-

AJCAA7 American Journal of Cancer. (New York, NY) V.15-40, 1931-40. For publisher information, see CNREA8

AJCNAC American Journal of Clinical Nutrition. (American Society for Clinical Nutrition, Inc., 9650 Rockville Pike, Bethesda, MD 20814) V.2- 1954-

AJCPAI American Journal of Clinical Pathology. (J.B. Lippincott Co., (Keystone Industrial Park, Scanton, PA 18512) V.1- 1931-

AJDEBP Australasian Journal of Dermatology. (Australasian College of Dermatologists, 271 Bridge Rd., Glebe, NSW 2037, Australia) V.9- 1967-

AJEBAK Australian Journal of Experimental Biology and Medical Science. (Univ. of Adelaide Registrar, Adelaide, S.A. 5000, Australia) V.1- 1924-

AJGAAR American Journal of Gastroenterology. (American College of Gastroenterology, Inc., 299 Broadway, New York, NY 10007) V.21- 1954-

AJHEAA American Journal of Public Health. (American Public Health Assoc., Inc., 1015 15th St., N.W., Washington, D.C. 20005) V.2-17, 1912-27; V.61- 1971-

AJIMD8 American Journal of Industrial Medicine. (Alan R. Liss, Inc., 150 Fifth Ave., New York, NY 10011) V.1- 1980-

AJMEAZ American Journal of Medicine. (Yorke Medical Group, 666 5th Ave., New York, NY 10103) V.1- 1946-

AJMSA9 American Journal of the Medical Sciences. (Charles B. Slack, Inc., 6900 Grove Rd., Thorofare, NJ 08086) V.1- 1841-

AJOGAH American Journal of Obstetrics and Gynecology. (C.V. Mosby Co., 11830 Westline Industrial Dr., St. Louis, MO 63141) V.1- 1920-

AJPAA4 American Journal of Pathology. (Harper & Row, Medical Dept., 2350 Virginia Ave., Hagerstown, MD 21740) V.1- 1925-

AJRRAV American Journal of Roentgenology, Radium Therapy and Nuclear Medicine. (Springfield, IL) V.67-125, 1952-75. For publisher information, see AAJRDX

AJVRAH American Journal of Veterinary Research. (American Veterinary Medical Association, 930 N. Meacham Road, Schaumburg, IL 60196) V.1- 1940-

AKBNAE Arkhiv Biologicheskikh Nauk. Archives of Biological Sciences. (Moscow, U.S.S.R.) V.1-64, 1892-1941. Discontinued

ALEPA8 Acta Leprol. (Publisher unknown) V.1- 1920(?)-

AMACCQ Antimicrobial Agents & Chemotherapy. (American Society for Microbiology, 1913 I St., N.W., Washington, DC 20006) V.1- 1972-

AMAHA5 Acta Microbiologica Academiae Scientiarum Hungaricae. (Akademiai Kiado, P.O. Box 24, Budapest 502, Hungary) V.1- 1954-

AMBNAS Acta Medica et Biologica. (Niigata University School of Medicine, 1 Asahi-machi-dori, Niigata 951, Japan) V.1- 1953-

AMBPBZ Acta Pathologica et Microbiologica Scandinavica, Section A: Pathology. (Copenhagen K, Denmark) V.78-89, 1970-81. For publisher information, see ACPADQ

AMBUCH Acta Medica Bulgarica. (Durzhavno Izdatelstvo Meditsina i Fizkultura, Pl. Slaveikov 11, Sofia, Bulgaria) V.1- 1973-

AMIHAB AMA Archives of Industrial Health. (Chicago, IL) V.11-21, 1955-60. For publisher information, see AEHLAU

AMIHBC AMA Archives of Industrial Hygiene & Occupational Medicine. (Chicago, IL) V.2-10, 1950-54. For publisher information, see AEHLAU

AMNTA4 American Naturalist. (University of Chicago Press, 5801 S. Ellis Ave., Chicago, IL 60637) V.1-1867-

AMOKAG Acta Medicia Okayama. (Okayama University Medical School, 2-5-1 Shikata-cho, Okayama 700, Japan) V.8- 1952-

AMONDS Applied Methods in Oncology. (Elsevier North Holland, Inc., 52 Vanderbilt Ave., New York, NY 10017) V.1- 1978-

AMPLAO AMA Archives of Pathology. (American Medical Association, 535 N. Dearborn St., Chicago, IL 60610) V.50,No.4-V.69, 1950-60. For publisher information, see APLMAS

AMRL** Aerospace Medical Research Laboratory Report. (Aerospace Technical Div., Air Force Systems Command, Wright-Patterson Air Force Base, OH 45433)

AMSHAR Acta Morphologica Academiae Scientiarum Hungaricae. (Akademiai Kiado, P.O. Box 24, H-1389 Budapest 502, Hungary) V.1- 1951-

AMSVAZ Acta Medica Scandinavica. (Almqvist & Wiksell, P.O. Box 62, 26 Gamla Brogatan, S-101, 20 Stockholm, Sweden) V.52- 1919-

AMTUA3 Acta Medica Turcica. (Dr. Ayhan Okcuoglu, Cocuk Hastalikari Klinig i, c/o Ankara University Tip Facultesi, PK 48, Cebeci, Ankara, Turkey) V.1- 1964-

AMUK** Acta Medica University Kioto. (Kioto, Japan)

ANBCB3 Antibiotics and Chemotherapy. (S. Karger, AG, Arnold-Boecklin-St 25, Postfach CH-4009 Basel, Switzerland) V.17- 1971-

ANESAV Anesthesiology. (J.B. Lippincott Co., Keystone Industrial Park, Scranton, PA 18512) V.1- 1940-

ANPTAL Acta Neuropathologica. (Springer-Verlag New York, Inc., Service Center, 44 Hartz Way, Secaucus, NJ 07094) V.1- 1961-

ANREAK Anatomical Record. (Alan R. Liss, Inc., 150 5th Ave., New York, NY 10011)V.1- 1906/08-

ANSUA5 Annals of Surgery. (J.B. Lippincott Co., Keystone Industrial Park, Scranton, PA 18512) V.1- 1885-

ANTBAL Antibiotiki. (Moscow, USSR) V.1-29, 1956-84. For publisher information, see AMBIEH

ANTRD4 Anticancer Research. (Anticancer Research, 5 Argyropoulou St., Kato Patissia, Athens, 907, Greece) V.1- 1981-

ANYAA9 Annals of the New York Academy of Sciences. (The Academy, Exec. Director, 2 E. 63rd St., New York, NY 10021) V.1- 1877-

ANZJA7 Australian and New Zealand Journal of Surgery. (Blackwell Scientific Publications, College of Surgeons' Gardens, 99 Barry St., Carlton 3053, Australia) V.1- 1931-

ANZJB8 Australian and New Zealand Journal of Medicine. (Modern Medicine of Australia Pty., Ltd., 100 Pacific Highway, North Sydney, 2060, Australia) V.1- 1971-

AOBIAR Archives of Oral Biology. (Pergamon Press, Headington Hill Hall, Oxford OX3 OBW, England) V.1- 1959-

AOHYA3 Annals of Occupational Hygiene. (Pergamon Press, Headington Hill Hall, Oxford OX3 OBW, England) V.1- 1958-

AOUNAZ Archiv fuer Orthopaedische und Unfall-Chirurgie. (Munich, Fed. Rep. Germany) V.1-90 1903-77. See AOTSDE

APAVAY Virchows Archiv fuer Pathologische, Anatomie und Physiologie, und fuer Klinische Medizin. (Berlin, Germany) V.1-343, 1847-1967. For publisher information, see VAAPB7

APDCDT Advances in Tumour Prevention, Detection and Characterization. (Elsevier North Holland, Inc., 52 Vanderbilt Ave., New York, NY 10017) V.1- 1974-

APHGBP Acta Pathologica (Belgrade). (Belgrade Univerzitet, Institute de Pathologie, Belgrade, Yugoslavia) V.2/3- 1938-

APJAAG Acta Pathologica Japonica. (Nippon Byori Gakkai, 7-3-1, Hongo, Bunkyo-Ku, Tokyo 113, Japan) V.1- 1951-

APLMAS Archives of Pathology and Laboratory Medicine. (American Medical Association, 535 N. Dearbon St., Chicago, Il. 60610) V.1-5, No. 2, 1926-28, V.100-1976-

APMBAY Applied Microbiology. (Washington, DC) V.1-30, 1953-75. For publisher information, see AEMIDF

APMIAL Acta Pathologica et Microbiologica Scandinavica. (Copenhagen, Denmark) V.1-77, 1924-69. For publisher information, see AMBPBZ

APSXAS Acta Pharmaceutica Suecica. (Apotekarsocieteten, Wallingatan 26, Box 1136, S-111, 81 Stockholm, Sweden) V.1- 1964-

APTOA6 Acta Pharmacologica et Toxicologica. (Munksgaard, 35 Noerre Soegade, DK-1370, Copenhagen K, Denmark) V.1- 1945-

APTOD9 Abstracts of Papers, Society of Toxicology. Annual Meetings. (Academic Press, 111 5th Ave., New York, NY 10003)

ARDEAC Archives of Dermatology. (American Medical Association, 535 N. Dearborn St., Chicago, IL 60610) V.82- 1960-

ARGEAR Archiv fuer Geschwulstforschung. (VEB Verlag Volk und Gesundheit Neue Gruenstr. 18, DDR-102 Berlin, German Democratic Republic) V.1- 1949-

ARHEAW Arthritis & Rheumatism. (Arthritis Foundation, 3400 Peachtree Road, N.E., Atlanta, Ga 30326) V.1- 1958-

ARMIAZ Annual Review of Microbiology. (Annual Reviews, Inc., 4139 El Camino Way, Palo Alto, CA 94306) V.1- 1947-

ARMKA7 Archiv fuer Mikrobiologie. (Springer (Berlin)) V.1-13, 1930-43; V.14-94, 1948-73. For publisher information, see AMICCW

ARPAAQ Archives of Pathology. (American Medical Assn., 535 N. Dearborn St., Chicago, IL 60610) V.5,no.3-V.50,no.3, 1928-50; V.70-99, 1960-75. For publisher information, see APLMAS

ARPTAF Arkhiv Patologii. Archives of Pathology. (v/o 'Mezhdunarodnaya Kniga,' Kuznetskii Most 18, Moscow G-200 U.S.S.R.) V.1- 1959-

ARSUAX Archives of Surgery. (American Medical Association, 535 N. Dearborn St., Chicago, IL 60610) V.1-61, 1920-50; V.81- 1960-

ARTODN Archives of Toxicology. (Springer-Verlag, Heidelberger, Pl. 3, D-1 Berlin 33, Germany) V.32- 1974-

ARZFAN Aerztliche Forschung. (Munich, Fed. Rep. Ger.) V.1-26, 1947-72. Discontinued.

ARZNAD Arzneimittel-Forschung. (Edition Cantor Verlag fur Medizin und Naturwissenschaften KG, D-7960 Aulendorf, Germany) V.1- 1951-

ASBUAN Archives des Sciences Biologiques. (Leningrad, U.S.S.R.) V.1-22, 1892-1922. Discontinued.

ATHBA3 Acta Radiologica, Therapy, Physics, Biology. (P.O. Box 7449, S-103 91 Stockholm, Sweden) V.1-16, No.6, 1963-77

ATSUDG Archives of Toxicology, Supplement. (Springer-Verlag, Heidelberger Pl. 3, D-1000 Berlin 33, Fed. Rep. Ger.) No. 1- 1978-

ATXKA8 Archiv fuer Toxikologie. (Berlin, Germany)

V.15-31, 1954-74. For publisher information, see ARTODN

AUODDK Acta Universitatis Ouluensis, Series D: Medica. (Oulu University Library, Box 186, SF-90101 Oulu 10, Finland) Number 1- 1972-

AVBIB9 Advances in the Biosciences. (Pergamon Press Ltd., Headington Hill Hall, Oxford OX3 0BW, England) V.1- 1969-

AVBNAN Arhiv Bioloskih Nauka. (Jugoslovenska Knjigu, P.O. Box 36, Terazije 27, 11001, Belgrade, Yugoslavia)

BAFEAG Bulletin de l'Association Francaise pour l'Etude du Cancer. (Paris, France) V.1-52, 1908-65. For publisher information, see BUCABS

BANRDU Banbury Report. (Cold Spring Harbor Laboratory, POB 100, Cold Spring Harbor, NY 11724) V.1- 1979-

BBACAQ Biochimica et Biophysica Acta. (Elsevier Publishing Co., POB 211, Amsterdam C, Netherlands) V.1- 1947-

BBRCA9 Biochemical and Biophysical Research Communications. (Academic Press Inc., 111 5th Ave., New York, NY 10003) V.1- 1959-

BCPCA6 Biochemical Pharmacology. (Pergamon Press, Headington Hill Hall, Oxford OX3 OBW, England) V.1- 1958-

BCSTB5 Biochemical Society Transactions. (Biochemical Society, P.O. Box 32, Commerce Way, Whitehall Rd., Industrial Estate, Colchester CO2 8HP, Essex, England) V.1- 1973-

BCSYDM Bristol-Myers Cancer Symposia. (Academic Press, 111 Fifth Ave., New York, NY 10003) V.1- 1979-

BCTRD6 Breast Cancer Research and Treatment. (Kluwer Academic Publishers Group, Distribution Center, POB 322, 3300 AH Dordrecht, Neth.) V.1- 1981-

BEBMAE Byulleten' Eksperimental'noi Biologii i Meditsiny. Bulletin of Experimental Biology and Medicine. (v/o 'Mezhdunarodnaya Kniga,' Kuznetskii Most 18, Moscow G-200, U.S.S.R.) V.1- 1936-

BECCAN British Empire Cancer Campaign Annual Report. (Cancer Research Campaign, 2 Carlton House Terrace, London SW1Y 5AR, England) V.1- 1924-

BECTA6 Bulletin of Environmental Contamination & Toxicology. (Springer- Verlag New York, Inc., Service Center, 44 Hartz Way, Secaucus, NJ 07094) V.1- 1966-

BEXBAN Bulletin of Experimental Biology & Medicine. Translation of BEBMAE. (Plenum Publishing Corp., 233 Spring St., New York, NY 10013) V.41- 1956-

BEXBBO Biochemistry and Experimental Biology. (Piccin Medical Books, Via Brunacci, 12, 35100 Padua, Italy) V.10- 1971/72-

BICHAW Biochemistry. (American Chemical Society Publications, 1155 16th St., N.W., Washington, DC 20036) V.1- 1962-

BICHBX Bioinorganic Chemistry. (Elsevier North Holland, Inc., 52 Vanderbilt Ave., New York, NY 10017) V.1-9, 1971-78

BIHAA2 Bibliotheca Haematologica. (S. Karger AG, Arnold-Boecklin-St 25, CH-4000, Basel 11, Switzerland) No.1- 1955-

BIJOAK Biochemical Journal. (Biochemical Society, P.O. Box 32, Commerce Way, Whitehall Rd., Industrial Estate, Colchester CO2 8HP, Essex, England) V.1- 1906-

BIMADU Biomaterials. (Quadrant Subscription Services Ltd., Oakfield House, Perrymount Rd., Haywards Heath, W. Sussex, RH16 3DH, U.K.) V.1- 1980-

BIMDB3 Biomedicine. (Masson et Cie, Editeurs, 120 Blvd. Saint-Germain, P-75280, Paris 06, France) V.18- 1973-

BIOJAU Biophysical Journal. (Rockefeller Univ. Press, 1230 York Ave., New York, NY 10021) V.1- 1960-

BIORAK Biochemistry. Translation of BIOHAO. (Plenum Publishing Corp., 233 Spring St., New York, NY 10013) V.21- 1956-

BIPMAA Biopolymers. (John Wiley & Sons, 605 3rd Ave., New York, NY 10158) V.1- 1963-

BIZNAT Biologisches Zentralblatt. (VEB Georg Thieme, Hainst 17/19, Postfach 946, 701 Leipzig, E. Germany) V.1- 1881-

BJCAAI British Journal of Cancer. (H.K. Lewis & Co., 136 Gower St., London WC1E 6BS, England) V.1- 1947-

BJDEAZ British Journal of Dermatology. (Blackwell Scientific Publications, Osney Mead, Oxford OX2 OEL, England) V.63- 1951-

BJEPA5 British Journal of Experimental Pathology. (H.K. Lewis & Co., 136 Gower St., London WC1E 6BS, England) V.1- 1920-

BJIMAG British Journal of Industrial Medicine. (British Medical Journal, 1172 Commonwealth Ave., Boston, MA 02134) V.1- 1944-

BJLSAF Botanical Journal of the Linnean Society. (Academic Press, 111 5th Ave., New York, NY 10003) V.62- 1969-

BJOGAS British Journal of Obstetrics and Gynaecology. (British Journal of Obstetrics and Gynaecology, 27 Sussex Place, Regent's Park, London NW1 4RG, England) V.82- 1975-

BJPCAL British Journal of Pharmacology & Chemotherapy. (London, England) V.1-33, 1946-68. For publisher information, see BJPCBM

BJSUAM British Journal of Surgery. (John Wright & Sons Ltd., 42-44 Triangle West, Bristol BS8 1EX, England) V.1- 1913-

BJURAN British Journal of Urology. (Williams & Wilkens Co., 428 E. Preston St., Baltimore, MD 21202) V.1- 1929-

BKNJA5 Biken Journal. (Research Institute for Microbial Diseases, Osaka Univ., Yamada-Kami, Suita, Osaka, Japan) V.1- 1958-

BLFSBY Basic Life Sciences. (Plenum Publishing Corp., 227 W. 17th St., New York, NY 10011) V.1- 1973-

BLOAAO Biologia (Bratislava). (PNS-Ustredna Expedicia Tlace, Gottwaldovo Namestie 48/7, CS-884 19 Bratislava, Czechoslovakia) V.24- 1969-

BLOOAW Blood. (Grune & Stratton, 111 5th Ave., New York, NY 10003) V.1- 1946-

BMBUAQ British Medical Bulletin. (Churchill Livingstone, Robert Stevenson House, 1-3 Baxter's Place, Leith Walk, Edinburgh, EH1 3AF, UK) V.1- 1943-

BMJOAE British Medical Journal. (British Medical Association, BMA House, Travistock Square, London WC1H 9JR, England) V.1- 1857-

BPYKAU Biophysik. (Berlin, Germany) V.1-10, 1963-73.

BSBSAS Boletin de la Sociedad de Biologia de Santiago de Chile. (Santiago, Chile) V.1-12, 1943-55. Discontinued.

BSIBAC Bolletino della Societe Italiana di Biologia Sperimentale. (Casa Editrice Libraria V. Idelson, Via Alcide De Gasperi, 55, 80133 Naples, Italy) V.2- 1927-

BSRSA6 Bulletin de la Society Royale des Sciences de Liege. (Societe Royale des Sciences de Liege, Universite de Liege, 15, Ave des Tilleuls, B-4000 Liege, Belgium) V.1- 1932-

BTDCAV Bulletin of Tokyo Dental College. (Tokyo Dental College, Misaki-cho, Chiyoda-Ku, Tokyo 101, Japan) V.1- 1960-

BTERDG Biological Trace Element Research. (The Humana Press, Inc., Crescent Manor, P.O. Box 2148, Clifton NJ 07015) V.1- 1979-

BTPGAZ Beitraege zur Pathologie. (Gustav Fischer Verlag, Postfach 72-0143 D-7000 Stuttgart 70, Germany) V.141- 1970-

BUCABS Bulletin du Cancer. (Masson et Cie, Editeurs, 120 Blvd. Saint- Germain, P-75280, Paris 06, France) V.53- 1966-

BWHOA6 Bulletin of the World Health Organization. (WHO, 1211 Geneva 27, Switzerland) V.1- 1947-

BZARAZ Biologicheskii Zhurnal Armenii. Biological Journal of Armenia. (v/o 'Mezhdunarodnaya Kniga', Kuznetskii Most 18, Moscow G-200, USSR) V.19- 1966-

CALEDQ Cancer Letters. (Elsevier Publishing, P.O. Box 211, Amsterdam C, Netherlands) V.1- 1975-

CAMEAS California Medicine. (San Francisco, CA) V.65-119, 1946-73.

CANCAR Cancer. (J. B. Lippincott Co., E. Washington Sq., Philadelphia, PA 19105) V.1- 1948-

CARYAB Caryologia. (Caryologia, Via Lamarmora 4, 50121 Florence, Italy) V.1- 1948-

CBINA8 Chemico-Biological Interactions. (Elsevier Publishing, P.O. Box 211, Amsterdam C, Netherlands) V.1- 1969-

CBPCBB Comparative Biochemistry and Physiology, C: Comparative Pharmacology. (Oxford, England) V.50-73, 1975-82.

CBTOE2 Cell Biology and Toxicology. (Princeton Scientific Publishers, Inc., 301 N. Harrison St., CN 5279, Princeton, NJ 08540) V.1- 1984-

CCLCDY Zhonghua Zhongliu Zazhi. Chinese Journal of Oncology. (Guozi Sudian, Beijing, Peop. Rep. China) V.1- 1978-

CCPHDZ Cancer Chemotherapy and Pharmacology. (Springer-Verlag, Heidelberger, Pl. 3, D-1 Berlin 33, Germany) V.1- 1978-

CCROBU Cancer Chemotherapy Reports, Part 1. (Washington, DC) V.52, no.6-V.59, 1968-75. For publisher information, see CTRRDO

CCSUDL Carcinogenesis - A Comprehensive Survey (Raven Press, 1140Ave. of the Americas, New York, NY 10036) V.1- 1976-

CDPRD4 Cancer Detection and Prevention. (Marcel Dekker, Inc., POB 11305, Church St. Station, New York, NY 10249) V.1- 1979-

CEDEDE Clinical and Experimental Dermatology. (Blackwell Scientific Publications Ltd., Osney Mead, Oxford OX2 0EL, England) V.1- 1976-

CGCGBR Cytogenetics and Cell Genetics. (S. Karger AG, Arnold-Boecklin Str. 25, CH-4011 Basel, Switzerland) V.12- 1973-

CGCYDF Cancer Genetics and Cytogenetics. (Elsevier North Holland, Inc., 52 Vanderbilt Ave., New York, NY 10017) V.1- 1979-

CHDDAT Comptes Rendus Hebdomadaires des Seances de l'Academie des Sciences, Serie D. (Centrale des Revues Dunod-Gauthier-Villars, 24-26 Blvd. de l'Hopital, 75005 Paris, France) V.262- 1966-

CHINAG Chemistry & Industry. (Society of Chemical Industry, 14 Belgrave Sq., London SW1X 8PS, England) V.1-21, 1923-43; No.1- 1944-

CHROAU Chromosoma. (Springer-Verlag, Heidelberger Platz 3, D-1000 Berlin 33, Federal Republic of Germany) V.1- 1939-

CHRTBC Chromosomes Today. (Elsevier Scientific Publishing Co., P.O. Box 211 Amsterdam, The Netherlands) V.1- 1966-

CHWKA9 Chemical Week. (McGraw-Hill, Inc., Distribution Center, Princeton Rd., Hightstown, NJ 08520) V.68- 1951-

CHYCDW Zhonghua Yufangyixue Zazhi. Chinese Journal of Preventive Medicine. (42 Tung Szu Hsi Ta Chieh, Beijing, Peop. Rep. China) Beginning history not known.

CIGZAF Chiba Igakkai Zasshi. Journal of the Chiba Medical Society. (Chiba, Japan) V.1-49, 1923-73. For publisher information, see CIZAAZ

CIHPDR Zhongguo Yixue Kexueyuan Xuebao. Journal of the Chinese Academy of Medicine. (China Book Trading Corp., POB 2820, Beijing, Peop. Rep. China) V.1- 1979-

CIIT** Chemical Industry Institute of Toxicology, Docket Reports. (POB 12137, Research Triangle Park, NC 27709)

CISCB7 CIS, Chromosome Information Service. (Maruzen Co. Ltd., POB 5050, Tokyo International, Tokyo 100-31, Japan) No.1- 1961-

CIZAAZ Chiba Igaku Zasshi. Chiba Medical Journal. (Chiba Igakkai, Inohana 1-8-8, Chiba 280, Japan) V.50- 1974-

CJBBDU Canadian Journal of Biochemistry and Cell Biology. (National Research Council of Canada, Ottawa, Canada ON KIA OR6) V.61- 1983-

CJBIAE Canadian Journal of Biochemistry. (Ontario, Canada) V.42-60, 1964-82. For publisher information, see CJBBDU

CJMIAZ Canadian Journal of Microbiology. (National Research Council of Canada, Administration, Ottawa, Canada K1A OR6) V.1- 1954-

CLONEA Clinics in Oncology. (W.B. Saunders Co., W. Washington Sq., Philadelphia, PA 19105) V.1- 1982-

CLREAS Clinical Research. (American Federation for Clinical Research, 6900 Grove Rd., Thorotare, NJ 08086) V.6- 1958-

CMAJAX Canadian Medical Association Journal. (CMA House, Box 8650, Ottawa K1G OG8, Ontario, Canada) V.1- 1911-

CMBID4 Cellular and Molecular Biology. (Pergamon Press Ltd., Headington Hill Hall, Oxford OX3 0BW, England) v.22- 1977-

CMJODS Chinese Medical Journal (Beijing, English Edition). New Series. (Guozi Shudian, Beijing, Peop. Rep. China) V.1- 1975- (Adopted vol. no. 92 in 1979)

CMMUAO Chemical Mutagens. Principles and Methods for Their Detection (Plenum Publishing Corp., 233 Spring St., New York, NY 10013) V.1- 1971-

CMSHAF Chemosphere. (Pergamon Press, Headington Hill Hall, Oxford OX3 OEW, England) V.1- 1971-

CNCRA6 Cancer Chemotherapy Reports. (Bethesda, MD) V.1-52, 1959-68. For publisher information, see CCROBU

CNJGA8 Canadian Journal of Genetics and Cytology. (Genetics Society of Canada, 151 Slater St., Suite 907, Ottawa, Ont. K1P 5H4, Canada) V.1- 1959-

CNREA8 Cancer Research. (Waverly Press, Inc., 428 E. Preston St. Baltimore, MD 21202) V.1- 1941-

COINAV Colloques Internationaux du Centre National de la Recherche Scientifique. (Centre National de la Recherche Scientifique, 15, Quai Anatole-France, F-75700 Paris, France) V.1- 1946-

COREAF Comptes Rendus Hebdomadaires des Seances, Academie des Sciences. (Paris, France) V.1-261, 1835-1965. For publisher information, see CHDDAT

CORTBR Clinical Orthopaedics and Related Research. (J. B. Lippincott Co., E. Washington Sq., Philadelphia, PA 19105) No.26- 1963-

CPBTAL Chemical & Pharmaceutical Bulletin. (Pharmaceutical Society of Japan, 12-15-501, Shibuya 2-chome, Shibuya-ku, Tokyo, 150, Japan) V.6- 1958-

CRNGDP Carcinogenesis. (Information Retrieval, 1911 Jefferson Davis Highway, Arlington, VA 22202) V.1- 1980-

CRSBAW Comptes Rendus des Seances de la Societe de Biologie et de Ses Filiales. (Masson et Cie, Editeurs, 120 Blvd. Saint-Germain, P-75280, Paris 06, France) V.1- 1849-

CRSUBM Cancer Research Supplement (Williams & Wilkins Company, 428 E. Preston St., Baltimore, MD 21202) No.1-4, 1953-56

CSHCAL Cold Spring Harbor Conferences on Cell Proliferation. (Cold Spring Harbor Laboratory, POB 100, Cold Spring Harbor, NY 11724) V.1- 1974-

CTKIAR Cell and Tissue Kinetics. (Blackwell Scientific Publications Ltd., Osney Mead, Oxford OX2 0EL, England) V.1- 1968-

CTOXAO Clinical Toxicology. (New York, NY) V.1-18, 1968-81. For publisher information, see JTCTDW

CTRRDO Cancer Treatment Reports. (U. S. Government Printing Office, Supt. of Doc., Washington, DC 20402) V.60- 1976-

CUSCAM Current Science. (Current Science Assoc., Mgr., Raman Research Institute, Bangalore 6, India) V.1- 1932-

CYGEDX Cytology and Genetics. English Translation of Tsitologiya i Genetika. (Allerton Press, Inc., 150 Fifth Ave., New York, NY 10011) V.8- 1974-

CYTBAI Cytobios. (The Faculty Press, 88 Regent St., Cambridge, England) V.1- 1969-

CYTOAN Cytologia. (Maruzen Co. Ltd., P.O. Box 5050, Tokyo International, Tokyo 100-31, Japan) V.1- 1929-

DABBBA Dissertation Abstracts International, B: The Sciences and Engineering. (University Microfilms, A Xerox Co., 300 N. Zeeb Rd., Ann Arbor, MI 48106) V.30- 1969-

DANKAS Doklady Akademii Nauk S.S.S.R. (v/o 'Mezhdunarodnaya Kniga,' Kuznetskii Most 18, Moscow G-200, U.S.S.R.) V.1- 1933-

DBABEF Doga Bilim Dergisi, Seri A2: Biyoloji. Natural Science Journal, Series A2. (Turkiye Bilimsel ve Teknik Arastirma Kurumu, Ataturk Bul. No. 221, Kavaklidere, Ankara, Turkey) V.8- 1984-

DBTEAD Diabete. (Le Raincy, France) V.1-22, 1953-1974

DEGEA3 Deutsche Gesundheitswesen. (VEB Verlag Volk und Gesundheit, Neue Gruenstr 18, 102 Berlin, E. Germany) V.1- 1946-

DHEFDK HEW Publication (FDA. United States). (Washington, DC) 19??-1979(?). For publisher information, see HPFSDS

DICRAG Diseases of the Colon and Rectum. (Harper & Row, Publishers, 10 E. 53rd St., New York, NY 10022) V.1- 1958-

DIGEBW Digestion. (S. Karger AG, Arnold-Boecklin Street 25, CH-4011 Basel, Switzerland) V.1- 1968-

DMBUAE Danish Medical Bulletin. (Ugeskrift for Laeger, Domus Medica, 2100 Copenhagen, Denmark) V.1- 1954-

DMWOAX Deutsche Medizinische Wochenschrift. (Georg Thieme Verlag, Herdweg 63, Postfach 732, 7000 Stuttgart 1, Federal Republic of Germany) V.1- 1875-

DOWCC* Dow Chemical Company Reports. (Dow Chemical U.S.A., Health and Environment Research, Toxicology Research Lab., Midland, MI 48640)

DRISAA Drosophila Information Service (Cold Spring Harbor Laboratory, POB 100, Cold Spring Harbor, NY 11724) No.1- 1934-

DTESD7 Developments in Toxicology and Environmental Science. (Elsevier, Scientific Publishing Co., POB 211, 1000 AE Amsterdam, Netherlands) V.1- 1977-

DUPON* E. I. Dupont de Nemours and Company, Technical Sheet. (1007 Market St., Wilmington, DE 19898)

EAGRDS Experimental Aging Research. (Beech Hill Publishing Co., P.O. Box 136, Southwest Harbor, ME 04679) V.1- 1975-

ECBUDQ Ecological Bulletins. (Swedish National Science Research Council, Stockholm) Number 19- 1975-

ECEBDI Experimental Cell Biology. (Phiebig Inc., POB 352, White Plains, NY 10602) V.44- 1976-

ECREAL Experimental Cell Research. (Academic Press, 111 5th. Ave., New York, NY 10003) V.1- 1950-

EESADV Ecotoxicology and Environmental Safety. (Academic Press, 111 5th Ave., New York, NY 10003) V.1- 1977-

EGJBAY Egyptian Journal of Botany. (National Information and Documentation Centre, Al-Tahrir St., Awgaf P.O. Dokki, Cairo, Egypt) V.1- 1958-

EJCAAH European Journal of Cancer. (Pergamon Press, Headington Hill Hall, Oxford OX3 OEW, England) V.1- 1965-

EJCBDN European Journal of Cell Biology. (Wissenschaftliche Verlagsgesellschaft mbH, Postfach 40, D-7000, Stuttgart 1, Fed. Rep. Ger.) V.19- 1979-

EJCODS European Journal of Cancer and Clinical Oncology. (Pergamon Press Ltd., Headington Hill Hall, Oxford OX3 0BW, England) V.17, No.7- 1981-

EJMBA2 Egyptian Journal of Microbiology. (National Information and Documentation Centre, A1-Tahrir St., Awqaf P.O. Dokki, Cairo, Egypt) V.7- 1972-

EJTXAZ European Journal of Toxicology and Environmental Hygiene. (Paris, France) v.7-9, 1974-76. For publisher information, see TOERD9

EKSODD Eksperimental'naya Onkologiya. Experimental Oncology. (V/O Mezhdunarodnaya Kniga, 121200 Moscow, USSR) V.1- 1979-

EMMUEG Environmental and Molecular Mutagenesis. (Alan R. Liss, Inc., 4 E. 11th St., New York, NY 10003) V.10- 1987-

EMPSAL Experimental and Molecular Pathology, Supplement. (Academic Press, 111 5th Ave., New York, NY 10003) No.1- 1963-

EMSUA8 Experimental Medicine & Surgery. (Brooklyn Medical Press, 600 Lafayette Ave., Brooklyn, NY 11216) V.1- 1943-

ENDOAO Endocrinology. (Williams & Wilkins Co., Dept. 260, P.O. Box 1496, Baltimore, MD 21203) V.1- 1917-

ENMUDM Environmental Mutagenesis. (Alan. R. Liss, Inc., 150 Fifth Ave., New York, NY 10011) V.1- 1979-

ENPBBC Environmental Physiology and Biochemistry. (Copenhagen, Denmark) V.2-5, No. 6, 1972-5, Discontinued.

ENVIDV Environmental Internationl. (Pergamon Press, Ltd., Headington Hill Hall, Oxford OX3 0BW, England) V.1- 1978-

ENVRAL Environmental Research. (Academic Press, 111 5th Ave., New York, NY 10003) V.1- 1967-

ENZYAS Enzymologica. (Dr. W. Junk bv Publishers, POB 13713, 2501 ES The Hague, Netherlands) V.1-43, 1936-72.

EPASR* United States Environmental Protection Agency, Office of Pesticides and Toxic Substances. (U.S. Environmental Protection Agency, 401 M St., S.W. Washington, DC 20460) History Unknown

ERNFA7 Ernaehrungsforschung. (Akademie-Verlag GmbH, Leipziger St. 3-4, 108 Berlin, E. Germany) V.1- 1956-

ESKGA2 Eisei Kagaku. (Nippon Yakugakkai, 2-12-15 Shibuya, Shibuya-Ku, Tokyo 150, Japan) V.1- 1953-

ESKHA5 Eisei Shikenjo Hokoku. Bulletin of the National Hygiene Sciences. (Kokuritsu Eisei Shikenjo, 18-1 Kamiyoga 1 chome, Setagaya-ku, Tokyo, Japan) V.1- 1886-

EUURAV European Urology. (S. Karger Publishers, Inc., 150 Fifth Ave., Suite 1105, New York, NY 10011) V.1- 1975-

EVHPAZ EHP, Environmental Health Perspectives. Subseries of DHEW Publications. (U.S. Government Printing Office, Superintendent of Documents, Washington, DC 20402) No.1- 1972-

EVSRBT Environmental Science Research. (Plenum Publishing Corp., 233 Spring St., New York, NY 10013) V.1- 1972-

EXERA6 Experimental Eye Research. (Academic Press, Inc. 1 E. 1st., Duluth, MN 55802) V.1- 1961-

EXMDA4 International Congress Series - Excerpta Medica. (Elsevier North Holland, Inc., 52 Vanderbilt Ave., New York, NY 10017) No.1- 1952-

EXMPA6 Experimental & Molecular Pathology. (Academic Press, 111 5th Ave., New York, NY 10003) V.1- 1962-

EXPADD Experimental Pathology. (Elsevier Scientific Publishers Ireland Ltd., POB 85, Limerick, Ireland) V.19- 1981-

EXPEAM Experientia. (Birkhaeuser Verlag, P.O. Box 34, Elisabethenst 19, CH-4010, Basel, Switzerland) V.1- 1945-

EXPTAX Experimentelle Pathologie. (Jena, Ger. Dem. Rep.) V.1-18, 1967-80. For publisher information, see EXPADD

FAATDF Fundamental and Applied Toxicology (Official Journal of the Society of Toxicology, 475 Wolf Ledges Parkway, Akron, OH 44311) V.1- 1981-

FACOEB Food Additives and Contaminants. (Taylor & Francis Inc., 242 Cherry St., Philadelphia, PA 19106) V.1- 1984-

FAONAU Food and Agriculture Organization of United Nations, Report Series. (FAO-United Nations, Room 101, 1776 F Street, NW, Washington, DC 20437)

FAVUAI Fiziologicheski Aktivnye Veshchestva. Physiologically Active Substances. (Akademiya Nauk Ukrainskoi S.S.R., Kiev, U.S.S.R.) No.1- 1966-

FCTOD7 Food and Chemical Toxicology. (Pergamon Press, Headington Hill Hall, Oxford OX3 OBW, England) V.20- 1982-

FCTXAV Food and Cosmetics Toxicology. (Pergamon Press Ltd., Maxwell House, Fairview Park Elmsford, NY 10523) V.1-19, 1963-81. For Publisher information, see FCTOD7

FEBLAL FEBS Letters. (Elsevier Scientific Publishing Co., POB 211, 1000 AE Amsterdam, Netherlands) V.1- 1968-

FEPRA7 Federation Proceedings, Federation of American Societies for Experimental Biology. (9650 Rockville Pike, Bethesda, MD 20014) V.1- 1942-

FESTAS Fertility & Sterility. (American Fertility Society, 1608 13th Ave. S. Birmingham, AL 35205) V.1- 1950-

FGIGDO Fujita Gakuen Igakkaishi. Journal of the Fujita Gakuen Medical Society. (Nagoya Hoken Eisei Daigaku Fujita Gakuen Igakkai, 1-98 Dengakuga, Kubo, Kutsukake-Cho, Toyoake, Aichi-Ken 470-11, Japan) V. 1-1977-

FKIZA4 Fukuoka Igaku Zasshi. (Fukuoka Igakkai, c/o Kyushu Daigaku Igakubu, Tatekasu, Fukuoka-shi, Fukuoka, Japan) V.33- 1940-

FLUOA4 Fluoride. (International Society for Fluoride Research, P.O. Box 692, Warren, MI 48090) V.3- 1970-

FMLED7 FEMS Microbiology Letters. (Elsevier Scientific Publishing Co., POB 211, Amsterdam, Neth.) V.1- 1977-

FOBLAN Folia Biologica (Prague). (Academic Press, 111 Fifth Ave., New York, NY 10003) V.1- 1955-

FOMIAZ Folia Microbiologica (Prague). (Academia, Vodickova 40, CS-112 29 Prague 1, (Czechoslavakia) V.4- 1959-

FOMOAJ Folia Morphologica (Warsaw). (Panstwowy Zaklad Wydawnictw Lekarskich, ul. Druga 38-40, P-00 238 Warsaw, Poland) V.1- 1929-

FRPPAO Farmaco, Edizione Pratica. (Casella Postale 114, 27100 Pavia, Italy) V.8- 1953-

FRPSAX Farmaco, Edizione Scientifica. (Casella Postale 114, 27100 Pavia, Italy) V.8- 1953-

FZPAAZ Frankfurter Zeitschrift fuer Pathologie. (Munich, Germany) V.1-77, 1907-67. For publisher information, see VAAZA2

GANMAX Gann Monograph. (Tokyo, Japan) No.1-10, 1966-71. For publisher information, see GMCRDC

GANNA2 Gann. Japanese Journal of Cancer Research. (Tokyo, Japan) V.1-75, 1907-84. For publisher information, see JJCREP

GANRAE Gan No Rinsho. Cancer Clinics. (Ishiyaku Publishers, Inc., 7-10 Honkomagome 1-chome, Bunkyo-ku, Tokyo, Japan) V.1- 1954-

GASTAB Gastroenterology. (Elsevier North Holland, Inc., 52 Vanderbilt Avenue, New York, NY 10017) V.1- 1943-

GENRA8 Genetical Research. (Cambridge University Press, P.O. Box 92, Bentley House, 200 Euston Rd., London NW1 2DB, England) V.1- 1960-

GENTAE Genetics. (P.O. Drawer U, University Station, Auston, TX 78712) V.1- 1916-

GERNDJ Gerontology. (S. Karger AG, Postfach CH-4009, Basel, Switzerland) V.22- 1976-

GESKAC Genetika i Selektsiya. Genetics and Plant Breeding. (Izdatelstvo na Naukite, ul. Akad. G. Bonchev, 1113 Sofia, Bulgaria) V.1- 1968-

GETRE8 Gematologiya i Transfuziologiya. Hematology and Transfusion Science. (V/O Mezhdunarodnaya Kniga, Kuznetskii Most 18,Moscow G-200, USSR) V.28- 1983-

GISAAA Gigiena i Sanitariya. (English Translation is HYSAAV). (v/o 'Mezhdunarodnaya Kniga,' Kuznetskii Most 18, Moscow G-200, U.S.S.R.) V.1- 1936-

GMCRDC Gann Monograph on Cancer Research. (Japan Scientific Societies Press, Hongo 6-2-10, Bunkyo-ku, Tokyo 113, Japan) No. 11- 1971-

GMJOAZ Glasgow Medical Journal. (Glasgow, Scotland) 1828-1955. For publisher information, see SMDJAK

GNKAA5 Genetika. (see SOGEBZ for English Translation) (v/o 'Mexhdunarodnaya Kniga,' Kuznetskii Most 18, Moscow G-200, USSR) No.1- 1965-

GROWAH Growth. (Southern Bio-Research Institute, Florida Southern College, Lakeland, FL 33802) V.1-1937-

GTKRDX Gan to Kagaku Ryoho. Cancer and Chemotherapy. (Gan to Kagaku Ryohosha, Yaesu Bldg., 1-8-9 Yaesu, Chuo-Ku, Tokyo 103, Japan) V.1- 1974-

GTPPAF Gigiena Truda i Professional'naya Patologiya v Estonskoi SSR. Labor Hygiene and Occupational Pathology in the Estonian SSR. (Institut Eksperimental'noi i Klinicheskoi Meditsiny Ministerstva Zdravookhraneniya Estonskoi SSR, Tallinn, USSR) V.8- 1972-

GTPZAB Gigiena Truda i Professional'nye Zabolevaniia. Labor Hygiene and Occupational Diseases. (v/o 'Mezhdunarodnaya Kniga,' Kuznetskii Most 18, Moscow G-200, U.S.S.R.) V.1- 1957-

GYNOA3 Gynecologic Oncology. (Academic Press, 111 Fifth Ave., New York, NY 10003) V.1- 1972-

HAEMAX Haematologica. (Il Pensiero Scientifico, Via Panama 48, I-00198, Rome, Italy) V.1- 1920-

HCKHDV Huanjing Kexue. Environmental Sciences. (China International Book Trading Corp., POB 2820, Beijing, Peop. Rep. China) 1976- (Adopted vol. no. with Vol. 1 in 1980)

HDSKEK Hiroshima Daigaku Sogo Kagakubu Kiyo, 4: Kiso, Kankyo Kagaku Kenkyu. Bulletin of the Faculty of Integrated Arts and Sciences, Hiroshima University, Series 4: Fundamental and Environmental Sciences. (1-1-89 Higashisenda-machi, Naka-ku, Hiroshima, 730, Japan) V.6- 1980-

HEGAD4 Hepatogastroenterology. (Georg Thieme Verlag, Postfach 732, Herdweg 63, D-7000 Stuttgart 1, Fed. Rep. Ger.) V.1- 1980-

HEREAY Hereditas. (J.L. Toernqvist Book Dealers, S-26122 Landskrona, Sweden) V.1- 1947-

HGANAO Haigan. Lung Cancer. (Nippon Haigan Gakkai, c/o Chiba Daigaku Igakubu Haigan Kenkyusho, 1-8-1 Inohona, Chiba 280, Japan)

HIKYAJ Hinyokika Kiyo. (Acta Urologica Japonica). (Kyoto University Hosp ital. Department of Urology) V.1- 1955-

HIUN** Department of Cancer Research, Research Institute for Nuclear Medicine and Biology, Hiroshima University, Kasumi 1-2-3, Hiroshima 734, Japan

HKXUDL Huanjing Kexue Xuebao. Environmental Sciences Journal. (Guoji Shudian, POB 399, Beijing, Peop. Rep. China) V.1- 1981-

HLSCAE Health Laboratory Science. (American Public Health Assoc., 1015 18th St., N.W., Washington, DC 20036) V.1- 1964-

HOIZAK Hokkaido Igaku Zasshi. Hokkaido Journal of Medical Science. (Hokkaido Daigaku Igakubu, Nishi-5-chome, Kita-12-jo, Sapporo, Japan) V.1- 1923-

HSZPAZ Hoppe-Seyler's Zeitschrift fuer Physiologische Chemie. (Walter de Gruyter & Co., Genthiner Street 13, D-1000, Berlin 30, Federal Republic of Germany) V.21- 1895/96-

HUGEDQ Human Genetics. (Springer-Verlag, Neuenheimer Landst 28-30, D-6900 Heidelberg 1, Germany) V.31- 1976-

HUHEAS Human Heredity. (S. Karger AG, Postfach, CH-4009 Basel, Switzerland) V.19- 1969-

HUMAA7 Humangenetik. (Heidelberg, Germany) V.1-30, 1964-1975. For publisher information, see HUGEDQ

HunNJ# Personal Communication from Nancy J. Hunt, E.I. DuPont de Nemours & Co., 1007 Market St., Wilmington, DE 19898, to Henry Lau, Tracor Jitco, Inc., May 10, 1977

HYSAAV Hygiene & Sanitation: English Translation of Gigiena Sanitariya. (Springfield, VA) V.29-36, 1964-71. Discontinued.

IAAAAM International Archives of Allergy and Applied Immunology. (S. Karger, Postfach CH-4009, Basel Switzerland) V.1- 1950-

IAEHDW International Archives of Occupational and Environmental Health. Springer-Verlag, Heidelberger, Platz 3, D-1000 Berlin 33, Federal Republic of Germany) V.35-1975-

IAPUDO IARC Publications. (World Health Organization, CH-1211 Geneva 27, Switzerland) No.27- 1979-

IARC** IARC Monographs on the Evaluation of Carcinogenic Risk of Chemicals to Man. (World Health Organization, Internation Agency for Research on Cancer, Lyon, France) (Single copies can be ordered from WHO Publications Centre U.S.A., 49 Sheridan Avenue, Albany, NY 12210)

IARCCD IARC Scientific Publications. (Geneva Switzerland) V.1-No.26, 1971-78, For publisher information, see IAPUDO

ICHUDW Yichuan. Heredity. (China International Book Trading Corp., POB 2820, Beijing, Peop. Rep. China) V.1- 1979-

IDZAAW Idengaku Zasshi. Japanese Journal of Genetics. (Genetics Society of Japan, Nippon Iden Gakkai, Tanida 111, Mishima-shi, Shizuoka 411, Japan) V.1-1921-

IGAYAY Igaku No Ayumi. Progress in Medicine. (Ishiyaku Shuppan K.K., 7-10, Honkomagone 1 chome, Bunkyo-ku, Tokyo, Japan) V.1- 1946-

IGKEAO Igaku Kenkyu. (Daido Gakkan Shuppanbu, Kyushu Daigaku Igakubu, Hoigaku Kyoshitsu, Fukuoka 812, Japan) V.1- 1927-

IGMPAX Igiene Moderna. Modern Hygiene. (Amministrazione de l'Igiene Moderna, Tipografia 'La Commerciale,' Piazza Pontida, 11, Fidenza, Parma, Italy) V.1-1908-

IGSBAL Igaku to Seibutsugaku. Medicine & Biology. (1-11-4 Higashi-Kanda, Chiyoda, Tokyo 101, Japan) V.1-1942-

IGSBDO Izvestiya Akademii Nauk Gruzinskoi SSR, Seriya Biologicheskaya. Proceedings of the Academy of Sciences of the Georgian SSR, Biological Series. (V/O Mezhdunarodnaya Kniga, Kuznetskii Most 18, Moscow G-200, USSR) V.1- 1975-

IJCAAR Indian Journal of Cancer. (Dr. D.J. Jussawalla, Hospital Ave, Parel, Bombay 12, India) V.1- 1963-

IJCNAW International Journal of Cancer. (International

Union Against Cancer, 3 rue du Conseil-General, 1205 Geneva, Switzerland) V.1- 1966-

IJEBA6 Indian Journal of Experimental Biology. V.1-1963- For publisher information, see IJBBBQ

IJEVAW International Journal of Environmental Studies. (Gordon & Breach Science Publishers Ltd., 41-42 William IV St., London WC2N 4DE, England) V.1- 1970-

IJLEAG International Journal of Leprosy. (Box 39088, Washington, DC 20016) V.1- 1933-

IJMRAQ Indian Journal of Medical Research. (Indian Council of Medical Research, P.O. Box 4508, New Delhi 110016, India) V.1- 1913-

IJPBAR Indian Journal of Pathology & Bacteriology. (Dr. S.G. Deodhare, Medical College, Miraj Maharashtra, India) V.1- 1958-

IMEMDT IARC Monographs on the Evaluation of Carcinogenic Risk of Chemicals to Man. (World Health Organization, Internation Agency for Research on Cancer, Lyon, France) (Single copies can be ordered from WHO Publications Centre U.S.A., 49 Sheridan Avenue, Albany, NY 12210)

IMMUAM Immunology. (Blackwell Scientific Publications, Osney Mead, Oxford OX2 OEL, England) V.1-1958-

IMSUAI Industrial Medicine & Surgery. (Chicago, IL/Miami, FL) V.18-42, 1949-73. For publisher information see IOHSA5

INFIBR Infection and Immunity. (American Society for Microbiology, 1913 I St., N.W., Washington, DC 20006) V.1- 1970-

INHEAO Industrial Health. (2051 Kizukisumiyoshi-cho, Nakahara-ku, Kawasaki, Japan) V.1- 1963-

INNDDK Investigational New Drugs. The Journal of New Anticancer Agents. (Kluwer Boston Inc., 190 Old Derby St., Hingham, MA 02043) V.1- 1983-

INSSDM INSERM Symposium. (Elsevier North Holland, Inc., 52 Vanderbilt Ave., New York, NY 10017) No.1-1975-

INTSAO International Surgery. (International College of Surgeons, 1516 N. Lake Shore Dr., Chicago, IL 60610) V.45- 1966-

INURAQ Investigative Urology. (Williams & Wilkins Co., 428 E. Preston St., Baltimore, MD 21202) V.1-1963-

IOVSDA Investigative Ophthalmology and Visual Science. (C.V. Mosby Co., 11830 Westline Industrial Dr., St. Louis, MO 63146) V.16- 1977-

IPPABX Iugoslavica Physiologica et Pharmacologica Acta. (Unija Bioloskih Naucnik Drustava Jugoslavije, Postanski fah 127, Belgrade-Zemun, Yugoslavia) V.1-1965-

IRLCDZ IRCS Medical Science: Library Compendium. (MTP Press Ltd., St. Leonards House, St. Leonards Gate, Lancaster LA1 3BR, England) V.3-11, 1975-83.

ISMJAV Israel Medical Journal. (Jerusalem, Israel) V.17-23, 1958-64. For publisher information, see IJMDAI

ITCSAF In Vitro. (Tissue Culture Association, 12111 Parklawn Dr., Rockville, MD 20852) V.1- 1965-

IUSMDJ ICN-UCLA Symposia on Molecular and Cellular

Biology. (Academic Press, 111 5th Ave., New York, NY 10003) V.1- 1974-

JACSAT Journal of the American Chemical Society. (American Chemical Society Publications, 1155 16th St., N.W., Washington, DC 20036) V.1- 1879-

JACTDZ Journal of the American College of Toxicology. (Mary Ann Liebert, Inc., 500 East 85th St., New York, NY 10028) V.1- 1982-

JAFCAU Journal of Agricultural & Food Chemistry. (American Chemical Society Publications, 1155 16th St., N.W., Washington, DC 20036) V.1- 1953-

JAJAAA Journal of Antibiotics, Series A. (Tokyo, Japan) V.6-20, 1953-67. For publisher information, see JANTAJ

JAMAAP JAMA, Journal of the American Medical Association. (American Medical Association, 535 N. Dearborn St., Chicago, IL 60610) V.1- 1883-

JANTAJ Journal of Antibiotics. (Japan Antibiotics Research Association, 2-20-8 Kamiosaki, Shinagawa-ku, Tokyo, Japan) V.2-5, 1948-52; V.21- 1968-

JAPMA8 Journal of the American Pharmaceutical Assoc., Scientific Edition. (Washington, DC) V.29-49, 1940-60. For publisher information, see JPMSAE

JAVMA4 Journal of the American Veterinary Medical Association. (American Veterinary Medical Assoc., 600 S. Michigan Ave, Chicago, IL 60605) V.48- 1915-

JBCHA3 Journal of Biological Chemistry. (American Society of Biological Chemists, Inc., 428 E. Preston St., Baltimore, MD 21202) V.1- 1905-

JBJSA3 Journal of Bone & Joint Surgery. American Volume. (10 Shattuck St., Boston, MA 02115) V.30- 1948-

JBJSB4 Journal of Bone and Joint Surgery. (Boston, MA) V.20-45, 1922-47. For publisher information, see JBJSA3

JBMRBG Journal of Biomedical Materials Research. (J. Wiley & Sons, 605 3rd Ave., New York, NY 10016) V.1- 1967-

JCEMAZ Journal of Clinical Endocrinology and Metabolism. (Williams & Wilkins Co., 428 East Preston St., Baltimore, MD 21202) V.12- 1952-

JCGEDO Journal of Cytology and Genetics. (Society of Cytologists and Geneticists, Treasurer, Professor M. S. Chennaveeraiah, Karnatak University, Department of Botany, Dharwar 580003, India) V.1- 1966-

JCHODP Journal of Clinical Hematology and Oncology. (Wadley Institutes of Molecular Medicine, 9000 Harry Hines Blvd., Dallas, Texas 75235) V.5, No.3- 1975-

JCINAO Journal of Clinical Investigation. (Rockefeller University Press, 1230 York Avenue, New York, NY 10021) V.1- 1924-

JCLBA3 Journal of Cell Biology. (Rockefeller University Press, 1230 York Avenue, New York, NY 10021) V.12- 1962-

JCPAAK Journal of Clinical Pathology. (British Medical Association, Tavistock Sq., London WC1H 9JR, England) V.1- 1947-

JCPCBR Journal of Clinical Pharmacology. (Hall Associates, P.O. Box 482, Stamford, CN 06904) V.13- 1973-

JCREA8 Journal of Cancer Research. (Baltimore, MD)

V.1-14, 1916-30. For publisher information, see CNREA8

JCROD7 Journal of Cancer Research and Clinical Oncology. (Springer-Verlag, Heidelberger Pl. 3, D-1 Berlin 33, Germany) V.93- 1979-

JCSOA9 Journal of the Chemical Society. (London, England) 1926-65. For publisher information, see JCPRB4

JCUPBN Journal of Cutaneous Pathology. (Munksgaard, 35 Noerre Soegade, DK-1370 Copenhagen K, Denmark) V.1- 1974-

JDREAF Journal of Dental Research. (American Association for Dental Research, 734 Fifteenth St., NW, Suite 809, Washington, D.C. 20005) V.1- 1919-

JELJA7 Journal of Electron Microscopy. (Japanese Society of Electron Microscopy, Japan Academy Societies Center, 2-4-16 Yayoi, Bunkyo-ku, Tokyo 113, Japan) V.1- 1953-

JEMEAV Journal of Experimental Medicine. (Rockefeller University Press, 1230 York Avenue, New York, NY 10021) V.1- 1896-

JEPTDQ Journal of Environmental Pathology and Toxicology. (Park Forest South, IL) V.1-5, 1977-81.

JETPEZ Journal of Engineering for Gas Turbines and Power. (American Society of Mechanical Engineers. Order Dept., POB 2300, Fairfield, NJ 07007) V.106- 1984-

JEZOAO Journal of Experimental Zoology (Alan. R. Liss, Inc., 150 Fifth Avenue, New York, NY 10011) V.1- 1904-

JFIBA9 Journal of Fish Biology. (Academic Press, 24-28 Oval Rd., London NW1 7DX, England) V.1- 1969-

JFLCAR Journal of Fluorine Chemistry. (Elsevier Sequoia SA, P.O. Box 851, CH 1001, Lausanne 1, Switzerland) V.1- 1971-

JGMIAN Journal of General Microbiology (P.O. Box 32, Commerce Way, Colchester CO2 8HP, UK) V.1- 1947-

JHMJAX Johns Hopkins Medical Journal. (Journals Dept., Johns Hopkins Univ. Press, Baltimore, MD 21218) V.120-151, 1967-82. Discontinued.

JIDEAE Journal of Investigative Dermatology. (Williams & Wilkins Co., 428 E. Preston St., Baltimore, MD 21202) V.1- 1938-

JIDZA9 Jinrui Idengaku Zasshi. Journal of Human Genetics. (Nippon Jinrui Iden Gakkai, c/o Tokyo Ika Shika Daigaku, 1-5-45 Yushima, Bunkyo-ku, Tokyo 113, Japan) V.1- 1956-

JIHTAB Journal of Industrial Hygiene and Toxicology. (Baltimore, MD/New York, NY) V.18-31, 1936-49. For publisher information, see AEHLAU

JJATDK JAT, Journal of Applied Toxicology. (Heyden and Son, Inc., 247 S. 41st St., Philadelphia, PA 19104) V.1- 1981-

JJCREP Japanese Journal of Cancer Research (Gann). (Elsevier Science Publishers B.V., POB 211, 1000 AE Amsterdam, Netherlands) V.76- 1985-

JJEMAG Japanese Journal of Experimental Medicine. (Editorial Office, The Institute of Medical Science, University of Tokyo, Shirokanedai, Minatoku, Tokyo, Japan) V.7- 1928-

JJIND8 JNCI, Journal of the National Cancer Institute.

(U.S. Government Printing Office, Superintendent of Documents, Washington, DC 20402) V.61- 1978-

JLCMAK Journal of Laboratory and Clinical Medicine. (C.V. Mosby Co., 11830 Westline Industrial Dr., St. Louis, MO 63141) V.1- 1915-

JMCMAR Journal of Medicinal Chemistry. (American Chemical Society Pub., 1155 16th St., N.W., Washington, DC 20036) V.6- 1963-

JMEJAS Jikeikai Medical Journal. (Pharmacological Institute, The Jikei University School of Medicine, Minato-Ku, Tokyo, Japan) V.1- 1954-

JMENA6 Journal of Medical Entomology. (Bishop Museum, Entomology Dept., POB 6037, Honolulu, Hawaii 96818) V.1- 1964-

JMIMDQ Journal of Microbiological Methods. (Elsevier Science Publishers B.V., POB 211, 1000 AE Amsterdam, Netherlands) V.1- 1983-

JMOBAK Journal of Molecular Biology. (Academic Press, 111 Fifth Ave., New York, NY 10003) V.1- 1959-

JMSUAT Journal of the Madras Agricultural Students' Union. (Madras Agricultural Journal, Tamil Nadu Agricultural University Campus, Coimbatore 641003, India) V.1-16, 1912-28

JNCIAM Journal of the National Cancer Institute. (Washington, DC) V.1-60, No.6, 1940-78. For publisher information, see JJIND8

JOBAAY Journal of Bacteriology. (American Society for Microbiology, 1913 I St., N.W., Washington, DC 20006) V.1- 1916-

JOCEAH Journal of Organic Chemistry. (American Chemical Society Pub., 1155 16th St., N.W., Washington, DC 20036) V.1- 1936-

JOCMA7 Journal of Occupational Medicine. (American Occupational Medical Association, 150 N. Wacker Dr., Chicago, IL 60606) V.1- 1959-

JOENAK Journal of Endocrinology. (Biochemical Society Publications, P.O. Box 32, Commerce Way, Whitehall Industrial Estate, Colchester CO2 8HP, Essex, England) V.1- 1939-

JOGNAU Journal of Genetics. (Asit Kr. Bhattacharyya, M. A., 18/1, Barrackpore Trunk Rd, Belghoria, India) V.1- 1910-

JOHEA8 Journal of Heredity. (American Genetic Association, 818 Eighteenth St., N.W. Washington, D.C. 20006) V.5- 1914-

JOIMA3 Journal of Immunology. (Williams & Wilkins Co., 428 E. Preston St., Baltimore, MD 21202) V.1- 1916-

JONUAI Journal of Nutrition. (Journal of Nutrition, Subscription Dept., 9650 Rockville Pike, Bethesda, MD 20014) V.1- 1928-

JOPDAB Journal of Pediatrics. (C.V. Mosby Co., 11830 Westline Industrial Dr., St. Louis, MO 63141) V.1- 1932-

JOPHDQ Journal of Pharmacobio-Dynamics. (Pharmaceutical Society of Japan, 12-15-501, Shibuya 2-chome, Shibuya-Ku, Tokyo 150, Japan) V.1- 1978-

JOUOD4 Journal of UOEH (University of Occupational Environmental Health). (University of Occupational &

Environmental Health, 1-1 Iseigaoka, Yahata-nishi-ku, Kitakyushu, 807, Japan) V.1- 1979-

JOURAA Journal of Urology. (Williams & Wilkins Co., 428 E. Preston St., Baltimore, MD 21202) V.1- 1917-

JPBAA7 Journal of Pathology & Bacteriology. (London, England) V.1-96, 1892-1968. For publisher information, see JPTLAS

JPETAB Journal of Pharmacology & Experimental Therapeutics. (Williams & Wilkins Co., 428 E. Preston St., Baltimore, MD 21202) V.1- 1909/10-

JPFCD2 Journal of Environmental Science and Health, Part B: Pesticides, Food Contaminants, and Agricultural Wastes. (Marcel Dekker, POB 11305, Church St. Station, New York, NY 10249) V.B11- 1976-

JPMSAE Journal of Pharmaceutical Sciences. (American Pharmaceutical Assoc., 2215 Constitution Ave., N.W., Washington, DC 20037) V.50- 1961-

JPPMAB Journal of Pharmacy & Pharmacology. (Pharmaceutical Society of Great Britain, 1 Lambeth High Street, London SEI 5JN, England) V.1- 1949-

JPROAR Journal of Protozoology. (Society of Protozoologists, P.O. Box 368, Lawrence, KS 66044) V.1- 1954-

JPTLAS Journal of Pathology. (Longman Group Ltd., Subscriptions (Journals Department, Fourth Avenue, Harlow, Essex, CM19 5AA, UK) V.97- 1969-

JRARAX Journal of Radiation Research. (c/o Tokai Daigaku Igakubu Bunshi Seibutsugaku Kyoshitsu, Tenbodai, Isehara, 259-11, Japan) V.1- 1960-

JRMSAS Journal of the Royal Microscopical Society. (London, England) V.47-88, 1927-68. For publisher information, see JMICAR

JRPFA4 Journal of Reproduction and Fertility. (Journal of Reproduction and Fertility Ltd., 22 New Market Rd., Cambridge CB5 8D7, England) V.1- 1960-

JSCCA5 Journal of the Society of Cosmetic Chemists. (Society of Cosmetic Chemists, 50 E. 41st St., New York, NY 10017) V.1- 1947-

JSFAAE Journal of the Science of Food and Agriculture. (Society of Chemical Industry, 14 Belgrave Sq., London SW1X 8PS, England) V.1- 1950-

JSGRA2 Journal of Surgical Research. (Academic Press, 111 Fifth Ave., New York, NY 10003) V.1- 1961-

JSOMBS Journal of the Society of Occupational Medicine. (John Wright & Sons, 42-44 Triangle W., Bristol BS8 1EX, England)

JSONAU Journal of Surgical Oncology. (Alan R. Liss, Inc., 150 5th Ave., New York, NY 10011) V.1- 1969-

JSONDX Journal of Soviet Oncology. (New York) V. 1-5, 1980-84.

JSTBBK Journal of Steroid Biochemistry. (Pergamon Press Ltd., Headington Hill Hall, Oxford OX3 0BW, England) V.1- 1969-

JTCSAQ Journal of Thoracic & Cardiovascular Surgery. (C.V. Mosby Co., 11830 Westline Industrial Dr., St. Louis, MO 63141) V.38- 1959-

JTEHD6 Journal of Toxicology and Environmental Health. (Hemisphere Publ., 1025 Vermont Ave., N.W., Washington, DC 20005) V.1- 1975/76-

JTSCDR Journal of Toxicological Sciences. (Editorial Office, Higashi Nippon Gakuen Univ., 7F Fuji Bldg., Kita 3, Nishi 3, Sapporo 060, Japan) V.1- 1976-

JUIZAG Juntendo Igaku. Juntendo Medicine. (Juntendo Igakkai, 2-1-1, Hongo, Bunkyo-ku, Tokyo, 113, Japan) V.1- 1955-

KAMJDW Kawasaki Medical Journal. (Kawasaki Medical School, Kurashiki 701-01, Japan) V.1- 1975-

KEKHB8 Kanagawa-ken Eisei Kenkyusho Kenkyu Hokoku. Bulletin of Kanagawa Prefectural Public Health Laboratories. (Kanagawa Prefectural Public Health Laboratories, 52-2, Nakao-cho, Asahi-ku, Yokohama 221, Japan) No.1- 1971-

KFIZAO Kyoto-furitsu Ika Daigaku Zasshi. Journal of the Kyoto Prefectural School of Medicine. (Kyoto-furitsu Ika Daigaku Igakkai, Hirokoji, Kawaramachidori, Kamiyoku, Kyoto, Japan) V.1- 1927-

KGGZAL Koku Geka Gakkai Zasshi. Oral Surgery. (Tokyo, Japan)

KIDZAK Kansai Ika Daigaku Zasshi. Journal of the Kansai Medical School. (Kansai Ika Daigaku Igakkai, 1, Fumizono-cho, Moriguchi 570, Osaka, Japan) V.8- 1956-

KIKNAJ Kokuritsu Idengaku Kenkyusho Nempo. Annual Report of the National Institute of Genetics. (Kokuritsu Idengaku Kenkyusho, 1111 Yata, Mishima, Shizuoka-ken 411, Japan) No. 1- 1949-

KJMSAH Kyushu Journal of Medical Science. (Fukuoka, Japan) V.6-15, 1955-64. Discontinued.

KLWOAZ Klinische Wochenscrift. (Springer-Verlag, Heidelberger Pl. 3, D-1 Berlin 33, Germany) V.1- 1922-

KNZOAU Kanzo. Liver. (Nippon Kanzo Gakkai, c/o Toyo Bunko, 28-21, 2-chome, Hon Komagome, Bunkyo-ku, Tokyo 113, Japan) V.1- 1960-

KRANAW Krankheitsforschung. (Leipzig, E. Germany) V.1-9, 1925-32. Discontinued.

KRMJAC Kurume Medical Journal. (Kurume Igakkai, c/o Kurume Daigaku Igakubu, 67, Asahi-machi, Kurume, Japan) V.1- 1954-

KSRNAM Kiso to Rinsho. Clinical Report. (Yubunsha Co., Ltd., 1-5, Kanda Suda-Cho, Chiyoda-ku, KS Bldg., Tokyo 101, Japan) V.1- 1960-

KTUNAA K'at'ollik Taehak Uihakpu Nonmunjip. Journal of Catholic Medical College. (Catholic Medical College, Seoul, South Korea) V.1- 1957-

LAINAW Laboratory Investigation. (Williams & Wilkins Co., 428 E. Preston St., Baltimore, MD 21202) V.1- 1952-

LANCAO Lancet. (7 Adam St., London WC2N 6AD, England) V.1- 1823-

LAPPA5 Lavori dell'Istituto di Anatomia e Istologia Patologica della Universita Degli Studi Perugia. (Istituto di Anatomia e Isologia Patologica, Caselle Postale 327, 06100 Perugia, Italy) V.1- 1939-

LBANAX Laboratory Animals. (Biochemical Society Book Depot, POB 32, Commerce Way, Colchester Essex CO2 8HP, England) V.1- 1967-

LBASAE Laboratory Animal Science. (American Association for Laboratory Animal Science, 210 N. Hammes Ave., Suite 205, Joliet, IL 60435) V.21- 1971-

LIFSAK Life Sciences. (Pergamon Press, Maxwell House,

Fairview Park, Elmsford, NY 10523) V.1-8, 1962-69; V.14- 1974-

LPDSAP Lipids. (American Oil Chemists' Society, 508 South Sixth St., Champaign, IL 61820) V.1- 1966-

MAIKD3 Maikotokishin (Tokyo). Mycotoxin. (Maikotokishin Kenkyukai, c/o Tokyo Rika Daigaku Yakugakubu, 12 Funagawara-machi, Ichigaya, Shinjuku-ku, Tokyo 162, Japan) No.1- 1975-

MCEBD4 Molecular and Cellular Biology. (American Society for Microbiology, 1913 I St., NW, Washington, DC 20006) V.1- 1981-

MDMIAZ Medycyna Doswiadczalna i Mikrobiologia. (Ars Polona-RUCH, POB 1001, 1, P-00068 Warsaw, 1, Poland) V.1- 1949- For English Translation, see EXMMAV

MEDIAV Medicine. (Williams & Wilkins, 428 E. Preston St., Baltimore, MD 21202) V.1- 1922-

MEHYDY Medical Hypotheses. (Churchill Livingstone Inc., 19 W. 44 St., New York, NY 10036) V.1- 1975-

MEIEDD Merck Index. (Merck & Co., Inc., Rahway, NJ 07065) 10th ed.- 1983- Previous eds. had individual CODENS

MELAAD Medicina del Lavoro. Industrial Medicine. (Via S. Barnaba, 8 Milan, Italy) V.16- 1925-

MEXPAG Medicina Experimentalis. (Basel, Switzerland) V.1-11, 1959-64; V.18-19, 1968-69. For publisher information, see JNMDBO

MFEPDX Methods and Findings in Experimental and Clinical Pharmacology. (Methods and Findings, Sub. Dept., Apartado Correos 1179, Barcelona, Spain) V.1- 1979-

MGBUA3 Microbial Genetics Bulletin. (Ohio State University, College of Biological Science, Dept. of Microbiology, 484 W. 12th Ave., Columbus, Ohio 43210) Number 1- 1950-

MGGEAE Molecular & General Genetics. (Springer-Verlag, Heidelberger Pl. 3, D-1 Berlin 33, Germany) V.99- 1967-

MGONAD Magyar Onkologia. Hungarian Onkology. (Kultura, P.O. Box 149, H-1389 Budapest, Hungary) V.1- 1957-

MIBLAO Microbiology (Moscow). (Plenum Publishing Corp., 233 Spring St., New York, NY 10013) V.26- 1957-

MIIMDV Microbiology and Immunology. (Center for Academic Publications Japan, 4-16, Yayoi 2-chome, Bunkyo-ku, Tokyo 113, Japan) V.21- 1977-

MILEDM Microbios Letters. (Faculty Press, 88 Regent St., Cambridge, England) V.1- 1976-

MJAUAJ Medical Journal of Australia. (P.O. Box 116, Glebe 2037, NSW 2037, Australia) V.1- 1914-

MJOUAL Medical Journal of Osaka University. (The University, 33, Joan-cho, Kita-Ku, Osaka, Japan) V.1- 1949-

MMAPAP Mycopathologia et Mycologia Applicata. (The Hague, Netherlands) V.5-54, No.4, 1950-74, For publisher information, see MYCPAH

MMJJAI Mie Medical Journal. (Mie Medical Society, Mie Prefectual Univ., School of Medicine, Tsu, Japan) V.3- 1952-

MOPMA3 Molecular Pharmacology. (The American Society for Pharmacology and Experimental Therapeutics, 9650 Rockville Pike, Bethesda, MD 20014) V.1-1965-

MRLEDH Mutation Research Letters. (Elsevier/North-Holland Biomedical Press, POB 211, 1000 AE Amsterdam, Netherlands)

MSERDS Microbiology Series. (Marcel Dekker, Inc., POB 11305, Church St. Station, New York, NY 10249) V.1- 1973-

MUREAV Mutation Research. (Elsevier/North Holland Biomedical Press, P.O. Box 211, 1000 AE Amsterdam, Netherlands) V.1- 1964-

MUTAEX Mutagenesis. (IRL Press Ltd. 1911 Jefferson Davis Highway, Suite 907, Arlington, VA 22202) V.1-1986-

MVMZA8 Monatshefte fuer Veterinaermedizin. (VEB Gustav Fischer Verlag, Postfach 176, Villengang 2, 69 Jena, E. Germany) V.1- 1946-

MYCPAH Mycopathologia. (Dr. W. Junk bv Publishers, POB 13713, 2501 ES The Hague, Netherlands) V.1-1938-

NAGZAC Nagasaki Igakkai Zasshi. Journal of Nagasaki Medical Association. (Nagasaki Igakkai, c/o Nagasaki Daigaku Igakubu, 12-4 Sakamoto-machi, Nagasaki 852, Japan) V.1- 1923-

NAIZAM Nara Igaku Zasshi. Journal of the Nara Medical Association. (Nara Kenritsu Ika Daigaku, Kashihara, Nara, Japan) V.1- 1950-

NARHAD Nucleic Acids Research. (Information Retrieval Inc., 1911 Jefferson Davis Highway, Arlington, VA 22202) V.1- 1974-

NASDA6 Nagoya Shiritsu Daigaku Igakkai Zasshi. Journal of the Nagoya City University Medical Association. (The University, Nagoya, Japan) V.1- 1950-

NATUAS Nature. (Macmillan Journals Ltd., Brunel Rd., Basingstoke RG21 2XS, UK) V.1- 1869-

NATWAY Naturwissenschaften. (Springer-Verlag, Heidelberger Platz 3, D-1000 Berlin 33, Federal Republic of Germany) V.1- 1913-

NCIBR* Progress Report for Contract No. NIH-NCI-E-68-1311, Submitted to the National Cancer Institute by Bio-Research Consultants, Inc. (9 Commercial Ave., Cambridge, MA 02141)

NCIMAV National Cancer Institute, Monograph. (U. S. Government Printing Office, Supt. of Doc., Washington, DC 20402) No.1- 1959-

NCISA* Progress Report for Contract No. PH-43-63-1132, Submitted to the National Cancer Institute by Scientific Associates, Inc. (6200 S. Lindberg Blvd., St. Louis, MO 63123)

NCITR* National Cancer Institute Carcinogenesis Technical Report Series. (Bethesda, MD 20014) No. 0-205. For publisher information, see NTPTR*

NCIUS* Progress Report for Contract NO. PH-43-64-886, Submitted to the National Cancer Institute by the Institute of Chemical Biology, University of San Francisco. (San Francisco, CA 94117)

NEJMAG New England Journal of Medicine. (Massachu-setts Medical Society, 10 Shattuck St., Boston, MA 02115) V.198- 1928-

NEOLA4 Neoplasma. (Karger-Libri AG, Scientific Booksellers, Arnold-Boecklin-Strasse 25, CH-4000 Basel 11, Switzerland) V.4- 1957-

NEURAI Neurology. (Modern Medicine Publications, Inc., 757 Third Avenue, New York, NY 10017) V.1-1951-

NEZAAQ Nippon Eiseigaku Zasshi. Japanese Journal of Hygiene. (Nippon Eisei Gakkai, c/o Kyoto Daigaku Igakubu Koshu Eisergaku Kyoshits, Yoshida Konoe-cho, Sakyo-ku, Kyoto, Japan) V.1- 1946-

NGCJAK Nippon Gan Chiryo Gakkai-shi. Journal of Japan Society for Cancer Therapy. (Nihon Gan Chiryo Gakkai, Kyoto, Japan) V.1- 1966-

NGGKED Nippon Gan Gakkai Sokai Kiji. Proceedings of the Annual Meeting of the Japanese Cancer Association. (Japanese Cancer Association, Tokyo, Japan) V.1-1956-

NGGZAK Nippon Geka Gakkai Zasshi. Journal of the Japanese Surgical Society. (Nippon Geka Gakkai, 2-3-10 Koraku, Bunkyo-ku, Tokyo, 112, Japan) V.8-1908-

NIBKAW Nippon Byori Gakkai Kaishi. Journal of the Japanese Pathological Society. (c/o Tokyo Daigaku Igakubu Byorigaku Kyoshitsu, 7-3-1 Hongo, Bunkyo-ku, Tokyo 113, Japan) V.1- 1911-

NIGHAE Archiv Fuer Japanische Chirurgie. (Nippon Geka Hokan Henshushitsu, c/o Kyoto Daigaku Igakubu Geka Seikei Geka Kyoshitsu, 54 Kawara- machi, Shogoin, Sakyo-ku, Kyoto 606, Japan) V.1- 1924-

NIOSH* National Institute for Occupational Safety and Health, U. S. Dept. of Health, Education, and Welfare, Reports and Memoranda.

NIPAA4 Nippon Shokakibyo Gakkai Zasshi. Journal of the Japanese Society of Gastroenterology. (Nippon Shokakibyo Gakkai, 4-12 7-Chome, Ginza, Chuo-Ku, Tokyo 104, Japan) V.1- 1899-

NISFAY Nippon Sanka Fujinka Gakkai Zasshi. Journal of Japanese Obstetrics and Gynecology. (Nippon Sanka Fujinka Gakkai, c/o Hoken Kaikan Building., 1-1 Sado-hara-cho, Ichigaya, Shinjuku-ku, Tokyo 162, Japan) V.1-1949-

NJUZA9 Japanese Journal of Veterinary Science. (Nippon Jui Gakkai, 1-37-20, Yoyogi, Shibuya-ku, Tokyo 151, Japan) V.1- 1939-

NKEZA4 Nippon Koshu Eisei Zasshi. Japanese Journal of Public Health. (Nippon Koshu Eisei Gakkai, 1-29-8 Shinjuku, Shinjuku-ku, Tokyo 160, Japan) V.1- 1954-

NKGZAE Nippon Ketsueki Gakkai Zasshi. Journal of Japan Haematological Society. (Kyoto Univ. Hospital, Faculty of Medicine, Kyoto, Japan) V.1- 1937-

NKRZAZ Chemotherapy (Tokyo). (Nippon Kagaku Ryoho Gakkai, 2-20-8 Kamiosaki, Shinagawa-Ku, Tokyo, 141, Japan) V.1- 1953-

NMJOAA Nagoya Medical Journal. (Nagoya City University Medical School, 2-38 Nagarekawa-machi, Naka-ku, Nagoya 460, Japan) V.1- 1953-

NNBYA7 Nature: New Biology. (Macmillan Journals Ltd.,

Houndmills Estate, Basingstoke, Hants RG21 2XS, England) V.229-246, 1971-73.

NNGZAZ Nippon Naibumpi Gakkai Zasshi. Journal of the Japan Endocrine Society. (Nippon Naibumpi Gakkai, c/o Kyoto-Furitsu Ika Daigaku, Kojinbashi Nishizume-Sagaru, Kamigyo-ku, Kyoto 602, Japan) V.1- 1925-

NPMDAD Nouvelle Presse Medicale. (Masson et Cie, Editeurs, 120 Blvd. Saint-Germain, P-75280, Paris 06, France) V.1- 1972-

NRTXDN Neurotoxicology. (Pathotox Publishers, Inc., 2405 Bond St., Park Forest South, IL 60464) V.1-1979-

NTIS** National Technical Information Service. (Springfield, VA 22161) (Formerly U. S. Clearinghouse for Scientific & Technical Information)

NTPTB* NTP Technical Bulletin. (National Toxicology Program, Landow Bldg. 3A-06, 7910 Woodmont Ave., Bethesda, Maryland 20205)

NTPTR* National Toxicology Program Technical Report Series. (Research Triangle Park, NC 27709) No.206-

NUCADQ Nutrition and Cancer. (Franklin Institute Press, POB 2266, Phildelphia, PA 19103) V.1- 1978-

NULSAK Nucleus (Calcutta). (Dr. A.K. Sharma, c/o Cytogenetics Laboratory, Department of Botany, University of Calcutta, 35 Ballygunge Circular Rd., Calcutta 700 019, India) V.1- 1958-

NYSJAM New York State Journal of Medicine. (Medical Society of the State of New York, 420 Lakeville Rd., Lake Success, NY 11040) V.1- 1901-

OBGNAS Obstetrics and Gynecology. (Elsevier/North Holland, Inc., 52 Vanderbilt Avenue, New York, NY 10017) V.1- 1953-

OGSUA8 Obstetrical and Gynecological Survey. (Williams and Wilkins, 428 E. Preston St., Baltimore, MD 21202) V.1- 1946-

OHSLAM Occupational Health and Safety Letter. (Environews, Inc., 1097 National Press Bldg. Washington, DC 20045) V.1- 1970-

OIGZDE Osaka-shi Igakkai Zasshi. Journal of Osaka City Medical Association. (Osaka-shi Igakkai, c/o Osaka-shiritsu Daigaku Igakubu, 1-4-54 Asahi-cho, Abeno-ku, Osaka, 545, Japan) V.24- 1975-

ONCOAR Oncologia. (Basel, Switzerland) V.1-20, 1948-66. For publisher information, see ONCOBS

ONCOBS Oncology. (S. Karger AG, Postfach CH-4009 Basel, Switzerland) V.21- 1967-

ONCODU Revista de Chirurgui, Oncologie, Radiologie, ORL, Oftalmologie, Stomatologie, Seria: Oncologia. (Rompresfilatelia, ILEXIM, POB 136-137, Bucharest, Romania) V.13, No.4- 1974-

ONKOD2 Onkologie. (S. Karger AG, Postfach CH-4009 Basel, Switzerland) V.1- 1978-

OSOMAE Oral Surgery, Oral Medicine and Oral Pathology. (C.V. Mosby Co., 11830 Westline Industrial Dr., St Louis, Mo. 63141) V.1- 1948-

OYYAA2 Oyo Yakuri. Pharmacometrics. (Oyo Yakuri Kenkyukai, Tohoku Daigaku, Kitayobancho, Sendai 980, Japan) V.1- 1967-

PAACA3 Proceedings of the American Association for

Cancer Research. (Waverly Press, 428 E. Preston St., Baltimore, MD 21202) V.1- 1954-

PAMIAD Pathologia et Microbiologia. V.23-43, 1960-75. For publisher information, see ECEBDI

PAPOAC Patologia Polska. (Ars-Polona-RUSH, POB 1001, 00-068 Warsaw 1, Poland) V.1- 1950-

PARPDS Pathology, Research and Practice. (Gustav Fisher Verlag, Postfach 72 01 43, D-7000 Stuttgart 70, Federal Republic of Germany) V.162- 1978-

PATHAB Pathologica. (Via Alessandro Volta, 8 Casella Postale 894, 16128 Genoa, Italy) V.1- 1908-

PBPHAW Progress in Biochemical Pharmacology. (S. Karger AG, Postfach CH-4009 Basel, Switzerland) V.1-1965-

PCBRD2 Progress in Clinical and Biological Research. (Allan R. Liss, Inc., 150 5th Ave., New York, NY 10011) V.1- 1975-

PCCRA4 Proceedings of the Canadian Cancer Research Conference. (Univ. of Toronto Press, Toronto, M55 1A6, Ontario, Canada) V.1- 1954-

PCJOAU Pharmaceutical Chemistry Journal. English Translation of KHFZAN. (Plenum Publishing Corp., 233 Spring St., New York, NY 10013) No.1- 1967-

PESTC* Pesticide & Toxic Chemical News. (Food Chemical News, Inc., 400 Wyatt Bldg., 777 14th St., N.W. Washington, DC 20005) V.1- 1972-

PESTD5 Proceedings of the European Society of Toxicology. (Amsterdam, Netherlands) V.16-18, 1975-77, Discontinued.

PEXTAR Progress in Experimental Tumor Research. (S. Karger AG, Postfach CH-4009 Basel, Switzerland) V.1-1960-

PGMJAO Postgraduate Medical Journal. (Blackwell Scientific Publications, Osney Mead, Oxford OX2 OEL, England) V.1- 1925-

PGPKA8 Problemy Gematologii i Perelivaniia Krovi. Problems of Hematology and Blood Transfusion. (v/o 'Mezhdunarodnaya Kniga,' Kuznetskii Most 18, Moscow G-200, U.S.S.R.) V.1- 1956-

PGTCA4 Pigment Cell. (S. Karger AG, Arnold-Boecklin St., 25 CH-4011 Basel, Switzerland) V.1- 1973-

PHARAT Pharmazie. (VEB Verlag Volk und Gesundheit, Neue Gruenstr 18, 102 Berlin, E. Germany) V.1-1946-

PHMCAA Pharmacologist. (American Society for Pharmacology and Experimental Therapeutics, 9650 Rockville Pike, Bethesda, MD 20014) V.1- 1959-

PHMGBN Pharmacology: International Journal of Experimental and Clinical Pharmacology. (S. Karger AG, Postfach CH-4009 Basel, Switzerland) V.1- 1968-

PHRPA6 Public Health Reports. (U.S. Government Printing Office, Supt. of Doc., Washington, DC 20402) V.1-1878-

PHTHDT Pharmacology & Therapeutics. (Pergamon Press Ltd., Headington Hall, Oxford OX3 0BW, England) V.4-1979-

PHYTAJ Phytopathology. (Phytopathological Society, 3340 Pilot Knob Rd., St. Paul, MN 55121) V.1- 1911-

PIATA8 Proceedings of the Imperial Academy of Tokyo.

(Tokyo, Japan) V.1-21, 1912-45. For publisher information, see PJACAW

PJABDW Proceedings of the Japan Academy, Series B: Physical and Biological Sciences. (Maruzen Co., Ltd., P.O. Box 5050, Tokyo International 100-31, Japan) V.53- 1977-

PJACAW Proceedings of the Japan Academy. (Tokyo, Japan) V.21-53, 1945-77. For publisher information, see PJABDW

PLMEAA Planta Medica. (Hippokrates-Verlag GmbH, Neckarstr 121, 7 Stuttgart, Germany) V.1- 1953-

PMDCAY Progress in Medical Chemistry. (American Elsevier Publishing Co., 52 Vanderbilt Ave., New York, NY 10017) V.1- 1961-

PMRSDJ Progress in Mutation Research. (Elsevier North Holland, Inc., 52 Vanderbilt Ave., New York, NY 10017) V.1- 1981-

PNASA6 Proceedings of the National Academy of Sciences of the United States of America. (The Academy, Printing & Publishing Office, 2101 Constitution Ave., Washington, DC 20418) V.1- 1915-

PNCCA2 Proceedings, National Cancer Conference. (Philadelphia, PA) V.1-7, 1949-72, For publisher information, see CANCAR

POASAD Proceedings of the Oklahoma Academy of Science. (Oklahoma Academy of Science, c/o James F. Lowell, Executive Secretary-Treasurer, Southwestern Oklahoma State University, Weatherford, Oklahoma 73096) V.1- 1910/1920-

PPTCBY Proceedings of the International Symposium of the Princess Takamatsu Cancer Research Fund. (Japan Scientific Societies Press, 2-10, Hongo 6-chome, Bunkyo-ku, Tokyo 113, Japan) (1st)- 1970(Pub. 1971)-

PREBA3 Proceedings of the Royal Society of Edinburgh, Section B. (Royal Society of Edinburgh, 22 George St., Edinburgh, Scotland) V.61- 1943-

PRLBA4 Proceedings of the Royal Society of London, Series B, Biological Sciences. (The Society, 6 Carlton House Terrace, London SW1Y 5AG, England) V.76- 1905-

PSDTAP Proceedings of the European Society for the Study of Drug Toxicity. (Princeton, NJ 08540) V.1-15, 1963-74. For publisher information, see PESTD5

PSEBAA Proceedings of the Society for Experimental Biology and Medicine. (Academic Press, 111 5th Ave., New York, NY 10003) V.1- 1903/04-

PSSCBG Pesticide Science. (Blackwell Scientific Publications Ltd., Osney Mead, Oxford OX2 OEL, England) V.1- 1970-

PTEUA6 Pathologia Europaea. (Presses Academiques Europeennes, 98, Chaussee de Charleroi, Brussels, Belgium) V.1- 1966-

PTLGAX Pathology. (Royal College of Pathologists of Australia, 82 Windmill St., Sydney, NSW 2000, Australia) V.1- 1969-

PTRMAD Philosophical Transactions of the Royal Society of London, Series A: Mathematical & Physical Sciences. (Royal Society of London, 6 Carlton House Terrace, London SW1Y 5AG, England) V.178- 1887-

PUMTAG Trace Substances in Environmental Health. Proceedings of University of Missouri's Annual Conference on Trace Substances in Environmental Health. (Environmental Trace Substances Research Center, Univ. of Missouri, Columbia, MO 65201) V.1- 1967-

PUOMA5 Proceedings of the University of Otago Medical School. (Otago Medical School Research Society, Box 913, Dunedin, New Zealand) V.1- 1922-

PWPSA8 Proceedings of the Western Pharmacology Society. (Univ. of California Dept. of Pharmacology, Los Angeles, CA 94122) V.1- 1958-

PYTCAS Phytochemistry. An International Journal of Plant Biochemistry. (Pergamon Press Ltd., Headington Hill Hall, Oxford OX3 OEW, England) V.1- 1961-

RABIDH Revista de Igiena, Bacteriologie, Virusologie, Parazitologie, Epidemiologie, Pneumoftiziologie, Seria: Igiena. (Editura Medicala, Str.13 Decembrie 14, Bucharest, Romania) V.23- 1974-

RAREAE Radiation Research. (Academic Press, 111 Fifth Ave., New York, NY 10003) V.1- 1954-

RARSAM Radiation Research, Supplement. (Academic Press, 111 5th Ave., New York, NY 10003) No.1- 1959-

RBBIAL Revista Brasileira de Biologia. (Caixa Postal 1587, ZC-00 Rio de Janeiro, Brazil) V.1- 1941-

RBPMB2 Revista Brasileira de Pesquisas Medicas e Biologicas. (Editora Medico -Biologica Brasileira, Rua Pedrosa de Alvarenga, 1255, Sao, Paulo, Brazil) V.1- 1968-

RCBIAS Revue Canadienne de Biologie. (Les Presses de l'Universite de Montreal, P.O. Box 6128, 101 Montreal 3, Quebec, Canada) V.1- 1942-

RCOCB8 Research Communications in Chemical Pathology and Pharmacology. (PJD Publications, P.O. Box 966, Westbury, NY 11590) V.1- 1970-

REEBB3 Revue Europeenne d'Etudes Cliniques et Biologiques. European Journal of Clinical and Biological Research. (Paris, France) V.15-17, 1970-72. For publisher information, see BIMDB3

REONBL Revista Espanola de Oncologia. (Instituto Nacional de Oncologia del Cancer, Ciudad Universitaria, Madrid 3, Spain) V.1- 1952-

REXMAS Research in Experimental Medicine. (Springer-Verlag, Heidelberger, Pl. 3, D-1 Berlin 33, Germany) V.157- 1972-

RFECAC Revue Francaise d'Etudes Cliniques et Biologiques. (Paris, France) V.1-14, 1956-69. For publisher information, see BIMDB3

RIHYAC Rinsho Hinyokika. Clinical Urology. (Igakushoin Medical Publishers, Inc., 1140 Avenue of the Americas, New York, NY 10036) V.21- 1967-

RKGEDW Rinsho Kyobu Geka. Japanese Annals of Thoracic Surgery.

RMCHAW Revista Medica de Chile. (Sociedad Medica de Santiago, Esmeralda 678, Casilla 23-d, Santiago, Chile) V.1- 1872-

RPZHAW Roczniki Panstwowego Zakladu Higieny. (Ars Polona-RUSH, POB 1001, 00-068 Warsaw 1, Poland) V.1- 1950-

RRBCAD Revue Roumaine de Biochimie. (Romprestilatelia, POB 2001, Calea Grivitei 64-66, Bucharest, Romania) V.1- 1964-

RRCRBU Recent Results in Cancer Research. (Springer Verlag New York, Inc., Service Center, 44 Hartz Way, Secaucus, NJ07094) V.1- 1965-

RRENAR Revue Roumaine d'Endocrinologie. (Bucharest, Romania) V.1-11, 1964-74. For publisher information, see RRENDU

RSABAC Revista de la Sociedad Argentina de Biologia. (Associacion Medica Argentina, Santa Fe 1171, Buenos Aires, Argentina) V.1- 1925-

RSTUDV Rivista di Scienza e Technologia degli Alimenti e di Nutrizione Umana. Review of Science and Technology of Food and Human Nutrition. (Bologna, Italy) V.5-6, 1975-76. Discontinued

SACAB7 South African Cancer Bulletin. (National Cancer Association of South Africa, 9 Jubillee Rd., Parktown, Johannesburg, South Africa) V.1- 1957-

SAIGAK Saishin Igaku. Modern Medicine. (Saishin Igakusha, Senchuri Bldg., 3-6-1 Hirano-machi, Higashi-ku, Osaka 541, Japan) V.19- 1945-

SAIGBL Sangyo Igaku. Japanese Journal of Industrial Health. (Japan Association of Industrial Health, c/o Public Health Building, 78Shinjuku 1-29-8, Shinjuku-Ku, Tokyo, Japan) V.1- 1959-

SBJODP Science of Biology Journal. (POB 2245, Springfield, Ill. 62705) V.1- 1975-

SCIEAS Science. (American Assoc. for the Advancement of Science, 1515 Massachusetts Ave., NW, Washington, DC 20005) V.1- 1895-

SCMGDN Somatic Cell and Molecular Genetics. (Plenum Publishing Corp., 233 Spring St., New York, NY 10013) V.10- 1984-

SCPHA4 Scientia Pharmaceutica. (Oesterreichische Apotheker- Verlagsgesellschaft MBH, Spitalgasse 31, 1094 Vienna 9, Austria) V.1- 1930-

SEIJBO Senten Ijo. Congenital Anomalies. (Nihon Senten Ijo Gakkai, Kyoto 606, Japan) V.1- 1960-

SEMEAS Semana Medica. (Sociedad Argentina de Gastroenterologica, Santa Fe 1171, Buenos Aires, Argentina) V.1- 1894-

SFCRAO Symposium on Fundamental Cancer Research (Williams and Wilkins Co., 428 E. Preston St., Baltimore, Md. 21202) V.1- 1947-

SHKKAN Shika Kiso Igakkai Zasshi. Journal of the Japanese Association for Basic Dentistry. (Shika Kiso Igakkai, Nihon Daigaku Shigakubu, 1-8 Surugadai, Kanda, Chiyoda-ku, Tokyo 101, Japan) V.1- 1959-

SHYCD4 Shengwu Huaxue Yu Shengwu Wuli Jinzhan. Progress in Biochemistry and Biophysics. (Kexue Chubanshe, 137 Zhaoyangmennei Dajie, Beijing, Peop. Rep. China) No.1- 1974(?)-

SinJF# Personal Communication from J.F. Sina, Merck Institute for Therapeutic Research, West Point, PA 19486, to the Editor of RTECS, Cincinnati, OH, on October 26, 1982

SJHAAQ Scandinavian Journal of Haematology. (Munksgaard, 35 Norre Sogade, DK 1370 Copenhagen K, Denmark) V.1- 1964-

SJRHAT Scandinavian Journal of Rheumatology. (Almqvist & Wiksell, POB 45150, S-10430 Stockholm, Sweden) V.1- 1972-

SJUNAS Scandinavian Journal of Urology and Nephrology. (Almqvist & Wiksell Periodical Co., POB 62, 26 Gamla Brogatan, S-101-20 Stockholm, Sweden) V.1- 1967-

SKEZAP Shokuhin Eiseigaku Zasshi. Journal of the Food Hygiene Society of Japan. (Nippon Shokuhin Eisei Gakkai, c/o Kokuritsu Eisei Shikenjo, 18-1, Kamiyoga 1-chome, Setagaya-Ku, Tokyo, Japan) V.1- 1960-

SMWOAS Schweizerische Medizinische Wochenschrift. (Schwabe & Co., Steintorst 13, 4000 Basel 10, Switzerland) V.50- 1920-

SOGEBZ Soviet Genetics. Translation of GNKAA5. (Plenum Publishing Corp., 233 Spring St., New York, NY 10013). V.2- 1966-

SSBSEF Scientia Sinica, Series B: Chemical, Biological, Agricultural, Medical, and Earth Sciences (English Edition). (Scientific and Technical Books Service Ltd., POB 197, London WC2N 4DE, England) V.25- 1982-

STBIBN Studia Biophysica. (Akademie-Verlag GmbH, Liepziger Str. 3-4, DDR-108 Berlin, German Democratic Republic) V.1- 1966-

STRAAA Strahlentherapie. (Urban & Schwarzenberg, Pattenkoferst 18, D-8000 Munich 15, Germany) V.1- 1912-

STRHAV Staub-Reinhaltung der Luft. (VDI-Verlag GmbH, Postfach 1139, D-4000 Duesseldorf 1, Fed. Rep. Germany) V.26- 1966-

SUFOAX Surgical Forum. (American College of Surgeons, 55E. Erie St., Chicago, IL 60611) V.1- 1950-

SURGAZ Surgery. (C.V. Mosby Co., 11830 Westline Industrial Dr., St. Louis, MO 63141) V.1- 1937-

SWEHDO Scandinavian Journal of Work, Environment and Health. (Haartmaninkatu 1, FIN-00290 Helsinki 29, Finland) V.1 1975-

SYSWAE Shiyan Shengwa Xuebao. Journal of Experimental Biology. (Guozi Shudian, China Publications Center, P.O. Box 399, Peking, Peop. Rep. China) V.1- 1953- (Suspended 1966-77)

TAKHAA Takeda Kenkyusho Ho. Journal of the Takeda Research Laboratories. (Takeda Yakuhin Kogyo K. K., 4-54 Juso-nishino-cho, Higashi Yodogawa-Ku, Osaka 532, Japan) V.29- 1970-

TCMUD8 Teratogenesis, Carcinogenesis, and Mutagenesis. (Alan R. Liss, Inc., 150 Fifth Ave., New York, NY 10011) V.1- 1980-

TCMUE9 Topics in Chemical Mutagenesis. (Plenum Publishing Corp., 233 Spring Street, New York, NY 10013) V.1- 1984-

TECSDY Toxicological and Environmental Chemistry. (Gordon and Breach Science Pub. Inc., 1 Park Ave., New York, NY 10016) V.3(3/4)- 1981-

TELEAY Tetrahedron Letters. (Pergamon Press Ltd., Headington Hill Hall, Oxford OX3 OBW, England) 1959-

TGANAK Tsitologiya i Genetika. (v/o 'Mezhdunarodnaya Kniga', Kuznetskii Most 18, Moscow G-200, USSR) V.1- 1967-

TIDZAH Tokyo Ika Daigaku Zasshi. Journal of Tokyo

Medical College. (Tokyo Ika Daigaku Igakkai, 1-412, Higashi Okubo, Shinjuku-ku, Tokyo, Japan) 1918-

TJADAB Teratology, A Journal of Abnormal Development. (Wistar Institute Press, 3631 Spruce St., Philadelphia, PA 19104) V.1- 1968-

TJEMAO Tohoku Journal of Experimental Medicine. (Maruzen Co., Export Dept., P.O. Box 5050, Tokyo Int., 100-31 Tokyo, Japan) V.1- 1920-

TJIDAH Tokyo Jikeikai Ika Daigaku Zasshi. Tokyo Jikeikai Medical Journal. (3-25-8, Nishi Shinbashi, Minato-ku, Tokyo, Japan) V.66- 1951-

TJXMAH Tokushima Journal of Experimental Medicine. (Tokushima Diagaku Igakubu, 3, Kuramoto-cho, Tokushima, Japan) V.1- 1954-

TKIZAM Tokyo Igaku Zasshi. Tokyo Journal of Medical Sciences. (Tokyo, Japan) V.59-76, 1951-68.

TKORAS Trudy Kazakhskogo Nauchno-Issledovatel'skogo Instituta Onkologii i Radiologii. (The Institute, Alma-Ata, U.S.S.R.) V.1- 1965-

TNICS* Toxicology of New Industrial Chemical Substances. (U.S.S.R. Academy of Medical Sciences, Moscow-Meditsina)

TOERD9 Toxicological European Research. (Editions Ouranos, 12 bis, rue Jean-Jaures, 92807 Puteaux, France) V.1- 1978-

TOFOD5 Tokishikoroji Foramu. Toxicology Forum. (Saiensu Foramu, c/o Kida Bldg., 1-2-13 Yushima, Bunkyo-ku, Tokyo, 113, Japan) V.6- 1983-

TOLED5 Toxicology Letters. (Elseveir Scientific Publishing Co., P.O. Box 211, Amsterdam, Netherlands) V.1- 1977-

TOPADD Toxicologic Pathology. (E.I. du Pont de Nemours Co., Inc., Elkton Rd., Newark, DE 19711) V.6(3/4)- 1978-

TOXID9 Toxicologist. (Society of Toxicology, Inc., 475 Wolf Ledge Parkway, Akron, OH 44311) V.1- 1981-

TPKVAL Toksikologiya Novykh Promyshlennykh Khimicheskikh Veshchestv. Toxicology of New Industrial Chemical Sciences. (Akademiya Meditsinskikh Nauk S.S.R., Moscow, U.S.S.R.) No.1- 1961-

TRBMAV Texas Reports on Biology and Medicine. (Texas Reports, University of Texas Medical Branch, Galveston, TX 77550) V.1- 1943-

TRENAF Kenkyu Nenpo - Tokyo-toritsu Eisei Kenkyusho. Annual Report of Tokyo Metropolitan Research Laboratory of Public Health. (24-1, 3 Chome, Hyakunin-cho, Shin-Juku-ku, Tokyo, Japan) V.1- 1949/50-

TRPLAU Transplantation. (Williams & Wilkins, Co., 428 E. Preston St., Baltimore, MD 21202) V.1- 1963-

TSITAQ Tsitologiya. Cytology. (v/o 'Mezhdunarodnaya Kniga', Kuznetskii Most 18, Moscow G-200, USSR) V.1 1959-

TUMOAB Tumori. (Casa Editrice Ambrosiana, Via G. Frua 6, 20146 Milan, Italy) V.1- 1911-

TXAPA9 Toxicology and Applied Pharmacology. (Academic Press, 111 5th Ave., New York, NY 10003) V.1- 1959-

TXCYAC Toxicology. (Elsevier/North-Holland Scientific

Publishers Ltd., 52 Vanderbilt Ave., New York, NY 10017) V.1- 1973-

UICMAI UICC Monograph Series. (Springer Verlag New York, Inc., Service Center, 44 Hartz Way, Secaucus, NJ 07094)

URGABW Urologe Ausgabe A. (Springer-Verlag, Heidelberger Pl.3, D-1000 Berlin 33, Fed. Rep. Ger.) V.9- 1970-

URLRA5 Urological Research. (Springer Verlag New York, Inc., Service Center, 44 Hartz Way, Secaucus, NJ 07094) V.1- 1973-

UROTAQ Urologia. (Libreria Editrice Canova, Via Panciera, 3b, 31100 Treviso, Italy) V.1- 1934

VAAZA2 Virchows Archiv, Abteilung B: Zellpathologie, Cell Pathology. (Springer-Verlag, Heidelberger Pl. 3, D-1 Berlin 33, Germany) V.1- 1968-

VAPHDQ Virchows Archiv, Abteilung A: Pathological Anatomy and Histology. (Springer-Verlag, Heidelberger pl.3, D-1 Berlin. 33, Germany) V.362- 1974-

VDGPAN Verhandlungen der Deutschen Gesellschaft fuer Pathologie. (Gustav Fischer Verlag, Postfach 53, Wollgrasweg 49, 7000 Stuttgart-Hohenheim, Germany) V.1- 1898-

VHTODE Veterinary and Human Toxicology. (American College of Veterinary Toxicologists, Office of the Secretary-Treasurer, Comparative Toxicology Laboratory, Kansas State University, Manhatten, Kansas 66506) V.19- 1977-

VINIT* Vsesoyuznyi Institut Nauchnoi i Tekhnicheskoi Informatsii (VINITI). All-Union Institute of Scientific and Technical Information. (Moscow, USSR)

VIRLAX Virology. (Academic Press, 111 Fifth Ave. New York, NY 10003) V.1- 1955-

VOONAW Voprosy Onkologii. Problems of Onkology. (v/o 'Mezhdunarodnaya Kniga,' Kuznetskii Most 18, Moscow G-200, U.S.S.R.) V.1- 1955-

VPITAR Voprosy Pitaniya. Problems of Nutrition. (v/o 'Mezhdunarodnaya Kniga,' Kuznetskii Most 18, Moscow G-200, U.S.S.R.) V.1- 1932-

VRDEA5 Vrachebnoe Delo. Medical Profession. (v/o 'Mezhdunarodnaya Kniga,' Kuznetskii Most 18, Moscow G-200, U.S.S.R.) No.1- 1918-

VRRAAT Vestnik Rentgenologii i Radiologii. Bulletin of Roentgenology and Radiology. (v/o 'Mezhdunarodnaya Kniga,' Kuznetskii Most 18, Moscow G-200, U.S.S.R.) V.1- 1920-

VTPHAK Veterinary Pathology. (S. Karger AG, Postfach CH-4009 Basel, Switzerland) V.8- 1971-

WATRAG Water Research. (Pergamon Press Ltd., Headington Hill Hall, Oxford OX3 0BW, England) V.1- 1967-

WMHMAP Wissenschaftliche Zeitschrift der Martin-Luther Universitaet, Halle- Wittenberg, Mathematisch-Naturwissenschaftliche Reihe. (Deutsche Buch-Export und-Import GmbH, Leninstr. 16, 701 Leipzig, E. Germany) V.1- 1951-

WTMOA3 Wiener Tieraerztliche Monatsschrift. (Ferdinand Berger & Soehne OHG, Wiene Str. 21-23, A-3580 Horn, Austria) V.1- 1914-

XENOBH Xenobiotica. (Taylor & Francis Ltd., 4 John St., London WC1N 2ET, England) V.1- 1971-

XPHCI* U.S. Public Health Service, Current Intelligence Bulletin. (National Institute for Occupational Safety and Health, 5600 Fishers Lane, Rockville, MD 20857)

XPHPAW U.S. Public Health Service Publication. (U.S. Government Printing Office, Supt. of Doc., Washington, DC 20402) No.1- 1950-

YACHDS Yakuri to Chiryo. Pharmacology and Therapeutics. (Raifu Saiensu Pub. Co., 5-3-3 Yaesu, Chuo-ku, Tokyo 104, Japan) V.1- 1973-

YJBMAU Yale Journal of Biology and Medicine. (The Yale Journal of Biology and Medicine, Inc., 333 Cedar Street, New Haven, Connecticut 06510) V.1- 1928-

YKKZAJ Yakugaku Zasshi. Journal of Pharmacy. (Nippon Yakugakkai, 12-15-501, Shibuya 2-chome, Shibuya-ku, Tokyo 150, Japan) No.1- 1881-

YMBUA7 Yokohama Medical Bulletin. (Npg. Yokohama Ika Daigaku, Urafune-cho, Minato-ku, Yokohama, Japan) V.1- 1950-

ZAPOAK Zeitschrift fuer Allgemeine Mikrobiologie. Morphologie, Physiologie, Genetik und Oekologie der Mikroorganismen. (Akademie-Verlag GmbH, Liepziger Str. 3-4, DDR-108 Berlin, German Democratic Republic) V.1- 1960-

ZAPPAN Zentralblatt fuer Allgemeine Pathologie und Pathologische Anatomie. (VEB Gustav Fischer Verlag, Postfach 176, Villengang 2, 69 Jena, E. Germany) V.1- 1890-

ZDVKAP Zdravookhranenie. Public Health. (v/o 'Mezhdunarodnaya Kniga', Kuznetskii Most 18, Moscow G-200, USSR) V.1- 1958-

ZEKBAI Zeitschrift fuer Krebsforschung. (Berlin, Germany) V.1-75, 1903-71. For publisher information, see JCROD7

ZENBAX Zeitschrift fuer Naturforschung, Ausgabe B, Chemie, Biochemie, Biophysik, Biologie und Verwandten Gebieten. (Verlag der Zeitschrift fuer Naturforschung, Postfach 2645, D-7400, Tuebingen, Federal Republic of Germany) V.2- 1947-

ZEVBA5 Zeitschrift fuer Verebungslehre. (Springer-Verlag, Heidelberger Pl.3, D-1 Berlin 33, Germany) V.89-98, 1958-66.

ZGASAX Zeitscrift fuer Gastroenterologie. (Karl Demeter Verlag und Anzeigen-Verwaltung, Wuermstr 13, 8032 Graefelfing/Munich, Federal Republic of Germany) V.1-1963-

ZHPMAT Zentralblatt fuer Bakteriologie, Parasitenkunde, Infektionskrankran- heiten und Hygiene, Abteilung 1: Originale, Reihe B: Hygiene, Praeventive Medizin. (Gustav Fischer Verlag, Postfach 72-01-43, D-7000 Stuttgart 70, Fed. Rep. Germany) V.155- 1971-

ZHYGAM Zeitschrift fuer die Gesamte Hygiene und Ihre Grenzgebiete. (VEB Georg Thieme, Hainst 17/19, Postfach 946, 701 Leipzig, E. Germany) V.1- 1955-

ZIETA2 Zeitschrift fuer Immunitaetsforschung und Experimentelle Therapie. (Stuttgart, Germany) 1924-V.124, 1962. For publisher information, see ZIEKBA

ZKKOBW Zeitschrift fuer Krebsforschung und Klinische Onkologie. (Berlin, Germany) V.76-92, 1971-78. For publisher information, see JCROD7

ZKMAAX Zhurnal Eksperimental'noi i Klinicheskoi Meditsiny. (V/O Mezhdunarodnaya Kniga, 121200 Moscow, USSR) V.2- 1962-

ZLUFAR Zeitschrift fuer Lebensmittel-Untersuchung und-Forschung. (Springer- Verlag, Heidelberger, Pl. 3, D-1 Berlin 33, Germany) V.86- 1943-

ZNCBDA Zeitschrift fuer Naturforschung, Section C: Biosciences. (Verlag der Zeitschrift fuer Naturforschung, Postfach 2645, D-7400 Tuebingen, Federal Republic of Germany) V.29C- 1974-

ZSNUAI Zeitschrift fuer Neurologie. (Berlin) V.198-206, 1970-74.

13BYAH 'Morphological Precursors of Cancer,' ed. Lucio Severi, Proceedings of an International Conference, Universita Degli Studi, Perugia, Italy, June 26-30, 1961, Perugia, Univ. of Perugia, 1962

14JTAF 'Mycotoxins in Foodstuffs,' Proceedings of the Symposium held at the Massachusetts Institute of Technology, Mar. 18-19, 1964, Wogan, G.N., ed., Cambridge, MA, MIT Press, 1965

22XWAN 'Chemical Mutagenesis in Mammals and Man,' F. Vogel and G. Roehrborn, eds., Berlin, Springer, 1970

23HZAR 'Carcinoma of the Colon and Antecedent Epithelium,' W.J. Burdette, Springfield, Illinois, C.C. Thomas, 1970

25NJAN 'International Cancer Congress, Abstracts, 10th,' Houston, Texas, May 22-29, 1970, Cumley, R.W. and J.E. McCay, eds., Chicago, IL., Year Book Medical Publishers, Inc., 1970

26QZAP 'Advances in Antimicrobial and Antineoplastic Chemotherapy, Progress in Research and Clinical Application,' 7th Proceedings of the International Congress of Chemotherapy, Hejzlar, M. et al., eds., Prague, Aug. 23-28, 1971, 3 Vols., Prague, Czecholovakia, University Press, 1972

26UYA8 'Psoriasis,' Proceedings of the International Symposium, Stanford, Calif., July 7-10, 1971, Farber, E.M. and A.J. Cox, eds., Stanford, Calif., Stanford University Press, 1971

27CWAL 'Medical Primatology,' Selected Papers from the 3rd Conference on Experimental Medicine and Surgery in Primates, Lyons, France, June 21-23, 1972, Goldsmith, E.I. and J. Moor-Jankowski, eds., White Plains, New York, Phiebig, 1972

29QKAZ 'Toxins of Animal and Plant Origin,' A. de Vries and E. Kochva, eds., New York, Gordon and Breach Science Publishers, 1971

31BYAP 'Experimental Lung Cancer: Carcinogenesis Bioassays, International Symposium, 1974,' New York, Springer, 1974

33AQAA 'Biology of Radiation Carcinogenesis,' J. M. Yuhas, et al., ed., New York, Raven Press, 1976

33IUAS 'Mycotoxins,' Purchase, I.F.H. ed., Amsterdam, Elsevier, 1974

34LXAP 'Insecticide Biochemistry and Physiology,' C.F. Wilkinson, ed., New York, Plenum, 1976

34ZRA9 'Proceedings Quadrennial Conference on Cancer,' L. Severi, ed., Perugia, Italy, University of Perugia, 1966

35WYAM 'In Vitro Metabolic Activation in Mutagenic Testing,' Proceedings of the Symposium on the Role of Metabolic Activation in Producing Mutagenic and Carcinogenic Environmental Chemicals, Research Triangle Park, N.C., Feb. 9-11, 1976, De Serres, F.J. et al., eds., New York, Elsevier North Holland, 1976

36PYAS 'Pharmacology of Steroid Contraceptive Drugs,' Garattini, S. and H.W. Berendes, eds., New York, Raven Press, 1977. (Monograph Mario Negri Inst. Pharm. Res.)

36YFAG 'Biological Reactive Intermediates, Formation, Toxicity and Inactivation,' Proceedings of the International Conference on Active Intermediates, Formation, Toxicity and Inactivation, University of Turku, Turku, Finland, July 26-27, 1975. New York, Plenum, 1977.

40RMA7 'Health and Sugar Substitutes,' Proceedings of the ERGOB Conference on Sugar Substitutes, Geneva, 1978, Guggenheim, B., ed., Basel, Switzerland, S. Karger AG, 1979

40YJAX 'Evaluation of Embryotoxicity, Mutagenicity and Carcinogenicity Risks In New Drugs,' Proceedings of the Symposium on Toxicological Testing for Safety of New Drugs, 3rd, Prague, Apr. 6-8, 1976, Benesova, O., et al., eds., Prague, Czechoslovakia, Univerzita Karlova, 1979

43GRAK 'Dusts and Disease,' Proceedings of the Conference on Occupational Exposures to Fibrous and Particulate Dust and Their Extension into the Environment, 1977, Lemen, R., and J.M. Dement, eds., Park Forest South, IL, Pathotox Publishers, 1979

43XWAI 'Brain Tumors and Chemical Injuries to the Central Nervous System,' Proceedings of the International Neuropathological Symposium, Warsaw, Sep. 23-26, 1976, Mossakowski, M.J., ed. Warsaw, Panstwowe Wydawnictwo Naukowe, 1978

45ICAX 'Nickel Toxicology,' 2nd International Conference on Nickel Toxicology. Swansea, U.K., 3-5 Sept., 1980. London, Academic Press, 1980

45KQAH 'Health Effects Investigation of Oil Shale Development,' Meeting, Gatlinburg, Tenn. USA, June 23-24, 1980, Editors: Griest, W.H., M.R. Guerin and D.L. Coffins, Ann Arbor Science Publishers, Inc., 1980

45OHAA 'Short-Term Test Systems for Detecting Carcinogens,' Proceedings of the Symposium, 1978, Norpoth, K.H., and R.G. Garner, eds., Berlin, Springer-Verlag, 1980

46GFA5 'Safety Problems Related to Chloramphenicol and Thiamphenicol Therapy,' Najean, Y., et al., eds., New York, Raven Press, 1981

46OJAN 'Chemical Analysis and Biological Fate: Polynuclear Aromatic Hydrocarbons,' 5th International Symposium, Battelle's Labs., Oct. 1980. Columbus, Ohio, Battelle Press, 1981

47JMAE 'Cytogenetic Assays of Environmental Mutagens,' Hsu, T.C., ed., Totowa, NJ, Allanheld, Osmun & Co., 1982

47YKAF 'Sporulation and Germination,' Proceedings of the Eighth International Spore Conference, 1980, Washington, DC, American Society of Microbiology, 1981

50EXAK 'Formaldehyde Toxicity,' Conference, 1980, Gibson, J.E., ed., Washington, DC, Hemisphere Publishing Corp., 1983

50EYAN 'Structure-Activity Correlation as a Predictive Tool in Toxicology,' Papers from a Symposium, 1981, Golberg, L., ed., Washington, DC, Hemisphere Publishing Corp., 1983

50NNAZ 'Polynuclear Aromatic Hydrocarbons,' International Symposium, 7th, 1982, Cooke, M., and A.J. Dennis, eds., Columbus, OH, Battelle Press, 1983

55DXAE 'Progress in Nickel Toxicology, Proceedings of the International Conference on Nickel Metabolism and Toxicology, 3rd, 1984,' Brown, S.S., and F.W. Sunderman, Jr., eds., Oxford, UK, Blackwell Scientific Pub. Ltd., 1985

85AGAF 'Effects and Dose-response Relationships of Toxic Metals,' G.F. Nordberg, ed., Proceedings from an International Meeting Organized by the Subcommittee on the Toxicology of Metals of the Permanent Commission and International Association on Occupational Health, Tokyo, November 18-23, 1974, New York, Elsevier Scientific, 1976

85CVA2 'Oncology 1970,' Proceedings of the Tenth International Cancer Congress, Chicago, Year Book Medical Publishers, 1971

85DAAC 'Bladder Cancer, A Symposium,' K.F. Lampe et al., eds., Fifth Inter-American Conference on Toxicology and Occupational Medicine, University of Miami, School of Medicine, Coral Gables, Florida, Aesculapius Pub., 1966

85DLAB 'Studies on Chemical Carcinogenesis by Diels-Alder Adducts of Carcinogenic Aromatic Hydrocarbons,' R.H. Earhart, Jr., Ann Arbor, Michigan, Xerox Univ. Microfilms, 1975

85DUA4 'Chemical Tumour Problems,' W. Nakahara, ed., Tokyo, Japanese Society for the Promotion of Science, 1970

85GMAT 'Toxicometric Parameters of Industrial Toxic Chemicals Under Single Exposure,' Izmerov, N.F., et al. Moscow, Centre of International Projects, GKNT, 1982

85JCAE 'Prehled Prumyslove Toxikologie; Organicke Latky,' Marhold, J., Prague, Czechoslovakia, Avicenum, 1986